GELLIS & KAGAN'S

CURRENT PEDIATRIC THERAPY

15

FREDRIC D. BURG, M.D.
Vice Dean for Education
University of Pennsylvania School of Medicine
Professor of Pediatrics
Children's Hospital of Philadelphia
Philadelphia, Pennsylvania

JULIE R. INGELFINGER, M.D.
Associate Professor of Pediatrics
Harvard Medical School
Chief, Pediatric Nephrology Unit
Massachusetts General Hospital
Boston, Massachusetts

ELLEN R. WALD, M.D.
Professor of Pediatrics
University of Pittsburgh School of Medicine
Chief, Division of Infectious Diseases
Vice Chairman, Department of Pediatrics
Children's Hospital of Pittsburgh
Pittsburgh, Pennsylvania

RICHARD A. POLIN, M.D.
Professor of Pediatrics
University of Pennsylvania School of Medicine
Division of Neonatology
Children's Hospital of Philadelphia
Philadelphia, Pennsylvania

GELLIS & KAGAN'S
CURRENT PEDIATRIC THERAPY

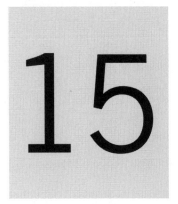

15

W.B. SAUNDERS COMPANY
A Division of Harcourt Brace & Company

Philadelphia   London   Toronto   Montreal   Sydney   Tokyo

W.B. SAUNDERS COMPANY
A Division of
Harcourt Brace & Company

The Curtis Center
Independence Square West
Philadelphia, Pennsylvania 19106

NOTICE

Medicine is an ever-changing field. Standard safety precautions must be followed, but as new research and clinical experience broaden our knowledge, changes in treatment and drug therapy become necessary or appropriate. The editors of this work have carefully checked the generic and trade drug names and verified drug dosages to ensure that the dosage information in this work is accurate and in accord with the standard accepted at the time of publication. Readers are advised, however, to check the product information currently provided by the manufacturer of each drug to be administered to be certain that changes have not been made in the recommended dose or in the contraindications for administration. This is of particular importance in regard to new or infrequently used drugs. It is the responsibility of the treating physician, relying on experience and knowledge of the patient, to determine dosages and the best treatment for the patient. The editors cannot be responsible for misuse or misapplication of the material in this work.

THE PUBLISHER

Managing Editor:
CARLA B. HULTMAN
Executive Assistant to the Vice Dean for Education
University of Pennsylvania School of Medicine

GELLIS AND KAGAN'S CURRENT PEDIATRIC THERAPY 15   ISBN 0–7216–5016–3

Contributors

SORAYA ABBASI, M.D.

Professor of Pediatrics, Jefferson Medical College, Thomas Jefferson University; Pediatrician, Pennsylvania Hospital, Philadelphia, Pennsylvania

Bronchopulmonary Dysplasia

STEVEN H. ABMAN, M.D.

Associate Professor, Section of Pulmonary Medicine, Department of Pediatrics, University of Colorado School of Medicine, Denver, Colorado

Persistent Pulmonary Hypertension

ISRAEL F. ABROMS, M.D.

Professor of Pediatrics and Neurology, University of Massachusetts Medical School; Division Director, Pediatric Neurology, University of Massachusetts Medical Center, Worcester, Massachusetts

Breath-Holding Spells

FESTUS O. ADEBONOJO, M.D.

Professor and Chairman, Department of Pediatrics, James H. Quillen College of Medicine, East Tennessee State University; Medical Director, Children's Hospital at Johnson City Medical Center, Johnson City, Tennessee

Undernutrition

RAYMOND D. ADELMAN, M.D.

Professor and Chairman, Department of Pediatrics, Eastern Virginia Medical School; Physician-in-Chief and Vice President of Medical Affairs, Children's Hospital of the King's Daughters, Norfolk, Virginia

Hydronephrosis; Perinephric and Intranephric Abscess

JOEL W. ADELSON, M.D., Ph.D.

Professor of Pediatrics and Physiology, Brown University School of Medicine; Director, Division of Pediatric Gastroenterology and Nutrition, Rhode Island Hospital, Providence, Rhode Island

Hirschsprung's Disease

BENOOSH AFGHANI, M.D.

Fellow, Pediatric Infectious Diseases, University of California Irvine, Irvine, California, and Memorial Miller Children's Hospital, Long Beach, California

Diphtheria

HASSAN HESHAM A-KADER, M.D.

Attending Physician, Samaritan Medical Center, Watertown, New York

Nonhemolytic Unconjugated Hyperbilirubinemia

EDWARD AKELMAN, M.D.

Associate Professor of Orthopedics, Brown University; Surgeon-in-Charge, Division of Hand, Upper Extremity, and Microvascular Surgery, Rhode Island Hospital, Providence, Rhode Island

Orthopedic Problems of the Extremities

STEVEN R. ALEXANDER, M.D.

Professor of Pediatrics, University of Texas Southwestern Medical Center; Director, Dialysis and Renal Transplantation, Children's Medical Center of Dallas, Dallas, Texas

Peritoneal Dialysis

CUNEYT M. ALPER, M.D.

Visiting Assistant Professor, University of Pittsburgh School of Medicine; Fellow, Department of Pediatric Otolaryngology, Children's Hospital of Pittsburgh, Pittsburgh, Pennsylvania

Salivary Gland Tumors

MARY G. AMPOLA, M.D.

Professor of Pediatrics, Tufts University School of Medicine; Acting Chief, Division of Clinical Genetics, Department of Pediatrics, New England Medical Center, Boston, Massachusetts

Phenylketonuria and Related Disorders

ALIA ANTOON, M.D.

Assistant Clinical Professor of Pediatrics, Harvard Medical School; Associate Pediatrician, Massachusetts General Hospital and Shriners Burns Institute, Boston, Massachusetts

Burns

ALLAN M. ARBETER, M.D.

Associate Professor of Pediatrics, Temple University School of Medicine; Chairman, Department of Pediatric and Adolescent Medicine, Albert Einstein Medical Center, Philadelphia, Pennsylvania

Varicella-Zoster Virus Infection

STEVEN ARKIN, M.D.

Assistant Professor of Pediatrics, Division of Pediatric Hematology/Oncology, Jack and Lucy Clark Department of Pediatrics, Mount Sinai School of Medicine, New York, New York

Anemia of Iron Deficiency

KENNETH A. ARNDT, M.D.

Professor of Dermatology, Harvard Medical School; Dermatologist-in-Chief, Beth Israel Hospital, Boston, Massachusetts

Chronic Nonhereditary Vesiculobullous Disorders

STEPHEN C. ARONOFF, M.D.

Professor, Department of Pediatrics, West Virginia University; Chief of Pediatrics, West Virginia University Hospitals, Morgantown, West Virginia

Histoplasmosis; Mucormycosis (Zygomycosis)

ANTHONY ATALA, M.D.

Assistant Professor, Department of Surgery, Harvard Medical School; Assistant in Surgery, Division of Urology, Children's Hospital, Boston, Massachusetts

Patent Urachus and Urachal Cysts; Disorders of the Bladder and Urethra

BALU H. ATHREYA, M.D.

Professor of Pediatrics, University of Pennsylvania School of Medicine; Director, Department of Rheumatology, Children's Hospital of Philadelphia and Children's Seashore House, Philadelphia, Pennsylvania

Systemic Lupus Erythematosus

BASSAM ATIYEH, M.D.

Associate Professor of Pediatrics, Wayne State University School of Medicine; Pediatric Nephrologist, Children's Hospital of Michigan, Detroit, Michigan

Systemic Hypertension; Fluid and Electrolyte Therapy in Children

CHARLES S. AUGUST, M.D.

Director, Division of Hematology-Oncology-Bone Marrow Transplantation, Miami Children's Hospital, Miami, Florida

Bone Marrow Transplantation

FELICIA B. AXELROD, M.D.

Professor of Dysautonomia Treatment and Research, Department of Pediatrics, and Professor, Department of Neurology, New York University School of Medicine; Director, Dysautonomia Treatment and Evaluation Center, New York University Medical Center, New York, New York

Familial Dysautonomia

WILLIAM F. BALISTRERI, M.D.

Dorothy M.M. Kersten Professor of Pediatrics, University of Cincinnati School of Medicine; Director, Division of Pediatric Gastroenterology and Nutrition, Children's Hospital Medical Center, Cincinnati, Ohio

Nonhemolytic Unconjugated Hyperbilirubinemia; Cholestasis (Conjugated Hyperbilirubinemia)

WILLIAM BANNER, Jr., M.D., Ph.D.

Attending Physician Pediatric Intensive Care Unit, St. Francis Hospital, Tulsa, Oklahoma

Arthropod Bites and Stings

MARK L. BATSHAW, M.D.

W.T. Grant Professor of Pediatrics and Professor of Neurology, University of Pennsylvania School of Medicine; Physician-in-Chief, Children's Seashore House, Philadelphia, Pennsylvania

Urea Cycle Disorders

STEPHEN BAUMGART, M.D.

Professor of Pediatrics, Jefferson Medical College, Thomas Jefferson University; Senior Staff Pediatrician, Division of Neonatology, Thomas Jefferson University Hospital, Philadelphia, Pennsylvania

Listeria monocytogenes; *Fluid and Electrolyte Therapeutics*

DIANA S. BEARDSLEY, M.D., Ph.D.

Associate Professor of Pediatrics and Internal Medicine, Yale University School of Medicine, New Haven, Connecticut

Platelet Disorders

LOUIS M. BELL, M.D.

Associate Professor of Pediatrics, University of Pennsylvania School of Medicine; Attending Physician, Emergency Medicine and Infectious Diseases, Children's Hospital of Philadelphia, Philadelphia, Pennsylvania

Fever

JERRY M. BERGSTEIN, M.D.

Professor, Department of Pediatrics, Indiana University School of Medicine; Director, Section of Nephrology, James Whitcomb Riley Hospital for Children, Indianapolis, Indiana

Hemolytic-Uremic Syndrome

RAHEL BERHANE, M.D.

Assistant Professor of Pediatrics, Tufts University School of Medicine; Assistant Pediatrician, New England Medical Center, Boston, Massachusetts

Acute and Chronic Diarrhea Syndromes

JUDY C. BERNBAUM, M.D.

Associate Professor of Pediatrics, University of Pennsylvania School of Medicine; Director, Neonatal Follow-Up Program and Senior Physician, Children's Hospital of Philadelphia, Philadelphia, Pennsylvania

Follow-up of the High-risk Infant

SHELLY C. BERNSTEIN, M.D., Ph.D.

Assistant Clinical Professor of Pediatrics, Harvard Medical School; Assistant in Medicine (Hematology/Oncology), Children's Hospital; Assistant Physician, Pediatric Oncology, Dana-Farber Cancer Institute, Boston, Massachusetts

Polycythemia

VINOD K. BHUTANI, M.D.

Professor of Pediatrics, Jefferson Medical College, Thomas Jefferson University; Pediatrician, Pennsylvania Hospital, Philadelphia, Pennsylvania

Bronchopulmonary Dysplasia

ROBERT J. BIDWELL, M.D.

Associate Professor of Pediatrics, John A. Burns School of Medicine, University of Hawaii; Director of Adolescent Medicine, Kapiolani Medical Center for Women and Children, Honolulu, Hawaii

Sexual Orientation and Gender Identity

AUDREY H. BIRNBAUM, M.D.

Assistant Professor of Pediatrics, Mount Sinai School of Medicine; Chief, Section of Hepatology, Division of Pediatric Gastroenterology, Mount Sinai Medical Center, New York, New York

Pancreatic Diseases

CHARLES D. BLUESTONE, M.D.

Professor of Otolaryngology, University of Pittsburgh School of Medicine; Director, Department of Pediatric Otolaryngology, Children's Hospital of Pittsburgh, Pittsburgh, Pennsylvania

Salivary Gland Tumors; Recurrent Parotitis

THOMAS F. BOAT, M.D.

Professor and Chair, Department of Pediatrics, University of Cincinnati College of Medicine and Children's Hospital Medical Center, Cincinnati, Ohio

Atelectasis

DRUCY BOROWITZ, M.D.

Clinical Assistant Professor of Pediatrics, State University of New York at Buffalo and Children's Hospital of Buffalo, Buffalo, New York

Childhood Obesity

KENNETH M. BOYER, M.D.

Professor and Associate Chairman, Department of Pediatrics, Rush Medical College; Director, Section of Pediatric Infectious Diseases, Rush-Presbyterian-St. Luke's Medical Center, Chicago, Illinois

Neonatal Sepsis and Meningitis; Group B Streptococcal Infections

DAVID W. BOYLE, M.D.

Assistant Professor of Pediatrics, Indiana University School of Medicine and Indiana University Medical Center, Indianapolis, Indiana

Disturbances of Intrauterine Growth

JOHN T. BOYLE, M.D.

Associate Professor of Pediatrics, Case Western Reserve University School of Medicine; Chief, Division of Pediatric Gastroenterology and Nutrition, Rainbow Babies and Children's Hospital, Cleveland, Ohio

Portal Hypertension

TIMOTHY J. BREI, M.D.

Assistant Professor of Pediatrics, Indiana University School of Medicine; Developmental Pediatrician , Section of Developmental Pediatrics, James Whitcomb Riley Hospital for Children, Indianapolis, Indiana

Meningomyelocele

PHILIP P. BREITFELD, M.D.

Associate Professor of Pediatrics and Biochemistry and Molecular Biology, Indiana University School of Medicine; Director, Pediatric Hematology-Oncology, James Whitcomb Riley Hospital for Children, Indianapolis, Indiana

Acute Leukemia

ANDREW S. BREM, M.D.

Associate Professor of Pediatrics, Brown University; Director, Division of Pediatric Nephrology, Rhode Island Hospital, Providence, Rhode Island

The Neurogenic Bladder

MATHIAS D. BRENDEL, M.D.

Senior Research Associate, Diabetes Research Institute, University of Miami School of Medicine, Miami, Florida

Organ Transplants: Pancreas and Islet Cells

NANCY B. BRENT, M.D., I.B.C.L.C.

Clinical Assistant Professor, University of Pittsburgh School of Medicine; Director, Maternal Infant Lactation Center, Mercy Hospital of Pittsburgh, Pittsburgh, Pennsylvania

Breastfeeding

NANCY D. BRIDGES, M.D.

Assistant Professor of Pediatrics, Washington University School of Medicine; Director, Cardiac Catheterization Laboratory, St. Louis Children's Hospital, St. Louis, Missouri

Congenital Heart Disease

ROSALIND S. BROWN, M.D., F.R.C.P.(C.)

Associate Professor of Pediatrics, University of Massachusetts Medical School; Director, Division of Pediatric Endocrinology/Diabetes, University of Massachusetts Medical Center, Worcester, Massachusetts

Thyroid Disorders

JAMES RUSSELL BUCK, M.D.

Assistant Professor of Pediatric Surgery and Pediatrics, Johns Hopkins University; Chief, Division of Pediatric Surgery, Sinai Hospital of Baltimore, Baltimore, Maryland

Disorders of the Esophagus

MARCIA L. BUCK, Pharm.D.

Clinical Assistant Professor of Pediatrics, University of Virginia; Clinical Pharmacy Specialist in Pediatrics, University of Virginia Health Sciences Center, Charlottesville, Virginia

Nutrition Support in the Very Ill Pediatric Patient

EDUARDO M. BUDGE, M.D.

Research Fellow, Harvard Medical School; Clinical and Research Fellow, Pediatric Pulmonary Unit, Massachusetts General Hospital, Boston, Massachusetts

Idiopathic Pulmonary Hemosiderosis

CHARLES A. BULLABOY, M.D.

Professor of Pediatrics, Eastern Virginia Medical School; Pediatric Cardiologist, Children's Hospital of the King's Daughters, Norfolk, Virginia

Mitral Valve Prolapse; Pericarditis

INA STEPHENS BURROWS, M.D.

Research Associate, Center for Immunization Research, Johns Hopkins University School of Hygiene and Public Health, Baltimore, Maryland

Cholera

KATHLEEN CALENDA, M.D.

Assistant Professor of Pediatrics, Tufts University School of Medicine, Boston, Massachusetts; Consultant Staff, Good Samaritan Hospital, Stoughton, Massachusetts

Inflammatory Bowel Disease

CHARLES E. CANTER, M.D.

Associate Professor of Pediatrics, Washington University School of Medicine; Medical Director, Cardiac Transplantation Service, and Director, Non-invasive Cardiac Laboratory, St. Louis Children's Hospital, St. Louis, Missouri

Congenital Heart Disease; Cardiomyopathies and Cardiac Transplantation

THOMAS O. CARPENTER, M.D.

Associate Professor of Pediatrics, Yale University School of Medicine; Attending Physician, Yale–New Haven Hospital, New Haven, Connecticut

Rickets; Idiopathic Hypercalcemia

MARY CARRASCO, M.D.

Associate Professor of Pediatrics, University of Pittsburgh School of Medicine; Assistant Professor of Health Services Administration, University of Pittsburgh School of Public Health; Director, Family Intervention Center, Children's Hospital of Pittsburgh, Pittsburgh, Pennsylvania

Sexual Abuse and Rape

GAIL H. CASSELL, Ph.D.

Charles H. McCauley Professor and Chairman, Department of Microbiology, University of Alabama at Birmingham Schools of Medicine and Dentistry, Birmingham, Alabama

Genital Mycoplasmal Infections

LYDIA CAVALES-OFTADEH, M.D.

Fellow-in-Training, Division of Allergy/Immunology, Harbor–University of California Los Angeles Medical Center, Torrance, California

Anaphylaxis

HARRY T. CHUGANI, M.D.

Professor, Departments of Radiology, Neurology, and Pediatrics, Wayne State University School of Medicine; Director, PET Center and Staff Neurologist, Children's Hospital of Michigan, Detroit, Michigan

Infantile Spasms

THOMAS G. CLEARY, M.D.

Professor of Pediatrics and Director, Pediatric Infectious Disease, University of Texas–Houston Health Science Center, Houston, Texas

Typhoid Fever

BERNARD A. COHEN, M.D.

Associate Professor of Pediatrics and Dermatology, Johns Hopkins University; Director, Pediatric Dermatology, Johns Hopkins Children's Center, Baltimore, Maryland

Discoid Lupus Erythematosus; Scabies and Lice

HARVEY J. COHEN, M.D., Ph.D.

Professor of Pediatrics and Chair, Department of Pediatrics, Stanford University School of Medicine, Stanford, California; Chief of Staff, Lucile Salter Packard Children's Hospital at Stanford, Palo Alto, California
Disseminated Intravascular Coagulation

BARBARA R. COLE, M.D.

Associate Professor of Pediatrics, Washington University School of Medicine; Director, Division of Pediatric Nephrology, St. Louis Children's Hospital, St. Louis, Missouri
Hematuria and Proteinuria

HARVEY R. COLTEN, M.D.

Professor and Chairman, Department of Pediatrics, Washington University School of Medicine; Pediatrician-in-Chief, St. Louis Children's Hospital, St. Louis, Missouri
Cystic Fibrosis

JAMES COPLAN, M.D.

Associate Professor of Pediatrics and Chief, Division of Child Development, State University of New York Health Science Center, Syracuse, New York
Disorders of Voice, Speech, or Language

W. THOMAS CORDER, M.D.

Associate Professor, Department of Pediatrics, West Virginia University; Section of Pediatrics, West Virginia University Hospitals, Morgantown, West Virginia
Mucormycosis (Zygomycosis)

MARVIN CORNBLATH, M.D.

Lecturer in Pediatrics, Johns Hopkins University School of Medicine; Clinical Professor of Pediatrics, University of Maryland School of Medicine, Baltimore, Maryland
Neonatal Hypoglycemia

ANDREW T. COSTARINO, Jr., M.D.

Assistant Professor, The University of Pennsylvania; Children's Hospital of Philadelphia, Philadelphia, Pennsylvania
Fluid and Electrolyte Therapeutics

WILLIAM M. CRIST, M.D.

Professor of Pediatrics, University of Tennessee College of Medicine; Chairman, Department of Hematology/Oncology and Deputy Director, St. Jude Children's Research Hospital, Memphis, Tennessee
Burkitt's Lymphoma

ALLEN C. CROCKER, M.D.

Associate Professor of Pediatrics, Harvard Medical School; Associate Professor of Maternal and Child Health, Harvard School of Public Health; Program Director, Institute for Community Inclusion/UAP, Children's Hospital, Boston, Massachusetts
Mental Retardation

PATRICIA K. CRUMRINE, M.D.

Associate Professor of Pediatrics and Neurology, University of Pittsburgh School of Medicine; Director, Pediatric Comprehensive Epilepsy Program, Children's Hospital of Pittsburgh, Pittsburgh, Pennsylvania
Seizure Therapy

MICHAEL J. CUNNINGHAM, M.D.

Assistant Professor of Otology and Laryngology, Harvard Medical School; Associate Surgeon in Otolaryngology, Massachusetts Eye and Ear Infirmary; Assistant in Pediatrics, Massachusetts General Hospital, Boston, Massachusetts
Acute Laryngotracheal Infections

SHERMINE DABBAGH, M.D.

Associate Professor of Pediatrics, Wayne State University School of Medicine; Director, Pediatric Nephrology and ESRD Program, Children's Hospital of Michigan, Detroit, Michigan
Systemic Hypertension; Fluid and Electrolyte Therapy in Children

IAN D. D'AGATA, M.D.

Fellow, Gastroenterology and Nutrition, Harvard Medical School; Fellow, Combined Program in Gastroenterology and Nutrition, Massachusetts General Hospital and Children's Hospital, Boston, Massachusetts
Chronic Active Hepatitis; Disorders of the Biliary Tree

RONALD E. DAHL, M.D.

Associate Professor of Psychiatry and Pediatrics, University of Pittsburgh School of Medicine; Director, Child and Adolescent Sleep Laboratory, Western Psychiatric Institute and Clinic, Pittsburgh, Pennsylvania
Common Sleep Disorders

ADNAN S. DAJANI, M.D.

Professor of Pediatrics, Wayne State University School of Medicine; Chief, Division of Infectious Diseases, Children's Hospital of Michigan, Detroit, Michigan
Acute Rheumatic Fever

GHALEB H. DAOUK, M.D., S.M.

Instructor in Pediatrics, Harvard Medical School; Assistant in Pediatric Nephrology, Massachusetts General Hospital, Boston, Massachusetts
Renal Hypoplasia and Dysplasia

BASIL T. DARRAS, M.D.

Associate Professor of Pediatrics and Neurology, Tufts University School of Medicine; Attending Physician, The Floating Hospital for Children, New England Medical Center, Boston, Massachusetts
Acute Ataxia

BARRY DASHEFSKY, M.D.

Associate Professor of Pediatrics, University of Pittsburgh School of Medicine; Staff, Division of Pediatric Infectious Diseases, Children's Hospital of Pittsburgh, Pittsburgh, Pennsylvania
Gonococcal Infections; Rat-bite Fever; Measles

ROBERT S. DAUM, M.D.

Professor of Pediatrics, University of Chicago Pritzker School of Medicine; Section Chief, Pediatric Infectious Diseases, The University of Chicago/Wyler Children's Hospital, Chicago, Illinois
Infections Caused by Haemophilus influenzae Type B

DAVID M. DAWSON, M.D.

Professor of Neurology, Harvard Medical School, Boston, Massachusetts; Chief of Neurology, Brockton-West Roxbury Veterans Administration Hospital, West Roxbury, Massachusetts
Myasthenia Gravis

VIRGINIA DELANEY-BLACK, M.D.

Associate Professor of Pediatrics, Wayne State University; Associate Neonatologist, Children's Hospital of Michigan, Hutzel Hospital, Detroit, Michigan
Neonatal Polycythemia and Hyperviscosity

DAVID RAY DeMASO, M.D.

Assistant Professor of Psychiatry, Harvard Medical School; Senior Associate in Psychiatry and Cardiology, Children's Hospital, Boston, Massachusetts
Depressive Disorders

J. CHRISTOPHER DiGIACOMO, M.D.

Lecturer in Surgery, Division of Traumatology and Surgical Critical Care, Department of Surgery, University of Pennsylvania School of Medicine and Medical Center, Philadelphia, Pennsylvania

Penetrating, Gunshot, and Knife Wounds in Children

CYNTHIA A. DOERR, M.D.

Fellow, Pediatric Infectious Disease, Baylor College of Medicine, Houston, Texas

Infective Endocarditis

STEPHEN E. DOLGIN, M.D.

Associate Professor of Surgery and Pediatrics, Mount Sinai Medical Center; Chief, Pediatric Surgery, Mount Sinai Medical Center, New York, New York

Malformations of the Intestine; Pyloric Stenosis; Inguinal Hernias and Hydroceles

ELIZABETH C. DOOLING, M.D.

Associate Professor of Neurology, Harvard Medical School; Neurologist and Associate Pediatrician, Massachusetts General Hospital, Boston, Massachusetts

Cerebrovascular Disease in Infancy and Childhood

JEFFREY S. DOVER, M.D., F.R.C.P.C.

Assistant Professor of Dermatology, Harvard Medical School; Chief of Dermatology, New England Deaconness Hospital, Boston, Massachusetts

Photodermatoses

DEBORAH A. DRISCOLL, M.D.

Assistant Professor, University of Pennsylvania School of Medicine and Division of Reproductive Genetics, Department of Obstetrics and Gynecology, Hospital of the University of Pennsylvania, Philadelphia, Pennsylvania

Intrauterine Diagnosis and Approach to the Malformed Infant

J. STEPHEN DUMLER, M.D.

Assistant Professor of Pathology, University of Maryland School of Medicine; Lecturer in Pathology, Johns Hopkins School of Medicine; Associate Director, Clinical Microbiology, and Staff Pathologist, University of Maryland Medical Systems Hospital, Baltimore, Maryland

Rickettsial Infections

LISA M. DUNKLE, M.D.

Executive Director, HIV Clinical Research, Bristol-Myers Squibb Pharmaceutical Research Institute, Wallingford, Connecticut

Infections due to Anaerobic Cocci and Gram-negative Bacilli

ADRÉ J. du PLESSIS, M.D.

Assistant Professor of Neurology, Harvard Medical School; Assistant in Neurology, Children's Hospital, Boston, Massachusetts

Neurologic Birth Trauma

PAUL G. DYMENT, M.D.

Professor of Pediatrics and Vice Chancellor for Academic Affairs, Tulane University Medical Center, New Orleans, Louisiana

The Hip

BETTY J. EDMOND, M.D.

Director, Pediatric Infectious Diseases, Brachenridge Hospital, Austin, Texas

Infectious Mononucleosis

MICHAEL G. EHRLICH, M.D.

Professor and Chairman, Department of Orthopaedics, Brown University School of Medicine; Surgeon-in-Chief, Department of Orthopaedics, Rhode Island Hospital, Providence, Rhode Island

Orthopedic Problems of the Extremities

LAWRENCE F. EICHENFIELD, M.D.

Assistant Professor, Pediatrics and Medicine (Dermatology), and Chief, Division of Pediatric Dermatology, University of California San Diego School of Medicine; Chief, Pediatric Dermatology, Children's Hospital of San Diego, San Diego, California

Disorders of Pigmentation

ELLIOT F. ELLIS, M.D.

Professor Emeritus, State University of New York at Buffalo, Buffalo, New York; Medical Director, MURO Pharmaceutical, Inc., Tewksbury, Massachusetts

Urticaria

S. JEAN EMANS, M.D.

Associate Professor of Pediatrics, Harvard Medical School; Co-Chief, Division of Adolescent Medicine, Children's Hospital, Boston, Massachusetts

Vulva and Vagina; Understanding and Assessing Adolescent Influences and Risk-taking Behavior

ELIZABETH C. ENGLE, M.D.

Instructor, Harvard Medical School; Assistant in Neurology, Children's Hospital, Boston, Massachusetts

Benign Intracranial Hypertension

TAHSIN M. ERGIN, M.D.

Private Practitioner, Essex Orthopaedics, North Andover, Massachusetts

Orthopedic Trauma

SCOTT A. ESTREM, M.D.

Associate Professor, University of Missouri School of Medicine, Columbia, Missouri

Middle Ear Trauma

OWEN B. EVANS, M.D.

Professor and Chairman, Department of Pediatrics, University of Mississippi Medical Center; Professor and Attending Physician, University Hospital, Jackson, Mississippi

Inflammatory Myopathies

JOEL E. FAGAN, M.D., F.R.C.P.C., M.Sc.

Professor, Department of Pediatrics, University of Calgary; Director, Developmental Clinic, Alberta Children's Hospital, Calgary, Alberta, Canada

Attention Deficit Disorder

RALPH D. FEIGIN, M.D.

J.S. Abercrombie Professor and Chairman, Department of Pediatrics, Baylor College of Medicine; Physician-in-Chief, Texas Children's Hospital; Pediatrician-in-Chief, Ben Taub General Hospital; Chief, Pediatric Services, The Methodist Hospital, Houston, Texas

Bacterial Meningitis and Septicemia Beyond the Neonatal Period

JO-DAVID FINE, M.D, M.P.H.

Professor of Dermatology, School of Medicine, and Adjunct Professor of Epidemiology, School of Public Health, University of North Carolina at Chapel Hill; Attending Physician, University of North Carolina Hospitals, Chapel Hill, North Carolina

Papulosquamous Disorders

LORETTA P. FINNEGAN, M.D.

Adjunct Professor of Pediatrics, Psychiatry and Human Behavior, Jefferson Medical College, Thomas Jefferson University; Director, Women's Health Initiative, National Institutes of Health, Bethesda, Maryland

Infants of Drug-dependent Mothers

LEWIS R. FIRST, M.D.
Professor and Chairman, Department of Pediatrics, University of Vermont, Burlington, Vermont
Foreign Bodies in the Nose and Pharynx; Nausea and Vomiting; Foreign Bodies in the Gastrointestinal Tract

MARGARET C. FISHER, M.D.
Associate Professor of Pediatrics and Associate Chair for Undergraduate Education, Department of Pediatrics, Medical College of Pennsylvania/Hahnemann University; Hospital Epidemiologist and Member, Section of Infectious Disease, St. Christopher's Hospital for Children, Philadelphia, Pennsylvania
Infant Botulism

COY D. FITCH, M.D.
Dref's Professor and Chairman, Department of Internal Medicine, St. Louis University School of Medicine; Chief of Medical Service, St. Louis University Hospital, St. Louis, Missouri
Malaria

RICHARD E. FITZPATRICK, M.D.
Assistant Clinical Professor, Division of Dermatology, Department of Medicine, University of California San Diego; Consultant, Scripps Hospital and Mercy Hospital, San Diego, California
Fungal Infections of the Skin

LARRY E. FLEISCHMANN, M.D.
Professor of Pediatrics, Wayne State University School of Medicine; Chief of Staff and Pediatric Nephrologist, Children's Hospital of Michigan, Detroit, Michigan
Systemic Hypertension; Fluid and Electrolyte Therapy in Children

MICHAEL L. FORBES, M.D.
Fellow, Pediatric Critical Care, and Former Chief Resident, Inpatient Services, Children's Hospital of Pittsburgh, Pittsburgh, Pennsylvania
Cellulitis

MARTIN T. FOSBURG, M.D.
Formerly, Assistant Professor of Pediatrics, Harvard Medical School; Associate Director, Transfusion Service, Children's Hospital, Boston, Massachusetts
Adverse Reactions to Blood Transfusion

WILLIAM W. FOX, M.D.
Professor of Pediatrics, University of Pennsylvania School of Medicine; Senior Physician, Children's Hospital of Philadelphia, Philadelphia, Pennsylvania
Meconium Aspiration Syndrome

KATHERINE B. FREEMAN, M.D.
Assistant Professor of Pediatrics, Brown University School of Medicine; Physician, Rhode Island Hospital, Providence, Rhode Island
Hirschsprung's Disease

GILBERT ANTHONY FRIDAY, Jr., M.D.
Professor of Pediatrics, University of Pittsburgh School of Medicine; Chief, Clinical Services, Asthma and Allergic Disease Center, Children's Hospital of Pittsburgh, Pittsburgh, Pennsylvania
Allergic Rhinitis; Insect Stings

ELLEN M. FRIEDMAN, M.D.
Professor of Otolaryngology, Head and Neck Surgery and Pediatrics, Baylor College of Medicine; Chief of Service, Pediatric Otolaryngology, Texas Children's Hospital, Houston, Texas
Foreign Bodies in External Auditory Canal

DONALD C. FYLER, M.D.
Professor Emeritus of Pediatrics, Harvard Medical School; Associate Chief of Cardiology Emeritus, Children's Hospital, Boston, Massachusetts
Cardiac Neoplasms and Other Intracardiac Masses

WILLIAM A. GAHL, M.D., Ph.D.
Head, Section on Human Biochemical Genetics, Human Genetics Branch, National Institute of Child Health and Human Development, National Institutes of Health, Bethesda, Maryland
Lysosomal Storage Disease

J. CARLTON GARTNER, Jr., M.D.
Professor of Pediatrics and Vice Chairman, Department of Pediatrics, University of Pittsburgh School of Medicine; Director, Pediatric Residency Program, Children's Hospital of Pittsburgh, Pittsburgh, Pennsylvania
Recurrent Abdominal Pain

ROBERT L. GEGGEL, M.D.
Associate Professor of Pediatrics, Tufts Medical School; Cardiologist and Director, Pediatric Cardiac Catheterization Laboratory, The Floating Hospital for Children at New England Medical Center, Boston, Massachusetts
Pulmonary Hypertension

ROBERT H. GELBER, M.D.
Clinical Professor of Medicine, University of California San Francisco, San Francisco, California
Leprosy (Hansen's Disease)

STEPHEN E. GELLIS, M.D.
Assistant Professor of Dermatology (Pediatrics), Harvard Medical School; Chief, Dermatology Program, Children's Hospital, Boston, Massachusetts
Disorders of the Hair and Scalp; Disorders of the Sebaceous Glands and Sweat Glands

MICHAEL K. GEORGIEFF, M.D.
Associate Professor of Pediatrics, University of Minnesota School of Medicine; Staff Neonatologist, University of Minnesota Hospital System, Minneapolis, Minnesota
Infants of Diabetic Mothers

JEFFREY S. GERDES, M.D.
Associate Professor of Pediatrics, Jefferson Medical College, Thomas Jefferson University; Chief, Section on Newborn Pediatrics, Pennsylvania Hospital, Philadelphia, Pennsylvania
Tetanus Neonatorum; Bronchopulmonary Dysplasia

ANNE A. GERSHON, M.D.
Professor of Pediatrics and Director, Division of Infectious Diseases, Columbia University College of Physicians and Surgeons, New York, New York
Varicella-Zoster Virus Infection

GERALD S. GILCHRIST, M.D.
Helen C. Levitt Professor and Chairman, Department of Pediatric and Adolescent Medicine, Mayo Medical School; Director, Comprehensive Hemophilia Center, Mayo Medical Center, Rochester, Minnesota
Congenital and Acquired Disorders of Coagulation

CHARLES M. GINSBURG, M.D.
Professor and Chairman and Marilyn R. Corrigan Distinguished Chair in Pediatric Research, University of Texas Southwestern Medical Center; Chief of Staff, Children's Medical Center of Dallas; Chief of Pediatrics, Parkland Memorial Hospital, Dallas, Texas
Erythema Multiforme; Human Parvovirus B19 Infections; Animal and Human Bites and Bite-related Infections

BRETT P. GIROIR, M.D.
Assistant Professor, Department of Pediatrics, Division of Critical Care Medicine, University of Texas Southwestern Medical Center; Attending Physician, Pediatric Intensive Care Unit, Children's Medical Center and Pediatric Trauma Unit, Parkland Memorial Hospital, Dallas, Texas
Erythema Multiforme

LAURENCE B. GIVNER, M.D.
Associate Professor of Pediatrics, Bowman Gray School of Medicine, Wake Forest University; Attending Physician, Brenner Children's Hospital, Winston-Salem, North Carolina
Aseptic Meningitis

MARY P. GLODE, M.D.
Professor of Pediatrics, University of Colorado Health Sciences Center; Director, Medical Education, The Children's Hospital, Denver, Colorado
Meningococcal Infections

BENJAMIN D. GOLD, M.D.
Assistant Professor of Pediatrics, Adjunct Assistant Professor of Microbiology and Immunology, and Attending Physician, Division of Pediatric Gastroenterology and Nutrition, Emory University School of Medicine. Atlanta, Georgia
Helicobacter pylori

RICHARD B. GOLDBLOOM, O.C., M.D., F.R.C.P.C.
Professor of Pediatrics, Dalhousie University; formerly Pediatrician-in-Chief, The Izaak Walton Killam Children's Hospital, Halifax, Nova Scotia, Canada
The Tonsil and Adenoid Problem

MARIA D. GOLDSTEIN, M.D.
Clinical Assistant Professor, Department of Pediatrics, University of New Mexico School of Medicine, Albuquerque, New Mexico
Plague

LINDA GRANOWETTER, M.D.
Assistant Professor of Pediatrics, Mount Sinai School of Medicine; Clinical Director of Pediatric Oncology, Mount Sinai Medical Center, New York, New York
Malignant Lymphomas

PETER GREALLY, M.D., M.R.C.P.I.
Honorary Senior Lecturer in Pediatrics, University of Dublin, Trinity College; Consultant in Pediatric Respiratory Medicine, National Children's Hospital, Dublin, Ireland
Right Middle Lobe Syndrome

ALEXANDER A. GREEN, M.D.
Professor of Pediatrics and Director, Section of Pediatric Hematology/Oncology, Rush Medical College; Senior Attending Physician, Rush-Presbyterian-St. Luke's Medical Center, Chicago, Illinois
Neuroblastoma

MICHAEL GREEN, M.D., M.P.H.
Assistant Professor of Pediatrics and Surgery, University of Pittsburgh School of Medicine; Division of Infectious Diseases, Children's Hospital of Pittsburgh, Pittsburgh, Pennsylvania
Leptospirosis; Viral Pneumonia

MORRIS GREEN, M.D.
Perry W. Lesh Professor of Pediatrics, Indiana University School of Medicine; Medical Staff, James Whitcomb Riley Hospital for Children, Indianapolis, Indiana
Psychosomatic Illnesses

JAY S. GREENSPAN, M.D.
Associate Professor of Pediatrics and Acting Director, Division of Neonatology, Department of Pediatrics, Jefferson Medical College, Thomas Jefferson University; Acting Director of Nurseries, Thomas Jefferson University Hospital, Philadelphia, Pennsylvania
Respiratory Distress Syndrome and Atelectasis

KATHERINE TEETS GRIMM, M.D.
Associate Professor of Pediatrics, Mount Sinai School of Medicine; Director, Divisions of Ambulatory Pediatrics and Pediatric Emergency Medicine, Mount Sinai Medical Center, New York, New York
Adverse Drug Reactions

CHARLES GROSE, M.D.
Professor of Pediatrics and Director of Infectious Diseases, University of Iowa Hospital, Iowa City, Iowa
Infectious Mononucleosis

KARYN L. GROSSMAN, M.D.
Resident in Dermatology, Harvard Medical School, Boston, Massachusetts
Chronic Nonhereditary Vesiculobullous Disorders

MOSES GROSSMAN, M.D.
Professor Emeritus of Pediatrics, University of California San Francisco and San Francisco General Hospital, San Francisco, California
Brucellosis

ALAN B. GRUSKIN, M.D.
Professor, Wayne State University School of Medicine; Chairman and Pediatrician-in-Chief, Children's Hospital of Michigan, Detroit, Michigan
Systemic Hypertension; Fluid and Electrolyte Therapy in Children

RICHARD L. GUERRANT, M.D.
Professor of Medicine, University of Virginia School of Medicine, Charlottesville, Virginia
Clostridium difficile

PAMELA J. GUEST, M.D.
Assistant Clinical Professor, Department of Dermatology, University of North Carolina at Chapel Hill; Attending Physician, University of North Carolina Hospitals, Chapel Hill, North Carolina
Papulosquamous Disorders

MARY ANNE GUGGENHEIM, M.D.
Board Member, Epilepsy Foundation of America; Pediatric Neurology Services, St. Peters Community Hospital, Helena, Montana
Febrile Seizures

ANN P. GUILLOT, M.D.
Associate Professor of Pediatrics, University of Vermont; Attending in Pediatrics, Fletcher Allen Health Care, Burlington, Vermont, and Dartmouth-Hitchcock Medical Center, Lebanon, New Hampshire
Renal Vein Thrombosis

RASHMI GUPTA, M.D.
Assistant Professor, Departments of Pediatrics and Neurology, Wayne State Univesity School of Medicine; Staff Neurologist, Children's Hospital of Michigan, Detroit, Michigan
Infantile Spasms

CYNTHIA GUZZO, M.D.
Assistant Professor, Department of Dermatology, University of Pennsylvania; Director, Psoriasis Center, Hospital of the University of Pennsylvania, Philadelphia, Pennsylvania
Atopic Dermatitis; Other Skin Tumors; Sun Protection

FOUAD M. HAJJAR, M.D.
Attending Physician, Pediatric Hematology-Oncology, Florida Hospital, Orlando, Florida
Indications for Splenectomy; Postsplenectomy Sepsis

MARGARET R. HAMMERSCHLAG, M.D.
Professor of Pediatrics and Medicine, State University of New York Health Science Center at Brooklyn; Active Attending, Kings County Hospital Center; Co-Director, Division of Pediatric Infectious Diseases, University Hospital of Brooklyn, Brooklyn, New York
Chlamydia

STEVEN D. HANDLER, M.D.
Associate Professor, Department of Otorhinolaryngology: Head and Neck Surgery, University of Pennsylvania School of Medicine; Associate Director of Otolaryngology, Children's Hospital of Philadelphia, Philadelphia, Pennsylvania
Developmental Cysts of the Neck; Lymphangioma

JANE N. HANNAH, Ed.D.
Assistant Professor of Pediatrics, Vanderbilt University Medical Center, Nashville, Tennessee
Disorders of Learning

MARY CATHERINE HARRIS, M.D.
Associate Professor of Pediatrics, University of Pennsylvania School of Medicine; Staff Neonatologist, Children's Hospital of Philadelphia, Philadelphia, Pennsylvania
Preparation for Transfer

ROBERT H.A. HASLAM, M.D., F.R.C.P.(C.)
Professor of Pediatrics and Neurology and Chairman of Pediatrics, University of Toronto; Pediatrician-in-Chief, Hospital for Sick Children, Toronto, Ontario, Canada
The Polyradiculoneuropathies

GREGORY F. HAYDEN, M.D.
Professor of Pediatrics, University of Virginia School of Medicine; Attending Pediatrician, Children's Medical Center of the University of Virginia, Charlottesville, Virginia
Mumps

SABRINA M. HEIDEMANN, M.D.
Assistant Professor of Pediatrics, Wayne State University School of Medicine; Staff Intensivist, Children's Hospital of Michigan, Detroit, Michigan
Respiratory Insufficiency

JONATHAN D. HEILICZER, M.D.
Associate Professor and Director of Pediatric Nephrology, Rush Medical College, Chicago, Illinois
Acute Renal Failure

DANN K. HEILMAN, M.D.
Fellow in Pediatric Allergy, Mayo Graduate School of Medicine, Rochester, Minnesota
Asthma

DOUGLAS C. HEINER, M.D., PH.D.
Professor of Pediatrics, Emeritus, Division of Immunology/Allergy, University of California Los Angeles School of Medicine, Los Angeles, California; Associate Medical Staff, Provo Asthma, Allergy and Immunology Clinic, Utah Valley Regional Medical Center, Provo, Utah
Anaphylaxis

WILLIAM C. HEIRD, M.D.
Professor of Pediatrics and Investigator, Children's Nutrition Research Center, Baylor College of Medicine, Houston, Texas
Feeding the Low Birth Weight Infant: Enteral and Parenteral

ROBERT A. HENDRIX, M.D.
Staff, Presbyterian Hospital, Charlotte, North Carolina
Epistaxis and Nasal Trauma

JULIANE HENTSCHEL, M.D.
Attending in Neonatology, UKRV Children's Clinic, Berlin, Federal Republic of Germany
Genital Mycoplasmal Infections

JOHN T. HERRIN, M.B.B.S.
Associate Clinical Professor of Pediatrics, Harvard Medical School; Director, Clinical Services, Division of Nephrology, Children's Hospital, Boston, Massachusetts
Hypocalcemia and Tetany

PETER T. HEYDEMANN, M.D.
Assistant Professor of Pediatrics and Neurology, Rush Medical College; Head, Division of Pediatric Neurology, Rush-Presbyterian-St. Luke's Medical Center, Chicago, Illinois
Muscular Dystrophy and Related Myopathies

RONALD B. HIRSCHL, M.D.
Assistant Professor of Surgery, Section of Pediatric Surgery, The University of Michigan Medical School, Ann Arbor, Michigan
Neonatal Intestinal Obstruction

DENA HOFKOSH, M.D.
Assistant Professor of Pediatrics, University of Pittsburgh School of Medicine; Coordinator, Infant Development Program, Child Development Unit, Children's Hospital of Pittsburgh, Pittsburgh, Pennsylvania
Effects of Maternal Alcohol Ingestion on the Developing Fetus

RONALD J. HOGG, M.D.
Director, Pediatric Nephrology, Baylor University Medical Center, Dallas, Texas
Vesicoureteral Reflux

PHILIP G. HOLTZAPPLE, M.D.
Professor of Medicine and Pediatrics and Interim Chief, Division of Gastroenterology, Department of Medicine, State University of New York Health Science Center, Syracuse, New York
Cirrhosis

DAVID HOLTZMAN, M.D., Ph.D.
Associate Professor, Harvard Medical School; Associate in Neurology, Children's Hospital, Boston, Massachusetts
Benign Intracranial Hypertension

IAN R. HOLZMAN, M.D.
Professor of Pediatrics, Obstetrics, Gynecology and Reproductive Sciences, Mount Sinai Medical Center; Chief, Division of Newborn Medicine and Acting Chair, Department of Pediatrics, Mount Sinai Hospital, New York, New York
Management of the Newborn Infant at Delivery

PAUL J. HONIG, M.D.
Professor of Pediatrics and Dermatology, University of Pennsylvania School of Medicine; Director, Pediatric Dermatology, Children's Hospital of Philadelphia, Philadelphia, Pennsylvania
Drug Reactions and the Skin; Erythema Nodosum; Diaper Dermatitis

BRENDA R. HOOK, M.D.
Assistant Professor of Pediatrics, University of Texas Medical School; Neonatologist, Hermann Hospital, Harris County Hospital District, and Lyndon B. Johnson Hospital, Houston, Texas
Pneumothorax and Other Air Leaks

PETER J. HOTEZ, M.D., Ph.D.

Assistant Professor, Departments of Pediatrics (Infectious Diseases Division) and Epidemiology and Public Health, Yale University School of Medicine; Associate Physician (Pediatrician), Yale–New Haven Hospital, New Haven, Connecticut

Toxocara canis

WALTER T. HUGHES, M.D.

Professor of Pediatrics, University of Tennessee College of Medicine; Chairman, Department of Infectious Diseases, St. Jude Children's Research Hospital, Memphis, Tennessee

Pneumocystis carinii *Pneumonitis*

CARL E. HUNT, M.D.

Professor and Chairman, Department of Pediatrics, Medical College of Ohio, Toledo, Ohio

Hypoventilation Syndromes

BARBARA IANNI, D.O.

Instructor in Pediatrics, Jefferson Medical College, Thomas Jefferson University; Senior Staff Pediatrician, Methodist Hospital, Philadelphia, Pennsylvania

Listeria monocytogenes

LILLY CHENG IMMERGLUCK, M.D.

Fellow, Pediatric Infectious Diseases, University of Chicago Priztker School of Medicine and Wyler Children's Hospital, Chicago, Illinois

Infections Caused by **Haemophilus influenzae** *Type B*

JULIE R. INGELFINGER, M.D.

Associate Professor of Pediatrics, Harvard Medical School; Chief, Pediatric Nephrology Unit, Massachusetts General Hospital, Boston, Massachusetts

Peripheral Vascular Disease; Renal Hypoplasia and Dysplasia

MIRA IRONS, M.D.

Assistant Professor of Pediatrics, Tufts University School of Medicine; Clinical and Biochemical Geneticist, Department of Pediatrics, The Floating Hospital for Infants and Children at New England Medical Center, Boston, Massachusetts

Carbohydrate Disorders

SHUNZABURO IWATSUKI, M.D., Ph.D.

Professor of Surgery, University of Pittsburgh School of Medicine and Medical Center, Pittsburgh, Pennsylvania

Tumors of the Liver

KATHY JABS, M.D.

Assistant Professor of Pediatrics, Harvard Medical School; Assistant in Nephrology, Children's Hospital, Boston, Massachusetts

Chronic Renal Failure

RICHARD F. JACOBS, M.D.

Horace C. Cabe Professor of Pediatrics, University of Arkansas for Medical Sciences; Chief, Pediatric Infectious Diseases, Arkansas Children's Hospital, Little Rock, Arkansas

Tuberculosis; Tularemia

DAVID S. JARDINE, M.D.

Assistant Professor of Anesthesiology and Pediatrics, University of Washington School of Medicine and Children's Hospital, Seattle, Washington

Malignant Hyperthermia; Heat-related Illnesses Including Hemorrhagic Shock and Encephalopathy Syndrome and Heat Stroke

BERNETT L. JOHNSON, Jr., M.D.

Professor of Dermatology and Associate Dean for Graduate Medical Education, University of Pennsylvania School of Medicine; Hospital of the University of Pennsylvania, Philadelphia, Pennsylvania

Nevi and Nevoid Tumors

HELEN S. JOHNSTONE, M.D.

Associate Professor of Pediatrics, University of Illinois School of Medicine; Attending Physician, University of Illinois Hospital, Chicago, Illinois

Thalassemia

SUE J. JUE, M.D.

Post-Doctoral Fellow, Division of Infectious Diseases, Department of Pediatrics, University of Alabama at Birmingham, Birmingham, Alabama; Assistant Professor of Pediatrics, Division of Infectious Diseases, Schumpert Medical Center, Shreveport, Louisiana

Herpes Simplex Virus Infections

HARALD JÜPPNER, M.D.

Associate Professor of Pediatrics, Harvard Medical School; Assistant in Pediatrics, Massachusetts General Hospital, Boston, Massachusetts

Parathyroid Disease

LEONARD B. KABAN, D.M.D., M.D.

Walte C. Guralnick Professor of Oral and Marillofacial Surgery and Chairman of Department of Oral and Marillofacial Surgery, Harvard School of Dental Medicine; Chief, Oral and Maxillofacial Surgery Service, Massachusetts General Hospital, Boston, Massachusetts

Craniofacial Malformations

PAIGE KAPLAN, M.B.B.Ch.

Associate Professor, University of Pennsylvania School of Medicine; Senior Physician, Division of Biochemical Development and Molecular Diseases, Children's Hospital of Philadelphia, Philadelphia, Pennsylvania

Amino Acid Disorders

SHELDON L. KAPLAN, M.D.

Professor and Vice-Chairman for Clinical Affairs, Baylor College of Medicine; Chief, Infectious Disease Service, Texas Children's Hospital, Houston, Texas

Lymph Node Infections

MANOOCHEHR KARJOO, M.D.

Professor and Chief, Pediatric Gastroenterology and Nutrition, State University of New York Health Science Center at Syracuse; Attending Physician, Department of Pediatrics, Crouse Irving Memorial Hospital, Syracuse, New York

Cirrhosis

SUDHA KASHYAP, M.D.

Associate Professor of Clinical Pediatrics, College of Physicians and Surgeons, Columbia University; Associate Attending Pediatrician, Babies and Children's (Presbyterian) Hospital, New York, New York

Feeding the Low Birth Weight Infant: Enteral and Parenteral

AUBREY J. KATZ, M.D.

Chief, Division of Pediatric Gastroenterology, Newton-Wellesley Hospital, Newton, Massachusetts

Gastroesophageal Reflux Disease

JULIE A. KATZ, M.D.

Assistant Professor of Pediatrics, Hematology/Oncology, University of Texas Southwestern Medical School, Dallas, Texas

Malignant Tumors of Bone and Limb Salvage

MICHAEL KATZ, M.D.

Reuben S. Carpentier Professor Emeritus of Pediatrics and Professor Emeritus of Public Health (Tropical Medicine), Columbia University; Consultant Emeritus, Presbyterian Hospital, New York, New York

Amebiasis; Enterobiasis; Giardiasis

MARGARET A. KENNA, M.D.
Appointment Pending, Harvard Medical School; Pediatric Otolaryngologist, Children's Hospital, Boston, Massachusetts
Labyrinthitis

DAVID W. KENNEDY, M.D.
Professor and Chairman of Otorhinolaryngology: Head and Neck Surgery, University of Pennsylvania School of Medicine; Hospital of the University of Pennsylvania, Philadelphia, Pennsylvania
Rhinitis and Sinusitis

KWANG SIK KIM, M.D.
Professor of Pediatrics, University of Southern California School of Medicine; Head, Division of Infectious Diseases and Attending Physician, Children's Hospital of Los Angeles, Los Angeles, California
Candidiasis

CHRISTOPHER L. KING, M.D., Ph.D.
Assistant Professor of Medicine, Division of Geographic Medicine, Case Western Reserve University; Staff Physician, Veterans Affairs, Wade Park Veterans Administration, Cleveland, Ohio
Schistosomiasis

JOHN P. KINSELLA, M.D.
Associate Professor, Section of Neonatology, Department of Pediatrics, University of Colorado School of Medicine; Assistant Director, Children's Emergency Transport Service, Children's Hospital, Denver, Colorado
Persistent Pulmonary Hypertension

MARTIN B. KLEIMAN, M.D.
Professor of Pediatrics and Director, Section of Pediatric Infectious Diseases, Indiana University School of Medicine; Attending Physician, Indiana University Hospitals and Wishard Memorial Hospital, Indianapolis, Indiana
Immunization Practice

JEROME O. KLEIN, M.D.
Professor of Pediatrics, Boston University School of Medicine; Director, Division of Pediatric Infectious Diseases, Boston City Hospital, Boston, Massachusetts
Pneumonias; **Mycoplasma**

RONALD E. KLEINMAN, M.D.
Associate Professor of Pediatrics, Harvard Medical School; Chief, Pediatric Gastroenterology and Nutrition, Massachusetts General Hospital, Boston, Massachusetts
Normal Nutrition; Chronic Active Hepatitis; Disorders of the Biliary Tree

ROBERT KLIEGMAN, M.D.
Professor and Chair, Department of Pediatrics, Medical College of Wisconsin; Pediatrician in Chief, Children's Hospital of Wisconsin, Milwaukee, Wisconsin
Necrotizing Enterocolitis

MARK W. KLINE, M.D.
Associate Professor of Pediatrics, Sections of Allergy/Immunology and Infectious Diseases, Baylor College of Medicine; Attending Physician, Texas Children's Hospital, Houston, Texas
Aspergillosis

SAMUEL A. KOCOSHIS, M.D.
Associate Professor of Pediatrics, University of Pittsburgh School of Medicine; Director, Pediatric Gastroenterology, Children's Hospital of Pittsburgh, Pittsburgh, Pennsylvania
Ascites

STEVE KOHL, M.D.
Professor of Pediatrics, University of California San Francisco; Chief, Pediatric Infectious Diseases, Moffit-Long Hospital and San Francisco General Hospital, San Francisco, California
Yersinia enterocolitica *Infection*

KATHERINE M. KONZEN, M.D., M.P.H.
Assistant Professor of Pediatrics and Consultant, Section of Pediatric Emergency Medicine, Mayo Medical Center, Rochester, Minnesota
Snakebites

BRUCE R. KORF, M.D., Ph.D.
Associate Professor of Neurology, Harvard Medical School; Director, Clinical Genetics Program, Children's Hospital, Boston, Massachusetts
Neurocutaneous Syndromes

KAREN L. KOTLOFF, M.D.
Associate Professor, Division of Infectious Disease and Tropical Pediatrics, Department of Pediatrics, University of Maryland School of Medicine, Baltimore, Maryland
Viral Hepatitis

RICHARD M. KRAVITZ, M.D.
Assistant Professor of Pediatrics, University of Pennsylvania School of Medicine; Attending Pulmonologist and Director, Asthma Care Program, Division of Pulmonary Medicine, Children's Hospital of Philadelphia, Philadelphia, Pennsylvania
Sarcoidosis

EDWARD P. KRENZELOK, Pharm.D., A.B.A.T.
Professor of Pharmacy and Pediatrics, University of Pittsburgh School of Medicine; Director, Pittsburgh Poison Center, Children's Hospital of Pittsburgh, Pittsburgh, Pennsylvania
Acute Poisonings

CYNTHIA S. KRETSCHMAR, M.D.
Assistant Professor of Pediatric Hematology-Oncology, Tufts University School of Medicine; Attending Physician, Division of Hematology-Oncology, Department of Pediatrics, The Floating Hospital for Children, New England Medical Center, Boston, Massachusetts
Childhood Brain Tumors

GEOFFREY KURLAND, M.D.
Associate Professor of Pediatrics, Division of Pediatric Pulmonology, Department of Pediatrics, University of Pittsburgh School of Medicine and Children's Hospital of Pittsburgh, Pittsburgh, Pennsylvania
Emphysema

DAVID LACOMIS, M.D.
Assistant Professor of Neurology and Pathology, University of Pittsburgh School of Medicine; Attending Physician, University of Pittsburgh Medical Center, Pittsburgh, Pennsylvania
Myasthenia Gravis

RONALD V. LACRO, M.D.
Instructor in Pediatrics, Harvard Medical School; Assistant in Cardiology, Children's Hospital, Boston, Massachusetts
Marfan Syndrome

ALAN M. LAKE, M.D.
Associate Professor of Pediatrics, Johns Hopkins University School of Medicine, Baltimore, Maryland
Disorders of the Esophagus

JOSEPH W. LANDAU, M.D.

Associate Clinical Professor of Medicine (Dermatology), Division of Dermatology, Department of Medicine, University of California Los Angeles School of Medicine, Los Angeles, California; Attending Physician, Dermatology Service, Santa Monica Hospital and St. John's Hospital, Santa Monica, California

Warts and Molluscum Contagiosum

PHILIP LANZKOWSKY, M.D., Sc.D., F.R.C.P., D.C.H.

Professor of Pediatrics, Albert Einstein College of Medicine; Chief of Staff and Chairman of Pediatrics, Schneider Children's Hospital, New Hyde Park, New York

Megaloblastic Anemia

ALLEN LAPEY, M.D.

Assistant Clinical Professor of Pediatrics, Harvard Medical School; Associate Pediatrician, Massachusetts General Hospital, Boston, Massachusetts

Urticaria and Angioedema

MARC R. LAUFER, M.D.

Instructor in Obstetrics, Gynecology, and Reproductive Biology, Harvard Medical School; Chief, Pediatric/Adolescent Gynecology, Assistant in Surgery (Gynecology), and Assistant in Medicine (Adolescent/Young Adult Medicine), Children's Hospital; Associate Obstetrician/Gynecologist, Division of Reproductive Endocrinology, Department of Obstetrics and Gynecology, Brigham and Women's Hospital, Boston, Massachusetts

Gynecology

MARY M. LEE, M.D.

Assistant Professor of Pediatrics, Harvard Medical School; Assistant Pediatrician and Biologist, Pediatric Endocrine Unit, Massachusetts General Hospital, Boston, Massachusetts

Tall Stature

PETER A. LEE, M.D., Ph.D.

Professor of Pediatrics, University of Pittsburgh School of Medicine; Attending Physician, Children's Hospital of Pittsburgh, Pittsburgh, Pennsylvania

Disorders of the Adrenal Gland

LAWRENCE G. LEICHTMAN, M.D.

Associate Professor of Pediatrics and Clinical Genetics, Eastern Virginia Medical School; Clinical Geneticist, Children's Hospital of the King's Daughters, Norfolk, Virginia

Hypoglycemia and Glycogen Storage Diseases; Hepatolenticular Degeneration (Wilson Disease)

NEAL S. LeLEIKO, M.D., Ph.D.

Professor of Pediatrics, Mount Sinai School of Medicine; Chief, Pediatric Gastroenterology, Nutrition, and Liver Diseases, Mount Sinai Medical Center, New York, New York

Pancreatic Diseases

JAMES A. LEMONS, M.D.

Hugh McK. Landon Professor of Pediatrics and Director, Section of Neonatal-Perinatal Medicine, Indiana University School of Medicine and Medical Center, Indianapolis, Indiana

Disturbances of Intrauterine Growth

MYRON M. LEVINE, M.D., D.T.P.H.

Professor of Medicine, University of Maryland at Baltimore, Center for Vaccine Development, Baltimore, Maryland

Cholera

LYNNE L. LEVITSKY, M.D.

Associate Professor of Pediatrics, Harvard Medical School; Chief, Pediatric Endocrine Unit, Massachusetts General Hospital, Boston, Massachusetts

Tall Stature; Insulin-dependent Diabetes Mellitus

JAMES M. LEWIS, M.D.

Associate Professor of Pediatrics, Marshall University School of Medicine, Huntington, West Virginia

Lymphedema

L. GLEN LEWIS, M.D.

Procter Research Scholar, Division of Pediatric Gastroenterology and Nutrition, Children's Hospital Medical Center, Cincinnati, Ohio

Cholestasis (Conjugated Hyperbilirubinemia)

MARY W. LIEH-LAI, M.D.

Assistant Professor, Department of Pediatrics, Wayne State University School of Medicine; Director, Intensive Care Unit, Children's Hospital of Michigan, Detroit, Michigan

Head Injury

CRAIG W. LILLEHEI, M.D.

Assistant Professor of Surgery, Harvard Medical School; Associate in Surgery, Children's Hospital, Boston, Massachusetts

Congenital Diaphragmatic Hernia

JEFFREY M. LIPTON, M.D., Ph.D.

Associate Professor of Pediatrics, Mount Sinai School of Medicine; Chief, Pediatric Hematology/Oncology, Mount Sinai Medical Center, New York, New York

Langerhans Cell Histiocytosis

CLIFFORD LO, M.D., M.P.H., Sc.D.

Assistant Professor of Pediatrics and Nutrition, Harvard Medical School and Harvard School of Public Health; Director, Nutrition Support Service, Children's Hospital, Boston, Massachusetts

Normal Nutrition

SARAH S. LONG, M.D.

Professor of Pediatrics, Temple University School of Medicine; Chief, Section of Infectious Diseases, St. Christopher's Hospital for Children, Philadelphia, Pennsylvania

Pertussis

MICHAEL T. LONGAKER, M.D.

Chief Resident in Plastic Surgery, New York University School of Medicine, New York, New York

Craniofacial Malformations

JOSEPH LOSCALZO, M.D., Ph.D.

Distinguished Professor of Medicine and Biochemistry, Director, Whitaker Cardiovascular Institute, and Vice Chairman, Department of Medicine, Boston University School of Medicine; Chief, Cardiovascular Medicine, Boston University Medical Center, Boston, Massachusetts

Hyperlipoproteinemia

JEFFREY L. LOUGHEAD, M.D.

Assistant Clinical Professor of Pediatrics, Wright State University School of Medicine; Medical Co-Director of Newborn Intensive Care, Children's Medical Center, Dayton, Ohio

Osteopenia of Prematurity

GERALD M. LOUGHLIN, M.D.

Associate Professor of Pediatrics, Johns Hopkins University School of Medicine; Director, Eudowood Division of Pediatric Respiratory Sciences, Johns Hopkins Hospital, Baltimore, Maryland

Bronchitis and Bronchiolitis

FREDERICK H. LOVEJOY, Jr., M.D.

William Berenberg Professor of Pediatrics, Harvard Medical School; Associate Physician-in-Chief, Children's Hospital, Boston, Massachusetts

Reye Syndrome

JANICE A. LOWE, M.D.
Instructor, Harvard Medical School; Associate Pediatrician, Massachusetts General Hospital, Boston, Massachusetts
Preventing Childhood Injuries

M. JEFFREY MAISELS, M.B., B.Ch.
Clinical Professor of Pediatrics, Wayne State University School of Medicine, Detroit, Michigan, and University of Michigan Medical School, Ann Arbor, Michigan; Chairman, Department of Pediatrics, William Beaumont Hospital, Royal Oak, Michigan
Neonatal Hyperbilirubinemia and Kernicterus

JOSEPH A. MAJZOUB, M.D.
Associate Professor of Pediatrics and Medicine, Harvard Medical School; Senior Associate in Medicine, Children's Hospital, Boston, Massachusetts
Diabetes Insipidus

SUDESH P. MAKKER, M.D.
Professor of Pediatrics and Chief, Division of Nephrology, University of California Davis; Director, Pediatric Nephrology, University of California Davis Medical Center, Sacramento, California
Acute and Chronic Glomerulonephritis

J. JEFFREY MALATACK, M.D.
Professor of Pediatrics, Temple University School of Medicine; Head, General Pediatrics, and Director, Diagnostic Referral Service, St. Christopher's Hospital for Children, Philadelphia, Pennsylvania
Cat-Scratch Disease

ERIC S. MALLER, M.D.
Assistant Professor of Pediatrics, University of Pennsylvania School of Medicine; Attending Physician, Division of Gastroenterology and Nutrition, and Medical Director, Liver Transplant Program, Children's Hospital of Philadelphia, Philadelphia, Pennsylvania
Malabsorptive Disorders

SUSAN BAYLISS MALLORY, M.D.
Associate Professor of Dermatology and Pediatrics, Washington University School of Medicine; Director, Pediatric Dermatology, St. Louis Children's Hospital, St. Louis, Missouri
Allergic Contact Dermatitis

KEITH E. MANDEL, M.D.
Assistant Instructor, Department of Pediatrics, University of Texas Southwestern Medical Center; Chief Resident, Children's Medical Center of Dallas, Dallas, Texas
Animal and Human Bites and Bite-related Infections

JAMES MANDELL, M.D.
Professor of Surgery and Pediatrics and Chief, Division of Urology, Albany Medical College, Albany, New York
Penis, Spermatic Cord, and Testes; Exstrophy of the Bladder

JOAN MANSFIELD, M.D.
Assistant Professor of Pediatrics, Harvard Medical School; Associate in Medicine (Endocrinology), Children's Hospital, Boston, Massachusetts
Gynecology

HERBERT C. MANSMANN, Jr., M.D.
Professor of Pediatrics and Associate Professor of Medicine, Jefferson Medical College, Thomas Jefferson University; Attending Physician, Thomas Jefferson University Hospital, Philadelphia, Pennsylvania
Magnesium Deficiency; Zinc Deficiency

PARIS TAYLOR MANSMANN, M.D.
Assistant Professor of Medicine, West Virginia University School of Medicine, Morgantown, West Virginia
Magnesium Deficiency; Zinc Deficiency

ANDREW M. MARGILETH, M.D.
Clinical Professor of Pediatrics, University of Virginia Health Sciences Center, Charlottesville, Virginia
Nontuberculous (Atypical) Mycobacterial Disease

MELVIN I. MARKS, M.D.
Vice Chairman, Department of Pediatrics, University of California Irvine, Irvine, California; Medical Director, Memorial Miller Children's Hospital, Long Beach, California
Yersinia enterocolitica Infection; Diphtheria

RICHARD J. MARTIN, M.D.
Professor of Pediatrics, Case Western Reserve University School of Medicine; Co-Director, Division of Neonatology, Rainbow Babies and Children's Hospital, Cleveland, Ohio
Pneumothorax and Other Air Leaks; Apnea of Prematurity

MARIA R. MASCARENHAS, M.B., B.S.
Assistant Professor of Pediatrics, University of Pennsylvania School of Medicine; Director, Nutrition Support Service, Children's Hospital of Philadelphia, Philadelphia, Pennsylvania
Vitamin Deficiencies and Excesses

ANN R. McGRAVEY, M.D.
Instructor, Harvard Medical School; Assistant in Medicine, Children's Hospital, Boston, Massachusetts
Nasopharyngitis

SARA C. McINTIRE, M.D.
Assistant Professor of Pediatrics, University of Pittsburgh School of Medicine and Children's Hospital of Pittsburgh, Pittsburgh, Pennsylvania
Headache

STEVEN E. McKENZIE, M.D., Ph.D.
Assistant Professor of Pediatrics and of Chemical and Biochemical Engineering, University of Pennsylvania School of Medicine; Attending Physician, Division of Hematology, and Member, Stokes Research Institute, Children's Hospital of Philadelphia, Philadelphia, Pennsylvania
Anemia and When to Transfuse

LINDA McKIBBEN, M.D., M.P.H.
Assistant Professor of Pediatrics and Project Director, The Pediatric Family Violence Awareness Project, Tufts University School of Medicine, Boston, Massachusetts; Preventive Medicine Resident, Carney Hospital, and Pediatrician, Neponset Health Center, Dorchester, Massachusetts
Children of Homeless and Battered Women

JULIA A. McMILLAN, M.D.
Associate Professor of Pediatrics, Johns Hopkins University School of Medicine; Director, Pediatric Residency Training Program, Johns Hopkins Hospital, Baltimore, Maryland
Encephalitis

DAN G. McNAMARA, M.D.
Professor of Pediatrics, Baylor College of Medicine; Emeritus Chief of Pediatric Cardiology, Texas Children's Hospital, Houston, Texas
Innocent Murmurs

LAURA F. McNICHOLAS, M.D., Ph.D.
Assistant Professor, Department of Psychiatry, University of Pennsylvania School of Medicine; Staff Physician, Philadelphia Veterans Affairs Medical Center, Philadelphia, Pennsylvania
Substance Abuse

MARIAN G. MICHAELS, M.D., M.P.H.

Assistant Professor of Pediatrics and Surgery, Division of Pediatric Infectious Diseases, University of Pittsburgh School of Medicine and Children's Hospital of Pittsburgh, Pittsburgh, Pennsylvania
Toxoplasmosis

RICHARD J. MIER, M.D.

Associate Professor of Pediatrics, University of Kentucky; Director, Pediatric Services, Shriners Hospital for Crippled Children, Lexington, Kentucky
Torticollis; Congenital Muscular Defects

LAURIE C. MILLER, M.D.

Assistant Professor of Pediatrics, Division of Pediatric Rheumatology, Tufts University School of Medicine; Pediatric Rheumatologist, The Floating Hospital for Children, Boston, Massachusetts
Dermatomyositis and Polymyositis

JAMES S. MISER, M.D.

Associate Professor of Pediatrics, University of Washington; Clinical Director, Pediatric Hematology/Oncology, Children's Hospital and Medical Center, Seattle, Washington
Malignant Tumors of the Kidney

THOMAS G. MITCHELL, Ph.D.

Associate Professor, Department of Microbiology, Duke University Medical Center, Durham, North Carolina
Blastomycosis

PHILLIP MOORE, M.D.

Assistant Professor of Pediatrics, University of California San Francisco, San Francisco, California
Cardiac Neoplasms and Other Intracardiac Masses

THOMAS MOSHANG, Jr., M.D.

Professor of Pediatrics, University of Pennsylvania School of Medicine; Acting Division Chief, Division of Endocrinology, Director, Endocrine Training Programs, and Director, Diagnostic and Research Growth Center, Children's Hospital of Philadelphia, Philadelphia, Pennsylvania
Short Stature

EUGENE MOWAD, M.D.

Resident, University of Pittsburgh School of Medicine, Pittsburgh, Pennsylvania
Cellulitis

LOUIS J. MUGLIA, M.D., Ph.D.

Instructor in Pediatrics, Harvard Medical School; Assistant in Medicine, Children's Hospital, Boston, Massachusetts
Diabetes Insipidus

PAMELA J. MURRAY, M.D., M.H.P.

Assistant Professor, Department of Pediatrics, University of Pittsburgh School of Medicine; Director, Section of Adolescent Medicine, Children's Hospital of Pittsburgh, Pittsburgh, Pennsylvania
Vulvitis, Vaginitis, and Urethritis; Sexuality Education and Contraception

HERBERT L. NEEDLEMAN, M.D.

Professor of Psychiatry and Pediatrics, University of Pittsburgh School of Medicine; Attending Physician, Children's Hospital of Pittsburgh, Pittsburgh, Pennsylvania
Lead Toxicity

JOHN D. NELSON, M.D.

Professor of Pediatrics, University of Texas Southwestern Medical Center at Dallas; Attending Staff, Children's Medical Center and Parkland Memorial Hospital, Dallas, Texas
Bone and Joint Infections

STEVEN W. NEUBAUER, M.D.

Assistant Professor of Dermatology and Pediatrics, University of Illinois at Chicago College of Medicine, Chicago, Illinois
Neonatal Skin Disorders

JANE W. NEWBURGER, M.D., M.P.H.

Associate Professor of Pediatrics, Harvard Medical School; Senior Associate in Cardiology, Children's Hospital, Boston, Massachusetts
Kawasaki Syndrome

MICHAEL A. NIGRO, D.O.

Professor of Neurology and Pediatrics, Wayne State University School of Medicine; Chief of Neurology, Children's Hospital of Michigan, Detroit, Michigan
Movement Disorders; Periodic Paralysis

JACQUELINE A. NOONAN, M.D.

Professor of Pediatrics and Chief of Pediatric Cardiology, University of Kentucky College of Medicine, Lexington, Kentucky
Congestive Heart Failure

CYNTHIA F. NORRIS, M.D.

Instructor in Pediatrics, University of Pennsylvania; Fellow, Pediatric Hematology-Oncology, Children's Hospital of Philadelphia, Philadelphia, Pennsylvania
Anemia and When to Transfuse

CHARLES P. O'BRIEN, M.D., Ph.D.

Professor and Vice Chairman, Department of Psychiatry, University of Pennsylvania; Chief, Psychiatry Service, Veterans Administration Medical Center, Philadelphia, Pennsylvania
Substance Abuse

REBECCA F. O'BRIEN, M.D.

Assistant Professor of Pediatrics, Tufts University School of Medicine; Attending Pediatrician, New England Medical Center, Boston, Massachusetts
Eating Disorders

HANS D. OCHS, M.D.

Professor of Pediatrics, University of Washington School of Medicine, Seattle, Washington
The Immunodeficiency Syndromes

EDWARD J. O'CONNELL, M.D.

Professor of Pediatrics, Mayo Medical School; Consultant, Section of General Pediatrics and Pediatric Allergy and Immunology, Mayo Clinic and Mayo Foundation, Rochester, Minnesota
Asthma

KWAKU OHENE-FREMPONG, M.D.

Associate Professor of Pediatrics, University of Pennsylvania School of Medicine; Director, Comprehensive Sickle Cell Center, The Children's Hospital of Philadelphia, Philadelphia, Pennsylvania
Management of Sickle Cell Disease

RICHARD D. OLSEN, M.D.

Assistant Professor of Pediatrics, Mayo Medical School; Consultant in Pediatrics, Mayo Clinic; Staff Physician, Rochester Methodist Hospital and St. Mary's Hospital, Rochester, Minnesota
Pica

JOSEPH OREN, M.D.

Assistant Professor of Pediatrics, Tufts University School of Medicine, New England Medical Center, Boston, Massachusetts
Pleural Effusion, Empyema, and Chylothorax

P. PEARL O'ROURKE, M.D.

Associate Professor of Anesthesiology (Pediatrics), University of Washington School of Medicine; Director, Pediatric Intensive Care Unit, and Attending Staff, Children's Hospital and Medical Center, Seattle, Washington

Septic Shock

ANN L. O'SULLIVAN, Ph.D., F.A.A.N.

University of Pennsylvania School of Nursing and The Children's Hospital of Philadelphia, Philadelphia, Pennsylvania

The Very Young Teen Parent

JAMES C. OVERALL, Jr., M.D.

Professor of Pediatrics and Pathology, Medical Director, Diagnostic Virology Laboratory, Associated Regional and University Pathologists, Pediatric Infectious Diseases Consultant, University of Utah and Primary Children's Medical Centers, Salt Lake City, Utah

Enteroviruses

JACK L. PARADISE, M.D.

Professor of Pediatrics, University of Pittsburgh School of Medicine; Active Staff, Division of General Academic Pediatrics, Children's Hospital of Pittsburgh, Pittsburgh, Pennsylvania

Otitis Media

DAVID S. PARSONS, M.D.

Professor of Surgery and Pediatrics, University of Missouri School of Medicine, Columbia, Missouri

Middle Ear Trauma

MARK S. PASTERNACK, M.D.

Associate Professor of Pediatrics, Harvard Medical School; Chief, Pediatric Infectious Disease Unit, Massachusetts General Hospital, Boston, Massachusetts

Peritonitis; Rabies

HOWARD A. PEARSON, M.D.

Professor of Pediatrics, Yale University School of Medicine; Attending Physician, Yale–New Haven Hospital, New Haven, Connecticut

Indications for Splenectomy; Postsplenectomy Sepsis

ALAN K. PERCY, M.D.

Professor and Director, Division of Pediatric Neurology, University of Alabama at Birmingham, Birmingham, Alabama

Degenerative Diseases of the Central Nervous System

GILBERTO R. PEREIRA, M.D.

Associate Professor of Pediatrics, University of Pennsylvania School of Medicine; Neonatologist, Children's Hospital of Philadelphia, Philadelphia, Pennsylvania

Nutritional Requirements of Low Birth Weight Infants

MICHAEL J. PETTEI, M.D., Ph.D.

Associate Professor of Pediatrics, Albert Einstein College of Medicine; Co-Chief, Division of Gastroenterology and Nutrition, Schneider Children's Hospital and Long Island Jewish Medical Center, New Hyde Park, New York

Constipation and Encopresis

DAVID A. PICCOLI, M.D.

Associate Professor of Pediatrics, University of Pennsylvania School of Medicine; Section Chief, Gastroenterology and Hepatology, Children's Hospital of Philadelphia, Philadelphia, Pennsylvania

Gastritis, Duodenitis, and Peptic Ulcer Disease

LARRY K. PICKERING, M.D.

Departments of Pediatrics and Microbiology/Immunology, Eastern Virginia Medical School; Director, Center for Pediatric Research, Children's Hospital of the King's Daughters, Norfolk, Virginia

Shigellosis; Campylobacter Infections

ROSITA S. PILDES, M.D.

Professor of Pediatrics, Finch University of Health Sciences/The Chicago Medical School; Neonatologist, Cook County Children's Hospital, Chicago, Illinois

Hemolytic Diseases of the Neonate

STANLEY A. PLOTKIN, M.D.

Medical and Scientific Director, Pasteur-Merieux-Connaught Laboratories, Marnes-la-Coquette, France; Professor Emeritus of Pediatrics, University of Pennsylvania School of Medicine; formerly Chief of Pediatric Infectious Diseases, Children's Hospital of Philadelphia, Philadelphia, Pennsylvania

Rubella and Congenital Rubella Syndrome

BARBARA R. POBER, M.D.

Assistant Professor of Genetics and Pediatrics, Yale University School of Medicine; Attending Physician, Yale–New Haven Hospital, New Haven, Connecticut

Idiopathic Hypercalcemia

MARGARET POLANECZKY, M.D.

Assistant Professor, Department of Obstetrics and Gynecology, Division of Women's Health, Cornell Medical College; Attending in Obstetrics and Gynecology, The New York Hospital/Cornell Medical Center, New York, New York

Uterus, Fallopian Tubes, and Ovaries

SCOTT L. POMEROY, M.D., Ph.D.

Assistant Professor of Neurology, Harvard Medical School; Assistant in Neurology, Children's Hospital, Boston, Massachusetts

Brain Abscess; Spinal Epidural Abscess; Cranial Subdural Empyema

J. CHRISTOPHER POST, M.D.

Assistant Professor of Otolaryngology, University of Pittsburgh School of Medicine; Director of Clinical Services, Children's Hospital of Pittsburgh, Pittsburgh, Pennsylvania

Tumors and Polyps of the Nose

WILLIAM P. POTSIC, M.D.

Professor of Otolaryngology: Head and Neck Surgery, University of Pennsylvania School of Medicine; Director, Division of Otolaryngology and Human Communication, Children's Hospital of Philadelphia, Philadelphia, Pennsylvania

Retropharyngeal and Peritonsillar Abscesses

CHARLES G. PROBER, M.D.

Professor of Pediatrics, Medicine, Microbiology, and Immunology and Associate Chairman, Department of Pediatrics, Stanford University School of Medicine, Stanford, California

Cytomegalovirus Infections

SUMA P. PYATI, M.D.

Associate Professor, Finch University of Health Sciences/The Chicago Medical School; Chairman, Division of Neonatology, Cook County Children's Hospital, Chicago, Illinois

Hemolytic Diseases of the Neonate

NEJIB RABOUDI, M.D.

Fellow in Pediatric Endocrinology, Harvard Medical School and Massachusetts General Hospital, Boston, Massachusetts

Insulin-dependent Diabetes Mellitus

WAYNE R. RACKOFF, M.D.

Assistant Professor of Pediatrics, Section of Hematology/Oncology, Indiana University School of Medicine and James Whitcomb Riley Hospital for Children, Indianapolis, Indiana

Aplastic Anemia

MICHAEL RADETSKY, M.D., C.M.
Clinical Professor of Pediatrics, University of New Mexico School of Medicine; Chairman, Department of Pediatrics, Lovelace Health System, Albuquerque, New Mexico
Staphylococcal Infections; Group A Streptococcal Infections

DIANA RADKOWSKI, M.D.
Assistant Professor, Case Western Reserve University School of Medicine and Departments of Otolaryngology/Head and Neck Surgery and Pediatrics, Rainbow Babies and Children's Hospital, Cleveland, Ohio
Disorders of the Larynx

JYOTI RAMAKRISHNA, M.D.
Fellow, Pediatric Gastroenterology and Nutrition, Tufts University School of Medicine, New England Medical Center, Boston, Massachusetts
Inflammatory Bowel Disease

JAMES E. RASMUSSEN, M.D.
Professor of Dermatology and Pediatrics, University of Michigan Medical Center and Ann Arbor Veterans Administration Hospital, Ann Arbor, Michigan
Genodermatosis

MARK REBER, M.D.
Clinical Assistant Professor of Psychiatry and Pediatrics, University of Pennsylvania School of Medicine; Consulting Psychiatrist, Children's Seashore House, Philadelphia, Pennsylvania
Autism

BEVERLY REDD, B.S., I.B.C.L.C.
Research Associate and Lactation Consultant, Maternal Infant Lactation Center, Mercy Children's Medical Center, Pittsburgh, Pennsylvania
Breastfeeding

MARGARET B. RENNELS, M.D.
Associate Professor, University of Maryland School of Medicine; Clinical Head, Infectious Diseases and Tropical Pediatrics, University Hospital, Baltimore, Maryland
Nontyphoidal Salmonellosis; Yersinia enterocolitica *Infection; Rotavirus*

FREDERICK J. RESCORLA, M.D.
Associate Professor of Surgery, Section of Pediatric Surgery, Indiana University School of Medicine; Pediatric Surgeon, James Whitcomb Riley Hospital for Children, Indianapolis, Indiana
Disorders of the Umbilicus

JEFFREY I. RESNICK, M.D.
Assistant Clinical Professor, Division of Plastic Surgery, University of California Los Angeles School of Medicine; Staff Surgeon, University of California Los Angeles Medical Center and Cedars-Sinai Medical Center, Los Angeles, California; Staff Surgeon, St. John's Hospital, Santa Monica, California
Diseases and Injuries of the Oral Region

ALAN B. RETIK, M.D.
Professor, Department of Surgery, Harvard Medical School; Chief, Division of Urology, Children's Hospital, Boston, Massachusetts
Patent Urachus and Urachal Cysts; Disorders of the Bladder and Urethra

JORGE REYES, M.D.
Assistant Professor of Surgery, University of Pittsburgh School of Medicine; Director, Pediatric Transplant Surgery, Pittsburgh Transplant Institution, Pittsburgh, Pennsylvania
Intestinal Transplantation

CAMILLO RICORDI, M.D.
Professor of Surgery, University of Miami School of Medicine Diabetes Research Institute, Miami, Florida
Organ Transplants: Pancreas and Islet Cells

RICHARD C. RINK, M.D.
Associate Professor of Urology, Indiana University School of Medicine; Chief of Pediatric Urology, James Whitcomb Riley Hospital for Children, Indianapolis, Indiana
Disorders of the Umbilicus

IDALIA R. RIVERA, M.D.
Fellow, Pediatric Infectious Disease, University of Texas–Houston Health Science Center, Hermann Hospital, and Lyndon B. Johnson Hospital, Houston, Texas
Typhoid Fever

DELIA M. RIVERA-HERNANDEZ, M.D.
Assistant Professor, Division of Pediatric Infectious Diseases and Immunology, University of Miami School of Medicine; Attending Pediatrician and Consultant in Pediatric Infectious Diseases, Children's Hospital Center, University of Miami Jackson Memorial Medical Center, Miami, Florida
HIV Infection

LIZ ROBERTS
Project Manager, Pediatric Family Violence Awareness Project, Women's Health Unit, Bureau of Family and Community Health, Massachusetts Department of Public Health, Boston, Massachusetts
Children of Battered and Homeless Women

ALBERT P. ROCCHINI, M.D.
Professor of Pediatrics, University of Minnesota; Director, Pediatric Cardiology, University of Minnesota Hospital and Clinic, Minneapolis, Minnesota
The Child at Risk of Coronary Artery Disease as an Adult

JOSE LUIS ROMERO, M.D.
Assistant Professor, Department of Microbiology, Universidad Autonoma de Mexico School of Medicine; Head, Clinical Parasitology Laboratory, Department of Infectious Diseases, Hospital Infantil de Mexico Federico Gomez, Mexico
Trichinosis

FERNANDO J. ROSAS, M.D.
Assistant Professor, Department of Pediatrics, West Virginia University School of Medicine; Neonatologist, West Virginia University Hospitals, Morgantown, West Virginia
Histoplasmosis

ELIZABETH ROSE, M.D.
Otolaryngologist, Royal Children's Hospital, Victoria, Australia
Recurrent Parotitis

BETH A. ROSEN, M.D.
Assistant Professor of Pediatrics and Neurology, University of Massachusetts Medical School; Pediatric Neurologist, University of Massachusetts Medical Center, Worcester, Massachusetts
Cerebral Palsy

NORMAN D. ROSENBLUM, M.D.
Assistant Professor of Pediatrics, University of Toronto; Associate in Pediatrics, The Hospital for Sick Children, Toronto, Ontario, Canada
The Nephrotic Syndrome

N. PAUL ROSMAN, M.D.
Professor of Pediatrics and Neurology, Tufts University School of Medicine; Chief, Division of Pediatric Neurology, The Floating Hospital for Children; Director, Center for Children with Special Needs, New England Medical Center, Boston, Massachusetts
Extradural and Subdural Hematoma; Acute Ataxia

BERTRAND A. ROSS, M.D.

Associate Professor of Pediatrics and Director, Section of Pediatric Cardiology, Eastern Virginia Medical School; Director of Pediatric Cardiology and of Electrophysiology and Pacing, Children's Hospital of the King's Daughters, Norfolk, Virginia
Syncope and Hypotension

ROBERT J. RUBEN, M.D.

Professor of Pediatric Otolaryngology, Albert Einstein College of Medicine, Yeshiva University; Chairman and Professor, Department of Otolaryngology, Montefiore Medical Center, Bronx, New York
Hearing Loss

TRENTON K. RUEBUSH II, M.D.

Chief, Malaria Epidemiology Section, Division of Parasitic Diseases, National Center for Infectious Diseases, Centers for Disease Control, Atlanta, Georgia
Babesiosis

GUILLERMO M. RUIZ-PALACIOS, M.D.

Head, Department of Infectious Diseases, Instituto Nacional de la Nutricion, Salvador Zubiran; Mexico City, Mexico
Shigellosis; Campylobacter *Infections*

BARRY H. RUMACK, M.D.

Clinical Professor of Pediatrics, University of Colorado Health Sciences Center; Director Emeritus, Rocky Mountain Poison and Drug Center, Denver, Colorado
Botulinal Food Poisoning

LAURIE S. SADLER, M.D.

Clinical Assistant Professor of Pediatrics, State University of New York at Buffalo School of Medicine and Biomedical Sciences; Associate Director, Clinical Genetics, and Clinical Director, Craniofacial Center of Western New York, The Children's Hospital of Buffalo, Buffalo, New York
Disorders of Porphyrin, Purine, and Pyrimidine Metabolism

PABLO J. SÁNCHEZ, M.D.

Assistant Professor of Pediatrics, Divisions of Neonatal-Perinatal Medicine and Pediatric Infectious Diseases, University of Texas Southwestern Medical Center; Attending Physician, Parkland Memorial Hospital and Children's Medical Center, Dallas, Texas
Syphilis

JOHN T. SANDLUND, M.D.

Associate Professor of Pediatrics, University of Tennessee College of Medicine; Assistant Member, Department of Hematology/Oncology, St. Jude Children's Research Hospital, Memphis, Tennessee
Burkitt's Lymphoma

JOSE IGNACIO SANTOS, M.D.

Professor of Infectious Diseases and Microbiology, Universidad Nacional Autonoma de Mexico School of Medicine; Head, Department of Infectious Diseases, Hospital Infantil de Mexico Federico Gomez, Mexico
Trichinosis

JOHN SARGENT, M.D.

Associate Professor of Psychiatry and Pediatrics, University of Pennsylvania School of Medicine; Director of General and Child and Adolescent Psychiatry Residency Training, University of Pennsylvania and Philadelphia Child Guidance Center, Philadelphia, Pennsylvania
Psychiatric Disorders and Mental Health Treatment

RICHARD M. SARLES, M.D.

Professor of Psychiatry and Pediatrics and Director, Division of Child and Adolescent Psychiatry, University of Maryland School of Medicine, Baltimore, Maryland
Tics and Tourette's Syndrome

ASHOK P. SARNAIK, M.D.

Professor of Pediatrics, Wayne State University School of Medicine; Chief, Critical Care Medicine, Children's Hospital of Michigan, Detroit, Michigan
Head Injury; Respiratory Insufficiency

JANE G. SCHALLER, M.D.

Pediatrician-in-Chief, Professor of Pediatrics, and Chief, Pediatric Rheumatology, Tufts University School of Medicine; Chairman, Department of Pediatrics, and David and Leona Karp Professor of Pediatrics, The Floating Hospital for Children, Boston, Massachusetts
Dermatomyositis and Polymyositis

KENNETH A. SCHENKMAN, M.D.

Acting Instructor, Department of Anesthesiology, University of Washington School of Medicine; Attending Physician, Department of Anesthesia and Critical Care Medicine, Children's Hospital and Medical Center, Seattle, Washington
Septic Shock

SELVA S. SCHENKMAN, M.D.

Formerly, Assistant Professor of Pediatrics, Seton Hall University of Graduate Medical Education, Orange, New Jersey; formerly, Chief, Pediatric Endocrine Section, St. Joseph's Hospital and Medical Center, Paterson, New Jersey
Ambiguous Genitalia

MARK S. SCHER, M.D.

Associate Professor of Pediatrics, Neurology, and Psychiatry, University of Pittsburgh School of Medicine; Director, Developmental Neurophysiology Laboratory, Magee-Women's Hospital, Pittsburgh, Pennsylvania
Neonatal Seizures

CRAIG M. SCHRAMM, M.D.

Assistant Professor of Pediatrics, Pediatric Pulmonary Division, University of Connecticut School of Medicine and University of Connecticut Health Center, Farmington, Connecticut
Pneumothorax and Pneumomediastinum

KENNETH SCHUIT, M.D.

Associate Professor of Pediatrics, University of Pittsburgh School of Medicine; Attending Physician, Pediatric Infectious Diseases, Children's Hospital of Pittsburgh, Pittsburgh, Pennsylvania
Cellulitis

ROBERT E. SCHUMACHER, M.D.

Associate Professor of Pediatrics, University of Michigan School and Department of Pediatrics and Communicable Diseases, Section of Newborn Services, Univeristy of Michigan Medical Center, Ann Arbor, Michigan
Extracorporeal Membrane Oxygenation

C. WILLIAM SCHWAB, M.D.

Professor of Surgery, University of Pennsylvania School of Medicine; Professor of Surgery and Chief, Division of Traumatology and Surgical Critical Care, University of Pennsylvania Medical Center, Philadelphia, Pennsylvania
Penetrating, Gunshot, and Knife Wounds in Children

MOLLY R. SCHWENN, M.D.

Associate Professor of Pediatrics, University of Massachusetts Medical School; Clinical Director, Division of Pediatric Hematology/Oncology, University of Massachusetts Medical Center, Worcester, Massachusetts
The Child Cured of Cancer

GWENDOLYN B. SCOTT, M.D.

Professor of Pediatrics and Director, Division of Pediatric Infectious Disease and Immunology, University of Miami School of Medicine; Attending Pediatrician, Children's Hospital Center, University of Miami/Jackson Memorial Medical Center, Miami, Florida
HIV Infection

JOHN H. SEASHORE, M.D.

Professor of Surgery and Pediatrics, Yale University School of Medicine; Attending Physician, Yale–New Haven Hospital, New Haven, Connecticut
Disorders of the Anus and Rectum

MICHAEL E. SELZER, M.D., Ph.D.

Professor of Neurology and Rehabilitation Medicine, University of Pennsylvania School of Medicine; Attending Neurologist, Hospital of the University of Pennsylvania, Philadelphia, Pennsylvania
Spinal Cord Disorders

ROBERT C. SHAMBERGER, M.D.

Associate Professor of Surgery, Harvard Medical School; Senior Associate in Surgery, Children's Hospital, Boston, Massachusetts
Congenital Deformities of the Anterior Chest Wall

EUGENE D. SHAPIRO, M.D.

Professor of Pediatrics and Epidemiology, Yale University School of Medicine and the Children's Clinical Research Center; Attending Pediatrician, The Children's Hospital at Yale–New Haven, New Haven, Connecticut
Infections of the Urinary Tract; Lyme Disease

STEPHEN R. SHAPIRO, M.D.

Pediatric Urologist, Sacramento, California
Perinephric and Intranephric Abscess

MONA SHEHAB, M.D.

Neonatologist, Group Neonatology Certified, Inc., Plantation, Florida
Apnea of Prematurity

JANE D. SIEGEL, M.D.

Professor of Pediatrics, University of Texas Southwestern Medical Center; Chairman, Infection Control Committee, Children's Medical Center; Medical Director, Pediatric Inpatient Service, Parkland Memorial Hospital, Dallas, Texas
Human Parvovirus B19 Infections

ERIC J. SIGEL, M.D.

Assistant Professor of Pediatrics, University of Colorado School of Medicine; Clinic Director, Adolescent Clinic, The Children's Hospital, Denver, Colorado
Understanding and Assessing Adolescent Influences and Risk-taking Behavior

BARRY P. SIMMONS, M.D.

Associate Professor, Harvard Medical School; Chief, Hand and Upper Extremity Service, Department of Orthopedics, Brigham and Women's Hospital, Boston, Masssachusetts
Congenital Hand and Upper Limb Deformities

ELISABETH SIMON, M.D.

Department of Pediatrics, New York Medical College, Westchester County Medical Center, Valhalla, New York
Chronic Renal Failure

ANA ABAD SINDEN, M.S., R.D., C.N.S.D.

Pediatric Nutritionist, University of Virginia and University of Virginia Health Sciences Center, Charlottesville, Virginia
Nutrition Support in the Very Ill Pediatric Patient

ANUP SINGH, M.D.

Assistant Professor, Children's Medical Center of Brooklyn, State University of New York Health Science Center, Brooklyn, New York
Renal Transplantation

JOHN T. SLADKY, M.D.

Associate Professor of Neurology and Pediatrics, University of Pennsylvania School of Medicine, Children's Hospital of Philadelphia, and Hospital of the University of Pennsylvania, Philadelphia, Pennsylvania
Near Drowning

DAVID S. SMITH, M.D.

Emeritus Professor of Pediatrics, Temple University School of Medicine and St. Christopher's Hospital for Children, Philadelphia, Pennsylvania
Pulmonary Thromboembolism

EVAN Y. SNYDER, M.D., Ph.D.

Assistant in Newborn Medicine (Joint Program in Neonatology) and Neurology, Children's Hospital, Boston, Massachusetts
Neonatal Intracranial Hemorrhage and Its Sequelae

EDNA H. SOBEL, M.D.

Professor Emerita of Pediatrics, Albert Einstein College of Medicine, Bronx, New York
Ambiguous Genitalia

SHAUL SOFER, M.D.

Associate Professor of Pediatrics, Ben-Gurion University of the Negev; Chairman of Pediatrics and Director, Pediatric Intensive Care Unit, Soroka Medical Center, Beer-Sheva, Israel
Rewarming and Hypothermia

LAWRENCE M. SOLOMON, M.D.

Professor and Head, Department of Dermatology, University of Illinois at Chicago College of Medicine, Chicago, Illinois
Neonatal Skin Disorders

JUAN RODRIGUEZ SORIANO, M.D.

Professor of Pediatrics, Basque University School of Medicine; Head, Department of Pediatrics, Hospital de Cruces, Bilbao, Spain
Renal Tubular Disorders

ALAN R. SPITZER, M.D.

Professor of Pediatrics and Chairman, Department of Pediatrics, Jefferson Medical College, Thomas Jefferson University, Philadelphia, Pennsylvania; Pediatrician-in-Chief, A.I. duPont Institute, Wilmington, Delaware
SIDS and Recurring Apnea; Respiratory Distress Syndrome and Atelectasis

JUDY BUCKMAN SPLAWSKI, M.D.

Associate Professor of Pediatrics, University of Texas Southwestern Medical Center; Medical Staff, Children's Medical Center of Dallas and Parkland Memorial Hospital, Dallas, Texas
Allergic Gastrointestinal Disorders

VIRGINIA A. STALLINGS, M.D.

Associate Professor of Pediatrics, University of Pennsylvania School of Medicine; Chief, Nutrition Section, Children's Hospital of Philadelphia, Philadelphia, Pennsylvania
Vitamin Deficiencies and Excesses

F. BRUDER STAPLETON, M.D.

A. Conger Goodyear Professor and Chairman, Department of Pediatrics, State University of New York at Buffalo; Pediatrician-in-Chief, Children's Hospital of Buffalo, Buffalo, New York

Disorders of Porphyrin, Purine, and Pyrimidine Metabolism; Urolithiasis

ANN R. STARK, M.D.

Associate Professor of Pediatrics, Harvard Medical School; Clinical Director, Joint Program in Neonatology, and Director, Newborn Intensive Care Unit, Children's Hospital, Boston, Massachusetts

Neonatal Intracranial Hemorrhage and Its Sequelae

JEFFREY R. STARKE, M.D.

Associate Professor of Pediatrics, Baylor College of Medicine, Houston, Texas

Infective Endocarditis

THOMAS E. STARZL, M.D., Ph.D.

Professor of Surgery, University of Pittsburgh School of Medicine; Director, Pittsburgh Transplantation Institute, Pittsburgh, Pennsylvania

Tumors of the Liver

RUTH E.K. STEIN, M.D.

Professor and Vice Chairman, Department of Pediatrics, Albert Einstein College of Medicine; Pediatrician-in-Chief, Bronx Municipal Hospital Center, Bronx, New York

The Child with a Serious Ongoing Condition

RONALD JAY STEINGARD, M.D.

Assistant Professor of Psychiatry, Harvard Medical School; Director of Psychopharmacology, Children's Hospital, Boston, Massachusetts

Depressive Disorders

MATTHEW J. STENZEL, M.D.

Acting Instructor, Department of Anesthesiology, University of Washington School of Medicine; Fellow, Pediatric Anesthesiology, Children's Hospital and Medical Center, Seattle, Washington

Malignant Hyperthermia; Heat-related Illnesses Including Hemorrhagic Shock and Encephalopathy Syndrome and Heat Stroke

ROBERT C. STERN, M.D.

Professor of Pediatrics, Case Western Reserve University School of Medicine; Associate Pediatrician, Rainbow Babies and Children's Hospital, Cleveland, Ohio

Bronchiectasis

JAMES A. STOCKMAN III, M.D.

Clinical Professor of Pediatrics, University of North Carolina School of Medicine; Consultant Professor, Department of Pediatrics, Duke University School of Medicine, Chapel Hill, North Carolina

Anemia of Chronic Disease

SYLVAN E. STOOL, M.D.

Professor of Otolaryngology and Pediatrics, University of Pittsburgh School of Medicine; Director of Education, Department of Pediatric Otolaryngology, Children's Hospital of Pittsburgh, Pittsburgh, Pennsylvania

Choanal Atresia

ARNOLD W. STRAUSS, M.D.

Professor of Pediatrics and Molecular Biology and Pharmacology, Washington University School of Medicine; Director, Pediatric Cardiology, St. Louis Children's Hospital, St. Louis, Missouri

Congenital Heart Disease; Cardiomyopathies and Cardiac Transplantation

†DENISE J. STRIEDER, M.D.

Associate Professor of Pediatrics, Harvard Medical School; Pediatrician, Massachusetts General Hospital, Boston, Massachusetts

Idiopathic Pulmonary Hemosiderosis

DENNIS M. STYNE, M.D.

Professor and Chair, Department of Pediatrics, University of California Davis; Chair of Pediatrics, University of California Davis Medical Center, Sacramento, California

Hypopituitarism and Growth Hormone Therapy; Precocious and Delayed Puberty

ROBERT P. SUNDEL, M.D.

Assistant Professor of Pediatrics, Harvard Medical School; Director of Rheumatology, Children's Hospital, Boston, Massachusetts

Kawasaki Syndrome

SUZANNE SUNDHEIM, M.D.

Instructor of Psychiatry, University of Colorado Medical School; Assistant Director, Services to Persons with Developmental Disabilities in Programs for Public Psychiatry, University of Colorado Health Sciences Center, Denver, Colorado

Autism

MICHAEL DAVID SUSSMAN, M.D.

Clinical Professor, Orthopedic Surgery, Oregon Health Science University; Chief of Staff, Shriners Hospital, Portland, Oregon

Disorders of the Spine and Shoulder Girdle

JAMES L. SUTPHEN, M.D., Ph.D.

Associate Professor of Pediatrics and Chief, Division of Pediatric Gastroenterology, University of Virginia Health Sciences Center, Charlottesville, Virginia

Nutrition Support in the Very Ill Pediatric Patient

MARY E. SUTTON, M.D.

Clinical Fellow in Neurology, Harvard Medical School; Senior Resident in Neurology, Children's Hospital, Boston, Massachusetts

Brain Abscess; Spinal Epidural Abscess; Cranial Subdural Empyema

RITA D. SWINFORD, M.D.

Fellow, Pediatric Nephrology, Massachusetts General Hospital, Boston, Massachusetts

Hypocalcemia and Tetany

ILONA S. SZER, M.D.

Associate (Adjunct) Professor in Pediatrics, University of California San Diego School of Medicine; Director, Pediatric Rheumatology, Children's Hospital of San Diego, San Diego, California

Juvenile Rheumatoid Arthritis and Spondyloarthropathy Syndromes

BRUCE TAUBMAN, M.D.

Clinical Associate Professor, Division of Gastroenterology and Nutrition, Department of Pediatrics, University of Pennsylvania Medical School, Philadelphia, Pennsylvania

Infant Colic Syndrome

RITA LITTLEWOOD TEELE, M.D.

Professor of Radiology, Christchurch School of Medicine, University of Otago; Pediatric Radiologist, Christchurch Hospital, Christchurch Women's Hospital, and Auckland Children's Hospital, Christchurch, New Zealand

Intussusception

---

†Deceased.

AMIR TEJANI, M.D.
Professor of Pediatrics, State University of New York Health Science Center at Brooklyn, Brooklyn, New York
Renal Transplantation

NATHAN M. THIELMAN, M.D., M.P.H.
Fellow in Infectious Diseases, University of Virginia School of Medicine, Charlottesville, Virginia
Clostridium difficile

CHARLES H. THORNE, M.D.
Assistant Professor of Surgery (Plastic), New York University School of Medicine; Chief of Plastic Surgery, Bellevue Hospital; Director, Ear Anomalies Program, New York University Medical Center, New York, New York; Chief of Plastic Surgery, Brooklyn Hospital, Brooklyn, New York
Craniofacial Malformations

SATORU TODO, M.D.
Professor of Surgery, University of Pittsburgh School of Medicine and Pittsburgh Transplantation Institute, Pittsburgh, Pennsylvania
Intestinal Transplantation

LAWRENCE W.C. TOM, M.D.
Assistant Professor of Otolaryngology: Head and Neck Surgery, University of Pennsylvania School of Medicine, Children's Hospital of Philadelphia, Philadelphia, Pennsylvania
Rhinitis and Sinusitis

R. FRANKLIN TRIMM III, M.D.
Assistant Professor of Pediatrics and Neurology, University of South Alabama College of Medicine, Mobile, Alabama
Children of Divorcing Parents; The Child and the Death of a Loved One

DEBRA A. TRISTRAM, M.D.
Assistant Professor of Pediatrics, State University of New York at Buffalo School of Medicine; Associate Attending Physician in Pediatrics, Children's Hospital of Buffalo, Buffalo, New York
Influenza Viruses

REGINALD C. TSANG, M.B.B.S.
Professor of Pediatrics and David G. and Priscilla R. Gamble Professor of Neonatology, University of Cincinnati College of Medicine; Director, Division of Neonatology, and Associate Chair of Academic Affairs and Research, Children's Hospital Medical Center, Cincinnati, Ohio
Osteopenia of Prematurity

LORI B. TUCKER, M.D.
Assistant Professor of Pediatrics, Division of Pediatric Rheumatology, Tufts University School of Medicine; Pediatric Rheumatologist, The Floating Hospital for Children, Boston, Massachusetts
Dermatomyositis and Polymyositis

NELSON L. TURCIOS, M.D.
Associate Professor of Pediatrics, New Jersey Medical School; Director, Pediatric Pulmonology, New Jersey Medical School–University Hospital, Newark, New Jersey
Intrathoracic Tumors and Cysts

TERI LEE TURNER, M.D.
Fellow, Academic General Pediatrics, Baylor College of Medicine, Houston, Texas
Bacterial Meningitis and Septicemia Beyond the Neonatal Period

FRANK J. TWAROG, M.D., Ph.D.
Assistant Clinical Professor, Harvard Medical School; Senior Associate in Medicine (Immunology), Children's Hospital, Boston, Massachusetts
Serum Sickness

ANDREAS TZAKIS, M.D.
Professor of Surgery and Chief, Division of Transplantation, University of Miami, Miami, Florida
Intestinal Transplantation

DAVID K. URION, M.D.
Assistant Professor of Neurology, Harvard Medical School; Director, Learning Disabilities/Behaviorial Neurology Program, Children's Hospital, Boston, Massachusetts
Hydrocephalus; Benign Congenital Hypotonia

ANDREA M. VANDEVEN, M.D., M.P.H.
Instructor in Pediatrics, Harvard Medical School; Assistant in Medicine, Division of General Pediatrics, Children's Hospital, Boston, Massachusetts
Vulva and Vagina

JOSEPH J. VOLPE, M.D.
Bronson Crothers Professor of Neurology, Harvard Medical School; Neurologist-in-Chief, Children's Hospital, Boston, Massachusetts
Neurologic Birth Trauma

KEN B. WAITES, M.D.
Associate Professor, Departments of Pathology, Microbiology and Rehabilitation Medicine, University of Alabama at Birmingham Schools of Medicine and Dentistry; Medical Director, Clinical Microbiology Laboratory, University of Alabama Hospital, Birmingham, Alabama
Genital Mycoplasmal Infections

EDWARD P. WALSH, M.D.
Associate Professor of Pediatrics, Harvard Medical School; Director, Electrophysiology Laboratories, Children's Hospital, Boston, Massachusetts
Acute Management of Cardiac Arrhythmias

DAVID S. WALTON, M.D.
Associate Clinical Professor, Harvard Medical School; Surgeon, Massachusetts Eye and Ear Infirmary, Boston, Massachusetts
The Eye

PETER M. WATERS, M.D.
Assistant Professor, Harvard Medical School; Clinical Director, Hand Surgery Clinic, Department of Orthopedic Surgery, Children's Hospital, Boston, Massachusetts
Congenital Hand and Upper Limb Deformities

JOHN B. WATKINS, M.D.
Professor of Pediatrics, Washington University School of Medicine and Divisions of Gastroenterology and Nutrition and Ambulatory Pediatrics, St. Louis Children's Hospital, St. Louis, Missouri
Malabsorptive Disorders

LOUIS M. WEISS, M.D., M.P.H.
Associate Professor of Medicine and Pathology, Albert Einstein College of Medicine; Attending Physician, Jack D. Weiler Hospital of the Albert Einstein College of Medicine and Bronx Municipal Hospital Corporation, Bronx, New York
Cysticercosis

ROBERT A. WEISS, M.D.
Associate Professor of Pediatrics and Director, Pediatric Nephrology, New York Medical College, Valhalla, New York
Hemodialysis

ROBERT C. WELLIVER, M.D.
Professor of Pediatrics, State University of New York at Buffalo School of Medicine; Attending Physician and Professor of Pediatrics, Children's Hospital of Buffalo, Buffalo, New York
Influenza Viruses

WILLIAM J. WENNER, Jr., M.D.
Assistant Professor of Pediatrics, University of Pennsylvania School of Medicine; Attending Physician in Gastroenterology and Nutrition, Children's Hospital of Philadelphia, Philadelphia, Pennsylvania
Gastritis, Duodenitis, and Peptic Ulcer Disease

RICHARD J. WHITLEY, M.D.
Loeb Eminent Scholar Chair in Pediatrics and Professor of Pediatrics, Microbiology and Medicine, University of Alabama at Birmingham, Birmingham, Alabama
Herpes Simplex Virus Infections

BERNHARD L. WIEDERMANN, M.D.
Associate Professor of Pediatrics, The George Washington University School of Medicine and Health Sciences; Attending Physician in Infectious Diseases and Director, Pediatric Residency Training Program, Children's National Medical Center, Washington, D.C.
Coccidioidomycosis

DAVID A. WILLIAMS, M.D.
Associate Professor of Pediatrics and Medical and Molecular Genetics and Kipp Investigator of Pediatrics, Indiana University School of Medicine, Indianapolis, Indiana; Associate Investigator, Howard Hughes Medical Institute, Ann Arbor, Michigan
Aplastic Anemia

JERRY A. WINKELSTEIN, M.D.
Professor of Pediatrics, Johns Hopkins University School of Medicine and Department of Pediatrics, Johns Hopkins Hospital, Baltimore, Maryland
The Immunodeficiency Syndromes

BOYD H. WINSLOW, M.D
Professor of Urology and Associate Professor of Pediatrics, Eastern Virginia Medical School; Surgical Director of Urology, Children's Hospital of the King's Daughters, Norfolk, Virginia
Hydronephrosis

PAUL H. WISE, M.D., M.P.H.
Assistant Professor, Department of Pediatrics, Harvard Medical School; Associate in Medicine, Children's Hospital, Boston, Massachusetts
Preventing Childhood Injuries

LAWRENCE S. WISSOW, M.D., M.P.H.
Associate Professor of Pediatrics, Johns Hopkins University School of Medicine, Baltimore, Maryland
Child Abuse and Neglect

THOMAS E. WISWELL, M.D.
Professor of Pediatrics and Director of Neonatal Research, Division of Neonatology, Jefferson Medical College, Thomas Jefferson University, Philadelphia, Pennsylvania
Meconium Aspiration Syndrome

SELMA SIEGEL WITCHEL, M.D.
Assistant Professor of Pediatrics, University of Pittsburgh School of Medicine and Children's Hospital of Pittsburgh, Pittsburgh, Pennsylvania
Disorders of the Adrenal Gland

MURRAY WITTNER, M.D., Ph.D.
Professor of Pathology and Parasitology, Albert Einstein College of Medicine; Attending Physician, Jack D. Weiler Hospital of the Albert Einstein College of Medicine and Bronx Municipal Hospital Corporation, Bronx, New York
Cysticercosis

LAWRENCE WOLFE, M.D.
Associate Professor of Pediatrics, Tufts University School of Medicine; Chief, Division of Pediatric Hematology Oncology, The Floating Hospital for Children, New England Medical Center, Boston, Massachusetts
Hemolytic Anemia; Neutropenia

JOSEPH I. WOLFSDORF, M.B., B.Ch.
Associate Professor of Pediatrics, Harvard Medical School; Clinical Director of Endocrinology, Children's Hospital, Boston, Massachusetts
Endocrine Disorders of the Testis; Gynecomastia

MARK L. WOLRAICH, M.D.
Professor of Pediatrics, Vanderbilt University; Director, Child Development Center, Vanderbilt University Medical Center, Nashville, Tennessee
Disorders of Learning

MICHAEL A. WOOD, M.D.
Assistant Professor of Pediatrics, Michigan State University, Lansing, Michigan; Director, Pediatric Endocrinology, DeVos Children's Hospital, Grand Rapids, Michigan
Endocrine Disorders of the Testis

WILLIAM F.H. YEE, M.D.
Assistant Professor of Pediatrics, Tufts University School of Medicine; Assistant Pediatrician, The Floating Hospital for Infants and Children, New England Medical Center, Boston, Massachusetts
Aspiration Syndromes

HARVEY A. ZAREM, M.D.
Professor Emeritus, University of California Los Angeles Medical School; Staff Surgeon, University of California Los Angeles Medical Center, Los Angeles, California; Staff Surgeon, St. John's Hospital and Santa Monica Hospital, Santa Monica, California
Diseases and Injuries of the Oral Region

BASIL J. ZITELLI, M.D.
Professor of Pediatrics, University of Pittsburgh School of Medicine and Children's Hospital of Pittsburgh, Pittsburgh, Pennsylvania
Ascaris lumbricoides

Preface

The challenge for all of us who are given the privilege of providing health care to infants, children, and adolescents is to be certain that we are offering our patients and their families the most effective therapy available during a period of enormous growth in knowledge about health and disease. *Current Pediatric Therapy* was developed by two outstanding pediatricians, Sydney S. Gellis, M.D., and Benjamin M. Kagan, M.D. For thirty years it served an immeasurable number of health care workers by providing expert advice on high-quality therapeutic care for our world's most precious asset, our children. Their success in working with thousands of pediatric experts to put together this book is a contribution that, when put into perspective, is probably one of the most important in the history of child care. It is both an honor and an enormous responsibility to embrace the challenge of guiding the future direction of this text and to work with pediatricians everywhere to continue to spread the word on how best to help the children of the world. As these children encounter diseases and a multitude of other health problems, proper management will allow more and more of them to thrive, to move into adulthood, and to face the next century with a promising chance to help our civilization move forward.

In planning the 15th edition it has been our goal to identify experts from multiple disciplines concerning the problems of infants, children, and adolescents. We approached this through a mailing to all pediatric department chairs in the United States and Canada. As a result the new text not only includes significant contributions from surgeons, psychiatrists, and specialists in child development but also reflects new developments in therapy that have grown from recent advances in molecular biology, bioengineering, and our understanding of the social sciences. Such advances are moving the field of child care forward at a remarkable pace, challenging us all to assimilate this new information, to integrate it into our practices, and to utilize it in the development of new approaches to child care. We hope you will find the organization and content of this book useful in meeting your needs in the provision of primary child health care and in facilitating your understanding of new developments at the cutting-edge of therapy.

For many contributions we have adopted the philosophy of Drs. Gellis and Kagan in assuming that a correct diagnosis has been made, so that the information presented in this text relates primarily to management. At times we have included other background information, especially in articles in which we believed such detail would provide a sound scientific base for understanding the proper management of a particular condition. Contributors have been asked to describe which treatments have worked for them rather than to present a review of therapies. As editors, we recognize that the *absolute truth* about how to treat certain conditions is not known, and thus approaches to some problems are described in various ways in different sections or articles. Clinical judgment is the cornerstone of a great practitioner's skill in enhancing outcomes, and the actual decisions made in planning the management of problems encountered lies in every pediatrician's hands. We hope that this book will be of help to you in making the best possible decisions.

In this edition we have tried to accomplish two new objectives. First, we have included more tables, which we hope will make it easier for you to manage each of these conditions. Second, as we are moving into a much more cost-conscious world, our authors have tried to present the most cost-effective therapies. We hope that the 16th edition will pay even greater attention to the cost of child care and outcomes data.

Current Pediatric Therapy offers the health care provider the latest information on how to manage the diseases of infants, children, and adolescents. All sections have been written by individuals who are nationally recognized experts in their topic areas. The approach to management is specific, with details about medical, surgical, and psychosocial interventions. Numerous tables and succinct presentations of approaches to therapy are intended to facilitate the use of this book while one is in the midst of caring for a patient. The problems addressed are the major medical and surgical problems that impact on the pediatric population. In addition, many psychosocial problems are now included, from the death of a loved one, to treating children of homeless and battered wormen, to a variety of significant psychiatric conditions. Because giving medications to children is more complicated than giving them to adults, careful attention has been paid to drugs by name, dosage, route, and timing.

Finally, we thank the many contributors to this volume who have taken time to write down and share with all of us their best ideas on how to provide health care for our children.

Fredric D. Burg, M.D.
Julie R. Ingelfinger, M.D.
Ellen R. Wald, M.D.
Richard A. Polin, M.D.

Contents

22 SPECIAL PROBLEMS IN THE ADOLESCENT 835

1

Nutrition

NORMAL NUTRITION

Clifford Lo, M.D., M.P.H., Sc.D.
Ronald E. Kleinman, M.D.

Nutrition provides the substrates that allow an embryo weighing a few grams to develop into an adult weighing tens of thousands of grams. It is used in a process in which millions of grams of carbohydrates, fats, proteins, minerals, and water are converted into muscle, bone, and functioning organ systems. Nutrition begins with the developing embryo and growing fetus during pregnancy and must support distinct growth patterns and unique needs at all ages. Nutrition in childhood may significantly influence health in later life, affecting the evolution of disorders, such as heart disease, cancer, and osteoporosis. Overnutrition and undernutrition of energy and many specific nutrients (especially saturated fat, cholesterol, and sodium) probably affect the majority of adult Americans today despite increased consciousness and concern about nutrition.

Historically, nutritionists have been particularly concerned with defining and quantifying the nutrients necessary to ensure optimal growth and development from infancy through adolescence. Although specific vitamin deficiency syndromes still occur in many parts of the world, such diseases as pellagra (niacin deficiency), beriberi (thiamine deficiency), scurvy (vitamin C deficiency), and rickets (vitamin D deficiency) are now quite uncommon in the United States. Although iron deficiency is still very common, the typical diet in the United States contains most nutrients in abundance. Thus, the focus for pediatric nutritionists has shifted to examining the effects of diet on long-term health, the management of obesity, and the nutritional support of premature infants and pediatric patients with chronic illnesses.

The Food and Nutrition Board of the National Research Council, National Academy of Science, has periodically issued revisions of its Recommended Dietary Allowances, which lists "levels of intake of essential nutrients . . . to be adequate to meet the known nutritional needs of practically all healthy persons." These age- and sex-specific guidelines (1989) are listed in Table 1. These levels have been set by expert panels who meet periodically, review published research of nutrient absorption and balance, and recommend daily nutrient intakes that intentionally exceed the nutrient requirements for most (but not all) people.

National nutrition surveys, such as the Ten-State Nutrition Survey (1972) and the Health and Nutrition Examination Surveys (HANES 1971–1974 and 1976–1980), have identified specific nutritional problems in the American population by analysis of dietary, biochemical, anthropometric, and other clinical characteristics of a large statistical sample of people (over 10,000), concentrating on low-income groups at greater nutritional risk. Although few overt clinical signs of specific nutritional deficiency were found, 95% of females of all ages consumed less than the recommended dietary intake of iron, and bio-

chemical evidence of iron deficiency was particularly prevalent in young children and adolescents, with as many as 22% of African American children under the age of 5 demonstrating abnormal transferrin saturation.

In 1980, the Surgeon-General of the U.S. Public Health Service issued a report that listed several dietary goals and guidelines for the diet of Americans. These goals are

1. Eat a variety of foods.
2. Maintain desirable weight.
3. Avoid too much fat, saturated fat, and cholesterol.
4. Eat foods with adequate starch and fiber.
5. Avoid too much sugar.
6. Avoid too much sodium.

In addition to recommending a varied diet and maintenance of a desirable weight, the report suggested avoiding excess total fat, saturated fat, cholesterol, sodium, sugar, and ethanol. In women and children, increased dietary intakes of calcium, iron, and fluoride were recommended.

BREAST FEEDING

It has long been accepted that human milk is the ideal food for the healthy mature human infant. Despite the wide variability of milk composition at different stages of lactation, time of day, or portion of feeding, breast-fed infants usually manage to satisfy all their nutrient requirements. Occasional failures of breast feeding may result in malnutrition and failure to thrive but are more likely caused by emotional factors or bad advice rather than nutritional inadequacy of the breast milk, even in malnourished mothers. Although exclusively breast-fed infants show a decrease in weight gain and length by about 6 months of age compared with their formula-fed counterparts, this probably represents a normal physiologic trend. Most recommendations stress the need for supplementation with solid foods by age 6 months.

There are many biochemical differences between human milk and infant formulas. Breast milk contains less total protein than whole cow's milk but more whey and less casein. Many nonnutritional substances found in breast milk play a role in host defense, such as lysozyme, lactoferrin, and secretory immunoglobulins. Many enzymes and hormones are also supplied in breast milk. The nonprotein nitrogen components of breast milk include greater amounts of taurine, nucleotides, and polyamines.

Fats provide a major source of energy for the newborn infant, and a lipase in breast milk complements the immature pancreatic exocrine system of neonates to aid in fat digestion and absorption. Palmitic acid, a saturated fatty acid found in abundance in human milk, is esterified, which facilitates hydrolysis by lipases. Human milk also contains significant amounts of long-chain desaturation products of omega-6 and omega-3 fatty acids, including docosahexanoic and arachidonic acids. The carnitine in breast milk may also aid in free fatty

1

TABLE 1. Food and Nutrition Board, National Academy of Sciences — National Research Council Recommended Dietary Allowances,* Revised 1989
Designed for the maintenance of good nutrition of practically all healthy people in the United States

CATEGORY	AGE (y) OR CONDITION	WEIGHT† (kg)	WEIGHT† (lb)	HEIGHT† (cm)	HEIGHT† (in)	PROTEIN (g)	FAT-SOLUBLE VITAMINS VITAMIN A (µg RE)‡	VITAMIN D (µg)§	VITAMIN E (mg α-TE)‖	VITAMIN K (µg)
Infants	0.0–0.5	6	13	60	24	13	375	7.5	3	5
	0.5–1.0	9	20	71	28	14	375	10	4	10
Children	1–3	13	29	90	35	16	400	10	6	15
	4–6	20	44	112	44	24	500	10	7	20
	7–10	28	62	132	52	28	700	10	7	30
Males	11–14	45	99	157	62	45	1,000	10	10	45
	15–18	66	145	176	69	59	1,000	10	10	65
	19–24	72	160	177	70	58	1,000	10	10	70
	25–50	79	174	176	70	63	1,000	5	10	80
	51+	77	170	173	68	63	1,000	5	10	80
Females	11–14	46	101	157	62	46	800	10	8	45
	15–18	55	120	163	64	44	800	10	8	55
	19–24	58	128	164	65	46	800	10	8	60
	25–50	63	138	163	64	50	800	5	8	65
	51+	65	143	160	63	50	800	5	8	65
Pregnant						60	800	10	10	65
Lactating	1st 6 mo					65	1,300	10	12	65
	2nd 6 mo					62	1,200	10	11	65

*The allowances, expressed as average daily intakes over time, are intended to provide for individual variations among most normal persons as they live in the United States under usual environmental stresses. Diets should be based on a variety of common foods in order to provide other nutrients for which human requirements have been less well defined. See text for detailed discussion of allowances and of nutrients not tabulated.
†Weights and heights of Reference Adults are actual medians for the U.S. population of the designated age, as reported by NHANES II. The median weights and heights of those under 19 years of age were taken from Hamill et al. (1979) (see pages 16–17). The use of these figures does not imply that the height/weight ratios are ideal.

acid oxidation of the absorbed triglycerides. Although breast milk contains lower concentrations of most vitamins and minerals than infant formulas, bioavailability of these nutrients (particularly iron, calcium, and zinc) is often much higher in human milk, facilitated by the presence of specific binding ligands. However, all breast-fed infants should be given supplemental vitamin K (at birth) to prevent rare but serious cases of newborn hemorrhagic disease. To prevent rickets, dark-skinned infants should be supplemented with vitamin D.

Low birth weight premature infants have special nutritional needs, some of which can be supplied by their own mother's milk, with its higher protein content. However, not all nutrient needs may be met by human milk, and this, along with the immaturity of organ systems, including the gastrointestinal tract, leads to the frequent use of parenteral nutrition and specialized infant formulas for premature infants. In addition, storage of expressed milk is complicated by bacterial contamination from skin flora. Refrigeration, freezing, or pasteurization may destroy many of the enzymes, vitamins, and protective factors in milk, but most other nutrients are not affected. Most drugs taken by the mother are excreted to some degree in breast milk, but relatively few are contraindicated during breast feeding.

Many of the advantages of breast feeding have only recently become understood, and studies of morbidity and mortality indicate that breast-fed infants are relatively spared from a wide range of gastrointestinal and infectious illnesses. Current recommendations in favor of breast feeding of full-term infants by a number of national and international organizations have resulted in the return of many mothers to breast feeding, at least for the first few months following birth.

WEANING

If and when breast feeding is no longer desired or possible, cow's milk-based infant formulas are suitable for the vast majority of American infants. For those who are intolerant to cow's milk, a diagnosis of cow's milk allergy may be entertained. Many infants are placed on soy-based or protein hydrolysate formulas when symptoms of intolerance to cow's milk-based formulas appear.

Although the age at which weaning foods are introduced has varied widely over the years, current recommendations are that solid foods be introduced gradually at about 4 to 6 months of age. At that point, the growth rate may slacken unless breast milk or formula feeds are supplemented by solids. Many parents feel that their infant demands supplementation at an earlier age for satiety or to permit them to sleep through the night. However, all nutrient needs can be met by exclusive breast milk or formula feeding until approximately 4 to 6 months of age, and early exposure to solid foods may provoke adverse reactions in infants predisposed to atopy. Furthermore, the complex process of feeding, including sucking, chewing, and swallowing a wide variety of textures, should be viewed as a series of tasks that mature gradually. The usual practice is to start with cereals, sequentially adding fruits, vegetables, then meats, as tolerated. Whole cow's milk should be introduced after 1 year of age, since it does not provide optimal nutrition for the rapidly growing infant.

CHILDHOOD

In childhood, frequent growth monitoring (every 6 to 12 months) is the best way to prevent either failure to thrive or obesity, as children's dietary habits and activity vary widely. At 1 to 2 years of age, parents often complain that their children suddenly have become "picky eaters," but that phenomenon corresponds with the normal physiologic flattening of the growth curve compared with the rapid rise in infancy. Emphasis should be placed on developing healthy eating habits, introducing a wide variety of foods, especially fruits and vegetables, during regular mealtimes and snacks. The addition of fluoride (in the water supply or as a supplement) and good dental hygiene will do much to prevent dental caries. A relatively high fat content in the diet is necessary for optimal growth and development in infants and young children, and lower fat diets should not be provided before the age of 2 years. For children who are found to be overweight for age or for height, early counseling involving the whole family and emphasizing regular meals, reduction of high calorie snacks, especially while watching television, and encouragement of

WATER-SOLUBLE VITAMINS						MINERALS						
THIA-MIN (mg)	RIBO-FLAVIN (mg)	NIACIN (mg NE)¶	VITA-MIN B₆ (mg)	FO-LATE (µg)	VITAMIN B₁₂ (µg)	CAL-CIUM (mg)	PHOS-PHORUS (mg)	MAG-NESIUM (mg)	IRON (mg)	ZINC (mg)	IODINE (µg)	SELE-NIUM (µg)
0.3	0.4	5	0.3	25	0.3	400	300	40	6	5	40	10
0.4	0.5	6	0.6	35	0.5	600	500	60	10	5	50	15
0.7	0.8	9	1.0	50	0.7	800	800	80	10	10	70	20
0.9	1.1	12	1.1	75	1.0	800	800	120	10	10	90	20
1.0	1.2	13	1.4	100	1.4	800	800	170	10	10	120	30
1.3	1.5	17	1.7	150	2.0	1,200	1,200	270	12	15	150	40
1.5	1.8	20	2.0	200	2.0	1,200	1,200	400	12	15	150	50
1.5	1.7	19	2.0	200	2.0	1,200	1,200	350	10	15	150	70
1.5	1.7	19	2.0	200	2.0	800	800	350	10	15	150	70
1.2	1.4	15	2.0	200	2.0	800	800	350	10	15	150	70
1.1	1.3	15	1.4	150	2.0	1,200	1,200	280	15	12	150	45
1.1	1.3	15	1.5	180	2.0	1,200	1,200	300	15	12	150	50
1.1	1.3	15	1.6	180	2.0	1,200	1,200	280	15	12	150	55
1.1	1.3	15	1.6	180	2.0	800	800	280	15	12	150	55
1.0	1.2	13	1.6	180	2.0	800	800	280	10	12	150	55
1.5	1.6	17	2.2	400	2.2	1,200	1,200	320	30	15	175	65
1.6	1.8	20	2.1	280	2.6	1,200	1,200	355	15	19	200	75
1.6	1.7	20	2.1	260	2.6	1,200	1,200	340	15	16	200	75

tinol equivalents. 1 RE = 1 µg retinol or 6 µg β-carotene. See text for calculation of vitamin A activity of diets as retinol equivalents.

cholecalciferol. 10 µg cholecalciferol = 400 IU of vitamin D.

Tocopherol equivalents. 1 mg d-α tocopherol = 1 α-TE. See text for variation in allowances and calculation of vitamin E activity of the diet as α-tocopherol equivalents.

NE (niacin equivalent) is equal to 1 mg of niacin or 60 mg of dietary tryptophan.

regular exercise and participation in sports is more appropriate than any dietary weight reduction program.

ADOLESCENCE

Adolescence is a period of rapid growth and changing dietary habits. Increased requirements for energy and protein for growth are often accompanied by an increased activity level. This is an important time to provide nutrition education and a range and volume of food appropriate to meet the adolescents' needs. Although eating habits rarely conform to those of more sedentary adults, behaviors such as frequent snacking permit adolescents to meet their needs. Recent evidence that precursors of atherosclerosis, as well as atherosclerotic lesions, are present in childhood has led to recommendations that adolescents with a family history of hyperlipidemia or premature coronary artery diseases should have a random determination of blood cholesterol. If this is elevated above 170 mg/dl, a fasting lipid profile including triglycerides, LDL, HDL, and VLDL cholesterol should be performed, and nutrition education with regard to limiting cholesterol and saturated fat in the diet should be provided, along with provision of regular exercise.

As they undergo the pubertal growth spurt and menarche, some adolescents develop cycles of binge eating, bulimia, and anorexia. A high percentage of these adolescents with eating disorders have severe psychologic problems, and psychiatric intervention is necessary before weight loss becomes severe. Iron deficiency is quite common among female adolescents, and a large percentage of adolescents do not obtain their recommended dietary allowance of 1200 mg/d of calcium, equivalent to 4 to 5 glasses of milk. This may put them at a relative disadvantage in achieving maximal peak bone mass and may predispose to later osteoporosis.

PROTEINS AND AMINO ACIDS

The typical American diet contains more than adequate protein to meet nutritional needs, and the excess protein is usually excreted as nitrogen in the urine. The requirement for protein ranges from 2.5 g/kg/d in newborns to 1.5 g/kg/d in childhood to 0.8 g/kg/d in adults and depends on the biologic value of the protein. Although amino groups are readily exchanged by transamination, certain essential amino acids cannot be synthesized by humans, including leucine, isoleucine, lysine, methionine, cystine, phenylalanine, tyrosine, tryptophan, threonine, valine, and possibly histidine, arginine, and taurine for infants. Vegetarians, especially lacto-ovovegetarians, can get enough protein in their diet by ingesting a wide variety of vegetables, cereals, and legumes. A wide variety will usually ensure a favorable amino acid balance that may not be achieved with a more limited selection, which may lack one or more of the essential amino acids.

CARBOHYDRATES AND FIBER

Carbohydrates make up a major portion (40% to 50%) of caloric intake in most diets. There is no absolute requirement for carbohydrates in the diet because glucose can be formed from glycerol or amino acids, but a carbohydrate-free diet often leads to ketosis and muscle protein breakdown. Dietary fibers are undigestible complex carbohydrates from plant cell walls, such as cellulose, hemicellulose, and pectin. They hold water in the colon and promote softer, bulky stools and, therefore, reduce the risk of constipation. Although controversial, fiber may also reduce the risk for the development of diverticulosis, colon cancer, and cardiovascular disease.

LIPIDS

Dietary lipids mainly consist of triglycerides and cholesterol and make up a large percentage of the caloric intake of infants, since they provide a concentrated form of energy, 9 kcal/g versus 4 kcal/g for carbohydrates and protein. The saturated fats contain no double bonds and come mainly from animal sources (meats, milk, butter, and eggs), whereas polyunsaturated fats come mainly from vegetable sources (such as corn oil, margarine, olive oil). Linoleic acid and linolenic acid are essential fatty acids for the formation of prostaglandins and cell membranes. Unlike other fatty acids, they cannot be synthesized by humans and must be supplied in the diet, although only 2% to 3% of total calories, or 3 to 6 g/d, is probably sufficient. Long-chain omega-3 fatty acid metabolites found in fish oils and human milk are critical components of developing visual and other cortical pathways.

Epidemiologic evidence in adult populations suggests that diets lower in total fats, saturated fats, and cholesterol reduce the risk of coronary artery disease. Recommendations to reduce total fat to 30% of dietary calories, saturated fat to less than 10% of total calories, and dietary cholesterol to less than 300 mg/d have been widely promoted. Children in the United States currently eat approximately 35% to 36% of their daily calories as fat. Although the risk of heart disease later in life must be considered, excessively fat restricted diets can have deleterious effects on nutrient intake and growth.

VITAMINS

Vitamins are a heterogeneous group of organic chemicals required in the diet in trace quantities because humans generally cannot synthesize them. They are present in most foods, especially in fresh fruits and vegetables, and in sufficient quantities in typical American diets to prevent any widespread deficiency syndromes. The classic vitamin deficiency disease, such as pellagra (niacin deficiency), beriberi (thiamine), rickets (vitamin D), and scurvy (vitamin C), are rarely seen in the United States but are still very prevalent in some developing countries, where there may be an insufficient variety of grains or availability of fresh vegetables. Many foods processed in the United States are fortified with vitamins. In an effort to decrease the risk of neural tube defects, processed flour in the United States will likely soon be fortified with folic acid. In most cases, excess water-soluble vitamins in the diet are excreted in the urine. Therefore, it is usually not necessary to provide any vitamin supplements for healthy children eating an unrestricted diet. Total vegetarian diets lack vitamin B_{12}, which is found only in foods of animal origin.

Considerable controversy has accompanied claims that vitamins prevent or treat some chronic illnesses, such as heart disease and certain cancer. Vitamin supplements are indicated for individuals with intestinal malabsorption syndromes and during pregnancy and lactation. Most multivitamin supplements are probably harmless, but vitamin A, which is stored in the liver, may be toxic if persistently ingested in excessive quantities. Excessive dietary carotene may cause yellowing of the skin but does not lead to vitamin A toxicity. Very large oral doses of vitamin D may cause hypercalcemia, although production of vitamin D by exposure of skin to sunlight does not. Megadoses of vitamin C may predispose to oxalate kidney stones. Toxicity from vitamin E and most of the water-soluble vitamins is very rare.

MINERALS

Minerals perform a wide variety of functions in the human body, from providing structural strength in the skeleton to serving as essential cofactors of metabolic reactions and intracellular messengers. Some, such as selenium and manganese, are trace elements present only in milligram quantities in the body. Others make up a large proportion of the bone mass. Most are consumed in quantities far above the necessary minimum, so that dietary deficiencies are extremely rare. With others, such as calcium, the RDAs are met only in a minority of the population.

Sodium is an example of a mineral that is ingested in quantities far above the necessary minimum, with American dietary intakes averaging 2 to 6 g/d (5 to 15 g of salt) and ranging up to 25 g (60 g salt) in some Asian diets. Almost all of the sodium is excreted by the kidney, with only a small percentage reabsorbed under hormonal control dictated by fluid needs. Without excessive sweating and with adequate renal conservation, only about 115 mg/d of sodium (300 mg salt) is absolutely necessary under most conditions, with the minimum RDA set at 500 mg sodium (1.2 g salt). Any excess usually can be excreted by the kidney, but compensatory mechanisms may be impaired in patients with hypertension or congestive heart failure. Current dietary goals suggest a reduction in the daily intake of sodium to 1 mg/kcal or to 2.4 g (5 g salt)/d.

Calcium forms the bulk of bone mineral where it is stored (about 1200 g) but is also required for many cellular processes, such as muscle contraction, nerve conduction, clotting, and enzyme function. Serum levels are regulated to a narrow range by several hormones, especially 1,25-dihydroxyvitamin D and parathyroid hormone, so that dietary calcium deficiency results not in hypocalcemia but in osteopenia. Adequate calcium intake in childhood and adolescence (800 to 1200 mg/d) is probably important in assuring maximal peak bone mass to prevent premature osteoporosis.

Magnesium and phosphorus are also major components of bone, as well as participating in many metabolic reactions. However, in contrast to calcium, they are widely distributed in most foods and are well absorbed in the intestinal tract, so dietary deficiencies are quite rare.

Iron deficiency is one of the most common nutrient deficiencies in childhood. Iron stores are much lower in infants, and anemia ensues when stores are depleted. Only 4% of women in national surveys actually had iron deficiency anemia with low hemoglobin levels, on an average intake of 10 to 11 mg/d elemental iron. Heme iron from animal sources is absorbed better than nonheme iron, so those on vegetarian diets may be at more risk. The RDA has been set at 10 mg in children.

Zinc and copper are essential components of many metalloenzymes. Although a syndrome of hypogonadism and growth retardation has been described in Iran, the most recognized form of zinc deficiency in the United States is in the rare inherited syndrome of acrodermatitis enteropathica. Likewise, copper deficiency is rarely seen, mostly in patients on parenteral nutrition or in the rare inherited Menkes kinky hair syndrome. The RDAs for the essential trace elements, including manganese, molybdenum, chromium, and fluoride, are listed in Table 2.

SUMMARY

The role of good nutrition in preventing later disease is again becoming increasingly appreciated, and both consumers and medical

TABLE 2. Estimated Safe and Adequate Daily Dietary Intakes of Trace Elements

CATEGORY	AGE (y)	COPPER (mg)	MANGANESE (mg)	FLUORIDE (mg)	CHROMIUM (µg)	MOLYBDENUM (µg)
Infants	0–0.5	0.4–0.6	0.3–0.6	0.1–0.5	10–40	15–30
	0.5–1	0.6–0.7	0.6–1.0	0.2–1.0	20–60	20–40
Children and adolescents	1–3	0.7–1.0	1.0–1.5	0.5–1.5	20–80	25–50
	4–6	1.0–1.5	1.5–2.0	1.0–2.5	30–120	30–75
	7–10	1.0–2.0	2.0–3.0	1.5–2.5	50–200	50–150
	11 +	1.5–2.5	2.0–5.0	1.5–2.5	50–200	75–250
Adults		1.5–3.0	2.0–5.0	1.5–4.0	50–200	75–250

professionals are eager for good advice. The American diet has shown signs of change in the past few years, but a continued emphasis on less total calories, sodium, sugar, and saturated fat and increased fruits, vegetables, and cereal grains will help reduce unnecessary overnutrition and later disease.

REFERENCES

1. American Academy of Pediatrics Committee on Nutrition: Pediatric Nutrition Handbook. Evanston, Ill, American Academy of Pediatrics, 1993.
2. National Cholesterol Education Program: Highlights of the report of the expert panel on blood cholesterol levels in children and adolescents. Pediatrics 89:495–501, 1992.
3. National Research Council Subcommittee on the Tenth Edition of the RDAs: Recommended Dietary Allowances, 10th ed. Washington, DC, National Academy of Sciences, 1989.

UNDERNUTRITION

Festus O. Adebonojo, m.d.

The term "undernutrition" has become a substitute for the term "malnutrition" and currently is being used interchangeably with the term "failure to thrive" in the pediatric literature. Undernutrition describes a state of negative energy balance that may be mild or severe, acute or chronic, and in which all five components of normal energy requirements are not met. Basal metabolism, the major component of energy requirement, accounts for about 55% to 60% and specific dynamic action for about 5%. Normal losses through the urine and stools account for another 5% to 8%. Of the remaining normal energy requirement, normal physical activities account for about half, or 15%, and normal growth in height and weight accounts for the remaining 15%. In a state of persistent, chronic negative energy balance, the first component to be sacrificed is growth, and weight gain is the first to cease. Indeed, the rate of weight gain slows fairly quickly, and if negative energy balance persists for a prolonged period, height growth slows or ceases.

In the developing countries where malnutrition (undernutrition) has remained a severe problem for a variety of reasons, it is referred to as "marasmus" in younger infants and "kwashiorkor" in older children with greater protein deficiency. Either description implies severe undernutrition with calorie or protein deficiency or both, characterized by a significant reduction in height and weight. In the young infant with marasmus, both height for age and weight for height are below the 5th percentile. In the older child with kwashiorkor, both height and weight are similarly compromised, but weight for height may appear mistakenly normal because of the hypoalbuminemic edema present in many of these children.

In the United States, undernutrition, often coded as "failure to thrive" in the hospital records, occurs in 2% to 4% of pediatric hospital admissions. About 75% to 80% of these are either psychosocial (50%) or combined organic/psychosocial (25%) in origin, and the rest have purely organic causes. It is estimated that varying degrees of undernutrition actually occur more frequently in hospitalized children, perhaps in as many as 20% to 30% of children admitted with various organic problems. Sixty to seventy percent of these are associated with neurologic and gastrointestinal disorders. The rest are found in association with such conditions as prolonged infections, malignancies, and cardiac, renal, and other diseases.

It has been difficult to clearly define the population at risk for undernutrition in the United States and, more importantly, to establish a consistent definition of undernutrition. Some definitions of undernutrition include a weight less than the 5th percentile on the growth chart or persistent decrease in the rate of weight gain. Other definitions have separated acute from chronic undernutrition and defined the former as a weight for height less than the 5th percentile and the latter as height for age less than the 5th percentile. The lack of consistency among definitions of undernutrition used for different public health purposes in the United States has hindered an effective diagnosis of the problem and the design of effective intervention to prevent and treat it.[3] Detection of the population at risk for undernutrition in the United States still appears to depend more on socioeconomic indicators than on physical or physiologic indexes.

MANAGEMENT

On a case by case basis, the management of undernutrition starts with an accurate complete assessment of the patient, including a complete history and detailed information about time of onset of the problem. Family history should explore family growth patterns and parental heights and weights. Nutritional history should include details of intakes, feeding behaviors, and problems associated with feeding. A complete and detailed psychosocial, behavioral, and developmental history should be obtained. Physical examination should be complete and include a search for findings suggesting the presence of organic diseases, edema, brittle, easily plucked hair, and other telltale signs of nutritional deficiencies. Accurate anthropometric measurement of height, weight, and head circumference should be made and plotted on a standard growth chart, such as the National Center for Health Statistics (NCHS) growth chart. Measurements of midarm circumference and skinfold thickness at different sites should be done by personnel skilled in these measurements. Otherwise, they may be of limited usefulness.

Initial laboratory tests include the standard urine analysis with microscopy, complete blood count with absolute lymphocyte count, and serum electrolytes, including bicarbonate and total protein with albumin. Decreased serum bicarbonate has been reported in some children with undernutrition of nonorganic origin.[2]

Undernutrition may be mild or severe. Determination of the degree of severity is aided by the history and physical examination. An infant whose height growth continues consistently along a normal curve on a growth chart when the rate of weight gain is rapidly declining should be suspected of having undernutrition, particularly when no apparent organic cause can be found. If identified early, mild undernutrition can be managed readily and successfully on an outpatient basis with an adequate diet designed with assistance from a nutritionist or dietitian. If managed on an outpatient basis, additional support should include home education for the mother and others who care for the child. Where available, the support of a home health team, social worker, nutritionist, and psychologist should be mobilized. In many cases, however, because of the underlying psychosocial family pathology, outpatient management is not feasible, and the child should be admitted to the hospital.

The first principle in the management of the child with undernutrition is "use the gut if it works." Infants with mild undernutrition from nonorganic causes usually will respond to oral feeding fairly promptly. Weight gain may be seen within 2 days of admission, and these children may show signs of "thriving," increased alertness, and responsiveness within 5 to 7 days. During the early renutrition phase, the child with mild undernutrition occasionally may develop vomiting or diarrhea. If the gastrointestinal tract is intact, simply slowing the rate of renutrition usually will succeed.

Children with severe undernutrition should be hospitalized. Not only does the severity of the problem require it, but also a temporary change of environment often helps to reduce family tensions. Hospitalization offers the opportunity to estimate accurately some of the factors that govern the child's net caloric intake and to observe the child's interactions with parents, hospital caregivers, and other children. Aggressive intervention in the hospital using trained personnel, actively involving the mother, and multidisciplinary support from social worker and nutritionist will help promote improved growth and development. Initial attention needs to be directed at the correction of associated dehydration when fluid and electrolyte imbalances are present. There may be significantly reduced serum albumin or bicarbonate, hypokalemia, hyponatremia, and other mineral imbalances.

TABLE 1. Selected Enteral Preparations

PRODUCT	MANUFACTURER	TOTAL ENERGY		PROTEIN		CARBOHYDRATE		FAT	
		kcal/L	kcal/oz	g/L	SOURCE	g/L	SOURCE	g/L	SOURCE
Standard formulas	——	670	20	15–16	Cow's milk protein	70–72	Lactose	36–37	Cow's milk fat
Attain	Sherwood	1000	30	40	Casein	135	Maltodextria	35	Medium chain tri-glycer-ides
Compleat	Sandoz	1070	32	43	Beef, Cas-ein	141	Cereal/fruit/vegeta-bles	37	Beef, corn oil
Ensure	Ross	1060	32	37.2	Casein, soy	145	Corn syrup, sucrose	37.2	Corn oil
Jevity	Ross	1060	32	44	Casein	151.7	Cornstarch, soy	36.8	MCT from coconut oil
Pediasure	Ross	1000	30	37	Casein, soy	145	Cornstarch	38	MCT, corn, soy
Portagen	Mead Johnson	1010	30	36	Casein	117	Corn syrup, sucrose	48	Corn oil, soy, lec-ithin
Sustacal	Mead Johnson	1000	30	61	Casein, soy	140	Lactose, sucrose, corn syrup	23	Soy oil
Ensure-Plus	Ross	1500	45	54.9	Casein, soy	200	Corn syrup, sucrose	53	Corn oil
Sustagen	Mead Johnson	1850	55	113	Milk, casein	318	Corn syrup, lactose, dextrose	17	Milk fat
Vivonex	Norwich-Eaton	1800	54	38	Amino acids	206	Maltodexdrins	3	Safflower

Initial treatment with intravenous fluids should be directed at correcting such imbalances. If infection is present, it should be treated appropriately. The ultimate objective of treatment, however, is to increase the level of the child's nutritional status as rapidly as possible without increasing the risks of complications associated with treatment. If the gastrointestinal tract is intact, the child should be fed by the oral route. Liquid formula preparations designed to provide the required nutrition should be instituted. The nutrient preparation employed depends on the status of the patient's gastrointestinal functions. Apart from the usual infant formulas, over 50 nutritional formulations containing appropriate mixtures of calories, proteins, minerals, and vitamins are now available. Table 1 summarizes the composition of some of these, and one formulation can be selected to meet the patient's nutritional requirements.

The renutrition regimen should be approached in three stages. During the first phase, lasting about 2 to 4 days, the child initially should be offered sufficient quantities of the appropriate liquid preparation to meet 100% of the daily requirement for calories and protein based on the actual weight on admission (Table 2). If the amount offered on the first day is well tolerated, the amount offered can be increased to provide on days 2 to 4 the calorie and protein intakes for 50th percentile weight for age. If the patient tolerates the increase well, she can be started on the second phase of renutrition therapy. This phase of treatment provides for catchup growth and is designed to provide the calories and proteins needed to reconstitute normal height and weight over a period of 1 week or more. To estimate the calorie and protein requirements for phase 2, the child is given the amount of formula provided in phase 1 multiplied by the patient's ideal body weight, divided by the actual admission weight. Care is exercised to avoid overhydration or overzealous renutrition, particularly with large fluid intake. Congestive heart failure may result. Following this phase, the third phase of renutrition, the consolidation phase, is initiated. During this phase, the child should be continued on the phase 2 regimen with additional caloric supplementation as needed to achieve full recovery. The diet should be tailored to meet the needs of the patient. If the patient is less than 6 months old, liquid formulas will suffice, but if over 6 months old, a variety of solids should be judiciously introduced. Phases 1 and 2 can be accomplished with liquid formulations, including regular infant formulas with or

TABLE 2. Recommended Protein/Energy Intakes for Children

AGE (y)	AVERAGE WEIGHT (kg)	PROTEIN (g)	TOTAL CALORIES (kcal/kg)
0.0–0.5	6	13	110–120
0.5–1.0	9	14	105
1–3	13	16	100
4–6	20	24	90
7–10	28	28	72

Adapted from the Recommended Dietary Allowances (1989). Food and Nutrition Board, National Academy of Sciences National Research Council.

without caloric supplementation or special formulas (Table 1). In phase 3, feedings should be varied to include a normal diet for age. Prolonged caloric supplementation may be required to achieve full recovery. Children with severe hypokalemia on initial diagnosis may require as much as two to three times the normal daily requirement for potassium during the first several days of rehydration and nutritional rehabilitation. Serum electrolytes should be monitored carefully.

If the gastrointestinal tract is functionally normal and if the oral route of renutrition produces significant vomiting or the child refuses oral feedings, nasogastric or nasojejunal tube feeding should be considered. The latter should be installed under x-ray guidance and should not be employed for more than 1 or 2 weeks during initial renutrition. Rarely, a gastrostomy or jejunostomy tube placement is required to feed the patient. Whether through oral route or tube feedings, the caloric concentration of the preparation employed may need to be increased, particularly if the volume of the standard preparations needed for adequate nutrition exceeds 200 to 250 ml/kg/d. In such circumstances, cautious use of more calorically concentrated preparations that can deliver 1 to 1.5 kcal/ml (Table 2) should be considered. These preparations, however, may produce an undesired osmotic diarrhea.

The nutritional rehabilitation of a severely undernourished child should provide 10% to 15% of total calories as protein, 50% to 60% as carbohydrate, and about 30% to 40% as fat. Several of the preparations available provide these proportions. However, adequate nutritional rehabilitation could be achieved with as little as 8% to 10% of total calories derived from protein even in the presence of hypoalbuminemia. The initial phase of renutrition usually lasts 3 days. Thereafter, total intake of as much as 150 kcal/kg/d can be provided and will produce measurable weight gain of about 10 to 15 g/kg/d. More body weight accretion can be achieved in the range of 20 to 25 g/kg/d by providing as much as 200 to 250 kcal/kg/d. In the absence of organic disease, most patients with severe undernutrition will progress to good recovery.

A child with severe undernutrition of nonorganic origin whose gastrointestinal tract is temporarily nonfunctional will rarely require parenteral nutrition. If parenteral nutrition will be required for less than a week, peripheral parenteral nutrition should be initiated. If the support will be required for more than a week, serious consideration should be given to establishing a central line and initiating central parenteral nutrition. Initially, the volume of parenteral fluid should be at the maintenance level, usually 100 ml/kg/d. Small quantities of supplemental oral nutrition should be provided as tolerated. The parenteral fluid initially should contain 5% to 10% dextrose and 0.5% to 1.0% protein, in the form of amino acid mixture, as well as appropriate concentrations of electrolytes, minerals, and vitamins. In peripheral parenteral administration, the maximum concentrations of dextrose and amino acids achievable over 1 or 2 days are 10% and 2.5%, respectively. Intravenous lipids at concentration of 10% to 20% can be infused in sufficient quantities to provide as much as 50% of total caloric requirements. The caloric density of these preparations renders them a very desirable source of calories, but hyperlipidemia should be carefully monitored, and if it occurs, the solutions should be stopped or the amount infused should be reduced. With a central line, the concentrations of dextrose and amino acids that can be administered can be as much as 50% and 4% to 5%, respectively. Hyperglycemia resulting from the high concentrations of dextrose can be treated with insulin.

Central parenteral nutrition may cause a number of problems, and these should be anticipated. Complications of catheter insertion include pneumothorax and thrombosis, catheter embolism, air embolism, thoracic duct injury, and others. Other complications, such as severe frontal headache, may result in unexplained irritability in a child who cannot express where the hurt is located. Usually, this is a transient disturbance that disappears in a few days. Hyperlipidemia or hyperglycemia, as previously mentioned, and other metabolic disturbances are not uncommon and should receive appropriate attention. Hypoglycemia, hypoalbuminemia, hypophosphatemia, hypomagnesemia, and other disturbances occur occasionally. Daily monitoring of serum biochemistry and biweekly monitoring of liver functions are necessary to assess the patient's progress. In 1% to 2% of patients with prolonged central line administration, significant bacterial sepsis occurs, and it is necessary to withdraw the line and vigorously treat the sepsis. A new line can be reinstated, if needed, within 24 to 48 hours, and treatment can be continued. It is now possible to provide adequate total nutrition through the parenteral route for several months. The ultimate goal in these patients, however, is to reinstate oral feedings and restore normal life as early as possible.

Regardless of the route of renutrition—oral, tube feedings, or parenteral—the child with severe undernutrition initially may lose weight for several days after treatment is initiated. This is usually a result of the loss of apparent or occult edema. The intestinal enzymes usually return to normal, and intestinal absorption of nutrients improves with resultant weight gain. Nutritional rehabilitation in severe undernutrition is a very protracted process. Continuing support must be provided to the family even after apparent full nutritional recovery. If indicated, the family should be assisted to enroll in programs designed to help needy families, such as the WIC, Commodity Supplemental Food, Summer Food Assistance, and Food Stamps programs. Appropriate frequent and regular follow-up visits in the office are essential to avoid relapse. At these visits, careful assessments of nutritional status are made, and the parents are offered continued supervision, encouragement, psychosocial and nutritional counseling, as well as proper parenting education.

PROGNOSIS

Severe undernutrition often is associated with generalized growth retardation and significant decrease in the rate of height and weight accretion. There are usually signs of developmental delay, withdrawal symptoms, physical and emotional deprivation, apathy, vomiting on feeding, and diarrhea. Neuromuscular hypotonia may be present. However, in most patients, the prognosis for the final outcome of treatment in childhood undernutrition is good. Nevertheless, if growth and development have been severely impaired, mental and physical retardation may persist.[1] Usually, the younger the infant at the onset of nutritional deprivation and the more prolonged the undernutrition, the more long lasting the devastating consequences will be. Deficits in visual perceptual and abstract abilities usually are longer lasting.

REFERENCES

1. Allen LH: Functional indicators and outcomes of undernutrition. J Nutr 120:924—932, 1990.
2. Bithony WG, Epstein D, Kim H: Decreased serum bicarbonate as a manifestation of undernutrition secondary to non-organic failure to thrive. J Dev Behav Pediatr 13:278–280, 1992.
3. Peterson KE, Chen LC: Defining undernutrition for public health purposes in the United States. J Nutr 120:933–942, 1990.

CHILDHOOD OBESITY

DRUCY BOROWITZ, M.D.

WHO CAN BE CARED FOR APPROPRIATELY BY THE GENERALIST?

Most overweight children can be cared for by a generalist who is willing to devote the time and energy. If the height age is appropriate or advanced for the weight age, a medical cause of the obesity is unlikely. Children whose height growth has slowed (thus, a normal increase in weight makes the weight-for-height inappropriately high) or those with short stature, particularly in the context of mental or behavioral disturbance, should be evaluated for the rare endocrinologic or genetic causes of obesity.

PREPARING TO MANAGE PEDIATRIC OBESITY

In larger communities, pediatric weight management programs may be available and are likely to be more effective than programs centered in a health practitioner's office. If such programs are unavailable, an office-based approach can be undertaken.

The medical practitioner must examine his or her own attitudes toward overweight patients before committing to treating them. Personal biases are strong, and one who views overweight children as lazy, weak-willed, or gluttonous should not be a part of a weight management program. Numerous dietary intake studies have failed to demonstrate that obese children consume more calories than their nonobese peers. When total energy expenditure is measured in the free-living state using the doubly labeled water method, obese children have been found to expend more calories than their nonobese counterparts, regardless of whether or not the study subjects gained or lost weight during the study period. Obesity has both genetic and environmental etiologic components. Our goals should be to optimize our patients' health, not to enable them to conform to the rather skewed ideal our society has for body size.

Pediatricians, family, and nurse practitioners who choose to take on the responsibility of treating childhood obesity should plan on using a multidisciplinary approach. Nutritionists (usually registered dietitians) can provide dietary counseling in greater depth than most medical practitioners. Mental health professionals who employ a family-centered approach should be identified, since some families may need referral.

INITIAL ASSESSMENT

The health care practitioner should set aside a *minimum* of one half-hour for the initial assessment. Initiation of weight management cannot be accomplished during a health maintenance appointment.

The health care practitioner should begin by assessing the family's motivation to effect change. Parents must be involved in any weight management strategy. It has been clearly shown that long-term success in weight management can be achieved if the family is actively involved. Nonspecific family involvement or a purely child-centered approach is unlikely to be effective over time. A program should not be undertaken if the physician or nurse practitioner is concerned about the child's weight but the family is not. In this circumstance, gentle counseling should be provided concerning long-term health issues, and the family should be left with an open-ended invitation to seek out the health care practitioner when they are more ready to address weight management.

A *history of the present illness* should be taken. If there is a clear point in time when the growth chart begins to deviate from the norm (reactive obesity), what events were happening in the child's life at that time? Does the child have any symptoms to suggest complications of obesity, such as snoring or frank sleep apnea, hip or knee pain, or constipation? These should be evaluated and treated. What is the child's social and school life like? Does the child participate in formal or informal sports? How much television does he or she watch? Does the child have friends? Contrary to myth, many overweight children are well adjusted socially. On the other hand, significant isolation or depression warrants referral to a mental health professional. In some instances, obesity may be a symptom of a more serious problem, such as parental neglect or abuse.

Concurrent chronic conditions in the *past medical history* can affect the treatment plan. For example, patients with diabetes will need close monitoring of blood sugar when exercise increases and the diet changes. Children with asthma should be managed aggressively so that exercise-induced bronchospasm does not interfere with a prescription of increased activity.

The practitioner should focus on the *family history* of obesity. If one or both parents are overweight, it should be determined when overweight became a problem for them, and when applicable, the issues associated with a parent's childhood onset of obesity should be explored. What experiences have overweight parents had with weight loss and weight gain? Are overweight parents ready to actively address their own weight problems at present? (Although family practitioners may care for both child and parents, pediatricians and pediatric nurse practitioners may want to suggest that overweight parents become involved with a balanced weight loss program during the time that the child is being seen. This can help to bring about real changes in the home food environment.) Are there other medical issues in the family that will interfere with an effective weight loss program? Examples would include significant psychiatric illness, severe acute or chronic illness, or death of a family member. The family history of cardiovascular morbidity and diabetes should be explored.

A complete *psychosocial history* and itemization of the family's strengths and weaknesses are necessary. Where does the child eat his meals? Do the parents have different views on food, weight, and exercise? What happens when the child is not in school? Does the child spend a significant amount of time in more than one household? If nonparental caretakers are involved, what are their attitudes about food, weight, and exercise? If the parents are divorced or separated, is the situation amicable or tense? What is the family style? Is the household rigid or chaotic? Is the child indulged, or are the parents distant? The family risk factors are determined at this initial interview. Many families of obese children are functional and supportive. However, if family counseling is indicated, a referral is made at the outset.

A standard *review of systems* will identify any other contributing medical factors.

The *physical examination* should include examination of the growth curve, an accurate weight on a balanced beam-type scale with the patient in underclothes or a hospital gown, height measured with a stadiometer (now widely available at reasonable cost), and blood pressure measured with an appropriately sized cuff. Those who plan to see overweight children on a regular basis need to have a selection of large blood pressure cuffs (including thigh cuffs, if necessary) to determine whether hypertension is a comorbidity. The examiner should especially note the presence or absence of enlarged tonsils, hepatomegaly, and acanthosis niger (indicative of chronic carbohydrate intolerance) and should determine the child's Tanner stage. Height growth will be limited in children who are already pubertal, thus making weight loss (as opposed to stabilization) more imperative. Males have an increase in their percent lean body mass as they progress through puberty, making weight loss somewhat easier than it is for females.

Laboratory assessment should be quite limited. A cholesterol and fasting triglyceride level are warranted to assess potential comorbidity. With a normal rate of height growth, thyroid function testing and other endocrinologic workup should be done only if the parents need assurance that their child does not have a "gland problem."

WEIGHT MANAGEMENT PROGRAM

The extent of psychosocial difficulties identified at the initial assessment will determine the course of action. If these issues are severe or acute, a recommendation to defer a weight loss program is warranted. If the assessment indicates that formal family counseling will be needed as part of the weight management program, modest goals for weight loss should be set (<1 pound/wk). Although these patients may not lose a great deal of weight in the short term, success of a program can be judged also by attainment of psychosocial goals, which sets the stage for long-term weight management. If psychosocial stressors are mild or absent, weight loss and behavioral goals should be set (1 pound/wk, short-term accountability for behavior changes).

The next step is referral to a dietitian for in-depth dietary history and counseling. The best approach with children is for them to learn specific concepts about foods (i.e., what is fat, what foods are high in fat) as opposed to counting calories per se. The dietitian should help with food-related education. However, education alone will not help most families. The patient and his family should be seen at least once a week for 10 to 12 weeks, with the themes of each visit defined (Table 1). Intervention will involve modifying behaviors centered around eating and activity and identification of emotional factors that interfere with behavioral changes. Weight should be measured at each visit, and blood pressure should be followed in patients with hypertension.

The health practitioner must define the behaviors related to eating and activity that are to change and determine how to keep the patient and family accountable for making these changes. Written logs can be used. Follow-through is necessary. For example, if "homework"

TABLE 1. Themes To Be Explored During Weight Management Visits

The patient's motivation for weight management

Nutrition education concerning meals versus snacks, foods low in fat and sugar, portion control, and other factors

Exercise habits, activity level, development of an exercise plan

Goals, limits, consequences, rewards

Identification of eating style, eating environment, eating cues, hunger and satiety

Understanding feelings, self-esteem, dealing with the way society views overweight people

Dealing with special occasions, binges, and cravings

Development of interests and sense of self unrelated to food is not done, what are the consequences? Modeling limit-setting behavior can help parents understand how to do likewise at home. The patient should be weighed on a weekly basis, but attaining behavioral goals (e.g., logs indicating increased family activity time or less television viewing time) may be as important as weight loss.

The physician or practitioner must be comfortable dealing with emotional issues and family dynamics and must help the child and family recognize the emotional factors related to eating and being overweight in order to defuse them. It is helpful to have specific teaching materials. The Shapedown Program has an age-appropriate syllabus based on weekly encounters and can be used for individuals or groups. This program emphasizes psychosocial interventions, as well as education concerning diet and exercise.

Medications

At the present time, appetite suppressants should not be a part of a weight management program. Although the pharmaceutical industry stands to make an enormous profit by developing a "weight loss pill," extensive research has not provided us with a safe medical adjunct to counseling and education. A balanced multivitamin can be taken daily while the child is actively losing weight as insurance against potential micronutrient deficiency.

Long-term Monitoring

The health professional in primary care will continue to follow patients they have treated intensively, as outlined previously. Follow-up visits can be scheduled at increasingly longer intervals but should be continued at least every 3 to 4 months until a stable pattern is established. Follow-up is especially important in patients with hypertension or hypercholesterolemia. The practitioner should be wary of extreme weight loss and continue to support families in which children regain lost weight.

Time, Reimbursement, and Reality

Weight management cannot be achieved in a few quick visits. Casual comments about weight or proffering of preprinted calorie sheets in the absence of follow-up often does more harm than good. A true weight management program takes time and effort but often will not be reimbursed by third party payers or even by health maintenance organizations whose philosophy touts preventive care. As a result, few obese children receive meaningful care. A recent position paper by the Center for Child and Adolescent Obesity outlines recommendations for preventing and treating childhood obesity in the United States.*

NUTRITION SUPPORT IN THE VERY ILL PEDIATRIC PATIENT

JAMES L. SUTPHEN, M.D., Ph.D.
ANA ABAD SINDEN, M.S., R.D., C.N.S.D.
MARCIA L. BUCK, Pharm. D.

With the introduction of specialized enteral and parenteral products, nutritional support has evolved into a complicated field over the past 25 years. Although these nutritional therapies have provided enormous benefits for sick people, they have also generated additional costs that can easily increase the daily cost of an inpatient hospitalization by several hundred dollars. If nutritional support becomes the only reason for an inpatient hospitalization, home treatment through

numerous outpatient pharmacies is advisable. Indeed, these home nutritional care companies have evolved into a highly specialized and lucrative industry. There are now hundreds of enteral and parenteral nutritional products, nearly all of which claim some special advantage. The clinician should always be wary of the claims advertised by the newest and, generally, most expensive products. As the medical–industrial complex lurches forward into nutritional support, one must always remember that a simple appetizing balanced diet remains the gold standard.

ENTERAL NUTRITION

Enteral nutrition support is the preferred modality for the critically ill pediatric patient. It provides a number of advantages over parenteral nutrition. Enteral nutrition more closely approximates the natural delivery of nutrients to the body and, by virtue of portal delivery, maintains the central metabolic function of the liver. It produces fewer metabolic and infectious complications. Nutrient provision is more complete and can easily include nutrients, such as trace elements, nucleotides, glutamine, fiber, and short chain fatty acids. Additional minerals can be added without concern for solubility factors that hamper delivery in parenteral nutrition. This is particularly important for calcium and phosphorous delivery for preterm infants, where requirement exceeds parenteral solution solubility. Enteral feedings also provide a trophic effect on the gut, thereby promoting intestinal adaptation and growth. Finally, but in this decade of cost containment perhaps most importantly, the expense of enteral feedings is a fraction of parenteral feedings.

There are a number of specific indications for enteral nutrition support in pediatric patients. Preterm infants present a unique challenge because of their gastrointestinal immaturity, fluid requirements, and increased requirements for specific nutrients. Before the coordination of their suck and swallow reflex at 32 to 34 weeks' gestation, they are fed via nasogastric (NG) or orogastric tubes, either intermittently every 1 to 3 hours or continuously for those infants unable to tolerate small frequent feeds. Infants and children with cardiorespiratory illness, in particular bronchopulmonary dysplasia, cystic fibrosis (CF), and congenital heart disease, often require supplemental tube feedings because of inadequate spontaneous intake. Acutely ill pediatric patients with gastrointestinal disease and dysfunction, such as Crohn's disease and short gut syndrome, benefit from enteral nutrition during the acute exacerbation period as well as for chronic nutrition management. Infants with end-stage renal, cardiac, or hepatic disease awaiting transplantation of organs may benefit from the provision of extra calories to induce growth and thereby facilitate surgical procedures. Pediatric patients with hypermetabolic conditions, including trauma, burn injury, or sepsis, can benefit from enteral nutrition as a modality to support the associated increased energy expenditure. Children with cerebral palsy or other devastating neuromuscular conditions who have limited spontaneous oral intake may benefit from intragastric enteral nutrition to improve nutritional status and lessen the demands on parents and health care providers presented by prolonged, often stressful attempts at oral feeding.

Delivery Modalities

In its simplest form, enteral nutrition supplementation is provided by eating additional food. High calorie foods, even junk foods, have the advantage of better patient compliance. It is useful to remember that the experts in weight gain (obese people) gain weight not from the boring, repetitive intake of a single supplement, but from a varied, often high fat, appetizing, and calorically dense diet. They eat during periods of inactivity, such as in front of the television or while reading. Also, they often eat another meal late at night when intake is generally not followed by activity, which can lessen the efficiency of weight gain. Therefore, if oral motor function is adequate but weight gain is a problem, eating additional appetizing high calorie foods is reasonable first advice.

---

*Mellin L, Brownell K, Dietz WH, et al: Child Obesity Recommendations for the United States. Center for Child and Adolescent Obesity, University of California, San Francisco, 1992.

If oral motor function is not adequate or appetite will not support a sufficient oral intake, it is necessary to bypass the mouth by NG or gastrostomy feedings. When this must be done, it is important to preserve some oral motor intake or stimulation to prevent atrophy of oral motor function. This can occur within a space of a few weeks in preterm or neurologically impaired children. For infants, if the suck and swallow reflex is lost early in life as a result of disuse, one must wait several months for sufficient skills to develop for cup feeding. Moreover, the attendant lack of oral stimulation may lead to tactile defensiveness and delayed acquisition of language skills. Nasogastric feedings are useful for short-term feedings (less than 2 to 3 months) and are a valuable first step for any invasive feeding regimen because they establish the tolerance of the gastrointestinal tract to the additional nutrient load. Intolerance may be manifest by gastroesophageal reflux or malabsorption or both. As a predictor of intestinal intolerance, the success of an empirical feeding trial is superior to any currently employed diagnostic test of gastroesophageal reflux or intestinal absorption. Continuous feeding with an elemental or fat modified, i.e., medium chain triglycerides (MCT), formula is used most commonly in children with short gut syndrome so as not to overwhelm limited mucosal and luminal digestive capacity with bolus feedings. Patients with minimal postcibal emesis also may benefit from continuous feedings because gastroesophageal reflux generally decreases with the smaller gastric feeding volumes. If malabsorption is severe and not correctable by dietary modifications, additional parenteral nutrition may be necessary. If total nutritional support is not feasible by enteral intake alone, this route should still be used to maximum capacity to speed the adaptation of enteral function to accommodate higher calorie loads.

If nasogastric feedings are prolonged, repeated daily passage of the tube eventually becomes intolerable. The newer soft tubes that are not made of polyvinyl chloride may be left in for several weeks. However, the tube ultimately must be switched from one nostril to another to prevent the development of sinus infection. Eventually, patients or their caretakers may want to consider gastrostomy feedings. Gastrostomies may be placed endoscopically, fluoroscopically, or surgically. Endoscopic or fluoroscopic gastrostomies are less involved than surgical gastrostomies and have a more rapid recovery period and shorter hospital stay. A surgical gastrostomy is performed if gastroesophageal reflux has been a problem during the empirical nasogastric feeding trial. During the surgical procedure, a Nissen fundoplication can be performed that can control the reflux. However, after the fundoplication, swallowing dysfunction, dumping syndrome, gas bloat, and episodes of retching and gagging are common complications that lead us to recommend a simple gastrostomy alone in most circumstances. Minimal gastroesophageal reflux observed during nasogastric feedings can be resolved by using continuous feedings. Also, with the switch to gastrostomy feedings, gastroesophageal reflux may decrease because nasopharyngeal tubes have been shown to stimulate reflux to some extent. If aspiration is an unavoidable risk, head-up positioning and chronic acid suppression with H_2-receptor antagonists or omeprazole are important to lessen the potential pulmonary reaction to aspirated acid gastric contents.

Another feeding technique that is useful if gastroesophageal reflux is a problem involves the passage of an NG tube beyond the pylorus. This generally can be done by inserting a weighted-tip tube, positioning the child in the right decubitus position, and administering metoclopramide to facilitate tube passage, which generally occurs within 1 day. Alternatively, the tube may be manually manipulated beyond the pylorus under fluoroscopy. Transpyloric placement can circumvent short-term pylorospasm with attendant problems with gastric emptying. However, if the patient is prone to chronic retching, the tube eventually will be vomited out of position. It is also possible to manipulate a transpyloric tube through an existing gastrostomy opening. This may require fluoroscopic guidance as the natural position of the gastrostomy opening is not in line with the pylorus. Finally, jejunostomy tubes can be placed surgically directly into the jejunum.

Enteral Formula Selection

Selection of the appropriate infant, pediatric, or adult enteral formula for use in the nutritional support of the critically ill child depends on a number of factors, including diagnosis, nutrient requirements, and gastrointestinal function. The formula's caloric density, osmolality, nutrient content, and distribution should all be taken into consideration before selecting a formula. Table 1 presents the nutrient content and sources of a variety of infant and pediatric formulas.

Preterm formulas have been developed to meet the physiologic needs and limitations of these infants, including lactase deficiency, limited bile salt pool, decreased energy and nutrient stores, limited gastric volume, and decreased intestinal motility. These formulas contain the following specific modifications: higher caloric density of 24 kcal/30 ml, a blend of lactose and glucose polymers as the carbohydrate source, 10% to 50% of the fat as MCT, an elevated protein content with a 60:40 whey/casein ratio, increased amounts of sodium, calcium, phosphorus, and both water-soluble and fat-soluble vitamins. When an infant is 6 to 8 weeks old, preterm formula supplemented with iron should be provided. When breast milk is used for the enteral nutrition support of a preterm infant, it should be fortified with a commercial fortifier, such as Enfamil Human Milk Fortifier (Mead Johnson, Evansville, IN) or Similac Natural Care (Ross Laboratories, Columbus, OH) to increase the nutrient density. See Normal Nutrition for information on regular infant formulas.

Pediatric and Adult Enteral Formulas

Pediatric patients between the ages of 1 and 6 years of age can be fed enterally with the pediatric formula, Pediasure (Ross Laboratories). The amount of protein, carbohydrate, and fat is between that of infant and adult formulas. The vitamin and mineral recommended dietary allowances for children ages 1 to 6 years of age can be met in 1100 ml of formula. Furthermore, at a caloric density of 1 kcal/ml, it often meets the elevated metabolic requirements of critically ill children with fluid restrictions. The formula contains 20% of its fat as MCT oil. Pediasure is also available with fiber (soy polysaccharide).

Formulas that contain hydrolyzed protein as peptides are useful when protein sensitivity is documented. Also, deficiencies in pancreatic digestion can be circumvented by the use of these hydrolysates. They are inherently less palatable and more expensive than intact protein products. MCT-containing products are particularly useful when bile salt deficiencies are present (biliary atresia, short bowel syndrome, preterm infants). These lipids can be absorbed with less bile solubilization than long chain triglycerides. Also, to some extent, they may be absorbed intact without pancreatic digestion, although presence of pancreatic enzymes will improve their absorption. Carbohydrate modification usually involves the use of glucose polymer products, which are less osmotically active than monosaccharides or disaccharides. These products can be absorbed without pancreatic digestion.

Adult enteral formulas can be used successfully in pediatric patients over the age of 7. Table 2 provides the nutrient content and source of a variety of adult enteral formulas that may be used successfully in pediatric patients. Standard adult formulas with low to moderate osmolality are well tolerated by children. Tube feeding formulas with added fiber, such as Jevity (Ross Laboratories) are often well tolerated in children with chronic constipation.

Specialized formulas designed for the nutritional support of patients with hypermetabolic or specific disease states are readily available. However, they are more expensive, and the clinician should weigh their often negligible advantage against the higher cost. High calorie, high protein formulas are readily available for the enteral nutrition support of children with hypermetabolic states. Some of these formulas contain nutrients, such as nucleotides, arginine, glutamine, and omega-3 fatty acid blends, considered to be conditionally essential in stressed and immunocompromised states. However, well-controlled clinical trials have yet to be appropriately conducted on these products. Therefore, their use in the pediatric population is unproven. Adult

TABLE 1. Infant Formulas and Pediatric Enteral Feedings

FORMULA	kcal/ml	(g/ml)			NUTRIENT SOURCE			Na⁺/K⁺ (mg/ml)	mOsm/kg
		CHO	FAT	PRO	CHO	FAT	PRO	Na⁺/K⁺ (mg/ml)	mOsm/kg
Human Milk	0.67	0.068	0.040	0.011	Lactose	Human milk	Lactalbumin casein	0.19/0.59	280
Standard									
Enfamil 20	0.67	0.069	0.038	0.015	Lactose	Soy, coconut oil	Whey, casein	0.18/0.73	300
Similac 20	0.67	0.072	0.036	0.015	Lactose	Soy, coconut oil	Casein, whey	0.22/0.81	290
SMA 20	0.67	0.071	0.035	0.015	Lactose	Soy, coconut oil, safflower, oleo	Whey, casein	0.15/0.55	290
SMA 24	0.80	0.086	0.043	0.018	Lactose	Soy, coconut oil, safflower, oleo	Whey, casein	0.18/0.67	360
SMA 27	0.90	0.097	0.047	0.020	Lactose	Soy, coconut oil	Whey, casein	0.20/0.76	416
Soy-based									
Prosobee 20	0.67	0.068	0.036	0.020	Corn syrup, solids	Coconut, soy oil	Soy protein, L-methionine	0.24/0.82	200
Isomil 20	0.67	0.068	0.037	0.018	Corn syrup, sucrose	Soy, coconut oil	Soy protein, L-methionine	0.32/0.95	250
Nursoy 20	0.67	0.068	0.036	0.021	Sucrose	Soy, coconut oil, safflower, oleo	Soy protein, L-methionine	0.20/0.71	296
Specialized									
Nutramigen	0.67	0.090	0.026	0.019	Corn syrup, tapioca starch	Corn oil	Casein hydrol.	0.32/0.73	320
Pregestimil	0.67	0.091	0.028	0.019	Corn syrup, tapioca starch	Corn oil (60%), MCT oil (40%)	Casein hydrol. & amino acids	0.32/0.73	348
Portagen	0.67	0.074	0.030	0.022	Corn syrup, lactose, sucrose	MCT oil (88%), corn oil (12%)	Sodium caseinate	0.35/0.80	236
Alimentum	0.67	0.068	0.038	0.019	Tapioca starch, sucrose	MCT oil (50%), safflower, soy	Casein hydrol. & amino acids	0.29/0.79	370
Preterm									
Enfamil Premature	0.80	0.089	0.041	0.024	Corn syrup, lactose	MCT, corn oil, coconut oil	Whey, casein	0.32/0.90	300
Similac Special Care	0.80	0.086	0.044	0.022	Corn syrup, lactose	MCT, corn oil, coconut oil	Whey, casein	0.41/1.14	300
"Preemie SMA"	0.80	0.086	0.044	0.020	Lactose, maltodextrins	Coconut, oleic, oleo, soy, MCT	Whey, casein	0.32/0.75	280
Pediatric Enteral									
Pediasure	1.0	0.110	0.050	0.030	Corn syrup, sucrose, lactose	Soy, safflower, MCT oil (20%)	Sodium caseinate	0.38/1.3	325

Note: Standard, soy, and specialized infant formulas with iron have between 1.1 and 1.5 mg iron per 100 ml. Preterm infant formulas with iron have 1.5 mg iron per 100 ml.

elemental formulas with predigested nutrients have a very limited use with pediatric patients because of their high osmolality and inappropriate mineral content. Their limited palatability means they are not useful as oral supplements for all but the most highly motivated patients. Controlled studies of oral supplementation do not compare these formulas to more palatable high calorie dietary items, such as sweets or snack food, that do not require as much parental prodding to promote their intake. Peptide-containing elemental formulas may be used during the intestinal adaptation phase of older pediatric patients with short gut syndrome or severe malabsorptive syndromes. The utility of these formulas as primary therapy for inflammatory bowel disease is marginal, and they should not replace medical therapy, although as adjunctive therapy for the treatment of coincident malnutrition, they can be very useful. Formulas with elevated branched-chain amino acids have been developed for the nutritional management of patients with liver failure and hepatic encephalopathy. Their use in pediatric patients, however, has not been evaluated.

Furthermore, their effectiveness in the resolution of encephalopathic symptoms is inconclusive. Renal formulas with lowered protein, electrolyte, and fast-soluble vitamin content but with elevated caloric densities can be used successfully in the pediatric patient with acute renal failure or end-stage renal disease. Because of their high osmolalities, however, these formulas often need to be diluted for optimal gastrointestinal tolerance.

It is worth emphasizing that the most critical nutrient in enteral nutrition is water. The provision of extra water to prevent slow dehydration, or tube feeding syndrome, is especially important for neurologically devastated or immature children who cannot communicate their thirst to the care provider. This problem is intensified during the hot summer months. Often, gastrointestinal tolerance is impaired by high calorie density of enteral feedings caused by its attendant effects of delayed gastric emptying and osmotic diarrhea. If used orally, these high calorie feedings will induce early satiety and decrease spontaneous fluid intake before adequate hydration is achieved. Unless there

TABLE 2. Selected Adult Formulas Used in Pediatric Patients

| PRODUCT NAME | kcal/ml | g/ml | | | mOsm/kg | COMMENTS/INDICATIONS |
		CHO	FAT	PRO		
Standard/Fiber Containing						
Osmolite	1.06	0.143	0.041	0.037	300	Standard tube feeding formulas: contain sodium and calcium caseinates, partial MCT, soy, corn oils: unflavored only
Isocal	1.06	0.130	0.044	0.034	300	Similar to Osmolite
Jevity	1.06	0.152	0.036	0.044	310	Fiber containing; meets 100% RDA adults at 1321 ml and 1400 calories; 1.36 g fiber per 100 calories; fiber source: soy polysaccharide
Ensure with Fiber	1.1	0.159	0.037	0.040	480	Oral or tube feeding formula with fiber
High-Caloric Density						
Isotein HN	1.2	0.156	0.035	0.067	300	High protein, isotonic formula; not meant for oral feeding
Perative	1.3	0.177	0.037	0.066	425	High calorie, high protein formula with added arginine and canola oil as omega-3 source
Nutren 1.5	1.5	0.170	0.067	0.060	410	Calorie dense, for patients with volume limitations
Elemental						
Peptamen	1.0	0.127	0.039	0.040	270	Peptide based, nutritionally complete; isotonic: contains part of fat content as MCT oil
Vital HN	1.0	0.180	0.010	0.042	500	Peptide based formula, low fat content with MCT; available in powdered form
Specialized Renal						
Suplena	2.0	0.252	0.095	0.030	615	Specialized formula for end-stage renal patients requiring protein/electrolyte restrictions
Nepro	2.0	0.215	0.096	0.069	635	For renal patients requiring dialysis
Travasorb Renal	1.35	0.270	0.018	0.023	590	Specialized renal formula as per above, available in powdered form

is a compelling reason to limit water intake, a caloric density of 0.67 to 1.0 kcal/ml of formula should be used. If an infant has short bowel syndrome or chronic diarrhea, there will be additional stool water losses. Output is often listed as "mixed" urine and stool on nursing flow sheets. As a screen to detect tube feeding dehydration, it is vital to follow daily weights and useful to check that there is some "urine only" output. If sequential chemistry screens are obtained, one should follow the ratio of blood urea nitrogen/creatinine and serum sodium levels to detect a slow, steady rise suggestive of tube feeding syndrome. If the child with short gut syndrome is not receiving parenteral fluids and is unable to maintain hydration with standard dilution formula, it may be useful to dilute the formula to levels less than 0.67 kcal/ml to preserve fluid balance. The goal of weight gain for neurologically devastated patients often leads to concentration of formulas, which can decrease gastrointestinal tolerance by promoting GER and malabsorption. Philosophically, determination of an optimal weight gain for these patients must take into account the priorities of the caregiver, who may have more modest goals of prevention of weight loss and dehydration as primary concerns. It may be inappropriate to strive for growth rates that are predicted by growth charts for healthy children, especially if feeding to the point of emesis, diarrhea, and intermittent dehydration is the result.

Modular Products

The importance of adequate water intake notwithstanding, infant, pediatric, and adult enteral formulas may need caloric or nutrient modification to meet special patient needs. A variety of carbohydrate, protein, and fat modular products is now readily available. Modular protein products, such as ProMod (Ross Laboratories, Columbus, OH), can be added to increase formula protein density, and lipid products, such as Microlipid (Chesebrough-Pond, Greenwich, CT), and carbohydrate products, such as Moducal (Mead Johnson, Evansville, IN), can be added to increase formula caloric density when

TABLE 3. Enteral Modular Products

PRODUCT	FORM	kcal	MAJOR NUTRIENT SOURCE	INDICATIONS
Protein Modules				
Casec	Powder	16 kcal/Tbsp	Protein, 4 g/Tbsp	Calcium, casein protein supplement, 75 mg Ca/Tbsp
ProMod	Powder	16.8 kcal/Tbsp	Protein, 3 g/Tbsp	Whey protein supplement
Fat Modules				
Microlipid	Liquid	4.5 kcal/ml	Safflower oil	50% fat emulsion caloric supplement for tube feedings
MCT Oil	Liquid	7.7 kcal/ml	Coconut oil	Bile salt deficiency; requires less pancreatic digestion; no essential fatty acids
Carbohydrate Modules				
Polycose	Powder	23 kcal/Tbsp	Glucose polymer	Caloric additive, low osmolality, minimum sweetness
Moducal	Powder	30 kcal/Tbsp	Glucose polymer	Same as above

formula concentration may be undesirable because of a resultant excess increase in renal solute load or osmolality. Before the addition of modular components, one must consider if the growth goal is appropriate for the child under consideration and whether the supplement can be given without risking tube feeding syndrome. Table 3 presents an overview of a variety of modular products commonly used.

Enteral Nutrition Administration

Enteral feedings may be administered continuously or intermittently (bolus). Continuous administration by infusion pump is often the method of choice for critically ill children, as this decreases the risk of aspiration. Continuous feedings are also beneficial for pediatric patients who have chronic diarrhea or short bowel syndrome or require transpyloric feedings. The continuous, slow delivery of nutrients is less likely to overwhelm absorption. Intermittent feedings deliver formula in a bolus over a period of time similar to oral feeds. This method of enteral formula delivery provides a more physiologic release of gastrointestinal hormones, such as gastrin, which can prove trophic to the gut. Furthermore, bolus feeding is vastly more convenient and allows for greater patient mobility. To preserve oral motor function, the optimal approach is to separate daytime bolus feedings by 3 to 4 hours to allow hunger to help stimulate oral intake. After an oral feeding attempt, the rest of the calories can be given by bolus as tolerated. If additional nutrition and fluid are required, they may be given overnight by a continuous infusion. If diarrhea, emesis, or dumping syndrome limits the size of the bolus feedings, some of the volume should be shifted to the overnight continuous feeding.

When indicated, enteral feedings should be started early following injury or surgery. Transpyloric feedings at slow rates of 0.5 ml/kg/h may be well tolerated even in the absence of audible bowel sounds. The time-honored practice of excruciatingly slow advancement of formulas through small adjustment in concentration, followed by gradual introduction of solids through sequential, minimally palatable fluid, full fluid, soft, and low residue stages is unproven and has been challenged recently for adult postoperative patients. Certainly, this practice is even more unpleasant for children. If fluid requirements are being met intravenously, infant, pediatric, and appropriately selected adult formulas with low to moderate osmolalities generally may be started at full strength and, thus, do not need to be diluted as is often practiced. Intragastric pediatric formulas generally may be started at 0.5 to 1 ml/kg/h for the first 8 to 12 hours and advanced by 0.5 to 2 ml/kg/h every 8 to 12 hours, as tolerated. Intermittent feedings may be begun at 2 to 5 ml/kg every 2 to 4 hours depending on the child's individual tolerance. Advancement may proceed at 2 to 5 ml/kg per feed every 8 to 12 hours, as tolerated. Checking gastric residuals is recommended before each intermittent feed or every 4 hours for continuous feeds. The significance of specific residual volumes and minimal spitting (in infants) in the determination of tolerance and advancement of the formula is often overemphasized. In many cases, persistent, small preprandial aspirates are noted that do not progressively increase with subsequent feeding. This finding need not preclude formula volume advancement.

Complications

Diarrhea, which is considered to be a common complication, is generally overemphasized. Often, more obvious causes, such as antibiotic administration, are overlooked in the rush to blame the enteral formula. Too often, formulas are changed in a mistaken, almost random search for the magic formula. With each change comes a delay in accommodation to the new formula. Other factors contributing to diarrhea can include malabsorption (inherent with short bowel syndrome), bacterial overgrowth, and malnutrition. In the presence of adequate weight gain and good hydration, it is often best to ignore a small amount of diarrhea, especially in infants. Tolerance of diarrhea is made easier if diaper rashes are treated aggressively or, preferably,

prevented by the chronic use of protective ointments and frequent diaper changes.

Metabolic abnormalities are common in malnourished patients, especially those with renal impairment or chronic diarrhea. Ongoing assessment of fluid, electrolyte, albumin, and prealbumin levels is useful. Mechanical complications, such as clogged or kinked tubes, also may occur. Flushing of the tube with a volume of water at least equal to the tube volume following formula or medication administration and every 4 to 6 hours during continuous feedings may help prevent the clogging of tubes. Medications should be used in the liquid or suspension form whenever possible or crushed to a fine powder and suspended in solution when a tablet form is required. These suspensions should be flushed through the tube with a bolus of water.

PARENTERAL NUTRITION

For children who are unable to satisfy their nutritional requirements for maintenance and growth by the enteral route, parenteral nutrition (PN) may be necessary. If it is feasible to meet maintenance nutritional requirements alone by the enteral route without any excess available for growth, the clinician should consider the possibility of meeting these requirements alone during limited illness rather than incurring the added risk, cost, and complexity of PN. Indeed, children do not always experience linear growth or weight gain during episodes of even mild illness. The hormonal milieu associated with acute trauma and stress renders actual linear growth difficult. In view of the child's capacity for catchup growth, the single-minded emphasis on excess calories during short periods of severe illness may be unwise, especially if it entails the risk of pulmonary aspiration or dehydrating diarrhea from enteral feedings or metabolic or infectious iatrogenia of parenteral feedings. Providing PN for the very ill child is based on the same principles as for any pediatric patient. The amount should be sufficient for maintenance and, if prolonged, for growth as well. Parenteral nutrition should be initiated slowly and titrated to patient response until optimal provision of calories can be achieved (Table 4).

Dextrose remains the primary source of carbohydrate in PN solutions. Concentrations up to 12.5% may be administered through a peripheral line. A central line is needed for higher concentration, hypertonic solutions to avoid phlebitis and infiltration problems. Therapy may be initiated with approximately 5 to 10 g/kg/d (4 to 6 mg/kg/min) and increased by increments of 2.5 to 5 g/kg/d as tolerated. Persistent glycosuria above 2+ should be avoided. Sepsis or steroid medications may hamper glucose tolerance. Excessive intravenous lipid intake will also hamper glucose tolerance.

Amino Acids

Children receiving total parenteral nutrition (TPN) will require approximately 1.5 to 2.5 g/kg/d of amino acids. Administration should begin with doses of 0.5 to 1 g/kg/d and be increased by 0.5 g/kg increments. Although developed to mimic serum amino acid patterns in infants, pediatric-specific amino acid solutions, such as TrophAmine (McGaw, Inc., Irvine, CA) and Aminosyn-PF (Abbott Laboratories, Abbott Park, IL) (Table 5), may provide desirable features in older pediatric patients as well. Standard adult amino acid solutions with concentrations up to 15% are available and may be desirable in severely fluid-restricted patients.

TABLE 4. Caloric Content of Parenteral Nutrition Components

1 g amino acid = 4 kcal
1 g dextrose (D-glucose monohydrate) = 3.4 kcal
1 g fat = 9 kcal
1 ml 10% fat emulsion = 1.1 kcal
1 ml 20% fat emulsion = 2.0 kcal

TABLE 5. Contents of Amino Acid Solutions

	TRAVASOL* (mg/dl)	TROPHAMINE* (mg/dl)	AMINOSYN-PF* (mg/dl)
Isoleucine	600	820	760
Leucine	730	1400	1200
Lysine	580	820	677
Methionine	400	340	180
Phenylalanine	560	480	427
Threonine	420	420	512
Tryptophan	180	200	180
Valine	580	780	673
Alanine	2070	540	698
Arginine	1150	1200	1227
Histidine	480	480	312
Proline	680	680	812
Serine	500	380	495
Taurine	0	25	70
Tyrosine	40	240	40
Glycine	1030	360	385
Glutamic acid	0	500	620
Aspartic acid	0	320	527
Cysteine	0	<16†	0†
Nitrogen (g/dl)	1.65	1.55	1.52

*Comparison of 10% solutions of Travasol (Clintec Nutrition, Deerfield, IL), TrophAmine (McGaw Inc., Irvine, CA), and Aminosyn-PF (Abbott Laboratories, Abbott Park, IL).
† Before addition of supplemental cysteine (40 mg/g of amino acid used).

Lipid

Intravenous fat emulsion provides calories, prevents essential fatty acids (EFA) deficiency, and may help to prolong catheter patency. Therapy should be initiated with a dose of 0.5 mg/kg/d and titrated upward at increments of 0.5 to 1 g/kg/d to a final dose of 1 to 3 g/kg/d. Products available for use are listed in Table 6. The use of 20% preparations is recommended in critically ill children to reduce fluid volume. If enteral intake is possible for a patient, it is best to avoid intravenous lipid and tailor the enteral intake to provide an adequate amount of enteral fat to prevent EFA deficiency. This is much less expensive, helps stimulate bile flow, and prevents cholestasis. By avoiding intravenous lipid, fewer intravenous lines are involved, and consequently there is less risk of infection.

Other Additives

Specific recommendations for intravenous vitamin dosages in pediatric patients are available (Table 7). The parenteral dosages of vitamins are generally higher than the oral recommended dietary allowances (RDA) because of concerns with their stability in PN so-

TABLE 7. Recommendations for Intravenous Vitamin Administration*

Lipid Soluble	
A	2,300 IU (700 μg RE)
D	400 IU
E	7 mg
K	200 μg
Water Soluble	
B₁ (thiamine)	1.2 mg
B₂ (riboflavin)	1.4 mg
B₃ (niacin)	17 mg
B₅ (pantothenic acid)	5 mg
B₆ (pyridoxine)	1 mg
B₁₂ (cyanocobalamin)	1 μg
C (ascorbic acid)	80 mg
Biotin	20 μg
Folic acid	0.14 mg

*Guidelines for children ages 1–11 years.

TABLE 6. Percent Fatty Acid Content of Intravenous Fat Emulsions

ACID	INTRALIPID*	LIPOSYN II*	LIPOSYN III*
Linoleic	50	65.8	54.5
Linolenic	9	4.2	8.3
Oleic	26	17.7	22.4
Palmitic	10	8.8	10.5
Stearic	3.5	3.4	4.2

*All available as 10% and 20% emulsions. Intralipid (Clintec Nutrition, Deerfield, IL), Liposyn II and III (Abbott Laboratories, Abbott Park, IL).

lutions. In addition, renal clearance of water-soluble vitamins is increased with parenteral administration. There is a commercially available multiple vitamin preparation (MVI Pediatric, Astra Pharmaceutical Products, Westborough, MA) that meets these recommended parenteral dosages in children.

Recommendations for electrolyte administration are listed in Table 8. Calcium and phosphate balance can be the most difficult component of preparing PN solutions. Infants and young children have high requirements, which are often difficult to meet when nutrition is provided solely by parenteral means. In higher concentrations and at higher temperature or pH, calcium and phosphate can form an insoluble precipitate. Pediatric amino acid solutions with supplemental cysteine may be preferable, since their lower pH facilitates administration of larger amounts of calcium and phosphate.

Copper, zinc, chromium, manganese, selenium, and iron are necessary for normal growth in children. Several trace element preparations containing copper, zinc, chromium, and manganese are marketed for pediatric use (Table 9). If selenium is not already included in the preparation, it can be added to the solution at a dose of 1 to 2 μg/kg/d. Iron may be needed in patients receiving chronic PN or in children with iron deficiency. A dose of 0.1 mg/kg iron dextran may be added to the PN on a chronic basis, or the dose may be calculated as

$$0.3 \times wt \ (lb) \times \left(100 - \frac{observed \ hemoglobin \times 100}{desired \ hemoglobin} \right)$$

This amount is divided and given over a 3 to 7 day period and repeated monthly, as needed. Ferritin levels should be monitored to prevent overload.

Considerations for Administration

Parenteral nutrition solutions not containing fat emulsion may be administered through a 0.22 μm filter. The need for filtration of solutions prepared in a laminar air-flow hood using aseptic technique is controversial. Intravenous fat emulsion cannot be filtered, as filtration may break or disrupt the physical characteristics of the oil-in-water emulsion. Components of PN solutions or medications may bind to the plastic of the bag or tubing used in PN delivery. A decrease in the concentration of vitamin A has been documented after prolonged contact with plastic equipment.

Monitoring of patients requiring long-term therapy is needed to assess the presence of nutritional deficiencies. Several vitamins, including cyanocobalamin, folic acid, pyridoxine, riboflavin, thiamine,

TABLE 8. Electrolyte Requirements for Pediatric Patients

Sodium	2–4 mEq/kg/d
Potassium	2–3 mEq/kg/d
Chloride	2–3 mEq/kg/d
Magnesium	0.25–2 mEq/kg/d
Calcium	0.5–3 mEq/kg/d
Phosphorus	0.5–2 mmol/kg/d

TABLE 9. Examples of Pediatric IV Trace Element Preparations

	PEDTRACE-4*	PEDTE-PAK-4*	MTE-PEDIATRIC*	PTE-4*	PTE-5*
Chromium (μg)	0.85	1	1	1	1
Copper (mg)	0.1	0.1	0.1	0.1	0.1
Manganese (mg)	0.025	0.025	0.03	0.025	0.025
Zinc (mg)	0.5	1	0.5	1	1
Selenium (μg)	0	0	0	0	15

*Contents given per milliliter of solution of Pedtrace-4 (Lyphomed, Deerfield, IL), PedTE-PA 4 (Smith & Nephew Solopak, Elk Grove Village, IL), Multiple Trace Element-Pediatric (American Regent, Shirley, NY), PTE-4 and PTE-5 (Lyphomed, Deerfield, IL).
Preparations designed for neonatal use are also available.

and ascorbic acid, degrade when exposed to light. Controversy exists as to the clinical significance of this degradation. Protection from light is needed during long-term storage of solutions but appears to be unnecessary during administration to the patient.

Parenteral nutrition solutions should be prepared and handled in an aseptic manner to avoid potential contamination. PN solutions and intravenous fat emulsions are excellent growth media for pathogens and must be kept sterile. Minimizing interruptions in the intravenous tubing and maintaining scrupulous sterile technique during administration also will help to reduce the risk of contamination.

When providing care to a critically ill child, limited intravenous access and fluid restriction may make administration of both nutrition and medications difficult. Several medications used in the intensive care setting may be mixed directly in the PN solution to reduce fluid volume. For example, heparin, insulin, albumin, and H_2-antagonists, such as ranitidine, are stable when mixed with PN solutions. More commonly, medications are injected into an access port where a PN solution is infusing. Reference materials providing information on the compatibility of medications with PN solutions should be available from pharmacies handling PN solutions.

Considerations for Special Patient Populations

Children with renal failure require optimal use of PN to maximize caloric intake while avoiding excessive fluid volumes. Conservative administration of protein is also recommended to avoid urea accumulation in the blood. Administration of histidine, usually considered a nonessential amino acid, may be of use, since de novo synthesis may be absent. Use of a pediatric amino acid solution will provide supplemental histidine (Table 5). Once dialysis has been initiated, there is no need to continue restricting fluid or protein, and use of standard nutrition guidelines may be resumed. Children with hepatic synthetic deficiency may not tolerate high amino acid intake. Pediatric amino acid formulations may be preferable to standard solutions for patients with hepatic failure, as they are higher in branched-chain amino acids and have slightly less methionine and phenylalanine.

Monitoring and Complications

Infection remains the most hazardous complication of intravenous nutrition. Fever without an obvious source is an indication for blood culture. Although *Staphylococcus epidermidis* infections may be treated without intravenous line removal, repeated infections mandate removal. Other infectious bacteria and fungi require line removal. Prevention through compulsive sterile technique is vital. Well-trained, motivated family members generally administer home PN with fewer infections than even the best medical centers.

Metabolic abnormalities should be screened routinely. Initially, electrolyte levels should be checked at least twice weekly and then at progressively longer intervals if no abnormalities are observed. Trace element levels and fat-soluble vitamin levels should be checked at 6 month intervals. Liver function test abnormalities are common and may include relatively benign transaminasemia or more severe cholestatic disease, as is more common in preterm infants and children with short gut syndrome. Cholestatic disease is best prevented by the provision of enteral intake, especially fat, to promote bile flow. Other

contributing factors may include small bowel bacterial overgrowth, with production of lithogenic bile acids and dehydration, which will increase the viscosity of bile. Periodic short courses of antibiotics (e.g., metronidazole) may be useful to treat bacterial overgrowth. Ursodeoxycholic acid also has been reported to be of use in the prevention of cholestasis. Kidney stones have been reported as a result of chronic intravenous alimentation, probably because of chronic hypercalciuria. It is useful to check urine calcium and phosphorus levels at intervals to see if there is excessive urinary loss. Adequate hydration will help prevent nephrolithiasis.

REFERENCES

1. Greene HL, Hambidge KM, Schanler R, Tsang RC: Guidelines for the use of vitamins, trace elements calcium, magnesium, and phosphorus in infants and children receiving total parenteral nutrition. Am J C Nutr 48:1324–1342, 1988.
2. Heird WC, Kashyap S, Gomez MR: Parenteral alimentation of the neonate. Semin Perinatol 15:493–502, 1991.
3. Koretz R: Selected summary: Postoperative feeding: Liquid versus solid fuel. Gastroenterology 104:32–236, 1993.
4. Sax HC, Souba WW: Enteral and parenteral feedings: Guidelines and recommendations. Med Clin North Am 77:863–880, 1993.

VITAMIN DEFICIENCIES AND EXCESSES

VIRGINIA A. STALLINGS, M.D.
MARIA R. MASCARENHAS, M.B.B.S.

Vitamins are dietary factors obtained from organic sources and are essential to life. Determining their optimal or adequate level of intake for infants, children, and adolescents is difficult because specific requirements are not known and levels producing toxic effects vary considerably. One population-based set of recommendations is the Recommended Dietary Allowances (RDA). The RDA are defined as "the levels of intake of essential nutrients that, on the basis of scientific knowledge, are judged by the Food and Nutrition Board to be adequate to meet the nutrient needs of practically all healthy persons."[3] On the basis of the most current scientific data, the RDA recommendations are considered safe levels of nutrients for maintaining good health and for evaluating the adequacy of food intakes of groups of people living in the United States. They are not intended to indicate adequacy for specific individuals or for sick individuals. To use the RDA to evaluate individual children, the average of several typical days of food intake should be reviewed and compared. This provides an estimate of the risk of nutrient deficiencies.

The RDA for infants is based on averages of nutrients consumed by healthy, growing infants breast fed by healthy mothers. Consumption of 750 ml of breast milk per day for the first 6 months and 600 ml/d for the second 6 months is considered minimal intake to meet the RDA recommendations. This suggests that infants consuming less than these amounts of breast milk or infant formula (patterned after human milk nutrient content) could be at risk for vitamin deficiencies.

TABLE 1. Diagnosis of Vitamin Deficiencies

VITAMIN	DIAGNOSTIC TEST	PREDISPOSING CONDITIONS	CLINICAL FEATURES
Water-Soluble Vitamins			
Thiamine	Whole blood thiamine/erythrocyte tran-sketolase levels	Breast-fed infants of malnourished or alcoholic mothers TPN Malnutrition Prematurity	Anorexia Irritability Vomiting Constipation Edema Cardiac symptoms Peripheral paralysis Neuropathy Coma
Riboflavin	Serum riboflavin/erythrocyte glutathione reductase levels	Malnutrition Prematurity TPN	Cheiloses Angular stomatitis Glossitis Dermatitis Photophobia
Pyridoxine	Plasma pyridoxal 5'-phosphate levels	Prematurity B_6 dependency syndromes Drugs (isoniazid)	Failure to thrive Irritability Seizures Anemia Cheilosis Glossitis GI disturbances
Niacin	Whole blood niacin levels	Prematurity High maize diets	Weakness Lassitude Dermatitis GI disturbances Dementia
Biotin	Serum biotin levels		Dermatitis Alopecia Irritability Lethargy
Folic acid	Serum or erythrocyte folate levels	Prematurity Breast-fed infants of folate-deficient mothers Infants on goat's milk Kwashiorkor Chronic hemolytic anemia Diarrhea Malignancies Hypermetabolic states Malabsorption Drug (sulfasalazine)	Megaloblastic anemia Neutropenia Thrombocytopenia Growth failure Diarrhea Glossitis
Vitamin B_{12}	Serum B_{12} levels	Breast-fed infants of vegetarian mothers or mothers with latent pernicious anemia Malabsorption Terminal ileal disease	Megaloblastic anemia Memory loss Paresthesias Confusion
Vitamin C	Serum or leukocyte ascorbate levels	Breast-fed infants of vitamin C-deficient mothers	Anorexia Megaloblastic anemia Memory loss Paresthesias Confusion Irritability Apathy Pallor Failure to thrive Hemorrhages Bone pain Costochondral beading
Fat-Soluble Vitamins			
Vitamin A	Serum retinol levels	Prematurity TPN Malnutrition Fat malabsorption Liver disease	Night blindness Xerophthalmia Xerosis Blindness Follicular hyperkeratosis Pruritis Growth retardation Anemia

TABLE 1. Diagnosis of Vitamin Deficiencies *Continued*

VITAMIN	DIAGNOSTIC TEST	PREDISPOSING CONDITIONS	CLINICAL FEATURES
Fat-Soluble Vitamins Cont'd			
Vitamin D	Serum 25-hydroxyvitamin D levels	No exposure to sun Children on milk not fortified with vitamin D Fat malabsorption Hepatic and renal disease Inborn errors of metabolism	Rickets Osteomalacia Craniotabes Rachitic rosary Pigeon breast Bowed legs Delayed eruption of teeth Painful bones Fractures Anorexia Weakness
Vitamin E	Serum vitamin E levels	Prematurity Liver disease Pancreatic insufficiency Short bowel syndrome Abetalipoprotemia	Hemolytic anemia Progressive neurologic disorder
Vitamin K	Prothrombin time, plasma PIVKA levels	Newborns who do not receive vitamin K Fat malabsorption Drugs (nonabsorbable antibiotics and anticoagulants)	Hemorrhage

TABLE 2. Treatment of Vitamin Deficiencies

	CLINICAL FEATURES	SUGGESTED DOSES
Fat-Soluble Vitamins		
Vitamin A	Severe deficiency with xerophthalmia	Child 1–8 y: 5,000 U/kg/d PO × 5 d or until recovery occurs; IM: 5,000–15,000 U/d × 10 d Child >8 y: 500,000 U/d PO × 3 d, then 50,000 U/d × 14 d, then 10,000–20,000 U/d × 2 mo; IM: 50,000–100,000 U/d × 3 d, then 50,000 U/d × 14 d
	Deficiency without corneal changes	Infants and children (1–8 y): initially 10,000 U IM followed by oral intermittent therapy: Infants: 50,000 U × 1; 6–12 mo: 100,000 U q4–6mo; 1–8 y: 200,000 U q4–6mo; Children >8 y: 100,000 U/d PO × 3 d, then 50,000 U/d × 14 d
Vitamin D	Liver disease and malabsorption	250–625 μg/d PO ergocalciferol
	Rickets and normal absorption	25–125 μg/d ergocalciferol for 6–12 wk
	Renal disease and failure	100 μg–1 mg/d ergocalciferol 0.25–2 μg/d PO calcitriol for patients not on hemodialysis and 0.01–0.05 μg/kg 3 times/wk if undergoing hemodialysis
Vitamin E	Premature infants	25–50 IU/d of D-α-tocopherol acid succinate
	Fat malabsorption and liver disease	15–25 IU/kg/d as tocopherol polyethylene glycol succinate
	Cystic fibrosis	Infants: 50 IU/d 1–2 y child: 50 IU b.i.d. >2 y child: 100 IU b.i.d. of D-α-tocopherol acetate
	Sickle cell disease and beta-thalassemia	450–750 IU/d
Vitamin K	Hemorrhagic disease of the newborn	0.5–1 mg IM/SC of phytonadione
	Fat malabsorption and vitamin K deficiency due to antibiotics	Infants and children: 2.5–5 mg d/PO or 1–2 mg/dose IM/IV Older children: 5–10 mg/d PO/IV/IM
Water-Soluble Vitamins		
Folic acid	Deficiency	Infants: 15 μg/kg/dose q.d. or 50 μg/q.d. Children: 1 mg/d initially, then 0.1–0.4 mg/d Children >11 y: 1 mg/d initially, then 0.5 mg/d
	Hemolytic anemia	May require higher dosages
Niacin	Pellagra	Niacin 100–300 mg/d in divided doses
Pyridoxine	Seizures	Infants: 10–100 mg IM/IV, then 2–100 mg PO daily
	Drug-induced deficiencies	10–50 mg/d × 3 wk, then 1–2 mg/kg/d
	Dietary deficiency	5–25 mg/d × 3 wk, then 1.5–2.5 mg/d in multivitamin product
Riboflavin		3–10 mg/d
Thiamine	Critically ill	10–25 mg/d IM/IV
	Not critically ill	10–50 mg/d PO in divided doses × 2 wk, then 5–10 mg/d × 1 mo
Vitamin B$_{12}$	Initially	100 μg/d IM/SC of cyanocobalamin for 10–15 d, then 100 μg/d once or twice per week for several months (total dose 1–5 mg)
	Maintenance	60 μg IM/SC once per month
Vitamin C	Scurvy	100–300 mg ascorbic acid per day in divided doses for several days

TABLE 3. Clinical Features of Vitamin Excesses

VITAMIN	SYMPTOMS
Vitamin A	Vomiting, pseudotumor cerebri, irritability, headache, insomnia, emotional instability, dry skin, myalgias, arthralgias, abdominal pain, hepatosplenomegaly and cortical thickening of hands and feet, bulging anterior fontanelle
Vitamin D	Hypercalcemia, vomiting, constipation, nephrocalcinosis, muscular weakness
Vitamin E	Hepatotoxicity
Vitamin K	Hemolytic anemia, hyperbilirubinemia
Pyridoxine	Sensory neuropathy

Deficiencies of vitamins occur when (1) intakes are inadequate, (2) physiologic requirements are high, (3) losses are excessive, or (4) nutrient-nutrient or drug-nutrient imbalances reduce efficacy. Although vitamin deficiency diseases are rarely seen today, pediatric health care professionals must be aware of those individual patients at risk and must be able to recognize symptoms of specific vitamin deficiency. Particularly suspect are patients with absorptive defects, narrow food choices, and acute illnesses necessitating medications that affect nutrients. Excessive intakes that may produce toxic effects also must be recognized, especially since some vitamins are used for therapeutic purposes, not just to maintain health. In such instances, the vitamins are considered to be drugs rather than vitamins, since the dosages are in the pharmacologic range. The safe level of intake of some vitamins is quite narrow, with little difference in the intake necessary to prevent deficiencies and to produce toxic effects. The amounts required to produce toxic effects may vary considerably in individual children of differing age groups, body sizes, and body compositions (amount of fat versus lean body mass). Tables 1 and 2 summarize the diagnostic tests, predisposing clinical conditions, clinical features, and treatment of vitamin deficiency diseases and syndromes. Table 3 summarizes the clinical symptoms of some vitamin toxicity syndromes.

WATER-SOLUBLE VITAMINS

Included in the list of water-soluble vitamins are the B complex vitamins—thiamine (B_1), riboflavin (B_2), niacin, pyridoxine (B_6), folate (folic acid and folacine), cyanocobalamin (B_{12}), biotin, and pantothenic acid—and ascorbic acid (vitamin C). The B complex vitamins generally function as coenzymes in metabolic processes. Vitamin C functions as an antioxidant, as well as a cofactor in several enzymatic processes.

Water-soluble vitamins must be consumed daily because there is limited storage in the body and amounts not used in metabolic processes are excreted in the urine. Only vitamin B_{12} is efficiently stored in the body. Careful diet histories that evaluate food consumed over time are useful in identifying individual patients at risk for deficiency before blood levels drop or deficiency disease symptoms are evident. Deficiencies of water-soluble vitamins are rarely seen in infants and children consuming adequate calories from a variety of foods.

Thiamin (B_1)

Prolonged deficiency of thiamine results in beriberi, a disease characterized by mental confusion, muscle weakness, anorexia, peripheral paralysis, muscle wasting, tachycardia, and enlarged heart. The occurrence of beriberi in the United States is extremely rare, since thiamine is widespread in whole grain products and refined cereals are fortified with thiamine. Wernicke-Korsakoff syndrome is a type of adult beriberi related to alcoholism. Infantile beriberi occurs in babies breast fed by mothers with a history of alcoholism or poor

dietary intake. Symptoms include cardiac failure, with aphonia, anorexia, vomiting, and irritability. The aphonia is related to recurrent laryneal nerve paralysis or vocal cord edema. Older infants may have a pseudomeningitic type of infantile beriberi, with seizures, fever, and ocular findings.

There are no documented cases of toxicity of thiamine ingested orally. However, there have been reports of sensitivity or toxicity from large amounts given in parenteral solutions. Pharmacologic doses of thiamine have been used in the treatment of some inborn errors of metabolism (e.g., maple syrup urine disease and thiamine-responsive lactic acidosis).

Riboflavin (B_2)

No specific deficiency disease is attributed to a lack of riboflavin, although symptoms are sometimes referred to as "ariboflavinosis." Clinical symptoms of deficiency are angular stomatitis, cheilosis, normocytic anemia, seborrheic dermatitis, and scrotal skin changes. Because riboflavin is used in the metabolism of niacin and pyridoxine, some deficiency symptoms may result from failure of metabolic processes requiring these nutrients.

There has been no documentation of toxic effects of excessive amounts of riboflavin. Neonates receiving high doses may develop hemolysis. Increased amounts of riboflavin given to well-nourished children have no positive health benefits.

Niacin

The requirement for niacin (nicotinic acid and nicotinamide) is complicated because much of the need for niacin is provided by the conversion of the amino acid tryptophan to niacin. Pellagra, the niacin-deficiency disease, is characterized by diarrhea, dermatitis, and dementia. Glossitis or inflammation of mucous membranes also may be present.

Large doses of nicotinic acid (>3 g/d) may cause flushing or vascular dilatation, decreased serum lipids, increased use of muscle glycogen stores, and decreased mobilization of fatty acids. Pharmacologic doses of niacin are used in treating hypercholesterolemia.

Pyridoxine (B_6)

Deficiency of pyridoxine rarely occurs in isolation but rather in conjunction with deficiencies of other B complex vitamins. In addition, the need for vitamin B_6 is closely related to the amount of dietary protein. As protein intake increases, the deficiency symptoms of pyridoxine are exacerbated. Symptoms of deficiency in infants and children include convulsions, abdominal distress, anemia, dermatitis, and hyperirritability.

There has been no documentation of toxicity from excessive intakes in infants and children. However, some adults treated with pharmacologic doses showed symptoms of ataxia and sensory neuropathy. Pyridoxine is used in large therapeutic doses to treat a variety of general symptoms (depression, muscular fatigue, heart disease) without documented efficacy. No benefit for supplementing the well-nourished child has been documented.

Vitamin B_{12}

Infants and young children in families practicing total vegetarianism may appear to be at risk for vitamin B_{12} deficiency, although no cases of deficiency symptoms have been documented. Breast-fed infants of vegetarian mothers with low levels of vitamin B_{12} have been shown to have low serum levels and symptoms of deficiency, such as macrocytic, megaloblastic anemia. Other symptoms of vitamin B_{12} deficiency are skin hypersensitivity, glossitis, and neurologic signs caused by demyelination in the central and peripheral nervous systems. Cases of pediatric vitamin B_{12} deficiency are rare, with most being the result of poor vitamin B_{12} absorption secondary to terminal ileal disease. No toxic effects of excessive amounts of vitamin B_{12} have been reported. In addition, no benefits have been documented in giving nondeficient children large doses.

Folate

The deficiency disease of macrocytic, megaloblastic anemia caused by folate deficiency is rare in infants and children because human and cow's milk are excellent sources of folate. Folate and vitamin B_{12} deficiencies cause megaloblastic anemia. Both must be evaluated to determine the proper diagnosis and treatment.

Excessive intakes of folic acid may inhibit the therapeutic effects of the anticonvulsant drug phenytoin, which calls for caution in supplementing folic acid in children with seizure disorders. Therefore, supplemental folate should not be given in large amounts. No documented benefits of supplementation have been seen in well-nourished children. Hypersensitivity reactions have been documented.

Biotin

Biotin deficiencies have been described rarely in infants and children and only in those receiving long-term parenteral nutrition. In adults, deficiency states have been produced by ingestion of large amounts of raw egg whites, which contain avidin, a biotin binder. Symptoms of biotin deficiency include dry, scaly dermatitis, anorexia, alopecia, glossitis, and vomiting.

There are no documented instances or reports of toxicity with ingestion of excessive amounts of biotin.

Pantothenic Acid

There has been no recognized deficiency of pantothenic acid in humans, although deficiency states have been described in animal models. The burning feet syndrome described in malnourished prisoners of war may be a form of pantothenic acid deficiency. Pantothenic acid is widespread in foodstuffs, making deficiency states unlikely. In addition, no toxic effects of pantothenic acid have been reported.

Vitamin C

Scurvy, the clinical presentation of ascorbic acid (vitamin C) deficiency, includes swollen or bleeding gums, petechial hemorrhages, and joint pain, with tenderness and swelling of the extremities. Loss of appetite and fatigue are common in older children. With supplementation of most fruit juices and the amount of vitamin C occurring naturally in fresh fruit and vegetables, the incidence of scurvy is rare in children eating a normally varied diet. Infants fed a cow's milk diet without vitamin C supplementation may develop infantile scurvy.

Toxicity of vitamin C has not been reported in children, although nausea and vomiting may occur with large doses. There is disagreement about the benefits, if any, of large doses of vitamin C on general health. Pharmacologic doses have been prescribed to enhance absorption of heme iron and as an antioxidant to prevent oxidative destruction of fat-soluble vitamins A and E.

FAT-SOLUBLE VITAMINS

The fat-soluble vitamins are vitamin A (retinol, retinal, retinoic acid), vitamin D (cholecalciferol-D_3, and ergosterol-D_2), vitamin E (tocopherols), and vitamin K (menaquinones and phylloquinones). Absorption and transport of these vitamins are associated with lipid absorption and transport. The presence of bile salts is required for adequate absorption. The fat-soluble vitamins are not excreted but are stored in the body in varying amounts. This storage allows for accumulation of these vitamins and eliminates the need for daily ingestion. It also creates the potential for toxicity when large amounts are ingested over time.

Vitamin A

Safe and adequate levels of vitamin A are derived from ingested vitamin A and from carotenoids that are converted to active forms of vitamin A in the body. Deficiency symptoms in children are growth failure, poor adaptation to darkness, conjunctival and corneal xerosis and ulceration (xerophthalmia), hyperkeratosis, increased susceptibility to infections, and keratinization of epithelial cells of the res-

piratory tract and other organs. Vitamin A deficiency is usually a result of fat malabsorption with gastrointestinal diseases or inadequate intake due to unusual dietary practices.

Numerous toxic signs are related to ingestion of high doses of vitamin A. Signs usually appear after long-term daily intakes greater than 20,000 IU. Included as signs of vitamin A toxicity are headaches, bone abnormalities, alopecia, vomiting, dryness of the mucous membranes, and liver damage.

The carotenoids (precursors of vitamin A) have not been shown to produce toxic effects, even at high doses. If taken in larger doses over time, they are absorbed into the subcutaneous fat and can color the skin. The skin appears yellow, but the color disappears when the high intakes are discontinued.

Vitamin D

The vitamin D deficiency disease in infants and children is rickets, which is manifested by poor bone mineralization, resulting in skeletal deformities. Rickets is rare in the United States because of fortification of milk and some other dairy products with vitamin D. However, some low birth weight and other infants who are breast fed may develop rickets when no supplement is provided or the infants receive inadequate exposure to sunlight. Other children at risk for deficiency include those with chronic fat malabsorption, nephrotic syndrome, and some African American infants with limited exposure to the sun.

Toxicity from ingestion of excessive amounts is more common with vitamin D than with the other fat-soluble vitamins. Clinical features include vomiting, hypertension, anorexia, renal failure, and failure to thrive. Hypercalcemia and hypercalciuria may lead to deposition of calcium in various soft tissues. Renal and cardiovascular damage is irreversible.

Vitamin E

Vitamin E deficiencies in children occur most commonly in premature or very low birth weight infants and in those who malabsorb fat (e.g., patients with cystic fibrosis, biliary atresia, other liver diseases, and lipid transport abnormalities). Clinical deficiency states have been characterized by neurologic defects and hemolytic anemias. The anemias were related to the relationship of vitamin E and dietary polyunsaturated fatty acids (PUFA). As intake of PUFA increases, the requirement for vitamin E increases. Most of the dietary oils supplying PUFA are also good sources of vitamin E.

Toxic effects from excessive oral intakes of vitamin E have not been substantiated. Pharmacologic doses given in treatment regimens over long periods have not resulted in serious side effects, although symptoms of nausea, headache, and fatigue have been reported. Because there are no known childhood health benefits associated with vitamin E supplementation, it is not recommended for well-nourished children.

Vitamin K

Vitamin K is sometimes defined as the antihemorrhagic vitamin because it is necessary for the synthesis of factors required for blood coagulation. Infants are at risk for vitamin K deficiency because the dietary intake is limited to milk-based products, which are a poor source. Therefore, most newborns are given a supplement of vitamin K (0.5 to 1.0 mg) soon after birth. Exclusively breast-fed and home-delivered infants require special attention. Other infants and children at risk for vitamin K deficiency are those who malabsorb fat and those treated with anticoagulant drugs or long courses of broad-spectrum antibiotics.

Excessive amounts of the natural forms of vitamin K have not been shown to cause toxic effects. However, the synthetic form (menadione) has produced toxic effects in neonates and patients with glucose-6-phosphatase deficiency when ingested in large amounts. These symptoms are manifested as hemolytic anemia, kernicterus, and hyperbilirubinemia.

SUMMARY

Because of the narrow range of safe levels of intake of most vitamins and the lack of clear benefit of supplementation, routine supplementation is not recommended in infants and children. Only those infants and children at risk of vitamin deficiency or showing clinical signs of deficiency disease require supplementation. Thus, parents should be cautioned against supplementation with vitamins. If vitamins are to be used in pharmacologic doses, careful monitoring of blood levels and side effects in individual children is required.

REFERENCES

1. American Hospital Formulary Service: Drug Information. McEvoy GK, Litvak K, Welsh OH (eds). Bethesda, Md, American Society of Hospital Pharmacists, 1994.
2. Grand JR, Sutphen JL, Dietz WH (eds): Pediatric Nutrition: Theory and Practice. Boston, Butterworths, 1987.
3. National Research Council: Recommended Dietary Allowances, 10th ed. Washington, DC, National Academy Press, 1989.
4. Shils ME, Olson JA, Shike M (eds): Modern Nutrition in Health and Disease, 8th ed. Philadelphia, Lea & Febiger, 1994.
5. Taketomo CK, Hodding JH, Kraus DM (eds): Pediatric Dosage Handbook, 2nd ed. Hudson, Oh, Lexi-Comp, Inc., 1993–1994.

MAGNESIUM DEFICIENCY

HERBERT C. MANSMANN, JR., M.D.
PARIS TAYLOR MANSMANN, M.D.

Magnesium is a dependent cofactor in the function of over 300 enzyme systems. It is essential for the synthesis of fat, protein, and nucleic acids, for muscle contraction, and for many transport systems. Many of the cytochrome P450 enzymes, which are responsible for biochemical metabolism, require Mg in a concentration-dependent amount for optimal electron transfer to metabolize drugs and toxins. Thus, any degree of Mg deficiency (MgD) puts the human at a significant disadvantage.

Mg homeostasis requires a daily oral intake that exceeds the 24-hour urinary Mg (uMg) output. Positive Mg balance (PMgB) is achieved by the assimilation of 30% to 50% of the Mg intake, with uMg equalling that amount. Negative Mg balance (NMgB) occurs whenever the intake is less than the amount eliminated. In the presence of a normal intake, there can be urinary wasting of Mg, which occurs because of the effect of many chemicals on renal tubular function. Table 1 lists substances known to cause uMg wasting.

It is also known that catecholamines result in an increase in free fatty acids (FFA), which bind Mg and cause a redistribution of Mg to nonaccessible sites, in effect, resulting in an MgD with a low uMg. Table 2 lists diseases that cause, and Table 3 lists drugs that cause,

TABLE 1. Substances Known to Cause Magnesium Wasting

Alcohol	Diuretics	Saline
Amiikacin	Ethacrynic acid	Sisomycin
Amphotericin B	Furosemide	Theophylline
Caffeine	Thiazides	Thyroid
Capreomycin	Epinephrine	Ticarcillin
Carbenicillin	Gentamicin	Tobacco
Cisplatin	Glucose	Tobramycin
Cyclosporine	Hydroxyurea	Urea
Digitalis	Mannitol	Vancomycin
	Mithramycin	Vitamin D
	Pentamidine	

From Mansmann HC Jr: Consider magnesium homeostasis: III: Cytochrome P450 enzymes and drug toxicity. Pediatr Asthma Allergy Immunol 8:7–28, 1994. Reprinted with permission.

TABLE 2. Diseases That Increase Serum Catecholamines

Central Nervous System	Cardiac
Acute disturbance	Acute myocardial infarction*
Encephalopathy	Mitral valve prolapse syndrome
Hemorrhage	
Infarct	**Miscellaneous**
Tumor	Heavy alcohol intake
Neural crest tumors*	Heavy exercise
Pheochromocytoma	Postsurgery
Stress	Renal disease
Emotional	Volume depletion
Physical	
Endocrine	
Diabetic ketoacidosis*	
Hyperglycemia	
Thyrotoxicosis	
Hypothyroidism	

*Markedly elevated
Normal epinephrine $\leq$ 110 pg/ml (supine), $\leq$ 140 pg/ml (sitting).
From Mansmann HC Jr: Consider magnesium homeostasis: III: Cytochrome P450 enzymes and drug toxicity. Pediatr Asthma Allergy Immunol 8:7–28, 1994. Reprinted with permission.

an increase in serum catecholamines. It should take little imagination to realize that the premature infant, term infant, child, and adolescent have sufficient exposure to these human conditions and substances to cause shifts in Mg balance even if only transient. However, any loss of body Mg needs to be compensated for. In MgD, more Mg is assimilated and there is renal conservation, which permits the bone to replace more Mg.

It has become increasingly apparent that MgD is underdiagnosed and, therefore, uncorrected. The progression from PMgB to NMgB has to follow a pathway through several stages of normomagnesemia MgD (NMgD), type I MgD (Table 4). This is because of the availability of Mg from storage sites, such as bone. The total serum Mg level (sMg) can be sustained in spite of considerable NMgB, except in rare acute situations where hypomagnesemia MgD (HMgD) (type II MgD) occurs without the initial loss of tissue Mg. An exchange transfusion could lead to acute HMgD due to the excess citrate binding of Mg. As the NMgB progresses the Mg storage sites become depleted and HMgD occurs, with its own stages and characteristics. Red blood cell Mg (rbcMg), uMg, and Mg load test (MgLT) are keys to this classification.

TISSUE CONSEQUENCE OF MgD

Experiments in rats have shown that selective Mg maternal malnutrition that started on day 2 of gestation resulted in survival of only

TABLE 3. Drugs That Increase Serum Catecholamines

Asthma Medications	Others
Epinephrine	Alpha$_1$-blockers
Theophylline	Beta-blockers
Isoproterenol (caffeine)	Chlorpromazine
	Diazoxide
Antibiotics	Drug withdrawal
Ampicillin	Alcohol
Tetracycline	Clonidine
	Labetalol
	MAO inhibitor
	Methyldopa
	Nicotine
	Quinidine

From Mansmann HC Jr: Consider magnesium homeostasis: III: Cytochrome P450 enzymes and drug toxicity. Pediatr Asthma Allergy Immunol 8:7–28, 1994. Reprinted with permission.

TABLE 4. Classification of Magnesium Deficiency—1994

TYPE	STAGE	DIAGNOSIS	sMg	rbcMg	μMg	Mg LOAD Test*
I		**Normomagnesemia**				
	1	Latent MgD	N†	N	N	>25%R
	2	Occult MgD	N	N	N	>50%R
	3	Subclinical MgD	N	D‡	N/D	>50%R
II		**Hypomagnesemia**				
	4	Acute MgD	D	N§	N/D	N/R
	5	Chronic MgD	D	D	D	>50%R
	6	Extreme MgD	D	D	D	>50%R
	7	Death due to MgD	D	N/D	N/D	N/R

*Mg load test: >25%R, retention is probable MgD.[13]
             >50%R, retention is definite MgD.
†N, normal; D, decreased; R, retention.
‡Younger RBC have less Mg and lower values over time.
§Mg enters RBC during maturation and is not lost suddenly.
From Mansmann HC Jr: Consider magnesium homeostasis: III: Cytochrome P450 enzymes and drug toxicity. Pediatr Asthma Allergy Immunol 8:7–28, 1994. Reprinted with permission.

13% of litters. If the Mg-free diet was started on day 10, there was an increased fetal reabsorption rate, and survivors were small, weak, and anemic. Edema was prominent in those with severe anemia.

Intrauterine growth retardation and fetal alcohol syndrome have to be MgD-induced in part, and the resultant HMgD can occur without a decrease in zinc. The associated protein calorie malnutrition can be corrected with magnesium supplement therapy (MgS) when a nutritious diet alone fails. If unrecognized, acquired MgD can lead to death.

CAUSES OF MgD

Table 5 lists the major mechanisms involved when patients go into NMgB. Three biochemical surges effect NMgB, glucose, catecholamine, and alcohol. These are part of daily life and, if sustained, lead to MgD.

MANAGEMENT OF MAGNESIUM DEFICIENCIES

Prevention

The RDA is the amount necessary to prevent manifestations of specific deficiencies. This should be considered the minimal quantity needed. In the case of Mg, the recommended doses if achieved daily should prevent tetany, a consequence of even NMgD. However, an individual optimal amount (IOA) will depend on the person's specific requirement to prevent chronic subtler signs and symptoms of NMgD. The IOA will vary from person to person and from time to time with individual daily variations in biochemical or pharmacologic surges, as described previously.

It is generally agreed that an oral elemental Mg dose of 6 mg/kg of lean body mass per day is sufficient to prevent MgD, provided the patient is in PMgB. When in PMgB, this dose must be maintained. Those with risk factors need to be treated expectantly, with an appropriate increase of two to three times the daily amount to prevent MgD.

In rare situations the maintenance oral doses may need to be slowly increased to between 20 and 40 mg/kg/d of elemental Mg in divided doses. This is why some have suggested that the IOA dose should be at least 10 mg/kg/d. During MgS therapy for those with known risk factors, the degree of control of the factor will determine the dose required to maintain PMgB, and frequent sMg should be obtained to ensure that the dose is sufficient and that the kidneys are handling the extra Mg load.

In patients with minimal or no symptoms who are treated with oral MgS it is impossible in the presence of normal renal function,

usually judged by a normal serum creatinine, to excessively increase the sMg because diarrhea will occur, limiting absorption from the gastrointestinal tract. The renal tubular maximum for Mg prevents excessive reabsorption.

Whenever a patient is to receive a substance that causes Mg renal wasting (Table 1) or develops one of the diseases listed in Table 2, the Mg maintenance dose should be increased, and sMg and rbcMg should be monitored. The same is true for patients who must receive a drug that increases serum catecholamines (Table 3). A specific example is the successful preventive use of $MgSO_4$ during surgery for pheochromocytoma to reduce the amount and peripheral effects of catecholamines.

Treatment of NMgD

NMgD treatment rarely has been addressed. This type of MgD may or may not be recognized clinically and occurs with and without subtle manifestations. In neonates, such symptoms may not be recognizable. The estimated Mg loss should be replaced regularly, and the sMg and rbcMg should be monitored. Oral MgS therapy is clearly indicated for asymptomatic patients, if for no other reason than to prevent progression to a more serious stage of MgD.

In the presence of any type of MgD, there frequently are abnormalities with Ca, P, Na, K, and Fe ions. Very often, these associated abnormalities are not correctable until the MgD has been adequately treated. For this reason, sMg should be routinely obtained in all hospitalized patients. One result of such a surveillance was the knowledge that persistent pulmonary hypertension of the newborn could be treated successfully with $MgSO_4$.

The oral treatment of choice for neonates and small children is Mg gluconate liquid (Fleming and Co.). It is palatable and causes one-third the frequency of diarrhea as MgCl. The dose is 1 ml/kg/d (0.9 mEq/kg/d of Mg) 1 hour before or 2 hours after a meal. Mg tablets of chloride, gluconate, and oxide salts are available for those old enough to swallow them. Mg chloride and oxide tablets should be taken with meals.

Treatment of HMgD

Patients Without Life-Threatening Symptoms

These patients can receive the oral therapy outlined for those with NMgD.

TABLE 5. Causes of Negative Magnesium Balance

CAUSE	EXAMPLES
Reduced intake	Mg-poor foods
	Dieting; starvation
	Infusion of IV fluids
	Vomiting
Reduced absorption	Chronic diarrhea
	Starvation diarrhea
	Gastrointestinal problems
	Intake of substances that bind Mg: phosphates in soda drinks, oxalates
Redistribution	Stress, acute or chronic
	Increased catecholamine release
	Increased serum-free fatty acids
	Hypoalbuminemia
Increased excretion	Multiple medications: diuretics, furosemide, chlorothiazides, sodium lactate, sodium bicarbonate, theophylline, caffeine, pentamidine
	During aciduria or glycosuria
	Citrate-containing blood products
	Hyperglycemia
	Alcoholism or as little as 2 oz/d alcohol

From Mansmann HC Jr: Consider magnesium homeostasis: III: Cytochrome P450 enzymes and drug toxicity. Pediatr Asthma Allergy Immunol 8:7–28, 1994. Reprinted with permission.

Patients With Life-Threatening Symptoms

These patients require intravenous MgSO₄. An Mg dose of 2 mEq/kg body weight b.i.d. should be given slowly (0.5 ml of a 50% MgSO₄ USP solution). This may be required for 3 to 5 days.

In infants, a 10% solution of MgSO₄ can be given during hemodynamic and electrocardiographic monitoring, observing for sinoatrial or atrioventricular heart block, systemic hypotension, or respiratory depression. The treatment of these complications is a 10% Ca gluconate slow intravenous infusion at a dose of 0.2 to 0.3 ml/kg body weight. Once the Mg dose and the patient are stabilized, the dose can be given intramuscularly and then orally. The intramuscular route has the advantage of a 3 to 4 hour effect, whereas the intravenous effect lasts for one-half hour. The objectives are to eliminate the symptoms, to prevent a recurrence, and to maintain the sMg at the upper end of normal by frequent monitoring.

Toxicity

Hypermagnesemia in the neonatal period is usually secondary to Mg therapy during maternal preeclampsia. After 8 to 16 mEq/h of MgSO₄ is given to the mother with pregnancy-induced hypertension, the infant's sMg is about 3.0 mEq/L. In infants, an sMg of 3 to 9 mEq/L is associated with nausea, vomiting, bradycardia, and hypotension, an sMg of 5 to 10 mEq/L is associated with hyporeflexia and variable electrocardiogram results, and an sMg above 10 mEq/L is associated with respiratory depression and asystolic cardiac arrest. In addition to the Ca gluconate infusion mentioned previously, respiratory support may be indicated. In severe situations, a double volume exchange transfusion with citrated blood to bind the free Mg has been recommended. In addition, the loop diuretics furosemide and ethacrinic acid facilitate Mg wasting, which can lower the sMg.

Major causes of hypermagnesemia are Mg-containing enemas, intravenous fluids, and intramuscular injection. In the presence of normal renal tubular function, hypermagnesemia due to the use of Mg cathartics has not been reported. It has been demonstrated in adults that giving 100 mEq over 12 hours results in an sMg less than 6.5 mEq/L.

CONCLUSION

NMgD is real, and the rbcMg, uMg, and MgLT all return to normal in 4 to 6 weeks after sufficient MgS to produce PMgB. HMgD is preventable and treatable, but both preventive and therapeutic measures must be aggressive.

REFERENCES

1. Mansmann HC Jr: Consider magnesium homeostasis: III: Cytochrome P450 enzymes and drug toxicity. Pediatr Asthma Allergy Immunol 8:7–28, 1994.
2. Mimouni F, Tsang RC: Perinatal magnesium metabolism: Personal data and challenges for the 1990s. Magnesium Res 4:109–117, 1991.
3. Seelig MS: Magnesium status in infants. *In* Seelig MS (ed): Magnesium Deficiency in the Pathogenesis of Disease. New York, Plenum Medical Book Co, 1980: 73–134.

ZINC DEFICIENCY

PARIS TAYLOR MANSMANN, M.D.
HERBERT C. MANSMANN, JR., M.D.

The physiologic effects of zinc (Zn) have been studied in various diseases and compared with effects in normal infants and children. Many clinical features of Zn deficiency (ZnD) are described, with alterations of serum, plasma, urine, and hair Zn content. Yet a common theme in these correlations is the usefulness of always suspecting ZnD in the presence of prematurity, hyperalimentation, diabetes, cirrhosis, renal insufficiency, sickle cells, pancreatic insufficiency, and inflammatory bowel. The therapy of ZnD varies with the number of risk factors, the clinical situation, the age of the patient, and the ZnD severity. An essential part is the administration of the Recommended Daily Allowance (RDA) to prevent additional ZnD, in addition to Zn replenishment.

Zn has been found as a component of over 200 metalloenzymes (at least 70 in humans), one being carbonic anhydrase. Zn has critical catalytic and regulatory roles. It is necessary for biomembrane structure and function. Zn does not transfer electrons, yet one example of its catalytic action is that it acts as a cofactor in insulin utilization.

TISSUE CONSEQUENCES OF ZnD

ZnD has profound effects during periods of rapid human growth. Therefore, its prevention and early correction is mandatory. Well over 95% of the total body Zn is found within cells, but these pools are generally unavailable to adequately maintain Zn homeostasis, which requires a daily intake of Zn. Although there appears to exist a small labile Zn pool, it cannot sustain for long the plasma Zn (pZn) concentration, even though the plasma contains only 0.1% of the Zn, in the presence of continued poor assimilation. Hypozincemia is diagnostic of ZnD, but erythrocyte Zn (eryZn), leukocyte Zn, and urinary Zn (uZn) levels are said to lack sensitivity and specificity. Hair Zn (hZn) reflects previous ZnD. Function tests currently are not practical in clinical practice.

Humans require daily optimal Zn intake, or there soon follows a ZnD-induced decrease in cell division. Impaired growth velocity is the likely consequence of mild ZnD, which is correctable by physiologic doses of supplemental Zn (ZnS) (in spite of the lack of a reliable, sensitive laboratory test for mild ZnD). Although the cornea contains the highest concentration of Zn, it is injured during ZnD. In severe ZnD, growth ceases in spite of an adequate calorie intake, and ZnD-induced secondary acrodermatitis enteropathica could develop. ZnD reduces the lymphoid tissues seen at autopsy, compromises the immune system, and results in a T cell immunodeficiency, which can be improved by ZnS, with a return of normal delayed cutaneous hypersensitivity and thymic restoration. It also causes other forms of generalized tissue dysfunction to develop rapidly.

RISK FACTORS FOR ZnD

Gestational Factors

Maternal

The Zn requirement is increased during pregnancy. ZnD is highly teratogenic and has been demonstrated in those with anencephaly and spina bifida. ZnD also causes intrauterine growth retardation, prematurity, and neonatal problems.

Pregnancy results in lower maternal pZn levels. Normal women should receive at least 12 mg/d of Zn and an additional 3 mg/d during pregnancy to prevent ZnD. Mothers with genetic acrodermatitis enteropathica should take their maintenance ZnS dose plus the 3 mg/d in order to have a normal infant.

Prematurity

The fetus receives two thirds of its total Zn during the last 10 to 12 weeks of gestation. Nevertheless, cord Zn levels have been reported as both normal and low in prematures. However, cord eryZn levels had a positive correlation with gestational age in one study, and gender was not a factor. It can be assumed, as expected, that the younger the premature, the more ZnS the infant requires for immediate growth to occur.

A full-term newborn has 140 mg of Zn. The Zn requirement for growth is about 300 μg/kg/d. The premature needs 438 μg/kg/d to replace the deficiency and to maintain positive Zn balance.

Maternal Diabetes

There is increased uZn excretion from the diabetic woman, whether pregnant or not. This suggests that infants of diabetic mothers will have low pZn and eryZn concentrations, as has been reported in premature infants of diabetic mothers.

Maternal Alcoholism

Hypozincemia and hyperzincuria have been reported in chronic alcoholism. Both lower pZn levels and lower cord pZn levels have been seen in women who drink compared with nondrinkers. The teratogenic effect seen in fetal alcohol syndrome supports the need to carefully monitor pZn levels. ZnS should be given until pZn has stabilized and replenishment has been completed.

Inborn Errors of Metabolism

Genetic Acrodermatitis Enteropathica

This is a rare, inherited, autosomal recessive defect occurring in both sexes. There is impaired absorption and transfer of Zn, correctable by a pharmacologic ZnS dose, which is usually required for life.

Mammary Gland Dysfunction

This has been described where decreased Zn milk secretion occurs in spite of a positive maternal Zn balance and with a lack of increased milk Zn following maternal ZnS.

Other Risk Factors

Known causes of ZnD are semistarvation due to anorexia, Zn-poor total parenteral nutrition (TPN), protein-energy malnutrition (PEM), insufficient intake, vegetarians on cereal-based diets, maternal smoking, cirrhosis, and gastrointestinal dysfunction due to many diseases, including short bowel syndrome and intestinal bypass surgery. ZnD has been reported in advanced HIV acquired immunodeficiency syndrome (AIDS), probably a result of PEM. Diuretics cause uZn excretion. Penicillamine, diethylene trianine pentaacetate, sodium valproate, and probably ethambutol may precipitate ZnD.

CLINICAL MANIFESTATIONS OF ZnD

In premature infants, anorexia, mood changes, diarrhea, and neurologic signs have been reported. Over time, the following signs are likely to occur: growth retardation, alopecia, poor wound healing, psoriasis-like skin lesions, recurrent boils, fragile fingernails, and impairment of cranial nerve senses of smell, taste, sight, and hearing. Behavioral changes, such as irritability, lethargy, and depression, have been reversed by ZnS.

LABORATORY ASSESSMENT OF ZnD

Measurement of serum Zn (sZn) is ideally done by flame atomic absorption spectrophotometry and will be shifted as much as 40% because of diurnal variation. It is recommended that a fasting level be obtained between 8:00 and 9:00 AM, with serum being separated within 60 minutes. Normal values are illustrated in Table 1. Zn in the circulation represents <1% of the total body pool. sZn roughly reflects the intake of Zn, yet most of the total body zinc in blood (75% to 80%) is in RBCs.

Measurement of pZn also is done by flame atomic absorption

TABLE 1. Normal Zinc Serum Levels as Determined by Atomic Absorption

AGE (y)	SEX	μmol/L (μg/dl)
0–1	M, F	9.9–21.4 (65–140)
1–5	M, F	10.3–18.1 (67–118)
6–9	M, F	11.8–16.4 (77–107)
10–14	M	12.1–18.0 (79–118)
	F	11.6–15.4 (76–101)
15–19	M	9.2–15.4 (60–101)
	F	9.8–17.9 (64–117)

TABLE 2. Zinc Plasma Levels as Determined by Atomic Absorption

Normal Adolescents	μmol/L	μg/dl
Male	12.8–13.5	(83.5–87.9)
Female	13.1–13.9	(83.3–90.5)
Children (0–15 y)		
Severely low	<10.7	(<69.7)
Low	10.7–13.2	(69.7–86)
Normal	13.2–16.4	(86.0–106.8)

spectrophotometry by specialized reference laboratories. Normal values are given in Table 2. Whole blood is obtained from heelstick, fingerstick, or venipuncture into special acid-washed (heparinized) tubes. Plasma should be separated as soon as possible, then stored at −20° C. pZn reflects metabolizable or exchangeable Zn that is delivered to metabolically active tissues.

hZn is measured by obtaining 20 to 50 mg of closely cut samples from the occipital area of the scalp with stainless steel scissors. After a nonionic detergent wash, they are analyzed by instrumental neutron activation. hZn has been proposed as an index of the chronic status of trace mineral nutrition. The values should be used with caution because they are influenced by the mean rate of hair growth and environmental contamination by external sources. The poor correlation between hZn content and pZn concentrations has been stressed.

MANAGEMENT OF ZnD

Prevention

Foremost in the physician's care is to think prevention of ZnD in mothers, infants, and children. For example, Zn concentrations should be checked for whichever formula is used for the infant. Pooled human milk is often poor in Zn content.

Treatment

Once confirmation of Zn status is obtained, ZnS should start. The U.S. RDA for infants varies between 5.5 and 6.3 mg Zn/d, and the World Health Organization (WHO) recommends 11 mg Zn/d for adult males. Higher doses should be used for ZnS, since replacement is also required. Various Zn compounds are available for oral administration, including the sulfates, gluconate, acetate, and oxide. Dosages of elemental Zn per tablet or capsule vary and range from 5 to 50 mg. Various claims for superiority in bioavailability, therapeutic efficacy, or tolerance have been made for one or another compound, but these are largely unsubstantiated. Although gastrointestinal irritation may be lessened by taking Zn at mealtimes, the absorption of therapeutic Zn is markedly reduced by food. It is best to administer Zn preparations between meals around 9:00 AM. ZnS does not appear to increase red cell or white cell Zn levels in research protocols, whereas pZn and sZn levels will reflect absorption even in severe illnesses of inflammation of the bowel.

The most consistent and notable changes observed postsupplementation were in the "Z scores" for triceps skinfold thickness and midarm circumference. Children who receive ZnS gain more fat and lose less muscle. A significant increase in linear growth is not expected for 4 to 5 months.

High Risk Patients

In spite of multiple analytic techniques, a clinical trial of ZnS is often the clinician's only accurate assessment, provided it is not used with other modalities of therapy. Treatment by ZnS for various age groups is as follows.

Prematures. Even though more risky, 0.35 or 0.4 mg/kg/d of intravenous ZnS should be used as part of the TPN.

Infants. An oral dose of 0.4 mg/kg/d should be used initially, then 0.5 mg/kg/d after 3 months, monitoring for anemia and irritability.

Young Children. Between 5 and 8 years of age, 10 mg/d is used.

Older Children. Doses as high as 50 to 150 mg/d are tolerated, but signs of toxicity must be kept in mind. In some older children with acrodermatitis enteropathica, lesser amounts of Zn may produce the desired therapeutic effect.

Zn TOXICITY

Acute

If Zn is given in high pharmacologic doses, it causes abdominal cramps, nausea, vomiting, headaches, dizziness, chills, flushing, blurred vision, and sweating. Premature infants are much more susceptible to Zn toxicity, responding with irritability, tremor, seizures, and tachyarrythmias.

Chronic

Since Zn interferes with copper bioavailability, copper deficiency has been reported with excessive Zn therapy, which is 25 mg/d for an infant over several weeks or 50 mg/d in adults. Copper deficiency has been associated with anemia and gastric erosion.

REFERENCES

1. Aggett PJ, Barclay SM: Neonatal trace element metabolism. *In* Cowett RM (ed): Principles of Perinatal-Neonatal Metabolism. New York, Springer-Verlag, 1991: 513–518.
2. Good RA, Fernandes G, West A: Nutrition, immunity and cancer. A review. Part I: Influence of protein and protein-calorie malnutrition, and zinc deficiency on immunity. Clin Bull 9:3–12, 1979.
3. King JC, Keen CL: Zinc. *In* Shils ME, Olson JA, Shika M (eds): Modern Nutrition in Health and Disease, 8th ed. Philadelphia, Lea & Febiger, 1994: 214–230.

2

Mental Development and Behavioral Disorders

DEPRESSIVE DISORDERS

RONALD JAY STEINGARD, M.D.
DAVID RAY DEMASO, M.D.

DIAGNOSIS

The diagnosis of major depressive disorder is based on the presence of cognitive and physiologic symptoms that co-occur and have persistence over time. Major depressive disorder requires the presence of either depressed or irritable mood and/or markedly diminished interest in all activities for at least 2 weeks. Associated symptoms (of which five are needed to make a diagnosis, in addition to depressed/irritable mood and loss of interest) include significant weight gain or loss, significant insomnia or hypersomnia, psychomotor agitation or retardation, fatigue or loss of energy, excessive feelings of worthlessness or inappropriate guilt, diminished ability to think, concentrate, or make decisions, and recurrent thoughts of death, suicidal ideation, suicide attempts, or a specific plan for committing suicide. These symptoms must represent a change from previous functioning and neither be caused nor maintained by an organic factor or represent a normal bereavement reaction. Delusions or hallucinations should not have developed before the mood symptoms or continue after they have remitted.

Dysthymia is a more chronic form of depression that has a less extensive symptom pattern. Dysthymia is characterized by the presence of depressed or irritable mood lasting at least 1 year without a cessation of symptoms for more than 2 months at a time. In addition, the mood change must be accompanied by at least two of the following additional symptoms: poor appetite or overeating, insomnia or hypersomnia, low energy or fatigue, low self-esteem, poor concentration or difficulty in making decisions, and feelings of hopelessness. As with major depressive disorder, dysthymia cannot be caused or maintained by an organic factor. Although there is some controversy regarding the point at which the distinction should be made between major depressive disorder and dysthymia, they are both serious and impairing emotional disorders in childhood and adolescence.

EPIDEMIOLOGY

Major depression occurs in approximately 2% of the prepubertal population, and the incidence increases to a prevalence rate of 5% in adolescence. Rates of depression are equal for males and females in childhood, but females predominate in adolescent samples. The incidence of the disorder is also affected by clinical site. Rates as high as 60% have been reported in hospitalized adolescents, whereas a 7% rate has been noted in a general pediatric population.

ETIOLOGY

Many etiologic models have been proposed. Genetic predisposition has been suggested by the higher likelihood of first degree relatives having depressive disorders, as well as the higher concordance rates for identical twins compared with fraternal twins. Biologic theories have focused on dysregulation of monoaminergic neurotransmitter systems, secondary to the fact that most of the effective pharmacologic treatments have been agents that effect monoaminergic transmission. The frontal lobes, temporal-limbic structures, and aspects of the basal ganglia have been most typically implicated neuroanatomically in depressive disorders, but the data are still preliminary. Social skill deficits, learned helplessness, cognitive distortions, and interpersonal loss have been suggested as important psychosocial factors. The presence of marital discord and depressive illness in a parent can negatively alter the prognosis.

DIFFERENTIAL DIAGNOSIS

The differential diagnosis of depressive disorders is important. All organic factors that may cause a depressivelike syndrome, such as AIDS, influenza, infectious mononucleosis, malignancies, thyroid abnormalities, drugs, and alcohol, must be considered. Comorbid psychiatric conditions, such as the disruptive behavior disorders (attention deficit hyperactivity disorder), anxiety disorders, learning disabilities, substance abuse, and child abuse, are common. A specific event, such as divorce or a new sibling, may precipitate an adjustment reaction with depressed mood. Over 35% of children who experience the death of a parent satisfy the criteria for a major depressive disorder in the 3 months following the loss. Bipolar (or manic) disorders may occur initially with a major depressive disorder. In fact, the presence of early onset major depressive disorder is a risk factor for the subsequent development of bipolar disorder.

TREATMENT

Chronic problems with depressive symptoms can lead to problems with self-esteem, interfere with the development of age-appropriate interactional skills, and adversely affect academic performance. Difficulties can also arise in peer and familial relationships. Therapies should be offered to address these difficulties when they occur.

Psychological Interventions

Psychotherapy has been one of the main approaches to treatment. Individual psychotherapy can address the issues of self-esteem, assist the patient in resolving issues of loss in the face of an acute precipitant to the depressive episode, explore alternative responses to life events and social interactions, provide support to the patient, and enhance self-understanding of depression.

Cognitive therapy has been shown to be effective in an adolescent population. This approach maintains that there are cognitive distortions that maintain the patient's depressive perceptions and that these can be corrected.

Family therapy can explore patterns of behavior that have evolved within a family system in response to a child's depression. Adaptive responses can then be supported and enhanced within the family. Given the familial nature of these disorders, the presence of mood disorders in the child's parents and siblings requires assessment for intervention. Preventative psychoeducational programs with families at high risk for depressive disorder are being developed.

Group therapy can provide remediation in the area of social skill development and enhance the child's capacity to negotiate peer relationships more successfully.

Although outpatient treatment is preferred, inpatient psychiatric hospitalization may be indicated when a youngster is suicidal and the family is unable to provide adequate monitoring. Psychosis (which can occur with severe depressive disorders), destructive acting out behavior, and drug abuse are other indications for hospitalization.

Consultation to the academic setting is another area of intervention. The school may need classroom intervention strategies, as well as a better understanding of the disorder. Psychologic testing may be needed to rule out the underlying and contributing learning disabilities.

Somatic symptomatology, such as recurrent headaches and abdominal pain, may accompany the presentation. The pediatrician's role in the assessment and management of these complaints along with the psychotherapist is important. The pediatrician plays an important ongoing supportive role to the child and family via their interest and support in the treatment program.

Pharmacology

A thorough psychiatric evaluation should be completed, and as indicated, adjunctive therapies should be initiated before the initiation of pharmacotherapy. Studies investigating the pharmacotherapy of depressive disorders in children and adolescents have been inconclusive. Early open trials and anecdotal experience have suggested a beneficial role for antidepressant therapy. However, well-designed, double-blind, placebo-controlled trials have failed to demonstrate the robust response seen in adults.

There have been five published studies employing DSM-III-R criteria for major depressive disorder in prepubertal children and six published reports in adolescents. Only seven of these studies have been double-blind controlled studies, and the total number of patients in these controlled trials is less than 100. Even within these better controlled studies, there are significant methodologic issues, in addition to the small sample size, that preclude any valid aggregate observations or conclusions. Ancillary treatments have been poorly controlled, placebo washout periods have been variable in duration, the duration of the clinical trials has varied in length, and there is some suggestion that they may have been too short to demonstrate an adequate treatment effect. Therefore, the efficacy of these interventions remains uncertain. Nevertheless, the significant morbidity associated with depressive disorders and the positive open trial experiences with antidepressants have led to the recommendation to use antidepressants when a child or adolescent experiences symptoms of a depressive disorder and functional incapacity as a result of these symptoms.

There are three classes of antidepressant available: cyclic, selective serotonin reuptake inhibitors, and the monoamine oxidase (MAO) inhibitors. The cyclic antidepressants include the tricyclic antidepressants, such as imipramine, amitriptyline, desipramine, and nortriptyline, and other cyclic compounds, such as maprotiline, trazadone, and bupropion. The tricyclic compounds have been studied more extensively than other antidepressant agents in the treatment of children and adolescents and are also used to treat attention deficit hyperactivity disorder, separation anxiety disorder, enuresis, and chronic pain in the pediatric population. The second class of antidepressants is selective serotonin reuptake inhibitors. These compounds include such agents as fluoxetine, sertraline, and paroxetine. Although newer than both the cyclic antidepressants and the MAO inhibitors, these compounds offer the possibility of less risk and comparable efficacy in children and adolescents. Unfortunately, very few reports have emerged regarding their use in childhood depressive disorders. The reports that have been published have generally been favorable, but the sizes of the samples have been small and the studies have generally been open in nature. The third class of compounds, the MAO inhibitors, include such compounds as phenelzine, isocarboxazid, and tranylcypromine. Although these compounds have shown some promise in the treatment of mood disorder and attention deficit hyperactivity disorder in the pediatric population, the strict dietary restrictions generally preclude their use in a pediatric population, and they are not discussed here.

Tricyclic Antidepressants

Tricyclic antidepressants have been the mainstay of pharmacotherapy of depressive disorders in children and adolescents. Amitriptyline and imipramine are tertiary amines, and their major metabolites are nortriptyline and desipramine, respectively. These metabolites are secondary amines and tend to be as effective and better tolerated than their parent compounds (Table 1). Tricyclic antidepressants are thought to work by blocking the reuptake of monoaminergic neurotransmitters (norepinephrine, serotonin) into the presynaptic nerve terminal and creating a functional increase in the availability of the neurotransmitters in the synaptic cleft. Their ability to affect other monoaminergic systems (histaminergic, muscarinergic or cholinergic, adrenergic) accounts for their side effect profile. Imipramine and nortriptyline are the only tricyclic agents approved by the FDA for investigational use in children under the age of 12.

As children tend to be more efficient metabolizers of these drugs and have shorter elimination half-lives than adults, these medications are typically given in a b.i.d. dose schedule in children but may be given once a day in older adolescents. These medications are usually started at small doses (0.5 mg/kg/d) and titrated slowly (0.5 mg/kg/d increase q4–5d as tolerated) to the lower end of the suggested dose range (Table 1). It is generally recommended that a clinical trial of a tricyclic antidepressant be continued at optimal doses for at least 6 to 8 weeks.

TABLE 1. Tricyclic Antidepressants

	RECOMMENDED DOSE RANGE (mg/kg/d)	ELIMINATION HALF-LIFE (h)	PLASMA LEVELS* (ng/ml)	MUSCURINIC BLOCKADE	SEDATION
Amitriptyline	2–5	16	NA†	+ + +	+ + +
Imipramine	2–5	16	125–250 (IMI + DMI)	+ +	+
Desipramine	2–5	22	NA‡	+	+
Nortriptyline	1–3	24	60–100	+	+ +

*Based on suggestions in current literature from small controlled studies.
†NA, not available; IMI, imipramine; DMI, desipramine.
‡Some sources suggest a maximum plasma level of 300 ng/ml in children with attention deficit disorder.

TABLE 2. Baseline Laboratory Studies

CBC with differential
BUN
Serum creatinine
Electrolytes
Liver function studies
Thyroid function studies
Electrocardiogram*

*Screening for tricyclic antidepressant.

TABLE 3. Selective Serotonin Reuptake Inhibitors

	STARTING DOSE (mg)	RECOMMENDED DOSE RANGE (mg)	CLINICAL HALF-LIFE (h)
Fluoxetine	5–10	5–40* 10–80†	24–72 (7–15 d for norfluoxetine)
Sertraline	25–50	25–200	25
Paroxetine	10–20	10–50	20

*Pediatric dose range used in published studies.
†Recommended adult dose range.

In addition to baseline laboratory studies (Table 2), plasma level monitoring is advised. The data regarding plasma levels and response are at best suggestive, but some guidelines have been made available (Table 1). It is possible that patients may respond to these agents at lower plasma levels. However, these guidelines are useful in treatment-resistant patients to ensure the adequacy of a clinical trial. Plasma levels can identify a patient who is an efficient metabolizer of these drugs and may require higher doses of the medication to achieve an adequate response. Although there is only the suggestion of a relationship between plasma level and response, cardiovascular toxicity increases with increasing plasma levels. Therefore, plasma level determinations early in treatment can alert the physician to the fact that a patient is a slow metabolizer and help avoid unnecessary risk.

The most common side effects are those associated with the anticholinergic effects of these drugs. Dry mouth and mild constipation are common in children and adolescents, whereas urinary hesitancy and blurred vision are reported less frequently than in adults. Sedation can also occur with these agents. Weight gain has been observed in children and adolescents. These agents carry a small risk of inducing seizures, but in patients who have no known risk factors, the incidence is less than 1% at therapeutic doses.

The most serious side effects of these agents are their cardiovascular effects. In addition to causing mild increase in pulse and diastolic blood pressure, these agents have a quinidine-like effect of cardiac conduction and can cause a prolongation of cardiac conduction. The FDA has provided a set of guidelines regarding cardiac monitoring in children being treated with either nortriptyline or imipramine. However, researchers in the psychiatry and cardiology departments at the University of Pittsburgh have provided a more extensive set of guidelines for the use of tricyclic antidepressants in children.

1. Obtain an electrocardiogram (ECG) at baseline before beginning cyclic antidepressants [to rule out a congenital conduction defect (e.g., Wolfe-Parkinson-White syndrome)]. Then obtain an ECG rhythm strip after each dosage increase and after reaching steady state on medication.
2. Reduce or discontinue cyclic antidepressants if the PR interval is greater than 0.18 seconds in patients under 10 years of age or greater than 0.2 seconds in patients over 10 years of age.
3. Reduce or discontinue medication if the QRS interval is greater than 0.12 seconds or widens more than 50% over the baseline QRS interval.
4. Reduce or discontinue medication if the corrected QT interval (QTc) is greater than 0.48 seconds.
5. Reduce or discontinue medication if the resting heart rate is greater than 110 beats per minutes (bpm) in children 10 years of age or under or greater than 100 bpm in children 10 years of age or older.
6. Reduce or discontinue medication if the resting blood pressure is greater than 140/90 or persistently greater than 130/85 in children under 10 and if the blood pressure is greater than 140/85 in children older than 10 years of age.

These guidelines are conservative, and other researchers have suggested less stringent guidelines for the use of tricyclic antidepressants in children. In addition, these guidelines are subject to revision as new research regarding the cardiovascular effects of the tricyclic antidepressants becomes available.

These guidelines take on added significance in the context of four reports of sudden death that have occurred in children receiving desipramine for the treatment of attention deficit hyperactivity disorder or depression. A full discussion of this issue is beyond the scope of this current review but warrants some comment. The association between desipramine and these occurrences remains unclear, as there is limited data available from some of these cases, and the total number of occurrences is small. However, given the quinidine-like effects of these agents, their use in children warrants a careful initial evaluation to rule out the presence of preexisting cardiac vulnerabilities and close monitoring of cardiac function during treatment. In the absence of prior cardiac abnormalities that might preclude the use of an agent with quinidine-like actions, serial ECGs are recommended at least during periods of active dose titration, and most investigators believe that monitoring ECGs during maintenance therapy is warranted as well, but the frequency of these evaluations is debated.

A flu-like withdrawal syndrome has been described and attributed to cholinergic rebound. It is advisable to taper, rather than abruptly withdraw, the medications following maintenance treatment.

Selective Serotonin Reuptake Inhibitors

The SSRIs have been shown in adults to have similar efficacy, a more tolerable side effect profile, and less risk in the event of an overdose when compared with either the tricyclic antidepressants or MAO inhibitors. There have been only a few studies of the use of these agents in children and adolescents, but those reports have been favorable. Larger well-controlled studies are warranted, but again, clinical practice often involves the use of these compounds in children and adolescents with depressive disorders. The agents work in a similar fashion to the tricyclics, but they have a greater affinity for serotonin reuptake sites and selectively block the reuptake of serotonin. These agents also have a much lower affinity for other monoaminergic systems and, therefore, have a lower side effect profile than the tricyclic antidepressants. These compounds are not approved by the FDA for use in children under the age of 12.

The dose range of these compounds is not well established for pediatric populations, and the dose range reported for fluoxetine has been extrapolated from the few reports of its use in this age range (Table 3). An adequate trial of these compounds is similar in duration to that recommended for the tricyclic antidepressants.

Baseline laboratory studies are comparable to those obtained with the tricyclic antidepressants. Unfortunately, there are no established plasma levels for these compounds, as it appears that there is no reliable relationship between plasma level and response. Therefore, the clinician is left to titrate the compound according to general dosing guidelines and in response to perceived benefits and emergent side effects. The major potential benefit of these compounds in a pediatric population is the decreased cardiovascular risk and diminished risk in overdose.

A major issue of concern with these compounds is their capacity to affect the liver cytochrome P450 enzyme system. This has implications for drug–drug interactions and suggests that dose changes and monitoring of plasma levels of other coadministered compounds that use this enzyme system may be warranted.

Adjunctive Strategies

A recent advance in adult psychopharmacology has been the attempt to augment the response to antidepressant medications in treatment-resistant patients by the coadministration of other neurologically active compounds. These strategies have included the coadministration of lithium carbonate, triiodothyronine (T_3), and stimulant compounds. In addition, investigators have reported on the coadministration of two different types of antidepressant compounds (*coadministration of MAOI with either tricyclic antidepressants or SSRIs is contraindicated*). Only lithium augmentation has been reported to date in children and adolescents. These are preliminary reports that have some promise but warrant further investigation.

PROGNOSIS

Studies of the natural history of depressive disorders without treatment in children and adolescents show that they may have an extended duration. The duration of a major depressive disorder is about 7½ months, with a 72% chance of recurrence within 5 years. Dysthymia has an average duration of 3 years. Typically, the younger the age at the time of diagnosis, the longer the course of the disturbance.

CONCLUSION

Major depressive disorder and dysthymia are associated with significant functional morbidity when they occur in children and adolescents. Evaluation requires careful study of coexisting psychosocial stressors and an appreciation for the impact of these disorders on children at different stages of development and their impact on the development of age-appropriate psychosocial and academic skills. Family evaluations must include an assessment of behavioral dynamics at play within the family system and also be alert to the presence of mood disorder in other family members.

Treatment strategies, therefore, need to be multimodal in nature and individualized to each child's needs and difficulties. As discussed, treatment may include a range of interventions, including individual psychotherapy, cognitive behavioral therapy, family therapy, social skills training and group therapies, and pharmacotherapy. Although there are only limited data about the efficacy of these interventions, the prevalence and morbidity of these disorders warrant active intervention.

REFERENCES

1. Diagnostic and Statistical Manual of Mental Disorders, 3rd ed, rev. Washington, DC, American Psychiatric Association, 1987:222–233.
2. Green WH: Child and Adolescent Clinical Psychopharmacology. Baltimore, Williams & Wilkins, 1991.
3. Work Group on Major Depressive Disorders, American Psychiatric Association: Practice guidelines for major depressive disorder in adults. Am J Psychiatry (suppl), 150:4, 1–26, 1993.

PSYCHIATRIC DISORDERS AND MENTAL HEALTH TREATMENT

JOHN SARGENT, M.D.

Pediatricians often are the initial professionals consulted when families, hospital staff, or school personnel have significant concerns about the emotional state or behavior of a child. The pediatrician also might note emotional difficulties or behavior problems during routine well child or illness-oriented office visits, as well as through concern raised during the inpatient medical hospitalization of a child he is treating. These concerns may take a variety of forms and can include withdrawal, excessive fearfulness, aggressive or impulsive behavior, or declining performance in school, activities, or athletic pursuits. Adult concerns about the child might have developed in early childhood or may develop acutely. The onset of difficulties could be abrupt, with an acute change in the child's behavior or emotional state, or might develop gradually, with persistent worsening of the child's emotional or behavioral status. It is essential that each pediatrician have a framework for evaluating the child's or adolescent's emotional state, behavioral status, and functional capacity, as well as have a method for classifying the child's difficulties, recommending appropriate treatment, and identifying the necessary resources to carry out that treatment. It is also necessary that each pediatrician have a method for directly informing involved adults about impressions of the child, necessary interventions, and what parents, school professionals, and other health care staff might expect as the child participates in the necessary treatment.

Several psychiatric disorders of children and adolescents are covered specifically in the other sections of this text, including depression, autism, attention deficit disorder, and psychosomatic disorders. Other sections address particular situations that may be stressful for a child or adolescent and require specific preventive support or therapeutic intervention. These include the child's response to the death of a loved one, chronic physical illness, physical and sexual abuse, and divorce. There are also sections on common behavioral difficulties of children, including tics, sleep disorders, breath-holding spells, learning disabilities, and pica, and a separate section on mental retardation. This section addresses both the general approach to understanding the child's emotional and behavioral status and an approach to identifying and beginning treatment for psychotic disorders, internalizing difficulties associated with anxiety and withdrawal, and externalizing disorders associated with aggressiveness and acting-out behavior.

ELEMENTS OF THE MENTAL HEALTH EVALUATION OF THE CHILD OR ADOLESCENT

The framework for understanding the child's emotional state and behavioral status includes assessment of history, the child's affect and behavior, and the child's response to the environment, including responses to family relationships, disruptions or stresses within the family, and difficulties in the child's and family's relationships with their community, including school, neighborhood, and extended family. Orienting data include the age of the child, grade in school, family background and composition, and the child's living situation, including with whom the child lives and any recent changes in the home.

Important history includes a description of what the problem has been, who has noticed it, where it has occurred, and how it developed. The psychosocial background of the child and family is important, including previous concerns about the child's emotional status, capacity to learn, behavior, and family history of psychiatric difficulties. Recent school performance, as well as information about the child's social relationships and participation in activities outside of school, is essential information.

A complete medical evaluation of the child is a necessary part of understanding any emotional or behavioral problem and includes an evaluation of the child's physical status and identification of any medications the child may be taking, as well as investigation of whether the ingestion of a toxic substance either purposely or inadvertently may have led to the child's current difficulties.

The child's mental status examination always includes an understanding of the child's ability to be oriented to person, place, and time, his appearance, including his ability to care for himself effectively, an appreciation of the child's memory and cognitive abilities, an assessment of the child's relating ability, speech, overall mood, and content and process of his thinking. It is essential that the pediatrician appreciate the child's behavior and his ability to control, modulate, and direct his behavior in association with expressed goals and the requirements of particular situations. As the child's behavior is evaluated, it is also important that his pediatrician attend to the child's ability to control impulses and to use judgment in directing behavior. A synthesis of the evaluation gives the pediatrician an overall impression of the nature of the difficulty, whether it affects the child's ability to maintain contact with reality, and a sense of whether the child's difficulties are primarily internally or externally directed.

The pediatrician must be able to develop a general impression of family functioning and family strengths, including the parents' ability to appreciate the child's difficulties, to provide direction and support, and to comfort the child when he or she is stressed. The family's ability to organize concerns about their child and to appreciate and use resources that might be necessary to assist their child also is an essential feature of the pediatrician's appreciation of the current difficulties and the level of intervention likely to be necessary. In evaluating the family, it is important for the pediatrician to pay attention to the level of concern of parental figures and their ability to develop shared impressions and to work together with extended family resources, neighborhood resources, and school professionals as they attempt to further identify their child's difficulties and structure effective treatment. After the pediatrician completes this evaluation, an overall impression of the nature of the child's difficulties will be gathered, and a diagnostic classification of the difficulties and a plan for appropriate treatment will become apparent. It is necessary that every pediatrician know the appropriate mental health resources available in the community and have trusted psychiatric and psychologic colleagues available for referral of difficult situations and consultation as needed. It is helpful if the pediatrician has an ongoing relationship with school personnel who will be able to identify difficulties the child is having in school and determine appropriate school placement for the child as mental health treatment proceeds. The more the pediatrician knows and trusts mental health resources, the more likely it is that a mental health referral will be accepted by a family and the resources will be used in an effective and straightforward fashion for the child's benefit.

PSYCHOTIC DISORDERS

Psychosis refers to a mental state in which major disturbances in thinking, relating, and reality testing occur. Psychotic patients do not express themselves clearly and have difficulty answering direct questions. They may be suspicious and hostile or acutely withdrawn and generally unresponsive. Psychosis may be the result of a psychiatric disorder or a medical problem. The child who becomes psychotic secondary to a medical problem is often likely to be disoriented with regard to time and place, there may be memory difficulties, and the child may be unable to describe the onset of his problems coherently. Hallucinations may be present and often include visual and tactile hallucinations in addition to or instead of auditory hallucinations. Medical conditions that may lead to psychosis are listed in Table 1. Some of these conditions are the result of acute infection or trauma, and some may develop acutely in a child, with severe emotional and behavioral symptoms being among the first identifying features of the illness. Other conditions may be chronic and known to the pediatrician and may be exacerbated by either current medical treatment or intercurrent difficulty, which leads to the development of psychotic thinking and behavior.

Table 2 lists drugs and substances that may lead to the development of psychotic behavior in a child or adolescent. Some of these may be used in the ongoing treatment of a known medical condition, for example, the use of steroids in the treatment of a child who then develops psychotic thinking and behavior as a result of steroid medication itself. Other toxic psychoses occur following ingestion by accident or for recreational or self-destructive purposes by a child or adolescent. The acute onset of psychotic behavior in a child or adolescent whose previous functioning had been generally normal is often indicative of the development of a medical condition or the ingestion of a toxic substance. Other causes of psychotic behavior in children and adolescents include the onset of schizophrenia, bipolar or manic depressive disorder, a continuation and worsening of an autistic state in a child, or the development of severe fearfulness and loss of appropriate recognition of reality in a child who has been severely traumatized. Autism is covered elsewhere in this chapter.

TABLE 1. Medical Conditions That May Lead to Psychosis

Central Nervous System Lesions
Tumor
Brain abscess
Cerebral hemorrhage
Meningitis or encephalitis
Temporal lobe epilepsy
Closed head trauma

Cerebral Hypoxia
Pulmonary insufficiency
Severe anemia
Cardiac failure
Carbon monoxide poisoning

Metabolic and Endocrine Disorders
Electrolyte imbalance
Hypoglycemia
Hypocalcemia
Thyroid disease (hyper- and hypo-)
Adrenal disease (hyper- and hypo-)
Uremia
Hepatic failure
Diabetes mellitus
Porphyria
Reye syndrome

Collagen-Vascular Diseases
Systemic lupus erythematosus
Polyarteritis nodosa

Infections
Malaria
Typhoid fever
Subacute bacterial endocarditis

Schizophrenia

Schizophrenia frequently has its onset in adolescence and occurs in approximately 0.5% of the population. It is equally common in males and females and is more prevalent among family members of known individuals with the disease. It is hypothesized that one feature of schizophrenia is an excess of dopamine activity in the brain.

Symptoms of schizophrenia involve impairment of basic psychologic processes, including perception, thinking, affect, and the capacity to relate. Impaired thought content includes delusions, strongly held beliefs with no basis in reality of persecution or external control. An adolescent with schizophrenia may feel that others can read his mind and insert thoughts into his mind and may imagine others as persecuting or pursuing him. Illogical thinking often occurs, speech frequently is characterized by loose associations where ideas shift

TABLE 2. Exogenous Substances Causing Psychosis Following Ingestion of Significant Quantity

Alcohol
Barbiturates
Antipsychotics (e.g., phenothiazines)
Amphetamines
Hallucinogens—LSD, peyote, mescaline
Marijuana
Phencyclidine (PCP)
Methaqualone (Quaalude)
Anticholinergic compounds
Heavy metals
Cocaine
Corticosteroids
Reserpine
Opioids (e.g., heroin, methadone)

from one subject to another, and auditory hallucinations are common, often including direct commands from the hallucinations. Affect may be blunted and flat or inappropriate and bizarre. Unpredictable changes in mood and behavior may occur. These teenagers often have neuropsychologic difficulties involving cognitive processes, perception, and memory and have significant difficulty in looking after themselves or directing their behavior. They may become incoherent and may appear to be talking to themselves, as well as losing interest in their usual activities and refusing to participate in hygiene and other normal behaviors. The child relates in an often bizarre fashion, and the pediatrician may note himself becoming uncomfortable in the presence of the child and unable to relate directly and effectively with him. Concern about this child may have developed over a long period of time, and there may be several months of gradual and insidious onset of these difficulties.

Psychiatric consultation and possible inpatient psychiatric hospitalization often are necessary acutely. For some children, one episode of this difficulty will occur, and on inception of appropriate treatment, further difficulties will be avoided. However, most adolescents with the onset of schizophrenia are likely to have a chronic course of serious difficulties that interfere significantly with the adolescent's education, development of social relationships, vocational functioning, and personal well-being. This is a very serious condition that generally requires ongoing psychiatric assistance and the development of a specific psychopharmacologic, psychotherapeutic, and vocational program for the child, with intensive support for the child's family. Neuroleptic medications generally are used in the treatment of schizophrenia and often are very helpful in reducing delusions, hallucinations, and bizarre thoughts and behaviors. These medications often have significant side effects, including acute extrapyramidal difficulties, such as oculogyric crisis, rigidity, and akathesia, and may lead to the development of long-term chronic difficulties, such as tardive dyskinesia. If the pediatrician needs to institute acute treatment before initiation of appropriate psychiatric treatment, the use of a benzodiazepine, such as lorazepam 1 to 2 mg and haloperidol 1 to 5 mg either by mouth or IM, often is helpful in calming the patient and inducing effective control of behavior, leading to the inception of appropriate and significant psychiatric treatment.

Bipolar Disorder

Bipolar disorder, or manic depressive illness, also occurs in approximately 0.5% of the population, with onset usually occurring before age 30 and infrequently during late childhood or adolescence. Since depression is discussed in a separate section, only manic psychosis is considered here.

A patient with mania has a distinct period of predominantly elevated, expansive, and irritable mood. There is often a marked decrease in the need for sleep, marked distractibility, hyperactivity, pressured speech, and emotional lability. These patients also exhibit what is called "flight of ideas," with a nearly continuous flow of accelerated speech and abrupt changes from topic to topic often based on understandable associations, distractions, or plays on words. This form of conversation, although bizarre and inappropriate, demonstrates a logical connection from one idea to the next but moves quickly from one topic to another. The manic patient may have inflated self-esteem and uncritical self-confidence and grandiosity. This grandiosity may include delusional ideas, leading the individual to become aggressive or combative. There may be a history of buying sprees or pursuit of other reckless behavior and also evidence of hypersexuality and markedly poor judgment and behavior control. These patients may have a history of previous depression, but often an acute manic episode is the initial presentation of this difficulty, which may result in cycling of the mood from mania to depression at different points in the teenager's course.

The differentiation of mania and schizophrenia in an initial episode of psychosis may be quite difficult. Distractibility, expansiveness, and marked irritability, as well as euphoric mood, often are helpful in identifying manic individuals. Both groups may have hallucinations and delusions. However, the speech of the manic patient usually demonstrates flight of ideas rather than loose associations and disconnections of ideas. Often, the schizophrenic patient is more likely to be inappropriate and withdrawn, shifting to suspicious and fearful, whereas the manic patient is more likely to be consistently expansive and demanding.

Management of manic patients requires psychiatric consultation and frequently may involve the need for acute voluntary or involuntary psychiatric hospitalization. The long-term treatment generally involves the use of lithium carbonate. This medication usually requires a period of time to develop its therapeutic effect. Regular monitoring of blood levels is essential to avoid toxic side effects. Psychiatric follow-up care for patients with defined bipolar disorder is an essential feature of their treatment and requires often chronic use of antimanic medication, as well as the development of specific resources to assist the family and identify and respond appropriately to the development of acute symptoms of either mania or depression. The use of antipsychotic medication, such as haloperidol (1 to 5 mg PO or IM every 4 to 6 hours), may be necessary to stabilize a patient who is acutely psychotic with manic depressive illness.

Reactive Psychosis

Occasionally, children who are acutely traumatized may develop the onset of psychotic behavior, including inappropriate affect, heightened arousability, significant fearfulness, and distortion of events in their lives. These children generally react in a highly bizarre fashion, with their behavior reflecting concern about being followed or being in significant danger. The history in these circumstances often reflects an acute onset of the child's disturbed behavior and the occurrence of an acute traumatic event or severely threatening circumstance. The child may have experienced severe physical or sexual abuse or may have been involved in an extraordinarily frightening episode. Not only do these children frighten themselves, but their behavior generally frightens their caretakers, leading to worsening of the child's condition and a significant level of concern about the child's safety, as well as confusion about controls for the child's unusual behavior.

It is essential in such situations that ingestion of an intoxicant or the acute development of a medical illness be ruled out. Once that has been accomplished, psychiatric consultation and inception of intensive psychiatric treatment is necessary. In the absence of identification of the precipitating event, psychiatric hospitalization may be necessary to ensure safety and to allow for time to identify what has been causing the child's difficulties.

Posttraumatic stress disorder (described later in this section) can lead to the development of acutely fluctuating behavior, auditory hallucinations, marked fearfulness, and misperception of one's circumstances, creating concern about the child's having developed a reactive psychosis. Acute management of these patients may involve the use of either neuroleptic or antianxiety medications, such as haloperidol or lorazepam, to establish a level of calm and relaxation in the child that will enable further evaluation and the inception of appropriate psychiatric treatment.

INTERNALIZING DISORDERS

Children who are experiencing either acute or long-standing stress may develop behavioral and emotional reactions characterized by anxiety, fearfulness, self-deprecation, and withdrawal. These children may further develop psychiatric syndromes that are characterized as internalizing disorders and are associated with marked preoccupation, decreased academic and social functioning, and resistance to new events, as well as fearfulness that is persistent and difficult to comfort. These disorders are more common in children who have a generally shy, slow-to-warm-up temperament and who may have demonstrated previously perfectionistic and anxious responses to new circumstances, mildly frightening events, or transitions or change in their lives. Such circumstances as moving, changing schools, or change from school to vacation or vacation to school may be the precipitant of worsening internalizing disorders in children or adolescents. These children may have been significantly close to one or both parents and may have difficulty with separation, particularly if the parent becomes ill or as the child starts a new program or begins school. Several internalizing disorders are recognized in children and are described here.

Obsessive-Compulsive Disorder

Obsessive-compulsive disorder is a persistent difficulty for children and adolescents that is manifested by obsessions, including recurrent or persistent ideas that are experienced as intrusive and outside of the child's control and that lead the child to attempt to neutralize or change these thoughts with other thoughts or behaviors. These behaviors may include compulsive rituals, such as handwashing, clapping, repetitively checking circumstances, or repeating in a patterned way the same behaviors ritualistically. The compulsive behaviors are pursued by the child in a conscious way to ward off or counteract the obsessional and fearful thoughts. These children and adolescents often pursue their compulsive behaviors secretly and are quite resistant to attempts at reassurance or control of their behavior. Children with this difficulty often are embarrassed by their problems and attempt to hide their obsessions and compulsions.

The most common obsessions are repeated thoughts about contamination, repeated doubts, the need to have to do things in a particular order, and aggressive or sexual impulses. These thoughts and impulses are not simply excessive concerns about real life problems and are unlikely to be related to real life situations. The anxiety that the child feels about the obsessions is significant and highly troublesome. It is important to note that children with obsessive-compulsive disorder frequently are very uncomfortable, feel very different from other children, and become easily isolated and develop poor self-esteem. They do not appreciate the difference in their thinking and worries as a disorder but rather experience their obsessions as real concerns that must be neutralized or warded off through their compulsive behavior. It is not uncommon to find parents' attempt to control the repetitive handwashing and patterned behavior with very little success, and the pediatrician may note marked parent–child conflict, mutual mistrust, and disappointment as he discusses these difficulties with the family.

Obsessive-compulsive disorder can lead to significant disturbance in academic performance, social relationships, and self-esteem, and accurate diagnosis and appropriate treatment are extremely important to prevent a persistent pattern of deteriorating function on the part of the child. The compulsions are often time consuming, and the obsessions often intrude on school work, homework, and those physical and intellectual activities the child might enjoy pursuing.

Often with this disorder, as with other childhood emotional difficulties, a pattern has developed where the child acts in a way that the parents perceive as strange and problematic. Parents attempt to control the child's behavior, and the child becomes more secretive and more isolated, and the parents become more frustrated, leading to a significant worsening of the problem. This disorder is usually persistent throughout childhood and often into adulthood, and it has a waxing and waning course, worsening usually at times of stress, transition, or other family difficulties. The waxing and waning course and the child's ability to control the compulsive behavior in some circumstances can lead the parents to be even less sure of what the problem is and more frustrated by its occurrence and persistence. Rapid accurate diagnosis is essential for both the child and family, as it can lead to increased understanding by everyone and decrease frustration and futile attempts at control in addition to providing appropriate treatment.

Obsessive-compulsive disorder usually has its onset in adolescence, although it can begin in the teenage years. It appears to have an earlier onset in boys than in girls and is more common in family members of individuals with the disorder. The degree to which these difficulties are present in different family members often varies. During assessment, it is important to realize that children and teenagers

with this difficulty often develop secondary problems, including depression, significant concerns about their health, other troubling worries, and other evidence of rigidly controlled behavior.

Referral for psychiatric care is essential. Education of both parents and the child as to the nature of the disorder and the fact that it is not controllable by the child and not the result of poor parenting often lessens the family conflicts concerning this difficulty and futile attempts to make it better. Children and adolescents when informed that they have a specific defined problem often feel much less distressed, and as they understand the nature of the problem, they can become less secretive and may feel less controlled by their problem.

Pharmacologic treatment for obsessive-compulsive disorder is indicated in situations where the disorder is persistent and the compulsions occupy a significant amount of the child's time and to reduce difficulties with self-esteem and social and academic adjustment. Medications used for obsessive-compulsive disorder include clomipramine, a tricyclic antidepressant that specifically increases serotonin levels in the central nervous system, or selective serotonin reuptake inhibitors, such as fluoxetine or sertraline. Appropriate doses of clomipramine are titrated to the level of 3 mg/kg or 100 mg/d. Fluoxetine can be used in the liquid form, giving 5 to 20 mg/d for children and adolescents. Fluoxetine is often chosen as the first drug to be used because of its low incidence of significant side effects. Family education, family therapy, and cognitive-behavioral therapy for the child often are necessary. These treatments are designed to help the child recognize the obsessive thoughts as symptoms of a disorder rather than representing real threats and to decrease the automatic attention to these thoughts and modulate the frequency and duration of compulsive behaviors. Other aspects of the treatment plan include specific attention to enhancing social relationships, maintaining academic achievement, and defining and reinforcing other strengths of the child.

Separation Anxiety Disorder

Separation anxiety disorder is a common problem in children of preschool and school age who demonstrate marked distress and anxiety on being separated from parents or parental figures. It is often persistent and is manifested by significant fears, dreams, or nightmares and can lead to both clinging behavior and severe difficulties at times of transition or separation. This includes being left at home with baby sitters, attending school or camp, or playing alone. The child exhibits his distress through complaints, expressions of fear, and finally through significantly upset, demanding, and distressed behavior. A wide range of physical symptoms and somatic concerns are common manifestations of the child's distress, and their occurrence often decreases the need for separation, and, therefore reduces, the child's anxiety.

This disorder occurs most commonly in close-knit and highly involved families. It is more common in children who are temperamentally reserved and slow to warm up and is readily reinforced by parental concern for the child, as well as parental stress. It is likely to be brought on by or exacerbated after a significant trauma or threat to the family or the household. As with other child mental health disorders, the disorder can readily lead to secondary difficulties, including poor social relationships, academic problems especially if school is missed, and family conflict. Often, one parent encourages the child to attend school and appears not to be concerned, while the other parent is worried about the child and believes that the best response is to decrease stress on the child and not require that the child pursue his usual activities. The ensuing family conflict becomes troubling to the family and leads to further isolation of the child, with worsening of the child's anxiety and difficulties with separation.

Other important clues to this diagnosis include the occurrence or exacerbation of the problem at the beginning of school, at the beginning of the school week, or after vacations. Often, these children are brought to pediatricians for physical evaluation after the development of symptoms, such as headache, stomachaches, syncopy, or limb pain. Medical evaluation usually does not reveal an organic pathology to explain the symptoms. Frequently, a family member has had similar physical symptoms. Also, often upon questioning the child and parents it is discovered that separation from parental figures is the precipitating factor in the development of the child's physical symptoms. Children with separation anxiety may have an underlying chronic physical illness, which increases the child's and parents' sense of the child's vulnerability and complicates the medical evaluation. The pediatrician's role is to accurately characterize the child's medical and physical status, to explain the results of the evaluation to the family, to acknowledge the child's distress and the fact that the child's concern leads to real physical symptoms, and to help the family and the child understand that concern about separation is the cause of both the child's anxiety and the physical symptoms and that the concern is significant and requires and will be improved by appropriate mental health treatment.

As in the case of all internalizing disorders in childhood, accurate diagnosis and comprehensive knowledge about the difficulty presented by the pediatrician to the child and family in a clear fashion is extremely helpful in reducing everyone's concern. They also can eliminate futile attempts at controlling the symptoms and familial distress caused by uncertainty and conflict about appropriate responses to the child's problem. As the family appreciates the position of the pediatrician and his reassurance that the child is physically in no danger, they can begin to develop a compassionate and comforting understanding of their child and can develop a firm approach to ensure their child's participation in normal academic and social activities.

Referral for family-oriented psychotherapy is indicated in situations of separation anxiety disorder when the pediatrician's reassurance about the child's physical well-being and definition of the problem is not enough to reduce the child's anxiety and to assist the family in helping the child pursue regular, normal activities. Psychotherapy for the family also can assist in identifying and decreasing other family stresses, resolving intrafamilial conflict, and assisting the family to develop a straightforward, patient, and consistent response to the child's concerns. Once the family learns to accept that expectations of separation will concern the child, they can develop methods of reassuring the child while decreasing their tendency to become upset when the child is anxious.

As the pediatrician stresses the importance of continuing with school and normal activities, he can reinforce the child's developing confidence as the child learns to manage the distress that occurs when separation is necessary. In some situations, the involvement and support of preschool or school personnel can be extremely important in assisting the child in calming and adapting to school. The school nurse will need to be informed and encouraged to allow the child a few moments to relax and return to class if anxiety leads to the development of functional physical symptoms within the school setting. This disorder occurs more commonly in families where apprehension and concern about the child's well-being are prevalent.

Although the severity of symptoms associated with this difficulty may decrease as the child gets older, these children might persist in becoming anxious and concerned at times of separation or significant parental difficulties. If the family understands that worry about separation is a feature of their child, they will be able to develop methods of planning for separations and responding to unexpected separations with patience and understanding. Psychopharmacology is rarely necessary in the treatment of this disorder. However, at times of severe persistent distress, tricyclic antidepressants, such as imipramine, are helpful in reducing the child's distress and assisting the child and family in pursuing appropriate individual and family psychotherapeutic treatments.

Posttraumatic Stress Disorder

In recent years, there has been increasing awareness of the impact of severe trauma on children and adolescents. Following the return of soldiers from Vietnam, there was recognition of a specific syndrome of persistent severe worry and psychiatric symptoms in combat survivors. It has become apparent in the last 20 years that children who are the victims of overwhelming unexpected trauma also experience persistent emotional symptoms. The traumatic occurrence is necessarily outside the realm of normal stresses and may either be a single catastrophic event, such as a kidnapping, the occurrence of threat of imminent physical violence, or a severe accident or violent event, or may be persistent, as in the case of repeated physical or sexual abuse.

Children who have experienced severe trauma may respond by developing a constellation of emotional and behavioral symptoms classified as posttraumatic stress disorder. These difficulties include excessive emotional response to change or minimal threat, development of nightmares and other sleep disturbances, hypervigilance and marked sensitivity to the environment, mistrust of others' motives or behavior, and intrusive, unexpected, and troubling recollections of the traumatic event. The child with posttraumatic stress disorder not only develops these symptoms but also attempts to avoid situations that remind the child of the traumatic event and makes a significant effort to avoid thinking about or discussing the traumatic event or its aftermath. The child may have difficulty recalling circumstances associated with the trauma or describing the events that occurred. These children may become markedly irritable and may have frequent unexpected outbursts of anger, especially in situations that remind them of the trauma. They may have trouble concentrating, and their school performance, social relationships, and participation in normal activities may decline. The child may develop depression and worsened self-esteem and become isolated.

The family usually is aware of the trauma that has occurred, and the traumatic circumstances have been extremely distressing for parents and siblings, thereby worsening the family's ability to discuss the trauma and support and comfort the child. Parental guilt may color the response to the traumatized child. The child's sleep disturbance, irritability, hypervigilance, and distress when reminded of the trauma unexpectedly can further worsen the family situation, leading everyone to become easily distressed, hyperresponsive, and difficult to calm. Often, children who have been seriously abused will experience hearing one or more extremely threatening voices in their head, usually involving threats if the abuse were to be revealed. The occurrence of these voices is further distressing for the child and may lead both parents and physicians to erroneously consider the child to be psychotic. Children with posttraumatic stress disorder do not have the difficulties in relating or appreciating reality that psychotic children have and are able to participate in conversations, activities, and social relationships when they do not feel threatened.

A thorough history is the essential feature of the evaluation of children with posttraumatic stress disorder. Suspicion of this diagnosis is raised when these difficulties are persistent, when the pediatrician sees the child as frightened but unable to explain why, and when the characteristic difficulties with sleep, hyperarousability, and marked irritability, as well as fluctuating behavior and emotional response, are present. It is important to remember that the child will find discussing the trauma extremely difficult and may indeed be unable to recall the event or describe specific aspects of the traumatic circumstance. In situations where the child's behavior and emotional response lead the pediatrician to consider posttraumatic stress disorder and there is no history of overwhelming trauma, the physician will need to be extremely suspicious of the possibility of abuse. Parents can be questioned concerning this possibility in a straightforward and sensitive fashion. Pediatricians can act in a preventive fashion when unexpected, overwhelming trauma occurs in their community or they are treating children who are victims of significant accidents or injuries. The experience of witnessing violence should lead pediatricians to develop a preventive and supportive response to the child along with the family and school personnel.

The pediatrician's role in the evaluation and treatment of posttraumatic stress disorder involves accurate diagnosis and referral for comprehensive individual and family psychotherapy. If the pediatrician suspects that posttraumatic stress disorder is the appropriate diagnosis, he will be able to inform both the family and the child that the child's reactions and behaviors are a common response to severe trauma and that with effective treatment and supportive care, children do recover from the effects of the traumatic events. It is important that family members participate actively and supportively in treatment and work together to reduce the impact of their distress and guilt on the child.

The central feature of the psychotherapeutic treatment for posttraumatic stress disorder is assisting the child in recognizing the intrusive memories, flashbacks, and nightmares to be a direct result of the traumatic occurrence, ensuring the child's safety, and developing soothing responses for the child when distressed or threatened. As the child begins to understand that the current emotional difficulties are the result of a previous trauma and is able to appreciate his and his family's ability to maintain his safety, he can develop methods of calming himself as well as experiencing the calming responses of others. This reduces the child's excessive arousal and vigilance. Another primary goal of treatment is to assist the child in developing an understandable account of the events of the trauma, which the child can discuss, and to assist him in gaining competence in mastering the emotional response to the memories and creating greater distance between himself and the horrifying experience. Since treatment and recovery will depend on the child's current experience of being accepted and safe, it is important that the pediatrician assist the parents in avoiding angry and excitable responses to the child's current distress and disturbing behavior. Medications may improve mood, reduce arousability, and decrease anxiety. Either tricyclic antidepressants, such as imipramine, or selective serotonin reuptake inhibitors, such as fluoxetine or sertraline, are helpful in reducing the child's emotional reactivity and promoting the child's participation in mental health treatment.

Children who have been severely traumatized or who experienced or witnessed events of violence and who have not yet developed the symptoms of posttraumatic stress disorder may be assisted by patient explanation of their current safety, by being given opportunities to discuss calmly what has happened, and by receiving the support and comfort of family members. It is essential that the pediatrician ensure to the fullest extent possible that the child is protected from further experiences of trauma or violence. If abuse is occurring, the pediatrician must file a report with the appropriate social service agency.

Phobias

It is not uncommon for children to experience fears associated with a specific object or situation. The feared object may include spiders, snakes, receiving injections, or concern about being in situations where they might embarrass themselves. The fears may be completely specific and have little impact on their behavior or development, or they may become generalized and lead to refusal to participate in normal and necessary activities. Exposure to the fear's stimulus almost invariably produces an immediate anxiety response on the part of the child that may be expressed through crying, tantrums, marked withdrawal, or clinging behavior and usually results in avoidance of the feared stimulus if at all possible. If the child is frightened in social circumstances, normal events, such as speaking in class, asking for dates, and interviewing for jobs, may become extremely distressing and may be avoided, thus interfering with further development.

As in other situations of excessive anxiety, pediatric evaluation and treatment require accurate recognition of the problem, involvement of the parents in effective treatment, and a clear explanation to the child of the nature of the problem and the goals of treatment. Treatment must include assisting the child in participating in normal activities, developing strategies for determining his own safety, and calming himself in order to be able to deal with the phobic stimulus as necessary. Parental responses will need to include firm insistence on continued participation in normal activities, clear understanding and explanation to the child about the nature of the fears, and calm reassurance of his safety.

For all internalizing disorders, education of the parent and appreciation of the child's temperamental tendency to become worried and patient emphasis on continuation with normal activities, coupled with calming and reassurance of the child, are essential parts of treatment. If the pediatrician recognizes that the child's fears are significantly interfering with daily life or development or the pediatrician experiences difficulty in assisting parents in developing a consistent response to the child's fearfulness, referral for family and individual psychotherapy is indicated. Also, in situations where significant family stresses or intrafamilial conflict complicates the family's response to the child's fears, family-oriented psychotherapy will be necessary. For all child mental health disorders, the presence of marital conflict or unresolved difficulties associated with separation and divorce can complicate and exacerbate the child's symptoms and make treatment more difficult.

EXTERNALIZING DISORDERS

Marked behavioral disturbances characterized by disregard for adult authority, defiance, and aggressive or destructive behaviors are among the most challenging and troubling psychiatric problems of children and adolescents. Children with marked conduct disorders often are difficult to trust and relate to, are unpredictable and threatening, and may be disruptive in a variety of settings, including home, school, and neighborhood. These children also create responses in adults that are rejecting and critical, worsening the child's situation. A temperamental tendency toward marked impulsivity, easy arousability, and heightened reactiveness often characterize these children and may lead to traumatizing and excessive responses on the part of parents or other important adults. These difficulties vary in severity, frequency of disturbed behavior, and the impact of the behavioral disturbance on others. Two forms are recognized in children and adolescents, oppositional defiant disorder and conduct disorder.

Oppositional Defiant Disorder

This difficulty is characterized by emotional and interpersonal disturbances that usually occur at times of adult imposition of control or direction over the child. The child frequently argues, acts defiantly, and is angry, resentful, and easy to upset. The child may act deliberately to annoy or disturb people, particularly parents or siblings, and may be spiteful or vindictive in behavior both when angry and when frustrated. This form of difficulty usually begins in the home, generally has a course of increasing frequency, and may extend to defiance and angry outbursts at school or in school or neighborhood activities. It is not associated with other behavioral disturbances or antisocial acts, and the results of the disorder may be poor self-esteem and worsening school performance. There may be progression to further difficulties with behavior and the development of a worsening antisocial style. Onset is usually during early to midchildhood, and it is more common in males than in females.

The pediatrician's role in families where a child is significantly oppositional is to identify the difficulty and ensure the family's participation in mental health treatment. Treatment will require consistent participation on the part of the entire family, a clear understanding and appreciation of the child's general behavioral style, and slow and steady imposition of consistent and patient parental setting of limits. Since oppositionality in a child occurs more commonly in families with at least one adult member with significant psychiatric difficulty, treatment of the parents and involvement of the parents in the treatment of the child are essential. Behavioral interventions, such as the consistent application of timeouts, expected consequences for misbehavior, and strategies to disconnect from arguments and refrain from excessive physical or verbal responses to the child's anger and defiance, are central features of treatment. Consistent supervision of the child is necessary to reduce the chance of worsening of the problem and development of further behavioral difficulties. Psychopharmacology is generally not effective in reducing the child's anger or defiance yet may be helpful in decreasing secondary symptoms, such as depression or anxiety, that may develop because of worsening of the child's self-esteem and of the child's failure in normal activities.

Conduct Disorder

As the child's behavioral disturbance extends beyond angry responses, tantrums, and verbal and behavioral defiance to include other antisocial, aggressive, or destructive events, the child or adolescent is considered to have a conduct disorder. This may have onset in either childhood or adolescence and consists of a persistent pattern of behavior in which the rights of others or rules and social norms are violated over a prolonged period of time. Behaviors that are frequently demonstrated by children and adolescents with conduct disorder include aggression to people and animals, intimidation, fighting, use of weapons, cruelty, and theft. The aggression also may include forcing sexual activities with the same or opposite sex victims. Other forms of disturbed behavior include destruction of property, theft, deceitfulness in order to obtain goods, or serious persistent violation of rules, including truancy, running away from home, or staying out late at night against parental direction. Conduct disorder is more commonly seen in males and seems to occur in as many as 5% of boys in some communities. In evaluating the child who demonstrates severely disturbed, violent, or destructive behavior, it is important to appreciate the cultural and community norms where the child is living and to appreciate the child's motivation in participating in the antisocial behavior.

Conduct disorder may occur in children with attention deficit disorder and may coexist with significant mood disorder, especially depression, in isolated adolescents. It is an extremely difficult problem to treat, and the prognosis for children with conduct disorder often is poor. A further problem that frequently complicates conduct disorder in late childhood and adolescence is substance abuse, and all children evaluated for behavioral disturbance or antisocial acts will need evaluation for the use of drugs and alcohol. Many children with conduct disorder have experienced excessive physical discipline or physical or sexual abuse, may have witnessed violence in their homes or neighborhoods, and may have experienced severe criticism, lack of effective supervision, and marked fluctuations in parental response, varying from permissiveness to neglect to excessive punishment. In evaluating the family of children with conduct disorder, one often finds significant psychopathology in parents, severe marital conflict, and parental antisocial behavior or substance abuse. Especially in adolescence, children with conduct disorder are at significant risk of self-inflicted harm or suicidal behavior, especially when caught after an antisocial act or incarcerated.

All children with conduct disorder will require referral for mental health treatment. They also may need special education services and may require assistance from the legal system in receiving treatment and developing consistent responses to disturbed and disturbing behavior. Children with conduct disorder may have coexisting learning disabilities and a history of academic failure as a result both of difficulties in learning and of poor school attendance caused by truancy.

Accurate diagnosis, rapid inception of consistent and persistent mental health treatment, involvement of parents, and effective supervision and follow-up are essential hallmarks of effective treatment of conduct disorders. No specific psychopharmacologic agent has been identified to reduce the incidence of disturbed behavior, although lithium carbonate may be useful in decreasing the explosiveness, and antidepressants may be helpful in decreasing secondary mood disturbances. If conduct disorder is occurring in association with either attention deficit disorder or substance abuse, effective treatment of these difficulties is essential. Generally, the treatment of conduct disorder is highly problematic, often associated with parental hopelessness and inconsistent participation. Family-oriented psychotherapy associated with parent effectiveness training and leading to the consistent application of discipline, effective supervision of the child, refusal to accept excuses for aggressive, destructive, or violent behavior, and strong encouragement of the child's participation in and success in academic and social activities are necessary. If effective supervision and parental consistency cannot be established, psychiatric hospitalization and long-term residential treatment are often used. For these children, however, frequent moves from one location to another and experiences of isolation and rejection often worsen the problem.

Pediatric care for children with externalizing disorders should always include effective education of parents, recognition of early responses to family stress that decrease parental consistency and availability, and preventive programs in school settings. The pediatrician should be aware of these children's responses to trauma and aggressiveness and work to support school and community collaboration in establishing and maintaining norms of behavior for all children.

SUICIDE

Suicide is the third leading cause of death among adolescents and young adults. The incidence of suicide has risen significantly in the last three decades, and the occurrence of suicidal behavior in children has increased significantly. Suicidal ideation and suicide attempts in children and adolescents represent a true medical emergency and require an immediate and concerted pediatric and psychiatric response. The evaluation and treatment of suicidal children and adolescents is often complicated by responses of family members and school and health care personnel. It is essential to recognize that any child or adolescent who is actively contemplating suicide or has made a suicide attempt is significantly troubled and in need of both effective medical treatment for the results of the suicide attempts and compassionate and effective mental health treatment for the underlying emotional and behavioral difficulties. Suicidality is frightening and disturbing to others, leading to impulsive and erratic responses, further worsening the clinical situation. Because children and adolescents who are considering suicide have felt isolated and unsupported and have experienced the distress of others, they often will request confidentiality or secrecy concerning their suicidal impulses and may be reluctant to discuss or disclose them or rapidly deny suicidality following disclosure or a suicide attempt. These children and adolescents often leave pediatricians and other health care personnel confused and disoriented as they engender compassion for their difficulties and reject help when it is provided. This typical response often is based on the experience of causing distress to already stressed family members and engendering criticism from parents concerning their distress.

Suicidal ideation often is persistent and may have been present for several months before a suicide attempt. However, usually the children do not discuss their self-destructive impulses and the suicide attempt can then appear to occur suddenly and inexplicably. Suicide attempts are often precipitated by an acute traumatic event, such as school failure, rejection by peers, failure to obtain a sought-after position, or incarceration following a behavioral transgression. Females attempt suicide more commonly than males, but males complete suicide more commonly than females. White males have the highest suicide rate in adolescence, followed by white and African American females, with African American males having lower suicide rates. Native American adolescents have a dramatically higher rate of completed suicides than other teenagers. Risk factors for suicidality in adolescence include previous suicide attempts, mood disorder, significant conduct disturbance, family history of attempted or completed suicide, and the presence of guns in the household. The pediatrician should be aware of the fact that 50% of American households have guns, and, therefore, an essential aspect of evaluating and treating children and adolescents who are suicidal includes inquiring about the presence of guns in the house and requiring that the parents remove the guns from the home so that they are not accessible to the child.

For children and adolescents, the degree of lethality of the suicide attempt is not an accurate gauge of the degree of suicidality on the part of the child or teenager, nor is it in any way an effective predictor of future suicidal behavior by that child or teenager. Therefore, the pediatrician should always respond in an involved and concerned manner to any child who admits to suicidal ideation or makes a suicide attempt. Pediatricians should be prepared to inquire about self-destructive thoughts or impulses in their evaluation of any child who has unexplained physical symptoms, appears sad or stressed, or demonstrates emotional or psychologic concerns. Inquiring about suicidality never increases the possibility of completed suicides, and not inquiring both reduces the possibility of effective treatment and increases the child's or adolescent's experience of isolation and distress. As the pediatrician learns of suicidal thoughts or becomes aware of suicidal behavior, it is important that he inquire about both chronic and acute stress, appreciate the nature of the child's concerns, and recognize the degree of hopelessness and impulsivity on the part of the child.

It is always essential that parents be informed of suicidal thoughts or behavior and that referral for effective mental health treatment be initiated. Studies of high school adolescents have demonstrated that less than 10% of children who make suicide attempts ever receive mental health treatment, and it is not uncommon for children to downplay the seriousness of their difficulties after admitting to suicidal ideation or making a suicide attempt. Teenagers, in particular, are fearful of mental health treatment and often work extremely hard to deny the existence of problems or minimize their seriousness until a significant acute stressor occurs that raises the possibility of an impulsive suicide attempt.

The pediatrician should be aware that as many as half of completed adolescent suicides occur under the influence of alcohol or drugs, and evaluation of any suicidal adolescent will, therefore, require consideration of substance abuse or use and monitoring to decrease the possibility that substance use will lead to disinhibition and a potentially lethal suicide attempt.

Suicidal children and adolescents often are exquisitely sensitive to the degree of stress and disruption in their household and feel that their best response to family stress is to keep their problems to themselves. Parents, therefore, may be unaware of the degree of distress that the child or adolescent may be experiencing and will be surprised and frightened by the child's suicidality. Often in these situations, the parents may have been working extremely hard to shield the child from their difficulties and experience a significant amount of guilt and failure as they become aware of their child's self-destructive thoughts or impulses. The parents may be extremely distressed by the child's actions, and parental anger at suicidal children and adolescents is not uncommon.

The pediatrician who finds himself in the middle of a frightening situation, such as upset parents with a disturbing child who denies his difficulties, may feel at a loss as to how to proceed and can be overwhelmed by the problem. In these circumstances it is essential that the pediatrician have trusted psychiatric consultants who are readily available, willing to provide assistance, and able to see the child and family in an emergent fashion. The pediatrician must provide supervision during necessary medical treatment, especially if the child needs hospitalization, and that supervision will need to be provided in a caring and humane fashion. Mental health treatment for suicidal children and adolescents may require psychiatric hospitalization depending on the degree of the child's impulse control and emotional support and supervision from the family.

The pediatrician's responsibility in these situations is to straightforwardly expect the family to participate in outpatient treatment throughout the course of resolution of the child's difficulties and to emphatically encourage the family to follow through with treatment regardless of its difficulty, cost, or disruption. Psychiatric treatment will always involve attention to family stresses and assistance in dealing with losses within the family, imposition of effective impulse control, and support for competence and achievement on the part of the child or adolescent. If a significant mood disorder is identified, psychopharmacology using either tricyclic antidepressants or selective serotonin reuptake inhibitors is an important part of treatment but not the only part of treatment. Because of the potential for overdose of antidepressant medication, it is essential that an effective partnership among family, child, and mental health professional be established before psychopharmacologic treatment.

Involvement of school personnel is a necessary part of treatment to provide the child with sufficient support, with reinforcement of

achievement and competency and opportunities to decrease the experience of isolation in school. The prognosis for suicidal adolescents depends to a great degree on the underlying disturbances identified and their effective treatment, as well as the consistent participation of the entire family in the treatment process. The pediatricians' role in the identification of suicidality in children and adolescents cannot be underestimated, and their effectiveness in arranging and supporting treatment is often instrumental in producing a successful outcome.

CONCLUSION

Pediatricians play many roles in the lives of children and their families. By compassionately understanding significant emotional and behavioral problems in children, providing accurate information, and optimistically encouraging and reinforcing mental health treatment, the pediatrician plays a most important role in promoting development and adaptation and reducing morbidity and stigma.

REFERENCES

1. American Psychiatric Association: Diagnostic and Statistical Manual of Mental Disorders, 4th ed. Washington, DC, American Psychiatric Association, 1994.
2. Lewis M (ed): Child and Adolescent Psychiatry: A Comprehensive Textbook. Baltimore, Williams & Wilkins, 1991.
3. Rutter M, Herson L: Child and Adolescent Psychiatry: Modern Approaches, 2nd ed. Oxford, Blackwell Scientific Publications, 1985.

AUTISM

SUZANNE SUNDHEIM, M.D.
MARK REBER, M.D.

Autism is a disorder characterized by striking deviations from the normal course of development in language, social interaction, play, and cognition. Strictly speaking, it is a behavioral syndrome defined by a number of characteristic, observable behaviors. The causes of autism are varied, and the neurodevelopmental abnormalities that give rise to the syndrome are still poorly understood. Treatment of this disorder is complex, multidisciplinary, and lifelong. Its efficacy depends on accurate, early diagnosis and the family's access to specialized services.

Autism is classified as a pervasive developmental disorder. It is defined and diagnosed using specific criteria from internationally recognized diagnostic systems (ICD-10, DSM-IV).

DIAGNOSIS

To make the diagnosis of autism in a child, there must be impairment beginning before age 36 months in three areas: reciprocal social interaction, communication, and behavior. Social deficits may be evident in difficulty with eye contact and mutual sharing of another's pleasure, lack of spontaneous imitation, absent or abnormal social play, and lack of interest in or awareness of others' thoughts and feelings.

In the domain of communication, there is a broad clinical spectrum. The child can be nonverbal (about half of autistic children do not develop speech). When language is present, it may lag behind other areas of development. Persisting echolalia is a common phenomenon. Pronoun reversals, for example saying "you" when "I" is intended, occur. Odd, stereotyped, and idiosyncratic usage may be meaningful only to those who are familiar with the child's past experiences. Prosody (rhythm, rate, and intonation of speech) may be affected. Speech pragmatics and the ability to sustain conversation may be impaired.

Behavior is characterized by rigidity, repetition, and restricted range of interests. The child may react to minor environmental changes, such as the furniture being moved, with severe distress or a tantrum. Motor stereotypies, including hand flapping, peculiar hand movements, rocking, dipping, and swaying movements of the whole body, may occur. Some children engage in self-injurious behaviors, such as head banging, biting, and scratching. There may be a fascination with movement or with the sound an object makes while it spins. A youngster can become oddly attached to specific objects, such as a piece of string or plastic tubing.

The pediatrician plays a critical role in helping autistic children receive proper treatment. Early diagnosis is associated with better prognosis if appropriate interventions are started promptly. At the same time, because of the profound social and emotional ramifications for the individual and the family, this is a diagnosis to be given only after serious consideration and evaluation. Very often, the diagnosis is made over time.

If autism is suspected, referral to a specialized center or to individual professionals experienced with autism is essential. The diagnostic process should be undertaken by a multidisciplinary team and include screening for specific neurologic disorders and sensory deficits, intelligence testing, and a speech and language assessment. Decisions about whether to obtain neuroimaging studies or an EEG or specific laboratory evaluations should be determined by the clinical picture and the need to rule out specific disorders. Associated medical conditions include neurofibromatosis, Goldenhar syndrome, Moebius syndrome, lactic acidosis, hypothyroidism, rubella embryopathy, herpes encephalitis, cytomegalovirus infection, congenital hydrocephalus, and infantile spasms.

Some genetic syndromes have an increased incidence of autism: fragile X syndrome, tuberous sclerosis, untreated phenylketonuria, Williams syndrome, XXY, and hypomelanosis of Ito.

It is important to note that standardized developmental and intelligence testing with autistic children is both possible—if appropriate instruments are used by skilled evaluators—and necessary. The presence of autistic features, such as stereotypies, must always be interpreted in terms of a child's developmental level. It is inappropriate to diagnose autism if a child's symptoms can be attributed to severe or profound mental retardation. Many children, however, have both autism and mental retardation. Two thirds of children with autism function in the mentally retarded range. Their treatment and prognosis are determined largely by their level of intellectual function.

The differential diagnosis of autism is broad and includes, in addition to mental retardation, neurodegenerative disorders, childhood schizophrenia, such other pervasive developmental disorders as Asperger syndrome and Rett syndrome, hearing impairments, specific developmental speech and language disorders, severe neglect and abuse, Tourette syndrome, and attention deficit hyperactivity disorder.

TREATMENT

There is no cure for autism. The goals of treatment are to support the most normal possible development and communication, to promote learning, to eliminate or modify behaviors that interfere with learning, such as rigidity, stereotypies, and social withdrawal, and to help the family cope with raising a child with a severe and devastating disorder. The role of the pediatrician is largely one of case manager: to follow the autistic child through life and ensure access to services as the child develops and family needs change. The pediatrician can also be a trusted counselor and friend and provide specific interventions, such as pharmacotherapy.

The best approach to treatment is a comprehensive treatment plan that includes treating the associated medical conditions, education, behavior management, and language and social skills training. Treatment must begin as soon as the diagnosis is made, whatever the age of the child.

Education

Under federal laws, children with autism are entitled to "zero to three" early intervention programs administered by a designated agency (either health, social service, or education) in each state and to special education in public school programs from age 3 through

21. Autism is recognized as a separate category under PL 101-476, The Individuals with Disabilities Education Act of 1990.

The education program must be in a highly structured environment with a high staff/child ratio. It must include teaching skills in socialization and language training. Through learning about how to socialize and communicate with others, some stereotypic behaviors may decrease. The education plan will need to meet the child at his current developmental level. For example, a 5-year old with an IQ of 50 with language skills of an 18-month old will need a program geared for a mental age of 2½ years with language skills of 18 months.

For the higher functioning, verbal school-aged autistic child, the decision of when and how much to mainstream should be based on the individual child's social and emotional development, as well as on academic skills. Many such children do better in learning support classes with children who have disorders of lesser severity rather than in self-contained classes for youngsters with severe autism and minimal language. They may also be partially integrated into regular classes, with close supervision and emotional support.

A multidisciplinary team that includes teachers and parents as collaborators in a partnership is a very successful strategy. A collaborative effort with open channels of communication among teacher, parent, and the specialists involved will facilitate the development of this alliance.

Speech–Language Therapy

Helping the autistic individual develop improved communication skills must start with an audiologic evaluation and a thorough speech and language assessment. Autism and deafness may occur in the same child. Once this assessment has been completed, specific interventions can be developed. Some children with autism are effective communicators by pointing to objects they want or by leading family members to what they need. Some become effective verbal communicators, and others develop proficiency with formal sign language. Many autistic children never develop verbal language.

Recently, two unproven therapies have been promoted for nonverbal or minimally verbal autistic children. These are facilitated communication and auditory integration training. At present, both interventions have weak scientific support and should be regarded as nonstandard treatments. In the case of facilitated communication, there is recent evidence from controlled studies that the facilitator (a trained adult who supports the autistic child's wrist as he types on a special keyboard) may be the initiator, if unconsciously, of the communications.

Behavior Modification

Of the specific interventions to reduce or eliminate maladaptive behaviors, therapy based on learning theory, or behavior modification, is the best established and most effective treatment. This treatment is generally carried out by teachers and parents under the guidance of psychologists or psychiatrists who have been trained in its use. Stereotypic, ritualistic, maladaptive, and self-injurious behaviors frequently are targeted for behavioral intervention. Behavior therapy can enhance the education program by identifying more adaptive coping strategies and effective communication strategies. Once a behavioral specialist has developed an intervention, consistent implementation at home and at school will be necessary.

Family Support

Family treatment begins with presentation of the diagnosis. Learning that one has a child with autism can be emotionally devastating. If information is not presented in a careful, supportive manner, with provision of time to answer questions (on multiple visits if needed) and suggestion of specific actions to be taken, the parents are likely to refuse to accept the diagnosis and begin a long and futile search for alternative diagnoses or easy cures. The pediatrician who refers a family to a specialized center or other professionals for diagnosis should follow up with that family to determine how they are coping with the news and to provide information and support.

Genetic counseling will be indicated for any specifically determined genetic cause of autism, such as tuberous sclerosis or fragile X syndrome. In addition, parents of children for whom no specific medical cause of autism can be found should be advised of the likely polygenic basis of inheritance and a risk of autism in a subsequent child of about 3%.

Most families will want to seek, and will benefit from, parent support groups. These are run in many communities by local branches of the Autism Society of America, whose national office is in Silver Spring, Maryland. There are, in addition, many other advocacy and support organizations for autistic children and their families.

For the family with an autistic member, there are additional emotional stresses that can impair marital and other family relationships. The family's ability to help members cope in general and achieve developmental goals can be seriously challenged. Supportive psychotherapy can be very helpful and is recommended at such times. Together with the consulting psychiatrist, the parents can determine whether family therapy, couples therapy, or individual therapy will be most helpful.

Medication

Although there is an increasing pharmacologic armamentarium available for the treatment of autism, there is no medication that will prevent or cure autism. In addition, medications alone are inadequate intervention. As part of a comprehensive approach, pharmacologic interventions have been used to treat specific targeted symptoms of autism or co-occurring psychiatric disorders. However, when used on target symptoms, medications should not be the first-line treatment. The context in which the disturbing symptom or behavior occurs must be carefully assessed. Does it occur only at home or at school? What happened before the behavior? How did those around respond? Does there appear to be environmental reinforcement, or is there no change in the behavior in different contexts (i.e., is it an *internally* driven behavior that may respond to medication)? Consultation with a behavioral psychologist should be obtained to clarify these questions. In the past, medications have been used to sedate patients in order to control disturbing behaviors, and this has interfered with the broader goals of treatment. It is more appropriate to use medications to treat target symptoms, such as anxiety and hyperactivity, or comorbid conditions, such as depression. Consultation with a psychiatrist experienced with autistic individuals will be helpful.

Although autism represents the expression of a final common pathway for many different brain-based problems, several different neurotransmitter systems appear to be involved. Intervention with medications that exert their effect on serotonin and dopamine pathways can bring clinical improvement to some people with autism.

Drugs that increase serotonin neurotransmission, such as selective serotonin reuptake inhibitors (SSRIs) and serotonin agonists, have been used successfully in autism. SSRIs include fluoxetine (Prozac), sertraline (Zoloft), and paroxetine (Paxil). Clomipramine (Anafranil) is a tricyclic antidepressant that also has a valence for serotonin neurotransmission. These medications are efficacious in the treatment of depression and obsessive-compulsive disorder. Decreased serotonin neurotransmission also has been associated with aggression. In some individuals with autism, SSRIs and clomipramine have been helpful in decreasing aggression directed toward self and others. Some studies have shown these medications to be useful in increasing social relatedness and decreasing repetitive behaviors. The SSRIs have few serious side effects and, in general, are well tolerated.

Fenfluramine is a short-term, indirect serotonin agonist that increases presynaptic serotonin release and blocks its reuptake from the synaptic cleft. Long-term administration, however, results in decreased neuronal serotonin. In the 1980s, fenfluramine was touted to be a potential general treatment for autism, but several large, controlled studies in children were completed that did not support its use. This drug is no longer recommended as a treatment for most autistic patients.

Other serotonergic medications, such as lithium and buspirone, occasionally have been helpful in the management of autism. Consultation with a psychiatrist who can supervise their use is recommended.

Dopamine neurotransmitter systems appear to be involved in autism. Dopamine antagonists have been shown to decrease disruptive, maladaptive behaviors in autistic children. Dopamine agonists, conversely, have been shown to exacerbate stereotypies. There is one major class of medications that targets the dopamine systems, the neuroleptics. In autistic individuals, neuroleptics, such as haloperidol (Haldol), pimozide (Orap), and thioridazine (Mellaril), have been efficacious in decreasing hyperactivity, irritability, social withdrawal, and aggressive behavior. However, they have a serious side effect profile. Short-term side effects include acute dystonia, which can be a frightening and, at times, life-threatening experience. Long-term risks include dyskinesias, which occur in about one fourth of autistic children treated for months to years and may not be reversible. Although neuroleptics have been found to decrease stereotypic behavior and social withdrawal and to increase orientation to requests in autistic individuals, the risks of excessive sedation, acute dystonia, and dyskinesia limit their use. In addition, neuroleptics lower the seizure threshold and can complicate seizure control.

Stimulants are dopamine agonists used to treat hyperactivity. They may also aggravate stereotyped behaviors and induce mood changes. Methylphenidate (Ritalin) has been shown to be helpful in controlling hyperactivity and improving attention in some children with autism.

Norepinephrine neurotransmitter systems have not been found to be primarily involved in autism. Tricyclic antidepressants affect norepinephrine systems (along with other systems) and can be helpful in the treatment of hyperactivity and anxiety in autism. Two other medications that act on norepinephrine systems, beta-blockers and clonidine, have had some limited success in managing the behavioral symptoms of autism. Beta-blockers have been used in the mentally retarded population to treat aggression. Studies have had small sample sizes, and usually the individual also has been on mood-stabilizing medications or neuroleptics. Beta-blockers are contraindicated in asthma, diabetes, and cardiac conditions. Clonidine (Catapres) is an alpha$_2$-noradrenergic agonist that acts centrally to inhibit norepinephrine neurotransmission. In autistic children, clonidine has had a modest effect in decreasing irritability and hyperactivity. Tolerance and loss of the clinical improvement may occur. Side effects include sedation, particularly in the early weeks of treatment, and hypotension. Clinical effects may not be evident until 4 to 6 weeks.

Neuropeptides are a new frontier in the treatment of autism that is currently being explored. One theory hypothesizes that self-injurious behaviors are internally driven events in individuals who have a decreased sensitivity to pain and who perform self-injurious behavior to provide sensory stimulation. Naltrexone (Trexan) is an opiate antagonist used in autism to treat self-injurious behavior. Studies with small groups of children receiving naltrexone have reported increased verbalization, attentiveness, eye contact, and decreased stereotypies.

A practical approach to pharmacotherapy of autism is to select medications for specific symptoms (Table 1). Seizures, which occur in 20% to 25% of autistic youngsters by adolescence, should be managed as in any other patient with seizures. Hyperactivity can be treated with methylphenidate, 0.3 to 1.0 mg/kg per dose in three doses per day. If stereotypies worsen or the child becomes cranky, clonidine, 0.15 to 0.3 mg/d in divided doses can be substituted or added. Tricyclic antidepressants are useful for anxiety and may serve as a third-line medication for hyperactivity. ECG monitoring is essential, especially as doses are titrated upward. Typical doses are 1.5 mg/kg/d of nortriptyline and 3 mg/kg/d of imipramine. Recommended ECG parameters and risks of tricyclic use are presented in texts of pediatric psychopharmacology.

Compulsive and repetitive behaviors can be treated with SSRIs, such as fluoxetine, 2 to 20 mg/d. The liquid preparation of this medicine makes low dosing possible. Self-injurious behavior may respond to SSRIs or can be treated with neuroleptics or opiate antagonists. Possible medications for severe aggression are beta-blockers

TABLE 1. Medications for Symptoms Associated with Autism

GENERIC NAME	TRADE NAME	DOSAGE*
Methylphenidate	Ritalin	0.9–3 mg/kg/d
Clonidine	Catapres	0.15–0.3 mg/d
Nortriptyline	Pamelor	1.5 mg/kg/d
Imipramine	Tofranil	3 mg/kg/d
Fluoxetine	Prozac	2–20 mg/d
Propranolol	Inderal	20–640 mg/d
Haloperidol	Haldol	0.5–4 mg/d
Thioridazine	Mellaril	20–200 mg/d

*These dosages represent typical daily doses and, depending on the medication, may be given at different intervals. Many of these medications need to begin at a lower dose and be gradually titrated up to the recommended dosages.

(propranolol, with dose titrated upward from 10 mg b.i.d. to as high as 640 mg/d in divided doses, as long as bradycardia and hypotension do not ensue) and neuroleptics (haloperidol, 0.5 to 4 mg/d, or thioridazine, 20 to 200 mg/d in one to three doses). Although useful for a wide range of symptoms, the neuroleptics generally should be reserved as agents of last choice.

SUMMARY

The pediatrician plays a crucial role in helping the individual with autism. As the primary care physician, the pediatrician is likely to be the first to suspect the diagnosis. Throughout the child's development, the physician will be there in an ongoing capacity as primary care provider, advocate, and as coordinator of treatment provided by the many specialists involved in the child's care. The pediatrician may also use medication to treat targeted symptoms of autism and comorbid conditions, with, and in support of, educational and behavioral interventions.

REFERENCES

1. Baron-Cohen S, Bolton P: Autism: The Facts. Oxford, Oxford University Press, 1993.
2. Werry JS, Aman MG: Practitioner's Guide to Psychoactive Drugs for Children and Adolescents. New York, Plenum, 1993.

TICS AND TOURETTE'S SYNDROME

RICHARD M. SARLES, M.D.

TICS

Tics are recurring, rapid, sudden, stereotyped, nonrhythmic, involuntary movements or vocalizations *(DSM-IV)*. There is, however, a broad range of movements and vocalizations encompassed in the total spectrum of tic disorders, ranging from simple transient tics to the complex chronic tics of Tourette's syndrome. In general, all tics are exacerbated and aggravated by emotions, may be voluntarily controlled to some degree, disappear during sleep, and are more common in boys than girls.

There seems to be some familial component in that families with one tic disorder are at higher risk for other tic disorders and obsessive-compulsive disorder.

Tic disorders occur in three distinct patterns, although there may be continuity from one to another in certain cases.

Transient tics may be seen in 5% to 10% of all school-age children. The tics usually are simple twitching, nose movements, and eye blinking or throat clearing and simple vocal noises. Such tics may last a few weeks or over a year and often come and go and are undiagnosed or mislabeled as attention deficit hyperactivity disorder or misdiagnosed as allergic rhinitis. Transient tics are diagnosed by clinical history and observation. The best treatment is reassurance and patience, as the great majority of such tics disappear with age.

Chronic tic disorders, in contrast, usually persist over many years and is generally unchanging in presentation. Chronic tics in childhood and adolescence may be relatively unnoticed by peers and teachers, since they are often disguised by the patient by incorporation into daily living habits. No treatment is particularly helpful for this disorder, although behavioral techniques, including hypnosis, may be useful to aid the patient in suppressing the tics during school or social situations. Anxiolytic medication and psychotherapy may be indicated during particularly stressful periods, which often accentuate tic disorder.

TOURETTE'S SYNDROME

Tourette's syndrome is characterized primarily by multiple motor and phonic tics. Symptoms often become manifest around puberty and generally are most intense and troublesome during adolescence. Symptoms of Tourette's syndrome generally lessen during adulthood, but the disorder usually persists throughout life, with exacerbations and remissions. Some cases become physically, socially, and emotionally crippling, and neuroleptics are then the treatment of choice. Tourette's syndrome has an association with attention deficit disorder with and without hyperactivity, specific learning disabilities, and affective disorder, and up to 40% of Tourette's syndrome patients have comorbid obsessive-compulsive disorder.

The treatment of Tourette's syndrome is primarily pharmacologic, although behavioral techniques, hypnosis, and psychotherapy often are very helpful to reduce anxiety and aid the patient in suppressing symptoms in social situations. The most efficacious medications are the neuroleptic dopamine blockers (such as haloperidol). Haloperidol is often effective at low doses, and patients are started at 0.5 mg/d, slowly increasing as necessary to 1 to 3 mg/d in two divided doses. For nonresponders, higher doses of 5 to 10 mg/d are required, but significant side effects, such as cognitive impairment, akathesia, drowsiness, weight gain, dystonic reactions, and the potential for tardive dyskinesia, at these higher doses usually restrict full therapeutic trials.

Pimozide, a neuroleptic derivative of diphenylbutylpiperidine, also is used to treat Tourette's syndrome, starting at 1 mg/d and increasing as necessary to a maximum of 6 to 10 mg/d. The side effects of pimozide are similar to those of haloperidol except for one important difference. Up to 20% of patients taking pimozide may manifest T-wave inversions, U waves, Q-T prolongation, and bradycardia on the ECG. It is recommended that pimozide be discontinued in such instances. Monitoring is required with pimozide and includes baseline ECG, routine periodic ECGs, and ECG whenever doses are increased.

Clonidine seems to be effective in about 40% of patients with Tourette's syndrome and is especially useful in diminishing complex motor or vocal symptoms and improving attention problems. Clonidine is an alpha-adrenergic agonist. It is generally started at a low dose of 0.05 mg/d and slowly titrated to 0.15 and 0.3 mg/d over a several week period. Beneficial effects on the tics may not be seen for several weeks, but a calming effect in temperament may be noticeable earlier. Sedation and irritability are major side effects, which may lessen after several weeks. Other psychosocial factors secondary to the tic disorder may require psychotherapeutic interventions to help the patient and family deal with the primary tic disorder and to minimize stress, which often exacerbates and exaggerates the disorder.

PSYCHOSOMATIC ILLNESS

MORRIS GREEN, M.D.

Psychosomatic symptoms in pediatric patients are most commonly caused by a psychogenic pain disorder, a conversion reaction, or an underlying emotional illness, such as depression. Psychogenic pain is defined in DSM-III-R as a "clinical picture in which the predominant feature is the complaint of pain, in the absence of adequate physical findings, and in association with evidence of the role of psychosocial factors." In children and adolescents, this disorder may be characterized by recurrent abdominal pain, chest pain, headache, or musculoskeletal complaints. It is essential that psychogenic pain be accepted as real. Any implication that the physician regards the symptom as imaginary or " in the child's head" should be studiously avoided.

Psychogenic pain disorders are most effectively approached through an assessment of the stressors that a child or adolescent is experiencing and through an understanding of the family and community context in which the patient lives. In these cases, the most effective diagnostic and psychotherapeutic tool is the pediatric interview. Parents and child may be seen together initially, but the older child and adolescent also should be interviewed alone. In addition to eliciting the data necessary to arrive at a diagnosis, the interview concurrently establishes the therapeutic alliance essential for success.

A conspicuously meticulous physical examination offers both diagnostically useful information and an opportunity for reassurance. A thorough examination also underlines the physician's serious attention to the complaint. Because parents and older children may talk more freely during or after the physical examination, important supplementary information may be forthcoming at this time.

When the physician suspects that the presenting complaint has a psychogenic etiology, it is important that this possibility be breached at the start of the visit with a comment such as, "In my experience, this symptom sometimes has a physical cause, but it may also be caused by the many stresses that children (adolescents) are experiencing these days. Sometimes both causes are operative. It's my practice to consider all these possibilities."

Both organic and psychosocial possibilities should be considered simultaneously. In most cases, ruling out an organic cause before exploring possible psychologic and developmental etiologic factors is not a useful approach. Since needless procedures tend to reinforce psychogenic pain, laboratory or x-ray examinations should be limited to those judged by the physician to be essential to clarify the diagnosis.

A psychogenic disorder is to be considered when the description of the complaint does not fit an established organic disease, when the reason for the patient's being seen remains unclear to the physician, when the symptom has been accompanied by frequent absence from school, when the report of the symptoms seems exaggerated, when somatic complaints involving several body systems are reported, and when the complaint has led to multiple investigations and hospitalizations.

The presence of current or recent stressors commonly associated with psychogenic pain disorder in children should be explored in the interview. These include such separation experiences as the death or the anticipated death of a significant person, parental separation, divorce, or remarriage, and a family move with loss of the child's friends and the need to enroll in a new school. Other family stressors include a physical or emotional illness of a parent, grandparent, or sibling, parental alcoholism, marital discord, family violence, lack of mutual understanding between parent and child, and economic hardship.

Possible etiologic factors include a child's inability to make friends, a lack of social skills, learning problems, difficulty expressing anger in a constructive fashion, pressure for achievement, long-term illness or handicap, being different, peer pressures, entrance to middle or junior high school, and physical or sexual abuse. The child may have learned that his parents will respond in a caring fashion to somatic complaints but seem unaware of feelings, such as depression, anxiety, or anger. The interview provides an opportunity for parents, who may have been preoccupied with other matters, to focus for a time on their child, the events in his or her life, and family interactions in a clarifying and, hopefully, insight-producing fashion.

These stressors are often spontaneously reported by the parents or child during the interview. Since parents are usually unaware of the historical data required to understand and manage psychologic problems or are hesitant to disclose such sensitive family matters as parental alcoholism or family violence, trigger questions may be used to augment the information initially volunteered. Also, many parents do not make the connection between the child's symptoms and stressful family events.

It is often useful to ask why the patient was brought in at the present time: "Mrs. Smith, Monica's pain has been present for some time, and I was just wondering why you wanted me to see her today?" To avoid having the parent leave the consultation believing that the physician overlooked a diagnosis or test, the following questions are often appropriate. "Susan has had this pain for some time now, and I'm sure that you have been thinking about what may have caused it. Although I realize that's why you brought her to see me, I was just wondering what you have thought might be the cause." "Usually patients come to see the doctor with some thoughts as to what will be done. What were your expectations?" If examinations mentioned by the parents are not to be ordered, the doctor should explain why he believes they are unnecessary. Because psychogenic pain may mask school resistance, the question, "Just how much school has her pain caused Susan to miss?" may identify the real problem that needs urgent attention.

It is also helpful if, in the course of the interview, it is the parent who first raises the possibility of a psychogenic etiology: "Could it be her nerves, Doctor?" Rather than reply immediately in the affirmative, even though that is the physician's initial impression, it is best to have the parents explain what they have in mind. "Well, I guess that's a possibility. You may be right. Tell me why you think that may be the case." This approach, in which the parent suggests a psychosocial cause, usually leads to a successful therapeutic outcome.

Once the contributory stresses have been identified in the interview and good communication and understanding exist in the family, improvement often ensues without further professional help. The findings may be presented in a summary statement, such as, "Mary is obviously a bright, sensitive girl. We wouldn't want to change that even if we could. But with her sensitivity, it's natural that some of the things that you have been telling me may have led to her pain. What we have to do now is try to lessen some of those stressors."

Another explanation may be presented as follows. "It sounds from what you have told me that this problem started with a viral infection. However, with the symptoms persisting so long, it's probable that some of the stresses that we've been talking about may have prolonged the problem." In other cases, when unalterable adverse circumstances, such as death or divorce, are etiologic, the physician can discuss with the parents and child how they might better cope with a situation that will not change.

Directive advice may be appropriate for other families. The parents may need to be referred for medical or psychiatric help or for marital counseling. A tutor may be suggested for the child with a learning problem. More involvement by the father with his son may be indicated. Ways to improve family communication may also be suggested. Increased sensitivity to the child's feelings may be another assignment for the parents.

Psychosomatic symptoms commonly accompany other childhood emotional disorders. Thus, depression may be the cause of a persistent headache, fatigue, anorexia, or insomnia. Anxiety may cause recurrent diarrhea or daytime enuresis. Anger may be associated with some instances of encopresis. In infants and young children, psychosomatic symptoms may include failure to thrive, rumination, anorexia, constipation, and hyperactivity.

Occurring most commonly in school-aged children and adolescents, the symptoms of a conversion disorder may be acute or insidious, persistent or intermittent. They include paralysis or weakness of an extremity, abnormal gait, aphonia, whispering, stridor, anesthesia, paraesthesia, pain, hyperventilation, dysphagia, and pseudoseizures. In some cases, identification with a significant person who has or has had a similar complaint may account for selection of the specific symptom. A precipitating stressful event, such as sexual abuse, a family crisis, a critical school examination, an acute illness, an injury, or surgery, often can be identified. Since the conversion mechanism is an unconscious one, the parents and the child usually do not spontaneously link the symptom with the precipitating stressor.

Diagnosis requires the simultaneous identification of psychologic factors consistent with a conversion reaction and the exclusion of an organic etiology. On the other hand, organic disease and a conversion disorder may coexist, and the symptoms suggestive of a conversion reaction may instead be an early manifestation of an organic disorder, such as a brain or spinal cord tumor. The attitude of la belle indifference is not a reliable diagnostic marker for a conversion reaction.

The prognosis is best when the onset of the conversion disorder is acute, a precipitating stressful experience can be clearly identified, the child has previously been emotionally healthy, and the family is able to accept a psychologic etiology. Psychiatric or psychologic consultation may help resolve the problem.

COMMON SLEEP DISORDERS

RONALD E. DAHL, M.D.

Sleep-related problems occur frequently in children and adolescents. Numerous well-controlled studies have documented prevalence rates for significant sleep problems ranging from 20% to 30% in community samples as well as pediatric clinic populations. In many cases, disturbed sleep is simply a mild behavioral problem in an otherwise healthy child. In other cases, however, sleep-related symptoms may represent a serious disorder, such as narcolepsy, or may be one component in a larger set of emotional or psychiatric symptoms. In addition, the relationship between sleep and behavioral/emotional problems appears complex. That is, behavioral and emotional problems can contribute to sleep disturbances, and, conversely, inadequate sleep can adversely affect mood and behavior. Given these complexities, treatment decisions should be balanced with consideration of further assessment, especially in the older child or adolescent with persistent sleep problems.

SLEEPLESSNESS IN THE VERY YOUNG CHILD

Difficulties in going to sleep and staying asleep are most often related to sleep-onset associations (learned and conditioned factors associated with going to sleep). Some infants learn self-comforting behaviors (such as thumb-sucking, face stroking, body rocking, hair twirling), others use transition objects (pacifier, teddy bear, blanket), and others cue to a parental behavior (such as being held or rocked). It is important to understand that all infants and children normally wake up multiple times at night but put themselves back to sleep uneventfully using the same self-comforting techniques or cues used to go to sleep initially. Children who fall asleep while being held, rocked, or fed may require the same parental interaction to go back to sleep following normal nighttime arousals. Optimal treatment for sleeplessness in the young child usually consists of behavioral techniques focused on helping the child develop *self-comforting behaviors* to substitute for parental comforting behaviors at sleep onset. This topic has been well reviewed by others.[2]

PARTIAL AROUSALS (NIGHT TERRORS, SLEEPWALKING, CONFUSIONAL AROUSALS)

Partial arousals from deep nonrapid eye movement (non-REM) sleep may manifest as night terrors, sleepwalking, sleeptalking, or confusional arousals. (Enuretic events occurring in the first 1 to 3 hours of the night also may be related to partial arousals.) Partial arousals occur commonly from age 3 to 8 years, developmental ages corresponding with the greatest amount of intensity of deep stage 4 sleep. Stage 4 sleep is the deepest sleep in humans, usually occurring in the first 1 to 3 hours after sleep onset. The transition out of stage 4 to light sleep can fragment into a mixed state of arousal (partially awake and partially in a deep sleep). The character of these partial

arousals can vary from mild events (a few awkward movements or calm mumbling) to intense events (a full-blown night terror with agitated running and screaming). The episodes typically last from 30 seconds to 10 minutes and usually terminate with an abrupt return to deep sleep, with the child having no memory of the event in the morning.

There are four important factors in treating partial arousals.

1. Reassuring the parents as to what these events are. (The events can be extremely frightening to parents because children can appear awake but confused and unresponsive.)
2. Explaining to the family that the events are physiologic, they terminate spontaneously with return to deep sleep, and there is no advantage to trying to awaken or shake the child during the event.
3. Instructing the family to ensure physical safety for children having frequent or intense events. (Although self-injury is rare, a safe physical environment is required, as these children are essentially asleep and can become agitated.)
4. Ensuring optimal nighttime sleep.

The role of adequate nighttime sleep in partial arousal events is a crucial point. Any factor that can result in "overtiredness" in a child (such as giving up a daytime nap, erratic changes in bedtime and wakeup time, the need to get up early for day care, or disturbed nighttime sleep) can contribute to partial arousal events. The physiologic adaptation to getting less sleep (or to chronically disturbed sleep) is an increase in the *depth* of stage 4 sleep. Increased depth of sleep makes the transition out of stage 4 more difficult and is more likely to result in a partial arousal event. *Thus, increasing the total amount of sleep (by 30 to 60 minutes a day) over 1 to 2 weeks can dramatically decrease the frequency of partial arousal events.* Similarly, removing the cause of a chronic sleep disturbance (such as a tonsillectomy in a child with sleep apnea) can produce a rapid resolution of partial arousals. Nighttime medications (e.g., theophylline) and medical conditions (e.g., atopic dermatitis or conditions with chronic pain) can also cause chronic sleep disturbances and resulting partial arousals.

One additional factor that can negatively feed into the cycle of partial arousals is the role of children being overly "wound up" during the day. Although the mechanism is unclear, children with a large degree of unexpressed anxieties and worries are more prone to partial arousals. Helping these children express their anxieties and concerns (therapeutically) has been documented to resolve partial arousals in some of these cases. There is also evidence that mental and emotional state just before falling asleep may be important in the occurrence of night terror. Thus, helping children feel safe, relaxed, and focused on positive thoughts and images as they are falling asleep can have a positive effect.

When optimal nighttime sleep has been achieved and intense partial arousals continue, medications can be an important adjunct to treatment. Benzodiazepines and tricyclic antidepressants are effective in decreasing the depth of stage 4 sleep and suppressing partial arousals. Diazepam (at a dosage between 1 and 2 mg at bedtime) and imipramine (10 to 50 mg at bedtime) have been used successfully in treating these events. At our center, we have had success using clonazepam (0.25 mg at bedtime) in some very severe cases (with multiple partial arousals every night). It is important to caution that there are no controlled trials to guide the use of pharmacotherapy for this disorder. Further, tolerance (the need to increase the dose over time) and rebound effects (severe partial arousals when the medication is discontinued) can be significant.

OBSTRUCTIVE SLEEP APNEA SYNDROME

Children with enlarged tonsils or adenoids often have increased breathing difficulties during sleep (especially during REM sleep, which causes a significant loss of muscle tone to airway and accessory muscles). Children with Down syndrome, micrognathia, hypotonia, some cleft palate repairs, and other maxillofacial conditions are at increased risk for obstructive sleep apnea syndrome (OSAS). Snoring, restless sleep, and signs of chronically disturbed sleep (daytime somnolence *or* irritability) are important signs suggesting OSAS.

Three important points are relevant to treatment decisions in OSAS in children.

1. The size of the tonsils and adenoids alone is *not* a good predictor of which children will have breathing difficulties during sleep.
2. The loudness of snoring is *not* a good predictor of respiratory difficulties, as some children with severe apnea are reported by parents as just "noisy" breathers.
3. There are two domains of disturbances in OSAS—the degree of breathing impairment (number and length of apneic events) *and* the degree of chronic sleep disturbance. This last point is often overlooked in treatment decisions. Chronically disturbed sleep in *prepubertal* children often occurs as irritability, difficulty with concentration, emotional lability, and impulsivity. These children are often difficult to awaken in the morning, but once up, they can appear hyperactive and may not look somnolent during the day. We have seen numerous children with OSAS receiving stimulant medication for their "attention deficits." Although stimulants do improve symptoms resulting from inadequate sleep, proper treatment requires removing the cause of sleep disturbance. *Tonsillectomy and/or adenoidectomy is the treatment of choice for most children with OSAS.* In other cases, nasal continuous-positive airway pressure (C-PAP) or oral devices to maintain airway patency may be indicated. More involved surgery, such as uvulopalatopharyngoplasty (as used in adult apnea), does not have a proven role in childhood OSAS.

SLEEP–WAKE SCHEDULE DISORDERS

Adolescents frequently develop very late sleep–wake schedules during summers, vacations, and weekends, often "sleeping in" until midday. For many of these adolescents, trying to realign their circadian systems to early school schedules is analogous to jet lag. Many of these adolescents have great difficulties falling asleep at night and are unable to get up on time for school. Severe problems can result in repeated school tardiness and school failure. In some cases, the problem is straightforward: the adolescent is having trouble consistently complying with an earlier bedtime. In other cases, however, even though the adolescent and family are highly motivated to shift to earlier hours, the adolescent has difficulty falling asleep because the circadian temperature rhythm (and timing of physiologic "tiredness") has not been successfully shifted to an earlier hour. A central concept in treating this problem is understanding the circadian regulatory system, which has difficulty adjusting to an *earlier* phase unless changes are small, gradual, and *consistent*. As with jet lag, different components of the system can readjust at different rates and may require 2 weeks on a new schedule to *stabilize* at the earlier time. The problem for many adolescents is that after working hard toward an earlier schedule for a few nights, they revert back to their late night (sleeping-in) schedule on weekends. *Successful treatment requires a structured behavioral contract specifying bedtimes (with lights, television, and music out), exact wakeup times, and avoidance of all naps for a 2- to 3-week period, including weekends*. Encouraging the adolescent to take responsibility for the schedule with appropriate rewards and consequences is important. Parents' roles should be simply enforcing the contract, not fighting with the adolescent to get up in the morning. Early morning activity and exposure to bright light (such as a walk outside) are important adjuncts to shifting rhythms to an earlier phase. In severe cases involving very late schedules, it can be easier to use successive *delays* in schedule by 3 hours a night (essentially going all the way around the clock until bedtime lines up with early clock time). This technique (called chronotherapy) has been used to treat many adults with delayed sleep phase syndrome. A detailed description of a program for adolescents has also been described.[1]

REFERENCES

1. Dahl RE: Child and adolescent sleep disorders. *In* Kaufman, DM (ed): Neurology for Child Psychiatrists. Baltimore, Williams & Wilkins, 1992:169–194.
2. Ferber R: Sleeplessness, night awakening, and night crying in the infant and toddler. Pediatr Rev 1987;9:69–82.

BREATH-HOLDING SPELLS

Israel F. Abroms, m.d.

Breath-holding spells occur in 4% to 5% of all children. The more common form is the cyanotic or "blue spell." This occurs following an emotional event and vigorous crying. The child holds his breath, becomes cyanotic, and loses consciousness. The last is probably caused by hypoxic ischemia involving the brainstem. Occasionally, a generalized tonic-clonic seizure may occur, followed by limpness. Breath-holding spells usually occur between the ages of 4 months and 4 years. Occasionally, they persist to 6 years of age. The frequency of cyanotic breath-holding spells can be reduced if a concomitant anemia (usually an iron deficiency anemia) is treated with oral iron preparations. A misdiagnosis of epilepsy can be made, but the electroencephalogram (EEG) in cyanotic breath-holding spells is normal.

There is no specific treatment for cyanotic breath-holding spells. Parents need to be reassured that these episodes will eventually disappear. Some parents are reluctant to discipline their child when necessary for fear of precipitating a cyanotic breath-holding episode. It is most important that the child's consultant address this issue by reassuring the family that they should treat this child as any other.

A less frequent type of breath-holding spell is the *pallid form*, also called a "vagal attack." The child often has a mild injury, and within seconds, even without any true breath-holding, pallor, bradycardia, and unconsciousness will develop. Because of cerebral hypoxic ischemia, a generalized tonic-clonic seizure may ensue, followed by limpness. Often there is a family history of syncope. Occasionally, prolonged seizures occur. This usually is associated with a family history of a lowered seizure threshold.

The EEG in these children is normal. With electrocardiographic (ECG) monitoring, ocular compression for 10 seconds performed during the ECG may result in bradycardia or even asystole that will last beyond 4 seconds. This test is not always confirmatory, however, and should be performed with care because prolonged asystole can occur.

A fair number of children exhibit both the cyanotic and pallid forms of breath-holding spells. An ECG or a prolonged period of Holter monitoring may be required to distinguish these from cardiac events.

In the pallid form, the differential diagnosis should include cardiac arrhythmias, such as sinus node dysfunction with either bradyarrhythmia or tachyarrhythmia. Sinus node disease occurs following surgical correction of congenital heart defects or may be associated with neuromuscular disorders, such as myotonic dystrophy, limb girdle muscular dystrophy, or Friedreich's ataxia in the older child. Cardiac inflammatory disorders need to be ruled out, such as acute rheumatic fever, viral myocarditis, and diphtheria. However, in many patients with sinus node disease, no definitive etiology is recognized. Intermittent atrial ventricular block may be present, and the syndrome of prolonged Q-T interval may be found on the ECG. The latter can be associated with congenital nerve deafness. It is frequently familial, with the disturbing history of recurrent seizures and sudden cardiac deaths.

If any of these cardiac conditions are suspected, the child requires a cardiologic consultation, an ECG, and an echocardiogram. Radiologic studies may be indicated.

If pallid breath-holding spells are occurring frequently, the infant or child may benefit from treatment with oral atropine sulfate (0.01

to 0.02 mg b.i.d. or t.i.d.). Occasionally, these spells are so prolonged that the infant requires a cardiac pacemaker.

ATTENTION DEFICIT DISORDER

JOEL E. FAGAN, M.D., F.R.C.P.(C.), M.Sc.

Children with attention deficit disorders may show a large number of problem behaviors and learning impediments. There is considerable clinical heterogeneity within this diagnosis. All children with this disorder share a weakness of selective attention, defined as a functionally significant inability to reliably and predictably choose as the focus of their attention that which most contributes to their success, learning, and pleasure. This attentional weakness most commonly manifests itself in a short attention span, abnormal distractibility, and impaired task completion. In addition, there are other symptoms, which often coexist but are not invariably present, that add to the functional disability and emotional burden borne by the child and shared by the parents and other family members, other caregivers, and teachers. These symptoms include hyperactivity, insatiability, impaired socialization, poor reinforcibility, impulsiveness, daydreaming, an exaggerated link between motivation and productivity, emotional lability, disturbed sleep patterns, and other impediments to learning, such as reading impairment. The lives of many affected children are marred by chronic success deprivation and conflict. Therefore, early recognition and effective treatment are important concerns, recognizing that at least 3% of children are affected, a significant majority of whom are males.

ISSUES IN THERAPY

Optimally, a multimodal treatment plan should be implemented that includes the following components: (1) establishment of a secure relationship with the patient and parents, (2) establishment of a good working relationship with the child's teachers, (3) taking of an advocacy role in communicating with the child's school, (4) teaching parental strategies to use with the child, (5) recognition of the possible need for involvement of other disciplines, and (6) medications.

The establishment of a secure relationship with the patient and the parents often requires considerable time spent in interpretation, consolation, alleviation of guilt and blame, explanation of treatment options, and reassurance about the safety and appropriateness of pharmacotherapy. This time is essential for ensuring trust and compliance.

It is necessary to establish a good working relationship with the child's teacher(s). Many teachers become fatigued and perplexed in response to the challenges of dealing with recurrent underproductivity and disruptiveness. They may conclude erroneously that the child has a primary disorder of character or motivation. The physician can be an invaluable ally to the child and family in reframing problematic behavior and academic performance as symptoms of this condition. The sharing of written material on attention deficit disorder can facilitate this process.

A treatment plan includes taking an advocacy role on behalf of the child in communicating with the school to ensure that the child receives suitable consideration for supportive services, which may include placement in a smaller class, special seating, subdivision or reduction of assignment size, remedial teaching, and measures to protect the child from humiliation in the classroom.

Parental strategies to lessen conflict and narrow the gap between performance and expectation might include ensuring eye contact during communication, providing the child with a quiet workplace at home, segmenting complex tasks into smaller components, acknowledging success systematically, formal behavioral modification techniques, sheltering the child from experiences that are predictably unsuccessful or humiliating, and providing the child with compensatory life experiences, such as sports or outdoor pursuits, that more strongly reflect the child's talents and interests. These practical strategies are useful in providing information that forms a framework for the establishment of more realistic expectations of the child and the lessening of environmental emotional stress, since such stress will further weaken selective attention and accentuate the symptoms of the attention deficit disorder. Mindful of this, the physician should seek to understand the meaningful stressors affecting the child and family and to assist in mobilizing available resources to relieve them. The impact of all forms of therapy will be blunted in the presence of pervasive environmental stress.

The physician must recognize that the concomitant problems and direct consequences of this condition may require the involvement of professional colleagues in other disciplines, particularly education, psychology, social work, and psychiatry. Some patients may require individual psychotherapy. Their parents may require marital therapy, or the larger family may be helped with family therapy. None of these counseling and situation-altering strategies will *directly* strengthen selective attention. The only therapy that may do this is pharmacotherapy.

MEDICATIONS

There are several types of medication that may be useful in this condition, but the stimulant medications, which include methylphenidate (Ritalin), dextroamphetamine sulfate (Dexedrine), and pemoline (Cylert), are the safest and most useful (Table 1). Of these, methylphenidate is prescribed most frequently. Stimulants strengthen selective attention directly, without primarily altering mood or other higher order processes. The stimulants provide a meaningful benefit to approximately 75% of children with a primary (endogenous) attention deficit. The symptoms that may potentially be helped are short attention span, distractibility, underproductivity, hyperactivity, impulsiveness, insatiability, internal distractibility (daydreaming), emotional lability, poor reinforcibility, and inconsistency. As a result, the quality of the child's life, both academically and socially, may improve to a meaningful degree.

Side Effects

As a group the stimulant medications are extremely safe and well tolerated. There are two relatively common side effects, appetite suppression and insomnia (Table 2). Less commonly, they produce

---

TABLE 1. Stimulant Medications Used in Attention Deficit Disorder

CHEMICAL NAME (Brand Name)	FORM	ONSET OF ACTION	DURATION OF ACTION (h)
Methylphenidate (Ritalin)	Tablets 5 (USA), 10, 20 mg	20 min	4
	Sustained release tablets (Ritalin SR) 20 mg	20 min	8
Dextroamphetamine sulfate (Dexedrine)	Tablets 5 mg	20 min	4–6
	Sustained release capsules (spansules) 10, 15 mg	20–30 min	12
Pemoline (Cylert)	Tablets 37.5, 75 mg	Gradual onset of action over 2–3 d	Approximately 24

TABLE 2. Common Problems in the Use of Stimulant Medication in Attention Deficit Disorder

PROBLEM	RECOMMENDATIONS
Stimulant-induced nausea or abdominal pain	Give medication with food or milk
Waning efficacy of medication	1. Review medication compliance 2. Inquire regarding increasing levels of emotional stress 3. If indicated, increase dosage
"Rebound" in symptoms of attention deficit disorder following medication effect	1. Consider an alternative stimulant 2. Extend period of medication action by adding an additional dose of short-acting form at 4–6 PM 3. Give sustained release form earlier in the day to extend duration of medication action
Stimulant-induced suboptimal weight gain	1. Offer additional food in nonmedicated hours 2. Offer high calorie dietary supplements in nonmedicated hours 3. Curtail use of medication on weekends, school vacations, and in evening hours
Stimulant-induced insomnia	1. Consider an alternative stimulant 2. Reduce dose of medication, particularly at noon and thereafter 3. When problem is severe and no alternative exists, consider phenothiazine (i.e., thioridazine) or clonidine in conjunction with stimulant
Suboptimal effectiveness or duration of action of sustained release form	1. Consider alternative sustained release product 2. Change to nonsustained release form

headache, nausea, abdominal discomfort, suboptimal weight gain, tachycardia (most evident in the standing position), and very occasionally, reversible slowing of linear growth. Symptoms indicating an excessive dose include undue quietude, passivity, withdrawal, or heightened emotional sensitivity. A dosage reduction will usually alleviate these symptoms, with preservation of the therapeutic effect of the drug.

Patients who are responsive to these medications usually remain so indefinitely. Physical addiction or dependency does not occur. Dosage adjustments are necessary with increasing body weight (Table 3). High levels of personal stress, often created by academic or social success deprivation, will blunt the effect of medication. If there is waning of the effect of a particular medication after a period of seemingly successful use, the physician should ask about stressful life circumstances. Although stimulant responsiveness or nonresponsiveness usually is present for all drugs in this family, occasionally a child who fails to respond to one drug may achieve a superior effect from another. Similarly, if one medication is losing its impact, changing to another in this category may be helpful.

Indications

In any child, if there is a meaningful degree of academic or social underachievement substantially because of a primary (endogenous)

attention deficit disorder, a medication trial should be considered. In the preschool child, a trial should be considered if weak selective attention is impeding the acquisition of school or life skills or if hyperactivity, impulsiveness, or behavioral noncompliance is posing a risk to the child's physical safety or emotional well-being.

Implementing Stimulants

In most instances, the initial drug tried is methylphenidate, in the regular acting (nonsustained release) formulation. A 2-week trial usually is sufficient to gauge its potential usefulness. Two doses may be compared in this interval, 0.4 mg/kg per dose and 0.6 mg/kg per dose, each dose given before breakfast and lunch.

It is most desirable that the anticipated benefits of medication be identified before implementing the trial and that these treatment effects are evaluated as objectively as possible. The input of the parents, teachers, and where possible, the patient should be sought, often through questionnaires. Based on a 2-week trial, further treatment decisions usually can be made. At times, additional dosage adjustments may be necessary to clarify future medication decisions.

Weekend and Vacation Use

If the decision is made to continue medication beyond the trial period, it must be decided whether to prescribe it on schooldays only

TABLE 3. Stimulant Medications Used in Attention Deficit Disorder

CHEMICAL NAME (Brand Name)	DOSAGE RANGE	USUAL MAXIMUM DOSAGE	MOST IMPORTANT SIDE EFFECTS
Methylphenidate (Ritalin)			
Tablets	0.3–1.0 mg/kg/DOSE* 2–3 doses per day	30 mg per dose 90 mg/d	Anorexia, insomnia, slow weight gain, nausea, abdominal discomfort, headache
Sustained release tablets	0.6–1.2 mg/kg/DOSE 1 dose per day	60 mg per dose	
Dextroamphetamine sulfate (Dexedrine)			
Tablets	0.2–0.45 mg/kg/DOSE 2–3 doses per day	20 mg per dose 45 mg/d	Anorexia, insomnia, slow weight gain, tachycardia, elevated blood pressure, restlessness
Capsules	0.45–0.9 mg/kg/DOSE 1 dose per day	45 mg/d	
Pemoline (Cylert)	37.5–112.5 mg/d 1 dose per day	112.5 mg/d	Insomnia, anorexia, slow weight gain, nausea, abdominal pain, headaches; elevations of AST (SGOT), ALT (SGPT), and serum LDH occur in up to 2% of children

*Most children require about 0.6 mg/kg/DOSE.

or on weekends as well. This decision should be made based on individual need. Some children struggle in the classroom but function comfortably in other settings. These children need medication on schooldays only. The majority of children, however, experience frustration, disappointment, and conflict in all settings and benefit from medication most days of the week. In many instances, individual weekend (or weekday evening) doses are best administered based on predictions of probable need, such as before team sports or music lessons.

Prolonging the Action of Stimulants

Both the nonsustained release form of methylphenidate and the tablets of dextroamphetamine sulfate are short acting, lasting 4 hours in the former case and 4 to 6 hours in the latter. The majority of children require two or three doses per day, which may be inconvenient for parents or school personnel and embarrassing for older children required to take medication while at school. In some children, there appears to be a rebound increase in inattention, impulsiveness, irritability, or hyperactivity after school when their medication wears off. Under these circumstances, there are benefits in terms of convenience and compliance in using a dosage form that has a longer duration of action, such as methylphenidate in the sustained release formulation (Ritalin SR: duration of action 8 hours), dextroamphetamine sulfate in the sustained release capsules (Dexedrine Spansules: duration of action 12 hours), or pemoline (Cylert tablets: duration 18 to 24 hours). See Tables 3 and 4 for dosage and precautions.

Compliance Issues

As in any long-term treatment, medication compliance is a potential concern. The following measures may be helpful.

1. Spending adequate time in explaining the diagnosis and the treatment plan
2. Involving the patient as fully as possible in the decision to treat
3. Directing questions regarding benefit and side effects to the patient
4. Advocating on behalf of the student with teachers to ensure that the school provides dignified (nonhumiliating) reminders to take medication at school in younger children and a private place to take the medication, such as the nurse's office or a locking washroom, in the case of older children, who fear the effect on their reputation of their peers knowing that medication therapy is necessary

TABLE 4. Precautions in Using Stimulant Medications in Attention Deficit Disorder

CHEMICAL NAME (Brand Name)	PRECAUTIONS RECOMMENDED
Methylphenidate (Ritalin)	Follow growth in height and weight, heart rate, blood pressure, caloric intake, sleep patterns; ask about the presence of tics or symptoms suggestive of overmedication (passivity, withdrawal, unusual or excessive quietude, and heightened emotional lability)
Dextroamphetamine sulfate (Dexedrine)	As for methylphenidate
Pemoline (Cylert)	As for methylphenidate; also obtain measurements of AST (SGOT), ALT (SGPT), and serum LDH before use and periodically thereafter; discontinue pemoline in the presence of abnormal liver function

5. Prescribing sustained release forms of medication for convenience and confidentiality
6. Providing adolescents an opportunity to discuss the advantages and disadvantages of medication in a confidential and nonjudgmental setting, recognizing that adherence to medical treatment may conflict with the age-appropriate need for independence

Follow-Up Measures

It is essential that children who require medication for attention deficit disorder be properly supervised by their physician. After the initial trial, the child might be seen again in 1 month, 3 months later, and at least twice yearly thereafter. These visits allow the physician to review the child's academic and interpersonal circumstances by means of parental description, report cards, and other written comments by teachers and others. The child's appetite, weight, height, pulse rate (lying and standing), and blood pressure should be measured at each visit, as well as the results of any relevant laboratory investigation. The physician should be reassured that medication remains necessary and is suitably effective in the dosage prescribed.

Since attention deficit disorder is a chronic condition, the physician should anticipate that there will be periods of relative stability and periods of increased difficulty. Dosage adjustments can be considered at these times.

Validating Long-Term Need for Medication

As with any medical regimen, it is most desirable that the treatment be given in the lowest effective dose for the minimum necessary duration. At regular intervals, confirmation should be sought that the medication remains necessary and effective. Often this fact is blatantly apparent from observing the child when one or more dosages are forgotten or omitted. When doubt exists, a short (1 to 2 week) drug holiday should be arranged at a time when the patient, parents, and teachers are in a position to comment on the contrasts between the medicated and nonmedicated states and at a time when the consequences of medication omission are apt to be minimized for the patient (i.e., the drug should not be stopped just before an important assignment or major examination). If it appears that the drug might be stopped indefinitely, the child's academic and social circumstances should be observed closely over many months by parents and teachers, since the impact of subtle changes in selective attention may take weeks or months to become fully apparent.

Adolescent Issues

Adolescence may be a particularly challenging time for individuals with an attention deficit disorder. To the usual tasks and stresses of this period of life are added the burdens of this condition. Deteriorations in mood and behavior may make extra demands on families and teachers and may require the involvement of mental health professionals. Parents should be reassured that medications remain safe and effective during this period and do not produce paradoxical accentuation of symptoms or addiction-dependency problems. Many adolescents develop a subtle emotional discomfort concerning medication use, which in some cases will weaken medication compliance. This discomfort, which is difficult for younger adolescents to articulate, may be rooted in fear of medication safety, apprehension regarding peer derision, or most commonly in the conscious or subconscious wish to be independent of the need for medication and related parental supervision.

In dealing with this discomfort, the physician should acknowledge its normalcy in a nonjudgmental and supportive manner and assist the adolescent noncoercively to compare the costs and potential benefits of further pharmacotherapy. The physician should make every effort to preserve the doctor–patient relationship, regardless of the decision reached.

Medicating Preschoolers

The substantial majority of children who require medication for attention deficit disorder have the criteria for therapy after beginning elementary school. There is, however, a small group of preschoolers with severe attention deficit disorders for whom medication is properly considered. These are children whose severe inattention, impulsiveness, insatiability, and poor reinforcibility create a distinct risk to safety and self-esteem. Others in this group will be hindered in terms of the acquisition of preschool academic skills. Some of these children will be greatly helped with stimulant medication (methylphenidate or dextroamphetamine sulfate).* It is best to start with the smallest doses and increase as necessary as determined by response and side effects. Commonly, formal behavioral management strategies should be added to the regimen, as well as parental respite, recognizing that the demands of these severely affected children may predispose to physical or emotional abuse. In the medicated state, many children will be more attentive and responsive to behavioral management strategies.

The Use of Stimulants in Children with Tic Disorders and Tourette's Syndrome

Current evidence suggests that stimulants do not cause tic disorders or Tourette's syndrome. It is possible that stimulants can prematurely trigger Tourette's disorder in a small number of vulnerable individuals who would have developed this condition in the future. In patients with preexisting simple or complex tics or Tourette's disorder, the introduction of stimulant medication will have no effect on the tics in approximately 60% of cases, will be followed by a lessening of tics in about 10% (presumably because of a reduction in the life stress of success deprivation), and will be followed by a worsening of tics in up to 30% of cases. It must be stressed that this exacerbation of tics is temporary and will be reversed promptly when the stimulant is discontinued or the dosage is reduced.

The question of stimulant use in the individual child with a tic disorder or Tourette's disorder is apt to be complex, necessitating a subjective comparison of risks and benefits. Nevertheless, there are many children with moderate or severe attentional problems, with a coexisting tic disorder, who can be helped to a meaningful degree with stimulants. Some of these children may require additional medication to control their tics.

Nonstimulant Medications

Since about 25% of children with fundamentally primary (endogenous) attention deficit disorder will be unresponsive to stimulant medications, it may be necessary to consider other medications for these children. Some children, particularly those who are highly anxious or depressed, may be helped by tricyclic antidepressants. Drugs in this family include desipramine (Norpramin, Pertofrane), and imipramine (Tofranil). There are certain potential risks associated with their use, including alterations in blood count and liver function, that necessitate periodic laboratory blood testing. This family of medications can have a very disruptive effect on the rhythm of the heart when overdosages are taken. These drugs should be dispensed in containers with childproof lids, and parents must be cautious in ensuring that the medication is given and stored safely.

Recently, there have been reports of four cases of sudden unexpected and unexplained death in children treated with conventional doses of desipramine, which has led many physicians to reconsider the criteria for employing this drug for this condition. It is presumed, but not proven, that the mode of death in these rare cases was cardiac arrhythmia. Consequently, Biederman has recommended that children receiving this drug have periodic blood level measurements, as well as repeated ECGs, in an effort to maximize the safety of its use.†

The potential benefits of the tricyclic antidepressants are their

continuous action throughout the day and the freedom from insomnia and appetite suppression in comparison with the stimulants.

Another family of medications that occasionally can be helpful in the child with severe aggressiveness, moodiness, or insomnia (either as a primary symptom of the attention deficit disorder or as a side effect of stimulant medication) is the phenothiazines. They occasionally can cause alterations in blood count and liver function, so that periodic laboratory tests should be performed.

REFERENCES

1. Levine MD: Developmental Variation and Learning Disorder. Educators Publishing Service, 1987, pp 15–67.
2. Shapiro AK, Shapiro ES, Young JG, Feinberg TE, eds: Gilles de la Tourette Syndrome, 2nd ed. New York, Raven Press, 1988, pp 402–413.
3. Stevenson R, Wolraich M: Stimulant medication therapy in the treatment of children with attention deficit hyperactivity disorder. Pediatr Clin North Am 36:1183–1197, 1989.
4. Wilens TE, Biederman J, Spencer T: Clonidine for sleep disturbances associated with attention-deficit hyperactivity disorder. J Am Acad Child Adolesc Psychiatr 33:424–426, 1994.

DISORDERS OF LEARNING

JANE N. HANNAH, Ed.D.
MARK L. WOLRAICH, M.D.

Within the last 20 years there have been increasing interest and concern for children with learning disabilities. Much of this is because of the increased number of children receiving a diagnosis of learning disability and the work of The Interagency Committee on Learning Disabilities, which presented a written report to Congress detailing their recommendations and findings in 1987. This agency estimated that 5% to 10% of the population has a learning disability. In the 1985–1986 school year, data collected under the Education of the Handicapped Act-Part B revealed that 42.8% of identified and served handicapped children were classified as having specific learning disabilities. This percent is equivalent to 1,872,399 children, as compared with only 120,000 students who were classified with a learning disability before P.L. 94-142, which was enacted in 1975.[1]

P.L. 94-142, entitled Individuals with Disabilities Education Act (IDEA), was the first federal law that recognized learning disabilities. This law mandated services for children between the ages of 3 and 18 (changed to age 21 in 1980) who met the criteria for a learning disability and allocated federal monies to public school systems to provide appropriate educational services. As the major provider of health care services to children, primary care physicians need to understand the nature of treatment for children with learning disabilities. It is of paramount importance for physicians to understand the inextricable relationship between school performance and the provision of health care services.

Because of the complexity and the wide spectrum of learning disabilities, it is imperative that a child be thoroughly evaluated before implementation of treatment. The school system in which the child is zoned, even if he is enrolled in a private school, is required by federal law to provide a multidisciplinary evaluation if a learning disability is suspected. Some parents, however, desire an independent or outside evaluation for the initial evaluation or as a second opinion if they have concerns about the evaluation provided by the school. The pediatrician can assist the parent in securing an evaluation, either by the school or an independent evaluation, by following the steps listed.

1. Take a careful developmental history of the child and rule out any physical problems that might interfere with the child's school performance, particularly auditory or visual impairments.
2. If the parents want the school system to test, the primary health care provider may write a letter to the school system requesting

---

*The manufacturer of methylphenidate has advised against its use in children under the age of 6 years, since safety and efficacy in this age group have not been established. The manufacturer of dextroamphetamine sulfate has recommended against its use in children under the age of 3 years.

†Biederman has proposed the following guidelines concerning desipramine: serum level <300 ng/ml (<1125 nmol/L); ECG PR interval <200 ms; ECG QRS duration <120 ms.

the evaluation, delineating specific concerns. Next, direct the parents to the Department of Special Education in their local school system, where they will submit a written request for the evaluation. The length of time between referral and placement should not exceed 40 schooldays, with interventions being attempted during the interim.

3. If the parents desire an independent evaluation, recommend a reputable professional to complete the assessment. This frequently requires a psychologist, educator, or speech and language pathologist. Health insurance plans may cover the cost of this evaluation, but the parents will need to clarify this. In the case of second opinions, the cost may or may not be covered by their school system.

DEFINITION

Controversies continue to exist in the educational, psychologic, and medical communities relative to the definition and criteria used to diagnose a learning disability, as well as the preferred form of treatment. Although there continues to be no one standardized or consistent definition of a learning disability, schools primarily identify children through psychometric procedures. Simply, a school makes the diagnosis of a learning disability when there is a significant discrepancy between the child's current level of academic attainment in reading, mathematics, written language, listening, or oral expression (based on the results of a standardized individual achievement test) and the child's intellectual ability, as measured on a recognized test of intelligence (e.g., Wechsler Intelligence Scale for Children-III, Stanford Binet, IV Edition). Even if a significant discrepancy does not exist between IQ and levels of achievement on standardized tests, the multidisciplinary team within the school can recommend certification of a learning disability. However, written evidence to support this recommendation must be made.

RISK FACTORS

Results of research support the finding that learning disabilities are associated with certain risk factors. Factors cited in the literature include (1) a very low birth weight, (2) head traumas, (3) seizure disorders, and (4) radiation therapy treatment for long-term survivors of acute lymphocytic leukemia. The primary factor that has been linked to learning disabilities, however, has been the presence of learning disabilities in other family members. Vellutino (1987) suggested that reading disabilities occur more often in near relatives than in the population at large and that they occur more often in twins than in other siblings.[5] Pennington (1991) found that family recurrence rates for dyslexia (a learning disability in reading) was as high as 35% to 45%, as compared with a 5% to 10% rate in the general population.[3]

Considering risk factors can help the primary care physician in identifying high-risk children before the child fails in school. The health care provider may decide to refer a child for testing when the following conditions are present.

1. Family history of reading and/or spelling problems and the patient is also struggling academically
2. Subtle language deficits that are more than developmental delays, despite adequate peripheral hearing and apparent average or above average intelligence
3. History of poor coordination, especially fine motor coordination; preschoolers may be less skilled at drawing and working puzzles and schoolaged children may perform poorly when asked to build things or complete art projects
4. Difficulty learning the letter names and associated sounds out of proportion to intelligence and age

TYPES OF LEARNING DISABILITIES

The type of interventions that are recommended depends on the type of learning disability.

Language Learning Disabilities

The largest group of children with learning disabilities are those with language-based deficits (i.e., reading, written language, listening comprehension, oral expression, mathematical reasoning, memory deficits). The link between language acquisition and language facility on learning to read and write cannot be over emphasized. In early childhood, a child may experience difficulty learning the spoken language. Subsequently, in the early grades, he may have problems learning phonics and in later grades do poorly in spelling and reading comprehension. It is clearly recognized that dyslexia is not the result of visual-spatial or visual perception problems as was once thought when introduced by Samuel Orton in 1925, and mirror writing or letter reversals are not considered to be the cause of dyslexia. Reading disability appears to be the "consequence of limited facility in using language to code other types of information."[5] Research further indicates that deficiencies in visual perception account for the inability to read in only a small group of children. In addition to problems with reading, most children with language-based learning disabilities have difficulty with some component of writing (e.g., written syntax, vocabulary, spelling, or organization).

Visual-Spatial Learning Disabilities

In addition to language-based learning problems, some children have a deficit in visual-spatial cognition and experience significant difficulty conceptually understanding mathematics. These children also often experience significant difficulty with handwriting and frequently are diagnosed with a developmental coordination disorder or motor clumsiness.

Social Skill Deficits

During the last 20 years, there has been growing concern over the number of children with difficulty interacting with peers. A high percentage of these children also have learning disabilities. High correlations exist between children with a social skill deficit and those who experience low self-esteem, poor school performance, juvenile delinquency, and school dropout. Although there is no separate diagnostic category for those with social skill deficits, professionals recognize that the quality of peer relationships may be impaired for the child with a learning disability.

TREATMENT

When making recommendations for treatment, the primary care physician can help the parent understand that there is no cure for a learning disability and there is no one way to offer remedial assistance. The condition is chronic, and every child demonstrates his own pattern of strengths and weaknesses. The course of treatment and progress can change significantly based on many factors (i.e., age treatment begins, intelligence, support from parents and school, motivation of child). There may be cases where it will be important for the primary care physician to work as the child's advocate and help the child's parents to advocate on his behalf, for example, to suggest that the child receive periodic reevaluations (federal law requires a reevaluation once every 3 years for those certified with a learning disability).

Remediation

The best-documented treatment to date for the child with a learning disability is direct educational remediation. This remediation can take the form of special education (e.g., resource placement) within the public school, where an individualized treatment plan will be written (individualized education plan, IEP). For the child with dyslexia, the remediation that has proved to be most effective is individual instruction (tutoring) using a phonics-based approach. Since the primary problem associated with dyslexia is phonologic coding and since it is central to reading development, this instruction cannot be circumvented. Parents are usually ineffective in tutoring or teaching their child with a learning disability, and pediatricians will want to discourage this practice unless it is provided as part of an overall program and is carefully monitored. As the child with dyslexia gets older, he would benefit from instruction in reading comprehension, study skill instruction, and metacognitive strategies (i.e., internal speech or talking himself through a problem, steps or checks on the product, written step-by-step procedure taped to his desk for solving problems) to facilitate learning. If the young child's fine motor skills are severely affected, the pediatrician may consider recommending an occupational therapy evaluation to determine the need for treatment for fine motor deficits.

Compensatory Treatments

There are times when it is more appropriate to recommend compensatory treatment rather than direct remediation. For example, spelling deficits are often less remediable. Thus, a recommended form of treatment includes use of Spell-check programs on word processors or the *Bad Speller's Dictionary*. The use of a word processor or typewriter is appropriate when handwriting deficits are prevalent. This use requires less fine motor or visual-spatial skills than does handwriting.

For the young child with difficulty understanding the concepts in mathematics, manipulables often are helpful. As the child gets older, the use of a calculator may be appropriate. In children with severe reading disabilities, functional reading may not be achievable, and adaptation to auditory means (tape-recorded notes, books on tape, oral examinations) may be required.

Long-Range Planning

Transition planning aimed at preparing the student for adult life is mandated in the Individuals with Disabilities Education Act (IDEA). IDEA requires that planning for secondary and postsecondary education be initiated in middle school and continue through high school for all students with learning disabilities. Domains to be addressed in this planning include education (planning for high school and, if appropriate, for college), personal responsibility, relationships, home and family, leisure pursuits, community involvement, and physical and emotional health. Contributors to this planning process should include the student, parent(s), and secondary and postsecondary education professionals. By being aware of this federal requirement, the primary care physician can inquire of the parent and student if this planning is occurring and, if not, recommend that the family begin the process before the child is an adolescent.

Retention

Physicians are frequently asked if a child should be retained if he is struggling in school. In a Supporting Paper on Retention presented in the National Association of School Psychologists *Communique'*, Rafoth et al. (1988) reviewed current literature on the policy of retention in schools.[4] They reported that retention can negatively affect achievement, social-emotional adjustment, and attitudes toward school. In addition, retention has been linked to later dropping out of school even when controlling for student background and achievement level. They further suggest that although retention may benefit a small percentage of students, it is extremely difficult to predict which students would benefit.

If it has been recommended that a patient be retained, the parents should be strongly encouraged to secure an evaluation first. If a learning problem is diagnosed, appropriate intervention should be planned rather than giving the child more of the same. McLeskey and Grizzle (1992) investigated the rate of grade retention of students with learning disabilities. Fifty-eight percent of the students in their study had been retained before being diagnosed with a learning disability. This rate was approximately twice that of students without learning disabilities. They conclude that "regardless of which alternative intervention is used, it is critical that professionals be aware that the data are overwhelming and nearly unequivocal that students with learning disabilities do not benefit from retention."[2] In light of the growing evidence against the practice of retention, pediatricians and other professionals are strongly encouraged to avoid this form of treatment when at all possible.

Controversial Treatments

The health care provider should be aware of controversial treatments endorsed by certain professions that make broad claims to success. The pediatrician can assist the parent in discerning the validity of certain treatments before they spend large sums of money and receive false hope that their child can be cured. Unsubstantiated treatments frequently recommended by certain groups include visual training, including muscle exercises, ocular pursuit or tracking exercises, neurologic organization training (policy statement from the American Academy of Ophthalmology, 1984), Irlen lenses or colored transparencies, sensory motor integration, chiropractic, medications intended to affect vestibular system functioning, and special diet or megavitamins. Often, parents are so desperate to help their child learn to read that they will spend large sums of money on well-publicized treatments when the efficacy of these treatments has not been scientifically proven.

It behooves each parent and professional interacting with a child diagnosed with a learning disability to help him improve feelings of self-worth. Although academic achievement is often strongly linked to self-worth, there are other skills or talents that need to be discovered. As the child matures, opportunities to openly and honestly discuss the learning disability and its impact on development should be grasped. A better understanding by the child of the diagnosed disability, as well as his pattern of strengths and weaknesses, facilitates more active participation and responsibility toward learning.

SUMMARY

It should be stressed that the characteristics of children with learning disabilities are variable, the condition is chronic, and each child demonstrates his own pattern of strengths and weaknesses.

The interventions should be school-based and tailored to the child's specific needs. Initially, the focus should be remediation, but this may need to shift to compensatory measures in more severe cases or as the child gets older. Retention is rarely helpful, and poor peer relations and self-esteem are major disabling aspects.

REFERENCES

1. Interagency Committee on Learning Disabilities: Learning Disabilities: A Report to the U.S. Congress. Washington, DC, U.S. Department of Health and Human Services, 1987:115.
2. McLeskey J, Grizzle KL: Grade retention rates among students with learning disabilities. Except Child 58:548–554, 1992.
3. Pennington BF: Diagnosing Learning Disorders: A Neuropsychological Framework. New York, Guilford Press, 1991, p 193.
4. Rafoth MA, Dawson P, Carey K: NASP Supporting Paper on Student Retention. Communiqué 1988.
5. Vellutino FR: Dyslexia. Sci Am 256:34–41, 1987.

CHILDREN OF DIVORCING PARENTS

R. Franklin Trimm III, M.D.

Children and divorce have been frequent companions for several decades. Between 1960 and the mid-1980s, the divorce rate in the United States tripled. More recently, information from the National Center for Health Statistics indicates a leveling of the divorce rate for the last several years. In spite of this, there are still 1 million children involved in family dissolution annually. This translates into a total of 12 million children under the age of 18 who have experienced the trauma of divorce at least once.

Although divorce may be the best solution for marital incompatibility and may ultimately provide a more optimal environment for the children in the family, it is also an ongoing loss for them. It initially involves the loss of one parent as a full-time family member. Subsequently, the remaining parent is often consumed with the trauma of the divorce and emotionally unable to meet the heightened needs of the children. At times, the custodial parent may turn to the children for the emotional support no longer available from the ex-spouse, resulting in the loss of yet another parent figure. The custodial parent often experiences a significant decrease in financial support after divorce and may need to return to work or increase the number of hours spent at work, further decreasing the availability to the children. As the custodial parent deals with her own grief and struggles to reorganize and financially support the family, routine discipline often becomes less consistent. The noncustodial parent may have limited contact with the children as a result of custody battles. Even in the absence of such conflicts, many noncustodial fathers become less available and involved as time passes, for a variety of reasons. As the children attempt to adjust with these losses, they often develop negative and disruptive behaviors as part of their coping. These behaviors further disrupt the parent–child bond, making emotional support less available.

Children of divorcing parents have been studied for several decades in an effort to address concerns about the detrimental impact divorce could have on them. In a review of a number of these studies, Long and Forehand indicate that research has taken two approaches: evaluation of the impact of being a child in a single-parent family and clinical research on those individuals who seek out mental health services for assistance in dealing with divorce.[1] Although the generalizability of the results of these approaches are somewhat limited by methodologic concerns, they do provide insights into the divorce process that are relevant to clinicians who take care of children.

It is clear that divorce is not a single crisis but rather a continuum of stress that begins with predivorce parental conflict, proceeds through the legal divorce process, and continues through family reorganization. Longitudinal studies indicate not only that children may have short-term problems dealing with the divorce but also that there may be other emotional upheavals years later as the maturing children begin to establish romantic relationships of their own, even if they initially appeared to adjust easily to the divorce situation. This suggests that assistance from clinicians may be needed over an extended period of time. An apparent uncomplicated adjustment to the divorce should not preclude additional follow-up.

It is also clear that not all children handle divorce in the same way, and neither do these children all have the same outcome. Factors that play a role in how well a child adapts to the family dissolution include a number of individual and situational variables. Important individual variables include age, developmental status, gender, temperament, and resiliency. Critical situational variables include the strength of the parent–child bond, the quality of the home environment throughout all phases of the divorce process, support resources available to the children and parents, the adjustment of the custodial parent to the divorce, and the level of parental conflicts. In order for the clinician to provide useful guidance that will help the parents minimize the emotional trauma of the child as well as anticipate the behavioral and developmental changes that occur as a result of divorce, both the individual and situational variables must be assessed. The relative importance of most of these factors varies from one child to another, but the level of parental conflict and how much of the conflict the child experiences is thought by many investigators to be the most universally significant factor. Children from divorced families that experience high levels of conflict show more pronounced symptoms of maladjustment than children from families whose divorce had low levels of conflict.

Of the individual variables noted, age and developmental status play a critical role in anticipating the needs and interpreting the symptoms of children experiencing divorce.

Although infants and toddlers (0 to 3 years of age) are not likely to be able to understand the complexities of divorce, they are sensitive to the emotional turmoil that is usually involved. The disintegration of the family may interfere with the developmental tasks of attachment and autonomy that are characteristic of this age range. Responses to divorce during this age period include sleeping difficulties, excessive crying, becoming withdrawn, overactivity, being demanding, and regression of emotional and self-help skills. The degree to which these problems occur often reflects the level of distress of the custodial parent.

Preschoolers (3 to 5 years of age) are rapidly developing their language and socialization skills and further refining their self-concept and gender identity. They have a strong perspective of right and wrong, are exceptionally egocentric, and freely incorporate fantasy into their reality. As a result, they will often have an erroneous perception of divorce. Children in this age range will usually blame themselves when a parent leaves, believing that if they had behaved better the parent would not have left. They may try to behave perfectly with the hope that the lost parent will return. They are unable to separate the loss of one parent from the fear that the other parent also will leave. They are also likely to deny that the separation has really occurred and attempt to live out a fantasy of family reunification. Responses to divorce during this age period include regression to earlier behaviors, such as thumbsucking and bedwetting, fear of the dark and being alone, physical and verbal aggression, sadness, confusion, and excessive neediness.

Children in the early elementary school years (6 to 9 years of age) have developed logical thought processes that are usually concrete in nature and enhance their self-concept by achieving academic and social goals and by being industrious. They usually view the divorce as being the fault of only one of the parents. They fully experience the pain and sorrow associated with the divorce and desperately desire the reunification of their parents. Additional responses during this age period include frequent crying, daydreaming, academic deterioration, and problems interacting with peers and superiors.

Children in the later elementary school years (10 to 12 years of age) are developing the ability of abstract thought and have developed a clear sense of moral standards. When confronted with divorce, they usually respond with anger, often toward one parent predominantly. They feel the need to have one parent be the "bad" parent so that they can choose the other one as deserving of their loyalty. Boys, in particular, are likely to exhibit significant hostility to the noncustodial parent. In addition to anger, children in this age range experience feelings of shame, embarrassment, rejection, and loneliness. They are likely to cover these feelings by presenting a front of being brave and strong, by excessively busying themselves in activities, or by becoming dictatorial in their attitude toward others. They may be torn between concerns about financial resources and resentment at having to take on additional chores.

Adolescents (13 + years of age) are shifting from a dependent to an interdependent role with their parents and making a transition into self-sufficiency in society. Responses to divorce during this period range from self-blame and regression to childish behaviors to excessive closeness with the same-sex parent. Adolescents experiencing family disruption struggle with conflicting feelings of anger toward one or both parents and worry about the well-being of the parents. They are at risk of repressing these conflicts by hiding behind a mask of pseudomaturity, numbing the pain with alcohol, drugs, and sex, becoming rebellious, or withdrawing because of depression.

Common to all developmental stages is somatization. All children and adolescents have a limit to the amount of stress they can effectively handle. In addition to the variety of coping mechanisms just described, disturbances in physical and physiologic functions can occur. Headaches, abdominal pain, and elimination and sleep disturbances that are inconsistent with recognized medical disorders may be the only indication to the clinician that a stress as serious as divorce may be occurring.

When a child experiencing divorce is identified, the clinician needs to perform an adequate psychosocial assessment. Issues that should be addressed include (1) parents' and children's concepts about divorce, (2) parents' understanding of children's expected responses to divorce, (3) changes in daily routine and living arrangements that are a result of the divorce, (4) degree of parental conflict, (5) degree of involvement of the noncustodial parent, and (6) availability of social and financial resources for parents and children.

Typically, intervention consists of providing support and accurate information aimed at minimizing the emotional damage the children experience. All knowledge deficits and areas of concern identified in the psychosocial assessment should be addressed. This should include giving the parents age-appropriate information about the likely responses to divorce they will encounter from their children and management suggestions. This can be done through giving advice, recommendation of reading materials, and referrals to mental health services as needed. The children can also benefit from direct exploration of their reactions and feelings to the divorce by a caring professional.

Some general recommendations for parents to consider should include the following. (1) Keep conflicting interactions to a minimum, especially in front of the children. (2) Tell the children about the separation or divorce before the actual departure of a parent, and tell all children at the same time. (3) Reassure the children that both parents love them. (4) Give specific details about plans for visitation with the noncustodial parent and ensure that the plans are carried out as much as possible. (5) Clarify that the divorce is final and that all has been done to reach reconciliation without success (if this has occurred). (6) Encourage the children to talk about their feelings. All expressed feelings should be honored and questions answered honestly. (7) Encourage the children's positive feelings about both parents. Avoid custody disputes that often require the children to take sides. Do not express negative comments about the ex-spouse or argue with the ex-spouse in front of the children. (8) Maintain discipline in both households as normally as possible. (9) Reassure the children that the divorce is not their fault. (10) Be patient in dealing with the children's behavioral problems. Remember that it is difficult for children to maintain self-control when their lives have been disrupted by divorce. (11) Obtain support needed to help themselves adjust to the divorce. Parents will not be able to provide the support their children need unless they take care of themselves as well.

Keeping in mind the developmental issues discussed earlier, the following developmental and age-specific recommendations can be offered. Infants experiencing distress from a divorce situation benefit from consistent and concerned care. The home environment should be kept as predictable as possible. Since the infant will experience the same emotional responses as the mother, it is essential that the mother get the social and emotional support she needs so that she can adequately nurture her infant.

Toddlers will benefit from consistency and predictable limit setting. An environment that is too restrictive or too lenient will likely result in worsening of behavioral problems. The custodial parent's adjustment to the divorce will be mirrored by the toddler. Therefore, the parents should avail themselves of needed help in adjusting to the divorce and the changes it has caused.

Preschool children may require repetitive explanations of the divorce, constant reassurance that they will be cared for, repetitive discussions about the plans for visitation with the noncustodial parent, and constant reassurance that the divorce is not their fault. Regressive behaviors should not be punished. High frequency positive attention given by both parents will help emotional stabilization to occur. A preschooler who shows few signs of adjustment problems or who is behaving much better than expected is probably fantasizing that this good behavior will bring the parents back together. This child needs encouragement and opportunity to discuss his real feelings about the divorce.

Early elementary schoolchildren will benefit from having easy access to the noncustodial parent. Frequent phone conversations that the children have permission to initiate on their own are helpful. Situations that would include both parents together might encourage the children's hopes for reconciliation and should be avoided if this is a problem. Consistent limits need to be set for children of this age. This should include limits on toys and gifts purchased by either parent,

since children may use the situation to manipulate either parent into buying more things than usual. Material objects will not substitute for quality time spent with each parent.

Later elementary schoolchildren will benefit from all the interventions suggested for early elementary schoolchildren. In addition, they need to be able to diffuse their anger about the divorce. This can be done by providing opportunities to discuss these feelings without fear of being punished or experiencing additional losses. A trusted, impartial family friend may be helpful in this. An appreciation of both parents should be encouraged to help deal with the natural anger toward one parent that is likely to occur.

Adolescents usually need a support system above and beyond what the family provides. Ongoing participation in school and social activities should be encouraged. The adolescent still needs the parent to be in a parenting role. Situations that would encourage the adolescent to be either parent's confidant should be avoided. Parents will need their own support systems to prevent this from occurring.

Primary care professionals are uniquely prepared to meet the needs of children of divorcing parents. They can incorporate the physical and psychosocial issues into a single assessment and treatment plan. They are experienced in giving anticipatory guidance, the primary treatment for this situation. They often have established a therapeutic alliance with the family that will enable their support to be effective and increase the probability that their advice will be taken seriously. They often have the opportunity to follow the family through the changes that divorce brings. Thus, a small amount of extra time spent with a family in crisis has the potential of minimizing the emotional trauma of the children and significantly enhancing their long-term outcome.

REFERENCE

1. Long N, Forehand R: The effects of parental divorce and parental conflict on children: An overview. J Develop Behav Pediatr 8:292–296, 1987.

THE CHILD AND THE DEATH OF A LOVED ONE

R. FRANKLIN TRIMM III, M.D.

Assisting in the care of a child who has lost a loved one through death not only is a challenging aspect of providing pediatric health care but also is something the provider can expect to encounter regularly. Few statistics are available to put the frequency into perspective, but obtainable data indicate that 93% of high school students have seen a dead person, 84% have experienced a personal, significant loss, and 10% have lost a parent through death. Among 10 year olds, 5% have lost a parent through death. Health care professionals are often approached for advice regarding child participation in funerals, frustration over and uncertainties about the child's mourning behaviors, and generalized support for dealing with a very difficult situation. Very often, the adult caretaker of the child is experiencing grief over the same loss.

The most important people in helping a child to cope with the loss of a loved one are other adults who are part of the child's immediate circle of support. These are adults who have helped nurture the child and who have established a relationship of mutual trust with the child before the loss—someone the child can turn to without hesitation. This could include a surviving parent, grandparents, aunts, uncles, adult siblings, or very close family friends. The most effective role professionals can play is in providing support and information to the sustaining adult who is attempting to help the child understand and cope with the tragedy and feelings of loss. The professional must realize what an overwhelming task this is for most adults.

Helping the sustaining adult(s) understand how the child conceptualizes death can assist them in addressing death at a level the child might understand, as well as helping them to appropriately interpret the child's responses to the loss. Not all children attain a mature understanding of death at the same age, and neither do all children mature in their understanding at the same rate. Children's grasp of death broadens and becomes more accurate or adultlike in parallel with the maturing of their cognitive abilities, as outlined by Piaget.

From birth to 2 years of age, the sensorimotor stage, the child's concepts of death are limited. However, it is during this time that the building blocks of future understanding are constructed. Experimenting with being and nonbeing through playing peek-a-boo and the mastering of separation anxiety are examples of these blocks.

As the child matures into the preoperational stage, which is usually from 2 to 7 years of age, death is interpreted through the tools of the stage: animism, egocentrism, and magical thinking, with little understanding of causality. Thus, the child may know the words "dead" and "death" but have little understanding of their meaning. Death is thought of as avoidable or reversible, much like sleep or a short separation (magical thinking). Attempting to explain death as "she's asleep" or "he's gone away" can thus be very confusing. As the reality of death becomes evident with time, the child may blame himself for the loss. The death can be interpreted only through the child's existing understanding, which usually centers around himself (egocentrism). The child may need multiple reassurances that he did not cause nor could he have prevented the death. Because of their limited understanding of death, children may not show signs of grief initially and may be viewed by adults as indifferent.

A child from 7 to 11 years of age, the concrete operations stage, develops an understanding of death as irreversible and inevitable for all living things. Children in the younger part of this age group are likely to view the cause of death in concrete terms, where something external to the person causes death as opposed to something intrinsic. Examples of accidents or murder are often given if the child is asked why someone died. Intrinsic causes, such as old age or an illness, are not likely to be given except by children in the older end of this age range. When discussing death with a child in this age range, the possibility of an incorrect understanding of the cause of death should be kept in mind and corrected as necessary.

As a child enters preadolescence and the formal operations stage, 12 + years of age, concepts of death mature to adult levels. The cause of death is understood to be the cessation of physiologic functions as opposed to an external action on the person. Death is viewed as a personal event, although not likely to occur to them until the distant future. When a child in this age range experiences a personal loss, he may show responses more typical of a younger child, since regression is a common response to stress.

There is no exact course of behavior a child should or should not demonstrate after experiencing the death of a loved one. However, there are some generalizations that can be useful in helping the child cope with this stressful experience. Although the acute phase of mourning occurs primarily during the first month after the loss, resolution of the grief may take from 6 months to 2 years.

The manifestations of the acute phase of mourning will vary based on the developmental stages, as described. Additional reactions may include sleep and appetite disturbances, temporary loss of previously gained developmental accomplishments, extreme reactions to separation from the sustaining adult, crying spells, a prevailing unhappy affect, and somatic pain complaints. Any new symptoms should be evaluated in the context of the child's grief and the family's grief without overlooking the possibility of a real organic problem. Signs of concern that should trigger a mental health consultation would include suicidal ideation, complete incapacitation, and persistence of any of the acute grief symptoms beyond 1 month.

A common practice that is often detrimental to the acute grief process is to send the child away until after the funeral. This is likely to cause confusion and prevent the mourning process from beginning normally. Sending a child away is usually done with the intent of

protecting him from the emotional trauma. In reality, the child can easily sense the emotional turmoil of his surroundings and the evasiveness or dishonesty that accompany the sendoff. He would best handle the situation by being told the truth and remaining around familiar surroundings, toys, and people. This may place additional burdens on the sustaining adult, but the sharing of grief can be beneficial for both the child and adult. Concerns about the availability of food and shelter and the well-being and possible loss of surviving family members may interfere with the acute grief process as well. Thus, it is important for the sustaining adult to provide the child with multiple assurances that he will be taken care of and that his remaining family will not abandon him. Remaining with the family in familiar surroundings will help provide these necessary reassurances.

An additional element that can play an important role in the acute stage of grief is the funeral of the loved one. This ritualistic activity is thought to play an important role in facilitating the grief process. In a review of children's reactions to a death in the family, Gardner recommends that children be allowed to attend the funeral because it can provide meaningful information about death and grief.[1] General guidelines for a child's participation in a funeral include the following. (1) An age-appropriate explanation of the activities involved with a funeral should be given to the child before the funeral. (2) The child should not be forced to attend, especially if he shows significant resistance during the explanation. (3) An adult who is not likely to be grief-stricken and with whom the child is comfortable should be with the child at all times during the funeral to provide explanations and comfort. This adult should be prepared to leave the funeral with the child should it become an overwhelming experience.

A child's long-term resolution of grief is not as dependent on a cognitive understanding of death as it is on long-term availability of a comforting, supporting, and understanding adult. The surviving adult family member is likely to be struggling with resolution also. This is an unpredictable and up-and-down process. There are times when the grief is overwhelming contrasting with short periods of apparent coping. It is unlikely that the child and adult will experience these peaks and troughs in unison. In addition, the entire process is overshadowed by a chronic sorrow that slowly improves with time. During this long-term phase, the health care provider may be contacted for a variety of concerns, often behavioral, for which there is no predictable antecedent or course. An explanation of the ups and downs of the long-term grieving process can help put the concerns into perspective. Additional recommendations that can be offered during this period include a variety of books on grief recovery that are available in libraries and bookstores and referral to any available grief recovery support groups in the area. Whereas the support group is most likely to assist the adult, there are books available for all age groups of children and adults. An excellent example is a book for parents by Grollman that teaches how to tell children about death.[2] It includes an example dialogue.

As painful as it may be for a grieving adult to focus on the needs of a grieving child, there is nothing else that can meet the child's needs as effectively. A health care provider who is consulted about a child who has lost a loved one may also find it difficult to focus on the needs of the child and family. This may be because of the presence of unresolved personal grief from the past or sadness related to the current family and its loss. The health care provider can play a supportive and informing role for the family that is unlikely to be matched by another source. Just as a grieving adult is likely to be helped by sharing in the grief of the child, so the professional's grief is likely to be helped by sharing in the sorrow of the child and family.

REFERENCES

1. Gardner RA: The child's reaction to a death in the family. *In* Schowalter JE, Patterson PR, Tallmer M, Kutscher AH, Gallo SV, Peretz D (eds): The Child and Death. New York, Columbia University Press, 1983, 104–124.
2. Grollman EA: Talking About Death: A Dialogue Between Parent and Child. Boston, Beacon Press, 1976.

CHILD ABUSE AND NEGLECT

LAWRENCE S. WISSOW, M.D., M.P.H.

Maltreatment by parents or other caretakers is one of the most prevalent threats to children's physical and mental health. By conservative estimates, about 1.5 million children in the United States suffer abuse or neglect each year. More than 20% of middle school and high school-age children report having been physically or sexually abused at some time in their lives. Maltreatment occurs to children of all ages. Serious physical injury is most common among infants, but the overall prevalence of maltreatment increases steadily throughout early childhood and adolescence.

Maltreatment frequently has immediate physical consequences, but it is also a serious threat to long-term social and emotional development. Maltreatment increases the child's lifetime risk of social and educational failures, major mental illness, substance abuse, and violent behavior.

Maltreatment is often conceptualized as falling into one of four categories: physical abuse, sexual abuse, emotional abuse, and neglect of necessary care. Neglect is thought to be the most common form of maltreatment, accounting for half or more of known cases throughout childhood. These categories, however, are inadequate guides for treatment of individual families and children. Child victims frequently suffer more than one form of maltreatment simultaneously or sequentially. Emotional abuse, in particular, occurs to a greater or lesser extent as a component of other forms of maltreatment. One useful approach to treatment is to view the presenting form of abuse, be it physical, sexual, or emotional, as only a symptom of some underlying disorder or disorders that must be uncovered before a long-term therapeutic plan can be devised. The search for treatable conditions involves examination of the child, the parents and extended family, and the family's environment. This section takes a general approach to the treatment of abuse and neglect. Sexual abuse and rape, the impact of domestic violence on children, and failure to thrive, which may sometimes be caused by emotional or physical neglect, are discussed in the following sections.

THERAPY DURING THE DIAGNOSTIC PROCESS

Although the purpose of this book is to describe therapy rather than diagnosis, the diagnostic process is a key part of therapy for cases of abuse and neglect. The process requires that families discuss sensitive and potentially incriminating details of their lives. The more this is done willingly, the more easily is subsequent therapy likely to be undertaken.

Demonstrating Interest in Psychosocial Topics

Primary care clinicians must create an environment in which family stresses can be discussed openly and honestly. Many parents do not feel that primary care providers are interested or competent to treat nonmedical conditions. Parents may also be concerned that disclosures of family discord will automatically trigger a referral to social service agencies, in the case of child abuse, or the police, in the case of domestic violence. Clinicians must demonstrate a willingness to listen to psychosocial concerns and a desire, before offering advice, to understand the family's situation in all of its complexity. Parents and children from violent families may need extra prompting to discuss personal issues. Both adults and children who have been abused may have difficulty verbalizing their own feelings or reading the social cues given by others. Beyond listening attentively and empathetically, clinicians must be ready to ask direct questions about psychosocial issues to demonstrate that these are acceptable topics (Table 1).

Visit Structure

Routine pediatric visits should be planned to give parents an opportunity to express concerns that may not have been stated openly

TABLE 1. Maneuvers to Demonstrate Receptivity to Discussion of Psychosocial Issues

Be alert for hidden agendas.
- Let patients complete their statement of the chief complaint.
- Ask "What else?"

Demonstrate attentive listening.
- Maintain good eye contact.
- Keep notetaking to a minimum.
- Give verbal cues that you are following the discussion.

Show empathy and support.
- Does not require condoning actions.
- Acknowledge feelings expressed by parents and child.
- Give praise and reinforcement where possible.

Ask direct questions about psychosocial issues.
- "Are things going smoothly at home?"
- "Do you have any concerns about her behavior?"

as the pretext for the visit. Families must be given time to complete their statement of the chief complaint. When they are finished, a prompt of "Is there anything else?" shows an interest in subjects the parent may have hesitated to bring up. Parents should be asked routinely whether home life is going smoothly or if there have been recent stresses. When possible, parents should be offered the opportunity to discuss concerns out of the hearing of their children. Likewise, beginning in late school age (10 to 12), children should also have the opportunity to speak privately with the clinician. Contrary to what might be assumed, these techniques do not lengthen visits. Instead, they serve to avoid prolonged discussions of vague medical problems while the parent or child waits for the clinician to deduce the true agenda.

Physical Examination

The physical examination also provides an opportunity for voluntary disclosures. Complete examinations, including the genitalia and perirectal area, demonstrate that these parts of the body, though sensitive and private, do not have to remain secret. The clinician demonstrates that they can be examined and talked about in the proper setting and in an unemotional way. The examination also offers a natural time for the clinician to mention the special circumstances in which someone is permitted to touch a child's body and to give age-appropriate counseling about what the child should do if touching occurs or has occurred in some other setting.

PRIMARY CARE PROVIDER'S ROLE IN MULTIDISCIPLINARY TREATMENT

Maltreatment always involves multiple members of a family and has causes that span generations as well as social and medical domains. Only in rare cases can the family be treated by a single clinician or even a single agency or institution. Primary care clinicians, however, play a vital role in treatment. They frequently are the only party able to maintain a neutral stance and advocate for the needs of the family as a whole. A central principle of abuse treatment is that the balance of a victim's vulnerabilities and strengths will shift over time and across developmental stages. The primary care clinician, whose care frequently is keyed to stages of the child's physical and cognitive development, is in a unique position to monitor progress and suggest when treatment may need to start, stop, or shift in intensity.

The Moment of Disclosure

Treatment of abused children and their families begins at the moment of disclosure. All family members usually experience a feeling of crisis and loss of control, regardless of whether a child has just been assaulted, has disclosed long-standing abuse, or is reporting a long-past incident. One of the primary care clinician's major roles is to demonstrate that the situation is indeed controllable, that similar events have happened to other families, and that constructive solutions can be found.

Often, the first opportunity to offer treatment comes with the physical examination of the suspected child victim. The child may have little sense of personal security or control, and a major goal of the examination is to help the child feel secure. The examination setting must be as quiet and calm as is consistent with the child's level of physical illness. Privacy and modesty are of paramount importance. The examination should be complete, both to uncover undisclosed injuries and to accustom the child to the clinician's touch before sensitive parts of the body are exposed. The examination also creates an opportunity to model an appropriate style of interaction with the child.

Ideally, the clinician takes a quiet, supportive, and methodical approach to the subsequent evaluation, balancing an open, collaborative tone with direction as it is needed (Table 2). Family members will need opportunities to express their feelings and to have procedures explained and, frequently, reexplained. Some expressions of feeling, however, will have to be redirected if they involve angry or deprecating statements about the victim or an alleged perpetrator. The family may want to be in control of decision making but is unable to agree among its members to anything the clinician proposes. One technique that can sometimes help break such an impasse is for the clinician to answer questions, such as, "What shall we do?" with "Let's go over your suggestions." In most cases, some elements of the family's proposals can be included in the treatment plan, increasing chances that the family will find the plan acceptable.

Parents are also likely to be sensitive about the appearance of being corrected, reprimanded, or outranked by a professional in front of their children. It may be reasonable to speak to the parents alone and to give them a chance to regain their composure before a final discussion involving the children. The ultimate goal of treatment is to enhance, rather than detract from, the parents' sense of competence and self-esteem.

Reporting to Civil Authorities

The obligation to report suspected maltreatment to civil authorities is one aspect of treatment that is out of the control of both clinicians and families. Throughout North America, Australia, New Zealand, and most of Europe, laws mandate that virtually any professional coming into contact with children must report "a reason to believe" that a child may have been abused or neglected by a permanent or temporary caretaker. Reporting laws are generally promulgated at the state/provincial level. They vary immensely in the detail with which they describe the acts of abuse or neglect to be reported and the amount of suspicion intended to trigger a report.

Clinicians often become confused about the level of certainty required before an abuse report becomes mandated. Laws vary but generally intend to trigger reporting of children who are suspected, but not known with certainty, to have been abused or neglected. Reporters do not have to be able to prove that abuse or neglect has taken place. The only requirement is that there be some clinically

sound reason for making the report. The observation or information that triggers the report should be verifiable and objective, and it should reflect reasonably established knowledge about the signs and symptoms of maltreatment.

This low threshold for reporting is a source of discomfort to many clinicians. Clinicians and parents frequently point out that it appears to reverse the usual direction of justice in that persons can be accused and actions taken that seem to presume guilt before anything can be proven. The process of reporting suspected abuse is not intended to be accusatory, however. It is designed to protect a child and provide urgent treatment services for a family. In fact, many states do not require that reports name a suspected abuser, and reporters may always choose to omit this information when they contact a social services agency. When police are involved in the response to a report, their decision to make an arrest is based on higher standards of proof or clearer evidence of an individual's dangerousness. Clinicians can help police officers by clearly stating when a report has been based on suspicions, which are unlikely to result in immediate police action, and when there is more certain knowledge of what has happened to a child.

Presenting parents with the need to report frequently is difficult, evoking feelings of guilt and anger in both the professional and the family members. Describing the reporting requirement as an onerous obligation or using it as a threat to obtain treatment compliance serves to undermine the clinician's authority and the potential that the report will serve a therapeutic purpose. As concerns for maltreatment grow, the clinician can determine his or her threshold for making a report and then announce that the point has been reached, explaining but not apologizing for the action. In most cases, it is best to inform parents before the report is made. Delayed disclosure involves a deception that, once discovered, can have negative consequences for the clinician–patient relationship. It also may send the family a message that the clinician cannot talk about the issue directly and, thus, tacitly establish an agreement that neither party will speak openly.

Clinicians often object that telling the family before reporting will lead to an uncooperative stance in which the family will become angry, refuse further evaluation, or take the child from the premises. There is no doubt that this can happen, although there is the hope that it can be avoided by an empathetic presentation of the clinician's differential diagnosis. The risks of deceit have to be weighed against the expected benefits. Deceit may be justified when injury has been serious or the parents appear to be seriously disturbed or dangerous.

Immediate Safety of the Child

Primary care clinicians often must participate in deciding if it is safe for a possibly maltreated child to return home with the family. Hospitalization is always an alternative given sufficiently serious medical problems or patients for whom adequate outpatient medical follow-up cannot be guaranteed.

When they have been involved, child protection agencies bear the final responsibility for permitting a discharge to home. The decision often involves weighing the risk to a child's physical safety in the home against the potential psychologic trauma of out-of-home placement. Several factors can be considered.

- Has the perpetrator been identified? How certain is the identification? Is he or she willing to leave the home and remain away?
- Will the victim be able to receive support and protection in the home? Are other family members so traumatized or angry that they will not support the victim?
- Is there any way to immediately ameliorate some of the circumstances that contributed to the abuse? For example, can a financial or housing crisis be remedied so that the general level of anxiety in the family is reduced?
- Are there any close family relatives or friends, well known to the child, who might be able to support the child in their home?
- Are there concerns for other forms of family violence that are as yet undisclosed (violence between spouses or siblings)?

TABLE 2. General Guidelines for Responding to Suspected Maltreatment

1. Resist the urge to propose or advocate for quick solutions. Family situations involving maltreatment are complex and chronic, with the status quo maintained by powerful forces. Take time to understand the situation and formulate a specific, individualized treatment plan.
2. Abusive families are no more or less likely than others to divulge all of their psychosocial concerns. Expect the process to take time.
3. Involve as many family members in treatment as possible.
4. Be prepared for a certain amount of passivity and helplessness. Avoid supplanting the parents but step in if needed to get the family into treatment.

If the child must be placed outside the home, even for a short period, great care must be taken that this does not appear to be a punitive action toward the family or child. Parents and children should be involved in the decision and should have an opportunity to understand the rationale and lack of alternatives. Placement with familiar friends or relatives is best, provided that the temporary caretakers understand the difficult role they are accepting and can take a supportive but neutral position. The child should be allowed to take familiar clothes and toys. Preliminary plans for visitation with the parents should be made and discussed with the child before separation takes place.

Anticipatory Guidance for Caretakers of Abused Children

Caretakers of the suspected victim should be prepared to cope with several potential behavioral symptoms, including regression, excessive noncompliance or dependency, rapid mood swings, fears, and disruption of sleep and appetite. The child should be encouraged to talk about feelings and allowed to talk freely about what has happened, but silence should be respected so long as caretakers make it clear that they are willing to listen should the child desire to speak. Caretakers should be careful not to make presumptions about the child's feelings, especially a dislike for the perpetrator or shame for what has happened. The child mostly needs assurance that he is loved, that disclosure of maltreatment was a good thing, and that his voice will be heard in decisions to be made about the family.

Short-Term Follow-Up

Another important role for primary care clinicians is to provide short-term follow-up (within a week to 10 days) for families grappling with maltreatment. The follow-up visit may be important for medical or diagnostic issues. It may be necessary to repeat cultures, obtain serologic samples, or reexamine skin lesions to look for evolution of color or bruising that might suggest a particular injury mechanism. The follow-up visit is also a good time for the clinician to assess how the family is coping with the disclosure, whether the child is being supported, and whether further diagnostic or supportive services have started to fall into place. Perhaps most importantly, it is a time for the primary care clinician to reinforce his role as an advocate for the family as a whole rather than as a person who has turned in the parents to protect the child.

Long-Term Treatment

Abusive families are sometimes treated at facilities dedicated to that purpose. Sometimes, treatment takes place in general medical or mental health settings. The choice often depends on local resources but also on the underlying causes of the maltreatment and the number of family members who must be involved. Only rare cases involve treatment of the child alone.

One way of approaching treatment decisions is to envision abuse and neglect as only the outward manifestations of one or more potentially treatable underlying problems. These problems can be divided into three large domains (parents/extended family, child, and community environment). The domains can be further subdivided into chronic and acute conditions (Tables 3 and 4).

Parent/Family Risk Factors and Behaviors

No single profile or set of behaviors serves to characterize parents and families in which maltreatment is taking place (Table 3). Potential chronic problems include poverty, parental medical or psychiatric impairment, distressed relations between parents, a parental history of abuse or serious emotional trauma in childhood, and a lack of appropriate models for adult–child interactions. Acute contributors to abuse include parents' workplace problems, sudden financial crises, the death of close relatives, ongoing victimization in a violent or emotionally abusive relationship, and failure to negotiate adult developmental milestones, such as marriage or a move away from the family of origin.

Abusive parents may have a number of undesirable ways in which

TABLE 3. Potentially Treatable Parental and Child Conditions and Behaviors

Parental

Enduring Traits
- History of abuse or trauma in childhood
- Chronic mental or physical illness
- Ongoing victimization by spouse/partner
- Poverty, chronic financial instability
- Inability to select supportive, nonviolent partners
- Social isolation

Recent Stresses
- Death or serious illness in family
- Financial or job-related crisis
- Legal difficulties
- Relationship with spouse/partner
- Failure to negotiate adult developmental milestone

Behaviors Toward Child
- Rejection or overly punitive
- Inability to modulate emotional response
- Insufficient verbal interaction
- Role reversal/failure to separate
- Inappropriate developmental expectations

Child

Enduring Traits
- Mental or physical conditions that impair normal responsiveness or developmental achievement
- Irritable, irregular, or difficult temperament
- Relative social isolation
- Chronic illness

Recent Stresses
- Passing through a new developmental level with which parent cannot cope
- Acute illness

Behaviors Resulting from Maltreatment
- Anxious or avoidant attachment
- Decreased empathy
- Decreased ability to decode nonverbal and verbal messages in social interaction
- Decreased ability to express own feelings
- Easy frustration
- Increased aggression
- Low self-esteem, self-blame for abuse
- School and social failure

they relate to their children. They often have difficulty responding to changes in their child's feelings. By overreacting or underreacting and by failing to verbalize how the child appears or the results of the child's behavior, they impair the child's ability to understand and label his own emotional states. In abusive families, parent–child interactions tend to have a more generally negative tone. Responses to child behaviors may be overly punitive, rejecting, or insufficiently supportive. These responses may stem from developmentally inappropriate expectations for a child's behavior or the parent's need to be supported and cared for by the child.

Treatment for abusing parents must be provided in a context of acceptance and approval. These individuals have primary problems

TABLE 4. Environmental Factors Contributing to Maltreatment

- Violence in the community
- Cultural values that condone violence toward children
- Lack of social supports or networks for children and adults
- Racial/culturally based discriminatory practices that detract from parental self-esteem
- Unresponsiveness of medical/school/community agencies to signs of intrafamilial distress
- Stigmatizing responses of medical/school/community agencies

with low self-esteem and fear of rejection. They may not be sufficiently trusting or mature for insight-oriented therapy. Often, a combination of emotionally supportive services with practical parenting aids can provide a basis on which to later explore more deep-seated issues. The following resources may be appropriate for parents who express an interest in changing their behavior.

Individual Therapy. Counseling or psychotherapy ultimately must involve both parents and later the entire family as a unit. Its goal is to aid the parents in developing new responses to dilemmas that they find overwhelming. Often, the therapy will have specific behavioral objectives, and sessions will focus on replays of situations that cause the parent to become anxious or angry. Parents who are open to insight therapy may be helped to explore personal issues that underlie their propensity to abuse. Such treatment is usually planned to last from 6 months to a year. It may extend indefinitely when the parent is found to have a specific psychiatric illness, such as depression or substance abuse.

Groups. Both supportive and explicitly psychotherapeutic groups can be effective means of helping parents confront their tendency to abuse and receive practical advice on the acquisition of new skills. The group is designed to be a major means of emotional support for the parent, in some instances substituting for a family when the abuser has none. In groups, parents are encouraged to express their feelings, deal with their poor self-esteem, and learn to accept some degree of social control. Parents Anonymous is one example of a successful group that combines support and therapy in a community-based setting. Groups are conducted under the coleadership of lay therapists and professionals and are open to both acknowledged abusers and parents who feel that they have the capacity to abuse. Group work is usually an adjunct to individual counseling.

Supportive Services. A variety of concrete services are available to help parents with the kinds of life stresses that seem to precipitate abuse. Lay therapists and parent aides often have the advantage of coming from a similar socioeconomic background as the parent. They may be able to model parenting and coping skills, as well as provide a secure and uncritical friendship. They give the parent a chance to build skills without exacerbating his or her feelings of inadequacy.

Emergency funds for food or clothing (or for decreasing isolation by paying for telephone service or transportation) may be available from community relief organizations. Transportation may be provided on a regular basis for medical visits or simply to allow parents the opportunity to go shopping or visit family members. The parents' own medical problems also need attention, ideally from a primary care provider with whom the parent can establish an ongoing relationship.

Hot Lines and Crisis Nurseries. These may serve two functions. Their very presence, even if not used, can help a parent feel more confident in facing stress knowing that help is always available. Alternatively, the parent may receive immediate support and concrete advice when required. Parents Anonymous members, for example, are urged to "pick up the phone" when they feel the impulse to harm a child. Crisis nurseries, facilities where parents can take their children for short periods (usually less than 72 hours), can provide a useful alternative to foster care for parents who suffer intermittent periods of dysfunction.

The Role of Legal Authorities. Child abuse is a felony offense in most jurisdictions. Jail may be an appropriate punishment for some instances of maltreatment, but it can have negative therapeutic implications for the perpetrator and the rest of the family. The family may suffer a loss of income and come to blame the child victim. The child may even feel guilt that the perpetrator's punishment is too severe. In many cases, however, the threat of prosecution or jail can be a very effective lever for enforcing treatment contracts. Prosecutors are generally very willing to work with clinicians to develop standards for the type and intensity of treatment that must be undertaken as a condition for a stay of legal action.

Family courts frequently develop treatment requirements for parents and children as part of their mandate to identify children in need of the state's protection. In this case, the penalties for noncompliance usually involve either a greater level of supervision of the family or the parents' loss of child custody. The clinician's best avenue for shaping these treatment strategies is to contact the attorney appointed to represent the child in family court hearings.

Child Factors Contributing to Maltreatment

Some children may be at increased risk of becoming victims (Table 3). Infants who are excessively irritable, irregular, or lethargic may present a challenge for parents. (These labels, however, must sometimes be seen through the parents' eyes.) Children with chronic illness or developmental disabilities may be at risk when paired with vulnerable parents. Socially isolated children may be so needy for affection that they are easily enticed into abusive and exploitive situations.

Abuse in infancy interferes with a child's ability to form secure and trusting attachments to caregivers. In healthy families, children come to count on caregivers for help and, thus, feel secure as they begin to separate and explore on their own. Many abused infants fail to form secure attachments. They falter in their exploration of the world around them and irritate their caregivers with seemingly unquenchable demands for nurturing. Abusive parents may then give the child ambiguous messages about the desired degree of attachment. The parent is gratified by the child's ongoing need for him or her but irritated by the child's failure to be independent and the often aversive ways of seeking attention.

In toddlers, main developmental tasks include acquisition of a sense of mastery over one's body and objects in the environment, as well as development of an ability to interact with people outside the parent–child dyad. Both of these tasks require the child to have a growing ability to identify his emotional states, understand their etiology, and identify them in other people. Children who fail this stage in development are likely to have subsequent problems adjusting to relationships outside the family and mastering the learning and social skills that will be required for success in school. Abused children are thus frequently caught in a downhill spiral of failure in and outside the family. The failure to negotiate early psychosocial milestones isolates them from potentially compensatory successes with friends, teachers, and other adults. They reach the later stages of childhood lacking emotional, social, and intellectual skills.

One contributor to the chronicity and increasing severity of abuse within families is that abuse in early childhood engenders child characteristics that make further abuse more likely. Abuse often creates children who are strongly but ambivalently attached to their parents. They have difficulty regulating simultaneous feelings of love and anger toward a parent. Such children may simultaneously cling to their parents at the same time as they are being physically aggressive. Boys, especially, may react to family stresses with aggressive or attention-demanding behaviors.

The following paragraphs outline some of the treatment options available for children from abusive families.

Crisis Intervention. In the short term, the child needs a chance to be relieved of any guilt or anxiety that he experiences for seemingly being at the center of the family's problems. The child may simultaneously be fearful of the parents' anger and frightened of losing the parents' love. Which professional helps to meet these needs will depend on the child's condition. If the child is hospitalized, it may be a nurse, social worker, or child life therapist. If the child is at home or in foster care, these issues must be addressed in a follow-up visit to a medical or counseling facility. That visit should be scheduled within a few days of the initial disclosure of abuse.

Specific Treatment for Chronic Medical Problems. At times, a child's chronic medical problems (asthma, a learning disability, a physical handicap) may put added stress on a family or serve as a trigger for abuse. Optimizing medical care of these conditions may help to reduce the risk of future injury.

Play Therapy for Preschool Children. Although preschool children usually are not able to verbally work through their reactions to abuse, they may benefit from individual play sessions that allow them to experience stable, understanding relationships with adults and to develop better social skills. Children who have become extremely withdrawn or overly aggressive may benefit most from this type of therapy.

Group Therapy. Groups address several goals. First and foremost, they offer the child a place of safety and acceptance. These qualities are often missing from the child's home environment. The child is helped to gain independence and self-confidence by separating from his parents and having a chance to try new skills without fear of being punished or ridiculed. The child also can learn better communication skills and more normal ways of interacting with other children. Head Start programs in the United States are a successful model of therapeutic preschool that allows younger abused children to contact other children from the community. Older children may benefit from a combination of group and individual psychotherapy.

Educational Assistance. Abused children frequently have done poorly in school, compounding their difficulties with social interaction. Some of their underlying behavioral problems may be rooted in learning disabilities or cognitive handicaps. After a thorough evaluation, specific remedial educational services should be provided as needed.

Preparation for Court Appearances. Participation in the legal process can be stressful for child victims. Many jurisdictions have specific programs, sometimes called a "court school," to prepare children to testify and to assure them that they are not the person who is on trial. At a minimum, children of all ages who will take part in a trial need an opportunity to understand the questions they will be asked and to become familiar with and comfortable in the courtroom.

Role Models and Individual Support in the Home. Programs such as Big Brothers may help a child who has had little chance to build self-esteem and appropriate social skills. They also help the child's parent get time away from child care responsibilities. It is important that volunteers commit themselves to work with a child for a fixed, extended period of time. Abused children are particularly vulnerable to feelings of loss and self-reproach when a meaningful relationship is unexpectedly ended.

Foster care is often considered as treatment for many kinds of abuse. Ideally, it combines the assurance of safety with the provision of a nurturing and stable environment. Foster care may be provided by a relative or by families selected by public or private agencies. Children entering foster care, however, may be more concerned over losing the only love and consistency they have ever known, even if it came in the context of abuse or neglect, than with their physical safety. Thus, the child may see foster care more as punishment than as rescue. When foster care is used, it is important for the child to understand the necessity and to know that contact with the biologic parents will not be cut off.

Abuse has been known to continue in foster care settings, and deaths of children in foster care have been reported. It is not known to what extent this is the fault of the foster families or protective service workers involved or to what extent the risk of abuse may have been increased by children's own behaviors. One of the most serious risks to children is that once placed in foster care they will enter a limbo state, where they are constantly shifted from one foster setting to another, never being returned to the family but never legally eligible for adoption or permanent placement. Children who remain in foster care for more than a short period of time are at a high risk for never being returned to their parents. Foster care is perhaps best seen as a treatment of last resort when no other alternatives are available and the risk to the child's safety is so great that it balances out the risks of placement.

Environmental Forces Promoting Child Abuse

Clinicians may not be able to directly change the environment in which a family lives, but they may help advocate for services or a change of neighborhood or provide support for families caught in a degrading or isolating social situation (Table 4). Perhaps the most important interventions open to primary care clinicians are to supportively and nonjudgmentally offer alternative norms for nonviolent, nonexploitive interpersonal relationships in general and parent–child relationships in particular. Clinicians can create an environment of respect and trust in their offices. Positive interactions during the medical visit may bolster resistance to negative community influences and provide the confidence parents need to make changes on their own.

WHEN IS TREATMENT COMPLETED?

Treatment for child maltreatment may never entirely end. Data from longitudinal studies suggest that maltreatment confers some degree of lifetime vulnerability on at least some of its victims. Adults and children alike will always need to be alert for a recrudescence of symptoms at times of increased stress or encounters with significant developmental milestones.

The major decision most often faced by therapists is at what point the various members of a family should be reunited by either returning a child to the home or allowing a perpetrator to rejoin the family. Such decisions ideally should be made by a consensus agreement of all the family members and professionals involved. Perpetrators must be willing to acknowledge to themselves and the family that they bear full responsibility for both past abuse and the prevention of further incidents. The perpetrator must generally have demonstrated some degree of insight into the causes of the abuse as well as a willingness to help the family even though he or she is temporarily living out of the home. This generally includes providing ongoing financial support and successfully negotiating visitations.

The period immediately after reunification frequently is marked by recurrence of maltreatment. Relationships that have been idealized from a distance are now reexperienced in all their complexity. Parents who were freed from day-to-day child care responsibilities are again limited by the need to care for children. The transition period thus requires close monitoring and possibly a temporary increase in the intensity of treatment.

Ultimately, termination of therapy involves considerations similar to those in other forms of mental health care. Patients and professionals come to a mutual assessment that close guidance is no longer needed. Markers for children can include good functioning with peers, in school, and within the family. Similarly, markers of adult functioning can include stability of relationships in and outside the family, steady job performance, and an increased sense of enjoyment of the parenting role. In-home or office observations may serve to demonstrate the improved nature of parent–child interactions and the parents' acquisition of age-appropriate behavior management skills. If child protection or criminal law authorities remain involved in a case, they may have some role in agreeing that therapy has been completed satisfactorily.

Some provision for long-term monitoring and support of the family should always be offered. Primary care providers can fulfill this role in many cases, since they will be seeing the child periodically for preventive medical care. Parents will want to have assurance that help will be available should they become vulnerable to abuse in the future. Only a handful of studies have examined the long-term response to treatment of abusive families. They suggest that relapses are relatively common but that many families benefit and report better functioning as a result of treatment.

REFERENCES

1. Bross D, Krugman RD, Lenherr MR: The New Child Protection Team Handbook, 2nd ed. New York, Garland Press, 1988.
2. Panel on Research on Child Abuse and Neglect: Understanding Child Abuse and Neglect. Washington, National Academy Press, 1993
3. Wissow LS: Child Advocacy for the Clinician: An Approach to Child Abuse and Neglect. Baltimore, Williams & Wilkins, 1990.

SEXUAL ABUSE AND RAPE

MARY CARRASCO, M.D.

Sexual abuse of children is a serious and common problem in the United States. According to the National Study on the Incidence of Child Abuse and Neglect done in 1988, 1% of children *experience* some form of sexual abuse and 2.5 children per 1000 are *reported* to be victims of sexual abuse each year. The true prevalence of sexual abuse is not known. Although with increased public awareness of sexual abuse, the rates of reporting have increased dramatically over the last few years, a significant percentage of cases still go unreported. The increase in reporting is probably a result of better understanding and awareness of the existence and frequency of sexual abuse rather than an actual increase in incidence. It should be noted that most children are abused by persons with whom they are familiar. The largest number of victims are girls, although in the younger age groups there are a significant number of boys. The largest percentage of perpetrators of reported abuse are male. This may represent some bias in both recognition and reporting.

All physicians who deal with children should have some knowledge about the diagnosis and initial management of children who make allegations of sexual abuse or have the many symptoms that may include sexual abuse in their differential diagnosis.

DEFINITION OF SEXUAL ABUSE

The National Center on Child Abuse and Neglect defines sexual abuse as follows.

> Sexual abuse consists of contact or interaction between a child and adult, when the child is being used for the sexual stimulation of that adult or another person. Sexual abuse may be committed by a person under the age of 18, when that person is either significantly older than the victim, or when the abuser is in a position of control over that child.

A "power differential" between the abuser and abused is an important element in sexual abuse, as well as other forms of abuse.

Note that sexual abuse does not necessarily require physical contact. It may include inappropriate exposure to sexually explicit materials or descriptions. Also, the degree of emotional trauma that a child may experience varies and is not necessarily related to the apparent extent of the abuse. Some children will experience significant trauma with what may seem to be a relatively minor abusive episode. Although the terms "sexual abuse" and "sexual assault" are often used interchangeably, the term "sexual abuse" is generally used for cases that are reportable to Child Protective Services (CPS) agencies.

By definition, it is considered sexual abuse when an adult engages in sexual activity with any child under the age of 14. One should also be concerned about abuse if there is a large difference in the ages of two children involved in sexual play or when activities, such as penetration or fellatio, are attempted by one of the children. In this case, one needs to be concerned that the child initiating the sexual activity has been abused.

Because it is common for the intensity of sexual interactions to escalate over time in sexual abuse, the boundary between normal and abusive activities may be difficult to define at the outset. Although the reaction of the child may help to define the difference, these vary from child to child.

It should be remembered that the initial disclosure is often incomplete. Complete disclosure may occur over an extended period, if at all. Certain parental behaviors, such as bathing or sleeping with a child, may sometimes be abusive.

INDICATORS OF POSSIBLE ABUSE

Certain indicators should make one highly suspicious of sexual abuse, including vaginal bleeding in a young child, vaginal or anal lacerations, sexually transmitted diseases (STDs), excessive or compulsive masturbation, and developmentally precocious sexual behavior. However, it is of great importance to note that many behaviors indicative of stress can be the only clue to sexual abuse. Although sexual abuse is one potential cause of stress, it should not necessarily be the first thing one thinks of when a child experiences symptoms of stress.

REPORTING

Abuse or gross neglect by a child's caretakers must be reported to the local CPS agency. Caretakers include parents, babysitters, teachers, or anyone else in a caretaking capacity. Abuse by adults who are noncaretakers is reportable to the police. In many jurisdictions, physicians have a legal obligation to report to the local police injuries inflicted in violation of any penal code. However, legal obligations vary, and it is important to become familiar with the reporting requirements in the jurisdictions where your patients reside. A report to the police does not mean that prosecution will occur. That is determined by the district attorney's office.

Reporting of sexual abuse is mandated by law. Immunity from civil liability is granted when mandated reports are made in good faith. Failure to report sexual abuse may result in a malpractice suit. The privileged communication between patient and physician does not apply to situations involving child abuse and does not constitute grounds for failure to report abuse. It is not necessary that a pediatrician be certain that abuse has occurred before a report is made to CPS. Suspected abuse reports are made when there is a high suspicion of abuse. If abuse is suspected, the law in most states allows the clinician to perform a complete physical examination, take x-rays, obtain appropriate specimens, and take photographs of areas of visible injury without parental consent.

If a parent appears to want to leave against medical advice and the child is deemed to be in imminent danger, the physician or hospital administrator may take temporary protective custody. CPS must be notified immediately, and in most areas, a hearing must be held within 24 hours to obtain a restraining order from a judge.

It is important to remember that the discovery of an STD in a young child is rarely followed initially by disclosure of the source of infection. Skilled interviews and team work are needed, considering both the probability of sexual and the possibility of nonsexual transmission.

FALSE ALLEGATIONS OF SEXUAL ASSAULT

Malicious false reports of sexual abuse are relatively uncommon, though they sometimes occur when parents or other relatives are all seeking custody of children. Sometimes, there is misinterpretation by an adult of normal childhood sexual behavior or of incomplete statements made by very young children that cannot be elaborated. It is very important not to confuse routine caretaking behavior, such as cleaning of the genital area in the course of bathing, washing, or diapering a child, with abuse, although sexual abuse sometimes begins in these situations.

IDENTIFICATION

Children come to medical attention for evaluation of possible sexual abuse via a large variety of sources. They may be brought for a medical examination after having disclosed sexual abuse, because of behavioral changes that lead adults to suspect sexual abuse, because of direct observation of sexual activity, or because of various complaints suggestive of sexual abuse, such as STDs. The number of behavioral and somatic complaints that include sexual abuse in the differential diagnosis is very large and includes many conditions that are merely indicators of stress. In many of these instances, sexual abuse should be considered in the differential but need not be considered the most likely cause. A child suspected of having been sexually abused must be interviewed and have a physical examination.

TREATMENT

Psychosocial Intervention

The primary issue that needs to be addressed is the child's safety and feeling of safety. It is important not to tell the child that all will be well now that he or she has disclosed abuse. One may convey that the child has done the right thing. However, because of the multiple people and systems involved, one cannot always predict the outcome for the child. Children respond to stress in a variety of ways, and their responses to sexual abuse may vary. Individual or group therapy usually is required, as is counseling for the nonoffending parent, when available, especially since the support provided to the child by the nonoffending parent is one of the major predictors of positive outcome for sexually abused children. When family reunification is a reasonable goal, individual and group therapy may be needed for the perpetrator.

Pregnancy Prevention

Pregnancies resulting from abuse rarely come to medical attention early, as abuse is often reported late by the child. Postcoital contraception should be discussed in postpubertal females seen within 72 hours of assault. A pregnancy test should be done to establish that the child is not currently pregnant. Two Ovral tablets given at once and two more tablets 12 hours later can be effective if started within 24 hours of the assault. Follow-up care should include a repeat pregnancy test within 2 weeks.

STD Prophylaxis and Treatment

Because children present most often with chronic abuse, the reported incidence of STDs in sexually abused children is low, and since gonorrhea and chlamydial infection are not generally ascending infections in prepubertal children, antibiotic prophylaxis is rarely indicated. In acute or recent rapes or when there are multiple assailants or perpetrators at high risk for STDs, prophylaxis may be desirable.

SEXUALLY TRANSMITTED DISEASE AND SEXUAL ABUSE

The presence of an STD may be the only indication of sexual abuse. A small number of infected children will readily disclose that they have been abused, and the alleged perpetrator is infected with the same organism. It then seems clear that sexual abuse was the source of the infection. Where there is no disclosure of abuse, those concerned often have difficulty accepting the possibility of sexual abuse and argue for nonsexual transmission, whereas others assume that any STD indicates sexual abuse.

According to the available scientific evidence, the likelihood of sexual abuse depends on which STD the child has. In some cases, such as gonorrhea, there is general agreement that virtually all cases are sexually transmitted. For other STDs, the evidence is less clear. The recommendations of the American Academy of Pediatrics' Committee on Child Abuse and Neglect for STDs confirmed by appropriate tests in the young child are listed in Table 1.

Gonorrhea

Gonorrhea is the most common STD seen in children, and there is general agreement that infection is spread by immediate physical contact with the mucosal surfaces of an infected person and that all cases in children are sexually transmitted. Because the gonococcus is a very fragile organism, infection through nonsexual contact is highly unlikely, and experimental studies of transmission have shown that the numbers of bacteria required to produce infection are unlikely to be present in nonsexual contact.

Transmission of genital or rectal gonorrhea by nonsexual means has not been shown to occur. Child-to-child infection through sexual play spread is rare but has been documented. Sexual transmission from an adult to a child is most common but is often difficult to document because of the reluctance of the child to disclose. It is important to culture other children who have had close contact with a child with gonorrhea, since they may also have positive cultures from abuse or sexual play.

TABLE 1. American Academy of Pediatrics Recommended Actions Following Diagnosis of STD

CONFIRMED	ABUSE	ACTION
Gonorrhea	Certain	Report*
Syphilis	Certain	Report*
Chlamydia	Probable	Report*
Condylomata	Probable	Report*
Trichomonas	Probable	Report
Herpes type 2	Probable	Report
Herpes type 1	Possible	Report†
Gardnerella	Uncertain	Follow
Candida (yeast)	Unlikely	Follow

*Unless perinatally acquired.
†If in genital area, report unless there is a clear history of autoinoculation.
From American Academy of Pediatrics Committee for Child Abuse and Neglect: Guidelines for the evaluation of the sexual abuse of children. Pediatrics 87(2):254–260, 1991.

Chlamydia

Chlamydia trachomatis is the second most common sexually transmitted cause of vaginal discharge in children. Maternal neonatal transmission clearly occurs, and the organism has been documented to persist for up to 2 years. In children over 2, a positive culture from vaginal discharge indicates a high probability of new acquisition and infection.

Human Papillomavirus (HPV)

HPV causes venereal warts, or condyloma acuminata, in the genital or anal area, and it is currently the most common STD in the United States. HPV in the larynx (laryngeal papillomatosis) in early childhood associated with a history of venereal warts in the mother is assumed to be transmitted during parturition. However, since this is also being diagnosed with increasing frequency in adults, presumably from oral–genital contact, it should not be assumed that all cases in children are the result of maternal–neonatal transfer, especially in the older child. After the age of 2, the possibility of sexual abuse should be strongly considered.

Herpes Simplex Virus (HSV)

HSV frequently causes recurrent infections of the lips (cold sores) or genitals. Genital infections may be caused by both types 1 and 2. In one study of HSV in children, sexual abuse was documented in most of the children with HSV genital infections.

TABLE 2. Recommended Treatment for STDs

Gonorrhea	Ceftriaxone
	125 mg IM (<45 kg)
	250 mg IM (>45 kg)
	Spectinomycin 40 mg/kg IM if allergic
Chlamydia infection	< age 8 y, erythromycin 50 mg/kg/d × 7 d
	> age 8 y, tetracycline 25–50 mg/kg/d PO
	q.i.d. × 7 d or doxycycline 100 mg PO
	b.i.d. × 7 d
Genital herpes	Acyclovir 200 mg PO 5 times a day for 10 d
	for an initial episode, for 5 d for recurrences
Trichomoniasis	Metronidazole 40 mg/kg (max 2 g) single dose
	or 15 mg/kg/d (max 1 g/d) b.i.d. × 7 d
HPV	Cryotherapy, surgical excision, laser, trichlor-acetic acid, or podophyllin
Bacterial vaginosis	Metronidazole 15 mg/kg/d PO b.i.d. (max 1 g)
	× 7 d or amoxicillin/clavulinic acid 500 mg
	t.i.d. × 7 d or clindamycin 300 mg PO
	b.i.d. × 7 d
Molluscum contagiosum	Often not necessary—curettage, cautery, or electrodesiccation

Trichomonas vaginalis

In adults, trichomoniasis is considered an STD, and it is rare before the onset of menses because the nonestrogenized vagina resists infection. Asymptomatic infection may occur in the newborn period and is usually acquired at delivery, when the newborn's vagina is stimulated by the mother's estrogen. Other than in newborns, the presence of trichomoniasis in a young child indicates a very high probability of sexual abuse.

Molluscum Contagiosum

This is a skin infection that may be transmitted sexually and nonsexually through direct contact with infected skin. If a child has lesions only in the genital area, the possibility of sexual abuse must be considered, but in other cases, it is reasonable to assume that transmission is nonsexual.

Gardnerella vaginalis

Data for this organism are incomplete. One study found it present in 4.2% in a control group of children, but children who had multiple episodes of sexual abuse were more likely to have *Gardnerella* infection.

Syphilis

If syphilis is found in the older child, it is most likely to be sexually transmitted. Maternal neonatal transmission does occur and usually occurs in infancy with a distinct set of signs and symptoms.

Pubic Lice

The presence of lice in the pubic area is most likely due to sexual transmission. However, if a child has pubic lice on the eye lashes and maculae cerulae (a blue discoloration of the eyelids), this is most likely from nonsexual transmission.

Mycoplasma hominis and Ureaplasma urealyticum

These organisms frequently are isolated from the genital tract, and infants may be infected during delivery. There has been no reported association with sexual abuse.

STD Treatment

Recommended treatment for STDs is given in Table 2.

REFERENCES

1. Bays J, Chadwick D: Medical diagnosis of the sexually abused child. Child Abuse Neglect 17:91–110, 1993.
2. Carrasco M: Sexually transmitted diseases in the young child: What do we know? Protective Serv Q vol 8, 1993.
3. Finkel AF, DeJong AR: Medical findings in child sexual abuse. *In* Reese RM (ed). Child Abuse: Medical Diagnosis and Treatment. Philadelphia, Lea & Febiger 1994.

CHILDREN OF HOMELESS AND BATTERED WOMEN

LINDA MCKIBBEN, M.D., M.P.H.
LIZ ROBERTS

Children of battered women and children of homeless women are two populations of children-at-risk with considerable overlap but also distinct issues. Dual advocacy for women and children is necessary for effective approaches to these complex and daunting problems. Both homeless children and the children of battered women are at increased risk of physical and sexual abuse and neglect. Increasingly, woman battering is being recognized as the single most important setting for child abuse. About 50% of children of battered women are likely to be directly abused. Conversely, 40% to 60% of mothers of abused children are also being victimized by adult partners. About 50% of homeless women have been physically abused.

THE PEDIATRICIAN'S ROLE

The role of the pediatrician is to be a resource to families struggling with the issues of homelessness or battering. According to the American Medical Association's protocol "Diagnostic and Treatment Guidelines on Domestic Violence" (an excellent resource), acquiring competence in this area is a matter of sound risk management, not simply good will. Pediatricians must first be ready to identify and respond appropriately to women and children whose lives have been disrupted by violence and homelessness. Identification should be through routine screening of mothers in primary care settings, as well as through skilled interviewing in higher-risk situations, such as emergency room presentations of child abuse. Women should always be interviewed privately, separate from their partners as well as any family members or friends who may accompany them to the health care setting. Information provided by the woman should never be divulged to her partner at any time. Direct interventions with an abusive partner are not recommended because of potential retribution to women and children. Confidentiality must be assured explicitly. Exceptions, such as mandated reporting of child abuse, should be stated up front. When asking about partner abuse, the use of neutral terminology is preferable. Such words or phrases as "abuse," "battered woman," "rape," and "domestic violence" should be avoided in the initial screening, since many abused women will not identify with these labels because of negative stereotypes about battered women and because denial and minimization are a normal reaction to abuse. Unless a patient has already disclosed her sexual identity, gender-neutral language should be used (i.e., "partner" rather than "husband" or "boyfriend").

Approaching violence as a health issue, a single question can be asked nonjudgmentally, such as, "Has your partner or expartner ever hurt or threatened you?" Following this question, one might ask more specifically about acts of violence: "Within the last year, have you been hit, slapped, kicked, or otherwise physically hurt by your partner or anyone else?" Additionally, the pediatric practitioner may ask about rape or sexual coercion, threats of harm by the abusive partner, use of and access to weapons by the partner, and possible escalation of the violence. The pediatrician must ask whether the children have been hurt or threatened or have seen their mothers being hurt physically or emotionally. Avoid victim-blaming questions, such as what the woman did to bring on the violence, why she has not left, and why she keeps returning. Battered women are at greatest risk of being killed when attempting to leave their partners. Many partners are successful at stalking and doggedly pursuing their victims. Expartners often continue to harass women and attempt to control them through the children. A woman and her children may not be safe despite leaving an abusive partner.

Clearly, a pediatrician's commitment to victims of family violence cannot rest on short-term, individual interventions. A pediatrician's interventions are to support a woman to be safe, a process that may take weeks to months. Once mothers are safe, they are usually more able to address the children's needs. Helping mothers to sort out complex questions regarding the effects of violence on the children is a service uniquely suited to the pediatrician. Until the mother is safe, direct inquiries to children about violence at home may endanger the children or their mother, as some children are used as spies on their mothers. Suspected child physical and sexual abuse and neglect are mandated as reportable to state authorities in the United States. When reporting suspected child abuse or neglect in a situation where the mother is battered or is homeless, the physician may be able to advocate for appropriate services and support that protect children without revictimizing their mothers. For example, in cases of suspected domestic abuse, the pediatrician's clear statement of concern about the mother's safety may contribute to a more accurate child protective investigation and a focus on protecting the mother as well.

Documentation

Physicians treating young adult and adolescent women should be suspicious of battering with the following findings.

- Any injury, especially to the face, central body, breasts, or genitals
- Bilateral or multiple injuries
- Delay between the occurrence of the injury and arrival at the health care site
- Explanation by the patient inconsistent with the injury
- Chronic pain symptoms with no clear etiology
- Prior use of emergency services for trauma
- Psychologic distress (i.e., suicide attempts, hyperventilation syndrome, panic attacks, depression, anxiety)
- Evidence of rape or sexual assault, unwanted pregnancy
- Pelvic inflammatory disease, STDs, especially when recurrent
- Substance abuse by the woman or her partner

Proper documentation of these signs in women's charts along with the diagnosis of "suspected partner abuse" when appropriate can be invaluable information for women if and when they are ready to pursue legal action. However, documenting adult domestic violence in the child's legal health record is not recommended if the mother's abuser has legal access to it (i.e., shares custody of the child). Laws on this vary from state to state. Physicians must know the law in their states.

Appropriate Referrals

Battered women's advocates/domestic violence specialists or skilled social workers usually are more prepared to offer crisis management services than are therapists. Crisis management includes lethality or danger assessments (to evaluate how likely an abusive partner is to kill) and safety planning (helping a battered woman get ready to leave if the violence escalates suddenly). Women not ready to leave can benefit from contact with domestic violence services, such as hotlines and peer support groups. Marriage or couples counseling and divorce mediation referrals are not appropriate for couples with a history of abuse because women often are further abused for telling their stories. Child witnesses to violence can benefit from support groups offered by battered women's shelters and other community resources. Once a woman is safe, abusive partners may be referred to batterers' treatment programs, but they rarely go unless court ordered. Programs that focus on anger management should be avoided. Instead, it is recommended that batterers' treatment programs clearly establish holding abusers accountable and promoting women's safety as their primary goals. When substance abuse is a factor, substance abuse treatment alone is not sufficient to stop the abuse. The violence and the addiction must be addressed as separate, though related, problems. Clinicians should become familiar with area resources, especially domestic violence hotlines, area shelters, victim advocacy services through local court systems, domestic violence units within police departments, and attorneys specializing in domestic violence or offering pro bono work for abuse victims. On some occasions, a woman and her children will be referred directly to a shelter from the clinical setting. The clinician should ask the woman if she feels safe to go home and be prepared to fully support her if she says no. To obtain accreditation, hospitals are now required to develop protocols to assist victims of abuse in crisis, specifying the roles of nursing, medicine, social work, and others. Office-based pediatricians and staff are recommended to develop an appropriate plan to assess and manage families in crisis in cooperation with local hospitals, community services, and family violence and homelessness specialists.

THE CHILD WITH A SERIOUS ONGOING CONDITION

RUTH E. K. STEIN, M.D.

Much of pediatrics is devoted to the care of children with acute conditions. However, a substantial fraction of children have serious ongoing conditions that persist over long periods of their lives. The care of these children can be both extremely challenging and rewarding.

Although some children carry the label of a past condition or of one that may develop in the future, we prefer to identify children based on the presence of

a disorder with a biologic, psychologic, or cognitive basis that has lasted or is virtually certain to last for at least one year and produces one or more of the following functional sequelae:
a) limitation of function, activities or social role in comparison with healthy age peers in the general areas of physical, cognitive, emotional, and social growth and development;
b) dependency on medications, special diet, medical technology, assistive device, or personal assistance to compensate for or minimize limitations of function, activities, or social role; or
c) need for medical care or related services, psychologic services or educational services over and above the usual for the child's age, or for special ongoing treatments, interventions or accommodations at home or in school[1]

These characteristics of the child's condition distinguish these children in functional terms from their healthy peers. These features also may require the pediatric practitioner to deal with special issues, and, therefore, a few pointers may be useful to those providing their care.

Children with ongoing conditions are prone to all the usual illnesses and normal developmental issues that their healthy age mates experience. Additionally, they may be predisposed to complications or illness as a result of their biologic condition. The specific nature of the problems that may develop is likely to vary with the biology of the health condition (e.g., pneumococcal infection in the presence of nephrotic syndrome or gallstones secondary to hemolytic anemia). These special considerations and vulnerabilities may make the delivery of their medical care more complex. The clinician must be aware of the range of problems that can arise and be alert to recognize when intervention is indicated.

Since so many of these children require the consultation of subspecialists, the primary care clinician is in the position of sharing care with the subspecialist rather than working independently. From the first referral to the subspecialist, there must be communication about concerns and plans so that the family experiences a cohesive care package. As the child enters school or early intervention programs, other types of service providers are likely to be involved. The primary practitioner can play an essential role in helping to coordinate the various issues that arise and helping to ensure that there are good communications between the members of the care team. Additionally, the primary practitioner can help ensure that the family has an opportunity to have questions answered and knows to whom to turn, if there are problems.

In caring for children who have serious ongoing health conditions, the goals of treatment are not only to handle the primary condition and the intercurrent issues but also to maximize the child's development and to normalize his function to the fullest extent possible. This requires that clinicians maintain a balanced approach and emphasize the child's strengths as well as deficits or limitations. It also is important to foster opportunities for increased independence as the child grows up.

One of the features that distinguishes long-term conditions from more acute ones is the need to know more about what family members think or believe in order to develop treatment priorities with their input. The large extent to which families assume ongoing responsibility for management of the child's condition on a daily basis requires the practitioner to step out of the prescriptive mode of care. Instead, it is useful to use a much more collaborative approach that recognizes the parents, and later the older child and adolescent, as partners in the care.

Sometimes, it is essential to know details of family life in order to solve logistic problems that accompany the challenges of providing home treatments. Although this may be uncomfortable initially for both practitioners and families, a nonjudgmental exploration of ways to make life easier often identifies key information that can lead to safe modifications of the treatment plan. It also may suggest the desirability of open communications with other key personnel, such as teachers and babysitters, whose greater involvement may facilitate care. Attention to details may make the difference between success and failure.

To maximize adherence to recommended management, it is critical to obtain a realistic sense of the family's understanding and beliefs about the condition and its etiology and prognosis, as well as their perceptions and preferences about alternatives to management. Forming a therapeutic alliance involves establishing trust and mutual respect and will have important long-term benefits. An essential ingredient in this process is honest and open sharing of information, including uncertainty when the answers to questions are not readily available.

Another area in which the primary care pediatrician can make important contributions is in helping the family to anticipate special problems that may arise and in preparing for potential emergency situations. It is helpful to provide the family with a letter summarizing key medical information, especially when they are travelling or away from their usual source of care. A convenient technique for assuring that children with serious ongoing conditions are never without access to lifesaving emergency care is the use of a medical alert bracelet, which allows easy identification of the child's essential medical information and emergency care needs.

Families often look to their practitioners for information about local and regional resources for children with special health conditions. These include a wide range of services, from suppliers of special equipment to recreational opportunities, from financial assistance programs to parent support groups and information about the school system. Familiarity with these resources will help the family to gain access to them.

Over time, many families are able to develop the skills to coordinate care and to be skilled managers of the many systems with which they must interact. Others may need help with case management. The clinician should help to enable the child and family to become as independent as they can but also provide some oversight and a safety net for those who need more assistance.

It is helpful to include multiple family members in discussions so that one adult is not left carrying questions and messages back and forth. This can be accomplished by planning to sit down even briefly on a periodic basis or around critical events in the child's development or disease. At these times, it is helpful to allow time for questions and to take stock of how the parents and other children are doing, since their needs may at times be inappropriately neglected in the focus on the child who has a special health condition. It is useful to inventory competing family and personal priorities that may affect the care of the child who has a special health condition, as well as the status of well siblings.

Having a child with any chronic condition has substantial impact on the family as individuals and as a unit. Typically, parents struggle with the questions of why their child has a health condition. They may have considerable guilt about a range of real and imagined things that may have contributed to the child's situation. Coupled with these emotions is the sense of burden of having to provide special care at home and through the health care system. This care has considerable costs in terms of time, energy, and money and often restricts individual and family options. Among the concerns families often raise are those relating to the cause of the condition, its prognosis, and its impact on daily life. It is helpful to be available to listen to these concerns but not to feel forced to provide solutions, especially when answers are uncertain. Families usually appreciate honesty more than guesses. Moreover, statistics only predict for groups of children, whereas the family cares about the specific outcome for the individual child. In the face of uncertainty, continued support and availability of the practitioner become the mainstays of a relationship.

All of these issues intensify the psychologic and social implications of caring for the condition and require the practitioner to address a range of issues. The nature of the psychologic and social issues is likely to be similar across a range of diverse medical conditions. This can be empowering to pediatric practitioners because experiences with patients with one condition may be useful for and have important implications when dealing with another. Although the vast majority of children and families do very well, some experience overwhelming difficulties and require intensive involvement of the pediatric practitioner. Assisting families to cope successfully with a chronic health condition can be extremely rewarding.

REFERENCE

1. Stein REK, Bauman LJ, Westbrook LE, et al: Framework for identifying children who have chronic conditions: The case for a new definition. J Pediatr 122:342–347, 1993.

MENTAL RETARDATION

ALLEN C. CROCKER, M.D.

The term "mental retardation," used as a descriptor of a personal trait, is a complex consideration, with many meanings and a potential for discriminatory interpretation. Mental retardation is not an absolute condition but rather is a construct, useful primarily to assist in procurement of educational and community services. A modern definition includes significantly subaverage intellectual functioning (I.Q. 70 or below), concurrent limitations in adaptive functioning, and onset of the features during the developmental period (before age 18). It is implicit that intelligence will be measured in an appropriate linguistic, cultural, and circumstantial setting. Determination of personal adaptation looks at context and relationships, noting achievement in daily living skills, play, work, and social interaction. Types and intensity of needed support functions are also factored in, per the latest definition of retardation from the American Association on Mental Retardation.

CAUSATION OF MENTAL RETARDATION

Deficits in intelligence, plus the attendant limitations in adaptive functioning, may derive from an extraordinarily diverse spread of sources, all in some fashion not supportive of full development of the central nervous system. An urgency exists to attempt at least a general etiologic hypothesis for the purposes of family counseling, most accurate health and other supports, anticipation of natural history, and long-range considerations regarding capacity for prevention. Consideration of causation in reference to developmental stage of origin suggests six general categories.

Hereditary Disorders

Hereditary disorders have a background that can be said to be preconceptual (determined by the genome of the parents). Family history may not provide an initial indication of these conditions. Most of the disorders have somatic abnormalities that are suggestive, though with variable expression. Many are progressive in their effects on the child. Included here are the inborn errors of metabolism, a variety of single-gene inherited neurologic syndromes, some chromosomal disorders with mendelian transmission (e.g., fragile X syndrome), and polygenic aberrations within families. Among children with mental retardation, heritable disorders do not constitute a large percentage.

Early Alterations of Embryonic Development

Early alterations of embryonic development, on the other hand, are a frequent background for the occurrence of mental retardation. These events are considered to be principally of sporadic occurrence, usually with an unknown ultimate cause. They produce phenotypic changes and a stable form of developmental impairment. In some instances, there are demonstrable chromosomal abnormalities present, such as trisomy 21 (Down syndrome) or 5p deletion (cri du chat syndrome). In many more, there is simply the presence of congenital anomalies, without markers, and these include many of the named syndromes. Fetal alcohol syndrome is an instance where causation can be documented.

Other Pregnancy Problems and Perinatal Morbidity

This refers to the continuing need for nutritional (placental) support for the fetus' progress and then salutary circumstances for birth. Intrauterine growth retardation may occur as the result of placental abnormalities. Significantly preterm delivery is the chief concern when birth circumstances are remarkable. Cerebral compromise may produce cognitive impairment, motor function problems (cerebral palsy), seizure or sensory disorder, or a combination of these. The timing varies considerably for clinical expression of such manifestations. The developmental delay should be stable, but the appearance of complications may influence the course. At present, perinatal issues are a relatively infrequent cause of mental retardation.

Acquired Childhood Diseases

Acquired childhood diseases occasionally result in intellectual impairment. The most important issues here are head injury and infection of the central nervous system (encephalitis, late-treated meningitis). Near-drowning, various toxins, and accidental asphyxia also may contribute, although the incidence of all of these is relatively low. The capacity for the return of some of the lost function with the passage of time is real but tenuous.

Environmental and Support Problems

Environmental and support problems are germane to normal developmental progress, and for the milder levels of retardation, they represent a major component. These include issues of cultural dyssynchrony, inadequate stimulation, child neglect, child abuse, and even matters of parental psychopathology. There are various *behavioral syndromes* of obscure origin, not environmental, such as hyperkinesis states, atypicality, and autism, where dynamic components of retardation exist, often with uncertain potential.

Unknown Origin

Finally, it is acknowledged that for many children, their retardation must be considered to be of truly unknown origin. This implies that in multifactorial circumstances, no single element can be declared to be ascendant and that, for others, useful clues regarding origin simply are not accessible.

THE SEARCH FOR ETIOLOGY

Final conclusions about the probable origin of serious developmental delay or mental retardation or both often require much deliberation and judgment. Important allies for the pediatrician in this regard include the child neurologist and the dysmorphologist/geneticist. The intensity of the exceptionality determines in some degree the level of investment in special studies that is justified. When there is evidence of notable organicity or of progressive disability, more aggressive investigation is required. Such ocular abnormalities as cloudy corneas, lens opacities, or retinal pathology, enlargement of the liver or spleen, or oppressive neurologic findings suggest a study of white blood cell lysosomal enzymes, urinary mucopolysaccharides,

bone and lung x-rays, and liver function tests. Some concurrent abnormalities of muscle texture or motor function justify enzymatic study for the muscular dystrophies. Poor growth should be evaluated by thyroid function. Blood or urine amino acid measurement is appropriate in certain organic settings, and other metabolites should be reviewed if there is evidence of acidosis or episodic relapses. Blood lead assay should be pursued in obscure attentional or learning problems.

The more common dilemmas involve when to use the relatively costly tools of chromosomal study and brain imaging. Again, the geneticist or neurologist can give good advice. It is clear that increasing numbers of children with birth defects are being found to have chromsomal aberrations, but for many of these, special study techniques are required (fragile X syndrome, Prader-Willi syndrome, other deletions). Unusual congenital anomaly syndromes (or phenotypic presentations) generally require karyotyping of the child for full description. Imaging studies of the central nervous system (CT scan, MRI) are likely to give useful results for children with (1) focal or shifting seizure patterns, (2) small or large or otherwise unusual configurations of the skull, (3) unexplained hemiplegia or other asymmetric neurologic syndromes, (4) a suspicion of tuberous sclerosis, or (5) serious retardation where no insights are available about etiology.

THE EXPRESSION OF MENTAL RETARDATION

It follows that the more serious the abnormality may be in the child's central nervous system, the earlier the exceptionality becomes apparent. Significant delay in achievement of the major motor milestones of the first year represents an unusual situation, except in the setting of cerebral palsy. Commonly, there is some delay in these events, but there is more concern as the complex developmental assignment of acquiring language and independence skills is noted to be slowed. Measurement of cortical function is less precise in children under 2 years of age, and diagnostic terminology is appropriately more cautious in that period.

Children with specific conditions can be considered to have *established disabilities,* with near certainty that developmental disability will be expressed. These include such conditions as Hurler syndrome and Down syndrome. Many more have a statistical risk of significant developmental aberration, but when they are first encountered, there is considerable uncertainty. Some children are referred to as having *biologic risk,* meaning that they have had experiences with possible pathologic effects (such as seriously preterm birth or severe asphyxia) or are showing personal courses with delays that cause pediatric concern. Beyond this, a very large number can be considered to have *environmental risk,* based on difficulties in support or nurturance (e.g., very young mother, serious psychosocial disadvantage, neglect, abuse, or other family difficulties). For these last two groups of children, the developmental effects of the past happenings are indeterminate. For them, the teaching, training, and family support elements of early intervention programs are of strategic value. Some of these children will proceed to normal or near-normal development, whereas others will have lasting delays (with retardation), although possibly less than might have been expected.

THE IMPACT OF MENTAL RETARDATION

With significant mental retardation, the element of greatest pressure for the child, the family, and the community is the matter of differentness. There are cultural and personal aspects of the exceptionality that require thoughtful accommodation. When that is accomplished with accuracy and love, substantial fulfillment can be expected. One aspect of differentness relates to *performance or achievement.* This can involve quantitative features (as measured) or qualitative facets. Another part of differentness is that of *services required.* Although all of us use community-based services, the urgency is greater for the child with mental retardation. There is also dissimilarity in *participation,* implying a danger of isolation regarding life activities. Our society is now more heedful of these concerns. Finally, there may be differentness in the attainment of *connectedness*, a more subtle concern for sharing and joining.

The children for whom meaningful support has been most challenging are those with progressive disorders (e.g., Rett syndrome, Niemann-Pick disease) or those with severe or profound retardation (I.Q.s below 35 or 20). Continuing lack of self-care or even survival skills, absence of language, bizarre or stereotypic behavior, and less clear capacity for learning cause confusion for educators and care providers. Fortunately, the last two decades have seen a growing commitment and sense of regard in work with these persons.

PEDIATRIC CARE FOR CHILDREN WITH MENTAL RETARDATION

The prevalence of mental retardation in children is around 2%. Surveys of pediatricians' offices generally have reported about 20 to 30 such patients being seen in individual practices. One can appropriately view the health care assignment for these young people as having *alike/unalike* aspects compared with that for typical children. Alike are the needs for treatment of infection, immunization, consideration of allergy, injuries, and general health maintenance. Unalike are the numerous special complications and vulnerabilities found in many of the syndromes that have mental retardation as a symptom. The child with Down syndrome, for example, often requires expert attention for cardiac, otologic, ocular, orthopedic, gastrointestinal, and endocrine concerns. The youngster with myelodysplasia may be troubled with hydrocephalus, paraplegia, scoliosis, complications of neurogenic bladder and bowel disability, skin trauma, and seizures. In the child with cerebral palsy, special attention may be needed for weakness, spasticity, contractures, dislocations, strabismus, seizures, hearing impairment, or nutritional problems.

The primary care pediatrician will need collaboration from relevant medical or surgical specialists or may wish to use a developmental pediatrician to provide coordination or supervision of particular aspects. Assistance is available in most metropolitan areas from child development centers, where both health and habilitative services can be guided. A close family relationship and the long and stable continuity given in child care are powerful contributions of the primary pediatrician in behalf of the best development of the child.

As could be anticipated, the presence of some degree of pathology in the central nervous system can produce other disabilities concurrent with the child's mental retardation. About 5% to 10% of children with retardation will have a seizure disorder, and up to 25% of those with epilepsy have mental retardation. Many children with mental retardation have motor function abnormalities (about 10% can appropriately be called cerebral palsy). In a service for children with cerebral palsy, 25% to 50% will have mental retardation. Hearing impairments (of diverse origins) are common in children with retardation (10% to 20%), and ocular difficulties are present in 5% to 10%. Issues of emotional disturbance, aberrant behavior, and attentional disorder are very common concerns.

In the field of developmental disabilities, there has been some reaction in recent years to the insinuation of a *medical model* for the guidance of care. This acknowledges that the health-related matters usually are only a portion of the child and family's challenge, and the vocabulary of illness should be minimized once the best supports are in place. The building of good self-concept and preparation for the most independence possible suggest that wellness beliefs are important. Medical personnel can be critically valuable team members in the care and training of young persons with mental retardation, although they are not usually the ultimate coordinators or managers.

THE PEDIATRICIAN AS ALLY AND ADVOCATE

The whole assignment in the service systems for children with significant mental retardation is very large. As noted in the adaptive skills section of the new definition of retardation by the American Association on Mental Retardation, assistance may be needed in communication, self-care, home living, social skills, community use, self-

direction, health and safety, functional academics, leisure, and work. These territories are given important attention over time by a wide range of providers and friends. There are three areas of overriding importance: family support, education and habilitative therapies, and community inclusion.

Family Support

Members of the child's family find themselves in compelling and unfamiliar roles, including the de facto requirement to be the case manager. Knowledge about educational and community services must be acquired quickly. If there are health care aspects, adjustments must be made for these. Transportation, special equipment, home adaptation, financial considerations, and respite care may need arrangements, plus attendance at seemingly endless conferences, planning meetings, hearings, and so on. Most important, there is a need to reach the best understanding possible about the background and nature of the child's exceptionality and to learn how to deal personally with the numerous points of differentness. It is often commented that at least four reactions are universal for parents—guilt, fear, loneliness, and anger—although with time they become modulated. Brothers and sisters have their own special needs as they deal with alterations in the normalcy of family rhythm, competition for parental resources and attention, possible misconceptions about the origins or outcome of the syndrome of the involved child, a requirement to act as a surrogate parent, and an obligation to meet enhanced parental expectations. They gain significantly by being provided meaningful information in suitable form, being involved in decision making, and having counseling or group activity with like peers when appropriate. For the parents, the value of sharing in practical matters and in activism with other mothers and fathers (in consumer groups) cannot be overstated.

Education and Habilitative Therapies

The last decade and a half has seen the flowering of appropriate education for all children with special needs, beginning as close to birth as identification of the need can be made. Enrollment in early intervention programs, from birth to 3 or 5 years, supported by Public Law 99-457, now involves about 3% to 5% of children in that age range. This is largely the at-risk group. Developmental training by physical, occupational, and speech therapists is the central element of service in the first 3 years. The arts therapies also are of great value. Social work assists in family support. Education from 5 to 21+ years is secured by Public Law 94-142 and its sequels. In that design, educational plans are being written for 10% to 14% of children in those years (for about 15% of children with plans, the issue is mental retardation). All of this has represented an authentic revolution, and the achievements go far beyond education. We are still learning about the degree to which integration can proceed for students with special needs and those who are typical, especially the potential for true inclusion in school. We falter sometimes at points of transition, such as from early intervention to preschool, and from high school to employment.

Community Inclusion

Beyond health and education lies a whole world of considerations and opportunities that have to do with making life be as rich as possible. Persons with disabilities, including mental retardation and related disorders, have a legal guarantee of access to public programs and activities per Section 504 of the Rehabilitation Act of 1973 and the Americans with Disabilities Act. Many children and adults with mental retardation, however, continue to feel out of joint (see discussion of differentness). In the larger sphere, it is now possible to look forward to community living (with support as needed), work for pay, opportunity for friendships and marriage, and voting in elections. Large congregate living arrangements (institutions) are rapidly declining in size and number, and admission of children to these facilities is virtually unknown now. Pediatric nursing homes for children with severe multiple disabilities are gradually learning a more dedicated habilitative philosophy.

The community pediatrician, in common with other child advocates, has shared in the excitement as services have improved, care has become more accurate, and basic rights have been affirmed. Pediatric contributions include creative use of medical and surgical specialist referral, support for needed habilitative therapies, prompt referral for early intervention services, family support in achieving cognitive coping, genetic counseling, and assistance in special needs adoption where sought. There is also the privilege of being able to provide warmth and hope along the child and family's journey.

A WORD ABOUT PREVENTION

As scientific gains have been achieved in molecular biology, genetics, infectious diseases, and neonatology, the capacity for prevention of discrete biomedical situations accompanied by mental retardation also has moved forward. Congenital rubella, measles encephalitis, kernicterus, Tay-Sachs disease, and retardation from phenylketonuria and congenital hypothyroidism are now largely eliminated. Improvements are occurring in morbidity from prematurity, lead intoxication, the incidence of neural tube defects, automobile head injury, and disorders detectable by prenatal diagnosis. Early intervention services and assistance to support families who have children with disabilities make a large difference in the child's ultimate situation. Where we are much less successful is in the new morbidity areas, where social disadvantage, joblessness, and poverty erode the nurturant base for child progress. Included here are the lack of improvement in teenage pregnancy rates and adequacy of prenatal care, substance abuse in pregnancy, preterm birth rates, congenital HIV infection, and child abuse. In all of these situations, developmental delay and mental retardation have increased in occurrence. Regrettably, we have not secured for all children the right to be born well.

REFERENCES

1. Batshaw ML, Perret YM: Children with Disabilities: A Medical Primer, 3rd ed. Baltimore, Paul H. Brookes Publishing Co, 1992.
2. Capute AJ, Accardo PJ: Developmental Disabilities in Infancy and Childhood. Baltimore, Paul H. Brookes Publishing Co, 1991.
3. Levine MD, Carey WB, Crocker AC: Developmental-Behavioral Pediatrics, 2nd ed. Philadelphia, WB Saunders Co, 1992.
4. Rubin IL, Crocker AC: Developmental Disabilities: Delivery of Medical Care for Children and Adults. Philadelphia, Lea & Febiger, 1989.

PICA

RICHARD D. OLSEN, M.D.

In the narrow definition, pica refers to the ingestion of nonedible substances. In the broader definition, it can include excessive ingestion of edible, but often unusual, substances (Table 1).

Pica is most common in children but may occur in other groups, most notably pregnant women and retarded individuals. The incidence of pica is 30% in African American children aged 1 to 6 years and 10% to 18% in white children. Approximately 30% of children with pica have lead poisoning.[1] Estimated daily soil ingestion in young children with pica in normal living conditions is 90 mg, with 190 mg representing the 90th percentile.[2]

Possible etiologic factors in pica have included nutritional and psychosocial factors. Iron, zinc, and trace mineral deficiencies have

TABLE 1. Substances Commonly Ingested

EDIBLE	INEDIBLE
Baking soda	Soil
Ice	Clay
Lettuce	Starch
Raw potatoes	Paint chips
Peanuts	Hair
Butter	Feces
Tomato seeds	

been implicated as nutritional factors. Other studies suggest insufficient or inappropriate maternal–child interaction as a cause. Cultural beliefs and practices may also play a role. No one etiologic factor explains childhood pica, and there may not be a single, underlying cause.

Depending on underlying etiology, complications of pica include anemia, lead poisoning, intestinal parasite infestation, visceral larva migrans, delayed development, and poor weight gain and growth.

Evaluation should include careful history and physical examination, complete blood count (CBC) with differential, and determination of serum ferritin levels. Depending on symptoms and endemic problems in a given geographic area, free erythrocyte protoporphyrin, serum lead, stool for ova and parasites, and serologic assessment for *Toxocara* may be indicated. If psychosocial factors are suspected as a possible cause of pica, an in-depth assessment of the child's development and parent–child interaction is indicated. On-site assessment of home and/or day care setting may be helpful.

Treatment of pica depends on the underlying etiology. If iron deficiency is found, treatment consists of oral iron at 4 to 6 mg/kg/d for 2 to 3 months, as well as dietary evaluation to determine whether contributing factors, such as excessive milk intake, are present. Prevention of recurrence includes dietary prescription of iron-rich foods, such as meats and poultry, as well as foods that promote iron absorption, including fruits and fruit juices.

If excessive lead levels are found, treatment will depend on the level of intoxication (class II through IV). Chelating agents are useful when lead intoxication falls into classes III and IV (lead levels greater than 50 μg/dl). Chelation may be done if the lead mobilization test is positive or if the patient is at class IV.

Treatment of intestinal and systemic parasite infections depends on the specific parasites.

Treatment of psychosocial factors, if they are contributing to the pica, is more complicated and requires a multidisciplinary approach, including developmental intervention, treatment of any underlying psychiatric disorder, and intensive support and education of parents. Involvement of social services and public health nursing often is helpful.

If pica is related to cultural practices, it is important to convey respect for cultural beliefs while providing education regarding the risk of pica.

Pica behavior often abates with correction of underlying iron deficiency. Improving mother–child interaction frequently reduces or resolves pica behavior if psychosocial factors are involved.

REFERENCE

1. Danford DE: Pica and nutrition. Ann Rev Nutr 2:308, 1982.
2. van Wijnen JH, Clausing P, Brunekreef B: Estimated soil ingestion by children. Environ Res 51:159, 1990.

3

Nervous System

HEAD INJURY

ASHOK P. SARNAIK, M.D.
MARY W. LIEH-LAI, M.D.

Trauma is the leading cause of death in children older than 1 year of age, and head injury accounts for 75% (4000 per year) of all such trauma-related deaths. Each year, approximately 100,000 children are admitted to hospitals in the United States for the treatment of traumatic head injury resulting from falls, pedestrian and motor vehicular accidents, intentional injuries, and other trauma. The mortality among children admitted for severe head injury varies between 9% and 35% in various series. Primary neuronal injury is caused by direct impact from the **initial** trauma, whereas secondary injury occurs from a variety of **ensuing** pathophysiologic events, such as hypoxia, ischemia, intracranial hypertension, and metabolic derangements. Although the management of the primary injury is of major importance, it is the secondary insults that often determine survival and neurologic outcome. Manifestations of secondary injury may occur within minutes or hours after the primary insult. Failure to recognize and manage this secondary injury can result in unnecessary death and neurologic morbidity.

Intracranial contents include fluid, brain parenchyma, and meninges. Intracranial fluid is partitioned into four compartments: the intravascular space, brain interstitium, intracellular fluid, and cerebrospinal fluid (CSF). The skull with its fused sutures is a rigid container filled with noncompressible fluid and solid tissue. For intracranial pressure (ICP) to remain constant, any increase in intracranial volume must be accompanied by an equivalent decrease in its preexisting contents. When enough volume cannot be displaced to compensate for a pathologic increase in one compartment, ICP begins to rise. Life-threatening intracranial hypertension with a relatively small increase in volume eventually occurs after spatial compensation is exhausted.

The driving force responsible for maintaining cerebral blood flow (CBF) is the cerebral perfusion pressure (CPP). CPP is measured clinically as mean arterial pressure minus ICP. Cerebral blood flow is normally autoregulated to remain constant by vasodilatation of the cerebral vasculature if CPP falls and vasoconstriction at a high CPP. Shortly after significant head injury, there is acute cerebrovascular engorgement, resulting in an increase in cerebral blood volume (CBV) and vasogenic cerebral edema. In severe head injury, cerebrovascular autoregulation is altered to such an extent that a marked decrease or increase in CBF may occur despite an apparently acceptable CPP. Within the usually encountered ranges of $Paco_2$ there is a 3% to 4% change in CBF per 1 mm Hg acute change in $Paco_2$. Hypercapnea results in increased CBV and CBF, whereas hypocapnea has the opposite effect.

Cerebral edema is an important consequence of head trauma. Based on its pathogenesis, cerebral edema is classified into vasogenic, cytotoxic, and interstitial edema. Disruption of the blood–brain barrier is a hallmark of vasogenic cerebral edema. Cytotoxic cerebral edema results from accumulation of excess water intracellularly. It occurs with increased intracellular osmolal content from impaired cellular metabolism (trauma, hypoxia) or from decreased extracellular osmolality (hyponatremia, syndrome of inappropriate antidiuretic hormone). Interstitial edema occurs when there is an increased hydrostatic gradient between the ventricular space and the brain interstitium (obstruction to the CSF flow), which results in transependymal movement of CSF into periventricular white matter. A consideration of pathogenic mechanisms in cerebral edema has important therapeutic significance. Osmotherapy is more effective in cytotoxic cerebral edema, hyperventilation is better applied in vasogenic edema, and relief of CSF obstruction is needed to treat interstitial cerebral edema. It is important to realize, however, that vasogenic, cytotoxic, and interstitial edema may occur concurrently in a child with head injury.

MANAGEMENT OF MINOR HEAD INJURY

Children with a history of loss of consciousness, changes in sensorium such as lethargy, confusion, amnesia, and irritability, repetitive vomiting, and visual disturbances require medical attention. Although skull radiographs commonly are obtained in such patients, they are useful only when the physical examination suggests (1) depressed skull fracture, (2) basilar skull fracture, (3) temporal/parietal hematoma, and (4) child abuse. Fractures involving the temporal bone and the sagittal suture should be further investigated with a CT scan. Patients with a Glasgow Coma Score (GCS) >13 can be discharged home with appropriate monitoring instructions. A period of observation over several hours in the office or the emergency room may be necessary to determine neurologic stability. A minor head injury with or without a skull fracture may be the initial manifestation of child abuse. Radiographic examination of the long bones and the chest and investigation of the social situation are warranted when nonaccidental trauma is suspected.

MANAGEMENT OF SKULL FRACTURES

Linear skull fractures require no treatment. Depressed skull fractures are classified as closed (simple) or compound depending on the presence or absence of scalp laceration overlying the fracture. Anteroposterior, lateral, and tangential radiographs are required to determine the extent of depression. An appropriately obtained CT scan with bone windows will accurately identify even small depressions. A closed, depressed skull fracture often is elevated electively with the rationale that this decreases the possibility of posttraumatic epilepsy and neurologic deficit. However, there are no data to support such a practice. On the other hand, compound depressed fractures carry a risk of CNS infection. These fractures are elevated as soon as the patient is stable. Basilar skull fractures often are associated with dural tears with or without a CSF fistula (CSF otorrhea or rhinorrhea). The incidence of CNS infection in basilar skull fracture without a CSF fistula is low and is not influenced by antibiotic prophylaxis. Such fractures require no therapeutic intervention. The efficacy of prophylactic antibiotics in decreasing the incidence of meningitis in CSF otorrhea and rhinorrhea is uncertain.

EMERGENCY ASSESSMENT AND MANAGEMENT

The initial steps in the management of a patient with severe head injury should include a brief, yet all encompassing history and physical examination that must proceed simultaneously with basic resuscitative procedures. The assessment must include an evaluation of the patency of the airway and the adequacy of ventilation and circulation. Rate and depth of respirations, air entry, heart rate, blood pressure, and capillary refill time should be determined immediately on presentation. The initial assessment also must include determination of associated injuries, particularly of the chest and abdomen. All children with traumatic head injury should be treated as if they have a spinal cord injury until proven otherwise. The severity of the head injury can be quantified by the GCS. Because of verbal limitations, a modified GCS has been proposed for young children (Table 1). A GCS ≤8 is indicative of severe head injury. The head should be examined carefully for lacerations and hematomas. The presence of CSF rhinorrhea, otorrhea, and hemotympanum indicates a basilar skull fracture. Focal neurologic deficits are important clues to localize the structural lesion. A funduscopic examination revealing retinal hemorrhages suggests intracranial hemorrhage and should raise the suspicion of child abuse in appropriate situations. Papilledema often does not develop in an acute setting, and its absence should not be taken as evidence against intracranial hypertension.

Maintaining airway patency, adequate ventilation and circulation must remain a constant priority. The neurologically compromised child is vulnerable to airway obstruction, hypoventilation, and aspiration. Hypercarbia and hypoxemia can occur in an unconscious child without clinical signs or symptoms. Sedatives should not be used in a combative patient without control of the airway and ventilation, since even small acute elevations in $PaCO_2$ may lead to serious intracranial hy-

TABLE 1. The Glasgow Coma Score Modification For Children

Eye Opening
4 Spontaneous
3 To speech
2 To pain
1 No response

Motor Response
6 Spontaneous (obeys verbal commands)
5 Localizes pain
4 Withdraws to pain
3 Decorticate posture
2 Decerebrate posture
1 No response

Best Verbal Response
5 Oriented
   Social smile, orients to sound, follows objects, cooing, converses; interacts appropriately with environment
4 Confused/disoriented
   Consolable cries; aware of environment, uncooperative interactions
3 Inappropriate words
   Inappropriate persistent cries, moaning, inconsistently aware of environment, or inconsistently consolable
2 Incomprehensible sounds
   Agitated, restless, inconsolable cries, unaware of environment
1 No response

From Rubenstein JS, Hageman JR: Monitoring of critically ill infants and children. Crit Care Clin 4:621, 1988.

pertension. Clearing the nasal, oral, and pharyngeal air passages and inserting an oral airway may be all that is required to establish a patent airway. Children with facial injuries and those with a suspected basilar skull fracture should not have gastric or endotracheal tubes passed via the nasal route. For reliable airway control beyond the immediate period, however, endotracheal intubation often is necessary. This should be performed under as controlled a setting as possible. In an emergency, the orotracheal route is preferred because of the ease of insertion. When cervical spinal injury is suspected, children should be intubated in a neutral position, with attention to cervical alignment and immobilization. Oral intubation with a standard laryngoscope and manual in-line axial traction is the most suitable technique in this situation. The patient should be given 100% oxygen and should be hyperventilated with a bag and mask device before intubation. Sedatives and a neuromuscular blocking agent often are needed in a struggling child to avoid intracranial hypertension and airway trauma. Morphine (0.1 mg/kg) or midazolam (0.1 mg/kg), along with a nondepolarizing neuromuscular blocker such as vecuronium (0.1 mg/ kg), is a reasonable combination. A persistent depolarizing agent, such as succinylcholine, provides a shorter duration of muscle paralysis. It can, however, result in an elevated ICP and hyperkalemia, both of which are poorly tolerated by children wth trauma and intracranial hypertension. In urgent situations, a rapid sequence consisting of orogastric suctioning, oxygenation, administration of sedative and muscle relaxant, laryngoscopy, cricoid pressure, and intubation may be necessary. Once the patient is intubated, a moderate level of hyperventilation ($PaCO_2$ 25 to 35 mm Hg) is appropriate in most situations.

Maintenance of cardiac output and organ perfusion is an integral component of initial resuscitation. Intravascular volume should be expanded using 20 ml/kg of isotonic crystalloid solution, such as 0.9% saline, or colloids, such as 5% albumin. Hemorrhagic shock should be treated with blood transfusion as soon as possible. Hypotonic solutions should never be used for intravascular expansion. Administration of such solutions can lead to dangerous intracellular fluid shifts, cerebral edema, and intracranial hypertension.

Secondary injury resulting from cerebral edema and intracranial hypertension poses a threat to neuronal survival. Prophylactic regimens to prevent intracranial hypertension may be more effective than initiating treatment only after increased ICP is demonstrated. Moderate hyperventilation is an effective way to lower a dangerously elevated ICP. The salutary effects of hyperventilation are due to cerebral vasoconstriction and a decrease in CBV. Excessive hyperventilation ($PaCO_2$ <20 mm Hg) should be avoided because a decrease in CBF below the ischemic threshold may occur. Osmotic diuretics, such as mannitol (0.5 g/kg), decrease brain water and, therefore, ICP. It has been argued that mannitol may increase CBV in patients with head injury who already have cerebral hyperemia. Subsequent studies, however, have shown that this concern is unfounded. We recommend the use of mannitol in combination with hyperventilation to treat suspected cerebral edema and intracranial hypertension. Because of its osmotic diuretic effect, the use of mannitol may result in hypovolemia and, therefore, an adequate circulation must be established **before** its use.

Approximately 9% of patients with head injury experience generalized tonic/clonic seizures. Undesirable effects of seizures include increase in cerebral metabolic rate, airway compromise, hypoventilation, aspiration, and exacerbation of intracranial hypertension. Lorazepam (0.1 mg/kg, maximum 5 mg) administered intravenously is the drug of choice for the immediate control of seizures. This dose may be repeated every 10 to 15 minutes for two additional doses. Patients with prolonged or repeated seizures should receive a loading dose of phenobarbital (20 mg/kg IV) or phenytoin (15 mg/kg IV) or both. The rate of administration should not exceed 1 mg/kg/min for phenobarbital and 0.5 mg/kg/min for phenytoin. The patient should be intubated and adequately ventilated while seizures are being controlled. The treatment of seizures may result in hypotension, which should be treated with volume expansion.

Transport Considerations

All unconscious patients with head injury should be considered to have a spinal injury. Extrication, immobilization, and transport of a child with suspected spinal cord injury should allow for rapid restoration of a neutral supine position and efficient access to the airway. Flexion, extension, or rotation of the head should be avoided. Gentle traction with hands locked under the jaw and neck should be used to align the patient's head and neck with the axis of the body. A backboard with cervical collar, sandbags, tape, and Velcro straps is useful for continued immobilization of the entire vertebral column until spinal injury can be reasonably excluded. Maintenance of a patent airway and adequate ventilation and circulation must be ensured continually during interhospital and intrahospital transport.

Laboratory and Radiologic Studies

A complete blood count and measurement of serum electrolytes, glucose, calcium, urea, and arterial blood gas should be obtained initially. Chest radiographs are important to determine proper endotracheal tube placement and to detect intrathoracic pathology. Initial evaluation of the spine should include anteroposterior and lateral radiographs of the cervical and upper thoracic vertebral column. **Emergency CT examination** is indicated when any of the following conditions is present:

- History of loss of consciousness
- Altered sensorium
- Focal neurologic deficits
- Penetrating craniocerebral wounds

Every attempt must be made to ensure airway patency, ventilation, circulation, and ICP control before and during the study.

IN-HOSPITAL MONITORING AND MANAGEMENT

Patients with a GCS <13 should be hospitalized in a facility where their vital signs and neurologic status can be monitored frequently. A decreasing level of responsiveness, confusion, restlessness, and agitation are early signs of worsening CNS functions. Bradycardia, hypertension, abnormal patterns of respiration, unilateral or bilateral dilatation of pupils with sluggish response to light, and dystonic movements or posturing represent progressive worsening of intracranial pathology. The clinical course of traumatic encephalopathy is best assessed by repeated GCS evaluation. Close attention to oxygenation/ventilation and fluid-electrolyte balance is essential. Hypotonic fluid overload and hyponatremia are very poorly tolerated by head-injured patients because of a preexistent pathologic increase in intracranial contents and elevated antidiuretic hormone levels. Fluid therapy should be aimed at maintaining normovolemia and electrolyte balance while restricting free water. A satisfactory daily maintenance fluid regimen in most cases is 1200 ml/m^2 containing 5% dextrose in 0.3% or 0.45% NaCl and 30 mEq potassium per liter. Any need for volume expansion should be met by using isotonic crystalloids or colloids.

Management of Intracranial Hypertension

Patients with severely compromised intracranial homeostasis of pressure and blood flow may suffer irreparable brain damage from intracranial hypertension and cerebral ischemia rather than from the primary disease process itself. Management of such patients is directed toward normalization of ICP and cerebral perfusion to allow sufficient time for cell repair. Patients with a GCS <9 should be managed in the intensive care unit. Many patients with cerebral injury have hemodynamic compromise, which is likely to be accentuated by therapeutic measures to reduce cerebral edema. All such patients should have continuous monitoring of their central venous pressure (CVP), arterial pressure, and urine output to determine the adequacy of blood volume. Patients with a GCS of 7 or less also require continuous monitoring of ICP to direct therapy for control of intracranial hypertension and to maintain CPP. An ICP below 15 mm Hg and a CPP above 50 mm Hg are the usually recommended therapeutic goals.

Epidural, intracerebral, or intraventricular placement of a fiberoptic pressure sensor is the most widely used method of ICP monitoring. Intraventricular catheters also allow removal of CSF as an additional means of controlling ICP, although this is more invasive and is associated with increased risk of infection.

Almost all the treatment modalities currently employed for cerebral support are controversial and lack appropriately controlled trials to prove their efficacy. We have shown that aggressive prophylactic and therapeutic interventions aimed to control ICP and CPP result in a better neurologic outcome than previously described in children with severe traumatic brain injury.

Mechanical Hyperventilation. Controlled hypocarbia (Paco$_2$ 25 to 35 mm Hg) should be maintained in all patients with suspected or confirmed intracranial hypertension. Excessive hyperventilation (Paco$_2$ <20 mm Hg), however, can be detrimental because of the resultant cerebral vasoconstriction and ischemia. Intermittent ICP spikes can be managed temporarily with additional hyperventilation. It is important to use relatively low tidal volumes or inflating pressures to avoid an excessive increase in intrathoracic pressure, which may impede cerebral venous return. To avoid increases in ICP, the use of sedatives and muscle paralysis is needed for a struggling and agitated patient. For this purpose, morphine (0.1 mg/kg), midazolam (0.1 mg/kg), and vecuronium (0.1 mg/kg) administered intravenously every hour are suitable agents. A positive end-expiratory pressure of 2 to 4 cm H$_2$O helps prevent atelectasis in a sedated, paralyzed patient.

Osmotherapy. An osmotic agent is most effective in reducing ICP in cytotoxic cerebral edema. Intravenous administration of 0.25 to 0.5 g/kg of mannitol every 4 to 6 hours is adequate in most patients. The dosage and frequency of mannitol should be adjusted according to ICP and clinical response. In some patients, up to 1 g/kg of mannitol may be needed every 2 to 3 hours. The aim of osmotherapy is to decrease brain bulk without causing total body dehydration and hypovolemia. Serum osmolality, serum electrolytes, BUN, urine output, and CVP should be carefully monitored in all patients receiving osmotherapy. To maintain a CVP between 3 and 7 mm Hg, judicious administration of isotonic crystalloids or colloids in 3 to 5 ml/kg boluses may be necessary. Mannitol should be withheld if serum osmolality is >310 mOsm/kg H$_2$O.

Barbiturates. Barbiturates decrease the cerebral metabolic rate, CBF, and ICP. The prophylactic use of barbiturate-induced coma to achieve burst suppression on EEG has not been shown to be of therapeutic benefit. Barbiturates should be considered as an adjuvant to other therapies to decrease ICP. For this purpose, pentobarbital (3 mg/kg IV bolus followed by a 1 to 3 mg/kg/h continuous infusion) is effective. The dose of pentobarbital should be adjusted according to the ICP response. A serum pentobarbital level >20 to 30 μg/ml is associated with myocardial depression, which may necessitate the use of an inotropic agent, such as dopamine.

Surgical Intervention. CSF drainage by an intraventricular catheter also can be used to lower ICP in patients with persistent intracranial hypertension. These catheters serve the dual purpose of intracranial decompression and ICP monitoring. Significant subdural and epidural hematomas require prompt evacuation. Removal of necrotic brain tissue and evacuation of an intraparenchymal hematoma may be necessary in selected cases.

Supportive Management. Patients with increased ICP are best managed with the head elevated at a 20- to 30-degree angle to facilitate cerebral venous drainage. The head should be in a neutral position to prevent jugular venous obstruction. Painful stimuli increase ICP and should be avoided. Local anesthesia should be used for invasive procedures even in those who appear unresponsive. Careful chest physiotherapy and suctioning should be performed every 1 to 2 hours, with intermittent manual hyperventilation to prevent a rise in Paco$_2$. Pulmonary toilet is best timed to coincide with the peak effects of sedatives and paralyzing agents to minimize ICP elevations. The routine use of therapeutic hypothermia has been shown to be of no benefit.

Hyperthermia, commonly observed in the brain-injured patient, should, however, be treated with antipyretics and, if necessary, a cooling blanket. Early institution of parenteral or enteral nutrition is important.

OUTCOME

The outcome of children with severe head injury has improved in recent years with a better understanding of the pathophysiologic response of the CNS to trauma, advances in diagnostic and monitoring techniques, and a team approach to neuroresuscitation. However, significant cognitive and psychomotor deficits are common in children with even relatively minor head injury. It has been suggested that some of these deficits may have been present before the head injury, thus making the child prone to injury. Neuropsychologic and rehabilitative interventions may improve the functional status of children with such residual deficits.

REFERENCES

1. Cooper PR (ed): Head Injury, 3rd ed. Baltimore, Williams & Wilkins, 1993.
2. Lieh-Lai MW, Theodorou AA, Sarnaik AP, et al: Limitations of the Glasgow coma scale in predicting outcome in children with traumatic brain injury. J Pediatr 120:195–199, 1992.

EXTRADURAL AND SUBDURAL HEMATOMA

N. Paul Rosman, M.D.

Most extradural and subdural hematomas in childhood follow head injuries. Extradural hematomas lie immediately beneath the skull and outside the dura, whereas subdural hematomas lie just below the dura. Both types of hematoma are located much more often above the tentorium (supratentorial) than in the posterior fossa (infratentorial). Such hematomas are classified as acute if accompanying symptoms appear within 48 hours, subacute when symptoms occur between 3 and 21 days, and chronic if they appear beyond 21 days.

ACUTE SUPRATENTORIAL EXTRADURAL AND SUBDURAL HEMATOMAS

Supratentorial, extradural hematomas are usually located in the temporoparietal area, and approximately 70% of affected individuals have an overlying skull fracture. Although they usually are caused by laceration of the underlying middle meningeal artery, at least 25% are of venous origin. Acute subdural hematomas are five to ten times more frequent than extradural hematomas and usually are caused by tearing of bridging meningeal veins. Occasionally, they are arterial in origin. Subdural hematomas usually are frontoparietal in location, and an accompanying skull fracture can be detected in 30% of affected children. An underlying brain contusion is frequently noted, and seizures often follow. The cranial CT scan is particularly valuable in distinguishing supratentorial extradural hematomas (usually lenticular) from subdural ones (usually curvilinear).

Acute subdural hematomas occur most often in early infancy, whereas extradural hematomas more often occur in older children (when the dura is less firmly adherent to the skull). Acute extradural hematomas are usually unilateral, and 75% of subdural hematomas are bilateral. Seizures occur in less than 25% of individuals with acute extradural hematomas but in 75% of children with subdural hematomas.

Signs and symptoms of intracranial hypertension are seen with both types of hematomas and include irritability or lethargy, vomiting, a full fontanelle, headache, papilledema, and altered vital signs (elevation of blood pressure, decreased or increased pulse rate, and slowed, irregular respirations). With sufficient elevation of pressure in the supratentorial compartment, unilateral transtentorial herniation may occur.

ACUTE INFRATENTORIAL EXTRADURAL AND SUBDURAL HEMATOMAS

Infratentorial hematomas occur much less frequently than those above the tentorium, and here, extradural hematomas occur more frequently than subdural hematomas do. Occipital skull fractures are frequent with both types of hematomas, and the bleeding is venous in both. Clinical signs include depressed consciousness, headache, vomiting, and altered respirations. Only half of affected children have posterior fossa signs. Hematomas here may be complicated by upward herniation of the cerebellum through the tentorial notch or, more often, by downward displacement of the cerebellar tonsils through the foramen magnum.

Treatment

Treatment of seizures complicating acute supratentorial hematomas is essentially the same as acute treatment of nontraumatic seizures. Phenytoin sodium (Dilantin) is the drug of choice because of its rapid entry into the brain and lack of sedation. It should be given intravenously in a dose of 15 to 18 mg/kg (at a rate of 25 to 50 mg/min) while the pulse and electrocardiogram are monitored. The total dose should not exceed 1000 mg. If phenytoin does not completely stop the seizures within a half-hour, paraldehyde in a dose of 0.1 to 0.25 ml/kg, or 1 to 1.5 ml per year of age (maximum dose of 7 ml), mixed with an equal volume of mineral oil, can be given rectally. If needed, the same dose can be repeated in 1 hour and every 2 to 4 hours thereafter. If seizure activity continues, intravenous diazepam (Valium) can be used as an alternative or adjunct to paraldehyde in a dose of 0.2 to 0.5 mg/kg (at a maximum rate of 1 to 2 mg/min). The total dose should not exceed 2 to 4 mg in the infant or 5 to 10 mg in the older child. This dose can be repeated every 15 to 30 minutes for a total of three doses if necessary. A benzodiazepine with a longer duration of action is lorazepam (Ativan). It is given intravenously in a dose of 0.05 to 0.1 mg/kg (at a maximum rate of 1 mg/min). If needed, an additional 0.05 mg/kg can be given 10 minutes later. The maximum total dose is 4 mg. Phenobarbital also can be used and is given intravenously in a dose of 15 to 20 mg/kg (at a rate of 30 to 100 mg/min). If needed, one-half the initial dose can be given 1 hour later and repeated every 4 to 6 hours thereafter. The maximum total dose is 300 mg. Phenobarbital and benzodiazepines given together may act synergistically to cause respiratory and cardiovascular depression.

With supratentorial hematomas, *treatment of increased ICP* by medical means is sometimes needed as a temporizing measure, especially when there is going to be a delay in surgical intervention. The airway must be cleared and patency ensured. If needed, ventilatory support should be provided. One hundred percent oxygen can be delivered by bag and mask or through nasal prongs. An intravenous line should be established, and circulatory support should be provided. With severe head injuries, a central venous line for fluid management should be placed, and an arterial line should be inserted to monitor blood pressure and facilitate measurement of blood gases. Hypovolemia can be corrected by intravenous administration of lactated ringer's solution, fresh frozen plasma, 5% albumin in normal saline, or blood. Circulatory failure can be treated with epinephrine, dobutamine, or dopamine. The head should be elevated to 30 degrees above the horizontal and stabilized in the midline. Fluid should be restricted to 100 ml/m^2/d (two thirds of daily maintenance). The bladder should be catheterized, and urinary output should be maintained at 1 ml/kg/h. Elevated temperatures should be lowered using antipyretics or cooling mattresses.

The most effective way to treat increased ICP rapidly is with passive hyperventilation, which does not potentiate intracranial bleeding or lead to a secondary increase in ICP (rebound). Hyperventilation lowers ICP by reducing the arterial carbon dioxide tension (PaCO_2), thereby inducing vasoconstriction. An acute reduction in arterial PaCO_2 of 5 to 10 mm Hg usually will lower the ICP by 25% to 30%. The PaCO_2 should not be reduced below 20 mm

Hg unless the jugular bulb Pao$_2$ is followed to ensure that cerebral ischemia has not ensued.

The intravenous administration of mannitol is another highly effective means of rapidly lowering elevated ICP. When given intravenously, mannitol remains in plasma and creates an osmotic gradient, which causes water to move from brain parenchyma into capillaries, thereby reducing ICP. Mannitol also slows production of CSF. When mannitol is given repeatedly, fluid and electrolyte imbalances and dehydration may result. Thus, the serum osmolality should be kept between 300 and 320 mOsm/L. Mannitol also increases CBF and, thus, may potentiate intracranial bleeding. Therefore, it should be given with caution during the first 2 to 3 days after a head injury (when brain swelling is caused primarily by hyperemia).

Glycerol is useful in the acute management of intracranial hypertension. Its administration, actions, and limitations are the same as with mannitol.

Induction of coma with barbiturates, usually pentobarbital, has been helpful in the management of intracranial hypertension following severe head injury when other measures have failed. Barbiturates reduce intracranial hypertension by inducing cerebral vasoconstriction, which secondarily lowers cerebral blood flow. They also reduce cerebral metabolism by up to 50%. Pentobarbital is given in an initial intravenous dose of 3 to 5 mg/kg over 10 to 20 minutes, followed by 1 to 3 mg/kg every 1 to 2 hours. Serum pentobarbital levels of 3 to 4.5 mg/dl should be maintained. The advantages of barbiturate coma include rapidity of onset and absence of rebound. Furthermore, it does not potentiate intracranial bleeding.

Hypothermia is an additional means of treating children with raised ICP. With lowering of body temperature to 30° C, the cerebral metabolic rate is decreased by almost 50%. The mechanisms of action, advantages, and limitations of hypothermia are similar to those with barbiturate coma. For each degree (C) that the temperature is lowered, there is approximately a 6% reduction in CBF.

Steroids act more slowly than hyperosmolar agents in reducing increased ICP. Further, despite their widespread use in head injuries, steroids, even in megadoses, have not been proven effective.

The *treatment of acute extradural hematomas* often is needed urgently, since these hematomas may enlarge rapidly and result in signs of acutely elevated ICP and worsening hemiparesis. In such instances, immediate neurosurgical treatment is required, including craniotomy, surgical removal of blood clot, and coagulation or clipping of the bleeding vessel. The mortality rate in children with acute extradural hematoma varies from 9% to 17%, but the survivors tend to be relatively free of neurologic sequelae.

The *treatment of acute subdural hematomas* generally is less urgent. When ICP is elevated in infants in whom a subdural hematoma is suspected (particularly in the absence of cranial CT), the subdural space should be tapped as a combined diagnostic and therapeutic measure. This is done at the two lateral corners of the anterior fontanelle. In older children, in whom the anterior fontanelle is closed, burr holes must first be placed. Subdural fluid should not be aspirated because of the risk of complicating rebleeding and hypovolemic shock. The taps should be repeated every 1 to 2 days until the fluid clears. If after 8 to 10 taps, the subdural fluid continues to reaccumulate, a shunt should be placed between the subdural space and the peritoneum or a pleural cavity. On those rare occasions when there is a marked increase in ICP complicating an acute subdural hemorrhage and when surgical intervention is not immediately possible, the intracranial hypertension should be treated by the medical measures described. Although the mortality rate with an acute subdural hematoma is usually less than with an extradural hematoma, the neurologic morbidity is greater because of the frequency with which the underlying brain is injured. The child may be left with recurrent seizures, weakness, spasticity or ataxia, speech difficulties, and learning, attentional, or behavioral problems. Depending on the sequelae, appropriate interventions should be prescribed.

On rare occasions, elevations in ICP cannot be reversed by the measures already discussed. When there is marked intracranial hypertension with signs of impending or evolving brain herniation, a ventricular tap with slow withdrawal of CSF may be lifesaving. If the raised ICP continues in an unremitting fashion, decompressive craniotomy may be needed.

SUBACUTE AND CHRONIC SUBDURAL HEMATOMAS

Most subacute and chronic hematomas occur in the older child and adolescent, in whom symptoms can include recurrent vomiting, boxlike macrocrania (reflecting a longer-standing increase in ICP), and patency/prominence of the anterior fontanelle. Seizures are frequent, and motor abnormalities are often found. Common systemic signs include irritability, vomiting, fever, anemia, and poor weight gain. These hematomas are best visualized with a cranial MRI.

Treatment of subacute and chronic subdural hematomas includes subdural taps with removal of subdural fluid, external drainage with shunting of subdural fluid to the peritoneum or pleural cavity, and aspiration or surgical removal of subdural clots through a burr hole or craniotomy.

BRAIN ABSCESS

MARY E. SUTTON, M.D.
SCOTT L. POMEROY, M.D. Ph.D.

Brain abscess is an intracranial suppurative infection resulting from contiguous spread of infection from the paranasal sinuses, middle ear, or mastoid or from hematogenous spread of infection from distant sites. Brain abscesses of hematogenous origin disseminate from pulmonary, dental, or skin infections, particularly in children with cyanotic congenital heart disease and a right-to-left shunt. Less often, brain abscess develops following penetrating head trauma, meningitis, or prior cranial surgery. In neonates, brain abscess occurs as a complication of purulent meningitis caused by *Proteus* or *Citrobacter* species.

The initial stage of brain abscess is focal cerebritis, characterized by an edematous area of inflammatory exudate with a necrotic center. Next, a capsule develops from inflammatory granulation tissue that is thickened by collagen fibers from proliferating fibroblasts. The adjacent brain tissue becomes increasingly edematous. Because of the risk of rapidly increasing mass effect and possible herniation, brain abscess must be diagnosed and treated rapidly with antibiotics and drainage or excision to avoid significant morbidity and mortality.

CLINICAL MANIFESTATIONS

The classic clinical triad of headache, fever, and focal neurologic signs and symptoms may occur in only one third of children with brain abscess. The most prominent clinical manifestations of brain abscess result from signs of increased ICP, including headache, vomiting, depression of mental status, and papilledema. Up to one half of children with brain abscess have focal neurologic signs or seizures, and three quarters of patients have fever. The presentation of brain abscess may be indolent or acute, but the majority of patients have symptoms of increased ICP for over 2 weeks prior to diagnosis. Neonates with brain abscess tend to have seizures, lethargy, and a bulging fontanelle and often have multiple abscesses.

DIAGNOSIS

Computed tomography (CT) scanning and magnetic resonance imaging (MRI) are the procedures of choice to establish the diagnosis of brain abscess. Contrast enhancement of the abscess rim and developing capsule surrounding a lucent nonenhancing center differentiates early abscess from infarct on CT. In infants with an open fontanelle, cranial ultrasonography can also be a useful diagnostic technique.

The peripheral white blood cell count may be normal in up to one third of cases of brain abscess, and an elevated erythrocyte sedimentation rate (ESR) is not consistently present. The etiologic organism is cultured from the blood in less than 10% of cases and usually only when endocarditis is the cause of the brain abscess. The CSF is a poor source for isolating the organism, and lumbar puncture is contraindicated because of the risk of cerebral herniation.

MICROORGANISMS ASSOCIATED WITH BRAIN ABSCESS

Culture of the abscess contents can isolate a wide range of microorganisms, including most bacteria and certain fungi and parasites. The abscess culture reveals a single organism in 70% of cases and multiple organisms in 30%. It is imperative that physicians collect specimens from the brain abscess in appropriate syringes or transport media and take them immediately to the microbiology laboratory for gram stain, fungal stain, and placement in culture media.

The type of microorganism isolated is dependent on the source of the brain abscess and host immunologic factors. Historically, the streptococci, especially alpha-hemolytic streptococci, such as *Streptococcus milleri*, and staphylococci have been the most common causative organisms. With improved culturing techniques, anaerobic bacteria have been isolated alone or in mixed infections in up to 80% of cases of brain abscess in children, particularly those resulting from sinusitis, otitis media, or dental infection. Other organisms, including *Haemophilus influenzae*, the pneumococcus, and *Staphylococcus aureus*, may be the causative organism in brain abscess related to sinusitis, otitis media, or mastoiditis. Otitis media and mastoiditis may be the source of brain abscess caused by Enterobacteriaceae, *Proteus* sp., *S. aureus*, or anaerobic species, such as *Bacteroides*.

Patients with cyanotic congenital heart disease most often have infections with *Streptococcus* sp., particularly alpha-hemolytic streptococci, and anaerobic gram-positive cocci. Brain abscess following meningitis occurs most commonly in infants less than 1 year of age and is caused by the pneumococcus or aerobic gram-negative rods, such as *Citrobacter diversus* or *Proteus* sp. In children with a ventriculoperitoneal shunt, *S. aureus*, *Staphylococcus epidermidis*, and gram-negative enteric rods are the most common causative pathogens of brain abscess. Immunosuppressed patients are at risk for brain abscess caused by a wide variety of aerobic and anaerobic bacteria, as well as fungi, such as *Candida* and *Aspergillus* sp., mycobacteria, and parasites (including *Entamoeba histolytica* and *Toxoplasma gondii*).

TREATMENT AND OUTCOME

Treatment of brain abscess generally requires intravenous antibiotic therapy and prompt aspiration or excision of the abscess. Patients who are unstable as a result of increased ICP should be intubated, hyperventilated, given mannitol, and taken to the operating room for surgical drainage or excision of the abscess. Steroid administration is controversial and should be used only for short-term control of cerebral edema. Aspiration or drainage of the abscess remains the definitive treatment for brain abscess. However, it is associated with a mortality rate of 10% to 15%. Surgical excision decreases the risk of abscess recurrence and decreases the duration of antibiotic therapy from a mean of 4 weeks to a mean of 2½ weeks. However, excision results in higher rates of neurologic sequelae (up to 70%) compared with rates seen in patients undergoing aspiration or surgical drainage (up to 50%).

Ideally, antimicrobial drug selection should be based on results of culture and sensitivity tests of pus obtained from the abscess cavity. Until culture results are known, empiric antibiotic therapy should be started in doses appropriate for meningitis and continued as long as the clinical status dictates (usually at least 4 weeks). Given the high frequency of polymicrobial brain abscesses, initial empiric antibiotic coverage should include a third-generation cephalosporin (cefotaxime or ceftazidime) and an antistaphylococcal agent, such as nafcillin. In patients with penicillin allergy, abscess secondary to ventriculoperitoneal shunt infection, or suspected methicillin-resistant staphylococ-

TABLE 1. Formulary

DRUG	DOSAGE*	COMMENTS
Cefotaxime	200 mg/kg/24 h IV, divided q6h	Max: 12 g/24 h
Ceftazidime	150 mg/kg/24 h IV, divided q8h	Max: 6 g/24 h
Ceftriaxone	100 mg/kg/24 h IV, divided q12h	Max: 4 g/24 h
Chloramphenicol	75–100 mg/kg/24 h IV, divided q6h	Max: 4 g/24 h Monitor serum peak and trough concentrations and CBC
Metronidazole	Loading dose: 15 mg/kg once, then 30 mg/kg/24 h IV, divided q6h	Max: 4 g/24 h
Mannitol	250 mg/kg/dose IV push	Repeat q5min as needed up to max 2 g/kg for increased ICP Monitor serum osmolarity
Nafcillin	200 mg/kg/24 h IV, divided q6h	Max: 10 g/24 h
Vancomycin	60 mg/kg/24 h IV, divided q6h	Max: 2 g/24 h Monitor serum peak and trough concentrations, renal function, hearing

*Dosages are reported for children and infants greater than 1 month of age.

cal infection, vancomycin may be substituted for the nafcillin. Metronidazole or chloramphenicol should be added when the source of infection is unknown or when an anaerobic infection is likely based on the site of primary infection, such as the paranasal sinuses, the middle ear, or the mouth. Immunosuppressed hosts with brain abscess should initially receive broad antibiotic coverage, including amphotericin B therapy if fungi are visible on fungal stain (Table 1).

Antibiotic coverage should be narrowed appropriately when the causative organism(s) and sensitivities are identified. The duration of antibiotic therapy generally ranges from 4 to 8 weeks and can be guided by follow-up CT scans. A small percentage of patients have been managed successfully with antibiotics alone. Typically, these patients have abscesses that are surgically inaccessible, multiple, or small. They should be followed closely by serial CT scans while receiving antibiotics.

With improved diagnosis by CT or MRI and rapid initiation of antibiotic therapy and abscess drainage, the mortality rate for brain abscess in children has declined in recent series to 10% to 15%. Findings that are associated with increased risk of mortality include age less than 2 years, coma on admission, a large abscess or multiple abscesses, performance of lumbar puncture, and rupture of the abscess into the ventricles.

One half of children surviving brain abscess experience neurologic sequelae, including epilepsy, hemiparesis, hydrocephalus, or cognitive impairment. Because neonatal brain abscess usually is associated wth multiple areas of infarction and necrosis, at least three fourths of neonates surviving brain abscess experience significant neurologic morbidity. Two thirds demonstrate mental retardation, and one half exhibit epilepsy.

REFERENCES

1. Brook I: Aerobic and anaerobic bacteriology of intracranial abscesses. Pediatr Neurol 8:210–214, 1992.
2. Patrick CC, Kaplan SL: Current concepts in the pathogenesis and management of brain abscesses in children. *In* New topics in pediatric infectious disease. Pediatr Clin North Am 35:625–636, 1988.
3. Renier D, Flandin C, Hirsch E, Hirsch J: Brain abscesses in neonates: A study of 30 cases. J Neurosurg 69:877–882, 1988.
4. Saez-Llorens XJ, Umana MA, Odio CM, McCracken GH, Nelson JD: Brain abscess in infants and children. Pediatr Infect Dis J 8:449–458, 1989.

SPINAL EPIDURAL ABSCESS

MARY E. SUTTON, M.D.
SCOTT L. POMEROY, M.D., Ph.D

Spinal epidural abscess is a rare pyogenic infection of the spinal epidural space that must be identified and treated urgently to prevent irreversible neurologic disability or death. In children, the rapid diagnosis of spinal epidural abscess may be delayed because of atypical presentations that vary from the classic triad of fever, back pain, and focal neurologic signs. Prompt antibiotic treatment and surgical drainage can lower the high rates of morbidity (up to 30%) and mortality (up to 30%) commonly seen with spinal epidural abscess in children.

CLINICAL MANIFESTATIONS

The classic phases of spinal epidural abscess include (1) localized back pain and fever, (2) pain radiating in a radicular pattern (because of inflammation or compression of the spinal nerves), (3) sensory loss and weakness (including bowel and bladder dysfunction), and (4) complete paralysis below the level of the abscess. Although the first three phases can progress rapidly over hours or slowly over weeks, the progression to paralysis can occur suddenly and irreversibly regardless of the previous tempo of the disease.

Infants and children often have atypical presentations of spinal epidural abscess that may delay diagnosis until after permanent neurologic damage has occurred. The earliest signs and symptoms in infants may be nonspecific, including fever, irritability, and poor feeding. Increased crying with handling, spine rigidity, decreased limb movement, or focal vertebral tenderness can help localize the problem to the spine. In older children, radiation of back pain to the chest, abdomen, or legs may lead to an erroneous initial diagnosis.

Localized back pain or tenderness, present in up to 90% of cases, appears to be the most sensitive indicator of spinal epidural abscess in childhood. However, diagnosis can be delayed because of the absence of one or more of the classic symptoms. Fever is seen in only 60% of children with spinal epidural abscess. Focal neurologic signs, such as weakness, sensory loss, or bowel/bladder dysfunction, are indications for immediate imaging of the spinal cord to rule out spinal epidural abscess.

DIAGNOSIS

A high index of suspicion and a careful history and physical examination are necessary for the rapid diagnosis of spinal epidural abscess before the onset of neurologic deficits. MRI of the spine is the imaging technique of choice owing to its lack of invasiveness and high sensitivity (91%), equal to that of CT myelography. In addition, MRI is the best technique for distinguishing other diseases, including spinal cord tumor, arteriovenous malformation, or transverse myelitis. Imaging the entire spine is advisable to avoid missing the rare possibility of multiple abscesses.

Lumbar puncture can cause neurologic deterioration if performed below a spinal block or result in meningitis if the needle traverses the epidural infection. The cerebrospinal fluid (CSF) may show evidence of a parameningeal focus with increased protein and pleocytosis. However, a normal CSF profile does not rule out spinal epidural abscess. CSF culture will be negative except for the unusual case in which leptomeningitis develops. A lumbar puncture is unnecessary unless it is clinically indicated to rule out meningitis or to perform CT myelography. Whenever possible, imaging should precede lumbar puncture to avoid passing the needle through the abscess.

Plain radiographs and bone scans are not usually helpful, even in the presence of an associated osteomyelitis. The causative organism can be cultured from the abscess in most cases, and blood cultures are positive for the offending organism in over 50% of cases. The erythrocyte sedimentation rate (ESR) is almost invariably elevated,

but the peripheral white blood cell count is not reliable as an indicator of this infection.

PATHOPHYSIOLOGY AND MICROBIOLOGY

The most common cause of spinal epidural abscess is hematogenous spread of bacteria from distant infections involving the skin and soft tissues, the upper and lower respiratory tract, or the urinary tract. It has been proposed that infected blood reaches the epidural space by shunting into the low pressure epidural network of veins (Batson's plexus) during a Valsalva maneuver.

Spinal epidural abscess also can be caused by local extension from osteomyelitis of the spine or from an infection after spinal surgery, epidural anesthesia, or multiple lumbar puncture attempts. A traumatic hematoma can create a nidus for infection. Rarely, inflammatory bowel disease results in fistulous tracts that extend into the epidural space. Spinal epidural abscess tends to occur in the posterior thoracic or lumbar region, where the epidural space is the largest, although it may occur focally or diffusely anywhere from the cervical to the sacral spine. Spinal cord pathology results from a combination of direct compression and ischemia.

Staphylococcus aureus causes over 50% of spinal epidural abscesses in adults and children. The next most common organisms are other aerobic gram-positive organisms, including *Streptococcus* sp., followed by gram-negative organisms (particularly in cases involving intravenous drug abuse, recent surgery, or urinary tract infections). Anaerobes, fungi, and mycobacteria also can cause spinal epidural abscess, and samples should be cultured for each of these types of organisms.

TREATMENT AND OUTCOME

Therapy for spinal epidural abscess consists of prompt administration of empiric broad-spectrum antibiotics and, in most cases, surgical drainage of the abscess. Weakness and bowel/bladder dysfunction can improve or resolve if surgery is performed within 24 hours of the onset of these neurologic deficits. Infants and children are at increased risk for spinal deformity following extensive laminectomy. Rarely, nonsurgical treatment of spinal epidural abscess (either antibiotics alone or antibiotics plus percutaneous aspiration of the abscess) has been successful. However, approximately one quarter of patients receiving appropriate antibiotic therapy develop sudden and often irreversible neurologic deterioration before surgical drainage. In general, nonoperative management should be reserved for patients who have high operative risks for other medical reasons.

Initial empiric systemic antibiotics should include an antistaphylococcal agent, such as nafcillin, and a third-generation cephalosporin, such as cefotaxime or ceftriaxone. Antibiotic coverage should be adjusted according to the identification and sensitivities of the organism and administered intravenously for 4 weeks. An additional 4 weeks of oral antibiotics is indicated when osteomyelitis is present.

Despite aggressive treatment, the morbidity and mortality of spinal epidural abscess remain high in infants and children. Up to one third of children with spinal epidural abscess die, and another one third are left with residual weakness, paralysis, incontinence, or spinal deformity. The prognosis of spinal epidural abscess in children improves with rapid diagnosis and treatment before the onset of significant neurologic disability.

REFERENCES

1. Hlavin MJ, Kaminski HJ, Ross JS, Ganz E: Spinal epidural abscess: A ten-year perspective. Neurosurgery 27:177–184, 1990.
2. Rubin G, Michowiz S, Ashkenasi A, Tadmor R, Rappaport Z: Spinal epidural abscess in the pediatric age group: Case report and review of the literature. Pediatr Infect Dis J 12:1007–1011, 1993.
3. Schweich PJ, Hurt TL: Spinal epidural abscess in children: Two illustrative cases. Pediatr Emerg Care 8:84–87, 1992.

CRANIAL SUBDURAL EMPYEMA

SCOTT L. POMEROY, M.D., Ph.D.
MARY E. SUTTON, M.D.

Subdural empyema, a pyogenic bacterial infection of the subdural space, is a rare intracranial infection. Although subdural empyema occurs less than once per 100 cases of bacterial meningitis, it must be considered in the differential diagnosis of a child with fever and neurologic signs. Once the diagnosis is established, it is a neurosurgical emergency with substantial mortality and neurologic morbidity. In infants, the infection occurs most frequently as a complication of meningitis. Among older children, subdural empyema arises following infection of the paranasal sinuses, from mastoiditis, or as a consequence of chronic otitis media. Less frequently, cranial trauma or surgical procedures precede the infection.

Because of the anatomy of the subdural space, subdural empyema often extends widely over the surface of one or both cerebral hemispheres. Occasionally, the empyema may be confined to the posterior fossa. The mass effect from progressive infection within this subdural space exerts pressure on the nervous system, which may lead to herniation. This perilous situation requires treatment with surgical drainage of the empyema in addition to systemic antibiotics for successful resolution.

CLINICAL MANIFESTATIONS

Clinical evidence of the primary source of infection may or may not be present. The principal signs and symptoms of subdural empyema include headache, fever, nuchal rigidity or other evidence of meningeal irritation, and focal neurologic signs referable to the site of infection. Seizures occur frequently and may be either focal or generalized. As the infection progresses, signs of increased intracranial pressure (ICP) become prominent. In infants, this is manifest as a bulging fontanelle with associated irritability, vomiting, and decreased responsiveness. Older children may develop papilledema in addition to progressive headache, vomiting, and mental status changes. These signs and symptoms progress as the ICP rises. In the most severe cases, marked elevation of ICP may lead to herniation of the cerebrum or cerebellum.

DIAGNOSIS

The diagnosis of subdural empyema is made either by computed tomography (CT) scanning or by magnetic resonance imaging (MRI). Characteristic findings on these studies include a thin, hypodense lesion within the subdural space, linear contrast enhancement most pronounced on the inner margin, and in advanced cases, inward displacement of the gray matter–white matter interface with mass effect. Laboratory investigations demonstrate a peripheral leukocytosis with predominance of polymorphonuclear cells, often with increased numbers of immature cells. If subdural empyema is considered a diagnostic possibility, lumbar puncture should be avoided because of the potential risk of cerebral herniation from the mass effect of the lesion. In cases where CSF is obtained, the fluid commonly reveals a pleocytosis, often with polymorphonuclear cell predominance, elevated protein, and decreased glucose. Cultures of the CSF frequently are negative. The use of angiography for diagnosis has largely been replaced by high-resolution CT and MRI.

MICROORGANISMS ASSOCIATED WITH SUBDURAL EMPYEMA

A wide variety of bacteria may be found within a subdural empyema. The causative organism varies with the site of the primary infection. Overall, aerobic and anaerobic *Streptococcus* sp. are the most common organisms. These microorganisms may be found in up to 70% of positive cultures. *Staphylococcus* sp. constitute 10% to 20% of isolates, and aerobic and anaerobic gram-negative bacteria may each be found in up to 5% of positive cultures. The incidence of sterile subdural collections is 15% to 25% in many series, whereas polymicrobial infections are found in up to 10% of cases.

TREATMENT AND OUTCOME

Treatment of subdural empyema requires both surgical drainage and administration of systemic antibiotics. The surgical approach for drainage is controversial but varies according to the extent and nature of the subdural lesion. Small collections without loculations may be drained by multiple burr holes, with irrigation. Most other cases require craniotomy for adequate exposure and drainage of the infection.

Systemic antibiotics should be administered at the time of diagnosis. Before identification of the causative organism and determination of antibiotic sensitivity, empiric therapy should be given. A gram stain of the empyema may guide the choice of antibiotics, but treatment with a third-generation cephalosporin (cefotaxime or ceftazidime) and an antistaphylococcal agent (nafcillin or oxacillin) will provide sufficiently broad coverage for most cases. If a methacillin-resistant staphylococcal infection is suspected or if the patient is allergic to penicillin, vancomycin may be substituted. Metronidazole should be added if anaerobic organisms are likely based on the site of the primary infection (sinusitis, otitis media, and dental infection).

With improvements in surgical technique and the widespread availability of CT and MRI scans, the mortality rate from subdural empyema has declined in most modern series to less than 10%. Significant neurologic sequelae may be found in up to 20% to 30% of survivors, although the incidence has been lower in more recent studies.

REFERENCES

1. Bok APL, Peter JC: Subdural empyema: Burr holes or craniotomy? A retrospective computerized tomography-era analysis of treatment in 90 cases. J Neurosurg 78:574–578, 1993.
2. Kaufman DM, Litman N, Miller MH: Sinusitis: Induced subdural empyema. Neurology 33:123–132, 1983.
3. Morgan DW, Williams B: Posterior fossa subdural empyema. Brain 108:983–992, 1985.

THE POLYRADICULONEUROPATHIES

ROBERT H. A. HASLAM, M.D., F.R.C.P.(C.)

GUILLAIN-BARRÉ SYNDROME

The Guillain-Barré syndrome (GBS), also known as acute inflammatory demyelinating polyradiculoneuropathy, is a demyelinating disease that targets peripheral nerves, producing a flaccid paralysis, sensory symptoms, and on occasion, autonomic abnormalities. GBS is the most common cause of acute loss of motor function in children except in those countries where poliomyelitis is still prevalent. The annual incidence is 0.75 to 2 cases per 100,000 population. The long-term prognosis in children, irrespective of specific treatment regimens, is generally favorable. The mortality rate is 3% to 5%, but most deaths result from preventable complications.

Diagnosis

The diagnosis of GBS should be considered when ascending paralysis of the legs and arms is associated with areflexia. The weakness is typically symmetric and progressive for up to 4 weeks. Although sensory symptoms or signs are generally mild, some children initially experience excruciating pain in the upper legs and back. There is often a history of an upper respiratory tract infection a few weeks preceding the onset of the disease, but fever is absent when the neurologic symptoms and signs develop. Bilateral facial nerve involvement is apparent in approximately 30% of cases. Autonomic dysfunction, including hypertension and cardiac arrhythmias, is not as common in children as in the adult patient. Examination of the cerebrospinal fluid (CSF) characteristically reveals an elevated protein concentration with fewer than 10 white blood cells per cubic millimeter. A markedly elevated CSF protein concentration (> 2.5 g/L) suggests a spinal cord tumor or an infectious process. Electrodiagnostic studies are typified by decreased motor nerve conduction velocities, an absent F response, and reduction of the distal compound muscle action potentials (CMAP). The diagnosis of GBS should be questioned if a sensory (spinal cord) level is demonstrated or if the symptoms and signs persist in an asymmetric distribution. Significant bowel and bladder dysfunction is rarely encountered in GBS, and CSF pleocytosis greater than 50 white blood cells per cubic millimeter makes the diagnosis of GBS doubtful.

Etiology

Although the precise etiology of GBS is unknown, an immunologic basis for the segmental demyelination of the peripheral nerves is the most likely cause. Immunohistochemical staining of lymphocytes infiltrating human peripheral nerve biopsies early in the course of the disease shows that the majority of these cells are T cells. Furthermore, serum from patients with acute GBS produces demyelination when injected into animals. It is quite likely that an antecedent viral or bacterial infection is responsible for triggering the destructive immunologic process. Agents that have been associated with GBS include the varicella-zoster virus, cytomegalovirus (CMV), hepatitis B virus, human immunodeficiency virus (HIV), and Epstein-Barr virus (EBV). More recently, *Campylobacter jejuni* and *Mycoplasma pneumoniae* have been implicated as possible causative agents. GBS is occasionally associated with autoimmune-mediated disorders, including lupus erythematosus, myasthenia gravis, and Hodgkin's disease.

Assessment

All children with suspected GBS should be hospitalized to monitor the rate of progression of motor weakness and to determine the presence of complications. Muscle strength should be recorded on a daily basis, using a scoring system that can be readily replicated. The scoring system used in the American plasmapheresis study of GBS has proven useful in monitoring patients, where $0 =$ normal power, $1 =$ minor symptoms and signs, $2 =$ able to walk ≥ 10 m without assistance, $3 =$ able to walk ≥ 10 m with a walker or support, $4 =$ bedridden or chairbound, unable to walk 10 m with a walker or support, $5 =$ requiring assisted ventilation for at least part of the day, and $6 =$ death.[1] Unfortunately, this scoring system is not adaptable to nonambulatory children and does not readily identify treatment-related fluctuations. If the course of the disease is mild and nonprogressive, the child may be discharged following a period of observation and examined regularly on an outpatient basis.

The immunization status of the child should be documented so that one can eliminate the possibility of poliomyelitis. The search for a causative agent should include culture of the urine for CMV the stool for *C. jejuni* and serologic studies for EBV, the hepatitis virus, and (if warranted) HIV. In addition, the history and physical and laboratory examination should be directed to detecting the possibility of an underlying systemic or immune-mediated disorder. A CSF specimen should be obtained for routine studies, with at least one vial stored and frozen for future use. An opening CSF pressure should be recorded. Nerve conduction velocities and an electromyogram are essential components of the diagnostic process. As cardiovascular dysautonomia may occur in the pediatric patient, cardiac monitoring and frequent blood pressure determinations must be obtained. Cardiac arrhythmias or significant alterations in the blood pressure demand observation and management in an intensive care unit.

Management

The most critical complication of GBS is respiratory failure. Impending respiratory failure is associated with rapid and shallow breathing, tachycardia, fatigue, and abdominal paradox. Delay in providing mechanical ventilation is associated with an increased complication

rate, including pneumonia, atelectasis, and pneumothorax, which can lead to death. If the child is able to cooperate, an expiratory vital capacity (VC) should be monitored every 4 to 6 hours, using a hand-held spirometer at the bedside. To gain maximal effort during the VC determination, the child can be encouraged to practice exhaling into a balloon, with the assistance and urging of the parents. Elective intubation is indicated if the VC is less than 20 ml/kg, the blood gas analysis demonstrates hypoxemia ($PO_2 < 60$ mm Hg in room air), or the child has difficulty clearing secretions associated with a weak or absent cough. As an elevated arterial PCO_2 is a late manifestation of respiratory failure, intervention by elective endotracheal intubation should take place before hypercapnia. The most common reason to intervene with an endotracheal tube is the presence of bulbar involvement, rather than mechanical respiratory failure. With bulbar paralysis (pooling of secretions, dysphagia, dysphonia), the arterial blood gases in room air may be normal or only marginally abnormal (PO_2 70 to 80 mm Hg). Intubation is accomplished nasally using a snugly fitting, noncuffed tube with the largest possible diameter for the patient's size. Cuffed endotracheal tubes are generally used in children 6 years of age and older.

The duration of ventilatory support required before return of intercostal muscle activity is variable but usually occurs before the recovery of bulbar function. Assessment of VC is relatively easy to perform in the intubated child by measuring the negative inspiratory force (NIF). The procedure is performed by occluding the endotracheal tube and determining the negative pressure generated distal to the occlusion. An NIF of greater than -30 cm H_2O usually indicates that the VC is adequate to generate an effective cough. At that point, extubation can be considered.

Although some centers recommend tracheostomy if neurologic recovery is not evident by the end of 1 week, there is no absolute rule as to when to perform a tracheostomy. We recommend placing a tracheostomy if the need for intubation exceeds 2 weeks duration, not because of concern about the safety of long-term nasotracheal intubation but rather for the psychologic benefit of the child. Not only does the removal of the nasotracheal tube improve the child's emotional outlook, but also a tracheostomy provides an additional degree of mobility and facilitates nursing, especially when caring for a child with long-term paralysis.

Exemplary nursing care is essential for the acutely ill child. Chest physiotherapy and skilled endotracheal suctioning are important components of pulmonary management. Parenteral or enteral alimentation using a feeding tube must be instituted for the child who cannot safely swallow. The choice of alimentation will depend on the severity of the bulbar signs, but, in general, total parenteral nutrition is the preferred method of alimentation for the ventilated child with poor deglutition. Physical therapy includes frequent passive range of motion exercises for all joints and the use of splints for the wrists and ankles to prevent contractures. Frequent turning and meticulous skin care are necessary to prevent decubitus ulcers. Severe pain occasionally is present during the initial few weeks of the disease. It is important to use a medication that does not significantly suppress respiratory function or interfere with the child's ability to cough. Analgesics that have proven useful include acetaminophen, nonsteroidal anti-inflammatory drugs, codeine, and morphine. The least toxic drugs should be used first. The most important principle in pain management, irrespective of the analgesic, is careful titration of the drug to achieve alleviation of pain without producing untoward side effects.

Autonomic dysfunction may be minimized by preventing sudden changes in body posture, by avoiding overly vigorous tracheal suctioning, and by maintaining adequate hydration. Atrial and ventricular arrhythmias should be treated by appropriate agents and wide excursions in blood pressure by short-acting pressors or antihypertensive drugs.

Finally, the emotional needs of the child must not be overlooked. A paralyzed child on a respirator who is unable to breathe or talk is terrified! The nursing and medical staff should make a special effort to constantly reassure the child. The parents must be encouraged to stay at the bedside and to provide support and reassurance for their child.

Specific Treatment Modalities

It is important to note that GBS is a reversible disease with a good prognosis for most children. However, approximately 10% to 20% of children develop respiratory failure secondary to muscle weakness or bulbar paralysis and require mechanical ventilation for periods up to 2 months. It is for these children that specific treatment modalities have been developed in an attempt to halt the progression of the disease and obviate the need for mechanical ventilation. Since GBS is considered to result from an autoimmune process, the therapeutic approaches have focused on the immune system.

Corticosteroids

Until recently, corticosteroids were the mainstay of treatment for GBS. However, two randomized controlled studies found no benefit of steroids as compared with placebo. Thus, the use of corticosteroids is no longer advocated for the treatment of GBS.

Plasmapheresis

The use of plasma exchange in adult patients with GBS has been thoroughly studied. There have been three major randomized controlled trials, primarily in adults, that have shown that plasmapheresis is beneficial. The duration of mechanical ventilation, time period to walking unassisted, and the 6 to 12 month morbidity outcomes were significantly enhanced in those patients who underwent plasma exchange. There have been no randomized controlled plasma exchange studies in children with GBS. Several retrospective studies and case reports indicate that the attainment of independent ambulation was enhanced and the duration of ventilatory assistance was decreased in the treated children. Plasmapheresis is not without risk in children, as vascular access can pose major difficulties. Aside from the mechanical problems associated with plasma exchange, volume overloading or hypotensive episodes may complicate the procedure, and there is a small but definite risk of blood-borne infection. Plasmapheresis is not recommended for routine use in children with GBS and, until randomized controlled studies are published, should be considered only for those patients with pending respiratory failure.

Intravenous Immune Globulin

The Dutch Guillain-Barré Study Group compared the efficacy of intravenous immune globulin and plasma exchange in adult GBS patients.[3] In that study, the use of intravenous immune globulin, shortened the time to recover independent locomotion, decreased the mean duration of ventilatory assistance, and lessened the complication rate in comparison with affected individuals treated with plasmapheresis. There have been several case reports of the effect of high-dose intravenous immunoglobulin in the pediatric literature, using approximately 0.4 to 1 g/kg/d for 2 to 5 consecutive days[2] (Table 1). In each case, significant and rapid neurologic recovery was reported. Intravenous immunoglobulin can be administered safely to children, including those with cardiovascular instability, at less cost than plasmapheresis. Until randomized controlled trials are reported for the pediatric age group, intravenous immune globulin is the preferred treatment for children with acute GBS and rapid neurologic deterioration.

TABLE 1. Treatments for GBS

TREATMENT	PROTOCOL
Plasmapheresis	200 ml/kg mean total plasma volume exchange on 4–5 successive days
Intravenous immune globulin	0.4–1 g/kg/d for 2–5 successive days

CHRONIC INFLAMMATORY DEMYELINATING POLYRADICULONEUROPATHY

Chronic inflammatory demyelinating polyradiculoneuropathy (CIDP) is a chronic neuropathy that has a slow and insidious onset. Because the weakness is symmetric and associated with diminished or absent deep tendon reflexes, the condition is often confused in the early stages with Guillain-Barré syndrome (GBS). However, the course and prognosis of CIDP is considerably different from those of GBS. Cranial nerve involvement is less common, and CIDP is rarely associated with a preceding viral infection. Although the condition has been reported during infancy, it is much more common in adults. The chronic course of CIDP is characterized by acute exacerbations of increased weakness, with occasional spontaneous remissions. Like GBS, CIDP is believed to be immune mediated.

CIDP in infants and children may occur with hypotonia, leading to a misdiagnosis of developmental delay or a familial demyelinating disorder. Exposure to toxins or heavy metals occasionally can result in a similar clinical picture, as can diabetes mellitus, porphyria, connective tissue diseases, or renal failure. CIDP should be suspected in a child with hypotonia who has an elevated CSF protein (without pleocytosis) and electrodiagnostic studies indicative of widespread demyelination and large fiber loss. The diagnosis of CIDP is confirmed by a sural nerve biopsy that shows segmental axonal demyelination and remyelination, with perivascular and endoneurial mononuclear infiltration associated with endoneurial edema and a tendency to onion-bulb formation.

Management

The management of CIDP is identical to that outlined for GBS. Meticulous attention must be directed to the respiratory system, with intervention by mechanical ventilation if impending respiratory failure is evident during an acute relapse. Permanent weakness and motor handicaps may be improved by the use of assistive devices. Furthermore, the chronic nature of the disorder demands ongoing psychosocial support and guidance.

Corticosteroids have been reported to be beneficial for the management of children and adults with CIDP, but their use has not been subjected to rigorous controlled trials in children.[2] Prednisone has been most commonly administered at an initial dose of 2 mg/kg/d. After 4 weeks, the dose is gradually tapered over an 8 to 10 week period to the lowest maintenance dose that stabilizes the child's motor function. In spite of alternate-day administration of prednisone to minimize the complications of the drug, the long-term use of steroids in children with CIDP is likely to cause serious side effects. Plasma exchange has proven useful in the management of CIDP in adults.[1] Since plasmapheresis usually is required on an ongoing basis and most young children will require placement of a central line, plasma exchange should be reserved for those children who are unresponsive to steroids and who cannot tolerate high-dose intravenous immunoglobulin. High-dose intravenous immunoglobulin is the treatment of choice for the management of CIPD in children.[3] The recommended dose is 0.4 to 1 g/kg/d intravenously for 5 consecutive days. Intravenous immunoglobulin does not prevent relapses, nor does it prolong the duration of a remission, but it can be administered repeatedly and safely in an outpatient setting, with minimal side effects and little discomfort.

REFERENCES

Guillain-Barré Syndrome

1. Guillain-Barré Syndrome Study Group: Plasmapheresis and acute Guillain-Barré syndrome. Neurology 35:1096–1104, 1985.
2. Shahar E, Murphy EG, Roifman CM: Benefit of intravenously administered immune serum globulin in patients with Guillain-Barré syndrome. J Pediatr 116:141–144, 1990.
3. Van Der Meche FGA, Schmitz PIM, Dutch Guillain-Barré Study Group: A randomized trial comparing intravenous immune globulin and plasma exchange in Guillain-Barré syndrome. N Engl J Med 326:1123–1129, 1992.

Chronic Inflammatory Demyelinating Polyradiculoneuropathy

1. Dyck PJ, Daube J, O'Brien P, et al: Plasma exchange in chronic inflammatory demyelinating polyradiculoneuropathy. N Engl J Med 314:461–465, 1986.
2. Sladky JT, Brown MJ, Berman PH: Chronic inflammatory demyelinating polyneuropathy of infancy: A corticosteroid-responsive disorder. Ann Neurol 20:76–81, 1986.
3. vanDoorn PA, Brand A, Strengers PFW, et al: High-dose intravenous immunoglobulin treatment in chronic inflammatory demyelinating polyneuropathy: A double-blind, placebo-controlled, crossover study. Neurology 40:209–212, 1990.

ACUTE ATAXIA

BASIL T. DARRAS, M.D.
N. PAUL ROSMAN, M.D.

Ataxia (Gr. *ataktos,* lacking order) refers to any disturbance in coordination of movement. Coordination is dependent on intact cerebellar, sensory, vestibular, and motor functions. Therefore, ataxia may result from disorders of the cerebellum (including cerebellar inflow and outflow pathways), sensory loss (especially that caused by spinal cord [posterior column], nerve root, or peripheral nerve disease), vestibular dysfunction, and motor abnormalities from disorders of the upper motor neuron (frontal lobe, corticospinal pathways) or lower motor neuron (particularly spinal cord, nerve root, or peripheral nerve). Paroxysmal disorders (such as seizures, migraine) and metabolic disturbances also can cause ataxia. In addition, ataxia can be functional, that is, without an organic basis, as seen with conversion hysteria. The presentation and course of ataxia can be acute, subacute, or chronic, progressive, static, or improving. Furthermore, it is not infrequent that a slowly progressive or static ataxia may worsen acutely, frequently from an intercurrent infection. Only new-onset acute ataxias are considered here.

Clinical features suggesting *cerebellar ataxia* include a wide-based, lurching, and often staggering gait (ataxic gait), incoordination of upper limb movements (dysmetria), constant to-and-fro movements of the body and/or head in the sitting position (titubation), intention tremor of the limbs, hypotonia, and at times, nystagmus. Signs of *sensory ataxia* include a cautious, wide-based gait (characterized by lifting each foot high, then slapping it down vigorously—steppage gait), a Romberg sign (worsening of station and gait with the eyes closed), decreased deep tendon reflexes, and loss of position and vibratory senses in the lower limbs. *Vestibular ataxia* usually occurs with vertigo (a sensation of spinning or rotation) and nausea. Nystagmus and hearing loss also may be observed. Weakness, with or without alterations in muscle tone and deep tendon reflexes, is a constant feature of *motor system ataxia.*

CEREBELLAR ATAXIA

Cerebellar ataxia may occur as a one-time acute event or may recur intermittently, with or without return to baseline after each attack. The causes of acute cerebellar ataxia are many. They include infectious and postinfectious (demyelinative) disorders, paraneoplastic syndromes, drug intoxication, trauma, increased intracranial pressure (ICP) (with or without tumor), tumor (unaccompanied by increased ICP), and primary demyelination (acute multiple sclerosis). Of these, the most common etiologies are primary infectious or postinfectious cerebellitis and drug intoxication.

Infections

Acute cerebellar ataxia may result from direct infection of the cerebellum or from postinfectious immune-mediated demyelination of the cerebellum. Direct infection has been inferred with echovirus type IX and coxsackievirus type B because these agents have been isolated from the CSF of patients with acute ataxia. Acute cerebellitis

also has been associated with infections caused by influenza A and B, herpes simplex, poliovirus type I, mumps, rubeola (measles), infectious mononucleosis, Japanese B encephalitis, and, most commonly, varicella. Systemic infections, not directly involving the cerebellum or other parts of the nervous system, such as typhoid fever, scarlet fever, diphtheria, leptospirosis, and *Mycoplasma pneumoniae* infection, may cause an acute cerebellar syndrome, probably mediated by circulating toxins. Effective therapies are available for many of these disorders (e.g., penicillin for scarlet fever, diphtheria, and leptospirosis; erythromycin for *M. pneumoniae*).

Acute cerebellar ataxia following an infectious illness usually occurs in children between 1 and 2 years of age but may occur as late as age 14 years. Although the time interval between the first sign of infection and the onset of the ataxia is typically briefer in a primary infection of cerebellum (a few days) than in a postinfectious cerebellitis (5 to 21 days), clinical distinction between the two frequently is difficult if not impossible. The ataxia in either instance typically occurs with acute gait difficulty, usually accompanied by hypotonia, dysmetria and tremor of the limbs, head and trunk titubation, scanning speech, and, sometimes, nystagmus. In some patients, the ocular movements can be chaotic [ocular flutter (horizontal) or opsoclonus (multidirectional)]. Mental status is normal. The CSF is usually unremarkable, although mild pleocytosis and elevation of CSF protein sometimes are seen. If the ataxia is postinfectious (demyelinative), CSF IgG may be elevated.

Acute infectious cerebellar ataxia can occur as a component of brainstem encephalitis, with the ataxia caused by involvement of cerebellar or brainstem pathways. In such cases, accompanying cranial nerve abnormalities usually are seen. The cause often has been viral, most often from coxsackie, echo, or adenovirus infections. Ataxia can be observed also during the course of and recovery from bacterial meningitis, usually caused by *Haemophilus influenzae* type B. Postvaccinial cerebellitis occurs rarely if at all.

The diagnosis of acute infectious or postinfectious cerebellitis is supported by the exclusion of other causes. A toxic screen should always be obtained. In cases with an uncertain relationship between an infection and the development of ataxia, a head MRI (or, less optimally, a head CT scan) should be done. The value of a lumbar puncture is controversial. Spontaneous remission generally begins a few days after the disorder peaks. Complete recovery occurs in two thirds of affected children but can take weeks to months. In the other one third, neurologic abnormalities, usually clumsiness and hypotonia, persist.

Treatment of acute infectious or immune-mediated postinfectious cerebellitis is symptomatic. There is no evidence that steroids are beneficial.

Paraneoplastic Syndromes

In rare instances, acute ataxia may be severe and associated with chaotic, jerky, multidirectional, conjugate eye movements (opsoclonus) and myoclonic jerks of the limbs, head, face, and trunk. This disorder, known as Kinsbourne's myoclonic encephalopathy or dancing eyes, dancing feet syndrome, may be associated with an occult neuroblastoma in a paraspinal or intraabdominal location. When this diagnosis is considered, the evaluation should include measurement of urinary catecholamines (VMA and HVA), serum metanephrines, plain radiographs, and ultrasonography of the chest and abdomen. A CT scan of the chest and abdomen is commonly obtained. Neuroblastoma, if found, must be removed surgically. Treatment with ACTH or oral prednisone will lessen symptoms in 80% of these cases. The course is usually prolonged, with residual motoric and intellectual deficits in one third to one half of affected children.

Drug Intoxication

Acute cerebellar ataxia may result from drug ingestion. The usual offending agents are anticonvulsants (such as phenytoin, barbiturates, and carbamazepine), diazepam, alcohol, and antihistamines (used in the treatment of allergies and upper respiratory tract infections). Less often, organic chemicals (such as ethyl chloride and toluene) and heavy metals (such as mercury and thallium-containing pesticides) are causative. Acute lead encephalopathy may occur with intracranial hypertension and cerebellar dysfunction. Cancer chemotherapeutic agents, such as methotrexate, 5-fluorouracil, and procarbazine, also have been implicated.

Ataxia caused by toxic ingestion is usually associated with changes in the child's alertness (e.g., lethargy) and personality (e.g., irritability). Nystagmus frequently is present. Other family members should be questioned about the use of anticonvulsants or psychotropic drugs. Urine and, at times, blood and gastric aspirate should be screened for intoxicating substances. Blood levels should be determined once a specific drug or other toxin has been identified. Treatment depends on the nature and amount of the ingested agent (e.g., chelation therapy for lead intoxication). Often, no specific treatment is available or needed. With drug intoxication, a reduction in dose or discontinuation of the offending agent (e.g., anticonvulsants) will usually improve the child's balance. In some cases, treatment should include administration of an antidote (if available) and supportive care in an intensive care unit.

Trauma

Even mild head injuries may be followed by ataxia, which is secondary to a cerebellar contusion or an extraparenchymal posterior fossa hematoma (extradural or subdural). In some cases, ataxia is seen as part of a postconcussion syndrome. In cervical injuries, ataxia may follow occlusive vertebrobasilar disease, with or without accompanying vertebral artery dissection.

Increased Intracranial Pressure

Intracranial tumors, particularly those located in the posterior fossa, usually cause increased ICP and, often, gait ataxia. Acute ataxia in such cases can be of new onset or may reflect acute worsening of a longer-standing, slowly progressive ataxia. In either circumstance, the ataxia may result from acute intracranial hypertension from hydrocephalus (caused by obstruction of CSF circulation by the tumor) or, less often, from hemorrhage into the tumor. Ruptured arteriovenous malformations or hydrocephalus related to nonneoplastic causes (such as an aqueductal stenosis or a Chiari I malformation) also can cause ataxia. With increased ICP, there usually are accompanying headache, early morning vomiting, paresis of lateral gaze, and papilledema. If a mass lesion is suspected, a brain-imaging study (CT or MRI) should be done. Occasionally, a brain tumor may cause ataxia without evidence of increased ICP. This is seen most often with brainstem glioma. Depending on its nature and location, treatment for brain tumor may include surgery, radiation, or chemotherapy, individually or in combination.

Acute elevation of ICP can be treated with intravenous mannitol (0.25 to 0.5 g/kg per dose), hyperventilation (lowering the P_{CO_2} to 20 to 25 mm Hg), fluid restriction, and head elevation (to about 30 degrees). Steroids, such as dexamethasone (0.25 mg/kg every 8 hours), are effective in alleviating edema surrounding brain tumors, but the onset of action is usually delayed (12 to 24 hours). Hydrocephalus can be treated surgically by ventriculoperitoneal shunting or medically with acetazolamide (50 to 100 mg/kg/d), with or without furosemide (1 mg/kg per dose), every 3 to 6 hours.

Demyelination

Ataxia may be the presenting feature of acute demyelinating disease (usually multiple sclerosis) involving the cerebellum or its major connections. Associated focal neurologic findings (particularly optic neuritis and internuclear ophthalmoplegia), elevated CSF protein (especially IgG), and CSF oligoclonal bands support the diagnosis. A 1-week course of ACTH (40 to 80 U/d) or prednisone (2 mg/kg/d), with slow tapering over the next 3 weeks, is often effective in managing such acute exacerbations. Very recently, interferon beta-1b has been shown to benefit relapsing-remitting multiple sclerosis.

SENSORY ATAXIA

Sensory ataxia is usually the result of longer-standing processes, such as demyelinating diseases (particularly multiple sclerosis), chronic inflammatory demyelinating neuropathies, Friedreich's ataxia, and subacute combined degeneration (from vitamin B_{12} deficiency). Therefore, sensory ataxia usually does not occur acutely. Exceptions are acute exacerbations of multiple sclerosis and the Miller Fisher variant of the Guillain-Barré syndrome (GBS). GBS would appear to be an immune-mediated disorder of peripheral myelin, with the Miller Fisher variant characterized clinically by ataxia, ophthalmoplegia, and areflexia. The distinction between Miller Fisher syndrome and brainstem encephalitis may be difficult. Mental status changes, CSF pleocytosis, and an abnormal EEG favor brainstem encephalitis, whereas in GBS, those findings are normal, and deep tendon reflexes are depressed or unobtainable. Conventional therapies used in the treatment of classic GBS (plasmapheresis, intravenous gamma globulin) are of unproven value in the Miller Fisher variant.

VESTIBULAR ATAXIA

Vertigo can be caused by disorders of the inner ear (labyrinth), vestibular division of the eighth cranial nerve, brainstem, or temporal lobe. Of these, labyrinthine causes occur most frequently. Patients with vertigo have difficulty maintaining balance and, thus, appear ataxic. Acute vertigo may result from labyrinthitis, trauma to the labyrinth (e.g., basal skull fracture with or without perilymphatic fistula), vestibular neuronitis, or drug toxicity or may represent benign paroxysmal vertigo. Nausea, vomiting, nystagmus (frequent), and hearing loss (occasional) are associated findings. Benign paroxysmal vertigo is considered a forerunner of migraine or a migraine equivalent and may be accompanied by headache. It is usually self-limited, but if it persists, symptomatic therapy with meclizine may be helpful. If headache becomes a disabling accompaniment, daily propranolol may reduce the frequency of recurrent attacks.

MOTOR SYSTEM ATAXIA

Weakness from an acute disorder affecting the spinal cord (such as transverse myelitis or spinal cord compression) may be manifested initially by ataxia caused by the weakness, with accompanying sensory loss, incontinence, and alterations in deep tendon reflexes. Acute weakness can also result from GBS, which is characterized by progressive symmetric ascending flaccid paralysis with accompanying areflexia. Here, the ataxia is secondary to weakness caused by demyelination of spinal nerve roots and peripheral nerves. Protein elevation in the CSF is usually seen within 1 to 2 weeks after onset. Steroids are not useful in the treatment of GBS, but plasmapheresis and intravenous gamma globulin both have been shown to be effective.

Another lower motor neuron cause of weakness, botulism, results from the neurotoxic effects of *Clostridium botulinum*. These children have cranial nerve paralysis and generalized weakness caused by inhibition of acetylcholine release at the neuromuscular junction. The treatment of children with botulism is discussed elsewhere in this text. An additional cause of weakness (of uncertain localization in the lower motor neuron) is tick bite paralysis. On occasion, ataxia can be secondary to cerebral disorders (particularly frontal and parietal in location) that cause weakness and sensory loss. Ischemic injury represents the most common etiology in affected children.

PAROXYSMAL ATAXIA

Epileptic Ataxia

Ataxia can be a major accompaniment of seizures during the ictal and postictal phases. Patients with Lennox-Gastaut syndrome, atypical absence, or complex partial seizures often manifest disturbances of posture and gait. Associated confusion, myoclonic jerks, and seizure activity on the EEG should indicate that such ataxia is epileptic in origin. The ataxia in such circumstances is usually responsive to anticonvulsant therapy.

Migraine

Gait ataxia is common in patients, frequently adolescents, with basilar migraine. Associated symptoms can include vertigo, visual loss, alternating hemiparesis, paresthesias, impaired consciousness, nausea, vomiting, and occipital headache. Treatment with propranolol (2 mg/kg/d), amitriptyline (2 mg/kg/d), cyproheptadine (0.2 to 0.4 mg/kg/d), or a calcium channel blocker, such as nifedipine (1 mg/kg/d), will usually reduce the frequency of recurrent attacks.

Metabolic Disorders

Acute ataxia can be a manifestation of many metabolic disorders where the ataxia is characteristically triggered by dietary intake (usually protein) or intercurrent illness (usually infections). In some of these diseases (e.g., maple syrup urine disease), protein restriction usually results in symptomatic improvement. In other disorders (e.g., biotinidase deficiency), vitamin administration may be helpful. Recurrent ataxia has been described in more than 20 families, transmitted as an autosomal-dominant trait. A metabolic defect has not been identified in affected individuals.

FUNCTIONAL ATAXIA

Astasia-abasia is a well-described hysterical gait disturbance, usually characterized by normal sitting balance but major swaying from the waist upward while standing. In spite of lurching and staggering, the gait is not wide-based, as seen in cerebellar ataxia. Hysterical ataxia can be diagnosed with confidence only after careful ongoing observation, which may have to be prolonged. It is particularly frequent in adolescent girls. Psychologic or psychiatric referral usually is indicated.

HYDROCEPHALUS

DAVID K. URION, M.D.

Hydrocephalus, or a pathologic collection of cerebrospinal fluid (CSF) within the intracranial spaces, is one of the most common causes of enlarged or enlarging head circumference (macrocephaly).

The causes of hydrocephalus may be divided into three physiologic origins.

1. Increased CSF production
2. Obstruction to the normal pattern of flow within the ventricular system
3. Decreased absorption of CSF at the level of the arachnoid granulations

During the era of radionuclide brain scans, it became common to talk of the second category as "noncommunicating" hydrocephalus and the third category as "communicating" hydrocephalus, the terms reflecting the patterns of isotope flow on introduction into the lumbosacral space (i.e., when the ventricular outflow was obstructed, the radioisotope did not communicate with the ventricles). These terms persist in clinical practice today, although the diagnostic technology that gave rise to them has been supplanted.

Increased CSF production is seen in children with choroid plexus papillomas and other tumors of the choroid plexus. Papillomas of the choroid plexus account for between 1% and 4% of most series of childhood intracranial tumors and, hence, are seen from time to time in practice. They usually occur in the first year of life as rapidly advancing hydrocephalus, occasionally with acute intraventricular hemorrhage. They may be associated with papilledema, otherwise a rare finding in infants. The choroid plexus appears intensely vascular on noncontrast CT scan.

Treatment may consist of drainage (through external or internalized shunt mechanisms) or attempts to decrease CSF production (such as the use of carbonic anhydrase inhibitors, e.g., acetazolamide). Production may be so robust (up to three or four times the usual) that

complications of shunting arise (cases of CSF ascites and biventricular heart failure from ventriculoperitoneal or ventriculoatrial shunts have been observed). In these instances, if medical techniques also fail, resection of the choroid plexus needs to be considered.

Obstructive hydrocephalus may be caused by intraventricular hemorrhage in the newborn period (producing a narrowing of the outflow tracts), compression or gliosis of the aqueduct, or a congenital aqueductal stenosis. Compression may be caused by a tumor or vascular anomaly, such as a vein of Galen aneurysm. Gliosis may be seen as a sequela of infection or in conjunction with neurofibromatosis. Chiari and Dandy-Walker malformations may compress the fourth ventricle and lead to hydrocephalus. Infection, such as meningitis, can lead to hydrocephalus by obstructing the foramina of Magendie or Luschka.

Treatment in these instances almost always requires creation of an alternative outflow pathway for the CSF, that is, a shunt. Most shunts in this setting begin as external drainage and are later internalized as either ventriculoperitoneal (VP) or ventriculoatrial (VA) shunts. Shunts are equipped with valves set to certain specified pressures, so that ventricles do not drain entirely by a siphon effect (creating a so-called *slit-ventricle syndrome*). The disadvantage of a single set pressure for shunt valves is their inflexibility in the face of a dynamic system, altered by patient growth. In the past, this has not infrequently required revision and replacement of the valves. Currently, experimental systems are being studied with externally programmable valves that can vary their pressure profiles.

Shunts also require revision as patients grow, since only a finite length of tube can be placed between head and abdominal cavity. In most all instances of obstructive hydrocephalus, patients remain shunt dependent for their lives and require two or three revisions based on growth.

Shunt infection and associated meningitis and ventriculitis were once a substantial problem in pediatric practice. The advent of intrathecal forms of antibiotics, as well as contemporary hygienic measures (such as a reluctance to tap shunts) have greatly reduced annual infection rates in most settings.

Nonobstructive hydrocephalus in childhood is caused by an imbalance between production and absorption, the latter in general being pathologically reduced. The reduction may be secondary to postinfectious inflammatory changes, posthemorrhagic changes, or a developmental immaturity of the arachnoid granulations. Although it has been traditional for infants with intraventricular hemorrhages to be treated with daily lumbar punctures (with or without the addition of loop diuretics and/or carbonic anhydrase inhibitors as an attempt to reduce CSF production), this has not been shown to decrease the number of children who ultimately require shunt placement. This procedure may be useful to temporize in the unstable newborn while awaiting a time when surgery may be more advantageous.

Most infants who are detected in infancy and survive until 2 years of age do not experience a reduction in life expectancy, nor do they exhibit major neurologic morbidities referable to the hydrocephalus itself. Associated CNS abnormalities may produce sequelae of their own, however.

MENINGOMYELOCELE

TIMOTHY J. BREI, M.D., F.A.A.P.

Meningomyelocele (spina bifida), one of the most frequent and complex birth defects associated with meaningful survival, is part of a heterogeneous group of neural tube defects and is characterized by a dysplastic spinal cord where nerve roots protrude through malformed vertebral arches into an external dural sac. Systemic manifestations include paralysis, sensory loss, and dysfunction of the bowel and bladder. Hydrocephalus occurs in nearly all such patients as a result of the Arnold-Chiari type II malformation.

EMBRYOLOGY AND EPIDEMIOLOGY

The embryologic defect occurs by the 28th day of gestation and is thought to result from either failure of primary closure of the neural tube or from secondary disruption of a closed neural tube. In the United States, the incidence is 0.4 to 1/1000 live births and has steadily decreased in recent decades. The incidence is lower in African Americans and higher for persons from the British Isles.

The etiology is thought to be multifactorial, involving both genetic and environmental factors. Meningomyelocele may be seen with trisomy 18, trisomy 13, or Meckel syndrome or associated with other anomalies, such as cleft lip/palate, tracheoesophageal fistula, omphalocele, diaphragmatic hernia, congenital heart disease, bladder exstrophy, or imperforate anus. Environmental factors implicated include maternal diabetes, use of valproic acid or alcohol, hyperthermia, and nutritional deficiencies. Increasing evidence indicates that folic acid deficiency plays a major role and that preconceptual and first trimester supplementation significantly reduces the incidence. It is recommended that women of childbearing age take 0.4 mg/d of folic acid in a multivitamin preparation and that women with a previous child with a neural tube defect increase the dose to 4 mg/d at least 1 month before conception and through the first trimester.[1]

Prenatal screening with maternal serum alpha-fetoprotein levels and targeted fetal ultrasound identify nearly all cases. Cesarean section is the preferred route of delivery if meningomyelocele is identified.

ASSESSMENT OF THE NEWBORN

Initial assessment includes determination of the size and position of the lesion, as well as the presence of CSF leak. The lesion is covered immediately with a sterile, saline-soaked, nonadhesive dressing. Evaluation of the lower extremities for deformities, hip dislocation, and motor function is important, but potential for ambulation cannot be predicted solely by the functional or anatomic level of the lesion. Head circumference is measured at the time of delivery and serially to evaluate for hydrocephalus. Definitive diagnosis of hydrocephalus relies on ultrasound or CT scan. An MRI scan, however, is a better way to define the posterior fossa anatomy and extent of the Arnold-Chiari malformation.

The primary care physician's role is equally important in providing basic information about meningomyelocele, facilitating smooth transition of care to the subspecialists, and lending support to the family undergoing the acute stresses of neonatal abnormalities, critical decision making, and separation.

Selection

The issue of selection for treatment has been furiously debated. Problems arise when trying to quantify factors, such as cost or pain and suffering, or to apply definitions of extraordinary or futile care to an individual child. Previous selection criteria have been both vague and unreliable in predicting outcome, and an accurate assessment of intellectual potential cannot be made. Experienced physicians advocate repair of the back lesion and shunting of hydrocephalus unless coexisting anomalies are incompatible with long-term survival.

Initial Subspecialty Management

The complex dysfunction inherent to meningomyelocele requires early comprehensive evaluation. Transfer to a tertiary care center is indicated if a multidisciplinary subspecialty team is not available.

Closure of the defect usually occurs on the first day of life. Repair may be delayed without adverse effect for up to 1 week if prophylactic antibiotics are given. Placement of a ventriculoperitoneal shunt for hydrocephalus is occasionally done in conjunction with surgical closure but most often is deferred to a second procedure to decrease the risk of infection.

Neonatal urologic evaluation is critical. Renal ultrasound and voiding cystourethrogram (VCUG) are recommended to evaluate kidney and bladder structure and to determine if vesicoureteral reflux is present. Assessments of voiding pattern and postvoid residual are beneficial. If urinary tract pathology is detected, additional studies may

be needed. Orthopedic assessment of lower extremity deformity and movement is made, and treatment of talipes equinovarus (clubfoot) and hip dislocation is initiated. If severe kyphosis is present, surgical repair may be needed at the time of closure. Most neonates do not require extensive orthopedic intervention and benefit primarily from physical therapy for stretching, positioning techniques, and developmental stimulation.

The pediatrician's role on the multidisciplinary team is to assist in coordinating care and to provide more detailed information, including etiology, recurrence risks, and preventive measures. Formal genetics consultation may be helpful.

LONGITUDINAL CARE

Multidisciplinary Team

The complex nature of meningomyelocele requires a team of physicians, therapists, and social workers to best meet the various medical and psychosocial concerns present from infancy through adulthood. The multidisciplinary team is designed to provide efficient, integrated services for persons with spina bifida. However, this team does not replace the primary care physician, who provides well child care, evaluates acute problems, and communicates knowledgeably with the subspecialists.

Neurosurgical Management

The most common neurosurgical problems are shunt malfunction and infection. Shunt malfunction in infants and younger children is manifested by bulging fontanelle, increasing head circumference, irritability, lethargy, or poor feeding. Personality changes, headaches, or worsening school performance suggest malfunction in the older child. Infections occur in about 5% of shunts, most within 2 months of initial placement. Fever, associated with signs of malfunction, is the most common presentation.

In addition to hydrocephalus, other complications of Arnold-Chiari II malformation may occur in the first month of life and almost always by 6 months. These signs of cranial nerve dysfunction include stridor, dysphagia, aspiration, vocal cord paralysis, hypoventilation, and apnea. Findings may be rapidly progressive or fairly insidious in onset, and all warrant immediate medical intervention. Posterior fossa decompression is done in an attempt to improve cranial nerve dysfunction, but its effectiveness remains controversial. If problems persist, some children may require gastrostomy tubes, tracheostomy, or long-term assisted ventilation.

Symptoms from a tethered spinal cord, which results from scar formation at the repair site, can develop at any time. Children who develop a change in gait, asymmetric loss of strength, spasticity, changes in bowel or bladder function, pain at the repair site, increasing scoliosis, worsening fatigability of the legs, or hyperlordosis should have neurosurgical evaluation.

Orthopedic Management

The goals of orthopedic management are to maintain joint alignment, achieve functional mobility, and prevent fractures and decubiti. Kyphosis and scoliosis occur frequently and may be secondary to vertebral anomalies, asymmetric muscle innervation, spasticity, tethered cord, or syringomyelia. Bracing is used initially, but almost all kyphosis or scoliosis ultimately requires surgical intervention.

Leg deformities are present in all but the lowest sacral lesions. Potential for ambulation determines long-term management. Initial attempts at upright positioning and bracing are made, with serial assessment of the child's ability to ambulate or the need for a wheelchair. Bracing is used to assist in functional ambulation and helps to reduce joint deformity. Children with low lumbar lesions may require an ankle foot orthosis, (AFO) and those with midlumbar lesions require knee support (KAFO). High lumbar and thoracic level lesions usually require hip and trunk support using the parapodium or reciprocating gait orthosis (RGO). Most children with midlumbar lesions or below will be able to ambulate, whereas those with higher lumbar and thoracic lesions most often rely on wheelchairs. Motivation, temperament, obesity, and spasticity also play significant roles in the success of ambulation. Surgery, including soft tissue release, tendon transfer, and osteotomy, may be required to correct anatomic defects and assist in alignment and function in severe deformities. Reduction of a dislocated hip is reserved for low lumbar and sacral levels of paralysis, where a stable hip improves mobility. In children with higher lesions, the hip abductors are absent, and hip dislocation does not interfere with functional mobility.

Loss of sensation due to injury of posterior nerve roots predisposes individuals to abrasions, burns, and decubiti. Anesthetic areas of skin need to be covered to reduce exposure to rough surfaces and sun. Anticipatory guidance regarding bath water temperature and avoidance of heat sources, such as registers, should be stressed. Braces may initiate skin breakdown, so contact sites must be examined regularly. Management of a decubitus includes removal of the causal agent, keeping the area clean and dry, and avoiding local pressure. Debridement may be necessary, but skin grafting rarely is required.

Urologic Management

Nearly all children with meningomyelocele will have some degree of neurogenic bladder and incontinence. Until recently, renal failure was the primary cause of death after infancy. Thus, close follow-up of the urinary system is essential. Upper tract anatomy is initially normal in 90% of affected children, but the lower tract is almost always damaged. Since the bladder and urethral sphincter are innervated by both sympathetic and parasympathetic nerves from the lumbosacral area, injury may result in hypotonia or spasticity of the sphincter and detrusor muscles. Morbidity is related to increased intravesicular bladder pressure predisposing to infection, ureteral reflux, hydronephrosis, and renal parenchymal damage. There is no correlation between the level of the lesion and the type of neurogenic bladder, nor is bladder function static over time.

The goals of urologic management are to prevent upper tract deterioration, provide functional continence, and reduce the frequency of infections. Most children require clean intermittent catheterization (CIC) for bladder dyssynergy or incomplete emptying. If bladder dynamics do not dictate a need for CIC in infancy, most children will initiate CIC during the schoolage years to provide functional continence. The addition of anticholinergic agents (oxybutynin) to reduce bladder contraction or alpha-adrenergic agents (pseudoephedrine) to increase outflow resistance may be helpful (Table 1). Prophylactic oral antibiotics or bladder irrigation with a urinary antiseptic agent may be used for recurrent infections. Although most children can achieve a reasonable degree of functional continence and prevent renal deterioration, those who continue to have significant incontinence may benefit from an artificial urethral sphincter. Bladder augmentation or vesicotomy may be indicated for bladders with poor compliance or small capacity. As augmentation uses a large or small bowel segment transplanted onto the bladder, regular CIC is mandatory or bladder rupture with peritonitis can result.

Routine urologic follow-up is necessary. Renal ultrasound is obtained every 6 to 12 months, and periodic VCUGs are performed if vesicoureteral reflux is present. Urodynamic studies are key to delineating bladder pathophysiology and determining the therapeutic measures necessary to attain continence and protect the upper tracts. The primary care physician, in conjunction with the pediatric urologist, is instrumental in surveillance and management of infections. Routine cultures or in-home use of nitrate or leukocyte esterase strips can be

done. Asymptomatic bacteriuria is common. Debate continues about the benefit of antibiotic treatment in these children.

Bowel Management

Bowel management is a critical factor for social integration. Goals of management are to prevent constipation and to achieve functional continence. Adequate fluid intake and a high fiber diet are essential. Most require regular use of stool softeners, and some also need cathartic suppositories or enemas. A regular pattern of toileting is crucial for success. By the developmental age of 2 to 3 years, children should be placed on the toilet after meals to take advantage of the gastrocolic reflex. Activities to increase abdominal pressure may improve effectiveness, but results are variable based on both degree of motivation and the level of lesion. For the few children who have rectal sensation, biofeedback may be useful. Many centers now use a daily enema with an incontinence catheter that has a balloon tip to facilitate retention of the enema fluid. High success rates are reported, but little is known about complications from long-term use.

PRIMARY CARE HEALTH CONCERNS

Children with meningomyelocele need age-appropriate general health care, including immunizations and anticipatory guidance for a variety of health care issues.

Seizures

Nearly 15% of children with meningomyelocele develop seizures, which generally are easy to control with a single anticonvulsant. Shunt malfunction must always be considered as an etiology of new or increasing seizures.

Cognition and School Performance

Cognition is normal in at least 70% of individuals with meningomyelocele. Mental retardation is more likely to occur in children with poorly controlled hydrocephalus, repeated episodes of shunt malfunction or infection, or a history of ventriculitis. Despite normal intelligence, specific learning disabilities in visual-motor or visual-perceptual skills, mathematics, reading, and auditory comprehension are common. Children struggling in school should receive appropriate psychometric testing. As strabismus and refraction errors are common, ophthalmologic evaluation should be done. Attention deficits are also prevalent and may require therapy with psychostimulants.

Obesity

Obesity occurs frequently, related to reduced energy requirements from limited mobility. Prevention of obesity is important to maintain ambulation and reduce the incidence of skin breakdown. Growth patterns should be monitored, and dietary instruction should be initiated in infancy. Arm span length may be a more accurate measurement than height in those with skeletal deformity. Once obesity has occurred, weight loss is extremely difficult given the decreased caloric requirements and limited opportunities or ability to exercise.

Puberty and Sexuality

Precocious puberty on a central basis may be seen in children with meningomyelocele and hydrocephalus. Anticipatory guidance is essential to prepare both the family and the child.

Concerns about limitations of sexual function and fertility begin early, and the adolescent will need many opportunities to discuss these issues. Females are capable of normal sexual function, including orgasm and fertility, but have high-risk pregnancies because of spinal deformities, exacerbation of bowel and bladder dysfunction, and shunt malfunction from increased abdominal pressure. Male sexual function is variable. About 75% have erections and may ejaculate, but fertility is decreased.

Psychosocial Effects

Children with meningomyelocele and their families undergo enormous stresses from birth into adulthood. Repeated hospitalizations,

TABLE 1. Formulary

Oxybutynin (Ditropan)	0.6 mg/kg/24 h PO tid
	Max 5 mg PO tid
	Do not give if child is less than 1 year of age
Pseudoephedrine (Sudafed)	2–5 years of age: 15 mg PO q6h
	6–12 years of age: 30 mg PO q6h

medical issues such as incontinence, increased and uninsured expenses, and school problems are especially difficult. Lack of acceptance by the community at large leads to ongoing barriers, especially for adolescents and adults. Families may need help in accessing school services, governmental assistance, or counseling. Failure to address psychosocial issues may interfere with care, manifested as poor compliance or missed appointments. The complex nature of meningomyelocele and altered family dynamics, combined with poor self-esteem, may impede the process of development toward independent, self-sufficient adulthood. Support by the primary physician can assist the family in identifying concerns and in maintaining long-term goals with an emphasis on the child's abilities rather than disabilities.

Latex Allergy

Latex allergy has been reported frequently in children with meningomyelocele. A careful history should be elicited at each visit regarding sensitivity to balloons, gloves, or urinary catheters. Protective measures, including avoidance of products containing latex in the hospital and at home and ready availability of epinephrine, should be taken, since anaphylaxis can occur.

SUMMARY

Optimal management of individuals with meningomyelocele requires knowledge of medical and surgical issues, as well as growth and development. Integration of care between pediatric subspecialists and the primary care physician is crucial to promote health, productivity, and independence.

REFERENCE

1. Centers for Disease Control: Recommendations for the use of folic acid to reduce the number of cases of spina bifida and other neural tube defects. MMWR 41 (No. RR-14):5–7, 1992.

CEREBRAL PALSY

BETH A. ROSEN, M.D.

Cerebral palsy is a term used to describe a heterogeneous group of disorders. The hallmark of cerebral palsy is abnormal control of movement and posture. It is caused by injury to the developing brain occurring early in life, usually before the age of 5. Cerebral malformations, prematurity, neonatal asphyxia, and postnatal events, such as trauma and meningitis, are known etiologies. Although the brain damage associated with cerebral palsy does not change over time, its manifestations often change as the child grows and develops. The most common form is spastic cerebral palsy, characterized by hypertonia and hyperreflexia. Other types of cerebral palsy include the dyskinetic and ataxic types. Almost all children with cerebral palsy have associated disorders, which can include mental retardation, learning disabilities, behavior problems, and seizures. These are often as disabling, if not more so, than the primary motor problems.

The initial diagnosis of cerebral palsy should be made as soon as possible because early intervention and treatment may improve outcome. In the majority of cases, the disorder is apparent by 1 year of age, though in milder cases, diagnosis may be delayed. Parents often suspect that there is a problem before it is clearly apparent to the physician. Nevertheless, they are frequently devastated when they hear the news. The physician should explain the findings on examination that led to making the diagnosis, using words that are easily understandable. A definitive prognosis should not be given at the time of initial diagnosis. Parents should be told that their child may acquire some skills at a slower rate than other children and is at risk for permanent disabilities. Specific areas of concern that parents can easily grasp, such as learning to walk and talk, should be identified. Such terms as "spasticity," "hemiparesis," "developmental delay," or "delayed milestones," should be avoided during the initial discussion because they are often meaningless to parents. Questions about the cause of cerebral palsy often arise, and this, as well as the guilt many parents feel, should be addressed.

It is important to present the family with a treatment plan as soon as the diagnosis is made, and this should include a referral to the early intervention program in their area. Early intervention is a family-centered, often home-based program available in every state that provides necessary developmental and support services for infants and toddlers at risk for developmental disabilities. The early intervention program will also help to move the child into the public school system at the age of 3. Several books are available in most larger bookstores for parents of children with cerebral palsy that directly address the questions that parents have but may be afraid to ask the physician.

There is no cure for cerebral palsy, but several treatments are available to improve function and prevent complications. A program should be instituted as soon as the diagnosis is made. The management of each child with cerebral palsy must be individualized, but in all cases, the input of many professionals is required, including physicians, physical, occupational, and speech therapists, and educators. In addition to the primary care pediatrician, physicians who most commonly care for children with cerebral palsy are developmental pediatricians, neurologists, physiatrists (specialists in physical medicine and rehabilitation), and orthopedic surgeons. Treatment of the child with cerebral palsy should always include adequate psychologic support for both the child and family members.

PHYSICAL THERAPY

The goal of physical therapy is to maximize the gross motor function and mobility of the child. Physical therapists work to strengthen functional muscles and to prevent fixed contractures. Passive and active stretching, range of motion exercises, and strengthening exercises are used. Physical therapists also use a variety of techniques to try to modify abnormal tone and postures, although whether it is actually possible to do this is controversial. Many different methods have been used, but the most common is the neurodevelopmental approach advocated by the Bobaths. In this type of therapy, the goal is to achieve normal patterns of movement while inhibiting primitive reflexes and postures. Various sensory inputs are used, including tactile, proprioceptive, and vestibular stimuli. It is important that all aspects of the physical therapy program be done at home by the parents, who should be taught to be active participants in their child's care.

OCCUPATIONAL THERAPY

The goal of occupational therapy is to assist the child in the development of skills necessary for activities of daily living. These include dressing, grooming, and other self-help skills. Feeding problems, which are commonly encountered in children with cerebral palsy, often are treated by occupational therapists. They also address fine motor and coordination delays involving the upper extremity, as well as cognitive and perceptual disabilities, especially in the visual-motor area. The occupational therapist adapts equipment and seating to allow better upper extremity use and promote functional independence.

SPEECH AND LANGUAGE THERAPY

Speech therapists have many roles in the treatment of the child with cerebral palsy. Evaluation of oral motor coordination, chewing, and swallowing is done early because abnormalities in these functions can lead to problems with feeding and speech production. They try to find an adequate method of communication for the child, whether it be speech, sign language, a communication board where a child points to pictures, letters, or words, or a computer-generated voice. Remarkable progress has been made over the past several years in the area of communication for the physically disabled, allowing many children the ability to express themselves as never possible before.

Finally, any child with cerebral palsy, no matter how mild, who has a delay in the acquisition of speech and language milestones should be referred to an experienced speech therapist. Both receptive and expressive language disorders are common and should receive treatment as early as possible.

ORTHOTICS AND ADAPTIVE EQUIPMENT

Orthotics are devices used by therapists and physicians to improve function and prevent deformity. The most commonly used orthotics are braces and splints. They can be made for the upper or lower extremity. In the past, these were bulky and cumbersome appliances made of metal and leather, but now they are constructed of a lightweight plastic material and Velcro.

Also included in this category are inhibitory casts. In this form of treatment, casts provide prolonged stretching to tight, spastic muscles to enhance range of motion and improve function. Unfortunately, the benefits of inhibitory casting often are only temporary.

There are many types of equipment available to aid the child with cerebral palsy. Some are designed specifically for the disabled child, whereas others are commonly used items, such as chairs, household items, and toys that are specially adapted. Positioning devices, including special seats and prone standers, can improve posture and upper extremity function. Walkers and wheelchairs can improve mobility. Modifications of everyday materials, such as weighting a spoon or tilting a dish, can provide greater independence. Computers, sophisticated electrical switches, and other devices can, for example, allow a severely impaired person to turn on a light with an eye blink or open a door with a head movement, leading to an improved quality of life.

MEDICATIONS

Various medications have been used in the treatment of children with cerebral palsy (Table 1), especially to relieve spasticity. The most commonly used antispasticity medications are the benzodiazepines (e.g., Valium), dantrolene, and baclofen. Both the benzodiazepines and baclofen act on GABA receptors in the CNS to inhibit excitatory neurotransmitters, especially at the spinal cord level. Dantrolene works directly on skeletal muscles by suppressing contractility. Results obtained using these medications generally have been disappointing. Effective doses are often undesirably sedating, and dantrolene can cause liver function abnormalities, requiring close monitoring. Furthermore, when the hypertonia of spasticity is removed, the underlying extremity is not normal but weak and poorly coordinated. When the medication is given orally, it is difficult to adjust the dosage to achieve a compromise between spasticity and weakness.

Recently, baclofen has been used intrathecally for the relief of intractable spasticity. The drug is delivered directly into the subarachnoid space of the spinal cord using a permanently implanted pump. This allows a lower, less sedating dose to be used and also allows for small, ongoing adjustments in dosage to be made. Early reports in adults with spinal cord injuries show promising results, although infection and malfunction of the implanted pump are potential problems. Studies in children with cerebral palsy are underway.

Reduction of spasticity in specific muscle groups can be achieved using peripheral nerve blocks. Phenol or alcohol is injected around motor nerves to cause partial denervation, leading to relief of spasticity for up to 4 to 6 months, occasionally longer. This can be especially useful in the hip adductors, where a nerve block can decrease scissoring and prevent hip subluxation. In turn, this can improve hygiene and sitting in a severely involved patient or improve gait in a patient with milder disabilities. Local nerve blocks can also be used to predict the type of response that will be obtained from orthopedic surgery.

Another important group of medications is the anticonvulsants used to treat seizure disorders. Seizures occur in one quarter to one third of children with cerebral palsy. The choice of anticonvulsant should depend on the type of seizure being treated and the side effects of medication.

Children with cerebral palsy may have behavioral problems or attention deficit disorder, which benefits from medication. Treatment should be individualized for each child.

SURGERY

Despite the use of therapy and orthotics, orthopedic surgery is often needed to correct deformities. The most common procedures

TABLE 1. Formulary

Generic name	Baclofen	Dantrolene	Diazepam	Benztropine
Brand name	Lioresal	Dantrium	Valium	Cogentin
Dosage	(To treat spasticity)	(To treat spasticity)	(To treat spasticity)	BENZTROPINE IS NOT RECOMMENDED FOR USE IN CHILDREN UNDER THE AGE OF 3. THERE ARE NO PUBLISHED GUIDELINES FOR THE USE OF BENZTROPINE TO CONTROL DROOLING. THE FOLLOWING ARE DOSES RECOMMENDED FOR DRUG-INDUCED EXTRAPYRAMIDAL REACTIONS.
	Initial dosage: 10–15 mg/d divided b.i.d. or t.i.d.	Children: Initial dosage: 0.5 mg/kg per dose b.i.d.	Children: Initial dosage: 1–2 mg per dose b.i.d.	
	Increase dose 5–15 mg/d q3–5d	Increase frequency to t.i.d.–q.i.d. at 4–7 d intervals, then increase doses by 0.5 mg/kg	Max: 0.8 mg/kg/d up to 40 mg/d divided t.i.d.–q.i.d.	
	Max:		Adults: 2–10 mg per dose b.i.d.–q.i.d.	
	Children 2–7: 30–40 mg/d divided t.i.d.	Max: 3 mg/kg per dose b.i.d.–q.i.d., up to 400 mg/d		
	Children 8 years and older: 60 mg/d divided t.i.d.	Adults: Initial dosage: 25 mg per dose q.d.		Children >3 y: 0.02–0.05 mg/kg per dose q.d.–b.i.d.
	Adults: 80 mg/d divided t.i.d. or q.i.d.	Increase frequency to t.i.d.–q.i.d., then increase dose by 25 mg q4–7d		Adults: 0.5–4 mg per dose q.d.–b.i.d.
		Max: 100 mg b.i.d.–q.i.d., up to 400 mg/d		
How supplied	Tablets, 10 and 20 mg	Capsules, 25, 50, and 100 mg	Solution, 1 mg/ml, 5 mg/ml Tablets, 2, 5, and 10 mg Capsule, sustained release, 15 mg	Tablets, 0.5, 1 and 2 mg
Side effects	Weakness, sedation, tremor, ataxia, hypotension, constipation, urinary frequency, withdrawal syndrome of seizures, and hallucinations	Weakness, confusion, sedation, *hepatotoxicity,* nausea; liver function tests should be monitored closely	Weakness, depression, memory disturbance, sedation, ataxia, nausea, rash; contraindicated in presence of glaucoma	Drowsiness, nervousness, irritability, weakness, dry mouth, palpitations

include heel cord lengthening and releases of hip adductors, hip flexors, and hamstrings. Unfortunately, the indications for, and the timing of, the procedures remain controversial. Many centers that specialize in the care of children with cerebral palsy have "gait labs," which use sophisticated equipment to analyze an individual child's gait to better understand which muscles are most functional. This is frequently used to assist in planning for orthopedic surgery.

Recently, a neurosurgical procedure called *selective dorsal rhizotomy* has been advocated as a method to relieve spasticity in some patients, especially those with spastic diplegia. This procedure involves the isolation and sectioning of selected posterior roots from the second lumbar to the first sacral spinal nerves. Intraoperative electrical stimulation of the nerves is performed, and those that appear to contribute most to spasticity are cut. Proponents claim that lower extremity spasticity and function, including gait, are improved. They have described gains in the areas of upper extremity and cognitive function not explained by the surgery. However, this procedure is quite controversial. Detractors believe that all improvements are a result of the extensive rehabilitation services provided postoperatively rather than the surgery itself. Much more work remains to be done in this area.

EDUCATION

Special education services are very important to the child with cerebral palsy. Up to 50% are mentally retarded, and many with normal intelligence have learning disabilities. Often, it is difficult to accurately assess the cognitive capability of children with cerebral palsy because their physical disabilities limit their ability to perform on intelligence tests.

Public law 99-457 guarantees a free public education and related services to all disabled children between the ages of 3 and 21 and mandates that these services be administered in the least restrictive environment. Parents and school personnel need to work together to determine how to provide the best environment for an individual child, whether it be in a mainstreamed or a self-contained classroom.

An important component of the educational process involves preparation for independent adult living to the greatest extent possible. This may include extra tutoring for the high functioning college-bound adolescent or vocational training to prepare for employment, whether it be in a competitive environment or in a sheltered workshop. Many schools offer programs for the more severely disabled that teach life skills, including shopping and meal preparation.

RECREATION

Recreation services are important to the well-being of the child with cerebral palsy. These should ideally involve activities with both disabled and nondisabled peers.

HEALTH MAINTENANCE

Perhaps the most important role of the primary care physician is that of coordinator of treatment and sounding board for the family, who may be overwhelmed by the large number of people involved in the care of their child.

Routine health maintenance is important for the child with cerebral palsy. In general, immunizations should be given according to the schedule outlined in the *Red Book* published by the American Academy of Pediatrics. Children with cerebral palsy may have abnormalities to other organ systems, and the physician should be attentive to this, especially during infancy. Commonly associated problems that require active surveillance include strabismus, visual impairment, hearing loss, hydrocephalus, and dental caries.

Abnormalities of the visual system occur in at least 50% of children with cerebral palsy and should be screened for at every visit. Strabismus is the most common, and early referral to an ophthalmologist is necessary to prevent amblyopia. Depending on the etiology and severity of cerebral palsy, other problems, such as cataracts, retinopathy of prematurity, nystagmus, and cortical visual impairment, may

occur. If there is any question about a child's vision, there should be prompt referral for further evaluation.

Hearing evaluation should be done in infancy. Certain types of cerebral palsy are associated with a high incidence of hearing loss, including cerebral palsy secondary to congenital viral infection and dyskinetic cerebral palsy secondary to bilirubin encephalopathy, but all children should be tested. In most cases, this should be done by an audiologist skilled in testing infants. If the results are equivocal or the child is not testable, brainstem auditory evoked responses should be performed.

Head circumference should be followed closely in infancy. Excessive head growth may indicate hydrocephalus, particularly in infants born prematurely. Plateauing of head circumference is indicative of poor brain growth and often is a prognostic indicator of poor intellectual function.

Dental care by a provider who is experienced in working with disabled children is very important. Routine cleanings and dental prophylaxis should begin when the child is a toddler. When this is neglected, children with cerebral palsy often ultimately need extensive dental work under general anesthesia.

FEEDING AND NUTRITION

Nutritional problems are very common. Chewing and swallowing difficulties lead to inadequate caloric intake in many children. Treatment can include working with a feeding specialist (usually an occupational or a speech therapist) to improve positioning and feeding techniques, dietary supplementation with high caloric foods, and if necessary, nasogastric or gastrostomy feedings. In addition, gastroesophageal reflux is often a problem, causing recurrent aspiration. The treatment of this complication is discussed elsewhere in this text.

Because of limited physical activity and the tendency for children who are socially isolated to overeat, some children become obese. The obesity can further impair their functional abilities and worsen the isolation.

Many children with cerebral palsy have problems with constipation that can be troublesome. Often, both nutritional interventions and medications are required.

Another common problem is excessive drooling. This is often considered socially unacceptable by the child and family, but effective treatment options are limited. A variety of interventions have been tried, including such behavioral techniques as biofeedback and such anticholinergic medications as benztropine (Cogentin). Surgical procedures to control excessive drooling are rarely used because of inconsistent results and postoperative complications.

PSYCHOSOCIAL SUPPORT

Children with cerebral palsy and their families require ongoing psychologic support. The most stressful time for a family is usually when the diagnosis is made and they recognize that their child will have a permanent disability. However, as the child grows, there will be other stressful times (e.g., the beginning of kindergarten and the onset of adolescence). These are important milestones when it can be quite obvious how different the child is from others of the same age. Parents have ongoing worries about what will happen to their child as an adult, particularly if the child is severely disabled. Children with cerebral palsy realize early on how different they are from their peers. The presence of both physical and learning disabilities can lead to social isolation and low self-esteem. Adolescents are particularly vulnerable to feelings of hopelessness and depression.

The physician should provide anticipatory guidance to both child and family. Recreational and social activities that the child enjoys should be encouraged. Realization that a disabled child can cause disruption to the family unit is important, and counseling for the family, as well as the child, often is indicated. During particularly stressful times, respite care for the child may be necessary.

NONSTANDARD TREATMENT

Despite the treatment modalities available for children with cerebral palsy, there is no cure, and many children remain severely disabled. Families who are understandably desperate often seek alternative therapies, including special diets, megavitamin therapies, and motor therapy regimens. Unfortunately, many of these unproven therapies are expensive and time consuming, and the emotional cost to the family of unsuccessful treatments is often great. The physician caring for the child should let families know that he or she is willing to discuss any therapeutic option and to help them choose those that are reasonable and safe.

RESOURCES FOR FAMILIES

Support Group

United Cerebral Palsy Associations
Seven Penn Plaza
Suite 804
New York, New York 10001

Books

1. Batshaw ML: Your Child Has a Disability. Boston, Little, Brown and Company, 1991.
2. Geralis E (ed): Children with Cerebral Palsy: A Parent's Guide. Rockville, MD, Woodbine House, 1991.

MOVEMENT DISORDERS

Michael A. Nigro, D.O.

Movement disorders of infancy and childhood are relatively common and represent a diagnostic and therapeutic challenge for the practitioner. A therapeutic approach can be developed from symptoms (e.g., chorea, dystonia), etiologic factors (infection, neoplastic), and age of onset. Dyskinesia (abnormal movement) results from some effect on the basal ganglia, that is, the putamen, globus pallidus, caudate nucleus, and their connections—red nucleus, substantia nigra, and the thalamic and cortical afferents. Tremor and myoclonus may be associated with abnormalities of the basal ganglia or cerebellum and interrelated systems.

Infantile dyskinesia is typically associated with cerebral palsy. The hyperkinetic dyskinesias are most common, including athetotic, choreic, and dystonic types. Most important, but quite rare, is the Segawa type or childhood onset idiopathic postural dystonia, characterized by diurnal worsening of dystonia and progressive motor and cognitive impairment. The Segawa type is very responsive to levodopa [typically administered as carbidopa-levodopa (Sinemet 10:100), beginning at one-half tablet daily and increasing weekly by one-half tablet to a maximum dosage of 400 mg levodopa daily]. The response should be definitive to warrant long-term use. Nonspecific symptomatic treatment (Tables 1 and 2) of dyskinetic cerebral palsy with trihexyphenidyl, propranolol, haloperidol, and clonazepam has not

been consistently effective. Seating orthosis, bracing, and tone-reducing restraints can be beneficial.

Progressive choreoathetosis of Lesch-Nyhan syndrome (LNS) is a hyperkinetic chorea characterized by self-abusive biting and hyperuricemia secondary to hypoxanthine-guanine phosphoribosyltransferase deficiency. Unfortunately, treatment with allopurinol to lower the uric acid levels does not result in an improvement in behavior. Carbidopa-levodopa, a high protein diet, and monosodium glutamate have been used to improve behavior and reduce dyskinesia but are not highly effective. Limb restraint has been effective in reducing self-mutilation and in diminishing the severity of dyskinesia.

Juvenile Huntington's chorea (Westphal variant) is an autosomal dominantly inherited disease that occurs in early childhood when the father is the affected parent. Affected children have parkinsonian features, dementia, and seizures. Instead of chorea, rigidity, tremor, and progressive bradykinesia are the predominant features. Symptomatic treatment with haloperidol and diazepam is marginally effective. Induction of chorea can result from levodopa use. Because of dementia, special education is required even at the preschool level. Seizures should be treated according to their type (see section on seizure disorders).

Toxic dyskinesias include those associated with prescriptive medication or poisonings, for example, antiepileptic drug-induced tics and chorea, antihistaminic-induced chorea, and dystonia caused by phenothiazine (Table 3). The primary treatment is removal of the offending agent. Phenothiazine-induced dystonia usually is responsive to parenteral diphenhydramine hydrochloride (Benadryl) (1 to 2 mg/kg, slowly IV) or benztropine mesylate (Cogentin) (0.5 to 1.5 mg per dose every 4 to 8 hours, with repeat oral dosages necessary for several days when the dyskinesia recurs). In severe idiosyncratic reactions, parenteral medication is required until the patient responds and can safely feed and take oral medication. Disulfiram-induced dyskinesia may be severe and permanent, and symptomatic treatment is usually minimally effective. Metoclopramide-induced akathisia and dystonia occur more prominently in children already affected by cerebral palsy (chronic motor disorder), and its treatment generally requires only withdrawal of the drug.

The **neuroleptic malignant syndrome** results from an idiosyncratic reaction to neuroleptic medication, usually within several weeks of initiation or abrupt change in dosage. It is heralded by bouts of rigidity, dystonia, impaired awareness, diaphoresis, myonecrosis, and hyperthermia. It is potentially fatal, and early recognition is imperative so that the neuroleptic can be discontinued and general medical support can be initiated (e.g., IV fluids, maintenance of airway and blood pressure). Dantrolene hydrochloride (2.5 mg/kg) should be administered intravenously over 1 hour. That dose may need to be repeated until the rigidity and temperature elevation have resolved. Oral dantrolene (4 to 8 mg/kg/d in four divided doses) may be used for several days following an acute crisis. Levodopa can be used in addition if dantrolene is ineffective.

Tics and Tourette's syndrome (TS) are the most common dyskinesias seen by physicians. Stimulant drug-induced (methylphenidate, pemoline, and dexedrine) tics are best treated by discontinuing

TABLE 1. Symptomatic Treatment

	HALOPERIDOL	TRIHEXYPHENIDYL	PIMOZIDE	CLONAZEPAM	CLONIDINE	LEVODOPA-CARBIDOPA	BENZTROPINE MESYLATE	VALPROATE	DIAZEPAM
Chorea	+	+	−	±	±	±	+	+	+
Athetosis	±	±	+	+	+	+	+	±	−
Dystonia	+	+	−	±	+	+	+	±	+
Ballismus	−	±	−	+	−	±	+	+	+
Myoclonus	−	+	−	+	−	+	−	+	+
Tourette's syndrome	+	−	+	+	+	−	−	−	−

+ Effective.
± Not known.
− Not indicated.

TABLE 2. Pharmacologic Agents Used For Dyskinesia

	STARTING DOSE	INCREMENT	MAXIMUM DOSE
Trihexyphenidyl (Artane)	2 mg b.i.d.	4 mg/d for 1 wk	80 mg/d
Benztropine mesylate (Cogentin)	0.5 mg	0.5 mg/d for 1 wk	2 mg/d
Clonazepam (Klonopin)	0.01 mg/kg/d	0.01–0.03 mg/kg/d	0.1 mg/kg/d
Haloperidol (Haldol)	0.25 mg b.i.d.	0.5 mg/d for 1 wk	10 mg/d
Clonidine (Catapres)	0.05 mg/d	0.05 mg/d for 1 wk	0.4 mg/d
Pimozide (Orap)	1 mg/d	1 mg/d for 1 wk	8 mg/d
Carbidopa-levodopa (Sinemet)	½ tablet 10:100 b.i.d	½ tablet per wk	25:100 q.i.d.
Propranolol (Inderal)	10 mg/d	10 mg/d for 1 wk	3 mg/kg/d
Baclofen (Lioresal)	5 mg/d	10 mg/d for 1 wk	80 mg/d
Primidone (Mysoline)	12.5 mg/d	12.5–25 mg/d for 1 wk	1000 mg/d
Clomipramine hydrochloride (Anafranil)	25 mg/d	12.5 mg/d for 1 wk	75 mg/d

the drug, but in some instances of preexisting TS, the tics may persist. Tics need treatment if they interfere with learning and social development or risk self-injury (e.g., brachial plexus injury, myelopathy). Effective treatment includes counseling, stress reduction, and medication. Drugs found to be highly effective include haloperidol, clonidine, and pimozide (Orap). Complete amelioration of vocal and motor tics is the goal but may not be feasible because of limitations of drug side effects. To minimize the likelihood of side effects, clonidine (Catapres), a centrally active alpha-adrenergic agonist, should be used initially. Treatment may be initiated 0.1 mg/d PO or via a Transderm patch and increased to 0.4 mg/d if necessary. Lethargy, however, may be a limiting factor with either route. Pimozide is highly effective and should be tried if clonidine is ineffective. It is a diphenylbutylpiperidine derivative and is a unique selective dopamine blocking agent. Side effects are less than those associated with haloperidol (Haldol). Sedation and cognitive impairment are more likely to be seen at higher dosages (>4 mg). Prolongation of the QT complex with resultant arrhythmia is a rare side effect of pimozide and is more likely in a patient with congenital prolonged QT syndrome. Therefore, a pretreatment ECG is warranted to rule out a conduction abnormality or other arrhythmia.

Haloperidol was the most commonly used drug and mainstay of treatment for TS for 25 years. Although haloperidol is highly effective, there are more side effects (impaired cognition, behavioral problems, dystonia, and sedation) associated with its use, especially at higher doses. Haloperidol may be used alone or in combination with clonidine. Clonazepam, an anticonvulsant benzodiazepam, is less effective and less frequently used. Clonazepam can also be highly sedating, and, therefore, the starting dosage should be 0.01 mg/kg/d.

The obsessive-compulsive behavior of TS can be very disruptive for the child but may respond to clomipramine hydrochloride (Anafanil 25 to 50 mg/d) or fluoxetine hydrochloride (Prozac 20 to 60 mg/d) in combination with clonidine, pimozide, or haloperidol. Stressful situations or difficulty dealing with stress should be identified and managed by appropriate counseling. Individual and family counseling is required in most instances and may be required periodically (e.g., transition to middle school or high school). Hyperactivity associated

with TS may be incompletely responsive to drugs used for tics, and, in rare instances, a stimulant drug will also be required. However, stimulant drugs have the potential to exacerbate tics. For this reason, behavior management, appropriate school placement, and counseling also should be used. TS support groups are helpful for the patient and family. A full range of services is available through the Tourette's Society. Inservice education programs at school may reduce peer pressure. Special education programs can be helpful in dealing with the central processing and emotional adjustment difficulties associated with TS.

Tardive dyskinesia in childhood is rare and often self-limiting. Withdrawal dyskinesia is the result of abrupt discontinuation of neuroleptic agents and usually remits spontaneously. Typical manifestations of tardive dyskinesia include orolinguimandibular, truncal, and limb choreic movements. Management of tardive dyskinesia begins with recognition of the etiology, gradual withdrawal or increase in dosage of the neuroleptic, and, when indicated, drug treatment. Clonazepam can be helpful in milder forms. Sodium valproate, baclofen, and trihexyphenidyl have been used with limited success.

Postviral opsoclonus polymyoclonus (OPMC) may be self-limiting, but when it is persistent and disabling, aggressive treatment with ACTH is warranted. A dosage of 20 to 80 units per day can be effective, and in some instances, treatment is required for several months or (rarely) several years. ACTH treatment requires attention to many potential side effects—hypertension, gastric ulcers and bleeding, irritability, hypertrophic cardiomyopathy, weight gain, lowered immune response, sleep disturbance, and hypercalciuria. Therefore, periodic assessment of blood pressure, occult blood loss in the stool, and the urine calcium/creatinine ratio (<0:21) are indicated. Ranitidine (Zantac) should be started prophylactically to decrease the risk of ulcer formation. Intravenous IgG (2 g/kg over 1 to 4 days) has at least limited benefit in OPMC, but repeated treatment becomes less effective. Plasmapheresis has been effective in several cases but warrants more evaluation before it is considered standard therapy (Table 4).

Postviral and idiopathic segmental myoclonus may be self-limiting but can last several weeks to a year. If it is disabling or persistent,

TABLE 3. Drug-induced Dyskinesias

TREMOR	DYSTONIA	CHOREA	TICS	MYOCLONUS
Phenytoin	Phenothiazine	Carbamazepine	Methylphenidate	Levodopa
Lithium	Metoclopramide	Antihistamine	Pemoline	Anticonvulsants
Amphetamines	Diphenhydramine	Ethosuximide	Dextroamphetamine	Tricyclic antidepressants
Bronchodilators		Metoclopramide	Carbamazepine	
Tricyclic antidepressants		Manganese		
Sodium valproate		Disulfiram (Antabuse)		
		Phenytoin		
		Lithium carbonate		
		Tricyclic antidepressants		
		Benzodiazepams		

TABLE 4. Immunomodulation Therapy

	ACTH	PREDNISONE	IVIG*	PHERESIS
Postviral myoclonus	+	+	+	+
Paraneoplastic myoclonus	+	+	±	±
Sydenham's chorea	—	+	±	±
Encephalitis	—	—	—	—

+ Effective.
± Not known.
—Not indicated.
*IVIG, intravenous IgG.

treatment may be helpful. Valproate and clonazepam have been inconsistently effective. In one instance, plasmapheresis produced a dramatic and immediate beneficial effect. However, further study is indicated.

Parainfectious dyskinesias can occur simultaneously with an infectious process or appear afterward. Sydenham's chorea is the classic postinfectious streptococcus-related movement disorder, characterized by progressive, usually asymmetric chorea that may be moderately to severely disabling. Treatment is aimed at preventing further streptococcal infection by the use of benzathine penicillin (1.2 million units per month) through adolescence. In the past 5 years, corticosteroid use has proven to be the quickest and most effective treatment, making it unnecessary to use antidyskinesia drugs. Prednisone 2 mg/kg/d is initiated and continued until there is complete amelioration of the chorea and then is tapered over the next 3 to 4 weeks. Exacerbation warrants repeat treatment over a longer period of time. Plasmapheresis is an incompletely effective and unproven treatment for Sydenham's chorea and warrants further evaluation. Cognitive and behavioral components accompanying Sydenham's chorea require specific medical treatment, and counseling may be necessary.

Systemic lupus erythematosus (SLE)–induced chorea is rare in this age group, and management of the autoimmune disease defines treatment. Symptomatic treatment commonly includes diazepam, haloperidol, and clonazepam.

Encephalitis can cause any of the acute hyperkinetic dyskinesias. They are usually transient and may require temporary symptomatic treatment (haloperidol, clonidine, trihyxyphenidyl, clonazepam). Less frequently, chronic therapy is necessary.

Trauma-induced dyskinesia can be seen after closed head injury and stroke. The movements can be choreic, dystonic, ballismic, athetotic, or tremor, and invariably the treatment is symptomatic (see specific symptom, Table 1). Rehabilitative treatment of ataxia and tremor requires gait and limb stabilization, oversized utensils, and ambulatory assistance devices.

Paraneoplastic dyskinesia, a remote effect of tumor, is typified by opsoclonus polymyoclonus (dancing eyes and dancing feet) and is associated with the presence of neuroblastoma. The onset of paraneoplastic dyskinesia may precede the appearance of the tumor by months. Although resection of the tumor, chemotherapy, and radiation therapy may result in reduction of the movements, ACTH is usually necessary to reduce persisting dyskinesias and gait instability. Intramuscular ACTH is initiated at 40 units per day and increased if necessary to 80 units per day to achieve a complete response. ACTH is then tapered over 4 to 8 weeks depending on dosage and duration. In some children, treatment may be required for many months.

Cerebral and cerebellar neoplasms can cause movement disorders, and treatment is aimed at tumor resection, radiation, and chemotherapy. Residual dyskinesia is then treated on a symptomatic basis (Table 1).

Postanoxic myoclonus (Lance Adams syndrome) and myoclonus associated with degenerative diseases (Lafora's disease, Ramsay Hunt syndrome) do not consistently respond to any one drug. Valproate, primidone, and clonazepam have been used with variable success. Treatment with L-tryptophan and carbidopa has produced improvement in several trials but remains investigational.

Kinesogenic chorea can be dominantly inherited, autosomal recessive, or isolated. Exercise or sudden movements usually induce the chorea, which may mimic seizures. In spite of a normal EEG, children usually respond to antiepileptic drugs, especially phenytoin (5 to 10 mg/kg/d) (see section on epilepsy). Unlike epilepsy, this disorder usually requires a lifetime of treatment.

Benign familial intention tremor inherited as an autosomal dominant trait usually affects the distal upper extremities and is exacerbated with volitional (especially terminal) movements. Treatment is indicated when the tremor affects performance or self-esteem. Two agents have been particularly helpful. Propranolol (10 to 20 mg t.i.d. in children <35 kg and 20 to 40 mg t.i.d. in children >35 kg) is effective in the majority of patients. Limiting side effects include lethargy and postural lightheadedness. Primidone (Mysoline), a barbiturate antiepileptic drug, is also effective at a low dosage (25 to 150 mg/d). Clonazepam (0.01 to 0.05 mg/kg/d) is indicated when primidone and propranolol are ineffective. Large-caliber writing utensils and wrist weights may help reduce the effect of tremor. Caffeinated beverages may exacerbate this condition.

Dominantly inherited focal dystonia can be relatively mild to profoundly disabling and commonly affects a distal extremity, the foot or wrist. Long-term carbamazepine therapy has been effective in treating this condition, and low to moderate therapeutic levels usually are effective. Trihexyphenidyl, diazepam, clonazepam, baclofen, and levodopa-carbidopa all have been used and may be effective in the treatment of focal dystonia and dystonia muscularum deformans. Trihexyphenidyl, diazepam, and baclofen are begun at low dosage, but very high dosages are well tolerated. Intramuscular injections of botulinum toxin (Botox) have been used in the past several years to treat the focal dystonias (laryngeal and limb dystonias) resistant to drug therapy.

Dyskinesias associated with metabolic disorders (e.g., phenylketonuria type II, glutaric aciduria, Wilson's disease, mitochondrial cytopathies, Leigh's disease) include chorea, dystonia, ballismus, and athetosis. Recognition of the etiology defines the treatment of these disorders. Dietary management, vitamin therapy (B_{12}, folate, thiamine, riboflavin, biotin), and nonspecific drug management (Table 1) may attenuate the movements.

Sandifer syndrome is an episodic dyskinesia caused by hiatal hernia and gastroesophageal reflux, resulting in stereotypic upper trunk, head, and neck movements that respond to surgical treatment (fundal plication) and/or metoclopramide. Dyskinesia can be a complication of metoclopramide. Ranitidine may be used if esophageal irritation is unresponsive to metoclopramide.

Shuddering attacks are best left untreated. They mimic and should be differentiated from seizures.

Paroxysmal torticollis of infancy is probably a result of vestibular dysfunction and results in head tilt lasting hours to days. Treatment is aimed at defining and treating middle and inner ear disease.

Sleep and arousal myoclonus is benign and does not warrant treatment.

SPINAL CORD DISORDERS

MICHAEL E. SELZER, M.D., Ph.D.

TRAUMATIC INJURY

Immediate Physical Diagnosis

Spinal cord injuries are uncommon in children, and most that do occur are in adolescence. The majority are the result of indirect trauma producing hyperextension or hyperflexion of the neck, as in motor vehicle or pedestrian/motor vehicle accidents, or vertical compression of the spine during falls, diving into shallow water, and other athletic injuries. In these settings, spinal cord injury is suspected in an awake child by the presence of weakness or paralysis and the loss of sensation below the level of the injury. In an unconscious or very young child, a spinal level can be suspected by the absence of withdrawal reflexes and myotatic reflexes below the level of injury (due to spinal shock) and by the dryness and warmth of the skin below the level of the injury (due to loss of autonomic responses). The neurologic deficits may worsen over the next 24 to 48 hours, as a cascade of metabolic and vascular changes produces secondary neuronal damage that is now believed to account for many of the ultimate pathologic changes.

Acute Treatment

The advent of trauma units has improved the immediate care of patients, who are transported where possible to a specialized spine trauma center without further movement of the spine. In cervical spine injuries, the neck should be maintained in a neutral position, and the limbs should be prevented from moving. The body should be placed on a rigid frame with shoulder and pelvic support. A supine position should be attained by careful rolling, using as many attendants as necessary to accomplish it without allowing the limbs and spine to move relative to one another. The neck should be supported by a soft collar, and sandbags should be placed on either side of the neck to prevent head rotation. A conscious patient should be warned not to move. These principles must be kept in mind especially during initial evaluation of patients with multiple injuries that might be more conveniently attended to if there were no restrictions on spine mobility. For example, if respiratory function deteriorates, an airway must be established. Nasotracheal intubation may not be possible if the head is immobilized, and tracheostomy would then have to be performed. Spinal cord-injured patients may have internal injuries and go into shock. Vital signs should be checked frequently.

In the emergency room, patients should have a hemoglobin level, serum electrolytes, and arterial blood gases determination, blood saved for type and crossmatch, vital capacity test, and chest x-ray. Blood loss and chest immobility are common causes of death. If vital capacity falls below 50% or the arterial oxygen saturation falls below 94%, ventilatory assistance may be required. Loss of autonomic regulation may lead to bradycardia or hypotension. These should be treated promptly (see section on syncope and hypotension).

Neurologic Assessment

A careful but rapid neurologic examination should be performed to assess the degree and level of spinal cord involvement and to monitor the patient's subsequent improvement. Neurologic evaluation should follow the International Standards for Neurological and Functional Classification of Spinal Cord Injury, which are now used in clinical studies. In awake patients, the sensory examination is particularly helpful in assessing the spinal level. Pin and light touch sensations are graded on a scale of 0 to 2 at key points in each of the 28 paired dermatomes: 0 = absent, 1 = impaired, 2 = normal, NT = not testable. In addition, sensation of the external anal sphincter to the examiner's inserted finger is graded as present or absent. If it is present, the injury is not complete regardless of other neurologic deficits, and this is associated with a better prognosis than a complete spinal cord injury. Strength is assessed on a 0 to 5 scale for key muscles in 10 paired myotomes from C5 to S1: 0 = total paralysis, 1 = palpable or visible contraction, 2 = full range of active movement (ROM) with gravity eliminated, 3 = full ROM against gravity, 4 = full ROM against moderate resistance, 5 = normal strength, NT = not testable. In addition, the ability of the external anal sphincter to contract around the examiner's inserted finger is graded as present or absent, again to determine completeness of the injury. The guidelines include methods for calculating sensory and motor scores, determining sensory and motor levels, and zones of partial preservation. These data are used to assign an overall score on the 5-point American Spinal Injury Association (ASIA) scale: A = complete impairment, E = normal motor and sensory function, and B, C, and D are grades of incomplete impairment below the neurologic level. Copies of these guidelines are available from Lesley M. Hudson,

M.A., 2020 Peachtree Road, N.W., Atlanta, GA 30309, tel. (404) 355-9772.

Methylprednisolone Treatment

Patients diagnosed with spinal cord injury should be treated as soon as possible with high-dose methylprednisolone. Based on the protocol of the Second National Spinal Cord Injury Study (NASCIS 2),[1] a bolus of 30 mg/kg should be given intravenously over 15 minutes. A pause of 45 minutes is then followed by administration of 5.4 mg/kg/h for the next 23 hours. This protocol resulted in statistically significant improvement of neurologic function over the next 6 months, which was maintained at 1 year. Initiation of treatment more than 8 hours after injury was ineffective. The influence of the improved neurologic status on functional independence has not been determined. This study excluded patients under the age of 13, but in the absence of a published clinical trial in the pediatric age group, the protocol is routinely followed in all children. Other pharmacologic approaches to restricting secondary neuronal damage following spinal cord injury are under intensive study. A small-scale trial of intravenous GM-1 ganglioside has suggested possible benefits, but this needs to be confirmed by a large-scale, multicenter trial.

Urinary retention is treated initially with an indwelling catheter, which, after the first day, can give way to intermittent catheterization. Enemas are required because of initial loss of bowel motility.

Radiologic Evaluation

Spinal cord-injured patients should be evaluated by CT with metrizamide myelography to determine the level or levels of injury, whether there is subluxation of vertebral bodies or disc herniation causing compression of the cord, and whether there are bone fragments in the spinal canal, a penetrating injury to the cord, or vertebral instability because of extensive disruption of the bony architecture in one or more vertebrae. Young children may have pseudosubluxations of the upper cervical spine, especially an anterior displacement of C2 on C3, which can confound the diagnosis of spinal cord injury. Because spinal cord injuries may involve multiple levels and may be accompanied by head injury, the entire spine and the head should be imaged. In most centers, MRI is not performed as readily as CT and may be difficult to perform on patients with multiple injuries requiring life support measures. It is also less accurate than CT in assessing bony damage. However, once the patient has been stabilized, MRI may be useful in imaging the spinal cord or intervertebral discs.

Spine injuries need not involve vertebral fracture or subluxation to produce spinal cord injury. In several recent studies, 29% to 35% of spinal cord-injured patients aged 0 to 17 years had no radiologic abnormality of the spine, and in patients below age 10, more than half had no abnormality. In approximately 25% of such patients, the neurologic deficits are delayed by up to 4 days.

Children with Down syndrome have hyperextensible joints, including hypermobility of the C1–2 (atlantoaxial) joint. This puts them at special risk for spinal cord injuries. Radiologic evaluation of these children is recommended at age 4 years before allowing them to engage in contact sports or other forms of strenuous exercise. A space of more than 5 mm between the odontoid process and the atlas indicates instability of the joint. Surgical repair may be required if there is clinical evidence of cord compression.

Surgical Treatment

A halo and tong traction device is usually used in cases of cervical hyperflexion injury. There is no evidence that surgical decompression is useful in cases of spinal cord injury where the spine itself is intact. Surgery is indicated in cases of open wounds, in incomplete lesions of the cord with CSF block to remove bony fragments or missiles that threaten the integrity of the cord, to stabilize a subluxed or shattered vertebral column that cannot be stabilized by traction and immobilization, and to explore reasons for delayed neurologic worsening.

Intermediate Care

The management of spinal cord-injured patients during the week following the injury involves standard though intense nursing and medical measures aimed at preventing pulmonary embolism and decubitus sores, initiation of bowel and bladder training, prevention of stress ulcers, and maintenance of nutrition. Decubitus sores are a special hazard if there is significant sensory loss because the patient is unaware of them. Patients should be placed on an air mattress once the spine is stabilized. Urinary tract infections frequently occur because of the need for indwelling or intermittent catheterization, and they should be treated with appropriate antibiotics (see section on urinary tract infections). Counseling and psychologic support should be provided to the patient and significant relations, emphasizing the need for their active participation in the process of recovery and providing a realistic view of the prognosis. According to NASCIS 2, patients given methylprednisolone within 8 hours after injury showed improvement in mean motor scores of 6.2 to 18.3 on a 70-point scale, depending on the completeness of initial impairment.[1] Patients with complete lesions improved least, and patients with some preservation of sensory and motor function below the level of injury improved most. Although specific comparisons are lacking, pediatric patients, especially those with incomplete lesions, appear to improve more than adults and are more likely to show good functional adjustments.

Rehabilitation

Long-term outcome will be best if the rehabilitation service is involved in the patient's evaluation and care from the beginning. Prolonged hospitalization in a facility with special expertise in rehabilitation of the spinal cord-injured patient is required for complete or near complete spinal cord injuries. It is a highly complex team activity that is beyond the scope of this text. Rehabilitation involves physical therapeutic approaches to strengthen spared muscles, occupational therapy to maximize function with regard to activities of daily living, continued bladder and bowel training, psychologic support, and counseling on a wide range of topics from sexuality to vocational rehabilitation. The functional independence measure (FIM) is used to monitor recovery of performance on daily life activities. Decubitus sores, pulmonary emboli, and urinary tract infections are continuing hazards. Recurrent urinary tract infections (more than three per year) require prophylactic antibiotic therapy with nitrofurantoin 1 to 2 mg/kg/d orally at bedtime or with trimethoprim-sulfamethoxazole 2 mg: 10 mg/kg PO every 1 to 2 days at bedtime.

TUMORS OF THE SPINAL CORD

Clinical Presentation

It is important to diagnose spinal cord tumors early because most of them are operable, even if their histologic appearance is malignant. Intramedullary tumors are generally of low-grade malignant histologic type. The most common are ependymomas and astrocytomas. Less common are glioblastomas, which have a worse prognosis. Extramedullary tumors (either intradural or extradural) are most often benign, except for metastatic tumors, which are discussed separately. Extramedullary tumors include neurofibromas (in children, seen most often in association with von Recklinghausen's disease), dermoid cysts, and teratomas. Meningiomas are rare in children. Both intramedullary and extramedullary tumors often cause pain and spinal rigidity, which allows time for diagnosis and treatment before neurologic deficits are severe. The pain of intramedullary tumors is frequently dull, aching, and referred symmetrically to the corresponding dermatomes (even the abdomen in the case of thoracic tumors), whereas that of extramedullary tumors is more intense, unilateral, segmental, often shooting, and accompanied by paresthesias.

As an intramedullary tumor grows, it produces gait disturbance by compression of the pyramidal tracts, which appear to be more sensitive to outward compression than are the sensory tracts. Stiffness and weakness of the legs develop more or less symmetrically, together with hyperreflexia, spasticity, and Babinski's signs. The motor deficits generally progress downward because of the organization of the pyramidal tracts with the sacralmost fibers located most laterally. Therefore, sphincter disturbance tends to be late. Occasionally, there is symmetric loss of pain and temperature sensation at the level of the tumor because of interruption of the decussating fibers of the anterolateral spinothalamic tract. When the tumor is in the cervical or lumbar enlargement, weakness and wasting of muscles may occur at the level of the lesion as a result of compression of the ventral gray matter, but this seems to be less common than spasticity. Approximately one third of children with intramedullary tumor present with scoliosis. Intramedullary tumors also may produce electric shocklike sensations running down the back and into the limbs, a sign of dorsal column involvement similar to Lhermitte's sign in multiple sclerosis. This is rarely seen with extramedullary tumors.

Extramedullary tumors often produce unilateral segmental weakness, muscle wasting, and sensory loss because of early involvement of nerve roots. Further expansion compresses the spinal cord. Once again, the arrangement of pyramidal and anterolateral tracts causes early sensory and motor symptoms of spinal cord compression to be manifest far from the site of spinal pain. One sees asymmetric ascending weakness and sensory deficits in the distribution of a Brown-Sequard syndrome, although usually not a complete one. The Brown-Sequard syndrome consists of ipsilateral weakness, spasticity, ataxia, and loss of vibration and joint position sensations, and contralateral loss of pain and temperature sensations.

Diagnostic Tests

The most important test is an MRI of the spinal cord with gadolinium enhancement, which easily distinguishes intramedullary from extramedullary lesions and can also distinguish intramedullary tumor from syrinx and cystic lesions from solid tumors. Additional radiologic procedures, such as angiography or CT, may be desirable in some circumstances. Intramedullary tumors may be confused with inflammatory lesions of the cord, since acute inflammatory lesions (multiple sclerosis and transverse myelitis) may also produce cord swelling and enhance with gadolinium. Decision about surgical exploration will depend on the clinical picture, primarily the time course of symptoms. In unusual cases, it may be advisable to wait a few weeks, as long as symptoms do not progress rapidly. A second MRI should then distinguish a chronic, nonenhancing plaque of demyelination from an expanding contrast-enhancing tumor. Lumbar puncture also may be helpful, since the CSF protein concentration will be elevated with an intramedullary tumor in proportion to the degree of CSF block, whereas in the case of demyelination, the protein will be elevated only in the acute phase.

Treatment

In most cases, the primary treatment is surgical excision of the tumor. Many extramedullary tumors can be totally excised. Those that cannot may respond well to radiation therapy. Neurofibromas do not respond to radiation therapy, and many cannot be totally excised, but neurologic outcome may be satisfactory following subtotal resection. Treatment of intramedullary tumors is more controversial. There is general agreement in favor of attempting total removal of ependymomas, almost half of which arise in the filum terminale. Astrocytomas traditionally have been treated by incomplete excision, followed by radiation. However, the development of microsurgical techniques has encouraged a more aggressive approach. Epstein and Farmer found that most intramedullary tumors, including astrocytomas, have a clear plane of dissection that allows their total removal.[4] Often, there is remarkable preservation of function despite the appearance of an almost totally atrophic shell of spinal cord surrounding the tumor, as long as surgery is performed before significant neurologic deficits have developed. Long-term survival has been high. Radiation is reserved for the minority of cases in which total excision was not possible. In many children, scoliosis and other spinal deformities develop after surgery and may require orthopedic stabilization procedures. Syringomyelia also may develop and produce symptoms similar to those produced by the original tumor. MRI is generally diagnostic, and the syrinx can be shunted.

METASTATIC SPINAL CORD TUMORS

Clinical Presentation

Metastatic spine disease, though less common in the pediatric population than in adults, is the most common nontraumatic cause of spinal cord compression in children. Often the tumor is found before there is significant cord compression. Sarcomas and neuroblastomas usually invade the spinal canal by direct extension from the paraspinous space through the epidural foramen or from the bone itself. Lymphomas and many other tumors enter the spinal canal by hematogenous spread through the paraspinal venous (Batson's) plexus to the vertebral body and then the epidural space. Intradural extramedullary metastases and intramedullary spinal cord metastases are rare. A picture of acute spinal cord compression can develop over 24 to 48 hours. Symptoms are similar to those of other extramedullary tumors, except for the accelerated course. They include radiating neck or back pain, asymmetric paraplegia and sensory levels, and bowel or bladder dysfunction.

Diagnostic Tests

Most often, the primary tumor is already known, so that the cause should be suspected. Plain x-rays of the spine may demonstrate lytic or blastic lesions, vertebral body collapse, or a paraspinous mass. CT myelography or MRI with gadolinium enhancement when available are the most important diagnostic tools. MRI is preferable because it does not entail lumbar puncture, which may accelerate spinal cord compression in the presence of complete CSF block. MRI is also much better at detecting intramedullary metastasis. On the other hand, if the primary tumor is not known and leptomeningeal metastasis is a possibility, myelography may provide CSF for cytologic identification of the tumor.

Treatment

Immediate therapy involves intravenous administration of 10 mg of dexamethasone, followed by 1 mg every 6 hours. This reduces edema and can result in rapid temporary improvement of symptoms. The next step is most often radiation, unless the tumor type is not known, in which case laminectomy with biopsy should be performed, followed by radiation and/or chemotherapy, depending on the tissue diagnosis. However, there is evidence that in children with spinal cord compression or greater than 50% CSF block, surgical decompression followed by radiation or chemotherapy gives a better result than radiation or chemotherapy alone. This is also true of sarcomas (e.g., Ewing's sarcoma, rhabdomyosarcoma, and osteosarcoma). Neuroblastoma invading the spinal canal is best treated by chemotherapy when the course is slowly progressive. When spinal cord compression is rapid, chemotherapy should be preceded by surgical decompression. Radiation therapy carries a significant risk of delayed ascending myelitis. Intrathecal chemotherapy may increase this risk.

POLIOMYELITIS AND OTHER ENTEROVIRAL INFECTIONS

Enteroviruses (small RNA viruses) commonly infect the CNS by hematogenous spread following an initial infection of the gastrointestinal tract. Included in this group are the poliovirus, coxsackievirus, and echoviruses and several unclassified enteroviruses designated by number only. These viruses may infect many parts of the nervous system, but the polioviruses show a predilection for spinal motor neurons and often the cranial nerve nuclei, the cerebellar vermis, and the deep cerebellar nuclei. Significant involvement of the diencephalon and telencephalon is unusual. Because of the widespread use of the oral vaccine, poliomyelitis is now rare in the developed world. However, it is still common in developing countries, and occasional cases occur in developed countries, usually in immunodeficient children receiving live poliovaccines. In addition, other enteroviruses can produce a paralytic illness identical to poliomyelitis.

Clinical Presentation

In most cases, poliomyelitis infection is asymptomatic. In 4% to 8%, there is a mild gastroenteritis manifested by headache, sore throat, vomiting, and other gastrointestinal symptoms lasting 1 to 2 days (abortive poliomyelitis). However, in 1% to 2% of infected children, the initial infection is followed in 2 to 5 days by the major illness, beginning with aseptic meningitis (nonparalytic poliomyelitis). This leads to flaccid paralysis in 0.1% of infected children. The aseptic meningitis lasts 1 to 2 days and is characterized by stiffness and pain in the neck and/or back, headache, fever, drowsiness, and irritability. Maximum paralysis often develops over a few hours, but occasionally it progresses over 2 to 5 days. It is heralded by muscle pain and twitching and is accompanied by fever. When the fever breaks, the progression of paralysis stops. Muscles are involved asymmetrically in any combination. The legs are involved in the majority of cases and the arms in approximately 40%, followed by the trunk and bulbar musculature (10% to 15%). Paralysis is accompanied by loss of myotatic reflexes. Autonomic involvement is common, and the bladder is paralyzed in 10% to 20% of cases. Sensory involvement is very rare and should suggest Guillain-Barré syndrome or acute transverse myelopathy. Recovery of muscle strength begins in a few weeks. Substantial improvement is seen in muscles that are not completely paralyzed at 1 month. The less the original weakness, the greater the degree of recovery, and in moderately weak muscles, near total recovery is the rule. Some improvement may continue even after 1 year, but this is not the rule.

In as many as 25% of patients, secondary deterioration, known as the postpolio syndrome, is seen 30 to 40 years later. This was originally confused with amyotrophic lateral sclerosis. However, the prognosis is much better because deterioration is limited to muscles involved in the original disease, and there is no upper motor neuron component. There is no evidence for persistence of the virus. The mechanism may involve the superimposition of normal age-related neuronal dropout on a background of a diminished number of abnormally larger motor units.

Diagnostic Tests

Spinal fluid shows a moderate pleocytosis of 20 to 500/mm³, which is predominantly polymorphonuclear in the nonparalytic phase and then becomes primarily mononuclear over the next week. CSF protein is initially only mildly elevated but rises to 100 to 200 mg/100 ml over the next 3 to 4 weeks. Virus can be cultured from the stool throughout the illness and for 1 to 3 months thereafter. Serologic diagnosis is based on an elevation of specific complement-fixation or neutralizing antibodies that can differentiate poliomyelitis from similar diseases caused by other enteroviruses.

Treatment

The most important treatment is prevention by administration of the oral attenuated live virus vaccine. Unimmunized adults and immunodeficient children are more susceptible and should be given the inactivated poliomyelitis vaccine rather than the oral vaccine. In India, where the incidence of poliomyelitis is still relatively high, an increased incidence of paralytic poliomyelitis has been observed in children who received intramuscular injections during the mild phase of the infection. The symptoms of gastroenteritis should be treated with oral medication, avoiding unnecessary intramuscular injections.

There is no specific treatment for the paralytic phase of the disease, but supportive treatment can be crucial. Vital capacity must be monitored closely as paralysis develops. Patients with a 50% reduction in vital capacity should receive respiratory assistance, with tracheostomy if necessary. Tube feedings may be required if swallowing is compromised. Urethral catheterization may be necessary if the bladder is paralyzed. These complications usually resolve, although continued ventilatory assistance is sometimes required.

ACUTE TRANSVERSE MYELOPATHY (TRANSVERSE MYELITIS)

Several syndromes that follow exanthematous (and rarely other) viral illnesses or vaccinations are lumped under the name "acute disseminated encephalomyelitis." Their pathology (except for post-mumps encephalitis, which is an active infection of the brain) is similar to that of experimental allergic encephalomyelitis and includes peri-vascular infiltrates, demyelination, and release of myelin basic protein into the spinal fluid. They are, therefore, thought to be cell-mediated autoimmune responses. The spinal cord may be involved as part of a general CNS process (discussed elsewhere in this text) or in isolation.

Clinical Presentation

Acute transverse myelopathy causes pain in the back, limbs, or abdomen, with loss of sensation and flaccid paralysis in the legs and loss of bowel and bladder control developing over 1 to 2 days. The fundamental pathologic condition is inflammation and demyelination in one or more contiguous segments, most often midthoracic. There is a variable amount of necrosis, but it is often severe. If the cervical cord is involved, arms can also be affected. Pain and temperature sensation are more involved than the dorsal quadrant sensations of joint position and vibration, suggesting that some cases might be due to anterior spinal artery occlusion, perhaps secondary to vasculitis. A history of recent vaccination or concurrent viral infection, including influenza, the viral exanthems, mononucleosis, herpesviruses, echo-viruses, and hepatitis B, is present in approximately 70% of cases, making distinction from acute postinfectious polyneuritis (Guillain-Barré syndrome) occasionally difficult in young children. In older children who can respond to questions, the sharp sensory level usually makes the diagnosis of transverse myelopathy obvious and, in addition, distinguishes it from poliomyelitis.

Course

The flaccid paralysis changes to spasticity over the first 2 weeks, during which symptoms begin to subside in the majority of patients. Little additional recovery occurs after 6 months, and 15% of patients do not recover at all. If the lesion affects the high cervical region, patients may be at risk of respiratory arrest. In young adults, an episode of transverse myelitis may be the first attack of multiple sclerosis in 30% of cases. However, multiple sclerosis is very rare in children below the age of 10 years and unusual in adolescents. Thus, most instances of acute transverse myelopathy in the pediatric age group remain isolated events.

Diagnostic Tests

The most important test is an MRI of the spinal cord, which easily excludes acute cord compression by metastasis or pyogenic abscess and differentiates an acute intraspinal lesion from acute polyneuritis. In the acute phase, transverse myelitis shows the swelling and in-creased signal intensity on T2-weighted images characteristic of edema fluid and may be mistaken for an intramedullary tumor or recent infarction. The value of lumbar puncture has been greatly diminished since the advent of MRI. The spinal fluid usually shows mild to moderate elevations in protein (up to 150 mg/100 ml) and white cell counts (up to 200/ml^3, primarily lymphocytes) but does not differentiate acute transverse myelitis from tumor. Because the dorsal columns are usually not greatly involved, sensory evoked po-tentials are not very helpful.

Treatment

High-dose corticosteroids usually are given, but the usefulness of this procedure has not been established. Methylprednisolone 2 mg/kg/d can be administered intravenously for 3 days and tapered over a 10-day period. Bladder and bowel management and prevention of decubitus sores are important elements of treatment. Patients should be placed on an air mattress and rotated frequently. Respiratory sup-port may be necessary. There is usually a need for rehabilitation, depending on the severity of the disabilities and the degree of early recovery.

REFERENCES

1. Bracken MB, Shepard MJ, Collins WF, et al: A randomized, controlled trial of methylprednisolone or naloxone in the treatment of acute spinal-cord injury. Results of the Second National Acute Spinal Cord Injury Study. N Engl J Med 322:1405–1411, 1990.
2. Dickman CA, Rekate HL, Sonntag VK, Zabramski JM: Pediatric spinal trauma: Vertebral column and spinal cord injuries in children. Pediatr Neurosci 15:237–255, 1989.
3. Dunne K, Hopkins IJ, Shield LK: Acute transverse myelopathy in childhood. Dev Med Child Neurol 28:198–204, 1986.
4. Epstein FJ, Farmer JP: Pediatric spinal cord tumor surgery. Neurosurg Clin North Am 1:569–590, 1990.
5. Klein SL, Sanford RA, Muhlbauer MS: Pediatric spinal epidural metastases. J Neurosurg 74:70–75, 1991.
6. Young W: Spine injury. In Johnson RT, Griffin JW (eds): Current Therapy in Neurologic Disease. St. Louis, Mosby-Year Book, 1993.

DEGENERATIVE DISEASES OF THE CENTRAL NERVOUS SYSTEM

ALAN K. PERCY, M.D.

Current concepts regarding degenerative diseases of the central nervous system (CNS) in infants and children have expanded dra-matically over the past decade. Significant advances in our under-standing of the molecular mechanisms of many of the inherited dis-eases associated with progressive neurologic and psychomotor dete-rioration are largely responsible for these new and broader concepts. In addition, the emergence of acquired immunodeficiency states and the aggressive treatment of neoplastic processes has resulted in in-creasing numbers of infants and children with declining CNS function. For example, the typical features of regression in psychomotor skills associated with CNS degeneration, including the loss of previously acquired milestones in the young child or personality changes and faltering school performance in the older child, are now recognized with alarming frequency in association with HIV infection in children. Furthermore, the implementation of high-dose radiation to the brain both for leukemia and for primary CNS neoplasms has been linked to a decrement in cognitive and motor skills. The immunocompro-mised child is also at risk for an opportunistic infection of the CNS, with concomitant deterioration in psychomotor performance. Thus, the differential diagnosis of a degenerative or progressive process affecting the CNS in the pediatric population has important impli-cations with respect to specific therapeutic intervention. The present discussion is limited to the inherited CNS degenerative disorders oc-curring in childhood.

The clinician is faced with a bewildering and ever expanding array of inherited disorders in which regression of CNS function is a hall-mark. These disorders (Table 1) may be considered from a number of points of reference. These include clinical features, principal patho-logic changes, and the relevant subcellular organelle or specific met-abolic abnormality where a biochemical or molecular abnormality is known. It is useful to separate this last group of disorders from those in which no molecular basis has been defined. Disorders associated with dysfunction at the subcellular organelle level include lysosomal, peroxisomal, and mitochondrial processes in which very unique, often organ-specific enzyme defects are involved. The identification of spe-cific biochemical abnormalities allows the development of rational treatment strategies. Currently available therapies include replacement of the missing enzyme or enzyme cofactor, elimination or minimi-zation of the relevant dietary precursor, and removal of the offending element by a chelating agent. Rapid progress in molecular genetics in recent years has provided the basis for replacing the defective gene. This has been accomplished in tissue culture in Gaucher disease and in relevant animal models of several storage diseases. Nevertheless, considerable work remains before gene replacement becomes standard therapy for inherited diseases.

TABLE 1. CNS Degenerative Diseases among Children

TYPE	DISEASE
Lysosomal	Mucopolysaccharidoses
	Sphingolipidoses
	Glycogen storage disease, type II
	Neuronal ceroid lipofuscinoses
Peroxisomal	Adrenoleukodystrophy complex
	Neonatal adrenoleukodystrophy
	Zellweger disease
	Refsum disease
	Neonatal Refsum disease
Mitochondrial	Leigh disease
	MELAS: mitochondrial myopathy, lactic acidosis, and strokelike episodes
	MERRF: myoclonic epilepsy with ragged-red fibers
	KSS: Kearns-Sayre syndrome
	LHON: Leber hereditary optic neuropathy
Systems degeneration	Juvenile parkinsonism
	Progressive dystonias
	Spinocerebellar ataxias
Specific diseases	Phenylketonuria
	Maple syrup urine disease
	Galactosemia
	Urea cycle defects
	Organic acidemias
	Biotinidase deficiency
	Wilson's disease
	Menkes' disease

Degenerative diseases for which the molecular defect is unknown generally are described by the principal neurologic features or by the systems involved. This group includes the neuronal lipofuscinoses (Batten disease), the disorders of movement, such as juvenile parkinsonism and the dystonias, and the spinocerebellar degenerations. Treatment strategies for these disorders are to provide symptomatic relief. For example, specific pharmacologic agents are used in children with one of the movement disorders to interrupt or reverse the movement abnormalities.

The treatment of degenerative CNS diseases may follow three avenues: (1) prevention, (2) specific treatment, or (3) supportive or symptomatic care.

PREVENTION

Prevention implies (1) the ability to identify individuals and families at risk for a particular disorder, (2) the availability of methodologies to detect and verify affected fetuses, and (3) the willingness of the family to consider interruption of a pregnancy involving an affected fetus. Neonatal screening programs are in place nationwide to identify infants with phenylketonuria and galactosemia. Through the use of advanced technology (mass spectrometry), screening programs can be expanded to include disorders, such as maple syrup urine disease. The feasibility of screening for biotinidase deficiency in the neonate has been demonstrated as well. At the present time (Table 2), carrier detection is feasible for disorders of lysosomal and mitochondrial origin and for adrenoleukodystrophy and for Refsum disease but not for other disorders of peroxisomal function. However, fetal diagnosis is possible for the other peroxisomal disorders, as well as for the neuronal ceroid lipofuscinoses using morphologic or chemical criteria. For disorders in which a specific diagnostic marker is lacking, it is important to provide the family with genetic counseling. This should include discussions regarding the risk of recurrence in the parents, in siblings, and in other family members. Despite the absence of a diagnostic test, it is still possible in most instances to define the genetic mechanism, whether dominant or recessive, autosomal or X-linked.

TABLE 2. Prevention of CNS Degenerative Diseases: Carrier Detection and Prenatal Diagnosis

DISORDER	CARRIER DETECTION	IN UTERO DETECTION
Lysosomal		
Mucopolysaccharidoses	Feasible	Feasible
Sphingolipidoses	Feasible	Feasible
Neuronal ceroid lipofuscinoses	Not feasible	Feasible
Peroxisomal		
Adrenoleukodystrophy complex	Feasible	Feasible
Refsum disease	Feasible	Feasible
Zellweger disease and neonatal forms	Not feasible	Feasible
Mitochondrial	Feasible	Feasible
Specific Diseases		
Biotinidase	Feasible	Feasible
Galactosemia	Feasible	Feasible

SPECIFIC THERAPIES

Specific therapies (Table 3) must be undertaken with the understanding that existing psychomotor dysfunction may not be reversible. The principal therapeutic goal is to stabilize the process and prevent further progression. The timing of therapeutic efforts is critically important, particularly for disorders that primarily involve neurons. Beyond the period of neuroblast proliferation at the end of the second trimester, neuronal regeneration or replacement is not likely to occur. For example, significant pathologic abnormalities have been noted in spinal cords from midgestation fetuses with GM-1 and GM-2 (Tay-Sachs disease) gangliosidoses. Thus, the effectiveness of specific treatments in such conditions may be directly related to early, even prenatal, intervention.

TABLE 3. Specific Therapies for CNS Degenerative Diseases

DISORDER	THERAPY
Lysosomal	Enzyme replacement
	Organ transplantation
	Gene therapy
Peroxisomal	
Adrenoleukodystrophy complex	Dietary modification
Refsum disease	Bone marrow transplantation
	Dietary restriction
Mitochondrial	Dichloroacetate
Leigh disease	L-Carnitine
	Thiamine
	Lipoic acid
	Coenzyme Q10
Specific Disease	
Phenylketonuria	Dietary restriction
Maple syrup urine disease	Dietary restriction
Galactosemia	Dietary restriction
Methylmalonic acidemia	Vitamin B_{12}
Biotinidase deficiency	Biotin
Wilson disease	Penicillamine
Menkes' disease	Copper histidinate
Urea cycle defects	Sodium benzoate; sodium phenylbutyrate
Juvenile parkinsonism	L-Dopa-carbidopa (Sinemet)
Progressive dystonias	L-Dopa-carbidopa
	Trihexyphenidyl (Artane)
	Amitriptyline (Elavil)

Specific therapies include replacement techniques via enzyme infusion, organ transplantation, including bone marrow transplantation (BMT), and gene therapies. Enzyme infusion has been very successful in the chronic, nonneuronopathic form of Gaucher disease but efficacy has yet to be demonstrated in progressive CNS disorders because of the difficulty inherent in delivering sufficient amounts of enzyme across the blood–brain barrier and into the targeted cells. Organ transplantation has been effective in a number of lysosomal storage diseases, including Gaucher disease (liver) and Fabry disease (kidney). Again, delivery of sufficient enzyme to the CNS is a problem. BMT has been employed successfully in neuronopathic Gaucher disease and the mucopolysaccharidoses (Hurler and Maroteaux-Lamy). BMT has been reported to be effective also in adrenoleukodystrophy and to slow disease progression in metachromatic leukodystrophy. Additional data are required before efficacy can be firmly established. Gene therapy is still in preclinical testing, with very encouraging results in Gaucher disease, Hurler disease, and type VII mucopolysaccharidosis. Despite the promise of these new techniques, a note of caution must be added. One should question the wisdom of converting a relatively rapidly progressive fatal disease into one that is more slowly progressive but still fatal.

Dietary approaches have been used for a number of disorders. The prototype disorder for dietary modification is phenylketonuria. Efficacy has been demonstrated with diets that limit the intake of offending compounds in Refsum disease (phytanic acid derived from chlorophyll conversion to phytol in ruminants), phenylketonuria (phenylalanine), and maple syrup urine disease (branched-chain amino acids). Important questions remain with respect to the duration of therapy and how precisely to regulate the level of the offending metabolite. In addition, hyperphenylalaninemia based on biopterin deficiency must be treated with both dietary restriction and biogenic amine neurotransmitter precursors (L-dopa for norepinephrine and L-tryptophan for serotonin). Dietary modification in the treatment of adrenoleukodystrophy is under intense study, using a diet with limited amounts of saturated long-chain fatty acids and increased amounts of triglycerides containing the unsaturated long-chain fatty acids, oleic and erucic acid. This is the diet publicized in the film *Lorenzo's Oil*. At present, a definite conclusion is not available as to its effectiveness in altering disease progression or, indeed, disease onset in presymptomatic children. It is ineffective in reversing existing neurologic dysfunction.

Treatment of mitochondrial diseases with dietary supplementation has not been established as effective with rigorous clinical trials. Conversely, biotinidase deficiency is very responsive to biotin replacement, as is the vitamin B_{12}-responsive form of methylmalonic acidemia. Hemodialysis or peritoneal dialysis may be required in the acute management of metabolic acidosis and/or hyperammonemia associated with the organic acidemias or urea cycle effects. Sodium benzoate and sodium phenylbutyrate may be helpful in children with urea cycle defects by providing alternate means for nitrogen elimination. Copper chelation in Wilson's disease can be achieved with penicillamine. However, copper replacement in Menkes' disease with copper histidinate is still under study.

Treatment of the movement disorders is often unsatisfactory. Clinical improvement following the respective pharmacologic agents may be transient at best. The drug combination L-dopa-carbidopa (Sinemet) was formulated for adults. Children often require additional carbidopa to counteract the gastrointestinal side effects. Thalamotomy performed with stereotactic surgery may also be effective, but when it is done bilaterally, significant speech impairment is possible.

SUPPORTIVE OR SYMPTOMATIC CARE

Supportive or symptomatic care is often the only approach available to the clinician in managing children with a CNS degenerative disease (Table 4). It is important at the outset to consider the needs of the family very carefully. This will require discussions of prognosis and long-term care requirements, realistic expectations regarding potential therapies, and clear understanding of genetic implications for

TABLE 4. General Therapies for CNS Degenerative Diseases

Family support	Counseling
	Respite care
	Long-term placement
Nutrition	Protein-calorie supplements
	Tube feedings
Respiratory care	Postural drainage
	Airway toileting
Bowel care	Stool softeners
	Suppositories
Bladder care	Intermittent catheterization
Skin care	Positioning
	Egg crate pad
	Sheepskin pad
Physical therapy	Positioning
	Stretching
	Orthotics
Occupational therapy	Daily skills
	Feeding techniques
	Interactive play
Orthopedic	
Scoliosis	Bracing
	Surgery
Pharmacologic	
Seizures	Antiepileptic agents
Spasticity	Baclofen, dantrolene
Behavior	Amitriptyline, thioridazine
Sleeping	Diphenhydramine, hydroxyzine, chloral hydrate, flurazepam

future pregnancies in the parents or siblings of the affected child. In addition, assistance must be provided to the family for establishing respite care, including parental acceptance of its importance. What is required frequently is to convince the parents that it is okay to take time off from what is essentially a full-time, 24-hour a day responsibility.

Except for the specific pharmacologic agents, the other elements of supportive or symptomatic care are standard and need not be discussed in detail. Orthopedic intervention does deserve mention. Surgical procedures should be considered only where daily care or activities are facilitated. Little is gained by tendon transfers or releases in the immobilized child. Surgery for progressive scoliosis is usually required when cardiopulmonary function is compromised. Effective management of seizures requires selection of the most appropriate agent(s) based on an analysis of clinical seizures and the EEG pattern. On occasion, it is difficult to differentiate between a clinical seizure and some other movement pattern. At such times, simultaneous video-EEG monitoring can be very helpful and may obviate the unnecessary use of antiepileptic agents. In many instances, a compromise will be required to achieve complete seizure control at the expense of unwanted drug toxicity.

Treatment of spasticity is difficult, and the available agents are problematic. Diazepam is not recommended, since the dosage needed to reduce spasticity is likely to produce sedation. The agents listed in Table 5, baclofen and dantrolene, are associated with significant side effects, particularly with chronic usage.

Behavior is often adverse and disruptive in children with CNS degenerative diseases. Amitriptyline may be effective therapy for undesirable behavior and has the added benefit of providing sedation when given at bedtime. Amitriptyline may also potentiate the muscle-relaxing effects of baclofen. Thioridazine should be considered also. As sleep is often erratic and interrupted, it is quite appropriate to use sedation for the benefit of both the child and other family members. Tolerance may develop to the recommended agents. Thus, it is sometimes necessary to rotate their use.

In summary, management of children with CNS degenerative diseases is difficult, but planning and forethought can obviate many potential problems. Attention must be given to both the child and the

TABLE 5. Recommended Dosing of Therapeutic Agents

	STARTING DOSE	MAINTENANCE DOSE
Antiepileptic Agents		
Carbamazepine	10 mg/kg/d t.i.d.	15–25 mg/kg/d t.i.d.
Valproic acid	15 mg/kg/d t.i.d.	30–50 mg/kg/d t.i.d.
Phenytoin	15–20 mg/kg IV	5–8 mg/kg/d b.i.d.
Phenobarbital	15–18 mg/kg IV	4–7 mg/kg/d b.i.d.
Spasticity		**Maximum Dose**
Baclofen	10–15 mg divided t.i.d.	<7 y: 20–40 mg divided t.i.d.
		≥8 y: 60 mg divided t.i.d.
Dantrolene	0.5 mg/kg per dose b.i.d.	2.5–3.0 mg/kg per dose 2–4 doses
Behavior		**Maximum Dose**
Amitriptyline	10–25 mg b.i.d.	25–50 mg t.i.d.
Thioridazine	—	1–2.5 mg/kg/d b.i.d.
Sedation		
Diphenhydramine	1–2 mg/kg per dose q6h p.r.n.	
Hydroxyzine	1 mg/kg per dose q6h	
Chloral hydrate	15–25 mg/kg per dose t.i.d. p.r.n.	
Flurazepam	≥10 y: 15 mg b.i.d. p.r.n.	
Movement Disorders		
L-Dopa-carbidopa (25–100)	½ tablet b.i.d. or t.i.d.	Increase q.o.d. as tolerated
Carbidopa		25 mg t.i.d. or q.i.d.
Trihexyphenidyl	5 mg b.i.d., extended use	60–80 mg/d b.i.d. Increase weekly as tolerated
Amitriptyline	10–25 mg b.i.d.	25–50 mg t.i.d.
Others		
Penicillamine	<10 y: 500 mg/d b.i.d.	
	≥10 y: 1 g/d b.i.d.	
Copper histidinate	600 mg/d	
Sodium phenyl-butyrate	0.45–0.6 g/kg/d	
Biotin	5–20 mg/d	
Vitamin B$_{12}$ (hydroxocobalamin)	1–2 mg/d IM initially; may decrease under monitoring	
L-Carnitine	50–100 mg/kg/d b.i.d. (max 3 g/d)	

family. For the child, emphasis must be placed on preserving function as long as possible, avoiding secondary complications, and assuring treatment with dignity. For the family, an open dialogue must be maintained throughout the course of the disease in order to address each question or management decision as it arises. Family support groups exist for many of these disorders, for example, the United Leukodystrophy Foundation, the National Tay Sachs and Allied Diseases Association, and the National Organization for Rare Diseases. Parents should be encouraged to contact such organizations. Finally, as the child's condition progresses, it is important to discuss critical care issues and agree on resuscitation status in the event of cardiorespiratory failure.

REFERENCE

1. Scriver CR, Beaudet AL, Sly WS, Valle D (eds): The Metabolic Basis of Inherited Disease, 6th ed. New York, McGraw-Hill, 1989.

FAMILIAL DYSAUTONOMIA

FELICIA B. AXELROD, M.D.

Familial dysautonomia (FD) is an inherited disease affecting the development and survival of sensory, sympathetic, and some parasympathetic neurons. Although the primary abnormality in FD is anatomic depletion of unmyelinated sensory and autonomic neurons, the clinical manifestations are the concern of the treating physician. The pervasive nature of the autonomic nervous system results in protean functional abnormalities. Signs of the disorder are present from birth, and neurologic function slowly deteriorates with age so that symptoms and problems will vary with time. Frequent manifestations include feeding difficulties, hypotonia, delayed developmental milestones, labile body temperature and blood pressure, absence of overflowing tears and corneal anesthesia, marked diaphoresis with excitement, recurrent aspiration pneumonia, breath-holding episodes, ataxia, spinal curvature, and intractable vomiting.

The disease process cannot be arrested. Treatment is preventative, symptomatic, and supportive. It must be directed toward specific problems, which can vary considerably among patients and at different ages.

FEEDING

Oropharyngeal incoordination is one of the earliest signs. Poor suck or discoordinated swallow is observed in 60% of infants in the neonatal period.[4] Feeding problems are treated with various maneuvers to improve feeding, prevent malnutrition, and avoid aspiration. Feeding therapy and experimentation with different nipples and thickened formula should be tried. If weight gain is not adequate, respiratory problems persist, or the infant has an elevated blood urea nitrogen, gastrostomy should be performed.

Oral incoordination can persist in the older patient and be manifested as a tendency to drool and eating with an open or overstuffed mouth. Cineradiographic swallowing studies using various food consistencies will determine if particular types are more apt to be aspirated. It is not uncommon that liquids will continue to be aspirated but that solids are consumed safely. Even when the patient is able to eat orally, it is not unusual to retain a preference for softer foods.

VOMITING

Dysautonomic patients have abnormal gastrointestinal motility, making them prone to vomiting. Vomiting occurs intermittently in some patients as part of a systemic reaction to infection or stress, either physical or emotional. Gastroesophageal reflux is also a common problem and should be considered in patients with frequent vomiting. About 40% of patients have a pernicious type of vomiting, prolonged episodes occurring in a cyclic pattern. These vomiting crises are often associated with hypertension, tachycardia, diffuse sweating, and even personality changes. The weekly or monthly cyclic pattern can be quite striking and is usually characteristic for a particular patient. Such crises can last from 3 to 72 hours. Dehydration and aspiration are ever present risks.

If gastroesophageal reflux is identified, medical management with prokinetic agents, H$_2$-antagonists, thickening of feeds, and positioning should be tried. However, if medical management is not successful, using the criteria of persistence of pneumonia, hematemesis, or apnea, surgical intervention (fundoplication) is recommended. After surgery, crises may continue. However, retching will be substituted for vomiting.

Vomiting or retching in a dysautonomic patient, irrespective of the cause, is managed with diazepam. *Diazepam is considered to be the most effective antiemetic for the dysautonomic crisis.* Diazepam can be administered orally, intravenously, or rectally at 0.2 mg/kg/per dose. The initial dose of diazepam should be effective in stopping the vomiting, normalizing the blood pressure, and decreasing agitation.

TABLE 1. Drugs

DRUG	DOSAGE
Chloral hydrate	30 mg/kg per dose
Clonidine	0.004 mg/kg per dose
Diazepam	0.1–0.2 mg/kg per dose
Florinef	0.1–0.2 mg/24 h
Ranitidine	2 mg/kg/24 h

If agitation or hypertension is not eliminated, chloral hydrate 30 mg/kg can be given as a rectal suppository. Subsequent doses of diazepam are repeated at 3-hour intervals until the crisis resolves. Chloral hydrate can be repeated at 6-hour intervals. Ranitidine (2 mg/kg/24 h) is a useful adjunct in reducing emesis volume. Cimetidine should not be used, as it slows the renal clearance of diazepam. If diastolic hypertension persists (>90 mm Hg), clonidine (0.004 mg/kg/per dose) is suggested. Clonidine can be repeated at 8-hour intervals (Table 1). The crisis usually resolves abruptly and is marked by normalization of personality and return of appetite. At this point, the patient may be allowed to resume a normal diet.

A crisis usually can be managed at home, especially if the child has a gastrostomy, which facilitates hydration and giving of medications. Hospitalization is indicated, however, if there is not the expected positive response to medication by 12 hours, if serious infection is suspected because of high fever or uncharacteristic behavior, if blood or coffee ground material is vomited, or if dehydration is suspected.

PNEUMONIA

Recurrent pneumonia is a common problem in affected children. *The major cause of lung infections is aspiration,* with most of the damage to the lung occurring during infancy and early childhood, when oral incoordination is extremely poor. If gastroesophageal reflux is present, the risk for aspiration increases.

The signs of pneumonia may be subtle. Cough is not consistently present and is rarely productive. The child is more likely to vomit increased pulmonary secretions. Tachypnea is generally not evident, and auscultation may be unrevealing because of decreased chest excursion. Initial radiographs may fail to document infection, and if aspiration is strongly suspected or symptoms persist, repeat radiographs should be done. Because of the increased likelihood of aspirating gastric contents, pathogens cultured from tracheal aspirations can be uncommon agents, such as *Escherichia coli* or *Proteus.* Broad-spectrum antibiotics should be used until bacteriologic study permits specific therapy. In the seriously ill child, blood gases must be monitored because respiratory control is abnormal in dysautonomic patients. Excessive CO_2 accumulation is not an uncommon problem, and it can be severe enough to cause coma and require assisted ventilation.

Because many of the respiratory problems are avoided when gastrointestinal dysfunction is well managed, patients who have had pneumonia require careful evaluation. For those individuals who misdirect swallows, barium studies should be done using varied consistencies to note which ones can be safely swallowed. *If liquids are aspirated, gastrostomy is indicated.* If the aspirations are believed secondary to gastroesophageal reflux, appropriate medications are started or fundoplication is performed.

Chest physiotherapy, consisting of postural drainage and inhalation of bronchodilators, is helpful not only in the acute situation but also as a daily routine for children with residual effects from previous aspirations or infections. Suctioning is often required in the individual who has an ineffective cough. Chest therapy should be administered at home by the parents on a regular basis. Chest surgery is rarely indicated, as the disease is usually diffuse. *In patients with gastroesophageal reflux, xanthine derivatives are avoided.*

Owing to the lack of appropriate response to hypoxia and hypercapnia, all dysautonomic patients must be cautious in settings where the partial pressure of oxygen is decreased, such as at high altitudes or during airplane travel. If the airplane's altitude exceeds 39,000 feet, the cabin pressure will be equivalent to more than 6000 feet, and supplemental oxygen probably will be necessary. Diving and underwater swimming also are potential hazards and should be done with care.

BREATH-HOLDING (SEIZURES)

The phenomenon of prolonged breath-holding with crying is frequent in the early years. It has occurred at least one time in 63% of patients. Breath-holding can be severe enough to result in cyanosis, syncope, and decerebrate posturing. Prolonged breath-holding results from lack of awareness that it is necessary for the next inspiration to be initiated; that is, the patients are manifesting insensitivity to hypoxia and hypercapnia. This may become a manipulative maneuver with some children. Such an episode is frightening but self-limited and, in our experience, has never been fatal. The cyanosis of breath-holding must be differentiated from that which occurs with mucous plugs. These spells occur suddenly and can be associated with choking. Often, the child will be pale and sweating and will require suctioning. Both types of cyanotic spells can produce seizurelike movements and decerebrate posturing. Electroencephalograms usually are normal or nonspecific, and the frequency of either type of spell is unaffected by anticonvulsant therapy.

About 25% of FD patients have abnormal EEGs, but less than 10% actually have a true seizure disorder. Within this special population of patients, the incidence of an abnormal EEG rises to 65%. The average age of onset of seizures is 12 years. Anticonvulsant therapy should be used in these cases. The dosage of anticonvulsants is the same as for any other child. Most of the anticonvulsants are tolerated well.

Metabolic seizures, induced by hyponatremia, have been observed during extremely hot weather when fluid and salt intake have failed to compensate for the excessive sweating manifested by these patients. Hyponatremic seizures also have occurred with severe infections.

FEVERS

Labile body temperatures result in brief episodic fevers in response to dehydration, mucous plugs in the bronchi, excessive external temperature, and even stress. *Fever is often preceded or accompanied by shaking chills, cold extremities, and gastroparesis.* With the first signs of shaking chills, antipyretics should be given. Cool extremities should be warmed and massaged while the trunk is cooled by sponging or the use of a hypothermic mattress. *The child should not be fed orally or by gastrostomy until the chills and the fever subside.*

In addition to antipyretics, a muscle relaxant often is helpful in reducing the anxiety and muscular spasms associated with hyperpyrexia. Diazepam (0.1 mg/kg/per dose) has been found effective.

Dysautonomic children are at greater risk for having febrile convulsions; 32% will have at least one febrile seizure. However, the shaking and muscle spasms should not be considered febrile convulsions and should not be treated with anticonvulsant therapy. A persistent fever lasting more than 24 hours requires a search for a source of infection.

SPINAL CURVATURE

Spinal curvature (kyphosis and/or scoliosis) develops in 95% of dysautonomic patients by adolescence. Spinal curvature may start as early as 3 years or as late as 14 years. There may be rapid progression at any time. The completion of puberty generally halts the progression of scoliosis, as it does in the idiopathic adolescent form, but puberty is commonly delayed in dysautonomia. Spinal curvature further compromises respiratory function, adding the component of restrictive lung disease to interstitial disease.

Annual examination of the spine will allow early diagnosis of scoliosis and permit appropriate institution of brace and exercise therapy. The latter is helpful in correcting or preventing secondary contractures in shoulders and hips. Extreme care is required in fitting of braces as decubiti may develop on the dysautonomic patient's insensitive skin at pressure points. Braces may also inhibit respiratory excursion and induce gastroesophageal reflux if there is a high epigastric projection. If the brace is not successful in halting progression or if the patient has a severe curve, spinal fusion is recommended.

CORNEAL ABRASIONS

Individuals with dysautonomia have diminished baseline eye moisture and do not cry with overflowing tears, which causes their eyes to be drier than normal eyes. Treatment is directed toward keeping the eye as moist as possible because drying results in corneal damage or ulceration.

Corneal complications have been decreasing with the regular use of topical lubricants as artificial tear solutions. These solutions often contain methylcellulose or are equivalent to hypotonic saline. Preparations without preservatives also are available. During sleep, a thicker preparation or an ointment may be used. The frequency with which tear solutions are instilled depends on the child's own baseline eye moisture and corneal sensitivity, which regulates the blink frequency. Environmental conditions and the child's state of health are other variables that affect the need for artificial tears. Moisture chamber spectacle attachments and goggles have been used to help retain eye moisture and protect the eye from wind and foreign bodies.

If an abrasion does occur, the frequency of artificial tear use should increase. Often, the eye will be helped by patching. Extreme care is necessary in applying a patch. To prevent the child from opening his eye under the patch and allowing the insensitive cornea to be damaged further by the patch, the eye should be taped closed first. An alternative to the patch is the soft contact lens, which applies gentle pressure and promotes healing.

For recurrent corneal problems or to promote tolerance of the hydrophilic soft contact lens, tear duct or punctal cautery has been very helpful because it increases baseline moisture. Tarsorrhapy can be done on a temporary basis by use of glue on the lashes. Permanent tarsorrhaphy has been reserved for unresponsive and chronic situations. Corneal transplants have not been successful.

BLOOD PRESSURE LABILITY

Orthostatic change in blood pressure is a cardinal sign of autonomic insufficiency and is present in all patients with dysautonomia. Patients demonstrate postural hypotension without compensatory tachycardia when they go from the supine to the erect position. Clinical manifestations of postural hypotension include episodes of lightheadedness or dizzy spells. Some patients complain of "weak legs." On occasion, there may be syncope. Symptoms tend to be worse in the morning, in hot or humid weather, when the bladder is full, before a large bowel movement, after a long car ride, coming out of a movie theater, or with fatigue. Generally, low blood pressure is more troublesome in the adult years and can limit function and mobility. Postural hypotension is treated by maintaining adequate hydration, as monitored by blood urea nitrogen levels. Lower extremity exercises are encouraged to increase muscle tone and promote venous return. Elastic stockings and florinef, a mineralocorticoid, have been of some benefit. Florinef 0.1 mg is given in the morning. A second dose is often added at midday.

Hypertension occurs intermittently in response to emotional stress or visceral pain or as part of the crisis constellation. Because blood pressure is so labile, treatment of hypertension should be directed to factors precipitating the hypertension rather than the use of blocking agents.

General anesthesia has caused profound hypotension and cardiac arrest. With greater attention to stabilization of the vascular bed by hydrating the patient before surgery and titrating the anesthetic, the risk of these problems has been greatly reduced.[2]

AZOTEMIA

It is not uncommon for patients to exhibit azotemia and variable values for creatinine clearance. Although clinical signs of dehydration may not be present, blood urea nitrogen values often can be reduced by simple hydration. Renal function appears to deteriorate with advancing age, so that about 20% of adult patients have reduced renal function. Pathologic studies reveal excess glomerulosclerosis. Renal biopsies performed on individuals with uncorrectable azotemia revealed significant ischemic-type glomerulosclerosis and deficient vascular innervation. The high prevalence of the renal lesion has been confirmed by retrospective analysis of autopsy material. Although the cause of the progressive renal disease is not certain, hypoperfusion of the kidney secondary to cardiovascular instability seems a likely explanation.[3]

Patients should be encouraged to maintain adequate hydration, especially during warm weather. Treatment of postural hypotension has become more aggressive, and blood pressures are carefully monitored during crises.

ANESTHESIA

Anesthesia for surgical procedures is associated with an increased risk because of extreme lability of blood pressure and diminished responsiveness to hypoxia and hypercapnia. Although local anesthesia with diazepam as preoperative sedation is preferred whenever possible, procedures requiring general anesthesia can be performed with less risk because homeostatic mechanisms in dysautonomia are now better understood.

Large amounts of epinephrine should not be infiltrated because of the exaggerated response to sympathomimetic drugs. Gas anesthetics have been useful because of the rapid reversibility of their effects. One of the most important factors in reducing risk is maintenance of an adequate circulating volume, as vasodilatation during anesthesia may be extreme. The patient is prehydrated the night before surgery with intravenous fluids. Arterial blood pressures and blood gases are monitored throughout surgery via an arterial line. Hypotension should be corrected by decreasing the percentage of gas anesthetic and administering volume expanders. Rarely, pressor agents, such as phenylephrine hydrochloride or epinephrine, are required. Postoperative management can be extremely challenging. Gastric secretions tend to be copious during excitatory anesthetic phases. To avoid postoperative aspiration, ranitidine can be given, and the stomach should be kept decompressed. This is facilitated if there is a gastrostomy present. Patients generally require vigorous chest physiotherapy, as there is a tendency toward development of mucous plugs and exacerbation of preexisting lung disease. The duration of intubation may need to be extended until the respiratory status stabilizes or there is less reliance on pain medication.

Visceral pain is appreciated and often causes hypertension, so narcotic pain medication may be required for intraabdominal or intrathoracic procedures. Orthopedic and ophthalmologic cases require minimal pain medication.

DECREASED SENSATION (INJURIES)

Although internal pain (e.g., stomachache, chest pain) is felt by dysautonomic children, skin and bone pain and temperature sensations are diminished. Burns, pressure sores, and even broken bones may go unnoticed. Pain insensitivity also results in inadvertent trauma to joints. Charcot joints and aseptic necrosis have been reported. *Swelling or mild discomfort with movement may be the only sign of a fracture.*

Since children with dysautonomia do not instinctively avoid harmful situations, they must be taught to protect themselves. For example, thermometers can be used to test bathtub water temperature, and they can look for steam from a coffee cup. If there is any reason to believe a fracture has occurred, a radiograph should be taken. Care must be taken in casting, as in bracing, to prevent the development of pressure sores. If possible, complete immobilization should be avoided, as children with neurologic problems develop muscle weakness rapidly with disuse. Chest physiotherapy during immobilization and physical therapy after the cast is removed are very important.

Dysautonomia can no longer be considered only a disease of childhood. With greater understanding of the disorder and development of treatment programs, survival statistics have markedly improved, and increasing numbers of patients are reaching adulthood.[1] For this type of success to occur, a great deal of effort is necessary. The parents must cope with the care of a chronically handicapped child, who may have repeated life-threatening crises. The physician has to become familiar with the varied manifestations of a multisystem disorder. The parents and child will rely on the long-term commitment of the physician for guidance, support, and reassurance.

REFERENCES

1. Axelrod FB, Abularrage JJ: Familial dysautonomia. A prospective study of survival. J Pediatr 101:234–236, 1982.
2. Axelrod FB, Donenfeld RF, Danziger F, Turndorf H: Anesthesia in familial dysautonomia. Anesthesiology 68:631–635, 1988.
3. Axelrod FB, Glickstein JS, Weider J, Gluck MC, Friedman D: The effects of postural change and exercise on renal haemodynamics in familial dysautonomia. Clin Autonom Res 3:195–200, 1993.
4. Axelrod FB, Porges RF, Sein ME: Neonatal recognition of familial dysautonomia. J Pediatr 110:946–948, 1987.

NEUROCUTANEOUS SYNDROMES

BRUCE R. KORF, M.D., Ph.D.

The neurocutaneous syndromes are a collection of diverse disorders whose clinical manifestations involve both the skin and the nervous system. This discussion reviews the management of some of the more common disorders of this type.

NEUROFIBROMATOSIS

There are at least two genetically distinct forms of neurofibromatosis, referred to as NF1 and NF2. NF1 affects about 1 in 4000 people and is characterized by café-au-lait spots, neurofibromas, learning disabilities, optic gliomas, other brain tumors, and skeletal dysplasias. NF2 is about tenfold less frequent and results in bilateral vestibular schwannomas, other schwannomas, meningiomas, brain tumors, and cataracts. Both are inherited as dominant traits, and both genes have been cloned. The NF1 gene is located on chromosome 17 and encodes a GTPase-activating protein (GAP). The NF2 gene is on chromosome 22 and encodes a cytoskeletal protein referred to as "merlin" or "schwannomin."

NF1

The diagnosis of NF1 is based on clinical criteria (Table 1). Many of the features are age dependent, making it difficult to establish a definitive diagnosis in young children. Children with NF1 most often

TABLE 1. Diagnostic Criteria for NF1

NF1 is diagnosed in any individual meeting two or more of the following criteria:
1. Six or more café-au-lait macules over 5 mm in greatest diameter in prepubertal individuals and over 15 mm in diameter in postpubertal individuals
2. Two or more neurofibromas of any type or one plexiform neurofibroma
3. Freckling in the axillary or inguinal regions
4. Two or more iris Lisch nodules
5. A distinctive osseous lesion, such as sphenoid dysplasia or thinning of lone bone cortex with or without pseudoarthrosis
6. A first-degree relative with NF1

From Stumpf DA, et al: NIH Consensus Development Conference on Neurofibromatosis, 1987. Arch Neurol 45:575–578, 1988.

have multiple café-au-lait spots. Those with more than six café-au-lait spots larger than 5 mm should be followed with at least annual physical examination and opthalmologic examination. The eye examination should include the use of a slit lamp to look for Lisch nodules, as well as an assessment of the optic nerve. Although the gene for NF1 has been cloned, no laboratory diagnostic test has been developed. Genetic linkage analysis can provide presymptomatic or prenatal diagnosis in some families with two or more generations of affected individuals.

Treatment

There is no definitive therapy for NF1. Affected individuals should be followed regularly (at least once a year) to detect and manage complications. Follow-up should include physical examination and ophthalmologic assessment. The use of routine neuroimaging in the asymptomatic patient with NF1 is controversial. Detection of asymptomatic lesions in the brain has not been demonstrated to improve outcome, and a normal scan at one time does not preclude a tumor from appearing months to years later. If an MRI scan is done, the family should be prepared for the possibility that regions of enhanced T2-weighted signal may be seen in the internal capsule, basal ganglia, brainstem, or cerebellum. These do not seem to represent tumors and are of no definite clinical significance.

Café-au-lait macules pose no medical risk, but pigment can be removed for cosmetic reasons using a laser. Cutaneous neurofibromas that cause discomfort or are cosmetically objectionable are managed by surgery. Plexiform neurofibromas can grow aggressively in the early years of life, sometimes causing physical deformity or airway obstruction. There is no treatment available other than surgery. Surgery for plexiform neurofibromas must be undertaken with caution because of the profuse vascularity of these lesions and a tendency to regrow. Surgery may be offered to relieve pain or to improve appearance. Ketotifen has been proposed for use in treating neurofibromas. This antihistamine may help relieve itching but has not been clearly demonstrated to reduce tumor growth. The drug is not available in the United States.

Orthopedic complications include tibial dysplasia and scoliosis. Tibial dysplasia usually is clinically apparent as anterolateral bowing of the lower leg. If this lesion is present, the limb should be placed in a brace to protect it against fracture. No really effective treatment has been devised to manage fractures associated with tibial dysplasia. Children with NF1 should be monitored for the development of scoliosis. Dystrophic thoracic scoliosis may require surgery.

The lifetime risk of malignancy related to NF1 is about 5%. Neurofibrosarcomas arise in plexiform neurofibromas or in deep subcutaneous neurofibromas attached to major nerves. Signs of malignant transformation include unexplained pain and sudden growth. Treatment usually involves a combination of surgery, radiation therapy, and chemotherapy. Optic gliomas may be asymptomatic or can lead to loss of vision and neuroendocrine disturbance. It is rarely necessary to biopsy an optic glioma to confirm the diagnosis. Asymptomatic optic gliomas are best observed without treatment. Precocious puberty can be treated by hormonal means and does not in itself constitute an indication to treat the glioma. For progressive optic gliomas, the standard treatment after 5 years of age is radiation therapy, but recently, chemotherapy has been used to treat younger children, with promising results.

A high proportion of children with NF1 have learning disabilities, and a small proportion will have more severe developmental delays. Children with NF1 should be monitored closely for learning disabilities and should be provided appropriate assistance in school. The learning problems are not progressive and are similar to learning disabilities in the general population. Seizures occur at slightly higher frequency than in the general population and are treated with standard antiepileptic medications. Seizures in NF1 rarely indicate the existence of brain tumor. Vascular headaches occur commonly in association with NF1 and respond to such treatment as propranolol.

Genetic counseling should be provided to all individuals with NF1

TABLE 2. Diagnostic Criteria for NF2

1. Bilateral vestibular schwannomas
2. First-degree relative with NF2 and either
   a. Unilateral eighth nerve mass, *or*
   b. Two of following
      (1) Schwannoma
      (2) Meningioma
      (3) Glioma
      (4) Juvenile posterior subcapsular cataract

From Stumpf DA, et al: NIH Consensus Development Conference on Neurofibromatosis, 1987. Arch Neurol 45:575–578, 1988.

and members of their families. An affected person has a 50% risk of transmitting the gene to any child, and the severity of the disorder in the next generation is unpredictable. Approximately 50% of cases occur sporadically resulting from new mutation. If both parents of a sporadically affected child are free of signs of NF1 (no skin or eye manifestations), their risk of having another affected child is very low (approximately the same as the general population).

NF2

Diagnostic criteria are listed in Table 2. Signs of NF2 can be subtle in young children, and those at risk of inheriting the disorder from an affected parent should be followed as though affected until proved otherwise. Genetic linkage studies now permit presymptomatic diagnosis in many families in which two or more generations are affected.

Treatment

Management of NF2 is aimed at early detection of complications. Vestibular schwannomas are best detected by gadolinium-enhanced cranial MRI. In the asymptomatic individual at 50% risk of inheriting NF2, this should be performed in adolescence, again before childbearing years, and at any time when signs or symptoms appear. An ophthalmologic evaluation to detect cataracts should be performed on young children at risk of NF2.

Most tumors associated with NF2 are managed surgically. Recently, experience has been reported using the gamma knife to treat vestibular schwannomas. This is a form of highly focused stereotactic radiotherapy. However, it is not clear that this approach offers an advantage over standard neurosurgical techniques. Paraspinal schwannomas can cause nerve root or spinal cord compression and should be ruled out before procedures involving cervical hyperextension (such as surgery) are done. Posterior subcapsular cataracts rarely impair vision but should be followed by an ophthalmologist and removed if necessary.

All patients with NF2 and members of their families should be provided genetic counseling regarding their risk of transmitting the trait. Genetic linkage-based diagnostic testing is available in some instances and can be useful in determining those who have inherited the gene and require medical follow-up.

TUBEROUS SCLEROSIS

Tuberous sclerosis is diagnosed by clinical criteria (Table 3). It is inherited as an autosomal dominant trait, but sporadic cases are common. Genetic linkage studies indicate at least two loci that may be involved in the etiology of tuberous sclerosis in different families. One of these genes has been identified. The pathology of tuberous sclerosis include hamartomas in the subependymal, subcortical, and cortical regions of the brain. Additional features include angiofibromas on the skin, angiomyolipomas and cysts in the kidney, phacomas in the retina, rhabdomyomas in the heart, and pulmonary fibrosis.

Treatment

The most common serious complication is seizures. All types of seizures can be seen in association with tuberous sclerosis, including

TABLE 3. Diagnostic Criteria for Tuberous Sclerosis

Definitive Diagnosis
Tuberous sclerosis diagnosed if any of these features are present:
   Cortical tuber
   Subependymal glial nodules
   Retinal hamartoma
   Facial angiofibroma
   Ungual fibroma
   Forehead/scalp fibrous plaques
   Multiple renal angiomyolipomas

Presumptive Diagnosis
Tuberous sclerosis is likely if any two of these features are present:
   Infantile spasms, myoclonic, tonic, or atonic seizures
   Hypomelanotic macules
   Shagreen patches
   Gingival fibroma
   Dental enamel pits
   Multiple renal tumors
   Cardiac rhabdomyoma
   Pulmonary lymphangiomyomatosis, or honeycomb lungs by x-ray
   Wedge-shaped cortical-subcortical calcification
   Multiple subcortical hypomyelinated lesions
   First-degree relative with tuberous sclerosis

From Gomez MR (ed): Tuberous Sclerosis, 2nd ed. New York, Raven Press, 1988.

infantile spasms. Developmental impairment is almost always associated with the onset of seizures in the first 2 years of life, but not all those with early onset seizures are developmentally impaired. Aggressive treatment of seizures with standard antiepileptic medications, including ACTH for infantile spasms, is indicated. Giant cell astrocytoma is a nonmalignant lesion that may cause obstruction of the foramen of Monro and hydrocephalus. This is managed by surgical removal and/or shunting.

Cardiac rhabdomyomas may be asymptomatic or cause ventricular outflow obstruction or arrhythmia. They may be present congenitally and, in some cases, may regress spontaneously. Surgery may be necessary to relieve obstruction. Renal angiomyolipomas increase in frequency with age and may be asymptomatic or cause hypertension, hematuria, or even renal failure. They are best detected by renal ultrasound. Therapy is symptomatic. Retinal phacomas are usually asymptomatic. In rare instances, life-threatening pulmonary fibrosis may occur, requiring symptomatic therapy.

Individuals with tuberous sclerosis should be counseled that there is a 50% risk of transmitting the gene to any offspring. The parents of a sporadically affected child should have skin and eye examination, renal ultrasound, and head CT or MRI scans. If no signs of tuberous sclerosis are found in either parent, the empiric recurrence risk is approximately 1%. Genetic testing is not available. In some cases, prenatal diagnosis has been accomplished by ultrasound scanning for cardiac rhabdomyoma, but the sensitivity of this approach has not been determined.

VON HIPPEL LINDAU DISEASE

This is a dominantly inherited disorder characterized by development of hemangioblastomas of the retina, cerebellum, and spinal cord, cysts of the kidney, pancreas, liver, epididymis, and adrenal, pheochromocytoma, and a variety of tumors, including renal and pancreatic carcinoma. Although it is often classified with the neurocutaneous disorders, there are no associated cutaneous manifestations. The gene is located on chromosome 3 and recently has been cloned. The diagnosis is established if both central nervous system and retinal hemangioblastomas are present or, if only one site is affected with hemangioblastoma, when there are characteristic cysts, pheochromocytoma, renal cancer, or an affected first-degree relative.

Treatment

Management is focused on early detection and surgical removal of hemangioblastomas. A program of regular medical, neurologic, and opthalmologic follow-up should be provided. This should include periodic abdominal ultrasound examination and MRI scan of the brain and spinal cord. Individuals with von Hippel Lindau disease should be provided genetic counseling. Gene linkage studies can be offered for presymptomatic diagnosis in some families.

NEVOID BASAL CELL CARCINOMA SYNDROME (GORLIN SYNDROME)

This is an autosomal dominant disorder recently linked to a locus on chromosome 9. It is characterized by macrocephaly, hypertelorism, frontal bossing, odontogenic cysts, palmar and plantar pits, and the appearance of basal cell nevi on the skin. The basal cell nevi usually appear from the second to the fourth decades and can lead to basal cell carcinoma. Odontogenic cysts appear in late childhood and are usually asymptomatic. There is an association with such tumors as ovarian fibroma and fibrosarcoma, rhabdomyoma and medulloblastoma.

Treatment

Basal cell nevi must be monitored for malignancy and can be removed surgically. Other tumors are managed by surgery. Radiation therapy may increase the likelihood of malignant transformation of skin lesions. Genetic counseling should be provided.

INCONTINENTIA PIGMENTI

Incontinentia pigmenti is a highly variable disorder transmitted as an X-linked dominant. It almost exclusively affects females. Males who inherit the gene are nonviable and are spontaneously aborted. The diagnosis is usually suspected on the basis of the characteristic skin lesions. These begin in the early days of life as regions of macular erythema that evolve into pustular or vesicular lesions. After several weeks, they become verrucous, and within months, they acquire a swirly brownish gray color. Lesions may be isolated or involve a substantial part of the body. The pigmentation may disappear during adult life, making it difficult to detect mildy affected carriers. Neurologic manifestations include early onset of seizures, microcephaly, and developmental delays. Retinal detachment, optic atrophy, bony malformations, and misshapen teeth may occur. It is likely that these complications are present in a minority of those with the disorder, however, and the majority have only mild cutaneous stigmata. Severe neurologic complications are generally apparent in the early days of life.

Treatment

The skin lesions require no specific treatment. Seizures are treated with antiepileptic medications. Dental and ophthalmologic follow-up is important for symptomatic management. Affected females have a 50% chance of passing the trait to any daughter. Sons who inherit the trait are likely to be aborted. Therefore, males at risk who survive to term are unlikely to be affected. The mother of an affected child should be examined carefully for signs of the disorder, but since the signs can be subtle, individuals found to have no signs may still be at risk of having other affected daughters. The gene(s) have not been identified, and genetic testing is not available.

DISORDERS OF DNA REPAIR

At least two disorders that involve defective DNA repair or DNA synthesis cause neurocutaneous manifestations. Xeroderma pigmentosum results from deficiency of the system responsible for repair of UV-irradiation-induced DNA damage. A number of genetically distinct subtypes exist. Cutaneous features include hyperpigmented spots, telangiectasia, atrophy, and bullous lesions following acute exposure to light. There is a markedly increased risk of skin cancer. Neurologic signs include, in some patients, microcephaly, choreoathetosis, ataxia, cognitive impairment, and peripheral neuropathy.

Ataxia telangiectasia is characterized by progressive ataxia and choreoathetosis, associated with cutaneous telangiectasias. The telangiectasias are most easily visible on the face, ear, and conjunctivae and appear in early childhood. There is an associated immune deficiency, particularly affecting IgA production, and an increased risk of cancer, mainly lymphoid malignancies. This is an autosomal recessive disorder, linked to a locus on chromosome 11.

Treatment

Neither disorder is amenable to definitive treatment. Patients with xeroderma pigmentosum should avoid exposure to UV light or direct sunlight and should be monitored for skin carcinoma or melanoma. Those with ataxia telangiectasia should be monitored for immune function and often require antibiotics for respiratory infections. Radiation therapy is contraindicated in these patients, since they display marked sensitivity to toxic effects of radiation.

STURGE-WEBER SYNDROME

This is a sporadic disorder characterized by the appearance of a portwine stain on the face and seizures. The cutaneous vascular lesion is usually unilateral, although it may be bilateral, and involves the trigeminal distribution. It is recognizable at birth. Neurologic sequelae correlate with the involvement of the first branch of the trigeminal nerve, involving the upper eyelid and forehead, although not all those with the cutaneous involvement develop neurologic complications. The neurologic manifestations result from vascular malformation of the leptomeninges, leading to venous infarction of the superficial cortex. The usual clinical manifestations are seizures occurring during the first year of life, along with neurologic deficits. In addition, there is a risk of glaucoma.

Treatment

Seizures are treated with antiepileptic medications. In some cases, intractable seizures have been treated by removal of damaged cerebral cortex. The eye must be monitored for development of glaucoma. Disfiguring skin lesions can be improved with laser treatments.

EPIDERMAL NEVUS SYNDROME

Epidermal nevi may be associated with neurologic problems in some individuals. The nevi may be hyperpigmented, verrucous lesions or may contain sebaceous elements (sebaceous nevus of Jadassohn). Sebaceous nevi are particularly characteristic of the facial lesions. Associated neurologic problems include seizures and developmental impairment. Presence of hyperostosis, limb asymmetry, or overgrowth of the hands or feet along with epidermal nevi is characteristic of proteus syndrome. Epidermal nevus syndrome is usually sporadic.

Treatment

Symptomatic treatment of the seizures with antiepileptic medications is the major form of therapy. Skin lesions may be unsightly but do not usually pose medical problems.

HYPOMELANOSIS OF ITO

This is a sporadic disorder in which streaky lines of hypopigmentation occur along with seizures and developmental delay. Patients may display mosaicism for various chromosomal abnormalities in peripheral blood or in skin fibroblasts taken from a lesion.

Treatment

Antiepileptic therapy is given for seizures as needed.

REFERENCES

1. Gomez MR (ed): Neurocutaneous Diseases. A Practical Approach. Boston, Butterworths, 1987.
2. Gomez MR (ed): Tuberous Sclerosis, 2nd ed. New York, Raven Press, 1988.
3. Rubenstein AE, Korf BR (eds): Neurofibromatosis: A Handbook for Patients, Families, and Health-Care Professionals. New York, Thieme, 1990.

SEIZURE THERAPY

PATRICIA K. CRUMRINE, M.D.

Seizures are common problems for children, their parents or care-takers, and their physicians. Epidemiologic studies have shown that about 3.5% of children will have at least a single seizure by the age of 15 years.[1] Most of these children will have a single event or have seizures for a limited period during their childhood years. Only a small percentage will have epilepsy (1%) or recurrent seizures, and of that group, only about 10% will have refractory seizures not responding to current antiepileptic therapy. The treating physician must be able to identify those events that are seizures, decide which require the initiation of antiepileptic drugs, assist patients and their families in dealing with a chronic illness, and work with an epilepsy specialist for those patients not responsive to standard therapy.

Seizures have been classified according to the 1981 international classification of the epilepsies (Table 1).[2] These various seizure patterns may be seen as single patterns in some of the age-related seizure syndromes or may occur in combination. There are many episodic or paroxysmal events that occur in young children that clinically resemble a seizure but may have an etiology other than an abnormal cerebral electrical discharge. It is important that the treating physician be able to exclude these events before committing a child to a chronic antiepileptic drug. Some of the more common of these disorders are listed in Table 2.

The evaluation and management of the child who has had a seizure will vary depending on the age at the first seizure, the suspected etiology, and the presence or absence of preexisting neurologic disorders. The primary care physician often is the first person the patient and family consults after a single seizure. The issues that the physician must consider are

- The age of the patient
- Association with fever or illness
- The type of seizure: partial or generalized
- Presence of preexisting neurologic disease
- Family history of epilepsy

If the child is a neonate or under 12 months of age, it is imperative to exclude a localized infection or sepsis as a cause. The evaluation should include a lumbar puncture and analysis of cerebrospinal fluid (CSF). Other diagnostic studies are listed in Table 3. The need for a metabolic evaluation, with serum or urine amino acids, organic acids,

TABLE 1. Seizure Classification

Partial
1. Simple: without loss of consciousness
   a. Sensory
   b. Motor
   c. Autonomic
   d. Psychic
2. Complex: with altered awareness/consciousness
3. Partial seizures becoming secondarily generalized

Generalized
1. Absence: both simple and atypical
2. Myoclonic
3. Clonic
4. Tonic
5. Tonic-clonic
6. Atonic

Unclassified
1. Some neonatal seizures
2. Unusual movements, such as eye movements and chewing

Adapted from Commission on Classification and Terminology of the International League Against Epilepsy. Proposal for revised clinical and electrographic classification of epileptic seizures. Epilepsia 1981;22:489–501.

TABLE 2. Nonepileptiform Paroxysmal Disorders

Those That Twitch or Move
Movement disorders
Gastrointestinal disorders
Sleep disorders
Episodic dyscontrol syndrome
Anxiety attacks

Those with Altered Consciousness/Respirations
Syncope
Migraine
Sleep disorders
Metabolic encephalopathies
Daydreaming
Breath-holding spell

Those with Both
Psychogenic seizures

and long-chain fatty acids, or imaging with MRI should be determined by clinical history, examination, and initial laboratory assessment.

If the child is over 12 months of age, has a brief febrile seizure with quick recovery, normal neurologic examination, and stable psychosocial environment, the initial CSF evaluation may not be necessary. The need for other studies can be determined by the treating physician, based on the history and examination. For the older child with an afebrile generalized seizure (tonic, clonic, or tonic-clonic), initial studies should be determined from the clinical history, examination, and family history. Head imaging with CT scan need only be done when there is concern about trauma, intracranial hemorrhage, or tumor as the precipitating cause. CSF analysis is necessary when meningitis or encephalitis is suspected. A lumbar tap should not be done if a brain abscess is part of the differential diagnosis (Table 3). An EEG should be obtained in all children with an abnormal neurologic examination, with the realization that a normal interictal EEG does not exclude the possibility of recurrent seizures. Focal or generalized epileptiform discharges (spikes or spike and waves) may be helpful in determining seizure types and the risk of seizure recurrence. Focal slowing plus focal epileptiform patterns suggest the possibility of underlying structural problems. Patients with these EEG features should have imaging studies, preferably an MRI.

It is helpful to consider some of the epileptic syndromes of childhood in chronologic order (Table 4). Many of these have similar characteristics:

- Occur within a certain age range
- Usually resolve
- ± characteristic EEG

TABLE 3. Evaluation of Febrile and Nonfebrile Seizures

EVALUATION	< 12 MO AFEBRILE	< 12 MO FEBRILE	1–5 Y AFEBRILE	1–5 Y FEBRILE
History	+	+	+	+
Examination	+	+	+	+
Electrolytes	+	+	±	+
Calcium	+	+	±	±
Magnesium	+	+	±	±
Glucose	+	+	±	±
Blood gases	+	+	±	±
BUN/creatinine	+	+	±	±
CSF	+	+	±	+
Cultures	±	+	−	+
EEG	+	±	+	±
Head imaging	±	−	±	±
Serum/urine amino acids	±	−	±	−
Organic acids	±	−	±	−
Long-chain fatty acids	±	−	±	−

TABLE 4. Features of Age-Dependent Epilepsies

	AGE AT ONSET	AGE RESOLUTION	EEG PATTERN
Neonatal seizures	Neonatal	Weeks–months	Variable
Benign infantile myoclonus	1–2 y	10–15 y	Generalized spike and wave
Febrile seizures	6–24 mo	5–6 y	Usually normal
Childhood absence	3–4 y	10–15 y	3 Hz spike and wave
Acquired epileptic aphasia	3–5 y	> 15 y	Multifocal spike and wave
Benign focal epilepsy	3–13 y	15–20 y	Central spikes
Benign occipital	3–13 y	15–20 y	Occipital spikes
Juvenile absence	Puberty	Persists	>3 Hz spike and wave
Juvenile myoclonic	Puberty	Persists	Generalized spike and wave
GTCS on awakening	2nd decade	Persists	Generalized spike and wave

GTCS = generalized tonic-clonic seizures.

- ± normal EEG background
- May have normal development

MYOCLONIC EPILEPSIES

Myoclonic events can occur in several different clinical settings in the young child. Not all myoclonus is epileptic. Myoclonus can have its origin from multiple areas in the nervous system, ranging from the spinal cord to the cerebral cortex. The phenomenon of myoclonus can be either physiologic or pathologic. Two relatively common clinical syndromes in infancy are mentioned here as the children come to the physician with a history of possible seizures. Some children will have multifocal myoclonic events during sleep in early infancy. The intensity and duration of these sleep-related events are of concern to parents and bring the child to the attention of the physician. An EEG recorded with the infant asleep frequently documents the benign nature of this problem when there is no associated EEG component to the movements. Most infants have decreased movements as they age. Medication is not required. The diagnosis can be made only by excluding other myoclonic syndromes and obtaining a normal EEG during the movements.

Another clinical pattern occurs in the older child between the ages of 1 and 2 years. These children develop intermittent symmetric myoclonic jerks that infrequently occur in clusters. These children are neurologically normal. EEGs usually are normal and do not show a hypsarrhythmic pattern, as is seen in children with infantile spasms. Most resolve by 2 years of age. They do not require antiepileptic drugs. For a discussion of infantile spasms, see later discussion in this chapter.

LENNOX-GASTAUT SYNDROME

Lennox-Gastaut syndrome (LGS) is a clinical syndrome in which there are seizures of multiple types (generalized tonic or tonic-clonic, atonic, atypical absence, and myoclonic). Seizures often begin between 1½ and 5 years of age. Additional clinical features include mental retardation and an EEG pattern that frequently demonstrates (1.5 to 2.5 Hz) slow spike and wave and slow waves maximum in the bifrontal regions. This syndrome may persist into adulthood. Although described as an epileptic syndrome, there is not one specific etiology. Many children with this syndrome have a prior history of infantile spasms, and a high percentage of affected children have an identifiable cause. Most of these children have static encephalopathies, but there is one progressive encephalopathy in which children may initially have a seizure pattern and EEG consistent with LGS. These are children with neuronal ceroid lipofuscinosis (NCL), a progressive degenerative disorder of unknown etiology that progresses slowly to a vegetative state and death over several years. Seizures may be the presenting symptom in children with NCL, particularly the childhood variant. The seizures are atonic, myoclonic, and atypical absence.

One of the more common seizure patterns in LGS is that of the atonic seizure (drop attack). These children have frequent falls, with facial injuries of eyelids, nose, and lips and may be taken frequently to an emergency room before parents or health care workers suspect seizures as the cause. Myoclonic seizures occur in about one third of the children. These seizures also may contribute to falls and drops. Convulsive status epilepticus occurs commonly in these children and may be the presenting event.

LGS is quite refractory to antiepileptic drugs. To date, the drugs and other therapies that have had some efficacy include valproic acid (Valproate), some of the benzodiazepines, prednisone, ketogenic diet, and immunoglobulin therapy. Carbamazepine can be effective for some of the tonic seizures but may exacerbate the atypical absence and myoclonic seizures. Other adjunctive therapies have included L-tryptophan and amantadine. A newly released antiepileptic drug, felbamate, a meprobamate derivative, has shown promise in the treatment of this population. Another drug under study in the United States, not yet released by the FDA, that has shown promise in Europe is lamotrigene. For those patients who have tried and failed all appropriate antiepileptic drugs, a surgical procedure in which the anterior two thirds of the corpus callosum is sectioned may reduce the frequency of atonic seizures. This procedure rarely eliminates all seizures but may improve those that are disabling to the patient and result in bodily injury.

Prognosis is grim in terms of intellect and seizures. If the children are normal at the outset of their illness, most have intellectual deterioration during the course. Seizures are difficult to control and usually last throughout adolescence and often into adulthood.

MYOCLONIC-ASTATIC SEIZURES (Syndrome of Doose)

This is another variation of myoclonic-atonic-astatic seizures that begins in childhood, usually between the ages of 1 and 5 years. Seizure patterns are very similar to those in the LGS. EEG patterns consist of 2.5 to 3 Hz generalized spike and wave discharges. These children are commonly normal at the onset of their seizures. Again, most undergo some deterioration in intellect. Treatment options are similar to those used for patients with LGS.

SIMPLE ABSENCE EPILEPSY

Seizures characterized by staring or altered awareness are referred to as absence seizures. It is important for the primary care physician to be aware that there are both absence seizures and absence syndromes, and the ability to identify and classify these is important in determining treatment regimens and providing prognostic information for families.

The different types of absence seizures are as follows:

- Simple absence
  Staring with impaired consciousness
  Without motor components
- Complex absence
  Altered consciousness
  With clonic motor components
  With automatisms
  With autonomic changes

- Atypical absence
  Prolonged altered awareness

Absence syndromes can be either idiopathic or symptomatic. The idiopathic disorders often are age-related syndromes and are classified as follows.

- Childhood absence
- Juvenile absence
- Juvenile myoclonic syndrome of Janz

Symptomatic absence syndromes are seen in children with LGS, syndrome of Doose, and myoclonic absences.

Children with absence seizures often are referred to a physician because of daydreaming or not paying attention in the classroom. The differential diagnosis must include not only absence seizures but also possible complex partial seizures and behavioral or attentional problems. Important features that may help distinguish among these seizures are shown in Table 5.

The average age of onset of typical simple absence seizures is between 3 and 4 years, although many children do not come to medical attention until they start school. The child briefly loses awareness and may or may not have some associated eye blinking or other motor activity. Automatisms may be seen in absence seizures, as well as in complex partial seizures. Thus, one may not use this feature to distinguish between the two types. If the seizure lasts more than 1 minute and has an associated postictal state, it is less likely to be an absence seizure and more likely to be a complex partial seizure. The physician may be able to induce a typical absence seizure in the office by having the patient hyperventilate for about 3 minutes by blowing on a pinwheel. When this is done concomitantly with an EEG, a typical generalized 3 Hz spike and wave pattern will be produced during the seizure. The interictal pattern on the EEG often is normal, and the EEG after the seizure immediately returns to normal.

About 30% to 50% of children with typical absence seizures also will have generalized tonic-clonic seizures. These may precede, coincide with, or follow the onset of absence seizures. There is a strong positive family history of epilepsy for those with idiopathic absence seizures.

Antiepileptic drugs that are effective in controlling absence seizures include ethosuximide, valproic acid, and clonazepam. Valproic acid and clonazepam also are effective against tonic-clonic seizures. For children who have only typical absence seizures, ethosuximide monotherapy is usually effective. If not, valproic acid may be substituted. For the rare patient who does not respond to either drug alone, the combination of ethosuximide and valproic acid may be effective. For children with symptomatic absence syndromes, valproic acid is often a more effective drug.

Outcome is good in those children with typical absence seizures, with about 80% resolving around 10 years of age. The group without associated generalized tonic-clonic seizures tends to have a somewhat

TABLE 5. Features That Distinguish Absence, Partial Complex, and Behavioral Seizures

	ABSENCE	PARTIAL COMPLEX	BEHAVIORAL
Duration	15–30 s	> 1 min	Variable
Frequency	Multiple per day	1–2/d	Multiple
Automatisms	Yes	Yes	No
Response to hyperventilation	Yes	Variable	No
Postictal	No	Frequent	No
EEG: ictal	3 Hz spikes and wave	Focal, often temporary	No changes

Adapted from Pearl PL, Holmes GL: Absence seizures. *In* Dodson WE, Pellock JM (eds): Pediatric Epilepsy: Diagnosis and Therapy. New York, Demos Publishers, 1993:157–169.

better prognosis. Once the patient has achieved a 2-year seizure-free interval and an EEG is normal with hyperventilation and sleep, antiepileptic drugs should be withdrawn gradually.

ACQUIRED EPILEPTIC APHASIA (Landau Kleffner Syndrome)

This is a disorder of verbal auditory agnosia, aphasia, and EEG abnormalities. About two thirds of the children have associated seizures, which may be either partial, complex partial, or generalized tonic-clonic. The EEGs of these children have multifocal spike and wave discharges, often in bitemporal areas. Although the seizures often respond well to appropriate antiepileptic medication, the aphasia and the EEG do not. In addition to treatment of seizures, these children should be placed in appropriate educational programs for hearing- and language-impaired children. The outcome for this syndrome is variable. Many of the children improve by the time they are in their adolescence, but persistent language deficits are commonly noted.

BENIGN FOCAL EPILEPSIES

There are some focal epilepsy syndromes that are age related and termed benign because of their disappearance in late adolescence. These seizure syndromes represent one of the most common epileptic syndromes of childhood, more so than typical absence seizures. EEGs are abnormal, with focal spikes usually seen in the centrotemporal areas on scalp-recorded EEGs. There is a certain morphology to the spike, with surface negativity greatest in the centrotemporal region but with a surface positive appearance in the frontal region. These increase in frequency with sleep onset. Although, they may originate from one hemisphere only, they more frequently appear independently from the two hemispheres. Spikes also may appear in frontal and occipital areas. Two specific syndromes are recognized, one with centrotemporal spikes and another with occipital spikes.

The clinical history in children with centrotemporal spikes is that of generalized tonic-clonic seizure on arising from sleep in the early morning. Daytime simple parietal seizures consisting of facial and arm clonic movements and difficulty with speaking also may occur. In most instances, it is believed that the seizure begins focally and is secondarily generalized. The problem with speech is not a true aphasia, but a motor problem secondary to facial weakness. Those with occipital spikes often have visual phenomena as part of the seizure. This latter disorder may be confused with migraine.

Although there are focal abnormalities on the EEG, background patterns are normal during the awake state. Most patients have normal neurologic examinations and a strong positive family history of epilepsy, especially those having centrotemporal spikes. The need for other diagnostic studies, such as head imaging, should be based on physical examination and clinical history. If the clinical history and EEG are characteristic for benign focal epilepsy with centrotemporal spikes, imaging is rarely necessary.

Benign focal epilepsy has its onset between 3 and 13 years of age. In most instances, the seizures disappear in late adolescence. For those having had a single seizure and a typical EEG pattern, it is reasonable to observe without treatment. If seizures occur frequently or during the daytime, treatment may be initiated and maintained for a 1 to 2 year period. Antiepileptic drugs that have been effective include carbamazepine, phenobarbital, and phenytoin. Carbamazepine has least effects on behavior and cognition. Prognosis is good following resolution of the seizures, as they rarely recur.

JUVENILE MYOCLONIC EPILEPSY

This is another age-related syndrome, with onset usually in the second decade of life. Clinical seizures consist of myoclonic jerks and tonic-clonic seizures beginning shortly after AM wakening. Many patients also have a history of absence seizures. This disorder has a strong familial association. Recent genetic studies have mapped the gene to the 6p21.3 locus. Typical age of onset is about 13 to 14 years, and male and females are affected equally. EEGs show generalized bilaterally synchronous polyspike and wave discharges in a frequency range of 4 to 6 Hz. If myoclonic jerks are recorded, polyspikes at 10 to 16 Hz appear.

These seizures respond well to antiepileptic drugs, particularly valproic acid, and most are well controlled with this drug. This is a lifetime disorder, and drugs need to be maintained. The seizure recurrence rate is about 95% with antiepileptic drug withdrawal.

REFRACTORY EPILEPSY

There is a small percentage of children whose seizures behave differently from many of the syndromes described previously. In this group, seizure patterns vary considerably, and many of the children exhibit symptomatic epilepsy, abnormal neurologic development, school and/or behavioral problems, and poor responses to antiepileptic drugs. Furthermore, many of these children have localization-related epilepsies, that is, epilepsies that have their origin in localized regions of the brain. Seizure patterns may be simple or complex, partial, or partial with secondarily generalization. Older terminology referred to those seizures that are now called complex partial as temporal lobe seizures. It is known that partial complex seizures can originate not only from temporal lobes but also from frontal, parietal, and occipital lobes. The clinical manifestation of the seizure sometimes is helpful in suggesting the region of origin. The seizure may begin as a simple partial seizure with a sensation the patient experiences; this is called the aura. There is an electrographic correlate to this sensation, although it may not always be recorded from scalp EEGs. Manifestations of complex partial seizures are varied. Automatisms are common and may consist of alimentary phenomena, such as gagging, chewing, swallowing, lip-smacking, and others, changes in facial expression with grimacing, expression of fear, and unusual smiling or laughter, walking or running, repetition of words or phrases, use of expletives, and crying or laughter. Autonomic changes are common and again varied. Gastrointestinal discomfort is a very common one, with ill-defined abdominal pain. Other manifestations may include color changes, heart rate changes, and occasionally apnea. Psychic and visual changes have been observed.

The differential diagnosis for complex partial seizures includes complicated migraine, absence seizures, and some behavioral disorders. The evaluation of a child with suspected complex partial seizures should include an EEG awake and asleep (and following sleep deprivation). If these are normal, a prolonged EEG with video monitoring may be necessary. Imaging of the head is indicated for those children with an abnormal neurologic examination or focal slowing with epileptiform discharges on their EEGs. MRI has greater resolution than CT and is the procedure of choice. Newer technologies, such as position emission tomography and single photon emission tomography, should not be used in the routine evaluation of epilepsy. They may, however, be of value in those children undergoing evaluation for epilepsy surgery.

Complex partial seizures may be associated with a variety of pathologic conditions, including such tumors as low-grade astrocytomas and oligodendrogliomas, encephalomalacia from prior traumatic brain injury, CNS infection or hypoxic ischemic injury, arteriovenous vascular malformations, and neurocutaneous diseases.

The most frequently used antiepileptic drugs are carbamazepine, valproic acid, phenobarbital, primidone, and phenytoin. Adjunctive drugs are methsuximide and clorazepate. New drugs available for partial seizures for older children are felbamate and gabapentin. Management of children with refractory epilepsies usually requires the involvement of an epileptologist and a health care team to work with drugs, school, and family. Because of the poor response that some of these children have to multiple drugs, surgery may be needed.

STATUS EPILEPTICUS

The term status epilepticus (SE) refers to a condition of continuous seizures lasting 30 minutes or longer or to a state of repetitive seizures. Status can occur with any seizure type and can be either convulsive or nonconvulsive. SE occurs more frequently in patients with symptomatic epilepsy.

Following is the **classification of status epilepticus.**
A. Convulsive
   1. Tonic
   2. Clonic
   3. Tonic-clonic
   4. Myoclonic
B. Nonconvulsive
   1. Absence
   2. Partial: complex
   3. Partial: simple motor

Convulsive SE is a medical emergency requiring immediate treatment and initiation of antiepileptic drugs. The morbidity and mortality of SE have decreased with improved intensive care support and aggressive antiepileptic drug treatment. The currently reported mortality figures in children range between 3% and 6% for convulsive SE. The outcome for these children is related to the underlying medical or neurologic problem. Causes of SE differ in pediatric and adult populations. In children, SE commonly results from infectious agents, metabolic disturbances, and preexisting neurologic disease. In older children and adults who have known epilepsy, drug withdrawal may play a role, because of either poor compliance or drug interactions resulting in lower drug levels.

The goals of treating a patient with convulsive SE are to (1) provide adequate oxygenation with an airway and oxygen as needed, (2) to stop the seizures both clinical and electrographic, (3) to identify and treat the underlying etiology, (4) to prevent recurrent seizures during the acute illness, and (5) to prevent other systemic complications from the SE, such as hypotension, hyperglycemia or hypoglycemia, lactic acidosis, or autonomic dysregulation.

Treatment should begin at the onset of the seizure by the patient's family or whoever is with the patient. Initial actions should consist of supportive measures, such as removing objects from the patient's path and loosening clothing from around the neck. The patient should be placed on his side, with the head extended to allow for secretions to roll out of the mouth. If seizures do not stop within 5 to 10 minutes, an emergency service should be contacted for further emergency treatment and transport to the nearest hospital.

On arrival in an emergency room, an adequate IV should be placed if one has not been inserted by paramedics. Blood should be drawn for glucose, electrolytes, BUN, arterial blood gases, calcium and magnesium, and antiepileptic drug levels if the patient has known epilepsy and is on treatment. Glucose (25%) should be administered at a dose of 2 to 4 ml/kg. Intravenous fluids should be given to correct any known existing deficits as they might relate to fever or dehydration, followed by maintenance appropriate for age. Antiepileptic therapy should be started at the same time. If an IV line cannot be placed, fluids and some of the antiepileptic drugs can be administered intraosseously.

Treatment of the seizures should be started with a benzodiazepine, either diazepam at 0.3 to 0.5 mg/kg or lorazepam at 0.1 mg/kg IV. Both are equally effective, but lorazepam has a much longer half-life (10 to 15 hours). The effect of diazepam diminishes after about 20 minutes, and a second dose often is required. However, its onset of action is somewhat faster. Another advantage of diazepam is that if IV access is not quickly established, the drug can be administered per rectum at a dose 0.5 mg/kg for younger children and 0.2 to 0.3 mg/kg for older children. Diazepam may also be administered intraosseously using the IV dose. A second longer-acting drug should be administered immediately following the benzodiazepine. This is more important when diazepam is the initial drug. Phenytoin and phenobarbital are both good second drugs. Phenytoin has the advantage over phenobarbital of not having sedative effects at the usual antiepileptic doses. Doses and routes of administration are listed in Table 6. Most children will respond to initial treatment with a benzodiazepine and phenytoin. When this does not occur, one must add a third line of drugs, either phenobarbital or a constant infusion with

TABLE 6. Drugs for Treatment of Convulsive Status Epilepticus

DRUG	DOSAGE
First-Line Therapy	
Benzodiazepines	
Diazepam	0.3–0.5 mg/kg slow IV push; can repeat in 20 min × 2
	Maximum doses
	Infant 1 mg/kg
	Child 5/10 mg
	Adolescent 10–15 mg
	Adult 15–20 mg
Lorazepam	0.1 mg/kg slow IV push
	Maximum dose: 8 mg
Phenytoin	Should be given after benzodiazepine 20/mg/kg IV at 50 mg/min
	Maximum dose: can give up to 30 mg/kg in first 8 h and up to 40 mg/kg within first 24 h
	Adult: 1000 mg
	Obtain serum level ½–1 h postload
Second-Line Therapy	When first line is not effective
Phenobarbital	20 mg/kg IV over 20 min; infusion rate about 100/mg/min
	Obtain serum level ½–1 h postload
	May need to consider intubation
Third-Line Therapy	
Anesthesia	General anesthesia with halothane, isoflurane, and barbiturates has been used; this should be done in an intensive care facility with adequate staff for intubation and subsequent nursing needs
Pentobarbital	Load with 5–10 mg/kg IV × 1 h
	Maintain with 0.25–1 mg/kg/h
	Maximum load: 30 mg/kg
	Hours 1–6: give additional boluses of 5 mg/kg up to maximum dose
	Hours 6–12: continue maintenance infusion
	>12 h: if clinical or electrical seizures persist, change rate to 0.5–1 mg/kg/h
	12–24 h: maintain
	24 h: stop infusion; monitor with EEG
Thiopental	Alternative drug
	Load with 30 mg/kg
	Maintain with 10–20 mg/kg/h IV
	Duration: 48–72 h
Phenobarbital	High dose: levels of ~100 µg/ml
Paraldehyde	No longer available

Alternative Methods of Antiepileptic Drug Administration

Rectal Diazepam or Lorazepam

Diazepam	0.3–0.5 mg/kg with equal amount saline
Lorazepam	0.05–0.1 mg/kg with equal amount saline

Rectal and Nasogastric Valproic Acid

Rectal	20 mg/kg with equal H$_2$O retention enema
Nasogastric	50–60 g/kg

Intranasal Midazolam

diazepam. At this point, it is usually necessary to electively intubate the patient so that the airway can be adequately protected and the patient can be ventilated. There is increasing sedation as more drugs are added and respiratory effort is diminished. Some patients do not respond to second-line and third-line therapies. For this small group, barbiturate coma can be induced. This should be done only in a pediatric intensive care unit, with a pediatric intensivist or pediatric anesthesiologist available. Both pentobarbital and thiopental have been used with about equal effectiveness. The goal of therapy is to stop the seizures and achieve a burst suppression or flat record on the EEG. Therefore, the drug should be given while an EEG is being recorded. The loading dose of the pentobarbital is 20 mg/kg, followed by a maintenance dose of 1 to 2 mg/kg/h as a constant infusion. Pentobarbital should be administered for 24 to 72 hours, depending on clinical and EEG response. Serum levels should be maintained at 20 to 40 µg/ml. At the end of 24 to 48 hours, the pentobarbital infusion can be decreased slowly if the EEG does not show electrographic seizures or repetitive epileptiform discharges. One of the complications of pentobarbital is its effect on blood pressure, often requiring administration of pressor agents. Other agents that have been used to treat SE include thiopental and high-dose phenobarbital. Thiopental has systemic effects similar to those of pentobarbital. High-dose phenobarbital has been administered IV, producing blood levels of 100 to 200 µg/ml without significant impact on respirations or blood pressure. Anesthetic agents (e.g., halothane and isoflurane) should be administered only by a pediatric anesthesiologist in an intensive care unit.

Nonconvulsive SE is not a medical emergency, but it should be treated aggressively once recognized. It accounts for about 25% of cases of SE. Children with this form of SE are still impaired. Absence status is one of the most common forms of nonconvulsive SE. Partial complex status is less common. Intravenous benzodiazepines may be effective acutely in breaking the clinical and electrographic SE. Long-term therapy may be more effective with valproic acid.

Management

For each child who has seizures, the treating physician needs to decide whether the seizure is one that requires an antiepileptic drug, and if so, which drug is most appropriate for the seizure type. As discussed previously, the child who has a single generalized tonic-clonic seizure and the child with isolated benign centrotemporal seizures may not require therapy. Most children with recurring seizures will be placed on drugs for a period of time. The current minimal time is 2 years. Studies are in progress to determine whether shorter treatment periods are equally effective. Certain principles should be considered when initiating therapy.

- Select antiepilectic drugs appropriate for the seizure type.
- Start with a single drug.
- Begin with the lowest dose needed to achieve a therapeutic level.
- Increase the dose as needed.
- Substitute a second drug if the first is not effective.
- Use polytherapy when monotherapy fails.

Drug dosing is another important issue. Most drugs are commercially available in several different forms. The physician should discuss with the parent (and child when possible) which form of the drug will be easiest to take. Many drugs have long half-lives, decreasing the necessity for multiple doses throughout the day (Table 7). Parents should have realistic expectations for the medication and understand

TABLE 7. Antiepileptic Drugs: Pharmacokinetics

DRUG	DOSE (mg/kg/d)	BIOLOGIC HALF-LIFE (h)	LEVEL (µg/ml)
Phenobarbital	4–5	50–150	10–40
Primidone	12–25	6–18	5–12
Phenytoin	5–10	10–40	10–20
Carbamazepine	15–20	8–20	4–12
Valproic acid (valproate)	15–50	8–12	50–100
Felbamate	15–45	14–22	Not determined
Ethosuximide	20–50	20–60	50–100
Clorazepate	0.3–3.0	50–150	Not determined
Clonazepam	0.1–0.2	22–33	40–100 ng/ml
Lorazepam	0.3–0.22 IV Maintenance dose not established	8–35	Not determined
Nitrazepam	0.2	20	Not determined
Gabapentin	20–30		Not determined

that a therapeutic level does not always guarantee 100% control. Families should also be informed about potential drug side effects. These should be discussed as dose-related and idiosyncratic side effects, and the families should be informed that the latter are uncommon. Adolescent women should be informed of the teratogenic effects of the drug as well. Some of the more common side effects are listed in Table 8.

The trend in treatment of the pediatric epilepsies has been to move from those drugs, which produce sedation, alter mood, and impair learning, to drugs with fewer of these side effects. None of the drugs are without side effects, and the treating physician must decide which drug is going to produce the best seizure control with the least number of side effects.

Since there are known toxicities associated with antiepileptic drug therapy, it is advisable to have routine blood studies drawn before beginning treatment. Such studies should always include a complete blood count, a differential count, and a platelet count. In addition, patients starting on phenytoin, carbamazepine, and valproic acid should have a specimen sent for AST and ALT determinations. A serum calcium level should be obtained in nonambulatory, neurologically impaired children. Follow-up studies should be determined by the clinical history and examination on follow-up visits. Drug-induced systemic side effects may not be detected during routine laboratory monitoring. Furthermore, studies have shown that routine monitoring of the blood counts and liver enzymes is not cost effective. Antiepileptic drug levels should be obtained when the patient reaches the initial steady-state after 4 to 5 half-lives of the drug, if the dose is changed, when a new drug is added (particularly if the new drug is known to compete for protein binding or enhance metabolism of the initial drug), or when there are suspected dose-related side effects.

The other aspect of management that the treating physician must address with the family is duration of therapy. Currently, most antiepileptics are continued for a 2-year period following seizure control. This period may vary for certain situations, such as neonatal seizures, seizures associated with an acute CNS illness, such as meningitis or encephalitis, and certain age-related epileptic syndromes. Once a child has achieved a 2-year period without seizures, the question should be raised whether antiepileptic drugs can be discontinued. The following information is helpful in making that decision:

1. Presence or absence of preexisting neurologic disorder
2. Positive family history of epilepsy
3. Known structural process, such as tumor, vascular malformation, encephalomalacia, which might be epileptogenic
4. Presence of epileptiform features on a routine and sleep-deprived EEG

For the child who has a normal neurologic examination, whose seizures were controlled with a single AED, who has no family history of epilepsy, and who has a normal wake or sleep-deprived EEG, the chance of seizure recurrence following discontinuation of AEDs is about 25%. The percentage will vary with seizure type, with higher recurrence rates seen in those with partial complex, juvenile myoclonic seizures and absence seizures with associated generalized tonic-clonic seizures.

The risks and benefits of discontinuing or continuing drug therapy should be discussed with the family. If all agree that drug discontinuation is appropriate, one drug at a time should be tapered and stopped. The maintenance dose may be tapered by 25% at intervals corresponding to 4 to 5 drug half-lives.

Recurrence is highest in the first 6 months of drug discontinuation, with about 80% of recurrences occurring in this period. Patients should be followed closely during this time period and for the next 2 years after the antiepileptic drug is stopped. If the patient is of driving age, it should be recommended to the patient and his parents that he not drive during the first 6 months of discontinuing the drug therapy. Other activities should be evaluated by the family and physician and discussed with all present (e.g., contact sports, swimming, diving).

TABLE 8. Antiepileptic Drug Side Effects

DRUG	DOSE-RELATED EFFECTS	IDIOSYNCRATIC EFFECTS
Phenobarbital	Lethargy	Hyperactivity Sleep problems Irritability Lability of mood Hepatitis SLE Allergic rashes
Primidone	Drowsiness Ataxia Nausea	Anemia Similar to phenobarbital
Phenytoin	Lethargy Drowsiness Nausea Ataxia Nystagmus	Gum hypertrophy Hirsutism Lymphadenopathy Hepatitis Behavioral changes Dementia Rashes/acne Involuntary movements
Carbamazepine	Drowsiness Headaches Ataxia Diplopia Behavioral effects Hyponatremia	Leukopenia Thrombocytopenia Aplastic anemia Hepatic changes Anemia Rashes Involuntary movements Psychoses
Valproic acid	Gastrointestinal distress Tremors Increased level of liver enzymes Tiredness	Hepatic failure Thrombocytopenia Alopecia Weight changes Anemia Leukopenia Pancreatitis
Felbamate	Nausea Vomiting Headache Drowsiness	Aplastic anemia Hepatic failure
Ethosuximide	Gastrointestinal distress Hiccoughs Headache Drowsiness	Leukopenia Pancytopenia SLE Involuntary movements Nephrotic syndrome Rashes
Clonazepam	Drowsiness Ataxia Nausea	Increased salivation Hyperactivity Behavioral effects Increased level of liver enzymes Skin pigmentation Hair loss Hematologic effects
Lorazepam Clorazepate	Similar to clonazepam Sedation Lethargy	
Nitrazepam	Similar to clonazepam	

Some modification of these is probably appropriate during the tapering and 6-month follow-up intervals.

Phenobarbital

This drug has been available as an antiepileptic drug since 1912. It is a relatively safe and effective anticonvulsant for generalized tonic-clonic, simple partial, and febrile seizures. However, recent studies have shown that the drug has significant effects on behavior, attention, memory, learning, and sleep patterns. Some studies cite figures as high as 70% for behavioral problems related to hyperactivity and inattention. Therefore, it is recommended that other drugs with similar efficacy for the seizure type be used first before resorting to phenobarbital. If selected as the most effective drug, it should be used at the lowest dose possible to sustain seizure control without behavioral or cognitive changes. The half-life of phenobarbital is about 96 hours. Therefore, the drug may be given one or two times per day. The child should be closely monitored for changes in behavior or school performance. Sometimes, these changes are subtle. Phenobarbital should be discontinued slowly, in increments of 20% to 25% at intervals no more frequent than 4 to 5 half-lives (about every 2 to 3 weeks). Withdrawal seizures can occur if the drug is tapered too rapidly.

Primidone

This drug is related to phenobarbital, and one of its metabolites is phenobarbital. Thus, many of the side effects that are seen with phenobarbital will occur with primidone. The anticonvulsant effect of primidone is in part a result of its metabolism to phenobarbital. However, another metabolite, phenylethylmalonamide (PEMA), and the unmetabolized drug itself both have anticonvulsant properties. There appears to be much more of a sedative effect with primidone than with phenobarbital. Primidone works best in children with generalized tonic-clonic seizures and partial seizures (both simple and complex).

Phenytoin

This drug was introduced in 1938 and has been an effective drug for the treatment of generalized tonic-clonic, tonic, and partial seizures. Phenytoin is a drug that follows nonlinear kinetics. Thus, as the enzyme systems become saturated with drug, small increases in dose will produce large increases in the serum level. Elimination of the drug is also affected by the concentration: the more drug in the system, the slower the rate of elimination. Phenytoin is highly bound to protein. The use of phenytoin with other protein-bound antiepileptic drugs, such as valproic acid, can affect the amount of free (active) drug available because it is highly protein bound. Half-lives are long and quite variable in the newborn infant, 5 to 18 hours in the young child, and 22 to 34 hours in the older child and adult. Because of these properties, phenytoin can be a difficult drug to use in the young child. Although phenytoin has a number of positive attributes (e.g., it is a very effective antiepileptic and is available as a suspension, a chewable tablet, and a parenteral preparation), it also has a number of undesirable side effects (Table 8). Chief among these are gingival hyperplasia and hirsutism. Gingival hyperplasia can be partially controlled with good oral hygiene and will resolve gradually after discontinuation of the drug. Hirsutism usually persists. Phenytoin also can have an impact on learning and school performance.

Although there are several forms of phenytoin available, the bioavailability of the drug varies among different forms and between the generic preparations and the parent drug. The phenytoin suspension should be used with caution. Although it does have good bioavailability, the amount of drug received per dose can be quite variable and is dependent on the vigor with which the bottle is shaken. Infants may require 8 to 10 mg/kg/d (administered b.i.d. or t.i.d.) to achieve therapeutic levels. Older children can be maintained on a dose of 5 mg/kg/d. For SE, the patient should be administered a loading dose of 20 mg/kg IV at a rate no greater than 3 mg/kg/min in the infant and 25 mg/kg/min in the older child. A 20 mg/kg bolus will achieve a serum level near 20 μg/ml.

Carbamazepine

Carbamazepine (CBZ) is another broad-spectrum antiepileptic drug effective in both generalized tonic-clonic and partial seizures. It is one of the more effective drugs for partial complex seizures. However, CBZ may worsen absence, atonic, and myoclonic seizures. In comparison with phenobarbital and phenytoin, it has significantly fewer side effects on learning, attention, and behavior, but CBZ commonly causes drowsiness. Dose-related side effects may occur 3 to 4 hours postdosing. These side effects frequently are visual ones of blurring or diplopia. Redistributing the dose during the day may eliminate this problem.

When CBZ is used as the first antiepileptic drug in a patient with seizures, the initial half-life can be as long as 20 to 30 hours. Therefore, the drug should be administered on a b.i.d. schedule for the first 1 to 2 weeks. CBZ induces its own metabolism, and the serum levels may drop after the first 3 to 4 weeks, requiring an increase in the dose. The half-life of CBZ ranges between 8 and 36 hours, with an average of about 14 hours. Therapeutic serum levels range between 4 and 12 μg/ml. Steady-state usually will be achieved by about 6 weeks. If the patient is receiving drugs, such as phenobarbital or phenytoin, the initial half-life of CBZ may be shorter, as these drugs also induce the metabolism of CBZ. Other drugs notable for their ability to increase serum CBZ levels include erythromycin, triacetyloleandomycin, and dextropropoxyphene.

When CBZ was introduced, there was concern about serious hematologic side effects, especially aplastic anemia. Therefore, it usually was recommended initially that patients receiving CBZ have and request blood counts. A number of patients may exhibit transient decreases in their white blood cell counts after initiation of treatment. Fortunately, these are neither long-lasting nor life threatening, and there is no need to discontinue the drug in such cases. Furthermore, there have been a number of studies that have shown that frequent monitoring of the blood count is neither helpful nor cost effective. Baseline studies should be obtained before drug initiation and then rechecked 6 to 12 weeks after starting the drug. An annual check of the blood count is reasonable.

CBZ may be started at a dose of 5 to 12 mg/kg/d (administered b.i.d.). Every 5 to 7 days, the dose can be increased by 5 mg/kg up to 20 mg/kg/d. A third dose is sometimes needed during the second or third week of therapy.

Valproic Acid

Valproic acid (valproate) (VPA) is a very effective drug for the generalized epilepsies, particularly absence, myoclonic, and generalized tonic-clonic. Recent studies have shown a beneficial effect in complex partial and secondarily generalized epilepsies. VPA is a drug with a relative short half-life and requires t.i.d. dosing or q.i.d. dosing on occasion. The drug is well absorbed, and levels peak 3 to 4 hours after a dose. Therapeutic levels range between 50 and 100 μg/ml, and some children require higher doses to achieve control. Serum levels may be increased to 125 to 150 μg/ml as long as there are no dose-related or systemic side effects. The enteric-coated tablet and sprinkle forms (Divalproex sodium) of VPA are more slowly absorbed than are other forms. One of the major advantages of VPA is that it does not impair cognition and learning. However, there are side effects to the drug, both dose dependent and idiosyncratic. Some of the more frequent side effects that patients experience include increased appetite with weight gain, hand tremors, and hair loss. Enteric-coated preparations can eliminate some of the gastrointestinal side effects experienced with the use of valproic acid capsule and syrup.

More serious side effects of VPA include thrombocytopenia, pancreatitis, and acute hepatic failure. On occasion, there are transient dose-related elevations in liver enzymes, which resolve with dose adjustment. In the initial reports, the risk of fatal hepatotoxicity was 1/500 in a child under 2 years on polytherapy and 1/7000 on monotherapy. By 1989, prescribing patterns had changed, and criteria were established to eliminate the risk of liver failure. Children on polytherapy with other antiepileptic drugs who were severely neurologically impaired or had a prior history of liver disease or a family history of liver disease were believed to be at risk for developing hepatotoxicity. By carefully selecting patients and evaluating for preexisting metabolic disease, the incidence declined to 1/800 on polytherapy and 0 on monotherapy in the 2 years and under group. The overall incidence of liver failure in a more recent study was 1/26,000 and

1/118,000 on polytherapy and monotherapy, respectively. Laboratory monitoring of liver enzymes is not helpful in predicting those children who will develop fatal hepatic failure. However, baseline determinations of AST and ALT, ammonia, prothrombin, and partial thromboplastin should be obtained and rechecked after the first month on therapy. Most children who develop fatal liver disease do so within the first 90 days of therapy. Parents should be carefully instructed to contact their physician with any flu-like illness, protracted nausea or vomiting, jaundice, or significant change in seizure pattern or frequency. The role of supplemental L-carnitine in decreasing VPA toxicity is controversial.

Felbamate

This is the newest antiepileptic drug released and the first in 14 years. It is a derivative of meprobamate and has been shown in clinical studies to be effective in adolescents and adults with partial seizures and in children with Lennox-Gastaut syndrome. It is chemically unrelated to existing antiepileptic drugs, and the mechanism of action is unknown. Dose forms come as 400 mg and 600 mg scored tablets and a suspension at 600 mg/5 ml. The half-life of felbamate varies from 2 to 13 hours. Doses should be initiated at 15 mg/kg/d on a t.i.d. or q.i.d. schedule and increased by 15 mg/kg/wk to a total dose of 45 mg/kg/d (maximal dose 3600 mg/d). Felbamate has been linked to several cases of acute liver failure and aplastic anemia in children and adults; some of these cases have been fatal. Liver failure occurred 1 to 12 months after initiation of therapy. It is recommended that felbamate be limited to those patients whose seizures have been refractory to existing antiepileptic drugs and whose seizures pose significant risks to them. Felbamate should not be used in those with a preexisting history of liver disease. Patients who receive felbamate should have baseline measurements of ALT, AST, and bilirubin and complete blood, differential, and platelet counts. Each of these should be assessed weekly while the patient is taking felbamate. Drowsiness, lethargy, nausea, and vomiting are the more common side effects experienced. There does not appear to be a correlation with serum level and seizure control, and therapeutic levels have not been determined. Drug interactions with coexisting antiepileptic drugs do occur. VPA inhibits the metabolism of felbamate, and levels of felbamate increase when the two are used together. CBZ and phenytoin accelerate the metabolism of felbamate. Current recommendations are to use felbamate as monotherapy in those children with life-threatening or refractory seizure disorders.

Ethosuximide

Ethosuximide is a derivative of a succinimide and is most effective in typical absence epilepsy. It has also been used as adjunctive therapy for treating absence seizures in patients with LGS, myoclonic/astatic epilepsies, and in combination with valproic acid for refractory absence epilepsy. The drug is well absorbed and reaches peak levels approximately 1 to 7 hours after dosing. Ethosuximide has a half-life in children ranging between 30 and 36 hours. In the adolescent and adult, the half-life is somewhat longer (55 hours). The drug should be started at 20 mg/kg/d and may be increased to 50 mg/kg/d. Most children tolerate a b.i.d. schedule better than a single daily dose, which tends to cause gastric irritation. Side effects are few, as are drug interactions. The most common side effects are gastric irritation and nausea. Ingestion of food with the drug helps to eliminate these symptoms.

Benzodiazepines: Clonazepam, Clorazepate, Diazepam, Lorazepam, and Nitrazepam

This class of drugs acts to enhance GABA. These drugs have similar pharmacokinetic properties and side effects. As a class of drugs, they have been most effective in the treatment of the generalized epilepsies. Diazepam and lorazepam have been used parenterally for the treatment of SE and are discussed under that section. Clorazepate has been used as an adjunctive drug in the treatment of partial seizures.

Nitrazepam has been used primarily for the treatment of myoclonic seizures in infantile spasms. Clonazepam is a broad-spectrum antiepileptic drug but is most commonly used in the treatment of LGS and myoclonic and atypical absence seizures. The development of tolerance limits the effectiveness of this class of drugs and requires increasing doses. The oral forms are well absorbed, and peak levels occur within 4 hours. Half-lives are long, usually 30 hours or longer. Although lorazepam has been used primarily to treat SE, there are some limited studies to indicate that it may be a good drug for maintenance therapy because of its shorter half-life (8 to 25 hours). In addition to tolerance, side effects also limit the effectiveness of benzodiazepines. Most produce moderate sedation, hypotonia, drooling, and behavioral changes. Furthermore, there is not a good correlation with seizure control and serum benzodiazepine levels. There are some recent studies documenting a new use for diazepam as a rectally administered drug (0.5 to 0.7 mg/kg) to control cluster seizures or prolonged seizures in the patient with known epilepsy. Diazepam is rapidly absorbed from the rectal mucosa, and blood levels peak within 15 minutes. The half-life of this form is much shorter than the others. There have been no reports of respiratory depression using this route. Additional studies are in progress to determine the effective unit doses and to obtain additional efficacy and safety information.

REFRACTORY EPILEPSY AND EPILEPSY SURGERY

Most patients will have significant to complete control of their seizures with appropriately selected and dosed antiepileptic drug therapy. Approximately 10% will fail drug therapy and be candidates for other treatment options. One nondrug regimen that is used for the treatment of children with LGS and other refractory epilepsies is a ketogenic diet high in fats and low in calories obtained from carbohydrates and protein. Other therapeutic options include steroids and epilepsy surgery. The trend in the field of epilepsy is to consider surgery at an earlier age, when it is clear that the child has failed to respond to at least three of the major antiepileptic drugs over a 2-year period. It is thought that earlier surgical intervention may prevent years of unnecessary treatment, avoid drug side effects, decrease school problems, and help to improve the adjustment period to adolescence and adulthood as functioning members of society.

Children considered candidates for epilepsy surgery are those who fail drug therapy, those with a history of complex partial seizures localized to a temporal lobe who have other objective information (e.g., MRI, SPECT, or PET) supporting abnormalities in the same region, those with localized seizures on EEG and evidence of a structural lesion such as a tumor or arteriovenous malformation (AVM), and children with generalized seizures resulting in bodily injury. These patients should be referred to a pediatric epileptologist and a medical center specializing in epilepsy surgery. The outcome for those patients undergoing temporal lobectomies is good, with some authors reporting postoperative seizure-free status of 80%. Epilepsies originating outside the temporal lobe do not have as favorable outcome, but many of these children do have a reduction in the number of seizures.

REFERENCES

1. Annegers JF: Epidemiology of childhood onset seizures. In Dodson WE, Pellock JM (eds): Pediatric Epilepsy, Diagnosis, and Treatment. New York, Demos Publishers, 1993:57–62.
2. Commission on Classification and Terminology of the International League Against Epilepsy: Proposal for revised clinical and electrographic classification for epileptic seizures. Epilepsia 1981;22:489–501.
3. Freeman JM, Vining EPG, Pilas DJ: Seizures and Epilepsy in Childhood: A Guide for Parents. Baltimore, Johns Hopkins University Press, 1990.

FEBRILE SEIZURES

MARY ANNE GUGGENHEIM, M.D.

DEFINITION AND BASIC FACTS

A febrile seizure (FS) occurs in 2% to 4% of all young children. Like other seizures, a FS is caused by a sudden excitatory neuronal discharge that results in abnormal motor activity and altered consciousness. Our current understanding of FS is that of a distinct developmentally determined syndrome, with an inherently benign course. The usual definition is a seizure related to fever (T > 101° F) in a child older than 1 month *not* due to primary central nervous system infection or metabolic imbalance. Most occur between 6 months and 5 years of age. The peak incidence occurs at 18 months. Most practitioners and researchers recognize that FS can occur in children older than these arbitrary limits. Children who have had a previous afebrile seizure and subsequently have a seizure with fever most likely have epilepsy. *Simple febrile seizures* are less than 15 minutes in duration and occur in 60% to 70% of all children with FS. *Complex febrile seizures* are those that are focal and/or last longer than 15 minutes and/or are multiple within the same illness. A child with preexisting neurologic abnormalities is at increased risk for having a complex FS. A complex FS, a positive family history of epilepsy, and preexisting neurologic abnormalities increase the statistical risk for that child to subsequently develop epilepsy.

PATHOGENESIS

FS are a convincing example of the developing brain's susceptibility to seizures and its tendency to outgrow this susceptibility. It has often been stated that a seizure is more likely to occur if the rate of temperature rise is unusually rapid. The only data supporting this claim are experimental studies performed in kittens several decades ago. Close inspection of these data is not very convincing. Other animal experiments showed the opposite: that *it is the degree of temperature elevation that determines the likelihood of a seizure's occurring.* This seems most compatible with clinical data and supports the concept that there is a normal range of temperature sensitivity of the developing brain to a seizure event. Moreover, this *threshold for seizures is determined both by the developmental state of brain maturation and genetic influences.* A positive family history for FS in a first-degree relative is found in approximately 25% of cases.

MANAGEMENT OF THE ACUTE FEBRILE SEIZURE EVENT

Acute management should include

1. Exclusion of a serious underlying and treatable condition
2. Stopping a prolonged seizure
3. Control of the fever and other general medical treatment
4. Initial parental reassurance and education

Exclusion of a Serious Underlying and Treatable Condition

Underlying conditions that require specific and urgent treatment include primary infections of the central nervous system, hypoglycemia, and hypo/hypernatremia. Only 1 in 1000 children who have FS have meningitis, but it must be seriously considered, even without signs of meningeal irritation. Preexisting history, prolonged lethargy, and the age of the child influence the decision as to whether or not to do a lumbar puncture. There is no absolute protocol for this decision; if in doubt, do a spinal tap. Hypoglycemia can be quickly and inexpensively detected by bedside testing and then confirmed by the laboratory. Electrolyte disturbances seldom occur outside a clinical setting of fluid imbalance and/or gastroenteritis. Transient hyperglycemia and leukocytosis may occur as a physiologic result of the seizure itself.

Stopping a Prolonged Seizure

If the seizure itself is prolonged (>10 minutes) and ongoing, it should be stopped with intravenous administration of an antiepileptic drug (AED). Diazepam (0.2 to 0.4 mg/kg) or lorazepam (0.05 to 0.1 mg/kg) usually is effective. Phenobarbital (20 mg/kg) or intravenous phenytoin (20 mg/kg) also may be used to stop an ongoing seizure. A combination of a barbiturate and benzodiazepine is more likely to cause respiratory depression than either alone. If it is not possible to obtain intravenous access promptly, rectal benzodiazepine administration results in quite rapid drug absorption, although never as effective as intravenous administration (see treatment of status epilepticus in discussion of seizure disorders). Long-term coverage with AEDs is not indicated.

Control of the Fever and Other General Medical Treatment

Antipyretic measures are important. Acetaminophen (10 to 15 mg/kg q4–6h), cold packs, removal of clothes, and other measures to facilitate reduction of elevated body temperature should be initiated promptly. Nasal oxygen and other general medical treatment for dehydration, respiratory problems, and other problems, as individually indicated, should be provided.

Initial Parental Reassurance and Education

Parents are usually extremely frightened by the seizure itself and often think that their child will either die or be damaged by the event. The clinician must reassure them (and there are facts to support this) that a febrile seizure does not cause death or neurologic sequelae.

Neuroimaging tests (skull x-rays, CT, or MRI) are *not* indicated unless there is a specific reason in the individual child, such as recent *severe* head injury. If the child has a preexisting neurologic abnormality, focal findings after the acute seizure has resolved, evidence of a neurodysgenic condition (i.e., tuberous sclerosis), or other indication of underlying structural brain abnormality, a scan can be done later. (Several studies have shown that routine skull x-rays give no useful information in FS.) A complex FS is not, in and of itself, an indication for neuroimaging studies. Tests for inborn errors of metabolism (disturbances of ammonia, carnitine, organic and amino acids, and other rare disorders) need not be done unless the child is encephalopathic longer than the usual postictal time period or has protracted vomiting or other unusual history or findings. An electroencephalogram (EEG) is not necessary for the acute management of FS.

MANAGEMENT AFTER THE ACUTE FEBRILE SEIZURE EVENT

The management of FS after the acute event and illness are resolved depends on understanding the natural history of this disorder, the possible benefits vs disadvantages of ongoing medical treatment, and discussing this information with the family to arrive at a mutually agreeable plan. Automatic institution of long-term AEDs, inappropriate diagnosis of epilepsy, or, conversely, lack of attention to underlying chronic disorders of the nervous system should be avoided. The cornerstone of appropriate medical management is effective communication with families.

Risk of Recurrence of Another Febrile Seizure After the First One

The recurrence risk of FS, whether simple or complex, is 30% to 35% over the child's lifetime and ~25% for the 12 months following the initial seizure. Thus, more than 60% of children have no further seizures after the initial FS. The risk of a second FS is increased if the child is <12 to 18 months old and/or if the fever at the time of the initial FS was <102° F (implying a lower than average threshold in that particular child). No other factors increase the inherent risk of recurrent FS. If there is a positive family history of epilepsy, preexisting neurodevelopmental abnormalities in the child, or if the FS was complex, the risk of developing epilepsy (but not recurrent FS) is slightly increased (~2%) compared with the incidence (~1%) in the general population.[1]

Risk of Developing Epilepsy

A small proportion (1% to 2%) of children whose initial clinical presentation is an FS have subsequent nonfebrile, recurrent seizures, that is, epilepsy. The consistent finding of a number of excellent studies done in the last 20 years is that an FS, even if complex, focal, prolonged, or otherwise atypical does not cause epilepsy. This is true even if the initial seizure was febrile status epilepticus. A child with FS who has a preexisting neurologic/developmental abnormality has an increased risk of subsequent epilepsy (~2% by age 7 years compared with ~1% in children in the general population). *Prophylactic continuous or intermittent AED treatment* of a child with FS, whether simple or complex, *does not alter the risk to that child of developing epilepsy.*

Risk of Neurologic or Developmental Abnormalities, Including Learning Disabilities

Although a small percentage of children who have FS also have identifiable neurologic abnormalities, there is no evidence that the FS plays any kind of causative role. In the NIH prospective study of 1706 children with FS, all children with chronic neurologic problems had evidence of this before their initial FS. Even children whose initial FS is febrile status epilepticus show no subsequent neurologic sequelae.

Does an EEG Give Any Useful Information?

In a word, no. Ictal EEGs in FS are rarely done but, not surprisingly, show epileptiform abnormalities during the actual seizure. EEGs done within 24 hours of the seizure show postictal slowing in 88%. Even 3 to 7 days later, slowing, sometimes focal, occurs in ~30%. This is a nonspecific postictal finding of no prognostic significance. The controversial issue in the past has been finding an abnormal, even overtly epileptiform EEG following a febrile seizure. Several European studies in which repeated EEGs have been done for years in children who originally had an FS have reported such abnormalities in >50%, *without any clear correlation with clinical epilepsy.* Conversely, children with normal EEGs following an FS may eventually develop epilepsy. The logical conclusion based on current data is that *an EEG in a child whose only clinical event is a febrile seizure provides neither positive nor negative predictive information.*[2]

What Is the Indication for Prophylactic Treatment with AEDs?

Two arguments are given for initiating chronic treatment with an AED in a child who has had an FS: (1) to prevent recurrent episodes of FS and (2) to prevent the development of epilepsy or chronic neurologic abnormalities. As discussed previously, recurrent febrile seizures, even when complex, *do not* increase an individual child's risk for epilepsy or neurodevelopmental problems. Thus, the only reasonable argument for prophylactic AED treatment after an initial FS is to prevent further episodes of FS. Therefore, let us consider the current data relative to this issue.

The natural history of FS indicates a recurrence risk of about 33%. The use of continuous phenobarbital, monitored with drug levels to ensure compliance and therapeutic blood levels, can reduce this to about 10%. Continuous prophylactic treatment with valproic acid has been popular in Europe, also with demonstrated effectiveness. Both clinical observations and recent controlled prospective studies have shown worrisome long-term consequences of continuous treatment with phenobarbital, consisting of adverse effects on behavior and learning. The known low but definite risk of serious or even fatal hepatic damage from valproic acid must be considered if one chooses to use this drug in young children. Intermittent use of an AED during febrile illness in children with a previous FS has been advocated. Intermittent phenobarbital produces little or no benefit (presumably because of the length of time required to achieve a therapeutic state).

A recent study using oral diazepam during febrile illnesses demonstrated a decreased recurrence of FS from the baseline rate of 31% to 21% over a 2-year follow-up period. However, since 60% to 65% of children have only a single febrile seizure, this one-third reduction in recurrent FS compared with the control group actually indicates an overall beneficial effect of only 10%. (Neither phenytoin nor carbamazepine provides protection from FS, yet another indication that the underlying pathogenesis of FS is different from that of epilepsy.)

Family Education and Counseling Issues

Since the only proven risk of a recurrent FS is another FS, each physician is obligated to understand and discuss clearly with the family the pros and cons of using either continuous or intermittent AEDs. Although it may seem gentler and kinder to suggest such treatment during the anxiety and emotion of an initial FS event, most physicians who have studied and considered this issue do not recommend preventive medical therapy, other than antipyretic intervention, during subsequent febrile illnesses. Most families who understand the benign nature of FS willingly accept this approach.

Since 60% to 65% of all children will remain seizure-free without any specific medical treatment, the economic implications of prophylactic treatment in all children with an initial FS (medication expense, laboratory monitoring, regular physician follow-up visits) vs emergency room or office expenses for those with recurrent seizures should also be considered. This has not yet been established.

REFERENCES

1. Berg AT, Shinnar S, Hauser WA, et al: A prospective study of recurrent febrile seizures. N Engl J Med 327:1122–1127, 1992.
2. Stores G: When does an EEG contribute to the management of febrile seizures? Arch Dis Child 66:554–557, 1991.

INFANTILE SPASMS

RASHMI GUPTA, M.D.
HARRY T. CHUGANI, M.D.

Infantile spasms are a unique form of seizures limited mostly to infants during the first 2 years of life. They are frequently refractory to conventional anticonvulsants and are associated with significant neurologic sequelae. Infantile spasms traditionally are divided into the symptomatic and cryptogenic groups, depending on whether an underlying cause can be determined. Patients in whom there is a clear-cut etiology (e.g., tuberous sclerosis, congenital brain malformations, perinatal asphyxia) belong to the symptomatic group. Those in whom no etiology can be found belong to the cryptogenic group.

Children with West syndrome have infantile spasms, psychomotor retardation, and a characteristic EEG pattern called *hypsarrythmia*. This EEG pattern consists of very high-voltage, slow waves with multifocal spikes, giving a picture of total chaotic disorganization. The clinical appearance of seizures depends on whether the flexor or extensor muscles are predominantly involved. Flexor spasms consist of sudden flexion of head, trunk, arms, and legs, giving rise to the *jackknife* or *salaam* seizures that are the hallmark of infantile spasms. Less severe flexor spasms with dropping of head and flexion at waist may resemble colic.

Extensor spasms consist of abrupt extension of the neck and trunk, with extension and abduction of the arms. The mixed flexor-extensor spasms combine flexion of the neck, trunk, and arms with extension of the legs. Of these, the mixed spasms are the most common, and the extensor spasms are the least common. Infantile spasms are often associated with a cry and occur in clusters several times a day, especially on awakening and when drowsy.

The prognosis for children with infantile spasms remains poor. The mortality rate is about 10% to 20%. Survivors are often left with significant neurologic sequelae. Mental retardation is found in 70% to 80% of patients and is severe in more than 50% of children, especially in the symptomatic group. Epilepsy following infantile spasms, in the form of other types of seizures, occurs in 50% to 60% of children.

It appears that the single most important factor affecting long-term outcome is whether the infantile spasms are classified as cryptogenic or symptomatic, with the latter having a poorer prognosis. The prognosis is best in children between 3 and 12 months of age, who are neurologically and developmentally normal at the onset of spasms, who do not display any other type of seizure, and in whom there is no identifiable etiology for the spasms.

MEDICAL TREATMENT

Infantile spasms are notoriously resistant to conventional antiepileptic drugs. Although there is controversy on whether early treatment of spasms affects the eventual outcome, most authors recommend that treatment be initiated as soon as possible. Of the therapies widely available, the benzodiazepines, valproic acid, adrenocorticotropic hormone (ACTH), and steroids have been found effective. ACTH or oral steroids have been the therapy of choice and are effective in controlling the seizures in 50% to 60% of patients. Once a diagnosis of infantile spasms is made, the child should be admitted to the hospital for a search for symptomatic causes and to begin ACTH therapy.

Baseline laboratory tests, such as complete blood count with differential, electrolytes, calcium, phosphorus, glucose, renal, and liver function tests, are obtained. A urinalysis, as well as urine for CMV, a TB test, and a chest x-ray are performed to rule out any underlying infection that may be exacerbated by the steroids. A baseline EEG with pyridoxine challenge is obtained to rule out a pyridoxine-dependent epilepsy.

Dosages of ACTH have ranged from 20 to 120 units per day, with most reports recommending smaller doses. We begin with a daily dose of 40 units per day of ACTH gel (Acthar gel) intramuscularly in children under 6 months of age and 60 to 80 units in older children. The usual duration of therapy is 4 weeks, with tapering doses and discontinuation over the subsequent 4 to 6 weeks. A therapeutic response is seen usually within a week and is either complete control or none at all. The child is started on antacids or ranitidine hydrochloride (Zantac) concurrent with the ACTH. While in the hospital, blood pressure and weight are monitored daily, and electrolytes and hemoglobin are monitored every other day. Parents are taught to give intramuscular injections and recognize spasms so that they can keep an accurate seizure calendar.

The patient is discharged home once the parent has successfully learned to give the ACTH intramuscularly and arrangements are made for a home nurse to measure blood pressure and weight at home. Parents are also taught to measure urine glucose with a dipstick and check stools for occult blood. Electrolytes and hemoglobin are monitored weekly on an outpatient basis. The patient is seen in follow-up weekly for the first month and biweekly for the next month. An EEG is obtained at 1 week, 4 weeks, and 2 months after initiation of therapy.

Oral corticosteroids can be used instead of ACTH for treating infantile spasms. The dose is 2 mg/kg/d in four divided doses for 4 weeks. That dose is then tapered over the following 4 weeks.

The side effects of ACTH and oral steroids are frequent and, at times, serious. In almost all children, cushingoid features develop. Hypertension, as well as extreme irritability, is seen in some. Electrolyte imbalance and sepsis are constant threats and should be appropriately treated when they occur. In addition, reversible cerebral atrophy (more likely a dehydration) can be observed. Therefore, it is important to obtain diagnostic CT scans in children before and after treatment with ACTH.

The benzodiazepine nitrazepam may be an acceptable alternative to steroid therapy, especially if side effects are troublesome. Most authors agree, however, that the benzodiazepines are less effective

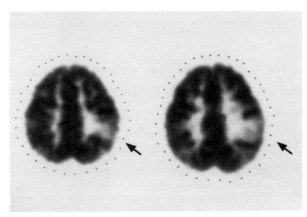

FIGURE 1. PET scan in a child with infantile spasms showing a well-demarcated left parietotemporal focus (*arrows*) of decreased glucose metabolism. An MRI scan was normal. The surgical specimen showed microscopic cortical dysplasia.

than steroids. The dose of nitrazepam is 0.5 to 1 mg/kg/d in two divided doses. Side effects include sedation and increased salivation. Nitrazepam is not approved for use in the United States, but is available in most epilepsy centers.

Valproic acid appears to control seizures in 20% to 40% of patients with infantile spasms. It may be used as maintenance therapy following hormonal treatment or when the latter has failed. We start with a dose of 20 mg/kg/d and increase as needed depending on the clinical response. The use of valproic acid is limited by potential hepatotoxicity, especially in the younger age group (under age 2 years). Valproic acid preferably should be used as a single agent, and liver function tests should be regularly monitored.

Other medical therapies that have been tried include pyridoxine, which is successful in pyridoxine-dependent patients, intravenous immunoglobulin and thyrotropin-releasing hormone (TRH). Vigabatrin, currently in clinical trials, has been reported to be useful in patients with infantile spasms, especially those with focal or multifocal EEG abnormalities such as would be seen in patients with tuberous sclerosis.

SURGICAL TREATMENT

Some patients with infantile spasms have focal cerebral lesions of various etiologies, and their resection has resulted in improvement of both seizures and cognitive development. Some of the lesions, such as astrocytoma, ganglioglioma, and porencephalic cyst, can be identified by CT or MRI. Others are more readily identified by positron emission tomography (PET) of cerebral glucose metabolism. PET has proven to be extremely sensitive in detecting focal functional cortical abnormalities (Fig. 1) associated with focal cortical dysplasias not visualized on CT or MRI. It is recommended that surgical intervention be considered in medically refractory cases to avoid the onset of an epileptic encephalopathy.

At present, it is recommended that the selection criteria for surgical treatment include the following.

1. Intractability of seizures—the child's seizures should be refractory to medical management, including the use of newer anticonvulsants.
2. Focal features on EEG—focal abnormalities should be present on interictal or ictal EEGs and should include focal slowing, focal epileptiform activity, focal decreased amplitude, and abnormal sodium thiopental activation.
3. Focal abnormalities on neuroimaging—all potential surgical candidates should show either an anatomic (CT or MRI) or metabolic (PET) lesion.

HEADACHE

SARA C. MCINTIRE, M.D.

Headache is a challenging complaint made regularly to physicians. The most important headache types for the practitioner are those that are most common—migraine and tension-type (formerly called muscle contraction or psychogenic headache)—and those headaches that are least common but most ominous: traction headaches. Families are often very anxious about chronic or recurrent headaches and may constrain pediatricians to order multiple studies or prescribe strong analgesics. However, migraine and tension-type headache account for the majority of chronic and recurrent headaches. Effective headache therapy depends on a correct diagnosis, and the key to an accurate and specific diagnosis is a detailed history and physical examination. Indiscriminate use of imaging studies is rarely helpful. This section delineates major clinical aspects of migraine, tension-type, and traction headaches and suggests therapy for migraine and tension-type headaches. Recommended doses of selected medications are shown in Table 1.

MIGRAINE

Migraine is a genetic disorder comprised of acute, recurrent attacks of headache. The pathogenesis of migraine as a primary vascular disorder is no longer in favor. Rather, neurogenic inflammation involving serotonin receptors may account for all migraine phenomena. Migraine can be clinically subdivided into migraine with aura (classic migraine), migraine without aura (common migraine), and complicated migraine (migraine with neurologic deficits). Clinical features include the occurrence of prodromes and auras, frontal or unilateral temporal pulsating pain that is moderate to severe, nausea, vomiting, abdominal pain, photophobia, exacerbation of the pain by motion, relief of the headache by rest or sleep, and a family history of migraine. Migraines usually last for several hours but may last longer or occur in clusters over several consecutive days. Other features include provocation by triggers, such as foods, menses, oral contraceptives, fatigue, or stress. A history of motion sickness or cyclic vomiting in early childhood is elicited frequently in patients with migraine. With the exception of the complicated migraine, the physical examination of the patient with migraine is normal.

TENSION-TYPE HEADACHE

The precise etiology of tension-type headache is unknown. The theory that it results from sustained contraction of the muscles of the head and neck has been disputed. The pain is dull or aching, mild to moderate in intensity, and located across the forehead or in both temples. The duration of the headache varies from hours to days. The frequency may be such that the patient will complain of headache for weeks to months at a time. Auras and prodromes are absent. Anorexia and nausea, but not vomiting, may be present. The physical examination is normal, although some patients may complain of discomfort on palpation of head and neck muscles.

TRACTION HEADACHES

Traction headaches arise from stress on pain-sensitive structures. They are the least common type but the most worrisome because they signify structural pathology. They are chronic and progress over weeks to months but, on occasion, occur acutely as a single or recurrent headache. Persistent pain located in the occiput or neck is common. A classic symptom is headache in the morning when the patient awakens but which then resolves. Valsalva maneuvers, such as coughing, straining, or squatting, may worsen the pain. The headache is rarely the only symptom or sign of the underlying disorder. A careful review of systems elicits typical symptoms, such as vomiting, weakness, double vision, ataxia, or personality changes, suggestive of tumors, hydrocephalus, and other causes of increased intracranial pressure. Eventually, the physical examination becomes appreciably abnormal.

THERAPY

For the patient with migraine or tension-type headache, reassurance that the pain is *not* due to a malignant cause is important to diminish anxiety. Next, children and their families must understand the basis for each type of treatment and the correct use of behavioral techniques and medications. Ample sleep, exercise, and a healthy diet are essential to any program of headache management. School attendance, despite headache, is imperative. Patients *must* have access to medications and a place to rest at school in the event of headache. Parents should downplay any secondary gain derived from complaints of pain and reward the child who functions as usual despite headache.

It is mandatory to identify triggers and overuse of medications that can cause or exacerbate headaches. A headache diary is invaluable in this regard. For 4 to 8 weeks, patients should record the number, severity, and duration of headaches, the time and circumstances in which they occurred, associated foods, drinks, and stresses, and all medications taken. The physician must then review this information and help the patient identify components that provoke or aggravate the headaches.

Therapy of Migraine

Medical treatment is divided into three phases: symptomatic relief when the headache is established, abortive treatment, and prophylactic measures for the patient with frequent or disabling migraines.

Symptomatic and Abortive Treatment

The child with a migraine should be allowed to rest or sleep in a dark and quiet room. Simple analgesics are preferred for the initial symptomatic treatment of migraine. Acetaminophen (Tylenol) and ibuprofen (Motrin) are effective, well tolerated, and available in liquid formulations for the child unwilling to swallow pills. Aspirin, although not routinely recommended for young children because of Reye syndrome, is effective and may be used safely in adolescents, with appropriate precautions. The medication should be taken *immediately* at the onset of the aura, prodrome, or headache. For older children and adolescents who fail to respond to simple analgesics, compound

TABLE 1. Pharmacotherapy of Migraine and Tension-type Headache

CATEGORY	DOSAGE
Analgesics	
Acetaminophen (Tylenol)	10–15 mg/kg per dose q4h
Ibuprofen (Motrin)	30–70 mg/kg/d t.i.d.
Acetaminophen/caffeine/butalbital* (Fioricet)	1–2 tablets at once, then 1 tablet q4h Max: 6 tablets per day
Isometheptene mucate/ dichloralphenazone/acetamino-phen* (Midrin)	1–2 capsules at once, then 1 capsule q1h Max: 4 capsules per day
Prophylactic Agents	
Propranolol (Inderal)	Under 35 kg: 10–20 mg per dose t.i.d. Over 35 kg: 20–40 mg per dose t.i.d.
Cyproheptadine (Periactin)	0.25–0.4 mg/kg/d divided q12h or q8h
Amitriptyline (Elavil)	25–50 mg qhs
Muscle Relaxant	
Diazepam (Valium)	Under 30 kg: 1–2 mg/d Over 30 kg: 2–5 mg/d

*Not recommended in young children: dosages are for children over 12 years.

analgesics containing acetaminophen, caffeine, and butalbital (Fioricet) or isometheptene mucate, dichloralphenazone, and acetaminophen (Midrin) are effective in both the acute treatment of established headaches and as abortive agents in patients experiencing auras.

Concurrent administration of an antiemetic is sometimes necessary in children with intense vomiting. Promethazine (Phenergan), trimethobenzamide hydrochloride (Tigan), and prochlorperazine (Compazine) can be used in children and adolescents and are available in oral and rectal preparations. Metoclopramide hydrochloride (Reglan), a prokinetic agent used for its antinausea effect in conjunction with analgesics, also has been shown in adults to be effective as a single analgesic agent in patients with migraine.[3]

Historically, ergot compounds have been used for abortive treatment of migraine in adults and adolescents but not in younger children. Dihydroergotamine mesylate (DHE 45) is a serotonin agonist that is useful for symptomatic and abortive treatment of severe migraine attacks in adults. Although it has not been studied extensively in children, it is now employed by some pediatric neurologists, especially for the treatment of severe or intractable migraine. For symptomatic or abortive treatment, sumatriptan succinate (Imitrex) is a serotonin receptor agonist useful in adult migraine and cluster headaches. However, its safety and efficacy in young children are unknown.

Finally, biofeedback and relaxation training clearly have a role in treatment of migraine.[1] The obvious benefits of such techniques include the avoidance of adverse drug effects and the sense of well-being patients derive from the feeling of mastery and control over their headaches. However, unless the primary physician is trained in these remedies, referral to an experienced physical therapist or psychologist is required.

Migraine Prophylaxis

Preventive therapy is indicated for the patient with frequent or disabling migraines. A headache diary may help identify triggers and prevent some, if not all, headaches. Propranolol (Inderal) is the drug of choice for many practitioners. It is contraindicated in patients with asthma and cardiac conduction defects. More cardioselective beta-blockers, such as metoprolol (Lopressor), may be used cautiously in patients with mild asthma. Cyproheptadine (Periactin) and amitriptyline (Elavil) are alternative agents for prophylaxis, although weight gain and sedation can be problematic with cyproheptadine, and asthma is a contraindication to its use. Documentation of a normal ECG is recommended before initiating therapy with amitriptyline. Patients and families must always be informed of its sedating effects and the consequences of overdose. An adequate trial of any prophylactic medicine will require 4 to 8 weeks of treatment. Furthermore, a headache diary should be kept during that time to monitor the response to therapy. Once good control is achieved, breakthrough episodes can be managed symptomatically. Prophylactic medicines should be tapered and discontinued after 3 to 6 months or during school vacations. Many children do not require a second trial. Again, biofeedback and relaxation training can play a primary role in migraine prophylaxis, particularly for those patients motivated by a desire to avoid medications.

Therapy of Tension-Type Headache

Symptomatic Treatment

The chronic nature of tension-type headaches makes treatment difficult. These patients need reassurance that the headache is not due to an organic process and that the pain is accepted as real. Depression is a feature in many children and adolescents with tension-type headache and is an indication to refer the patient for psychologic evaluation and therapy. Although medications play a role in treatment, the importance of psychologic therapy, biofeedback, relaxation training, and physical therapy cannot be underestimated and may be more effective than medication alone.

Tension-type headaches may be treated with the same analgesics used for migraine. Even though sustained muscle contraction may not be the primary disturbance in tension-type headache, muscle relaxants, such as diazepam (Valium), often are helpful. In patients with depression as a component of their headaches, amitriptyline offers antidepressant as well as analgesic effects. Although codeine may be effective, narcotic use in general should be avoided.

The management of tension-type, analgesic-rebound headache is particularly challenging. These increasingly severe headaches result from overuse of analgesics. Patients need a clear explanation of this phenomenon and must also understand that overuse of analgesics may diminish the effects of other medications, such as antidepressants.[2]

GOALS OF THERAPY AND PROGNOSIS

The goals of therapy are to prevent headaches, to treat exacerbations effectively, and to allow the child or adolescent to lead a normal life. Ultimately, the prognosis for both migraine and tension-type headaches is good. For patients with migraine, there is a high rate of spontaneous remission even in patients with severe or frequent attacks. Patients with tension-type headaches have a moderate rate of spontaneous remission and are at no increased risk of epilepsy or organic disease.

REFERENCES

1. Duckro P, Cantwell-Simmons E: A review of studies evaluating biofeedback and relaxation training in the management of pediatric headache. Headache 29:428–433, 1989.
2. Kudrow L: Paradoxical effects of frequent analgesic use. Adv Neurol 33:335–341, 1982.
3. Tek DS, McClellan DS, Olshaker JS, et al: A prospective, double-blind study of metoclopramide hydrochloride for the control of migraine in the emergency department. Ann Emerg Med 19:1083–1087, 1990.

BENIGN INTRACRANIAL HYPERTENSION

ELIZABETH C. ENGLE, M.D.
DAVID HOLTZMAN, M.D., Ph.D.

The syndrome of benign intracranial hypertension (BIH), or pseudotumor cerebri, is diagnosed when an alert child has elevated intracranial pressure (ICP > 200 mm H_2O), normal cerebrospinal fluid (CSF), and normal scans of the brain (no mass or hydrocephalus) by computed tomography (CT) or magnetic resonance imaging (MRI). *BIH is a misnomer, since these children are at significant risk for visual loss and require close neurologic and ophthalmologic care.* Evaluation and rational treatment of BIH require an understanding of etiology, diagnosis, and therapeutic options.

BIH of childhood occurs at all ages and affects males and females equally. Children usually present with a combination of headache, blurred vision, transient visual obscurations, and diplopia. The headache is characteristic of increased ICP and is often associated with vomiting. Signs of BIH include papilledema, unilateral or bilateral sixth nerve palsy (a false localizing sign), and deterioration in visual acuity and visual fields. Infants may present only with irritability, lethargy, vomiting, and split sutures and/or a bulging fontanelle without papilledema.

Table 1 lists conditions associated with BIH. In most cases, the etiology remains unknown. Before the advent of aggressive antibiotic therapy, BIH often was associated with otitis media and mastoiditis, with secondary venous sinus thrombosis. Today, it is more commonly associated with obesity, chronic steroid use and withdrawal, malnourishment and refeeding, anemia, antibiotics, or megavitamins. One of the first steps in therapy is to eliminate any potential etiologic factors.

In most children the prognosis of BIH is good. A significant percentage recover after a single diagnostic lumbar puncture (LP), and approximately half are normal by 6 months. Some children experience

TABLE 1. Conditions Associated with Benign Intracranial Hypertension

Intracranial Venous Drainage Obstruction
Mastoiditis and lateral (sigmoid) sinus obstruction
Extracerebral mass lesions
Congenital atresia or stenosis of venous sinuses
Head trauma
Cryofibrinogenemia
Polycythemia vera
Paranasal sinus and pharyngeal infections

Cervical or Thoracic Venous Drainage Obstruction
Intrathoracic mass lesions and postoperative obstruction of venous return

Endocrine Dysfunction
Pregnancy
Menarche
Marked menstrual irregularities
Oral contraceptives
Obesity
Withdrawal of corticosteroid therapy
Addison's disease
Hypoparathyroidism
Catchup growth after deprivation, treatment of cystic fibrosis, correction of heart anomaly
Initiation of thyroxine treatment for hypothyroidism
Adrenal hyperplasia
Adrenal adenoma

Hematologic Disorders
Acute iron deficiency anemia
Pernicious anemia
Thrombocytopenia
Wiskott-Aldrich syndrome

Vitamin Metabolism
Chronic hypervitaminosis A
Acute hypervitaminosis A
Hypovitaminosis A
Cystic fibrosis and hypovitaminosis A
Vitamin D-deficiency rickets

Drug Reaction
Tetracycline
Perhexiline maleate
Nalidixic acid
Sulfamethoxazole
Indomethacin
Penicillin

Prophylactic Antisera

Miscellaneous
Galactosemia
Galactokinase deficiency
Sydenham's chorea
Sarcoidosis
Roseola infantum
Hypophosphatasia
Paget's disease
Maple syrup urine disease
Turner's syndrome

a progressive or recurrent syndrome and are refractory to medical therapy. Early clinical series found no visual loss in pediatric patients and concluded that children are protected from optic nerve damage. However, subsequent reports have firmly established that children, like adults, are at significant risk for optic neuropathy. The CSF, which is contained within the subarachnoid space between the optic nerve and surrounding dural sheath, transmits the elevated pressure to this compartment. Visual loss occurs when the increased CSF pressure compresses the nerve. The early changes of optic neuropathy are increased size of the physiologic blind spot and constriction of visual fields. Later, decreased visual acuity and blindness develop. Ophthalmologic testing, therefore, must include formal visual field and contrast and color desaturation testing. Visual evoked potentials (VEPs) are abnormal, with decreased visual acuity, and do not detect the early changes of optic neuropathy. The occurrence and progression of visual loss are unpredictable. Visual loss can progress insidiously or occur suddenly. It may be present at diagnosis, may occur during treatment, or may be found only late in the disease. It does not correlate with the degree of papilledema, the presence of diplopia, or the extent of visual symptoms. Visual loss can improve or can be completely reversed with treatment, even after optic atrophy has developed.

The patient in whom BIH is suspected must undergo neuroimaging for the presence of hydrocephalus, a mass lesion, subarachnoid or intraparenchymal hemorrhage, or demyelination. MRI is recommended over CT because it provides information about the patency of the venous sinuses and abnormalities in the brain.

If the imaging study is normal, a lumbar puncture should be performed. The first LP has both diagnostic and therapeutic benefits. The opening pressure must be recorded with the patient horizontal, breathing comfortably, and relaxed, with neck and legs extended. Although premedication and patience may be required, this technique ensures that the pressure is not falsely elevated. Fluid should be determined for cell count and differential, protein, and glucose. Normal CSF is

evidence against meningeal infection or inflammation, subarachnoid hemorrhage, or a demyelinating process. Enough fluid must be removed to lower the closing pressure to less than 100 mm H_2O. This usually ranges from 10 to 30 ml and depends on the size of the patient.

TREATMENT

The two goals of treatment of BIH are relief of symptoms and preservation of visual function. Symptomatic complaints can often be controlled medically by the use of serial LPs, carbonic anhydrase inhibitors, corticosteroids and analgesics, and surgery. *Neuroophthalmologists generally agree that a lumboperitoneal shunt or optic nerve sheath fenestration should be performed with any deterioration of vision.* The choice of treatment options is patient dependent, but general guidelines for each are discussed here.

Lumbar Puncture

The LP provides a nonspecific CSF leak that, if the dura is torn slightly, may continue to drain slowly and lower CSF pressure. Some patients have lasting symptomatic relief. Most clinicians repeat the LP after a day in order to document a persistent elevation in pressure. After two or three taps, however, LPs become painful and frightening to children. Single pressure recordings may not be accurate. If the patient is asymptomatic and frequent ophthalmologic findings remain normal, there is no indication for serial LPs or other treatment. Such a patient still needs monthly neuroophthalmologic evaluation.

Medications

When a patient has persistently elevated pressure on two taps and is symptomatic without visual deterioration, it is appropriate to begin acetazolamide (up to a maximum of 60 mg/kg/d), a carbonic acid inhibitor that decreases CSF production. Side effects include acid-base and electrolyte imbalances, renal calculi, gastrointestinal upset, and appetite suppression. Occasionally, furosemide (2 mg/kg three times a day) is used also. Headaches may be controlled by conventional analgesics for tension or vascular pain (nonsteroidal anti-inflammatories, amitriptyline, beta-blockers, periactin). It is essential that these be used only if the patient complies with frequent ophthalmologic appointments. Freedom from headache does not ensure lack of optic nerve damage.

Steroids

The use of steroids for treatment of BIH in children is controversial. It is generally agreed that steroids should not be used for more than several weeks. Long-term use is associated with severe side effects, including weight gain, cushingoid features, acne, and proximal myopathy. If prolonged use appears necessary to control symptoms or if visual deterioration occurs during steroid therapy, the patient should be evaluated for surgery.

Surgery

Surgery is indicated as initial therapy in a patient who presents with visual loss. The first surgical treatment for BIH was a subtemporal decompression. This was abandoned because of failures and complications. *Lumboperitoneal shunts* have been effective for patients with headaches refractory to medical management and no visual loss. The shunt allows CSF to flow down a pressure gradient from the lumbar subarachnoid space into the peritoneum, where it is reabsorbed. When constant drainage is provided, the optic nerve is protected from intermittent pressure spikes. Shunts have the disadvantage of necessitating revisions and serving as a nidus for infection. Low-pressure headaches can occur in shunted patients in whom BIH has resolved.

The most recent advance in treatment of BIH is *optic nerve sheath fenestration*. If the dura and meninges surrounding the optic nerve are opened just behind the globe, CSF can continuously escape, and pressure within the subarachnoid space around the nerve is decompressed. In most adults this procedure has yielded stable to improved visual acuity and visual fields, with relief of headache in more than 50%. Unilateral surgery has improved papilledema bilaterally. Optic atrophy preoperatively does not predict a poor outcome. This procedure is becoming the treatment of choice in any child whose visual acuity or visual fields show deterioration.

REFERENCE

1. Lessell S, Rosman NP: Permanent visual impairment in childhood pseudotumor cerebri. Arch Neurol 43:801-804, 1986.

CEREBROVASCULAR DISEASE

ELIZABETH C. DOOLING, M.D.

Cerebrovascular disease affects about 3700 infants and children each year. Often, the stroke is preceded by an apparently mild febrile or afebrile illness or develops after a prolonged seizure or injury in a previously healthy infant or child. Mortality is low in most acutely hemiplegic infants and children, but morbidity is high. Hemiparesis or quadriparesis, epilepsy, visual or speech disorders, learning disabilities, and behavior disorders are the usual sequelae. The prognosis for normal intelligence may be better when the event is not associated with status epilepticus and fever and the child is over 2 years of age.

Although diverse in etiology, cerebrovascular diseases may be classified broadly as either occlusive, resulting in ischemia in a vascular territory, or hemorrhagic with dissection of blood into the surrounding tissue. The categories of cerebrovascular disorders in order of their incidence are occlusion (thrombotic or embolic), hemorrhage, hemoglobinopathy, vasculopathy, and coagulopathy. Trauma, metabolic disorders, and neoplasm may make these conditions manifest, or the disorders may arise de novo. For patients with refractory posthemiplegic seizure or movement disorders, surgical intervention, for

example, hemispherectomy or thalamotomy, may be indicated when medical, that is, pharmacologic, means are exhausted.

Advances in neuroimaging technology (CT scans and MRI) not only have allowed the visualization of acute intracranial hemorrhages and cerebral infarctions but also have shown previously unrecognized vascular malformations or earlier undiagnosed or asymptomatic hemorrhages. Whereas both kinds of scans can easily demonstrate areas of hemorrhage or infarction after an acute injury, MRI sequences for magnetic susceptibility can identify blood products for several months after the initial hemorrhage. Magnetic resonance imaging-angiography (MRA), using 3-D time-of-flight or phase contrast sequences, is a sensitive way to detect vascular abnormalities in the anterior and posterior cerebral circulations. The advantages of MRA are twofold: contrast medium is not necessary, and general anesthesia usually can be avoided. As MRA becomes more widely used and the results are compared with traditional invasive angiography, the use of transfemoral angiography should decrease.

Insults to the developing infant brain may be sustained in the prenatal and perinatal periods but may not become manifest until the patient is several months old and disuse or weakness of the arm(s) and leg(s) is recognized. Acute events will be heralded postnatally by fever, vomiting, headache, loss of consciousness, gait changes, dysphasia, visual complaints, weakness, or seizures.

ARTERIAL OR VENOUS OCCLUSIVE DISORDERS

Patients with acute or subacute occlusive cerebrovascular disease experience weakness, slurred speech, visual disturbances (visual scotoma or hemianopia), and focal or generalized seizures associated with headache, nausea, vomiting, lethargy, somnolence, and obtundation. Table 1 lists conditions in which arterial or venous occlusions may be observed.

The underlying disorder must be identified, and appropriate therapy must be started to increase collateral circulation and minimize tissue damage in the hypoperfused region. Whenever feasible, heart disease should be corrected if the patient weighs enough and is clinically stable. If vascular occlusion has resulted from thrombus or embolus, anticoagulation with heparin in the acute phase followed by warfarin or aspirin for 6 to 12 months or more should be considered. Thrombectomy, surgical bypass of stenotic areas, or endarterectomy may be indicated in certain cases. Embolization of fistulas with Gelfoam or other sealants may be useful in children with inoperable arteriovenous malformations. The use of streptokinase or tissue plasminogen activator may not be appropriate for lysing clots in intracranial vessels because propagation of smaller clot fragments may cause additional neurologic deficits. Similarly, angioplasty may compromise already damaged tissue, and revascularization may result in hemorrhage in a previously underperfused area. If aggressive antibiotic therapy does not resolve the infection in a child with endocarditis, replacement of the infected valve may prevent further embolic events. There is controversy about the value of anticoagulation in hemolytic-uremic syndrome.

HEMORRHAGIC DISORDERS

Patients with acute intracranial hemorrhage have severe headache, meningismus with nuchal rigidity, diplopia, hemianopia, speech disturbance, vomiting, cranial nerve palsies, disorientation, agitation, somnolence or obtundation, or seizures. Intracranial vascular malformations occur ten times more frequently than cerebral aneurysms in infants and children. When aneurysms rupture, there may be sudden or apoplectic loss of consciousness and fulminant clinical deterioration. Some causes of intracranial hemorrhage are shown in Table 1.

Supportive care in the first hours of the hemorrhage is needed. After consultation with the neurosurgeon, a decision can be made about the risks and benefits of surgical excision of a vascular malformation, clipping of an aneurysm, or evacuation of a symptomatic hematoma. In some cases, radiosurgery with the gamma knife or single or fractionated proton beam therapy in conjunction with pre-

TABLE 1. Cerebrovascular Diseases

Arterial and Venous Occlusive Disorders
1. Porencephalic cysts secondary to an embolus or thrombus in a major intracranial vessel, such as the middle cerebral artery; in neonates, the embolus may originate in a placental vessel
2. Cyanotic congenital heart disease resulting in polycythemia and hypoxia, such as occurs in tetralogy of Fallot or transposition of the great vessels
3. Vascular malformations, e.g., vein of Galen malformation
4. Infarcts caused by emboli from indwelling arterial catheters or extracorporeal membrane oxygenation (ECMO)
5. Vasculitis secondary to intrauterine or postnatal CNS infections
6. Dysgenetic states, such as schizencephaly
7. Dehydration, mastoiditis, or otitis resulting in sagittal or lateral sinus thrombosis
8. Hemolytic-uremic syndrome and thrombotic thrombocytopenic purpura
9. Vascular stenosis secondary to cocaine or amphetamine use
10. Infectious endocarditis with or without vegetations
11. Postchemotherapy, e.g., after use of asparaginase
12. Postradiation vascular necrosis resulting in major vessel thrombosis
13. Aminoacidopathies, e.g., homocystinuria
14. Mitochondrial disorders including mitochondrial encephalopathy-lactic acidosis-strokelike syndrome (MELAS)
15. Migraine
16. Fat or air embolus
17. Trauma, e.g., tears of internal carotid artery resulting from soft palate or peritonsillar injury or carotid-cavernous fistula

Hemorrhagic Disorders
1. Intraventricular or intraparenchymal hemorrhage in prematurity
2. Rupture of arteriovenous malformation
3. Rupture of intracranial congenital or mycotic aneurysm
4. Rupture of venous or cavernous angioma, or hemangioma in von Hippel-Lindau disease
5. Pial-cortical bleeding in Sturge-Weber disease
6. Epidural hematoma, accidentally or purposely incurred
7. Subdural hematoma, accidentally or purposely incurred
8. Cerebral hematoma or contusion, accidentally or purposely incurred
9. Idiosyncratic reaction to diet pills containing phenylpropylamine
10. Thrombocytopenia or coagulopathies
11. Hemorrhage into vascular tumors, e.g., PNET, medulloblastoma
12. Acute hemorrhagic necrotizing encephalitis

Vasculopathies
1. Fibromuscular disease with or without neurofibromatosis
2. Moyamoya disease, idiopathic or postradiation
3. Dissection of media of internal carotid or vertebral artery because of blunt trauma or congenital dysplasia
4. Loops and kinks of internal carotid artery

Hemoglobinopathies
1. Sickle-cell aenmia
2. Hemoglobin C
3. Bart's hemoglobin

Coagulation Disorders
1. Hemophilia
2. Protein C deficiency
3. Protein S deficiency
4. Antithrombin III deficiency
5. von Willebrand's disease
6. Idiopathic thrombocytopenia purpura
7. Fanconi's anemia
8. Wiskott-Aldrich syndrome

---

operative and postoperative embolization may be superior to a neurosurgical procedure. Antifibrinolytic agents and calcium-channel blockers have also been used in selected cases. Administration of fresh platelets or fresh frozen plasma may be needed in patients with thrombocytopenia and coagulation disorders.

VASCULOPATHIES

These disorders result from structural abnormalities of one or more cerebral blood vessels. Table 1 lists frequently encountered types.

Surgical revascularization using grafting of the superior temporal artery to the dura has been used with success in many cases of moyamoya disease where collaterals supply some of the involved areas. Patients with dissection are treated with anticoagulation. Fibrinolytic agents have been used in a few patients with fixed deficits, without worsening of their condition.

HEMOGLOBINOPATHIES

The disorders listed in Table 1 result from inherited variants of hemoglobin synthesis (e.g., valine for glutamic acid in sickle-cell disease).

Doppler ultrasonography has been used to monitor the occurrence of thromboses in patients with sickle-cell disease. MRA does not require contrast material and decreases the risk of sickling in sickle-cell patients. Regular transfusion of sickle-cell disease patients to maintain the hemoglobin above 11 g/dl has been recommended as a way to decrease the incidence of strokes.

COAGULOPATHIES

These disorders (Table 1) result from inherited or immune-mediated deficiencies of platelets or soluble coagulation factors necessary for clot formation.

Administration of the deficient product, for example, factor VIII concentrate in hemophiliacs, or platelets is necessary.

REYE SYNDROME

FREDERICK H. LOVEJOY, JR., M.D.

In 1963, Reye and colleagues described a constellation of autopsy findings in children, consisting of cerebral edema (without perivascular or meningeal inflammation) and fatty infiltration of the liver (and, to a lesser extent, the pancreas, kidneys, and heart). The disease, Reye syndrome, even today is of unclear etiology. Cases were recognized with increasing frequency throughout the 1970s, reached a peak incidence of 0.88 cases per 100,000 in 1980, and progressively declined to 0.15 cases per 100,000 in 1985. Case fatality rates range from 10% to 40%, with reduced mortality ascribed to early recognition and improved intensive care management.

Predominantly a childhood illness, the median age of patients is 8 years. A viral illness, generally varicella or influenza A or B, precedes by several days the onset of the syndrome. Since 1980, attention has focused on the strong association observed between Reye syndrome and the use of aspirin, with the result that labeling of aspirin noting this association is now required by federal law.

Criteria for the diagnosis of Reye syndrome include the following.

1. A mild antecedent respiratory or gastrointestinal illness
2. Hepatic dysfunction defined by a blood ammonia greater than 50 μ/dl or an increase in serum liver enzymes and a prolonged prothrombin time

3. Objective evidence of CNS dysfunction (abnormalities on neurologic examination and a consistent electroencephalographic pattern, with *normal* cerebrospinal fluid findings)
4. Liver biopsy revealing microvesicular fat with no displacement of the central nucleus and diagnostic mitochondrial alterations seen under electron microscopy
5. Exclusion of other diseases with a similar clinical presentation (chronic salicylate and acute acetaminophen poisoning, viral encephalitis, lead poisoning, viral hepatitis)

A national staging system has been useful in describing the clinical and biochemical course and in following and grading its severity.

Stage I—lethargy, drowsiness, vomiting, elevation in serum liver enzymes, normal blood ammonia level, and grade I EEG (Lombroso grading)

Stage II—disorientation, combativeness, hyperventilation, tachycardia, pupillary dilation, hyperactive reflexes, purposeful response to painful stimuli, bilateral Babinski reflex, elevation in blood ammonia and serum liver enzymes, and grade II or III EEG

Stage III—coma, upper midbrain involvement (loss of ciliospinal reflex, pupillary dilation, decorticate posturing in response to painful stimuli, bilateral Babinski reflex), persistent elevation in blood ammonia and serum liver enzymes, and grade III or IV EEG

Stage IV—coma, further rostrocaudal progression of midbrain involvement (loss of doll's head maneuver, sluggish pupillary response to light, decerebrate rigidity and posturing to painful stimuli, bilateral Babinski reflex), decreased blood ammonia and serum liver enzyme activity, and grade III or IV EEG

Stage V—coma, loss of response to stimuli and to light or doll's head maneuver, cessation of spontaneous respiration, continued improvement in blood ammonia and serum liver enzyme activity, and grade IV or electrocerebral silence on EEG

The disease occurs in several discrete stages and can be limited in severity to any stage. Recovery occurs when illness is limited to stage I through III, and recovery from stage V does not occur. Other indices associated with poor outcome include rapid passage through clinical stages, a blood ammonia level greater than 300 μ/dl, a prothrombin time two times greater than control, and an increase in liver *and* skeletal creatine phosphokinase.

Diagnosis is made by clinical and laboratory findings. A lumbar puncture is relatively contraindicated and should be preceded by cranial tomography to rule out cerebral edema. Liver biopsy should be reserved for patients in whom the diagnosis is unclear. Early diagnosis appears to improve clinical outcome. Suspicion for the disease should be raised in children who have altered mental status and severe vomiting after a viral illness (varicella) or use of aspirin.

TREATMENT

There is no specific treatment for Reye syndrome. Because of the striking increase in arterial blood ammonia, lactulose and neomycin to decrease its generation by enteric bacteria and administration of citrulline and arginine have been used. There are no data indicating that these maneuvers affect outcome. Exchange transfusion and peritoneal dialysis have also been used and subsequently abandoned because of lack of a beneficial change in outcome. Children with Reye syndrome are best cared for in a pediatric intensive care unit.

With the basic pathophysiologic derangement and cause of death being cerebral edema, therapy directed toward correcting this abnormal physiology has been pursued. Monitoring of increased intracranial pressure should be performed. The use of intracranial monitoring devices has made assessment of intracranial pressure more objective. With such devices, mannitol to maintain serum osmolarity between 300 and 320 mOSM/kg and nasotracheal intubation with ventilatory control to maintain P_{CO_2} between 20 and 30 mm Hg can maintain the intracranial pressure below 15 mm Hg and the cerebral perfusion pressure at 40 mm Hg or better. These maneuvers are ideally instituted in stage II patients with ominous prognostic signs or in stage III patients. Steroids have not proven useful in managing cerebral edema.

Barbiturate-induced coma has been used in cases of uncontrolled cerebral edema in an effort to decrease cerebral metabolic demands. A clear benefit from this approach has not been shown.

Other therapies for Reye syndrome include judicious use of fluids with 10% dextrose concentrations, vitamin K to correct prolonged prothrombin time, and phenytoin to control seizures. Children must have careful outpatient follow-up. They may recover fully neurologically, but many have subsequent behavioral and adverse educational sequelae.

REFERENCES

1. Aoki Y, Lombroso CT: Prognostic value of electroencephalography in Reye's syndrome. Neurology 23:33, 1973.
2. Consensus Conference. Diagnosis and treatment of Reye's syndrome. JAMA 246:2441–2444, 1981.

NEUROBLASTOMA

ALEXANDER A. GREEN, M.D.

Neuroblastoma is the most common tumor seen in young children. The age at the time of diagnosis ranges from prenatal recognition to rare occurrences in teenagers. Nearly 30% of cases will be diagnosed before 1 year of age, the median age is 22 months, and between 80% and 90% will be found before the child is 6 years old. Its incidence is approximately 1 case per 100,000 children per year worldwide. Neuroblastoma arises from neural crest cells within the adrenal gland (40%) or sympathetic ganglia in paraspinal locations from the neck to the pelvis. Its cause is still unknown and seems unrelated to environmental or genetic factors. It is speculated, however, that genetic factors may play a role, since familial cases have been documented. Furthermore, epidemiologic surveys have suggested environmental exposures, but none have been confirmed by other studies. The unique biologic behavior of this disease has led to wide speculation regarding cause and optimum treatment.

Children with the benign tumor, ganglioneuroma, are thought to represent cases of spontaneous maturation of neuroblastoma. It is common to find some degree of differentiation expressed at the time of diagnosis and even during treatment of neuroblastoma. The impact of this unique feature on a child's prognosis, as well as the phenomenon of spontaneous regression, unfortunately cannot be predicted or measured at the time of diagnosis.

Today, infants and children less than 1 year old when diagnosed, regardless of stage, and older children with localized disease have an excellent prognosis. In contrast, children older than 1 year of age with disseminated disease have a very poor prognosis even with modern multimodality therapy. Our goal has always been early diagnosis and accurate determination of the extent of disease (stage). However, the sites of origin are silent, and it is usually the symptoms of metastatic disease that bring the child to medical attention. These complaints unfortunately are nonspecific (e.g., fever and irritability) and usually are ascribed to more common disorders.

DIAGNOSIS

The diagnosis of neuroblastoma usually follows a period of illness ascribed to other more common disorders and is uncovered when studies are performed to better characterize why the child has not responded to common treatments. There are no unique early findings. Thus, the disease is disseminated when first recognized in over 50% of children. However, its treatment and the child's prognosis are largely dependent on the stage of disease and the child's age. Tumor begins within the adrenal gland in approximately 40% and elsewhere in the abdomen in another 20%. Less than 5% occur within the neck or pelvis, and the rest begin within the thoracic cavity. The location of these sites close to the spinal canal explains the frequent occurrence

TABLE 1. Workup of Child with Neuroblastoma

TEST	PRIMARY VALUE
Diagnostic imaging	Measurement of tumor volume and organ involvement
Ultrasound	At best a screening study
CT scan	Excellent study to demonstrate extent of tumor
MR scan	Useful to evaluate spinal cord compression
Skeletal radiographs	In young children localized bone scan of abnormal sites may be necessary
Nuclear medicine	Can evaluate many sites at the same time
^{99m}Tc bone scan	Needed as initial study of all children with this tumor
MIBG scan	Of little practical use (positive with ganglioneuroma)
Urine catecholamines	If elevated can be useful follow-up tool; however, positive with ganglioneuroma.
Bone marrow aspirate and biopsy	Several sites must be sampled; positive in >50%
Clinical chemistries	Needed to evaluate multiple organ function
BUN, creatinine, uric acid	Renal function
Serum enzymes	Liver function
Special tumor tissue analysis	Needed for planning treatment and estimating prognosis
DNA ploidy	Essential in infants with disseminated disease
N-*myc* copy number	Prognostic importance for infants and older children
Lymph node involvement	Accurate staging

of neurologic abnormalities associated with neuroblastoma. The location also explains its silent enlargement and dissemination before the child is recognized to be seriously ill. Fever without a recognized focus, pain and skeletal complaints without injury, ecchymoses about the eyes, and proptosis without trauma all are frequently present at the time of diagnosis. It is seldom that significant weight loss or poor appetite is a reason for seeking medical care, although these are frequently recorded for children with advanced disease. Horner syndrome often is associated with neck and upper thoracic primary sites.

Typically, the child will be found to have a calcified mass (70%) in a paraspinal location, be less than 3 years old, and have generalized constitutional complaints of more than 4 months duration. Once suspected, neuroblastoma frequently is easily diagnosed from the clinical findings and confirmed by biopsy. Table 1 suggests the most useful tests for evaluating the child suspected or demonstrated to have neuroblastoma. Since the prognosis and treatment rely on extent of disease, this initial workup is the most important set of studies to perform and should be completed before surgical intervention is planned. If neuroblastoma is suspected, an appropriate workup should be performed by the clinical team that will eventually plan treatment and care for the child. A panel of blood studies should be obtained, but none is specific for neuroblastoma. The serum LDH is high because of frequent intralesional trapping and destruction of red blood cells, as well as tumor cell necrosis. If neuroblastoma is suspected, a bone marrow aspirate, which will be positive in 50%, may preclude an initial surgical procedure and permit a tissue diagnosis by biopsy.

STAGING

Neuroblastoma disseminates by hematogenous as well as lymphatic spread and by direct extension. Thus the primary site as well as known metastatic sites (lymph node, bone marrow, liver, and skeleton) must be carefully evaluated. Extensive surgical resection of a child with disseminated disease is not necessary before beginning treatment and is best reserved for later to aid in assessment of response. Table 2 outlines the current staging criteria for children with neuroblastoma. The International System was proposed recently to better link the surgical-pathologic staging system of the Pediatric Oncology Group (POG) and the clinical staging system used by the Children's Cancer Study Group (CCSG). Until treatment outcome improves for older children with disseminated disease, the fundamental criteria for stag-

TABLE 2. Staging Systems for Neuroblastoma

INTERNATIONAL (INSS)	PEDIATRIC ONCOLOGY GROUP (POG) SYSTEM	CHILDREN'S CANCER STUDY GROUP (CCSG) SYSTEM
Stage 1. Localized tumor confined to the area of origin; complete gross excision, with or without microscopic residual disease; identifiable ipsilateral and contralateral lymph nodes negative microscopically	**Stage A.** Complete gross resection of the primary tumor, with or without microscopic residual disease. Intracavitary lymph nodes not adhered to the primary tumor must be histologically free of tumor. Nodes adhered to the surface of or within the primary may be positive	**Stage I.** Tumor confined to the organ or structure of origin
Stage 2A. Unilateral tumor with incomplete gross excision; identifiable ipsilateral and contralateral lymph nodes negative microscopically	**Stage B.** Grossly unresected primary tumor. Nodes and nodules the same as in stage A	**Stage II.** Tumor extending in continuity beyond the organ or structure of origin, but not crossing the midline. Regional lymph nodes on the ipsilateral side may be involved
Stage 2B. Unilateral tumor with complete or incomplete gross excision; with positive ipsilateral regional lymph nodes; identifiable contralateral lymph nodes negative microscopically		
Stage 3. Tumor infiltrating across the midline with or without regional lymph node involvement; or, unilateral tumor with contralateral regional lymph node involvement; or, midline tumor with bilateral lymph node involvement	**Stage C.** Complete or incomplete resection of primary. Intracavitary nodes not adhered to primary must be histologically positive for tumor. Liver as in stage A	**Stage III.** Tumor extending in continuity beyond the midline. Regional lymph nodes may be involved bilaterally
Stage 4. Dissemination of tumor to distant lymph nodes, bone, bone marrow, liver and/or other organs (except as defined in stage 4S)	**Stage D.** Dissemination of disease beyond intracavitary nodes (i.e., extracavitary nodes, liver, skin, bone marrow, etc.)	**Stage IV.** Remote disease involving the skeleton, bone marrow, soft tissue and distant lymph node groups (see stage IV-S)
Stage 4S. Localized primary tumor as defined for stage 1 or 2 with dissemination limited to liver, skin, and/or bone marrow	**Stage DS.** Infants <1 year of age with stage 4S disease (see INSS)	**Stage IV-S.** As defined in stage I or II, except for the presence of remote disease confined to the liver, skin, or marrow (without bone metastases)

ing are localized, regional, or disseminated disease and age less than or greater than 1 year of age.

Assessment of the child's liver, kidney, and cardiovascular function is performed by the blood study panel and physical assessment. Symptomatic and supportive therapy for abnormal findings may be necessary before active therapy for neuroblastoma is started.

TREATMENT

Because of the high likelihood of dissemination of disease before diagnosis, chemotherapy is administered to nearly all children with neuroblastoma. However, supportive therapy to control pain, nutritional deficits, hypertension, and infection frequently is necessary. General recommendations for the use of the major treatment modalities and current treatment for disease focused by stage and age follow.

Surgery

As mentioned previously, the clinical findings suggest the correct diagnosis in nearly all cases. These findings, along with a positive bone marrow biopsy, are adequate to initiate treatment. However, surgical biopsy or even surgical resection of the primary tumor site may be required if localized disease is suggested by the initial workup. In patients with localized disease, surgical removal of tumor is curative without other therapy. Neuroblastoma has only a pseudocapsule around it at best, and when there is local lymph node dissemination, complete resection at the time of diagnosis often is not possible (less than 25%). More frequently, the role of surgery is to confirm the response and remove residual tumor after a period of chemotherapy. This delayed procedure can be curative for patients with regional or initially nonmetastatic but unresectable localized disease. The placement of a central venous access device is almost always required in these children.

Radiation Therapy

The use of radiation therapy remains controversial in the treatment of children with this disease. It can, however, aid in the cure of children with localized masses that have responded incompletely to drug therapy and remain unresectable.

Chemotherapy

A number of drugs are active against neuroblastoma (cyclophosphamide, doxorubicin, cisplatin, etoposide, ifosfamide, carboplatin, and vincristine). Many combinations and dosage schedules are being administered. Each child with neuroblastoma should be treated by one of the current clinical research protocols available at the time of diagnosis. Treatment should be administered by a team familiar with the clinical behavior of neuroblastoma who have the facilities of a pediatric center available to them.

Localized Disease (Stage A)

If localized disease is suspected from presurgical staging studies and confirmed at the time of surgery, these children need no other therapy. Careful follow-up is required, but 90% are expected to remain free of disease.

Localized Disease (Stage B)

Generally, cyclophosphamide and doxorubicin are administered for a period of 4 months, with possibly a second surgical procedure. This treatment is expected to lead to long-term disease-free survival in approximately 90% of patients.

Disseminated Disease (Stages C and D)

If the child is less than 1 year of age and has an aneuploid DNA index, administration of cyclophosphamide and doxorubicin for 4 months is curative in over 80%. If the infant's tumor has a normal DNA index, multiagent chemotherapy similar to that used in older children should be administered. Although the prognosis for infants with diploid tumors remains better than that for older children, it is much poorer than that for infants with aneuploid tumors.

Children over 1 year of age with disseminated disease have the poorest prognosis. Multiple combinations or high-dose chemotherapy are administered. Some current protocols advocate autologous or allogeneic bone marrow stem cell infusion as a consolidation therapy. Treatment for this group should be considered experimental, in that only 25% to 30% will survive the disease. The challenge is to maintain a positive aggressive approach through initial therapy, since no study can identify the small percentage who will be cured by therapy. In addition, long periods of disease-free survival are achieved even in those who will eventually die.

Evans Stage IV-S and POG Stage DS

The treatment of this small group of infants with disseminated neuroblastoma to skin, liver, and possibly bone marrow, without a large primary tumor or bone involvement, continues to be widely debated more than 20 years after they were identified as a subgroup. Some will undergo spontaneous regression. It is my opinion that since they all respond quickly to cyclophosphamide and doxorubicin, they should be treated with chemotherapy. Spontaneous regression, when it occurs (approximately 50% of the time), requires months for the disease to disappear, and these children are frequently quite ill with their tumors and require extensive supportive care until the tumor regresses.

Supportive Therapy

Supportive therapy of children with neuroblastoma frequently becomes the most important aspect of their therapy. Cancer in children can be devastating to a family, and the proper care of a child with neuroblastoma requires psychologic support for the entire family. The pediatric oncologist frequently becomes the child's primary care physician and must constantly assess normal growth and development expectations and be available to aid in the management of normal pediatric conditions. The management of pain in small children requires a close assessment of the child. Narcotics should be administered when required, since pain is a primary problem in all children with bone and bone marrow involvement (>50%).

It is recommended that all infants undergoing chemotherapy receive trimethoprim-sulfamethoxazole prophylaxis at least 3 days a week to prevent *Pneumocystis carinii* infections. Even with intensive therapy, older children do not appear at unusual risk for this organism. However, they have extended periods of neutropenia frequently associated with fever. At the first sign of fever, these children require aggressive antibiotic management until it is proven that sepsis does not exist. The use of central venous access devices only increases the risk of blood-borne infections.

Although uncommon, hypertension, most frequently from renal vessel involvement, must be managed aggressively. The frequent involvement of the spinal cord requires careful neurologic assessment and supportive care when paresis or plegia is present. Neurogenic bladder requires aggressive management to prevent upper tract problems and urinary tract infections. As previously mentioned, nutritional support frequently is required. Nasogastric feeding and even venous alimentation may be necessary. A weight loss of 10% or more requires immediate intervention. The needs of these children and their families require the availability of a cancer team usually only present in a center focused on tertiary pediatric care.

CHILDHOOD BRAIN TUMORS

CYNTHIA S. KRETSCHMAR, M.D.

The management of a child with a suspected tumor of the central nervous system (CNS) requires a multimodality team approach, which includes a pediatric oncologist, neuroendocrine and neuropsychologic subspecialists, a neurosurgeon, neurologist, and radiation therapist.

DIAGNOSIS

Two thirds of childhood brain tumors occur infratentorially, with pressure effects on the posterior fossa, CSF pathways, and brainstem. Common symptoms include headache, morning vomiting, ataxia, diplopia with sixth nerve compromise, facial asymmetry, head tilt, and drooling. Older adolescents more commonly develop supratentorial tumors with headache, paralysis, or seizures. Infants may develop large supratentorial masses with increased head size, lethargy, irritability, or failure to thrive. Radiologic evaluation always includes CT and/or MRI imaging. Furthermore, children with posterior fossa or germ cell tumors should have spinal MRI with gadolinium contrast or spinal myelography, since approximately 40% of children and 60% of infants less than 2 years of age may have tumor seeding. Bone scan and bone marrow biopsy are recommended in patients with medulloblastoma, and serum and CSF alpha-fetoprotein and beta-hCG should be determined in patients with suspected germ cell tumors in the pineal or suprasellar regions.

SURGERY

Since there is evidence that the extent of surgical resection is a determinant of prognosis, particularly for such tumors as medulloblastoma, children should be evaluated by a pediatric neurosurgeon familiar with microsurgical laser techniques and cavitron ultrasonic surgical aspiration (CUSA). Deep-seated tumors in the thalamic, hypothalamic, or pineal regions should be biopsied to differentiate germ cell neoplasms from low-grade or high-grade gliomas. Children with brainstem tumors may benefit from excision of partially cystic or exophytic lesions, although controversy remains as to whether biopsy of pontine lesions is useful because of sampling inconsistency and poor prognosis regardless of malignant grade.

CLASSIFICATION

Pediatric brain tumors may be classified purely according to the putative cell of origin (WHO criteria) or may include tumor location as a determinant of prognosis. The WHO system divides neuroepithelial tumors into subgroups whose cell lineage is (1) glial, for example, astrocytomas, ependymomas, and choroid plexus neoplasms, (2) neuronal, for example, gangliogliomas, (3) primitive neuroectodermal (described globally in this system as PNET), for example, medulloblastoma, and (4) pineal. Tumors arising from germ cells, meninges, or nerve sheath are classified separately. Alternatively, investigators have used medulloblastoma to describe the common primitive neuroepithelial tumor of the posterior fossa and PNET to describe the highly malignant primitive neuroectodermal tumor or variant cerebral neuroblastoma, arising above the tentorium. The term "cerebellar astrocytoma" may be used to describe cystic or pilocystic low-grade cerebellar lesions that often are cured by surgical excision, whereas supratentorial astrocytomas are either low grade or high grade, the latter designation including anaplastic astrocytoma and glioblastoma multiforme (GBM). The differentiation of low-grade from high-grade gliomas is most frequently made by the presence or absence of anaplastic features and necrosis.

TREATMENT

Medulloblastoma

The treatment of this most common (approximately 25% incidence) malignant childhood brain tumor has evolved markedly over the past decade with widespread use of an oncology staging system, national chemotherapy trials, and high-dose, experimental, ablation therapies for relapsed disease. The Chang staging system has proven valuable in differentiating those children with good prognosis, circumscribed lesions, which may be completely excised (stage T1 or T2), from those with invasive tumors that extend into the brainstem or seed or both along the neuraxis (T3, T4, M1, M2). Early stage lesions are reported to have 5-year progression-free survivals (PFS) of 70%, with radiotherapy as the standard treatment. Children with more invasive, incompletely resected, or metastatic lesions have benefited from the addition of adjuvant vincristine and CCNU (with or without prednisone). In national trials in the United States and Europe, the PFS has been 56% to 59% using this regimen. In a recent Philadelphia study, the addition of cisplatin to vincristine plus CCNU after radiotherapy resulted in a projected PFS for poor-risk patients greater than that of early stage patients treated with radiation alone.

Chemotherapeutic agents, such as cisplatin, cyclophosphamide, and etoposide, have been effective (approximately 50% to 80% response rate) in shrinking tumors when given before radiation therapy. Therefore, they should be considered for any child with advanced disease. National trials are investigating the effectiveness of chemotherapy and the timing of radiation treatment. Children with T1–T2 lesions may be candidates for a proposed randomized national trial of reduced neuraxis radiation, with adjuvant chemotherapy.

Low-Grade Astrocytomas

Gross resection is curative for children with cerebellar astrocytomas (cystic, pilocytic, or fibrillary). Those patients with residual disease may benefit from radiation therapy, although close observation (scans every 6 months) without radiation is appropriate management, particularly for a young child. There are preliminary data to suggest that patients with predominantly exophytic brainstem lesions may do well after surgery alone. Supratentorial low-grade gliomas are not usually amenable to total resection. Radiation therapy for residual disease is commonly advised, although it is not clear that the addition and the timing of radiation change the 5-year PFS (60% to 70%). Older children with progressive symptoms, however, should be considered candidates for radiation.

Low-grade tumors of the optic tract, particularly in children with neurofibromatosis, may remain quiescent without therapy for years. Young children (less than 6 years of age) with progressive disease should be offered the option of initial chemotherapy instead of radiation therapy. Regimens of vincristine plus dactinomycin, vincristine plus etoposide, or monthly carboplatinum have been effective in halting or shrinking growing tumors, allowing postponement of radiation.

High-Grade Gliomas and PNET

The median survival with radiation therapy for children with anaplastic astrocytoma is less than 3 years and for children with GBM is less than 18 months. These patients should be considered candidates for intensive chemotherapy and/or innovative high-dose radiation therapy. A recent national study of adjuvant vincristine, CCNU, plus prednisone demonstrated a 5-year PFS of 46% for patients with anaplastic astrocytoma. The Pediatric Oncology Group (POG) is conducting a therapeutic trial comparing the preradiation response of high-grade gliomas and PNETs to either BCNU plus cisplatin or cyclophosphamide plus etoposide. The chemotherapy is followed by twice-daily (hyperfractionated) radiotherapy. These high-risk children should be treated maximally on a dose-intensive protocol with combinations of these agents, in conjunction with radiation treatment of the involved field.

Brainstem Gliomas

Children with intrinsic pontine gliomas have a median survival of less than 1 year, with little improvement despite hyperfractionated radiotherapy dose escalation. The addition of cisplatin as a radiation sensitizer is being evaluated in a current POG study. A few patients have benefited from multiagent preradiation chemotherapy.

Ependymoma

Although children with low-grade lesions have been managed with gross surgical excision without radiotherapy, more recent studies suggest that such patients ultimately fail and that all patients with ependymoma (particularly those with ependymoblastoma) should be treated intensively. Because of the propensity for spinal axis seeding, standard therapy has included craniospinal radiotherapy for patients with posterior fossa tumors, although hyperfractionated radiation therapy may be more effective in providing local control. The addition of effective chemotherapy, particularly the platinum compounds, may improve survival for these children. However, there have been no national trials of this treatment.

Pineal and Germ Cell Tumors

Historically, children with pineal or suprasellar tumors were radiated without biopsy, since germ cell tumors responded rapidly to radiation, and high-grade gliomas were not treated with other therapies. In the 1990s, however, a patient with tumor in this region should be considered a candidate for biopsy, particularly if germ cell marker studies are negative. Young children with pure germinomas may benefit from reduced radiation following platinum-based chemotherapy, whereas children with nongerminomatous germ cell tumors, malignant teratomas, or gliomas should be offered multiagent chemotherapy appropriate to the histology. A recent international trial has reported on 12 children with germinomas who have remained progression free at a median 12 months after receiving chemotherapy without radiation therapy. Children with tumors in the pineal or suprasellar regions should have a careful endocrine evaluation for possible hypothalamic or pituitary dysfunction.

Craniopharyngiomas

Patients with these localized, often cystic, lesions are managed initially by surgery. Long-term survival with decreased morbidity may be better with conservative, subtotal resection followed by adjuvant radiation therapy.

Choroid Plexus Tumors

Children with benign papillomas may be cured by excision, but infants with malignant carcinomatous tumors should be treated with multiagent drug and radiation treatments.

Treatment of Very Young Children

An attempt should be made to defer or avoid high-dose cranial radiation in children less than 4 or 5 years of age. Radiation affects cognition, personality, growth, and developing neuroendocrine pathways. IQ deficits of 20 points or more have been documented for children treated before age 5 years. The POG has reported that chemotherapy with vincristine-cyclophosphamide plus cisplatin-etoposide has allowed postponement of radiation with a 40% PFS at 1 and 2 years for infants aged 24 to 36 months and less than 24 months, respectively. Children who had complete responses to chemotherapy had a PFS similar to those with gross surgical resection, and 11 of 13 children whose parents declined radiation therapy were disease free at 1 year median follow-up. Tumor response to initial vincristine-cyclophosphamide was documented in 48% of patients with medulloblastoma or ependymoma and in 60% of children with malignant glioma. A 2-year PFS of 54% for these young children with malignant glioma exceeds that of older children treated with radiation alone and suggests that chemotherapy may significantly improve the prognosis for infants.

As these young children continue to survive, it is critical that the pediatrician assist in late effects monitoring of thyroid function, growth and pubertal development, and neuropsychologic and cognitive status.

Future Developments

Improvements in microsurgical techniques and stereotactic biopsy have provided the literal framework for stereotactic radiotherapy, which offers single high-dose treatment of well-localized ($\leq$ 3 cm) lesions. This therapy may benefit the occasional patient with a small, high-grade lesion. Surgical placement of radioactive implants (brachytherapy) has been practiced in adults with gliomas. Similar implantation of chemotherapy-impregnated polymers may be appropriate for circumscribed tumors in adults and children. There is some evidence that immunotherapeutic techniques may be effective in children with microscopic disease. Systemic administration of interferons and localized treatment with lymphocyte activated killer (LAK) cells and with monoclonal antibodies are being evaluated. Several investigators are exploring whether using genetically engineered mutant herpesviruses, which are cytotoxic in animal models, will be effective against glioma.

In the last few years, oncologists have extrapolated from the effectiveness of chemotherapy documented in young children to the concept of high-dose ablation chemotherapy, followed by hematopoietic stem cell rescue with autologous reinfusion of the patient's bone marrow (autologous bone marrow transplant, ABMT). Using two to three times the dose levels of such agents as cyclophosphamide, melphalan, BCNU, carboplatinum, thiotepa, or etoposide, several ABMT programs have provided prolongation of life to some patients with refractory disease and are now treating patients with highly malignant gliomas at diagnosis.

In conclusion, pediatricians, working together with pediatric oncologists, need to be cognizant of the rapidly evolving treatment options in the new field of neurooncology. There must be careful consideration of the late effects of treatment on the developing child and the critical coordination of subspecialists before initiation of therapy.

REFERENCES

1. Duffner PK, Horowitz ME, Krischer JP, et al: Postoperative chemotherapy and delayed radiation in children less than three years of age with malignant brain tumors. N Engl J Med 328:1725–1731, 1993.
2. Kovnar EH, Kellie SJ, Horowitz ME, et al: Preirradiation cisplatin and etoposide in the treatment of high-risk medulloblastoma and other malignant embryonal tumors of the central nervous system: A phase II study. J Clin Oncol 8:330–336, 1990.
3. Packer RJ, Sutton LN, Atkins TE, et al: A prospective study of cognitive function in children receiving whole-brain radiotherapy and chemotherapy: 2-year results. J Neurosurg 70:707–713, 1989.

4

Respiratory Tract

DISORDERS OF VOICE, SPEECH, OR LANGUAGE

JAMES COPLAN, M.D.

Language consists of any symbol system for the storage or exchange of information, *speech* consists of symbolically meaningful vocalizations (i.e., words), and *voice* refers to the phonatory quality of the pharynx and larynx. Disorders of speech, language, or voice may be caused by hearing loss, focal or diffuse central nervous system (CNS) dysfunction, or anatomic abnormalities of the vocal tract. Prompt recognition of speech or language delay is facilitated through the incorporation of a structured measure of early language development as one component of well child care (Fig. 1). Medical management includes determining the correct *developmental diagnosis,* determining the underlying *organic etiology,* providing the family with information regarding *prognosis,* and *monitoring the child's progress.*

HEARING LOSS

Otitis Media with Effusion (OME)

Chronic or recurrent OME during infancy is associated with an increased risk of delayed speech development and subtle defects of central auditory processing and classroom performance in later childhood. Human and animal studies strongly suggest a critical period for postnatal maturation of brainstem auditory pathways during the first 12 to 18 months of life. Insertion of pressure equalization (PE) tubes alleviates the fluctuating, mild to moderate conductive hearing loss associated with OME and may protect the developing CNS during this critical period. Infants below 6 months of age are candidates for PE tube insertion at the time of their second episode of acute otitis media (AOM) or after 60 days (cumulative) with OME, since CNS maturation is proceeding most rapidly during this time and because infants who experience AOM/OME below 6 months of age are at high risk for chronic or recurrent OME throughout childhood. Infants between 6 and 18 months of age are candidates for PE tube insertion after their third episode of AOM or after 90 days (cumulative) with OME. PE tube insertion beyond 18 months of age may be indicated for medical management of middle ear disease per se but probably has little impact on CNS maturation or speech and language development.

Permanent Hearing Loss

Hearing loss (HL) is extremely difficult to recognize on physical examination during infancy and early childhood. Profound congenital HL is not diagnosed, on average, until 24 to 30 months, and moderate or unilateral congenital HL is not diagnosed until school entry at age 5. To eliminate this deplorable delay, the National Institutes of Health recently recommended universal audiologic screening for all infants.

Unless or until such a program is implemented, all children who meet defined high-risk criteria should be referred for formal audiologic assessment, *no matter how well the child seems to hear during the physical examination* (Table 1). If HL is found, annual audiologic reevaluation must be performed to rule out progressive HL. Genetic counseling must be obtained regarding all children with congenital HL of undetermined etiology. Infant or preschool siblings of a child with newly diagnosed congenital HL must be referred for audiologic evaluation to rule out a familial form of HL. A negative family history does *not* exclude genetic factors. The family history is typically negative in cases of autosomal recessive deafness and may be negative in dominantly transmitted disorders with variable expressivity.

Habilitation includes amplification and some combination of orally based speech therapy and sign language instruction. Classroom instruction may include the use of an "interpretutor," who interprets spoken material into sign language for the child. Children with severe to profound sensorineural HL may be candidates for cochlear implantation. Children with moderate to severe conductive HL as a result of malformations of the ossicles may be candidates for reconstructive middle ear surgery.

Prognosis for speech depends on the age at onset of HL, the age at recognition of HL and institution of appropriate habilitative measures, the presence of coexisting cognitive impairment, and the severity of the hearing loss. A threshold greater than 90 decibels at and above 1000 cycles per second is generally associated with a poor prognosis for oral communication.

DISORDERS OF LANGUAGE OR SPEECH RESULTING FROM CNS DYSFUNCTION

Mental Retardation

Three percent of children are mentally retarded, and all children with mental retardation (MR) have language delay. Medical management includes determining the etiology of the MR and exclusion of coexisting developmental disabilities. HL often coexists with MR (as in congenital cytomegalovirus infection or neonatal intracranial hemorrhage). Therefore, it is incorrect to assume that language delay is exclusively caused by MR until hearing has been evaluated by an audiologist. Habilitation includes an infant or preschool stimulation program. Prognosis for language development is a function of the degree of MR.

Developmental Language Disorders

Developmental language disorders (DLD) affect at least 5% of preschool children. DLDs are characterized by varying degrees of expressive and receptive oral language development. Unclear speech and reduction in the total amount of speech are the most common initial signs. Speech may be fluent (though unintelligible) or labored, but pure types analogous to the Wernicke or Broca type aphasia of adulthood are rare.

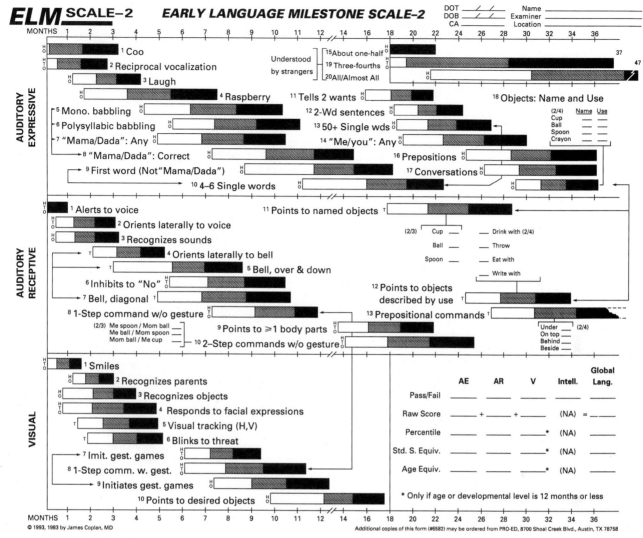

FIGURE 1. The Early Language Milestone Scale, 2nd ed. (ELM Scale-2). The ELM Scale-2 is an easy way to monitor language development from birth to 36 months and intelligibility of speech from 18 to 48 months of age. The ELM Scale-2 is available from PRO-ED, 8700 Shoal Creek Boulevard, Austin, TX 78757. Copyright PRO-ED, 1983, 1993. Reprinted by permission.

TABLE 1. Indications for Audiologic Evaluation

All neonatal intensive care unit (NICU) patients
Congenital infection with agents known or suspected of causing hearing loss (cytomegalovirus, rubella, syphilis, toxoplasmosis, herpes)
Anomalies
    Mesodermal: Abnormalities of first or second branchial arches (auricles, mandible, other craniofacial)
    Ectodermal: Abnormalities of neural crest (iris heterochromia, albinism, piebaldness)
    Presence of syndrome known to be associated with hearing loss (Usher syndrome, Waardenberg syndrome)
Family history of congenital or childhood-onset hearing loss
Bacterial meningitis
Other infectious disease known to be associated with hearing loss (mumps, measles, Epstein-Barr virus)
Ototoxic drugs (including but not limited to aminoglycosides, loop diuretics)
Radiation therapy when auditory pathways lie in radiation field
Neurodegenerative disorder known to be associated with hearing loss
Head trauma, especially with fracture through temporal bone
Parental concern about child's hearing
Speech or language delay
Other developmental disability (mental retardation, autism, cerebral palsy, developmental language disorder)

Adapted from Coplan J: Deafness: Ever heard of it? Delayed recognition of permanent hearing loss. Pediatrics 82:447–452, 1988, and from Early identification of hearing impairment in infants and young children. NIH Consensus Statement, March 1–3, 1993, 11(1):1–24.

Management includes determination of the underlying organic etiology when possible and exclusion of HL. Habilitation includes enrollment in a language-based infant stimulation or preschool special education program. In addition to orally based speech therapy, manual sign language may be used to good effect as a temporary measure (typically for 1 or 2 years) to give the preschool child with DLD an adequate means of expression until intelligibility and total oral output improve. Parents must be reassured that the temporary use of sign language does *not* delay the emergence of speech. On the contrary, sign language may stimulate the emergence of speech and reduces the child's frustration level. Intelligibility of speech typically improves greatly by ages 4 to 6, often revealing an expressive *language* disorder with abnormalities of word order, omission of tense endings, pluralization markers, and conjunctions, word retrieval difficulties (anomia), and subtle defects in listening comprehension. Children with DLD are at increased risk for the presence of learning disabilities.

Acquired Epileptic Aphasia

Acquired epileptic aphasia, or Landau-Kleffner syndrome, is a rare disorder characterized by sudden cessation of speech accompanied by auditory agnosia that may mimic deafness as a result of epileptogenic activity in one or both temporal lobes. If seizures are present, the patient is treated with anticonvulsants. There is no good evidence to support the use of anticonvulsants for the treatment of the language disturbance per se. Prognosis for speech and language development is guarded, compared with children with idiopathic DLD.

Autism

Autism is characterized by delayed and *deviant* language development, with echolalia, verbal perseveration, impaired ability to use language for communicative purposes, and stilted or sing-song inflection. Visual communication also is impaired, with reduced or absent eye contact, failure to imitate or initiate gesture games, and failure to point to desired objects. If possible, the underlying organic etiology for the autism should be determined and coexisting disabilities (MR, HL) should be sought. Drug treatment remains empiric and symptomatic. Improvement has been reported with narcotic antagonists and with clomipramine, a tricyclic antidepressant used to treat obsessive-compulsive disorder (which shares with autism a propensity for repetitive, ritualistic behavior).[2]

Habilitation is aimed at improving communication and socialization skills. The technique of facilitated communication (FC) currently enjoys great popularity in educational circles. Unfortunately, controlled studies have shown unconscious facilitator influence over the typed output represented as originating with the autistic individual in most instances (the subject of several articles in the *Journal of Autism and Developmental Disorders*, 24:3, June 1994). Parents may be encouraged to explore FC, but claims made on its behalf should be subject to proof, particularly when the child's output via FC is drastically discordant from his or her apparent level of function as measured by conventional methods.

Prognosis is governed by the severity of the autism and the presence of MR, if any. The high-functioning autistic child (i.e., non-MR, with mild autism) usually undergoes remarkable improvement, to the point where he or she is no longer easily recognizable as autistic, although subtle autistic traits, such as verbal literalism and difficulty with spontaneous socialization, remain. The child with severe autism, or autism plus MR, usually remains overtly autistic and severely disabled for life.

Dysarthria

Dysarthria is caused by impairment of the muscles of speech production and usually is encountered as one facet of a generalized, static upper motor neuron encephalopathy (i.e., cerebral palsy). Speech is unintelligible or absent. Receptive language is normal unless there is coexisting intellectual impairment or HL. Dysarthria often is accompanied by feeding difficulties, such as poor suck, excess drooling, difficulty chewing, or choking during feedings. There may be asso-

ciated developmental disabilities (MR, HL). Hearing should be assessed via brainstem auditory evoked response testing if the child's voluntary motor responses are too limited to permit conventional behavioral response audiometry. Children with dysarthria should be referred to a speech pathologist. If feeding problems are severe, a modified barium swallow with fluoroscopic visualization of the swallowing process should be obtained.[3]

Habilitation may include orally based speech therapy or an alternative communication system, such as a picture board or a computer with speech synthesis capability. Devices are available with speech recognition capability that can be trained to translate the output of the dysarthric individual into intelligible form. Prognosis for speech is guarded, particularly in the presence of coexisting disabilities (MR, HL).

Stuttering

Stuttering is an abnormality of fluency (rate and rhythm) of speech. Language is unimpaired. Transient, intermittent loss of fluency is normal between 30 and 48 months of life. This is also the age, however, when stuttering first appears. Transient, physiologic loss of fluency usually involves whole-word repetitions and is not troubling to the child. In contrast, stuttering typically involves part-word repetitions or prolongations and is a source of distress to the child. Transient, physiologic loss of fluency should be distinguished from stuttering, and the young stutterer should be referred promptly to a speech pathologist if any of the following are present: loss of fluency for more than 6 months, struggle behavior while dysfluent (grimacing, change in respiratory pattern, loss of eye contact with the listener), stuttering in a sibling or parent, or concern on the parents' part. Admonishing the child to slow down is unhelpful, since this is apt to make the child even more self-conscious and dysfluent. Prognosis is variable. If there are no long-term stutterers in the family, there is a good chance that the child's stuttering will partially or totally remit by adolescence. If a first-degree relative has lifelong stuttering, however, the child is more likely to do the same.

DISORDERS OF VOICE

Hypernasality and Hyponasality

Hypernasality indicates *excess* nasal emission of air during speech because of incomplete closure of the palate against the posterior pharyngeal wall. Hypernasality can be caused by cleft palate, occult or submucous cleft palate, short palate, or impaired movement of the velopharyngeal musculature on a neurogenic basis. In contrast, hyponasality indicates *insufficient* nasal emission of air during speech because of obstruction to the nasal cavity. The hyponasal child often has a history of mouth breathing, snoring, or obstructive sleep apnea. The most common cause of hyponasal speech is adenoidal hypertrophy. The child with hypernasality or hyponasality should be referred to a speech pathologist and an otorhinolaryngologist. Adenoidectomy usually alleviates hyponasality, but it exacerbates hypernasality and should be avoided in hypernasal children.

Hoarseness

Hoarseness, or weak, breathy cry, in an infant may be caused by laryngomalacia, vocal cord paresis, or congenital anatomic abnormality of the larynx or airway. Stridor may be a clue to the presence of gastroesophogeal reflux. In older children, chronic hoarseness is most often caused by vocal cord nodules. Rarely, brainstem tumor or Arnold-Chiari malformation with slowly progressive cranial nerve dysfunction may give rise to changes in voice quality. Voice abnormalities must be assessed by careful neurologic examination and consultation with an otorhinolaryngologist[1] and (in children old enough to speak) a speech pathologist.

ETIOLOGIC CONSIDERATIONS

Fragile X syndrome, sex chromosome aneuploidy, and minor chromosomal translocations and deletions are common causes of MR,

DLD, and autism. A G-banded karyotype will detect most chromosomal abnormalities. High-resolution banding should be obtained if a specific interstitial deletion is suspected. Fragile X syndrome should be excluded by DNA analysis, since cytogenetic methods are much less sensitive. The physician should ask explicitly about teratogenic exposure (alcohol, anticonvulsants, illicit drugs) in any child with language or cognitive impairment. HIV encephalopathy should be considered in any child with developmental delay, even in the absence of identified risk factors. Duchenne's muscular dystrophy should be considered in any boy with mild global developmental delay. Perinatal distress should not be assumed to establish a perinatal cause for a developmental disability, since perinatal distress often signifies a preexisting fetal abnormality. Perinatal events can give rise to cerebral palsy and/or HL, which may be associated with MR, DLD, or autism. Isolated cognitive disability is unlikely to be caused by perinatal events, however.

REFERENCES

1. Choi SS, Cotton RT: Surgical management of voice disorders. Pediatr Clin North Am 36:1535–1549, 1989.
2. Mauk JE: Autism and pervasive developmental disorders. Pediatr Clin North Am 40:567–578, 1993.
3. Stevenson RD, Allaire JH: The development of normal feeding and swallowing. Pediatr Clin North Am 38:1439–1453, 1991.

CHOANAL ATRESIA

SYLVAN STOOL, M.D.

Choanal atresia is an infrequent cause of neonatal respiratory distress. Its estimated occurrence is 1 in 8000 deliveries. Although it may be the only birth defect, more than 50% of children who have bilateral atresia have another major birth defect, and it is part of several syndromes or associations, such as CHARGE. The child with bilateral choanal atresia experiences respiratory distress that occurs when the mouth is closed and is relieved with crying. Unilateral atresia may be much more cryptic and, indeed, may be missed until the child is much older. The newborn is an obligate nose breather, so anything that causes nasal obstruction will result in suffocation unless the mouth is opened. With bilateral atresia, the child closes his mouth and tries to breath but cannot unless he cries. If an oral airway is not provided, the child will soon become exhausted.

Therapy should be applied immediately to provide an adequate airway and prevent anoxia. A simple and effective method is to insert a large red rubber catheter through the mouth into the stomach. This accomplishes two purposes: it breaks the glossopalatine seal and provides a method for nutrition. Catheters usually are available in the delivery room. Alternate methods are to use a neonatal plastic airway and tape it in. However, such airways are rigid and may cause erosion of the palate if used for a prolonged period. A McGovern nipple may be used. This simply is a nipple in which the opening has been enlarged. It is held in the mouth with tape.

After the airway is secure, the diagnosis can be confirmed. The simplest method is to auscultate the nose for airway sounds. A catheter can be inserted through the nasal space along the floor of the nose. If an obstruction is met at about 3 cm, atresia is suspected. A potential error occurs if the catheter curls, giving a false impression of patency. The passage of the catheter can be confirmed by palpating the oral cavity and pharynx or visualizing directly.

Radiographic examination offers further information. Before the study, mucus should be suctioned from the nose. The use of radiopaque dye demonstrates lack of passage. At present, the most informative study is CT in the horizontal plane. The relationship of nasal walls and the extent of the bony and membranous atresia can be accurately determined.

Repair of the atresia will depend on its extent and the condition of the child. Simple membranous atresias are rare and can be opened by inserting a urethral sound to break the membrane and to dilate the orifice. The decision to perform a transnasal or transpalatal operation will depend on the surgeon. I prefer a transpalatal approach as early as possible after the child is stabilized.

Several decisions will have to be made by the surgeon. Will stents be inserted, and if so how large and what type? After a transpalatal procedure, I usually insert a transnasal airway for 24 to 48 hours and then remove it. Most infants do well and start to feed. In the ideal case, dilatation of the nasal space and choanal area may be necessary once or twice to remove granulation tissue. However, only about half of my cases are ideal, and reoperation or insertion of an indwelling stent may be necessary.

Unilateral choanal atresia may not be apparent in the newborn who does not manifest respiratory obstruction. The most frequent sign is persistent thick mucoid unilateral nasal discharge in the absence of a respiratory infection. Occasionally, the patent side is occluded by the septum or secretions, and the child becomes symptomatic. If this does not occur, the surgical correction may be delayed.

TUMORS AND POLYPS OF THE NOSE

J. CHRISTOPHER POST, M.D.

Nasal masses require careful evaluation to ensure appropriate management. Anterior nasal rhinoscopy can be performed with an otoscope and ear speculum, but examination of the posterior nasal cavity and nasopharynx requires a flexible or rigid fiberoptic nasopharyngoscope. Headlight and mirror examination of the nasopharynx in a young child is generally unproductive.

Imaging studies should be performed before biopsy is undertaken. Plain films are of limited value when compared with computed tomography (CT) or magnetic resonance imaging (MRI) studies. CT demonstrates the relationship of the mass to bony structures. Bone erosion is indicative of a malignancy, whereas bony remodeling and expansion are more characteristic of benign lesions. MRI is very helpful in determining soft tissue extent and is the study of choice to evaluate intracranial extension. Biopsy should be performed in the operating room under general anesthesia after the potential for bleeding or intracranial extension has been carefully evaluated. Biopsy of a hemangioma or a mass with an intracranial component can be disastrous in the office setting.

BENIGN LESIONS

Nasal polyps result from chronic inflammation or infection and can have an allergic component. Children with polyps have nasal obstruction and hyponasal speech and may complain of a loss of the senses of smell and taste. Polyps are smooth and bluish gray in appearance. Cystic fibrosis should be ruled out in a pediatric patient with nasal polyps. Samter's syndrome should be considered in a child with nasal polyposis, asthma, and aspirin intolerance.

Topical nasal steroid sprays are useful in controlling nasal polyps and should be considered before surgical management. Care should be taken in prescribing these medications to children who have not had varicella. Local side effects include mucosal drying, with epistaxis and burning. Most children prefer the aqueous preparation (designated AQ) as there is less of a burning sensation than with the alcohol preparation. Short courses of systemically administered steroids may provide temporary relief from symptoms but should be used with caution in children, and they are not suitable for long-term management.

Surgical resection will relieve symptoms, but the patient and family should be cautioned that recurrence is likely. CT evaluation is quite helpful in determining the extent of disease. A physician experienced in pediatric nasal surgery should perform the surgical excision under direct vision using endoscopes. Anterior ethmoidectomy appears to reduce the frequency of recurrence by allowing a more complete removal of the polyps. Complications are not common in experienced hands but can be serious, given the close proximity of the eye and brain to the surgical site. Nasal steroids are helpful in controlling disease recurrence after surgical resection.

Antrochoanal polyps originate in the maxillary sinus and extend through the maxillary ostium into the nasal cavity and nasopharynx, with subsequent nasal obstruction. On examination, a bulging soft palate or mass extending from the nasopharynx into the oropharynx may be noted. Transoral and transnasal endoscopic removal is indicated, and the maxillary ostium should be examined carefully for residual disease. The maxillary antrum may be entered endoscopically, but complete resection may require a Caldwell-Luc approach. This should be avoided in young children to avoid disruption of the permanent dentition.

Hemangiomas can occur in the nasal cavity. These tumors will be intensely enhancing on CT or MRI studies with contrast, which is helpful in distinguishing hemangiomas from polyps. Surgical excision, with or without preoperative embolization, is curative. *Lymphangiomas* also occur in the nasal cavity and should be managed by excision to improve the nasal airway.

Nasal dermoids, encephaloceles, and *gliomas* result from aberrant embryologic development of the anterior base of the skull and nose. These may cause nasal obstruction, recurrent infections, or meningitis. Nasal dermoids contain ectodermal elements and often are associated with a midline pit. Dermoids are nonpulsatile, do not transilluminate, and do not enlarge with crying. Approximately 25% extend intracranially. Encephaloceles appear as translucent, pulsatile masses in the nasal airway or externally at or near the midline and contain meninges, CSF, and brain. The mass may expand with crying. There is, by definition, intracranial involvement. Unjudicious biopsies may result in meningitis and a persistent CSF leak. Nasal gliomas are uncommon midline masses that should be considered in a neonate with respiratory distress. These also contain neural tissue but do not connect with the subarachnoid space. However, intracranial extension is present in 15% to 25% of patients. Surgical excision of these lesions is curative. Excision may require a combined otolaryngologic and neurosurgical approach, either in a single or a staged procedure.

Juvenile nasopharyngeal angiofibromas are vascular neoplasms that arise from the superior margin of the sphenopalatine foramen in the nasopharynx and occur almost exclusively in adolescent males. This diagnosis should be considered in any young man with nasal obstruction and recurrent epistaxis. Therapy consists of surgical resection, with preoperative embolization used to decrease intraoperative bleeding. Radiation therapy can be curative, but long-term effects on skeletal growth and the potential for tumor induction should be considered. Hormonal therapy and chemotherapy have also been advocated but are not considered the treatments of choice.

Papillomas occur as exophytic nasal masses and can be excised, cauterized, or removed with a CO_2 laser. Close follow-up is necessary, given their propensity for recurrence. Inverting schneiderian papillomas are very rare in children and generally occur on the lateral nasal wall. Simple excision generally results in recurrence, whereas a wider surgical excision through a lateral nasal rhinotomy can be curative. These lesions may be associated with malignancy.

Other rare tumors include minor salivary gland tumors, teratomas, epignathi, hemangiopericytoma, and melanotic neuroectodermal tumor of infancy. Wegener's granulomatosis may occur as a granulomatous mass on the nasal septum. Rhinoliths are calcified masses associated with foreign bodies present in the nose for long periods of time. They show up well on plain films and should be managed by removal.

MALIGNANT LESIONS

Malignant nasal tumors may remain undiagnosed for long periods of time, as these tumors can originate in clinically silent areas or cause such nonspecific findings as nasal obstruction, nasal discharge,

hyponasal speech, epistaxis, and eustachian tube dysfunction with middle ear effusion. Since these findings are so common in children, multiple courses of symptomatic treatment may be administered before arriving at the correct diagnosis. More advanced lesions may cause facial remodeling, visual changes, loss of teeth, cranial nerve findings, neck masses, or constitutional symptoms from metastatic disease. These tumors can involve the paranasal sinuses or intracranial vault and may be unresectable at the time of diagnosis.

A pathologist experienced in pediatric tumors should be consulted before biopsy to ensure that adequate tissue is delivered in proper condition for any special studies that may be necessary. A metastatic workup is essential before aggressive surgical approaches are considered.

Rhabdomyosarcoma is the most common malignant nasal tumor in children. Combination therapy, consisting of surgical excision if possible, radiation therapy, and chemotherapy, has increased survival rates. Lymphomas are initially diagnosed through surgical biopsy but are then managed with chemotherapy and radiation therapy. Nasopharyngeal carcinoma generally has an excellent initial response to radiation therapy and may require systemic chemotherapy to control distant disease. Esthesioneuroblastomas arise high in the nasal vault and may be controlled with surgery and radiation therapy, with a craniofacial approach potentially offering better resection of the tumor margins.

Other, more rare tumors may arise in the pediatric nasal cavity. Chondrosarcomas, Ewing's sarcoma, angiosarcomas, Burkitt's lymphoma, and chordomas all have been reported as occurring in the pediatric population. Specific treatment depends not only on the histologic type of tumor as determined by biopsy but also on the limits of the tumor as determined by imaging studies and an examination under anesthesia. Surgical debulking or excision, radiation therapy, and chemotherapy are all potential modalities. These patients are best served by a multidisciplinary approach in a specialty setting. Staged or combined surgical procedures with close cooperation between the otolaryngology and neurosurgery services may be necessary.

EPISTAXIS AND NASAL TRAUMA

ROBERT A. HENDRIX, M.D., F.A.C.S.

EPISTAXIS

Spontaneous epistaxis is a common childhood disorder that often requires medical attention. In 80% of cases, bleeding arises from Little's area of the anterior septum. The anterior and posterior ethmoidal arteries, the nasal branches of the internal maxillary artery, and the septal branch of the facial artery supply Kiesselbach's plexus of vessels at this site.

The etiology of anterior epistaxis may be trauma or combinations of rhinitis, nose picking, and low humidity. In teenagers, epistaxis may be associated with pregnancy. Systematic consideration of sinus and nasopharyngeal abnormalities occasionally is necessary. Juvenile angiofibroma, usually found in male teenagers, often occur with epistaxis. Epistaxis may be an initial sign or a manifestation of a serious systemic disease. Gaucher disease, a disturbance of lipid storage resulting in accumulation of histiocytes filled with glucosyl ceramide in various organs and bones, is associated with epistaxis, hemoptysis, and spontaneous gingival hemorrhage.

Patients with coagulopathy, leukemia, or renal failure are at high risk for refractory epistaxis and may require transfusion of appropriate blood or serum products. In the presence of such disorders, epistaxis can even mimic gastrointestinal bleeding.

Osler-Weber-Rendu syndrome, or hereditary hemorrhagic telangiectasia, is another cause of epistaxis. It occurs in 90% of affected patients before age 21. The mean onset age is 12 years, and symptoms progress with age. The average patient experiences more than 18 episodes of epistaxis per month, with each episode averaging 7.5 minutes. Screening for pulmonary and cerebral arteriovenous malformations in children and affected parents should be considered. Laser therapy combined with standard septodermoplasty enables patients to gain excellent control of epistaxis for several years.

Iatrogenic epistaxis can occur during nasotracheal intubation. Decongestion of the nasal mucosa before manipulation is advised. Oxymetazoline (0.05%) is reportedly as effective for prevention of epistaxis with intubation as 10% cocaine (which was associated with mild systemic cardiovascular effects) and more effective than 4% lidocaine with 1:100,000 epinephrine. However, other manipulation, such as dilation with nasopharyngeal airways, needlessly add time, trauma, and hemorrhage to routine nasotracheal intubation of healthy patients.

Management

Simple pressure to the nasal alae and septum is an effective treatment for most children. It is also appropriate to instruct the patient and family in techniques for effective self-treatment of common, anterior nosebleeds: Tilt the head forward, take note of which nostril is bleeding, apply a 5-minute pinch to the entire external cartilaginous nose, and seek medical attention if bleeding persists despite two 5-minute periods of continuous pressure. Humidification and well-trimmed fingernails help prevent further bleeds.

Refractory nosebleed requires progressively more involved intervention. Cautery of an identifiable source of epistaxis is commonly performed with topically applied silver nitrate. The less commonly used electrical or thermal cautery must be used with caution. Cautery of both sides of the septum can result in perforation if the cautery sites are in apposition to one another. Some practitioners recommend the use of antiseptic cream to the nasal septum as the primary treatment of epistaxis in children. One author found no statistically significant difference between treatments with silver nitrate cautery and antiseptic nasal cream.

Several materials are available for packing the nasal cavity. Calcium sodium alginate fiber is described as an acceptable alternative to traditional gauze packing, Gelfoam, NuGauze strips, and Merocel.

Gelfoam (The Upjohn Company, Kalamazoo, MI) is a hemostatic, absorbable gelatin sterile sponge. Gelfoam is prepared from purified pork skin gelatin as a water-insoluble, nonelastic, porous, pliable product. Gelfoam may be left in contact with mucosal surfaces until it liquefies.

Hemostatic agents are sometimes used in combination to provide more effective hemostasis. However, allergic reactions can occur with the use of topical hemostatic agents. Bovine topical thrombin (BTT) is a heterologous plasma thrombin concentrate that has been used frequently for hemostasis since the 1940s. IgE-mediated anaphylaxis has been reported in Japan with the use of topical bovine thrombin. The prick test with 1000 U/ml (1 g/ml) appears to be useful to detect highly sensitive patients. Commercially available thrombin of human origin also may be hazardous. Immunologic analysis revealed that one thrombin preparation (human origin) contained IgG, hepatitis B surface (HBs) antibody, and human immunodeficiency virus (HIV) antibody.[3] Documentation should be made of any hemostatic agent left in situ with any packing. The manufacturer of Gelfoam advises against combining thrombin and Gelfoam because thrombin is antigenic, and, further, the hemostatic properties of Gelfoam are not enhanced by thrombin.

Merocel nasal tampon (American Corporation, Mystic, CT) is a synthetic open-cell foam polymer of hydroxylated polyvinyl acetal. The Merocel sponge is useful for anterior or posterior epistaxis. Application of this product requires wetting the compressed sponge and inserting it into the nasal cavity within 5 seconds after its becoming wet. Merocel expands fully within 7 seconds after wetting. I prefer to coat the Merocel sponge with bacitracin ointment before placement. Subsequently, the substance of the packing is soaked with sterile saline dripped onto or injected into the sponge. The sponge should be left in place at least 2 hours.[2] The Merocel nasal tampon is one of the easiest to apply and most effective for control of epistaxis.

Toxic shock syndrome (TSS) is a systemic disease characterized by fever and erythroderma, with subsequent desquamation and shock. TSS is mediated by staphylococcal exoproteins, including TSST-1 (the primary toxin identified with TSS). The nasal carriage rate for *Staphylococcus aureus* varies from 18% to 50%.

NuGauze strips (Johnson & Johnson, New Brunswick, NJ) are made from a special narrow woven cotton gauze. One author reports the recovery of substantially more *S. aureus* isolated on plated NuGauze postoperative material than from Merocel. It is suggested that the thick aggregates of microscopic fibrils in NuGauze support a larger population of microorganisms. Of interest, TSS has been observed when Gelfoam had been used. In contrast, Merocel nasal packing appears to inhibit bacterial proliferation and offer some protection against TSS.[1]

NASAL TRAUMA

Soft tissue injury to the external nose is managed according to general principles. Contusions usually heal spontaneously, though hematoma may require evacuation by aspiration. Abrasions contaminated with particulate matter should be irrigated or debrided by scrubbing to avoid tattooing. An organic solvent, such as ether, may be required to remove tar, grease, or oil from a wound. Lacerations from inanimate objects or animal bites and scratches generally can be closed within 8 hours after thorough cleaning. The risk of tetanus and rabies must be assessed. Human bites require thorough cleaning and, in general, should not be closed primarily. Burns should be managed with antiseptic technique, but reconstruction should be delayed to allow demarcation of tissue loss. Full-thickness skin loss should be repaired by an experienced reconstructive surgeon.

Nasal trauma must be assessed in relation to associated injuries and the patient's condition. For example, severe head injury or a gunshot wound can be associated with carotid-cavernous sinus fistula. Such a pathologic communication between the internal carotid artery and the surrounding cavernous sinus at the base of skull may result in permanent impairment of vision and, rarely, fatal epistaxis. Diagnosis is confirmed by carotid angiography or CT scan. Packing the nasal cavity blindly before assessment of the skull base can result in intracranial injury.

Prompt management of airway, cardiovascular function, and ocular or CNS injury must always take priority. Even the patient complaining of an isolated nasal trauma can have unrecognized, associated injuries. Direct questioning can indicate involvement of other systems, for example, loss or alteration of consciousness, hearing loss, tinnitus or dysequilibrium, diplopia or visual disturbance, and neck pain. The standard of care requires a thorough examination of the head and neck: tympanic membranes to rule out hemotympanum, eye examination for visual acuity, pupillary response, eye grounds, and extraocular motion, palpation of the facial skeleton with demonstration of stability of the premaxilla, range of motion of the mandible and dental occlusion, and palpation of the cervical spine for point tenderness.

The history of an isolated nasal injury should document the physical vectors of trauma and patient observations regarding the injuries, the presence and site of epistaxis or rhinorrhea, and impairment of the nasal airway. The patient's perception of the nasal appearance is pertinent. A thorough examination of the nasal cavity is critical to rule out septal hematoma or anatomic rearrangement.

Nasal trauma with disruption of the ethmoidal arteries results in severe epistaxis. This requires surgical intervention with ligation of the ethmoidal arteries by a Lynch incision. Epistaxis from mucosal lacerations is generally controlled with packing. Septal hematoma requires prompt drainage, packing, and antibiotics. Unrecognized septal hematoma can become abscessed, with risk of septal resorption and development of saddle nose, that is, collapse and concavity of the nasal dorsum.

External nasal fracture is best diagnosed clinically by the appearance of the nose and palpation of the nasal bones. On occasion, a simple closed reduction can be achieved in the immediate posttraumatic period. It is noteworthy that recognition and treatment of nasal injury and displacement in the newborn can reduce the chance of subsequent deformity, particularly of the septum. In most cases, the degree of acute swelling and tenderness prevents an adequate assessment of the nasal configuration. Medical textbooks frequently recommend nasal x-rays at presentation. However, such studies rarely have any influence on the management of nasal trauma. With the exception of facial x-rays to evaluate for other fractures of the facial skeleton, nasal x-rays constitute a needless and unjustifiable expense.

With septal hematoma ruled out, subsequent examination by an otolaryngologist is recommended 4 to 7 days posttrauma. The patient's (or family's) perception of deformity of the nose as a result of the trauma is a necessary but not sufficient basis for surgical reduction. In children, it may be impossible to effectively reduce a displaced nasal fracture beyond 10 days after the injury. Stabilization with intranasal packing or postoperative splinting may be necessary.

Open reduction is sometimes recommended for external fracture in the acute posttrauma period. However, open reduction may adversely affect future growth of nasal structures. Whereas closed reduction usually achieves an acceptable outcome for the external nose, the nasal septum is usually manipulated with limited success. Further, closed reduction of a displaced septum risks intraseptal bleeding and hematoma.

REFERENCES

1. Breda SD, Jacobs JB, Lebowitz AS, Tierno PM Jr: Toxic shock syndrome in nasal surgery: A physiochemical and microbiologic evaluation of Merocel and NuGauze nasal packing. Laryngoscope 97:1388–1391, 1987.
2. Doyle DE: Anterior epistaxis: A new nasal tampon for fast, effective control. Laryngoscope 96:279–281, 1986.
3. Suzuki S, Sakuragawa N: A study on the properties of commercial thrombin preparations. Thromb Res 53:271–277, 1989.

FOREIGN BODIES IN THE NOSE AND PHARYNX

LEWIS R. FIRST, M.D.

The most important concept in diagnosing and subsequently removing a foreign body from the nose or pharynx is to consider the possibility that an ingestion, aspiration, or foreign body insertion has occurred regardless of the history. The sooner the diagnosis is entertained, the quicker and often easier the removal can be.

The average age for inserting a foreign object into the nose is 2 to 3 years, with most case reports ranging from 1 to 6 years. Girls are more apt to insert beads, whereas boys will more often place paper and toy parts into their nostrils. Both sexes will equally insert food items. The most common site for lodging a foreign body in the nose includes the floor just below the inferior turbinate or anterior to the middle turbinate.

The classic symptoms of a nasal foreign body (usually an organic or porous substance) can include discomfort, foul odor, or discharge. The presence of a unilateral yellow or green, foul-smelling nasal discharge is classic for such a nasal foreign body, but a bilateral nasal discharge also is possible. Bleeding can result if the object is sharp. Inorganic metallic or plastic objects may lodge for prolonged periods without producing a malodorous inflammatory discharge until, eventually, obstruction and bleeding occur from buildup of granulation tissue around the inorganic item. Pain is unusual in the setting of an uncomplicated nasal foreign body, and its presence should suggest complications, such as an associated sinusitis.

Radiographs are usually not helpful with nasal foreign bodies, since most are radiolucent, although some toys and beads appear on radiographic views of the sinuses and nasal cavity. Therefore confirmation of the diagnosis rests on the physical examination. A good examination requires the use of a nasal speculum and head lamp or other form of indirect illumination to visualize the nasal cavity. Indirect laryngoscopy using a nasopharyngeal mirror and adequate illumination of the pharynx may be needed to view the posterior aspects of the nose, should the anterior approach be unrevealing.

The vast majority of nasal foreign bodies can be removed in the office or emergency room setting without referral to an otorhinolaryngologist. In fact, referrals to such a specialist usually are those that result from failed home attempts before reaching an office or emergency room setting. The use of a topical vasoconstrictor-anesthetic agent (e.g., topical lidocaine, phenylephrine, and cocaine) can help with the vasoconstriction of the turbinates and provide pain relief during the procedure. A first-line, often successful approach in a cooperative child is to compress the contralateral naris (following administration of the topical anesthetic) and ask the child to blow out through the naris that contains the foreign body. If this maneuver is unsuccessful, or if the child is too young to follow directions, the next step is proper immobilization of the patient and subsequent good visualization of the object. Restraining the child with a papoose board can be extremely useful. Removal of a nasal foreign body in the office or emergency room setting requires a nasal speculum (or a wide speculum from an otoscope) along with appropriate illumination from a head lamp or floor spotlight lamp. Alligator, mosquito, or bayonet forceps should be available for removal of objects with edges. Wire loops, right-angle hooks, or even a cerumen curet may be all that is needed to remove a round object from the nose. The instrument selected should be inserted alongside and then behind the round object and then pulled forward, bringing the object out in front of it. A suction catheter if available may be successful in removing or at least pulling a smooth round object anteriorly for easier removal. Suction also can be useful to remove purulent secretions that prevent visualization of the foreign body.

An alternative method is to place an 8F Fogarty catheter behind the object, inflate the catheter balloon, and pull the object forward in front of the balloon. Insertion of such a catheter can also force the object more posteriorly into the nasopharynx, where it might be aspirated down an unprotected airway, and thus should be considered only as a last resort or be performed only under the guidance of someone experienced with this technique.

It is not recommended that foreign body removal be undertaken by irrigation of the nasopharynx as a means of washing out the object. This maneuver may either force the object more posteriorly, even into the airway, or result in swelling of the object (e.g., a sponge, paper, pea, or bean), further obstructing the airway cavity.

Complications of removing a nasal foreign body can include subsequent rhinosinusitis, mucosal laceration, epistaxis, aspiration, or even incomplete removal of the object. The other nostril should always be explored as well to ensure that no other objects are present. If bleeding occurs during the removal, the use of an oral antibiotic, such as amoxicillin, has been suggested in some studies to prevent possible infection.

Button disc batteries are more notorious for causing problems in the gastrointestinal tract, but they have been known to lodge in the nose as well. If left in the nasal cavity, a disc battery can generate an electrical current or leak its contents, resulting in superficial electrical or chemical burns to the nasal turbinates (within 1 hour of placement) and, in extreme cases, even septal erosion and perforation. In addition, pressure necrosis can occur at the nasal septum simply from prolonged impaction with the battery. Therefore, one should never overlook the nose in the diagnostic evaluation of a disc battery ingestion.

The oral pharynx can harbor foreign bodies, and again, one should entertain the suspicion even if the child denies it. Most pharyngeal and hypopharyngeal foreign bodies occur in children between 6 months to 6 years, often because they lack molars to help with chewing. Although less common than nasal foreign bodies (because of the presence of a gag reflex, as well as the tongue, which can eject an unwanted object), the complications of a foreign body in the pharynx or most notably in the hypopharynx can be life threatening. In fact, 500 deaths occur yearly in the United States as a result of asphyxiation from an obstructing foreign body. One of the most notorious culprits is a balloon, which if popped or bitten into by a child can propel itself to the back of the pharynx and block the airway. In addition, such items as fish bones, pins, and pieces of plastic can get caught in the oral mucosa, tonsils, or hypopharynx. Most fatalities, however, result from blockage from food products rather than from pieces of toys or other objects.

The clinical presentation of a foreign body in the hypopharynx can simulate that of a foreign body in the trachea by causing extrinsic compression of the airway. Choking, hoarseness, stridor, pain, drooling, and inability to swallow, as well as bad breath, all can be indicators of a hypopharyngeal foreign body. Infants may refuse to eat.

If respiratory obstruction occurs, appropriate protocols for a blocked airway should be followed (e.g., the Heimlich maneuver in children over 10 kg, back blows and chest thrusts in children under 10 kg). In an emergency setting, a blocked airway requires emergency intubation (with removal of the object using Magill forceps) or, if the physician is unable to visualize the obstruction, an emergency tracheostomy must be performed.

If only partial airway obstruction is noted, indirect laryngoscopy should be performed, which may allow visualization and removal of a foreign body lodged in a tonsillar fossa. Such a body could then be removed with an alligator forceps without the need for a radiograph. If the object cannot be seen with indirect laryngoscopy or direct visualization, anteroposterior and lateral radiographic views of the airway and nasopharynx should be obtained, since more objects may be radiopaque in this area than in the nose.

Removal again requires immobilization and good visualization. A Magill forceps can be extremely useful for removal of a well-visualized object. A Foley catheter can be inserted into the hypopharynx beyond the object, and the balloon can be inflated and then withdrawn only if the suspected object is smooth. If the object is sharp, complications, such as scratches and tears of the mucosa, may occur as the object is removed. A safer mode of removal is intubation to protect the airway and removal of the object under general anesthesia. A recent development has been the use by otorhinolaryngologists of the flexible nasopharyngoscope to remove fishbones in the oropharynx or hypopharynx using local anesthesia with conscious sedation.

Following removal of any object from the nose or pharynx, the area should be reexamined. This ensures that the entire object has been evacuated and documents whether any further trauma to the area has occurred in the process of removing the foreign body.

REFERENCES

1. Jone NS, Lannigan FJ, Salama NY: Foreign bodies in the throat: A prospective study of 388 cases. J Laryngol Otolaryngol 105:104–108, 1991.
2. Tong MC, Van Hasselt CA, Woo JK: The hazards of button batteries in the nose. J Otolaryngol 21:458–460, 1992.

NASOPHARYNGITIS

ANN R. MCGRAVEY, M.D.

Nasopharyngitis is inflammation and congestion of the nasal passages and oral pharynx. The majority of cases are acute and viral in nature, and, thus, the term is used interchangeably with the common cold.

This entity is quite common, affecting the average child three to eight times per year. Children in day care may have up to 50% more colds (as well as otitis media), and the incidence may also increase in the setting of parental smoking, crowding, and malnutrition. More than 200 viruses can cause a cold, and rhinovirus accounts for more than one third.

Transmission usually occurs via a symptomatic person who sheds virus in nasal secretions. Contacts innoculate themselves by touching their nose or conjunctivae with contaminated hands. The virus then invades the upper respiratory tract, causing release of inflammatory mediators (probably not histamine). These cause increased vascular permeability, edema, and hence nasal stuffiness. Stimulation of cholinergic nerves leads to increased mucus production (rhinorrhea) and sometimes to bronchoconstriction, which causes coughing. Cough also occurs as a reflex mechanism to clear secretions. Direct cellular damage is probably the cause of the sore throat.

The nasopharyngeal symptoms may be accompanied by myalgia, malaise, decreased appetite, headache, eye irritation, and fever. Infants may have high fever and are often irritable and restless and have difficulty with feeding or sleeping. They may have posttussive vomiting.

By the second or third day, the child starts to feel better but may start to cough, particularly at night. Systemic symptoms usually subside within 5 to 7 days, but the rhinitis, often quite purulent by this point because of shedding of epithelial and white blood cells, may persist for another week until the nasal epithelial cells have regenerated.

DIFFERENTIAL DIAGNOSIS

The natural history of the disease is important to keep in mind in differentiating viral nasopharyngitis from bacterial entities, such as sinusitis, that require antibiotic treatment. Mucopurulent nasal discharge does not always imply bacterial superinfection, as it is commonly seen in colds with little or no change in bacterial flora.

Sinusitis should be considered when rhinorrhea has persisted for more than 10 days, when a cold has not improved but worsened, or when a child with cold symptoms appears very ill.[2] Young children do not usually complain of facial pain or headaches, and rhinorrhea and chronic cough may be the only symptoms. Physical examination may reveal nasal or postnasal mucopurulent discharge and foul breath. In addition to the lack of specificity of symptoms and signs, the radiologic findings may be equivocal. Culture of the nasal discharge is not helpful, since the bacteria responsible for sinusitis are also normal nasopharyngeal flora. These difficulties in diagnosis are probably responsible for overtreatment of colds with antibiotics for fear of missing a diagnosis of sinusitis.

An even more common complication of a cold is otitis media. Many viral upper respiratory infections may be associated with serous otitis media. Whether or not all of these require antibiotic treatment is debatable.

Other entities exist in the differential diagnosis of the child with nasal congestion and discharge. Allergic rhinitis may be hard to differentiate from recurrent viral nasopharyngitis. Its diagnosis should be suggested by a seasonal incidence, an atopic family history, recurrent or persistent watery rhinorrhea, frequent sneezing, itchy eyes, nose, or throat, eczema, asthma, or frequent nighttime cough. Physical findings may include allergic facies and edematous, pale nasal turbinates. A stained swab of nasal secretions may reveal eosinophils.

A unilateral foul-smelling nasal discharge suggests a foreign body, and chronic purulent rhinorrhea suggests polyps, adenoidal hypertrophy, or immune deficiencies.

Pharyngitis caused by group A *Streptococcus* occasionally is associated with rhinorrhea in children less than 3 to 4 years of age. Accordingly, nasopharyngeal cultures may be useful in this age group. The older child with a streptococcal throat infection will not usually have rhinorrhea as a symptom. Viral cultures and immunofluorescent tests are available, but since most children recover uneventfully, such tests are rarely cost effective.

TREATMENT

Most children with colds or viral nasopharyngitis need no treatment. Nonpharmacologic therapy may make the child feel better without the risk of side effects. Good hydration and the use of a cool mist vaporizer or humidifier can loosen secretions and decrease nasal obstruction. Secretions can be removed by use of a bulb syringe. To aid the removal, saline nose drops, either purchased over-the-counter or made at home using ¼ to 1 teaspoon of salt in 8 ounces of water may be used. Two drops can be instilled in a nostril approximately 2 minutes before suctioning. This is particularly helpful in infants (who may be unable to mouth breathe effectively) before meals and sleep. Additionally, one may elevate the head of the bed to enhance posterior nasal drainage during sleep. There have been no formal studies on the efficacy of chicken soup. Vitamins have not been found to decrease the duration of symptoms.

Pharmacologic treatment probably should be used only if the child is particularly uncomfortable or if the child does not respond to nonpharmacologic measures. If the child is febrile, acetaminophen at a dose of 10 to 15 mg/kg per dose every 4 to 6 hours may reduce the body temperature and improve how the child feels. The nature of pharmacotherapy should be symptom-specific. The various classes of pharmacotherapies are shown in Table 1.

For the relief of nasal obstruction, locally applied or orally administered systemically active decongestants are used frequently, but neither their true efficacy nor their adverse effects have been evaluated carefully in children. Their use should probably be restricted to infants and children older than 4 to 6 months of age, since younger infants may develop tachycardia and irritability. They should be used only for 3 to 5 days, preferably at times of greatest need (bed, meal, and school times). They should perhaps be recommended on a 1-day trial basis and discontinued if no benefit is observed. Topical decongestants produce a prompt vasoconstriction but more temporary relief than oral agents. They are associated with fewer side effects than oral preparations but can only be used for a maximum of 3 days before rebound vasodilatation occurs.

For rhinorrhea, antihistamines with their anticholinergic effects often are tried. However, this activity may be very weak or even insignificant at dosage levels found in cold preparations, and sedation is a major side effect. Their use should probably be reserved for allergic rhinitis.

Very often, children will be bothered by a dry hacking cough. Antitussives of three types (Table 1) are available. These agents are probably not indicated in the first few days of a cold, when the cough is useful in clearing secretions, but may be helpful when the cough becomes excessive, especially the dry, nonproductive type that can be discomforting, interfere with sleep, and become self-perpetuating. Dextromethorphan is probably the most useful of the three types, being equipotent to codeine without the CNS and respiratory depression.

Expectorants have been proposed to loosen respiratory secretions, but no studies document their efficacy. Good hydration is probably a more reasonable approach.

TABLE 1. Classification of Over-the-Counter Cold Medicines

CLASS	EXAMPLES	SIDE EFFECTS
Sympathomimetics	Phenylpropanolamine Pseudoephedrine Phenylephrine	Excess stimulation Irritability Hypertension Insomnia
Antihistamines	Ethanolamines (diphenhydramine) Ethylenediamines Alkylamines (chlorpheniramine, brompheniramine)	Sedation Paradoxical CNS stimulation
Expectorants	Guaifenesin	Gastric upset
Cough expectorants	Dextromethorphan	Sedation, gastrointestinal upset
	Codeine	Drowsiness, respiratory depression

Antiviral drugs have been found useful for specific viruses, for example, amantadine or rimantidine for influenza A. For other viruses, especially rhinovirus, the most common agent in the common cold, no therapy is available.

PREVENTION

Since colds are so difficult to treat, attempts at prevention have been tried. Avoidance, such as keeping children out of day care, is impractical. Frequent handwashing after contact with an infected person reduces the risk of secondary infection. Use of disinfectants, such as tincture of iodine and phenol alcohol (Lysol) can interrupt transmission, but the compounds have no residual virucidal activity. Use of iodine-impregnated disposable handkerchiefs has been postulated to decrease spread. Avoidance of smoking may decrease the number of infections. Breast feeding has not been proven conclusively to reduce the frequency or duration of viral nasopharyngitis.

Vaccines have been difficult to produce, in part because of the large number of antigenic types, the poor responsiveness of nasal IgA production to the inactivated antigens, and short-lived immunity. A recent study has demonstrated a significant reduction in the incidence of otitis media with the use of influenza vaccine among children in day care. The new live attenuated vaccine for intranasal administration may be more effective and better accepted. A cold recombinant vaccine would probably have greatest usefulness for universal immunization of children under 10 years of age.

REFERENCES

1. Glezen WP: Viral respiratory infections. Pediatr Ann 20:8, 407–410, 1991.
2. Wald ER, Guerra N, Byers C: Upper respiratory tract infections in young children—Duration of and frequency of complications. Pediatrics 87:129–133, 1991.

RHINITIS AND SINUSITIS

LAWRENCE W.C. TOM, M.D.
DAVID W. KENNEDY, M.D.

Although rhinitis and sinusitis are typically considered in many texts as separate disease processes, the two disorders are closely related. Studies have demonstrated that viral rhinitis may result in radiographic changes in the sinuses (mucosal thickening and air–fluid levels) for several weeks following the infection. Similarly, chronic rhinitis is typically associated with some degree of sinus involvement, and conversely, sinusitis may cause intranasal edema and obstruction. In this section, rhinitis and sinusitis are differentiated in the traditional manner. However, the treating physician should always keep the intimate relationship between the two disorders in mind.

RHINITIS

Viral infections of the upper respiratory tract are the most common cause of rhinitis. These infections are self-limited, require no specific therapy, and usually resolve within 2 weeks. When the rhinitis persists beyond 2 weeks, other possible causes, including bacterial sinusitis, must be considered.

Rhinitis in infants, even secondary to viral respiratory tract infections, may cause serious problems. Newborns are obligate nose breathers, and the rhinitis may restrict their ability to breathe. These children may require vigorous suctioning to maintain the airway. Saline nasal drops and topical decongestants may provide additional relief. In infants and young children, group A beta-hemolytic streptococcal infections may occur as persistent upper respiratory tract infections. In these children, a 10-day course of phenoxymethyl penicillin (125 mg q.i.d. for children weighing less than 25 kg or 250 mg q.i.d. for those weighing more than 25 kg) or, in penicillin-allergic children, erythromycin (40 mg/kg/d in four divided doses) is recommended (Table 1).

Allergies are a frequent cause of rhinitis and should be considered in cases where rhinitis fails to improve after antibiotic therapy. Children with seasonal symptoms and the physical stigmata of allergies, such as sneezing, watery eyes, and dark rings under their eyes (allergic shiners), are not difficult to diagnose. On the other hand, the diagnosis may be challenging in children with perennial symptoms and isolated nasal complaints. Characteristically, children with allergic rhinitis have pale, bluish purple nasal mucosa with watery rhinorrhea. Symptomatic relief may be obtained with an oral antihistamine-decongestant and a topical intranasal steroid, such as beclomethasone (1 inhalation or spray 2 to 3 times a day) or flunisolide (1 spray 3 times a day). The effects of the nasal steroids, however, are not immediate, and parents should be warned that it may take 3 weeks to achieve maximum relief. If the allergen can be identified, avoidance is advised. If these measures fail, desensitization may be needed.

Both chronic rhinitis of childhood and vasomotor rhinitis may be difficult to distinguish from allergic and infectious rhinitis. Chronic rhinitis of childhood is characterized by regular episodes of nasal congestion and mucopurlent rhinorrhea. It usually appears about age 6, decreases in severity with time, and disappears by age 10. Systemic decongestants provide effective relief. Vasomotor rhinitis is a hyperactive cholinergic response to stimulants, such as temperature changes, irritants, and recumbent positioning, resulting in swelling of the nasal turbinates and rhinorrhea. It may be precipitated or worsened by a low-grade sinusitis. Treatment is directed at avoidance of the stimulant. Antihistamines should not be prescribed because they impair nasal ciliary motility and may worsen the condition. If symptoms persist, the child should be evaluated for the presence of sinusitis, and, if present, this should be treated.

Other causes of rhinitis include intranasal foreign bodies and rhinitis medicamentosa. Foreign bodies should be suspected when the discharge is unilateral, foul smelling, purulent, and/or bloody. Removal of the foreign body is curative. Rhinitis medicamentosa occurs after the prolonged use of topical decongestants. A rebound develops causing edema, erythema, and thickening of the nasal mucosa. Parents and children must be cautioned to avoid using these decongestants for more than 3 to 5 days. Treatment consists of elimination of topical decongestants and a short course of systemic steroids or an intranasal steroid spray.

SINUSITIS

Acute sinusitis most commonly occurs following upper respiratory tract infections. Children have six to eight upper respiratory tract infections per year, and it is estimated that 0.5% to 5.0% will develop acute bacterial sinusitis. Acute sinusitis should be suspected when an upper respiratory tract infection lasts beyond 10 to 14 days.

Although 40% of cases of acute sinusitis will resolve spontaneously, all patients should be treated to achieve a rapid clinical cure, eradicate microorganisms from the sinuses, prevent chronic disease, and prevent complications. The most common pathogens causing pediatric sinusitis are *Streptococcus pneumoniae* (30%), *Haemophilus influenzae* (20%), and *Moxarella catarrhalis* (20%). In most cases, amoxicillin (40 mg/kg/d in three divided doses) is the initial antibiotic

TABLE 1. Drugs and Dosages: Rhinitis and Sinusitis

Rhinitis	
Oral Antibiotics for Group A Streptococcus	
Phenoxymethyl penicillin	Children < 25 kg: 125 mg q.i.d.
	Children > 25 kg: 250 mg q.i.d.
Erythromycin	40 mg/kg/d in 4 divided doses
Intranasal Steroid Sprays	
Beclomethasone	1 inhalation or spray b.i.d. or t.i.d.
Flunisolide	1 spray t.i.d.
Sinusitis	
Oral Antibiotics	
Amoxicillin	40 mg/kg/d in 3 divided doses
Trimethoprim-sulfamethoxazole	8 mg and 40 mg/kg/d respectively in two divided doses
Erythromycin-sulfisoxazole	50 and 150 mg/kg/d, respectively, in 4 divided doses
Cefaclor	40 mg/kg/d in 3 divided doses
Loracarbef	30 mg/kg/day in two divided doses
Cefuroxime axetil	Children < 12 y: 125–250 mg b.i.d.
	Children > 12 y: 250–500 mg b.i.d.
Amoxicillin with clavulanate	Children < 40 kg: 40 mg/kg/d in 3 divided doses
	Children > 40 kg: 250–500 mg with a maximum dose of 1.5 g
Intravenous Antibiotics	
Cefuroxime	150 mg/kg/d in 3 divided doses
Oxacillin and chloramphenicol	150 mg/kg/d and 50–75 mg/kg/d, respectively, in 4 divided doses
Intranasal Steroid Sprays	
Beclomethasone	1 inhalation or spray b.i.d. or t.i.d.
Flunisolide	1 spray t.i.d.
Osteomyelitis and Orbital Complications	
Intravenous Antibiotics	
Oxacillin and chloramphenicol	150 mg/kg/d and 75 mg/kg/d, respectively, in 4 divided doses
Clindamycin and chloramphenicol	40 mg/kg/d and 75 mg/kg/d, respectively, in 4 divided doses
Ampicillin with sulbactam (Unasyn)	200 mg/kg/d in 4 divided doses
Oxacillin and metronidazole	150 mg/kg/d and 30 mg/kg/d, respectively, in 4 divided doses
Intracranial Complications	
Intravenous Antibiotics	
Oxacillin and chloramphenicol	150 mg/kg/d and 75 mg/kg/d, respectively, in 4 divided doses
Oxacillin and metronidazole	150 mg/kg/d and 30 mg/kg/d, respectively, in 4 divided doses
Imipenem	100 mg/kg/d in 4 divided doses

of choice. It is relatively safe, inexpensive, active against the common pathogens, and well tolerated. If the child is allergic to penicillin or a beta-lactamase-producing organism is suspected, alternative medications include trimethoprim-sulfamethoxazole (8 and 40 mg/kg/d, respectively, in two divided doses), erythromycin-sulfisoxazole (50 and 150 mg/kg/d, respectively, in four divided doses), cefaclor (40 mg/kg/d in three divided doses), loracarbef (30 mg/kg/d in two divided doses), and in children able to swallow tablets, cefuroxime axetil (125 to 250 mg twice daily). Amoxicillin with potassium clavulanate (40 mg/kg/d in three divided doses, with a maximum dose of 1.5 g) also is effective against beta-lactamase-producing bacteria. Topical and systemic decongestants, steam, mucolytic agents, and saline nose sprays are adjunctive measures that will help to decongest the mucosa, moisturize the nose, and promote drainage. *In acute sinusitis, antihistamines should be avoided*. They can impair ciliary motility and increase the viscosity of the secretions, impeding the drainage of sinus secretions.

Most patients will respond to this conservative medical management, but *if there is no response or a worsening of the condition after 48 to 72 hours, a broader-spectrum antibiotic appropriate for beta-lactamase-producing organisms is indicated*. Plain sinus radiographs will help determine the extent of disease. These films are helpful for evaluation of the maxillary sinuses but may underestimate the presence and extent of ethmoid disease. A normal sinus x-ray does not rule out ethmoid sinusitis.

If the child does not improve despite a broad-spectrum oral antibiotic, intravenous antibiotics are required. Cefuroxime (150 mg/kg/d in three divided doses) and a combination of chloramphenicol (75 mg/kg/d) and oxacillin (150 mg/kg/d) in four divided doses are excellent choices. Intravenous antibiotics must also be considered for children with acute frontal or sphenoidal sinusitis. These sinuses are in close proximity to intracranial structures, and there is the potential for intracranial complications.

When identification of the microorganism is necessary, such as in children who have not responded to conventional therapy, are immunocompromised, or have significant complications, sinus aspiration is performed. Aspiration also provides relief from pressure and discomfort. Although puncture of the maxillary sinus may be performed with sedation in cooperative children with maxillary sinusitis, this is a difficult office procedure. Most otolaryngologists prefer to perform maxillary sinus punctures under general anesthesia. The *endoscopic approach* is becoming an increasingly popular technique for aspiration. Under direct telescopic visualization, the ostia of the affected sinuses can be identified. Secretions can be suctioned and cultured, and the sinuses can be opened to facilitate drainage. Although all the sinuses can be approached endoscopically, caution must be taken with frontal sinusitis. For isolated frontal sinus disease, trephination is an excellent technique for aspiration.

In children with recurrent episodes of acute sinusitis and chronic sinusitis, identification and treatment of any predisposing factors are important. These underlying conditions include immunodeficiencies, immotile cilia syndrome, cystic fibrosis, allergies, day care, pollution especially second-hand smoke, and anatomic abnormalities, such as nasal septal deviations, infected adenoids, and polyps.

Chronic sinusitis occurs when the clinical presentation persists beyond 8 weeks. *Chronic sinusitis tends to be a polymicrobial infection*. Children with cystic fibrosis and chronic sinusitis have a high incidence of *Pseudomonas aeruginosa. A 4- to 6-week course of a broad-spectrum antibiotic and an intranasal steroid spray is the preferred treatment for chronic sinusitis*.

If the symptoms persist despite this management, CT of the sinuses with coronal views and bone windows is performed. Sinus CT provides an excellent view of the sinuses and surrounding bony structures and is the study of choice for evaluation of the sinuses. MRI does not display bony landmarks, provides too many false positives, and is not used routinely for evaluation of sinus disease. MRI may be performed to assess the extension of disease beyond the sinuses or to differentiate soft tissue masses from infection in the sinuses.

If the symptoms continue and there is objective evidence of sinusitis despite adequate medical therapy, surgery should be considered. The specific procedure depends on the individual circumstances and pathologic condition. *Functional endoscopic sinus surgery (FESS)* has supplanted more traditional operations, such as nasal antral windows, the Caldwell-Luc, and external ethmoidectomy, as the procedure of choice for patients with chronic sinusitis. FESS relies on direct telescopic visualization to remove diseased sinus mucosa and improve sinus drainage. The procedure is well tolerated by most children, and there is little postoperative discomfort. It is beneficial in approximately 80% of children.

Complications of Sinusitis

Antibiotic treatment has reduced the incidence and altered the presentation of the complications of sinusitis. Children with acute sinusitis and deficiencies of their immune system are more likely to develop complications, which can be classified as local, orbital, and intracranial.

Local complications include mucoceles and osteomyelitis. A mucocele is a cystic lesion that becomes filled with mucus and eventually will expand to distort the involved sinus and surrounding tissue. FESS is ideal for removal and drainage of the mucocele.

Osteomyelitis is an infection of the marrow spaces of the bones surrounding the sinuses. The infection spreads to the overlying soft tissue, causing a cellulitis. Osteomyelitis of the ethmoid is most common in young children, whereas osteomyelitis of the frontal bone may occur in older children and adolescents. Therapy consists of a 4 to 6 week course of intravenous antibiotics, sinus drainage, and in many cases, debridement of the infected bone. The combination of oxacillin and chloramphenicol is the treatment of choice. In penicillin-allergic children, clindamycin can be substituted for oxacillin. Other choices include the combination of ampicillin and sulbactam (Unasyn) and oxacillin combined with metronidazole.

Orbital infections are the most common complication of sinusitis in children and are usually a result of ethmoid disease. In order of increasing severity, these complications are periorbital cellulitis, orbital cellulitis, subperiosteal abscess, orbital abscess, and cavernous sinus thrombosis.

Sinus CT is performed to establish the type and extent of disease. Blood cultures are rarely positive, but drainage of a subperiosteal abscess will often yield a positive culture. The usual bacterial isolates in children with subperiosteal abscesses are *Staphylococcus aureus*, streptococci, and anaerobes of the upper respiratory tract.

Periorbital cellulitis without chemosis may be treated initially with a broad-spectrum oral antibiotic if the child appears well and the eye is still at least 50% opened. Intravenous antibiotics, however, are necessary if the response to oral medication is sluggish and for all other orbital complications. Cefuroxime (150 mg/kg in three divided doses) is a good selection for periorbital cellulitis. For the more severe complications, the antibiotics are as indicated for osteomyelitis.

Children who develop abscesses require surgical drainage of the abscess and underlying sinus disease. This can be achieved with an external ethmoidectomy and, in selected cases, the nasal endoscopic approach. Cavernous sinus thrombosis is associated with significant morbidity and mortality. In addition to high-dose intravenous antibiotics, anticoagulants may be necessary. Surgery to eradicate the sinus disease is performed only after the patient is stable. Antibiotics must be continued for at least 2 to 3 weeks after the sinus procedure.

Intracranial infections are the second most common complications of sinusitis and include meningitis, epidural abscess, subdural abscess, and brain abscess. Most of these infections develop from frontal sinusitis, and since the frontal sinus does not develop until age 6 or older, these complications are usually seen in older children and adolescents. Intracranial complications occur in adolescent males more frequently than in any other age group, and frontal sinusitis in adolescents should be treated aggressively. The clinical presentations of these infections are varied, but an intracranial complication should be suspected in any child with acute sinusitis and signs of a CNS complication, such meningeal irritation, increased intracranial pressure, cranial nerve deficit, or change in mental status. A sinus CT scan should be performed.

All patients with an intracranial complication should be managed by a team consisting of a pediatrician, neurosurgeon, and otolaryngologist. The antibiotic treatment is similar to that for children with significant orbital complications except that clindamycin is generally not used for CNS infections. Imipenem may be a useful alternative to oxacillin and chloramphenicol or oxacillin and metronidazole. The antibiotics may be changed depending on the culture results. Drainage of any intracranial abscess is performed as soon as possible, and definitive surgical treatment of the sinus disease is performed as soon as the neurologic status permits.

RETROPHARYNGEAL AND PERITONSILLAR ABSCESSES

WILLIAM P. POTSIC, M.D.

Retropharyngeal and peritonsillar abscesses are fairly common in children and adolescents. Both create considerable morbidity and are potentially life threatening when they are severe and produce airway obstruction.

RETROPHARYNGEAL ABSCESS

Retropharyngeal abscess is usually diagnosed in a child who has a stiff neck, difficulty swallowing, and neck fullness. *Stertorous breathing* also may be present, indicating impingement on the airway. A lateral neck radiograph with widening of the retropharyngeal space suggests the diagnosis, but computed tomography (CT) or magnetic resonance imaging (MRI) is required to confirm the presence and extent of retropharyngeal abscess.

Retropharyngeal abscesses require intravenous antimicrobial therapy directed at polymicrobial infection, including aerobic and anaerobic organisms, for 7 to 10 days. A first-generation cephalosporin or clindamycin usually is effective (Table 1). Patients who do not respond as expected to intravenous antimicrobial therapy or have *stertorous respiration* require surgical drainage using general anesthesia. A transoral or lateral cervical approach is selected based on the CT or MRI findings. Complete recovery is expected, and recurrence is extremely rare. No specific follow-up evaluations are required.

PERITONSILLAR ABSCESS

Peritonsillar abscess is more common in adolescents than in young children but occurs at all ages. Signs and symptoms of pharyngotonsillitis are accompanied by displacement of the involved tonsil and uvula to the opposite side and varying degrees of *trismus*. The severity of trismus usually correlates with the size of the abscess.

When the degree of trismus does not prevent adequate visualization of the peritonsillar area, needle aspiration with an 18-gauge needle usually provides immediate relief of discomfort and trismus. Patients who are able to swallow adequately to maintain hydration and take oral antibiotics are treated with a first- or second-generation cephalosporin for 10 days as an outpatient. The patient is rehydrated in the

TABLE 1. Formulary

DRUG	DOSAGE
Cephalexin (Keflex)	50–100 mg/kg/24 h PO in 4 divided doses q6h
Cefazolin (Ancef)	50–150 mg/kg/24 h IV in 3 divided doses q8h
Cefaclor (Ceclor)	40 mg/kg/24 PO in 3 divided doses q8h
Clindamycin	30 mg/kg/24 h IV in 4 divided doses q6h

emergency room, given a dose of intravenous antimicrobial therapy before discharge, and instructed to return in 5 days or sooner if not improving.

Patients who fulfilled the criteria for tonsillectomy before having a peritonsillar abscess treated by needle aspiration and antimicrobial therapy should be considered for an elective tonsillectomy.

Patients with a poor clinical response to oral antimicrobials, recurrent peritonsillar abscess, or severe trismus or who are too young to participate in peritonsillar abscess needle aspiration require general anesthesia for incision and drainage. A concurrent tonsillectomy provides wide drainage, prevents recurrence, and permits discharge from the hospital in 12 to 24 hours. Intravenous antimicrobial therapy is given with a first-generation cephalosporin during the hospitalization and continued orally for 7 to 10 days after discharge. Complete recovery is expected, and follow-up examination beyond the usual for patients undergoing tonsillectomy is not required.

REFERENCES

1. Asmar BI: Bacteriology of retropharyngeal abscess in children. Pediatr Infect Dis J 9:595–597, 1990.
2. Ravindranath T, Janakiraman N, Harris V: Computed tomography in diagnosing retropharyngeal abscess in children. Clin Pediatr 32:242–244, 1993.
3. Savolainen S, Jousimies-Somer J, Makitie AA, Ylikoski JS: Peritonsillar abscess: Clinical and microbiologic aspects and treatment regimens. Arch Otolaryngol Head Neck Surg 119:521–524, 1993.

THE TONSIL AND ADENOID PROBLEM

RICHARD B. GOLDBLOOM, O.C., M.D., F.R.C.P.C.

It has been estimated that some 250,000 tonsil and adenoid (T & A) removals are performed each year in the United States. This represents a progressive reduction from the approximately 1 million performed annually 20 years ago. This decline has been attributed to several factors, including lack of conclusive evidence of effectiveness, availability of alternative therapeutic options, and concerns about complications. Curiously, the decline in T & As has been mirrored by a progressive increase in the rate of performance of myringotomy and ventilating tube insertions under general anesthesia. As a result, the combined annual total of the two most frequently performed otolaryngologic surgical procedures has not changed substantially.

A decision for surgical removal of tonsils and/or adenoids should never be undertaken lightly. A small but significant number of fatalities associated with T & A continue to occur. Postoperative hemorrhage is not uncommon, but doubts have been raised about the value of routine preoperative screening for coagulopathies because of the large number of false positive laboratory tests and bleeding histories as compared with the relatively rare incidence of inherited and acquired coagulopathies. Other unanticipated serious complications, such as malignant hyperthermia, can turn an ostensibly simple procedure into a major catastrophe. T & A should never be considered minor surgery and should be carried out in hospitals that offer skilled pediatric anesthesia and attentive postoperative care. In most instances, a decision to perform elective T & A is one that selects a procedure that carries a small but definite mortality rate to correct a condition that carries some.

The list of what once were considered absolute indications for T & A has been shrinking in recent years. The rare combination of documented obstructive sleep apnea with carbon dioxide retention, hypoxia, and cor pulmonale is a definite indication for the procedure. In less severe instances of obstructive sleep apnea, documentation of clinical benefit is less clear. Other possible indications include the uncommon association of tonsil or adenoid dysphagia, weight loss, and failure to thrive, the presence of persistent or recurrent tonsillar hemorrhage, and the rare instances of tonsillar malignancy in which surgery may be required for histologic diagnosis. In combination, however, these indications represent only a tiny fraction of all tonsillectomies currently performed.

Peritonsillar abscess (quinsy) formerly was considered an absolute indication for tonsillectomy, often performed some time after the initial infection had subsided. It has now been documented, however, that the recurrence rate of peritonsillitis is low and the need for tonsillectomy after a single episode of quinsy has been seriously questioned. In older children, needle aspiration coupled with parenteral antibiotic therapy (oxacillin, clindamycin, or a cephalosporin) is efficacious and safe. Tonsillectomy is reserved for the few nonresponders. In younger children, incision and drainage or needle aspiration should be carried out in the operating room, at which time tonsillectomy can be performed if judged necessary.

The need for tonsillectomy in children with recurrent tonsillitis is much more problematic. On follow-up of such children, many have not had the frequency or severity of tonsillitis described by their parents. Further, in a randomized, controlled clinical trial of surgical vs medical management of children with recurrent tonsillitis, a significant reduction in the incidence of sore throats was found in the first and second years after surgery but not in the third. On the other hand, many of those who did not have surgery also had markedly fewer sore throats during follow-up, and most of those were minor. Thus, in individual children, the modest, short-term benefits of tonsillectomy must be weighed against the risks of the procedure. It has been estimated that at most only 1 or 2 children with throat infections of the frequency and severity required for inclusion in the cited clinical trial would be seen annually in a pediatric or family practice.

For most children, surgery should be considered only after truly adequate antibiotic treatment has failed. In many instances, a trial of antibiotic prophylaxis may be a desirable alternative. It has been speculated that since β-lactamase-producing organisms may be involved in recurrent tonsillitis, the condition may be more effectively treated with a β-lactamase-stable or β-lactamase-inhibiting antimicrobial agent to eliminate an underlying streptococcal infection.

Adenoidectomy is most often recommended for the relief of obstruction (often manifested as snoring at night) or for the treatment of recurrent otitis, with or without myringotomy and ventilating tube insertion. When adenoids are obstructive, causing mouth breathing, snoring, and hyponasal speech, removal may relieve such symptoms. However, the overall health benefits of surgery for this purpose have not been clearly documented. Parenthetically, it is interesting to note how many children are subjected to surgery to correct snoring, whereas adults whose snoring is usually much louder often are tolerated indulgently. The benefit of adenoidectomy for children with recurrent sinusitis has not been established.

In the treatment of recurrent otitis media, adenoidectomy with or without myringotomy has been shown to be more effective than no surgery in reducing recurrences, but tonsillectomy does not increase the efficacy of adenoidectomy alone. One absolute contraindication to adenoidectomy is the presence of a cleft palate or of any palatal condition that may permit nasal escape of air during speech. In such instances, removal of the adenoid further exaggerates the defect in palatopharyngeal closure, increasing the nasal escape of air and creating more serious speech problems. The presence of a bifid or notched uvula also should be regarded as a potential contraindication, since these minor anomalies often are accompanied by a submucous cleft or related palatal abnormalities.

Physicians sometimes feel pressured by parents' insistence that something be done for their child who has recurrent throat or ear infections, snores at night, or has other symptoms attributed to enlarged or infected tonsils or adenoids. It has now been well documented that parental perceptions of the frequency of antecedent sore throats in their child are unreliable predictors of the subsequent frequency of sore throats under close observation. From the physician's viewpoint, it may be easier and quicker to recommend surgery than to discuss the pros and cons of surgery with patients (or guardians), defer a decision, or attempt less dramatic alternatives. The temptation to take this path should be resisted.

Parents' tolerance for recurrent respiratory infections in their children varies greatly. Diminished tolerance or exasperation may be conditioned by familial factors unrelated to the child or by anecdotal reports of dramatic improvements following surgery. A thorough understanding of the family is essential to making a joint decision that is in the child's best long-term interest. When the basis for conservatism is fully explained to parents, they usually will accept and respect such caution.

At present, tonsil and adenoid removal frequently is performed as an outpatient procedure (day surgery). The following reasonable criteria have been evaluated and are recommended in selecting children who are suitable to undergo such procedures on an outpatient basis.

1. Home less than 30 miles (50 km) from hospital
2. Presence of an adult (besides the driver) in the car
3. A positive parental attitude toward caring for the child
4. No history of bleeding tendency
5. No major or chronic health problems
6. Surgery performed no less than 4 weeks after a respiratory infection or tonsillitis
7. No evidence of severe respiratory infection in the family
8. No seasonal allergies at the time
9. No smokers at home
10. No children with Down syndrome

The natural process of involution of tonsillar and adenoidal lymphoid tissue in the prepubertal years is usually associated with decreasing frequency of throat and ear infections. In this age group, a decision to defer surgery often is rewarded by progressive and spontaneous clinical improvement.

Aside from any beneficial impact that tonsillectomy and adenoidectomy might have on the frequency of throat and ear infections, our knowledge about possible deleterious effects of such surgery on the immune system is fragmentary. Before the advent of the polio vaccine, it had been demonstrated that previously tonsillectomized children who contracted poliomyelitis were at increased risk for bulbar involvement. Children who underwent tonsillectomy have been shown to be at increased risk for colonization by *Neisseria meningitidis*, but it is not yet known whether children thus colonized (or their associates) are at increased risk for invasive meningococcal disease. The presence of virus-specific cellular reactivity in tonsillar lymphocytes is associated with significant clinical protection during close household contact with varicella-zoster virus. These observations are mentioned here simply to underline the possibility that the long-term effects of tonsillectomy and adenoidectomy may extend well beyond the pharynx and are still poorly understood. Taken together, the foregoing considerations favor caution and conservatism in recommending tonsillectomy or adenoidectomy in the majority of children.

REFERENCES

1. Paradise JL, Bluestone CD, Backman RZ, et al: Efficacy of tonsillectomy for recurrent throat infection in severely affected children: Results of parallel randomized and nonrandomized trials. N Engl J Med 310:674–683, 1984.
2. Paradise JL, Bluestone CD, Rogers KD: Efficacy of adenoidectomy for recurrent otitis media in children previously treated with tympanostomy tube placement: Results of parallel randomized and nonrandomized trials, JAMA 263:2066–2073, 1990.

DISORDERS OF THE LARYNX

DIANA RADKOWSKI, M.D.

A spectrum of diseases may affect the pediatric larynx, ranging from congenital to acquired, infectious to oncologic. Although the clinical presentation often is similar, subtle variations in signs and symptoms may aid the physician in arriving at the appropriate diagnosis and, ultimately, the necessary intervention.

Anatomically, the larynx may be subdivided into three components: supraglottis, glottis, and subglottis. Disorders in one of these components will produce a unique set of symptoms that allows the physician to begin narrowing the field of possible causes of the airway distress in the child.

Embryologically, the larynx has three primary functions: airway protection, respiratory modulation, and voice production. The pediatric larynx has unique features, when contrasted with that of an adult, that affect its ability to perform these three primary functions in both the normal and the diseased state. Although the pediatric larynx is only one-third the size of the adult larynx, the arytenoid cartilages are adult size at birth. This relationship between the supraglottic structures and the laryngeal inlet may contribute to the development of laryngomalacia in some infants. The subglottis is the smallest component of the pediatric larynx, whereas in the adult, the glottic aperture is the size-limiting factor. The development of subglottic stenosis in the pediatric patient following endotracheal intubation is directly related to the small size of the subglottic opening. In addition to differences in size, the pediatric larynx differs in its position in the neck relative to the cervical and facial skeleton. At birth, the larynx may be found at approximately the level of the C4 vertebra. As the child grows, the larynx begins its inferior descent, ultimately resting at the level of C7. The high location of the larynx in the young child provides some protection against external trauma. The cephalad location of the larynx also affords additional protection to the lower airway of the neonate, who has not fully developed the necessary protective reflexes to prevent aspiration during swallowing. In the young infant, the epiglottis rests on the nasopharyngeal surface of the soft palate. This position allows the infant to suckle without danger of aspiration and to breathe with the mouth closed.

For the clinician with a basic understanding of pediatric laryngeal embryology, anatomy, and functional requirements, a careful history of the child with airway symptoms often will lead to the correct diagnosis. Of primary importance in evaluating the pediatric airway is determining the degree of emergency and the need for the establishment of an artificial airway (i.e., endotracheal intubation or tracheotomy). A rapid assessment of the child's overall airway status should take less than 1 minute and can be done while investigating the history of the child's symptoms. The duration and severity of the child's symptoms and the progressiveness of the airway distress may direct the examiner toward either a congenital or an acquired disorder. An attempt should be made to characterize the stridor, if present, as either inspiratory, expiratory, or biphasic. Although not uniformly true, the level of obstruction often is reflected in the character of the stridor. Supraglottic lesions tend to produce a coarse, inspiratory stridor, whereas glottic and subglottic disorders are more musical in quality and often biphasic in nature. Pure tracheal lesions frequently will occur with a prolonged expiratory phase and expiratory stridor. A parent often can quite accurately describe the nature of the child's stridor if it is not present at the time of initial evaluation. Changes in the quality of the stridor with the level of activity of the child and the position of the young infant are crucial aspects of the history. The quality of the child's cry (normal, weak, or aphonic) may direct the examiner to a glottic lesion, although severe subglottic narrowing may produce an abnormal cry because of limited air movement. The presence or absence of cough should be documented. A feeding history is critical especially in the young infant and child. Symptoms of aspiration, cyanosis, or "dying spells" with feeds may signal a specific disorder. Failure to thrive or other signs of systemic illness may indicate a more chronic disorder. The child's prenatal and perinatal history may reveal an unsuspected history of traumatic delivery or neonatal intubation.

If the child is in extremis or there are signs to suggest significant airway compromise, extreme caution should be exercised. Manipulation of the child should be minimized until the airway can be secured. The child can be observed for tachypnea, tachycardia, retractions (supraclavicular, subcostal, intercostal), nasal flaring, cyanosis, drooling, cough, and level of consciousness (restless, agitated, stuporous) without increasing the level of the child's anxiety.

Laryngeal examination should not be performed in the child with an unstable airway unless the appropriate personnel and equipment are available for urgent airway access when necessary. In most institutions, these patients should be handled in the operating room so that endotracheal intubation or tracheotomy may be performed expeditiously when necessary. In the stable child, a more careful history and physical examination may be possible. Flexible fiberoptic nasolaryngoscopy is widely available and allows direct inspection of the larynx. Evaluation of the awake child has several distinct advantages. The larynx can be viewed in a dynamic fashion so that the degree of laryngeal collapse during active respiration is appreciated. In addition, vocal cord motion can be assessed. Flexible bronchoscopy allows for further dynamic evaluation of the subglottic airway and lower tracheobronchial tree. For more controlled laryngeal evaluation, direct laryngoscopy and rigid bronchoscopy under general anesthesia are necessary. If a deep inhalational anesthetic technique is used, dynamic laryngeal and tracheal function can be assessed using this method as well. Direct laryngoscopy with rigid bronchoscopy is the method of choice in evaluating a child with air hunger, cyanosis, or any critical symptoms that may necessitate intubation.

Ancillary testing in the child with a *stable airway* is useful in further identifying the site of lesion before possible endoscopy and surgical intervention. Radiographic evaluation of the upper airway (anteroposterior and lateral neck films) is useful in suspected supraglottitis, croup, subglottic stenosis (either congenital or iatrogenic), soft tissue laryngeal tumors (hemangiomas, papillomas), and laryngeal foreign bodies and when there are esophageal foreign bodies producing airway symptoms. Ballooning of the hypopharynx is frequently seen on the lateral neck film in a child with significant airway obstruction. Reversal of the cervical lordotic curvature is suggestive of a retropharyngeal process. Airway fluoroscopy allows for a dynamic assessment of the airway and may be done in conjunction with a modified barium swallow to evaluate for vascular anomalies or tracheoesophageal fistula or to better define the contribution of a swallowing disorder to the airway symptoms. Computed tomography (CT scan) is reserved for evaluation of the child with a suspected laryngeal tumor or in the case of suspected laryngeal trauma.

Disorders of the pediatric larynx are best subdivided into congenital and acquired lesions. Severe congenital laryngeal anomalies are quite rare and, in general, manifest themselves within the first few minutes of life. These include atresia, severe stenosis, and near total laryngeal webs. If such disorders are recognized, tracheotomy may be a lifesaving procedure. Often, however, these severe laryngeal anomalies are found in conjunction with various other life-threatening neurologic, cardiac, gastrointestinal, and lower airway lesions. The overall prognosis for these neonates is dependent not only on the laryngeal problem but also on the infant's overall development and the impact of other concomitant lesions.

CONGENITAL LARYNGEAL DISORDERS

Supraglottis

Laryngomalacia

Laryngomalacia (congenital flaccid larynx, congenital laryngeal stridor) is the most common cause of stridor in the infant and accounts for up to 60% of laryngeal problems in the pediatric population. Clinically, the stridor develops between the second and fourth weeks of life. The stridor is typically characterized as coarse, inspiratory noise. The patients are generally better in the prone position, as this serves to decrease the degree of supraglottic collapse on inspiration. Agitation tends to exacerbate the stridor, and it may disappear completely during rest. Feeding difficulties are unusual. Cry is normal. Severe airway obstruction is unusual and generally is seen in children with underlying neuromuscular disorders. The natural history of the disease is one of progression until 8 to 12 months of age, with complete resolution in most children by 2 years of age. The etiology of laryngomalacia remains elusive, although generalized neurologic immaturity of the infant's aerodigestive tract is believed to play a role. Gastroesophageal reflux frequently is present in these children and may affect the severity of the laryngeal symptoms.

When the stridor is not associated with any severe cyanotic spells, fiberoptic nasolaryngoscopy is useful in confirming the diagnosis of laryngomalacia. During inspiration, the supraglottic structures collapse into the laryngeal inlet, narrowing the air passage and creating the classic coarse stridor. Collapse of the arytenoids is a key component to the development of clinically significant obstruction rather than isolated epiglottic prolapse as initially hypothesized. Airway fluoroscopy and modified barium swallow are useful adjuvants in the evaluation of these children. Often, the skilled airway fluoroscopist can support the diagnosis of laryngomalacia. The subglottic airway may be indirectly evaluated using this technique, and a search can be made for possible vascular anomalies affecting the integrity of the airway. Up to 10% of infants with laryngomalacia will have a second airway lesion, most commonly congenital subglottic stenosis. Direct laryngoscopy/rigid bronchoscopy is indicated in the atypical patient to confirm the suspected diagnosis of laryngomalacia and to evaluate for the possible existence of a secondary lesion below the level of the glottis.

In most cases, therapy for laryngomalacia is observation and reassurance. In more severe cases, endoscopic laser aryepiglottic fold excision (epiglottoplasty) has been reported to provide symptomatic relief without the need for tracheotomy. Tracheotomy, however, remains the gold standard for severe laryngomalacia resulting in significant airway obstruction.

Bifid Epiglottis and Absent Epiglottis

Both bifid epiglottis and absent epiglottis are rare. Severe subglottic stenosis frequently is seen with these unusual supraglottic anomalies. Tracheotomy is necessary because of the associated subglottic lesion. Aspiration is variable.

Supraglottic Cysts

Most cysts of the larynx develop in the supraglottic location (aryepiglottic fold, epiglottis, vallecula) and gradually increase in size during the first few months of life. Because of the location of these lesions, as well as their slowly progressive course, they may be indistinguishable clinically from laryngomalacia. These patients often have inspiratory stridor that worsens with agitation and when in the supine position. In older children, the voice may become muffled as the cyst enlarges. Progressive dysphagia with aspiration is more commonly seen in these patients than in patients with classic laryngomalacia. If undetected and untreated, these cysts may become quite large and result in complete laryngeal obstruction. Fiberoptic evaluation will confirm the presence of a supraglottic cyst and is the minimum requirement for all infants with new onset, progressive inspiratory stridor. The treatment involves either endoscopic marsupialization or complete excision (either endoscopically or externally) of the cyst. Attempts to aspirate or uncap the dome of the cyst inevitably will lead to cyst recurrence.

Glottis

Vocal Cord Paralysis

Vocal cord paralysis is second only to laryngomalacias as a cause of stridor in the pediatric patient, accounting for 10% to 15% of new cases. Although the paralysis may not be a true congenital lesion, it frequently is present at birth and is, therefore, grouped with other congenital anomalies of the larynx. The majority of these lesions are unilateral.

Clinically, the infant often is symptomatic within the first week of life. In the case of unilateral injury, the infant may have a weak cry and develop stridor only when stressed (agitation, infection). The stridor is typically either inspiratory or biphasic in character. The

child may have a history of choking, coughing, or brief cyanotic spells during feeds, which is indicative of aspiration. Roentgenographic evaluation remains an important step in the management of these patients. Unilateral paralysis may be associated with atrial enlargement or anomalous great vessels, which can be detected on chest x-ray and barium swallow. In the absence of a history of traumatic delivery or cardiac/thoracic surgery (i.e., patent ductus arteriosus ligation, tracheoesophageal fistula repair) that may have resulted in injury to the vagus or recurrent laryngeal nerve, the course of the vagus nerve should be investigated. Fiberoptic evaluation to confirm the diagnosis of vocal cord paralysis may be difficult if significant laryngomalacia is present obscuring visualization of the laryngeal inlet during vocalization (crying). Ultrasound imaging is a new, alternative technique for assessing vocal cord function in the difficult patient. The treatment of unilateral vocal cord paralysis depends on the severity of the child's symptoms. Often, the respiratory symptoms are minimal, and adjustments in the infant's diet may eliminate the problem with aspiration. The majority of cases of unilateral paralysis will resolve spontaneously over 6 to 12 months. Direct surgical management of the paralyzed cord is, therefore, generally not recommended. Tracheotomy is rarely necessary in unilateral cord paralysis.

Bilateral paralysis creates more severe respiratory symptoms because of significant encroachment on the glottic aperture. Often, there are associated neurologic abnormalities, such as Arnold-Chiari malformation and hydrocephalus, in infants with bilateral vocal cord paralysis. Evaluation of the infant with bilateral cord paralysis should, therefore, include CT or MRI imaging of the central nervous system and the base of skull. Unlike the infant with unilateral paralysis, bilateral cord paralysis often necessitates tracheotomy.

Glottic Web

A laryngeal web is the result of failure to recanalize the laryngeal inlet at approximately 10 weeks gestation. The web is a membrane of varying thickness and most frequently involves the glottis from the anterior commissure to the vocal process. The infant may not be symptomatic at birth. As the level of activity increases between 4 and 6 weeks of age, the child usually develops biphasic stridor. The cry often is weak, and in severe cases the child may be nearly aphonic. Feeding is not affected. Treatment of a laryngeal web depends on the thickness of the web itself and the degree of subglottic extension. Thin webs can often be treated endoscopically with the laser. Thicker, more fibrotic webs may require tracheotomy and an external approach with stent or keel placement.

Subglottis

Subglottic Stenosis

The normal subglottis measures between 5 and 7 mm in the neonate. Congenital subglottic stenosis occurs when the subglottic diameter is less than 4 mm. Congenital stenosis often results from an abnormally shaped cricoid ring, elliptical rather than circular, or from excessive thickening of the subglottic tissue. Rarely, the first tracheal ring may be displaced superiorly and come to lie within the cricoid itself. In mild forms, the stenosis may go undetected until the child is 2 to 3 years of age, when recurrent crouplike episodes prompt endoscopic evaluation. In more severe cases, biphasic stridor is present with a classic croupy cough in the absence of any systemic signs of a viral illness. The cry usually is normal and feeding is only an issue in cases of significant shortness of breath caused by airway compromise. In general, congenital stenosis is concentric. Roentgenographic evaluation usually will demonstrate symmetric subglottic narrowing. Management of these lesions depends on the severity of the child's symptoms and the age at presentation. Congenital subglottic stenosis usually is less severe than the iatrogenic form following endotracheal intubation. In select cases, an anterior cricoid split may avoid the need for tracheotomy in infants up to 18 months of age. In more severe cases of stenosis or in the older child, laryngotracheal reconstruction using rib for augmentation is the treatment of choice.

Subglottic Hemangioma

Subglottic hemangioma is a rare lesion of the airway that can lead to significant airway compromise if untreated. A hemangioma is a vascular neoplasm characterized by proliferation of the capillary endothelium. The hemangioma is the most common tumor of infancy, usually occurring in the skin. In the larynx, the lesion generally appears as a smooth, eccentric, compressible mass in the subglottis. Up to 50% of infants with a documented subglottic hemangioma will have a cutaneous lesion as well. The clinical presentation of a subglottic hemangioma is similar to that of subglottic stenosis. The infant typically has progressive biphasic stridor beginning at 4 to 6 weeks of age. Unlike the static subglottic lesion, the symptoms associated with a hemangioma may fluctuate in severity from day to day. The fluctuating character of symptoms is strongly diagnostic of subglottic hemangioma. The stridor is worse with crying or agitation because of vascular engorgement of the hemangioma. Feeding difficulties are unusual unless severe airway obstruction exists. The cry is generally normal. Roentgenographic evaluation (anteroposterior soft tissue neck film) may show an asymmetric narrowing of the subglottis. The diagnosis of a subglottic hemangioma is confirmed at the time of direct laryngoscopy/rigid bronchoscopy.

The treatment of subglottic hemangiomas must take into account the natural history of the neoplasm. Initially, the lesion undergoes rapid postnatal growth for 8 to 18 months (proliferative phase), followed by very slow but inevitable regression for the next 5 to 8 years (involutive phase). Systemic steroids on a daily or every other day schedule may control the proliferative phase of the hemangioma and obviate the need for further surgical intervention. The carbon dioxide laser is a valuable tool in the treatment of larger lesions and those less responsive to systemic steroid therapy. In cases of extensive airway involvement, a tracheotomy will provide a secure airway until the tumor involutes. Recent investigations into possible alternative treatment options for extensive cervicofacial and airway hemangiomas have shown preliminary success in the use of interferon alfa-2a for growth control. Use of this agent, however, is still controlled by experimental protocol.

Posterior Laryngeal Cleft

Failure of fusion of the posterior cricoid lamina results in a posterior laryngeal cleft. This rare developmental anomaly usually causes respiratory distress precipitated by feeding. Multiple other congenital anomalies are known to be associated with this lesion. If the cleft is mild, dietary changes (thickened feeds) often will be sufficient to prevent aspiration. A gastrostomy is recommended if thickened feeds do not prevent aspiration, and open repair with a posterior rib graft is advocated.

ACQUIRED LARYNGEAL DISORDERS

Supraglottis

Angioneurotic Edema

Angioedema is either a hereditary (C1 esterase inhibitor deficiency) or an idiopathic disorder (allergic, immune complex related, physical stimuli) that results in increased vascular permeability and subsequent subcutaneous/submucosal swelling. Laryngeal involvement may lead to rapid airway obstruction if not recognized and treated appropriately. Fortunately, the occurrence of angioedema in the pediatric patient is uncommon. Initial treatment focuses on airway stabilization, with supplemental oxygen, subcutaneous epinephrine, and systemic steroids if an allergic component is suspected.

Malignant Tumors

Malignant laryngeal tumors are extremely uncommon in the pediatric population. Rhabdomyosarcoma, fibrosarcoma, and squamous cell carcinoma are the lesions most frequently reported. Because of the rarity of these lesions, treatment is individualized and often based on established adult protocols.

Glottis

Vocal Cord Nodules

Vocal cord nodules (singer's nodules, screamer's nodules) are the most common cause of hoarseness in the young child. The nodules are fibrous aggregates and arise at the junction of the anterior and middle thirds of the true vocal cords. The nodules are believed to result from vocal abuse. The nodules typically involute during puberty, and, therefore, surgical excision is generally not advised before age 15 or 16 years. If the nodules persist into adulthood, endoscopic surgical excision should be combined with preoperative and postoperative speech therapy to prevent recurrence.

Recurrent Laryngeal Papillomatosis

Although rare, benign squamous papilloma remains the most common tumor of the pediatric larynx. The disease generally occurs before the age of 15 years, and most patients are diagnosed at less than 3 years of age. Hoarseness is the primary presenting symptom. Stridor and airway obstruction are seen if the lesions are allowed to progress. Although histologically benign, these lesions are relentless in their propensity to recur despite apparently adequate surgical removal and are responsible for significant morbidity and occasional mortality in the affected child. The causative agent is human papillomavirus (HPV-6 and HPV-11) in over 90% of cases. Interestingly, the virus has been isolated from histologically normal neighboring respiratory epithelium. Harboring of the virus within normal respiratory epithelial cells may account in part for the propensity for these lesions to recur. A strong association exists between vaginal condyloma accuminatum and laryngeal papillomatosis, and 50% to 60% of affected children have a known association with active maternal infection at the time of delivery. Less than 1% of children with papillomatosis are delivered by cesarean section. Although not entirely protective (suggesting more than one route of transmission), cesarean section effectively decreases the risk of laryngeal papillomatosis in children born to infected mothers.

Papillomatosis can involve any part of the airway from nasal vestibule to distal bronchi. The laryngeal inlet is the site most frequently involved. Lesions of the distal airway are uncommon and occur almost exclusively in children who have required a tracheotomy for extensive laryngeal disease. Soft tissue lateral neck films may demonstrate several ill-defined pedunculated masses at the level of the glottis. In the stable child, fiberoptic nasolaryngoscopy preoperatively will confirm the diagnosis.

Treatment of laryngeal papillomatosis is directed at maintaining airway patency. Carbon dioxide vaporization is the gold standard for treatment of these lesions. Repeated procedures are frequently necessary. Intervals range from 5 days to several months depending on the rate of regrowth in the individual case. Interferon is of limited use in patients with recurrent laryngeal papillomatosis. Although initial reports were favorable regarding the efficacy of interferon, long-term studies have shown only limited success. Spontaneous regression is unusual before puberty, and the disease is known to persist into adulthood. Malignant conversion is exceedingly rare, but intermittent biopsy for histologic inspection probably is warranted, especially in cases of aggressive disease.

Intubation Granuloma

Granuloma formation may result following endotracheal tube intubation. The child is often hoarse following extubation, with progression rather than improvement of the symptoms with time. Evaluation of the larynx reveals a yellow-red pedunculated mass arising from the vocal process of the arytenoid. Microlaryngoscopy and removal of the lesion often result in resolution of the child's symptoms. Repeat evaluation is recommended at 2 to 3 weeks to ensure that the granuloma has not recurred.

Subglottitis

Laryngotracheal Bronchitis (Croup)

Croup is the most common infection causing airway obstruction in the pediatric patient. The etiology and management of this disorder are discussed elsewhere in this text. Recurrent croup in children less than 12 months of age may be indicative of undetected congenital subglottic stenosis and should be investigated endoscopically when the child is stable.

Iatrogenic Subglottic Stenosis

The use of endotracheal intubation to secure the airway in the pediatric patient and to allow for mechanical ventilation has become the standard of care in the critically ill child and the premature infant. Despite recent efforts to reduce the risk of subglottic stenosis secondary to endotracheal intubation, complications of airway manipulation, primarily subglottic stenosis, continue to occur. Several factors exist in the pediatric airway that predispose the intubated child to subglottic stenosis. The subglottic lumen is the narrowest aspect of the pediatric larynx. Premature infants and children with Down syndrome tend to have smaller cricoid rings than normal, thus increasing the overall risk of subglottic stenosis.

Gastroesophageal reflux is an important factor in the pathogenesis of subglottic stenosis and is encountered more frequently in the premature infant and young child. Difficulty in stabilizing the endotracheal tube in the neonate often results in repeated intubations and increased injury to the subglottis. Extreme immaturity requiring intubation for periods of several months predisposes to subglottic injury. Hypoxia and sepsis are important variables in the development of subglottic tissue damage and are commonly seen in the neonatal intensive care setting.

Injury to the subglottis may be reduced by the following procedures:

1. Use of smaller endotracheal tubes
2. Keeping air leakage at less than 20 mm H_2O pressure
3. Avoiding cuffed endotracheal tubes in the infant and young child
4. Aggressive treatment of gastroesophageal reflux
5. Aggressive treatment of systemic infection
6. Minimizing patient movement to prevent accidental extubation (sedation and paralysis as necessary)
7. Considering tracheotomy if prolonged intubation is anticipated (greater than 10 to 14 days) (Of note, the neonate tolerates endotracheal intubation for much longer periods of time than the child or young adult.)
8. Extubating under ideal conditions (In the difficult airway, high-dose systemic steroids for 24 to 48 hours before and after extubation may result in successful extubation. The use of racemic epinephrine immediately after extubation helps to reduce airway edema.)

The treatment of iatrogenic subglottic stenosis depends on the severity of the stenosis, the age of the child, and concomitant medical problems. Tracheotomy remains the cornerstone of treatment, especially in the child with multisystem failure or the child with significant pulmonary disease. The anterior cricoid split may be used in the neonate up to 18 months of age if mild stenosis exists. As in congenital subglottic stenosis, laryngotracheal reconstruction using rib cartilage is the method most commonly employed for treatment of significant pediatric subglottic stenosis.

REFERENCES

1. Belmont J, Grundfast K: Congenital laryngeal stridor (laryngomalacia): Etiologic factors and associated disorders. Ann Otol Rhinol Laryngol 93:430–437, 1984.
2. Benjamin B: Prolonged intubation injuries of the larynx: Endoscopic diagnosis, classification, and treatment. Ann Otol Rhinol Laryngol 102(4/2):1–15(suppl), 1993.
3. Hollinger L: Etiology of stridor in the neonate, infant and child. Ann Otol 89:397–400, 1980.

ACUTE LARYNGOTRACHEAL INFECTIONS

MICHAEL J. CUNNINGHAM, M.D.

Acute laryngotracheal infections in childhood may rapidly result in airway obstruction, the major symptom of which is stridor. The primary aims of management are to establish a diagnosis rapidly and to maintain or secure the child's airway. Medical treatment and airway stabilization measures vary for the three most prevalent laryngotracheal infections, supraglottitis, laryngotracheitis, and bacterial tracheitis, as well as for older and newer infectious airway entities.

DIPHTHERITIC LARYNGITIS

Corynebacterium diphtheriae was the principal etiologic agent of acute airway obstruction in children at the turn of the century. The nonimmunized immigrant population remains at risk for this disease in the United States today.

Diphtheritic laryngitis differs from the majority of acute laryngotracheal infections in that pharyngeal involvement occurs first. A characteristic gray membrane appears covering the tonsillar fossae and posterior pharyngeal and hypopharyngeal structures. The onset of laryngeal infection is typically insidious, with an initial barking cough, soon followed by inspiratory stridor and eventual respiratory distress. The morbidity of this disease results from both airway obstruction and endotoxin-induced systemic effects, such as myocarditis and peripheral neuritis.

Treatment includes erythromycin or penicillin and the administration of diphtheria antitoxin. Relief of the airway obstruction requires operative endoscopic removal of the membranous exudate, with endotracheal intubation or tracheotomy often necessary for airway maintenance. The prognosis primarily relates to the clinical stage or severity of disease at the time of diagnosis.

SUPRAGLOTTITIS (EPIGLOTTITIS)

The entity of supraglottitis is caused by *Haemophilus influenzae* type B (HiB). Supraglottitis is the preferred term for this clinical condition because it appropriately describes the observed inflammation of all supraglottic structures in addition to the epiglottis.

Supraglottitis occurs in children from 1 to 6 years of age, with a particular affinity for the 3- to 4-year-old age group. The disease incidence is approximately 14/100,000 children, and the annual mortality in this pediatric population is estimated at 1.3/1 million. Virtually all these children have respiratory distress and require airway management.

The characteristic signs and symptoms of supraglottitis are best described as four "Ds and an "S"—dysphagia, dysphonia, drooling, distress, and stridor. The stridor is inspiratory in nature. There is associated fever, rapid clinical progression, and an absence of cough. The child often sits upright with the jaw jutted forward and the mouth open in a spontaneous attempt to maintain the airway.

The clinical presentation of this disease typically is classic enough to immediately initiate definitive treatment. A radiologic workup is warranted *only* when the diagnosis is in doubt. A lateral neck radiograph will be positive in only approximately 50% of children with endoscopically proven supraglottitis. Nonspecific hypopharyngeal dilatation may be the only roentgenographic indicator of disease.

Ambulatory blood work should be avoided in these children so as not to increase anxiety and precipitate further respiratory distress. The white blood cell count is typically elevated in a range greater than 10,000/mm³. Laryngeal cultures obtained at the time of endoscopic examination typically reveal HiB, and blood cultures are positive for HiB in approximately 50% of pediatric cases. There have been few atypical childhood cases in which both laryngeal and blood cultures have grown an organism other than HiB.

Despite the high incidence of supraglottitis-associated HiB bacteremia, few extraepiglottic infections occur. Pneumonia and cervical adenitis have been reported in 5% to 25% of children. There is a strikingly low incidence of concomitant meningitis.

Noninfectious complications are more frequent. Airway obstruction can lead to respiratory and subsequent cardiac arrest. Anoxic encephalopathy may occur when intervention in such cases is delayed. Even appropriate intervention by endotracheal intubation may result in pulmonary edema following the acute relief of airway obstruction.

The medical treatment of supraglottitis is principally antibiotic therapy. The initial antibiotic choice(s) must take into account the fact that 10% to 20% of HiB are β-lactamase-producing organisms. The traditional regimen of ampicillin plus chloramphenicol has been replaced in recent years by second- and third-generation cephalosporins.

Rifampin prophylaxis for elimination of the carrier state is indicated in all children with this disease. Household contacts should be treated if there are other children in the home less than 4 years of age, and school contacts should be treated if there are schoolmates less than 2 years of age.

Endotracheal intubation is the airway management technique of choice in treating supraglottitis. All young children with this disease require airway securement. Adolescents with endoscopically documented supraglottitis and mild symptoms may sometimes be treated without intubation as long as they can be observed in an intensive care setting. Any suggestion of progressive airway obstruction in these older patients should likewise be managed by endotracheal intubation.

Determining the duration of intubation remains controversial. Elective extubation may be dictated by the presence of an air leak around the endotracheal tube, the resolution of systemic symptoms, or laryngeal visualization. The last may be performed by flexible bedside laryngoscopy or by rigid laryngoscopy in an operating room.

The most promising change in the management of supraglottitis is the recent availability of conjugated HiB vaccines that can be administered to children as young as 2 months of age. Elevated antibody responses in young children suggest the conjugated vaccines will be of potential benefit in decreasing the incidence of this disease entity.

CROUP SYNDROME

The use of the term "croup" requires a distinction between acute viral laryngotracheitis and so-called spasmodic croup. Spasmodic croup has minimal to no viral prodrome, characteristically occurs at night, and is typically a transient clinical entity, readily responding to conservative measures. Those cases that have come to endoscopic examination typically demonstrate pale, boggy, subglottic tissues attributed to noninflammatory submucosal edema. The etiology of spasmodic croup appears to be more allergic or angioneurotic in nature than infectious.

Children with acute viral laryngotracheitis or classic croup characteristically have a prodromal respiratory tract infection, after which they develop a hoarse cry and barking cough. Their associated stridor is initially inspiratory in nature, becoming biphasic with progressive severity of disease. Associated signs and symptoms of respiratory distress likewise vary with disease progression.

The age range for acute laryngotracheitis overlaps that of supraglottitis, although younger children are afflicted more typically. The mean age of involvement is 18 months. In contrast to supraglottitis, there is a fall/winter predominance of this disease because of its viral etiology.

Children who experience acute stridor and in whom there is any question of supraglottitis should have direct endoscopic examination. When the more classic clinical presentation of acute laryngotracheitis is present and the degree of respiratory distress is mild to moderate, an outpatient workup can be conducted. Radiographic evaluation consists of anteroposterior (AP) and lateral plain neck films. The classic subglottic steeple sign is noted in only approximately 40% to 50% of children with acute laryngotracheitis. As in supraglottitis, nonspecific hypopharyngeal widening reflecting upper airway obstruction is observed commonly. An accompanying chest x-ray is important to rule

out associated lower respiratory tract infection. One AP and one lateral view often can be used to visualize both the neck and chest in young children.

Children with acute laryngotracheitis typically have normal or mildly elevated white blood cell counts. Viral and bacterial cultures are used principally for investigational purposes, as the etiology of acute laryngotracheitis is well established. Parainfluenza viruses account for the majority of cases. In very young children, respiratory syncytial virus plays an important role. Influenzae viruses types A and B and *Mycoplasma pneumoniae* may be causative agents in children 5 to 6 years of age or older.

There is an increasing body of evidence supporting an immunologic or reactive airway disease component in children who suffer from recurrent acute laryngotracheitis. Parainfluenza virus-specific IgE has been documented in such children, and children followed long term have demonstrated an increased frequency of lower respiratory tract reactive airway disease in later years.

The management of acute laryngotracheitis is principally an outpatient endeavor. Only 5% to 10% of children with moderate to severe disease require hospitalization. Monitoring vital signs and oxygen saturation can sometimes be difficult in a restless young child. Humidified room air is commonly administered, and oxygen may be necessary, depending on saturation readings. Sedation should be absolutely avoided. Properly diagnosed, acute laryngotracheitis requires no antibiotic therapy. Nebulized racemic epinephrine appears to provide temporary benefit in treating acute respiratory decompensation. However, its administration by means of intermittent positive pressure breathing has been shown to be of limited additional value.

The use of a single intramuscular or intravenous dose of steroid (0.6 to 1.0 mg/kg of dexamethasone [Decadron] equivalent) has been shown to decrease both the duration and the severity of respiratory symptoms compared with placebo in children with acute laryngotracheitis. The maximum effect of steroid administration occurs approximately 6 hours after administration. There is no evidence to show that repeated administration of steroid is of benefit in this disease.

Airway intervention is necessary in children with acute laryngotracheitis who fail to respond to medical management or in whom there is clinical suspicion of an alternative etiology. Failure of medical management may reflect diffuse upper and lower airway involvement (laryngotracheobronchitis) or associated parenchymal disease (pneumonitis/pneumonia). Alternative etiologies include supraglottitis, bacterial tracheitis, or foreign body.

In those children who do require airway management, the potential adverse effect of endotracheal intubation in the inflamed subglottic area has been debated relative to the alternative choice of tracheotomy. Several factors must be taken into consideration. The major one is the child's risk of post-extubation subglottic stenosis. Children who are less than 1 year of age and those who may have already experienced a degree of subglottic trauma as a result of a difficult intubation or an inappropriately large endotracheal tube size may be candidates for tracheotomy. The support staff available at the institution is of crucial importance. If no suitably trained person is available to reintubate the child in the event of accidental extubation, tracheotomy may be a safer mode of therapy.

The size of the endotracheal tube chosen in those who require airway management is crucial. An adequate airway as opposed to the largest possible airway is desirable. The endotracheal tube size chosen should be at least one and perhaps two sizes smaller than the appropriate size for that child under normal intubation circumstances.

In the child who has required endotracheal intubation, endoscopic airway evaluation may be indicated if the child demonstrates no air leak at 5 to 7 days or fails extubation by this time. Children with a previously known traumatic intubation may require endoscopic evaluation during their acute hospitalization.

In children who have recurrent episodes of croup requiring hospitalization or who have atypical croup, endoscopy is indicated after several weeks to allow time for inflammation to resolve. Atypical croup is defined as a clinical course lasting longer than 1 week in the standard age group or croup occurring in infants less than 6 months of age or in children older than 5 to 6 years. An endoscopic evaluation is especially indicated if there are persistent radiologic airway abnormalities on follow-up fluoroscopy. A noninfectious lesion predisposing to episodes of acute airway obstruction should be suspected in such children.

BACTERIAL TRACHEITIS

Bacterial tracheitis is also known as pseudomembranous croup or membranous laryngotracheitis. Children with bacterial tracheitis have both a barking cough and inspiratory stridor. A gradual progression of mild airway symptoms is typically followed by an acute febrile phase of rapid respiratory decompensation. In contrast to supraglottitis, such children tend to lie flat as opposed to sitting up, and they do not drool.

AP and lateral neck radiographs typically demonstrate a normal supraglottic shadow and subglottic narrowing. The classic roentgenographic finding is clouding of the tracheal air column or, more specifically, an irregular tracheal margin on high-resolution, soft-density films. Approximately 50% of children with bacterial tracheitis also demonstrate pneumonic infiltrates on chest x-ray. This is especially true if the duration of illness is greater than 24 hours.

In contrast to children with acute laryngotracheitis, there is an elevated white blood cell count. Tracheal cultures are typically positive for bacterial pathogens, whereas blood cultures are usually negative.

In the United States the etiologic agent of bacterial tracheitis is predominantly *Staphylococcus aureus*. Cases due to *Streptococcus pneumoniae, Branhamella catarrhalis,* group A streptococci, and HiB have been reported.

Bacterial tracheitis is likely a secondary bacterial infection complicating a primary viral disease. Concomitant positive parainfluenza viral cultures have been documented in some studies. The mucosal destruction and/or local immunodeficiency caused by the viral illness may predispose to the bacterial suprainfection.

The most common complication of bacterial tracheitis is pneumonia. Cardiorespiratory arrest secondary to airway obstruction may occur. Toxic shock syndrome (TSS) also has been described secondary to toxin-producing staphylococci.

The medical management of bacterial tracheitis includes hydration, humidification, and antibiotics. Early intervention is crucial. Initial antibiotic therapy typically includes nafcillin plus cefuroxime or cefotaxime. Clindamycin plus chloramphenicol is an alternative regimen in penicillin-allergic children.

Endoscopic airway assessment is diagnostic and potentially therapeutic. The removal of an obstructive membranous exudate may obviate the need for subsequent endotracheal intubation or tracheotomy. The need for airway support appears to be related to both the age of the patient (younger patients with smaller airways are at greater risk) and the presence or absence of associated pulmonary involvement. Tracheotomy may be considered when there is obstruction of the endotracheal tube by thick secretions or, in cases of prolonged intubation, where there is concern that subglottic stenosis will develop.

LARYNGEAL CANDIDIASIS

Laryngeal candidiasis has been reported in children with acquired immunodeficiency syndrome (AIDS) and other forms of immunosuppression and also in healthy newborns apparently secondary to perinatal acquisition. In the latter group, isolated laryngeal involvement is typical, whereas it is more commonly associated with generalized mucocutaneous candidiasis in the immunosuppressed population. The typical endoscopic finding is that of an erythematous, edematous larynx with an overlying, thick, white exudate. Both laryngeal swab cultures placed in Sabouraud's agar and mucosal biopsy specimens stained for fungal identification are often required for diagnosis. Airway management measures include endoscopic removal of exudate and endotracheal intubation in severe cases. Parenteral amphotericin B therapy often is required, especially in immunodeficient patients.

REFERENCES

Diphtheritic Laryngitis
1. Freeland AP: Acute laryngeal infections in childhood. *In* Evans JNG, (ed): Pediatric Otolaryngology. London, Butterworth & Co., 1987:453–454.

Supraglottitis (Epiglottitis)
1. Baker AS, Eavey RD: Adult supraglottitis (epiglottitis). N Engl J Med 314:1185–1186, 1986.
2. Gonzalez C, Gartner JC, Casselbrant ML, Kenna MA: Complications of acute epiglottitis. Int J Pediatr Otorhinolaryngol 11:67–71, 1986.
3. Sendi K, Crysdale WS: Acute epiglottitis: Decade of change—A ten-year experience with 242 children. J Otolaryngol 16:196–202, 1987.

Croup Syndrome
1. Cherry JD: The treatment of croup: Continued controversy due to failure of recognition of historic, ecologic, etiologic and clinical perspectives. J Pediatr 94(2):352–354, 1979.
2. McEniery J, Gillis J. Kilham H, Benjamin B: Review of intubation in severe laryngotracheobronchitis. Pediatrics 87:847–853, 1991.
3. Postma DS, Jones RO, Pillsbury HC: Severe hospitalized croup: Treatment trends and prognosis. Laryngoscope 94:1170–1175, 1984.

Bacterial Tracheitis
1. Friedman EM, Jorgensen K, Healy GB, McGill TJI: Bacterial tracheitis—Two-year experience. Laryngoscope 95:9–11, 1985.
2. Jones R, Santos JI, Overall JC: Bacterial tracheitis. JAMA, 242:721–726, 1979.

Laryngeal Candidiasis
1. Hass A, Hyatt AC, Kattan M, Weiner MA, Hodes DS: Hoarseness in immunocompromised children: Association with invasive fungal infection. J Pediatr 111:731–733, 1987.
2. Jacobs RF, Yasuda K, Smith AL, Benjamin DR: Laryngeal candidiasis presenting as inspiratory stridor. Pediatrics 69:234–236, 1982.

BRONCHITIS AND BRONCHIOLITIS

GERALD M. LOUGHLIN, M.D.

Although bronchitis is a common diagnosis made by both parents and pediatrician, it is a condition for which there is no precise definition. Therefore, the pediatrician should guard against accepting a parent's report of bronchitis at face value. Since bronchitis means different things to different people, parents should be asked to define the symptoms and not simply provide a diagnosis. Symptoms arise from inflammation of the trachea and major bronchi. Bronchitis occurs in both acute and chronic forms, with cough as the primary manifestation of either condition.

ACUTE BRONCHITIS

Bronchitis typically results from infection, although aspiration of gastric contents or inhalation of noxious agents can also produce an acute tracheobronchitis (Table 1). Common pathogens include parainfluenza virus, adenovirus, influenza virus, and respiratory syncytial virus (RSV). Except for *Mycoplasma pneumoniae*, primary bacterial infection is an unusual cause of bronchitis in a normal host.

Therapy for acute bronchitis is largely supportive, since the cause is most often a virus. Avoidance of irritants, such as cigarette smoke, is important to minimize coughing. If the air is particularly dry in the home, some children appear to benefit from the use of a vaporizer, although support for its use is largely anecdotal. Antitussives *are not* indicated, especially in the child with a productive cough. Mucolytics are of unproven efficacy, and their use most likely only adds to the costs of care. In patients with known or suspected asthma or in those who have associated small airway obstruction (hyperinflation) or wheezing, consideration should be given to bronchodilator therapy. A trial of an oral or inhaled beta-agonist may be beneficial. Oral steroids should be considered in children with significant symptoms or wheezing incompletely responsive to bronchodilators. Antibiotics are generally not indicated for uncomplicated acute bronchitis. Even for *M. pneumoniae* infections, antibiotics may not be helpful.

TABLE 1. Causes of Bronchitis

Acute Bronchitis
Viral
  Parainfluenza, influenza, adenovirus, respiratory syncytial virus (RSV)
Bacterial
  Mycoplasma pneumoniae, Haemophilus influenzae, Branhamella catarrhalis, Streptococcus pneumoniae, Bordetella pertussis, Chlamydia trachomatis, Corynebacterium diphtheriae
Chemical injury
  Aspiration, toxic exposure

Chronic Bronchitis
Asthma
  Wheezy bronchitis, asthmatic bronchitis
Cystic fibrosis
Chronic recurrent aspiration
  Gastroesophageal reflux, dysfunctional swallowing, tracheoesophageal fistula
Dyskinetic cilia syndrome
Immune deficiency states
  IgG, IgG subclasses, IgA
Chemical irritants
  Cigarette smoke and other sources of indoor pollution
Retained foreign body
Tuberculosis

CHRONIC BRONCHITIS

For purposes of this discussion, chronic bronchitis in children is defined as the persistence or recurrence of a productive cough with or without wheezing for longer than 3 weeks. The differential diagnosis of chronic bronchitis in children is presented in Table 1. Asthma is by far the most frequent cause of chronic cough in children. In fact, symptoms of asthma should be considered as a spectrum ranging from isolated cough without evidence of airway obstruction to wheezing with airflow limitation and respiratory distress.

Beta-agonists (oral or inhaled depending on the age of the patient) usually are used first. If symptoms are particularly severe or do not respond to beta-agonists, consideration should be given to a short course of oral steroids and/or a trial of oral theophylline. Theophylline has been shown to be effective in treating cough variant asthma, but its use has been limited by concern over side effects. Nonetheless, a trial of theophylline should be attempted before deciding that the cough is not caused by asthma. The recommended starting dose is 10 to 12 mg/kg/d. Although this dose is low and may need to be increased to achieve a therapeutic level, starting low may help minimize side effects that interfere with compliance.

Exposure to environmental irritants (e.g., passive smoking, wood-burning stove) is an infrequent cause of chronic cough (bronchitis) in infants and young children. A smoking history should be obtained from the family as part of well child care, as well as when evaluating the child with chronic bronchitis. This history should be obtained from both the parent and the older child or adolescent, as many children begin to smoke while still in middle school or high school. The child should be questioned in privacy. Otherwise, the veracity of the response may be suspect. Treatment of bronchitis caused by both active and passive smoking is smoking cessation. At a minimum, cessation of smoking in the home and automobile can result in resolution of symptoms in those exposed involuntarily.

BRONCHIOLITIS

Bronchiolitis is an acute inflammatory process primarily involving the small airways. Infants under 1 year of age are particularly at risk. RSV infections are responsible for the majority of the cases. However, parainfluenza virus, adenovirus, influenza virus, and *M. pneumoniae* can cause bronchiolitis. Certain adenovirus subtypes are capable of causing a severe necrotizing bronchiolitis that can result in permanent lung damage (bronchiolitis obliterans).

Treatment of bronchiolitis is largely supportive. Most patients are mildly symptomatic and can be managed quite easily at home with simple maintenance of adequate hydration. If the infant is experiencing wheezing and increased work of breathing, an oral beta$_2$-agonist can be tried. Oxygen saturation should be assessed in the infant with marked respiratory distress or unexplained tachycardia. If saturation readings are normal, no other therapy is indicated other than provision of close follow-up and instructions to parents on how to detect a worsening clinical status. Respiratory symptoms resolve gradually over 10 to 14 days, although in very young infants, tachypnea may persist for some time.

The infant in more severe distress or who is found to be hypoxemic should be admitted to the hospital for supplemental oxygen, observation, and additional therapy. Intravenous hydration should be strongly considered, since the infant breathing at rates approaching 60 bpm is at significant risk of aspiration during oral feeding. It is not necessary to give extra fluid, as this will have no effect on the consistency of the secretions and may increase the risk of developing pulmonary edema. Oxygen should be administered for all infants with saturation values on pulse oximetry of less than 92%. Oxygen can be delivered by nasal cannula or by oxyhood. The inspiratory oxygen concentration (FiO$_2$) should be titrated to maintain the saturation value above 95%. Patency of the nasal passage and the cannula must be monitored, since these pathways may become occluded by excessive nasal secretions. Furthermore, nasal obstruction may lead to mouth breathing with entrainment of room air. An oxyhood often provides a more consistent source of supplemental oxygen.

Monitoring is imperative, since these infants are at risk of respiratory failure from ventilatory muscle fatigue. However, it is important to remember that there is no substitute for close observation by nursing and medical personnel. Arterial blood determinations are necessary to confirm the clinical impression of respiratory failure, although in most instances, it is quite evident.

Bronchiolitis results in small airway obstruction primarily by mucosal edema and desquamation of airway epithelium. This obstruction generally is unresponsive to pharmacologic manipulation. Antibiotics are unnecessary. Steroids have been tried in a number of instances, but they have not been consistently helpful. The clinical benefit of bronchodilators (including theophylline) is controversial. In most studies, although the group mean data may not demonstrate improvement, individual subjects do show benefit. Sympathomimetics (albuterol, epinephrine) have been shown to be effective. One study demonstrated improvement in symptoms with the use of a combination of albuterol and dexamethasone. Considering the association between bronchiolitis and subsequent airway hyperreactivity and asthma, it is not surprising that this therapy may be useful in some infants. Since it is impossible to predict who will respond to bronchodilators, all infants who are sick enough to be admitted to the hospital should be given a trial of nebulized albuterol 0.1 to 0.15 mg/kg in 2 ml saline (maximum dose 5 mg) and steroids. Oxygen should be used as the driving gas for the nebulizer, since beta-agonist therapy may induce transient worsening of hypoxemia. Steroids should be administered intravenously in divided doses.

Ribavirin, a synthetic nucleoside analog, is a recently developed antiviral agent that has been demonstrated in clinical studies to be modestly effective in reducing symptoms in children with severe RSV bronchiolitis. Although its use is not universally accepted, the Infectious Disease Committee of the American Academy of Pediatrics in a recent update of its original policy statement said that ribavirin treatment is recommended for infants with underlying congenital heart disease, immune deficiency, severe chronic lung disease, or "severe" bronchiolitis.[1] Controversy has surrounded the use of ribavirin because most of the studies demonstrating efficacy have based improvement predominantly on clinical scoring systems. Furthermore, the drug is expensive, and it has not consistently reduced the length of hospital stay. Ribavirin must be administered in a tent, with the medication delivered by a small particle aerosol generator (Spage) for about 14 to 18 hours a day.

Appropriate monitoring of the infant by both electronic techniques and human contact must be maintained while the child is shrouded in the mist. Precautions should be taken to limit exposure of staff to the medication, so that human contact is not compromised by concern over exposure to the drug. Recent experience has shown that this medication can be administered safely to patients receiving mechanical ventilation as long as there is meticulous attention to respiratory care. However, its efficacy in this setting is unestablished. In infants without underlying disease, ribavirin has been shown to shorten the duration of mechanical ventilation.

REFERENCES

1. American Academy of Pediatrics Committee on Infectious Diseases: Use of ribavirin in the treatment of respiratory syncytial virus infection. Pediatrics 92:501–504, 1993.
2. Loughlin GM: Bronchitis. *In* Kendig E, Chernick V (eds): Disorders of the Respiratory Tract in Children, 4th ed. Philadelphia, WB Saunders Co, 1990:349–359.
3. Morgan WT, Taussig LM: The chronic bronchitis complex in childhood. Pediatr Clin North Am 31:851, 1984.
4. Tal A, Bavilski C, Yohai D, et al: Dexamethasone and salbutamol in the treatment of acute wheezing in infants. Pediatrics 71:13, 1983.
5. Wohl MEB, Chernick V: Bronchiolitis. Am Rev Respir Dis 118:759, 1978.

BRONCHIECTASIS

ROBERT C. STERN, M.D.

Bronchiectasis (permanent dilatation of the subsegmental airways, usually associated with noneradicable infection) is a final common pathway of many lung diseases and virtually always represents a medical or psychosocioeconomic failure. For example, the patient may have a disease for which available treatment is inadequate (e.g., cystic fibrosis), may have a long-neglected problem (e.g., an aspirated foreign body), or may not have complied with medical advice (e.g., failure to obtain adequate protection from pertussis or rubeola). Thus, in all patients with bronchiectasis, there are two general goals: (1) optimal treatment of the underlying disease (e.g., removal of foreign body, comprehensive treatment of cystic fibrosis, correction of hypogammaglobulinemia) and (2) treatment directed at the bronchiectasis itself. The first goal is not discussed here. The reader is directed to other sections of this text for discussion of individual disease entities. Achieving the second goal, direct treatment of the bronchiectasis itself, requires interruption of the vicious cycle that tends to perpetuate and aggravate the lesion. This cycle should be attacked in every possible way.

ANTIBIOTIC TREATMENT

Infection should be aggressively treated. It can lead to additional direct injury to the airway wall, to the establishment of a hypersecretory state (with further accumulation of retained secretions), and to local and occasionally systemic hypoxia. Infection also is associated with various systemic manifestations, such as fever, anorexia, and fatigue. Furthermore, spread of infection to adjacent airways is an ever present threat.

Sputum cultures, gram stains, and cytologic examination should be undertaken as part of the initial workup. In some diseases, such as cystic fibrosis, sputum cultures at regular intervals may be helpful. Since the infection in bronchiectasis is largely within the airway (and not in a tissue that has a true blood supply), large doses of antibiotics may be needed to achieve sufficient antibiotic penetration into the respiratory secretions. In many patients, chronic (even continuous) antibiotic use may be necessary, since the infection can never be totally eradicated. Trimethoprim-sulfamethoxazole, tetracycline (for older children), oral cephalosporins, or antistaphylococcal penicillins may be indicated. Empiric treatment for anaerobes with clindamycin should be considered if the patient complains of foul breath coincident with a flareup of symptoms or if the patient has responded to this treatment previously. As a rule, concern about the emergence of future resistant

organisms in these patients is subordinate to the importance of controlling the infection that is already there.

GAMMA GLOBULIN

The use of gamma globulin for patients with global immunodeficiency states is evident. However, intravenous immune globulin (IVIG) may benefit other patients, including some with defects that are less severe but are demonstrable on specialized testing. The use of IVIG in patients with no demonstrable immune defect is still controversial.

MUCUS CLEARANCE

Measures to facilitate expectoration of secretions benefit most of these patients. Once limited to traditional postural drainage (usually with vibration, clapping, and voluntary cough) mucus clearance measures now include newer techniques (e.g., autogenic drainage/huffing) and ancillary equipment (e.g., positive expiratory pressure [PEP] devices).

Postural drainage with vibration and clapping should be taught to the family and patient. Some authorities are satisfied with relatively short treatment sessions that involve treating entire lobes, but segmental positioning may be more effective, either because the positions themselves are more accurate or because the treatment period is longer. In the case of young children, initiation of chest physiotherapy generally requires hospitalization so that a respiratory or physical therapist can demonstrate the proper technique to the family. Parents can gradually take over their child's treatments in a carefully supervised setting. Patients with severe disease may need one or more daily treatments for long periods of time, perhaps for life. Other children improve, and may reach a point where they need the treatment only during exacerbations of infection or when they have acute upper respiratory infections. Children who have problems with gastroesophageal reflux may have a difficult time with postural drainage, particularly the head-down positions. In these children, postural therapy may have to be modified to accommodate the fine line between achieving optimal clearance of secretions and avoiding the risks of aspiration of gastric contents and the nutritional stress of vomiting meals.

Autogenic drainage is very effective for some patients and can be taught to children as young as 5 years of age. Some PEP devices (including a standard PEP mask and the Flutter device, which has received clearance by the U.S. FDA for marketing to cystic fibrosis patients) also hold considerable promise. In all likelihood, the ideal overall treatment will consist of blending the options and tailoring the treatment program to the individual patient's lifestyle and needs.

The efficacy of repeated bronchoscopic lavage (washouts) has not been definitely proven. Similarly, although maintenance of normal hydration is important, no expectorant (including iodides and glyceryl guaiacolate) has been shown to be clinically effective in patients who are not dehydrated. Furthermore, the possibility of inducing thyroid disease with chronic iodide therapy is an additional reason not to use them.

AEROSOL TREATMENT

Aerosols may be useful, particularly in patients with hyperreactive airways. These treatments probably are most effective if done just before postural drainage/clapping treatments. However, in patients with gastroesophageal reflux, care must be taken to minimize the problems caused by the tendency of most bronchodilators to aggravate reflux. The clinician must remember that in some patients a paradoxical worsening of pulmonary status may occur with aerosolized bronchodilator use. The administration of aerosolized antibiotics has limited usefulness except in children with cystic fibrosis, where their effectiveness has been convincingly demonstrated. The use of mucolytic drugs is tempting in view of the tenacious mucus occasionally seen in these patients. However, acetylcysteine (Mucomyst), the major mucolytic agent for aerosol use commercially available, may cause bronchospasm and has not proven worthwhile except in some patients with cystic fibrosis. Recombinant human DNase (rhDNase, Pulmo-zyme) seems more promising in that it is more effective and generally better tolerated. However, its long-term toxicity is not known, and it should be used with caution in patients who are doing well without it. In December 1993 the U.S. FDA cleared rhDNAse for use in cystic fibrosis patients.

SURGERY

Surgical resection may be indicated, especially for localized sac-cular bronchiectasis (which is less likely to show anatomic reversal than the cylindrical type). Surgery is ideal for the patient who does not have a progressive underlying disease (e.g., a patient with a foreign body that has been removed), who has excellent overall pulmonary function, and who has severe but localized disease that is responding poorly to medical management. Poor surgical candidates are those individuals who have severe underlying disease (e.g., cystic fibrosis, diffuse bilateral involvement, and marginal pulmonary function).

OTHER TREATMENTS

Routine immunizations should be kept current, particularly for those diseases (e.g., rubeola) that are known to cause or aggravate chronic pulmonary disease. Most patients with bronchiectasis should receive influenza vaccine every year. Amantadine, which is active against type A influenza, should be considered for acute febrile ill-nesses in patients who have not received influenza vaccine and during the years when there is a high incidence of vaccine failures. Aman-tadine must be used very early in the illness, before confirmation of influenza virus disease is possible.

In the patient with bronchiectasis, active sinus disease should al-ways be considered. If it is present, aggressive local treatment (e.g., decongestants, surgical drainage) may be useful. Detailed advice about the dangers of smoking and its potential additive effect on the bronchiectasis should be reinforced intermittently. Adverse pulmonary effects of other types of substance abuse (e.g., inhalation of any chemical, intravenous injection of capsule drugs containing talc) should be explained. Similarly, career counseling (avoidance of jobs that involve regular exposure to industrial fumes or smoke) may be appropriate. With the resurgence of tuberculosis and the difficulty in radiologic identification of early tuberculous lesions in patients with very abnormal chest radiographs, routine testing with purified protein derivative (PPD) is indicated. Finally, patients in whom cystic fibrosis has been excluded but in whom Young's syndrome (early onset chronic pulmonary disease with bronchiectasis, associated with progressive aspermia) is being considered should be offered the opportunity to bank their sperm for future use (if semen analysis shows that sper-matozoa are still present).

ASPIRATION SYNDROMES

WILLIAM F. H. YEE, M.D.

Aspiration is a clinical syndrome characterized by the abnormal entry of liquids or solids into the tracheobronchial tree, resulting in pulmonary injury, respiratory compromise, and possible long-term sequelae. It is comprised of three major clinical categories:

1. Pneumonia initiated predominantly by infection due to aspiration of nonsterile liquids or solids or infection acquired secondarily in the milieu of impaired clearance and altered local pulmonary de-fense mechanisms
2. Pneumonia characterized by an inflammatory response to foreign substances in the airway and alveoli
3. Foreign body aspiration leading to airway obstruction, atelectasis, asphyxia, or possibly pneumonia.

The pathophysiology of aspiration may involve significant overlap of these categories. The severity of resultant pneumonia is a function of the frequency, volume, acidity, and composition of the aspirate, as well as the defense mechanisms of the host. As a rule, evidence of bacterial infection is not clinically apparent in the first 48 hours following aspiration.

In the pediatric patient, aspiration may be caused by any of the following conditions:

1. Gastroesophageal dysfunction: gastroesophageal reflux, tube feed-ing, delayed gastric emptying with distention, hiatal hernia, con-genital and acquired disorders of esophageal motility
2. Altered levels of consciousness: sedation, anesthesia, coma, sei-zure
3. Neurodevelopmental immaturity and delay: prematurity, cerebral palsy
4. Craniofacial and foregut malformations (palatal and laryngeal clefts, esophageal strictures, esophageal atresia with or without tracheoesophageal fistula
5. Swallowing dysfunction: tracheostomy, dermatomyositis, poly-myositis
6. Neuromuscular disorders: muscular dystrophy, Werdnig-Hoff-mann disease, myasthenia gravis, Guillain-Barré syndrome

One should have a high index of suspicion for diagnosing **aspi-ration** in a child with any of the following conditions:

1. Predisposing risk factors
2. Unexplained chronic respiratory findings, such as recurrent pneu-monias, repeat abnormal chest examinations, chronic cough, or apnea
3. Unexplained changes in the chest roentgenogram
4. A feeding history suggestive of aspiration or choking

The presence of a gag reflux does not invalidate the diagnosis since healthy children do aspirate.

ASPIRATION OF INFECTIOUS SECRETIONS

The most common of the aspiration syndromes is pulmonary in-fection caused by aspiration of oropharyngeal secretions high in bac-terial concentration. The organisms indigenous to the oral cavity, which are predominantly anaerobes (*Peptostreptococcus* sp., *Fuso-bacterium* sp., and *Bacteroides* sp.) and, to a lesser extent, the mi-croaerophilic streptococci are the major pathogens. Anaerobes are recovered in over 90% of cases of aspiration pneumonia acquired in the community setting. In the hospital setting, however, as many as two thirds of aspiration pneumonias are mixed infections (i.e., both anaerobes and aerobes are recovered) involving indigenous flora and nosocomial pathogens (*Staphylococcus aureus*, organisms in the fam-ily Enterobacteriaceae, *Pseudomonas* sp., and *Streptococcus* sp.). As a rule, most infectious aspirations are polymicrobial, and the vast majority involve anaerobes. Regardless of setting, they are clinically indistinguishable.

Patients with infectious aspiration may have fever, cough, purulent sputum production, respiratory distress including pleuritic pain, and hypoxemia acutely. However, other patients may have an indolent course, with low-grade fever, mild cough and chest pain, malaise, weight loss, night sweats, and anemia. Rarely, there may be hemop-tysis or pyopneumothorax. This history may predate the diagnosis by 1 to 2 weeks. The physical examination findings are entirely consistent with bacterial pneumonia, and the laboratory findings usually reveal a modest leukocytosis and an elevated erythrocyte sedimentation rate. Blood cultures are usually negative, and expectorated sputum cultures are not useful because of oropharyngeal contamination and the in-ability to culture anaerobes. For patients with parapneumonic effu-sions, diagnostic thoracentesis before antibiotic therapy is critical for successful recovery of a pathogen and subsequent analysis for anti-biotic sensitivities.

Classically, the chest roentgenogram will reveal infiltrates in the posterior segments of the upper lobes and superior segments of the lower lobes if the aspiration occurred in the supine position. If aspiration occurred in the upright position, the basal segments of the lower lobes would be involved. Air fluid levels usually indicate abscess formation. Lateral decubiti films are useful in detecting pleural effusions and may be augmented by chest ultrasonography for localization and aspiration of fluid, especially if loculations are present. Serial chest films may show progression of disease during the first week of antimicrobial therapy and, therefore, are not reliable early indicators of clinical response. Although not usually indicated in initial management, computed tomography (CT) of the chest may help distinguish pulmonary from pleural and mediastinal pathology and help guide therapy, especially if there is clinical deterioration.

Invasive diagnostic procedures, such as (1) transtracheal aspiration, (2) transthoracic needle aspiration under CT scan guidance, (3) bronchoscopy for diagnostic lavage, protected brush specimens for culture, and transbronchial biopsy, and (4) open lung biopsy, are unnecessary. However, the immunocompromised patient who does not respond to standard therapy may require a more aggressive approach. In instances where foreign body aspiration is a consideration, rigid bronchoscopy is indicated. Antimicrobial therapy is the foundation of management and ideally should be guided by the culture and antibiotic sensitivity testing of the appropriate pathogens. However, because of the impracticality of recovery and culture of anaerobes, one must assume that they are always present in infectious aspirations and that the expected clinical response of the patient on antibiotic therapy must be determined empirically.

High-dose parenteral penicillin as a single agent has been used for many years in the treatment of community-acquired aspiration pneumonia. However, as many as 15% of anaerobes, especially *Bacteroides* sp., are penicillin resistant, thereby possibly accounting for treatment failures. As a result, the addition of metronidazole has been encouraged to broaden anaerobic coverage. Clindamycin as an alternative single agent has been shown to be more effective than penicillin. Although experience in the pediatric population is limited, monotherapy using agents effective against anaerobes has been effective in the management of aspiration pneumonia in the community setting. Such agents include the extended carboxyl penicillins (especially ticarcillin-clavulanate), the carbapenems (imipenem-cilastatin), the extended penicillins (ampicillin-sulbactam), the second generation cephalosporin cefoxitin, and to a lesser extent chloramphenicol.

However, in nosocomial infection, one must be concerned about gram-negative bacilli, and an aminoglycoside or possibly ciprofloxacin (in children greater than 16 years of age) should be empirically added to a β-lactam or clindamycin to extend coverage against the Enterobacteriaceae and *Pseudomonas* sp.

In general, the clinical course is determined by the degree of pulmonary involvement. Simple aspirations may require only 2 to 3 weeks of antibiotic therapy, with defervescence of fever within 5 to 7 days of treatment. Necrotizing pneumonitis (multiple radiologic densities less than or equal to 1 cm in diameter representing tissue necrosis), abscess formation (>1 cm densities or ≥1 cm cavitations in communication with the bronchial tree), and empyema are complications that usually develop 7 to 14 days after the aspiration event and may require prolonged parenteral therapy (a minimum of 4 to 6 weeks), with defervescence occurring as late as 1 month into treatment. Empyemas require thoracentesis, surgical evaluation, and often closed chest tube drainage. In thick empyemas, thoracoscopic drainage is useful, and thoracotomy and decortication rarely are necessary. Ideally, abscesses respond to medical management and rarely require percutaneous drainage or resection. Treatment duration is determined clinically and requires individual judgment. As a practical guide, patients should be treated with parenteral antibiotics until they are afebrile and clinically improved. Oral antibiotic therapy is continued until substantial radiologic improvement has been achieved. Chest physical therapy and postural drainage or encouragement of vigorous coughing to assist in clearance of secretions have not been proven to shorten the clinical course. Such maneuvers may be deleterious, in fact, in the presence of pulmonary abscess, since soilage of unaffected areas of lung with infective secretions is a possibility. Nebulized bronchodilators may be helpful in the setting of reactive airways.

ASPIRATION OF TOXIC FLUIDS

Aspiration of fluids toxic to the lung (e.g., acids, especially gastric acid, hydrocarbons, mineral oil, milk) may result in an intense inflammatory reaction of the airways and alveolar spaces. The most common chemical aspiration (and potentially the most serious of all the aspiration syndromes) is caused by gastric acid and has been the most extensively studied in experimental models. Initially, acid aspiration results in exudation of fluid and protein into the interstitium, causing pulmonary edema with early intraalveolar and peribronchial hemorrhage. Atelectasis ensues, accompanied within hours by desquamation of the bronchial epithelium and infiltration of polymorphonuclear leukocytes first into the submucosa and then ultimately into the alveolar spaces. The airways fill with desquamative epithelium and inflammatory cells. The net result is an intense alveolitis and bronchiolitis followed by hyaline membrane formation.

Pathophysiologically, lung compliance and diffusing capacity decline, and there is severe ventilation and perfusion mismatching, resulting in venous admixture and intrapulmonary shunting. Pulmonary vascular resistance increases. Physical findings include the acute onset of respiratory distress (within 1 to 2 hours) characterized by hypoxemia and occasional cyanosis, tachypnea, and hyperventilation. These changes result in respiratory alkalosis, dyspnea, and bronchospasm. Other findings include cough, crackles, wheezing, low-grade fever in the absence of infection, hypotension, and tachycardia. Classically, multifocal alveolar infiltrates are seen on chest roentgenogram within hours, with greater involvement of the lower lobes and right-sided predominance. In uncomplicated cases, the patient stabilizes within 24 to 48 hours and completely recovers in 4 to 5 days. The chest film shows clearing within 4 to 7 days, with resolution within 2 weeks. Based on experimental evidence, clinical severity is dependent on the pH, composition, and volume of the aspirate.

Hydrocarbon aspiration (kerosene, gasoline, turpentine) is usually the result of ingestion followed by vomiting. The clinical presentation and management are similar to those of gastric acid aspiration. Induction of vomiting or gastric lavage usually is contraindicated to prevent further aspiration. Food particle aspiration differs from gastric aspiration and is characterized by a widespread granulomatous reaction with a predominant mononuclear cell infiltrate of the interstitium. The clinical course is less severe than the course of gastric aspiration.

The acute treatment of chemical aspiration is primarily supportive and consists of supplemental oxygen, chest physical therapy, and postural drainage with suctioning. Hemodynamic support includes hydration. Electrolyte abnormalities should be corrected. Bronchodilators may help if reactive airways disease is present. Positive pressure ventilation and positive end-expiratory pressure are indicated for respiratory failure.

Bronchoscopy is indicated if there is a suspicion that large particulate matter or a foreign body is causing obstruction. Lavage for removal of toxic fluids or neutralization of acid has no proven benefit and may result in harm. Prophylactic antibiotics and administration of steroids to reduce inflammation have not affected the clinical outcome and cannot be recommended. Recovery is usually complete, but respiratory sequelae, including chronic cough, wheeze, dyspnea, bronchial hyperreactivity, and bronchiectasis, may result. Rarely, the pulmonary course may progress to adult respiratory distress syndrome (ARDS), resulting in pulmonary fibrosis, bronchiolitis obliterans, or even death. The major complication of chemical aspiration, especially gastric, is bacterial pneumonia, which usually develops longer than 72 hours after the initial aspiration. It is estimated to occur in 25% to 50% of all acid aspirations and is the major cause of clinical deterioration after initial improvement. Clinically, there is a new onset of fever with purulent sputum production, leukocytosis, progressive infiltrates on chest roentgenogram, and worsening hypoxemia. The offending microbial pathogens are almost always nosocomial, and antibiotic therapy is similar to that for nosocomial bacterial aspiration pneumonia.

In the absence of observed aspiration, the diagnosis is based on index of suspicion and clinical findings. In gastric aspiration, the feeding history and the neurodevelopmental examination (including a swallowing assessment) are critical. Appropriate diagnostic studies may include a modified barium swallow to assess oropharyngeal function and an esophagram with an upper gastrointestinal series to evaluate the structure and function of the esophagus, stomach, and proximal small bowel. Intraesophageal pH monitoring is a specific and sensitive measure to assess gastroesophageal reflux and may be followed by endoscopy with esophageal biopsy or by esophageal manometry to evaluate lower esophageal sphincter histology and function. Radionuclide scanning of the lungs (the gastric scintiscan) following ingestion of technetium-labeled milk is a specific but often insensitive tool to document aspiration. Quantitation of lipid-laden macrophages collected from bronchoscopic lavage has been reported to be a sensitive and relatively specific marker of aspiration, specifically in the pediatric age group. Identification of food particles confirms the diagnosis. It is important to note that these diagnostic studies assess the risk factors for aspiration and infrequently prove a causal relationship between respiratory symptoms and aspiration pneumonia.

In the absence of specific therapies for chronic gastroesophageal reflux and aspiration, medical management should be implemented, consisting of positioning (prone with elevation of the head), a feeding protocol (thickened feedings, limitation of volumes), and possibly medications (H_2-receptor antagonists and cholinergics). If such conservative measures fail and the risk of pulmonary morbidity and potential mortality is significant, antireflux surgery should be considered (fundoplication with possible gastrostomy tube placement and pyloroplasty). Under extreme circumstances in which intractable aspiration is associated with laryngeal incompetence, procedures to isolate the tracheobronchial tree from the alimentary system have been performed (laryngotracheal closure, tracheoesophageal diversion, epiglottopexy, and laryngectomy). There is little if any pediatric experience with these procedures. Several result in tracheostomy and loss of speech, and laryngectomy is irreversible.

Foreign Body Aspiration

Foreign body aspiration is subcategorized as aspiration of inert or potable fluids (usually nonacidic or clear fluids such as water or saline) or solids such as food or inert substances (metal, teeth, bone, plastic). Drowning as a form of foreign body aspiration is discussed elsewhere.

Aspiration of inert fluids leads to laryngospasm and bronchospasm, resulting in acute dyspnea, transient hypoxemia, and occasionally pulmonary edema. Airway obstruction is the pathophysiologic event. Respiratory distress is usually short-lived and reversible, and pulmonary inflammation is much less intense compared with acid aspiration. Treatment is supportive and consists of supplemental oxygen, chest physical therapy with postural drainage and suctioning, and bronchodilators. Steroids may be helpful, and bronchoscopy is indicated diagnostically and therapeutically for evaluation of persistent atelectasis.

The clinical presentation of aspiration of solids depends on particle size. As a rule, aspiration of food (especially nuts and seeds) is the most common variety. Right-sided aspirations occur nearly twice as frequently as left-sided aspirations. The disturbed respiratory physiology results from mechanical obstruction of the airways.

Aspiration of a large foreign body results in obstruction at the level of the larynx or central airway and is characterized clinically by choking, severe sudden respiratory distress, aphonia, dysphagia, asphyxia, and occasionally severe stridor. This form of aspiration may be rapidly fatal and should be treated promptly with back blows and chest thrusts in the infant or the Heimlich maneuver in the child and adolescent if respiratory arrest is imminent.

Aspirated small foreign bodies affect the peripheral airways and result in cough, focal wheezing, and focal decrease in breath sounds. There may be a history of gagging or choking, and the patient may complain of dyspnea or chest pain. Occasionally, the patient may be hypoxemic. If the foreign body is radiopaque, the diagnosis is obvious on chest roentgenography. Standard diagnostic studies include inspiratory and expiratory chest films, decubitus views of the chest, and chest fluoroscopy. One most commonly finds obstructive emphysema (classically, air trapping on the affected side with shift of the mediastinum especially accentuated on expiration) and, less commonly, atelectasis.

The diagnosis is based on the history and a strong index of suspicion. One should always consider this diagnosis in any patient with persistent infiltrates at the same location that may clear only partially on antimicrobial therapy or in any patient with unexplained persistent cough or wheeze.

Rigid bronchoscopy under general anesthesia is necessary for diagnosis and removal of the foreign body. As a rule, antibiotics are unnecessary both before and after extraction unless respiratory signs and symptoms suggest infection. Humidification, bronchodilation, and administration of steroids 24 to 48 hours after foreign body extraction may be helpful. Attempts at foreign body removal using inhaled bronchodilators, followed by percussion and postural drainage cannot be recommended because of the risk of central airway obstruction and cardiopulmonary arrest. Under extreme conditions, thoracotomy with bronchotomy may be required to remove a foreign body. Failure of foreign body extraction may result in recurrent pneumonias (onset usually 1 to 2 weeks after the initial aspiration), hemoptysis, persistent atelectasis, bronchiectasis, pulmonary abscess, and chronic respiratory findings. Treatment of pneumonia is similar to treatment of bacterial aspirations. Prevention is the best treatment for foreign body aspiration, since 80% of such aspirations occur in the under 3-year-old age group.

ATELECTASIS

THOMAS F. BOAT, M.D.

Atelectasis is incomplete lung expansion or collapse of previously expanded lung tissue. Both normal and diseased lung can be involved. Atelectasis usually reflects dysfunction in the airways or surrounding tissues but is not a primary disorder. Its distribution can be either diffuse, as in respiratory distress syndrome of the newborn or hydrocarbon ingestion, or focal, usually a manifestation of airways obstruction or compression. Focal atelectasis is further characterized by the extent of the problem: subsegmental, segmental, lobar, or total lung. Furthermore, atelectasis may be an isolated event, recur infrequently in a number of disease states, or occasionally be chronic or persistent. Avoidance of persistent atelectasis by preventive or early treatment measures is a universal therapeutic goal.

ETIOLOGIC FACTORS

Recognition of etiologic factors in the development of atelectasis is important so that the responsible factor(s) can, if possible, be treated successfully. A list of pathologic processes contributing to atelectasis and disease states associated with this condition is presented in Table 1.

DIAGNOSIS

Large areas of atelectasis may be detected on physical examination by diminished breath sounds and a hyperresonant percussion tone. However, in many instances, atelectasis is not detected on physical examination. Diffuse atelectasis or decrease in lung volume can be diagnosed on routine chest roentgenograms by noting elevated diaphragms and a decreased cross-sectional area of the thorax. Subseg-

TABLE 1. Causes of Atelectasis in Childhood

Endobronchial Obstruction
Foreign body
Granuloma (e.g., endobronchial tuberculosis)
Endobronchial tumors
Papillomatosis
Mucous plugging
  Cystic fibrosis
  Other bronchiectasis
  Asthma
  Allergic bronchopulmonary aspergillosis
  Bronchopulmonary dysplasia
Improperly placed endotracheal tube

Bronchial Wall Abnormalities or Injury
Airway stenosis
  Congenital
  Acquired (e.g., suction injury)
Aspiration or inhalation injury
Infection (e.g., bronchitis, bronchiolitis)
Asthma

Extrinsic Bronchial Compression
Lymph nodes
Tumors
Cardiomegaly (especially large left atrium)
Vascular anomalies (e.g., pulmonary artery sling)
Lung cysts

Deficiency or Dysfunction of Surfactant
Respiratory distress syndrome
  Newborn
  Adult
Hydrocarbon ingestion
Near drowning
Pneumonia
Pulmonary edema
Alveolar proteinosis
Diffuse alveolar hemorrhage

Compression of Normal Lung Tissue
Lobar emphysema
Cardiomegaly
Pleural fluid or air
Tumors
Lung cysts

Hypoventilation
Postoperative failure to cough, deep-breathe
Neuromuscular weakness
Diaphragm dysfunction

mental atelectasis may occur as a platelike density anywhere in the lung fields. Segmental and lobar atelectasis can be diagnosed based on their characteristic roentgenographic patterns and distribution. Chest CT may provide additional information about location and extent of atelectasis but is not indicated routinely. The need for special studies to determine the etiology of atelectasis is highly dependent on the clinical information available in each case.

TREATMENT

Successful therapy usually depends on identification of the specific etiologic process.

Intrabronchial Obstruction

Foreign bodies must be suspected, detected and removed by rigid bronchoscopy. Granulomas, intrabronchial tumors, and airway papillomas similarly are detected and often removed bronchoscopically. Mucous plugging should be suspected based on certain underlying disease processes, such as asthma, allergic bronchopulmonary aspergillosis, or cystic fibrosis, and typical findings on chest roentgeno-

grams. Lobar and segmental mucous plugging can be confirmed by fiberoptic bronchoscopy. In these cases, aggressive treatment of airways infection or reactive airways disease may resolve the problem. Atelectasis caused by allergic bronchopulmonary aspergillosis often responds to corticosteroid therapy. Refractory atelectasis may disappear after removal of a mucous plug bronchoscopically. Mucolytic agents, such as DNase (dornase alpha), may be a useful adjunct, particularly if applied directly to a mucous plug via the bronchoscope. An intratracheal tube that is positioned in one of the mainstem bronchi, causing atelectasis of the opposite lung, can easily be repositioned, usually resulting in prompt lung expansion.

Bronchial Wall Abnormalities or Injury

Airway injury caused by infection or reactive airways disease can be treated with antibiotics or with bronchodilators and anti-inflammatory agents, respectively. Viral disease caused by the respiratory syncytial virus is more difficult to treat but, in severe cases, may improve with the use of aerosolized ribavirin.

Extrinsic Bronchial Compression

Cardiomegaly, especially with a large left atrium, occasionally causes left mainstem bronchus compression and collapse of the entire lung. Treatment of left heart failure may be enough to diminish the size of the left atrium and reduce compression. Compression by lymph nodes, tumors, vascular abnormalities, and lung cysts often requires surgical intervention.

Surfactant Deficiency States

Previously, mechanical ventilation was required until spontaneous generation of surfactant was achieved in the dysfunctional lung. Surfactant replacement therapy is now a routine treatment for anticipated or early respiratory distress syndrome in the newborn. Adult-type respiratory distress syndrome may also respond to this approach. Pneumonia and pulmonary edema are treated by well-known, standard measures. Alveolar proteinosis has been treated successfully by large-volume alveolar lavage to remove the accumulated alveolar lipids.

Compression of Normal Lung Tissue

When patients are symptomatic because of poor lung ventilation as a result of pleural disease, evacuation of fluid (pus, noninfected fluid, blood) or air under tension usually allows lung reexpansion. When lobar emphysema is symptomatic and has caused extensive compression of surrounding lung tissue, surgical removal of the emphysematous segment or lobe is indicated. Lung tumors of all types should be removed if they cause symptomatic atelectasis.

Hypoventilation Resulting from Mechanical Abnormalities

Postoperative use of analgesics may allow deep breathing and coughing, thus preventing atelectasis. Early ambulation, other activity, and the use of incentive spirometry also has a salient effect. Severe neuromuscular weakness may require intermittent positive pressure breathing or even periods of mechanical ventilation with an endotracheal tube.

Symptomatic Therapy

Symptomatic therapy should be considered. Hypoxemia secondary to shunting through a poorly ventilated region of the lung should be treated with oxygen therapy. Fluid replacement in a dehydrated child with mucous plugging is theoretically useful, but its efficacy is unproven. Chest physical therapy and voluntary coughing are often prescribed, but their efficacy has not been systematically demonstrated. Similarly, the use of inhaled recombinant DNase when mucous plugging is identified has not been studied but might be tried for several days.

Persistent atelectasis, as in the right middle lobe syndrome, especially if attended by bronchiectases and chronic focal infection, may require lobectomy. This approach should be considered only if the patient is persistently symptomatic despite aggressive medical therapy. Persistent atelectasis for weeks or even several months has been shown to expand without apparent subsequent dysfunction of the involved lung. Therefore, every attempt to expand atelectatic lung tissue should be made before considering surgery.

RIGHT MIDDLE LOBE SYNDROME

PETER GREALLY, M.D., M.R.C.P.I.

DEFINITION

Right middle lobe syndrome (RMLS) is characterized by persistent or recurrent atelectasis of that lobe. In children, it is the site most commonly affected by chronic atelectasis. The middle lobe bronchus is longer and diverges from the bronchus intermedius at a relatively sharp angle and is encircled by mediastinal lymph nodes draining the middle and lower lobes. The lobe is also separated by fissures from both the upper and lower lobes and, therefore, lacks the aerating effects of collateral ventilation. These anatomic features allow the retention of mucous secretions and facilitate bronchial compression by enlarged hilar nodes. Thus, a cycle consisting of mucus retention, secondary bacterial infection, and reactive hilar adenopathy can develop that specifically predisposes the middle lobe to atelectasis.

ETIOLOGY

Airway obstruction, external compression of lung parenchyma, and increased surface tension at the air–lung interface are the mechanisms by which atelectasis occurs. Of these, airway obstruction plays the major role in the pathogenesis of RMLS. Airway obstruction can be classified according to the site of the lesion as intrinsic (within the airway) or extrinsic (outside the airway). When originally described, the syndrome was commonly associated with hilar node enlargement secondary to pulmonary tuberculosis. Now, the most common cause of childhood RMLS in developed countries is bronchial mucosal inflammation secondary to asthma. However, other diagnostic possibilities should always be entertained (Table 1).

NATURAL HISTORY

The natural history of RML atelectasis is dependent on the underlying cause. Commonly, it is the result of asthma, in which case the atelectasis is likely to resolve spontaneously with time. However, persistent atelectasis is associated with an increased risk of infection, bronchiectasis, and fibrosis in affected lobes.

DIAGNOSIS

RMLS may be manifest by recurrent pneumonia in that area. The presence of a chronic productive cough raises the possibility of bronchiectasis. However, atelectasis may be completely asymptomatic, in which case symptoms are caused by the underlying disorder. If atelectasis is caused by asthma, symptoms may be chronic cough, recurrent wheeze, and exercise-induced dyspnea. A history of growth retardation, recurrent sinusitis, pale bulky stools, or serious systemic infections in the presence of RMLS should prompt a search for alternative diagnoses (Table 1). Physical examination may reveal dullness to percussion and reduced breath sounds in the right axilla or over the anterior portion of the lower right thorax.

Radiologically, anteroposterior views of the chest may be unremarkable, often only exhibiting some irregularity of the right heart border and downward displacement of the transverse fissure. More information often can be derived from the lateral view, in which volume loss and opacification of the right middle lobe will be apparent. A CT scan of the chest may help distinguish chronic atelectasis from fibrosis or bronchiectasis. When clinically indicated, a sweat chloride estimation, sinus films, skin tests (PPD, *Candida*, mumps), spirometry (pre- and postbronchodilator), complete blood count and differential leukocyte count, serum immunoglobulins, serum immunoglobulin G subclasses, and ciliary studies should be performed. Patients should undergo flexible fiberoptic bronchoscopy to exclude structural abnormalities, unsuspected foreign body aspiration, or underlying infection, particularly if a trial of conservative management has failed. Bronchoalveolar lavage demonstrates a preponderance of neutrophils and respiratory pathogens (*Haemophilus influenzae* and *Streptococcus pneumoniae*) in 40% to 50% of cases of RMLS caused by asthma.

THERAPY

Treatment modalities depend on the diagnosis and should address the underlying mechanisms. For instance, if the atelectasis is caused by tuberculous lymph nodes, it should resolve with appropriate antituberculosis therapy. RMLS caused by asthma should respond to allergen avoidance, inhaled bronchodilators combined with inhaled anti-inflammatory drugs, and if necessary, short courses of oral corticosteroids. The beta$_2$-agonists possess the additional properties of enhancing ciliary beat frequency and promoting better mucociliary clearance. Antibiotics should be used if bacterial infection is suspected. Parents can be taught chest physical therapy, which may dislodge mucous plugs, accelerate reexpansion, and prevent recurrence. Flexible bronchoscopy also may be used therapeutically to remove mucous plugs. However, there is no convincing evidence to suggest that bronchoscopy alters the natural history of the condition. Surgical removal of the affected lobe is now rarely indicated and is necessary only when significant bronchiectasis has supervened despite optimum medical management.

REFERENCES

1. Livingston GL, Holinger LD, Luck SR: Right middle lobe syndrome in children. Int Pediatr Otolaryngol 13:11–23, 1987.
2. Redding GJ: Atelectasis in childhood. Pediatr Clin North Am 31:891–906, 1984.
3. Springer C, Avital A, Noviski N, Maayan C, Ariel I, Mogel P, Godfrey S: Role of infection in the middle lobe syndrome in asthma. Arch Dis Child 67:592–594, 1992.

TABLE 1. Site and Etiology for Right Middle Lobe Syndrome

SITE OF OBSTRUCTION	DIAGNOSIS
Intrinsic	Asthma
	Bronchitis, bacterial or viral
	Bronchiectasis
	Chronic aspiration
	Cystic fibrosis
	Ciliary disease
	Endobronchial tuberculosis
	Endobronchial tumors
	Foreign body
	Immunodeficiency
Extrinsic	Tuberculous nodes
	Lymphoma
	Bronchogenic cyst

EMPHYSEMA

GEOFFREY KURLAND, M.D.

Pulmonary emphysema, as defined by the American Thoracic Society, is a condition of the lung characterized by abnormal permanent enlargement of the air spaces distal to the terminal bronchioles, accompanied by destruction of their walls. The physiologic consequences of this pathologic condition are the loss of elastic recoil of the lung, obstruction of air flow, and trapped gas in the lung. Pulmonary emphysema leads to radiographic abnormalities, including hyperlucency, air trapping, and diminished vascularity. Although the

TABLE 1. Pulmonary Emphysema in Children: Diagnostic Entities

Congenital lobar emphysema
Cystic adenomatoid malformation
Emphysema secondary to airway obstruction
Swyer-James syndrome
Alpha$_1$-antiprotease deficiency

exact diagnosis of emphysema relies on pathologic (tissue) findings, the clinician often will be confronted with a chest radiograph showing hyperlucency and decreased vascularity of the lung. Several different entities will thus result in the radiographic diagnosis of emphysema.

It must be emphasized that classic emphysema involving the entire lung, as often seen in adult smokers, is distinctly uncommon in children. Indeed, most pediatric conditions included in a discussion of emphysema do not meet the pathologic criteria of emphysema. Rather, they are labeled emphysema because of the radiographic finding of hyperlucency, which itself may be secondary to air trapping in the lung or interstitial space, a decrease in blood flow, or, rarely, tissue destruction (true emphysema). The most common diagnostic entities that lead to radiographic hyperlucency are outlined in Table 1.

CONGENITAL LOBAR EMPHYSEMA

Congenital lobar emphysema (CLE) is a misnomer, as it does not fit the pathologic definition of emphysema. CLE is characterized by overinflation and air trapping of the affected lobe, and it is unusual to see destruction of the airway wall to the degree seen in emphysema. The causes of CLE include absent or diminished bronchial wall cartilage, extrinsic compression of the affected lobar bronchus, and other intrinsic abnormalities of the lobar bronchus. In up to 50% of cases, no distinct abnormality is identified. The majority of cases involve the left upper lobe, with the right middle and upper lobes being the next most common sites. Most children with CLE show evidence of respiratory compromise within the first week of life.

In the immediate neonatal period, the affected lobe may show increased radiodensity because of delayed clearance of pulmonary fluid. Subsequently, the affected lobe usually shows progressive overdistention, leading to compression of adjacent lobes. In extreme cases, herniation of the affected lobe across the mediastinum, with compression of adjacent lung, will lead to respiratory distress early in the neonatal period. Occasionally, overdistention may not be as severe, leading to more subtle signs, such as progressive tachypnea and wheezing.

When CLE leads to respiratory distress, especially with impingement on vital structures in the thorax, surgical extirpation is the treatment of choice. In less severely affected cases, it is not unreasonable to observe rather than move directly to surgery. In such instances, bronchoscopy can help rule out reversible lesions, such as bronchial obstruction or compression, as the cause of the air trapping. Some patients with CLE have done well without surgery. Some case reports suggest that corticosteroids may be useful in CLE, although these may be best reserved for those with obstructive inflammatory bronchial lesions.

CYSTIC ADENOMATOID MALFORMATION OF THE LUNG

Cystic adenomatoid malformation of the lung (CAM), as its name implies, is characterized by a collection of thin-walled cystic lesions that usually are unilobar in distribution. Like CLE, it may show radiographic density in the immediate neonatal period because of delayed clearance of fetal lung fluid. Thereafter, progressive hyperlucency and overinflation, with the appearance of multiple cysts, usually lead to the diagnosis. Rarely, the lesion may have adenomatous changes without cysts and, thus, will appear more radiodense. A thoracic CT or MRI scan can help delineate the nature of the lesion.

The most dramatic cases involve the onset of respiratory distress in the neonatal period and are associated with large malformations.

Older children, usually with smaller areas of the lung affected, may have recurrent pneumonia or abscess.

Surgical resection is the treatment of choice for CAM and is especially important in those infants affected with respiratory distress.

EMPHYSEMA SECONDARY TO AIRWAY OBSTRUCTION

The presence of partial airway obstruction may lead to a ball-valve phenomenon, wherein air can enter the lung distal to the partial obstruction but is trapped because of obstruction during exhalation. This leads to progressive, local (usually lobar) air trapping, with radiolucency consistent with emphysema. Complete obstruction of an airway usually leads to atelectasis and volume loss in the affected lobe, with compensatory hyperinflation of adjacent lung. Either of these two mechanisms will lead to the radiographic diagnosis of emphysema, although in the former case, it is the affected lobe that is hyperlucent, whereas in the latter case, it is the unaffected lobe that is hyperlucent. This form of compensatory emphysema is the most common form of emphysema seen in childhood.

The causes of secondary emphysema are numerous, since anything that can obstruct an airway may lead to localized overexpansion. Extrinsic masses, such as bronchogenic cysts, enlarged lymph nodes, or tumors, may compress an airway, leading to partial or complete obstruction. Intrinsic airway lesions, such as thick secretions in asthma and cystic fibrosis, airway foreign bodies, or endobronchial tumors, such as adenomas or carcinoid, also can cause obstruction. Either instance may lead to the radiographic appearance of hyperinflation and decreased pulmonary vascularity.

The diagnostic evaluation should be directed by the history and physical findings. Chest fluoroscopy, inspiratory-expiratory chest x-rays, or bilateral decubitus chest x-rays may help determine the presence of air trapping. Flexible fiberoptic bronchoscopy is useful for documenting extrinsic airway compression or for aspiration of thick secretions. Rigid bronchoscopy should be used for foreign body removal. When asthma or cystic fibrosis leads to secondary emphysema, medical management rather than bronchoscopy is preferable as initial treatment.

SWYER-JAMES SYNDROME

The Swyer-James syndrome, also known as the unilateral hyperlucent lung syndrome, is a form of bronchiolitis obliterans, an uncommon pathologic response to severe pulmonary insult in infancy. Infectious agents associated with the syndrome have included adenovirus, rubeola virus, influenza virus, and *Mycoplasma pneumoniae*. Hydrocarbon aspiration is another cause. The syndrome is characterized by progressive obliterative destruction of the small airways (bronchiolitis obliterans) and distal air trapping, which in turn leads to compression of the accompanying vasculature and decreased blood flow. In most instances, one lung is predominantly affected. The radiographic hallmark of Swyer-James syndrome is the presence of a unilateral hyperlucent lung that is small in size. There is no compression of normal thoracic structures by the affected lung. A ventilation-perfusion scan will help confirm the decreased perfusion and ventilation to the affected lung. There is no specific therapy for Swyer-James syndrome, but it must be differentiated from other entities, such as CLE or foreign body aspiration, congenital unilateral absence of a pulmonary artery, or pulmonary thromboembolism.

ALPHA$_1$-ANTIPROTEASE DEFICIENCY

Alpha$_1$-antiprotease (A$_1$-AP), also known as alpha$_1$-antitrypsin, is a glycoprotein (MW 52 kD) produced mainly by hepatocytes. Its principal function is to bind and inactivate neutrophil elastase (NE), a protease that is released from neutrophils during phagocytosis, membrane perturbation, or cell lysis. If unopposed, NE will degrade elastin, a molecule responsible for elastic recoil of the lung, as well as other lung matrix proteins. A$_1$-AP is the most important antiprotease in the lower respiratory tract and, as such, protects the lung from damage by neutrophils. In the normal lung, there is a constant, chronic, low-grade burden of NE secondary to the presence of small numbers of neutrophils. With inflammation, smoke exposure, or infection, the number of neutrophils and NE in the lung increases.

The expression of A_1-AP is determined by codominant alleles, which are polymorphic. The major forms of A_1-AP, known as Pi types, are differentiated by their electrophoretic mobility, and are designated as F (fast), S (slow), M (midrange), and Z (slowest). Null mutations (no A_1-AP produced), as well as numerous less common phenotypes, have been described. Because of the codominance, individuals may have two allelic forms of A_1-AP (e.g., MM, ZZ, MZ, MS). Most individuals have an MM genotype and normal A_1-AP activity, whereas the ZZ genotype is associated with a severe reduction in activity. The development of emphysema in people with A_1-AP deficiency is associated with serum levels of A_1-AP < 11 μmol, whereas the serum A_1-AP levels seen in MM individual are 20 to 53 μmol. The ZZ genotype is associated with the development of emphysema, usually in the third to fourth decade of life, and is also responsible for the development of liver disease because of the accumulation of the abnormal protein within the hepatocyte. Other less common genotypes are associated with emphysema but may not lead to liver disease. The development of emphysema in individuals at risk (i.e., those with the ZZ genotype) in childhood or adolescence is extremely unusual.

Unlike the other forms of emphysema discussed in this chapter, the emphysema associated with A_1-AP deficiency is a true, panacinar form of emphysema and tends to occur initially in the lung bases. Cigarette smoking is a major risk factor for emphysema in ZZ individuals, as smoking leads to an increase in neutrophils in the lung.

The treatment of A_1-AP deficiency is dependent on the genotype and the age of the patient when the problem is diagnosed. In childhood, individuals noted to have the ZZ genotype and minimal or no symptoms should be counseled to avoid cigarette smoking. Patients with liver disease may require liver transplantation. Because many patients with A_1-AP deficiency have wheezing and evidence of airway obstruction, a trial of aerosolized bronchodilators is indicated, especially if pulmonary function testing confirms a positive response to bronchodilator administration. Intravenous augmentation therapy with concentrated A_1-AP is available on an experimental basis. There is evidence that this material can effectively raise serum A_1-AP levels and protect the lung from the effects of NE. An ongoing clinical trial, organized by the National Institutes of Health, is designed to study a large cohort of patients and confirm the protective role of A_1-AP in these patients.

REFERENCES

1. Crystal RG: Alpha$_1$-antitrypsin deficiency, emphysema, and liver disease. J Clin Invest 85:1343–1352, 1990.
2. Lierl M: Congenital abnormalities. *In* Hilman BC (ed): Pediatric Respiratory Disease: Diagnosis and Treatment. Philadelphia, WB Saunders Co, 1993:457–498.

PNEUMOTHORAX AND PNEUMOMEDIASTINUM

CRAIG M. SCHRAMM, M.D.

ETIOLOGY

Normally, the pleural space is gasless and is under a resting pressure of -3 to -5 cm H_2O at functional residual capacity (FRC) because of the balance of opposing inward and outward recoil forces of the lung and chest wall. Pleural pressure becomes more negative during inspiration, when the thoracic cavity expands and the lung elastic recoil pressure increases. This negative pleural pressure allows,

under certain traumatic, iatrogenic, or spontaneous conditions, for the entry of gas into the pleural space, a pathophysiologic condition termed pneumothorax. Traumatic pneumothoraces develop following alveolar or airway rupture from blunt trauma or after lung or chest wall laceration. Iatrogenic pneumothoraces may be deliberate, as in thoracoscopy, or may result from accidental medical trauma, as may occur with thoracentesis, transbronchial or transthoracic lung biopsy, cardiopulmonary resuscitation, or subclavian venous catheterization. Pneumothoraces also can arise spontaneously, 20% of which develop secondarily in patients with preexisting chronic lung disease (Table 1) and the rest occurring unexpectedly in otherwise healthy individuals.

Primary spontaneous pneumothoraces develop most frequently in young (16 to 34-year-old) men (6:1 male/female ratio), with a reported annual incidence of 9 cases per 100,000 population. There is no predilection for the left or right hemithorax. Patients are generally taller and thinner than age-matched controls, and their ratio of lung height to body height is high (although their total lung capacity is usually normal). Familial clusterings of spontaneous pneumothorax have been reported, and HLA haplotype A2B40 may be a risk factor. The air leak is thought to occur as a result of rupture of a subpleural bleb or cyst usually located near the apex of the upper lobe. Such blebs can be demonstrated by conventional radiography in only 20% of cases but can be found by CT or on thoracotomy in 85% of patients. Although the exact pathogenesis of bleb formation is unknown, it is speculated that it is related to the gravitational gradient of pleural pressure. Pleural pressure is most negative at the apices. Hence, apical alveoli are subjected to greater mean distending pressures than are alveoli at the bases of the lung. This increased distending pressure would be exaggerated in taller individuals and could cause apical alveoli to rupture, allowing gas to collect as subpleural accumulations (blebs).

TABLE 1. Lung Diseases Associated with Secondary Spontaneous Pneumothorax

Chronic Obstructive Disorders
Asthma
Bronchopulmonary dysplasia
Cystic fibrosis
Emphysema
Histiocytosis X
Sarcoidosis

Infectious Disorders
Pneumonia
Lung abscess
AIDS and *Pneumocystis carinii* infection
Tuberculosis
Coccidioidomycosis
Hydatid disease

Connective Tissue Disorders
Ehlers-Danlos syndrome
Marfan syndrome
Straight back syndrome

Parenchymal Disorders
Idiopathic pulmonary fibrosis
Pulmonary alveolar proteinosis
Pulmonary hemosiderosis
Pulmonary infarction
Rheumatoid disease
Scleroderma

Neoplastic Disorders
Primary lung cancer
Secondary cancer (adrenal, osteogenic sarcoma, Wilms' tumor)

Drug Abuse
Inhaled free-base or crack cocaine
Attempted central venous injection

TABLE 2. Disorders Associated with Pneumomediastinum

Pulmonary Injuries
Alveolar-interstitial air leak
Tracheal or bronchial rupture
Inhalational drug abuse
    Cocaine
    Methylenedioxyamphetamine ("Ecstasy")

Gastrointestinal Disorders
Esophageal perforation
Gastrointestinal perforation
Bacillary dysentery
Laparoscopy

Head and Neck Injuries
Tonsillectomy
Dental extractions
Zygomatic-maxillary fractures

In addition to dissecting peripherally to form subpleural blebs (which may rupture to cause pneumothorax), gas leaking from alveoli into the pulmonary interstitium can move centrally along perivascular lymphatic and bronchiolar sheaths until it reaches the mediastinum. Air reaching the mediastinal space may remain there to form a pneumomediastinum, or it may dissect into subcutaneous tissue, the retroperitoneal space, or the pericardium. Spontaneous pneumomediastinum can occur in healthy young men, typically during the third decade of life, in whom a presumed local parenchymal scar results in alveolar rupture during coughing or straining. Pneumomediastinum is more frequently seen, however, in patients with chronic lung disease and in abusers of inhaled drugs, in whom the initial lung rupture may occur in sites other than a subpleural location. Pneumomediastinum also can arise secondary to gas leakage from other sites (Table 2).

DIAGNOSIS

Patients developing a spontaneous pneumothorax usually experience sudden chest pain and dyspnea. Ipsilateral chest pain is reported by up to 90% of pneumothorax patients. The pain typically is pleuritic at onset but later becomes a persistent dull ache. The dyspnea is dependent on the previous condition of the lungs and the size of the pneumothorax. Therefore, it often progresses as the pneumothorax expands. Physical examination may be normal, particularly in patients with small ($\leq$ 25%) pneumothoraces or chronic lung disease. Larger pneumothoraces may cause rapid, shallow respirations and ipsilateral hyperinflation of the hemithorax, absent vocal fremitus, and diminished or absent breath sounds. A pleural friction rub may be present. The trachea may be deviated to the contralateral side if a tension pneumothorax exists. More than 80% of patients with spontaneous pneumothorax are also hypoxemic because of ventilation-perfusion mismatch and anatomic shunting in the partially atelectatic lung.

Tension pneumothorax is a potentially life-threatening condition that is seen most commonly in patients with traumatic pneumothoraces and those receiving mechanical ventilation, especially when positive end-expiratory pressure (PEEP) is employed. It rarely occurs with a primary spontaneous pneumothorax. A tension pneumothorax can originate from even a small defect in the lung if a flap of tissue at the site of air leak begins to function as a one-way ball valve, allowing air to flow into the pleural space during inspiration but closing during expiration. By this mechanism, air is essentially pumped into the pleural space, and the intrapleural pressure quickly begins to exceed atmospheric pressure. As the pressure increases, the diaphragm is flattened, and the mediastinum is displaced away from the tension. Compression of the contralateral lung further impairs already compromised ventilation, and compression of the great vessels reduces venous return. The conscious patient will become acutely dyspneic and cyanotic and often will develop diaphoresis, tachycardia, jugular venous distention, and arterial hypotension. Once the diagnosis of tension pneumothorax is made or even highly suspected, it must be treated immediately with supplemental oxygen (to lessen the severity of the hypoxemia) and insertion of a needle into the pleural cavity anteriorly through the second intercostal space to release the pressure. These procedures should not be delayed for any radiographic studies that would prolong the time to release of the positive pleural pressure and increase the patient's risk of cardiopulmonary collapse.

In most other situations, the diagnosis of pneumothorax is confirmed by chest radiography, which demonstrates a space of air density devoid of lung markings between the lung and the chest wall. This delineation is seen most easily in erect patients, in whom the pleural gas collects over the apex of the lung. When the degree of pulmonary collapse is minimal, conventional inspiratory radiographs may not show the pneumothorax, and a frontal chest film taken during maximal expiration may more clearly demonstrate pleural air around the collapsed lung. Estimating the size of a pneumothorax from inspection of chest radiographs notoriously underestimates the amount of pleural air present. Since the volumes of the lung and hemithorax are fairly proportional to the cubes of their diameters, a more accurate estimate of the size of the pneumothorax can be obtained by cubing the diameters of the lung and hemithorax and subtracting the ratio from 100%.

Pneumomediastinum, isolated or in combination with a pneumothorax, may occur with little signs or symptoms in a patient with chronic lung disease. In contrast, a spontaneous pneumomediastinum arising in an otherwise healthy individual is heralded by the sudden onset of severe retrosternal pain in 90% of patients, possibly radiating to the arms or neck. Sixty percent of patients experience dyspnea, and 40% have dysphagia. Physical signs suggestive of a pneumomediastinum include subcutaneous emphysema, crepitation in the suprasternal notch, distant heart sounds, and crunching or clicking noises synchronous with the heartbeat (Hamman's sign). The last two findings are not limited to pneumomediastinum, as either can occur with left-sided pneumothoraces as well. The diagnosis of pneumomediastinum is established radiographically. In infants, the mediastinal air lifts one or both lobes of the thymus off the anterior mediastinum and results in a characteristic spinnaker or sail sign. Older patients will demonstrate mediastinal and subcutaneous emphysema.

THERAPY

By the time a patient with a primary spontaneous pneumothorax seeks medical attention, the site of rupture often is closed. Patients with little or no chest pain and dyspnea may be followed without treatment by obtaining periodic chest radiographs until the pleural gas is absorbed. Absorption occurs at an average daily rate of 1.25% of the original lung volume and can be accelerated to about 5% by O_2 breathing. Breathing pure O_2 lowers total gas pressure in mixed venous blood and tissue from ~645 mm Hg ($P_{CO_2} = 45$, $P_{O_2} = 40$, $P_{N_2} = 560$ mm Hg) to ~120 mm Hg ($P_{CO_2} = 50$, $P_{O_2} = 70$, $P_{N_2} = 0$ mm Hg), thereby increasing the pressure gradient confronting the pneumothorax and facilitating its reabsorption. In practice, O_2 breathing is rarely performed because of the concern for O_2 toxicity in asymptomatic patients and the desire for more rapid resolution in symptomatic patients. From the noted rate of absorption of pleural air, it can be seen that a pneumothorax occupying 15% to 20% of the hemithorax would require 12 to 16 days to resolve passively. This conservative management approach has a high failure rate, however, with 33% to 50% of patients eventually requiring tube thoracostomy. It should be noted that the rare deaths resulting from primary spontaneous pneumothorax occur *only* in patients treated with observation alone.

Because of protracted resolution, patients with larger pneumothoraces and patients with dyspnea or progressive air leak need to be treated more actively. One consideration for the initial treatment of a patient's first primary spontaneous pneumothorax is simple needle aspiration. Since primary spontaneous pneumothoraces are rarely life threatening and the air leak is typically closed by the time of presentation, needle aspiration can be an effective procedure, with minimal morbidity. An 18- or 16-gauge needle with an internal polyethylene catheter is inserted into the second anterior intercostal space at the midclavicular line following local anesthesia. Air is withdrawn manually with a 60-ml syringe connected to the catheter via a three-way stopcock until no more can be aspirated. The stopcock is closed off for several hours, whereupon if there has been no radiographic reaccumulation of the pleural air, the catheter is removed, and the patient is discharged. Simple aspiration can resolve up to 70% of primary spontaneous pneumothoraces but is less successful in cases of secondary spontaneous pneumothorax, which have only about a 30% resolution rate with this technique.

More commonly, however, patients with more severe symptoms or extensive air accumulation are treated with tube thoracostomy and suction to evacuate their pneumothoraces. Tube thoracostomy is the treatment of choice in all patients with tension pneumothorax, in patients with significant lung disease, and in patients who are receiving mechanical ventilation. In those groups of individuals, even small pneumothoraces can markedly impair lung function. Furthermore, the likelihood of early spontaneous closure of the site of lung rupture is not very high. Traumatic and iatrogenic pneumothoraces also are almost always treated by tube thoracostomy. Tube thoracostomy is performed by placement of a small to medium sized (10 F in an infant to 25 F in an adult) chest tube into the anteroapical portion of the pleural space. The tube may be inserted into the second anterior intercostal space in the midclavicular line, but it is more often inserted into the fifth intercostal space in the midaxillary line. Under local anesthesia, a small incision is made at least one intercostal space below the space to be entered. A tunnel is made through the subcutaneous tissue, and the pleural space is entered over the superior margin of the cephalad rib, thereby avoiding injury to the neurovascular bundle along the rib's inferior margin. An oblique subcutaneous tunnel usually closes readily and lessens the chance of recurrent pneumothorax after the tube is removed. In larger patients, the inserter's finger can be advanced through the tract to ensure that the pleural space has been entered. Although chest tubes are sometimes inserted over trocars, it is preferable to insert them using a large hemostat to reduce the risk of impaling the lung parenchyma. Once in position and operating properly, the thoracostomy tube is secured with heavy pursestring suture and tape. A simple pneumothorax may only require waterseal for lung reexpansion, but gentle suction of 10 to 20 cm H_2O generally is applied to the chest tube for more rapid reexpansion. The intrathoracic position of the tube should be verified radiographically as soon as possible after insertion. Thereafter, serial chest films are essential for monitoring the function of the thoracostomy tube and resolution of the pneumothorax.

Technical complications of chest tube insertion occur in about 1% of patients. These include puncture of the lung, laceration of the intercostal or internal mammary artery, penetration of the mediastinum or diaphragm, and laceration of the liver or spleen. Ipsilateral pulmonary edema can develop following rapid reexpansion of a collapsed lung, and it may be potentiated by excessive suction. Postthoracostomy empyema has been reported in 3% to 6% of patients with traumatic pneumothoraces but rarely occurs in nontraumatic cases. Accordingly, routine antibiotic prophylaxis is not recommended in patients with spontaneous pneumothorax but may be indicated in patients with traumatic pneumothorax following penetrating chest wall injuries.

Once the air leak stops, the thoracostomy tube is clamped or placed to waterseal for 24 hours to guarantee that lung collapse will not recur. If the pneumothorax does not redevelop, the chest tube may be removed, and the thoracostomy site may be closed with the pursestring sutures. Over 95% of primary spontaneous pneumothoraces resolve within 24 to 48 hours if the lung is completely reexpanded and the visceral and parietal pleura are in approximation. Persistence of the air leak beyond 5 to 7 days of therapy is more common in patients

with underlying lung disease or in those receiving mechanical positive pressure ventilation. If the risk of thoracotomy is high in such a patient, tube drainage may be continued for more than 7 days, perhaps with placement of a second chest tube to aid in air evacuation. Extended thoracostomy treatment is warranted in patients with continued risk for air leak because of ongoing mechanical ventilation or with treatable pulmonary conditions, such as status asthmaticus or ARDS.

Patients who have persistent air leaks or collapsed lungs after 7 days of thoracostomy suction or who have had a recurrent pneumothorax are candidates for surgical exploration. With recent technologic innovations, all procedures previously requiring open thoracotomy—including ablation or resection of ruptured blebs or lung tissue, pleural abrasion, parietal pleurectomy, and instillation of sclerosing agents—can be performed through a thoracoscope in larger children and adults. Thoracoscopy is associated with considerably less morbidity than thoracotomy and results in reduction in the risk of recurrent pneumothorax to less than 10%. Although some authors advocate that all patients with a primary spontaneous pneumothorax undergo thoracoscopic evaluation and removal of blebs, it may be more reasonable to wait for the second episode, since over 50% of patients with a first primary spontaneous pneumothorax will never have a recurrence.

Nevertheless, 30% to 50% of patients with primary spontaneous pneumothorax treated without pleurodesis will have a recurrent pneumothorax, 75% of which are on the same side and most of which occur within 2 years of the initial episode. The recurrence risk is similar whether the initial pneumothorax was untreated or whether it was evacuated by tube thoracostomy and pleural suction. Furthermore, it is increased in patients with secondary spontaneous pneumothoraces and in patients who already have had one recurrence. Accordingly, obliteration of the pleural space usually is considered after two ipsilateral episodes of spontaneous pneumothorax. Pleurodesis may be performed surgically as described or chemically by instillation of various compounds through the chest tube placed to evacuate the pneumothorax. Compounds employed for this purpose include talc, quinacrine, silver nitrate, kaolin, and tetracycline derivatives. Because of its ready availability, low cost, and low morbidity, a tetracycline may be the agent of choice. The recommended adult dose is 1 ml/kg of a solution containing 20 mg/kg tetracycline or 5 mg/kg minocycline. Chemical pleurodesis is associated with severe pain, and patients often are given intrapleural lidocaine (up to 3 mg/kg in 1 ml/kg total volume) before injection of the sclerosing agent.

Special consideration is needed in patients who are candidates for lung transplantation, such as young adults with cystic fibrosis. Tube thoracostomy is acceptable in such patients, but chemical or surgical pleurodesis can make patients less desirable transplant candidates because of increased surgical difficulty and excess bleeding. More recently, however, some centers have begun to accept patients for transplantation even though they have received pleurodesis. Chemical pleurodesis is nearly as effective as surgical pleurodesis in preventing recurrences of primary spontaneous pneumothorax and is less invasive. Thoracoscopic pleurodesis is relatively noninvasive, however, and offers several advantages over chemical pleurodesis, including the ability to directly ablate or resect blebs or cysts, direct visualization of sites of mechanical or chemical pleural abrasion, and the ability to close a persisting bronchopleural fistula and reexpand a partially collapsed lung, thereby improving the chances for successful subsequent pleurodesis.

Simple pneumomediastinum rarely requires treatment, even when air dissects into the subcutaneous tissues of the neck. However, surgical decompression may be necessary occasionally to alleviate severe pain or dyspnea or to relieve hemodynamic compromise because of the mediastinal pressure. This is usually accomplished by needle aspiration or mediastinotomy, with a small transverse incision just above the suprasternal notch. Recurrent spontaneous pneumomediastinum can occur in up to 10% of patients.

PLEURAL EFFUSION, EMPYEMA, AND CHYLOTHORAX

JOSEPH OREN, M.D.

The pleural cavity is a potential space between the visceral pleura, which covers the lung, and the parietal pleura, which covers the inner surface of the thoracic cage. Normally, only a thin layer of fluid is present between the two layers of pleura. A variety of clinical disorders can lead to pleural effusion, which is characterized by excessive fluid accumulation in the pleural cavity.

DIAGNOSIS

The most common clinical signs of pleural disease are shortness of breath, pleuritic chest pain, and cough. Occasionally, the patient is asymptomatic, and finding of an effusion is the result of a chest roentgenogram obtained for other reasons. The findings on physical examination depend on the size of the effusion. Large effusions usually produce decreased breath sounds, decreased or absent tactile and vocal fremitus, and dullness to percussion.

Chest Roentgenogram

Frontal and lateral chest roentgenograms, augmented by decubitus views, should be obtained to determine the amount of fluid, whether the fluid is free flowing or loculated, and the presence of adjacent parenchymal lung disease.

Thoracocentesis

In all confirmed pleural effusions of unexplained etiology, the pleural fluid should be examined. If the effusion is free flowing and its thickness is more than 1 cm on the lateral decubitus view, diagnostic thoracocentesis should be performed. If the fluid is loculated, thoracocentesis should be performed under ultrasound guidance. Contraindications to thoracocentesis include an insufficient quantity of pleural fluid, chest wall skin infection, or hemorrhagic diathesis. Potential complications include pneumothorax, bleeding from an intercostal artery, infection in the pleural space, and injury to the liver, spleen, or kidney.

Pleural Fluid Analysis

The pleural fluid should be examined for color and turbidity. Specific studies on the pleural fluid should include:

1. A complete blood cell count with differential
2. Chemistry studies, including protein, lactic acid dehydrogenase, glucose, and pH (the fluid sample for pH should be handled as an arterial pH and drawn into a heparinized syringe and placed on ice)
3. Stains and cultures for aerobic and anaerobic bacteria, fungi, and mycobacteria.

Other studies, such as cytology, amylase, triglycerides, rheumatoid factor, antinuclear antibody, and countercurrent immunoelectropho-

TABLE 1. Etiology of Pleural Effusions

Transudates
Increased hydrostatic pressure
  Congestive heart failure
  Systemic or pulmonary venous hypertension
Decreased oncotic pressure
  Cirrhosis
  Nephrosis
  Hypoalbuminemia

Exudates
Increased capillary permeability
  Pleuropulmonary infections
  Noncardiogenic pulmonary edema (ARDS)
  Collagen vascular diseases
  Neoplasms
  Intraabdominal diseases (pancreatitis, subphrenic abscess)
  Pulmonary infarction
  Hemothorax
  Chronic atelectasis or trapped lung
Impaired lymphatic flow
  Chylothorax

resis, should be obtained if clinically indicated. The first diagnostic step is to determine if the fluid represents a transudate or exudate. Transudates result from an imbalance between the hydrostatic and osmotic forces in the pleural capillaries, leading to the accumulation of low protein fluid (<3 g/dl) in the pleural space. Exudates result from increased permeability of the capillaries in the pleura, leading to an increased flow of high protein fluid (>3 g/dl) into the pleural space. The information obtained from studying the pleural fluid should be used in classifying the pleural effusion (Tables 1 and 2).

TREATMENT

General supportive measures include supplemental oxygen when the patient is hypoxemic, relief of chest pain with appropriate analgesics, and drainage of large pleural effusions when dyspnea is present.

Transudates

The treatment of children with transudative pleural effusions should be focused on correction of the underlying disease. Congestive heart failure is the most common cause of a transudative pleural effusion. The effusion is caused by the elevated systemic and pulmonary venous pressures, which favor increased formation and decreased absorption of pleural fluid. When the congestive heart failure is appropriately treated, the pleural effusion will disappear. Cirrhosis, complicated by ascites, is another cause of a transudative pleural effusion. Treatment of this condition should be directed primarily toward management of the ascites. Rarely, a large pleural effusion may cause dyspnea, which will require removal of fluid by thoracocentesis. In most cases, however, the risks imposed by thoracocentesis outweigh the temporary benefits achieved by removal of fluid.

TABLE 2. Classification of Pleural Effusions

| TYPE OF EFFUSION | APPEARANCE | PROTEIN (g/dl) | LDH[a] (U/L) | PLEURAL/SERUM RATIO | | | GLUCOSE (mg/dl) |
				PROTEIN	LDH	pH	
Transudate	Straw colored	<3	<200	<0.5	<0.6	≥7.3	S[b]
Exudate	Turbid	≥3	>200	≥0.5	≥0.6	≥7.2	S;>40
Empyema	Turbid to purulent	≥3	>1000	≥0.5	≥0.6	<7.1	<40
Chylothorax	Milky or turbid	≥3	S	≥0.5	≥0.6	≥7.4	S

[a]LDH, lactic acid dehydrogenase.
[b]S, same as serum.

Exudates

Noninfectious exudates usually resolve with appropriate treatment of the underlying disease. In contrast, parapneumonic effusions, which are the most common exudative pleural effusions, should be treated early in their course to avoid progression into empyema. If the patient has a free-flowing, nonpurulent pleural fluid with biochemical parameters that are consistent with an exudate (Table 2), empiric antibiotic treatment should be started after all the appropriate specimens have been examined and sent for cultures. Selection of the initial antibiotic treatment should be based on the results of the gram stain and on the predominant bacterial pathogens that cause pneumonia in the patient's particular age group. There is no reason to perform serial therapeutic thoracocentesis in these patients because the effusion usually resolves spontaneously, leaving little or no pleural disease. If the patient remains febrile or if the pleural effusion increases in size, a repeat thoracocentesis should be performed to verify that the effusion has not progressed into empyema.

Empyema

This complicated parapneumonic effusion is characterized by thick pleural fluid, positive pleural fluid Gram stain or bacterial cultures, and typical biochemical parameters (Table 2). During the acute phase of empyema, the exudate is free flowing and should be drained promptly with a large-bore chest tube, in addition to being treated with appropriate antibiotics. Medical management should be continued for 10 to 14 days if the patient responds favorably, as evidenced by resolution of fever, dyspnea, oxygen requirement, and leukocytosis. The chest tube should be removed when output is under 30 to 50 ml/24 h. The chest roentgenogram may reveal pleural thickening even months after the acute episode and should not serve as an indication for surgical intervention. If, however, there is no improvement in the patient's clinical status in 48 hours, a chest CT or ultrasound study should be obtained. If the pleural space is found to be inadequately drained, another chest tube should be inserted. In those instances where chest tube drainage is not sufficient because of multiple loculations, trapped lung, or an organized peel, thoracotomy with lung decortication may be indicated. This procedure involves removal of a constricting fibrous peel and reexpansion of entrapped lung parenchyma.

Chylothorax

Chylothorax is the accumulation of pleural fluid, rich in chylomicrons and triglycerides. Congenital chylothorax is the most common cause of pleural effusion in the neonatal period. It is usually associated with birth trauma or with developmental anomalies of the lymphatic system. Beyond the neonatal period, the leading cause of chylothorax is trauma during cardiopulmonary surgery. Other less common causes are listed in Table 3. Initial management consists of decompression of the pleural space by repeated thoracocentesis, with replacement of protein and electrolyte losses. However, rapid reaccumulation of fluid necessitates insertion of a chest tube, followed by continuous low pressure aspiration. Chest tube drainage allows the parietal and visceral pleura to appose and to eventually adhere to each other (pleuredesis). To minimize thoracic lymphatic flow, enteral fat intake should be replaced by medium-chain triglycerides that are absorbed directly into the portal system rather than by the intestinal lymphatic system. If despite this regimen the pleural effusion persists, total

TABLE 3. Causes of Chylothorax

Trauma (accidental or surgical)
Pulmonary or intestinal lymphangiectasia
Congenital anomalies of thoracic duct system
Fetal hydrops
Superior vena cava syndrome
Malignancy
Idiopathic

parenteral nutrition should be instituted. Chylothorax can be treated successfully using a nonoperative approach for several weeks, provided the nutritional and metabolic status of the patient is not adversely affected. If effusion recurs or persists after 4 to 6 weeks of medical treatment, surgical intervention may be considered, especially if severe nutritional or metabolic complications appear imminent. The surgical approach to refractory chylothorax includes pleuroperitoneal shunting, thoracic duct ligation, or thoracotomy with pleurodesis.

INTRATHORACIC TUMORS AND CYSTS

Nelson L. Turcios, m.d.

Most primary intrathoracic tumors and cysts in infants and children are located in, or are adjacent to, the mediastinum. Occasionally, they occur in the pulmonary parenchyma. These lesions are a heterogeneous group of congenital, neoplastic, and infectious disorders. Many are potentially life threatening and malignant.

DIAGNOSIS

The vast majority of children with intrathoracic masses are symptomatic. Cough, respiratory distress, and neurologic manifestations are the most commonly observed complaints. The variety of signs and symptoms is related to the patient's age, the nature of the lesion, and the anatomic location of the mass. Children younger than 2 years and children who have malignant lesions are most likely to be symptomatic.

The physical examination is rarely helpful in localizing the lesion. If lymphadenopathy or organomegaly is present, the most likely diagnosis is malignant lymphoma, and the workup should proceed accordingly. If the neurologic examination reveals evidence of spinal cord compression, the tumor is probably neurogenic.

Newborns with respiratory distress and children who have chronic cough, recurrent wheezing, or neurologic symptoms require roentgenographic evaluation. The plain chest x-ray (posteroanterior and lateral views) is the most valuable tool for demonstrating the presence of a mass and localizing it. When a mass lesion is demonstrated, computed tomography (CT) becomes an important study because it further defines the precise anatomic location of the lesion, distinguishes cystic lesions from solid tumors, and demonstrates the extent of involvement of vital structures. The last information is most helpful to the surgeon in determining the resectability of the mediastinal mass.

Magnetic resonance imaging (MRI) can discriminate masses in the mediastinum from vascular structures better than CT and is more sensitive in detecting intraspinal extension. Other radiographic procedures, such as barium swallow and angiography, may be useful in evaluating specific lesions that are not otherwise well demarcated.

Once the presence of a mediastinal mass has been established, it is necessary to consult a surgeon because in the majority of cases, tissue must be obtained to make a definitive diagnosis. Cervical or supraclavicular lymphadenopathy, if present, provides an easily accessible area for biopsy. Thoracotomy permits excellent visualization of the lesion and provides access for removal of adequate tissue for diagnosis. It is the procedure of choice when complete excision of the mass is contemplated.

Mediastinoscopy, which is generally associated with lower morbidity, also may provide sufficient tissue for diagnosis in the majority of cases. Thoracoscopy provides a unique opportunity to examine the entire hemithorax and is useful in evaluating parenchymal abnormalities and pleural disease in addition to the mediastinal mass.

If CT of the chest suggests a malignant neoplasm, such as lymphoma, CT scanning of the abdomen and pelvis should be obtained to expedite the staging workup. An oncologist should be consulted, and bone marrow aspiration should be performed. Infiltration of the marrow with malignant lymphoblasts will confirm the diagnosis. However, the absence of marrow involvement does not exclude the diagnosis.

TUMORS AND CYSTS OF THE MEDIASTINUM

Since the mediastinal organs are in relatively fixed positions, the mediastinum has been arbitrarily divided into three compartments based on anatomic structures discerned on lateral chest films. Because most masses arise from structures that are normally present, there is a remarkable predilection for anatomic localization of mediastinal masses according to pathologic type.

The *anterior mediastinum* contains the thymus, anterior mediastinal lymph nodes, and the anterior portions of the heart and pericardium. The *middle mediastinum* contains the heart and great vessels, the trachea, and the bulk of the mediastinal lymph nodes. The *posterior mediastinum* contains the esophagus, the thoracic duct, the vagus and splanchnic nerves, and the descending thoracic aorta.

Once a mediastinal mass is identified, localization to one of these three compartments aids in the differential diagnosis (Table 1). Approximately 30% of mediastinal masses in children are located in the anterior mediastinum, 30% in the middle mediastinum, and 40% in the posterior mediastinum.

Anterior Mediastinal Masses

The most common masses of the anterior mediastinum are thymic lesions, angiomatous tumors, and teratomas. Intubation or tracheostomy may not bypass the obstruction if the mass is extensive. Emergency surgical intervention to decompress the airway occasionally is required.

Thymic Lesions

Thymic enlargement is the most common cause of a widened anterior mediastinum in young infants, an age when malignant lymphoma is very unusual. Thymic hyperplasia rarely if ever causes symptoms and will generally regress spontaneously with age.

Benign thymic cysts often originate in the cervical portion of the thymus and may be palpable in the supraclavicular and suprasternal areas. CT will confirm the cystic nature of this lesion. Surgical excision is recommended to avoid tracheal compression.

Malignant thymoma is very rare in children. This entity is best treated by surgical resection. Some experts also recommend local radiation.

TABLE 1. Mediastinal Masses in Children

COMMON	RARE
Anterior Mediastinum	
Thymic lesion	Substernal thyroid
Hyperplasia	Thymic mass
Angiomatous tumor	
Hemangioma	
Lymphangioma	
Teratoma	
Middle Mediastinum	
Lymphoma	
Hodgkin disease	
Non-Hodgkin lymphoma	
Lymphadenopathy	Pericardial cyst
Bronchogenic cyst	
Posterior Mediastinum	
Neurogenic tumor	Neurolemomas
Duplication cyst	Neurofibromas
	Pheochromocytoma
	Anterior meningocele

Angiomatous Tumors

Approximately 75% of mediastinal hemangiomas and lymphangiomas occur in the anterior compartment. Both lesions may cause tracheal compression, especially in children younger than 2 years.

Hemangiomas in the anterior mediastinum may occur in association with similar cutaneous lesions. Angiography may be useful for confirming the vascular nature of the lesion and outlining involvement. Laser therapy is the treatment of choice for patients with hemangiomas who are symptomatic. Interferon alfa has been used with some success when complete surgical removal is not possible because of involvement of major vessels or when the hemangioma is recurrent.

Lymphangiomas (cystic hygromas) represent a failure in development of the lymphatic channels that drain lymph sacs into the venous system. The lesion may be confined to the mediastinum, or it may represent an extension of a cervical lesion. Lymphangiomas usually are found in children younger than 3 years. They are often large and involve more than one mediastinal compartment. Intrathoracic extension should be looked for in all cases of cervical or axillary cystic hygroma. Surgical excision is the treatment of choice. If the mediastinal component is not large, the entire mass can sometimes be removed through a cervical incision.

Teratomas

Teratoid tumors of the mediastinum may be classified as benign cystic teratoma, benign solid teratoma, or malignant teratoma. Presumably, they arise when fetal tissue of one type becomes displaced and embedded in tissue of another type. Most teratomas are cystic and contain elements derived from all three germ layers. However, dermoid tumors, consisting primarily of ectodermal elements, also occur. Calcification is frequently present. In fact, it is the presence of teeth and/or calcification in an anterior mediastinal mass that suggests a diagnosis of teratoma. Eighty percent of these lesions are benign, and surgical excision usually is curative. The treatment of choice for the benign solid or malignant teratoma (more commonly seen in infants and young children) is surgical resection.

Pericardial Cysts

These cysts are usually located anteriorly in the cardiophrenic angles, more frequently on the right side, and occasionally on or in the diaphragm. They are usually asymptomatic and are discovered on routine x-ray. Resection by open thoracotomy is the procedure of choice.

Middle Mediastinal Masses

The key question in evaluating radiographic findings is if lymphadenopathy alone is present or if the child has bronchopulmonary and foregut malformations. Lymphadenopathy is more common.

Although enlarged lymph nodes of the middle mediastinum most often represent malignant lymphoma, infectious causes must also be considered, especially tuberculosis and histoplasmosis. It is unusual for these disorders to cause enlargement of the mediastinal lymph nodes in the absence of pulmonary involvement, but the lymphadenopathy may be far more prominent than is suggested by the parenchymal lesions alone. Sarcoidosis, although rare in children, must be considered in the differential diagnosis when hilar lymphadenopathy predominates, especially in African-American teenagers.

Lymphomas

By far the most common malignant neoplasms arising within the middle mediastinum are lymphomas, which may involve the anterior mediastinum as well. Lymphomas are the most frequent cause of mediastinal masses in older children and adolescents. They are often associated with generalized lymphadenopathy, hepatosplenomegaly, and systemic symptoms, such as fever, night sweats, and weight loss.

A histologic diagnosis must be obtained because treatment and prognosis vary with the histologic subtype. In the absence of cervical or supraclavicular lymph node enlargement, biopsy of scalene nodes often provides tissue for diagnosis. Otherwise, tissue from an intrathoracic tumor should be obtained using one of the biopsy methods described previously. Complete resection should not be attempted. Surgery is required primarily for diagnosis and does not play a role in the treatment of mediastinal lymphomas.

On rare occasions, a rapidly growing lymphoma produces life-threatening respiratory distress. In such cases, emergency treatment with mediastinal radiation or chemotherapy may be necessary to relieve the airway obstruction before tissue can be obtained for pathologic diagnosis.

Hodgkin disease frequently involves the mediastinum and may occur primarily as a mediastinal mass. This disorder is found most commonly in adolescents and young adults. It is rare in young children. Hodgkin disease is one of the few malignancies that may represent a truly localized process. In the localized variety, patients frequently can be cured by radiation therapy alone. Advanced disease is managed with a variety of chemotherapeutic drugs, with or without radiation of areas of bulk disease.

Non-Hodgkin lymphoma of the mediastinum may occur at any age, but it is seen more frequently in older children and adolescents than in infants and young children. These lesions tend to grow much more rapidly than those of Hodgkin disease, so the duration of symptoms is usually brief. Patients with non-Hodgkin lymphoma are more likely to experience severe respiratory distress or the superior vena cava syndrome.

As is the case with Hodgkin disease, a complete workup to determine the extent of the disease is mandatory. This should include evaluation of the bone marrow and cerebrospinal fluid (CSF), two common sites of spread of malignant lymphomas.

In contrast to Hodgkin disease, mediastinal non-Hodgkin lymphoma in children is invariably more widespread than is apparent clinically or radiographically. Therefore, aggressive systemic therapy is always required. Newer combination chemotherapy programs have produced cure rates in excess of 70% for patients in whom the CNS is free of tumor at diagnosis.

Bronchogenic Cysts

These malformations usually occur singly in the middle mediastinum near the carina and adjacent to the bronchi, but they may be found in the lungs as well. They are more frequent on the right side than on the left and more common in boys than in girls. The majority of bronchogenic cysts range in size between 2 cm and 10 cm in diameter and are unilocular. Usually, these mucus-containing cysts have a thick wall and are lined by respiratory epithelium. Bronchogenic cysts are believed to result from abnormal lung budding in the primitive foregut. They do not contain distal lung parenchyma. Since these cysts originate before formation of the bronchi, few, if any, of these lesions communicate with the airway.

Symptoms are caused by compression of the adjacent portion of the tracheobronchial tree, with resultant air trapping and overdistention of the portion of the lung distal to the lesion. Severe respiratory distress may occur in neonates and young infants, who may have localized wheezing, persistent infiltrates, or atelectasis. Older children often are asymptomatic.

Small cysts may not be visible on plain chest roentgenograms, but the diagnosis should be suspected in any child who has recurrent lobar pneumonia or roentgenographic signs of bronchial obstruction. An esophagogram may demonstrate indentation of the anterior wall of the esophagus by the cyst.

Surgical excision of the cyst, without pulmonary resection, is curative.

Posterior Mediastinal Masses

More than 90% of these masses are neurogenic tumors. Duplication cysts of the foregut account for most of the rest.

Neurogenic Tumors

These tumors are the most common cause of posterior mediastinal masses in young children. In children younger than 4 years, neurogenic tumors are usually malignant neuroblastomas or ganglioneuroblastomas. Older children are more likely to have benign ganglioneuromas. Benign neurilemomas, neurofibromas, and pheochromocytomas also may occur in the posterior mediastinum.

Patients with large lesions that extend anteriorly may experience respiratory distress as a result of airway compression. Children also may have pain, irritability, and symptoms of spinal cord compression, including increased deep tendon reflexes, bowel or bladder dysfunction, and even paraplegia, when there is intervertebral extension of a lesion.

The rare neurologic syndrome of opsoclonus-myoclonus has been associated with a form of neuroblastoma arising within the mediastinum, although its pathogenesis remains unclear. Horner syndrome is present at diagnosis in a small number of patients.

Chest roentgenography usually reveals a well-defined, smooth-bordered, soft tissue mass in the posterior mediastinum. Because these tumors arise from sympathetic ganglia, they tend to orient themselves along a vertical axis. Calcification frequently is present. Erosion and spreading of the posterior ribs are seen commonly.

Urinary catecholamines, such as vanillylmandelic acid (VMA) and norepinephrine, should be evaluated because they suggest the neurogenic origin of the lesion and are useful tumor markers for evaluating the success of therapy. However, only a minority of mediastinal neuroblastomas secrete catecholamines, so that negative results do not exclude the diagnosis.

The diagnostic workup should include a skeletal survey, bone scan, and bone marrow aspiration and biopsy. In the absence of demonstrable metastases, an attempt should be made to surgically excise the primary tumor. If indicated because of symptoms, MRI should be done before surgery to rule out intraspinal extension of the tumor. If the results are abnormal, the patient should undergo a decompressive laminectomy before thoracotomy for tumor resection to prevent neurologic morbidity related to bleeding from residual extradural tumor.

Although radiation therapy has been used frequently to eradicate residual tumor following incomplete resection, it has not been documented that the use of radiation improves the survival rate. Furthermore, laminectomy and spinal radiation may predispose the child to develop scoliosis.

The prognosis is much more favorable for patients with mediastinal neuroblastoma than for those with primary tumors in the abdomen or pelvis. If the tumor is localized, the majority of children survive their disease. Even patients whose tumors are only partially excised often do well. As is true of neuroblastoma arising in other sites, infants younger than 1 year do better than older children. Patients with histologic evidence of maturation tend to have a more favorable prognosis than those with completely undifferentiated neuroblastomas. Unfortunately, the outlook for older children with disseminated disease at diagnosis remains poor.

Duplication Cysts

Esophageal duplication cysts are usually asymptomatic. However, they may cause respiratory symptoms or swallowing difficulty. When symptoms are present, distortion of the esophagus is demonstrable by esophagography. About two thirds of these lesions are right-sided and are in intimate contact with the wall of the esophagus. Removal by thoracotomy is indicated.

Gastroenteric duplications may be lined by esophageal epithelium or by gastric or enteric mucosa. Some share a common muscle wall with the esophagus, although they rarely communicate with the esophageal lumen. Other cysts are distinctly separate from the esophagus but may traverse the diaphragm and communicate with the intestinal tract. These may be demonstrable on an upper gastrointestinal series, and late films may confirm filling of the mass from the upper gastro-intestinal tract. Patients who have one duplication often are found to have a second elsewhere in the gastrointestinal tract.

Duplication cysts occasionally rupture into the pleural cavity. When they do, patients may have pleural effusion or empyema. Upper gastrointestinal bleeding may occur if acid secretions from the cyst enter the small intestine and cause ulceration, but such bleeding is rare. Duplication cysts of the mediastinum are almost always associated with abnormalities of the lower cervical or upper thoracic vertebrae, including hemivertebrae, incomplete fusion of neural arches, and spina bifida. The association of any of these vertebral anomalies with a posterior mediastinal mass strongly suggests the diagnosis.

The proper management of a duplication cyst is surgical excision. The surgeon must be aware that the cyst may connect with the alimentary tract below the diaphragm or may involve the dura at the site of the vertebral anomaly. Orthopedic treatment may be required for the vertebral anomaly or resultant scoliosis.

PULMONARY TUMORS

Benign Pulmonary Tumors

Hamartoma

This tumorlike malformation consists mostly of cartilage and variable amounts of epithelium, fat, and muscle. Although the appearance of a solid mass on the chest x-ray may lead one to suspect a hamartoma, the diagnosis usually is made after excision.

Bronchial Adenoma

This neoplasm arises from either the cells of the mucous glands of the bronchi or the cells lining the excretory ducts of these glands. Both carcinoid and cylindromatous type adenomas are described. The carcinoid tumor accounts for the greatest number of bronchial adenomas and most commonly affects the right main bronchus. Bronchial adenomas are more common in males. Since the adenoma is intraluminal, recurrent or persistent chest infiltrates may be a manifestation. The diagnosis is made by bronchoscopy, and the treatment is surgical resection.

Malignant Pulmonary Tumors

Bronchogenic Carcinoma

Primary pulmonary neoplasms are very rare in children, but this diagnosis should be considered in young patients with solitary pulmonary masses. Every cell type except alveolar cell carcinoma, giant cell carcinoma, and carcinosarcoma has been reported in children. Lobectomy is required.

Metastatic Pulmonary Tumors

Primary sarcoma of the kidney (Wilms), primary malignant skeletal tumors (chondrosarcoma and osteogenic sarcoma), Ewing tumor, reticulum cell sarcoma, and soft tissue sarcomas (fibrosarcoma, rhabdomyosarcoma, liposarcoma, malignant neurilemoma, and synovioma) may metastasize to the lung.

Aggressive treatment, which employs surgical resection, radiation, and chemotherapy, of unilateral or bilateral pulmonary metastases is now advocated, regardless of the interval between diagnosis of the primary sarcoma and recognition of the pulmonary metastases. Repeated thoracotomies for removal of recurrent lesions are acceptable.

PULMONARY CYSTS

Congenital Cysts

Pulmonary Bronchogenic Cysts

Bronchogenic cysts arise when there is an anomalous lung budding later in the course of bronchial branching. They are more common in the lower lobes. A chest x-ray obtained before infection demonstrates an oval, thin-walled, air-filled cyst occupying a portion of one pulmonary lobe. Communications with the bronchial tree allow for bacterial contamination. Thus, persistent or recurrent infection is a common presentation for a bronchogenic cyst. In addition, the cyst airway connection may lead to air trapping, which compresses the ipsilateral lung, depresses the diaphragm, shifts the mediastinum to the contralateral side and affects pulmonary function in that lung. Thoracotomy with lobectomy is the recommended treatment.

Cystic Adenomatoid Malformation (CAM)

This malformation results from an abnormality of alveolar development that leads to an overgrowth of terminal bronchiolar structures. Histopathologically, they consist of cystic lesions of different sizes, lined by ciliated columnar epithelium without cartilage.

Three distinct types of congenital adenomatoid malformation are described:

- *Type I*, comprising 70% of CAMs, has the best survival rate. It is characterized by multiple large cysts or by a predominant large cyst with smaller cysts that mimic infantile lobar emphysema. The cysts are usually 3 to 5 cm in size.
- *Type II*, occurring in 20% of patients with CAMs, has a poor survival rate because of the high frequency of other congenital anomalies, such as renal agenesis or dysgenesis, cardiac defects, and intestinal atresia. The cysts range in size from 0.5 to 1.2 cm.
- *Type III* is the rarest and has a 50% survival rate. Type III is composed of multiple small (0.5 cm) cysts, and this type is almost exclusively seen in males. The vast majority of CAMs are diagnosed prenatally or during the newborn period. Prematurity, anasarca, and polyhydramnios are frequently associated findings.

The chest x-ray will demonstrate a cystic appearance of one or more lobes. The differential diagnosis includes diaphragmatic hernia, bronchogenic cysts, and pulmonary lymphangiectasia. CT, ultrasonography, or gastrointestinal studies can be used to establish the preoperative diagnosis. Early surgical excision is the treatment of choice, and lobectomy is curative.

PULMONARY SEQUESTRATION

Pulmonary sequestration is a localized mass of nonfunctioning tissue that is classified as either extralobar or intralobar.

Extralobar sequestration, as its name implies, is separated from the normal lung, and it is encompassed by its own pleura. There is no communication with the bronchial tree. Its blood supply is systemic in origin, and its venous drainage is predominantly to the systemic circulation. It is more common on the left side. The association of extralobar sequestration with gastrointestinal anomalies, heart defects, and diaphragmatic hernia is a helpful aid to diagnosis. The chest x-ray shows a mass of uniform density.

Intralobar sequestrations are contained within normal lung tissue and are encased by the same pleura. There may be communication with the bronchial tree. The blood supply is often provided by one or more arteries arising from the aorta or its branches. Venous drainage is into the pulmonary venous system. Intralobar sequestrations seem to be more common on the right side, and they are rarely associated with congenital defects. They have never been reported in the newborn period. Some have hypothesized that the intralobar sequestration is an acquired lesion secondary to chronic infection. The chest x-ray may reveal cystic lesions in the lower lobes.

Aortography remains the preferred method of confirming the diagnosis of sequestration, since it identifies both the arterial supply and the venous drainage. Surgical excision is the treatment of choice.

PULMONARY ARTERIOVENOUS MALFORMATION

Small, direct arteriovenous communications exist in the normal lung. However, the presence of large or multiple interconnections can lead to cyanosis, digital clubbing, and polycythemia in the absence of right-to-left intracardiac shunting. This malformation occurs as part of the syndrome of hereditary hemorrhagic telangiectasia.

In newborn infants, this malformation is one cause of cyanosis and congestive heart failure. The lack of an increase in PaO_2 while breathing 100% oxygen will help identify the presence of a fixed right-to-left shunt. Chest radiographs demonstrate cardiac enlargement and tortuosity of pulmonary vessels. A contrast CT can confirm the presence of a blood density structure in the thorax. Radionuclide angiocardiography and contrast echocardiography may reveal the presence of a right-to-left shunt, but these are not specific. Pulmonary angiography remains the definitive diagnostic study. The therapeutics modalities available include ligation of feeding vessels, excision of the lesion and surrounding segment, lobe, or lung, and embolization.

ACQUIRED CYSTS

Acquired cysts of the lung (pneumatoceles) are lesions that usually follow pulmonary infections with *Staphylococcus aureus* and *Klebsiella pneumoniae*. Acquired cysts can also follow blunt trauma. Occasionally, penetrating injuries of the lung result in a hematoma, which leaves a pneumatocele that will eventually disappear. Rarely, an acquired cyst may rupture into the pleural space, giving rise to a pneumothorax and the necessity for chest tube insertion.

PRIMARY CARDIAC AND PERICARDIAL TUMORS

Myxoma is by far the most common primary tumor of the heart. It may be encountered at almost any age. Most myxomas are located in the atria (left > right) and arise from the septa. Surgical removal is indicated.

Rhabdomyoma appears to be the only cardiac tumor showing a definite predilection for the younger age groups. This is particularly true of children with tuberous sclerosis. Rhabdomyoma may regress spontaneously without causing significant cardiac dysfunction.

Primary sarcoma of the heart is less common than myxoma. It tends to infiltrate the wall of the myocardium and extends into the pericardial cavity but does not proliferate into the lumina of the heart.

Primary tumors of the pericardium are rare. The predominant tumors are mesotheliomas and sarcomas. The treatment of choice is removal by thoracotomy.

REFERENCES

1. Brecher ML: Pediatric mediastinal masses: Your role in management. J Respir Dis 7(11):73–87, 1986.
2. Pizzo PA, et al: Principles and Practice of Pediatric Oncology, 2nd ed. Philadelphia, JB Lippincott, 1993.
3. Turcios NL, et al: When a neonate has a cystic lung disease. J Respir Dis 8(8):85–96, 1987.

PULMONARY THROMBOEMBOLISM

DAVID S. SMITH, M.D.

In contrast to adults, nearly all children with deep venous thrombosis (DVT) and pulmonary embolism have a recognizable and often treatable underlying disorder. Predisposing conditions to thrombotic complications have changed in recent years. Nearly one quarter are associated with the use of central venous catheters in children receiving total parenteral feedings or intravenous medications. Thrombotic events may complicate renal and hepatic transplantation. There is increasing recognition of congenital, as well as autoimmune, deficiencies of vitamin K–dependent plasma proteins that inhibit coagulation, such as protein C, protein S, and heparin cofactor II. Use

of granulocyte-macrophage colony-stimulating factor has been associated with venous thrombosis and pulmonary embolism. In adolescents, causes of venous thrombosis include trauma, drug abuse, use of oral contraceptives, and recent abortion. Infants and small children receiving long-term parenteral nutrition and children requiring hemodialysis may be at increased risk of developing DVT because of the need for indwelling catheters. Fatal pulmonary embolism has been less frequent following venous thrombosis in the upper versus the lower extremities.

Pulmonary embolism is accompanied by dyspnea, tachypnea, cyanosis, chest pain, and tachycardia. Clinical evidence of deep venous obstruction is more often found in children than in adults. Angiography has been more reliable than Doppler ultrasonography in confirming the diagnosis of DVT. A ventilation-perfusion scan should be performed to confirm a suspected embolism.

PROPHYLACTIC THERAPY FOR DEEP VENOUS THROMBOSIS

In contrast to adults, there are no data supporting the use of prophylactic anticoagulant therapy in children undergoing surgical procedures. Most children with central venous catheters, however, receive prophylactic catheter flushes with heparin-containing solutions once or twice daily. Although low-dose warfarin therapy is of proven value in adults as prophylaxis, no data exist to recommend this therapy in children.

TREATMENT OF DEEP VENOUS THROMBOSIS AND PULMONARY EMBOLISM

There are few data on the use of thrombolytic and anticoagulant drugs in children despite apparent differences in pharmacokinetics between adults and children. Recommendations for treatment of deep venous thrombosis and pulmonary embolism in children are based on data derived from adults. The physician should assume that DVT in children poses as great a risk to the child as to the adult.

Heparin therapy should be initiated in a dose of 75 U/kg over 10 minutes, followed by infusion of 22 U/kg/h. Heparin activity should be monitored 4 to 6 hours after the initial dose by determination of an activated partial thromboplastin time (APTT) or a heparin level. Five to seven days of heparin therapy usually is adequate, except in cases of extensive thrombosis or pulmonary embolism. Therapy with warfarin can be initiated within 48 hours of starting heparin, with a single daily dose of 0.2 mg/kg (maximum of 10 mg). Dosage should be modified after 48 hours depending on the international normalized ratio (therapeutic range of 2 to 3). Therapy with warfarin should be continued for 3 months unless the DVT is recurrent. Infants receiving formulas fortified with vitamin K may be difficult to manage. Thrombolytic therapy is controversial. Streptokinase should not be used for catheter obstruction because of the frequency of allergic reactions.

Systemic thrombolytic therapy may be useful for treatment of massive pulmonary embolism not responding to heparin therapy. Urokinase is administered in a loading dose of 4400 U/kg and then infused in the same dose hourly for 6 to 12 hours. The patient receiving urokinase should be monitored closely by measurements of fibrinogen, thrombin clotting time, prothrombin time, APTT, and fibrinogen degradation products. Tissue plasminogen activator may be substituted at a dosage of 0.1 mg/kg/h for 6 hours. Patients receiving tissue plasminogen activator should be monitored in a similar fashion. Heparin therapy should be initiated when maintenance thrombolytic therapy is completed.

General supportive treatment for the patient with pulmonary thromboembolism should include oxygen to maintain arterial hemoglobin saturation above 90%, the use of inotropic agents in patients with hypotension, and the judicious use of analgesics for pain. Attention should be paid to the underlying disease process. Emergency surgical procedures, such as pulmonary artery embolectomy and interruption of the inferior vena cava, should be considered in desperately ill patients whose embolus occurred less than 72 hours previously.

IDIOPATHIC PULMONARY HEMOSIDEROSIS

†DENISE J. STRIEDER, M.D.
EDUARDO M. BUDGE, M.D.

Idiopathic pulmonary hemosiderosis (IPH) is a rare disease with a variable course and an uncertain pathogenesis.[4] It follows, therefore, that there is no specific therapy and that no empirical therapy has been proven efficacious in a controlled clinical trial.

Patients who have mild disease or who have benefited from an early diagnosis mostly need iron supplements and close follow-up. Exacerbations are treated symptomatically. The established practice of prescribing corticosteroids for both acute and maintenance therapies is based on a reasoning by analogy: a number of other diseases causing pulmonary hemorrhage are known to be mediated by autoimmune processes and to respond to corticosteroid therapy. The prescription of a second immunosuppressive drug, such as cyclophosphamide or azathioprine, represents an extension of the same reasoning. Both practices are supported by a good number of case reports describing successful outcomes.

MILD OR SUBACUTE PRESENTATION

Infants and toddlers usually are started on a milk-free diet because of the known association of pulmonary hemosiderosis with cow's milk allergy (Heiner's syndrome). Milk-free diets are tried even when the patients have no demonstrable antibodies to milk proteins. When such a diet is effective, it works rapidly. The cough and low-grade fever disappear in a few days. On chest roentgenogram, alveolar infiltrates resolve in 1 or 2 weeks, but diffuse reticulations may persist. Such resolution of pulmonary hemorrhage can be attributed to the avoidance diet only if a cow's milk challenge triggers a recurrence. Such challenge is not necessarily in the interest of the child and often is omitted because the severity of the response to the challenge cannot be predicted. The milk-free diet is continued as long as a continuing remission supports the impression of efficacy. Milk is reintroduced cautiously 2 or 3 years later.

Symptomatic children, including the young ones in whom the avoidance diet fails, usually are started on oral prednisone 1 mg/kg/d. Once a remission has been induced, the dose is tapered toward an every other day regimen, as allowed by the clinical course. For all patients, an iron supplement is given as needed. Careful follow-up should include frequent physical examinations, hematocrit determinations, and chest roentgenograms, looking for evidence of disease activity. A urinalysis should be included routinely, as progression to one of the pulmonary-renal syndromes is a constant concern. Follow-up examinations should occur monthly at first, then progressively less often. Hematocrit determinations should be obtained monthly for at least 1 year.

Mild or moderate exacerbations are treated with reinstitution of prednisone therapy, followed by careful dose tapering and resumption of the recommended follow-up schedule. In a single case report, one such exacerbation was managed with administration of intravenous immunoglobulin (IVIg) 400 mg/kg/d for 5 days. Tachypnea, tachycardia, and hypoxemia resolved 48 hours after the start of therapy. For maintenance, the same dose of IVIg was given every 2 weeks for 3 months. Remission was sustained during a 1-year follow-up. We mention this report only because it suggests a low-risk and low-cost alternative in the event that immunosuppression is contraindicated, poorly tolerated, or opposed by the child's parents.

LIFE-THREATENING HEMORRHAGE

Acute alveolar hemorrhage causes cough with or without hemoptysis, respiratory distress, and hypoxemia and has the potential to progress to respiratory failure and shock. Because this progression can be very rapid, affected patients should be managed in a pediatric intensive care unit generally at a tertiary care medical center. Symptomatic management begins with oxygen supplementation and infusion of packed red blood cells to correct the anemia. Only if the patient is in shock should fresh frozen plasma be added. Careful monitoring aimed at avoiding fluid overload and elevation of pulmonary venous pressure is as important as restoring effective circulation. Placement of a Swan-Ganz catheter is helpful in this respect. Separate access sites for drug administration and provision of maintenance fluids should be secured. Initial therapy generally consists of corticosteroids, given as methylprednisolone pulses 1 mg/kg q6h or q8h. The concurrent administration of cyclophosphamide 1 mg/kg q6h should be considered as well because it may be of value in the treatment of catastrophic hemorrhage occurring in the course of IPH[2] and it is difficult to rule out the possibility of another disease with similar manifestations, such as Goodpasture's syndrome,[1] systemic lupus erythematosus,[3] or Wegener's granulomatosis. These and other aggressive vasculitides can have an initial phase consistent with IPH. Full clinical expression of the systemic disease may be delayed for months or years.

In the event of progressive respiratory distress, the need for endotracheal intubation and positive pressure ventilation is indicated more often by worsening hypoxemia than by CO_2 retention. Changes in blood pressure should be interpreted and managed with due concern for the risk of corticosteroid-induced hypertension. Once corticosteroids are started, an H_2-receptor blocker and an antacid should be started as well.

Case reports suggest that with symptomatic management plus corticosteroids (with or without cyclophosphamide), many patients will stabilize in 24 to 48 hours and successfully extubate within a few days. The incidence of such success versus that of failure is not known. There is a consensus, however, that the dose of corticosteroids should be reduced after 3 days. For patients who still exhibit recurrent bleeding at that time, the addition of either azathioprine 2 to 4 mg/kg/d or cyclophosphamide may be indicated. In a case report, plasmapheresis was credited with remission of acute hemorrhage. Eventually, one can reduce the corticosteroid dose without incurring a clinical setback. When the dose has been reduced to 1 mg/kg/d, it should be administered as a single morning dose, in preparation for maintenance therapy.

MAINTENANCE THERAPY

Various maintenance regimens have been tried with the aim of preventing bleeding recurrences and progressive lung fibrosis. There is a majority opinion that oral prednisone should be instituted and continued at decreasing daily morning doses for 3 to 12 months. At our institution, we prefer to administer prednisone for 12 months. The dose is reduced relatively quickly during the first 3 months and then more cautiously for the rest of the year, during which time an every other day regimen is employed. The patients should be followed very closely to ensure early detection of recurrent bleeding. Pulmonary function tests may be helpful in that regard. Bronchoalveolar lavage (BAL) also has been used for monitoring patients, as intact erythrocytes, neutrophils, and eosinophils in BAL fluid are markers of disease activity, whereas the number of hemosiderin laden macrophages is not. Assessment of diffusing capacity for carbon monoxide is of no value for therapeutic decision making.

If the prednisone dose cannot be decreased below 1 mg/kg/d without triggering an exacerbation, the addition of a cytotoxic drug should be considered. A regimen of alternate-day oral prednisone and azathioprine[5] is likely to limit or even avoid the side effects of either drug and can be well tolerated for years.

Once a patient has been weaned from immunosuppressive drugs, ongoing follow-up is mandatory. One should look not only for recurrent bleeding in the lung but also for evidence of renal disease, signs of vasculitic involvement at other sites, and when indicated, biologic markers of systemic disease (antinuclear antibodies, anti-

†Dr Strieder died October 17, 1994.

basement membrane antibodies, antineutrophil cytoplasmic antibodies). It is not known how long such surveillance should be continued. We consider 2 or 3 years to be a minimum amount of time.

Alternate maintenance regimens make use of inhaled corticosteroids and/or cromolyn. The latter is worthy of consideration when numerous mast cells are evident in a lung biopsy. Splenectomy has been tried and found of no benefit. Desferoxamine does not succeed in mobilizing the iron stored by macrophages in the alveoli, the lung interstitium, and the pulmonary lymph nodes.

In the long term, many patients enjoy a durable remission off drugs. Others, over a period of years, will develop pulmonary fibrosis, progressive hypoxemia, and cor pulmonale. This unfavorable outcome is commonly cited in the literature, but the frequency of its occurrence is unknown. In such cases, the accepted management is symptomatic. We think that patients who have a significant restrictive defect of lung function after surviving IPH should have frequent (every 2 or 3 months at first) pulmonary function tests. Without evidence of disease activity, progressive restriction means progressive fibrosis, which may be checked by modest doses of oral prednisone, as corticosteroids have been shown to inhibit collagen deposition in the lungs.

REFERENCES

1. Case Records of the Massachusetts General Hospital: A 13-year-old girl with gross hematuria four years after a diagnosis of idiopathic pulmonary hemosiderosis. N Engl J Med 328:1183–1190, 1993.
2. Columbo JL, Stolz SM: Treatment of life-threatening primary pulmonary hemosiderosis with cyclophosphamide. Chest 102:959–960, 1992.
3. Kuhn C: Systemic lupus erythematosus in a patient with ultrastructural lesions of the pulmonary capillaries previously reported in the Review as due to idiopathic pulmonary hemosiderosis. Am Rev Respir Dis 106:931–932, 1972.
4. Levy J, Wilmott RW: Pulmonary hemosiderosis (clinical review). Pediatr Pulmonol 2:384–391, 1986.
5. Rossi GA, Balzano E, Battistini E, et al: Long-term prednisone and azathioprine treatment of a patient with idiopathic pulmonary hemosiderosis. Pediatr Pulmonol 13:176–180, 1992.

CYSTIC FIBROSIS

HARVEY R. COLTEN, M.D.

Cystic fibrosis (CF) is a relatively common (1/2500 live births in American whites, 1/17,000 in African Americans) genetic disorder in epithelial electrolyte and water transport. Cystic fibrosis is a multisystem disease, but the morbidity and mortality of cystic fibrosis are predominantly a consequence of chronic inflammation of airways, leading ultimately to respiratory failure in nearly all patients. Recent advances in diagnosis and therapy have markedly improved the life span (median survival late 20s) and quality of life for patients with CF. The rate of change in outlook for these patients has accelerated following discovery of the cystic fibrosis transmembrane conductance regulator *(CFTR)* gene and the subsequent studies that have elucidated the genetic, molecular, and cellular biology of cystic fibrosis.

More than 200 mutations have been identified in the *CFTR* gene. Among these, a deletion of phenylalanine at residue 508 (ΔF_{508}) accounts for some 70% of chromosomes in northern European populations. Approximately 80% of patients recorded in the U.S. Cystic Fibrosis Foundation registry carry the ΔF_{508} mutation on at least one chromosome (more than half of these are homozygous for ΔF_{508}). The presence of this mutation (and several others) prevents normal processing and delivery of the CFTR protein to the cell membrane. Genotyping has become an important tool for family studies/genetic counseling, reproductive decision-making, and to some extent for ascertaining prognosis. There is accumulating evidence that certain disease manifestations and the clinical course correlate with certain genotypes. For example, pancreatic insufficiency is correlated with ΔF_{508} and several other mutations, but some other mutations are found more frequently in patients with intact pancreatic exocrine function.

Hence, the assessment of patients with CF increasingly makes use of modern molecular biologic tools for evaluation of patients and their families. It should be noted, however, that factors other than genotype (e.g., bacterial colonization, airway reactivity) also influence the severity of disease.

The clinical diagnosis of CF still primarily depends on the recognition of typical signs and symptoms, together with elevated electrolyte concentrations in sweat. Measurements of sweat electrolytes should be performed in laboratories with good quality control and large sample numbers because technical difficulties otherwise substantially increase test errors. Two values for chloride that exceed 60 mEq/L with elevated Na (>70 mEq/L) in the context of signs and symptoms of cystic fibrosis suffice to establish the diagnosis. False negative tests (even in qualified laboratories) may be the result of severe hyponatremia, edema, or both. Based on genotyping, CF has been diagnosed in patients with borderline or even normal sweat electrolytes. Hence, if CF is strongly suspected on clinical grounds and the sweat test is normal, genotyping is indicated.

Signs and symptoms of CF can be recognized at birth (or before) in patients with meconium ileus or somewhat later in infancy or early childhood. In the latter groups, gastrointestinal/nutritional or respiratory symptoms often are manifestations of the disease. Nearly 80% of CF patients are diagnosed before the age of 2 years. Rarely, CF is diagnosed later in life, usually because of the presence of mucoid *Pseudomonas* infection associated with chronic respiratory disease or male infertility.

The diagnosis of CF should prompt referral to one of the many established Cystic Fibrosis Centers throughout the United States, where the initial assessment and management plan can be developed. The appropriate plan involves input from professionals, including many, if not all, of the following specialists: geneticists, genetic counselors, pulmonologists, gastroenterologists, surgeons, physiotherapists, social workers, specialized laboratory technicians (e.g., pulmonary function laboratory), and others. Input from these specialists must be synthesized and interpreted for the family so that the impact of the diagnosis can be assimilated and the long-term treatment can be understood. In general, the support and care given by the CF team should be coordinated with the primary care physician (pediatrician, family practitioner, or general practitioner).

GASTROINTESTINAL SYMPTOMS

The majority of the gastrointestinal features of CF can be treated successfully. The earliest gastrointestinal manifestation, meconium ileus, generally is recognized at birth or within the first 2 days of life, with signs and symptoms of obstruction and failure to pass meconium. On rare occasions, it is identified prenatally. Provided that intestinal perforation has not occurred, treatment is medical (e.g., hyperosmolar enemas). Whether medical or surgical therapy is indicated, both require the services of highly skilled, experienced pediatric specialists. Later in infancy, gastrointestinal signs and symptoms include steatorrhea, failure to thrive, protein-calorie malnutrition in spite of a usually large food intake, and fat-soluble vitamin deficiencies, specifically A, E, K, and rarely D.

Treatment of pancreatic insufficiency depends on administration of exogenous enteric-coated pancreatic enzymes. For infants, a portion of the granules from a capsule may be mixed with fruit or cereal and given before each feed. The dose is usually titrated according to stool frequency, consistency, absence of abdominal pain, flatus, and improved weight gain. Patients failing to respond to pancreatic enzyme replacement should undergo studies for the presence of other coexisting gastrointestinal disorders. Elemental formulas are used frequently, but these are not mandatory, and breast milk or cow's milk formula is acceptable and less expensive. Patients generally should receive 130% to 150% of the recommended daily allowance of calories, well balanced in protein, carbohydrate, and fat. Low-fat diets are *not* recommended. Vitamins A, D, and E should be administered daily, and vitamin K (5 mg) should be given once weekly. Judicious salt supplementation is sometimes required in infants with CF, especially in hot weather, or hyponatremic dehydration may supervene.

Among CF patients, significant gastrointestinal complications are recognized with varying frequency.

- **Rectal prolapse** is observed in more than 10% of patients, especially early in life and in patients with poorly controlled steatorrhea. Manual reduction is usually successful and can be effected by the parent after adequate education. Surgical intervention is almost never required.
- **Recurrent severe intestinal obstruction,** noted in older children and young adults, is now referred to as DIOS (distal intestinal obstruction syndrome). This syndrome is a consequence of thick intestinal secretions and poorly digested intestinal contents. Vomiting, abdominal pain and distention, and a palpable stool mass are observed frequently in the acute disorder. This complication requires nasogastric decompression, acetylcysteine (Mucomyst) orally and rectally, or hyperosmotic enemas to relieve the obstruction. Intussusception should be ruled out. Chronic management depends on adjustment of exogenous pancreatic enzymes (usually an increase is needed, but sometimes just better compliance with the recommended dosage is effective). Stool softeners may be useful as adjunctive therapy.
- **Gastroesophageal reflux and esophagitis** are common in CF patients, especially in those with advanced obstructive pulmonary disease. Treatment of this problem is not specific for CF (see Chapter 6).
- **Pancreatitis** is a frequent finding, especially in CF patients with retention of exocrine pancreatic function. Treatment of this condition is not specific for CF and is described elsewhere (see Chapter 6).
- **Diabetes mellitus** is tenfold more common in CF patients than in the general population at the same age. Onset is usually gradual because of the progressive destruction of islets. The high incidence of diabetes prompts many clinicians to periodically screen for incipient glucose intolerance by measuring glycosylated hemoglobin. Diabetes should be considered in a CF patient who loses weight or whose growth rate slows in the absence of a change in food intake, stool pattern, or a pulmonary exacerbation. Ketoacidosis is extremely rare even in the presence of high blood glucose levels. The increasing life span of CF patients warrants treatment with insulin with an aim to achieve stringent control of blood sugar, thereby diminishing diabetic complications.
- **Severe biliary cirrhosis** is uncommon, but histologic evidence of asymptomatic biliary obstruction has been noted in infants and children. Serologic monitoring for evidence of hepatobiliary disease (e.g., liver enzymes, bilirubin) should be undertaken at the initial evaluation and at least annually because about one third of patients with CF liver disease will be without overt symptoms. No specific therapy is available for the primary liver disease, but such complications as portal hypertension, liver failure (2% to 5% of CF patients), and cholelithiasis are managed as they are in non-CF patients. The ethical issues regarding liver transplantation in patients with end-stage CF liver disease are more complex than for many other causes of liver failure because many patients have coexisting lung disease.

PULMONARY SYMPTOMS

The pulmonary disease associated with CF initially consists of inflammation in small airways and recurrent bacterial infection and/or colonization. Among the bacteria most commonly isolated are a mucoid form of *Pseudomonas aeruginosa* (90% of all CF patients), *Staphylococcus aureus,* and *Haemophilus influenzae.* A minority of patients have been infected with *Pseudomonas cepacia,* an organism believed to be associated with a poor prognosis. With time, progressively larger airways are involved, and parenchymal tissue is affected intermittently. Respiratory symptoms, appearing in infancy or later, usually consist of cough, tachypnea, and wheezing. Progressive ob-

structive pulmonary disease usually supervenes, but the rate at which this occurs is highly variable. Secondary effects of the chronic pulmonary disease include pulmonary hypertension, cor pulmonale, congestive heart failure, hemoptysis, and pneumothorax. In general, the management of these complications is not specific to CF.

Several different approaches to the management of CF pulmonary disease have emerged, but few have been subjected to rigorous study. The objective of maintenance therapy is to slow progression of the respiratory disease. This is accomplished by promoting more effective clearance of secretions from airways and limiting the amount of secondary tissue injury. Chest physiotherapy is an important modality in achieving this objective. Several different methods are employed, including postural drainage, forced expiratory maneuvers, and manual or mechanical percussion techniques. Families should be instructed in the use of one of these methods. Chest physiotherapy is most critical during exacerbations of pulmonary disease because normal exercise regimens and activities are decreased at the same time that sputum amount and viscosity are increased. Most clinicians recommend chest physiotherapy about once daily, with increased frequency during exacerbations. This approach helps in promoting good compliance with the prescribed regimen. In conjunction with a regular exercise program, this modality usually is successful in promoting reasonable airway toilet. In patients with reactive airway disease, bronchodilators may be of substantial aid, and some prescribe these agents even in the absence of solid functional data to support their use. Inhaled beta$_2$-adrenergic or anticholinergic agents are most often employed. The use of theophylline for chronic management of reversible airway obstruction has some proponents, but many reserve this drug for more acute therapy. In addition to bronchodilation, theophylline effects improvement in respiratory muscle function, but exacerbation of gastroesophageal reflux by theophylline can be a substantial limiting side effect. Cromolyn sodium and inhaled corticosteroids also are used for maintenance therapy, as in the management of asthma.

Antibiotic therapy plays an important role in the management of CF lung disease. The efficacy of maintenance therapy with oral antibiotics (trimethoprim-sulfamethoxazole and cephalosporins or semisynthetic penicillins) to control *H. influenzae* and *S. aureus* infections has not been proven, but some clinicians employ this approach. The chronic administration of aerosolized aminoglycosides (usually in b.i.d. dose schedules) has been shown to be effective, but the long-term effect of this approach has not been determined. Acute management of pulmonary exacerbations with intravenous antibiotics (usually a cephalosporin or semisynthetic penicillin plus an aminoglycoside), coupled with more aggressive chest physiotherapy for 2 to 3 weeks, usually is successful in decreasing signs and symptoms, as well as objectively improving pulmonary function. Such therapy may be given in hospital or at home, depending on the age of the child, the family circumstances, and the severity of the exacerbation. Newer oral agents effective against *Pseudomonas* (e.g., ciprofloxacin) are being used in older children and adults with CF pulmonary exacerbations. This therapy may forestall the need for intravenous antibiotic treatment.

Most clinicians obtain sputum culture and sensitivity data to guide antibiotic therapy. Systematic studies suggest that these data are unreliable. Hence, the clinical course may prompt changes in therapy that are not substantiated by the culture and antibiotic sensitivity testing. Nevertheless, the initial choice of antibiotic therapy often is based on these sputum culture data.

Recently, controlled clinical studies of two new therapeutic approaches for increased clearance of airway secretions suggest the potential for an improvement in maintenance therapy. The first of these, recombinant generated human DNAse (Dornase alpha), is administered by aerosol to decrease sputum viscosity and thereby promote clearance of CF secretions. The rationale for this therapy is based on observations that the high sputum viscosity in CF is caused in large part by its content of DNA (mostly derived from inflammatory cell debris). Dornase alpha delivered by aerosol about twice daily is effective, but the cost of therapy may be a limiting factor in its widespread use.

The second major approach now under study is designed to lower sputum viscosity by increasing hydration of the secretions. Amiloride, a diuretic that affects sodium transport, has been administered by inhalation in controlled trials and appears to be effective. Studies of this agent and others that control chloride transport are under active investigation. These will likely be available for clinical use in the near future.

Lung transplantation offers promise to some patients with respiratory failure. Only a few centers worldwide have sufficient experience with this procedure, and even fewer have experience with bilateral lung transplantation in young children. Nevertheless, the results in these major centers are encouraging, although the long-term benefits cannot yet be ascertained. Careful case selection based on physiologic, psychologic, ethical, and social parameters must be done to make optimal use of the scarce supply of organs from suitable donor lungs. Recently, the use of living related donors (lobectomy in parent used for transplantation) has been advocated so as to bypass the limited organ supply problem. This procedure generates additional medical and ethical problems, and consensus regarding its use has not been achieved.

Gene therapy provides the promise of a definitive cure of CF lung disease. Early experimental data suggest that this will be clinically useful, but many problems remain. Progress has been rapid, however, and it is likely that these problems will be resolved.

Pulmonary complications of CF that deserve special mention include the following:

- **Hemoptysis:** Blood-streaked sputum is observed frequently in patients with advanced pulmonary disease. This finding rarely requires specific therapy, provided it is not a reflection of a platelet or clotting disorder. An acute episode of hemoptysis is a relatively rare but potentially life-threatening condition. It is treated most effectively by selective bronchial artery embolization. Massive hemoptysis or recurrent hemoptysis (100 ml over several days) is usually controlled by this method. Complications of this therapy are rare but are major (e.g., transverse myelitis, small bowel necrosis), so that skilled interventional radiologists or cardiologists should perform the procedure.
- **Pneumothorax:** The severity of pulmonary disease in patients with pneumothorax may limit therapy to the most conservative procedures (needle aspiration, observation, or chest tube thoracostomy). However, with these approaches, the recurrence rate has been reported to be 50% to 80%. The recurrence rate of pneumothorax can be reduced to approximately 10% by intrapleural instillation of the sclerosing agent quinacrine. An even greater reduction in recurrence rate may result from surgical therapy. Pulmonary function after either sclerosing therapy or pleurectomy is generally similar to that before the pneumothorax, but at some later date lung transplantation (if indicated) may be technically more challenging.
- **Allergic bronchopulmonary aspergillosis (ABPA)** has been reported in about 10% to 15% of CF patients. The diagnosis of ABPA is difficult in the CF population because of overlapping clinical and laboratory findings between the two disorders. The additive pathophysiologic effects from these diseases make it essential to establish the diagnosis and treat ABPA as soon as possible. Treatment of ABPA with daily systemic corticosteroids (prednisone) is effective. Return of the serum IgE to baseline offers the best guide to effective therapy because other clinical signs and symptoms of CF lung disease and ABPA are so similar.
- **Chronic respiratory failure** with hypoxemia, hypercapnia, and cardiovascular complications is a common problem in the later stages of the disease. Night oxygen therapy when the Pao_2 decreases below 60 mm Hg may slow progression of the cardiac disease. Continuous O_2 supplementation, diuretics, and occasionally digitalis are employed in the later stages of cardiopulmonary decompensation.

OTHER SYMPTOMS

- **Sinusitis/nasal polyposis:** Chronic sinusitis is extremely common in CF patients but is infrequently a cause of significant discomfort. When symptoms are persistent and severe, surgical therapy may be indicated. Medical therapy with antibiotics, decongestants, nasal cromolyn, or corticosteroids is of uncertain benefit but is often employed. Nasal polyps are noted in about 15% of patients. In teenage patients, the nasal polyposis, aspirin sensitivity, and asthma triad must be ruled out. Surgical removal of polyps provides temporary relief. Recurrence is frequent. Nevertheless, surgery is indicated if the polyps are unsightly, disfigure the nasal bridge, or contribute to acute sinusitis.
- **Cutaneous venulitis:** In CF patients, cutaneous venulitis is a painful, purpuric, episodic lesion localized to dependent areas of the body and often found during pulmonary exacerbations. Immune complex deposition has been noted in postcapillary venules in association with cutaneous venulitis. In addition to immune complex deposition, a diffuse, generalized inflammatory cell infiltrate is found on histologic examination. This condition responds to corticosteroid therapy (prednisone 1 mg/kg/d in AM). Maintenance therapy (prednisone q.o.d. in the AM) usually is required to prevent exacerbations.
- **Male infertility:** Nearly all males with CF are azospermic because of obstruction/involution of wolffian duct structures. There is no therapy for this condition, but teenage boys should be counseled and reassured that sexual maturation and potency usually are normal (depending on nutritional and pulmonary status).

SARCOIDOSIS

RICHARD M. KRAVITZ, M.D.

Sarcoidosis is a granulomatous disease of unknown etiology. It is characterized by the presence of noncaseating granulomas that can appear in any tissue in the body. The lungs are the most common organ involved, although other systems are frequently affected, including the lymphatics, skin, eyes, kidney, liver, spleen, heart, nervous system, and bone. Sarcoidosis is usually thought of as an adult-onset illness, with most cases occurring between 20 and 50 years of age. Children, however, can be affected, most commonly between the ages of 8 and 15 years. Sarcoidosis is rare in young children, though isolated cases in children under 4 years of age have been reported. These youngest children usually do not have pulmonary disease but instead have skin rashes, ocular findings, and joint involvement. In the United States, this illness is endemic to the southeastern and southcentral regions of the country and affects African Americans more than whites. There is no sexual predominance.

The cause of sarcoidosis is unknown, but it is believed to be the immunologic response to an exogenous agent that enters the body through the lungs. Initially, an intense alveolitis is seen. Macrophages release interleukin 1 (IL-1), which causes a cascade of events notable for lymphocyte migration (especially T4 helper cells) to the affected site, T cell activation, and IL-2 production. These cells and lymphokines initiate monocyte migration to the area of inflammation and subsequent macrophage activation. Ultimately, this leads to giant cell formation and the appearance of the noncaseating granulomas that define the disease. In addition, the T4 cells stimulate B cells, which produce IgG, IgA, and IgM. Increased levels of these immunoglobulins are found both in lung tissue and the peripheral circulation. This immune reaction is partially downregulated by the production of 1,25-dihydroxyvitamin D_3 by activated macrophages, which inhibits IL-2 and immunoglobulin production. The production of this mediator leads to the hypercalcemia (and occasional hypercalciuria) seen in sarcoidosis.

The lungs are the most common organ system affected, with pulmonary disease present in 90% of patients. Frequently, the child has no respiratory symptoms. In the adult population, up to 45% of cases are discovered on a chest film obtained for another indication. Pulmonary symptoms vary but usually include a dry cough, dyspnea, and chest pain. Radiographic findings are divided into four stages: stage 0 is a normal film, stage I shows bilateral hilar adenopathy with right-sided paratracheal nodes, stage II shows hilar adenopathy with parenchymal disease, and stage III shows parenchymal changes alone, with frequent evidence of fibrosis and bullae formation. Pulmonary function testing reveals a restrictive pattern, with a decrease in the forced vital capacity (FVC), diffusing capacity, and lung compliance. Serial pulmonary function studies and chest x-rays can be useful parameters in following the progression of the pulmonary aspects of this disease.

Other manifestations of sarcoidosis depend on the organ system involved. Infiltrates in the peripheral lymphatics can lead to the appearance of painless, freely movable, rubbery lymph nodes. Any chain can be involved, but sarcoidosis is one of the few illnesses that can cause epitrochlear adenopathy. Ocular disease can affect the anterior chamber (i.e., iritis, uveitis, conjunctival granulomas), the posterior chamber (i.e., optic nerve granulomas), or rarely, the orbit. Untreated eye disease can lead to cataract formation, glaucoma, and blindness, so a thorough eye examination, including slit-lamp examination, is always needed. If ocular findings are present, serial ophthalmologic examinations will be required. Skin involvement can vary from non-specific findings, such as erythema nodosum (commonly seen in adults but less frequent in children) to more specific lesions, such as papules, plaques, and subcutaneous nodules. Granulomatous infiltrates in the spleen can lead to an enlarged spleen and occasionally hypersplenism. Involvement of the liver is clinically asymptomatic, but an elevation in alkaline phosphatase and the transaminases can be seen. Renal involvement is usually secondary to the hypercalcemia described earlier and the resultant hypercalciuria. Neurologic involvement can include central and peripheral neuropathies, with a temporary seventh nerve palsy being the most common finding. The central nervous system can also be affected, with space-occupying masses, hydrocephalus, seizures, and occasionally, aseptic meningitis. Bone infiltration leads to the characteristic lytic lesions affecting the metacarpals, metatarsals, and distal phalanges. These lesions are asymptomatic and usually are found only on radiographs. Sarcoidosis can affect the myocardium, producing a cardiomyopathy that diminishes cardiac function. If the conduction system is involved, arrhythmias may occur. Many times, the child will have only nonspecific constitutional symptoms, such as a low-grade fever, weight loss, and malaise.

The diagnosis of sarcoidosis is based on clinical evidence of disease, along with the presence of noncaseating granulomas in biopsy samples of affected organs. In the absence of a biopsy, useful adjuvant testing includes a white blood cell count (demonstrating leukocytosis and eosinophilia), an erythrocyte sedimentation rate, serum immunoglobulin levels (demonstrating hypergammaglobulinemia), serum and urine calcium determinations (demonstrating hypercalcemia with or without hypercalciuria), and an angioensin-converting enzyme (ACE) level (demonstrating an increase). Skin testing reveals a depression in the delayed-type hypersensitivity reaction. Chest x-ray findings and pulmonary function testing have been described previously. Although not performed routinely, bronchial alveolar lavage fluid will show a lymphocytic predominance. Gallium-67 scanning demonstrates an increased uptake in the affected organs. Because of its expense, nonspecificity, and large radiation dosage, however, gallium scanning is not recommended unless the diagnosis is difficult to make.

Because the etiology is unknown, treatment is controversial. Many patients (up to 60% to 70% of cases) will have a spontaneous resolution of their disease. If treatment is necessary, the medication of choice is an adrenocorticosteroid, such as prednisone or prednisolone (Table 1). These drugs have been found to be highly effective in reversing the progression of the disease. Indications for initiating systemic steroid therapy include symptomatic stage II or stage III pulmonary disease, any pulmonary disease (stage I, II, III) that is progressive,

TABLE 1. Drugs for Treating Sarcoidosis

DRUG	DOSAGE	COMMENTS
Prednisone	1 mg/kg/d until symptoms improve (usually several weeks)	Wean over several months to low daily or every other day dosage (total therapy should last at least 6 months)
Chloroquine	250 mg PO b.i.d. for 2 weeks 250 mg PO daily for long-term suppression	*Note:* Keep maintenance dosage <3.5–4.0 mg/kg (ideal body weight) per day to avoid retinopathy side effects

ocular findings unresponsive to local steroids, disfiguring skin lesions, deterioration of renal function secondary to hypercalcemia, constitutional symptoms, massive splenomegaly with hypersplenism, the onset of liver failure, cardiac involvement of any type, and central neurologic involvement, especially if there is a space-occupying lesion or new onset seizure disorder.

There is no set treatment protocol, and duration of therapy should be individualized to the patient's specific symptoms. Prednisone is usually started at a dose of 1 mg/kg/d for several weeks until the symptoms come under control. At that time, the dosage should be slowly weaned to a low daily or every other day schedule. Therapy should be continued for at least 6 months or for however long it takes to control the patient's symptoms. Parameters that can be followed to assess the effectiveness of steroid therapy include serial chest x-rays, pulmonary function testing, and measurement of ACE levels. Although these parameters do not reflect the patient's prognosis, they can indicate the response to treatment.

Frequently, the patient may have a flareup of the disease during the tapering of the steroid or at some time after the steroid has been discontinued. This commonly resolves without increasing the dosage back to the initial 1 mg/kg/d level or restarting therapy. If, however, an increase in the dosage or reinstitution of therapy is required, one only needs to resume the steroid at the most recent effective dosage. Once symptoms are again under control, tapering can be resumed, but at a slower pace.

Steroid drops or ointment (0.5% to 1% concentration) can be effective in the treatment of ocular lesions, and steroid ointments can be effective in the treatment of skin disease. Both are more effective, however, when combined with systemic steroids.

Other drugs are available as alternatives to steroids in the treatment of sarcoidosis, although there is little experience with these medications in the pediatric population. Chloroquine (and to a lesser extent, hydroxychloroquine) is useful for treating skin lesions. No pediatric dosage has been established, but a dose of 250 mg b.i.d. for 2 weeks, tapered to 250 mg/d for maintenance therapy has been found to be effective in treating adults. If the total daily maintenance dose is kept to <4 mg/kg/d, the risk for the well-described side effect of retinopathy is minimized. Methotrexate, cyclosporine, chlorambucil, and azathioprine have been tried in resistant cases of sarcoidosis, with variable results.

HYPOVENTILATION SYNDROMES

CARL E. HUNT, M.D.

Hypoventilation disorders in children can be classified as either congenital or acquired. The congenital disorders include central hypoventilation syndrome (CHS) and a milder form labeled alveolar hypoventilation (AH). By definition, CHS patients require mechanical ventilatory support (at least during sleep), whereas AH patients do not require any treatment other than a respiratory stimulant. CHS may be observed in association with central nervous system malformations (e.g., Moebius syndrome or Chiari II malformation) or metabolic disease (Leigh disease, pyruvate dehydrogenase deficiency, carnitine deficiency), or they may result from asphyxia, central nervous system infection, trauma, tumor, or infarction.

Under normal conditions, the rate and depth of breathing are controlled automatically to maintain appropriate levels of carbon dioxide (Pco_2) and oxygen (Po_2). Central (alveolar) hypoventilation occurs when the output from the brainstem centers is deficient. The deficit in respiratory control in AH is, by definition, mild and affects only the automatic control of breathing during sleep. Voluntary or awake control of breathing is spared. Patients labeled as CHS have a more significant degree of hypoventilation during sleep, but the range of severity encompasses milder forms in which ventilation is sufficient to avoid acute symptomatology (but insufficient to avoid progressive cor pulmonale) and more severe forms in which the extent of hypoventilation is incompatible with acute survival in the absence of ventilatory support. CHS subjects typically have normal respiratory rates associated with shallow breathing (hypopnea). In less severe cases, this occurs only during sleep, whereas in the most severe instances, it extends into wakefulness to a variable degree. The normal rates do not increase in response to the progressive asphyxia that develops because of the absence of automatic control of respiration and failure of response (recognition). Overt (central) apnea is uncommon in CHS, but the extent of hypopnea can be quite substantial, with measured tidal volumes less than physiologic dead space. The extent of hypopnea is state dependent and may be evident only during stages 3 and 4 of quiet sleep in the milder cases, during REM and quiet sleep in moderately severe cases, and during wakefulness as well as sleep in the most severely affected cases. Even in this last group, the respiratory control deficit will follow the usual progression of severity: maximal in quiet sleep, less severe in REM sleep, and still less severe during wakefulness. The respiratory control abnormalities characteristic of CHS thus include all of the following.

- Hypoventilation (hypopnea) during quiet sleep, all sleep, or all states depending on severity of the condition, leading to progressive hypercarbia and hypoxemia
- Absent or negligible ventilatory and arousal sensitivity to hypercarbia during sleep
- Absent or negligible hypercarbic ventilatory responsiveness while awake regardless of the adequacy of awake ventilation
- Variable deficiency in hypoxic ventilatory responsiveness in all states (absent in the most severe cases)
- Absent or negligible hypoxic arousal responsiveness during sleep
- General unresponsiveness to respiratory stimulants (especially during sleep)
- Absence of autoresuscitation or gasping (asleep) and inability to perceive asphyxia or to experience dyspnea

CLINICAL PRESENTATION

The age at presentation varies as a function of severity of the underlying respiratory control deficit and ranges from the newborn period to older childhood. Even when there is a congenital etiology for the CHS, the diagnosis occasionally is delayed until later infancy or childhood. Acquired disorders will occur following the imposed event, with the delay in symptoms depending on the severity of the resultant respiratory control impairment.

Most subjects with a hypoventilation syndrome initially have symptomatology suggesting a clinical diagnosis of primary cardiac disease, acute respiratory failure, or a primary neuromuscular disorder. In milder forms, patients may experience unexplained pulmonary edema or cor pulmonale, recurrent acute respiratory failure, or pneumonia.

Symptoms may occur in all states of arousal. However, they are typically most severe during sleep, especially quiet sleep. By clinical report, the invariable and most obvious symptom is color change (generally cyanosis but occasionally pallor). Acute neurologic symptoms also may be part of the presentation, including but not restricted to seizures, hypersomnolence, coma, or neurodevelopmental delay.

Infants with congenital CHS often have one or more associated conditions that may affect the age and nature of the clinical presentation. Hirschsprung's disease occurs in approximately 18% of patients. Some patients have prominent symptoms related to autonomic instability, manifested as vagal hyperresponsiveness and/or bradyarrhythmia. Congenital neuroblastoma, ganglioneuroblastoma, and benign ganglioneuroma all have been observed in association with CHS. CHS can be related to a more diffuse central neurologic deficit that also affects endocrine functions. Hypothalamic dysfunction and growth hormone deficiency have both been observed in affected children.

DIAGNOSIS

The diagnosis of CHS requires a high index of suspicion based on the medical history and generally can be suspected by examination of the patient during sleep. To confirm the diagnosis, it is necessary to exclude other disorders capable of causing hypoventilation, such as primary lung disease, airway obstruction, phrenic nerve paralysis, diaphragmatic abnormalities, focal brainstem pathology, neuropathy, and myopathy.

Although the clinical diagnosis may be substantially established by the pediatrician, referral to an experienced pediatric sleep laboratory is still necessary to quantify the severity of the condition and to implement an appropriate treatment plan. The adequacy of ventilation should be assessed during wakefulness, REM sleep, and quiet sleep and documented by appropriate electrophysiologic and behavioral criteria during polysomnography (PSG). Invasive blood gas sampling generally is not necessary or desirable. End-tidal Pco_2 and pulse oximetry are suitable modalities for assessment of ventilatory status and for determination of hypoxic and hypercapnic responsiveness. The PSG should also include measurements of tidal volume during all states of arousal. In combination with noninvasive blood gas sampling, the severity of the alveolar hypoventilation can thus be determined precisely.

To complement the PSG quantification of acute ventilatory status, it is generally necessary to determine the extent of chronic hypoventilation. Since a major complication of chronic asphyxia is cor pulmonale, a chest roentgenogram, ECG, and echocardiogram all need to be performed. The presence and extent of polycythemia should be assessed.

TREATMENT

Pharmacotherapy

Drug therapy is invariably effective only in milder degrees of alveolar hypoventilation. Methylxanthines, such as theophylline and caffeine (Table 1),[2] may normalize sleep ventilation in AH patients who have normal awake ventilation and modest sleep-related hypoventilation, especially when the abnormality is limited to quiet sleep. For the same degree of ventilatory stimulation, caffeine will yield fewer side effects. Progesterone is also a central respiratory stimulant, although the mechanism is not understood. It has been very effective in some AH patients and has the potential to improve central ventilatory drive without any adrenergic stimulation. Therefore, in girls of any age and in prepubertal boys, progesterone should be considered for the chronic treatment of the AH patient. Methylphenidate has been beneficial in some children with AH but requires precise titration to avoid sleep deprivation. The longer-acting form, pemoline, is better suited for chronic use but has the same limitation related to narrow therapeutic range. None of these drugs has been effective in CHS patients in decreasing the extent of mechanical ventilatory support. However, they may be of some benefit in ameliorating awake hypoventilation in CHS subjects who require ventilatory support during sleep.

Doxapram is the only drug proven effective for CHS patients who require ventilatory support. Intravenous doxapram will improve sleep ventilation in the majority of CHS patients but generally will not

TABLE 1. Pharmacotherapy for Hypoventilation Syndromes

DRUG	DOSE*	BLOOD LEVEL (mg/L)	COMMENTS
Methylxanthines			All peripheral side effects are less with caffeine than with theophylline
Theophylline	2.5 mg/kg per dose q6–8h	10–20	
Caffeine	2.5 mg/kg per dose q.d.	10–20	
Progesterone	2–4 mg/kg/d divided t.i.d.		Depending on age, may be contraindicated in boys; no adrenergic side effects
Pemoline	1.9–3.3 mg/kg/d divided q12h		Negligible peripheral side effects
Doxapram	1–2.5 mg/kg/h IV	2–5	No enteral preparation available in United States

*Except for doxapram, all doses are oral.

permit weaning from ventilatory support. Further, even though intravenous doxapram has been acutely helpful in some patients, the nonspecific adrenergic stimulation and resultant nonrespiratory side effects may be incompatible with long-term use.

The customary doses and blood levels for each drug are summarized in Table 1. The beneficial effect of methylxanthine treatment on hypoventilation can be achieved at blood levels of 10 to 12 mg/L or less. If the extent of improvement in ventilation is insufficient, the dose should be increased until a blood level of 13 to 15 mg/L is attained. Levels >15 mg/L do not generally yield any further benefit. Blood levels are not available for pemoline or progesterone. No systematic data are available correlating doxapram blood levels with the extent of ventilatory improvement. Levels of 2 to 5 mg/L have been reported as adequate for treatment of apnea of prematurity and should be regarded as a safe initial goal for treatment of CHS.

Mechanical Ventilatory Support

The evaluation of CHS patients will always require the resources of an experienced pediatric sleep laboratory not only for the necessary PSGs but also for the establishment and chronic reassessment of clinical ventilatory status and efficacy of the selected method of mechanical ventilatory support.

The treatment options include positive pressure ventilation, negative pressure ventilation, and diaphragm pacing (Table 2). In infants and young children, negative pressure methods will probably not be practical. Therefore, insertion of a tracheostomy generally will be necessary.

Positive Pressure Ventilation

In combination with chronic tracheostomy, this method has been the most commonly used long-term treatment for CHS. The recommended home ventilators[3] are battery operated and, thus, permit reasonable age-appropriate mobility as long as awake ventilation is adequate without mechanical ventilatory support and O_2 supplementation is not necessary. Since cuffed tracheostomy tubes are not suitable for home use, the ventilator should be pressure controlled to minimize problems related to (variable) tracheostomy leaks. In children requiring ventilatory support 24 h/d, the activity limitations caused by attachment to the ventilator during wakefulness will severely restrict age-appropriate activities. Home ventilators are thus most effective and least intrusive in patients who require support only during sleep.

TABLE 2. Ventilatory Treatment for Hypoventilation Syndromes

> **Positive Pressure**
> Tracheostomy
> Nasal mask
> **Negative Pressure**
> Chest shell (cuirass)
> Wrap ventilator (jumpsuit)
> Tank ventilator (iron lung)
> **Diaphragm Pacing**

As an alternative to chronic tracheostomy, limited success with positive pressure ventilation has been achieved in a few older children using a nasal mask. The obvious potential advantage of the nasal mask is avoidance of a tracheostomy, but there are two practical limitations. First, intercurrent respiratory infections that may be managed at home easily with a tracheostomy will likely require admission and intubation. Second, the nasal mask requires a greater degree of family support and patient cooperation and a closer extent of family and medical surveillance to ensure successful long-term use.

Negative Pressure Ventilation

Depending on age and referral center preference, success has been achieved in children using either a chest shell (cuirass) or a wrap ventilator. Tank ventilators (iron lungs) also have been used successfully, especially in older children. For reasons of availability, simplicity, comfort, convenience, and overall child/family preference, however, the iron lung has been generally supplanted by the cuirass or jump suit.

All negative pressure techniques rely on a negative inspiratory pressure generated inside the container. The negative pressure allows the chest and upper abdomen to passively expand in an amount proportional to tidal volume. The distinct advantage of negative pressure over conventional positive pressure ventilators is that most older children can be successfully ventilated during sleep without a tracheostomy. Infants and young children, however, generally still require a tracheostomy to avoid negative pressure-related upper airway collapse. Limitations of these techniques include decreased effectiveness in patients with reduced lung compliance, frequent refitting with growth to maintain appropriate ventilation, and decreased portability because the systems are cumbersome and are not battery operated.

Diaphragm Pacing

Substantial clinical experience is available in infants as well as older children.[5] Bilateral pacing generally is required to achieve adequate ventilation, especially in infants and younger children. A tracheostomy usually is necessary (at least until school age) to compensate for the absence of activation of upper airway dilator muscles associated with the noncentrally mediated inspiratory stimulation provided by the pacers.

The preoperative evaluation, surgical placement, establishing of the pacer regimen after surgery, and long-term follow-up of paced subjects all require referral to a pediatric sleep laboratory experienced in the clinical applications of diaphragm pacing. The diaphragm pacer system includes an external transmitter and a loop antenna and three internal components: a receiver, unipolar phrenic nerve electrode, and an indifferent electrode (anode). The transmitter radio frequency signal is emitted from the antenna placed on the skin overlying the subcutaneously implanted receiver. The receiver converts the radiofrequency signal to an electrical impulse, which is carried by hard wire from the receiver to the stimulating electrode on the (thoracic) phrenic nerve. As a result of the electrical stimulation of the phrenic nerve, the diaphragm contracts.

The primary complication of pacing is periodic failure of an implanted pacemaker component. The collective experience to date indicates a mean time to failure of about 56 months. It is noteworthy, however, that there has not been any evidence of chronic phrenic nerve or diaphragm damage or burnout. This is an issue of particular concern in children because of the additional years of anticipated exposure to the pacing stimulus.

Diaphragm pacing offers clear-cut benefits in infants and children with CHS who require awake ventilatory support, providing the opportunity for optimum mobility during wakefulness. The resultant enhancement of age-appropriate activities permits a more normal lifestyle or quality of life. Pacing also offers substantial potential benefits for those patients requiring ventilatory support only during sleep, enabling the family to minimize the inherent inconveniences of home ventilator support, maximize the potential for normal mobility and overall lifestyle, and potentially eliminate the need for the tracheostomy. These benefits of pacing are not outweighed by the potential inconvenience of receiver or electrode malfunction or brief rehospitalization for replacement of components.

OUTCOME

The morbidity and mortality associated with a hypoventilation syndrome can be negligible if the clinician has a high index of suspicion and appropriately uses the resources of a state-of-the-art pediatric sleep laboratory. With the exception of congenital CHS patients who have associated abnormalities, optimum long-term outcome appears to be related primarily to the avoidance of cor pulmonale. Timely diagnosis, establishment of an effective home ventilation program and effective long-term surveillance should be sufficient to prevent the later development of cor pulmonale.

The neurodevelopmental outcome should be normal for patients with hypoventilation syndrome sufficiently mild to be corrected pharmacologically (Table 1). Although the neurodevelopmental data are limited and variable in CHS children requiring long-term ventilatory support, full-scale IQ scores are typically above 70. More extensive assessments of neurodevelopmental and neuropsychologic status have revealed a broad spectrum of subtle abnormalities, suggesting either a more generalized central disturbance of nervous system function or injury secondary to severe pretreatment hypoventilation-related asphyxia or chronic intermittent asphyxia in patients with severely impaired or absent perception/responsiveness to asphyxia.

There is no evidence that any child with a congenital hypoventilation syndrome will later outgrow the respiratory control deficiency or that an acquired syndrome will resolve after the ventilatory control deficit has been stable for 3 to 6 months. There is, however, a tendency for predictable changes to occur in the overall adequacy of automatic control of breathing in the congenitally acquired conditions. Therefore, although young subjects with a hypoventilation syndrome may experience some later stabilization of their ventilatory deficit, they do not appear to have any potential for full recovery of automatic ventilatory control.

REFERENCES

1. Beckerman RC, Brouillette RT, Hunt CE (eds): Respiratory Control Disorders in Infants and Children. Baltimore, Williams & Wilkins, 1992:231–241, 352–399.
2. Blanchard PW, Aranda JV: Pharmacotherapy of respiratory control disorders. *In* Beckerman RC, Brouillette RT, Hunt CE (eds): Respiratory Control Disorders in Infants and Children. Baltimore, Williams & Wilkins, 1992:352–370.
3. Keens TG, Davidson Ward SL: Ventilatory treatment at home. *In* Beckerman RC, Brouillette RT, Hunt CE (eds): Respiratory Control Disorders in Infants and Children. Baltimore, Williams & Wilkins, 1992:371–385.
4. Silvestri JM, Weese-Mayer DE, Nelson MN: Neuropsychologic abnormalities in children with congenital central hypoventilation syndrome. J Pediatr 120:388–393, 1992.
5. Weese-Mayer DE, Hunt CE, Brouillette RT: Diaphragm pacing in infants and children. *In* Beckerman RC, Brouillette RT, Hunt CE (eds): Respiratory Control Disorders in Infants and Children. Baltimore, Williams & Wilkins, 1992:386–399.

SIDS AND RECURRING APNEA

ALAN R. SPITZER, M.D.

Sudden infant death syndrome (SIDS) refers to the sudden, unexpected death of a child between 1 month and 1 year of age that cannot be explained by postmortem examination, death scene investigation, or review of the past medical records of the child. SIDS is responsible for approximately 6,000 to 10,000 infant deaths in the United States annually and is the leading cause of death between 1 month and 1 year of life. For reasons that are not completely clear, the incidence of SIDS in this country has decreased slightly during the past several years.

By definition, SIDS is a disease of exclusion. If a death can be adequately explained, it cannot be a SIDS death. Consequently, the etiology of SIDS is unknown. It appears likely that SIDS represents a final common pathway for a variety of triggering elements, all of which may lead to sudden cessation of heart rate and respiration. Prematurity, infant apnea, cardiac rhythm disturbances, gastroesophageal reflux, seizures, neurodevelopmental maturation irregularities, carbon dioxide rebreathing, and infant overheating are but a few of the factors that have been proposed as important etiologic mechanisms. To date, however, support for these theories is primarily circumstantial.

Prevention of SIDS has been a concern in pediatrics for the past several decades. Recent evidence suggests that sleeping position of infants may be an important consideration in reducing SIDS deaths. In a number of studies from around the world, placement of young infants in the supine position has resulted in a dramatic decrease in the incidence of SIDS. The American Academy of Pediatrics (AAP) issued a policy statement in 1992, recently reemphasized (May 1994), supporting the use of the supine position as the optimal sleeping position for full-term, healthy infants. The incidence of complications, such as gastroesophageal reflux or aspiration, does not appear to be increased in infants who sleep supine. Excluded from this AAP policy statement are preterm infants and infants with medical problems that may be aggravated by supine sleeping. Such infants include those with gastroesophageal reflux and craniofacial abnormalities. It is postulated that supine sleeping may avoid positions in which carbon dioxide rebreathing or infant self-suffocation is more likely to occur. Overheating may be an important factor that places the SIDS-susceptible child at greater risk in the prone position. Further investigation is needed to define why supine positioning does reduce SIDS. It should be noted, however, that SIDS is not completely eliminated by supine positioning and that children have died of SIDS while supine.

Since SIDS remains a mystery with respect to etiology, it is unclear if any intervention can completely eliminate it. If one assumes, however, that breathing must cease and that heart rate must decrease before death, one can legitimately ask whether cardiorespiratory monitoring can be used to prevent SIDS. Although cardiorespiratory monitoring has long been available in the hospital setting, its use in the home environment as a device has become widespread only during the past decade. Home cardiorespiratory monitors that are available are essentially similar in design. Two channels are used, one that measures averaged heart rate and the other that detects thoracic impedance and uses this value as a measure of respiratory effort. With most monitors, electrodes are attached to the chest by either stick-on leads or by means of a belt that extends around the chest. One electrode from the monitor emits a continuous signal, whereas the second electrode detects the duration of time for the signal to be received. With inspiration, the thorax expands and impedance increases. During expiration, a decrease in impedance is noted. This variation in signal is recorded by the device as a breath. If inadequate chest movement results in an insufficient degree of positional change in the electrodes, an alarm of 90 to 110 decibels is triggered.

The heart rate on these monitors is detected in a manner similar

TABLE 1. General Screening Evaluation for Infants with Apparent Life-Threatening Episodes (ALTE)

All Infants
In-hospital observation with cardiorespiratory monitoring
Careful physical and neurologic examination
Complete blood count
Blood glucose, electrolytes, calcium, phosphate, and magnesium determination
Chest roentgenogram
Electrocardiogram
Electroencephalogram
Evaluation of cardiorespiratory function; multichannel recording with pulse oximetry is essential in such instances

Selected Infants Under Certain Clinical Circumstances
Septic workup (blood, urine, CSF cultures)
Barium swallow
Lateral neck roentgenogram; otolaryngology evaluation
Radionuclide milk scan of swallowing
Esophageal pH study with multichannel recording
Ultrasound or CT scan of the brain
Arterial blood gases, especially after the ALTE event
Echocardiogram

TABLE 3. Drug Dosages for Apnea Treatment

DRUG	DOSAGE
Caffeine	10 mg/kg PO of caffeine base (2 mg caffeine citrate = 1 mg caffeine base) as a loading dose, followed by 2.5–5 mg/kg/d in one dose PO; after the child is 3 months of age, caffeine may have to be given two or three times daily to maintain blood levels. A serum concentration of between 5 and 20 μg/ml is desirable after 48 h of treatment
Theophylline	Loading dose of 5–10 mg/kg PO is given, followed by a dose of 5–8 mg/kg/d in three divided doses PO; serum levels should be checked after 48 h of therapy, with a level of 6–12 μg/ml being optimal for management of apnea

to that used in an electrocardiogram (ECG). The electrical activity of the heart is conducted to the surface of the skin, where it registers as a typical QRS complex. The monitor averages the heart rate and will alarm if the heart rate falls below a preset value. As with an ECG, if there is excessive bodily movement, the skin conductivity is disrupted. The monitor then fails to detect sequential cardiac impulses, and the mean heart rate falls below the threshold limit. An alarm is triggered in such cases, although it is obviously a false alarm.

With the standard home cardiorespiratory monitors, settings can be changed depending on the circumstances and needs of the child. In general, low heart rate alarms are set depending on the age and resting heart rate of the child, averaging about 70 to 80 bpm as the low limit for a neonate, whereas a 6-month-old infant may have a low heart rate limit of 60 bpm. If the heart rate drops below this level, an audible alarm is triggered. The monitor also allows for a time delay before sounding an apnea alarm. The delay recommended is usually 15 to 20 seconds to start. If a shorter delay is established, frequent false alarms will occur. In addition, many individuals will have 10 to 12 second apnea as a normal part of their respiratory pattern. With the institution of 15- to 20-second delays, if apnea does occur, the child will be relatively early into the episode. Therefore, resuscitation will rarely require more than simple tactile stimulation. Often, the sound of the monitor alarm itself is sufficient to arouse the infant. In our experience, CPR is rarely needed for apnea patients at these suggested monitor settings.

Before institution of monitoring, all children should be evaluated to determine if the etiology of their apnea can be more precisely diagnosed and more accurately treated. Recommended studies in these infants include those indicated in Table 1. The child who has apnea

accompanying seizures, hypoglycemia, or gastroesophageal reflux is better treated by pursuing those etiologies rather than treating the apnea alone. In some of these cases, however, monitoring may still be an important adjunct to therapy. Home monitoring should be considered in children for the indications outlined in Table 2. Methylxanthines (caffeine or theophylline) are used for frequent episodes of central apnea and bradycardia (>3/6 hour recording) or if oxygen desaturation (<85%) is observed. Periodic breathing greater than 10% of total sleep time should also be treated, especially if it is accompanied by bradycardia or oxygen desaturation. Caffeine should be administered PO in a dose of 10 mg/kg of caffeine base (2 mg caffeine citrate = 1 mg caffeine base) as a loading dose, followed by 2.5 to 5 mg/kg/d administered as a single daily dose. After 3 months of age, caffeine may have to be given two or three times daily to maintain blood levels. A serum concentration of between 5 and 20 μg/ml is desirable after 48 hours of treatment. If theophylline is used, a loading dose of 5 to 10 mg/kg (PO) is given, followed by a dose of 5 to 8 mg/kg/d in three divided doses. Serum levels should be checked after 48 hours of therapy, with a level of 6 to 12 μg/ml being optimal for management of apnea with theophylline (Table 3). These drugs initially may cause tachycardia, irritability, restlessness, or decreased sleep in some infants. These effects usually resolve within 2 weeks, but reduction of apnea frequency persists. For children with obstructive apnea, methylxanthines generally are ineffective.

As can be seen, one of the primary problems with home cardiorespiratory monitoring is the ease with which false alarms are triggered. For some families, these events may significantly interfere with the technique of home monitoring. Usually, however, parents or caretakers can be counseled about lead placement with these monitors to reduce the incidence of such false alarms to an absolute minimum. Other problems commonly seen with the use of home cardiorespiratory monitoring include monitor malfunctions, increased numbers of false alarms during intercurrent illnesses, skin irritation from electrodes, overdependence on the monitor, sibling jealously over monitor use, and lack of compliance with monitoring instructions.

Compliance concerns have improved with the introduction of smart monitors. These units contain a computer memory that records daily and hourly monitor use, allowing the clinician to determine the accuracy of compliance with instructions. In addition, these units store events so that the physician can review episodes experienced by the family and decide whether they represent true apnea and bradycardia or false alarms triggered by bodily movement or lack of movement of the chest electrodes.

The management of the monitored child is indicated in Figure 1. It is crucial that families have a clear support structure and contact people defined *before* the child is discharged. On average, home monitoring is used in our program for approximately 3 months. Preterm infants who require monitoring usually are treated for shorter periods, whereas children with recurring episodes of apnea or apparent life-threatening events may need longer treatment.

TABLE 2. Indications for Home Cardiorespiratory Monitoring

History of severe life-threatening event or apneic episode
Multichannel recording documentation of apnea
Documentation of increased periodic breathing (>5% of total sleep time)
Sibling of a SIDS victim
Twin of a SIDS victim
Severe feeding difficulties with apnea and bradycardia
Gastroesophageal reflux-associated apnea
The technology-dependent child (e.g., ventilator dependency, bronchopulmonary dysplasia)
The child with certain pulmonary, cardiac, or neurologic problems
Some infants exposed to cocaine or opiates in utero

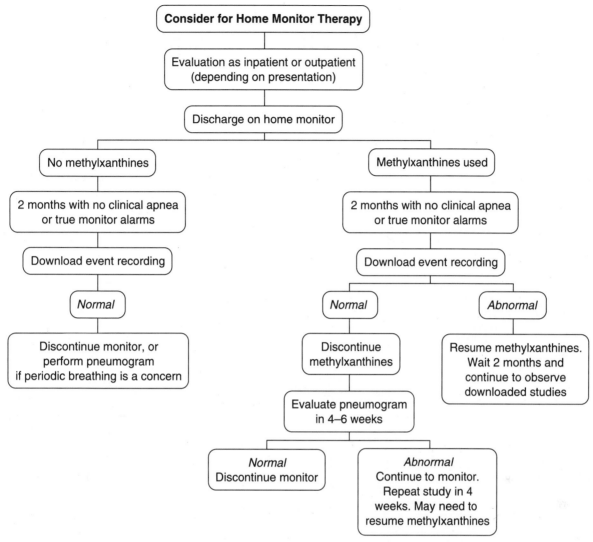

FIGURE 1. An approach to the child who requires home cardiorespiratory monitoring.

RESPIRATORY INSUFFICIENCY

Ashok P. Sarnaik, m.d.
Sabrina M. Heidemann, m.d.

Respiratory insufficiency is defined as the inability to maintain adequate alveolocapillary gas exchange to meet metabolic demands. There is a great deal of interdependence between the respiratory system and other systems. An otherwise well-tolerated pulmonary pathologic state may readily progress to decompensation in the presence of cold stress, fluid overload, sepsis, or myocardial dysfunction. Respiratory insufficiency in such situations cannot be managed effectively without attention to coexistent pathophysiologic processes. The causes of respiratory insufficiency can be categorized as diseases of airways and pulmonary parenchyma, neuromuscular and chest wall abnormalities, diseases associated with an inadequate respiratory center drive, and those characterized by excessive metabolic demands.

DIAGNOSIS

Appropriate interpretation of clinical findings and blood gas values is the first step in establishing the diagnosis and formulating a treatment plan. Severe respiratory failure may occur in the absence of significant respiratory distress. For example, patients with neuromuscular diseases, such as Guillain-Barré syndrome or myasthenia gravis, and those with an abnormal respiratory center drive may develop severe respiratory failure but will not respond with increased effort. In these patients, respirations are either ineffective or may even appear normal in the presence of respiratory acidosis and hypoxemia. Respiratory tract abnormalities can be classified as extrathoracic airway obstruction (e.g., supraglottitis and viral croup), intrathoracic-extrapulmonary airway obstruction (e.g., vascular ring and mediastinal tumors), intrapulmonary airway obstruction (e.g., asthma and bronchiolitis), and parenchymal lesions (e.g., pneumonia and pulmonary edema). Clinical observations especially important in determining the site of abnormality of airways and pulmonary parenchyma are the rate and depth of respirations and the presence of retractions, inspiratory stridor, expiratory wheezing, and grunting (Table 1).

Interpretation of blood gas values is important in localizing the site of the lesion and estimating its severity, especially when considered with clinical observations. In airway obstruction above the carina, blood gases reflect overall alveolar hypoventilation, manifested by an elevated $Paco_2$ and a proportionate decrease in Pao_2. Since there is no parenchymal disease with right to left shunting, hypoxemia responds very well to supplemental O_2. In intrapulmonary airway obstruction, blood gases reflect ventilation-perfusion imbalance and venous admixture. In these diseases, the obstruction is not uniform

TABLE 1. Interpreting the Clinical Signs of Respiratory Disease

	EXTRATHORACIC AIRWAY OBSTRUCTION	INTRATHORACIC-EXTRAPULMONARY AIRWAY OBSTRUCTION	INTRAPULMONARY AIRWAY OBSTRUCTION	PARENCHYMAL PATHOLOGY
Tachypnea	+	+	+ +	+ + + +
Retraction	+ + + +	+ +	+ +	+ + +
Stridor	+ + + +	+ +	−	−
Grunting	±	±	+ +	+ + + +
Wheezing	±	+ + +	+ + + +	+

throughout the lungs, resulting in areas that are hyperventilated and others that are hypoventilated. In mild disease, the hyperventilated areas predominate, resulting in hypocarbia. Because of the shape of the oxygen-hemoglobin dissociation curve, however, an elevated Po_2 in hyperventilated areas cannot compensate for the decreased Po_2 in hypoventilated areas. This results in venous admixture and a lowering of Po_2. With increasing disease severity, more areas become hypoventilated, resulting in normalization of $Paco_2$ with further decrease in Pao_2. A normal or slightly elevated $Paco_2$ in a patient with asthma should be viewed with concern as a possible indicator of impending respiratory failure. In severe airway obstruction, hypoventilated areas predominate, leading to respiratory acidosis and increasing hypoxemia. The degree to which supplemental O_2 raises Pao_2 depends on the severity of the illness and the degree of venous admixture. In alveolar and interstitial diseases, blood gas values reflect both right to left shunting and a diffusion barrier. Such conditions are associated with hypoxia and either normocarbia or hypocarbia. Elevated $Paco_2$ is usually a late occurrence and reflects muscle fatigue, leading to hypoventilation.

MANAGEMENT

The goal of management of respiratory insufficiency is to maintain alveolar ventilation and oxygenation appropriate to the metabolic needs, with minimum complications. Several pathophysiologic considerations need to be taken into account when managing children with respiratory insufficiency. The soft chest wall of an infant readily retracts when subjected to increasingly negative intrathoracic pressure, resulting in reduced functional residual capacity (FRC) and, therefore, a greater risk of hypoxemia. The respiratory muscles of young children are poorly equipped to sustain large workloads. They are more easily fatigued than in adults, and this significantly limits their ability to maintain adequate ventilation in lung disease. The soft airway of a child is excessively susceptible to collapse when subjected to either negative intramural pressure or positive extramural pressure. Infants have twice the oxygen consumption as adults, and their response to hypoxemia by hyperventilation is short-lived, with subsequent depression of the respiratory center. Sudden respiratory arrests are, therefore, common in hypoxemic infants.

Monitoring

The clinical status and the adequacy of therapeutic interventions must be monitored continuously during treatment of respiratory insufficiency. In addition to heart rate, respiratory rate, and blood pressure, various invasive and noninvasive methods often are necessary. Noninvasive methods include pulse oximetry, transcutaneous gas analysis, and capnography. Pulse oximetry uses two wavelengths (660 and 940 nm) of light to determine the percentage of oxyhemoglobin (Sao_2) compared with deoxygenated hemoglobin. In most situations, an Sao_2 >95% is a reasonable treatment goal. However, pulse oximetry has certain limitations. Because of the nature of the O_2-hemoglobin dissociation curve, changes in $Pao_2 > 70$ mm Hg are not readily identified by oximetry. Additionally, at the same Pao_2 level, there may be a significant change in Sao_2 at different blood pH values. Significant elevations of $Paco_2$ may occur in patients with satisfactory Sao_2 levels, especially in those receiving supplemental oxygen. Pulse

oximetry, therefore, cannot be relied on to ensure adequate ventilatory status. Pulse oximetry yields falsely high Sao_2 levels in the presence of carboxyhemoglobin and methemoglobin. Furthermore, for pulse oximetry to be accurate, the probe must detect pulsatile flow. Despite these limitations, pulse oximetry is a noninvasive, easily applicable, and readily available means of evaluating oxyhemoglobin level.

Transcutaneous measurement of O_2 and CO_2 levels with the use of a heated sensor offers the advantage of continuous monitoring of oxygenation and ventilation. Adequate cutaneous perfusion and periodic correlation with arterial blood gas values are necessary for accurate interpretation. The monitoring site needs to be changed intermittently to avoid thermal injury to the skin. Capnography (end-tidal CO_2 measurement) is a helpful indicator of alveolar ventilation in intubated patients.

Measurement of arterial blood gases remains the gold standard for laboratory monitoring of respiratory failure. The risk/benefit ratio of an indwelling arterial catheter must be considered in the individual patient. Capillary blood gas analysis performed on a sample obtained from a warm digit is a reasonable alternative. However, it may considerably underestimate Pao_2 in a child with poor peripheral perfusion. Patients with severe pathophysiologic derangements requiring extensive respiratory support may benefit from determination of oxygen delivery and oxygen consumption with the use of indwelling arterial and pulmonary artery catheters.

Oxygen Administration

Providing supplemental O_2 to treat or prevent hypoxemia is the first step in the management of respiratory insufficiency. The major determinants of arterial oxygen content are the level of hemoglobin and the extent to which it is saturated with O_2. Maintenance of an adequate hemoglobin level is, therefore, important. In an acute situation, O_2 should be administered in as high a concentration as possible, the risk of toxicity notwithstanding. When monitoring is available, O_2 therapy should be directed to attain a Pao_2 sufficient to ensure an Sao_2 above 95%. Further increase in Pao_2 will not significantly improve O_2 delivery and may increase the risk of O_2 toxicity from prolonged exposure to high inspiratory oxygen concentration (Fio_2). Several O_2 delivery systems are available for a spontaneously breathing patient, and the choice should depend on patient tolerance and the amount of Fio_2 necessary. A nasal cannula allows for a simple, low flow oxygen delivery through two short plastic prongs that are inserted into the nares. It is a relatively well tolerated system, although nasopharyngeal irritation can occur at high flows. It is useful for children requiring only a modest amount of supplemental O_2. To administer a higher Fio_2, a hood is preferred in infants and young children. The inspired gas must be warmed and humidified. Maintaining a flow rate above 10 to 15 L/min raises Fio_2 inside the hood close to that of the gas source and also prevents CO_2 rebreathing. The O_2 mask is the most common device used in older children. A simple mask delivers 35% to 60% O_2 at a flow rate of 6 to 10 L/min. A partial rebreathing mask has an added reservoir bag that can reliably deliver up to 60% O_2 with a flow of 10 to 12 L/min. A nonrebreathing mask with one-way valves between exhalation port and the exterior and between the bag and the reservoir allows for O_2 delivery as high as 95% and prevents CO_2 rebreathing.

Helium-Oxygen Mixture

Gas flow in an obstructed airway results in considerable turbulence. Airway resistance in such situations is dependent on gas density rather than on viscosity as it is in an unobstructed airway with a laminar flow. Replacing nitrogen with the less dense helium in the inspired gas thus reduces resistance to gas flow in an obstructed airway. Heliox (79% helium with 21% oxygen) can be used alone or blended with supplemental O_2 to decrease airway resistance. However, when greater than 40% O_2 is required, the reduction in airway resistance by helium is probably not clinically useful. Both spontaneously breathing and mechanically ventilated patients can be treated with helium-oxygen administration. Patients with tracheal as well as peripheral airway obstruction may have improved ventilation with this therapy.

Endotracheal Intubation

The four major indications for endotracheal (ET) intubation are (1) to maintain a patent airway, (2) to protect from aspiration lung injury, (3) to facilitate pulmonary toilet, and (4) to institute mechanical ventilation. Emergency intubation is required in relatively few patients. In almost all cases, a short period of preparation and stabilization (including the attachment of appropriate monitors and alarms) is essential. O_2 should be administered in as high a concentration as possible, and the patient should have ECG, heart rate, and preferably pulse oximetry monitoring before and during intubation. An appropriate-sized bag and mask and suction equipment should be readily available. In the event of inadequate respirations or unsatisfactory oxygenation, positive pressure ventilation should be instituted with the bag and mask.

An alpha-adrenergic agent, such as topical phenylephrine, and a lubricant facilitate passage of the tube and minimize nasopharyngeal trauma. For children over 2 years of age, the ET tube size can be estimated by the formula

$$\frac{\text{Age in years}}{4} + 4 = \text{Internal diameter of ET tube in millimeters}$$

Table 2 represents a useful reference for the size and approximate length of ET tube to reach the midtracheal level.

Intubation in a conscious, struggling child results in unnecessary pain and anxiety and carries the risk of airway trauma, aspiration, and cardiopulmonary instability. Adequate sedation and muscle paralysis are necessary for most planned intubations. The choice of sedative and paralytic agent depends on the onset and duration of action, elimination, and side effects. These are summarized in Table 3. In controlled circumstances, preoxygenation should be followed by sedation, bag and mask ventilation, and paralysis before intubation. Satisfactory tube position should be established initially by chest auscultation to determine equal breath sounds and should be confirmed subsequently by a chest radiograph.

TABLE 2. Average Dimensions of Endotracheal Tubes

AGE	INTERNAL DIAMETER (mm)	ORAL: MOUTH TO MIDTRACHEA (cm)	NASAL: NARE TO MIDTRACHEA (cm)
Premature	2.5–3	9	10
Full-term	3–3.5	10	11
6 mo	4	11	13
12–24 mo	4.5	13–14	16–17
4 y	5	15	17–18
6 y	5.5	17	19–20
8 y	6	19	21–22
10 y	6.5	20	22–23
12 y	7	21	23–24
14 y	7.5	22	24–25
Adults	8–9.5	23–25	25–28

Mechanical Ventilation

The decision to institute mechanical ventilation is based on derangements of gas exchange, as well as a clinical impression of patient fatigue and impending exhaustion. Although there are no absolute laboratory criteria for instituting mechanical ventilation, a $PaO_2 < 60$ mm Hg with an $FIO_2 > 0.6$ and a $PaCO_2 > 60$ mm Hg and a pH < 7.25 often are reasons for ventilatory support. The choice of the respirator and ventilatory technique depends on patient characteristics and altered pulmonary pathophysiology. When planning a ventilatory strategy, four phases of the respiratory cycle need to be considered separately: (1) initiation of inspiration, (2) inspiratory flow characteristics, (3) termination of inspiration, and (4) expiratory flow maneuvers.

Initiation of Inspiration (Mode)

Intermittent mandatory ventilation (IMV) is the most commonly used ventilator mode in clinical practice. The inspiration is initiated at a set frequency with a timing mechanism regardless of patient effort. In between machine-delivered breaths, the patient can breathe spontaneously from a source of fresh gas. IMV allows adjustment in ventilator support according to the patient's need and is, therefore, very useful at initial institution of mechanical ventilation as well as during weaning. The disadvantage of IMV is that the patient cannot determine the timing of inspiration. Thus, asynchronous respiration results, especially at a high ventilator rate. Asynchronous respiration may lead to wasted effort, ineffective mechanical ventilation, and barotrauma. Patients with severe abnormalities of compliance and resistance may need heavy sedation and/or muscle paralysis when they are ventilated in IMV mode at a high rate. To obviate this problem, synchronized IMV (SIMV) is now available as an option, with many respirators designed for older infants and children. With

TABLE 3. Drugs Used for Endotracheal Intubation

DRUG	DOSE	ONSET	DURATION	ELIMINATION	COMMENTS
Sedatives					
Midazolam	0.1 mg/kg	3–5 min	1–2 h	Liver, kidney	Amnesia
Diazepam	0.1 mg/kg	15 min	2–4 h	Liver, kidney	Amnesia
Morphine	0.1 mg/kg	10–15 min	2–4 h	Liver, kidney	Analgesia, hypotension
Fentanyl	2–10 μg/kg	3–5 min	0.5–1.5 h	Liver	Analgesia, chest wall rigidity
Paralytic Agents					
Succinylcholine	1 mg/kg	45–60 sec	5–10 min	Pseudocholinesterase	Dysrhythmias, malignant hyperthermia, hyperkalemia in neuromuscular disease, severe burns, and trauma
Pancuronium	0.1 mg/kg	3–5 min	60–90 min	Urine (60%–80%)	Tachycardia
Vecuronium	0.1 mg/kg	2–3 min	35–75 min	Bile (80%)	
Atracurium	0.5 mg/kg	2–3 min	20–30 min	Hoffman elimination Ester hydrolysis	Histamine release, hypotension

SIMV, the machine-delivered breaths are synchronized with the patient's inspiratory effort. However, with many of these respirators, the patient has to open a demand valve by generating sufficient inspiratory pressure for spontaneous respiration. This represents a significantly increased work of breathing, especially in young infants, and can cause fatigue. To overcome this problem, a pressure support mode is now available on newer respirators that allows a rapid rise in ventilatory circuit pressure to a preselected level to assist spontaneous inspiration. The newly introduced microprocessor-controlled ventilation system also has the ability to vary the flow rate of the gas during spontaneous respiration to reduce the work of breathing. Assist/control is another mode used to synchronize initiation of inspiration with patient effort, with a backup total (patient and ventilator) obligatory rate. Unlike SIMV, however, all of the patient's inspiratory efforts trigger a machine-delivered breath in assist/control mode. Though useful in some patients, the assist/control mode cannot be used in the weaning process.

Inspiratory Flow Characteristics

A constant inspiratory flow produces a square wave flow pattern, whereas a variable flow produces a sine wave pattern. It is debatable which flow pattern is better in a given disease. The technique of inspiratory pause holds inspiration either after a certain amount of volume has been delivered or when a preset level of pressure has been reached in the ventilator circuit. This allows for a more even distribution of ventilation. However, it can also result in increased mean airway pressure, barotrauma, and decreased cardiac output.

Termination of Inspiration (Cycle)

The two most commonly used inspiratory terminating mechanisms are time cycled and volume cycled. With a time-cycled mechanical breath, inspiration is terminated after a preselected amount of inspiratory time has elapsed, whereas with a volume-cycled breath, the inspiration ends after a preselected amount of volume has been delivered by the machine into the ventilator circuit and the patient's respiratory tract. A time-cycled breath is almost always pressure limited where the peak inflation pressure (PIP) is held for a certain length of time. A volume-cycled breath can be pressure limited as a safety mechanism to avoid barotrauma. Time-cycled, pressure-limited ventilation allows for precise regulation of the inspiratory/expiratory ratio (I:E) and provides a certain degree of ET tube leak compensation. With this cycling mechanism, the tidal volume delivered depends on the lung compliance and airway resistance. Since PIP is limited at a relatively low preset level, any changes in the lung's compliance or resistance will greatly affect the tidal volume delivered to the child. With volume-cycled ventilation, a constant amount of tidal volume is delivered by the machine with each breath. Part of this volume is lost because of gas compression, tube distention in the ventilator circuit and ET tube leak. The rest of the volume is delivered to the patient. I:E ratios can be adjusted only within the limits of inspiratory flow rate capabilities. With a volume-cycled breath, changes in PIP are indicative of changing compliance and resistance of the patient's respiratory system, offering useful diagnostic information. It must be emphasized that although the machine-delivered volume is constant with volume-cycled ventilation, the tidal volume the patient receives will change with alterations in compliance and resistance affecting both the peak inspiratory pressure and volume of gas lost in the ventilator circuit. Additionally, endotracheal tube leak is not compensated for with a volume cycled breath.

Expiratory Flow Maneuvers

The most clinically useful expiratory flow maneuver is the application of positive end-expiratory pressure (PEEP), which can be applied for both machine-delivered and spontaneous breaths. The most important clinical effect of PEEP is an increase in FRC, which minimizes fluctuations in alveolar gas tension during inspiration and expiration. PEEP is most useful in improving oxygenation in disease states associated with decreased FRC and hypoxemia. Other salutary effects of PEEP include redistribution of extravascular lung water away from gas-exchanging areas, improved ventilation-perfusion relationship, prevention of early airway closure, and stabilization of the chest wall. Excessive amounts of PEEP can result in barotrauma and decreased venous return and cardiac output. The effect of PEEP on pulmonary compliance is variable depending on the level of PEEP provided. Excessive PEEP may lead to overdistention of alveoli and reduced lung compliance, whereas appropriate levels of PEEP may recruit more alveoli, delay airway closure, and improve lung compliance.

Ventilator Settings

The most efficient mechanical ventilatory support is the one that ensures adequate O_2 delivery and CO_2 removal with the lowest possible risk of barotrauma and O_2 toxicity. Strategies for improving gas exchange must take into account the pathophysiologic alterations encountered. The effect of any therapeutic manipulation must be assessed continually by clinical and laboratory parameters.

Tidal Volume and Rate

Machine-delivered tidal volume is the primary setting when using a volume-cycled ventilator. The tidal volume received by the patient is estimated by subtracting the volume loss in the ventilator circuit from the machine-delivered tidal volume. The choice of tidal volume and rate depends on the time constant, which is a reflection of time needed for pressure (and, therefore, volume) equilibration between proximal airway and alveoli to occur. The time constant is the product of compliance and resistance. Diseases characterized by decreased static compliance (e.g., pneumonia, pulmonary edema, atelectasis) are associated with a shortened time constant and, therefore, require less time for alveolar inflation and deflation. Diseases associated with increased resistance (e.g., asthma, bronchiolitis, aspiration syndromes) have a prolonged time constant and, therefore, require more time for alveolar inflation and deflation. Commonly used initial settings for a patient on a volume ventilator are a tidal volume of 7 to 10 ml/kg and a rate of 20 to 40 breaths per minute. Patients with reduced lung compliance and, therefore, shorter time constants are best ventilated with relatively lower tidal volumes and faster rates to minimize peak inflation pressure. In patients with increased airway resistance, an excessively rapid rate does not allow enough pressure equilibration to occur between the proximal airway and the alveoli. Such patients are, therefore, best ventilated with relatively slower rates and larger tidal volumes.

Peak Inflation Pressure (PIP)

When using a time-cycled respirator, the inspiratory flow is often set to reach a predetermined inflation pressure limit early during inspiration, thus resulting in an inspiratory hold. The tidal volume received by the patient depends on the PIP and respiratory compliance and resistance. A PIP of 25 to 30 cm H_2O is a reasonable initial setting for most patients. Higher pressures are necessary for patients with severely decreased lung compliance. In a volume-cycled respirator, PIP is a secondary variable determined by the tidal volume, respiratory compliance, and resistance. To avoid barotrauma from excessive PIP, a pressure limit can be set at 40 to 60 cm H_2O with a popoff valve during volume-cycled ventilation.

Inspiratory Time (Ti) and Expiratory Time (Te)

Ventilator rate and I:E ratio determine inspiratory and expiratory time. I:E ratios can be precisely adjusted with time-cycled respirators, whereas the duration of inspiration is determined by adjusting the inspiratory flow rate in a volume-cycled respirator. Ti and Te should be determined by the nature of the pulmonary abnormality. An I:E ratio of 1:2 is reasonable for most patients and allows for adequate inflation and deflation. In diseases with low FRC and decreased lung compliance, a prolonged inspiration can improve oxygenation. In severe cases, oxygenation may be improved by adjusting Ti to exceed Te. This strategy is referred to as inverse ratio ventilation. In pulmonary diseases characterized by decreased lung compliance and a shortened time constant, the reduced Te is still sufficient to allow for adequate deflation. The disadvantage of prolonged Ti is an elevation in mean intrathoracic pressure resulting in decreased cardiac output and barotrauma.

Diseases with intrathoracic airway obstruction, such as asthma, are characterized by a greater prolongation of the expiratory time constant compared with the inspiratory time constant. In addition to ventilating at a relatively slow rate, such patients require prolongation of Te for sufficient deflation to occur to minimize air trapping. I:E ratios of 1:3 or 1:4 may be appropriate in such situations.

PEEP

PEEP is used in infants who are mechanically ventilated to improve O_2 delivery and to maximize O_2 consumption. In most children, measurements of O_2 delivery and O_2 consumption are not available, and serial determination of Pao_2 is the most commonly used guide for PEEP therapy. Application of a minimum of 2 to 4 cm H_2O of PEEP is beneficial for all mechanically ventilated patients to prevent atelectasis. The benefit of improved Pao_2 from PEEP must be weighed against the risk of decreasing cardiac output and barotrauma. As a general rule, a gradual increase in PEEP up to 8 to 10 cm H_2O is considered reasonable if each stepwise increase in PEEP is associated with an increase in Pao_2. If the use of PEEP permits a reduction in the Fio_2, the risk of oxygen toxicity may be decreased.

High-Frequency Ventilation (HFV)

Mechanical ventilation at supraphysiologic rates and low tidal volumes has been shown to improve gas exchange in a selected group of patients who do not respond to conventional mechanical ventilation. The major advantage of HFV is the ability to use a reduced airway pressure for effective ventilation. Two most commonly employed techniques are high-frequency jet ventilation (HFJV) and high-frequency oscillation (HFO). In HFJV, a high-frequency flow interrupter is interposed between a high-pressure gas source and a small cannula that is incorporated in an ET tube. The cannula propels tiny amounts of gas at high velocity and frequency through the ET tube. An additional amount of gas is dragged in (entrainment) from a parallel circuit by the Venturi effect. Expiration occurs passively as a result of the elastic recoil of the lungs and chest wall. The respiratory rate (60 to 1600/min), PIP, and inspiratory time can be adjusted independently.

HFO uses a vibrating loudspeaker or a piston and flywheel combination to generate to-and-fro air movement. Additional air is entrained through a parallel circuit by the Venturi effect. Unlike HFJV, air is actively sucked out during expiration with the use of HFO. Respiratory rate (60 to 3600/min), I:E ratio, mean airway pressure, and change in proximal airway pressure (amplitude) can be adjusted independently.

At this time, HFV is not used as an initial method of ventilatory support for patients with respiratory insufficiency. It may, however, represent an important rescue therapy when conventional ventilation has been ineffective. HFV is especially helpful in patients with bronchopulmonary fistulas and persistent air leaks.

Extracorporeal Life Support (ECLS)

Selected patients with severe respiratory failure with potentially reversible pulmonary parenchymal disease may benefit from extracorporeal oxygenation and CO_2 removal. ECLS has to be considered as a temporary means of cardiopulmonary support, allowing sufficient time for recovery to occur while preventing additional lung injury from pressure and oxygen. For ECLS to be beneficial, it should be instituted before the occurrence of severe irreversible pulmonary injury. However, reasonable entry criteria have not been established outside the neonatal period to select patients who would most benefit from ECLS. The place of ECLS in the therapeutic armamentarium for nonneonatal respiratory failure is still not established.

5

Cardiovascular System

CONGENITAL HEART DISEASE

Nancy D. Bridges, m.d.
Charles E. Canter, m.d.
Arnold W. Strauss, m.d.

Congenital heart disease occurs in approximately 8 of 1000 live births in the United States. The variations in cardiac malformations are legion, and the diagnosis of congenital heart disease may be made at any age from fetal life to senescence. Congenital heart disease frequently is the most visible sign of multisystem congenital malformations. Associations of specific genetic defects with congenital heart lesions have been established in a few cases, and our understanding of the developing myocardium is increasing. Improvements in ultrasound technology have allowed detection of congenital heart disease in utero. Thus, therapy for congenital heart disease includes not only therapy for the specific lesion but also screening for underlying genetic or multisystem anomalies, prenatal counseling, and counseling for the risk of recurrence. Continued research into the control mechanisms affecting the developing heart and the etiologies of congenital malformations may bring us closer to the goal of true prevention of congenital heart disease.

Medical therapy for congenital heart malformations includes both palliative and preventive measures. Digitalis, diuretics, vasodilators, and antiarrhythmic medications are all employed for control of symptoms of cardiac insufficiency. Preventive medical therapy includes antibiotic prophylaxis against bacterial endocarditis at the time of dental, gastrointestinal, and genitourinary instrumentation, activity restrictions for children with cyanotic or obstructive lesions or myocardial disease, and careful monitoring of the hematocrit and iron status in children with compensatory polycythemia. Although many congenital heart lesions will resolve spontaneously or remain hemodynamically insignificant, most will require surgical and/or transcatheter intervention for definitive therapy. *Corrective interventions* restore normal or near normal cardiovascular physiology. *Palliative interventions* improve symptomatology when correction is not possible or is believed to involve prohibitive risk. Heart, lung, and heart-lung transplantation have been employed as therapies for children with congenital heart disease with increasing frequency and variable success. Thus, in the 1990s, there is no child who is inoperable, but the life expectancy, cumulative morbidity, and quality of life after some interventions remain uncertain.

Most operations and transcatheter therapies for congenital heart disease are associated with a very low mortality risk. At centers where a large volume of congenital heart surgery is performed, the overall surgical mortality rate is generally about 5%. Restoration of normal physiology is undertaken as early as possible, based on the premise that this offers the patient the best chance of a good long-term outcome. Thus, repair in the newborn period or during the first year of life is the rule, rather than the exception, for almost all lesions amenable to biventricular repair. This is true even for those children who are well palliated or well compensated without surgical palliation.

LESIONS CHARACTERIZED BY SYSTEMIC-TO-PULMONARY ARTERY SHUNTING

Lesions characterized by systemic-to-pulmonary artery shunting are associated with ventricular volume overload early in life and the development of increased pulmonary vascular resistance as a later consequence. The goal of management is timely referral of those requiring surgical therapy to minimize deleterious effects on the ventricles and avoid the development of irreversible pulmonary vascular disease.

Ventricular Septal Defects

The clinical importance of a ventricular septal defect (VSD) is a function of its size and its location in the ventricular septum. Most small defects, that is, those associated with low right ventricular pressure and a pulmonic/systemic flow ratio less than 2:1, require no therapy other than subacute bacterial endocarditis (SBE) prophylaxis. However, some small paramembranous and subpulmonary VSDs are associated with aortic insufficiency and are surgically closed in an attempt to prevent progression of the aortic valve involvement. Many paramembranous and muscular VSDs will diminish in size or close completely with time. Thus, even if these defects are associated with symptoms of congestive heart failure, medical management may be attempted. Defects in the inlet septum (VSDs of the AV canal type), malalignment-type VSDs (which result from anterior or posterior malalignment of the infundibular septum), and VSDs resulting from conal septal hypoplasia are usually large and do not close spontaneously. Transcatheter closure of VSDs that cannot be closed surgically via the right ventricle or semilunar valves has been performed but remains investigational.

The vast majority of VSDs can be surgically corrected at very low risk, even in small infants. For this reason, almost any infant with a large VSD who has growth failure or other symptoms of congestive heart failure unresponsive to medical management is referred for surgical repair. This is true even in very small infants or for defects that might theoretically close spontaneously over time. In almost all cases, primary repair is preferred over banding of the pulmonary artery.

Absence of symptoms of congestive heart failure in the presence of an unrestrictive VSD suggests an increase in pulmonary vascular resistance. In this circumstance, repair within the first 6 to 12 months of life may minimize the risk of developing irreversible pulmonary vascular disease. VSDs associated with subsystemic pulmonary artery pressure but with a pulmonary/systemic flow ratio ≥2:1 are generally repaired in early childhood, preferably by 2 years of age.

When the findings on clinical examination are consistent with those of the echocardiogram and when the acoustic windows are adequate for a complete echocardiographic diagnosis, surgery may be performed without a prior diagnostic cardiac catheterization. When the magnitude of the shunt or degree of pulmonary hypertension is in doubt, when irreversible pulmonary vascular disease is suspected, or when there are multiple muscular defects, cardiac catheterization is indicated before surgery.

Atrial Septal Defects

The signs and symptoms of an atrial septal defect (ASD) are usually quite subtle in childhood. However, patients whose defects are associated with significant left-to-right shunting will usually become symptomatic at some point during adult life if the lesion is not repaired, and a small fraction of these patients will develop irreversible pulmonary vascular disease. About 25% of ASDs will close spontaneously before 3 years of age. For these reasons, all ASDs that are associated with signs of right ventricular volume overload are repaired in early childhood (age 3 to 5 years) or at the time of diagnosis in older children. When the findings on physical examination are consistent with those of the echocardiogram, cardiac catheterization is not necessary before surgery. Small defects or patent foramina that are not associated with right ventricular volume overload are generally not repaired. However, such defects may be implicated in the etiology of embolic stroke in young patients, and in that setting, they may be closed in the hope of preventing recurrent stroke. During the last several years, umbrella devices that can be delivered through a sheath have been developed for the nonsurgical repair of atrial septal defects, but these devices remain investigational.

Patent Ductus Arteriosus

Persistent patency of the arterial duct (patent ductus arteriosus, PDA) is a frequent complication of prematurity. If it is associated with respiratory distress or signs of cardiac failure, medical treatment with indomethacin frequently is the primary intervention. However, the risk of PDA ligation, even in very small premature infants, is very low. Thus, surgery may be performed as the initial treatment and certainly is indicated where indomethacin has failed or is contraindicated. For the full-term infant or older child, a PDA is generally electively closed regardless of size. The combination of a characteristic continuous murmur and the demonstration of left-to-right ductal flow by echocardiography is sufficient to establish the diagnosis and proceed with surgery or transcatheter closure. Recently, high-resolution color flow mapping techniques have resulted in the demonstration of tiny PDAs that are not associated with murmurs. Whether these silent PDAs require treatment remains controversial.

Atrioventricular Canal Defects

Abnormalities in the atrioventricular canal portion of the heart result in a spectrum of defects: a primum-type atrial septal defect with a cleft mitral valve, a transitional AV canal defect in which there is a restrictive ventricular septal defect in the AV canal portion of the ventricular septum along with the primum ASD, or a complete common atrioventricular canal defect in which both the ASD and VSD are large and there is a single atrioventricular valve entering both ventricles. These defects never resolve spontaneously.

The timing of repair of a primum ASD may be affected by the degree of involvement of the mitral valve but is generally performed before 3 years of age. Complete common AV canal defects are associated with symptoms of congestive heart failure, and if they are unrepaired, irreversible pulmonary vascular disease develops at an early age. For these reasons, complete atrioventricular canal defects are generally repaired within the first year of life. Although operative mortality is slightly higher than for repair of a simple VSD, primary repair is almost always preferable to pulmonary artery banding, even in very small infants. Symptomatic insufficiency of the left atrioventricular valve is a complication of repair of AV canal defects and will lead to reoperation and valve replacement in some patients.

MALFORMATIONS WITH OBSTRUCTION TO RIGHT OR LEFT VENTRICULAR OUTFLOW

Double-Chambered Right Ventricle

In this lesion, there is right ventricular outflow tract obstruction at the level of the os infundibulum. This defect is almost invariably associated with a paramembranous ventricular septal defect and less commonly with a subaortic membrane. The obstructive muscle bundles in the right ventricle become increasingly obstructive with time. They may be inapparent when the VSD is diagnosed early in life and later become the dominant lesion. Surgical repair is generally performed once the gradient is greater than 40 mm Hg, with closure of the VSD and resection of the subaortic membrane (if present) being done at the same time as resection of the anomalous RV muscle bundles. Surgery is almost always curative as far as the right ventricular muscle bundles are concerned, but the subaortic membrane may recur.

Valvar Pulmonic Stenosis

Valvar pulmonic stenosis may occur as an asymptomatic lesion in an older child or as a life-threatening cyanotic lesion in the newborn with critical pulmonic stenosis. In the latter, treatment consists of palliation with an infusion of prostaglandin E_1, followed by transcatheter or surgical pulmonary valvotomy. In older children, transcatheter valvotomy has become the treatment of choice and is indicated for a gradient ≥ 40 mm Hg. In children older than 1 year of age, valvotomy is essentially curative, whereas in those treated at less than 1 year of age, recurrence is more likely. Infants and children with dysplastic pulmonary valves have a less favorable response to either surgical or transcatheter valvotomy and may require more extensive surgical treatment.

Supravalvar Pulmonic Stenosis and Peripheral Pulmonic Stenosis

Congenital discrete supravalvar pulmonic stenosis may occur as an isolated lesion or in association with a dysplastic pulmonary valve. Discrete or diffuse supravalvar pulmonic stenosis also may be seen as a complication of the arterial switch operation. Congenital supravalvar pulmonic stenosis is rarely if ever amenable to transcatheter therapy. Acquired supravalvar pulmonic stenosis can be treated by transcatheter techniques in some cases.

Peripheral pulmonic stenosis takes many forms. Most commonly, it is a benign developmental phenomenon seen in infants in the first 6 months of life. Unilateral congenital branch pulmonary artery stenosis involving the left pulmonary artery (sometimes referred to as coarctation of the left pulmonary artery) may be the result of the contraction of ductal tissue extending into the left pulmonary artery. Multiple, bilateral sites of peripheral pulmonic stenosis may be a component of tetralogy of Fallot, may exist as an isolated lesion, or may coexist with supravalvar aortic stenosis, with or without other features of Williams or Alagille's syndrome. It can be a life-threatening entity resistant to both transcatheter and surgical therapy.

Subaortic Stenosis

Subaortic stenosis may be membranous or muscular. It may exist as an isolated lesion or in association with hypertrophic cardiomyopathy, multiple sites of left heart obstruction, or some degree of left heart hypoplasia. Subaortic membrane may be associated with progressive aortic valve insufficiency. Although there have been reports of successful transcatheter treatment of subaortic membrane, surgery remains the treatment of choice at most centers. The timing and technique of surgery depend on the anatomy and severity of the obstruction, the degree of aortic valve involvement, and the nature of the associated lesions. Recurrence or subtotal correction is not uncommon. Thus, surgery is likely to be palliative rather than curative.

Valvar Aortic Stenosis

Valvar aortic stenosis may occur as severe or critical aortic stenosis in the newborn, as asymptomatic valvar stenosis in the child, or as late onset aortic stenosis in adults as a result of calcification of a bicuspid aortic valve. Severe aortic stenosis in the newborn is often associated with some degree of left heart hypoplasia and/or dysfunction. The infant requires intensive support with prostaglandin E_1 and pressors until obstruction is relieved (either by surgical or transcatheter valvotomy) and there is some recovery of ventricular function. The distinction between aortic stenosis and hypoplastic left heart syndrome is not always obvious. The size of all of the left heart structures must be considered when choosing between biventricular and univentricular palliation. All treatment is palliative in this entity, with most patients ultimately requiring valve replacement.

In childhood aortic stenosis, in contrast, the other left heart structures usually are normal, and the child is usually asymptomatic. Valvotomy is indicated for a gradient greater than or equal to 50 mm Hg. In most centers where there is an experienced catheter interventionist, balloon dilatation has become the treatment of choice initially. Both transcatheter and surgical treatment of valvar aortic stenosis are associated with an increase in aortic insufficiency. When valve replacement is indicated either because of combined stenosis and insufficiency of the valve or because valvotomy has been unsuccessful, several surgical approaches are possible: transplantation of the patient's own pulmonary valve to the aortic position with placement of a right ventricular-to-pulmonary artery conduit (pulmonary autograft or Ross procedure), aortic root replacement with an aortic homograft, or replacement of the valve with a mechanical prosthesis. In the last case, anticoagulation is indicated.

Supravalvar Aortic Stenosis

Discrete supravalvar aortic stenosis may occur as an isolated lesion or in association with supravalvar pulmonic stenosis. It may occur in normal children or as part of Williams syndrome. It is occasionally associated with coronary insufficiency as a result of obstruction of inflow into one or both coronary arteries and rarely is seen in association with complete atresia of the orifice of one of the coronary arteries. In the absence of coronary insufficiency, surgery is indicated for a gradient ≥50 mm Hg. Coronary insufficiency is an indication for surgery regardless of gradient.

Coarctation of the Aorta

Coarctation may occur as an isolated lesion or in association with other sites of left heart obstruction. It is also seen in association with Turner's syndrome. Coarctation may occur as critical left heart obstruction in the newborn, requiring intensive support with prostaglandin E_1 and pressors until surgical relief of obstruction can be carried out, or as an asymptomatic lesion of infancy or childhood. In the latter case, indications for surgery include a gradient between the upper and lower extremities of ≥20 mm Hg and/or upper extremity hypertension. Opinions are divided as to whether balloon angioplasty is an appropriate therapy for native coarctation of the aorta. Even in centers where there is an experienced catheter interventionist, these children may be referred for surgical repair. In contrast, balloon angioplasty generally is considered the treatment of choice for recurrent coarctation of the aorta.

MALFORMATIONS WITH ARTERIAL DESATURATION AMENABLE TO REPARATIVE SURGERY

Tetralogy of Fallot

The combination of an unrestrictive interventricular communication and pulmonary outflow obstruction is seen in a number of different cardiac malformations, of which tetralogy of Fallot is the most common. The right ventricular outflow tract obstruction in tetralogy of Fallot is the result of anterior malalignment of the infundibular septum. Obstruction may exist at the subvalvar, valvar, and supravalvar level. The combination of an unrestrictive VSD with right ventricular outflow tract obstruction allows hypercyanotic, or Tet, spells to occur. These are characterized by hyperpnea and severe cyanosis. Severe

spells can result in loss of consciousness, brain damage, and rarely, death. These spells are a medical emergency. Therapy includes sedation and suppression of hyperpnea with morphine, augmentation of venous return with crystalloid and use of the knee-chest position, and elevation of systemic vascular resistance with alpha-agonists. The occurrence of hypercyanotic spells is an indication for surgical intervention regardless of age.

Most children with tetralogy of Fallot have the malformation repaired by the age of 2 years, and more recently, the trend has been to refer children for repair by the age of 6 months. Repair may be delayed, or a palliative procedure (i.e., an aortopulmonary shunt) may be performed if there is an aberrant left anterior descending coronary artery (which interferes with the usual method of repair and necessitates the use of a right ventricle to pulmonary artery conduit) or if the pulmonary arteries are thought to be prohibitively small.

In its most severe form, tetralogy of Fallot includes atresia of the pulmonary valve. This is frequently associated with severe, diffuse hypoplasia of the pulmonary arteries and multiple systemic-to-pulmonary artery collateral vessels. The ability to accomplish a complete repair is dependent on the presence of a pulmonary vascular bed that can accept a full cardiac output from the right ventricle (via a surgically placed conduit) at subsystemic pressure. If the pulmonary arteries are of adequate size and supply most or all of both lungs, this can be accomplished in a single operation. When the pulmonary arteries are diminutive or do not communicate with a large portion of the pulmonary vascular bed, repair, if possible, must be carried out in several staged procedures. It is generally accepted that growth of the pulmonary arteries is promoted by the presence of antegrade flow early in life. Thus, a right ventricular-to-pulmonary artery conduit is placed within the first year of life when possible. In the absence of recruitable pulmonary arteries, the only repair possible is heart-lung transplant or heart repair with lung transplant.

Transposition of the Great Vessels

Patients with transposition of the great vessels (TGV) and an intact ventricular septum have severe cyanosis shortly after birth. Those with TGV, VSD, and no left ventricular outflow tract obstruction either may have cyanosis or may develop symptoms of congestive heart failure. Patients with TGV, VSD, and pulmonic stenosis generally are cyanotic but not in overt congestive heart failure. Newborns with TGV and severe cyanosis are emergently palliated with infusion of prostaglandin E_1 and/or a balloon atrial septostomy (Rashkind procedure). Anatomic repair of TGV (the arterial switch procedure) has become the surgical procedure of choice for this lesion. It is performed during the first days of life in patients with intact ventricular septum and may be delayed a little longer in those with a large VSD. Although the presence of a large VSD and/or a patent ductus arteriosus will be associated with adequate arterial oxygenation, repair within the first weeks of life is indicated to prevent pulmonary vascular disease, which may develop quite early in these patients.

Truncus Arteriosus

Truncus arteriosus generally occurs with signs of pulmonary overcirculation and heart failure rather than severe cyanosis. Reparative surgery is performed at the time of presentation, usually within the first 2 weeks of life. A valved human homograft is used to establish right ventricle-to-pulmonary artery continuity in most cases. Thus, reoperation for replacement of the conduit is anticipated in the first years of life. Insufficiency or stenosis of the truncal valve, if present, is often progressive, and replacement of the valve may be necessary. Surgical repair of truncus arteriosus carries a higher mortality risk (10% to 20%) than many other lesions.

Total Anomalous Pulmonary Venous Return

Total anomalous pulmonary venous return (TAPVR) causes symptoms of congestive heart failure when the pulmonary venous return is unobstructed and of severe cyanosis when the pulmonary venous return is obstructed. In the former case, the pulmonary venous pathway is usually supradiaphragmatic, and in the latter, it is subdiaphragmatic. In some patients, the pulmonary venous return can be mixed (i.e., partially supradiaphragmatic and partially subdiaphragmatic). In most cases, the diagnosis can be made echocardiographically. However, this is probably the most commonly missed cardiac diagnosis in the sick newborn, with obstructed TAPVR being mistaken for pulmonary disease. Surgical repair is performed at the time of diagnosis, usually with an excellent outcome.

MALFORMATIONS WITH ARTERIAL DESATURATION NOT AMENABLE TO BIVENTRICULAR REPAIR

When there is only one ventricle or atrioventricular valve of adequate size or when the configuration of the heart precludes septation of two adequate-sized ventricles, the goal of medical and surgical management is to accomplish a Fontan palliation. Anatomic lesions that fall into this category include single ventricle of all types, tricuspid or mitral atresia, some cases of pulmonary atresia with intact ventricular septum, and many complex lesions, such as malaligned atrioventricular canal defects, superoinferior ventricles, and criss-cross hearts.

Although there are many technical modifications of the Fontan operation, all rely on the principle that the systemic venous return can be directed to flow passively into the pulmonary arteries without a pulmonary ventricle. This may be accomplished with an intracardiac baffle or conduit or an extracardiac conduit, depending on the patient's anatomy and the surgeon's preference. For this to work, the pulmonary vascular resistance must be low and the pulmonary pathway must be unobstructed. The normal state of increased pulmonary vascular resistance in infancy precludes carrying out this surgery very early in life. Thus, early management of infants with functional single ventricle has as its goal the preservation of characteristics that will make the patient a good candidate for the Fontan operation, which is generally performed some time after 12 months of age.

Some patients will be perfectly balanced at birth, that is, have enough pulmonic stenosis to keep the pulmonary artery pressure low, but with enough pulmonary blood flow to maintain adequate arterial oxygen saturations. These patients can undergo the Fontan operation as their first (and perhaps only) cardiac operation. However, many others will need interim palliation before the Fontan operation. Palliative operations include a pulmonary artery band to reduce pulmonary flow and pressure or an aortopulmonary or cavopulmonary shunt to provide adequate pulmonary flow. The combination of subaortic stenosis and unrestricted pulmonary flow may be palliated by division of the main pulmonary artery, with end-to-side anastomosis of the proximal portion to the ascending aorta (thus bypassing the aortic stenosis), and closure of the distal end of the divided main pulmonary artery with sutures or a patch. Either an aortopulmonary shunt or a cavopulmonary shunt is created for pulmonary blood flow. Any of these interventions may result in distortion of the pulmonary arteries or excessive pulmonary artery pressure and flow. Thus, any infant who has either a band or a shunt needs to have a cardiac catheterization within 6 months to assess the effects of these interventions. The emphasis during the first few years of life is on vigilant monitoring of the state of the pulmonary vascular bed and ventricle. The outward appearance of wellness is not an adequate indicator of the child's condition in terms of his or her ultimate suitability for Fontan palliation. Children who are not candidates for Fontan palliation generally will be referred for heart or heart-lung transplantation.

Operative survival after the Fontan operation has improved greatly over the last decade, so that at present the surgical mortality risk is 3% to 10%, and the short-term outcome is excellent. Postoperative pleural effusions are a common complication and are difficult to treat. The intentional creation of an atrial level right-to-left shunt (adjustable ASD or fenestrated Fontan) is a modification that appears to reduce mortality and morbidity at the expense of a period of continued cyanosis and the need (for most patients) of a subsequent procedure to close the hole. Early survivors of the Fontan operation (that is, those

who underwent surgery before 1985) have been shown to have significant late morbidity and a decreased life expectancy. The long-term outcome of patients undergoing surgery in the current era remains to be seen.

REFERENCES

1. Allen HD, Driscoll DJ, Fricker FJ, Herndon P, Mullins CE, Snider AR, Taubert KA: Guidelines for pediatric therapeutic cardiac catheterization. Circulation 84:2248–2258, 1991.
2. Cohen DM: Surgical management of congenital heart disease in the 1990s. Am J Dis Child 146:1447–1452, 1992.

MARFAN SYNDROME

RONALD V. LACRO, M.D.

Marfan syndrome is an autosomal dominant disorder of connective tissue affecting approximately 1 in 10,000 individuals. The most important life-threatening complications include aneurysm of the aorta and aortic dissection. Recent genetic studies have identified abnormalities in the gene encoding for the connective tissue protein fibrillin. Mutations in the fibrillin gene exert a pleiotropic effect, producing multiple, seemingly unrelated phenotypic features that stem from a single genetic change. These features exhibit age dependency and extensive variability, not only between families but also within families. Although the gene responsible for Marfan syndrome has been identified, there is no readily available laboratory test to confirm or exclude this diagnosis. Rather, the diagnosis is made *clinically,* based on characteristic abnormalities of the musculoskeletal, ocular, and cardiovascular systems and a positive family history for the syndrome (Table 1). Early diagnosis is essential for optimal management, which focuses on recognizing abnormalities and altering the natural history of each clinical manifestation as early as possible.

The diagnosis, evaluation, and management of Marfan syndrome require coordinated, multidisciplinary skills. Patients and families are best served in Marfan syndrome clinics with demonstrated interest and expertise in heritable disorders of connective tissue. Multidisciplinary Marfan syndrome clinics are becoming more common. However, when these are unavailable to the family, the primary care physician may assume the responsibility of coordinating complex, multidisciplinary medical care. Even when a Marfan syndrome clinic is available, the pediatrician plays a number of important roles in the management of affected individuals. The primary physician should be familiar with the major features of the syndrome and must make the appropriate initial referrals for diagnosis. Once the diagnosis has been confirmed, the primary care physician can help to screen for age-dependent manifestations, particularly scoliosis. The pediatrician also provides ongoing support and advocacy for the family. Families, as well as clinicians caring for them, benefit greatly from the resources of the National Marfan Foundation.

NATURAL HISTORY AND MANAGEMENT

General guidelines for the management of patients with Marfan syndrome are given in Table 2. All patients should undergo a comprehensive medical evaluation at least annually, with more frequent examinations depending on the severity of clinical manifestations.

Cardiac Features

Up to a third of patients have normal cardiac findings on physical examination, yet nearly all affected individuals have abnormal echocardiograms, most often showing aortic root dilatation and mitral valve prolapse. Aortic dissection and rupture occur against a background of progressive aortic dilatation. A significant amount of dilatation may occur before any clinical symptoms or signs are evident, highlighting the need for early diagnosis of the syndrome, presymptomatic screen-

TABLE 1. Marfan Syndrome: Criteria for Diagnosis*

Skeletal System
Anterior chest deformity, especially asymmetric pectus excavatum/carinatum
Dolichostenomelia (long arms and legs)
Arachnodactyly (long fingers)
Vertebral column deformity
  Scoliosis
  Thoracic lordosis
  Reduced thoracic kyphosis (straight back)
Tall stature
High, narrowly arched palate and dental crowding
Protrusio acetabulae
Abnormal joint mobility
  Congenital flexion contractures
  Hypermobility

Ocular System
Ectopia lentis (subluxation of the lens)†
Flat cornea
Elongated globe
Retinal detachment (much more common after lens removal)
Myopia

Cardiovascular System
Dilatation of the ascending aorta†
Aortic dissection†
Aortic regurgitation
Mitral regurgitation due to mitral valve prolapse
Calcification of the mitral annulus
Mitral valve prolapse
Abdominal aortic aneurysm
Dysrhythmia
Endocarditis

Pulmonary System
Spontaneous pneumothorax
Apical bleb

Skin and Integument
Striae distensae
Inguinal hernia
Other hernia (umbilical, diaphragmatic, incisional)

Central Nervous System
Dural ectasia† (lumbosacral meningocele)
Dilated cisterna magna
Learning disability (verbal-performance discrepancy)
Hyperactivity with or without attention deficit disorder

Genetics
Autosomal dominant inheritance (25%–30% of cases are sporadic, i.e., no family history)

Requirements for Diagnosis
In the absence of an unequivocally affected first-degree relative: involvement of the skeleton and at least two other systems; at least one major manifestation
In the presence of at least one unequivocally affected first-degree relative: involvement of at least two systems; at least one major manifestation preferred, but this will depend somewhat on the family's phenotype
Urine amino acid analysis in the absence of pyridoxine supplementation confirms absence of homocystinuria

Adapted from Beighton P, de Paepe A, Danks D, et al: International nosology of heritable disorders of connective tissue, Berlin, 1986. Am J Med Genet 29:581–594, 1988. Copyright © 1988. Reprinted by permission of Wiley-Liss, a Division of John Wiley and Sons, Inc.
*Listed in approximate order of decreasing specificity.
†Major manifestation.

TABLE 2. Management of Patients with Marfan Syndrome

Regular examinations (at least annually)
  General medical
  Cardiologic, including echocardiography
  Ophthalmologic (more often for those with ectopia lentis or retinal detachment)
  Scoliosis screening until skeletal maturity
  Orthopedic (if indicated)
Examinations as needed
  Neurologic/behavioral
  Physical therapy
  Computed tomographic (CT) scanning or magnetic resonance imaging (MRI) of the aorta or the vertebral column (when echocardiographic imaging is inadequate or when aortic aneurysm distal to the root, aortic dissection, or dural ectasia is suspected)
Discussion with parents, patient, spouse, or significant other regarding psychosocial concerns, genetic counseling, and any new advances in treatment or research
Activity restriction depending on age and cardiovascular features
Antibiotic prophylaxis for bacterial endocarditis (regardless of evident valve pathology)
Therapy with beta-blockers
Prophylactic composite graft or homograft repair of ascending aorta

Adapted from Pyeritz RE: The diagnosis and management of the Marfan syndrome. Am Fam Phys 34:83–94, 1986. Reprinted by permission of the American Academy of Family Physicians.

ing, and careful, long-term follow-up. The prevalence and degree of aortic regurgitation, as well as the risks for dissection and rupture, are proportional to the size of the aortic root. The presence of an aortic root of normal size does not exclude the syndrome completely but makes it less likely and rules out the main life-threatening complication of the disorder.

Individuals with Marfan syndrome should avoid contact sports (including basketball), isometric exercises, weightlifting, and participation in physical activity at maximal exertion or to the point of exhaustion.

All patients should receive prophylaxis for subacute bacterial endocarditis, regardless of evident valve pathology.

Beta-blockers have been effective in slowing the rate of aortic root dilatation, as well as in decreasing the incidence of aortic regurgitation and dissection. The objective of beta-blockade therapy is to reduce the abruptness of ventricular ejection, thereby reducing the physiologic impact on the ascending aorta. Atenolol has the advantages of increased cardiac selectivity and once or twice daily dosing, but propranolol and other beta-blockers are also effective. Counting a patient's heart rate after several minutes of moderate exercise is an easy way to monitor drug compliance and efficacy. In older children, adolescents, and adults, heart rate during exercise should not exceed 100 bpm.

Composite graft operation, in which the ascending aorta and aortic valve are replaced by a synthetic tube that has an artificial valve sewn into the proximal end, is recommended when the aortic root diameter is about 5 to 6 cm. More recently, aortic root replacement with an aortic homograft rather than a prosthetic valve has obviated the need for long-term anticoagulant (coumarin) therapy.

Ophthalmologic Features

All patients should undergo an initial ophthalmologic examination with continued follow-up on at least a yearly basis and more frequently for those with ectopia lentis or retinal detachment. The latter complication is much more common in those who have undergone lens removal.

Skeletal Features

Scoliosis is common and may worsen rapidly during growth spurts. Scoliosis screening should be performed regularly until skeletal maturity has been achieved. Other skeletal findings that may necessitate orthopedic intervention include chest wall abnormalities, flat feet, and joint dislocations.

Neurologic and Behavioral Features

Learning disability and hyperactivity, with or without attention deficit disorder, may lead to school and behavioral difficulties. Pemoline (Cylert) and methylphenidate HCl (Ritalin) therapy have been beneficial in some cases, with the former probably having fewer cardiovascular effects.

Counseling

Prudent management should include regular discussions with parents, patient, spouse, or significant other regarding psychosocial concerns, genetic counseling, and any new advances in treatment or research.

DIFFERENTIAL DIAGNOSIS

Conditions most often considered in the differential diagnosis include homocystinuria, familial or isolated mitral valve prolapse syndrome, familial or isolated annuloaortic ectasia (aortic dissection without clear features of Marfan syndrome), congenital contractural arachnodactyly (Beals syndrome), and Stickler syndrome.

Aortic root dilatation can be seen in a number of other syndromes, including other heritable connective tissue disorders: annuloaortic ectasia, Ehlers-Danlos syndrome types I, II, III, and X, autosomal dominant cutis laxa syndrome, osteogenesis imperfecta types I, III, and IV, and Larsen syndrome. In addition, aortic root dilatation is seen occasionally in Noonan syndrome and Turner's syndrome. The natural history of the aortic manifestations in these other disorders is less well defined, but the recommended follow-up and treatment are essentially the same as for Marfan syndrome.

REFERENCES

1. McKusick VA: The defect in Marfan syndrome. Nature 352:279–281, 1991.
2. Shores J, Berger KR, Murphy EA, Pyeritz RE: Progression of aortic dilatation and the benefit of long-term beta-adrenergic blockade in Marfan's syndrome. N Engl J Med 330:1384–1385, 1994.

CONGESTIVE HEART FAILURE

JACQUELINE A. NOONAN, M.D.

The heart is essentially a pump whose main function is to deliver oxygen to tissues at a rate sufficient to meet metabolic needs. Whenever the pump is unable to meet these needs, heart failure results. Treatment of heart failure depends primarily on the underlying cause and should be directed also at secondary effects of heart failure, namely, fluid and sodium retention. Homeostatic mechanisms come into play whenever metabolic demands are not met, and the syndrome of congestive heart failure results from a variety of compensatory mechanisms. Decrease in oxygen delivery causes the kidneys to increase angiotensin II. There is also an increase in circulatory catecholamines and alpha-adrenergic neural activity. These factors, in turn, cause renal vasoconstriction, with a decrease in glomerular filtration rate and a resultant increase in sodium and fluid reabsorption in the proximal tubules. Another effect is an increase in aldosterone secretion because of an increase in renin angiotensin system activity. This causes the distal tubules of the kidney to increase sodium and fluid reabsorption and to increase potassium excretion. This compensatory mechanism of sodium and fluid retention helps to maintain cardiac output but, unfortunately, leads to undesirable effects of pulmonary congestion, as well as liver congestion and edema.

Heart failure can occur from intrinsic heart muscle dysfunction, with decreased contractility leading to decreased cardiac output. Myocardial ischemia, metabolic derangement, or inflammation can cause primary myocardial dysfunction. Structural heart disease caused by congenital heart disease is a frequent cause of cardiac failure in children. This may result from an abnormal afterload because of pressure overload caused by aortic stenosis, coarctation of the aorta, or pulmonary stenosis. There may be an abnormal excessive preload because of increased volume in the heart as a result of a large left-to-right shunt or AV fistula. Cardiac failure may be caused by obstruction to inflow, as occurs with mitral stenosis, cor triatriatum, or constrictive pericarditis. Reduced afterload and an increase in metabolic needs, caused by hyperthyroidism, anemia, or malnutrition, places a high volume load on the heart and results in so-called high-output heart failure. Respiratory insufficiency from upper airway obstruction, muscle weakness, or severe lung disease with resulting hypoxia may cause pulmonary hypertension and lead to cor pulmonale with cardiac failure. Rapid sustained tachycardia may lead to cardiac failure. In children, there may be a combination of several causes acting in combination, for example, an infant with a ventricular septal defect who is also anemic. An understanding of the basic pathophysiology is essential in choosing the most appropriate therapy for heart failure.

INOTROPIC AGENTS

Myocardial dysfunction may cause an acute reduction in cardiac output, leading to a shocklike picture easily confused with sepsis. Prompt recognition and appropriate treatment are essential, and such patients are best treated in an intensive care unit. Intravenous inotropic agents are most appropriate. Dopamine and dobutamine are used most frequently in children because of their rapid onset of action, their predictable alpha-adrenergic effect on the peripheral vasculature, and their minimal risk of inducing arrhythmia. Dopamine at a dose of 3 to 5 µg/kg/min causes renal vasodilatation, which can improve renal blood flow and increase diuresis. An intermediate dose of 10 to 20 µg/kg/min of dopamine has primarily beta-adrenergic effects, which increase inotropic stimulation of the heart. At higher doses, dopamine has the disadvantage of causing vasoconstriction and may actually limit the increase in cardiac output. Dobutamine is a synthetic sympathomimetic agent that, at recommended dosage, exerts primarily an inotropic effect on the heart and helps increase cardiac output. A combination, therefore, of dopamine to enhance renal blood flow and dobutamine (5 to 10 µg/kg/min) to improve cardiac contractility is used frequently in all pediatric age groups. Isoproterenol has an inotropic effect but also causes peripheral and pulmonary vasodilatation. Unfortunately, isoproterenol has the disadvantage of causing tachycardia and arrhythmia. *All of these potent drugs require close monitoring. They should be administered by an infusion pump, with monitoring of systemic blood pressure, as well as central venous pressure and wedge pressure. Urinary output and peripheral perfusion should be carefully monitored.*

Amiodarone is a nonglycosidic phosphodiesterase inhibitor that improves contractility by increasing cyclic AMP, which causes a subsequent increase in intracellular calcium. Amiodarone results in vasodilatation and reduction in afterload. An intravenous form at a dose of 0.75 µg/kg over several minutes is given to load the patient, followed by a maintenance infusion of 5 to 10 µg/kg/min. This drug has potent vasodilatory effect, so that blood pressure and intravascular volume must be carefully monitored. Thrombocytopenia may occur. Thus, platelet counts must be monitored.

Digoxin is a fundamental therapeutic agent in the treatment of heart failure because of its inotropic effect on the myocardium. Although intravenous digoxin therapy is available and can be used in instances of acute severe heart failure, other parenteral inotropics already mentioned may be safer and more efficacious in the acute situation. Digoxin therapy is perhaps best used when the medication can be given by the oral route. It is widely used in the treatment of heart failure after initial stabilization has occurred or for initial treatment when heart failure occurs more gradually and can be managed at home or in the noncritical care hospital setting. In the premature and newborn infant, digoxin should be used with caution. I generally give neonates a maintenance dose of 5 μg/kg q12h *without* a loading dose. In the older infant or child, 40 μg/kg is a reasonable digitalizing dose and can be given in divided doses (one half given at the onset and one quarter given q6–8h for two additional doses). Maintenance is usually 10 μg/kg given once a day or divided into q12h doses. Newborns may have an endogenous digitalis-like substance in the blood, making digoxin levels difficult to interpret. Determination of digoxin levels is not necessary for the routine management of patients with cardiac failure. The electrocardiogram and clinical status should be sufficient. Levels may be useful in patients with impaired renal function or electrolyte disturbance or when drugs known to alter digoxin levels, such as verapamil, quinidine, and amiodarone, also are prescribed. If any dysarrhythmia occurs, digoxin toxicity should be considered, and a digoxin level should be obtained.

AFTERLOAD REDUCTION

When myocardial function is impaired, with resulting low cardiac output and elevated systemic vascular resistance, the use of an arterial dilator or vasodilator may be very beneficial. Intravenous sodium nitroprusside at 0.25 to 5.0 μg/kg/min, with adequate monitoring, will result in a decrease in systemic resistance. If falls in blood pressure and filling pressures result, it may be necessary to give adequate volume to raise the filling pressures to sustain cardiac preload. For this reason, measurement of cardiac output during nitroprusside infusion can be very helpful. Measurement of both cardiac output and systemic vascular resistance will allow the appropriate titration of inotropic agents, vasodilators, and fluid replacement. Nitroprusside, if used beyond 24 hours, must be monitored for serum thiocyanide levels (toxic metabolite).

Other effective vasodilators include hydralazine and captopril. Hydralazine acts directly on smooth muscle and is available on both IV and PO forms. Captopril is an angiotensin-converting enzyme inhibitor (the enzyme that converts angiotensin I to angiotensin II). With blocking of the formation of angiotensin II, a powerful vasoconstrictor, vasodilatation occurs, aldosterone secretion is lowered, renal blood flow is increased, and sodium diuresis occurs. The result is a decrease in systemic resistance, a lowering of ventricular filling, and a rise in cardiac output. Captopril is used commonly in hypertensive patients following coarctation surgery, as well as in postoperative patients undergoing a Fontan operation. This medication is usually well tolerated if blood pressure is monitored. The captopril dose for an infant under 6 months is 0.05 to 1 mg/kg/d divided into two to three doses. (In neonates, captopril has caused renal failure and must be used with caution.) In children above 6 months, the dose is 1 to 5 mg/kg/d divided into two to three doses. The onset of action is fairly rapid (within minutes in some individuals). Thus, blood pressure and renal function should be monitored.

DIURETICS

In acute heart failure, diuretics should be used with caution. If there is evidence of pulmonary edema, furosemide at 1 mg/kg per dose may improve the congestive symptoms and decrease preload, especially in volume overload lesions, such as large left-to-right shunts

or severe anemia. With pressure overload lesions, such as critical aortic stenosis or coarctation of the aorta, or with primary myocardial dysfunction, furosemide should be used cautiously in case volume preservation is needed to maintain adequate cadiac output. Diuretics should be used only when there is evidence of volume overload. In chronic heart failure, fluid retention is frequent, and diuretics often are helpful in management. Furosemide may be given IV, IM, or PO. The usual oral dose is 1 to 2 mg/kg per dose. Hypokalemia may occur, and potassium supplementation may be required. The addition of spironolactone 1.5 to 3 mg/kg/d in two to three divided doses often is used along with furosemide as an aldosterone blocker to increase potassium retention. When spironolactone is used with furosemide, additional potassium supplementation should be avoided. Both chlorothiazide and hydrochlorothiazide are less potent diuretics than furosemide, and both require concomitant potassium supplementation. When fluid retention becomes a problem in spite of adequate furosemide, the addition of metolazone PO at 0.2 to 0.4 mg/kg/d often will cause a brisk diuresis. Electrolytes and liver function studies should be followed closely when this potent diuretic is used.

PROSTAGLANDIN E₁

In the newborn with severe left ventricular outflow obstruction, acute cardiac failure may result when the ductus arteriosus narrows and cardiac output falls. This is particularly true in infants with interrupted aortic arch or severe coarctation of the aorta and may also occur in severe aortic stenosis. Diminished cardiac output results in metabolic acidosis, with poor renal perfusion, decreased urinary output, and possible rise in potassium. It is important to recognize this cause of heart failure, which can be established by echocardiography. Once the diagnosis is made, prostaglandin E_1 (PGE_1) should be started immediately at 0.05 to 0.1 μg/kg/min to dilate the ductus and improve the cardiac output and perfusion. An endotracheal tube for intubation and a ventilator should be available in case apnea occurs during the early use of PGE_1.

SURGICAL TREATMENT

If the primary cause of congestive heart failure is identified as severe obstruction, either cardiac catheter interventional therapy or surgical treatment is indicated. Balloon dilatation or surgical valvotomy for critical aortic stenosis or repair of coarctation of the aorta or interrupted aortic arch should be planned on an urgent basis. The patient should be stabilized with an inotropic agent and an infusion of PGE_1. Acid-base balance should be corrected while the patient is awaiting the surgical procedure. In any infant or child who develops cardiac failure secondary to a cardiac defect, surgical repair should be recommended if feasible. Palliative surgeries, such as pulmonary artery banding, may be helpful in those patients who have a cardiac lesion, such as a single ventricle, not amenable to total correction. Unless there is prompt resolution of the cardiac failure and the natural history of the cardiac lesion is favorable, surgical repair should be carried out in a timely fashion. A moderate-size ventricular septal defect may cause cardiac failure, but with appropriate medical treatment and close follow-up, it may become smaller, with complete recovery from heart failure and with a benign long-term prognosis. Surgical repair in such patients may not be necessary. If and when cardiac failure occurs in a patient with a congenital heart defect, it is a serious complication, often requiring surgical treatment for a good outcome.

TRANSFUSION

An increase in hematocrit in patients with congestive heart failure will improve the oxygen-carrying capacity to tissues and may be particularly helpful in improving heart failure in infants with large left-to-right shunts. The cautious use of packed red cells may be helpful for such patients. If acute heart failure is a result of severe anemia, it is essential to determine whether the anemia is acute or long standing. In the case of severe, chronic anemia, such as that due to iron deficiency, partial exchange transfusion should be given to avoid even further volume overload in an already failing heart.

PERICARDIOCENTESIS

Cardiac tamponade is an uncommon cause of acute cardiac failure in children. This may occur secondary to injury, as a postoperative complication, or as the result of acute pericarditis, particularly of a bacterial infectious etiology. Accumulation of blood or fluid in the pericardium will compress the cardiac chambers, leading to impaired diastolic ventricular filling and a markedly decreased cardiac output. Pericardiocentesis may be life saving and should be performed by a skilled operator.

RESPIRATORY SUPPORT

Acute cor pulmonale from respiratory insufficiency may result from upper airway obstruction, muscle weakness, or severe lung disease. Correction of hypoxia and hypercarbia by ventilatory support is essential, since successful treatment of the respiratory problem often will relieve the heart failure.

OTHER SUPPORTIVE MEASURES

Infants in cardiac failure often have respiratory compromise, and the use of an infant seat may cause symptomatic improvement. In the older child, elevation of the head of the bed or the use of a cardiac chair may be of benefit. Oxygen supplementation may help tissue perfusion, particularly when pulmonary congestion is present. It is important to maintain normal body temperature. If respiratory insufficiency develops, mechanical ventilation may be necessary.

Since many infants with chronic heart failure have failure to thrive, an adequate diet is essential. Digoxin and diuretics often are effective in controlling congestion, so that milk formulas can be prescribed not to exceed 24 kcal/oz. Low-salt formulas are not usually necessary. Tube feedings may be necessary to supply adequate calories for growth. In children with venous congestion and peripheral edema, a no-added-salt diet is recommended. This may need to be modified to satisfy the child's food preference.

Patients with cardiomyopathy sometimes benefit from L-carnitine supplementation. Metabolic defects are being recognized with increasing frequency so that in all patients with cardiomyopathy, determination of the carnitine level may be useful, and L-carnitine can be prescribed if indicated.

PROGNOSIS

Prognosis depends on the underlying cause of the heart failure. If the cardiac failure is the result of a heart lesion amenable to surgical correction and a successful operation is carried out, prognosis usually is excellent. Cardiac failure may occur in the postoperative period but usually resolves with appropriate treatment if the surgical procedure has been successful. Successful treatment of anemia, hypertension, or respiratory insufficiency also leads to a good prognosis. In those patients where the underlying cause of heart failure persists, as in some patients with cardiomyopathy, the long-term prognosis is more uncertain. Some patients may remain fairly asymptomatic, with prolonged medical treatment for congestive heart failure, but if poor myocardial function persists, the long-term prognosis is poor. Fortunately, cardiac transplantation is available for some of these patients.

REFERENCES

1. Artman M, Graham TP, Jr: Guidelines for vasodilator therapy of congestive heart failure in infants and children. Am Heart J 1987, 113:994.
2. Talner NS: Heart failure. *In* Adams FH, Emmanouilides GC, Riemenschneider TA (eds): Moss' Heart Disease in Infants, Children and Adolescents, 4th ed. Baltimore, Williams & Wilkins, 1989:660–675.

MITRAL VALVE PROLAPSE

CHARLES A. BULLABOY, M.D.

The mitral valve prolapse (MVP) conundrum began in the early 1960s, with phonocardiographic documentation that midsystolic clicks and late systolic murmurs emanated from the mitral valve apparatus. Known by 44 synonyms and associated with at least 62 clinical entities, MVP is the most common congenital cardiac abnormality, with a conservative pediatric prevalence of 2% to 4%. An autosomal dominant pattern of inheritance with variable expressivity is postulated with a female/male ratio of approximately 2:1. Pathologically, myxomatous proliferation of the mitral valve matrix is present, along with alterations in the collagen substrate of the chordae tendineae and mitral annulus, perhaps as a manifestation of a generalized mesenchymal or connective tissue disorder.

The overwhelming majority of patients with MVP are asymptomatic, but some may have complaints of fatigue, exercise intolerance, palpitations, dizziness, presyncope (rarely syncope), and chest pain. The chest pain is typically nonanginal, nonexertional, sharp, fleeting, and localized over the left precordial area. This symptom complex may represent a hyperadrenergic state with autonomic imbalance. The body habitus frequently is gracile, with associated skeletal findings of pectus excavatum or carinatum, thoracic scoliosis, and ligamentous laxity. The variability in timing, intensity, and duration of the auscultatory findings are best conceptualized by the ventriculovalvar disproportion. Provocative maneuvers that decrease the left ventricular end-diastolic volume or increase the rate of left ventricular contractility move the midlate systolic click(s) or murmur closer to the first heart sound. A unique apical honk or whoop, occasionally audible to the naked ear with the patient upright, may be unappreciated if auscultation is performed only with the patient supine.

A resting electrocardiogram is recommended for all patients to evaluate the rhythm, corrected QT interval, and presence of any ST-T changes (T-wave flattening or inversion in leads II, III, aVF, V_5, and V_6). In the absence of mitral regurgitation or associated cardiac defects, chest roentgenography generally is unnecessary and unrevealing, except for the possible skeletal findings. Systolic superior displacement of either mitral valve leaflet above the atrioventricular junction into the left atrium on cross-sectional echocardiography in the parasternal long axis view is both sensitive and specific for MVP. Symptomatic patients, those desiring to participate in competitive athletics, and those at high risk (i.e., family history of sudden premature death, T wave, or QT_c abnormalities, dysrhythmias, or moderate to greater mitral regurgitation) should be evaluated with 24-hour ambulatory electrocardiography and exercise stress testing.

The natural history of the low-risk patient with only an isolated click is typically benign and nonprogressive. Patient education, family counseling, and reassurance about the favorable outcome is mandatory to prevent cardiac neurosis. Sudden death is rare. Only the presence of malignant dysrhythmias, Marfan syndrome or other connective tissue disorders, or significant mitral regurgitation should disqualify such patients from strenuous physical endeavors. The symptomatic patient with a nonrevealing diagnostic evaluation should have a trial of observation with avoidance of volume depletion and any stimulants before resorting to beta-blocker therapy with propranolol (1 to 3 mg/kg/d PO divided q6–8h) or, in the older patient, atenolol (1 to 2 mg/kg/d PO, maximum 50 to 100 mg). These agents should be stepped down or weaned after a reasonable, symptom-free interval (3 to 6 months). The criteria for treatment of dysrhythmias are the same as for any patients with dysrhythmia. Beta-blockers have been found to be extremely effective in these individuals (Table 1). The MVP patient with transient ischemic attacks and no other forthcoming diagnosis should be treated with platelet inhibitors, either acetylsalicylic acid (ASA) (3 to 5 mg/kg/d PO, maximum 325 mg) or dipyridamole (3 to 5 mg/kg/d PO; typical adult dosage 25 mg t.i.d.). Progressive

TABLE 1. Drug Treatment for Mitral Valve Prolapse

DRUG	DOSE	COMMENT
Acetylsalicylic acid (ASA)	3–5 mg/kg/d PO Max: 325 mg	For antiplatelet effect
Atenolol	1–3 mg/kg/d PO Max: 50–100 mg	Less CNS side effects than propranolol; beta-1 selective
Captopril	0.1–2.0 mg/kg per dose PO q8–12h 6.25–25 mg per dose PO q8–12h for adolescent	Hypotension, cough, dysgeusia, neutropenia, proteinuria, renal failure in sodium-depleted patient
Dipyridamole	3–5 mg/kg/d PO, up to 25–50 mg 1–3 times/d	
Enalapril	0.04–0.10 mg/kg per dose PO q12–24h	Same as captopril
Propranolol	1–3 mg/kg/d PO divided q6–8h	Depression, nightmares, hypoglycemia, decreased cardiac contractility, conduction disturbances, increased LDL and VDL; contraindicated in asthma

mitral regurgitation is treated medically with digoxin, diuretics, vasodilator therapy with angiotensin-converting enzyme inhibitors (captopril or enalapril), and, if necessary, definitive surgery, either valvuloplasty or replacement. Endocarditis prophylaxis is recommended for all until the divergent opinions concerning this subject are resolved.

REFERENCE

1. Judd VE: Mitral valve prolapse. *In* Garson A Jr, Bricker JT, McNamara DG (eds): The Science and Practice of Pediatric Cardiology. Philadelphia, Lea & Febiger, 1990:1973–1986.

ACUTE MANAGEMENT OF CARDIAC ARRHYTHMIAS

EDWARD P. WALSH, M.D.

The spectrum of cardiac rhythm disturbances is quite diverse (Table 1), and the key to effective long-term management is accurate diagnosis of the precise arrhythmia mechanism. Therefore, with the exception of premature beats and a few common forms of supraventricular tachycardia, children with rhythm disturbances should be referred to a pediatric cardiologist for more detailed evaluation after initial stabilization. The long-term management plan will be strongly influenced by an in-depth analysis that can pinpoint the arrhythmia mechanism and evaluate the patient for underlying organic heart disease. For the practicing pediatrician, this chapter focuses primarily on acute therapy for cardiac arrhythmias at the time of initial presentation.

PREMATURE BEATS

Occasional premature beats are fairly common in the pediatric age group. When extrasystoles are detected on a physical examination, an electrocardiogram (ECG) should be performed to determine whether they are of atrial or ventricular origin.

Atrial premature beats may occur at any age, including fetal life. In an asymptomatic young patient, isolated atrial extrasystoles do not require therapy.

Occasional *ventricular premature beats* (VPBs) are likewise most often benign, but a small subset of these patients may have serious underlying organic heart disease as the substrate for their ventricular ectopy. Therefore, a more concentrated effort must be made to exclude the possibility of underlying cardiac disease, which involves careful history and physical examination, a formal 12-lead ECG, and possibly a chest x-ray. If any question remains, even in the absence of symptoms, the patient should be referred to a cardiologist. Ventricular ectopy occurring in a patient with a potentially abnormal heart should be investigated further with Holter monitoring, exercise stress testing, and echocardiography. In an otherwise healthy and asymptomatic patient, occasional isolated ventricular premature beats do not require treatment. The benign forms of ventricular ectopy typically occur in a teenage patient, are generally suppressed with exercise, show no repetitive activity (i.e., no couplets or salvos), and have one uniform QRS morphology.

TACHYCARDIAS

When a patient first experiences a sustained tachycardia, the proper first step is to perform a 12-lead ECG and determine whether the QRS complex is narrow or wide. Tachycardias with a narrow QRS complex that is identical to normal sinus rhythm can be safely assumed to be the result of a supraventricular mechanism and are associated with a good prognosis. On the other hand, if the tachycardia has a wide QRS complex, ventricular tachycardia (VT) should be considered as the primary diagnosis, and the prognosis is much more guarded. Some forms of supraventricular tachycardia (SVT) can cause a wide QRS complex if bundle-branch aberration or an accessory pathway, such as Wolff-Parkinson White (WPW) syndrome, is present. However, it is difficult to distinguish these atypical forms of SVT from VT in the acute setting.

Supraventricular Tachycardia

By far the most common mechanism for SVT in the pediatric age group involves reentry, either via an accessory pathway or within the AV node. Acute treatment of these disorders is similar and begins with physical maneuvers aimed at increasing vagal tone, such as application of ice to the face, immersion of the face in very cold water (for older patients able to hold their breath), an intense Valsalva maneuver with strain lasting at least 10 seconds (for patients old enough to cooperate), or carotid sinus massage. Vagal maneuvers are

TABLE 1. Classification of Arrhythmias

Premature Beats
Atrial premature beats
Ventricular premature beats

Tachycardias
Supraventricular tachycardia (SVT)
 Atrial flutter
 Atrial fibrillation
 Ectopic atrial tachycardia
 Multifocal atrial tachycardia
 AV nodal reentry
 Reentry via Wolff-Parkinson-White (WPW) accessory pathway
 Reentry via concealed accessory pathway
Ventricular tachycardia (VT)
 Monomorphic reentry
 Polymorphic reentry
 Automatic focus
 Torsade de pointes

Bradycardias
Sinus bradycardia
Tachybrady syndrome
AV block
 First degree
 Second degree (Mobitz I type)
 Second degree (Mobitz II type)
 Third degree (congenital)
 Third degree (acquired)

effective in acutely terminating these forms of SVT in about 20% to 30% of cases. If this fails, an intravenous line should be placed for administration of adenosine. Adenosine acts by transiently blocking conduction within the AV node and terminates almost all of the common forms of SVT. It has a very short half-life (about 10 seconds) because of its rapid metabolism by endothelial cells and blood cells. Thus, in order for an effective bolus to reach the heart, the drug must be administered very quickly in a vein as close to the central circulation as possible (such as the antecubital vein). The starting dose in children is 0.1 mg/kg given by rapid IV push and followed by a generous flush of saline. An effect should be seen within 30 seconds. If tachycardia persists, a second dose of 0.2 mg/kg can be tried.

If tachycardia does not terminate with administration of adenosine, consultation with a cardiologist usually is indicated. It may be that the SVT is caused by one of the less common mechanisms listed in Table 1, many of which respond to adenosine with only transient AV block but persistence of the rapid atrial rate. Examples include atrial flutter or ectopic atrial tachycardia, where adenosine has minimal effect on atrial tissue but can serve to unmask the abnormal atrial activity during the brief period of blocked conduction to the ventricles. Adenosine may be of more diagnostic than therapeutic use in this setting. After consultation, other pharmacologic maneuvers may be attempted for some of the less common forms of SVT, including verapamil (to be used only in children over 1 year of age), procainamide, or esmolol. Alternatively, overdrive pacing with a transesophageal electrode can be attempted if equipment is available and an experienced individual is on hand. If at any time a patient appears to have either compromised arterial blood pressure, advanced congestive heart failure, or altered consciousness, a synchronized DC cardioversion should be performed. An energy of 0.25 to 0.5 J/kg is usually a sufficient starting dose for SVT. Since cardioversion is a painful procedure, patients should be properly sedated before delivery of the energy.

Following successful conversion of SVT, a repeat 12-lead ECG should be obtained immediately, with the patient in sinus rhythm. The presence of anterograde preexcitation (the delta wave of WPW syndrome) is important to note on the sinus rhythm ECG, since the long-term management of this disorder may differ from that of other forms of SVT. If the sinus rhythm ECG is entirely normal, it may be necessary to refer the patient for electrophysiology testing with either transesophageal or intracardiac catheters to determine the precise cause of the tachycardia.

Long-term management of the tachycardia should be chosen in consultation with the cardiologist. This may begin with simple coaching of vagal techniques so that the patient or family can manage SVT themselves. This course of action is appropriate for cases where SVT is infrequent and does not cause severe symptoms. In cases of frequently recurring SVT, consideration is often given to transcatheter ablation procedures using radiofrequency electrical current delivered through an intracardiac catheter. The success rate of this procedure exceeds 95% at centers with experienced operators. In very young patients who may be at slightly higher risk of complications from an interventional catheterization, chronic antiarrhythmic medications may be used instead.

It should, above all, be remembered that SVT is rarely if ever a life-threatening rhythm disturbance. Acute episodes should be approached calmly and carefully, concentrating on obtaining good quality data with 12-lead ECGs in both SVT and normal sinus rhythm. The mode of chronic therapy is likewise chosen carefully after considering patient age, severity of symptoms, the presence or absence of underlying heart disease, and the exact arrhythmia mechanism.

Ventricular Tachycardia

An acute episode of VT should be treated as an emergency. It typically occurs in the setting of organic heart disease (such as repaired congenital heart defects or cardiomyopathy) or a primary electrical abnormality of the heart (such as the long QT syndrome). VT is much less predictable than SVT, and the patients are at risk for abrupt degeneration into ventricular fibrillation. Although some forms of SVT may mimic VT in terms of a wide QRS complex on ECG, it is extremely difficult to make the distinction in an acute setting. Thus, all tachycardias with a wide QRS should be treated as ventricular tachycardia until definitely proven otherwise.

At initial presentation, basic stabilization with attention to airway and breathing should be instituted promptly, and it is once again important that a 12-lead ECG be obtained. Any patient who is hypotensive or unresponsive should be treated immediately with direct current cardioversion. If the patient is awake and has adequate perfusion, an initial attempt at pharmacologic conversion can be made with lidocaine, using a dose of 1 mg/kg administered by rapid IV push. This dose may be repeated at 10-minute intervals for two subsequent doses.

In addition to lidocaine, medications for VT must be chosen based on the ECG appearance of the tachycardia. If the QRS has one single morphology (monomorphic VT), IV procainamide is the most reasonable second-line drug choice. However, if the QRS has a varying morphology where the direction of the QRS varies and seems to twist around the isoelectric baseline (torsade de pointes related to QT prolongation), procainamide should be avoided, and the patient should be treated instead with magnesium sulfate at a dose of 25 mg/kg by slow IV push over 10 minutes.

If at any time during initial treatment the patient has deterioration in perfusion or consciousness, DC cardioversion should be used. An energy dose of 1 J/kg can be tried initially, with the energy doubled on each subsequent attempt. If the tachycardia accelerates or degenerates into ventricular fibrillation, higher energy shocks in the range of 2 J/kg should be used.

Consultation with a cardiologist should be sought for every patient with a wide QRS tachycardia. Formal electrophysiologic testing in the catheterization laboratory usually is required to arrive at an accurate determination of the arrhythmia mechanism and to choose long-term therapy. Chronic management of VT is difficult. If there is underlying organic heart disease that can be improved by medical or surgical techniques, aggressive efforts should be made to improve the underlying hemodynamic status. Specific therapy for the VT usually begins with serial trials of chronic oral medications. In patients with life-threatening VT who do not respond to drugs, implantation of an automatic internal defibrillator may be necessary. Some specific forms of VT caused by a discrete automatic focus or reentry within the His-Purkinje system may be treated with transcatheter ablation techniques.

BRADYCARDIAS

Slow heart rhythm can result from disorders of impulse generation (sinus bradycardia) or impulse conduction (atrioventricular block). *Sinus bradycardia* is usually a secondary phenomenon in the pediatric age group, resulting from hypoxia, sepsis, or hypoglycemia. Treatment of the underlying cause is usually the only necessary therapy. Primary disease of the sinus node may be observed in patients who have undergone surgery for congenital heart disease, particularly the Mustard, Senning, and Fontan operations. Dysfunction of the sinus node may be further complicated by intermittent tachyarrhythmias, such as atrial fibrillation and atrial flutter, and this clinical picture is often referred to as the *tachybrady syndrome*. Symptoms in these patients are more generally caused by the fast heart rhythms rather than the slow sinus rhythm, but in some situations, it may be necessary to accelerate the underlying heart rate transiently. This usually can be accomplished with atropine or isoproterenol. Artificial pacing can be employed, using either temporary pacing from a transesophageal electrode or permanent pacing with an implanted pacemaker generator. Permanent pacing often is necessary in patients with the tachybrady syndrome when chronic antiarrhythmic drugs are needed to control recurrent tachyarrhythmias. In this setting, medications often slow down the already compromised rhythm, and this effect can be offset only by the concomitant implantation of a pacemaker.

AV conduction disturbances are divided into three grades (Table 1). *First degree AV block* is generally benign and does not require treatment. Occasional *second degree heart block* may be a normal

TABLE 2. Antiarrhythmic Drugs and Cardioversion

DRUG	DOSE
Adenosine	0.1–0.2 mg/kg rapid IV push
Esmolol	0.5 mg/kg rapid IV push, followed by infusion of 50–250 µg/kg/min
Verapamil	0.05–0.1 mg/kg rapid IV push (not for use in infants or any patient taking beta-blocker)
Lidocaine	1 mg/kg rapid IV push, may repeat to total of 3 doses at 10-min intervals, followed by infusion of 20–50 µg/kg/min
Procainamide	7–15 mg/kg IV over 15 min, followed by infusion of 20–60 µg/kg/min
Magnesium sulfate	25 mg/kg IV over 10–15 min
Cardioversion	SVT: 0.5 J/kg, double and repeat if needed VT: 1 J/kg, double and repeat if needed VF: 2 J/kg, double and repeat if needed

finding in otherwise healthy patients, particularly while asleep. Second degree block that occurs in the setting of organic heart disease or is associated with symptoms may require implantation of a permanent pacemaker.

Third degree block may be subdivided into either congenital or acquired forms. Congenital heart block is typically first diagnosed in utero and is most often the result of exposure to maternal lupus antibodies. Most of these patients require a pacemaker by the time they reach adulthood, but, in general, the prognosis is excellent. Most patients with congenital heart block can be followed conservatively for many years until they have reached an age and size where implantation of a permanent transvenous pacemaker is a fairly easy undertaking. Acquired third degree AV block may be seen after repair of congenital heart disease or after certain infections (Lyme disease, myocarditis, endocarditis). Postoperative patients with third degree heart block that persists for more than 10 days after surgery should be treated with a pacemaker. Likewise, persistent third degree heart block caused by infection should be treated with a permanent pacemaker.

ANTIARRHYTHMIC MEDICATIONS AND ELECTRICAL CARDIOVERSION

Drug doses and energy requirements for cardioversion are reviewed in Table 2 for quick reference. This list is restricted to medications used in the acute setting by intravenous administration. Chronic oral medications should be chosen after consultation with a cardiologist.

REFERENCES

1. Moak JP: Pharmacology and electrophysiology of antiarrhythmic drugs. *In* Gillette PC, Garson A (eds): Pediatric Arrhythmias: Electrophysiology and Pacing. Philadelphia, WB Saunders, 1990:37–118.
2. Walsh EP, Saul JP: Transcatheter ablation for pediatric tachyarrhythmias using radiofrequency electrical energy. Pediatr Ann. 1991;20:386–392.
3. Walsh EP, Saul JP: Cardiac arrhythmias. *In* Fyler DC (ed): Nadas's Pediatric Cardiology. Philadelphia, Hanley and Belfus, 1992:377–435.

THE CHILD AT RISK OF CORONARY DISEASE AS AN ADULT

ALBERT P. ROCCHINI, M.D.

Coronary artery disease has its origin in childhood. Coronary atherosclerotic fatty streaks appear in Americans as early as the second decade of life, and fibrous plaques have been found at autopsy in adolescents and young adults who have died accidentally. Epidemiologic and clinical studies in adults with coronary heart disease have made it possible to develop a list of risk factors that can help to identify individuals susceptible to the development of coronary heart disease. The risk factors identified are increased blood levels of cholesterol, elevated blood pressure, cigarette smoking, obesity and poor physical fitness. This section focuses on how four of these risk factors (lipids, cigarette smoking, reduced physical activity, and obesity) affect the development of cardiovascular disease and the types of therapy currently being used to modify them.

SMOKING

Cigarette smoking is the major avoidable cardiovascular risk factor. One of the most disturbing features about smoking is that since 1964 over 30 million Americans have stopped cigarette smoking, yet cigarette smoking has not decreased in its prevalence rate among adolescents. Thus, adolescent subjects represent the largest group of individuals at risk to start cigarette smoking. Smoking is known to increase cardiovascular risk directly by altering blood pressure regulation, by increasing total serum cholesterol, and by decreasing HDL-cholesterol levels.

The most effective way of treating smoking is through prevention. Since the incidence of smoking is highest among adolescents, it is this age group for whom smoking prevention is most critical. Most studies have shown that a school-based prevention program, beginning in grade 6 with booster sessions throughout the remaining 6 years of secondary education, can result in a significant reduction in the incidence of adolescent smoking.

LIPIDS

Based on numerous epidemiologic surveys, hyperlipidemia is known to be an important risk factor for the development of adult onset heart disease. To understand abnormalities of lipid metabolism and their treatment, it is important to understand the process by which the body handles cholesterol. Cholesterol from dietary fat is digested, absorbed, and reprocessed in the liver. The liver then secretes the reprocessed cholesterol into either the intestine as bile or into the bloodstream in combination with triglycerides as very low-density lipoprotein (VLDL) particles. The VLDL particles are converted in the plasma to low-density lipoproteins (LDL), which can then be taken up by the cells and reconverted back into cholesterol. The LDL particles are guided by apoproteins, lipoprotein surface proteins, to the LDL receptor sites on the cell. *The number of LDL receptors and their affinity for apoproteins determine the level of cholesterol in the blood.*

Cells prefer to use exogenous cholesterol rather than to manufacture it. This preferential usage depends on a biochemical feedback system whereby raising intracellular cholesterol levels reduces cholesterol production by inhibiting the enzyme 3-hydroxy-3-methylglutaryl coenzyme A (HMG CoA) reductase and by activating the enzyme acyl coenzyme A transferase (ACAT), which esterfies cholesterol for storage. Increased intracellular cholesterol also reduces cellular LDL-cholesterol uptake by blocking formation of LDL receptor proteins and by inhibiting LDL receptor gene expression.

Intracellular cholesterol that is not used or stored by the cell is passed out of the cell and combines with recycled LDL particles to form high-density lipoprotein (HDL) particles. These HDL particles eventually are removed from the circulation by the liver. The formation of HDL-cholesterol is the major way in which excess cholesterol is removed from cells.

Abnormalities in the method by which the cell handles LDL receptor formation is the cause of one of the common genetic forms of hyperlipidemia, familial hypercholesterolemia. In this disease, there is an alteration in either the number or function of LDL receptors, leading to a reduced binding of LDL-cholesterol to the receptors, a higher serum LDL-cholesterol concentration, a higher plasma cholesterol, and atherogenesis.

Historical information is of prime importance in determining which child should be screened for hyperlipidemia. The most important feature is a family history (parent or grandparent) of premature atherosclerotic disease, defined as the appearance of clinical manifestations of atherosclerosis before 50 years of age for men and 60 years in women. Several other historical features also can suggest the presence of hyperlipidemia. These include a history of recurrent unexplained pancreatitis or abdominal pain (seen with exogenous hyperchylomicronemia, familial hypertriglyceridemia, or familial combined hyperlipidemia), a history of an abnormal glucose tolerance or hyperuricemia (seen with all types of hypertriglyceridemia), a history of xanthoma (seen with familial hypercholesterolemia), and information suggesting a systemic disease that is secondarily associated with hyperlipoproteinemia, such as thyroid disease, liver disease, renal disease, or diabetes. *Lipid screening is recommended only if a child has a history compatible with hyperlipidemia* (Figs. 1 to 3).

Determination of plasma levels of lipoproteins ultimately is the method for finding the presence or absence of hyperlipidemia. Ideally, a blood sample should be drawn after a 12 to 14 hour fast. Interpretation of the plasma values of these lipoproteins should be made with consideration of what constitutes normality. As with most clinical laboratory tests, normals are based on a statistical distribution of values in the general population. Traditionally, values greater than the 90th percentile cutoff have been employed for defining abnormal cholesterol and triglycerides (Table 1).

The cornerstone of lipid management regardless of cause is diet. Both the saturated fat content and the cholesterol content of the diet must be reduced to obtain and maintain maximum dietary benefit. Saturated fat appears to increase the synthesis of LDL-cholesterol and decrease LDL-cholesterol disposal. Polyunsaturated fat decreases VLDL-triglyceride, cholesterol, and apoprotein-B synthesis. Monounsaturated fats, such as olive oil and peanut oil, are especially beneficial in that they not only reduce LDL-cholesterol but also reduce the LDL-cholesterol/HDL-cholesterol ratio. Another way in which changes in diet can lower cholesterol is to increase the intake of high fiber food, such as oatbran, beans, and other-water soluble fibers. Marine or omega-3 fatty acids also can cause a reduction in VLDL triglycerides, primarily by decreasing VLDL synthesis. With dietary management alone, one can expect a 5% to 20% decrease in choles-

terol. The standard dietary recommendation is an American Heart Association phase I diet, which contains 30% of calories as fat, 55% as carbohydrates, and 15% as protein. The fat should be approximately equally divided among polyunsaturated, monounsaturated, and saturated fats. The major source of carbohydrates should be complex carbohydrates, and the cholesterol intake should be below 300 mg/d. If cholesterol elevation persists, the next approach involves a phased reduction in cholesterol intake to 100 mg/d, with 20% of the calories as fat with equal components of saturated, monounsaturated, and polyunsaturated, 65% as carbohydrates, and 15% as protein. Other than diet, the other two nonpharmacologic forms of therapy for hyperlipidemia are weight reduction and exercise.

The goal of therapy should be to reduce total cholesterol below 200 mg/dl and LDL-cholesterol below 120 mg/dl while maintaining HDL-cholesterol greater than 40 mg/dl. If these goals cannot be reached by nonpharmacologic therapy alone, pharmacologic agents must be considered. However, because pharmacologic agents are not without side effects, especially in the growing child, most pediatric lipid specialists do not recommend adding lipid-lowering drugs unless dietary means are unable to reduce total cholesterol below 250 mg/dl and LDL-cholesterol to below 175 mg/dl.

Table 2 lists some of the drugs used to treat hyperlipidemia. In the pediatric population, bile acid resins are the most commonly used first-line lipid-lowering drug. The bile acid resins bind bile acids in the intestines and prevent their reabsorption. As a result, there is increased conversion in the liver of cholesterol to bile acid, which ultimately leads to the reduction in hepatic cholesterol content and to an up regulation of LDL receptor synthesis and an increased disposal of LDL-cholesterol from plasma. Unfortunately, as the intracellular content of cholesterol decreases, cellular cholesterol synthesis increases, thus reducing the cholesterol-lowering efficacy of the resins. Therefore, to lower the LDL-cholesterol level further, it may be necessary to use a resin in combination with one of the other drugs that block cholesterol synthesis, such as niacin or lovastatin (Mevacor).

It is important to remember that although there is increasing evidence in the adult that treatment of hyperlipidemia can result in a reduction in coronary mortality and even regression of atherosclerotic

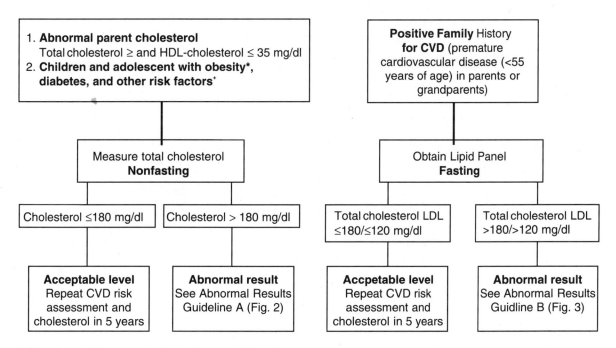

* Obesity = 30% overweight for height. ⁺ High blood pressure, diabetes mellitius, oral contraceptives, unobtainable family history.

FIGURE 1. Screening children (>5 years of age) and adolescents for hypercholesterolemia.

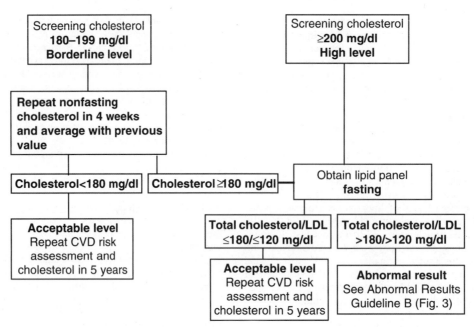

FIGURE 2. Abnormal results: Abnormal nonfasting cholesterol.

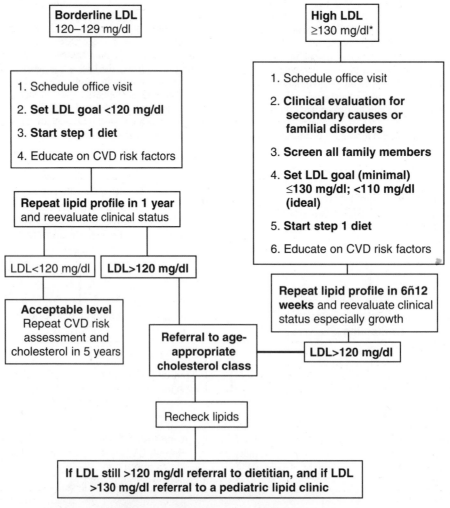

FIGURE 3. Abnormal results: abnormal LDL-cholesterol.

TABLE 1. 90th Percentile by Age and Sex for Cholesterol, LDL-Cholesterol, and Triglycerides and 10th Percentile for HDL-Cholesterol

AGE (y)	WHITE MALES				WHITE FEMALES			
	5–9	10–14	15–19	20–24	5–9	10–14	15–19	20–24
Total cholesterol (mg/dl)	191	190	183	204	195	190	191	214
LDL-cholesterol (mg/dl)	117	122	123	138	125	126	129	141
Triglycerides (mg/dl)	85	102	120	165	90	114	114	141
HDL-cholesterol* (mg/dl)	42	40	34	32	38	40	38	37

*10th percentile.
From the lipid research clinics's population studies data book, vol 1. The prevalence study. Lipid Metabolism Branch Division of Heart, Lung and Vascular Disease, National Heart, Lung and Blood Institute, U.S. Department of Health and Human Services, Public Health Services, NIH publication No. 80-1527, Washington, DC, Government Printing Office, 1980.

lesions, few or no data are available in the pediatric age group on the efficacy of long-term treatment of mild to moderately elevated cholesterol to prevent atherosclerosis later in life.

PHYSICAL EXERCISE

A reduced amount of physical exercise has been documented to be an important cardiovascular risk factor. The amount of exercise an individual regularly performs inversely correlates with cholesterol and triglyceride levels and with obesity. In addition, habitual exercise can normalize triglyceride levels, increase HDL-cholesterol levels, and, in some individuals, reduce LDL-cholesterol levels. Although it is clear in the adult that physical activity can reduce coronary risk, there is little information concerning the long-term effect of childhood exercise programs to reduce the risk of developing cardiovascular disease.

For children, 30 to 60 minutes of exercise four times per week is sufficient to maintain cardiovascular fitness. The exercise must be individualized by considering the type of exercise the child best enjoys and the facilities and equipment available. Not all types of exercise are equally useful for becoming cardiovascularly fit. Activities requiring effort against heavy resistance, such as weightlifting, can cause increased efficiency of certain muscle groups but do little to improve cardiovascular fitness. To achieve the desired degree of cardiovascular adaptation and conditioning, aerobic exercise is necessary. Any activity that can be maintained continuously, is rhythmic, and uses large groups of muscles is aerobic. A few recommended activities are vigorous walking, jogging, skating, skiing, aerobic dance, and bicycling. Despite the reported benefits of regular aerobic exercise training, the dropout rate among those beginning regular exercise is high. Support from family and friends is critical to maintaining continued compliance.

TABLE 2. Therapy of Hyperlipidemia

TYPE	MECHANISM	REDUCTION IN CHOLESTEROL (%)	EFFECT ON VLDL	EFFECT ON HDL	SIDE EFFECTS	DOSE
Nonpharmacologic Therapy						
AHA Prudent diet	Limits exogenous cholesterol	10–15	Decrease	Decrease		
Exercise	Improves insulin resistance	Some decrease	Decrease	Increase		
Weight loss	Improves insulin resistance	Some decrease	Decrease	Mild increase		
Pharmacologic Therapy						
Bile acid resins	Accelerates LDL disposal	20–30	Mild decrease	Mild increase	Epigastric distress, constipation, bloating, interferes with some drug absorption	Up to 24 g/d of cholestyramine in divided doses
Nicotinic acid or niacin	Reduces VLDL and LDL synthesis; increases HDL	25	50% decrease	30%–40% increase	Flushing, headache, tachycardia, gastrointestinal distress, activation of peptic ulcer disease and inflammatory bowel disease, hepatic dysfunction	Titrate up to 1 g 3 t.i.d.
Probucol (Lorelco)	Increases LDL disposal; reduces HDL/LDL	5–15	—	Decrease	Nausea, diarrhea, flatulence, eosinophilia, hepatic dysfunction, prolongs QT interval	0.5 g b.i.d.
Gemfibrozil (Lopid)	Enhances VLDL breakdown and decreased VLDL production	Decrease	40%–50% decrease	20%–30% increase	Rarely myositis, should not be used in patients with renal disease, cholelithiasis, or liver dysfunction	600 mg b.i.d. twice/day
HMG-CoA reductase inhibitor, Lovastatin (Mevacor)	Inhibits cholesterol synthesis and increases LDL disposal	30–40	—	—	Elevated liver enzymes, myositis, cataracts in animals	20–40 mg b.i.d.

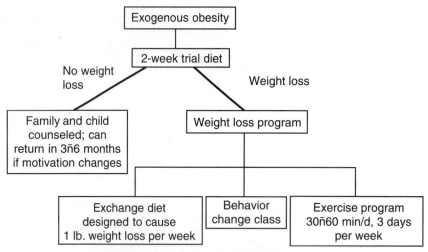

FIGURE 4. Outline of a pediatric weight loss program.

OBESITY

Obesity is a complex and difficult clinical problem. It is probably the most prevalent and serious nutritional disease in the United States. Childhood obesity is known to exert a major impact on cardiovascular risk. We have documented that 97% of obese adolescents had four or more of the following risk factors: elevated serum triglyceride levels, decreased HDL-cholesterol levels, increased total cholesterol level, elevated systolic and/or diastolic blood pressure, diminished maximum work capacity, and a strong family history of coronary heart disease.

Before describing how to treat obesity, it is important to give a brief definition of obesity. In both adults and adolescents, obesity is defined as an accumulation of body fat greater than 22% of total body weight for men and greater than 30% of total body weight for women. Weight for height standards also are useful in defining obesity. A commonly accepted definition for childhood obesity is the combination of triceps and subscapular skinfolds being greater than the 80th percentile and weight for height being greater than the 75th percentile for age and sex. Obesity defined by these criteria is present in 15% to 20% of all schoolage children.

Treatment modalities employed in obese children and adolescents can be categorized into one of a combination of six basic approaches: caloric restriction, appetite-reducing drugs, increased physical activity, therapeutic starvation, bypass surgery, and habit pattern changes based on social learning therapy. Certainly, drugs, starvation, and surgery are unacceptable treatment strategies for the majority of children.

A practical weight loss program is outlined in Figure 4. To assess the child's ability to comply with a weight loss program, we believe it is advisable to place the child on a trial diet for 2 to 3 weeks. If the child is successful with this trial diet, loses at least 1 to 2 pounds in 2 to 3 weeks, he or she is likely to benefit from a weight loss program. If the child is unsuccessful, the family and child should be counseled and asked to return in 3 to 6 months, or sooner if there is a change in attitude toward weight loss.

The weight loss program consists of three components: diet, behavior change, and exercise. The caloric requirements necessary for a child to lose 1 to 2 pounds per week are determined by reducing the current level of calories by 500 to 1000 calories per day. We believe that adolescent weight reduction diets should not go below 1200 calories per day, since it then becomes difficult to provide adequate vitamins and nutrients to promote normal growth and development. On the other hand, calorie levels should never exceed 2500 calories per day, since the child is unlikely to take the diet seriously if allowed too large a calorie intake. An exchange type diet is recommended, since it teaches the child the essentials of good nutrition and gets the child actively involved in determining his own diet. The behavior change component of the program includes a weekly, 1 hour

class for 20 weeks, then every other week until the weight goal has been maintained for at least 1 month. The classes should center around (1) nutrition education, (2) record keeping, (3) stimulus control for restricting the external cues that set the occasion for eating, and (4) reinforcement of altered behavior. The purpose of the behavior change component is to help the obese child learn to eat like a nonobese person, become aware of current habits, and normalize and accept responsibility for eating behavior. All children are also encouraged to exercise for 30 to 60 min/d on at least 3 days per week. The weight loss program should have a built-in reinforcement system to help the child establish and maintain the new habits. Finally, in addition to the child's structured portion of the program, family support is critical. The child's family needs to be taught how to give the child positive support without nagging or taking over the child's weight loss program.

Using this type of program, we have been able to achieve adequate weight loss in those adolescents who are motivated to lose weight. When dealing with childhood obesity, it is important to remember that if the child does not want to lose weight, no weight loss program, regardless of its approach, organization, or cost, will be successful.

SUMMARY

Since coronary artery disease has its origins in childhood, it is critical that the pediatrician become involved in the identification and treatment of the child at risk for early development of cardiovascular disease.

REFERENCES

1. National Cholesterol Education Program: Report of the Expert Panel on Blood Cholesterol Levels in children and adolescents. Pediatrics 1992;89 (suppl 3, part 2).
2. Rocchini AP: Adolescent obesity and hypertension. Pediatr Clin North Am 1993;40:81–92.
3. Simons-Morton BG, Pate RR, Simons-Morton DG: Prescribing physical activity to prevent disease. Postgrad Med 1988;83:165–176.

PERIPHERAL VASCULAR DISEASE

JULIE R. INGELFINGER, M.D.

A rapid and considered approach to diagnosis and therapy is necessary for the management of peripheral vascular disease in children, in that certain findings need only environmental manipulation, whereas others need surgical intervention. Obstruction to blood flow may occur in both peripheral arterial disease and venous disease.

This fact must be kept in mind during assessment and therapy. Several categories of peripheral vascular disease or injury are discussed.

FROSTBITE

In frostbite, it is critical to restore heat to the affected limb(s), with careful attention to hemodynamics, to obtain complete recovery.[1,2] When the extremity is still frozen or is very cold, moderately warm water (40 to 42° C) should be used promptly for fairly rapid rewarming, with the proviso that this should be done only when the danger of freezing again has been eliminated. Time for rewarming should depend on the depth of frozen tissue, since deeper tissue layers may require more than an hour (if there has been through-and-through freezing). If freezing has occurred over 24 hours before the onset of medical care, rewarming should not be done. In cases of severe frostbite occurring far from medical facilities, the physician may be taking consultation by radio and telephone. It is crucial that the remote consultant be sure that those doing the rewarming understand the instructions. Subsequent to rewarming, the care mandates impeccable hygiene for a lengthy period of time. At the present time, rapid rewarming plus antiinflammatory agents and aloe vera cream are the main components of care. Aloe vera appears to help remove high concentrations of thromboxane and is applied topically in an aqueous solution (70% aloe vera or greater). Blisters may develop and should be managed aseptically. Blisters that are white or clear should be debrided, and 70% aloe vera cream should be applied topically every 6 hours. More severe, hemorrhagic blisters should be left intact, since debridement in this case exposes deep structures that may then become desiccated or necrotic. The frostbitten parts should be elevated and splinted as needed. Analgesia with meperidine (Demerol) should be administered as needed. Hydrotherapy on a daily basis should be provided. Tetanus toxoid should be administered prophylactically, and immune globulin should be supplied if the patient has not previously been immunized or is overdue for a booster. Antibiotic coverage is important, generally penicillin at 50,000 IU/kg/d in four divided doses. Anti-inflammatory medication, such as ibuprofen (12 mg/kg/d) is especially helpful in blocking the effects of thromboxane.

Surprisingly, with conservative management alone, recovery is quite frequent. Thus, amputation or extirpation should be delayed. Following the acute stage, physical therapy is important to permit restoration of full function of the affected part. It is especially helpful to include physicians who have experience with frostbite injury in the management team.

PERIPHERAL VASCULAR DISORDERS

Vasoactive Disorders

Raynaud Syndrome

The characteristic sequence of pallor, cyanosis, and rubor defines Raynaud phenomenon, which is a vasospastic disorder of fingers and toes.[3] When there is an underlying disorder, Raynaud phenomenon is the appropriate term, but when there is not, it is called Raynaud disease. A variety of events (often related to cold temperature or emotional changes) precipitate episodes. In general, the condition is bilateral, without gangrene. Raynaud phenomenon is associated with collagen diseases, such as scleroderma, systemic lupus erythematosus, and mixed connective tissue disease. It may also occur in vasculitis, obstructive arterial diseases, and hypothyroidism and with hepatitis B antigenemia. Medications associated with Raynaud phenomenon include beta-adrenergic blockers, cyclosporine, amphetamines, imipramine, vinblastine, and bleomycin.

If a child is in good health and has isolated, mild vasospastic complaints, an exhaustive medical evaluation is not in order. Primary Raynaud disease tends to be a benign disorder. The secondary form, however, may lead to arterial occlusion and fingertip ulcers and may even progress to gangrene on occasion. Occlusion should be evaluated by measuring systolic pressures in the involved finger(s) using ultra-

sound or plethysmography. It is important to evaluate the possibility of progression to tissue loss. Finger pressures of less than 70 mm Hg, wrist/digit ratios of over 30 mm Hg, and brachial artery/finger differences of over 40 mm Hg are indications that occlusive disease is likely to be present.

Since primary Raynaud disease is generally a mild problem, all that is usually required for treatment is environmental change. If possible, affected individuals should live within a warm, dry climate and wear warm clothing that conserves rather than dissipates heat. Increasing physical activity may help in preventing episodes. Likewise, biofeedback may be of benefit. In severe cases, it may be helpful to use calcium channel blockers, e.g., nifedipine (0.2 mg/kg three times a day generally suffices). Fifty percent to seventy-five percent of severely affected patients seem to improve with this regimen. Long-acting calcium channel blockers, such as nifedipine (Procardia XL, 30 to 90 mg), given once per day may prevent episodes. Alpha-adrenergic blockers, such as phenoxybenzamine (5 to 10 mg/d) or prazosin (Minipress) (0.01 to 0.05 mg/kg/d), also have been reported to be effective. Older hypotensive agents, such as guanethidine or reserpine, have been used to treat Raynaud phenomenon. Ketanserin, a 5-HT-2 receptor antagonist, may relieve symptoms. Most of these agents have substantial side effects. Thus, management without medications should be the preferred approach.

Chilblains

In some susceptible individuals, cold leads to erythema, itching, and occasionally blisters over the proximal phalanges, fingers, toes, and the back of the hand. This is termed chilblains or pernio.[4] Such findings also may occur over the lower legs and heel. Chilblains occurs particularly in children who live in damp, cool climates. It is generally a mild disease, more a nuisance than anything else. Treatment should consist of antipruritics and soothing ointments, such as lanolin-petrolatum. In severe, chronic cases, a treatment approach similar to that for Raynaud phenomenon, with alpha-adrenergic blockade is especially effective.

Acrocyanosis

Acrocyanosis consists of a stocking and glove pattern of cyanosis in response to cold. The pale and red phases seen with Raynaud disease do not occur, and ulcerations are rare. Therapy is usually not needed unless cosmetic therapy is desired. Acrocyanosis is virtually never related to systemic diseases. Thus, an evaluation for collagen disease is not needed.

Livedo Reticularis

Livedo reticularis and cutis marmorata (marble skin) are very mild, peripheral vascular reactions to cold. Netlike or reticulated patterns of cyanosis occur in the arms and legs. This pattern is often seen when a child becomes cold after, for example, being in a cool bath for a very high fever. No therapy is needed.

Erythromelalgia

Erythromelalgia is a rare condition, occurring only occasionally in children, and is characterized by warmth of local skin, edema, redness, and burning.[5] The feet tend to be affected more frequently than the hands. Treatment should aim at controlling precipitating physical factors and providing medication for relief. Cooling soaks and cooling the body in general may ameliorate symptoms. Administering ephedrine (0.5 mg/kg q4–6h) may be helpful, along with a sedative or tranquilizer. The use of aspirin on a routine basis may be useful, since endogenous bradykinin may participate in the pathogenesis of erythromelalgia. Antiserotoninergic agents have been advocated because of the concept that erythromelalgia is associated with serotonin release, a type of peripheral migraine. Thus, such agents as cyproheptadine (0.08 mg/kg per dose t.i.d.) have been administered. Additionally, propranolol (1 to 2 mg/kg twice daily) has been used as therapy.

Causalgia

Causalgia is defined as burning pain, often associated with trophic skin changes because of peripheral nerve injury. In the absence of an obvious wound with accompanying deep tissue injury leading to nerve trunk disruption, causalgia can be confused with a primary vascular disorder. Often, a history of trauma may exist, and therapy is paravertebral sympathetic blockade (by injecting 1% lidocaine). If diagnosis is accurate, the relief will be striking and last for several hours. Subsequent to such blockade, vigorous physical therapy is important to achieve a more long-term improvement. It is rarely necessary to do sympathectomy in the treatment of causalgia.

OBSTRUCTIVE DISORDERS

Trauma

When trauma interrupts arterial flow to tissue and limb, therapy should be directed at preserving tissue and preventing limb loss. Thus, as soon as possible, arterial continuity and flow must be reestablished, clots must be removed and further ones prevented, any spasm must be relieved, and tissue edema must be controlled so as not to compromise flow. Restoring the patient's circulating blood volume systemically and locally is critical both for the obvious preservation of life and to ensure local circulation. Gangrene is rare in childhood, but a vascular injury managed without an operative approach beyond 6 to 8 hours often leads to ultimate limb weakness and atrophy.

The eventual function of every involved limb must be considered from the outset. Flow must be assessed initially and, depending on the situation, serially. Transcutaneous Doppler flow is less traumatic than classic arteriography and may be repeated with ease. In the future, magnetic resonance angiography, which is noninvasive, may be helpful. There is insufficient experience with this modality at present to recommend it for routine assessment of traumatic interruption of arterial flow.

Fastidious debridement and removal of distal clots are crucial. End-to-end vascular anastomosis should be done if there is adequate arterial length. Otherwise engraftment with autogenous or autologous veins should be performed. Fasciotomy may be necessary to avoid edema and hematoma. Anticoagulation with heparin should be considered.

Complications as a result of vascular cannulation are an increasingly common cause of arterial problems. The overly long presence of indwelling lines or inadequate technique can cause embolism and frank vascular occlusion. It is important to remember that catheterization through the femoral or iliac arteries to examine the left heart or renal vessels can lead to leg shortening if there is subsequent clotting. After such a procedure, instillation of heparin and/or the use of aspirin for 1 to 2 days may be helpful. Both arterial pulses and leg growth should be followed in individuals who have undergone such procedures.

Congenital Arterial Stenosis

It is rare for peripheral arterial stenoses to occur, and they rarely produce any symptoms or signs in the very young. Collateral circulation will develop in childhood and usually circumvents any difficulties.

Arteritis

Major vessel arteritis may require bypass grafting or transluminal angioplasty if blood flow is obstructed. It is important to identify and stop any sensitizing medical agents, to remove and treat toxins, and to avoid renal allergens. Steroids are the most commonly used agent in treating severe generalized arteritis. A full discussion is found later in this chapter.

When small arteries and arterioles are involved, muscle biopsy is important for diagnosis. Inflammatory arteritis can occur locally or be part of a systemic disorder, such as polyarteritis. Such entities as Kawasaki disease and moyamoya are considered later in this chapter.

FISTULAS

Congenital Fistulas

Congenital arteriovenous (AV) fistulas can be extremely difficult to treat and may be impossible to remove easily. Sometimes, treatment with sclerotic agents or embolization may ablate or control the size of the malformation. However, in large AV malformations, there may be extension into the abdominal cavity. Afflicted individuals may be susceptible to recurrent deep tissue infections or sepsis. Local management may be helpful for control of edema and superficial venous incompetence. Thus, support stockings and elevation may prevent stasis changes.

Traumatic Fistulas

Iatrogenic fistulas as a result of needle puncture are among the most common traumatic peripheral vascular fistulas. When these occur, closure should be surgical, taking great care to avoid arterial compromise. Additionally, an arteriovenous fistula may be intentionally created to achieve access for hemodialysis. Once the patient no longer needs hemodialysis, closure may be indicated, taking care to preserve arterial flow.

Thrombophlebitis

Superficial thrombophlebitis is often an iatrogenic result of intravenous therapy in hospitalized patients. Deep thrombophlebitis, however, is unusual in children. Its presence is a serious event, associated with considerable morbidity and even mortality. Treatment should be prompt and effective and aggressive, dictated by the extent of the problem. In a patient who has thrombophlebitis, it is important to search for markers of coagulation, including plasminogen activator inhibitor (PAI), and decreases in antithrombin II, protein C, or protein S. The use of fibrinolytic agents, such as streptokinase or urokinase or the recombinant human plasminogen activator (rtPA), may promote lysis of clot and resorption. There is much more experience with rtPA in adults than in children. Additionally, IV heparin and bedrest with heat and elevation are standard management. Heparin should be given by a continuous infusion so that the whole blood clotting time is elevated 2 to 2½ times and PTT is at 50 to 80 seconds. It is very important to have a good constant speed infusion pump to avoid pulses of the anticoagulant. Following recovery, anticoagulation with warfarin is useful to keep the prothrombin time 1.2 to 1.5 times normal. Therapy should continue for at least 3 months. If there has been a pulmonary embolism, an even longer period of anticoagulation is worthwhile. Thrombophlebitis is more common in children with nephrotic syndrome, as deficiencies in protein C and protein S and increases in PAI may be present. Thus, a physician must monitor such individuals carefully.

Occasionally, massive deep thrombophlebitis may occur. This is called phlegmasia cerulea dolens. In this instance, there can be associated arterial spasm. If it is present, thrombectomy should be attempted only if limb viability is questioned. In this circumstance, venous ligation is performed intraabdominally. Additionally, such maneuvers as placement of an inferior vena caval filter, which is permanent and must remain for the life of the patient, should be entertained only if all other options have failed.

Once the patient has had deep thrombophlebitis, subsequent edema should be controlled with tailormade gradient stockings that go from the foot to the upper thigh.

REFERENCES

1. Britt LD, Dascombe WH, Rodriguez A: New horizons in management of hypothermia and frostbite injury. Surg Clin North Am 1991;71:345–370.
2. Crouch C, Smith WL: Long-term sequelae of frostbite. Pediatr Radiol 1990;20:365–366.
3. Duffy CM, Laxer RM, Lee P, Ramsay C, Fritzler M, Silverman ED: Raynaud syndrome in childhood. J Pediatr 1989;114:73–78.
4. Spittell JA Jr, Spittell PC: Chronic pernio: Another cause of blue toes. Int Angiol 1992;11:46–50.
5. Strozik K, Lis GT, Krzanowska-Dyras M: Case of primary erythromelalgia in a child [Letter]. Clin Pediatr 1992;31:378–379.

CARDIAC NEOPLASMS AND OTHER INTRACARDIAC MASSES

PHILLIP MOORE, M.D.
DONALD C. FYLER, M.D.

In preparation for this report computer files extending over 40 years at the Children's Hospital, Boston, were reviewed. It was a surprise to discover that one half of all cardiac masses were recorded in the period from 1989 to the present. The experience with cardiac neoplasms (5/y) has stabilized over the past 15 years, while new patients with intracardiac thrombi (30/y), vegetations (6/y), and foreign bodies in the heart (6/y) have been increasing. The profusion of clinically recognized cardiac masses is the result of improved echocardiographic equipment and greater experience in its use.

Protocols for the management of these newly recognized abnormalities are under development and are not yet firmly established. Similarly, protocols for the most productive scheduling of echocardiograms to discover thrombi are evolving. Still, our experiences may be of some use to those facing these problems.

THROMBI

Thrombi are the most common cardiac masses. When discovered within the heart and great vessels, thrombi are almost invariably associated with other fundamental problems, such as prior cardiac surgery, foreign bodies within the heart (i.e., an inlying catheter), bacterial endocarditis, infected thrombi, myocarditis, atrial fibrillation, and nonpulsatile flow, as seen after Fontan surgery. These associations usually are present when the mass is a thrombus but are rarely encountered when the mass is a cardiac neoplasm—a point of some significance in differential diagnosis. It follows that treatment of the thrombus may confound the management of the underlying problem, occasionally raising difficult treatment choices.

Many clinically recognized thrombi are small, are located in the *right heart,* resolve spontaneously, and cause few clinical problems. There is rarely evidence of pulmonary embolism. Treatment consists of periodic observation. Larger thrombi are more of a problem, often requiring anticoagulation, usually with warfarin or (rarely) streptokinase. Surgical removal is used when the thrombus is infected or threatens obstruction of the circulation.

Atrial or caval thrombi may be the source of paradoxical embolization to the systemic circulation if there is an atrial septal defect or a patent foramen ovale. When there has been paradoxical embolization, prompt closure of the atrial septum is indicated by either surgery or catheter technique.

Thrombi in the *left heart* chambers that have been the source of emboli or threaten to embolize are more dangerous. When there has been an embolus, surgical removal of the left heart thrombi often is undertaken, and multiple or large thrombi, particularly if mobile, are removed. Small and fixed thrombi in the left heart are treated with anticoagulants. In either case, repeated echocardiograms will guide therapy.

Chronic anticoagulation is used to prevent emboli in patients with atrial fibrillation. The longer atrial fibrillation has persisted and the larger the size of the left atrial chamber, the more likely it is that thrombi and emboli will occur.

FOREIGN BODIES

Foreign bodies serving as a nidus for thrombosis, usually a catheter left for a long time or an escaped intravenous line, are removed either by snaring with a second catheter or by surgical exploration. Artificial materials used in surgical repair of the heart or devices, such as artificial valves, occasionally develop thrombi. These may persist despite anticoagulation and require thrombectomy or sometimes removal of the device itself. When thrombus development has been documented on an umbilical catheter, the catheter should be removed. Catheters left in the circulation more than a few days are checked regularly because of the tendency to develop clots.

VEGETATIONS

The vegetations of bacterial endocarditis are treated with prolonged and specific antibiotic therapy. With effective antibiotics, complete resolution is the rule. Antibiotics are continued as long as vegetations can be visualized. When there has been embolization or the vegetations are large, surgical removal may be indicated.

EXCRESCENCES

Another result of the technologic improvement in echocardiographic machines is the discovery of congenital excrescences of tissue attached to cardiac structures, usually at the root of a valve. These curiosities, often labeled as aberrant endocardial cushion tissue, are found increasingly during routine echocardiography for other cardiac disease. How often they occur in otherwise normal hearts remains to be determined. Some are cystic, and others are on a stalk flopping loosely with the flow of blood. Concern arises that a large excrescence may obstruct a valve or even break loose as an embolus, but these problems are very rare. Since removal requires manipulation of valvar tissue, intervention is rarely justified. These bits of congenitally misplaced tissue must be distinguished from true neoplasm.

CARDIAC NEOPLASMS

Cardiac tumors in children are extremely rare, and, fortunately, the vast majority are benign. Our files list 67 children with cardiac tumors. Only 6 of these were malignant; 2 were primary cardiac tumors; and 4 were metastases to the heart. In our series, the most common cardiac tumor was rhabdomyoma (42%), followed by unspecified tumors (diagnosis made by echocardiography or catheterization without features of a specific tumor type) (22%), myxoma (9%), fibroma (6%), malignant metastases (6%), pericardial cysts (3%), and fibrosarcoma (3%). Transient atrial septal swelling was seen in 2 neonates, and there was 1 patient with a fungal mass in the right atrium. In addition to these patients, 7 children had mediastinal tumors that caused direct compression of the heart or had direct extension to the pericardium. Of these 7, 4 had Hodgkin's lymphoma, 1 had acute lymphocytic leukemia, 1 had a lymphangioma that compressed the pulmonary veins, and 1 had a chest wall sarcoma.

Treatment of cardiac tumors depends primarily on the tumor type and the physiologic derangements attributable to the tumor, e.g., obstruction to blood flow, decreased myocardial contractility, or arrhythmias. In general, benign tumors can be left alone unless they are causing significant symptoms. Malignant tumors, however, require intervention by surgical resection, chemotherapy, or both.

Rhabdomyoma

Of the 28 patients with rhabdomyoma in our series, 4 were diagnosed by fetal echocardiography (27 to 36 weeks gestation), 2 because of tuberous sclerosis in the mother, and 2 because tumors were seen on a screening fetal echocardiogram. Only 4 of the 28 patients were over 1 year of age at the time of diagnosis (range 27 weeks gestation to 18.5 years). Seventeen of the 28 children (60%) had associated tuberous sclerosis, which is similar to the statistics in other reports. Over one half of the patients had multiple tumors, with nearly one quarter having tumors in two or more chambers. Tumors were located most often in the right ventricular free wall, followed by the left ventricle, and then the right atrium. No patients had a rhabdomyoma in the left atrium. On echocardiographic examination, the tumor is usually a nonpedunculated mass in the ventricular or atrial wall, with or without protrusion into the chamber cavity.

Nine children had surgical resection for symptoms of obstruction, most often right or left ventricular outflow tract obstruction. Two patients had associated arrhythmias, 1 with supraventricular tachycardia, and the other with third degree heart block. At least 3 patients had documented regression of their tumors. Spontaneous complete regression has been reported in up to 80% of tumors. Of interest, 2 patients developed a discrete subaortic fibrous ridge as a rhabdomyoma regressed in the left ventricular outflow tract. Because of the high probability of tumor regression, surgical resection should be performed only when significant outflow tract obstruction exists.

Myxoma

Myxoma is the most common cardiac tumor in adults, and usually occurs in children during adolescence, though 3 of our patients were less than 12 years old. The tumors are typically pedunculated masses attached to the atrial septum, most often on the left side near the foramen ovale, although they occasionally are found in the right ventricle. One of our younger patients had a myoma attached to the noncoronary cusp of the aortic valve. Exertional dyspnea, palpitations, or syncope can result from mitral or tricuspid inflow obstruction. Embolization to either the pulmonary or systemic circulation occurs in up to 25% of patients. Four of our 6 patients had surgical resection, and 2 of these 4 required repeat operation for recurrence of tumor before age 20 years. An operative mortality of 3.7% has been reported, with an actuarial survival of 91% ± 4%. Because of the potential for tumor embolization and the excellent surgical results, surgical resection is the treatment of choice for cardiac myxoma.

Fibroma

Over 80% of all reported cases of fibromas occur in children. The average age in our series was 4.2 years, with a range of 2 days to 8 years. Unlike rhabdomyomas, fibromas usually are solitary masses found in the left ventricular free wall, although they do occur in the right ventricular septum or the atrium. Symptoms are caused by arrhythmias or obstruction to blood flow. Surgical resection is the treatment of choice in symptomatic patients, with excellent long-term survival.

Other Benign Tumors

Other more unusual benign cardiac tumors that occur in childhood include hamartomas, teratomas, pericardial cysts, and mesotheliomas of the AV node. Hamartomas, also known as Purkinje cell tumors, occur in infants generally less than 20 months of age. These are associated with incessant ventricular tachycardia. Intraoperative electrophysiologic mapping and surgical excision are the preferred treatment because the arrhythmia is refractory to medical therapy. Teratomas occur within the pericardium at the base of the great vessels and, as with pericardiac cysts, are associated with pericardial effusions and, thus, should be surgically removed if they are causing hemodynamic compromise. Mesotheliomas occur during adolescence, are localized to the AV node, and may cause heart block.

Malignant Tumors

Primary malignant cardiac tumors in children are extremely rare and include angiosarcoma, rhabdomyosarcoma, fibrosarcoma, leiomyosarcoma, mesothelioma, and lymphoma. Treatment consists of aggressive surgical resection and chemotherapy, with or without radiotherapy. Despite aggressive treatment most patients die within 1 year of diagnosis.

REFERENCES

1. Bortolotti U, Maraglino G, Rubino M, et al: Surgical excision of intracardiac myxomas: A 20-year follow-up. Ann Thorac Surg 1990;49:449–453.
2. Smythe JF, Dyck JD, Smallhorn MD, et al: Natural history of cardiac rhabdomyoma in infancy and childhood. Am J Cardiol 1990;66:1247–1249.
3. Thomas CR, Johnson GW, Stoddard MF, et al: Primary malignant cardiac tumors: Update 1992. Med Pediatr Oncol 1992;20:519–531.

PERICARDITIS

CHARLES A. BULLABOY, M.D.

The pericardium is susceptible to a myriad of diseases that can convert this normally helpful protector into a bad neighbor of the heart (Table 1). Pericardial responses to inciting events include inflammation, effusion, and fibrosis. Since it is reported only once per 850 hospital admissions, a high index of suspicion concerning pericardial involvement is necessary to make the diagnosis of pericarditis. Appropriate therapy begins with establishing a firm diagnosis based on all available information.

The pericardial space normally contains 10 to 15 ml of an ultrafiltrate of plasma. The clinical significance of any abnormal fluid depends on its physical composition, rapidity of progression, and absolute fluid volume and the physical compliance of the pericardium. A tense pericardial space restricts diastolic heart filling, causing the hemodynamic embarrassment of tamponade. Kussmaul's sign—an inspiratory increase of jugular venous pressure—is truly paradoxical [as opposed to pulsus paradoxus, which is an exaggeration of the normal inspiratory decrease in systemic arterial pressure (not exceeding 10 mm Hg)]. Compression of the left lower lung lobe produces bronchial breath sounds below the angle of the left scapula (Ewart's sign) and also produces dyspnea. Classically, the discomfort from pericardial pain is exacerbated by lying supine and ameliorated by sitting up and leaning forward. On auscultation, the often evanescent rub sounds similar to the squeak of new leather. Heart tones may be distant and muffled.

Large effusions smooth out the cardiac borders, causing a water bottle configuration of the cardiac silhouette on roentgenography and low voltage and electrical alternans on electrocardiography. The pericardium is electrically silent. Thus, the serial ECG findings of ST segment elevation with return to baseline followed by T-wave flattening, inversion, and resolution reflect alterations of the underlying involved myocardium. Echocardiography is of indispensable value in detecting, quantifying, and serially following the accumulation or resolution of pericardial fluid. Fluoroscopy, carbon dioxide angiography, and radionuclide gated blood pool scanning are essentially obsolete and of historical interest only.

Diastolic collapse of the right atrium, right ventricle, and left

TABLE 1. Common Etiologies of Pericarditis

Autoimmune disorders	Rheumatic fever, rheumatoid arthritis, systemic lupus erythematosus
Drugs	Anticoagulants, daunorubicin, hydralazine, isoniazid, minoxidil, phenytoin, procainamide
Idiopathic	
Infections	
Anaerobes	
Bacterial	In decreasing order of frequency: *Staphylococcus aureus, Haemophilus influenzae*, pneumococcus, streptococcus, meningococcus, gram-negative coliform bacteria
Fungal	*Candida* sp., histoplasmosis
Mycobacterial	Tuberculosis
Parasites/protozoal	Amebiasis, echinococcosis, toxoplasmosis
Viral	Coxsackievirus A or B, echovirus, HIV, influenza, infectious mononucleosis, varicella
Metabolic/endocrine	Myxedema, uremia
Neoplastic	Non-Hodgkin's lymphoma, neuroblastoma, sarcoma, Wilms' tumor
Postcardiac injury syndromes	Chest trauma, chylopericardium, hemopericardium, postpericardiotomy
Radiation	

atrium are signs of *cardiac tamponade* and correlate directly with its clinical diagnosis. Stroke volume is limited in cardiac tamponade, and cardiac output and blood pressure are maintained by reflex tachycardia and vasoconstriction. These compensatory mechanisms are vital and must not be corrected but, indeed, should be augmented by judiciously avoiding diuretics, maintaining high filling pressures (approximately 15 mm Hg), using normal saline or other effective volume expanders, and supporting myocardial function by the positive inotropic and chronotropic actions of isoproterenol (0.05 to 1 μg/kg/min IV). Fluid should be drained from the pericardial space for both diagnostic and therapeutic purposes. Pericardiocentesis, not an innocuous procedure, is optimally performed by experienced personnel in a setting with available echocardiographic, hemodynamic, and radiographic capabilities. Anesthetic agents that depress myocardial contractility should be avoided. Midazolam (0.05 to 0.15 mg/kg IV) and ketamine (0.5 to 1 mg/kg parenterally) are particularly useful in this clinical scenario. Positive pressure ventilation will increase the afterload on an already struggling cardiovascular system. The mainstay percutaneous subxiphoid catheter over needle approach is usually futile if the effusion is small, posterior, loculated, or densely reflective on ultrasonography. Such findings suggest either a purulent pericardial peel or a coagulated thrombus. Bloody fluid, the enigma of all pericardial tappers, does not clot and has a lower hematocrit than that of the intravascular space. If monitored under echocardiographic guidance, 3 to 5 ml of agitated saline injected through the exploring needle confirms proper position if a cloud of echoes envelops the pericardial space. Fluid should be handled and examined in the same manner as that obtained from the lumbar or pleural spaces. Additional studies depend on the perceived clinical diagnosis. Unstained smears and fluid are held in reserve for any special or controversial issues.

Idiopathic pericarditis (often benign and presumed viral by default) is the form most commonly occurring in children. *Viral pericarditis* has been described with at least 27 different nonpolio enteroviruses, frequently coxsackievirus B5 and echovirus 6 in the older child. The purported viral etiology of the well-described *postpericardiotomy syndrome* following open heart surgery has not been substantiated using the powerful diagnostic tools of ELISA and polymerase chain reaction. These self-limited processes, usually lasting 2 to 6 weeks, are managed with the following therapeutic guidelines.

Tamponade is rare, and unless therapy would be altered, pericardiocentesis is not justified. Bedrest is prudent initially as early physical activity frequently exacerbates the clinical symptomatology. The inflammatory/immune response is quieted by daily, oral nonsteroidal anti-inflammatory drugs (NSAID): acetylsalicylic acid (ASA) 80 to 100 mg/kg (maximum 3.6 g divided q4-6h tapered to maintain a level of 15 to 20 mg/dl), ibuprofen 30 to 40 mg/kg (maximum 2.4 g divided q6-8h), or indomethacin 1 to 2.5 mg/kg (maximum 200 mg divided q6-12h, frequently used in the older child or with uremic pericarditis). Corticosteroids (prednisone 1 to 2 mg/kg/day, maximum 60 mg divided q6-8h) are a last resort in refractory cases but generally are best avoided because of the frequent rebound phenomenon when tapered and the masking of other illnesses, of which the pericardial component may be only coincidental. Pain usually responds to the NSAID therapy or, if needed, codeine 2 to 3 mg/kg/d divided q4-6h PO (maximum 1.5 mg/kg per dose), meperidine 6 mg/kg/d divided q4-6h (maximum 2 mg/kg per dose up to 100 mg), or morphine sulfate 0.1-0.2 mg/kg per dose q4-6h (maximum 10 mg). Experience is limited in courses with multiple relapses with once daily PO azathioprine 1 to 2 mg/kg or colchicine 1 mg/kg (Table 2). Creation of a pericardial window may be necessary to effect a cure in chronic unremittent effusions.

Purulent pericarditis mandates an intensive search for the offending organism and its source. Since the pericardium is unable to absorb either a transudate or exudate, the obligatory 2 to 6 weeks course of appropriate antibiotic therapy in septic/meningitic doses will prove futile unless this closed abscess is initially surgically decompressed. After surgery, drains are usually left in situ for 3 to 5 days. Instillation of antibiotics into the pericardial space itself is unwarranted and un-

TABLE 2. Drugs Used in Treating Pericarditis

DRUG*	DOSE	COMMENT
Acetylsalicylic acid (ASA)	80–100 mg/kg/d PO divided q4-6h Max: 3.6 g/d	Optimal serum concentration: 15–20 mg/dl
Azathioprine	1–2 mg/kg/d PO	Limited experience in refractory pericardial effusion
Codeine	2–3 mg/kg/d PO, IM, or SC divided q4-6h Max: 5 mg/kg/d, 1.5 mg/kg per dose	May cause constipation or CNS depression
Colchicine	1 mg/kg/d PO	Limited experience in refractory pericardial effusion
Ibuprofen	30–40 mg/kg/d PO divided q6-8h Max: 2.4 g/d	
Indomethacin	1–2.5 mg/kg/d PO divided q6-12h Max: 200 mg/d	
Isoproterenol	0.05–1 μg/kg/min IV	
Ketamine	0.5–1 mg/kg IM or IV	
Meperidine	6 mg/kg/d PO, IM, SC, or IV divided q4-6h Max: 100 mg per dose	
Midazolam	0.05–0.15 mg/kg per dose IV	
Morphine	0.1–0.2 mg/kg per dose PO, IM, SC, or IV q4-6h	
Prednisone	1–2 mg/kg/d PO divided q6-8h Max: 60 mg/d	
Triamcinolone hexacetonide	1–2 mg/kg per dose Max: 50–100 mg	Instilled into pericardial space in uremic pericarditis

*Indications for these various agents are found in the text.

necessary, as adequate antibiotic concentrations are achievable with systemic administration. The pericarditis seen in the convalescent stage of appropriately managed meningococcal infection is immune related, sterile, and self-limited.

Traumatic pericarditis following an acute pericardial bleed from cardiac trauma, rupture, or postoperative surgery occurs with Beck's triad of increasing systemic venous pressure, decreasing systemic arterial pressure, and a small quiet heart. Immediate surgical evacuation of the bloody pericardial space is indicated.

Uremic pericarditis responds to intensification of the dialysis regimen and, if needed, a one-time instillation of a nonabsorbable corticosteroid (triamcinolone hexacetonide 1 to 2 mg/kg) into the pericardial space. *Drug-related toxic pericarditis* typically abates when the offending medication is discontinued. Percutaneous catheter drainage and catheter balloon pericardiotomy are viable, nonsurgical alternatives in selective persistent effusions, especially *neoplastic pericarditis* in which sclerosing agents are used to obliterate the pericardial space postevacuation.

Constrictive pericarditis can be a sequela of initial appropriate therapy of any of the previously mentioned entities. In the past, constriction frequently complicated tuberculosis, but now pericardial injury following mediastinal radiation or cardiac surgery is more common. The thickened, scarred, fibrotic, and occasionally calcified pericardium resists late diastolic heart filling. Hepatomegaly, ascites, protein-losing enteropathy, and occasionally a nephrotic picture dominate and confound the clinical presentation. Computed tomography, magnetic resonance imaging (modalities particularly valuable in evaluating pericardial thickness and geometry), and cardiac catheterization frequently are necessary to distinguish this confusing state from a restrictive cardiomyopathy. Medical therapy to reduce systemic venous hypertension by diuretics and salt restriction must be viewed as temporizing until pericardiectomy (usually via median sternotomy) is undertaken.

REFERENCES

1. Lowell BH, Braunwald E: Pericardial disease. *In* Braunwald E, (ed.): Heart Disease: A Textbook of Cardiovascular Disease. Philadelphia, WB Saunders, 1988:1484–1534.
2. Pinsky WW, Friedman RA: Pericarditis. *In* Garson A Jr, Bricker JT, McNamara DG (eds.): The Science and Practice of Pediatric Cardiology. Philadelphia, Lea & Febiger, 1990:1590–1599.

INFECTIVE ENDOCARDITIS

CYNTHIA A. DOERR, M.D.
JEFFREY R. STARKE, M.D.

Infective endocarditis results when microorganisms adhere to the endocardial surface of the heart. Although it is difficult to obtain accurate statistics for children, it appears that endocarditis occurs in approximately 1 in 1300 to 4500 pediatric hospital admissions and that the incidence has increased in the last decade. About 80% of children who develop endocarditis have underlying congenital heart disease. An increasing number of children with endocarditis have prosthetic valves or shunts and grafts constructed with artificial materials. The average age of children with infective endocarditis has increased to early adolescence, which is likely a result of increased survival and life expectancy of those with congenital heart disease. An increasing number of cases also are being noted in premature infants and ill neonates without congenital heart disease.

Most established principles of endocarditis diagnosis and management are derived from studies in adults, who more often develop endocarditis complicating damaged native or prosthetic heart valves. It has not been established definitively if treatment regimens for endocarditis in adults are equally successful in children with endocarditis after surgical repair or palliation of congenital heart defects. However, it appears that currently advocated regimens are generally safe and effective in children with infective endocarditis.

Management of infectious endocarditis requires prompt and appropriate antimicrobial therapy. Often, endocarditis is suspected clinically before a causative organism is cultured, and initial empiric treatment is directed at the most likely etiologic agents.

Traditionally, infective endocarditis has been classified as *subacute* or *acute* based on the progression of disease. Subacute endocarditis may be community acquired or postoperative and usually occurs in patients with underlying structural heart disease. It has an indolent course over weeks to months characterized by low-grade fever, vague systemic complaints, and mild embolic phenomena. Table 1 lists the etiologic agents of infectious endocarditis in children. Viridans streptococci are the most frequent cause of subacute disease, but *Staphylococcus aureus* also can cause a subacute presentation. Acute endocarditis has a more fulminant course, with higher fever, systemic toxicity, sepsis, and major embolic events. It is more often community acquired and affects previously normal hearts but can complicate cardiac surgery or placement of a central venous catheter. *Staphylococcus aureus* is the most frequent etiologic agent. This classification has become less useful since there is increasing overlap of clinical appearance for a variety of organisms. The approach to treating endocarditis should involve selection of initial empiric therapy based on the clinical situation and pertinent medical history and definitive therapy based on identification and the antimicrobial susceptibilities of the causative organism.

TABLE 1. Etiologic Agents of Infective Endocarditis in Children

AGENT	CASES (%)
Streptococci	
Viridans	40
Enterococci	4
Pneumococci	3
Beta-hemolytic	3
Other	1
Staphylococci	
Coagulase-positive (*Staphylococcus aureus*)	24
Coagulase-negative	5
Gram-negative bacilli	4
Fungi	1
Others or mixed	2
Culture negative	13

CULTURES AND OTHER TESTS

When a patient is suspected of having infective endocarditis, the most important laboratory test is the blood culture. The bacteremia associated with endocarditis is usually low grade and continuous. In untreated infection, the first two blood cultures yield the causative organisms in 90% of cases. Culture positivity drops to 60% when there has been previous antibiotic treatment. Cultures should be obtained through any indwelling vascular catheters, as well as from a meticulously prepared venipuncture site. If the patient is clinically stable, two to three blood cultures should be obtained 1 to several hours apart before starting antimicrobial therapy. At least 1 ml of blood, and preferably more, should be sampled. Some of the specimen may be inoculated into thioglycollate broth and held for several weeks to detect slow-growing organisms. Nutritionally variant streptococci should be suspected if growth in broth fails to yield an organism on subculture to standard solid medium. These organisms may be L-cysteine deficient or pyridoxal phosphate deficient and should be subcultured again on the appropriate media. Blood cultures should be obtained every 24 to 48 hours after initiation of treatment until two or three consecutive specimens are sterile.

Transthoracic echocardiography, when performed by a skilled examiner, can detect vegetations in many pediatric patients with valvular or mural endocarditis, but the yield is lower when shunts or graft material is infected. Transesophageal echocardiography increases the detection rate, but the need for heavy sedation is a drawback to its use. In many cases, echocardiographic abnormalities persist for weeks to months after completion of ultimately successful antibiotic therapy, so the prognostic benefit of serial examinations is limited in the absence of embolic phenomena.

Antimicrobial susceptibility testing for the causative organism of endocarditis, in general, should be determined by the minimal inhibitory concentration (MIC) and minimal bactericidal concentration (MBC). Some experts recommend obtaining a serum inhibitory concentration (SIC) and serum bactericidal concentration (SBC) once a bacterium has been isolated and the patient is on appropriate antimicrobial therapy. For these tests, patient serum containing the antibiotic is added in serial twofold dilutions to a standard inoculum of the infecting organism. After incubation, the lowest dilution resulting in inhibition or killing of the organism can be determined. Many reference laboratories perform this test, but there are variations among laboratories in the inoculum size, composition of the broth medium, timing of samples, methods of dilution, and determination of end points. Most experts agree that an SBC at peak antibiotic concentration of ≥1:8 is desirable (although not always adequate), and most patients treated with the antibiotic doses listed in Table 2 will achieve these levels. Determination of the SIC and SBC may be most helpful for unusual organisms or antibiotics or if the clinical response to treatment is slow.

TABLE 2. Antimicrobial Therapy for Infective Endocarditis in Children

ETIOLOGIC AGENT	PRIMARY ANTIBIOTIC(S)	DURATION (weeks)	ALTERNATIVE ANTIBIOTIC(S)
Unknown (Start of Therapy or Culture Negative)			
Community acquired or late postsurgery	Nafcillin[1]	4–6	Vancomycin[3]
	+ gentamicin[2]	1–2	+ gentamicin
Nosocomial or early (≤ 60 d) postsurgery	Vancomycin	4–6	Add rifampin[4] if poor or slow clinical
	+ gentamicin	1–2	response
Streptococci			
Native valve, MIC < 0.1 μg/ml	Penicillin[5]	4	Vancomycin
	Penicillin[5]	2–4	+ gentamicin
	+ gentamicin	2	
Native valve, MIC ≥ 0.1 μg/ml (includes enterococci)	Penicillin	4–6	Vancomycin
	+ gentamicin	4–6	+ gentamicin
Prosthetic valve, graft, or surgical shunt	Penicillin	4–6	Vancomycin
	+ gentamicin	2–6	+ gentamicin
Staphylococci			
Methicillin-susceptible	Nafcillin	4–6	Vancomycin
	+ gentamicin	1–2	+ gentamicin
	± rifampin	2–4	± rifampin
Methicillin-resistant	Vancomycin	4–6	
	+ gentamicin	1–2	
	± rifampin	2–4	
Gram-Negative Bacilli	Use antimicrobial susceptibility patterns	6	
Fungi	Amphotericin B[6] ± 5-fluorocytosine[7] or rifampin	Minimum 40–50 mg/kg total dose	

[1] Naficillin 150–200 mg/kg/d (max: 12–20 g/d); oxacillin or methicillin may be substituted.
[2] Gentamicin 5–7.5 mg/kg/d; tobramycin or amikacin (15–30 mg/kg/d) may be substituted. Must check serum levels.
[3] Vancomycin 40–60 mg/kg/d (max: 2 g/d). Must check serum levels.
[4] Rifampin 10–20 mg/kg/d in 2 doses PO or IV; use if slow clinical response or staphylococcal infection of a prosthetic valve.
[5] Penicillin G 200,000–300,000 U/kg/d (max: 12–24 million U).
[6] Amphotericin B 1 mg/kg/d.
[7] 5-Fluorocytosine 50–100 mg/kg/d divided q6h. Must check serum levels.

SPECIAL CONSIDERATIONS

Neonates

The incidence of endocarditis in the neonate has increased dramatically over the past decade, probably because of improved survival and the increased use of indwelling vascular catheters. The relative immaturity of the neonate's immune system also may contribute to the higher incidence. Neonates are most likely to have involvement of previously normal right-sided heart structures and less frequently develop endocarditis on congenital heart defects. Since most neonatal endocarditis is nosocomial, the most frequently encountered organisms are *S. aureus,* coagulase-negative staphylococci (CONS), and *Candida* sps. Persistent isolation of an organism from a neonate's blood cultures should suggest the possibility of endocarditis. In general, neonatal endocarditis has a good prognosis unless *Candida* is the causative organism.

Postoperative Endocarditis

Early postoperative endocarditis (≤ 60 days after the operation) is usually a nosocomial infection resulting from contamination at the time of surgery or bacteremia that occurs in the hospital. Early endocarditis is most often caused by CONS, *S. aureus,* gram-negative bacilli, or fungi, especially *Candida* and *Aspergillus.* Patients often experience bacteremia and nonspecific systemic signs and symptoms, but clinical and immunologic features that are common in community-acquired subacute endocarditis often are absent. Late postoperative endocarditis is more often community acquired, although nosocomial infections due to CONS can have a long delay in clinical presentation. The distinction between early and late postoperative endocarditis is somewhat arbitrary and less apparent because of better sterilization

and surgical techniques and improved artificial materials. In general, the risk of postoperative endocarditis is greatest in the 2 months after surgery, then decreases steadily during the first year. Palliative systemic-to-pulmonary shunting has the greatest risk for postoperative endocarditis, followed by prosthetic valve placement and valve conduit repairs. Noncardiac procedures that predispose the patient to endocarditis include placement of indwelling vascular catheters into the right atrium, ventriculoatrial shunt placement to manage hydrocephalus, and surgically created arteriovenous fistulas.

MEDICAL THERAPY

The typical lesion of infective endocarditis is a dense, multilayered collection of platelets, thrombin, and other clotting components that has been invaded by large numbers of slowly proliferating organisms. Penetration of antimicrobial agents into this lesion is difficult and erratic, and the treatment period usually must be long. It is important that the antibiotics used are bactericidal for the causative organism. The drugs and regimens recommended here have been well studied in adults and used extensively in children. Some newer antibiotics may offer treatment advantages. For instance, ceftriaxone, which has been effective in the treatment of endocarditis in adults, can be given only once or twice per day. Although there is little experience with this drug in children with endocarditis and it cannot, at this time, be recommended generally, there may be children for whom its use would be a reasonable alternative to standard regimens.

Traditionally, infective endocarditis has been treated in the hospital. Economic and patient comfort considerations have increased the desire to use outpatient treatment for endocarditis. We always treat patients in the hospital for the first 1 to 2 weeks, when complication rates are highest and the need for clinical and laboratory monitoring is most intense. After this period of time, some patients may complete parenteral therapy at home if frequent visits can be arranged, the family has rapid access to appropriate medical facilities, the child has had a rapid response to initial therapy, and no complications have occurred or are expected.

Although some adult patients with endocarditis have been treated successfully with oral antimicrobial therapy, this approach cannot be recommended in children at this time.

Initial Therapy

Initial therapy is usually empiric, based on knowledge of the usual pathogens (Table 1) and the clinical circumstances. For community-acquired endocarditis in patients with rheumatic heart disease, those with congenital heart disease who have not recently undergone surgery, or those with no known heart disease, the most likely causative organisms are viridans streptococci, *S. aureus,* and fastidious gram-negative rods (HACEK bacilli—*Haemophilus, Actinobacillus, Cardiobacterium, Eikenella,* and *Kingella*). Since most community-acquired *S. aureus* is methicillin susceptible, the usual initial regimen is an antistaphylococcal semisynthetic penicillin (nafcillin, oxacillin, or methicillin) and an aminoglycoside (gentamicin usually is preferred because of its much lower cost). However, if the patient has been hospitalized recently in a unit where methicillin-resistant *S. aureus* (MRSA) is prevalent, vancomycin should be substituted for the semisynthetic penicillin (Table 2). Some experts add penicillin to the initial regimen, since it may have a higher bactericidal activity against viridans streptococci. However, the activity of the semisynthetic penicillins against viridans streptococci is usually adequate for initial therapy. If there is a strong suspicion of enterococcal endocarditis, however, it would be prudent to use penicillin in the initial regimen. Vancomycin can be used in place of penicillin or a semisynthetic penicillin in penicillin-allergic patients.

In early postoperative endocarditis, especially after placement of a prosthetic valve, the most common causative organism is CONS. Since most community-acquired and hospital-acquired CONS are resistant to semisynthetic penicillins, vancomycin and an aminoglycoside are most often used initially for early postoperative endocarditis.

Streptococci

Therapy for streptococcal endocarditis is determined by the clinical course and the antimicrobial susceptibility of the organism. Most viridans streptococci are highly susceptible to penicillin (MIC < 0.1 µg/ml). The most common treatment for these organisms has been 4 weeks of penicillin with or without the addition of gentamicin during the first 2 weeks of therapy. Clinical trials in adults with uncomplicated viridans streptococcal endocarditis, with 2 weeks total of combined penicillin and aminoglycoside treatment, have demonstrated success, but most of these patients had native valve endocarditis without foreign material in place. Endocarditis caused by viridans streptococci occurring on a prosthetic valve, graft, or surgical shunt usually should be treated with 4 to 6 weeks of penicillin combined with initial aminoglycoside therapy. Although *Streptococcus bovis,* Lancefield groups A, B, C, and G streptococci, and pneumococci usually are highly susceptible to penicillin, they often cause a more fulminant and destructive form of endocarditis, which requires 4 to 6 weeks of treatment.

Some streptococci and all enterococci are relatively resistant to penicillin (MIC ≥ 0.1 µg/ml). The usual penicillin MIC for enterococcus is > 2.0 µg/ml, but the combination of penicillin (or ampicillin) and an aminoglycoside is synergistic for enterococci. The usual treatment for endocarditis caused by these relatively resistant streptococci and enterococci is 4 to 6 weeks of penicillin or ampicillin and gentamicin. Some enterococci have become highly resistant to gentamicin. Streptomycin can be used if the streptomycin MIC is ≤ 2000 µg/ml. For beta-lactamase-producing enterococci, vancomycin should be substituted for penicillin.

Staphylococci

Staphylococcus aureus is the most common cause of an acute occurrence of endocarditis, especially when it occurs in a previously normal heart. Most isolates remain susceptible to semisynthetic penicillins, which are the drugs of choice. Although animal studies indicate that combination therapy using an antistaphylococcal penicillin and a low-dose aminoglycoside leads to more rapid sterilization of the blood and cardiac lesions than use of a beta-lactam drug alone, there are limited data from humans that support this concept. Most experts recommend combination therapy for the first 1 to 2 weeks of treatment. Rifampin is also an effective second drug and is often used in combination with vancomycin for penicillin-allergic patients, especially if the clinical course becomes complicated. Uncomplicated endocarditis due to *S. aureus* can be treated for 4 weeks. Treatment is extended to 6 weeks or longer if the patient has a slow clinical response, persistently positive blood cultures in the initial phase of treatment, intracardiac extension of infection, or significant embolic infection.

Endocarditis caused by methicillin-resistant *S. aureus* is increasing in frequency in many secondary and tertiary care centers. Vancomycin is the primary antibiotic, used in combination with gentamicin and/or rifampin. Although MRSA has not been associated with increased morbidity or mortality compared with susceptible strains of *S. aureus,* treatment usually is extended to 6 weeks.

The incidence of CONS endocarditis appears to be increasing in neonates and in the early postoperative period, especially after placement of a prosthetic valve. The CONS are usually resistant to antistaphylococcal penicillins, and vancomycin in combination with gentamicin and/or rifampin for 4 to 6 weeks is the regimen of choice. However, if the isolate is susceptible to the semisynthetic penicillins, they are the preferred drugs. The addition of rifampin may be particularly helpful if blood cultures are persistently positive or a myocardial abscess is suspected. When CONS endocarditis occurs on a prosthetic valve, the infected valve usually must be replaced.

Fungi

Fungal endocarditis is rare but usually has a devastating clinical course. It is most often found in premature infants and immunocompromised hosts who have had indwelling vascular catheters or as a postoperative complication of cardiac surgery. *Candida albicans* is the most frequent cause, but other *Candida* species can cause endocarditis. Blood cultures often are positive only intermittently. When *Aspergillus* causes endocarditis, blood cultures are negative, and the infection is usually discovered at autopsy. Therapy of fungal endocarditis usually requires a combined medical and surgical approach, although sporadic case reports have demonstrated cures with medical therapy alone. Amphotericin B is the usual treatment, and combination therapy with 5-fluorocytosine or rifampin is often used, although no clinical trials have documented their effectiveness. The optimal length of therapy has not been established, but a total amphotericin B dose of 40 to 50 mg/kg is a reasonable goal. If possible, surgery should be delayed until the patient has received 7 to 10 mg/kg of amphotericin B.

Gram-Negative Organisms

Gram-negative bacillary endocarditis occurs most often in immunosuppressed patients, injection drug users, and patients with prosthetic valves. About one half of cases are caused by the HACEK bacilli, which are fastidious and often require 2 to 3 weeks for culture isolation. The other cases are caused by enteric bacilli and more unusual organisms. Treatment should be dictated by the susceptibility patterns, and, in general, two-drug combination therapy is given for about 6 weeks.

Culture-Negative Endocarditis

About 10% of pediatric patients with clinical endocarditis have negative blood cultures. The incidence of culture-negative endocarditis increases in patients who have been treated with outpatient oral antibiotics. It is important to instruct the microbiology laboratory to hold blood cultures for 3 to 4 weeks so that fastidious, slow-growing organisms (HACEK bacilli, *Brucella,* fungi, nutritionally variant streptococci) can be isolated. Rare causes of culture-negative endocarditis in children are *Coxiella burnettii* (the agent of Q fever), chlamydiae, and possibly viruses.

In general, treatment for culture-negative endocarditis is similar to the initial empiric regimens, depending on the epidemiologic setting for the patient (Table 2). An important prognostic feature is the patient's response to the initial treatment. Ongoing surveillance to find an organism or to detect relapse or nonresponse to therapy is a critical part of treatment. If the initial response to therapy is good, the prognosis usually is excellent.

Evaluation of Therapy and Complications

The patient must be monitored for the effectiveness and safety of antimicrobial therapy. The most common side effect of long-term use of penicillins is bone marrow suppression, most notably neutropenia. Nafcillin and oxacillin can cause hepatitis, and methicillin most often causes interstitial nephritis. A weekly complete blood count and white blood cell differential and periodic liver enzyme tests and urinalysis should be obtained when these drugs are used. Vancomycin and aminoglycosides can cause eighth cranial nerve damage or renal dysfunction. The peak and trough serum levels of these drugs should be measured weekly.

Daily or every-other-day blood cultures should be obtained from patients being treated for endocarditis until several consecutive cultures are sterile. Echocardiographic assessment usually is obtained at diagnosis. Routine serial echocardiographic evaluation is not necessary if the patient has a rapid initial response to treatment and an uncomplicated course. However, repeat evaluation should occur if during treatment there is a new or changing murmur, hemodynamic instability, new embolic phenomena, or new positive blood cultures.

Complications of endocarditis can be cardiac or extracardiac. The most common cardiac complication is congestive heart failure caused by a dysfunctional valve or significant hemodynamic change. Other cardiac complications include pericarditis, myocardial abscess, rupture of the chordae, or myocardial infarction. Evidence of dysrhythmia or conduction defect may be the first clue to intracardiac extension of infection from the perivalvular area. Cardiac complications are most common when endocarditis is caused by staphylococci. Extracardiac complications, which usually arise from infected emboli, occur in 20% to 40% of children with endocarditis. Therapy with aspirin or other anticoagulants to attempt to decrease the incidence of embolic events (especially in patients who already have had one major or several minor embolic complications) has been advocated sporadically. The limited number of studies has included only adults, and the results have been conflicting. In general, anticoagulation therapy should not be used, especially if the need for surgical intervention is judged to be appreciable.

SURGICAL THERAPY

The use of surgery as adjunctive treatment for endocarditis appears to be increasing. There are several clear indications for surgery: intractable heart failure caused by valvular obstruction; prosthetic valve dehiscence; intracardiac extension of infection causing myocardial abscess, rupture of the chordae, papillary muscles, or ventricular septum, or uncontrollable dysrhythmia; most cases of fungal endocarditis; recurrent major emboli; and persistently (>1 week) positive blood cultures despite appropriate antimicrobial therapy. Early postoperative prosthetic valve endocarditis, especially when the organism is CONS, is usually an indication for surgery. Mortality from surgery ranges from 10% to 40% depending on the type of infection, condition of the patient, and type of procedure required.

The presence of a large vegetation, even on left-sided heart structures, is not by itself an indication for surgical intervention. The size of the vegetation is not predictive of early or late embolization. Although some organisms are more likely to be associated with endocarditis that results in embolization, with the exception of fungi, the identity of the infecting organism does not dictate the need for surgery. Because of the great risk of cardiac surgery in patients with endocarditis, most experts recommend surgically removing a vegetation only after a second major embolic event, usually to the central nervous system. Right-sided heart lesions that can embolize to the lungs rarely require removal of vegetations, since even multiple pulmonary emboli are rarely life threatening.

PREVENTION

Endocarditis can be prevented by either repairing the underlying cardiac defect or reducing the likelihood of significant bacteremia in patients at risk. The rationale for antimicrobial prophylaxis of endocarditis is based on many assumptions, and there are no adequately controlled clinical trials to validate the effectiveness of the suggested regimens. The American Heart Association regimens are based on in vitro studies, clinical experience, experimental animal models, and expert opinion. Of course, endocarditis can still occur despite the correct use of prophylactic regimens.

The conditions and procedures for which endocarditis prophylaxis is recommended are listed in Table 3. The American Heart Association recommendations for prophylactic regimens are shown in Table 4. The choice of regimen is determined by the most likely organism, relative risk of the patient for endocarditis, tolerance of oral antibiotics, and physician preference. In several clinical situations, these recommendations may not be optimal. Surgical procedures through infected body fluids or tissues require antimicrobial therapy directed against the causative organisms. Children who receive penicillin for prevention of rheumatic fever recurrences should receive erythromycin or clindamycin for endocarditis prophylaxis, since the previous penicillin treatment may have selected for relatively resistant viridans streptococci. Children at risk for endocarditis who undergo cardiac surgery should receive prophylaxis aimed against staphylococci. A first-generation cephalosporin or vancomycin would be an adequate choice.

TABLE 3. Conditions and Procedures for Which Endocarditis Prophylaxis is Recommended

Cardiac Conditions
Prosthetic cardiac valves
Most congenital cardiac malformations[1]
Rheumatic or other acquired valvular dysfunction
Hypertrophic cardiomyopathy
Mitral valve prolapse with valvular regurgitation
Previous infective endocarditis

Procedures[2]
Dental procedures that produce gingival or mucosal bleeding
Tonsillectomy and/or adenoidectomy
Surgery involving the intestinal or respiratory mucosa
Rigid bronchoscopy
Sclerotherapy for esophageal varices
Esophageal dilatation
Gallbladder surgery
Cystoscopy or urethral dilatation
Urethral catheterization or surgery if urinary tract infection is present[3]
Prostatic surgery
Incision and drainage of infected tissue[3]
Vaginal delivery if infection is present[3]

[1] Congenital cardiac malformations not requiring prophylaxis include isolated secundum atrial septal defect, surgical repair without residua beyond 6 months of secundum atrial septal defect, ventricular septal defect or patent ductus arteriosus, previous coronary artery bypass graft surgery, and mitral valve prolapse without valvular regurgitation.
[2] Selected procedures, not meant to be all-inclusive.
[3] Antibiotic therapy should be directed against the most likely bacterial pathogen(s).

TABLE 4. American Heart Association Recommendations for Endocarditis Prophylaxis

Regimens for Dental, Oral, or Upper Respiratory Tract Procedures

Standard

Amoxicillin PO	50 mg/kg 1 h before procedure, then 25 mg/kg 6 h after initial dose

Standard Penicillin-Allergic Patients

Erythromycin PO	20 mg/kg 1 h before procedure, then 10 mg/kg 6 h after initial dose
or clindamycin PO	10 mg/kg 1 h before procedure, then 5 mg/kg 6 h after initial dose

Patient Cannot Take Oral Medications

Ampicillin IM or IV	50 mg/kg 30 min before procedure, then 25 mg/kg 6 h after initial dose
or clindamycin IV	10 mg/kg 1 h before procedure, then 5 mg/kg 6 h after initial dose

High-Risk Patients

Ampicillin, gentamicin, and amoxicillin	Ampicillin IM or IV 50 mg/kg + gentamicin 2 mg/kg 30 min before procedure, then amoxicillin PO 25 mg/kg 6 h after initial dose or repeat parental regimen 8 h after initial dose
or vancomycin IV	20 mg/kg starting 1 h before procedure, no repeat dose necessary

Regimens for Genitourinary/Gastrointestional Procedures

Standard

Ampicillin, gentamicin, and amoxicillin	See High-Risk Patients

Penicillin-Allergic Patients

Vancomycin and gentamicin	Vancomycin IV 20 mg/kg and gentamicin 2 mg/kg 1 h before procedure, may be repeated 8 h after initial doses

Alternate Low-Risk Patient

Amoxicillin PO	50 mg/kg 1 h before procedure, then 25 mg/kg 6 h after initial dose

REFERENCES

1. Baltimore RS: Infective endocarditis in children. Pediatr Infect Dis J 1992; 11:907–913.
2. Bisno AL, Dismukes WE, Durack DT, et al: Antimicrobial treatment of infective endocarditis due to viridans streptococci, enterococci, and staphylococci. JAMA 1989;261:1471–1477.
3. Dajani AS, Bisno AL, Chung KJ, et al: Prevention of bacterial endocarditis: Recommendations by the American Heart Association. JAMA 1990;264:2919–2922.
4. Saiman L, Prince A, Gersony WM: Pediatric infective endocarditis in the modern era. J Pediatr 1993;122:897–853.
5. Tolan RW Jr, Kleiman MB, Frank M, et al: Operative intervention in active endocarditis in children: Report of a series of cases and review. Clin Infect Dis 1992;14:852–862.

CARDIOMYOPATHIES AND CARDIAC TRANSPLANTATION

CHARLES E. CANTER, M.D.
ARNOLD W. STRAUSS, M.D.

CARDIOMYOPATHY

The term cardiomyopathy encompasses heart disease originating primarily from defective cardiac muscle. Cardiomyopathies are generally divided into dilated, hypertrophic, and restrictive subtypes based on anatomy and hemodynamic characteristics. Treatment has traditionally been directed at symptomatic relief of the effects of congestive heart failure and arrhythmias. An increasing number of inborn errors of metabolism involving energy production and use (glycogeneses, beta-oxidative and mitochondrial respiratory chain disorders) that may result in a clinical picture of hypertrophic and/or dilated cardiomyopathy have been identified and are associated with other signs, such as hypotonia, hypoglycemia, sudden infant death syndrome, and Reye-like syndrome. Although these known genetic diseases are responsible for a minority of pediatric cardiomyopathies, identification is important, since some are treatable with dietary modification, and many are preventable with genetic counseling.

Dilated Cardiomyopathy

Dilated cardiomyopathies are characterized by increased left ventricular volume, an insufficient compensatory increase in wall thickness, and impaired systolic function. A large number of conditions have been associated with dilated cardiomyopathy: metabolic (thiamine, selenium, or magnesium deficiency), inflammatory (viral, bacterial, or protozoal myocarditis), neuromyopathic (muscular dystrophy), endocrinologic (hyperthyroidism and catecholamine excess), and toxic (anthracyclines). Other conditions that may be mistakenly diagnosed as a dilated cardiomyopathy include incessant atrial tachycardia and anomalous origin of the left coronary artery from the pulmonary artery. In these conditions, cardiac muscle dysfunction can be reversed with appropriate medical and surgical treatment of the underlying disorder. Nutritional and electrolyte deficiencies leading to dilated cardiomyopathy must particularly be suspected in patients who also have been supported with long-term parenteral nutrition. Some pediatric patients with myocarditis and dilated cardiomyopathy may improve with immunosuppressive medications, such as prednisone and azathioprine. A recent study has suggested that intravenous gamma globulin may promote myocardial recovery in children with myocarditis. Identification of a pediatric patient with an idiopathic dilated cardiomyopathy should be followed by a careful family history and evaluation of family members. Recent epidemiologic studies have demonstrated evidence of a familial cardiomyopathy in over 20% of patients with dilated cardiomyopathy. Echocardiographic evidence of dilated cardiomyopathy can be identified in asymptomatic family members.

Specific, curative medical treatment cannot be directed to most dilated cardiomyopathies observed in pediatric patients. Therefore, the goals of therapy are to (1) maximize cardiac function and exercise tolerance, (2) minimize embolic complications, and (3) control symptomatic arrhythmias. Angiotensin-converting enzyme (ACE) inhibitors, such as captopril and enalapril, prolong survival in adult patients with cardiomyopathy and congestive heart failure. These drugs, along with digoxin and diuretics, are also the cornerstone of therapy in pediatric patients with congestive heart failure. In advanced heart failure, combinations of ACE inhibitors and other vasodilators, such as isosorbide dinitrate and/or hydralazine, are useful (see discussion of congestive heart failure). There is a growing body of evidence indicating that beta-blockers, such as metoprolol, improve cardiac performance in adults with dilated cardiomyopathy. Beta-blockers are started at extremely low doses and are titrated carefully to avoid exacerbation of symptoms of congestive heart failure. Weeks of treatment may be needed before a beneficial effect is observed. Beta-blocker therapy has been started in dilated cardiomyopathy patients with mild symptomatology and must still be considered investigational for the pediatric patient.

Dilated, poorly contracting left ventricles commonly develop thrombi. Anticoagulation with warfarin is indicated to minimize the risk of pulmonic and systemic embolism. Ventricular arrhythmias are observed frequently in patients with dilated cardiomyopathy, but antiarrhythmic therapy is generally reserved for those with symptoms of syncope or near syncope. Atrial fibrillation or flutter should be controlled to maximize ventricular stroke volume. Antiarrhythmics should be used cautiously in these patients with dilated cardiomyopathy because of the proarrhythmic and negative inotropic effects of these medications.

In spite of optimal medical therapy, however, the prognosis for patients with dilated cardiomyopathy is poor. Myocarditis is often associated with recovery of heart function but has been associated with chronic, idiopathic dilated cardiomyopathies. There is some evidence that occurrence at a young age (less than 2 years) carries a better prognosis, but this has not been observed in all natural history studies. When medication cannot effectively palliate symptoms, orthotopic cardiac transplantation becomes the final therapeutic option.

Hypertrophic Cardiomyopathy

Hypertrophic cardiomyopathy is characterized by massive myocardial hypertrophy usually in an asymmetric manner involving the midportion and upper portion of the interventricular septum. However, symmetric, concentric hypertrophy also may occur. The most characteristic pathophysiologic abnormality is diastolic dysfunction, leading to elevated left ventricular end-diastolic pressure. The left ventricular outflow obstruction classically associated with the disease is not observed in all cases. Hypertrophic cardiomyopathy present in infants of diabetic mothers generally resolves spontaneously. Other conditions, including Noonan's syndrome and Friedreich's ataxia, have been associated with hypertrophic cardiomyopathy. Familial hypertrophic cardiomyopathy has been associated with mutations in the beta-myosin heavy chain, tropomyosin, or troponin T genes. It has an autosomal dominant inheritance pattern and a variable expression and penetrance. The majority of, but not all, pediatric cases of these contractile protein mutations are first clinically identified in adolescence.

Hypertrophic cardiomyopathy carries a 2% to 4% annual mortality rate in adults, and this rate in children is somewhat higher (3% to 6%). The goals of treatment of hypertrophic cardiomyopathy are primarily symptomatic relief of exercise intolerance, chest pain, and syncope. Sudden death is the most dreaded complication of hypertrophic cardiomyopathy, and adverse family history and syncope are clear risk factors in children. All patients with hypertrophic cardiomyopathy should be prohibited from athletics and activities involving strenuous effort.

Beta-blockers, such as propranolol, and calcium channel antagonists, such as verapamil, have been demonstrated to improve symptoms of exercise intolerance and chest pain in pediatric patients but apparently do *not* decrease the incidence of arrhythmias or the risk of sudden death. Thus, the benefits of treating asymptomatic patients with medication are not obvious. Surgical myectomy is contemplated when medical therapy is ineffective and may relieve symptoms, but it does not eliminate arrhythmias or sudden death. Recent investigation has indicated that implantation of an atrial rate-responsive (DDD) pacemaker will relieve symptoms and left ventricular outflow systolic pressure gradients in patients with hypertrophic cardiomyopathy who are resistant to medical therapy. Ventricular arrhythmias and atrial fibrillation may exacerbate symptoms in hypertrophic cardiomyopathy and can be treated with amiodarone. Transplantation is performed in patients with hypertrophic cardiomyopathy for intractable symptoms of heart failure or life-threatening arrhythmias unresponsive to medical therapy.

Restrictive Cardiomyopathy

Restrictive cardiomyopathies are unusual in the pediatric population and are characterized by normal ventricular size and systolic function, with elevated end-diastolic pressure, diastolic dysfunction, and marked atrial enlargement. Diuretics may be used to relieve symptoms of vascular congestion but must be employed cautiously, since these patients do not tolerate acute, marked reductions in intravascular volume. Vasodilators, such as ACE inhibitors, may reduce blood pressure without increasing cardiac output and probably should be avoided.

CARDIAC TRANSPLANTATION

Pediatric cardiac transplantation has been used increasingly as the final therapeutic option for both cardiomyopathies and congenital heart disease. The International Society for Heart and Lung Transplantation registry reveals that only 20 pediatric heart transplants were performed in 1984, but more than 250 were performed in 1992. Heart transplantation is considered in any pediatric patient with cardiac disease who (1) has progressive deterioration of ventricular function or functional status despite optimal medical and/or surgical therapy, (2) has growth failure secondary to congestive heart failure unresponsive to other treatment, (3) has a malignant arrhythmia or is a survivor of cardiac arrest unresponsive to medical treatment and unlikely to be treated successfully with an implantable defibrillator, (4) has a need for ongoing intravenous inotropic support, or (5) has an unacceptably poor quality of life. Because of the high mortality associated with staged, palliative surgery for hypoplastic left heart syndrome, we and others have offered transplantation as primary therapy for that lesion. Candidates for heart transplantation must generally (1) be free of chronic infection and major untreatable primary disease in other organ systems, (2) demonstrate an absence of irreversible pulmonary vascular disease as measured by pulmonary vascular resistance or transpulmonary pressure gradients, and (3) have evidence for an optimal social support structure to facilitate chronic care. Patients are listed for transplant based on blood type, acceptable donor weight range, and severity of illness.

Once transplantation has been performed, patients must remain on lifelong immunosuppression. Combinations of a number of immunosuppressive agents are used. We have employed a common combination termed "triple therapy," consisting of prednisone, azathioprine, and cyclosporine, with excellent results. Other centers have begun to use another immunosuppressant drug, FK506, as monotherapy. Cellular rejection and serious infections from bacteria or viruses, such as cytomegalovirus, occur most frequently within the first 6 months after transplantation. Side effects of immunosuppressive therapy include hypertension, hirsutism, renal toxicity, and gingival hyperplasia (cyclosporine), leukopenia (azathioprine), and growth retardation (steroids). Cyclosporine has a number of drug interactions that can both increase (erythromycin, ketoconazole, metoclopramide) and decrease (trimethoprim-sulfamethoxazole, phenobarbital, phenytoin, carbamazepine) cyclosporine blood levels and, thus, either increase the risk of side effects or reduce the level of immunosuppression. Diarrheal illnesses may lead to malabsorption of cyclosporine and lower blood levels, requiring transient increases in dosage. Live virus vaccines, such as the MMR and oral poliovaccines, should not be given to immunosuppressed patients, but other vaccines, such as DPT, HiB, and Salk poliovaccine, can be used safely. Varicella infection can be severe. Exposures frequently are treated with varicella hyperimmune globulin, and infections are treated with oral and intravenous acyclovir.

Despite the need for lifelong medications and careful surveillance, pediatric patients with heart transplants generally lead normal lives, with good somatic and cardiac growth. The overall survival for pediatric heart transplant recipients, especially infants, is lower than for adult recipients. We and others have achieved 5-year survival rates of over 80%. The major long-term complications of pediatric heart transplant recipients are neoplasia and coronary arteriopathy. Coronary disease in transplant recipients involves a diffuse narrowing of the coronary vasculature, especially affecting the small coronary arteries. The disease is common (demonstrable in 30% to 50% of adult transplant recipients 5 years after transplantation), progressive, and likely a manifestation of chronic rejection different from cellular rejection. The major symptoms of transplant coronary arteriopathy are heart failure and sudden death. Angina is generally not present, as the heart is denervated. To date, the only effective treatment for substantial coronary disease is retransplantation. Coronary arteriopathy has been observed in pediatric heart transplant recipients, but it remains unclear if it occurs with the same frequency as in adult heart transplant recipients. These long-term complications emphasize the uncertain future for pediatric heart transplant recipients.

REFERENCES

1. Drucker NA, Colan SD, Lewis AB, Beiser AS, Wessel DL, Takahashi M, Baker AL, Perez-Atayde AR, Newburger JW: Gamma-globulin treatment of acute myocarditis in the pediatric population. Circulation 1994;89:252–257.
2. Kelly DP, Strauss AW: Inherited cardiomyopathies. N Engl J Med 1994;330: 913–919.
3. O'Connell JB, Bourge RC, Costanzo-Nordin MR, Driscoll DJ, Morgan JP, Rose EA, Uretsky BF: Cardiac transplantation: Recipient selection, donor procurement, medical follow-up. Circulation 1992;86:1061–1079.

ACUTE RHEUMATIC FEVER

ADNAN S. DAJANI, M.D.

GENERAL THERAPY

When possible, a patient with the presumptive diagnosis of acute rheumatic fever should be admitted to a hospital for close observation and appropriate workup. Initial evaluations should include a throat culture, complete blood count, erythrocyte sedimentation rate, streptococcal antibody titers, chest roentgenogram, electrocardiogram, and echocardiogram.

Bedrest reduces physical activity and may lessen joint pain. The duration of bedrest is variable and individually determined. Ambulation may be attempted once fever abates and acute phase reactants return to normal. The patient should be allowed to return to reasonably normal physical activity. Strenuous physical exercise should be avoided, however, particularly if carditis is present.

Although throat cultures are rarely positive for group A streptococci at the onset of rheumatic fever, a 10 day course of penicillin therapy should be given. Patients allergic to penicillin should be treated with erythromycin (Table 1).

If heart failure is present, the patient should receive oxygen, diuretics, and digitalis and be on a restricted salt intake. Digitalis preparations should be used cautiously because cardiac toxicity may occur with conventional dosages.

ANTIRHEUMATIC THERAPY

There is *no specific* therapy for the inflammatory reactions in acute rheumatic fever. Supportive therapy is aimed at reducing constitutional symptoms, controlling toxic manifestations, and improving cardiac function.

TABLE 1. Primary Prevention of Rheumatic Fever (Treatment of Streptococcal Pharyngitis)

AGENT	DOSE	MODE	DURATION
Benzathine penicillin G	600,000 units for patients <60 lb 1,200,000 units for patients >60 lb *or*	IM	Once
Penicillin V (phenoxymethyl penicillin)	250 mg t.i.d.	PO	10 days
For Individuals Allergic to Penicillin			
Erythromycin estolate	20–40 mg/kg/d b.i.d.– q.i.d. (maximum 1 g/d) *or*	PO	10 days
Erythromycin ethylsuccinate	40 mg/kg/d b.i.d.– q.i.d. (maximum 1 g/d)	PO	10 days

Adapted with permission from Dajani AS, Bisno AL, Chung KJ, Durack DT, Gerber MA, Kaplan EL, Millard D, Randolph MF, Shulman ST, Watanakunakorn C: Special report. Prevention of rheumatic fever. Circulation 1988;78:1082–1086. Copyright 1988 American Heart Association.

Patients with mild or no carditis usually respond well to salicylates. Salicylates are particularly effective in relieving joint pain. Such pain usually subsides within 24 hours of starting salicylates. Indeed, if joint pain persists after salicylate treatment, the diagnosis of rheumatic fever may be questionable, and the patient should be reevaluated. Because there are no specific diagnostic tests for rheumatic fever,[1] anti-inflammatory therapy should be withheld until the clinical picture has become sufficiently clear to allow for a diagnosis. Early administration of anti-inflammatory agents may suppress clinical manifestations and prevent appropriate diagnosis.

For optimal anti-inflammatory effect, serum salicylate levels of approximately 20 mg/dl are desirable. Aspirin, in a dose of 100 mg/kg/d, given 3 to 4 times daily, usually results in adequate serum levels for a clinical response. Optimal aspirin therapy must be individualized, however, to ensure adequate response and avoid toxicity. Tinnitus, nausea, and vomiting are common dose-related toxicities associated with salicylism.

Children with significant cardiac involvement, particularly pericarditis or congestive heart failure, may respond more promptly to corticosteroids, and an occasional patient who does not respond to adequate doses of aspirin may benefit from a trial course of corticosteroids. The usual dose of prednisone is 1 to 2 mg/kg/d divided into 2 or 3 doses.

There is no evidence that salicylate or corticosteroid therapy affects the course of carditis, shortens the duration of the illness, or diminishes residual heart disease. Therefore, the duration of therapy with anti-inflammatory agents is arbitrarily based on the severity of the episode and the promptness of the clinical response. Mild attacks with little or no cardiac involvement may be treated with aspirin for about 1 month or until there is sufficient clinical and laboratory evidence of inflammatory inactivity. In more severe cases, therapy with corticosteroids may be continued for 2 to 3 months. Corticosteroids are then gradually reduced over the next 2 weeks. Even with prolonged treatment, approximately 5% of patients will continue to demonstrate evidence of rheumatic activity for several months.

A rebound, manifested by the reappearance of mild symptoms or of elevated acute phase reactants, may occur in some patients after anti-inflammatory medications have been discontinued, usually within 2 weeks. Mild symptoms usually subside without further treatment, but more severe symptoms may require treatment with salicylates. Some recommend the use of salicylates during the period when corticosteroids are being tapered and believe that such an approach may reduce the likelihood of a rebound.

Information about the use of salicylates other than aspirin is very limited. There is no evidence that nonsteroidal anti-inflammatory agents are more effective than aspirin. In children who are allergic to aspirin or cannot tolerate it, a trial of a nonsteroidal agent may be warranted. Aspirin preparations that are coated or that contain alkali or buffers also may be tried. However, there is little evidence that such preparations are better tolerated.

PRIMARY PREVENTION

Prevention of primary attacks of rheumatic fever depends on the prompt recognition and proper treatment of group A streptococcal pharyngitis. Eradication of group A streptococci from the throat is essential. Although appropriate antimicrobial therapy started several days after the onset of acute streptococcal pharyngitis is effective in preventing primary attacks of rheumatic fever, early therapy is advisable because it reduces both the morbidity and the period of infectivity. Usually, patients are considered noncontagious after 24 hours of initiation of therapy.

Table 1 outlines modified recommendations for the primary prevention of rheumatic fever as established by the Committee on Rheumatic Fever, Endocarditis, and Kawasaki Disease of the American Heart Association. Penicillin remains the agent of choice. Amoxicillin (with or without clavulanate), oral cephalosporins, and clindamycin are also acceptable agents. In individuals allergic to penicillin, erythromycin is recommended. Although a few recent reports suggest that some oral cephalosporins eradicate group A streptococci from the pharynx more effectively than penicillin, the role of these agents in the prevention of rheumatic fever has not been established. Sulfonamides, trimethoprim, tetracyclines, and chloramphenicol are *not* acceptable agents for the treatment of streptococcal pharyngitis.

Routine posttreatment throat cultures are generally not indicated except in individuals who are at high risk for rheumatic fever, who remain symptomatic, or who develop recurrent symptoms. Asymptomatic individuals who continue to have group A streptococci in the throat after appropriate antimicrobial therapy do not need repeated courses of therapy unless they or a family member have rheumatic fever. If a repeated course is necessary, it may be advisable to select a different acceptable antimicrobial agent rather than a second trial with the same agent.

SECONDARY PREVENTION

A patient who has an attack of rheumatic fever is inordinately susceptible to recurrent attacks following subsequent group A streptococcal infections of the upper respiratory tract. Such infections need not be symptomatic to cause a recurrence. *The most effective protection from rheumatic fever recurrences is provided by continuous antimicrobial prophylaxis.*

The risk of recurrences depends on several factors. The risk decreases as the interval since the most recent attack increases. Multiple previous attacks increase the risk. Individuals who are more likely to be exposed to group A streptococci, such as school teachers, parents of young children, physicians, nurses, and military recruits and other individuals living in crowded conditions, are at an increased risk for recurrences. The risk of recurrent carditis is particularly high in individuals who have had rheumatic carditis, and each recurrence is likely to cause further cardiac involvement and damage.

The American Heart Association regimens for antibiotic prophylaxis are listed in Table 2. Benzathine penicillin has an advantage because it does not depend on the patient's compliance. However, it requires a painful injection, and measurable levels of penicillin in serum may not persist beyond 18 days after administration in some individuals. Sulfadiazine is comparable to penicillin as a prophylactic agent but is not readily available. Other sulfonamides may be acceptable as prophylactic agents, but little information is available about their efficacy. Erythromycin may be used in individuals allergic to penicillin. Unfortunately, no data are available about the efficacy of erythromycin, oral cephalosporins, other beta-lactams, or clindamycin as prophylactic agents.

Patients who develop rheumatic carditis should receive long-term antibiotic prophylaxis well into adulthood and perhaps for life. Prophylaxis should continue even after valve surgery or valve replacement because the risk of rheumatic fever recurrence remains. Patients who do not develop carditis should receive prophylaxis for at least 5 years

after the last attack of rheumatic fever and until they are 20 years old. Prophylaxis beyond that should be determined on an individual basis after assessing the various factors mentioned. *No single regimen is totally effective in either eradicating streptococci from the pharynx or preventing recurrent attacks of rheumatic fever.*

REFERENCE

1. Dajani AS, Ayoub E, Bierman FZ, Bisno AL, Denny FW, Durack ST, Ferrieri P, Freed M, Gerber M, Kaplan EL, Karchmer AW, Markowitz M, Rahimtoola SH, Shulman ST, Stollerman G, Takahashi M, Taranta A, Taubert KA, Wilson W: Guidelines for the diagnosis of rheumatic fever. Jones criteria, 1992 update. JAMA 1992;268:2069–2073.

KAWASAKI SYNDROME

ROBERT P. SUNDEL, M.D.
JANE W. NEWBURGER, M.D., M.P.H.

Kawasaki syndrome (KS) is an idiopathic childhood vasculitis of small and medium-sized vessels that has become one of the leading causes of acquired heart disease in American children. The syndrome is characterized by fever, conjunctivitis, rash, mucosal inflammation, lymphadenopathy, and extremity changes, but the major morbidity involves the heart. Coronary artery aneurysms or ectasia develop in approximately 15% to 25% of untreated children with the disease and may lead to ischemic heart disease with angina, myocardial infarction, or sudden death. *Intravenous gamma globulin decreases the incidence of coronary artery aneurysms by threefold to fivefold if given within 10 days of disease onset.* Management of children with suspected KS, therefore, requires accurate and expeditious diagnosis and close monitoring of the cardiovascular system.

DIAGNOSIS

The diagnosis of KS rests on fulfilling at least five of six clinical criteria of mucocutaneous inflammation (Table 1). These criteria vary considerably in their frequency. Lymphadenopathy is most likely to be absent at diagnosis. Up to one half of children with KS do not have lymphadenopathy at presentation, and this is especially common in younger children. Fever, on the other hand, is a virtual sine qua non for the diagnosis. No laboratory values are included in the criteria for KS, but in ambiguous cases, certain trends may be helpful. Early in the disease course, acute phase reactants (e.g., ESR, CRP) tend to be elevated, and there is often a leukocytosis and left shift in the white blood count. The hematocrit is frequently more than 2 SD below normal, even early in the disease course. Urethritis, aseptic meningitis, and hepatitis are common features of the illness.

TABLE 2. Secondary Prevention of Rheumatic Fever (Prevention of Recurrent Attacks)

AGENT	DOSE/FREQUENCY	MODE
Benzathine penicillin G	1,200,000 U q3–4 wk*	IM
	or	
Penicillin V (phenoxymethyl penicillin)	250 mg b.i.d.	PO
For Individuals Allergic to Penicillin		
Erythromycin estolate	250 mg b.i.d.	PO

*Report of a WHO Study Group. Rheumatic Fever and Rheumatic Heart Disease. Technical Report Series 764. Geneva, World Health Organization, 1988.
Adapted with permission from Dajani AS, Bisno AL, Chung KJ, Durack DT, Gerber MA, Kaplan EL, Millard D, Randolph MF, Shulman ST, Watanakunakorn C: Special report. Prevention of rheumatic fever. Circulation 1988;78:1082–1086. Copyright 1988 American Heart Association.

TABLE 1. Diagnostic Criteria for Kawasaki Disease

I. Fever ≥5 days unresponsive to antibiotics
If the fever disappears because of IV gammaglobulin (IVGG) therapy before the fifth day of illness, a fever of <5 days duration fulfills fever criterion for case definition.
II. At least four of the five following physical findings with no other more reasonable explanation for the observed clinical findings
  A. Bilateral conjunctival injection
  B. Changes in the oropharyngeal mucous membranes (erythematous and/or fissured lips, strawberry tongue, injected pharynx)
  C. Changes of peripheral extremities, including erythema and/or edema of the hands or feet (acute phase) or periungual desquamation (convalescent phase).
  D. Polymorphous rash, primarily truncal
  E. Cervical lymphadenopathy ≥1.5 cm diameter

Modified from Centers for Disease Control: Kawasaki disease—New York. MMWR 1990;39 (No. RR-13):17–18.

The criteria for KS do not identify all cases of the illness and may be particularly insensitive in infants less than 12 months of age. Children of any age who subsequently develop coronary artery abnormalities might not fulfill the criteria (so-called atypical KS), so pediatricians should suspect KS in any child with prolonged, unexplained fever. On the other hand, certain conditions might mimic KS, including viral infections (measles, enteroviruses, adenovirus), toxin-mediated illnesses (toxic shock syndrome, beta-hemolytic streptococcal infection), drug reactions, and autoimmune diseases (juvenile rheumatoid arthritis). Although there is no definitive test for KS, exclusion of alternatives will allow a presumptive diagnosis in most situations.

THERAPY

Aspirin

Aspirin was the first medication to be used for the treatment of KS because of its anti-inflammatory and antithrombotic effects. Experts vary in their dosage recommendations in KS because of the paucity of objective data concerning an ideal regimen and different perceptions of theoretical and potential risks, such as Reye syndrome. Additionally, aspirin-binding studies suggest that the hypoalbuminemia of children with KS predisposes them to toxic free-salicylate levels despite measured (bound) values within the therapeutic range. Many clinicians have the impression that high-dose aspirin makes children less uncomfortable and benefits the associated arthritis seen in up to one third of cases of KS. Trials comparing high-dose and low-dose aspirin in KS are being conducted. Preliminary results show a trend toward more rapid normalization of signs of systemic inflammation (fever, leukocytosis) in children receiving higher salicylate doses.

Typically, high aspirin doses are employed during the inflammatory phase of illness, and salicylate levels are monitored to avoid toxicity. Once the child has been afebrile for 2 or 3 days, aspirin may be decreased to antithrombotic doses. If the coronary arteries remain normal, salicylates may be discontinued approximately 7 weeks after the onset of fever. Following the acute inflammatory stage of KS, platelet counts may remain elevated for weeks, and coronary artery endothelium is thought to have diminished antiaggregatory potential. Accordingly, low-dose aspirin is conventionally continued in order to provide some antithrombotic effects. Thus, our typical regimen consists of aspirin at a dose of 80 to 100 mg/kg/d in four divided doses until the child is afebrile for 48 hours. We then decrease the aspirin dose to 3 to 5 mg/kg/d, and if joint symptoms return, we add naproxen (7 to 10 mg/kg per dose b.i.d.) or ibuprofen (8 to 10 mg/kg per dose t.i.d. or q.i.d.) on an as-needed basis. All medications are discontinued once the platelet count and ESR return to normal.

Intravenous Gamma Globulin

Prospective, randomized, multicenter controlled trials in Japan and the United States have demonstrated a significant decrease in coronary artery abnormalities when treatment is initiated within 10 days of onset of fever. Therapy with gamma globulin has additional benefits as well. Treatment results in a reduced prevalence of giant aneurysms (internal diameter at least 8 mm), the most serious form of coronary abnormality caused by the disease, and accelerates normalization of abnormalities of left ventricular systolic function and contractility. High-dose IVGG also reduces fever and laboratory indices of inflammation, suggesting a rapid, generalized anti-inflammatory effect. Standard treatment for KS is a single infusion of 2 g/kg over 8 to 12 hours. In a recently concluded multicenter, randomized, controlled trial of 549 children with KS, the overall prevalence of coronary artery abnormalities was lower than with the former regimen of four daily infusions of 400 mg/kg/d (12/260 versus 24/263 at 2 weeks of illness, $p = 0.042$).[1] Furthermore, resolution of fever and systemic inflammation is faster, allowing earlier discharge from the hospital. Adverse effects are unusual. Although fluid overload and development of congestive heart failure pose a theoretical concern, experience shows that these complications are quite rare. Five to ten percent of children might experience mild reactions during the gamma globulin infusion (fever, chills, headache), but these usually resolve when the infusion rate is decreased.

Antithrombotic Therapy

The risk of coronary artery thrombosis is greatest during the subacute phase of the disease. At that point, usually beginning approximately 2 to 3 weeks after disease onset, smoldering coronary vasculitis coincides with marked thrombocytosis and hypercoagulability because of both endothelial and fluid phase abnormalities. Low-dose aspirin (<5 mg/kg/d given as a single dose) is the mainstay of antithrombotic therapy in KS. Dipyridamole (3 to 6 mg/kg/d in three divided doses) may be substituted for aspirin when salicylates are contraindicated (e.g., following varicella exposure in a nonimmune child). For children without evidence of coronary artery ectasia or aneurysms, antiplatelet therapy is usually discontinued approximately 2 months after onset of illness, once the platelet count and ESR have normalized.

Children with coronary artery abnormalities require chronic antithrombotic therapy, usually with low-dose aspirin. Dipyridamole is sometimes added to aspirin therapy, although its value in this setting is controversial. The risk of coronary thrombosis and myocardial infarction is especially great in children with rapidly increasing coronary dimension or with giant aneurysms. In these children, treatment options include antiplatelet therapy (aspirin with or without dipyridamole), anticoagulation using warfarin (at doses adequate to achieve a 1.5-fold prolongation of the PT), or a combination of antiplatelet and anticoagulant therapy. No prospective data exist to guide the clinician in choosing an optimal regimen, and anecdotal reports suggest cases of thrombosis despite treatment with each of these drug combinations.

Thrombolytic Therapy

Despite the use of antithrombotic agents, myocardial infarction secondary to thrombotic occlusion of coronary aneurysms may develop in some children, especially in those with giant aneurysms. In others, the presence of a coronary artery thrombus may be detected on serial two-dimensional echocardiography. Thrombolytic agents (e.g., urokinase or streptokinase), either intravenous or intracoronary, have been used with variable success. Thrombolytic therapy for coronary artery thrombosis is most effective if begun within 3 to 4 hours of the onset of symptoms. Immediately following clot lysis, systemic heparin is begun in combination with aspirin. Maintenance of reperfusion then requires chronic oral antithrombotic therapy (e.g., warfarin with dipyridamole), although the ideal regimen has not been established.

Surgical Management

Surgery in KS consists primarily of coronary artery bypass grafts (CABG) for obstructive lesions, although mitral valve replacement occasionally is necessary in children with papillary muscle dysfunction or valvulitis. The indications for CABG procedures in children have not been established definitively, but such surgery should be considered when stenosis is demonstrated to be progressive, the myocardium to be perfused through the graft is still viable, and no appreciable lesions are present in the artery peripheral to the planned graft site. When these conditions are satisfied, surgery is an option if arteriography demonstrates critical stenosis of the left main coronary artery or occlusions or progressive critical stenosis are present in two or more of the other coronary vessels. Isolated stenotic lesions in the proximal left anterior descending artery or the right coronary artery probably are not an indication for bypass grafting. Optimal results are obtained with the use of internal mammary artery grafts, which increase in both diameter and length as the children grow.

Other Treatment

Data are inadequate to allow firm recommendations concerning treatment of two groups of children, those who fail to respond to IVGG and those who have fever more than 10 days after the onset of KS. In both instances, aggressive management seems warranted in view of the association of prolonged fever with increased risk of developing coronary artery abnormalities. We recently reviewed our experience with retreating persistent or recrudescent fever caused by KS. During the 5-year period analyzed, 13 children who failed to defervesce after their initial dose of IVGG or whose fevers recurred within 72 hours were reinfused with IVGG, 1 g/kg. Ten of the 13 responded promptly, and 1 other child defervesced after a third dose of IVGG. The risk of retreatment was minimal, so retreatment seems to be appropriate in a subset of severe or nonresponsive KS. Nonetheless, clinicians must be careful to rule out alternative explanations for the fever before any dose of IVGG, and complete assessment of the efficacy of IVGG retreatment awaits randomized, controlled studies.

No other specific second-line therapy has been tested in patients for whom gamma globulin is ineffective. A potential role for corticosteroids is controversial. Similarly, there are no controlled trials of IVGG treatment in patients appearing after the tenth day of fever. Nonetheless, most clinicians with experience in KS treat such children with gamma globulin if they are still febrile or if they have coronary artery disease and any signs of active inflammation.

MONITORING

Coronary artery lesions resulting from KS change dynamically over time. The first echocardiogram and laboratory studies (especially CBC, platelet count, and ESR) are obtained on admission for IVGG treatment. Follow-up studies and examinations are performed by a pediatric cardiologist approximately 2 and 4 to 8 weeks later unless evidence of a rapidly expanding aneurysm necessitates more frequent evaluations. Despite IVGG therapy, 5% to 10% of children will have echocardiographically demonstrable coronary artery abnormalities 2 weeks after the onset of fever. At least one half of these will regress within 12 to 24 months. Healing occurs by myointimal proliferation or organization of thrombus. In addition to histologic abnormalities, regressed aneurysmal segments show abnormalities of function. The long-term prognosis for children with regressed coronary abnormalities is unknown, so we prefer to follow these children indefinitely at regular intervals. The frequency of cardiologic evaluations in children with coronary artery aneurysms is individualized depending on the patient's condition.

If coronary arteries remain normal throughout the first month after acute KS, subsequent development of new lesions is extremely unusual. On the other hand, abnormalities in prostaglandin and lipid metabolism may persist for months after clinical resolution of the disease, suggesting long-term endothelial cell dysfunction. Therefore, repeat cardiology evaluations are obtained 1 year after onset of KS and then at 5-year intervals. At these appointments, lipid profiles are also evaluated, and prudent diet and exercise regimens are discussed. From the purely clinical perspective, however, children without known cardiac sequelae during the first month of KS appear to return to their previous state of health without signs or symptoms of cardiac impairment, and their overall prognosis appears to be excellent.

REFERENCE

1. Newburger JW, Takahashi M, Beiser AS, et al: A single intravenous infusion of gamma globulin as compared with four infusions in the treatment of acute Kawasaki syndrome. N Engl J Med 1991;324:1633–1639.

PULMONARY HYPERTENSION

ROBERT L. GEGGEL, M.D.

Pulmonary hypertension can be caused by a variety of conditions (Table 1). Before instituting treatment, the clinician must establish a precise diagnosis, since timely therapy for some conditions can resolve or significantly reduce the elevation in pulmonary pressure. A complete evaluation includes a detailed history and physical examination, followed by appropriate laboratory tests, which may include a chest radiograph, arterial blood gas, pulmonary function tests, ventilation-perfusion scan, echocardiogram, electrocardiogram, cardiac catheterization with pulmonary angiography, collagen vascular screen, liver function tests, and occasionally a lung biopsy. Frequently missed diagnoses include thromboembolic disease, pulmonary interstitial fibrosis, sleep disorder associated with hypoxic vasoconstriction, venoocclusive disease, partial anomalous pulmonary venous connection, and pulmonary vein stenosis or atresia.

GENERAL MEASURES

Patients with near systemic levels of pulmonary pressure should be restricted from strenuous exercise to decrease the risk of syncope. The increased cardiac output associated with exertion produces further elevation in pulmonary pressure in patients with fixed vascular obstruction and can lead to ventricular dysfunction. Women of childbearing age with moderate to severe pulmonary hypertension should avoid pregnancy, since ventricular dysfunction and aggravation of

TABLE 1. Causes of Pulmonary Hypertension

Cardiac
Increased pulmonary blood flow associated with left-to-right shunts at the atrial, ventricular, or great vessel level
  Examples: atrial septal defect, ventricular septal defect, complete atrioventricular canal, patent ductus arteriosus, transposition of the great arteries, truncus arteriosus
Left-sided obstructive lesions associated with pulmonary venous congestion
  Examples: coarctation of the aorta, aortic stenosis, mitral stenosis, pulmonary vein stenosis or atresia, cor triatriatum, atrial myxoma
Cardiomyopathy

Pulmonary
Idiopathic: primary pulmonary hypertension, venoocclusive disease
Hypoxic vasoconstriction
  Alveolar hypoventilation: sleep disorders, upper airway obstruction, neuromuscular disorder, chest wall deformity
  Obstructive or restrictive lung disease: cystic fibrosis, broncopulmonary dysplasia, interstitial fibrosis
  Pneumonia
  High altitude
Pulmonary hypoplasia: primary; associated with congenital diaphragmatic hernia or renal dysplasia
Peripheral pulmonary stenosis
Persistent pulmonary hypertension of the newborn

Thromboembolic
Ventriculoatrial shunt, indwelling catheters, deep vein thrombosis
Parasitic disease: filariasis, schistosomiasis
Hematologic: sickle cell disease, polycythemia

Hepatic Disease
Cirrhosis, portal hypertension

Collagen Vascular Disease
Scleroderma, systemic lupus erythematosus, rheumatoid arthritis, mixed connective tissue disease

Granulomatous Disease
Sarcoidosis

pulmonary hypertension can result from the increased cardiac output during gestation or with significant fluid shifts in the peripartum period. Maternal or fetal death has been reported in this setting. In patients with right-to-left shunting, pregnancy increases the risk of deep vein thrombosis and paradoxical embolus. To minimize the risk of paradoxical embolus at other times, nonhormonal forms of birth control are preferred.

Digoxin augments right ventricular contractility against the elevated afterload and is also useful if there is coexisting left ventricular dysfunction. Patients with pulmonary hypertension associated with pulmonary parenchymal disease can be more susceptible to toxic effects of digoxin even at therapeutic serum levels, so that careful monitoring is necessary.

Diuretics relieve symptoms of right ventricular failure, such as congestive hepatosplenomegaly, ascites, and edema. There can be left ventricular diastolic dysfunction because of posterior interventricular septal displacement from a pressure overloaded right ventricle, producing dyspnea and orthopnea. Diuretics can ameliorate these symptoms. However, diuretics can produce an electrolyte imbalance, which could increase the risk of toxicity if digoxin is used concomitantly.

Anticoagulation with warfarin is necessary in pulmonary hypertension associated with thromboembolic disease and may be beneficial in moderate to severe pulmonary hypertension from other causes. Severe pulmonary hypertension produces progressive luminal narrowing of pulmonary arteries from medial hypertrophy and intimal hyperplasia, which may contribute to in situ thrombosis. However, pulmonary hemorrhage is a complication of severe chronic pulmonary hypertension, and it is unclear whether anticoagulation increases the risk of this event.

Severe polycythemia requires partial erythrophoresis. Central hematocrit values in excess of 70% are associated with markedly elevated blood viscosity, which decreases cardiac output, decreases perfusion to organs including the heart, increases the risk of thrombosis, and produces symptoms including headache, fatigue, or chest pain. Reducing the hematocrit from these values by approximately 10% increases cardiac output and relieves symptoms. The following formula can be used to estimate the amount of whole blood to withdraw.

Blood volume to remove (ml)
$$= \frac{\text{Estimated blood volume (ml)} \times (\text{Hct}_i - \text{Hct}_d)}{\text{Hct}_i}$$

where Hct_i is the initial central venous hematocrit and Hct_d is the desired central venous hematocrit. For children greater than 1 year of age, the blood volume is approximately 70 ml/kg and for adults approximately 65 ml/kg. It is safest to replace any withdrawn blood with an equal volume of either normal saline, fresh frozen plasma, or 5% salt-poor albumin or to use a pheresis machine that returns the patient's plasma to the opposite arm from which blood is withdrawn.

Patients with pulmonary hypertension should receive the annual winter flu vaccine. Pneumonitis in such patients will elevate pulmonary pressure further, which may be poorly tolerated.

PRIMARY PULMONARY HYPERTENSION

Primary pulmonary hypertension is a rare disease, especially in patients less than 20 years of age. In addition to the general principles outlined, a trial of vasodilator therapy is offered. All vasodilator testing needs to be performed with intravascular hemodynamic monitoring. With the exception of inhalational nitric oxide, all available agents are nonselective and can cause systemic hypotension, more profound cyanosis from increased right-to-left shunting via a patent foramen ovale, exacerbation of pulmonary hypertension because of increased cardiac output in a nonreactive pulmonary vascular bed, and occasionally death.

There is spontaneous variability in pulmonary hemodynamics in patients with primary pulmonary hypertension. Changes can be attributed to a vasodilator if pulmonary pressure decreases by more than 22% and calculated pulmonary resistance decreases by more than 36%

when vasodilator therapy is used. Yet the benefits to a patient in whom a vasodilator increases cardiac output, decreases calculated pulmonary resistance, and does not affect pulmonary pressure are unclear. In such a situation, right ventricular work load is increased, and pulmonary vascular disease may progress because of increased shear forces. Also, in this circumstance, the interpretation of a reduction in pulmonary vascular resistance is difficult. Vascular resistance is a calculated rather than a measured value and assumes a linear relationship between pressure and flow. An increased cardiac output may lead to recruitment or passive distention of blood vessels rather than reduction in pulmonary vascular tone. Criteria for a beneficial effect include a significant reduction in pulmonary pressure, reduction in the ratio of pulmonary/systemic vascular resistance indicating a predominant pulmonary effect, and no clinically significant change in systemic pressure.

A wide variety of vasodilator agents have been used in patients with primary pulmonary hypertension. Children and young adults are more likely to respond favorably, since vasoconstriction is an early component, followed later by fixed vascular obstructive changes. Unfortunately, the majority of patients with primary pulmonary hypertension do not benefit from currently available vasodilators.

Initial screening is performed most safely with short-acting intravenous agents to avoid prolonged systemic effects. Adenosine, a purine nucleoside, provides safe and rapid assessment of vascular reactivity. Adenosine has a short half-life (2 to 10 seconds) because of metabolism by adenosine deaminase in endothelial cells and erythrocytes. Adenosine increases vascular smooth muscle levels of adenosine 3′, 5′-cyclic monophosphate, which mediates vasodilation. The initial infusion rate is 50 μg/kg/min, and it is increased by 50 μg/kg/min at 2-minute intervals to a maximum rate of 500 μg/kg/min. Ideally, the infusion should be into the right ventricle or main pulmonary artery to minimize systemic effects. The infusion is discontinued if the pulse rate increases by more than 50% or the systemic pressure decreases by more than 30%. Side effects include a sensation of chest pressure, headache, tingling or numbness of the extremities, nausea, dyspnea, and heart block. These effects resolve within 30 seconds of discontinuation of the infusion. Adults with primary pulmonary hypertension do not respond favorably to nifedipine if a beneficial response to adenosine has not been demonstrated. Studies in the pediatric population are not available.

Prostacyclin (prostaglandin I₂), a metabolite of arachidonic acid produced by vascular endothelial cells is a useful screening agent. The use of prostacyclin is under protocol, so that general availability is limited. The half-life of prostacyclin is 3 minutes, with the peak effect occurring within the first 3 minutes. The initial infusion rate is 1 to 2 ng/kg/min, and it is increased by 1 to 2 ng/kg/min every 5 to 15 minutes to a maximum rate of 40 ng/kg/min. The infusion is discontinued if the pulse rate increases by more than 50%, the systemic pressure decreases by more than 30%, no further pulmonary vasodilation occurs with a higher infusion rate, or intolerable side effects occur. Side effects, in addition to systemic hypotension, include cutaneous flushing, headache, pulmonary edema, and nausea or vomiting. Adult and pediatric patients have not had a favorable response to other vasodilators (nifedipine, diltiazem, hydralazine, phentolamine, isoproterenol, or sodium nitroprusside) without also having a beneficial response to prostacyclin. Small numbers of adult patients have been treated with prolonged (up to 18 month) infusions of prostacyclin via a central venous line using a portable syringe pump with persistent hemodynamic benefit. Over extended periods, some tachyphylaxis develops so that higher infusion rates are necessary. This therapy has not been used in children. Because the equipment is cumbersome, such an approach should be used only if oral agents are ineffective. Prolonged prostacyclin use may have a role as a bridge to heart-lung or lung transplantation in selected patients.

Nitric oxide is an endothelial-derived relaxing factor synthesized from L-arginine in vascular endothelial cells. Nitric oxide is lipophilic and readily diffuses into the adjacent smooth muscle cell, where it mediates vasodilation by increasing intracellular levels of guanosine

3',5'-cyclic monophosphate. The half-life of nitric oxide is 3 to 6 seconds. Nitric oxide rapidly binds to hemoglobin and is inactivated, so that it produces no systemic effects. When inhaled in a concentration of 40 parts per million (ppm) in adults with primary pulmonary hypertension, nitric oxide selectively decreases pulmonary vascular resistance by 5% to 68%. This agent may become a useful screening tool. The methemoglobin produced in the inactivation of nitric oxide has not reached clinically significant levels in inhaled concentrations of 40 to 80 ppm for 30 minutes or 6 to 20 ppm for 1 to 53 days. Nitric oxide in the presence of oxygen is oxidized to nitrogen dioxide and higher orders of nitrogen that potentially can be toxic to the lung. Further work is needed to ensure that no oxidant injury occurs.

The most commonly used vasodilator in patients with primary pulmonary hypertension is the calcium channel blocking agent nifedipine. High-dose therapy in adults has been documented to lower pulmonary pressure and improve survival. When administered sublingually, the half-life is 2 hours, and the peak effect occurs in 20 to 30 minutes. When administered PO, the half-life is 3 hours, and the peak effect occurs in 20 to 45 minutes. Acute testing in adults consists of giving 20 mg PO on an hourly basis until the pulse rate increases by more than 50%, systemic pressure decreases by more than 30%, intolerable side effects occur (dizziness, flushing, headache), or no further reduction in pulmonary pressure or resistance is noted with an additional dose. In children, a 10 mg dose is used, which can be repeated in a similar manner. The total cumulative dose is halved, and this amount is given every 6 to 8 hours. Nifedipine has a negative inotropic effect, and, therefore, careful monitoring of ventricular function is required.

Phentolamine, an alpha-adrenergic blocking agent, has reduced pulmonary pressure and resistance in a small number of patients. The half-life is 19 minutes. The initial infusion rate is 5 μg/kg/min, and this is increased by 5 μg/kg/min every 15 minutes to a maximum rate of 15 μg/kg/min. The infusion is discontinued if the pulse rate increases by more than 50% or systemic pressure decreases by more than 30%. Side effects include tachycardia, arrhythmia, or gastrointestinal stimulation. Oral therapy can be continued with prazosin. The initial dose is 25 to 40 μg/kg every 12 hours, and this is increased slowly to a maximum daily dose of 20 mg divided in two to three doses. Tachyphylaxis to prazosin occurs frequently with long-term therapy.

The clinical utility of other vasodilation agents reported in the literature in patients with primary pulmonary hypertension is questionable. Tolazoline is associated with multiple side effects and is ineffective as a chronic oral agent. Isoproterenol frequently increases pulmonary artery pressure because of a higher cardiac output and is arrhythmogenic. Its sublingual absorption is unreliable. Diazoxide, a direct smooth muscle relaxant, frequently causes significant systemic hypotension when tested acutely (1 to 5 mg/kg bolus infusion). Its chronic use (3 to 8 mg/kg/d divided in two to three doses) is associated often with fluid and sodium retention, hyperuricemia, hyperglycemia, hirsutism, arrhythmia, gastrointestinal intolerance, and postural hypotension. There is limited experience with sodium nitroprusside. Oral therapy with isosorbide dinitrate in some patients reduces cardiac output. Hydralazine is a potent systemic vasodilator that increases cardiac output and usually minimally reduces pulmonary pressure. In many patients with primary pulmonary hypertension, symptoms of right ventricular failure develop as a result. The injectable form of hydralazine is no longer manufactured. Captopril, an angiotensin-converting enzyme inhibitor, has not produced long-term hemodynamic benefit in patients with primary pulmonary hypertension. It may benefit patients with pulmonary hypertension secondary to left ventricular dysfunction.

PERSISTENT PULMONARY HYPERTENSION OF THE NEWBORN

Neonates with persistent pulmonary hypertension of the newborn can have underdevelopment of the lung (associated most commonly with congenital diaphragmatic hernia or renal dysplasia or agenesis),

maladaptation with failure of normal neonatal pulmonary vasodilation, maldevelopment with excessive muscularization of the pulmonary arteries, or a combination of these abnormalities. Surgical correction of a diaphragmatic hernia is required. Conventional medical management to promote pulmonary vasodilation includes measures to relieve hypoxia and acidosis, which contribute to the elevated pulmonary vascular resistance. Mechanical ventilation with high concentrations of inspired oxygen and hyperventilation, combined with infusion of sodium bicarbonate, is used. Neuromuscular blockade can limit an acute rise in peak inspiratory pressure in an agitated neonate and decrease the risk of pneumothorax. Nonselective pulmonary vasodilators (tolazoline, isoproterenol) are useful in an occasional patient but usually are ineffective or associated with systemic side effects, including hypotension. Metabolic or hematologic abnormalities are corrected, and intravenous inotropic support (dopamine, dobutamine) is added if needed. In selected centers, extracorporeal membrane oxygenation (ECMO) is available. Critically ill neonates are assigned this therapy, and, therefore, precise determination of complications is difficult. However, many patients have significant neurologic, hemorrhagic, cardiovascular, and renal complications.

The recent use of inhalational nitric oxide (see previous section) for this condition may represent a significant advancement. Concentrations of 80 ppm have been used for 1 day and 6 to 20 ppm for as long as 3 days, with selective reduction in pulmonary artery pressure and resistance. Therapy of sufficient duration can lead to permanent reduction in these values even after the nitric oxide is discontinued. Some centers have noted a marked reduction in the frequency of use of extracorporeal membrane oxygenation since offering nitric oxide therapy. Further studies are necessary to ensure that no important side effects occur.

CONGENITAL HEART DISEASE

Pulmonary hypertension complicates a variety of congenital heart defects. If the pulmonary circulation is exposed to increased flow or pressure or both for too long, nonreversible and progressive obstructive anatomic changes occur in the pulmonary vessels. The only effective treatment is timely surgical repair of the cardiac defect to avoid the development of such vascular changes. Certain lesions cannot be repaired definitively in infancy and require palliation with a pulmonary artery band. The level of pressure and rate of progression depend on the lesion and individual variation. Those defects associated with both increased pulmonary flow and pulmonary pressure (e.g., large ventricular septal defect, large patent ductus arteriosus, transposition of the great arteries with ventricular septal defect, complete atrioventricular canal, truncus arteriosus, single ventricle without pulmonary stenosis) are at greatest risk for pulmonary vascular obstructive disease developing as early as 4 months to 2 years. Such patients require surgical repair or palliation within that time period. A minority of patients with defects associated with increased pulmonary flow (10% to 17% of patients with large atrial septal defect) develop pulmonary hypertension, usually in adult life although exceptions occur in the pediatric age range. Repair of such lesions usually can safely be deferred until 4 to 8 years of age. The pulmonary hypertension associated with pulmonary venous obstruction (left-sided obstructive lesions) usually normalizes after surgery, especially if repair is performed during infancy. Patients with congenital heart disease and Down syndrome are at increased risk for early pulmonary vascular obstructive disease because of possible coexisting pulmonary hypoplasia, chronic upper airway obstruction, or sleep-induced ventilatory dysfunction. Patients living at high altitudes also have earlier onset of pulmonary hypertension.

The decision about the suitability for operation of patients with elevated pulmonary vascular resistance can be difficult. The reactivity of the pulmonary vascular bed is assessed by administering 100% oxygen. Inhaled nitric oxide (80 ppm for 30 minutes) has additive effects to hyperoxia and unmasks additional reversible vasoconstriction. Usually infants 6 to 12 months of age are offered surgery, since advanced pulmonary vascular obstructive disease is unusual in this age range. Older patients often are offered surgery if pulmonary resistance is less than 8 to 10 $U \cdot m^2$, there is a predominant left-to-right shunt, and the ratio of pulmonary/systemic resistance is less than 0.5. An occasional patient with higher pulmonary vascular resistance values (e.g., less than 15 $U \cdot m^2$ in atrial septal defects) may benefit from surgery.

OTHER CONDITIONS

Patients who have pulmonary hypertension associated with pulmonary parenchymal disease, collagen vascular disease, upper airway obstruction, and other conditions outlined in Table 1 require treatment of the underlying disease. Vasodilators have been tried in patients with chronic obstructive pulmonary disease, including cystic fibrosis, and generally have produced little if any clinical benefit. Vasodilators in this setting may adversely affect ventilation-perfusion matching because of relief of vasoconstriction in poorly ventilated regions of the lung and produce decreased systemic oxygenation.

SEVERE PULMONARY VASCULAR OBSTRUCTIVE DISEASE

Patients with marked elevation in pulmonary vascular resistance associated with ventricular dysfunction may benefit from the creation of an atrial septal defect. This can be accomplished nonsurgically in the cardiac catheterization laboratory (Park blade septostomy). By creating a right-to-left shunt, systemic cardiac output is increased and right-sided congestion is relieved at the expense of systemic cyanosis and the risk of paradoxical embolus.

Such patients also are candidates for transplantation procedures. Cardiac radionuclide studies are useful in assessing right and left ventricular function. If these studies show reasonable right and left ventricular function, these patients may require a single or double lung transplantation rather than a heart-lung transplantation procedure. The waiting time for organ procurement is long, and many patients die before surgical opportunity. Complications include the development of atherosclerotic heart disease, bronchiolitis obliterans, infection, rejection of the transplanted organs, and systemic hypertension and renal dysfunction caused by chronic use of immunosuppressive medication.

REFERENCES

1. Geggel RL: Inhalational nitric oxide: A selective pulmonary vasodilator for treatment of persistent pulmonary hypertension of the newborn. J Pediatr 1993;123:76–79.
2. Rich S: Primary pulmonary hypertension. Prog Cardiovasc Dis 1988;31:205–238.

SYSTEMIC HYPERTENSION

BASSAM ATIYEH, M.D.
SHERMINE DABBAGH, M.D.
LARRY E. FLEISCHMANN, M.D.
ALAN B. GRUSKIN, M.D.

It is estimated that in the United States, hypertension affects approximately 20 to 25 million people and that about 250,000 die each year from its complications. The pediatrician's interest in hypertension and its related complications has grown considerably over the past decade because of increasing evidence that childhood hypertension may predict the later development of sustained hypertension and its related complications. Until a few years ago, there was no universal agreement regarding the limits of normal blood pressure (BP) in children, which made the task of defining hypertension difficult. In 1987, however, the Second Task Force on Blood Pressure Control in Children reported BP data from samples of 70,000 children from nine major

national and international studies.[3] The curves showing age-specific distributions of systolic and diastolic BP for boys and girls provide guidelines to use in the detection of hypertension.

Definitions of normal BP or hypertension are somewhat arbitrary. BP is considered normal if it falls below the 90th percentile for age. Hypertension is defined as the persistence of BP at or above the 95th percentile on at least three separate occasions. However, one exception is that with marked BP elevation, it is important to initiate evaluation and therapy immediately. Borderline hypertension is defined as systolic or diastolic BP between the 90th and 95th percentile for age and sex. The borderline group presents a dilemma to the clinician, since such patients may be at higher risk for developing hypertension or its sequelae at a later time. However, the risk to the patient with borderline hypertension is thought to be low over the short term and does not usually warrant treatment with antihypertensive medications. When BP values exceed the upper limit of normal by the 50th percentile, a hypertensive emergency exists. This unfortunate situation usually results from delay in the recognition of hypertension, inadequate treatment, or noncompliance with a treatment regimen in a known hypertensive. Based on this definition of high BP, the prevalence of hypertension is 5%. Significant hypertension is defined as BP that falls between the 95th and 99th percentile for age, and severe hypertension is defined as BP that falls at or above the 99th percentile for age (Table 1).

Traditionally, hypertension has been classified as either primary (essential) when the cause is unknown or secondary when it is related to an underlying definable renal, neurologic, endocrine, or cardiovascular disease. The pathophysiology of essential hypertension is still not clear. However, essential hypertension may really be a syndrome with multiple etiologies. These multifactorial mechanisms include genetic tendency, increased systemic vascular resistance, high cardiac index, and environmental factors.

Several studies have established that a renal etiology is the most common cause of secondary hypertension in preadolescent children. Reflux nephropathy, pyelonephritis, and glomerulonephritis are the most common renal causes. The classification of hypertension into primary and secondary types is important because it profoundly affects the course of and response to therapy. Treatment of primary hypertension is usually symptomatic. Treatment of secondary hypertension, on the other hand, may be curative if the underlying etiology can be corrected. Primary hypertension, the most common cause of high BP in adults, is uncommon in young children. The prevalence of primary hypertension, however, rises with age, and in older children and young adolescents, it may be responsible for more than one third of the cases of high blood pressure. In neonates, the most common cause of severe hypertension is renovascular (secondary to renal artery thrombosis). The rise in the incidence of neonatal renal artery thrombosis is related to the widespread use of indwelling umbilical catheters.

TABLE 1. Classification of Hypertension by Age Group

AGE GROUP	SIGNIFICANT HYPERTENSION (mm Hg)	SEVERE HYPERTENSION (mm Hg)
Newborn		
7 d	SBP ≥ 96	SBP ≥ 106
8–30 d	SBP ≥ 104	SBP ≥ 110
Infants (<2 y)	SBP ≥ 112	SBP ≥ 118
	DBP ≥ 74	DBP ≥ 82
Children (3–12 y)	SBP ≥ 116	SBP ≥ 124
	DBP ≥ 76	DBP ≥ 84
Adolescents (13–18 y)	SBP ≥ 136	SBP ≥ 144
	DBP ≥ 86	DBP ≥ 92

Abbreviations: SBP, systolic blood pressure; DBP, diastolic blood pressure.
Modified from the report of the Second Task Force on Blood Pressure in Children. Pediatrics 1987;79:1. Reproduced by permission of Pediatrics. Copyright 1987.

TREATMENT

There is general agreement that coronary artery disease begins in childhood and that hypertension is a major risk factor. There is also a prevalent belief that therapeutic intervention at an early age may favorably modify the long-term outcome of hypertension. The goal of therapy of hypertension is to reduce the risk of end-organ damage induced by BP elevation without allowing side effects of therapy to aggravate other risks. Table 2 describes some of the therapeutic objectives of treating hypertension in children. The level to which elevated BP is to be lowered remains an arbitrary decision. It is generally accepted that a drop to levels between the 80th and 90th percentile for age is desirable.

Two modalities of therapy for the treatment of high BP in children are employed, nonpharmacologic and pharmacologic. It is generally accepted that patients with BP between the 95th and 99th percentile without end-organ damage should be treated with nonpharmacologic therapy.

Nonpharmacologic Therapy

Weight Reduction

Several studies have shown that more than half of the patients with primary hypertension are obese. A positive relationship between weight and BP is present by the age of 2 years and peaks between the second and third decades of life. The pathogenesis of obesity-related hypertension is unknown, but increased sympathetic nervous system activity, enhanced renal sodium absorption, insulin resistance, and hyperinsulinemia are some of the factors implicated. In adults, significant reductions in both systolic and diastolic BP are achieved with weight loss. Although there are few similar studies in children, weight loss is still recommended for obese hypertensive children. The effect of weight loss on the sensitivity of BP to sodium has been evaluated in obese adolescents. A significantly larger drop in mean arterial BP was achieved when obese adolescents' diets were switched from a high to a low salt content than when the diets of nonobese adolescents were switched. Although the success rate of weight reduction has been variable, its effectiveness may be enhanced in consultation with a nutritionist, a social worker, and perhaps a psychologist or psychiatrist.

Physical Conditioning

Exercise and physical fitness have gained popularity over the last few decades as an important adjunct to overall well-being and protection against cardiovascular disease. Dynamic exercise (aerobics, swimming, walking, bicycling) has been shown to reduce BP in chronically hypertensive adolescents after approximately 6 months. The effect of static or isometric exercise (such as weight lifting and hand gripping) on BP is still controversial. During isometric muscular contraction, there is a marked increase in diastolic BP. Weight training that increases muscle mass may contribute to an increase in BP. In the absence of data to determine the long-term outcome of isometric exercise on BP, it is recommended that exercise programs be developed around aerobic forms. The mechanism whereby dynamic exercise lowers BP is not well understood. It may be related to a decrease in heart rate and catecholamine release.

TABLE 2. Therapeutic Objectives for Treating Hypertension in Children

1. Lower BP to <90th percentile for age and sex
2. Control hypertension with nonpharmacologic means if possible
3. Use the least amount of drug to control BP
4. Use drugs with the fewest side effects
5. Use a simplified regimen to ensure patient compliance
6. Use inexpensive drugs if possible

Dietary Modification

Dietary modification usually has focused on sodium restriction. The etiologic relationship between sodium restriction and hypertension continues to be debated. Several studies, however, have demonstrated a lower prevalence of hypertension and its related complications in societies thriving on relatively lower sodium diets. It has been found that systolic BP was 2.1 mm Hg higher in 245 infants fed a normal sodium diet from birth through 25 weeks of age than in 231 infants fed a low sodium diet for the same time period ($p < 0.001$). Severe salt restriction may make food unpalatable and may interfere with the child's nutrition and growth. We, therefore, suggest that mothers do not add salt to food and restrict food with a high salt content.

There is evidence that potassium supplementation reduces BP. In one study of hypertensive adolescents, sodium restriction alone did not lower BP until the diet was supplemented with potassium. Potassium supplementation, however, should be restricted to patients with normal renal function who are not taking medications that can produce hyperkalemia (such as angiotensin-converting enzyme, ACE, inhibitors or potassium-sparing diuretics).

The role of calcium intake in high BP in adults has been controversial. Several studies have shown an inverse relationship between high calcium diets and BP, whereas others have shown no effect. Still others have shown a positive relationship.

Vegetarians in general have lower BP than meat eaters, although what it is in their diet that lowers the BP is not known. It may be related to the higher dietary content of monounsaturated and polyunsaturated fatty acids (olive oil and safflower oil) ingested by vegetarians. These have been shown to alter favorably the composition and cation transport of cell membranes and, hence, to lower BP.

Although caffeine is a mild sympathomimetic, tolerance develops quickly, so that little if any effect on BP has been seen over fairly large ranges of consumption of caffeinated beverages. The manner by which coffee is brewed however, may make a difference. Boiled Turkish coffee, as compared with filtered coffee, significantly raised BP in 64 men and women during a 79-day controlled study.

Cessation of Smoking

Cigarette smoking is a major killer in the United States. The relationship between cigarette smoking and BP has been underestimated because most BP measurements are taken after the patient has not smoked for an hour or longer while waiting in the physician's office. The application of ambulatory BP monitoring in the smoking population has shown that while the smoker puffs away, repeated rises in pressure are noted. No tolerance was observed, and the overall pressure level is definitely higher than in nonsmokers. In addition, cessation of smoking promotes energy expenditure, especially during exercise that keeps body weight down. Despite the multiple hazards of smoking, very few physicians advise their patients to quit. In a survey of patients in Michigan, only 44% of smokers who had seen a physician in the previous year were counseled to quit smoking. It is believed that even a smaller number of pediatricians counsel about the bad effects of smoking.

Role of Alcohol

Excessive alcohol consumption is responsible for 5% to 10% of hypertension in adult men. A chronic pressor effect takes place only when the average daily consumption is greater than two drinks, the equivalent of 1 ounce of 95% ethanol. On the other hand, moderate alcohol intake will likely prevent a considerable amount of hypertension and, at the same time, provide the protection from coronary disease that comes from excessive drinking.

Stress Management

Although stress-induced activation of the sympathetic nervous system is probably involved in the pathogenesis of hypertension, it has not been possible to show that relief of stress provided by various relaxation methods will prevent hypertension, much less provide more than a placebo effect in lowering BP in those with established hypertension. In contrast, stress has been shown to raise BP acutely.

Pharmacologic Therapy

Drug therapy is required in (1) the presence of severe hypertension, (2) the presence of end-organ damage, (3) signs or symptoms attributable to hypertension, or (4) when nonpharmacologic therapy alone fails to achieve normotension after several weeks to months of monitoring. The issue of risk versus benefit should be considered carefully before pharmacologic therapy is initiated. Major questions with regard to the long-term effects of antihypertensive drug treatment on growth and cognitive function in children remain to be answered, and, therefore, a definite need must be established before any of these agents is used. Even if drug therapy is used, nonpharmacologic therapy should be continued because it usually reduces the dose of the medication required to control the hypertension.

The stepped-care approach has traditionally been used to treat essential hypertension in adults. In this approach, drug therapy is usually started with a small dose of a single drug, usually a diuretic, and the dose is increased till BP is controlled or side effects develop. If, after checking for compliance, BP is still not controlled, a second drug is added or substituted. Recently, a more individualized approach has been used. Our better understanding of the pathophysiologic mechanisms leading to hypertension and the availability of newer drugs with different mechanisms of action allow for targeting therapy to obtain better control of high blood pressure. Often, combination therapy from different antihypertensive classes is needed to achieve adequate BP control. A drug is selected based on the pathophysiology of hypertension. When adding a second drug, there is no therapeutic benefit from using a second drug from the same category.

A large number of antihypertensive agents with various sites and mechanisms of action are commercially available (Table 3).

Vasodilators

This group of agents produces direct vasodilation of vascular smooth muscle cells probably by stimulating production of vasodilator prostaglandin and prostacycline by endothelial cells. Such drugs act mainly on the arterial beds.

Hydralazine. Hydralazine has long been approved for use in children. When given orally, its antihypertensive effects are modest, and, therefore, it is often combined with another antihypertensive agent. Because hydralazine causes fluid retention and reflex tachycardia, it is commonly used in association with a beta-blocker or a diuretic. Side effects include a lupuslike syndrome that is usually reversible when the drug is discontinued. Other side effects include headache, flushing, nausea, vomiting, easy fatigability, and hypotension.

Minoxidil. Use is usually limited to patients with refractory hypertension. The onset of action of minoxidil is 2 to 3 hours, and its hypotensive effects last for 48 to 72 hours. As with other vasodilators, its hypotensive effect is associated with reflex tachycardia and fluid retention secondary to activation of the renin-angiotensin-aldosterone system and the peripheral sympathetic nervous system. Hence, this drug is contraindicated in patients with pheochromocytoma. The side effect that is most distressing to the patient, especially female adolescents, is severe hypertrichosis. Hair growth is most prominent on the forehead, trunk, and upper arms. It usually appears during the first month of therapy and disappears 2 to 4 months after minoxidil is discontinued. Other side effects occasionally include pericardial effusion and rebound hypertension following rapid withdrawal of the drug.

Beta-Blockers

Several beta-blockers are available. They differ in potency, lipophilicity, and pharmacokinetics. The mechanisms of action of beta-blockers are listed in Table 4. Common side effects include hyperlipidemia, bradycardia, masking of the symptoms of hypoglycemia, hyperglycemia, and bronchoconstriction.

TABLE 3. Oral Antihypertensive Medications Most Commonly Used in Children

CLASS: GENERIC NAME	TRADE NAME	DOSE RANGE/kg	FREQUENCY
Diuretics			
Chlorothiazide	Diuril	10–20 mg	q.d., b.i.d.
Hydrochlorothiazide	HydroDiuril	1–2 mg	q.d., b.i.d.
Furosemide	Lasix	0.5–5 mg	q.d., q.i.d.
Spironolactone	Aldactone	0.5–3 mg	q.d., b.i.d.
Triamterene	Dyazide	1–2 mg	b.i.d.
Bumetanide	Bumex	0.01–0.2 mg	q.d., b.i.d.
Metolazone	Zaroxolin	0.05–0.3 mg	q.d.
Beta-Blockers			
Propranolol	Inderal	0.5–2 mg	t.i.d., q.i.d.
Atenolol	Tenormin	1–2 mg	q.d.
Metoprolol	Lopressor	1–4 mg	b.i.d.
Labetalol (alpha and beta)	Trandate	1–6 mg	q.d., b.i.d.
Calcium Channel Blockers			
Nifedipine	Procardia	0.25–1 mg	t.i.d., q.i.d.
Diltiazem	Cardizem	1–3 mg	q.d., t.i.d.
Verapamil	Calan	1–3 mg	q.d., t.i.d.
ACE Inhibitors			
Captopril	Capoten	0.3–5 mg	t.i.d., q.i.d.
Enalapril	Vasotec	0.1–0.5 mg	q.d., b.i.d.
Lisinopril	Zestril	0.2–1 mg	q.d., b.i.d.
Central Adrenergic Inhibitors			
Clonidine	Catapres	5–30 μg	q.d., b.i.d.
Methyldopa	Aldomet	5–40 mg	b.i.d., t.i.d.
Vasodilators			
Hydralazine	Apresoline	0.5–1.5 mg	t.i.d., q.i.d.
Minoxidil	Loniten	0.1–1.0 mg	q.d., b.i.d.
Alpha-Blockers			
Prazosin	Minipress	0.05–0.2 mg	b.i.d., t.i.d.

Propranolol. Propranolol is a nonselective beta-adrenergic antagonist that has been used extensively in the treatment of pediatric hypertension. It is available in the liquid form (20 and 40 mg/5 ml), which makes it easier to administer to young children. It has a rapid onset of action of 1 hour and a half life of 4 to 6 hours. Because of its lipid solubility, propranolol crosses the blood–brain barrier and can produce somnolence, drowsiness, lethargy, night terrors, and depression. Its use is contraindicated in patients with reactive airway disease.

Atenolol. Atenolol is a new beta₁-adrenergic antagonist. Its longer half-life permits once a day dosage. It is the least lipophilic agent among the beta-blockers. Consequently, fewer central nervous system side effects are observed. It may be used cautiously in the patient with mild, but not severe, reactive airway disease.

Labetalol. Labetalol is the first antihypertensive agent with both alpha- and beta-adrenergic blocking properties, with a beta/alpha blocking activity of 7:1. In addition to the oral preparation, intravenous labetalol is available and is used to treat severe hypertension

TABLE 4. Antihypertensive Mechanisms of Beta-Adrenergic Blocking Drugs

1. Decreased cardiac output
2. Antagonism of the effects of norepinephrine on vascular smooth muscle cells
3. Decrease in renin release
4. Decrease in tyrosine hydroxylase and dopamine beta-hydroxylase activity in the central nervous system (particularly lipophilic drugs, such as propranolol)

or hypertensive emergencies. It can be given as bolus infusion of 0.25 to 0.5 mg/kg per dose two to three times at 10-minutes intervals or as a continuous infusion at a rate of 1 to 3 mg/kg/h. Labetalol offers special advantage in treating patients with thyrotoxicosis, pheochromocytoma, and other catecholamine-producing tumors and patients with renal insufficiency, where nitroprusside use is associated with a higher toxicity.

Calcium Channel Blockers (CCB)

Calcium influx leads to depolarization of vascular smooth muscle cells. Increase in intracellular calcium concentration causes calcium to bind to calmodulin. This promotes phosphorylation of actomyosin and, hence, bridging of actin/myosin filaments. CCB mainly prevent the influx of calcium into the intracellular space and, to a lesser extent, prevent release of calcium from the sarcoplasmic reticulum.

CCB are powerful antihypertensive drugs with few side effects and are commonly used as initial therapy in the treatment of hypertension. In contrast to beta-blockers, CCB do not depress cardiac output or cause bronchoconstriction. Hence, CCB may be used in patients with reactive airway disease. Unlike diuretics, CCB do not cause serum electrolyte, lipid, or uric acid abnormalities and do not cause carbohydrate intolerance. Unlike vasodilators, CCB are usually not accompanied by significant tachycardia. A small percentage of patients, however, may experience vasodilation, peripheral edema, facial flushing, paresthesia, hypotension, headache, and nausea or vomiting. These side effects usually diminish with time.

Nifedipine. Nifedipine is the most potent vasodilator among the CCB. It has few negative inotropic or chronotropic effects. The sublingual dose or the bite-and-swallow approach is used frequently in the treatment of hypertensive emergencies. Its onset of action is 15 to 20 minutes, and it peaks at 60 to 90 minutes. The dose can be repeated in 30 to 60 minutes if additional lowering of BP is required. The BP lowering effect lasts 2 to 3 hours with the sublingual route and 4 to 6 hours with the oral route. As with many antihypertensive agents, nifedipine is not available in the liquid form. The 0.34 ml of oily liquid contained in the 10 mg gelatinous capsule can be aspirated into a tuberculin syringe and the required dose obtained for use in young children. In addition, a sustained-release formulation is available (nifedipine 30, 60, and 90 mg XL). When the tablet is exposed to gastrointestinal fluid, it expands and releases a constant amount of the drug over a 24-hour period. This system permits once a day dosing. Because the tablet must be swallowed whole, it has limited application in infants.

Verapamil. Verapamil was used initially in the treatment of supraventricular tachycardia, since this drug increases atrioventricular conduction delay. It also exerts a negative inotropic effect and, hence, should be used with caution in patients with AV conduction delay, Wolff-Parkinson-White syndrome, congestive heart failure, or sick sinus syndrome. Combinations of a beta-blocker and verapamil should be avoided, since they may produce a significant decrease in cardiac output. Verapamil is also available as a sustained-release form. Its antihypertensive effect is less than that of nifedipine.

Diltiazem. The potency of diltiazem as a hypertensive drug is midway between nifedipine and verapamil. Diltiazem also exerts a negative inotropic and chronotropic effect but to a milder extent than verapamil. It has the advantage of slowing down the metabolism of cyclosporine, allowing the use of a smaller dose of cyclosporine in transplant recipients.

Angiotensin-Converting Enzyme Inhibitors

Angiotensin-converting enzyme (ACE) inhibitors were discovered during the search for an antidote for the venom of pit vipers. These peptides inhibit not only the conversion of angiotensin I to angiotensin II but also the inactivation of vasodilatory prostaglandins and bradykinin. This is because ACE (which converts angiotensin I to angiotensin II) and kininase II (which inactivates kinins) are identical. Like CCB, ACE inhibitors do not raise lipid, glucose, or uric acid

concentrations. ACE inhibitors are the first line of treatment in patients with unilateral renovascular hypertension and high renin states, such as reflux nephropathy. Caution is warranted when ACE inhibitors are used in patients with bilateral renal artery stenosis or in patients with renal artery stenosis of a solitary kidney. Under these circumstances, acute renal failure may develop because of a preferential dilatation of the glomerular efferent arterioles and consequent reduction in intraglomerular hydrostatic pressure. In addition, ACE inhibitors should be used with care in patients with renal insufficiency because these medications, which are excreted by the kidney, may accumulate and can result in granulocytopenia by an effect on the bone marrow or significant hyperkalemia by decrease in aldosterone production. Other side effects include skin rash, dysgeusia, cough, dizziness, proteinuria, glycosuria, and interstitial nephritis. Because of their afterload reduction effect, ACE inhibitors are frequently used in patients with hypertension and congestive heart failure. ACE inhibitors have the advantage of reducing intraglomerular hydrostatic pressure by preferential vasodilation of the efferent arteriole. Hence, these drugs may delay the progression of renal damage in patients with renal hypertension and also may decrease proteinuria in patients with nephrotic syndrome and other glomerulonephritides. Because of a preferential action on arterial rather than venous smooth muscle cells, ACE inhibitors improve blood flow to the heart, brain, and kidneys despite lowering BP. ACE inhibitors are toxic to the fetus and *should not* be used in pregnancy. Information on the two ACE inhibitors most often used in children follows.

Captopril. Captopril was the first orally available ACE inhibitor to be used in children. Captopril has a rapid onset of action of 60 to 90 minutes, and its antihypertensive effect lasts 6 to 8 hours. The recommended starting dose is 0.3 mg/kg t.i.d. Like many other antihypertensive agents, captopril is not available in liquid form. It is often dissolved in tap water for administration to young children. It should be noted, however, that the drug is not stable in solution, and when suspended in tap water, captopril's activity declines from 90% at 24 hours to 29% at 48 hours and no activity detectable at 96 hours. It is reported that when captopril is dissolved in sterile, distilled water, it may retain its activity for a few days. We recommend that it is best for individual doses to be prepared fresh daily if sterile water is used or before each individual dose if tap water is used. In addition, captopril has a sulfhydryl group that is associated with side effects yet has been shown to have some anti-inflammatory activity. Hence, captopril is of particular benefit to the hypertensive patient with such conditions as scleroderma renal disease where anti-inflammatory activity is important.

Enalapril. Enalapril lacks the sulfhydryl group present in captopril and, hence, has a lower incidence of side effects. Enalapril has a longer half-life and can be used as a single q.d. or b.i.d. dosage. Unlike captopril, its gastrointestinal absorption is not affected by food. Moreover, hydrolyzed enalapril (enalaprilat) can be used intravenously at a dose of 0.05 to 0.25 mg/kg q6h.

Alpha₁-Adrenergic Blocking Agents

Alpha$_1$-adrenergic blocking agents exert their hypotensive effect by competitively blocking vascular postsynaptic alpha$_1$-adrenergic receptors. This produces a decrease in arterial resistance, venous tone, and mean arterial pressure without a significant tachycardia. The relative lack of tachycardia with chronic use may, in part, be related to the combined action of these agents on both the arteriolar and venous sides of the circulation, preventing the marked increase in venous return and cardiac output observed with agents that act primarily on arterial vascular smooth muscle. On the other hand, profound hypotension, syncope, and loss of consciousness can occur with the first dose of alpha$_1$-adrenergic blockers. Hence, they are usually used in patients with refractory hypertension. Prazosin is the alpha-adrenergic agent most often used, but phenoxybenzamine and phentolamine are also used in patients with pheochromocytoma and other catecholamine-producing tumors.

Central Sympatholytics

Central sympatholytics stimulate central alpha$_2$-adrenoceptors, resulting in reduction of norepinephrine release and total sympathetic outflow from the brainstem. Clonidine, alpha-methyldopa, and guanabenz are agents in this category. Clonidine is the most commonly used drug.

Clonidine. Because of its frequent side effects, clonidine is usually used when other drugs fail to control the high BP. In addition to the oral route, clonidine is available in transdermal patches of 0.1 mg, 0.2 mg, and 0.3 mg strengths, which are equivalent to a daily dose of 0.1 mg, 0.2 mg, and 0.3 mg, respectively. Because the patch needs to be changed only once a week, compliance is improved. As the medicine is uniformly distributed, the patch can be cut into several pieces, and the dose can be graded to the patient's weight. Contact dermatitis occasionally develops and can be treated with hydrocortisone ointment and by changing the site of application. Other side effects include drowsiness, depression, dryness of the mouth, nausea, and constipation. These effects, however, usually improve within 1 to 2 weeks. The drug should be tapered gradually, usually over a 7 to 10 day period, since abrupt discontinuation may result in rebound hypertension and signs and symptoms of sympathetic hyperactivity.

Diuretics

Three groups of diuretic agents are used to treat childhood hypertension, thiazides, loop diuretics, and distal tubular diuretics. They are the drug class of choice in patients with volume-dependent hypertension and are commonly used with other drugs, such as beta-blockers and vasodilators.

Thiazides. Thiazides, such as hydrochlorothiazide and chlorothiazide, inhibit sodium transport in the early distal tubule. Major adverse affects include hypokalemia, hyponatremia, and metabolic alkalosis. Hyperglycemia, hyperuricemia, hyperlipidemia, and hypercalcemia are less common complications. Thiazides also interfere with the diluting ability of the kidney and decrease free water clearance. Most importantly, because thiazides become ineffective if the GFR is less than 50% of normal, a loop diuretic should be substituted in renal failure.

Loop Diuretics. Loop diuretics have their major site of action in the ascending loop of Henle by causing inhibition of Na$^+$-K$^+$-Cl^{2+}-transporter. Furosemide, ethacrynic acid, and bumetanide are loop diuretics. Ethacrynic acid is not commonly used because it has been associated with irreversible ototoxicity. Bumetanide is 40 times more potent than furosemide on a milligram/milligram basis and also has proximal tubular action manifested by its phosphaturic effect.

Furosemide is the most common agent used. It is available in both oral and intravenous forms. Its principal side effects are hypokalemia, hyponatremia, metabolic alkalosis, interstitial nephritis, and volume depletion. Because of their site of action, loop diuretics interfere not only with the diluting ability of the kidney but also with its concentrating capacity. Although usually reversible, ototoxicity may be irreversible, especially in patients with renal insufficiency. Furosemide increases urinary calcium excretion, which can result in nephrocalcinosis and bone demineralization, especially in infants.

Potassium-Sparing Diuretics. Potassium-sparing diuretics are the least potent diuretics because less than 5% of sodium reabsorption occurs in the distal tubule. These drugs usually are used in combination with thiazides and loop diuretics as an adjunct to control hypokalemia. Spironolactone is a stoichiometric competitive inhibitor of aldosterone. It is especially useful in conditions with mineralocorticoid excess, such as primary hyperaldosteronism, Cushing's syndrome, and glucocorticoid remediable aldosteronism. Its major side effects include hyperkalemia, gynecomastia, and menstrual irregularities. The effect of the drug may not be seen for 3 or more days, and it may take as many as 10 days before maximum effectiveness develops.

Triamterene and amiloride are nonsteroidal potassium-sparing agents with an action independent of aldosterone antagonism.

Duration of Pharmacotherapy

One should remember that once an extensive course of adequate BP control has been achieved (3 to 6 months), an attempt at gradual reduction or withdrawal of medications should be made. During tapering, the BP should be closely monitored for rebound hypertension that can occur in particular with ACE inhibitors, beta-blockers, and central adrenergic agonists.

HYPERTENSIVE CRISIS

When BP increases rapidly or exceeds the upper limit of normal for age by 50%, a hypertensive emergency situation exists. Malignant hypertension is accompanied by papilledema, along with retinal hemorrhages and exudates, whereas in accelerated hypertension, there is retinopathy but not papilledema. Malignant hypertension is usually associated with necrotizing arteriolitis that involves several organs, including the retina (exudates and hemorrhage), kidney (proteinuria, hematuria, and decreased renal function), heart (congestive heart failure), vascular system (thrombosis and hemolysis), and central nervous system (encephalopathy). Hypertensive crisis in a child usually results from delayed recognition of high BP, inadequate treatment or noncompliance with medications, dietary therapy, or dialysis therapy.

After a brief history and physical examination, the patient is best managed in an intensive care unit with an intraarterial catheter for continuous BP monitoring. The speed and the level of reduction in BP remain a clinical decision. In severely hypertensive asymptomatic patients, an acceptable therapeutic plan is to reduce the BP by one third over the initial 6 hours and another one third over the next 12 hours, with normalization within 48 to 72 hours. Internists are always concerned about too rapid normalization of high BP because of the risk of reducing cerebral, cardiac, or renal perfusion. In children with hypertensive emergencies associated with end-organ damage, the risk of rapid normalization of BP appears to be less than the risk of continued vascular damage.

The therapy of hypertensive convulsions that we recommend consists of stopping the seizure with anticonvulsant medications, such as diazepam or dilantin, and lowering the BP with antihypertensive agents. If the seizure is short with no sequelae, anticonvulsants should be tapered within 1 to 2 weeks. If the seizure is prolonged or associated with focal deficits or electroencephalographic changes, anticonvulsants should be used for 6 months, and then their use should be reevaluated.

A variety of antihypertensive agents can be used in a hypertensive emergency (Table 5). It is advisable to begin treatment with one antihypertensive agent and to add another agent only if the initial one is not sufficient in controlling BP after the maximum dose is given.

TABLE 5. Drugs Used in the Treatment of Hypertensive Emergencies

DRUG	DOSE RANGE AND ROUTE	COMMENTS
Hydralazine	0.1–0.5 mg/kg IV	Can be repeated in 5–10 min
Sodium nitroprusside	0.5–8 µg/kg/min IV	Protect lines from light
Nifedipine	0.25–0.5 mg/kg PO/SL	One dose can be repeated in 30 min
Diazoxide	1–5 mg/kg IV	Can be repeated in 5–10 min; maximum dose is 300 mg
Labetalol	1–3 mg/kg/h IV	Can be used as bolus of 0.25–0.5 mg/kg q10–15min
Nitroglycerine	0.5–10 µg/kg/min IV	Use is limited to postoperative patients

In this section, we consider only those agents that have not been discussed earlier.

Diazoxide

Diazoxide is a benzothiadiazine derivative related to thiazide diuretic in structure but without diuretic activity. It relaxes arterial smooth muscle cells, most likely by stimulating prostacycline synthesis. It is given by rapid infusion of less than 1 to 2 minutes at doses of 1 to 5 mg/kg. (A slower infusion rate is often ineffective because the drug is protein bound and can lose its potency.) The onset of action is within 1 to 3 minutes, and the action may last for 12 to 18 hours. The dose can be repeated in 5 to 10 minutes if there is no response. Side effects include nausea, vomiting, hypotension, fluid retention, metallic taste in the mouth, hyperuricemia, and hypertrichosis. With repeated doses, hyperglycemia and nonketotic hyperglycemic coma develop as the drug interferes with pancreatic insulin release. A continuous infusion regimen has been developed to try to avoid the complication of hypotension associated with a bolus injection. The infusion rate is 0.25 µg/kg/min, with a maximum dose of 5 µg/kg/min over 20 minutes.

Sodium Nitroprusside

Sodium nitroprusside is a direct vasodilator of both arterial and venous beds and is used in the treatment of acute hypertensive crisis. It is given by continuous intravenous infusion at a dose of 0.5 to 8 µg/kg/min. The rate of the infusion is titrated according to the BP response. Its onset of action occurs within a few minutes. It is necessary to cover the pump and the infusion lines with aluminum foil because the drug becomes unstable when exposed to light. Nitroprusside is rapidly degraded into cyanide ions and nitroso- group. The latter is responsible for the antihypertensive effect of the drug. Cyanide ions are then metabolized to thiocyanate, a process dependent on the liver enzyme rhodanase and the availability of thiosulfate or other sulfur-containing substrates. Nitroprusside should be used cautiously in patients with renal insufficiency because thiocyanate is excreted in the kidney. Blood thiocyanate levels should be monitored if the drug is to be used for more than 48 hours. Serum thiocyanate levels should be kept under 10 mg/dl. Impaired thiocyanate production may lead to toxic cyanide levels in patients with hepatic insufficiency (because of deficient rhodanase activity) and in malnourished patients (because of thiosulfate substrate unavailability). Metabolic acidosis and tachyphylaxis are the earliest signs of nitroprusside toxicity. Other side effects include muscle twitching, sweating, apprehension, and vomiting. Since nitroprusside causes venous dilatation, there is no increase in cardiac output or reflex tachycardia as is seen with other vasodilators.

Nitroglycerine

Nitroglycerine is a vasodilator of both arterial and venous beds. It is rapidly degraded by the liver, and, therefore, the dose can be titrated quickly when it is given intravenously. Nitroglycerine can be used only in a glass bottle, as it loses its potency in a plastic bag. Its use in children has been limited to perioperative control of BP during heart surgery and in control of ECMO-related hypertension. It is also used in patients with impaired renal function, as it is hepatically degraded.

Once BP is controlled, one should consider if there is a surgically correctable lesion, such as coarctation of the aorta, renal artery stenosis, renal tumors, or catecholamine-producing tumors, causing the hypertensive emergency.

NEONATAL HYPERTENSION

Interest in neonatal hypertension has increased considerably over the past decade owing to the availability of norms for newborns and the survival of many very ill infants. Techniques for measuring BP in infants and curves showing age-specific distributions of BP for

TABLE 6. Antihypertensive Medications Used in Neonates

NAME	DOSE RANGE	FREQUENCY/ROUTE
Captopril	0.05–0.2 mg/kg	t.i.d., q.i.d./PO
Chlorothiazide	20–50 mg/kg	q.d., b.i.d./PO
Furosemide	1–3 mg/kg	q.d., t.i.d./IV, PO
Methyldopa	5–50 mg/kg	b.i.d., t.i.d./PO
Propranolol	0.5–2 mg/kg	t.i.d., q.i.d./PO
Labetalol	0.5 mg/kg/h	Continuous infusion q2–4h/IV
	1 mg/kg	
Enalaprilat	5–10 µg/kg	q.d., b.i.d., t.i.d./IV
Nifedipine	0.25 mg/kg	q1–2h/SL

both premature and full-term infants are now available. Symptoms of neonatal hypertension are usually nonspecific and include irritability, poor appetite, failure to grow, signs and symptoms of congestive heart failure, and respiratory distress.

As in older children and adolescents, treatment is indicated for persistent systolic or diastolic BP above the 95th percentile for age and weight. Transient elevations in BP are usually not treated unless they are very marked or occur in babies who may be at high risk for cardiovascular or cerebral injury. Mild degrees of hypertension are treated with a diuretic or hydralazine, but if BP continues to be poorly controlled a beta-adrenergic blocking agent, such as propranolol, or a centrally acting agent, such as methyldopa, may be used. Infants with renovascular hypertension can be treated with captopril. However, side effects are more common in infants compared with older children when the usual dose of 0.3 mg/kg is used. Hence, a lower dose of 0.15 mg/kg is recommended. Intravenous enalaprilat has been used in neonates who cannot take oral medications.

For severe hypertension in the neonate, sublingual nifedipine is being used at a dose of 0.25 mg/kg every 1 to 2 hours. The drug is relatively safe and effective on most occasions. Intravenous labetalol also has been used for symptomatic hypertension in the neonatal period. It provides a smooth and stepwise reduction in BP as opposed to the precipitous drop seen with diazoxide. Labetalol can be given as a bolus infusion every 2 to 4 hours or as a continuous intravenous infusion. Table 6 lists the more commonly used agents to manage neonatal hypertension.

REFERENCES

1. Adelman RD: Hypertension in the neonatal period. Clin Perinatol 1988;15:567–585.
2. Jung FF, Ingelfinger JR: Hypertension in childhood and adolescence. Pediatr Rev 1993;14:169–179.
3. Task Force on Blood Pressure Control in Children (1987): Report of the Second Task Force on Blood Pressure Control in Children. National Heart, Lung and Blood Institute, Bethesda, Maryland. Pediatrics 1987;79:1–25.

SYNCOPE AND HYPOTENSION

Bertrand A. Ross, M.D.

Syncope describes a physiologic event with varied causes, so the proper therapy is predicated on ensuring the correct diagnosis. However, the diagnostic process is neither as daunting nor as difficult as it has been portrayed in the past. Indications for treatment to prevent syncope are based on preventing symptoms that adversely affect lifestyle or preventing episodes that place the patient at risk of serious morbidity or even mortality.

From a practical point, the treatment of syncope can be divided into two categories, cardiac and noncardiac. Cardiac causes of syncope and appropriate treatment are well known and, therefore, are discussed only in a summary fashion. Structural cardiac defects that decrease cardiac output can lead to syncopal episodes. Left-sided obstructive lesions are the time-honored example of this phenomenon (particularly aortic stenosis and idiopathic hypertrophic subaortic stenosis). However, right-sided obstructive lesions may produce a similar physiologic event. In patients with such defects, changes in ventricular filling and vascular resistance can episodically interact to produce a sudden fall in cardiac output, leading to a syncopal event. The acute treatment is fluid expansion to maintain blood pressure plus atropine in those patients with an associated vagal reflex response. This type of episode can either be self-limited or progress to sudden death either from a malignant vagal reflex producing asystole or from ventricular tachycardia/fibrillation. The immediate treatment in such a situation obviously is cardiopulmonary resuscitation. Subsequent prevention then consists of correcting the anatomic defect. Fortunately, modern pediatric cardiac practice has made anatomic defects associated with syncope uncommon, since surgical correction is undertaken successfully at such young ages.

Arrhythmias, as a cardiac cause of syncope, have always been of great concern because of the lethality of the episodes. However, the likelihood of an arrhythmia contributing to a syncopal event is directly associated with the presence of structural or functional abnormalities. In other words, the likelihood of a patient with a totally normal heart having an arrhythmia as a cause of syncope is quite small. Conversely, the patient with an abnormal heart who has a syncopal event should be considered at great risk of sudden death until proven otherwise. Therefore, the key to treatment in such patients is to ascertain *cardiac normality*. The treatment of such cardiac arrhythmias is dealt with elsewhere and is not the subject of this section.

Over the last several years, investigations of syncope have centered on neurally mediated cardiovascular reflexes and their contribution to the production of syncope. A number of terms have been used to describe these physiologic responses and the complex interactions that then produce syncope: autonomic dysfunction, autonomic syncope, and, most recently, neurocardiogenic syncope. Neurocardiogenic syncope is by far the most common cause of noncardiac syncope. The difficulty in differential diagnosis between neurocardiogenic syncope and a lethal arrhythmia was indicated in the case of the basketball star Reggie Lewis, who died of the latter.

Maintenance of blood pressure involves peripheral vascular receptor and effector response, myocardial receptor and effector response, and central processing of receptor input and effector response. At the peripheral level, vascular neuroreceptors may be unable to produce constriction or may inappropriately produce dilatation, leading to a decrease in venous return and ventricular filling. Mechanoreceptors in the ventricular myocardium may have increased sensitivity to stimulation during contraction or may be stimulated excessively by a hypercontractile state from decreased ventricular filling. This then leads to a central monosynaptic vagal reflex at the level of the autonomic center, producing sympathetic withdrawal and increased vagal tone. The sympathetic withdrawal and increased vagal tone result in varying degrees of bradycardia and hypotension from peripheral vasodilatation, producing the syncopal event. Various treatments have become available based on therapeutic effect at different points along the physiologic chain of events just described.

VOLUME EXPANSION

Fludrocortisone alone or with salt has been used successfully to treat recurrent neurocardiogenic syncope. Salt alone also has been employed successfully (Table 1). We have treated over 56 patients with fludrocortisone alone or in combination with salt loading and have a success rate of over 90%. The mechanism of action appears to be volume expansion, although increased vasoconstriction may also play a role in long-term treatment.

Side effects rarely occur in the pediatric age range. Peripheral edema and headaches may be experienced transiently during the beginning of volume expansion. Patients are checked weekly for the

TABLE 1. Formulary for Treatment of Syncope and Hypotension

DRUG	DOSE	COMMENTS
Fludrocortisone	0.1–0.3 mg q.d. × 3 d, then 0.1 mg q.d. Daily dosage range 0.1–0.3 mg	Volume expansion; can cause headaches, hypertension
Salt	250–500 mg t.i.d. with meals	Difficult to swallow
Beta-blockers	Propranolol 2–4 mg/kg/d divided q6h Long-acting preparation atenolol 1–2 mg/kg/d	Can exacerbate tiredness
Disopyramide	6–10 mg/kg/d divided q6h Sustained release divided q12h	Can cause dry mouth, tremulousness; should be started in hospital
Fluoxetine hydrochloride (Prozac)	10–20 mg/d adult dosage	New treatment for this problem; data are limited

first month and then monthly to ensure that there is neither hypertension (supine) nor electrolyte abnormalities. We have had no electrolyte abnormalities and only 2 cases of transient hypertension. Some patients who are severely affected require continued treatment for several years, but most patients appear to have the problem of syncope transiently, and, thus, can be taken off therapy after 1 year. An association of hypertension and long-term use of fludrocortisone-salt therapy (>1 year) has been reported in several adults.

RECEPTOR LEVEL TREATMENT

Beta-Blocker Drugs

Beta-blocker drugs have been among the most commonly used in the treatment of patients with neurocardiogenic syncope (Table 1). The precise localization of the beta-blocker effect is speculative, but receptors at several places along the reflex chain may be affected. Peripherally, there is some evidence that these patients may have hypersensitive beta-receptors that produce peripheral vasodilatation or venodilatation, which the beta-blockers may help prevent. Additionally, the contractile force of the cardiac ventricles, as well as the mechanoreceptors in the myocardium, may be blunted by beta-blockers.

Side effects are the same as those known to be associated with beta-blocker therapy, with fatigue being the most common.

Theophylline Therapy

Desensitization of the supersensitive beta-receptors has been proposed as the mechanism for successful treatment with theophylline preparations.

Side effects generally are due to the increased beta-receptor sensitivity in these patients, which produces tremulousness and agitation when the patient undergoes desensitization with theophylline.

VAGOLYTIC DRUGS

Vagolytic drugs exert their effect by blunting or preventing the vagus nerve from participating in the reflex. Ephedrine, propantheline bromide (Pro-Banthine), and disopyramide (an antiarrhythmic drug with anticholinergic effects) have been used most frequently (Table 1). As with all of the treatments for syncope except fludrocortisone, vagolytic agents have been used mainly in adults.

Side effects consist mainly of anticholinergic symptoms, such as tremulousness, dry mouth, and irritability. However, disopyramide can be proarrhythmic, producing ventricular arrhythmias. Therefore, it is started in a hospital setting. It should be noted that the proarrhythmia effect generally has occurred in patients requiring the medication for control of arrhythmia.

CENTRAL NERVOUS SYSTEM LEVEL TREATMENT

Higher nervous system centers, such as the cerebellum and the limbic area, have input into the reticular area and the nucleus ambiguous, where many of the peripheral impulses in this reflex phenomenon are processed. It has been shown that these higher centers can affect or exaggerate the reflex response. Invasive monitoring of blood pressure with an arterial line during testing of these patients can increase the number of positive test results, presumably by increasing the innervation from such areas as the limbic cortex to the autonomic center. We have had success with imipramine in 2 patients who appeared to have a very high anxiety level in association with these episodes. More recently, investigators have found fluoxetine hydrochloride (Prozac) to have beneficial effects in the treatment of neurocardiogenic syncope and speculate that the fluoxetine hydrochloride may blunt the response to rapid shifts in serotonin, which may play a role in the development of hypotension. However, given the recent concerns about this medication, especially as detailed in the lay press, one should be judicious in its use (Table 1). As more becomes known, centrally acting agents may assume a greater role in our treatment armamentarium for this problem.

CARDIAC PACING

Because of the exaggerated vagal reflex response in these patients, severe bradycardia and, not infrequently, asystole have been seen during testing. The asystole may be as short as several seconds or as long as 30 to 45 seconds or more. Bradycardia pacing has been advocated in the treatment of such patients. There are two issues regarding choosing pacing. The first is that by preventing bradycardia and asystole by pacing, the syncopal episodes can be blunted or aborted by maintaining an adequate heart rate and, therefore, sustaining cardiac output. The second is that by pacing, the concern of prolonged asystole producing ventricular fibrillation and sudden death is averted. Although the literature is divided, it appears that the great majority of patients do not require permanent pacing. Treatment with pacing should be reserved for a select few who cannot be treated successfully medically or who are at risk of sudden death from prolonged asystole. Temporary pacing during testing in patients proven to have neurocardiogenic syncope has not shown pacing to be efficacious in preventing syncope. This seems understandable, since the physiologic phenomenon is well underway when the vagal response ushers in the bradycardia just before the syncopal event. We have had success without pacing in treating patients with syncope and reflex asystolic periods of over 20 seconds. Preventing the reflex phenomenon, which then triggers the asystole, should be the first treatment approach, with permanent pacing reserved for those patients thought to be at significant risk from prolonged asystole.

ORTHOSTATIC SUPPORT

Since a number of patients exhibit signs of venous pooling during orthostatic testing, the issue of treatment directed at venous pooling must be considered. Often, the patient's history is not suggestive of venous pooling as a contributor to the syncopal event. In several patients who have continued to have significant symptoms on a variety of oral medications, we have employed vascular compression hose, with surprisingly good success. These stockings should be ordered at thigh length or longer and come in a variety of colors and compression pressures. Compression pressures can be varied from 20 to 40 mm Hg, although we generally have used 20 to 30 mm Hg.

REFERENCES

1. Grubb B, Wolfe D, Samoil D, et al: Usefulness of fluoxetine hydrochloride for prevention of resistant upright tilt-induced syncope. PACE 1993;16:458–463.
2. Milstein S, Buetikofer J, Dunnigan A, et al: Usefulness of disopyramide for prevention of upright tilt-induced hypotension-bradycardia. Am J Cardiol 1990;65:1339–1344.
3. Sra J, Murthy V, Jazayeri M, et al: Use of intravenous esmolol to predict efficacy of oral beta-adrenergic blocker therapy in patients with neurocardiogenic syncope. J Am Coll Cardiol 1992;19:402–408.

INNOCENT MURMURS

DAN G. MCNAMARA, M.D.

Having consulted on patients with "innocent" murmurs for some 35 years, I have often heard about the logistical problems that pediatricians face in dealing with a "new" unexpected murmur in the midst of a busy day seeing well and sick young people. It takes more than a cursory listen to the heart to be reasonably sure that a murmur is innocent. However, pediatricians, accustomed to hearing these normal sounds, generally ignore those that are faint or transient—and rightly so. Probably there is no need to mention every innocent murmur to the parent any more than the many normal variants found in other organs and systems on routine physical examination of the developing individual.

When a murmur is quite prominent or somewhat puzzling to the examiner, however, one has to decide at that time whether it indicates congenital or acquired heart disease or only a normal variant. The examiner must also decide whether the parents should be told about it before they are told by someone else. A prolonged and more-detailed-than-usual auscultation of the heart without some explanation is likely to alarm the parent who is accustomed to seeing only a fairly brief cardiac examination. If doctors inform a parent about an innocent murmur, they are obliged to explain the phenomenon, a simple enough thing to do except for the time involved to do it well.

It is for these reasons that a discussion of the management of innocent murmurs is timely and appropriate for this volume on therapy in pediatric practice.

MAGNITUDE OF THE PROBLEM

Innocent murmurs comprised 18.5% (100 of 540 consecutive new patients under the age of 18 years in the first 4 months of 1990) referred to the cardiology service at Texas Children's Hospital, Houston, for known or possible congenital or acquired heart disease. It is certainly the single most frequent final diagnosis made in new patients beyond infancy in the outpatient clinic.

I do not know the percentage of presumed healthy infants, children, or adolescents in whom pediatricians hear a new murmur that calls for a return visit, prompts the ordering of graphic tests, or necessitates a consultation with a pediatric cardiologist. Probably it is a daily problem in a busy practice.

Referring the patient for another opinion is a perfectly reasonable and certainly expedient way to handle a problematic innocent murmur, and aside from the time and expense and the possible parental anxiety in waiting for an appointment, there is no reason not to order a consultation.

Throughout the United States, pediatric cardiologists, including the author, have not really been discouraging these welcome referrals! Frankly, we enjoy seeing patients with a normal heart and innocent murmur. For one thing, such patients provide an excellent teaching opportunity for residents in pediatrics and fellows in a pediatric cardiology training program. Also, because parents bringing their child to a cardiology clinic for that first visit usually arrive fearing that there is important heart disease that might limit physical activity, require surgical repair, or shorten the child's life, it is professionally very satisfying to be able to give the good report that the heart is normal.

The ideal for all concerned is for pediatricians to manage innocent murmurs themselves. This can usually be achieved without graphic tests, and, by following some simple steps that require no more than a few extra minutes of time per week, one can learn to become expert at recognizing innocent murmurs. For a description of the four common innocent murmurs, see Table 1.

Many times, patients with innocent murmurs are referred by pe-

diatricians who are reasonably certain, by physical examination alone, that a murmur is innocent. Nevertheless, a parent insists on a second opinion. In discussing this matter with parents, I have concluded that parents ask for another opinion when one of the following has occurred:

1. They have perceived, and may have been told, that the pediatrician is uncertain about the importance of the murmur.
2. The diagnosis is rendered after only a hurried and limited auscultation of the heart.

TABLE 1. Physicians' Guide to Normal Variants in Heart Sounds Often Heard in Young People and Some Common Pathologic Conditions That They May Resemble

1. **Neonatal Pulmonary Artery Branch Murmur**
   a. Age first heard: newborn to 6 wk of age
   b. Age murmur disappears: 2–4 mo
   c. Location: midaxillary region, infraclavicular area; right or left side or both, posterior chest
   d. Patient position that amplifies murmur: supine or prone
   e. Character: soft, high pitched, short, and grade I–II/VI
   f. Phase of cardiac cycle: midsystole
   g. Confused with:
      (1) Pathologic pulmonary artery branch stenosis, which produces a louder murmur
      (2) Very mild pulmonary or aortic valve stenosis
   h. Murmur produced by: turbulence in pulmonary artery branches before maturation of pulmonary vascular bed

2. **Venous Hum**
   a. Age first heard: 2–3 y
   b. Age hum disappears: 7–8 y
   c. Location: right, left, or both infraclavicular areas near sternum and over manubrium sternum and base of neck over jugular veins
   d. Patient position that amplifies murmur: sitting or standing patient with head tilted up
   e. Patient position that obliterates venous hum: supine
   f. Character: soft, blowing grade I–III/VI
   g. Phase of cardiac cycle: continuous throughout systole and diastole
   h. Confused with: small patent ductus, but PDA murmur persists and is often louder with patient supine; PDA murmur sharper and localized to pulmonary valve area
   i. Murmur produced by: turbulent flow of blood in jugular—left innominate vein and superior vena caval junction

3. **Still's Aortic Valve Vibratory Murmur (the most common innocent murmur referred for cardiac consultation. Venous hum is more prevalent but seldom prompts referral)**
   a. Age first heard: neonate, infant; 3–7 y
   b. Age murmur disappears: early to midadolescence
   c. Location: sternal edge, third and fourth spaces with weak transmission to apex; murmur may transmit to right carotid artery
   d. Patient position that amplifies murmur: best heard in supine position during held expiration but may persist with standing position; murmur attenuated or obliterated by forced Valsalva maneuver or deep held inspiration
   e. Character: low-pitched, groaning, or musical; short, grade I–III
   f. Phase of cardiac cycle: midsystole
   g. Confused with:
      (1) Left ventricular false tendon; the inconsequential false tendon usually has less variation with change in body position and is heard over a wider area on the chest wall, including the apex
      (2) Left ventricular HOCM with subaortic pressure gradient, but HOCM murmur persists with all positions
      (3) MR murmur of acute rheumatic valvulitis, but MR murmur is high-pitched and at the apex of the heart; it is unlikely to disappear entirely with erect position
      (4) Small VSD; murmur of small VSD is actually not very similar to Still's murmur, but some patients are referred with a possible diagnosis of VSD; VSD murmur is long and harsh and persists in all patient positions
   h. Murmur produced by: aortic valve leaflet vibration during midsystole

4. **Pulmonary Valve Flow Murmur**
   a. Age first heard: late childhood, early adolescence
   b. Age murmur disappears: early adult life; murmur may be heard in adult pregnant women or in adults with a thin chest wall and with increased cardiac output
   c. Location: left second intercostal space at sternal edge
   d. Patient position that amplifies murmur: murmur invariably heard best with patient supine, especially after exercise and during held expiration; murmur attenuated or obliterated by deep held inspiration and often simply with patient standing
   e. Character of murmur: high frequency, blowing, occasionally scratchy
   f. Phase of cardiac cycle: systole
   g. Murmur confused with:
      (1) ASD of the secundum type, but ASD has wide splitting of S_2
      (2) Mild pulmonary valve stenosis, but pulmonary stenosis is usually preceded by an ejection click and persists in all positions and with held inspiration

5. **Normal Heart Sounds That May Prompt Referral for Cardiac Evaluation**
   Prominent Physiologic Splitting of S_2
   a. Age first heard: early to midchildhood, rarely heard in young infants because heart rate is usually too fast to detect splitting
   b. Age sound disappears: S_2 splitting remains throughout life but is often hard to hear in adults with a thick chest wall
   c. Location: left second and third intercostal spaces and sternal edge
   d. Position which amplifies sound: S_2 splitting enhanced by supine position and during slow inspiration; S_2 splitting less prominent in standing position, during tachycardia, and during Valsalva maneuver held for 3–4 s
   e. Confused with: *fixed splitting* of S_2 found in ASD defect and with complete right bundle branch block; *physiologic splitting* is very similar to pathologic fixed splitting, but in a cooperative child with a heart rate less than 120 beats/min, lack of movement of S_2 is very clear when compared with normal splitting; in physiologic splitting, the "lub-dub" in expiration changes during slow inspiration to "lub-trrup"

   Physiologic Splitting of S_1
   a. Age first heard: late childhood, adolescence, or an age that the heart rate slows to 60–80 beats/min
   b. Age sound disappears: physiologic splitting remains throughout adult life but is harder to hear in obese or thick-chested individuals
   c. Location: left sternal border and third, fourth, and fifth spaces (tricuspid area); less prominent at apex
   d. Patient position that amplifies S_1 splitting: either supine or standing
   e. Sound attenuated or obliterated by: tachycardia 110–120 beats/min or more
   f. Sound confused with:
      (1) Midsystolic click of mitral leaflet prolapse—the split sounds like "trrup'dub" and midsystolic click sounds like "lub-ip-dub"
      (2) Aortic ejection click of bicuspid aortic valve; ejection click has a sharper, snappier sound than duller components of physiologically split first sound; ejection click best heard at apex with transmission to sternal edge

PDA, patent ductus arteriosus; HOCM, hypertrophic obstructive cardiomyopathy; MR, mitral regurgitation; VSD, ventricular septal defect; ASD, atrial septal defect.

3. The physician recommends return visits to check the murmur again later.
4. The physician's explanation of innocent murmurs seems perfunctory to the parents or has been phrased in medical jargon.

Thus, an approach to management of innocent murmurs by pediatricians in the office is one that avoids management practices that unwittingly leave parents or teenaged patients feeling uneasy or confused.

MANAGEMENT BY PEDIATRICIANS

Keeping the Ear Trained To Recognize Innocent Murmurs with Confidence

By the end of residency training, pediatricians have learned to recognize the several innocent murmurs peculiar to the young. Some months or years after entering practice, however, physicians may find that they have lost their once mastered skill of auscultation. Probably this can be largely avoided or rectified by taking advantage of the daily opportunity that a busy practice affords to refresh on hearing these normal variants of heart sounds that may appear transiently or may be elicited at one time or another in virtually all young people. A good time to search for innocent murmurs is on an occasion in which the patient has increased cardiac output, for example, immediately after vigorous exercise (enough to raise the heart rate to 120 to 130 beats per minute), in the infant shortly after a full feeding, when there is fever, infection, anxiety, or excitement, or with mild anemia. Each of these situations increases the intensity of latent or existing physiologic murmurs (as well as pathologic ones, for that matter).

One obstacle to a prompt and accurate evaluation of heart murmurs or unusual sounds is listening too long at only one valve area and with the subject placed in only one position. It is actually better to listen to only three to five cardiac cycles at each of the valve areas, moving back to the site where the murmur is loudest for a second brief listen if needed. This ought to be done with the child placed in each of the traditionally prescribed positions: supine, sitting, and

---

TABLE 2. Information for Parents and Patients*

Misconceptions about innocent murmurs in the young can cause a lot of unnecessary trouble and anxiety for the family. Some people are perfectly satisfied to accept a hurried dismissal of an innocent murmur: "It's nothing. Forget about it." But others, despite full trust in their doctor, want more details. Although physicians certainly want to take the time to explain an innocent heart murmur, the demands of a busy practice sometimes make this impractical. This table can assist the physician in discussing a heart murmur with the family.

Heart Murmurs and Heart Sounds

What is the difference between a *heart murmur* and a *heart sound?* Usually, when the physician listens to the normal heart with a stethoscope, two heart sounds occur in each cardiac cycle and resemble something like "lub-dub." These two sounds occur with closure of the heart valves: the first sound, with closure of the valves between the upper and lower heart chambers (tricuspid valve on the right side and mitral valve on the left), and the second sound, with closure of the valves opening into the great vessels that leave the heart (pulmonary and aortic valves). Usually, while the heart pumps blood out and while it fills with blood, no sound is heard with a stethoscope, except in a high percentage of normal healthy young people, in whom prolonged sounds (called murmurs) may occur during the usually silent pumping phase of the heart cycle *(systole)* and sometimes also during the filling phase *(diastole).*

What makes the term *murmur* confusing is that some birth defects of the heart or acquired diseases also produce murmurs. Thus, physicians must specify whether the murmur is *innocent* (benign or functional), implying no recognizable abnormality or disease of the heart, or *organic,* indicating that the prolonged sound is caused by some abnormality of the heart or its blood vessels.

What is the importance of an innocent murmur? The only importance of an innocent murmur lies in the fact that it may be mistaken for an organic murmur. One or more of these insignificant noises can be heard at one time or another in most, but not all, young people. These murmurs usually disappear before adult life. They cause no harm, require no follow-up, call for no restriction of physical activity, and should be considered normal variants.

One reason that so many young people but few adults have these sounds emanating from the normal heart is that the thin chest wall of the child transmits sound to the chest surface very readily. Also, the heart in the child is relatively close to the chest wall, which allows heart sounds as well as murmurs to be readily heard. The parent can borrow the doctor's stethoscope and listen to the heart of the fully grown adult and then to that of the infant, child, or adolescent. Even without medical training, the parent will realize how much louder the child's heart is.

Young people are often examined by the doctor when there is an increased rate of blood flow through the heart because of fever, infection, or simply the anxiety that goes with a visit to the doctor. This faster blood flow through the circulation brings out murmurs that may not be present at rest and makes existing murmurs louder.

Types of Innocent Murmurs

There are four common innocent murmurs and at least two variants of normal heart sounds that may sometimes lead to suspicion of an organic murmur or pathologic sound.

Neonatal Pulmonary Artery Murmur

In some newborns (perhaps 15% to 20%) during the first few weeks of life, a short, high-pitched murmur can be heard in the sides of the chest under the arms, in the front of the chest just below the collar bones, or in the back between the "wings" (scapulae). These murmurs disappear within a few weeks and are unassociated with any enlargement of the heart or other sign of difficulty.

Still's Murmur (Aortic Valve Vibratory Murmur)

Still's murmur (named for Dr. Still, the English physician who first described it) arises from normal aortic valve vibration produced by the rapid movement of the aortic valve leaflets when the heart pumps blood through the valve. The more rapidly blood moves through the valve during fever, exercise, or the anxiety associated with a doctor's examination, the greater the vibration and the more likely that the vibrations will be transmitted to the surface of the chest as a heart murmur.

Pulmonary Valve Flow Murmur

Production of this murmur, like that of Still's murmur, results from vibration of a valve, but at the pulmonary instead of the aortic valve.

Venous Hum

This is a continuous "whirring" sound heard in both phases of the cardiac cycle (systole and diastole). Venous hum occurs as blood flows through the large veins in the neck en route to the heart. In almost all young children, a venous hum can be brought out by sitting the child up and raising the chin.

Normal Variants of Heart Sound

The first heart sound is produced by closure of tricuspid and mitral valves, and the second heart sound is produced by closure of pulmonic and aortic valves. The valves close so nearly simultaneously that in children we usually hear only two single sounds, lub'-dub, but when the heart slows down with increasing age of the child, the tricuspid and mitral valve closure times separate slightly and we hear each valve closure separately; the lub'-dub becomes trrup'-dub. Although this is not a murmur, it can give the impression that it is either a murmur or an abnormal click of the mitral valve or the aortic valve.

Management of Innocent Murmurs by Physicians and Parents

Once the physician determines that a heart murmur or an unusual sound is innocent, it is no longer necessary to check it. The child should not be restricted, and no special precautions need be taken. Substituting the word "normal" for "innocent" may be the best way to think about it. That alone should guide the management of a young person who has one of these sounds, which can plague his or her life if not appropriately ignored.

---

*For further information, you may contact Dan G. McNamara, MD, at Pediatric Cardiology, Texas Children's Hospital, Houston, Texas 77030. Phone (713) 770-5600. FAX (713) 770-5630.

standing, first at rest and then, when possible, immediately after exercise, which turns up the volume (intensity) of heart sounds and existing or latent murmurs.

In addition, it helps to note the effect of deep continuous, quiet, unforced respiration, the effect of deep held inspiration, and, finally, deep held expiration, with the patient supine. Of course, auscultation must be performed while the patient and the examining room are perfectly quiet, not always an easy thing to achieve in a busy office or with talkative onlookers. With practice, however, a complete auscultation can be accomplished in a quiet, cooperative patient in 2½ to 3 minutes.

This full cardiac examination is hardly practical and indeed unnecessary in every well child examined, but if one tries to elicit these murmurs once or twice per week, the examiner becomes and remains expert at it. The auscultatory skills developed in this way are then available when needed to evaluate a new unexpected murmur.

Gaining the Confidence of the Family and Patient

If the examiner has decided that a murmur is benign and tells the family about it, the diagnosis, which sometimes causes alarm, is far better accepted if the physician has performed a complete cardiovascular auscultation using the several maneuvers and putting the patient in the different positions cited previously.

The topic described in this section pertains only to murmurs. A complete cardiovascular examination, of course, includes pulses, blood pressure, and palpation of the precordium—all too well known to most readers of this volume to itemize in detail.

Avoiding the Temptation To Make Return Appointments To Check on the Murmur

Once it has been determined by the primary care physician or the consultant that the murmur is innocent, it need not, and in fact, should not, be "checked on," at least ostensibly, at subsequent office visits. Parents are best advised that although the sound usually disappears as the patient matures, it need not disappear entirely in order to confirm that the sound is innocent. These murmurs often appear and disappear inexplicably. In fact, the two most common innocent murmurs (*Still's aortic valve vibratory murmur* of childhood and *pulmonary valve flow murmur* of adolescence) are very likely to reappear intermittently or become louder whenever situations arise that increase cardiac output and when examining conditions are ideal (quiet, cooperative patient and quiet examining room).

Explaining Innocent Murmurs To the Family Orally and in Writing

The term *murmur* is so much a part of our medical vocabulary that physicians forget that many people do not know what the term means—let alone know the difference between an "innocent" and "pathologic" murmur. It helps family members to understand and accept the diagnosis if they have been informed on the elementary facts about innocent murmurs and how these sounds are produced, to

some extent, in all individuals but heard more readily in children. They may not know that "normal" murmurs are prevalent in children because the chest wall is thinner and the heart relatively closer to the anterior chest wall than in the adult. Also, children are more likely than adults to experience events that increase the cardiac output (fever, infection, excitement, or anxiety in the doctor's office), which makes the murmur louder.

It helps to name the particular murmur(s) found in the patient. Naming the murmur adds credibility to the diagnosis and makes explanation easier. Also, parents are more readily convinced about innocent murmurs when they learn that research studies using intracardiac phonocardiography have shown that in healthy adults, blood turbulence is created at the great vessel valves during the ejection phase of the cardiac cycle. This turbulence at the pulmonary valve can be heard as a pulmonary flow murmur and at the aortic valve as Still's aortic vibratory murmur under certain physiologic conditions. Similarly, turbulence in the jugular–superior vena caval junction in young children produces a venous hum. Pulmonary artery branch turbulence in the maturing neonate causes the neonatal transient murmur.

Because an oral explanation may take 15 to 20 minutes, not including time for questions, and because anxiety about a murmur on the part of parents may interfere with their paying full attention in the doctor's office, it has proved helpful, in my experience, to draft an explanation in lay terms for the family to take home to read and reread and share with family members who were not present at the doctor's office. The explanation used by several of the pediatric cardiologists at Texas Children's Hospital in Houston is presented in Table 2.

Allowing Normal Physical Activity (Including Competitive Sports and Avoiding Any Special Precautions for Handling Infection or Surgical Procedures)

Despite identification of the murmur as a purely innocent one, parents may nevertheless restrict the child from physical exertion or may worry needlessly if the child needs anesthesia unless they are informed that the only consequence of an innocent murmur is an inordinate concern about it.

CONCLUSION

If the pediatrician wishes to refer the patient with a troublesome, but most likely innocent, murmur to the pediatric cardiologist, this is a reasonable plan of management that is evidently in widespread use throughout this country, and, except for the time, expense, and possible anxiety for the parents and child associated with a visit to the consultant, this method of management can be quite satisfactory and definitive. For those physicians who prefer to handle these patients themselves in their office, the steps outlined in Table 2 should provide the means to accomplish this successfully and expeditiously.

6

Digestive Tract

MALFORMATIONS OF THE INTESTINE

Stephen E. Dolgin, M.D.

PROXIMAL INTESTINAL OBSTRUCTION

If duodenal obstruction is diagnosed in a fetus by prenatal sonography, care should be directed to a team that can provide the proper counseling and perinatal steps for further evaluation and treatment. Coordination among the obstetrician, pediatric surgeon, neonatologist, and pediatric anesthesiologist is important. Since about one third of newborns with duodenal atresia have Down syndrome, fetal karyotype is critical. The fetus should be screened for other malformations.

Duodenal obstruction is initially managed postnatally with gastric decompression. A large (10F or 12F) oral gastric tube is well tolerated by even the smallest premature newborn. The small feeding tubes common in the neonatal units are not effective for draining thick secretions. Plentiful gastric secretions, especially if bilious, are confirmatory of obstruction. An upright plain film taken after allowing a short time for air swallowing will establish the presence of duodenal obstruction. The classic double bubble, two upper abdominal air-fluid levels with no air distally, establishes complete duodenal obstruction. The same findings with a paucity of air distally suggest partial duodenal obstruction. Contrast studies are not usually indicated. If the apparent duodenal obstruction is partial, the plain film may be equivocal, and a barium swallow is indicated. Otherwise, further studies to elucidate the specific cause of duodenal obstruction are not needed, since this is resolved in the operating room.

Operative repair is an emergency if malrotation cannot be excluded because of the risk of volvulus causing midgut infarction. Otherwise, time can be spent assessing other anomalies. If the baby is extremely small, a period of preoperative intravenous alimentation can be considered.

Ordinarily, operative repair is performed shortly after diagnosis, with the patient appropriately hydrated and in metabolic balance. Under the guidance of a pediatric anesthesiologist and with proper monitoring, general anesthesia is induced, and the abdomen is opened through a transverse supraumbilical incision on the right side.

Dudodenal atresia and annular pancreas are treated by an anastomosis from the duodenum proximal to the obstruction to the duodenum or jejunum just distal to the obstruction. A duodenal web can be treated by excision, but the distal common bile duct must be protected. An intraoperative cholangiogram may be helpful.

When correcting duodenal obstruction, the surgeon must exclude any other intestinal obstruction. A more distal obstruction is excluded if saline is instilled into the distal intestine and milked to the recto-sigmoid. If the anesthesiologist can advance a gastric tube to the proximal duodenotomy, a more proximal obstruction is excluded.

Postoperative Course

When a baby is born with duodenal obstruction, the condition is chronic. Swallowed amniotic fluid results in a thick, dilated, floppy proximal duodenum. For this reason, recovery after duodenal anastomosis for congenital obstruction often has been slow, requiring prolonged gastric drainage and intravenous feeds. With careful operative technique, recovery and the resumption of feeds often can be accomplished within a week. The anastomosis should be fashioned on the dependent part of the duodenum just proximal to the obstruction. The intestine just beyond the obstruction is used for the distal end of the anastomosis. It must not be twisted or kinked. Because the pylorus has been so chronically stretched and rendered ineffective, bilious duodenal secretions freely enter the stomach. Therefore, the continued presence of bile in the stomach should not be used as a reason to continue gastric drainage. When the abdomen is scaphoid and the gastric drainage decreases, the gastric tube can be removed and replaced 12 hours later. If the stomach remains empty during this 12 hour trial, feeds can be initiated the next day. Parents should expect a 3 to 4 week hospitalization, but discharge often can be accomplished much sooner (1 to 2 weeks).

MALROTATION

Of all the congenital causes of intestinal obstruction, malrotation is the most critical because of the risk of midgut infarction from volvulus. Volvulus can occur at any age. If volvulus is suspected clinically, emergency abdominal exploration is necessary after rapid fluid resuscitation and gastric decompression. Resection for massive infarction results in the short gut syndrome, which requires a very prolonged hospitalization, intravenous calories, and slow resumption of drip feeds. The course is likely complicated by cholestasis and bouts of sepsis. If there is scant viable intestine, especially if there are other serious morbid conditions, a more rational approach is to close the abdomen and allow the patient to die comfortably. The family is not given false expectations, and the misery is not prolonged. This requires clear preoperative communication, with documentation of the family's wishes. The absolute minimum amount of intestine necessary for recovery is not clear and varies with the postconceptual age and the level of prematurity (the premature's intestine has considerable potential growth).

Frequently, malrotation becomes evident because of abnormal bands causing duodenal obstruction. Delay is not acceptable in this setting because the operation should be done before volvulus occurs. The operation for malrotation, the Ladd procedure, includes reducing the volvulus if present, lysing any abnormal bands, excluding intrinsic intestinal obstruction, and, if the baby is stable, removing the appendix. The intestines are left in the malrotated but untwisted position.

SMALL BOWEL ATRESIA

Small bowel atresia has multiple dilated loops of intestine by examination and abdominal roentgenogram. A barium enema may be needed to exclude other causes of distal obstruction, some of which may not require an immediate operation (such as meconium plug, small left colon, uncomplicated meconium ileus, Hirschsprung's disease).

The operation for small bowel atresia is complicated by the size discrepancy between the intestine proximal and distal to the atresia. At times, stomas and staged reconstruction are appropriate. In some babies, enteroplasty to narrow the proximal intestines has been useful. Multiple atresias can result in the short gut syndrome.

MAJOR ABDOMINAL WALL DEFECTS

If diagnosis of a major abdominal wall defect is made in the fetus, care should be transferred to a team experienced in major newborn malformations. Amniocentesis with determination of fetal karyotype is important because of the association with major chromosome abnormalities. The fetus should be screened for other malformations that are common with omphalocele and uncommon with gastroschisis. The type and timing of delivery can be individualized. The surgeon should meet the parents well before the delivery.

An orogastric tube should be placed in the delivery room, and the baby should be kept warm. The exposed intestines, which are unprotected in gastroschisis and covered by a sac in the omphalocele, should be covered with warm saline-soaked gauze and wrapped in Kerlix. An overhead warmer during the period of exposure is important to protect against hypothermia. There is usually no great advantage in delaying the operative repair.

Intragastric or intravesical pressure can be measured intraoperatively to help decide if primary closure is safe. Too high intraabdominal pressure interferes with renal vein blood return, respiratory function, and perfusion of the intestine. Primary closure of the defect in gastroschisis is made easier if the intestinal contents are washed out with dilute acetylcysteine, if the abdominal wall is stretched by a kneading action, and, occasionally, if a small fascial hernia is permitted. If primary closure cannot be safely accomplished, the surgeon employs a delayed closure with a prosthetic silo sewn to the fascial edges of the defect. An indwelling central line for intravenous feeding often is needed in babies with gastroschisis because about 3 weeks are required for the intestines, which have been bathing in amniotic fluid, to recover good function. One of twenty patients with gastroschisis has intestinal atresia, which is managed with either stomas or primary reconstruction.

The small and medium-size omphaloceles usually can be closed primarily. The more difficult omphalocele is large, with the liver often herniated, and is frequently associated with other anomalies. Here, a delayed closure is necessary.

INTESTINAL DUPLICATIONS

Intestinal duplications, although rare, vary in their size, shape, and location. They may cause intestinal obstruction by encroaching on the adjoining lumen or acting as the lead point of an intussusception. They can cause gastrointestinal bleeding secondary to ectopic acid-secreting gastric mucosa. They can arise in the abdominal or thoracic cavity, cross the diaphragm, and be very extensive. They may be noted by prenatal sonography, most often as an intraabdominal cyst. Because duplications often have ectopic gastric mucosa, they can be demonstrated at times on a scan done for a Meckel's diverticulum.

The most common site of duplication is at the distal ileum, and it usually is managed by resection and primary anastomosis. Since the typical duplication arises within the leaves of the mesentery, resection of the adjoining intestine is usually needed. No single operative approach can be dictated for all intestinal duplications. At the duodenum, partial excision of the duplication may be appropriate. At the rectum, dividing the shared septum between the presacral duplication and the

rectum may be the best approach. Long duplications occasionally have been managed with multiple incisions in the duplicated segment and stripping out of the abnormal mucosa.

REFERENCES

1. Grosfeld JL, Rescorla FJ: Duodenal atresia and stenosis: Reassessment of the treatment and outcome based on antenatal diagnosis, pathologic variance, and long-term follow-up. World J Surg 1993;17:301–309.
2. Molenaar JC, Tibboel D: Gastroschisis and omphalocele. World J Surg 1993;17:337–341.

HIRSCHSPRUNG'S DISEASE

KATHERINE B. FREEMAN, M.D.
JOEL W. ADELSON, M.D., Ph.D.

DEFINITION, PATHOPHYSIOLOGY, AND EPIDEMIOLOGY

Hirschsprung's disease, or congenital aganglionic megacolon, results from the absence of the ganglion cells of the parasympathetic system in the intestinal wall. The condition always includes the anus plus a variable length of intestine extending proximally. This lack of intestinal innervation results in permanent tonic contraction of the affected intestine, with an inability to relax in response to proximal dilatation. The absence of ganglion cells is thought to be because of an in utero failure of the normal caudal migration of neural crest cells down the gastrointestinal tract during the fifth through the twelfth week of gestation. The earlier in gestation this migratory failure occurs, the longer the affected segment. The disease is usually limited to the colon, with 75% of cases limited to the rectosigmoid, although occasional cases include the small bowel.

The incidence is 1 in 5000 live births, with an overall male/female ratio of about 4:1. There is no reported racial predilection. There is a familial association, with an elevated risk to siblings of 4%. The longer the involved segment, the greater the risk of familial recurrence. There is a tenfold increase in the incidence of Hirschsprung's disease in patients with Down syndrome, and there are reports of an association with the Waardenburg and other syndromes, as well as with cardiac and genitourinary defects.

The majority (80%) of patients are diagnosed in the first year of life, with 15% diagnosed within the first month and 64% diagnosed by the third month. A few are not diagnosed until later, even into adulthood. The shorter the involved segment, the longer it may take to be recognized.

CLINICAL CHARACTERISTICS

The cardinal feature of Hirschsprung's disease is constipation. In neonates, this frequently occurs with delayed passage of meconium. In normal infants, 94% pass the first meconium stool by 24 hours of life, and 99% by 48 hours. Hirschsprung's disease should be strongly suspected in any infant who has not had a first stool by that time. Within the first 48 to 72 hours, these neonates are likely to develop anorexia, vomiting, and abdominal distention. Some infants may exhibit temporary relief of the obstruction after stimulation with a rectal thermometer or suppository, but they go on to have chronically poor intake and failure to thrive.

During the first 3 months of life, infants with Hirschsprung's disease are at particular risk for the development of enterocolitis, a serious complication and the leading cause of death in children with this condition. The enterocolitis causes severe abdominal distention, explosive watery diarrhea, and fever. Protein-losing enteropathy, hypovolemic shock, and perforation of the appendix or colon may develop.

Older children with Hirschsprung's disease often have significant abdominal distention, fecal retention, recurrent fecal impaction, and poor appetite and growth. They may also have rectal bleeding because of fissures, as well as urinary retention, hydroureters, or hydronephrosis caused by ureteral compression (additionally, concomitant genitourinary anomalies may occur). They usually do *not* have fecal soiling (except, in some authors' opinion, patients with short-segment Hirschsprung's disease). This difference can be an important diagnostic clue in differentiating these patients from patients with functional constipation and encopresis.

DIAGNOSIS AND DIAGNOSTIC MANAGEMENT

Physical Examination

The abdomen is usually distended, and dilated loops of stool-filled bowel may be palpated. On rectal examination, the sphincter tone may be increased or normal. Usually, the rectal vault is empty and not dilated (except, in some authors' opinion, in patients with short-segment disease), which can be another important clue in differentiating Hirschsprung's disease from functional constipation.

Radiologic Studies

In infants, a plain film of the abdomen with the child in the prone position may show absence of gas in the rectum and a dilated proximal intestine. A standard diagnostic test is the single-contrast barium enema in the child who has not received preparatory evacuating enemas (an "unprepped" barium enema). In up to 80% of patients, the enema will show the classic findings of Hirschsprung's disease—a transition zone between the proximal dilated intestine and the distal aganglionic contracted segment. The transition zone is seen most clearly on lateral films. Rectal manipulation with a suppository, examining finger, rectal thermometer, or enema before the study may temporarily dilate the aganglionic area to a normal caliber and mask the transition zone. This should be avoided. Infants less than 1 month of age and children with either short-segment disease or total colonic involvement are more likely to have a normal-appearing barium enema. A postevacuation film should be obtained, since over 50% of patients with Hirschsprung's disease are reported to show a delay in the passage of the barium up to 24 to 48 hours. In a child with constipation and a normal-appearing barium enema, an additional clue to Hirschsprung's disease may be the caliber of the rectum. In patients with Hirschsprung's disease, the rectum may appear narrower than the sigmoid colon, whereas in functional constipation, the rectum may be very dilated.

Manometry

Anorectal manometry is a valuable diagnostic tool. The normal response to balloon dilatation of the rectum is a reflex relaxation of the internal sphincter, with a drop in the pressure tracing. In Hirschsprung's disease, this relaxation is absent, and a paradoxical contraction of the internal sphincter may occur instead. Rectal manometry may be falsely abnormal in normal newborns as a result of the lack of development of reflex relaxation of the internal sphincter.

Rectal Biopsy

Whenever Hirschprung's disease is suspected, histologic confirmation should be made by rectal biopsy. Suction rectal biopsies are usually satisfactory for this purpose and are less invasive than full-thickness surgical biopsies. Ten percent to thirty percent of suction biopsies, however, may not be deep enough to show the myenteric and submucosal plexus. Further, biopsies may be inaccurate if obtained too high or too low in the rectum. Various biopsy regimens have been suggested because of these concerns. A commonly accepted protocol recommends biopsies at 3, 4, and 5 cm from the anal margin. The biopsy should demonstrate the absence of ganglion cells in the myenteric (Auerbach) plexus and the submucosal (Meissner) plexus. Hypertrophied nerve bundles between the circular and longitudinal muscles in the submucosa are found. Histochemical staining for acetylcholinesterase can be very helpful in illuminating these findings.

TREATMENT

If enterocolitis occurs, it should be treated aggressively with nasogastric and colonic decompression, intravenous fluid resuscitation, broad-spectrum antibiotics, colonic irrigation with normal saline, and monitoring for perforation. A colostomy can be performed when the surgeons think that the child has improved and is stable. The definitive pullthrough may be delayed for a year.

Surgery

The definitive treatment for Hirschsprung's disease is surgical resection of the abnormal aganglionic segment of the intestine, with an anastomosis of the normal intestine to the rectum. In North America, most surgeons elect to perform a temporary leveling colostomy in the normal intestine proximal to the aganglionic segment while confirming the presence of ganglion cells in the normal segment with intraoperative frozen sections. The definitive pullthrough operation is performed when the child is 6 to 12 months old and weighs 15 pounds or more. In older children, a temporary colostomy may not be done. Several definitive surgical approaches have been used. The Swenson procedure involves the anastomosis between normal colon and a diagonally fashioned cuff of aganglionic distal rectum. In the Duhamel procedure, the aganglionic rectum is left anteriorly, and normal colon is anastomosed posteriorly in an end-to-side fashion. In the Soave and Boley endorectal pullthrough procedures, the aganglionic mucosa is dissected from the rectum, and the normal colon is brought down through the retained muscular rectal tube and anastomosed to the anus.

Postoperative Complications

Patients with an ostomy may have significant fluid and electrolyte losses with subsequent imbalances, such as hyponatremic, hypochloremic, metabolic alkalosis and poor growth.

The long-term complications of Hirschsprung's disease after a pullthrough procedure are variable and depend on the amount of intestine resected, the condition of the child before surgery, and the type of procedure chosen by the surgeon. Potential complications include stricture at the surgical site, recurrent enterocolitis, recurrent constipation, and fecal impaction. The most common problem seen after surgery is fecal incontinence. The majority of children do quite well postoperatively and have regular bowel movements without difficulty.

NEONATAL INTESTINAL OBSTRUCTION

RONALD B. HIRSCHL, M.D.

Intestinal obstruction in the neonate occurs secondary to a number of congenital and acquired abnormalities (Table 1). In this section, we review the approach to and treatment of the most commonly seen causes of gastrointestinal obstruction in the neonate. Pyloric stenosis, necrotizing enterocolitis, and Hirschsprung's disease are covered extensively in other sections of this book and, therefore, are not discussed here.

Although often accompanied by a variety of symptoms, bilious vomiting or bilious nasogastric tube aspirate with or without abdominal distention is the hallmark of surgically important bowel obstruction in the newborn period. Because of the possibility of malrotation with volvulus and associated bowel ischemia and necrosis, all workup for bowel obstruction in the neonate should be performed emergently until this diagnosis has been excluded. Sequential radiographic evaluation with plain upright and flat x-rays of the abdomen, contrast enema evaluation, and an upper gastrointestinal contrast series should be performed to ascertain the presence, etiology, and location of an obstruction. The preoperative management for all newborns with bowel obstruction should include placement of an orogastric or nasogastric tube on continuous suction. The fluid and electrolyte status

TABLE 1. Common Causes of Neonatal Gastrointestinal Obstruction

> Esophageal atresia
> Pyloric stenosis
> Duodenal atresia/stenosis
> Annular pancreas
> Duodenal web
> Malrotation with Ladd's bands
> Malrotation with volvulus
> Jejunoileocolic atresia
> Meconium ileus
> Small left colon syndrome
> Meconium plug syndrome
> Hirschsprung's disease
> Imperforate anus

should be evaluated, and appropriate resuscitation should be performed to ensure appropriate urine flow (1 to 2 ml/kg/h). If a dose has not been given, vitamin K (AquaMEPHYTON 1 mg IM) is administered routinely, as are IV antibiotics. Care is taken to maintain the newborn in a warm environment.

ESOPHAGEAL ATRESIA AND TRACHEOESOPHAGEAL FISTULA

Patients with esophageal atresia frequently have an in utero history of polyhydramnios. Evidence of drooling is often present after birth and is accompanied by choking and coughing with feeding. Usually, an unsuccessful attempt is made at passing a nasogastric or orogastric tube. Curling of the tube in the dilated proximal esophageal pouch is pathognomonic for esophageal atresia. Radiologic evaluation, performed with careful administration of contrast medium into the upper pouch with the patient sitting upright to avoid aspiration, will verify the diagnosis of esophageal atresia and exclude the presence of a rarely present proximal tracheoesophageal fistula (TEF). Examination of the plain abdominal radiograph will document the presence of air within the gastrointestinal tract and distinguish, therefore, an esophageal atresia with a distal TEF (85%) from pure esophageal atresia (7%).

Initial management should include placement of a suction tube into the proximal esophageal pouch to prevent aspiration of secretions (Replogle tube). The patient with a TEF should be maintained in a 30- to 45-degree upright position to inhibit gastric secretions from refluxing into the tracheobronchial tree. Intravenous antibiotics should be administered prophylactically because of the risk of pneumonia. The newborn should be evaluated for those anomalies that are part of the VATER or VACTERL association preoperatively.

In general, patients with esophageal atresia and a distal TEF have adequate esophageal length to allow primary reconstruction. A retropleural approach through the right chest is used. The distal TEF is identified in the region of the carina and is divided. The proximal esophageal pouch is mobilized in the upper mediastinum, and an esophagoesophagostomy is performed. In most cases, this anastomosis may be performed under mild to moderate levels of tension. A retropleural chest tube is placed to allow drainage should an anastomotic leak occur. A Hypaque swallow is performed 7 days after operation. If the anastomosis appears intact, feedings are initiated, antibiotics are discontinued, and the retropleural chest tube is removed.

In patients with esophageal atresia without a TEF, the distal segment is quite short and precludes immediate repair. A decision must be made whether to attempt to salvage the native esophagus. Options for management, therefore, include (1) placement of an upper pouch Replogle suction tube and a gastrostomy with daily dilatation of the upper pouch; after 8 to 10 weeks, growth of the proximal and distal esophageal segments will typically allow an esophagoesophagostomy to be performed; or (2) creation of a cervical esophagostomy with gastrostomy tube placement in the newborn that will allow stable management until reconstruction of the esophagus with stomach, colon, or small bowel may be performed at 1 year of life.

Patients with a TEF but no esophageal atresia (4%) often have episodes of gastric distention during crying and choking and cyanotic spells during feeding. Diagnosis is best made by bronchoscopy and esophagoscopy, which demonstrates the H-type fistula between the trachea and esophagus. Occasionally, a barium swallow is necessary for documentation of the fistula. A Fogarty catheter may be placed through the fistula at the time of bronchoscopy, with ligation performed usually via a cervical approach.

Current overall survival rates are generally in the 85% to 90% range. Mortality is usually secondary to associated anomalies. Immediate postoperative complications include anastomotic leak in 15% of cases. Almost all leaks will resolve spontaneously with continuation of IV antibiotics and chest tube drainage. Stricture formation occurs in approximately 15% of cases and is often associated with an anastomotic leak. Most strictures are responsive to repeated dilatations. Recurrent TEF occurs in 5% of cases and requires reoperation, with division and ligation of the fistula. The most common long-term problems associated with esophageal atresia include gastroesophageal reflux (up to 70% of patients) and tracheomalacia (approximately 25% of patients).

CONGENITAL DUODENAL OBSTRUCTION

Congenital duodenal obstruction with duodenal dilatation may be appreciated on in utero ultrasound done when polyhydramnios is observed. In the first 24 to 48 hours of life, feeding intolerance and bilious vomiting often are noted. If the obstruction is proximal to the ampulla of Vater, as it is in 5% to 10% of cases, the vomitus may be nonbilious. Abdominal distention is *not* typical. Classic plain abdominal radiographs demonstrate a double-bubble, with an air-filled, dilated stomach and proximal duodenum. The double-bubble sign may be enhanced by instillation of approximately 20 ml of air via the orogastric or nasogastric tube. The distal small intestine and colon will remain gasless unless *partial* duodenal obstruction is present. If a classic double-bubble is observed, further radiographic study usually is unnecessary, since the specific etiology of the obstruction may be determined at the time of operation. Approximately 30% of newborns with congenital duodenal obstruction will have trisomy 21, and, therefore, appropriate blood samples for chromosomal analysis should be obtained preoperatively should intraoperative transfusion become necessary. As long as intestinal malrotation has been excluded, emergent operation is not mandatory. However, in most cases, prompt surgical intervention is appropriate.

Congenital duodenal obstruction typically is induced by one of the following lesions: (1) an *annular pancreas* in which a ring of pancreatic tissue either completely or partially surrounds the duodenum inducing complete or partial obstruction, (2) a *duodenal atresia,* or (3) *stenosis* secondary to either Ladd's bands in the setting of intestinal malrotation or a mucosal web with an opening of variable size. Atresias and stenoses most commonly occur at the site of the ampulla of Vater in the second portion of the duodenum. Other bowel atresias concomitant with duodenal atresia are quite rare. A right supraumbilical incision with mobilization of the duodenum allows identification of the markedly dilated duodenum proximal to and the decompressed duodenum distal to the site of obstruction. In general, bypass of the obstructing lesion with a duodenoduodenostomy, an anastamosis of the proximal to the distal duodenum around the obstructing lesion, is the best approach. If a relatively wide gap between the two ends of the duodenum makes duodenoduodenostomy difficult, a loop of proximal jejunum may be brought in retrocolic fashion up to the duodenum, and a duodenojejunostomy may be performed between the end of the proximal duodenum and the side of the jejunum.

Morbidity and mortality usually are due to associated complications from prematurity, trisomy 21, or congenital heart disease. It frequently takes several days to weeks until the dilated proximal duodenum functions appropriately and allows enteral feeds to be tolerated. For this reason, some surgeons suggest placement of a gastrostomy tube and a transgastric feeding jejunostomy tube at the time of correction of the duodenal atresia to allow early initiation of feeding.

MALROTATION OF THE INTESTINE

During development, the intestines undergo a 270-degree counterclockwise rotation, which results in proper fixation of the bowel at the ligament of Treitz and in the area of the cecum and right colon. If this rotation fails to occur, the small intestine remains on the right side of the abdomen and the colon on the left. The normal broad fixation of the midgut thus fails to occur. The fairly mobile midgut is quite easily able to twist, or volvulize, which may compromise superior mesenteric artery and venous blood flow, with potentially catastrophic ischemia or necrosis of the entire small intestine and right and transverse colon.

The primary symptom is bilious vomiting. Abdominal distention often is *not* present. Newborns may have obstructive symptoms as a result of midgut volvulus or compression from peritoneal bands, termed Ladd's bands, when malrotation is present. These bands extend from the abnormally placed cecum to the right posterior body wall, crossing the distal duodenum and inducing partial obstruction. Physical examination is surprisingly unremarkable unless midgut volvulus with intestinal compromise is present. Radiologic plain film of the abdomen often will demonstrate a dilated stomach and a distended duodenum, with distal small bowel air present. These findings are in contrast to duodenal atresia, where complete absence of distal air is typical. The upper gastrointestinal series is diagnostic and demonstrates the duodenojejunal junction to the right of the midline, along with absence of the normal posterior and cephalad fixation of the duodenum at the ligment of Treitz.

Midgut volvulus is one of the most serious emergencies seen in the neonate. Approximately 90% of patients will be brought to the physician in the first year of life, with 50% in the first month of life. Bilious vomiting in the newborn, therefore, should be regarded as potentially life threatening and requires immediate evaluation to rule out this anomaly. Once the diagnosis of malrotation has been made, immediate operation is indicated. Exploratory laprotomy should be the only means used to distinguish whether volvulus is present. Patients should be expeditiously fluid resuscitated, and any electrolyte or hematologic derangements should be corrected. After a right, supraumbilical transverse incision is performed, midgut volvulus is relieved by detorsion of the bowel in a counterclockwise direction. The duodenum is mobilized, and the Ladd's bands are divided. The transverse colon and the proximal jujenum are separated so that a broadbased mesentery is formed. Subsequent adhesion formation will prevent recurrent volvulus. An appendectomy is performed to eliminate future confusion in the setting of appendicitis (because of the anticipated unusual location of the appendix). If compromised bowel is identified, resection with primary anastomosis or enterostomy formation may be performed. Necrosis of the entire midgut makes long-term survival unlikely, and excessive morbidity should be expected. Many factors must be taken into account before a decision to perform resection in this setting is made.

Mortality is minimal and is primarily associated with extensive intestinal necrosis in the setting of midgut volvulus. Recurrent volvulus or duodenal obstruction is rare. Approximately 1% to 10% of patients will develop subsequent small bowel obstruction from adhesions.

INTESTINAL ATRESIA OR STENOSIS

Occasionally, the diagnosis of jejunoileal atresia may be suspected in utero when dilated loops of bowel are observed on ultrasound done in the setting of polyhydramnios. Typically, however, a newborn with jejunoileal atresia experiences bilious vomiting, abdominal distention, and failure to pass meconium on the first day of life. Abdominal distention may vary depending on the level of obstruction and is often acquired, in contrast to the distention obvious *at birth* in patients with meconium ileus. Although atypical, passage of bile-stained meconium with or without rectal stimulation may occur in the setting of a jejunoileal atresia that has developed later in gestation. Plain abdominal radiographs often demonstrate a single large loop of dilated, air-filled bowel just proximal to the site of the atresia. The rule of thumb, the presence of thumb-sized or greater loops of dilated bowel on the newborn abdominal radiograph, indicates a complete intestinal obstruction, most often secondary to an atresia. Peritoneal calcification is noted in 12% of cases and indicates the presence of an in utero perforation with localized saponification of fat and subsequent calcification because of the presence of pancreatic enzymes in the sterile, extraluminal meconium. Contrast enema demonstrates a diminutive and unused colon unless the intrauterine vascular catastrophe resulting in the atresia occurred late in gestation. Contrast enema evaluation also eliminates the possibility of colonic atresia (and precludes the need for intraoperative colonic evaluation).

Three different types of jejunoileal atresia are observed: type I (19%) consists of an intraluminal diaphragm; type II (31%) is an atresia with a fibrous cord between the proximal and distal segments; and type III (50%) is an atresia in which a segment of the intestine and often the associated mesentery are absent. All are treated similarly. As long as malrotation with volvulus is excluded by radiologic findings, a timely, but not emergent, operation may be performed. A transverse supraumbilical incision typically reveals a massively dilated proximal bowel segment and a decompressed distal segment. The dilated proximal segment must be resected back to a reasonable caliber of bowel to prevent subsequent anastomotic dysfunction. A discrepancy in size will still be present, and, therefore, a proximal end to distal oblique anastomosis is performed. Since between 6% and 20% of newborns may have more than one atresia, the distal small bowel must be insufflated with saline or with air and examined carefully to rule out the presence of another atretic segment of bowel. Colonic atresia is rarely observed, but the treatment is similar to that of jejunoileal atresia.

Morbidity and mortality generally are limited to that imposed by associated problems, such as prematurity, congenital heart disease, or short gut syndrome. Anastomotic problems, such as leak or stricture, occur in approximately 5% of cases. Prolonged dysfunction of the proximal dilated intestine is quite common, and a number of days to weeks may be needed before enteral feeds may be established. Most infants with more than 15 cm of remaining small bowel and an intact ileocecal valve (or more than 40 cm of proximal bowel if the ileocecal valve has been resected) will survive.

MECONIUM ILEUS

Meconium ileus consists of distal obstruction of the small intestine by meconium and is present in 10% to 20% of newborns with cystic fibrosis. Abnormal, hyperviscous intestinal secretions, enhanced by impaired pancreatic enzyme secretion, result in obstruction because of the presence of thick, tenacious, tarry meconium in the midileum and pellets of gray, inspissated meconium in the distal ileum. The hallmark of the newborn with meconium ileus is *abdominal distention at birth,* with multiple doughy loops of dilated bowel noted on palpation. The heavy meconium-filled bowel may twist in 30% to 50% of patients and produce a volvulus resulting in ischemic necrosis and perforation. Complicated meconium ileus with a stricture or an atresia may result. Perforation, with intraperitoneal dissemination of sterile meconium, may lead to the formation of isolated regions of calcification (meconium peritonitis) or even the development of a large meconium-containing cyst. Meconium ileus is not usually associated with nonintestinal malformations.

Plain radiograph of the abdomen classically reveals multiple dilated loops of bowel of varying size. A ground-glass effect because of the presence of large amounts of intestinal meconium often is observed in the right lower quadrant of the abdomen. Air-fluid levels are rarely identified because the tenacious, adherent meconium within the lumen of the bowel precludes formation of an air-fluid level. In utero perforation and meconium peritonitis may be identified by the presence of intraperitoneal calcification. Contrast enema can be both diagnostic and therapeutic, demonstrating the presence of a small, unused microcolon with the presence of thick, inspissated meconium in the terminal ileum.

Nonoperative therapy with radiologic contrast enema and mechanical lavage of meconium from the distal ileum is successful in approximately 30% of cases. Repeated contrast enemas and irrigations may be necessary and may be continued as long as progress is demonstrated radiologically. Care should be taken to keep the newborn warm while in the radiology suite and to provide adequate fluid resuscitation, especially when hyperosmolar contrast agents are used. Failure to pass meconium within a few hours of the enema, progressive distention, and evidence of complicated meconium ileus are indications for operation.

Operation in the setting of meconium ileus mainly entails evacuation of the obstructing meconium from the terminal ileum. This is accomplished by irrigating the intestine through an enterotomy placed in the dilated ileum proximal to the obstruction. Meconium may be milked by external massage and by irrigation with warm saline or N-acetylcysteine into the colon. If the meconium cannot be successfully evacuated, if the bowel has been compromised, or if an atretic or stenotic segment is identified, the involved segment of ileum is resected. In general, a simple end-to-end anastomosis is preferable. If associated peritonitis, bowel compromise, or concurrent medical problems make an anastomosis risky, formation of an ileostomy with an adjacent mucous fistula may be performed, with plans for establishing bowel continuity 4 to 6 weeks later.

Recent improvements in perioperative care and management of patients with cystic fibrosis have resulted in increased survival rates in the 70% to 100% range. Postoperative care is specifically aimed at treatment of pulmonary problems. Dilute N-acetylcysteine is administered through the nasogastric tube to prevent recurrent ileal obstruction. Oral pancreatic enzyme administration is necessary with the initiation of feeding.

MECONIUM PLUG SYNDROME

Patients with the meconium plug syndrome often have abdominal distention and bilious vomiting. Enema contrast study demonstrates thick meconium plugs in the colon and/or rectum and may be therapeutic by providing mechanical evacuation of the meconium plugs. In general, meconium plug syndrome is observed in preterm neonates who are otherwise normal. However, cystic fibrosis and Hirschsprung's disease may be associated with this process and should be excluded by cystic fibrosis screening and suction rectal biopsy.

NEONATAL SMALL LEFT COLON SYNDROME

Newborns with this process have signs and symptoms consistent with intestinal obstruction. Barium enema demonstrates a small-caliber, smooth, rounded left colon with a normal large intestine proximal to the splenic flexure. This abnormality is often found in infants of diabetic mothers. Barium enema is often curative, and the caliber of the left colon normalizes over the ensuing weeks to months.

IMPERFORATE ANUS

Imperforate anus consists of an arrest of the normal descent of the rectum to the perineum. Patients are divided into those in whom the end of the rectum is above the sphincter muscles (high), partially through the sphincter mechanism (intermediate), or fully through the sphincter mechanism (low). From a clinical point of view, it is only necessary to distinguish low anomalies from intermediate/high anomalies. It is important to note that males frequently have high/intermediate lesions, whereas females have a preponderance of low malformations. A low lesion in a male may be discerned by the presence of a thin membrane covering the anus (often with visible dark meconium underneath or an anocutaneous fistula in the midline along the perineal or scrotal raphe). In the female patient, a perineal or vaginal vestibular fistula most always indicates the presence of a low lesion. Therefore, in both males and females, the absence of a fistula or anal membrane suggests the presence of an intermediate/high lesion. The majority of those patients with an intermediate/high anomaly will have an associated fistula to the genitourinary tract, a rec-

toprostatic or rectobulbar urethral fistula in the male and a rectovaginal or rectovestibular fistula in the female.

The presence of imperforate anus should be apparent at the initial newborn examination, although lesions associated with a large perineal fistula or ectopic anus can be missed easily. If a low malformation is present, passage of meconium via a sizable perineal or vestibular fistula may allow adequate decompression of the gastrointestinal tract. If not, symptoms of obstruction, with abdominal distention and bilious vomiting, may occur. Diagnostic documentation of the presence of a low lesion may be ascertained by (1) needle aspiration of the perineum, with documentation of return of meconium from the rectum within 1 to 2 cm of the perineum, or (2) ultrasound evaluation of the perineum, allowing visualization of a distal rectal pouch and documentation of the distance between the anal dimple and rectum. Radiologic evaluation in conjunction with physical examination will allow a low lesion to be discerned in most cases. However, if diagnosis of a low lesion cannot be established, the newborn should be considered to have an intermediate/high anomaly.

As many as 70% of newborns with imperforate anus will have associated additional anomalies. Specifically, those malformations that constitute the VATER or VACTERL association should be ruled out in all patients with imperforate anus.

Treatment of imperforate anus depends on the level and type of lesion identified in the diagnostic studies. If an obstructive anomaly is present, orogastric or nasogastric suction should be used, along with administration of antibiotics. Operation may await the completion of diagnostic studies. All intermediate/high lesions are managed initially with a colostomy, followed by elective performance of a distal colostogram to ascertain the specific lesion and to document the presence and location of a fistula. Corrective operation by performance of a posterior sagittal anorectoplasty is often accomplished at 8 to 12 months of life, although some surgeons are now performing definitive repair in children who are younger. This procedure involves division of the perineum from the anterior border of the external sphincter muscle to the coccyx, with division of all muscles of continence, including the levator ani, in the midline. The rectum is identified, and the rectourethral, rectovaginal, or rectovestibular fistula is divided and closed. The rectum is approximated to the anus as the levator ani and associated muscles of continence are reconstructed in the midline around the rectum.

Most low malformations may be definitively repaired in the newborn period. In both males and females, an anal membrane may be punctured and dilated. A perineal fistula is addressed by incision of the skin and rectum back to the posterior margin of the external sphincter, with suture approximation of the rectal mucosa to the skin (cutback anoplasty). In the female, mobilization of a vestibular fistula requires posterior transposition of the fistula to the proper site of the anus. This latter procedure is somewhat more complex and, therefore, is not usually performed in the immediate newborn period.

The postoperative mortality of 10% to 30% is usually the result of associated anomalies. Problems with rectal prolapse or anal stenosis may be observed in 5% to 10% of infants. All patients should undergo progressive anal dilatation beginning 3 weeks after operation and continuing through the following year. Patients should be followed carefully for evidence of genitourinary problems and should be placed on prophylactic antibiotics in the initial newborn period if an intermediate/high lesion is identified. Evaluation for sacral anomalies and evidence of a thethered spinal cord should be performed.

Newborns with low malformations have an excellent outlook, with fecal continence documented in 95% of patients. Constipation may, however, be a problem in females with low lesions and vestibular fistulas. Approximately 50% to 70% of patients with intermediate/high anomalies have good results, with only occasional soiling noted in some patients. The remaining 30% to 50% of patients have fair to poor results, with varying degrees of continence. The majority of these patients may be managed with a bowel program consisting of enemas, laxatives, or constipating agents. The functional results are mostly related to the presence of sphincter muscle hypoplasia and abnormal sacral innervation, which is observed in patients with intermediate or high anomalies.

REFERENCES

1. DelPin CA, Czyrko C, Ziegler MM, Scanlin TF, Bishop HC: Management and survival of meconium ileus: A 30 year review. Ann Surg 1992;215:179–185.
2. Ford EG, Senac MO, Srikanth MS, Weitzman JJ: Malrotation of the intestine in children. Ann Surg 1992;215:172–178.
3. Grosfeld JL, Rescorla FJ: Duodenal atresia and stenosis: Reassessment of treatment and outcome based on antenatal diagnosis, pathologic variance, and long-term follow-up. World J Surg 1993;17:301–309.
4. Manning PB, Morgan RA, Coran AG, Wesley JR, Polley TZ Jr, Behrendt DM, Kirsh MM, Sloan HE: Fifty years' experience with esophageal atresia and tracheoesophageal fistula. Ann Surg 1986;204:446–453.
5. Pena A: Atlas of Surgical Management of Anorectal Malformations. New York, Springer-Verlag, 1990.
6. Rescorla FJ, Grosfeld JL: Intestinal atresia and stenosis: Analysis of survival in 120 cases. Surgery 1985;98:668–676.

NECROTIZING ENTEROCOLITIS

ROBERT KLIEGMAN, M.D.

Necrotizing enterocolitis (NEC) is the most common neonatal gastrointestinal emergency. It occurs predominantly in premature infants in neonatal intensive care units. NEC affects between 2000 and 4000 neonates each year in the United States. The incidence of NEC and the susceptibility to NEC are inversely related to gestational age. Thus, infants weighing less than 1000 g are at greater risk of developing NEC for a longer period of time than more mature infants are. The mean birth weight of affected infants varies between 1250 and 1500 g, and 10% of affected patients weigh more than 2500 g.

NEC usually develops after the onset of enteral alimentation. The mean day of onset varies between day 12 and day 16 of life, usually after the infant has recovered from the common diseases of prematurity, such as respiratory distress syndrome (RDS) and patent ductus arteriosus (PDA), and often when the infant had been tolerating enteral feedings.

The most obvious risk factor for NEC is prematurity. Rapid feeding protocols (daily increments of greater than 20 to 30 ml/kg/d), various identified and unidentified infectious agents (NEC may be endemic or epidemic), in utero exposure to cocaine, and polycythemia have been proposed as additional risk factors. RDS, PDA, birth asphyxia, anemia, shock, and the presence of umbilical vessel catheters are not consistently reported to be risks for NEC.

DIAGNOSIS

NEC causes a broad spectrum of systemic, gastrointestinal, and radiologic manifestations described as follows in the modified Bell staging criteria (Table 1). Stage I NEC may represent subclinical or mild NEC but also may represent feeding intolerance or other more benign gastrointestinal processes. Nonetheless, the incidence of stage I NEC increases in parallel with those of more advanced stages of NEC during epidemics of this disease. Stage I is characterized by systemic signs of temperature instability, apnea and bradycardia, and mild lethargy. The gastrointestinal signs include elevated pregavage gastric residuals, mild abdominal distention, and minimal to no abdominal tenderness, emesis, and occult or gross blood in the stool. Radiologic signs may be absent or demonstrate mildly dilated loops of bowel. Stage I rarely progresses and lasts for approximately 72 hours.

TABLE 1. Modified Bell Staging Criteria for Neonatal Necrotizing Enterocolitis

	STAGE	SYSTEMIC SIGNS	INTESTINAL SIGNS	RADIOLOGIC SIGNS	TREATMENT
IA	Suspected NEC	Temperature instability, apnea, bradycardia, lethargy	Elevated pregavage residuals, mild abdominal distention, emesis, guaiac-positive stool	Normal or intestinal dilatation; mild ileus	NPO, antibiotics for 3 d pending cultures, gastric decompression
IB	Suspected NEC	Same as IA	Bright red blood from rectum	Same as IA	Same as IA
IIA	Definite NEC, mildly ill	Same as IA	Same as IA and IB plus diminished or absent bowel sounds ± abdominal tenderness	Intestinal dilatation, ileus, pneumatosis intestinalis	Same as IA plus NPO, antibiotics for 7–10 d if examination is normal in 24–48 h
IIB	Definite NEC, moderately ill	Same as IIA plus mild metabolic acidosis and mild thrombocytopenia	Same as IIA plus definite abdominal tenderness, ± abdominal cellulitis, or right lower quadrant mass, absent bowel sounds	Same as IIA ± portal vein gas, ± ascites	Same as IIA plus NPO, antibiotics for 14 d, NaHCO₃ for acidosis, volume replacement
IIIA	Advanced NEC, severely ill, bowel intact	Same as IIB plus hypotension, bradycardia, severe apnea, combined respiratory and metabolic acidosis, DIC, neutropenia, anuria	Same as IIB plus signs of generalized peritonitis, marked tenderness, distention, and abdominal wall erythema	Same as IIB, definite ascites	Same as IIB plus as much as 200 ml/kg fluids, fresh frozen plasma, inotropic agents, intubation, ventilation therapy, paracentesis; surgical intervention if patient fails to improve with medical management within 24–48 h
IIIB	Advanced NEC, severely ill, bowel perforated	Same as IIIA, sudden deterioration	Same as IIIA, sudden increased distention	Same as IIB plus pneumoperitoneum	Same as IIIA plus surgical intervention

Data from Bell MJ, Ternberg JL, Feigin RD, et al: Neonatal necrotizing enterocolitis: Therapeutic decisions based upon clinical staging. Ann Surg 1978;187:1–7, and Kliegman R, Walsh M: Neonatal necrotizing enterocolitis: Pathogenesis, classification, and spectrum of illness. Curr Prob Pediatr 1987;17:213–288.

Stage II NEC is documented and confirmed NEC. The systemic signs may be mild as in stage I (stage IIa) but may progress (stage IIb) to a mild metabolic acidosis and thrombocytopenia. Stage IIa demonstrates diminished to absent bowel sounds with or without abdominal wall tenderness and pneumatosis intestinalis on abdominal x-rays. This latter finding correlates anatomically with grape-sized, gas-filled cysts along the submucosal and subserosal areas of the small and large bowel. Stage IIb demonstrates a progression to definite abdominal tenderness, absent bowel sounds with or without abdominal wall cellulitis, a right lower quadrant mass, and portal vein gas or ascites.

Stage III NEC is a severe and particularly lethal disease characterized by unstable vital signs (hypotension, tachycardia, bradycardia, apnea, hypothermia), a metabolic acidosis, disseminated intravascular coagulation, neutropenia, and multiple organ system dysfunction. Sudden deterioration may herald the onset of gastrointestinal perforation, which is confirmed by the presence of pneumoperitoneum on abdominal x-ray. Peritonitis is suggested by the presence of marked abdominal distention and abdominal wall erythema and extreme abdominal wall tenderness.

Overall, the most common gastrointestinal manifestations of NEC, in order of frequency, include abdominal distention, abdominal tenderness, occult or gross blood in stools, and larger than normal gastric residuals. Pneumatosis intestinalis is the most common diagnostic x-ray finding, followed by a fixed sentinel loop of bowel, portal venous gas, ascites, and pneumoperitoneum.

DIFFERENTIAL DIAGNOSIS

Initially, it may be difficult to distinguish NEC from sepsis. Because the initial evaluation (blood, urine, and CSF culture, CBC, x-rays) and initial management (Table 2) are similar, this may not be important. Nonetheless, with time, the gastrointestinal manifestations of NEC will dominate the clinical picture.

Pneumatosis intestinalis is rarely associated with other gastrointestinal diseases in the neonatal period. Pneumatosis intestinalis has been associated with acute and chronic infectious diarrhea, predominantly in malnourished term infants in developing countries.

Malrotation with midgut volvulus rarely may produce pneumatosis intestinalis (1% to 2%). Volvulus is an acute surgical emergency, whereas only 20% to 25% of patients with NEC require immediate or any surgical intervention. Volvulus may be distinguished from NEC by being more common in term infants, occurring later in life, and having associated anomalies, marked bilious emesis, and marked proximal duodenal obstruction on x-ray. If there is any question of the presence of volvulus, a water-soluble contrast, upper gastrointestinal x-ray series with small bowel follow-through should be performed to exclude an abnormal rotation of the duodenum.

NEC is the most common cause of pneumoperitoneum in the premature infant. NEC must be distinguished from a pneumoperitoneum secondary to gas that dissects to the abdominal cavity following pulmonary interstitial emphysema, a pneumothorax, or pneumomediastinum. The last is seen predominantly in patients receiving aggressive mechanical ventilation. If there is any uncertainty, paracentesis and/or an upper gastrointestinal contrast study should be performed to exclude the possibility of an intestinal perforation.

Pneumoperitoneum may result from intestinal perforation associated with dexamethasone or indomethacin therapy. The latter drug-induced gastrointestinal perforation has been characterized as focal and thus causes fewer of the more severe manifestations of NEC. Nonetheless, surgery is indicated for repair of these perforations.

PATHOPHYSIOLOGY

The pathogenesis of NEC is unknown. Although a hypothetical interrelationship among the intestinal bacterial flora, possible gastrointestinal pathogens, intestinal ischemia, neonatal feeding practices, and immature gastrointestinal host defense mechanisms has been proposed, the precise role of each of these factors and their relative importance in initiating or propagating the disease has yet to be determined.

The pathophysiology of NEC is similar to that of the systemic inflammatory response syndrome (SIRS) in adults. SIRS is defined by having two or more signs of a systemic reaction to endothelial cell inflammation (hyper-hypothermia, tachycardia, tachypnea-hyperventilation, leukocytosis-neutropenia) in the setting of a known cause of endothelial cell inflammation (infection, pancreatitis, ischemia, trauma, hemorrhagic shock, immune-mediated tissue injury, or exogenous administration of interleukins). Severe SIRS is associated with multiorgan system dysfunction (renal—ATN, hepatic—jaundice, hematologic—DIC, CNS—coma, cardiac—shock, pulmonary—ARDS), which includes hypoperfusion (lactic acidosis, oliguria, reduced mental status) and inflammation-induced hypotension. SIRS is due, in part, to the activation of endogenous mediators of inflammation, such as cytokines (tumor necrosis factor [TNF], platelet-activating factor [PAF], interleukin 1 and 2 [IL-1 IL-2]), leukotrienes, prostaglandins, complement, and various kinins. Such agents produce profound hypotension, capillary leak syndrome, neutropenia,

TABLE 2. Approach to Management of Patients with Necrotizing Enterocolitis

ABNORMALITY	INTERVENTIONS	GOALS
Presumed infection	Broad-spectrum antibiotics	Eradicate infection
Peritonitis/intestinal perforation	Antibiotics plus surgery (paracentesis with drain placement)	Eradicate nidus of infection; remove necrotic bowel, ascites
Intestinal distention/ileus	NPO; nasogastric tube drainage	Decrease intestinal gas production; remove intestinal secretions; decompress abdomen
Hypotension	Volume expansion, vasopressor agents	Restore gestational and postnatal age-appropriate blood pressure
Hypoperfusion/oxygen delivery	Volume expansion, vasopressor and inotropic agents; mechanical ventilation, oxygen, packed red blood cell transfusions	Hemoglobin 12–14 g/dl Oxygen saturation >95% Normal blood lactate level (pH) Above normal cardiac index
Organ system dysfunction	Volume expansion, vasopressor and inotropic agents; mechanical ventilation, oxygen; packed red blood cell, platelet, fresh frozen plasma transfusion; diuretics	Normalize or reverse abnormalities: *Renal:* urine output, BUN, creatinine *Hepatic:* bilirubin, coagulopathy, albumin *Pulmonary:* alveolar-arterial gradient, hypercapnia *Cardiac:* blood pressure, cardiac index *CNS:* level of consciousness *Hematologic:* correct anemia, DIC (if active bleeding)
Poor nutritional intake	Parenteral alimentation (central or peripheral)	Reverse catabolism; improve nitrogen balance and healing; prevent hypoglycemia

thrombocytopenia, intestinal hemorrhage, shock, myocardial depression, and tissue necrosis. In both animal models and human cases of NEC, TNF and PAF have been implicated in the pathophysiology of the disease. A rational management plan of therapy would be based on reversing and correcting the multiorgan system dysfunction associated with the SIRS that accompanies severe NEC (Table 2).

In addition to the presence of the SIRS, the mechanical problems of marked intraabdominal pressure (ileus, distention, ascites) contribute to complicating features of NEC. Distention can produce additional bowel injury, reduce renal blood flow, and interfere with diaphragm function, thus producing a respiratory acidosis with or without apnea.

TREATMENT

Medical Management

Most patients with NEC can be managed with a combination of broad-spectrum intravenous antibiotics, gastrointestinal decompression with a nasogastric tube, and good supportive care to reverse the multiorgan system dysfunction that accompanies the SIRS. The amount, duration, and complexity of therapies increase as the stage of NEC progresses from stage I to stage III.

Patients with stage I NEC must be placed NPO, undergo nasogastric tube (Replogle-type) intestinal decompression, and receive broad-spectrum intravenous antibiotics. This antimicrobial therapy is empiric as there are few randomized controlled trials comparing different antibiotic regimens. Current recommendations include a combination of an extended-spectrum penicillin (ampicillin, ticarcillin, carbencillin) and an aminoglycoside (gentamicin, kanamycin, amikacin) or a combination of vancomycin and cefotaxime. The latter combination produced a greater suppression of the gastrointestinal flora, a lower incidence of thrombocytopenia, and an improved survival in infants less than 2200 g in one report (uncontrolled, nonrandomized) when compared with ampicillin and gentamicin. If the patient has stage II or III NEC, some authors add a third antibiotic (clindamycin or metronidazole) for greater coverage of anaerobes. The traditional triple-drug regimen is ampicillin, gentamicin, and clindamycin, which is effective against most gram-negative bacteria found in the intestine, in addition to enterococci and the enteric anaerobic bacteria.

Patients with stage I NEC usually receive antibiotics and remain NPO for 72 hours unless blood, urine, or CSF cultures are positive or the patient develops pneumatosis intestinalis.

Patients with stage II NEC are initially treated as are those with stage I disease. If they have stable vital signs, rapid improvement in gastrointestinal manifestations with normal bowel sounds and resolution of ileus, they may be treated (NPO, decompression, antibiotics) for 7 to 10 days. If they have unstable vital signs, acidosis, or signs of peritonitis, they are acutely treated as for stage III and are treated for a minimum of 14 days.

Patients with stage III NEC are critically ill and have the highest mortality, morbidity, and risk of gastrointestinal perforation, or development of NEC totalis, which is the most severe and lethal form of NEC, characterized by irreversible intestinal necrosis from the duodenum to the rectum. Patients with stage III NEC require the same antibiotic therapy as discussed previously, as well as nasogastric tube intestinal decompression while being NPO. Frequent (q6h) abdominal x-rays (left lateral decubitus or cross-table laterals) are taken to detect pneumoperitoneum, which indicates intestinal perforation. In addition, serial blood gases, coagulation profiles, electrolytes with BUN and creatinine, and aminoglycoside or vancomycin levels must be determined to optimize care, detect early deterioration, and avoid toxicity. The critical aspects of managing NEC-associated SIRS are to avoid or reverse organ system dysfunction and to prevent permanent sequelae. This predominantly involves close monitoring of cardiac, pulmonary, and hematologic function to avoid deficits in oxygen delivery to vital organs, as well as the intestine, which needs adequate blood flow to potentially reverse NEC and to eventually heal (Table

2). Poor perfusion should be managed with a combination of volume resuscitation and inotropic vasopressor agents. Volume replacement includes the use of crystalloid (normal saline) or colloid (albumin, hetastarch, or dextrans). Fresh frozen plasma should not be used for volume replacement alone. If DIC is documented and bleeding is evident, fresh frozen plasma and platelet transfusions can improve volume status and simultaneously treat the coagulopathy. Platelet transfusions are not indicated for isolated thrombocytopenia in the absence of bleeding. In acutely ill hypotensive patients, volume resuscitation may require large amounts of fluids (in excess of 40 ml/kg in the first hour or 100 ml/kg in the first 6 to 12 hours of therapy). All patients with NEC and SIRS will develop peripheral edema, which has little prognostic significance or obvious morbidity. Nonetheless, volume status must be monitored carefully, preferably with CVP monitoring or by clinical assessment to avoid opening a PDA or producing iatrogenic pulmonary edema. Strict attention to blood pressure, urine output, and cutaneous perfusion must be balanced by the possible complicating development of rales, hypercarbia, and hypoxia. However, the latter two blood gas abnormalities may develop independently of the patient's volume status, thus heralding the presence of ARDS, which is the pulmonary complication of SIRS and is due to nonhydrostatic leaky capillary-induced pulmonary edema.

Any patients with significant cardiovascular instability, plus those who demonstrate any apnea, new-onset hypercapnia (Pco_2 >50), or hypoxia, require endotracheal intubation and mechanical ventilation to reverse hypoventilation (CNS depression, poor diaphragmatic contraction) and hypoxia (ARDS, hydrostatic pulmonary edema). Positive end-expiratory pressure is also a beneficial treatment for both these causes of hypoxia.

If significant hypotension or poor perfusion persists despite aggressive fluid management, vasopressor inotropic agents must be added to reverse the myocardial depression associated with SIRS. Echocardiograms may demonstrate a normal cardiac index but a greatly reduced ejection (shortening) fraction and increased left ventricular end-diastolic volume. Dopamine or dobutamine is started alone or in combination at a dose of 5 μg/kg/min and titrated to 20 to 30 μg/kg/min as needed. Epinephrine is rarely needed.

Additional interventions and their goals are noted in Table 2. Total duration of therapy for patients with stage III NEC who respond to medical management ranges from 14 to 21 days and is dependent on the return of normal bowel function, defecation, bowel sounds, and a nondistended, nontender abdomen.

Surgical Management

Because NEC may require a surgical procedure, all suspected cases must have an early surgical consultation. Pneumoperitoneum is an absolute indication for a surgical procedure. Relative and harder to define indications for a surgical procedure include failure to respond to medical management (usually 24 to 48 hours of such treatment) and a persistent fixed sentinel loop of bowel noted on serial abdominal x-rays. Another indication is the presence of free flowing, brown-colored, cloudy fluid with multiple species of microorganisms and neutrophils present in the gram stain of paracentesis fluid of a patient when there is a high index of suspicion for bowel perforation but no evidence of pneumoperitoneum on abdominal x-rays. The paracentesis is performed with an 18- or 20-gauge angiocath, with side holes cut out along the distal length of the catheter. The catheter is placed in the left lower quadrant along the anterior to midaxillary line or in the midline below the umbilicus. Additionally suggested but not universally accepted indications for a surgical procedure include portal venous gas, a right lower quadrant mass, and anterior abdominal wall erythema.

Surgical procedures usually depend on the severity and extent of necrosis of the involved bowel and the clinical condition of the patient. Most patients requiring surgery for acute NEC undergo exploratory laparotomy through an upper abdominal transverse incision. The surgeon must avoid excessive resection of marginally involved tissue and must only resect bowel that demonstrate total necrosis. Excessive resection of potentially viable bowel may produce significant morbidity with the short bowel syndrome (10% to 15% of surgical cases). If the surgeon is unsure of the distinction between areas with total gangrene and marginal perfusion or if there is NEC totalis (10% to 15% of surgical cases), a second-look operation within 24 to 48 hours may help to identify the true extent of necrosis.

Most surgeons perform enterostomies after resection of the necrotic bowel. The conjoined Mikulicz, or a side-to-side enterostomy, provides ample stoma visualization and function and facilitates early (at 2500 g) reanastomosis of the bowel. A primary anastomosis at the time of the initial surgery is indicated in patients with limited localized disease who have no distal bowel involvement and in patients who have demonstrated a walled-off perforation who are no longer manifesting the SIRS.

An alternate approach to exploratory laparotomy, bowel resection, and enterostomy formation is the use of paracenteses and peritoneal drainage (with or without lavage) performed under local anesthesia, followed by an exploratory laparotomy within 24 to 48 hours if the patient does not improve. A one-quarter-inch Penrose drain is placed in the right lower quadrant and permitted to drain peritoneal contents and decompress the abdomen. This procedure has been employed predominantly in infants less than 1000 g who have severe SIRS and are viewed as too unstable to be transported or to undergo exploratory laparotomy. In experienced hands, one third of patients require only drain placement, whereas the others require acute exploratory laparotomy for ongoing SIRS or delayed laparotomy for the resection of a stricture, which occurs in 10% to 30% of patients recovering from NEC.

Solitary or multiple strictures usually occur 2 to 8 weeks after recovery from the acute NEC episode and manifest signs of intestinal obstruction (emesis, distention, obstipation), persistent or recurrent rectal bleeding, perforation, or sepsis. All patients treated surgically for NEC must have a contrast x-ray study to determine the presence of distal strictures before reanastomosis. Medically managed patients are not consistently screened for strictures with a barium enema. When symptoms herald the onset of obstruction, a barium enema is performed.

Therapy of obstructing strictures traditionally is performed by resection and a primary anastomosis. Partially obstructing strictures also may be managed by stricturoplasty.

PROGNOSIS

The overall mortality of NEC is 10% to 30%. Long-term prognosis is excellent for stages I and II NEC. The highest risk for mortality is among the most immature infants who require surgery for intestinal perforation. The mortality may be as high as 30% to 50%.

Patients with surgical resection may develop failure to thrive secondary to a functional short bowel syndrome. True short bowel syndrome is associated with significant mortality and morbidity because of sepsis, cirrhosis, and complications of central venous hyperalimentation. The prognosis for short bowel syndrome is best for patients who retain their ileocecal valve and who have an intestinal length of greater than 10 cm. Without an ileocecal valve, bowel length greater than 25 cm usually predicts the eventual ability to receive all nutrients by the gastrointestinal tract. However, central venous alimentation may be required for 6 to 18 months while intestinal adaptation permits increasing volumes of oral nutrients.

REFERENCES

1. Ein SH, Shandling B, Wesson D, et al: A 13-year experience with peritoneal drainage under local anesthesia for necrotizing enterocolitis perforation. J Pediatr Surg 1990;25:1034–1037.
2. Kleinhaus S, Weinberg G, Gregor MB: Necrotizing enterocolitis in infancy. Surg Clin North Am 1992;72:261–276.
3. Kliegman RM, Walsh MC: Neonatal necrotizing enterocolitis: Pathogenesis, classification, and spectrum of illness. Curr Probl Pediatr 1987;17:219–288.
4. Parrillo JE: Pathogenetic mechanisms of septic shock. N Engl J Med 1993; 328:1471–1477.

PYLORIC STENOSIS

STEPHEN E. DOLGIN, M.D.

PREOPERATIVE MANAGEMENT

The management of a baby with pyloric stenosis begins with correction of the accompanying fluid, electrolyte, and metabolic derangement. This takes precedence even over establishing the diagnosis. No matter what the cause of the vomiting, a dehydrated neonate or young infant requires intravenous resuscitation. The operative correction of pyloric stenosis cannot be executed safely until there is evidence of normal fluid and electrolyte balance.

When an "olive" (a term less upsetting than "tumor" when overheard by parents at the crib) is palpated, usually in the right upper quadrant, by the responsible surgeon, the diagnosis is confirmed. If imaging is required, sonography is replacing the barium swallow as the first-line diagnostic study.

When the diagnosis is suspected, the baby should not be allowed anything by mouth. A clear and logical approach to managing the electrolyte and fluid depletion is mandatory. Often, these patients have been weighed frequently before admission to the hospital so the deficit can readily be quantified if a documented weight loss is consistent with the degree of clinical dehydration. It should be remembered that a deficit less than 5% of body water is not clinically evident but should still be corrected before administering the anesthetic.

I estimate the fluid deficit by taking into account a combination of the weight loss and the clinical signs and begin replacing with intravenous bolus therapy with normal saline. Once the baby urinates, the rest of the deficit is replaced over 24 to 48 hours depending on the degree of dehydration. A wide-bore (10 or 12 F) orogastric tube should be placed to keep the stomach empty. Any measured gastric drainage must be replaced (ongoing loss). A solution of D 5½ NS plus 10 to 20 mg KCl/L can be used to replace the ongoing gastric losses as well as the rest of the deficit after initial bolus therapy in a baby with mild to moderate dehydration. This replacement solution can be run as a piggyback into an IV providing maintenance fluid. In an infant with severe dehydration, urine output must be established before KCl administration.

WHEN TO DELAY THE OPERATION

Patients with long-term partial gastric outlet obstruction can have the most severe derangements, especially when parents have maintained the babies with water, apple juice, or other hypotonic fluids. Although the fluid deficit may not be severe in such cases, the electrolyte, pH, and nutritional status may be markedly deranged, in which case several days may be needed for correction before pyloromyotomy.

A mild intercurrent upper respiratory infection need not delay operation. However, pneumonia (which may have developed from aspiration) is best treated and the baby rendered asymptomatic before administration of the anesthetic.

Marked jaundice because of unconjugated hyperbilirubinemia has a well-known association with pyloric stenosis. It will resolve quite quickly after pyloromyotomy and does not warrant delay for extensive investigations provided the bilirubin is largely unconjugated. Coffee ground (bloody) gastric drainage or vomiting is common as a result of gastritis or esophagitis and also will resolve postoperatively.

ANESTHESIA FOR PYLOROMYOTOMY

Pyloromyotomy is usually performed under general anesthesia. Inhalation induction, as is commonplace for elective inguinal hernia repair, is contraindicated. Because of gastric outlet obstruction, a rapid sequence induction or awake intubation is required. The safety of this undertaking is only assured with a properly trained anesthesiologist comfortable with the anesthetic management of small infants.

THE OPERATION

The pyloromyotomy itself has not changed much since originally described in 1912. The operation takes little time, requires only a small incision, involves no gastric suturing, and is highly effective. The hypertrophied muscularis is split longitudinally, which relieves the stenosis. Since wound infections with *Staphylococcus aureus* are reported in about 10% of cases, a dose of antistaphylococcal intravenous antibiotics just before the skin incision is warranted.

POSTOPERATIVE MANAGEMENT

Dilute feeds in small volumes are begun the morning after the operation and gradually advanced in amount and concentration. Discharge is usually accomplished on the second or third postoperative day. Vomiting is not uncommon in the immediate postoperative period and ordinarily resolves after a little gastric rest. It is wise to have warned the parents preoperatively about such vomiting so they are not needlessly worried if this happens. Rarely, surgeons have had to reoperate for an incomplete pyloromyotomy. The condition does not recur, however. The laparoscopic approach is not an improvement.

PYLOROSPASM

Pylorospasm is defined clinically. In pylorospasm, the pylorus seems to close more intensely than usual, suggesting a functional abnormality in gastric motility and emptying. This diagnosis is suspected in those infants under 3 months of age with recurrent vomiting but without pyloric stenosis. Generally, such infants do not have marked caloric and nutritional impairment and grow well. Treatment is with small frequent feedings, and, additionally, antispasmodic therapy has been tried. Some children with pylorospasm have underlying peptic ulcer disease. Milk protein allergy may also contribute to pylorospasm.

If a newborn or young infant appears clinically to have pyloric stenosis, which is not confirmed by sonogram, a barium swallow may be helpful. The radiologist must watch esophageal function, look for gastroesophageal reflux, and observe gastric emptying. Pylorospasm can be diagnosed by the barium swallow but is not a common finding.

REFERENCE

1. Garcia VF, Randolph JG: Pyloric stenosis: Diagnosis and management. Pediatr Rev 1990;11:292–295.

DISEASES AND INJURIES OF THE ORAL REGION

JEFFREY I. RESNICK, M.D.
HARVEY A. ZAREM, M.D.

CLEFT LIP AND PALATE

The spectrum of facial deformity in congenital clefts runs from the minimal microform cleft lip to the severe complete bilateral cleft lip and palate. Classification of these deformities takes into account the variable involvement of the lip and palate and whether unilateral or bilateral clefting is present.

The parents of a child born with a cleft lip and palate need a great deal of information that addresses both the immediate treatment and long-term expectations. Over the past two decades, multidisciplinary cleft palate teams have emerged in most major medical centers as a resource for treating the complex problems associated with cleft lip and palate. These teams include pediatricians, plastic surgeons, otolaryngologists, medical geneticists, speech and hearing therapists, dentists and orthodontists, and social workers. Although the primary pediatrician will assume care of the child with cleft lip and palate,

the cleft palate team will provide guidance in ensuring that the proper interventions are carried out in a timely fashion. Whether or not a cleft palate team is available, the primary pediatrician needs to coordinate the care of the child with a cleft.

In the newborn period, the evaluation of infant feeding, and the search for other congenital anomalies take precedence. Associated defects are noted in approximately 15% of involved infants. Feeding problems are associated with clefts of the palate, since many infants are unable to generate an adequate suck. The infant should not be discharged from the hospital until it is clear that he or she is feeding well. In the presence of a cleft palate, adequate feeding can be ensured with the use of a cross-cut nipple or a long, soft lamb's nipple, each of which empties by gravity. Breast feeding, although not impossible, requires extraordinary effort by the mother to express milk in the absence of an adequate suck. By ensuring that the mother is feeding the infant well before hospital discharge, problems with failure to thrive should be minimized. However, close follow-up is necessary to ensure that weight gain is normal.

Timing of surgical repair of a cleft lip is somewhat variable, with lip repairs being done anywhere from the newborn period to 3 to 6 months of age. Most surgeons recommend repair of cleft lips at approximately 3 months of age, when the infant tolerates general anesthesia well and when the anatomic landmarks are better defined. The infant should be thriving, and a general guideline is the "rule of 10": weight over 10 pounds, hemoglobin over 10 g, age over 10 weeks. When a wide unilateral cleft lip is present, a preliminary lip adhesion procedure can be done at 4 to 6 weeks of age to align the lip segments better before definitive lip repair. However, this preliminary step is optional and is considered to be unnecessary by many surgeons.

Repair of cleft palate is necessary for proper development of speech. Speech pathologists would like to see restoration of normal anatomy as early as possible to maximize the chances for normal speech. *Most teams are now recommending repair of cleft palates at 1 year of age or earlier, assuming that no upper airway problems are present.* There are some theoretic concerns that early palate repair can lead to diminished growth potential for the maxilla, but the goal of normal speech outweighs these concerns.

Children with a cleft of the palate show an extremely high incidence of chronic otitis media. Many otologists have recommended that children with cleft palate undergo routine myringotomy with insertion of tubes to reduce the incidence of chronic otitis media with subsequent hearing loss. This is usually done at the same time as cleft palate repair when indicated. In any infant with cleft palate and a chronic middle ear effusion, ventilation tubes should be inserted. The family must be alerted to the incidence of otitis media to facilitate early diagnosis and treatment in order to minimize the chances of long-term scarring and hearing loss.

Parents of a child with cleft lip and palate will benefit from genetic counseling. Although most cases of cleft lip and palate are sporadic in nature, many syndromes and inheritance patterns may be present. A medical geneticist can best address the possible risks for future offspring, as well as deal with the possible guilt associated with the affected child.

By the age of 1 year, most children with clefts will have undergone repair of the lip and palate. Close attention must then be paid to speech development. Any speech delay must be investigated, with both receptive (hearing) and expressive components examined. An anatomic basis for poor speech can be present, with the most common problem being inadequate closure of the soft palate to the posterior and lateral pharyngeal walls. If this velopharyngeal incompetence is present, secondary surgery in the form of a pharyngoplasty or pharyngeal flap will be required if speech therapy does not correct the problem.

Residual palatal fistulas with communication between the oral and nasal cavities can result in problems. Large fistulas can cause escape of fluid or food particles through the nose and can, less frequently, affect speech. Small fistulas are rarely symptomatic. Closure of oral–nasal fistulas often can be combined with other revisional procedures in the child with a cleft.

Routine tonsillectomy and adenoidectomy should not be performed in the child who has undergone cleft palate repair. Frequently, the hypertrophic adenoids and tonsils aid in the occlusion of the velopharynx, improving speech quality by minimizing velopharyngeal incompetence. In some cases, a submucous cleft palate may become symptomatic after tonsillectomy and adenoidectomy. A submucous cleft may be recognized by a bifid uvula, the presence of a thin blue midline in the soft palate, and a notch in the posterior border of the hard palate in the midline. Before tonsillectomy and adenoidectomy are recommended, adequate soft palate length and function must be ascertained.

The child born with a unilateral or bilateral cleft lip and palate may expect a normal life pattern in view of the high quality of surgical, orthodontic, otologic, and speech therapy that has evolved. However, a significant number of developmental deformities will produce problems even with excellent surgical and dental care. Soft tissue problems, such as lip scars and soft tissue deficiency, will need to be addressed as the child grows. Bone grafting of alveolar clefts should proceed during the stage of mixed dentition to stabilize the maxilla. Orthognathic surgery may be required to optimize the dental occlusion in maxillary hypoplasia. One of the most difficult problems is correction of the associated nasal deformity that accompanies both unilateral and, especially, bilateral clefts. Multiple surgical procedures and orthodontics can be expected to achieve a satisfactory functional and aesthetic result into adolescence. Timing of these procedures will depend on the specific stage of development of the child, as well as on the specific symptoms that arise.

RARE CRANIOFACIAL CLEFTS

As in the more common cleft lip and palate, rare craniofacial clefts may be quite subtle or may cause severe and often grotesque facial anomalies. Involvement of the perioral region is often in the form of macrostomia or the presence of confluence of the oral cavity with the nasal cavity, maxillary sinus, or orbital region. Classification and treatment of these rare anomalies are beyond the scope of this text, but referral to a regional craniofacial team is indicated to optimize the complex care required.

MACROGLOSSIA

Macroglossia, or tongue enlargement, may be symmetric or asymmetric, with a unilateral form being the most common type. Primary macroglossia may be related to hyperthyroidism, glycogen storage disease, cretinism, or amyloidosis. A rare congenital cause is Beckwith-Wiedemann syndrome, associated with abdominal wall defects and hypoglycemia. Secondary causes include lymphangioma, hemangioma, neurofibroma, cystic lesions, and solid tumors. In the infant, the primary concern with macroglossia is the potential for mechanical airway obstruction. In the young child with significant macroglossia, an open bite and drooling are strong indications for partial tongue excision.

PIERRE ROBIN SEQUENCE

The primary problem in children with the Robin sequence is *retrognathia,* an underdeveloped mandible that is posteriorly displaced. This leads to glossoptosis, or inferior displacement of the tongue. Cleft palate is present in about half of the affected children. Children with Robin sequence often have respiratory and feeding difficulties, manifested shortly after birth or as late as 1 to 2 months of age. Prone positioning of the infant usually improves both breathing and feeding. Frequent aspiration can accompany the Robin sequence. When the child is supine, upper airway obstruction from the tongue can cause asphyxiation. When the deformity is severe or when conservative

positioning maneuvers fail, an operative procedure to secure the tongue forward (a tongue-lip adhesion) can be lifesaving. This adhesion is temporary and may be reversed after the neonatal period, when the danger of respiratory obstruction has passed.

Many children with Robin sequence ultimately attain normal dental occlusal relationships, but close follow-up of mandibular growth is indicated. Cleft palate repair is usually delayed to about 18 months of age to allow for development of the upper airway.

TONGUE-TIE

Infants born with a short frenulum extending from the tongue to the central incisor area of the mandible are generally asymptomatic. If there are suspicions that a tongue-tie is leading to speech difficulties, evaluation by an experienced speech pathologist is warranted. Surgical release of the tongue with lengthening of the frenulum is a simple operative procedure that is effective in the rare symptomatic patient.

MACROSTOMIA

The diagnosis of macrostomia, or greatly exaggerated mouth width, is occasionally missed because it is associated with underdevelopment of the mandible. The distance between the midline of the upper or lower lip and the oral commissure is greater on the affected side than on the normal side (except in rare bilateral cases). Macrostomia is commonly associated with the first and second branchial arch syndrome (hemifacial microsomia), with variable hypoplasia of the entire half of the face, including the ear, temporal muscle, masseter muscle, parotid gland, zygoma, maxilla, and mandible. The macrostomia can be surgically corrected by Z-plasty. The management of the jaw and other related deformities is complex and best treated in a craniofacial center.

JAW DEFORMITIES

Micrognathia and Macrognathia

Micrognathia, or small jaw, may occur separately or in association with syndromes, such as Pierre Robin sequence, Treacher-Collins syndrome, or hemifacial microsomia. Macrognathia, an enlargement of the mandible or mandibular prognathism, is characterized by an obtuse angle between the ramus of the mandible and the body of the mandible, often with an open bite deformity. A significant number of small and large mandibles occur as hereditary features and not necessarily as part of a specific syndrome. Unless jaw developmental deformities are extreme, they are usually not apparent until the child is 5 to 6 years of age. The child should be evaluated by an experienced orthodontist, who is most capable of assessing dental and jaw development.

Treatment of the majority of children who require operative correction is deferred to the late teens, after full dental eruption. Severe facial deformities due to extreme jaw abnormalities are treated earlier, with treatment influenced by the dentition.

Bony Overgrowth of Jaws

A number of disorders with overgrowth of either the maxilla or mandible are not common but present a problem of diagnosis and treatment.

Arteriovenous Malformation

Overgrowth of the jaw may be the result of arteriovenous malformation, which is usually apparent by the increased prominence of the vessels, by a bruit in the external carotid and its branches to the involved area, and by increased warmth of the soft tissues. The management of an arteriovenous malformation involving the maxilla or mandible is difficult. The disease is invariably progressive and may be punctuated by bleeding episodes that require blood transfusions. Frequently, it is necessary to ligate the external carotid artery to control the bleeding, but the ultimate treatment is radical excision of the involved parts. This decision is difficult because the surgery and resulting deformities can be extensive. However, once the diagnosis is established and the progressive risk of serious hemorrhage has been clarified, definitive treatment should be instituted.

Neurofibromatosis

The face may be involved in patients with neurofibromatosis, either local or diffuse (as in *von Recklinghausen's disease*). Overgrowth of the soft tissues and bones on the involved side of the face may be a consequence. There is increased bulk of the maxilla or mandible, with gingival hypertrophy and displacement of the teeth. Management centers on the excision of offending tissues and sculpturing tissues to correct the deformity. To "cure" the disease with radical resection would entail an extensive operative procedure with removal of many normal structures and is never advisable. The course of this disease depends on the progression and age of onset of symptoms. The earlier the age of onset and the more rapid the course in youth, the worse the prognosis. Hemifacial hypertrophy, with enlargement of all the facial structures unilaterally (including jaws and teeth) presents a similar picture but lacks the soft tissue neurofibromas.

Fibrous Dysplasia

Fibrous dysplasia of the jaws is an unusual condition involving the mandible or maxilla, which is enlarged because of the fibrous and noncalcified tissue within the bone. Fibrous dysplasia is usually not evident until late childhood and is usually self-limited as the child passes puberty and growth ceases. This disorder must be recognized to avoid a radical excision of tissues. Conservative contouring of bone to reduce the deformity can be done to tide the child over until skeletal maturation occurs. In many instances, bony deformities will recur, requiring further operative intervention.

Infantile Cortical Hyperostosis

Infantile cortical hyperostosis (*Caffey's disease)* is a self-limiting disease of children seen with the onset of fever, soft tissue swelling, and periosteal new bone formation of the mandible. It occurs most commonly in the neonatal period (2 to 4 months of age) and may be mistaken for osteomyelitis of the mandible. The clavicles are often involved with overlying brawny induration of the soft tissues. The radiographic picture is one of increased density on the surface of the bone as a result of new bone formation.

In mild cases, no treatment is necessary except comfort measures. With severe involvement, treatment with corticosteroids is indicated. It is recommended that the steroids be continued over several months because exacerbations have occurred with early withdrawal of steroids.

Tumors

Tumors of the facial skeleton include benign and malignant odontogenic tumors (arising from primitive tooth elements) and osteogenic tumors. These tumors are uncommon in children. Treatment depends on the specific histologic diagnosis, with radical resections reserved for the malignant lesions.

TRAUMA

Most injuries about the oral region are minor, and hospitalization is not required. For the occasional severe injury, the most immediate concerns are control of the airway, ventilation, and control of major hemorrhage. Airway obstruction may be caused by the tongue, laryngeal edema, or foreign material, including blood, vomitus, or teeth. Airway control may require tracheal intubation or emergency cricothyroidotomy. Most bleeding can be stopped by direct pressure. An adequate airway must be ensured, and a detailed search for other injuries, such as skull facture, closed head injury, and cervical spine injury, must be undertaken. Evaluation of the thoracic cavity, abdomen, and extremities is mandatory before treatment of facial injuries is instituted.

Fractures

Fractures of the facial skeleton should be suspected in the presence of obvious deformity, asymmetry, bony instability or stepoffs, tenderness or crepitance with palpation, dental malocclusion, intraoral lacerations, or visual disturbances. Definitive diagnosis of facial fractures in children will require x-ray evaluation. Plain radiographs, accompanied by panoramic films in selected cases, are most appropriate for the evaluation of the lower facial skeleton. A computed tomographic (CT) scan is essential for the detailed identification of fractures involving the midface and upper facial skeleton.

Fractures of the mandible in children are less common than in adults. Treatment of mandibular fractures in children depends on the site of the fracture, as well as the state of the dentition, whether primary or mixed. Mandibular growth must be closely observed after a fracture, especially one involving the condylar and subcondylar regions.

Dental Injuries

Trauma to the teeth may involve the tooth itself, as well as surrounding periodontal structures. Injuries to teeth can result in fractures of the enamel and dentin, with or without exposure of the underlying tooth pulp. If only the dental crown is fractured, restoration is straightforward. For root involvement or pulp exposure in the primary dentition, tooth extraction is the best course. In the permanent dentition, root involvement or pulp exposure will require restoration with probable endodontic (root canal) treatment.

Periodontal injuries are manifested by loosened or avulsed teeth. Mobility may be horizontal or vertical, and the tooth may be malpositioned. Loosened permanent teeth need to be immobilized as soon as possible to minimize the chance of tooth loss. Avulsed teeth may be replanted, but unless replantation occurs soon after injury, success is unlikely. After gentle rinsing, the avulsed tooth should be loosely placed back in its socket while enroute to the dentist.

Lacerations

Most lacerations around the mouth and face can be repaired using local anesthesia, often with the addition of mild sedation. Anesthesia in the face is accomplished by direct infiltration of lidocaine (Xylocaine) 1% with 1:100,000 epinephrine or by regional nerve blocks. The entire upper lip can be anesthetized by injecting the infraorbital nerve bilaterally, and the entire lower lip can be anesthetized with bilateral mental nerve blocks. These simple nerve blocks are effective, and the child is usually cooperative once the area is anesthetized.

With the use of antibiotics, it is appropriate to close all facial wounds that are not overly contaminated, despite the fact that many hours have elapsed from the time of injury to the time of treatment. In animal bites or severe contamination, the use of tetanus toxoid, antibiotics, and judicious initial closure or delayed primary closure (within several days of injury) is indicated. An oral first-generation cephalosporin should be used in most instances. In selected cases, intramuscular or intravenous cephalosporins should be considered. It is rarely advisable to allow a wound of the face or oral region to heal secondarily because of the resulting scar deformity. If a wound is closed with the degree of contamination underestimated, close follow-up will allow for drainage of any resulting infection and prevent a serious consequence.

A large number of wounds seen in children in the emergency room are puncture wounds of the lower lip from the incisors. This through-and-through wound lacerates the mucosa, lower lip musculature, and skin. It is best cleansed with saline irrigation after local anesthesia and closed primarily. A two- or three-layer closure may be necessary, depending on the size of the wound.

Sutures on the face should be placed close to the edge of the wound and not tied overly tight to avoid suture marks. They should be removed approximately 4 to 5 days following the injury. The wound can be supported after suture removal with a porous adhesive tape, such as Steri-strips. These paper tape closures should remain on the skin for about 5 days.

When the laceration about the lip extends across the mucocutaneous junction (the white line between the vermilion of the mucosa and the skin), care must be taken to align the edges of the wound. This is best done with the aid of magnifying loupes by aligning the fine white roll that is apparent because of the thick sebaceous glands at the juncture. A small malalignment will be conspicuous. When there is significant loss of mucosa, it is often advisable to excise the wound in a V fashion and close the wound primarily. Other methods of addressing mucosal loss include rotation of an adjacent mucosal flap or harvesting a mucosal graft. Injuries in which there is a significant loss of lip tissue are difficult, and the reconstruction to restore mucosa, muscle, and skin is complex. Sometimes, it is best to close the wounds in a simple fashion and defer extensive reconstructive procedures. When the immediate treating physician is not adequately experienced or if associated injuries prevent extensive primary surgery, it is always wisest to do a simple wound closure. Secondary procedures, which include mucosal flaps, cross-lip flaps, and tongue flaps, should be undertaken only by an experienced surgeon.

Lacerations of the tongue are usually a problem because of extensive bleeding. When necessary, bleeding can be controlled by large sutures encompassing a moderate amount of tongue tissue.

Injuries to Mucosa

In all significant injuries of the mucosa of the mouth, including lips, gingiva, tongue, soft palate, and pharynx, several steps have resulted in diminished infection and improved results. The child should be kept on a clear liquid diet for a minimum of 3 days. This prevents food particles from entering the wound as a nidus for infection. After resuming solid foods, it is wise to rinse the mouth after each meal with water or a mild salt solution (1 teaspoon of salt in a quart of water). Frequent washing of the mouth and irrigation of the wounds in this manner have resulted in excellent wound healing. Most surgeons agree that the use of an oral penicillin or first-generation cephalosporin for 5 days is safe and has resulted in a diminished incidence of wound infection and inflammation.

Injuries to the Parotid Duct

In all significant injuries about the mouth, the treating physician should be aware of possible injury to the parotid duct and facial nerve. Parotid duct injury, if not recognized, can result in parotid secretions into the tissues or in a parotid fistula, which is difficult to manage and often requires secondary procedures. If, on the other hand, the injury to the parotid duct is recognized at the time of injury, repair of the duct is simple and effective and is best accomplished with general anesthesia in the young child.

Injuries to Facial Musculature or Facial Nerve

Injuries to the facial musculature or to the facial nerve should be appreciated before treatment, especially before the administration of local anesthetics. The child should be asked to activate all of the muscles of facial expression, and asymmetry should be carefully noted. If injury to the facial nerve occurs anterior to a vertical line through the lateral canthus of the eye, the likelihood of recovery of function without surgical repair of the nerve is excellent. However, if the injury occurs proximal to this line, which is proximal to the anterior border of the masseter muscle, it is prudent to undertake nerve exploration. This must be done using general anesthesia with magnification and microsurgical repair.

Electrical Burns

Electrical burns of the mouth are unusual. They occur most commonly when a toddler places the juncture of an electrical appliance and an extension cord into the mouth. The saliva acts as a conductor and causes an electrical burn. Severe electrical burns can result in a loss of major portions of the upper and lower lip, with the most severe cases involving gingiva, tooth buds, and mandible. Fortunately, most of these injuries involve only the lips and oral commissure. Electrical

injuries to the midportion of the upper and lower lip usually heal without severe deformity.

Immediately after the electrical burn, the degree of trauma is usually not evident. The child should be given sedation and antibiotics (oral penicillin or first-generation cephalosporin), and the family must watch the child carefully. *Late bleeding from the labial artery can be dramatic, and if it occurs, it does so 5 to 7 days following injury.* Parents are instructed to watch for bleeding and, if bleeding is present, to pinch the lip between the fingers and bring the child to the emergency room immediately.

Most surgeons prefer to treat electrical burns with antibiotic therapy and to allow secondary healing. This course is followed because it is often difficult to determine the extent of soft tissue loss in the early postinjury phase. By 3 weeks after the burn, demarcation has occurred, and the degree of tissue loss is evident. If a late deformity occurs, reconstruction is undertaken electively.

SALIVARY GLAND TUMORS

CUNEYT M. ALPER, M.D.
CHARLES D. BLUESTONE, M.D.

Salivary neoplasms in children account for 8% of all pediatric head and neck tumors. However, fewer than 5% of all salivary gland tumors occur in children and in young adults.[3]

The best chance for long-term control of neoplasms arising in a salivary gland is achieved by adequate initial treatment. The method of management for the majority of cases is by excisional biopsy (i.e., removal of the salivary gland), which is also the method for establishing the diagnosis.[2] A firm mass in a salivary gland should be considered a neoplasm unless proven otherwise. When a neoplasm is suspected, the definitive diagnosis is made by biopsy, despite the availability of advanced imaging techniques that can predict the nature of the salivary gland mass in many instances. Fine needle aspiration biopsy may be useful in distinguishing tumors from inflammatory disease and in planning surgery. Using needle biopsy, the accuracy in differentiating histologic types of tumors can be as high as 75%.[3] However, the pathologist usually needs to study the entire tumor to make the definitive diagnosis. Incisional biopsy of salivary gland tumors is to be condemned because of the risk to the facial nerve and tumor spillage. Having established the histologic type of tumor by excisional biopsy, a decision is made whether to add other therapeutic measures, such as more radical surgery (e.g., neck dissection), radiotherapy, or chemotherapy.

Vascular lesions of the salivary gland, such as hemangiomas and lymphangiomas, are considered to be hamartomas rather than neoplasms. Diagnosis of such masses is usually evident from the physical examination, but magnetic resonance imaging (MRI) is helpful in confirming the diagnosis. Hemangiomas are the most common cause of a parotid mass in the infant. The median age at the time of diagnosis is 4 months. Rapid growth during the first 6 months of life usually precedes involution, which occurs soon after. Resection of the hemangioma is usually not necessary, since most will regress. Indications for surgical intervention of hemangiomas in infants and children are rapid increase in tumor size, failure of tumor to involute, hemorrhage into the lesion, or doubts about the correct diagnosis. Lymphangiomas involving the salivary gland should be treated conservatively. Surgery may be necessary for debulking purposes (i.e., to reduce the size and extent). The usual indication is when the mass interferes with function (e.g., airway obstruction).

The treatment and outcome of children with primary epithelial tumors are influenced by tumor size and location but most importantly by the histopathologic type of the tumor. If vascular lesions are excluded, only half of salivary gland tumors are benign. A benign tumor usually is a unilateral, painless, slowly enlarging mass anterior or inferior to the auricle or just below the angle of the mandible, without signs and symptoms of infection. Pleomorphic adenoma (mixed tumor) is the type of benign neoplasm encountered in the pediatric age group.[1] Superficial parotidectomy (i.e., removal/excision of superficial lobe) is the treatment for this benign tumor. Imaging studies help in determining the location and extent of these benign tumors. Most are limited to the superficial lobe. However, to provide safe margins during resection to prevent recurrence, total parotidectomy (i.e., removal of both superficial and deep lobes) is performed, even when the tumor appears to be within a superficial lobe. Pleomorphic adenoma arising in the submandibular gland requires total excision of the gland.

Rapid growth, pain, cranial nerve involvement, fixation to surrounding tissues, and the presence of cervical lymphadenopathy are the criteria for suspicion of malignancy. Mucoepidermoid carcinoma is the most common salivary gland malignancy in childhood. Approximately half of the malignant salivary tumors are of this cell type, followed by acinic cell carcinoma, adenoid cystic carcinoma, and adenocarcinoma. Total parotidectomy, performed as the initial definitive diagnostic and therapeutic procedure, is sufficient for low or intermediate grade malignancies, which constitute the majority of cases. Excision of the facial nerve is not necessary unless the nerve is directly invaded or an intact nerve limits the necessary resection. When nerves are invaded, they should be traced back to clear margins of tumor confirmed by frozen section at the time of surgical resection. Facial nerve grafting can restore the functional and cosmetic sequelae after facial nerve resection. Neck dissection is not necessary unless there are clinically positive lymph nodes. A modified radical neck dissection rather than radical neck dissection, is the recommended method of management.

Postoperative radiotherapy may be employed for the following: (1) high grade malignancies, (2) possible residual disease after radical resection of extensive tumors, (3) tumor noted histologically at the surgical resection margins, and (4) evidence of perineural invasion or multiple level involvement of cervical lymph nodes. However, radiotherapy should be used with caution in children who have a long-term life expectancy, since there is the possibility of late serious sequelae, such as radiation-induced malignancy. Since there is no strong evidence that chemotherapy as a primary modality increases the survival rate in salivary gland tumors, it should be reserved for palliation or adjuvant therapy when an extensive malignancy is present.

REFERENCES

1. Callender DL, Frankenthaler RA, Luna MA, et al: Salivary gland neoplasms in children. Head Neck Surg 1992;118:472–476.
2. Seibert RW: Diseases of salivary glands. *In* Bluestone CD, Stool SE (eds): Pediatric Otolaryngology. Philadelphia, WB Saunders, 1990:948–960.
3. Shikhani AH, Johns ME: Tumors of the major salivary glands in children. Head Neck Surg 1988;10:257–263.

RECURRENT PAROTITIS

ELIZABETH ROSE, M.D.
CHARLES D. BLUESTONE, M.D.

Recurrent parotitis in children is characterized by multiple episodes of parotid swelling that may affect both glands. There is associated pain and fever, with purulent sialorrhea, but suppuration of the gland is rare. There are several different causes for this disease, and the investigation and therapy for affected children should, therefore, be varied appropriately.

CLINICAL FEATURES

Most children experience parotitis before the age of 5 years, and often in infancy.[2] Each attack lasts 2 to 5 days, with a mean exacerbation rate of five per year, although some children have monthly

TABLE 1. Causes of Parotid and Nonparotid Swelling in Children

Causes of Parotid Swelling
Sialectasia, possibly congenital
Heredity
Immunodeficiency of serum IgG or IgA or salivary IgA
HIV
    Diffuse infiltrative lymphocytosis
    Recurrent viral infections, especially with Epstein-Barr virus
Autoimmune diseases, especially Sjögren's syndrome
Allergy to specific foods, e.g., strawberries
Bulimia
Pneumatic inflation of the parotid, e.g., by trumpet playing
Medications
    Antihistamines
    Phenothiazines
    Cytotoxics (cytarabine)
Sialolithiasis

Causes of Nonparotid Swelling
Hemangioma
Cystic hygroma
Masseter hypertrophy

attacks. There is a tendency for the interval between attacks to lengthen as the child becomes older, but 10% still have episodes after the age of 20. In older children, an autoimmune disease, such as Sjögren's syndrome, should be suspected,[3] and in adolescents, bulimia or self-induced pneumatic inflation of the parotid may cause recurrent parotid swelling.

ETIOLOGY (TABLES 1 AND 2)

The organism most commonly cultured from the parotid secretion is *Staphylococcus aureus,* although anaerobes and mixed organisms often are isolated.[1] Several different viruses can cause parotitis, which explains recurrent infections in some cases. Epstein-Barr virus (EBV) may cause recurrent infections.

If sialography is performed, sialectasis is demonstrated often in both glands even when one side only is affected clinically. These changes may represent a congenital abnormality of the duct system rather than being the result of recurrent infection. Such changes have been demonstrated in infants. There are several reports of familial cases.

Some children have deficiencies of IgG or of serum or secretory IgA, which predispose them to recurrent parotitis. Sialograms generally are normal in these cases. Children with HIV frequently have recurrent parotid swelling from either diffuse infiltrative lymphocytosis or recurrent viral infections, especially from EBV.

Rare cases of recurrent parotitis in patients with a specific food allergy to strawberries or seafood have been reported.

TABLE 2. Microbiology of Recurrent Parotitis in Children

Bacteria
Aerobes
    Staphylococcus aureus
    Streptococcus sp.
    Escherichia coli

Anaerobes
    Bacteroides sp.
    Peptostreptococcus sp.

Viruses
Paramyxovirus (mumps)
Epstein-Barr virus
Coxsackie virus
Influenza A virus
Parainfluenza virus

TABLE 3. Investigation for Recurrent Parotitis

Collection of secretions from Stensen's duct for
  Gram stain
  Culture—aerobic and anaerobic
  Susceptibility testing
Antinuclear antibody (ANA) in older children
Serum IgG with subclasses, serum IgA
Salivary IgA
Sialography when quiescent

TABLE 4. Therapy for Recurrent Parotitis

Nonspecific Therapy
Hydration
Massage and warm compresses to the gland
Stimulation of salivary flow with citrus juices

Antibiotic Therapy
Amoxicillin-clavulanate
  40 mg/kg/d PO q8h
Clindamycin 25 mg/kg/d PO q6–8h
  or 25–40 mg/kg/d IV q6h
Cefoxitin
  50–150 mg/kg/d IV q6–8h
Imipenem
  50 mg/kg/d IV q6–8h
Metronidazole
  15–30 mg/kg/d PO q6–8h
  with
Vancomycin
  50 mg/kg/d IV q6h

Surgery
Intraoral ligation of Stensen's duct
Total parotidectomy

MANAGEMENT (TABLES 3 AND 4)

Saliva from the parotid duct should be cultured, and therapy should be started. Therapy includes hydration, massage of the gland, sialogogues, such as citrus juice, to stimulate salivary flow, and analgesics, as well as antibiotic therapy. In many cases, there is a good response to amoxicillin-clavulanate, but the antimicrobial agent can and should be altered according to the clinical progress and the results of cultures and susceptibility testing. Many children appear to benefit from prophylactic antibiotics. Although the length of the course is not easily determined, prophylaxis may be necessary until puberty.

Further evaluation includes investigation for underlying immune deficiencies or autoimmune diseases. In some children, there is a reduced recurrence rate of the parotitis after sialography.

Surgical therapy is reserved for those patients with severe and frequent infections and for those whose episodes recur despite antimicrobial prophylaxis. Ligation of Stensen's duct is relatively easy and has good results. Total parotidectomy risks damage to the facial nerve but may be necessary if a lesser procedure fails.

REFERENCES

1. Brook I, Frazier EH, Thompson DH: Aerobic and anaerobic microbiology of acute suppurative parotitis. Laryngoscope 1991;101:170–172.
2. Ericson S, Zetterlund B, Öhman J: Recurrent parotitis and sialectasis in childhood. Clinical, radiologic, immunologic, bacteriologic, and histologic study. Ann Otol Rhinol Laryngol 1991;100:527–535.
3. Hara T, Nagata M, Mizuno Y, Ura Y, Ueda K: Recurrent parotid swelling in children: Clinical features useful for differential diagnosis of Sjögren's syndrome. Acta Paediatr 1992;81:547–549.

DEVELOPMENTAL CYSTS OF THE NECK

STEVEN D. HANDLER, M.D.

BRANCHIAL ARCH CYSTS AND SINUSES

Branchial arch cysts and sinuses represent failure of obliteration of the embryologic branchial arch system. These lesions classically occur as a smooth, round swelling at the anterior border of the sternocleidomastoid muscle. If an external opening is present, the diagnosis of branchial cleft sinus or fistula is obvious. (A branchial cleft sinus connects to the overlying skin, whereas a fistula communicates with both the overlying skin and the pharynx medially.) Ultrasound, computed tomography (CT), and magnetic resonance imaging (MRI) are often helpful in differentiating a cyst from a lymph node or other type of neck mass.

Surgical excision is the treatment of choice for these lesions. Sinus and fistula tracts drain continually and are a constant source of local irritation to the neck. Although small cysts may remain asymptomatic, they contain fluid and epithelial debris that have the potential to become infected. Infection of a branchial cleft cyst causes inflammation and scarring that can make surgical excision more difficult. If a lesion becomes infected, systemic antibiotics are administered until the infection subsides (usually 2 to 3 weeks), allowing surgical excision. Rarely, incision and drainage or needle aspiration of an acutely infected cyst may be required to control the infection before surgical excision.

Radiographic dye studies of the sinus or fistula tract are unnecessary and, often, misleading. The dye may not outline the full extent of the tract, or it may extravasate and give an inaccurate picture of the lesion. Similarly, injecting methylene blue into the tract before the procedure has the same drawbacks.

The operating surgeon must be familiar with the potential course and connections of the branchial arch anomaly and its relationship to adjacent structures. A second incision may be required to excise long tracts that may enter the pharynx in the tonsillar fossa or pyriform sinus. Any connection to the pharynx must be excised, and the opening must be ligated securely. Incomplete excision of the lesion will result in recurrence of the anomaly.

A first branchial arch anomaly presents added difficulties in both diagnosis and management. These lesions occur above the level of the hyoid bone and may course medially to the external auditory canal or the middle ear. If a first branchial arch anomaly is suspected, CT scanning is strongly recommended before surgical excision. Since these lesions will often pass in close proximity to the branches of the facial nerve, the operating surgeon must begin the operation with a superficial parotidectomy and facial nerve dissection so that these neural elements can be protected during excision of the first branchial arch sinus tract.

THYROGLOSSAL DUCT CYSTS

Thyroglossal duct cysts are epithelial remnants of the embryologic descent of the thyroid gland. They may occur anywhere along its course from the base of the tongue to the anterior neck. The typical appearance is that of a smooth, round mass in the midline of the neck at the level of the hyoid bone. The lesion usually moves with protrusion of the tongue and with swallowing. There is no opening to the skin unless the lesion has become infected and drained spontaneously or has been incised and drained.

The diagnosis of a thyroglossal duct cyst is usually obvious on clinical examination. Ultrasound, CT, or MRI may prove helpful in differentiating the lesion from other midline masses, such as dermoid cysts or lymph nodes. Imaging of the thyroid gland is mandatory before surgical excision of a suspected thyroglossal duct cyst to ensure that the lesion is not, in reality, ectopic thyroid or the child's only functioning thyroid tissue. Although a thyroid scan has been the traditional imaging technique, we have found that an ultrasound study of the neck will identify the thyroid gland in its normal position and has the advantage of avoiding radioactive isotopes. The ultrasound study can be done on one visit to the hospital compared with the two visits required for a thyroid scan.

Surgical excision of a suspected thyroglossal duct cyst is the treatment of choice. Infection of a thyroglossal duct cyst causes inflammation and scarring that can make surgical excision more difficult. If a lesion becomes infected, systemic antibiotics are administered until the infection subsides (usually 2 to 3 weeks), permitting surgical excision. Rarely, incision and drainage or needle aspiration of an acutely infected cyst may be required to control the infection before surgical excision. Since the descent of the thyroid gland may leave epithelial remnants adjacent to or within the hyoid bone, the central portion of the hyoid bone is removed (Sistrunk procedure) with the surgical specimen. This does not create any disability in the child and decreases the chance of incomplete excision and subsequent recurrence of the lesion.

REFERENCES

1. Doi O, Hutson JM, Myers NA, McKelvie PA: Branchial remnants: A review of 58 cases, J Pediatr Surg 1988;23:789–792.
2. Radkowski D, Arnold J, Healy GB, et al.: Thyroglossal duct remnants. Arch Otolaryngol Head Neck Surg 1991;117:1378–1381.
3. Torsiglieri AJ Jr, Tom LWC, Ross AJ, Wetmore RF, Handler SD, Potsic WP: Pediatric neck masses: Guidelines for evaluation. Int J Pediatr Otorhinolaryngol 1988;16:199–210.

LYMPHANGIOMA

STEVEN D. HANDLER, M.D.

Lymphangiomas are congenital malformations of the lymphatic system, although some consider them to be benign neoplasms. They are divided into three categories based on histologic appearance: *lymphangioma simplex,* composed of thin-walled capillary sized lymph channels; *cavernous lymphangioma,* composed of dilated lymphatic spaces; and *cystic hygroma,* composed of cysts of varying sizes. Some investigators believe that these distinctions are artificial and that the differences in appearance really represent a continuum of the same disease process. The clinical and histologic occurrence of a lesion is most likely related to the location of the lesion. For example, cystic hygroma is more common in the cervical area, where the loose areolar tissue permits development of cystic spaces. In the tongue, on the other hand, the compact muscle tissue encourages development of smaller channels consistent with lymphangioma simplex.

These lesions commonly appear in the head and neck, especially the posterior triangle of the neck. Over half of the lesions are present at birth, and over 90% are apparent by the end of the second year of life. The diagnosis usually is obvious, with a large fluctuant, cystic cervical mass that will transilluminate. In the oral cavity, these lesions may appear as rubbery, irregular masses in or on the tongue or oral mucosa.

Lymphangiomas usually demonstrate a pattern of slow growth as the child grows. Small, localized lesions that are not causing any cosmetic or functional problems may be managed with close observation. Small lymphangiomas of the oral cavity may cause local discomfort or be associated with episodes of bleeding as the child bites or chews the mucosa overlying it. These lesions are usually amenable to local surgical excision. Diffuse lesions on the surface of the tongue are shaved with a laser or electrocautery.

Cystic lymphangiomas may manifest episodes of rapid enlargement secondary to lymphadenitis associated with upper respiratory infections or as a result of hemorrhage into the cystic spaces. If a lesion becomes infected, systemic antibiotics are administered until the infection subsides (usually 2 to 3 weeks), permitting surgical excision. Rarely, incision and drainage or needle aspiration of an acutely infected cyst may be required to control the infection before surgical excision. Needle aspiration of large or infected cystic lesions will lead to short-term decompression of the lymphangioma and may relieve pressure on the adjacent structures, such as the airway or esophagus, but will not provide any long-lasting benefit in the management of the hygroma.

Surgical excision is the required treatment for the large cystic lesions of the head and neck area. Observation of large lymphangiomas is not indicated, since these do not undergo spontaneous regression, as seen in hemangiomas. Large cystic hygromas of the neck in infants are often associated with feeding and breathing difficulties as the lesion compresses and displaces the esophagus and upper airway (larynx and trachea). Preoperatively, radiographic evaluation (CT, MRI, or ultrasound) is helpful in determining the extent of the lesion.

The fact that these lesions often insinuate into tissue planes of the head and neck may make it impossible to accomplish total surgical excision. Therefore, multiple staged procedures may be required in their treatment. An attempt should be made to excise as much of the lymphangioma as possible, taking care to avoid injury to vital neural and vascular structures. Radical excision of these lesions is never indicated. It is important to incise as many septae and to open as many cysts as possible in order to decompress the lesion and to help induce involution. Recurrence of the lesion is rare if total removal is accomplished. The reported recurrence rate of 5% to 15% after incomplete excision reflects the fact that involution can occur after removing many of the septae and allowing the cystic spaces to contract. Tracheostomy and/or gastrostomy may be necessary in the management of neonates with large lymphangiomas compressing the trachea and/or esophagus.

Sclerosing agents and radiation therapy have been used to treat extensive lesions, but these modalities have the potential to cause further damage to the child and are not recommended. Malignant degeneration of these lesions is extremely rare.

REFERENCES

1. Kennedy TL: Cystic hygroma-lymphangioma: A rare and still unclear entity. Laryngoscope 1989;99:1–10.
2. Torsiglieri AJ Jr, Tom LWC, Ross AJ, Wetmore RF, Handler SD, Potsic WP: Pediatric neck masses: Guidelines for evaluation. Int J Pediatr Otorhinolaryngol 1988;16:199–210.
3. Yuh WTC, Buehner LS, Kao SCS, Robinson RA, Dolan KD, Phillips JJ: Magnetic resonance imaging of pediatric head and neck cystic hygromas. Ann Otol Rhinol Laryngol 1991;100:737–742.

DISORDERS OF THE ESOPHAGUS

ALAN M. LAKE, M.D.
JAMES RUSSELL BUCK, M.D.

This discussion of the disorders of the esophagus is divided into three categories: congenital disorders causing obstruction, motility disorders causing impaired swallow, and mucosal disorders produced by infection, trauma, or other acquired disease. The emphasis is on recognition, therapy, and long-term complications. Discussion of gastroesophageal reflux and the esophageal complications of reflux esophagitis follows this discussion. Portal hypertension is reviewed later in this chapter.

CONGENITAL DISORDERS

Esophageal Atresia

Esophageal atresia occurs in approximately 1 in 3500 births. Fifty percent of affected babies have intrauterine polyhydramnios, and 40% of involved infants are born prematurely. There is an equal incidence in males and females. Only 10% of involved neonates have isolated esophageal atresia, as 85% have a proximal esophageal pouch with distal tracheoesophageal fistula (TEF) and 3% to 5% have a H-type TEF. Approximately 50% have other midline anomalies, such as cardiac ventricular defect or atrial septal defect (25%), gastrointestinal duodenal atresia or imperforate anus (15%), or urologic hypospadias (5%). Between 10% and 20% have trisomy chromosomal disorders, predominantly trisomy 21.

Presentation is primarily with frothy saliva in the nose and mouth or an aspiration episode following the first feeding. Evidence of right upper lobe aspiration and consolidation is frequent in the setting of TEF if the diagnosis is delayed.

Diagnosis is established by the impossibility of advancing a 10F radiopaque tube beyond 10 to 12 cm. The tube should then be left in place to suction oral secretions. A radiograph is obtained documenting the level of atresia and the presence or absence of a distal TEF by the presence of air in the stomach or intestine. Contrast studies are rarely required. If transport to a tertiary care site is required, the neonate is transported upright, with intravenous fluids and antibiotics. On rare occasions, an emergency gastrostomy is required to decompress the stomach. Intubation and ventilator support may be required but must be used judiciously, since severe gastric distention will complicate positive pressure breathing.

Primary repair of esophageal atresia with division of any associated TEF is usually possible in the neonate. An extrapleural approach by right thoracotomy is employed. If the gap is greater than 3 cm, the primary repair is benefited by upper esophageal lengthening by circular myotomy. If a primary anastomosis is not possible, the TEF is divided. A delayed esophageal anastomosis is performed after weeks of esophageal lengthening by bouginage. This is the initial therapy for complete atresia without TEF.

Following repair, ventilatory and nutritional support often are required. A postoperative anastomotic leak, if seen, is controlled by the chest tube placed at surgery and usually closes spontaneously.

Because the distal esophagus, below the original atresia, does not have normal motility, gastroesophageal reflux is nearly universal, and 30% of affected infants will require a fundoplication within 6 months of repair. One clue to severe reflux is recurrent stricture formation at the anastomotic site. Because of the dysmotility of the anastomotic site, some dysphagia is expected when solid foods are begun, as well as recurring frustrations with food impactions when the patient is a toddler and young child. Repeated dilatation is required in 20% of children. Protracted stridor because of tracheomalacia may also occur.

In the setting of an H-type TEF, the diagnosis is often delayed for months to years until repeated pneumonias occur. Infants with H-type TEF rarely have associated anomalies. Diagnosis is established at bronchoscopy or by esophagram performed by a tube placed in the proximal esophagus. The major operative complication is trauma to the recurrent laryngeal nerve.

Esophageal Stenosis and Web

Originally attributed to a complication of reflux, these rare disorders occur in 1:25,000 to 1:50,000 live births. A fibromuscular stenosis develops as a localized segmental hypertrophy. If the segmental region is composed of only mucosa and submucosa, in the absence of muscle, it is termed a *web*. Both are often attributed to a failure of complete recanalization of the esophagus, which normally occurs during the tenth week of gestation. Associated esophageal atresia and TEF may be present.

Symptoms generally occur at the time of introduction of more solid foods, with dysphagia, emesis, aspiration pneumonia, or failure to thrive. Neonatal presentation is possible with high-grade obstruction and mimics atresia. On endoscopy or contrast radiography, the stenosis is often irregular, and the web appears as an intraluminal shelf. Endoscopic lysis of a diaphragmatic web is possible. Unless there is a tracheobronchial remnant in the stenosis, success with dilatation is expected. Surgical resection is, thus, rarely required. If a distal esophageal stenosis requires resection, consideration of a concomitant fundoplication to prevent postoperative iatrogenic reflux is appropriate.

Esophageal Compression by Vascular Ring

Vascular anomalies within the thorax may compress and partially obstruct the esophagus. Usually, tracheal compression occurs as well, producing stridor or impaired clearance of pulmonary secretions. Compression may occur from a full ring, such as the double aortic arch, or a partial ring of a vessel combined with a fibrous remnant, as with right aortic arch and ligamentum arteriosus. The most common cause of esophageal compression is from an aberrant right subclavian artery. This may not be symptomatic for years. The compression is pulsatile and can be documented radiographically or endoscopically. The peculiar swallowing sensation is termed "dysphagia lusoria." Confirmation by MRI precludes the need for arteriography. Surgical intervention is required for symptomatic esophageal compression.

Esophageal Duplication

Duplications of the esophagus are often multiple, cystic, and associated with vertebral anomalies. There may be emesis, dysphagia, partial obstruction, or chronic respiratory signs. Confirmation is by MRI, and surgical dissection and removal of the duplicated mucosa are required.

Esophageal Diverticula

Congenital diverticula may occur with or without associated TEF. They usually consist of mucosa and submucosa without a muscular component. Diverticula above the upper esophageal sphincter are termed "Zenker's diverticula," whereas those in the midesophagus are called "traction diverticula," and those above the lower esophageal sphincter are called "epiphrenic diverticula."

Zenker's diverticula are removed, often with a myotomy of the cricopharyngeal muscle to reduce proximal esophageal pressure and prevent premature closure of the upper esophageal sphincter. Traction diverticula, often multiple and attributed to primary motor disease of the esophagus, are not removed unless they are very large. Epiphrenic diverticula also may be attributed to abnormal motor function, as in achalasia or diffuse esophageal spasm. Surgical resection, when required, is accompanied by myotomy or other treatment of the associated dysmotility in the distal esophagus.

MOTILITY DISORDERS

Disorders of esophageal motility can occur in a variety of ways, often with intermittent signs or symptoms, including dysphagia, reflux, failure to thrive, chest pain, or recurrent aspiration. Understanding these disorders requires a brief background on normal physiology of the three functional regions of the esophagus.

The upper esophageal sphincter (UES) is a 2 to 4 cm segment composed of the lower pharyngeal constrictors and upper cricopharyngeal striated muscles. They generate an asymmetric resting pressure that ranges from 20 mm Hg as a newborn to more than 100 mm Hg as an adult. The UES relaxes during swallow, emesis, or belch.

The body of the esophagus is a 20 to 22 cm tube of skeletal and smooth muscle. The proximal 5% is striated skeletal muscle. The middle 30% to 40% is mixed with an increasing proportion of smooth muscle distally. The distal 50% to 60% is entirely smooth muscle. Primary peristalsis progresses at 2 to 4 cm/s, with a smaller amplitude to the wave at the middle than at either end. A key component of the peristaltic mechanism is deglutitive inhibition, the second swallow inhibiting the first. Whereas stimulation of the vagus nerve produces primary peristalsis, secondary peristalsis can be initiated at any level of the esophagus by luminal distention from air, fluid, or bolus even after vagotomy.

The lower esophageal sphincter (LES) is a 3 to 4 cm segment of tonically contracted smooth muscle at the distal end of the esophagus. This tonic contraction generates an intraluminal pressure that, beyond the newborn period, averages 15 to 30 mm Hg. The resting LES pressure is greatest at night and lowest in the postprandial period. Transient LES relaxation is a component of the belch reflex and is greatly increased by gastric distention. LES relaxation is mediated by preganglionic cholinergic vagal fibers and postganglionic noncholinergic, nonadrenergic (probably nitric oxide) nerves.

The functional assessment of each region of the esophagus can be documented by cineradiography (best for oral and UES function) and by manometry (best for tubular and LES function).

Cricopharyngeal Dysfunction

The failure of the cricopharyngeus to relax produces UES achalasia or spasm. Manometric studies may remain normal. The infant experiences impaired swallow, choking, cough, and nasal reflux of feedings. This condition is especially prominent in trisomy 21 syndrome. Delayed relaxation of UES is a feature of familial dysautonomia (Riley-Day). Premature closure of the UES is believed to induce Zenker's diverticulum.

Although the cricopharyngeus can be dilated, most infants can be managed conservatively with gavage feedings for 4 to 6 months because maturational improvement in UES relaxation often occurs.

The failure to sustain UES pressure, termed "UES hypotension," is a feature of myoneural disease and contributes to recurrent aspiration. UES hypotension often complicates the course of children with a spectrum of diagnoses, such as esophageal atresia, botulism, cerebral palsy, poliomyelitis, myasthenia gravis, and the inflammatory myositis of connective tissue disease. When the primary etiology is untreatable, the use of thickened feedings or even gastrostomy feedings may provide some relief.

Diffuse Esophageal Spasm

Diffuse spasm of the esophagus, caused by tertiary contractions of the esophagus, is seen primarily in moderate to severely retarded children. It may occur with irritability, peculiar posturing (Sandifer sign), chest pain, and dysphagia. The distal 10 to 15 cm of the esophagus will demonstrate abnormal manometric contractions that may be seen on radiographic contrast studies as segmentation of barium (nutcracker esophagus). The LES pressure usually is normal.

Although most common in children with retardation and adults with psychiatric concerns, this form of dysmotility may be seen also in children with pseudoobstruction syndrome, scleroderma, graft-versus-host disease, or diabetes or following caustic ingestion or chronic reflux peptic esophagitis.

Over the years, management with pneumatic dilatation has been attempted, with inconsistent results. Calcium channel blockers, such as nifedipine, are now employed. With severe chronic pain and dysmotility, a long esophageal myotomy to the level of the aortic arch is advised.

Achalasia

Achalasia is incomplete relaxation of the LES on swallowing. It is usually associated with ineffective or absent peristalsis of the distal esophagus and elevated LES pressure. It is uncommon in childhood, with less than 10% of affected individuals diagnosed before 18 years of age. Two variants exist in early childhood. The first is an autosomal recessive form in infancy associated with retardation, vitiligo, muscle wasting, and nerve deafness. The second is achalasia in the context of familial glucocorticoid and mineralocorticoid deficiency.

The most common signs are dysphagia, slow eating, retrosternal pain, sensation of food sticking, and regurgitation of undigested food. Symptoms are usually slowly progressive, producing weight loss or failure to thrive. Patients must sleep with the head of the bed elevated. An air-fluid level may be seen on chest x-ray, and the barium swallow is diagnostic, with a beaked distal esophagus, dilated midesophagus, and impaired esophageal emptying. Early in the disease, particularly in adolescents, the barium study may be normal. On manometry, the UES is normal, with elevated resting pressure in the LES and body.

Pneumatic dilatation will be successful in 60% to 80% of affected children. A second dilatation may be required in up to 20%. Esophageal perforation occurs in 1% to 2% of dilatations. Short-term relief has been reported with calcium channel blockers, such as nifedipine given as 10 mg t.i.d. before meals in adolescents. Continued symptoms after two dilatations are an indication for surgical esophagomyotomy. Excellent long-term results are achieved by experienced surgeons in 70% to 85% of children. Postoperative gastroesophageal reflux may be expected in 20% to 30% of patients. In light of the impaired esophageal clearance, an antireflux procedure at the time of myotomy is recommended. Prolonged postoperative dysphagia is the rule.

Disorders of Suck and Swallow

The coordination of suck and swallow is a complex neuromuscular process. Oral liquids can be swallowed with only impetus from the tongue and gravity. Oral solids require the additional action of the pharyngeal constrictors.

Oral motor dysfunction, termed "oral apraxia," is a common feature in neonates, especially the premature. Gradual resolution over 3 to 6 months is the norm. Perinatal neurologic insults induce a more profound and prolonged incoordination of swallowing. Direct laryngeal penetration and aspiration contribute to recurrent reactive airway disease, pneumonia, or cough.

After exclusion of specific treatable oral conditions, such as cleft palate, feeding gastrostomy is required. Antireflux fundoplication is not routinely employed. Most infants can continue oral stimulation, if not significant caloric intake, with the use of advancing textured solids. Ongoing therapy with an experienced occupational therapist should be done to prevent the child's forgetting how to eat.

ACQUIRED ESOPHAGEAL DISEASE

Caustic Ingestion

At least 5000 caustic ingestions occur yearly in the United States, most by children between 1 and 3 years of age. Regrettably, the presence or absence of oral injury does not predict esophageal injury. If there is any question, water is immediately given to wash the caustic material from the esophagus.

Ingestion of acid is infrequent, and esophageal damage is unusual. Strong acids, such as battery fluid, may cause coagulation necrosis of the esophagus, but the major sites of injury are the stomach and duodenum. The esophageal injury induced by alkali varies with pH, with modest injury at pH 9 to 11 and severe injury if the pH exceeds 11. As little as 1 ml of 30% sodium hydroxide can cause transmural necrosis of the esophagus within 1 second. Penetration to the point of mediastinitis can be seen. Fibrosis of the injured esophagus develops within 14 days, and stricture develops within 1 month. Ulcerations may last for months.

Esophageal injury is most commonly noted at the four sites of anatomic narrowing: the cricopharyngeus, aortic arch, left mainstem bronchus, and diaphragm. During the first 48 hours, dysphagia is due to inflammatory edema, often closing the lumen. Although symptoms may not correlate with extent of injury, in the presence of two or more of the symptoms of emesis, drooling, or stridor, 50% of the children have severe injury.

Vomiting should *not* be induced, and barium contrast studies are not performed. Neither adsorption by charcoal nor neutralization by weak acid or alkali should be attempted. Chest x-ray is the initial study. Intravenous fluids are given. *Early endoscopy is advised*, ideally within 12 hours, to document the extent of injury as first, second, or third degree injury.

If no esophageal burn is seen, the child is discharged home, taking broad-spectrum antibiotics for 7 days, and advancing to a soft diet at 72 hours. Patients with first degree burns receive a course of IV fluids until the oral burn is resolved, along with antibiotics, and are advanced to a soft diet over 72 hours. If the patient is asymptomatic, no further studies are performed. Children with second or third degree caustic burns are handled in the same way and, in addition, have a contrast swallow 4 days after injury. If significant motility disturbance is present at this point, they are followed again at 6 weeks to ascertain the presence of stricture formation. If severe motility disturbance is present at 4 days, a gastrostomy may be placed, as well as an esophageal stent. Rarely, with ingestion of commercial strength alkalis, mediastinitis and abdominal findings are present initially, and radical surgery is indicated in the initial stabilization. The routine use of steroids in esophageal burns is no longer recommended, although controversy persists in this area.

Complications include aspiration pneumonia, gastric perforation, and bleeding, which usually develop in the first 36 hours. Tracheomalacia may develop as a late finding. Strictures are seen in 25% of children with second or third degree esophageal burns and are managed by a dilatation program beginning 6 weeks after injury. Though repeated dilatation is often required, long-term symptomatic relief is achieved in more than 90%. Esophageal dysmotility may persist for years. Following significant caustic ingestion, patients have a 1000-fold increased risk for squamous carcinoma of the midesophagus. This is generally noted 20 to 40 years later but has been described as soon as 10 years postinjury. Recommendations are made to the family for long-term follow-up after resolution of the acute injury.

Esophageal Replacement

The use of esophageal replacement has been greatly diminished by the use of esophageal myotomies to lengthen the upper esophagus in long segment atresias in the neonate, recognition and aggressive management of reflux, preventing severe stricture disease, and the regulated disappearance of highly concentrated alkali from the consumer market. The problem seen in the long-term follow-up of esophageal replacement patients has reinforced the salvage of the damaged esophagus at nearly all costs. When required, the stomach is the favorite replacement. In older children, the entire stomach is mobilized by laparotomy and brought through the chest posteriorly, with the esophageal gastric anastomosis being performed in the neck. For infants, a gastric tube is created, since intrathoracic gastric distention with the whole stomach may compromise lung development. This gastric tube, created from the fundus, is brought up posteriorly, and the anastomosis is performed in the neck. Some surgeons use the colon as an esophageal replacement, and a few have used jejunum by either pedicle graft or free graft.

Foreign Body

The approach to ingested foreign bodies should not be casual. More than 1500 people die each year in the United States from complications of foreign body ingestion. Eighty percent of ingestions occur in children, usually under 3 years of age. The sudden onset of dysphagia, stridor, or wheeze suggests foreign body ingestion. Do *not* induce emesis. If ingestion is suspected, the first study is the chest x-ray. Up to 20% of ingested foreign bodies enter the bronchial tree. If the foreign body is not radiopaque and the patient is symptomatic, a thin barium swallow is done. Of objects that reach the stomach, 95% will pass uneventfully, usually within 4 days. If a small foreign body remains in the esophagus, an underlying stricture is suspected. The major foreign bodies noted in children are coins, small batteries, and food.

The most important component of treatment is maintenance of the airway. Esophageal foreign bodies should be removed under direct visualization with intubation of the airway. Many times, the relaxation of general anesthesia causes a distal small object, such as a dime or penny, to fall into the stomach. These usually will pass through the rest of the intestine easily. Blind retrieval of esophageal foreign bodies by balloon catheters, although reported to be successful, is no longer advised because of the risk of aspiration and the inability to assess any mucosal injury.

Disc batteries that remain in the esophagus should be removed immediately, since esophageal transmural injury can occur within 4 hours. If the battery enters the stomach, batteries greater than 20 mm in diameter or persisting greater than 72 hours should be removed.

Impaction of meat is commonly noted in children after esophageal surgery, such as esophageal atresia with TEF. If the child is very uncomfortable or there are respiratory concerns, endoscopic removal

is performed. If the child is minimally symptomatic and an x-ray shows no bone component, the patient may be observed for 12 to 18 hours. During that interval, meat tenderizer or papain 5 ml orally every 30 minutes for 4 hours may be employed. Meat tenderizer should not be employed for longer intervals because it may cause mucosal ulceration and hypernatremia.

Traumatic Perforation or Tear

Perforation or rupture of the esophagus may be seen in the neonate as a spontaneous rupture or in older children as an induced rupture from emesis, foreign bodies, tube placement, or blunt trauma. The signs may be acute esophageal obstruction, cervical hematoma, subcutaneous emphysema, or tension pneumothorax.

Spontaneous neonatal perforation is attributed to the intrauterine rupture of a fluid-filled esophagus during uterine contraction. It may be seen also after aggressive suctioning. A right-sided tension hydropneumothorax may develop. Conservative management with intravenous fluids, antibiotics, and evacuation of the pleural space usually is successful. Surgical intervention is reserved for mediastinitis or mediastinal abscess. A few neonates will be shown later to have developed pseudodiverticula of the esophagus.

Esophageal rupture from blunt trauma usually involves the left lateral wall and is often associated with tracheal injury as well. Perforation from a foreign body is commonly complicated by mediastinitis. Surgical two-layer closure and irrigating tube drainage are nearly always required.

The Mallory-Weiss tear of the distal esophagus from protracted forceful emesis usually causes hematemesis. Following stabilization, endoscopic confirmation of the degree of tear and bleeding determine the level of intervention. Most tears are 1 to 2 cm in length and can be managed conservatively with intravenous fluids, bowel rest, and observation, with expected resolution within 48 hours. Infusion of the left gastric artery with vasopressin or an embolizing agent usually is attempted before surgery. Tamponade is of no value.

Perforation of the esophagus during endoscopic evaluation is very uncommon, occurring in 0.03% of flexible endoscopies. It occurs most commonly during dilatation, sclerotherapy, or foreign body removal. The three cardinal symptoms of endoscopic perforation are fever, pain, and emphysema. Pleural effusion will complicate mediastinal involvement. Although operative treatment usually is advised, nonoperative treatment is considered with mild symptoms. This treatment consists of nasoesophageal suction, broad-spectrum antibiotics, and parenteral alimentation, with Gastrografin swallows performed every 3 to 5 days to confirm healing. In children, the operative procedure is nearly always drainage and repair.

Epidermolysis Bullosa

Esophageal traumatic injury frequently complicates the course of epidermolysis bullosa (EB) in children. There are several forms. The recessive lethalis form is associated with universal early death from sepsis and fluid loss. The autosomal dominant form has moderate bullous lesions of skin, mouth, esophagus, and anus, but without risk for stricture. The acquired form is mild.

Esophageal concerns thus occur primarily in the recessive dystrophic form (RDEB). Esophageal bullae may develop spontaneously or from ingestion of coarse food. Acute esophageal obstruction may occur. Strictures are common, with 50% located high in the esophagus.

Treatment is with the use of pureed diets to minimize trauma. Acute bullae are treated with high-dose steroids to reduce dysphagia. There is some evidence that phenytoin given orally and monitored by blood levels to 10 mg/dl may reduce development of stricture. Esophageal dilatation must be done with extreme care. Extensive stricture formation will mandate interposition by colon or gastric tube.

Dysphagia may also complicate other skin diseases, such as Behcet's syndrome, benign mucosal pemphigoid, psoriasis, Stevens-Johnson syndrome, and chronic graft-versus-host disease.

Connective Tissue Disease

Scleroderma is the major connective tissue disease affecting the esophagus, with dysphagia developing in 75% to 95% of patients. This is due to loss of primary and secondary peristalsis, producing dysphagia, anorexia, and weight loss. In the context of associated LES hypotension, reflux, heartburn, and esophagitis ensue. Both Barrett's epithelium and adenocarcinoma are seen in scleroderma and are attributed to chronic reflux. Patients with Raynaud phenomenon have the greatest frequency of dysphagia.

Treatment is symptomatic and designed to reduce complicating reflux esophagitis. H_2-blockers, such as cimetidine and ranitidine, are employed, usually with prokinetic drugs, such as cisapride, erythromycin, and metoclopramide.

Recently, an abnormal motility syndrome identical to that seen in scleroderma was described in children who were breast-fed by mothers having silicone breast implants. None of the children had Raynaud phenomenon or autoantibodies. The children ranged in age from 18 months to 6 years. None had breast-fed more than 7 months.

Abnormal esophageal motility and variable degrees of dysphagia are reported to a lesser degree in patients with systemic lupus erythematosus, dermatomyositis, polymyositis, mixed connective tissue disease, and rheumatoid arthritis. Amyloid infiltration of the esophageal muscle wall has been reported also.

Drug-Induced Esophagitis

Medications capable of direct esophageal injury include doxycycline, slow-release potassium, quinidine, ferrous sulfate, ascorbic acid, and nonsteroidal anti-inflammatory drugs. The site of injury is nearly always at the level of the aortic arch, where an extrinsic compression is noted and a reduction in peristalsis occurs in the transition from skeletal to smooth muscle. The child senses the dysmotility that ensues, describing the sensation that food or medication "sticks" on the way down. Endoscopy confirms acute mucosal erosions, sparing the distal esophagus.

Treatment is cessation of the medication or conversion to a liquid form. Topical therapy with a sucralfate slurry is advised.

Candida Esophagitis

Candida is the most common organism implicated in infectious esophagitis. It does not require any predisposing condition. The diagnosis is usually made endoscopically with the finding of discrete, white, raised lesions, although macroscopic features range from patchy erythema to diffuse ulceration.

Therapy is dictated by the severity and the degree of immune competence. Mild to moderate disease in the immune-competent host responds to 14 days of oral nystatin, clotrimazole troches q.i.d., or oral ketoconazole 3 to 6 mg/kg/d. In children with AIDS, the presence of oral thrush and esophageal symptoms is 95% predictive of esophageal candidiasis. Treatment is usually presumptive with either ketoconazole or fluconazole for at least 2 weeks after symptoms clear. Prophylaxis is justified only in the presence of recurrent relapses. Patients not responding clinically within 7 to 10 days are studied endoscopically to confirm the diagnosis and obtain biopsies to exclude herpes, CMV, or idiopathic ulcerative esophagitis. Patients on treatment with zidovudine (AZT) or zalcitabine (ddC) may develop a drug-induced esophagitis. If *Candida* infection is confirmed, intravenous amphotericin B is initiated.

Infectious Esophagitis

Once rare in childhood, infectious esophagitis now is frequently encountered in immunosuppressed children who are posttransplant or have leukemia, ethanol abuse, diabetes mellitus, and especially acquired immunodeficiency syndrome (AIDS). Patients have severe pain on swallowing (odynophagia), atypical chest pain, dysphagia, hoarseness, or a sense of food sticking.

In children with AIDS, four factors predispose to infectious esophagitis. First, the esophagus is in direct continuity with the outside environment. Second, there is a failure of mucosal immune surveillance. Third, reactivation of disease by pathogens that affect the esophagus, such as herpes and cytomegalovirus (CMV). Fourth, multiple simultaneous infections may occur, clouding the diagnosis and complicating therapeutic decisions.

Although barium swallow investigation frequently is used first, it rarely establishes a diagnosis. Endoscopy with brushings and biopsy for histology and culture is the definitive procedure.

Herpes Simplex Virus (HSV)

Herpes esophagitis causes acute odynophagia, retrosternal pain, and hematemesis. Most HSV esophagitis reflects a reactivation of disease. Ulceration of the esophagus is restricted to squamous epithelium. Associated features may include oral ulcers, stricture formation, and viral pneumonia.

The immune-competent patient with mild herpes infection can be managed supportively. More symptomatic patients and all immune-suppressed patients are treated with oral acyclovir 10 mg/kg/d up to 200 mg q4h, ideally begun early in the symptomatic phase.

Cytomegalovirus

CMV esophagitis occurs less acutely than HSV esophagitis, with nausea, emesis, weight loss, and moderate pain. In children with reduced cell-mediated immunity, reactivation and esophagitis can occur even in the presence of high levels of antibody. Furthermore, CMV esophagitis can be simultaneous with both HSV and *Candida* infection. Diagnosis is by endoscopic biopsy.

Approximately 50% of patients respond to treatment with 2 to 3 weeks of intravenous ganciclovir 5 mg/kg b.i.d. Maintenance therapy is continued in the presence of retinitis.

Tuberculosis

Tuberculosis also occurs with esophagitis in the context of AIDS-related reactivation. Symptoms include dysphagia, fever, and weight loss. Radiographic features include striking extrinsic compression from mediastinal adenopathy. Pseudodiverticuli are noted, as well as sinus tracts extending into the mediastinum. Standard antituberculosis therapy is effective in compliant patients.

Chagas Disease

Chagas disease, caused by *Trypanosoma cruzi,* destroys ganglion cells in the esophagus, producing achalasia. The process may take up to 10 to 30 years after infection, so occurrence in early childhood is unusual. Patients respond to dilatation and, ultimately, myectomy.

Other Infections

Other organisms isolated by culture or biopsy from the esophagus, generally in AIDS patients, include *Cryptosporidium, Aspergillus, Histoplasma,* and human papillomavirus.

Tumors

Most esophageal tumors are benign, including neurofibromas, lipomas, inflammatory polyps, hamartomas, and hemangiomas. Rare cases of leiomyosarcoma, lymphoma, or carcinoma are distinguished by endoscopic biopsy and surgical resection.

REFERENCES

1. Anderson KD, Rouse TM, Randolph JG: A controlled trial of corticosteroids in children with corrosive injury of the esophagus. N Engl J Med 1990;323:637–640.
2. Lovejoy FH: Corrosive injury of the esophagus in children. N Engl J Med 1990;323:668–669.

GASTROESOPHAGEAL REFLUX DISEASE

AUBREY J. KATZ, M.D.

Gastroesophageal reflux disease (GERD) is one of the most common medical conditions in both pediatric and adult populations. It is appropriate to divide gastroesophageal reflux occurring in infancy from GERD in later childhood, adolescence, and adulthood.

GASTROESOPHAGEAL REFLUX DISEASE IN INFANTS

The two categories of gastroesophageal reflux have been described by Boyle[1]: physiologic reflux, so-called normal spitting, and pathologic reflux, which must be evaluated and treated.

Physiologic Gastroesophageal Reflux

Physiologic gastroesophageal reflux, or vomiting, is common in infants. Infants with physiologic reflux are otherwise normal, healthy infants who are happy, eat well, thrive, do not have evidence of gastrointestinal bleeding, have no pulmonary symptoms, and have no irritability or fussiness suggesting heartburn. Parents are extremely upset about babies who vomit all the time, but it is merely vomiting of inconvenience and having to change clothes, both parents' and child's. In this case, reassurance and feeds thickened with cereal are all that is needed. Physiologic reflux may last up to 15 months of age. Patients with vomiting alone after the age of 15 months should be evaluated at least with an upper gastrointestinal series and further evaluation as needed.

Pathologic Reflux in Infants

Pathologic reflux means that the babies have vomiting with one or more of the following features: failure to thrive; irritability and fussiness either postprandially or at night; evidence of bleeding, such as guaiac-positive stools or hematemesis; and pulmonary symptoms, which include apnea, recurrent pneumonia, wheezing, and upper airway disease, specifically stridor. It is important to remember that some of these infants have all these features, with the exception of vomiting, and, therefore, GERD should be considered in the differential diagnosis.

Symptoms of GERD in older children and adolescents may be similar to those in adults, with certain exceptions. Some children complain of recurrent abdominal pain rather than heartburn; intermittent vomiting or regurgitation; chest pain; recurrent pulmonary symptoms, including asthma and recurrent pneumonias, gastrointestinal bleeding, lack of weight gain, anorexia, dysphagia or odynophagia, halitosis, or excessive dental caries. Sandifer syndrome, which occurs in infants and young children with peculiar extending movements of the head associated with feeding, is due to gastroesophageal reflux and certainly may not be associated with vomiting.

ETIOLOGY

The etiology of GERD is not known. It appears that acid and motility of the esophagus, stomach, and duodenum, in varying combinations, are important initiators of GERD. Inapparent, transient relaxation of the lower esophageal sphincter, coupled with delayed gastric emptying, appear to be important in the etiology of GERD. Anatomic factors, such as abnormalities in the crura of the diaphragm and the presence of hiatal hernia, also appear to play a part in the pathogenesis of GERD. Antroduodenal dysmotility may be the prime problem in some patients with reflux disease. An assessment of motility disorders is gradually being recognized to be important in patients with GERD.

EVALUATION

Limitations in diagnostic testing by the constraints of modern managed medicine appear to be interfering with adequate diagnostic evaluations in patients with GERD. It is our belief that adequate evaluation not only is essential to effective therapy but also is cost effective in the long term. Tests for GERD include a variety of studies.

Barium Swallow

Barium swallow defines anatomic abnormalities. The degree of reflux indicated on a barium swallow may not necessarily correlate with the presence or absence or the degree of GERD. The same rule applies to the absence of reflux on a barium swallow. Such abnormalities as esophageal stricture, pyloric stenosis, and intestinal malrotation are certainly found this way, and because of the increased incidence of anatomic abnormalities in the pediatric age group, an upper gastrointestinal study is still mandatory in the initial evaluation of GERD in infancy and childhood.

Endoscopy

Endoscopy can determine if esophagitis is absent or present. Esophageal biopsy to ascertain the presence of esophagitis is important and can assess the degree of GERD. Esophageal biopsy classically shows basal cell hyperplasia and eosinophilic and polymorphic infiltration. It is important to recognize that allergic esophagitis is indistinguishable from gastroesophageal reflux esophagitis pathologically.

24 Hour pH Monitoring

pH monitoring still remains an important tool for the measurement of the degree of reflux in both the distal and the proximal esophagus. It should be used in patients with atypical reflux, where the diagnosis needs to be confirmed, in patients with resistant GERD, or as a tool to evaluate the efficacy of antacid therapy.

Technetium Study

A technetium study to assess gastric emptying is used in the solid and liquid phase. It is an important tool to assess patients with chronic reflux.

Esophageal Motility Studies

Esophageal motility studies are important in patients with intractable reflux to assess lower esophageal sphincter pressure and to rule out associated esophageal dysmotility.

Antroduodenal Motility Studies

Antroduodenal motility studies are now coming into their own and appear to be important in selecting patients with intractable GERD who may be candidates for fundoplication. Patients with significant antroduodenal dysmotility, including postprandial hypomotility, probably should be treated medically rather than undergo surgery. Many of these patients appear to develop significant problems following fundoplication.

TREATMENT

Diet and Positional Alternations

Dietary changes may be helpful. In infants with physiologic reflux, thickening the formula with cereal (1 teaspoon per oz or more if needed), together with a liquid antacid, such as Mylanta or Amphojel, if the patient has associated irritability, will help most patients.

In older patients, the avoidance of acids such as citric acid, and spicy foods is recommended. Fatty foods also should be avoided, since they accentuate delays in gastric emptying and aggravate the gastroesophageal reflux. Chocolates and peppermints have been known to decrease lower esophageal sphincter pressure.

In patients above 6 months of age, raising the head of the bed at night decreases reflux, although this appears not to be the case in infants under 6 months of age.

Drug Therapy

Drug therapy consists of two types of drugs, antacids and prokinetic agents. Antacids are of several types: classic antacids, H_2-blocking agents, and proton pump inhibitors. Types and doses are as follows.

1. Antacids: liquid antacids, such as magnesium- and aluminum-containing antacids
2. H$_2$-blocking agents
   a. Cimetidine (Tagamet) 10 mg/kg per dose q.i.d.
   b. Ranitidine (Zantac) 2 to 4 mg/kg/d divided t.i.d. rather than b.i.d. for reflux disease
   c. Famotidine (Pepcid) 0.6–0.8 mg/kg/d b.i.d.
3. Proton pump inhibitors
   a. Omeprazole: the dose for adults is 20 mg q.d.–b.i.d. and can be used for significant esophagitis. There is no liquid preparation available, but in infants and young children with severe GERD, opening the capsule and placing it in an acid medium appears to be effective.

Side effects may occur. Cimetidine may cause irritability, change in personality, and muscle aches. Impotence is described in older males. Ranitidine has been associated with headaches and also with change in personality. Omeprazole has been associated with hypergastrinemia. Experience in Australia for over 15 years with the use of the drug appears to show no evidence for the development of gastrinoma.

The commonly used prokinetic agents are metoclopramide (Reglan), cisapride (Propulsid), and bethanechol. Metoclopramide was the first drug to be introduced as a prokinetic agent, at a dose of 0.1 mg/kg t.i.d. or q.i.d. given half an hour before meals. Side effects are related to the fact that the drug crosses the blood–brain barrier and predisposes to extrapyramidal side effects, including irritability. Reports of tardive dyskinesia have been described in older women.

Cisapride has been introduced recently in the United States, although it has been used in Europe for many years. It does not cross the blood–brain barrier and has a selective effect on the gastrointestinal tract. It, therefore, does not have the extrapyramidal side effects of metoclopramide and obviously will be the first choice for a prokinetic agent. Side effects include some degree of drowsiness, which usually is not persistent, and abdominal discomfort and intermittent diarrhea. Enuresis or increased urination in the day may occur as a result of bladder stimulation (tapering the dose in this situation may resolve the problem). The usual dose is 0.3 mg/kg per dose t.i.d. or q.i.d.

Bethanechol at a dose of 0.01 mg/kg q.i.d. before meals has also been shown to be helpful. In some cases, combinations of bethanechol with either cisapride or metoclopramide may be used.

Duration of Therapy

With the advent of new drugs, such as omeprazole and cisapride, a more aggressive and longer period of medical therapy is indicated before surgery is used.

Surgery

Nissen fundoplication appears to be the standard operation for patients with intractable reflux disease. Pediatric gastroenterologists and surgeons appear to be more conservative in selecting patients for this operation. We have become more aware that patients with significant antroduodenal dysmotility are probably those patients who suffer and develop postprandial hypomotility following fundoplication. Patient selection, therefore, should be done carefully. It is important that patients should have gastric emptying studies and antroduodenal motility studies performed before they are selected for fundoplication.

PROGNOSIS

Seventy to eighty percent of infants with physiologic reflux outgrow it by 10 to 12 months of age. Patients with persistent vomiting beyond 15 months of age should be evaluated for GERD. Patients with GERD and esophagitis over the age of 2 years are likely to be chronic refluxers in adulthood.

NEUROLOGICALLY IMPAIRED CHILDREN

There is an extremely high incidence of GERD in patients who are neurologically impaired. Therefore, such patients with any of the other symptoms described should be evaluated aggressively for GERD. Shorter terms of medical therapy may be indicated, and Nissen fundoplication appears to be associated with less complications than in neurologically normal patients.

COMPLICATIONS

Complications of GERD may be serious and include esophageal stricture, Barrett's esophagus, and autonomic nervous system dysfunction. It has become apparent that some patients with GERD show evidence of autonomic nervous system dysfunction, perhaps associated with excessive vagal tone. This remains to be proven. These patients may have gastroesophageal reflux in association with episodes of pallor, cyanosis, sweating, or syncope.

REFERENCES

1. Boyle JT: Gastroesophageal reflux in the pediatric patient. Gastroenterol Clin North Am 1989;18:315–338.
2. DiLorenzo C, Flores AF, Hyman PE: Intestinal motility in symptomatic children with fundoplication. J Pediatr Gastroenterol 1991;12:169–173.
3. Hyman PE, Napolitano JA, Diego A, Patel S, Flores AF, Grill BB, Reddy SN, Garvey TQ, Tomomasa T: Antroduodenal manometry in the evaluation of chronic functional gastrointestinal symptoms. Pediatrics 1990;86:39–44.

GASTRITIS, DUODENITIS, AND PEPTIC ULCER DISEASE

WILLIAM J. WENNER, JR., M.D.
DAVID A. PICCOLI, M.D.

The knowledge of acquired lesions of the upper gastrointestinal tract in both children and adults has increased dramatically in the past decade. It is recognized not only that inflammatory lesions are caused by acid-mediated damage but also that infections, toxins, medications, hormones, bile reflux, and allergic and autoinflammatory processes play important roles in the etiology of these lesions. An understanding of the etiology of the lesion must guide therapy. Although controlled studies in children are limited, there is extensive information in adults about acid-blocking therapy, acid-neutralizing therapy, antibiotics, surface binding agents, and medications that modify prostaglandin metabolism. Therapeutic decisions in pediatrics have been guided predominantly by the experience in adults. However, there is increasing information about the pharmacokinetics and efficacy of each of these agents in pediatric populations. The use of these agents in infants and children is extensive, although formal guidelines for use and dosage in children have not been established.

Acquired lesions of the upper gastrointestinal tract generally are classified by three criteria: type of lesion, anatomic location, and duration. Differentiation by type of lesion, that is, inflammation or ulcer disease, generally will not alter the therapy. Differentiation by anatomic location assists in determining the etiologic agent and specific therapeutic needs. Surgical and angiographic options, which are used as last resorts, are generally site specific. Differentiation by duration, that is, acute from chronic disease, is made from the history or histology or certain findings on endoscopy or upper gastrointestinal series. Duration of disease alters therapy.

GASTRITIS

Endoscopic and histologic evidence of mucosal inflammation define gastritis. Radiologic studies are sometimes useful but are not sensitive. Gastritis occurs when the mucosal barrier is damaged, as happens with *Helicobacter pylori* infection and many medications. Therapy is designed to limit further mucosal damage and augment protective responses that promote healing. Gastritis has been differentiated by its chronologic pattern. Generally, the causes of acute gastritis differ from the etiologies of chronic gastritis. These differences have important implications for therapy and rate of relapse.

Acute Gastritis

Acute damage to the mucosal cells and blood vessels of the lamina propria can occur from medications, toxic ingestions, stress, trauma, or infections. Therapeutic agents, such as aspirin, acetaminophen, nonsteroidal anti-inflammatory drugs (NSAIDs), chemotherapy, and erythromycin, can cause acute gastritis. Ingestion of caustic agents, such as ethanol, lye, hydrochloric acid, formaldehyde, button batteries, and magnets, can also cause acute gastritis. Acute gastritis has been observed after viral infections, severe trauma, major surgery, septic shock, and portal hypertension.

Acute gastritis commonly occurs with vomiting or hematemesis. Pain is the most common symptom but may not always be present, and its absence does not rule out acute gastritis. The diagnosis may be inferred clinically, but a confirmation of the diagnosis generally will require endoscopy with biopsy and culture. Barium studies are of limited value because of their low sensitivity. Some lesions occurring with hematemesis (peptic ulcer disease and esophagitis) are treated in a similar fashion to gastritis, but others (variceal bleeding and Mallory-Weiss tear) have different therapy and implications. Definitive diagnosis is therefore strongly encouraged.

Acute gastritis generally will resolve with supportive therapy. Vital signs with orthostatic measurements, nasogastric lavage, rectal examination, hemoglobin determination, and reticulocyte count assess the amount and duration of bleeding. A platelet count, a prothrombin time, and a partial thromboplastin time assess coagulation status. Large volume bleeding from any cause requires immediate resuscitation with crystalloid solutions and rapid procurement of appropriate blood and plasma products.

After the initial evacuation of the stomach, low-pressure, intermittent suction may be continued. Repeated lavage with room temperature saline will provide ongoing estimation of further bleeding. There is no role for iced saline lavage as a therapy.

The initial therapy for gastritis should neutralize existing gastric acidity and prevent further acid secretion. The efficacy of therapy should be assessed by monitoring the pH of nasogastric aspirates, which should be maintained at a pH > 4.0. Oral H_2-receptor antagonist therapy is adequate for mild cases. In severe acute gastritis, intravenous H_2-receptor antagonist therapy provides better results. Histamine receptor blockers have been shown to reduce acid output and promote healing. They also offer the theoretical benefit of protection of mucosal blood flow during hypotensive events.

When hemodynamic stability cannot be maintained with medical and fluid therapy, specific invasive measures must be instituted to stop recurrent bleeding. Uncontrolled bleeding may require systemic venous or localized arterial infusion of vasopressin, with intensive care monitoring for peripheral vascular, cardiac, and electrolyte complications. Arterial embolization, effective in localized lesions, is usually ineffective in diffuse lesions, such as acute gastritis. Occasionally, focal bleeding gastritis can be controlled endoscopically with heater probe, bicap, or laser coagulation.

Chronic Gastritis, Duodenitis, and Peptic Ulcer Disease

Chronic gastritis is distinguished from acute gastritis by the time course of symptoms and by histologic features in the mucosa and submucosa. Chronic gastritis is defined by a predominant lymphocytic and plasma cell infiltration of the lamina propria and/or the presence of neutrophils in a flattened or irregular epithelium. The major symptom is pain, and the etiology is unclear. A possible relationship to acute gastritis and a progression to peptic ulcer disease has been postulated but is unconfirmed. Treatment is similar to that of duodenitis and peptic ulcer disease.

Duodenitis is a diagnosis that requires tissue for pathologic confirmation. Radiographic changes are often missed or misinterpreted,

and visual changes seen on endoscopy are often not supported by pathologic findings. These pathologic findings are similar to those of chronic gastritis and include invasion of lymphocytes, neutrophils, and plasma cells, with loss of the normal architecture. In the absence of a primary etiology, such as Crohn's disease, treatment is similar to that of peptic ulcer disease.

Peptic ulcers are classified as either primary or secondary according to the etiology. Primary ulcers appear in otherwise healthy children on no medication. Secondary ulcers are linked to medication or a primary systemic disease. In the adult, gastric ulcers are the most common primary ulcers. They are usually multiple and antral in location. In the child, the most common primary ulcer is found in the duodenum and is usually solitary and in the bulb. Multiple duodenal ulcers should suggest Zollinger-Ellison syndrome.

Because it requires unique therapy, *H. pylori* must be considered in the evaluation of chronic gastritis, duodenitis, and peptic ulcer disease. It has been reported as a finding in each of these inflammations and in esophagitis. *Helicobacter* is the major cause of chronic gastritis and is associated with peptic ulcer diseases. Some reports suggest that over half of the chronic acquired lesions of the pediatric gastrointestinal tract are associated with *H. pylori*. Other reports suggest up to 100% of duodenal ulcers in children are associated with *H. pylori*.

The diagnosis can be made by identification of the organism in H & E-, silver-, or acridine-stained biopsy specimens, by growth on special culture media, or by the presence of bacterial urease activity. Serologic tests for anti-*Helicobacter* antibody are available, but the significance of a positive result is uncertain. The incidence of positive antibody by serologic tests for *H. pylori* in patients under 20 years of age is 5%, but it increases dramatically with age.

As *H. pylori* is spread by close contact, a positive family history should raise suspicion of its presence.

THERAPY

The therapeutic end point in all acquired lesions of the pediatric gastrointestinal tract is healing of the lesion and prevention of recurrence. The pharmacopeia available to obtain this end point is varied (Table 1) and includes antacids, H_2-receptor antagonists, H^+-K^+-ATPase antagonists, synthetic prostaglandins, ulcer-coating sucrose phosphate polymers, and antibiotics and bismuth salts for *H. pylori* infection.

Antacids

As the first line of therapy, antacids neutralize gastric acid. Consisting of salts of calcium, aluminum, or magnesium, they are effective in providing temporary pain relief. They have limited value in the healing and in the prevention of recurrence. Standard doses for children are 5 to 30 ml per dose of liquid antacid up to 7 times per day for a maximum of 10 days. A further need for antacid use should require endoscopy and other evaluation for the etiology of the symptoms. Aluminum salts should be used with caution with any renal compromise.

Histamine Antagonists

These agents work by blocking histamine-induced acid release. There are several products available for use, including cimetidine (Tagamet), ranitidine (Zantac), and famotidine (Pepcid). Each has been used in varying degrees in the pediatric population. The longest experience has been with cimetidine, although the use of the other agents is increasing. All are cleared by the kidneys. Numerous side effects have been reported. Cimetidine interferes with cytochrome P450 activity and may be associated with hepatotoxicity, lowering of mean arterial pressure when administered by intravenous route, gynecomastia, abnormalities of sperm count, and increased prolactin levels. Ranitidine and famotidine appear not to interfere with P450 activity, nor are antiandrogenic effects noted. H_2-antagonists have been shown to affect pulmonary vasculature. They block the tolazoline-induced pulmonary vasodilatation in newborn and fetal sheep.

TABLE 1. Formulary

	SCHEDULE	LENGTH OF THERAPY	
Antacids			
5–30 ml per dose	Up to 7× per day	10 d	
Histamine Antagonists			
Cimetidine			
20–30 mg/kg/d	Divided q6–8h	8 wk	
Ranitidine			
2–4 mg/kg/d	Divided q12h	8 wk	
H⁺-K⁺-ATPase Antagonists			
Omeprazole			
0.2–3.3 mg/kg/d	q.d.	8 wk	
Synthetic Prostaglandins			
Misoprostol			
Pediatric dose not defined			
Sucrose Phosphate			
0.5–1 g per dose	q.i.d.	8 wk	
Helicobacter pylori Therapy			
Bismuth subsalicylate			
Weight–Age Dependent			
6.4–8 kg:	43.6 mg per dose	q6–8h	2 wk
>13 kg and <6 y:	87.5 mg per dose	q6–8h	2 wk
6–9 y:	175 mg per dose	q6–8h	2 wk
9–12 y:	265.5 mg per dose	q6–8h	2 wk
>12 y:	265.5–525 mg per dose	q6–8h	2 wk
Ampicillin			
50–100 mg/kg/d	Divided q6h	2 wk	
Amoxicillin			
40–70 mg/kg/d	Divided q8h	2 wk	
Erythromycin ethylsuccinate			
50 mg/kg/d	Divided q6h	2 wk	
Metronidazole			
5–10 mg/kg per dose	q8h	2 wk	

A significant antagonism to the effects of tolazoline by ranitidine has been reported in children. Therefore, it has been recommended that in children with known or potential pulmonary hypertension, ranitidine should be used only with patients who have a pulmonary vascular resistance index (PVRI) of < 5 dyne·sec/cm⁵·m². It should not be used with tolazoline. Similar caution may be appropriate with all H₂-antagonists.

Standard doses for H₂-antagonists vary with the agent. Cimetidine is given orally, intramuscularly, or intravenously at a dose of 20 to 30 mg/kg/d divided in 6 to 8-hour intervals. It is available as a liquid preparation of 300 mg in 5 ml. The adult oral dose is 300 to 400 mg per dose 3 to 4 times per day. Ranitidine is given orally at a dose of 2 to 4 mg/kg/d divided in 12-hour intervals. It is available as a liquid preparation of 75 mg in 5 ml. The adult dose is 150 mg per dose every 12 hours. The intravenous or intramuscular dose in the child is 1 to 2 mg/kg/d divided in 6 or 8-hour intervals. The duration of therapy with H₂-antagonists should be a minimum of 6 to 8 weeks. Therapy of longer duration should be closely monitored and followed.

H⁺-K⁺-ATPase Antagonists

Omeprazole (Prilosec) inhibits gastric acid production by interfering with the function of the H⁺-K⁺-ATPase of the secretory membrane of the parietal cell. This agent suppresses both histamine-stimulated and vagal-stimulated acid secretion. Omeprazole is more potent than H₂-antagonists and has been found effective in the treatment of H₂-antagonist-resistant lesions. Its use in the pediatric population has been documented in the literature, but the experience is limited. Reported side effects occur in 1% to 6% of patients. These are mostly gastrointestinal symptoms, such as diarrhea, abdominal pain, and constipation. Less frequently reported side effects include elevation

of serum transaminases, hepatic failure, peripheral neuropathy, skin rash, and the proliferation of enterochromaffin-like cells in omeprazole-treated rats, raising a concern about dysplastic or neoplastic changes. There have been no confirmatory findings of these enterochromaffin-like cell changes in humans.

Omeprazole is administered by a single daily oral dose. A pediatric dose has not been established for omeprazole. Dosages in the range of 0.2 to 3.3 mg/kg/d have been reported. Because of the lack of experience, caution should be used in pediatric patients, and initial administration should begin with a low dose. The adult dose is 20 mg/d. The drug is acid labile and can be rendered ineffective if the capsule is opened. The duration of therapy has been up to 3 months. Therapy of longer duration may be necessary but should be closely monitored.

Synthetic Prostaglandins

Misoprostol (Cytotec), a synthetic prostaglandin E₁ (PGE₁), works by decreasing acid production and by a cytoprotective effect. It binds to PGE receptor sites of the parietal cell, but the cytoprotective action has not been defined. It has a demonstrated benefit in the prevention and perhaps the treatment of gastrointestinal lesions secondary to NSAIDs. Side effects include abdominal pain, diarrhea, and uterine contractions and bleeding. Use in the pediatric population is limited to individual experiences, and there are no published trials in this age group. The standard dose in the pediatric age group has not been defined. The adult dose range is 100 to 200 μg per dose four times per day.

Sucrose Phosphate

The aluminum salt of sucrose phosphate, sucralfate (Carafate) reacts with the proteinaceous exudate of damaged mucosa and binds to the lesion. This barrier prevents further damage by preventing acid, peptic, or bile activity. It does not raise the pH of the gastric environment. It has been found effective in promoting the healing of gastric and duodenal ulcers, and it may be effective for healing of gastritis and esophagitis. The side effects are constipation and possible interference with the absorption of other medications. The standard dose is 0.5 to 1 g per dose up to 4 times per day. It is available as a 1g tablet and as a liquid preparation (1g/10 ml).

Helicobacter pylori Therapy

The simultaneous use of bismuth and an antibiotic appears to be successful in children in the eradication of *H. pylori*. This approach seems to be more successful in the pediatric population than in adults, where the use of three-drug therapy has been advocated because of the rapid development of drug resistance. Bismuth subsalicylate or subcitrate (not currently available in the United States) has been used in combination with ampicillin or amoxicillin. There are reports of the use of erythromycin as the antibiotic and also reports in children of dual therapy with amoxicillin and tinidazole. The duration of therapy has not been well defined. In cases nonresponsive to dual therapy, metronidazole (Flagyl) may be added for a short course of triple-drug therapy. Recent reports in the adult population suggest a combination of omeprazole and an antibiotic may be effective. As this may be a less toxic therapy, the reader is advised to monitor current publications for changes in recommendations.

Bismuth toxicity has been reported in adults, but no cases have been seen in children. Toxicity includes encephalopathy and renal dysfunction. Bismuth subsalicylate places the child at risk for salicylate toxicity. Thirty milliliters of bismuth subsalicylate contain 263 mg of salicylate, equivalent to an adult aspirin. The salicylate component is rapidly and completely absorbed, but little bismuth is absorbed (<0.005%). Although no cases of Reye syndrome have been reported in children treated for *H. pylori* infection, this may be a risk to consider, and parents must be informed of the use of salicylate.

Published doses for bismuth subcitrate are 275 mg/m² body surface area per day divided in 3 or 4 doses. The standard dose of bismuth subsalicylate is weight dependent and shown in Table 1. The recommended ampicillin dose is 50 to 100 mg/kg/d in 4 doses. The amoxicillin dose is 40 to 70 mg/kg/d in 3 doses. The erythromycin ethylsuccinate dose is 50 mg/kg/d divided in 4 doses. Metronidazole is supplied in 250-mg tablets, which can be crushed and suspended in cherry syrup NF at a concentration per 5 ml of the dose calculated for a particular patient. The pediatric dose is 5 to 10 mg/kg to a maximum of 250 mg per dose every 8 hours. It is stable for 30 days at room temperature or when refrigerated. The solution should be shaken before administration. Metronidazole has a disulfiram-like effect, and the intake of alcohol must be avoided. Metronidazole interacts with cimetidine, phenobarbital, anticoagulants, phenytoin, and other medications.

MONITORING AND RESOLUTION

Response to therapy should be closely monitored. Symptoms indirectly correlate and are of value in monitoring response. Improvement or resolution of symptoms indicates that healing is occurring. Although symptoms may resolve early in therapy, no improvement may be reported until the end of a course of therapy. The precise role of histologic monitoring has not been defined. Histologic improvement can be seen after a few days of therapy, but in some upper intestinal inflammations, such as that caused by *H. pylori*, plasma cell and lymphocytic infiltration may not resolve for over a year. Completion of the course of therapy is important in preventing relapses.

Failure of therapy is signaled by worsening or continued symptoms. A failure in therapy may be resolved by a second course of the initial regimen, by increasing the dosage to the high end of the accepted range, or by using a different agent. There are no studies to guide the choice of second-line therapy. However, persistent symptoms after two therapeutic courses should prompt a reevaluation of the initial diagnosis.

New therapeutic approaches for the treatment of upper intestinal inflammation are in continual evolution. Similarly, experience in the treatment of pediatric upper intestinal inflammation is accumulating. Periodic review of the recent literature may be of value.

REFERENCES

1. Bush A, Busst CM, Knight WB, Shinebourne EA: Cardiovascular effects of tolazoline and ranitidine. Arch Dis Child 1991;62:241–246.
2. Gryboski JD: Peptic disease in children. Med Clin North Am 1991;75:889–902.

ACUTE AND CHRONIC DIARRHEA SYNDROMES

RAHEL BERHANE, M.D.

Classifications of diarrhea based on pathophysiologic mechanisms commonly describe two broad categories, osmotic and secretory. *Osmotic diarrhea* defines a malabsorption resulting from the osmotic load created by the presence of unabsorbed, small, osmotically active particles in the gastrointestinal lumen. The diarrhea secondary to carbohydrate malabsorption is a classic example: Stools tend to have an acid pH; stool electrolytes usually show a fecal sodium of less than 50 mEq/L; and a significant osmolar gap is noted. Normally 2(stool Na$^+$ + stool K$^+$) equals measured fecal osmolality. In osmotic diarrhea, however, the product falls short of measured fecal osmolality, suggesting the presence of some other solute contributing to osmolality. Osmotic diarrhea stops when feeding is discontinued. *Secretory diarrhea*, on the other hand, persists even when the patient is fasted. Unlike osmotic diarrhea, the osmolality of the stool of patients with secretory diarrhea can be accounted for by normal ionic constituents. Classically, secretory diarrheas are mediated by vasoactive intestinal peptide (VIP)–secreting tumors, such as ganglioneuromas. Bacterial enterotoxins (such as those of *Vibrio cholerae* or *Escherichia coli*) and congenital disorders of electrolyte transport (such as congenital chloridorrhea) also may produce secretory diarrhea.

Unfortunately, most acute and chronic diarrhea syndromes do not lend themselves to classification into these simple categories. In many conditions, both secretory and osmotic mechanisms may be involved. For example, inflammatory diarrheas of the small bowel have a secretory component driven by prostaglandins and other mediators, as well as an osmotic component as a result of loss of brush border enzymes involved in disaccharide hydrolysis. The classification in Figure 1 provides an alternative, practical algorithm by which most diarrhea syndromes in pediatrics can be approached.

ACUTE DIARRHEA

The duration of acute diarrhea is arbitrarily defined at less than 2 weeks and often is considerably shorter. Most often, acute diarrhea

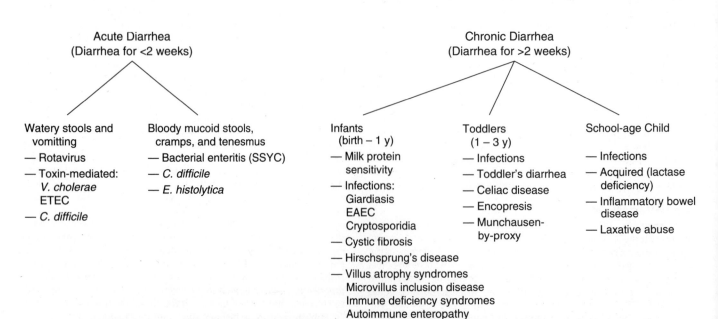

FIGURE 1. Acute and chronic diarrhea syndromes. ETEC = enterotoxigenic *Escherichia coli*; SSYC = *Shigella, Salmonella, Yersinia, Campylobacter*; EAEC = enteroadherent *E. coli*; Crypto = *Cryptosporidium*; IBD = inflammatory bowel disease.

is caused by an enteric infection. In general, viral pathogens produce injury to the proximal small intestine, causing watery diarrhea and vomiting, whereas bacterial pathogens tend to involve distal small bowel colonic inflammation, causing dysentery-like symptoms. However, in cases where toxin-producing bacterial pathogens, such as enterotoxigenic *E. coli,* are involved, watery diarrhea may be the sole manifestation.

In the United States rotavirus is the most commonly isolated organism causing acute gastroenteritis. Other viral pathogens include the Norwalk agent, enteroviruses, and enteric adenoviruses. Protozoal pathogens, such as *Cryptosporidium,* may also produce acute self-limited diarrhea with nausea and vomiting. Of the diarrhea syndromes of bacterial origin causing watery diarrhea, cholera is the prototype and should be considered when the travel history makes it relevant. Certain species of *Aeromonas* and *Pleisomonas shigelloides* may also produce toxin-mediated diarrhea.

Dehydration, the most common complication of acute diarrhea, is the prime cause of diarrhea-related morbidity and mortality. Glucose-based oral rehydration solutions (ORS) have been shown to be effective in the initial rehydration and subsequent replacement of ongoing losses, regardless of the cause of diarrhea. The basis for the efficacy of these oral glucose-electrolyte solutions is the phenomenon of sodium-glucose cotransport, by which sodium ions travel with glucose (and certain other organic molecules, such as amino acids) from the lumen of the intestine across the villous epithelium into the body fluids. The great majority of trials that showed unquestioned efficacy of these solutions were done using the oral rehydration salt formula recommended by the World Health Organization and UNICEF, which includes (in millimoles per liter) Na^+, 90; K^+, 20; Cl^-, 80; base, 30; and glucose, 111. The American Academy of Pediatrics Committee on Nutrition recommends a ratio of carbohydrates/sodium in these solutions of less than 2:1. WHO guidelines use the more stringent ratio of 1.4:1. Surveys have shown that most of the fluids used for oral rehydration by practicing physicians in the United States are suboptimal. Cola drinks and apple juice, for example, are low in sodium and have a CHO:Na ratio greater than 200. The commercial glucose-electrolyte solutions, such as Pedialyte and Rehydralyte, are closer to the recommended composition and should be used whenever possible.

For mild dehydration (slightly dry buccal membranes and increased thirst), 50 ml/kg of oral rehydration solution should be administered in the first 4 hours to replace the deficit. Ongoing losses should be replaced by giving 10 ml/kg (or ½ to 1 cup) of oral rehydration solution for each stool. For moderate dehydration (sunken eyes and fontanel with loss of skin turgor), initial deficit replacement with 100 ml/kg of oral rehydration solution is recommended. Periodic monitoring of the patient's state of hydration and attention to replacement of ongoing stool losses are crucial to a successful outcome. Patients with evidence of severe dehydration (with evidence of a fast pulse with diminished volume, hypotension, and lethargy) should receive initial resuscitation with intravenous saline 20 ml/kg. Therapy can then be continuous using ORS.

The glucose-based solutions, although effective in rehydration and maintenance of ongoing losses, do not decrease stool volume. This is a significant drawback, especially in the mind of the users, who expect some improvement in stool output. Recent studies have indicated that oral rehydration solutions in which rice and other food sources of starch are substituted for glucose reduce the severity and duration of diarrhea, are well accepted by infants, and result in significant improvement in mean weight gain. Research is underway to develop various food-based oral rehydration solutions using starch from cereal, rice, or corn or protein sources that can be produced inexpensively and maintain adequate stability during prolonged storage.

Feeding should be resumed as soon as the initial phase of rehydration is completed. The American Academy of Pediatrics' latest recommendations are for initiation of feeds with a full-strength lactose-free formula or half-strength cow's milk (with gradual progression to full strength). Many authors recommend the use of full-strength lactose-free formula in the first 48 hours because of the high incidence of symptomatic lactase deficiency, especially in very young patients, and the easy availability of lactose-free formulas in the United States. For the weaned child, solids beginning with readily absorbed complex carbohydrates, such as rice and wheat noodles, should be provided and advanced as the child improves. Heavily sweetened fruit juices and carbonated and caffeine-containing beverages should be avoided.

Acute self-limited bloody diarrhea is usually caused by a bacterial pathogen. *Shigella, Salmonella, Campylobacter,* and *Yersinia* are typical examples. Antimicrobial treatment of uncomplicated cases of *Salmonella* gastroenteritis is not recommended because of the increased prevalence of the carrier state following such therapy. However, patients at high risk for development of disseminated disease (immunocompromised patients, patients with hematologic disease, and infants less than 1 year of age) should be treated. Most *Salmonella* are sensitive to a variety of commonly used antibiotics, such as ampicillin, chloramphenicol, trimethoprim-sulfamethoxazole, and third-generation cephalosporins.

Antibiotic treatment of *Shigella* infections has been shown to shorten the course of disease and the time period of organism excretion. It also decreases the secondary attack rate. Routine treatment, however, may facilitate the emergence of resistant strains and should be reserved for those with severe symptoms at initial examination. Similarly, the need for routine treatment of *Campylobacter* and *Yersinia* infections is controversial. Treatment is generally recommended for patients who are very symptomatic. Erythromycin is the antibiotic of choice for *Campylobacter.* Most *Yersinia* species are sensitive to trimethoprim-sulfamethoxazole and to third-generation cephalosporins.

PROTRACTED DIARRHEA

Infants (Birth–1 Year)

The conditions causing protracted diarrhea change markedly with age. In the young infant, the differential diagnosis includes cow's milk protein intolerance, infections (*Giardia,* enteroadherent *E. coli*), congenital transport defects, and idiopathic villous atrophy syndromes.

Milk protein sensitivity is a significant cause of persistent diarrhea in infants. In original reports, such infants have had persistent diarrhea, often with anemia, protein-losing enteropathy, and failure to thrive. The histologic changes are nonspecific, consisting mainly of partial villous atrophy, infiltration of lamina propria with lymphocytes, and varying degrees of crypt hyperplasia. The gold standard of diagnosis is an elimination diet with double-blind milk protein challenge. Intolerance to soy proteins in cow's milk-allergic patients has been reported to range from 11% to 35%. This has led the American Academy of Pediatrics to recommend that soy protein not be used in the management of documented allergic reactions to cow's milk proteins. Contrary to common belief about the hypoallergenic potentials of goat's milk, there are reports showing that 57% to 73% of patients allergic to cow's milk also react to goat's milk. Casein hydrolysate formulas are effective in the vast majority of patients and should be used. However, some patients will continue to be sensitive even to these formulas. In refractory patients, switching to a different hydrolysate (whey instead of casein) or recourse to using noncommercial preparations with comminuted chicken or lamb is advised.

Infections, such as those by *Giardia, Cryptosporidium, Yersinia,* and some strains of enteroadherent *E. coli* may cause persistent diarrhea in infants. Giardiasis can cause acute watery diarrhea, nausea, and abdominal pain or chronic intermittent symptoms that include steatorrhea, weight loss, lactose intolerance, or protein-losing enteropathy. Asymptomatic occurrence where the presence of *Giardia* cysts in the stool is the sole manifestation is also not uncommon. The treatment of choice is metronidazole in doses of 15 to 20 mg/kg divided into three doses for 1 week or 250 mg three times a day for adults. Furazolidone (Furoxone) 100 mg four times a day for 7 to 10 days in adults or 6 mg/kg/d divided into four doses for children also can be used.

Closely related to this group with infectious diarrhea are those patients who continue to have diarrhea after eradication of a diarrheal pathogen. Such patients appear to have postenteritis enteropathy, a condition of unclear pathophysiology that may be caused partly by transient disaccharidase deficiency and postinfectious milk protein sensitivity. Most of the studies reporting the occurrence of milk protein sensitivity following infectious diarrhea, however, have serious methodologic flaws. Thus, routine use of protein hydrolysate formulas is not recommended.

Congenital transport defects, such as congenital chloridorrhea, generally represent autosomal recessive disorders of the chloride-bicarbonate exchange mechanism in epithelial membranes. Severe secretory diarrhea usually starts at birth. Patients have a hypochloremic alkalosis, and stool chloride concentrations are very high. With supplemental oral electrolyte replacement, patients will achieve normal growth and development. Other rare brush border enzyme deficiencies, such as congenital lactase deficiency, also may cause chronic osmotic diarrhea in early infancy.

Idiopathic villous atrophy syndromes, also known as intractable diarrhea of infancy, are the most severe forms of chronic diarrhea in infants. The villous atrophy probably represents the final common pathway for a number of pathogenic mechanisms. At least three different syndromes are defined by this category.

Congenital Microvillous Atrophy

Also known as "microvillus inclusion disease," congenital microvillous atrophy probably represents a failure of normal maturation and differentiation of crypts. Recent reports of electron microscopic findings of inverted microvilli suggest an abnormality in microvillus assembly. Usually, diarrhea starts shortly after birth and runs an unremitting course. Affected infants are universally TPN dependent, and most eventually succumb to complications of long-term TPN therapy.

Autoimmune Enteropathy

Autoimmune enteropathy usually begins somewhat later in life than microvillus inclusion disease, anywhere from 2 to 6 months of age. The diarrhea may not be fulminant initially but progresses to full-blown secretory diarrhea. Histologic study shows severe proximal intestinal mucosal injury, with villus flattening and nonspecific inflammatory cell infiltration of the lamina propria. Some patients may have enterocyte autoantibodies. Evidence of other autoimmune diseases has been reported in some patients. Sporadic reports suggest a role for immunosuppressive treatment with prednisone and cyclosporine.

Immunologic Deficiency Syndromes

Protracted diarrhea in some infants may be the first manifestation of either a congenital or an acquired immunodeficiency syndrome. Cultures for common enteric pathogens may be persistently positive. Evaluation of the humoral and cellular immune systems is, therefore, justified in the evaluation of such patients. Treatment is directed at eradicating pathogens and adjusting nutritional intake.

Other Causes

Other causes of protracted diarrhea in infants include undiagnosed Hirschsprung's disease. The mechanism of protracted diarrhea in Hirschsprung's disease is unknown, although bacterial stasis in a proximal adynamic segment with resultant inflammation has been postulated. Enterocolitis may occur in patients with Hirschsprung's disease even after surgical repair. History of delayed passage of meconium and family history should be sought. In fulminant cases, prompt decompression either by rectal tube or by a surgical ostomy is indicated to prevent serious complications of toxic megacolon, perforation, and death.

Toddlers (1–3 Years)

The infections listed for infants are important in the differential diagnosis of protracted diarrhea in toddlers and should be considered in the first stages of the evaluation. Other conditions in the differential diagnosis include celiac disease, toddler's diarrhea, drug-induced diarrheas, such as Munchausen syndrome, and encopresis.

Toddler's Diarrhea

This condition has been known variably as irritable colon of childhood and idiopathic persistent diarrhea. It is defined as diarrhea occurring for at least 3 weeks, with no evidence of enteric pathogens in children generally less than 3 years of age. The children typically have normal growth and development, although a small percentage fail to gain weight adequately because of inadequate caloric intake. The first stools of the day tend to be more formed than subsequent ones throughout the day. Several pathogenetic mechanisms have been suggested for this condition, ranging from altered intestinal motility (as evidenced by lack of disruption of migrating motor complexes in response to dextrose) to various food intolerances. In one recent report, almost one fifth of the patients with chronic nonspecific diarrhea were consuming more than 2.5 times their fluid requirement per day. Reducing their fluid intake to calculated maintenance requirements resulted in a resolution of symptoms. Other studies have suggested a role for unabsorbed fructose and sorbitol in fruit juices as a mechanism for toddler's diarrhea. Studies have shown that glucose-dependent cotransport of fructose is an important mechanism of fructose absorption, and significant fructose malabsorption was reported in both healthy children and adults when a fructose solution was given by itself. Thus, fruit juices with a fructose/glucose ratio approaching 1:1 (such as orange juice and white grape juice) are better absorbed than juices with a high fructose/glucose ratio (such as pear and apple juice). Although the mechanism is unknown, the presence of sorbitol in some fruit juices has been shown to exacerbate fructose malabsorption. Juices with low sorbitol content (orange, whole grape juice) were found to be better tolerated than those with a high sorbitol content (pear, apple juice). Careful history with a particular emphasis on the amount of fluid intake and the type of fruit juices, with appropriate therapeutic trials of elimination, should always be undertaken before embarking on an extensive workup for malabsorption.

Other Causes

Children with chronic diarrhea should be evaluated for classic causes of malabsorption, such as celiac disease and pancreatic insufficiency, as in cystic fibrosis. In the management of these conditions, particular attention should be paid to nutritional rehabilitation, with respect to protein and calories as well as fat-soluble vitamins.

Small bowel bacterial overgrowth syndromes are a common cause of diarrhea in children with predisposing conditions (e.g., anatomic abnormalities, such as blind loop, duplication, stricture, and ileocecal valve; motility disorders, such as pseudoobstruction or excessive bacterial load secondary to achlorhydria). Enteric bacteria have enzymes that deconjugate bile salts and convert them to secondary bile acids. This decreases the critical micellar concentration, leading to fat malabsorption and steatorrhea. The presence of $> 10^5$ colony-forming units of facultative anaerobes in duodenal aspirates is diagnostic. Less invasive tests include determination of serum conjugated and free bile acids. Total serum bile acids are often elevated in patients with small bowel bacterial overgrowth, and almost all of the increase is represented by free bile acids, which are normally present in only trace amounts. Measurement of breath H_2 production following glucose or lactulose load is being used increasingly. This test is attractive in its simplicity. In a very small number of people, its sensitivity is limited by the absence of hydrogen-producing flora.

Management of small bowel bacterial overgrowth should focus on treatment of the underlying predisposing conditions and correction of both undernutrition and iron deficiency anemia. Vitamin B_{12} deficiency is a concern in children because of relatively lower stores than in adults. Metronidazole and trimethoprim-sulfamethoxazole are effective in significantly reducing the bacterial count and achieving resolution of symptoms.

School-Aged Child

The differential diagnosis for protracted diarrhea in the school-aged child includes (in addition to infections) acquired lactase deficiency, inflammatory bowel disease, irritable bowel syndrome, and laxative abuse. Laxative abuse should be suspected if the social history suggests the potential for abuse, especially in the preteen child and the adolescent with a profile suggestive of an eating disorder. Lactase deficiency occurs as a normal maturational process in most of the world's adult population, with the exception of those from northern Europe. Symptoms develop when sufficient amounts of lactose are ingested to overwhelm normal colonic conservation mechanisms. Fresh yogurt may be well tolerated in affected patients, as it has considerable bacterial lactase activity. Milk with lactase added is now available in many food stores.

DISORDERS OF THE ANUS AND RECTUM

JOHN H. SEASHORE, M.D.

ANORECTAL MALFORMATIONS

Imperforate anus is a complex spectrum of malformations resulting from arrested development at any stage of embryogenesis of the hindgut. Clinically, these anomalies can be divided into three main categories depending on the relationship of the rectum to the puborectalis muscle. In *low anomalies*, the rectum has descended normally through the puborectalis muscle, there is no connection to the genitourinary tract, and meconium is usually discharged from an external perineal fistula. In *intermediate anomalies*, the rectum is at or below the level of the puborectalis muscle but is often displaced anteriorly, and there may be a persistent connection to the genitourinary tract. In *high anomalies*, the rectum ends above the puborectalis muscle, frequently as a fistula to the urinary tract or vagina. These distinctions are important in planning treatment and determining prognosis, since the puborectalis muscle is essential to achieve continence.

A renal ultrasound study should be performed before discharge in all children who have anorectal malformations in order to search for major structural abnormalities of the urinary tract. Further evaluation (such as voiding cystourethrography) is indicated if there is evidence of urinary tract infection, neurogenic bladder, or other symptoms. Ultrasound examination of the spine also is indicated to evaluate the infant for cord anomalies, particularly tethered cord, which have been identified with increasing frequency. If this study is not done in the neonatal period, magnetic resonance imaging (MRI) should be performed later.

Low Anorectal Malformations

Imperforate anal membrane is ruptured with a probe or small dilator, and the accompanying anal stenosis is treated by serial dilatations over several weeks until the anus accepts a 12 mm Hegar dilator without difficulty. *Anal stenosis* without an obstructing membrane may not be diagnosed until later in infancy and is also treated by serial dilatation. In *anterior ectopic anus*, the anus is perfectly normal but is displaced anteriorly. These children have severe constipation and straining because of the sharp angulation of the anorectal canal. Generous doses of mineral oil usually relieve the symptoms, but if constipation persists, a posterior anoplasty is indicated. *Covered anus*, with or without *anocutaneous or anovestibular fistula*, is treated by perineal anoplasty. A cruciate incision through the anal dimple opens directly into the rectum, which is then sutured to the skin. The anus is dilated for several weeks postoperatively to prevent stricture.

Intermediate Anomalies

In *ectopic perineal anus*, the anal dimple and external sphincter are in the normal position, but the anal opening is located anteriorly in the perineum. The anus is stenotic and is treated initially by dilatation. At about 6 months of age, an anal transposition is performed. The rectum is dissected from the surrounding soft tissues for several centimeters, then tunneled posteriorly and sutured to a cruciate incision in the anal dimple. The treatment of *rectovestibular fistula* in girls is the same, but special care is taken to avoid injury to the posterior vaginal wall. Boys who have the rare *rectourethral fistula* to the membranous urethra are treated by a diverting colostomy at birth. Posterior sagittal anorectoplasty and division of the fistula are performed at 6 months of age.

High Anomalies

All high anomalies are treated by double-barreled transverse colostomy at birth. Barium studies through the distal limb of the colostomy are helpful to define the anatomy. Imaging of the pelvic muscles by MRI or computed tomography (CT) may be helpful to define the anatomy and plan reconstructive surgery.

Posterior sagittal anorectoplasty reconstruction is performed at 6 months of age. The anomaly is first approached posteriorly through a midline incision from the distal sacrum down through the anal dimple, which can be identified with a muscle stimulator if necessary. The levator muscles and the deep and superficial external sphincter muscles are divided in the midline. The coccyx is removed to facilitate identification of the distal rectum in the presacral space. The anterior wall of the rectum is carefully dissected to look for a fistula to the urethra or vagina. If a fistula is present, it is divided, and both ends are oversewn. The rectum is mobilized circumferentially up to the peritoneal reflection, taking care to keep the dissection right on the rectal wall. In most patients, the rectum will then reach the perineum without tension. The distal end is opened and sutured to the skin at the inferior part of the incision. Moderate tapering of the distal 2 cm of rectum may be necessary to make it fit inside the external sphincter, but the bulbous nature of the rectum is preserved above this level to create an ampulla. The various components of the external sphincter and levator ani muscles are individually sutured together posterior to the rectum to complete reconstruction. The skin incision is closed with subcuticular sutures. If the rectum cannot be located easily in the presacral space or if the mobilized rectum does not reach the perineum, the wound is loosely closed, and the infant is turned to the supine position. Laparotomy is performed, and the rectosigmoid and sigmoid colon are mobilized to allow the rectum to reach the perineum without tension. The abdomen is closed, the patient is turned back to the prone position, the incision is reopened, and the operation is completed as described previously.

Girls who have a single perineal orifice have a *cloacal anomaly*. There are many anatomic variations of cloacal anomalies, and reconstruction can be very complex. In general, one-stage rectal and vaginal pullthrough is preferred. The urogenital sinus is preserved as a urethra. Reflux of urine through large fistulas into the colon or vagina may lead to persistent urinary tract infection or hyperchloremic acidosis. Early definitive surgery or division of the fistula may be necessary.

Long-term follow-up of children with high anorectal malformations is essential. Toilet training is difficult, and complete continence by age 3 or 4 is the exception. Bowel control slowly improves with time, but many children do not achieve an optimal result until the teenage years. Habit toilet training, dietary modification, and stool softeners are often helpful. Many of these children have sensory and motor deficits that make it difficult to achieve continence, but it appears that they gradually become aware of alternative sensory pathways, and develop the perineal muscles to aid in bowel control. Coercive toilet training is discouraged. Ultimately, about 80% of these children achieve normal or at least socially acceptable continence. Permanent colostomy may be the best solution for a few patients who have total failure of bowel control.

ANAL FISSURES

Fissures are treated by warm baths and liberal doses of mineral oil to soften and lubricate the stool. The dose of mineral oil ranges from 1 to 2 teaspoons a day in infants to 3 to 4 tablespoons a day in older children. For infants under 6 months of age, corn syrup or molasses extract accomplishes the same purpose and may be safer than mineral oil because of the risk of aspiration. The dose is adjusted to keep stools soft but not to the point of oozing. Treatment is continued for 1 or 2 weeks after the fissure heals. Vigorous treatment of fissures is indicated, since inadequately treated anal fissure is a common cause of chronic constipation and encopresis.

PERIANAL AND PERIRECTAL ABSCESS AND FISTULA

Superficial abscesses are incised and drained in the office, but deep abscesses should be opened under general anesthesia to allow adequate drainage. Anal fistulas, manifested by persistent drainage or recurrent abscess, may require anal fistulectomy. A probe is inserted into the cutaneous opening of the fistula, and with the aid of proctoscopy, an attempt is made to identify the internal end of the fistula, which is usually in an abnormal anal crypt. The fistula is opened throughout its length. This may require cutting the external sphincter, but most fistulas in children are superficial to the sphincter. The lining of the sinus tract is excised, and the wound is packed open. Complete healing in 7 to 10 days is expected. Persistent perianal disease in an older child may be a manifestation of Crohn's disease.

RECTAL PROLAPSE

Rectal prolapse is most common in toddlers and is usually caused by straining to pass a large, hard stool that overstretches the sphincter. The lax sphincter then allows prolapse to occur even without straining, and this prevents the sphincter from regaining its normal tone. Thus, treatment is directed toward preventing prolapse until tone is restored. Generous doses of mineral oil may be sufficient. Tight strapping of the buttocks with tape is also effective. Children who are toilet trained should use an appropriate size potty chair to prevent spreading of the buttocks and to provide a firm platform for their feet. As long as the prolapse is easily reducible, persistence in these simple measures is indicated, since they almost always work. If the condition is progressive or does not resolve, several operations are available, but none is totally satisfactory.

TRAUMA

Most *foreign bodies* in the rectum pass spontaneously. The most common foreign body encountered in children is a broken rectal thermometer. More harm may be done by vigorous rectal examination or proctoscopy than by the foreign body itself. Careful observation and administration of mineral oil by mouth to facilitate passage are indicated. Large impacted foreign bodies should be removed. General anesthesia may be necessary to achieve adequate relaxation and dilatation of the anus.

Careful observation after any kind of rectal trauma is indicated, since initial examination may fail to reveal the full extent of the injury. The rectum is so short, especially in infants, that thermometers, sticks, and other pointed objects may cause intraperitoneal *perforation*. Unrecognized extraperitoneal perforations may also have serious consequences. The urinary tract and the vagina may be involved. If a more serious injury is suspected, examination under general anesthesia is performed. If gross or microscopic hematuria is present, a retrograde urethrogram and voiding cystourethrogram are performed preoperatively. Rectal perforations and lacerations are repaired as accurately as possible, and the perirectal space is drained. Most patients who have major rectal injuries require a temporary loop colostomy to divert the fecal stream while the wound heals. Urinary tract injuries are repaired, and suprapubic urinary drainage is established.

INTUSSUSCEPTION

RITA LITTLEWOOD TEELE, M.D.

Intussusception is the clinical condition where proximal bowel telescopes into distal bowel. Typically, ileum telescopes into colon. Idiopathic intussusception affects babies and young children. It is most common in the first year of life. Boys are more frequently affected than girls; 1.5:1 to 4:1 male/female ratios are quoted, depending on the series. Seasonal variation in the prevalence of intussusception is likely not significant, although patients do seem to appear in clusters, making an infectious association attractive. Although enlarged Peyer's patches may be the lead point for idiopathic intussusception, they may be the sequelae. Ravitch[3] noted enlargement of adjacent lymph nodes as a result of intussusception produced experimentally in dogs. However, the association of previous upper respiratory illness with lymphadenopathy, the abundant lymphoid tissue in infants compared with older children, the actual visual impression at surgery that lymphoid tissue can be virtually intraluminal, and the lack of any other reasonable theory have combined to indict enlarged Peyer's patches as the primary cause of intussusception in babies and young children. A child who is younger than 2 months or older than 4 years of age and who has signs and symptoms of intussusception is likely to have a definable lesion acting as a lead point. Meckel diverticulum, polyp, duplication cyst, hemangioma, hemorrhage associated with Henoch-Schönlein purpura or hemophilia, lymphoma, inspissated stool associated with cystic fibrosis, appendiceal stump following appendectomy, and postoperative ileus all have been associated with intussusception.

CLINICAL PRESENTATION

The clinical presentation of intussusception is similar for those with and without a definable lead point. Vomiting, colicky abdominal pain, which is typically manifest by the child drawing up the legs, and currant jelly stool are the classic signs and symptoms, but they are not invariably present. Bilious vomiting is usually a sign of significant obstruction. The currant jelly appearance of the stool results from blood mixed with mucus. Veins and lymphatics draining the intussusceptum are compressed, and the mucosal surface oozes blood into the lumen. On examination, the baby is usually well nourished and quite sleepy between paroxysms of pain. Depending on the state of hydration and blood loss, there may be pallor, tachycardia, and hypotension. Fever to 38° C is common. If symptoms have been present for longer than 24 hours, the baby may be extremely lethargic. The abdomen may be distended from small bowel obstruction. Physical examination usually reveals a sausage-shaped palpable mass in the right upper or midabdomen. A complete intussusception may present as a palpable mass via rectal examination.

DIAGNOSIS

Diagnosis and therapy of intussusception go hand in hand. Supine and erect or decubitus radiographs are routine for babies and children suspected of having intussusception or other obstructing surgical lesion.[1,2,4] Signs of intussusception include a soft tissue mass, the crescent sign (air outlining the intussusceptum), the target sign (crescenteric lucencies associated with soft tissue mass because mesenteric fat is sandwiched between bowel wall during the invagination), dilatation of small bowel from the obstruction, and lack of stool in colon distal to the intussusception. Free intraperitoneal gas indicates perforation proximal to the obstructing lesion and is an indication for immediate surgery.

If intussusception is suspected from the combination of clinical and plain radiographic information, there are two possible courses of action. One can move immediately to radiographic performance of an enema for diagnosis and subsequent therapy, or one can use ultra-

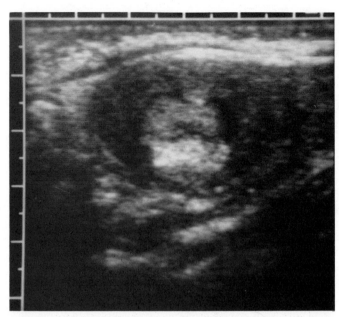

FIGURE 1. This longitudinal scan of the abdomen in an 8-month-old girl shows the typical target appearance of ileocolic intussusception.

sonography for diagnosis. The mass of intussuscepted bowel has a characteristic target appearance on ultrasonograms (Fig. 1). Authors of recent studies[5] have stated that ultrasonographic diagnosis is very accurate. Accuracy undoubtedly varies with local expertise and experience in pediatric ultrasonography.

THERAPY

Contrast enema is both diagnostic and therapeutic. In western nations 10 years ago, there would have been little discussion about the type of contrast used. Barium was almost universally employed for diagnosis of intussusception and its subsequent reduction. In China, however, reduction with air was the procedure of choice, and there gradually appeared reports of large series of patients treated thus in the American pediatric surgical literature of the mid-1980s. Pneumatic reduction of intussusception was initiated at several large pediatric centers in North America and Australia, and articles began appearing that compared air with barium. Adding yet another option to the choice of therapeutic pathways, authors from China and Korea suggested that ultrasonography be used to monitor reduction of intussusception during retrograde instillation of saline or tap water.

This plethora of choices has resulted in there being some disagreement within the radiologic ranks about the best method for reduction of intussusception.[1,3] Over the next 2 to 5 years, a general consensus undoubtedly will evolve. In the meantime, the following comments should serve as a guide for clinicians.

First, intussusception is a surgical problem. If the reduction cannot be achieved with enema or if there are complications during an enema, the surgeon is the person who is ultimately responsible for the child's care. Therefore, he or she has to be notified when the diagnosis of intussusception is being considered. Furthermore, children should not be brought to radiology without an intravenous line being placed and resuscitative efforts being initiated. This can be done with pediatric and/or surgical help.

The reader is referred to Chapter 1, therapy for dehydration. In general, mild dehydration is treated with 10 ml/kg of normal saline or lactated Ringer's solution as an intravenous bolus and followed with maintenance fluids. Moderate to severe dehydration requires 20 ml/kg of intravenous fluids as a bolus.

There are several optional measures that depend on local practice and consultation between the physicians involved. Placement of a nasogastric tube for decompression can be done. Broad-spectrum antibiotics are initiated by some but are dismissed as unnecessary by others. If given, they should include coverage for aerobic and anaerobic bacteria. Combinations could be ampicillin, an aminoglyoside such as gentamicin, and clindamycin or cefotaxime and metronidazole.

Sedation is given by many and spurned by others, and analgesia is likely more useful than sedation. If a child is medicated, there have to be monitoring equipment and personnel available during and after the procedure. Agents used for sedation include pentobarbital sodium (Nembutol) 3 mg/kg IV, repeated if necessary. Meperidine (Demerol) 1 mg/kg IM may be added for analgesia. Meperidine 25 mg/ml, promethazine (Phenergan) 6.25 mg/ml, and chlorpromazine (Thorazine) 6.25 mg/ml can be given to children who are older than 2 years for an intramuscular dose of 1 ml/10 kg to a maximal total dose of 2 ml.

Recent experimental evidence suggests that the Valsalva maneuver is a protective mechanism against perforation during an enema with air. A sedated child would be less likely to maintain a Valsalva maneuver. The use of glucagon as an enteric relaxant during reduction is not warranted, and a trial with and without glucagon showed no difference in outcome.[3]

Assuming that the child has finally reached the radiographic table after resuscitative efforts have been initiated, the following are my suggestions for the performance of contrast enemas.

1. Ultrasonographic reduction (that is, using ultrasonography to monitor a reduction as water or saline is instilled into the colon) requires skills that may or may not be universally available and should be done only by someone who is practiced in the technique.
2. When the child appears to have classic intussusception, air is the most efficacious reducing agent (Fig. 2).
3. Because the contrast provided by water-soluble material is perfectly adequate, I prefer to use it for reduction in all cases where I choose positive contrast over air. Meglumine sodium diatrizoate (Gastrografin or Urografin 76%) diluted 1:3 or 1:4 with warm tap water provides good contrast and is easy to mix. In the unlikely event of a perforation, intraperitoneal spill of water-soluble agent results in fewer long-term problems compared with barium. Many centers, however, have a long experience with the traditional barium enema and feel comfortable with its use in intussusception.
4. When the diagnosis is uncertain, either water-soluble contrast or barium can be used. For example, the subtle edema or ulceration of colitis can be completely missed without positive contrast.
5. If there is overt small bowel obstruction and a long (greater than 24 hours) history of symptoms, sterile water-soluble contrast is my agent of choice. One can use it for diagnosis and then for therapy if the intussusception is not impacted. In my experience, regurgitation of contrast into small bowel that is filled with air is much easier to document when it is positive contrast than if it is air.
6. When there is a high likelihood of a lead point in an otherwise typical case of intussusception (child younger than 2 months or older than 4 to 5 years), an enema of water-soluble contrast or barium is more likely than air to demonstrate the lead point. Reduction is not attempted when there is an obvious lead point because surgery will be inevitable.
7. Documentation of informed consent from the parent(s) may be required in some institutions, and the local policy should be followed.

For all enemas, the catheter is introduced into the child's rectum and taped firmly in place or kept from being expelled by inflating the balloon. I prefer using a 14 or 16 F Foley catheter with a 30 cc balloon. A bag of barium 60% w/v, hung 1 meter above the table, has been shown to produce an intracolonic pressure of approximately

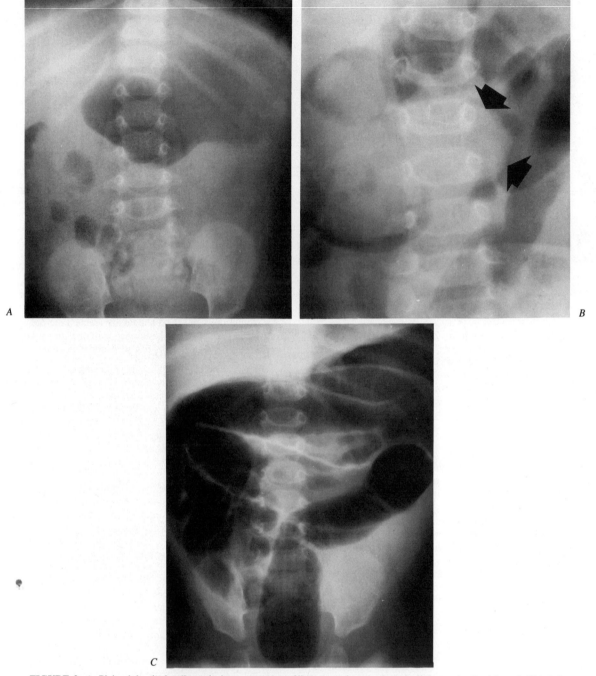

FIGURE 2. *A,* Plain abdominal radiograph demonstrates gas-filled stomach and relatively little gas in distal bowel. This baby had typical clinical features of intussusception and had a palpable upper abdominal mass. Therefore, enema with air was performed. *B,* The intussusceptum *(arrows)* is outlined by air. *C,* Reduction is proven by air refluxing into loops of small bowel.

110 mm Hg. To achieve the same intracolonic pressure, a bag of water-soluble contrast is hung at 1.5 meters or 5 feet above the table. Contrast is introduced under fluoroscopy, and the first film is taken when the intussusceptum is outlined. This documents the diagnosis. Contrast is kept flowing as long as reduction is ongoing. When liquid contrast is being used, three attempts of 3 to 5 minutes per attempt at reducing the intussusception is the traditional rule of thumb. Free reflux of contrast into small bowel indicates reduction. When gas is used, an intracolonic pressure of 80 mm Hg is maintained by squeezing

the bulb of a modified sphygmomanometer. If reduction does not occur with this pressure, the system is switched so that the intracolonic pressure can reach 120 mm Hg. If reduction of the intussusception has not occurred by 3 to 6 minutes of maintaining this pressure, the procedure is unlikely to be successful.

The major complication of both liquid and gaseous reduction of intussusception is perforation of the bowel. Experience suggests that the rate of perforation is slightly higher with air, but this may reflect the higher intracolonic pressure achieved with air. Perforation typically

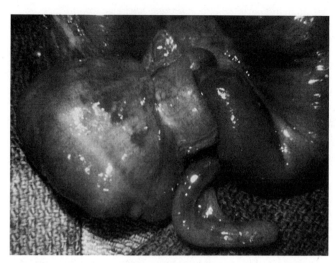

FIGURE 3. Operative photograph is of a typical ileocecal intussusception.

occurs as ischemic bowel is uncovered by the intussusceptum being pushed retrograde. Perforation with air results in fewer long-term complications than perforation with liquid.

If an intussusception has been reduced successfully by the radiologist, the child is watched in hospital for approximately 24 hours. The child should be passing stool or flatus, should be taking food by mouth, and should be without pain or other symptoms before discharge. Re-intussusception occurs in approximately 3% to 5% of patients and generally happens within 24 hours of the initial occurrence. If a child has three successive episodes, surgery is considered because of the possibility of a lead point being present.

Unsuccessful radiologic reduction is followed by operative management by a surgeon (Fig. 3). Operation consists of approaching the bowel through an incision in the right lower quadrant, identifying the intussusception, and milking the intussusceptum retrograde by gentle compression of bowel just distal to it. An appendectomy is usually performed after reduction. Unsuccessful manual reduction or the presence of necrotic bowel necessitates resection of the involved segment and ileocolonic anastomosis.

CONCLUSION

Intussusception is one of the more common surgical situations encountered in the practice of pediatrics. Its diagnosis and therapy are primarily radiologic, but surgical involvement in the patient's care should be organized when the diagnosis is suspected. Local practice dictates the ancillary medical care, such as sedation, analgesia, and antibiotics. Local radiologic experience in the therapeutic approach should be encouraged and maintained, and techniques should be updated as experience increases.

REFERENCES

1. Katz ME, Kolm P: Intussusception reduction 1991: An international survey of pediatric radiologists. Pediatr Radiol 1992;22:318–322.
2. Meyer JS: The current radiologic management of intussusception: A survey and review. Pediatr Radiol 1992;22:323–325.
3. Ravitch MM: Intussusception. In Welch KJ, Randolph JG, Ravitch MM, O'Neill JA, Rowe MI (eds): Pediatric Surgery, 4th ed. Chicago, Year Book Medical, 1986;868.
4. Skucas J: Pharmacoradiology. In Gore RM, Levine MS, Laufer I (eds): Textbook of Gastrointestinal Radiology. Philadelphia, WB Saunders Co, 1994;33.
5. Weinberger E, Winters WD: Intussusception in children: The role of sonography. Radiology 1992;184:601–602.

INFLAMMATORY BOWEL DISEASE

JYOTI RAMAKRISHNA, M.D.
KATHLEEN CALENDA, M.D.

Inflammatory bowel disease is now recognized as a common diagnosis in the pediatric age group. In fact, 25% to 30% of all patients with Crohn's disease and about 20% with ulcerative colitis are diagnosed with inflammatory bowel disease before the age of 20 years. Inflammatory bowel disease has been diagnosed as early as the first few months of life. In addition to the usual gastrointestinal symptoms, diarrhea, abdominal pain, and rectal bleeding, children sometimes have extraintestinal manifestations, such as growth failure, weight loss, anemia, and joint symptoms. The etiology of these disorders remains unknown.

Although the treatment of ulcerative colitis and the treatment of Crohn's disease are similar in many ways and the disorders have many features in common, it is important to bear in mind that these two entities are considered to be separate disorders. Hence, there are some points of difference in their therapy.

THERAPY (TABLE 1)

Corticosteroids are still the mainstay of treatment for active inflammatory bowel disease. They are not recommended for long-term low-dose treatment, however, not only because of their adverse effects but also because they are ineffective in maintaining a remission. An

TABLE 1. Drug Therapy for Inflammatory Bowel Disease

DRUG	DOSE
Methylprednisolone (Solu-Medrol)	1–2 mg/kg/d IV in 2 or 3 divided doses
Cyclosporine (Sandimmune)	2–4 mg/kg/d IV as continuous infusion or in 2 or 3 divided doses
25, 100 mg capsules	4–8 mg/kg/d in 2 or 3 divided doses
100 mg/ml oral solution	Monitor blood levels closely
Metronidazole (Flagyl)	15–20 mg/kg/d in 3 divided doses
250 mg tablets	IV or PO
Prednisone (Deltasone)	1–2 mg/kg/d initially as single
2.5, 5, 10, 20 mg tablets	morning dose; taper as per text
Sulfasalazine (Azulfidine)	50–75 mg/kg/d in 3 or 4 divided
500 mg tablets	doses; start at lower dose, advance over 5–7 d
Olsalazine (Dipentum)	20–40 mg/kg/d in 2 or 3 divided
250 mg tablets	doses with meals; advance to full dose over 5–7 d
Olsalazine (Asacol)	4.8 g/d in 2 or 3 divided doses for
400 mg tablets	treatment of acute phase; 2.4 g/d for maintenance therapy in adults; in children, 30–60 mg/kg/d in 2 or 3 divided doses recommended
6-MP or mercaptopurine (Purinethol)	1–1.5 mg/kg/d in single dose; advance to full dose over 7–10 d
50 mg tablets	
Azathioprine (Imuran)	1.5–2 mg/kg/d in 1 or 2 doses; advance to full dose over 7–10 d
50 mg tablets	
Hydrocortisone enemas	Daily at bedtime
Cortenema: 100 mg/60 ml	
Cortifoam: 90 mg/applicator full	
Mesalamine enema (Rowasa enema)	Daily at bedtime
4 g/60 ml	
Mesalamine suppositories (Rowasa suppositories)	b.i.d.
500 mg each	

algorithm for the management of inflammatory bowel disease is shown in Figure 1.

Patients with acute severe disease or moderately severe disease that remains unresponsive to oral therapy are given intravenous methylprednisolone 1 to 2 mg/kg/d in divided doses, often in conjunction with bowel rest and parenteral nutrition. Once clinical improvement is achieved, treatment can be switched to oral prednisone at the same dose. This higher dose is given for 4 to 6 weeks and then tapered by 5 mg/wk, initially to an alternate-day dose, and then tapered completely under cover of a maintenance drug. Alternate-day dosage is associated with fewer side effects and also allows for linear growth.

In moderately active disease, oral corticosteroids, such as prednisone 1 to 2 mg/kg/d, are given in a single morning dose for 4 to 6 weeks, and then tapered as for severe disease. Some patients relapse during the tapering and need to receive a higher dose. They may then tolerate a slower tapering. On occasion, this also will fail, and this is the setting in which immunosuppressive therapy with 6-mercaptopurine or azathioprine is useful. Since the average time to efficacy of immunosuppressives is 4 months, patients can be held in remission with alternate-day steroids until the immunosuppressives begin to act.

Side effects of using steroids long term and at a high dose include increased risk of infections, weight gain and striae, cataracts, glaucoma, hypertension, diabetes mellitus, osteopenia, and mood changes. When daily steroids are used for extended periods, there is a risk of growth failure that increases with time.

For distal disease, retention enemas of hydrocortisone and/or prednisolone are used. Steroid suppositories and foams are available for treatment of proctitis. In addition to these, newer steroid preparations with lower systemic bioavailability, such as beclomethasone, prednisolone metasulfobenzoate, tixocortol pivalate, and budesonide, eventually may be shown to be useful for topical therapy. Many of these are under investigation for oral use. In general, they are poorly absorbed and rapidly cleared by first-pass metabolism by the liver.

Sulfasalazine consists of 5-aminosalicylic acid (5-ASA) linked to sulfapyridine by an azo-bond. About 10% to 20% is absorbed intact from the gastrointestinal tract, most of which is excreted in bile. On reaching the colon, the azo-bond is broken by bacterial action, and

the sulfapyridine is rapidly absorbed, whereas 70% to 80% of the salicylate is excreted in the feces. Studies have shown that 5-ASA is the therapeutically active component.

Sulfasalazine is used in the initial treatment of mild inflammatory bowel disease in a dose of 50 to 75 mg/kg/d in divided doses to a maximum of 4 to 6 g/d. There is a lower incidence of dose-related side effects if the drug is started at a lower dose and increased to the desired dose over 6 to 8 days. Studies in adults have shown a 60% to 70% response rate in mild to moderate attacks. The response is seen at a mean interval of 3 to 4 weeks after the start of treatment.

Sulfasalazine is also useful in the maintenance of remission in all forms of inflammatory bowel disease and brings down the relapse rate from 60% to 70% to approximately 30%. Its beneficial effect in patients with Crohn's ileitis is not clear.

Side effects are seen in 10% to 40% of patients who take sulfasalazine. Dose-dependent side effects include nausea, vomiting, and anorexia. Idiosyncratic reactions, such as hepatitis, pancreatitis, hemolysis, fever, exacerbation of colitic symptoms, and rashes (ranging from mild to Stevens-Johnson syndrome), require cessation of use. Sulfasalazine also reversibly reduces sperm count and alters morphology. These return to normal after discontinuation of the drug. Folate absorption is impaired during sulfasalazine therapy but not so much as to justify routine supplementation. If patients receiving sulfasalazine are not taking daily multivitamin supplements, the folate level should be checked occasionally.

The dose-dependent side effects and male infertility are caused by the sulfapyridine molecule, leading to the development of newer drugs that deliver 5-ASA, the therapeutically active component, without the sulfapyridine carrier.

5-ASA taken orally in a nonprotected form is rapidly absorbed in the proximal small intestine. Therefore, delivery systems have been developed to facilitate its release in the distal small bowel or colon.

There are three groups of products available. *Olsalazine* (Dipentum) (250 mg capsules) is made up of two 5-ASA molecules linked by an azo-bond that requires cleavage by colonic bacteria before it is active. *Mesalazine* (Salofalk, Claversal) and *mesalamine* (Asacol, Rowasa) are delayed-release preparations coated with different resins

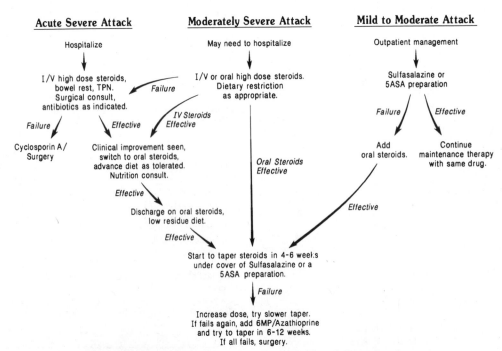

FIGURE 1. Treatment guidelines for inflammatory bowel disease based on disease severity.

designed to be released at a set pH. Asacol and Rowasa (400 mg tablets) are released at a pH over 7 in the distal ileum and colon. Salofalk and Claversal (250 mg tablets) are released at a pH over 5.6 from the mid-small bowel distally. *Pentasa* (250 mg tablets) is a timed-release preparation in the form of microgranules coated with a semi-permeable membrane of ethyl cellulose. Release occurs continuously throughout the small bowel and colon, but the rate is affected by pH. The commercial availability of these products differs around the world.

5-ASA preparations are an alternative to sulfasalazine in the treatment of mild to moderate colitis and in the maintenance of remission. The beneficial effect on small bowel disease in Crohn's disease is probably related to local bioavailability of the active drug. These preparations have been found to be equal in efficacy to sulfasalazine. The main advantage is reduced toxicity.

5-ASA is also available in topical form. Rowasa enemas contain 4 g of 5-ASA in a 60 ml suspension. Suppositories of 250 mg are available and are well tolerated even in children. Topical treatment with these can be used alone as first-line therapy in distal disease or for tenesmus accompanying more extensive colonic disease. Mesalamine enemas have been shown to be at least as efficacious as hydrocortisone for distal disease.

Metronidazole is useful in the treatment of Crohn's disease, where it has been found to be at least as effective as sulfasalazine. It is particularly useful in perineal/perianal lesions of Crohn's disease, where it induces healing in over 80% of cases. It is also used as an adjunct to therapy when suppurative lesions are suspected or detected. It is given at a dose of 15 to 20 mg/kg/d intravenously or orally in divided doses.

Unfortunately, metronidazole has certain unpleasant side effects, such as a metallic taste, furry tongue, nausea, dyspepsia, and anorexia, that limit its use in a fair number of patients. Adolescents should be warned of its disulfiram-like action. Long-term use is not recommended, since it may cause a peripheral neuropathy and/or paresthesias in as many as 50% of patients. This is usually dose related and reversible but may persist long after the drug is discontinued.

Ciprofloxacin is another antibiotic that has been used recently and seems effective for the same indications as metronidazole.

6-Mercaptopurine (6-MP) and azathioprine are the two *immunosuppressives* most extensively used and studied in patients with inflammatory bowel disease. These have been in use for over 20 years and have been shown to be safe and effective. Azathioprine is metabolized to 6-MP in vivo, and it is presumably the active component. Immunosuppressive agents are cytotoxic, destroy stimulated lymphoid cells, and thus, suppress inflammation. However, at the doses used in the treatment of inflammatory bowel disease, recurrent systemic infections are uncommon.

Immunosuppressives are used when repeated (two or three) attempts to taper steroids fail or prolonged steroid use becomes an issue. In 75% of patients previously dependent on steroids, immunosuppressives offer a steroid-sparing effect, allowing steroid reduction and eventual discontinuation. They are also useful when frequent relapses prompt the physician to look for alternate treatment options.

6-MP is given at 1.5 mg/kg/d, and azathioprine is given at 2 mg/kg/d, each in two divided doses. They are usually started at a lower dose and increased over 7 to 10 days to the full dose. The beneficial effect is delayed and is seen between 6 weeks and 6 months, with an average of 4 months in pediatric patients. Though these are relatively low doses, potential toxicity and the extremely small potential risk of a secondary neoplasm must be kept in mind. However, inflammatory bowel disease itself may predispose to malignancy, and there is no evidence that immunosuppressives increase that risk. It is recommended to stop therapy with these agents within a few years, although many patients require, or want to remain on, this form of therapy because of its efficacy.

Immediate side effects include allergic reactions and acute pancreatitis. The latter reverses completely on stopping the drug but precludes further use. Rarer side effects include leukopenia and hep-

atitis, which can occur at any time. Infectious complications have been seen, but no deaths are reported.

Cyclosporine A has been used recently for acute severe refractory inflammatory bowel disease. It suppresses various components of cell-mediated immunity. It is used when high-dose intravenous steroids fail to bring about clinical improvement in 7 to 10 days or when the patient's condition worsens in spite of them. Cyclosporine is started intravenously at 2 to 3 mg/kg/d, either continuously or in divided doses, and then switched to the oral form at 4 to 8 mg/kg/d. Absorption may be erratic, and levels may be hard to follow. Its usefulness has now been demonstrated in various studies, especially for patients who would have undergone surgery if they had not received it.

Side effects include hypertension, renal and hepatic dysfunction, hirsutism, peripheral neuropathy, and seizures. Malignancies, such as non-Hodgkin's lymphoma, can occur with long-term use. In inflammatory bowel disease, a short course of 6 to 8 weeks is recommended to allow recovery from the acute phase of disease. Cyclosporine is then slowly tapered as other immunosuppressive therapy is begun. Methotrexate and FK 506 also are being tried for similar indications, but data in pediatric patients are only anecdotal.

NUTRITION

Nutritional therapy is a very important adjunct to drug therapy. One of the major concerns in pediatric patients with inflammatory bowel disease is to achieve optimal growth. In children with growth failure, caloric supplementation in the form of commercially available high-calorie formulas/drinks is given either orally or as nighttime nasogastric infusions. Many teenagers can learn how to pass their own nasogastric tube. Nutrition especially is an issue with small bowel Crohn's disease. Up to 150% of recommended daily caloric and protein intakes may be needed for catchup growth. Those patients who have multiple surgeries with a residual short gut may need parenteral nutrition via a central line. This can be done at home overnight. However, the complications of a central line must be weighed against the necessity for such therapy.

In the acute severe form of inflammatory bowel disease, oral nutrition may be virtually impossible and parenteral nutrition becomes necessary. The enteral route is still the preferred one, and patients should be switched to this at the earliest possible time. Although elemental and polymeric liquid diets have been useful in inducing a remission in patients with Crohn's disease, they are seldom well tolerated long term. Also, they are not useful in maintaining a remission. There have been comparative studies of nutritional therapy alone versus drug therapy in which the latter has been shown to be superior.

Patients with luminal narrowing benefit from a low-residue diet. Lactose intolerance occurs in the same percentage (20% in the white population; higher in other groups) as in the general population, and a lactose breath hydrogen test should be performed where this is suspected. A suitable diet can then be instituted, providing replacement calories, protein, and calcium.

SURGICAL THERAPY

Surgery is the first line of management in the presence of massive uncontrollable bleeding, abscess, toxic megacolon, and bowel perforation. It is also indicated when medical therapy fails in acute severe disease and in cases of bowel obstruction that do not resolve with conservative management. Patients with nonhealing fistulas eventually may need surgery, as may those patients who are unable to come off steroids and are suffering from steroid side effects.

In Crohn's disease, the resections are more conservative in an attempt to save as much bowel as possible. Strictures often can be treated with strictureplasty. In ulcerative colitis, total proctocolectomy is curative. In children, such surgery is done only when all other therapy fails. This can be done as a two- or three-stage procedure, depending on the severity of illness. In the two-stage procedure, an initial colostomy is performed with defunctionalizing ileostomy and a rectal pouch, with rectal mucosal stripping, an ileal pullthrough, and ileorectal anastomosis and creation of an ileorectal reservoir. In the three-stage procedure, the colectomy and ileostomy are performed first, and then the other two stages are performed electively. An alternative is proctocolectomy with a continent ileostomy (Koch's pouch). These procedures are not usually performed in patients with Crohn's disease. It must be kept in mind that the failure rate of these procedures is 10% to 15% in the best hands. The pouch or reservoir evacuates 4 to 8 times a day and excoriation of the surrounding skin may occur. Inflammation of the pouch (pouchitis) is a known complication and can be treated effectively with metronidazole. Recurrent pouchitis should raise the suspicion of Crohn's disease. It is obviously better to undergo surgery electively when the patient is in relatively good health, but this may not always be an option. However, the decision to operate must not be taken lightly. In patients with longstanding ulcerative colitis, especially those whose disease began in childhood, prophylactic colectomy should be recommended, as the risk of colon cancer increases dramatically over time.

LONG-TERM ISSUES

The aim of treatment is to induce and maintain remissions, to ensure adequate growth, and to give the child as normal a life as possible. Most patients will have intermittent attacks, the length of the remission varying from weeks to years.

As many as 70% of Crohn's disease patients require surgery during their lifetime. Some may require surgery more than once. In ulcerative colitis, 20% to 30% of patients with an acute severe attack may require surgery at the time. Almost all will eventually undergo total proctocolectomy.

Ulcerative colitis is known to be associated with a significant cancer risk 10 years after the initial attack, and this risk increases with each decade of life. Hence, surveillance colonoscopy and biopsies are recommended every 6 to 12 months after 10 years of disease. Crohn's disease is also associated with a high relative risk for both small and large bowel adenocarcinoma. Though the absolute risk for small bowel cancer is low, the risk for colon cancer over time is now thought to be almost as high as that in ulcerative colitis.

Patients undergoing prolonged or repeated hospitalizations or surgery are often under considerable stress, as are those who are newly diagnosed or chronically ill. Because of the long-term nature of the disease, a good physician–patient relationship is important. The need for psychologic support should be recognized and met when it arises. Support groups are helpful for patients to interact with others with similar problems. Organizations, such as the Crohn's and Colitis Foundation (386 Park Avenue South, New York, NY 10016), are useful sources of patient information and education regarding these diseases.

REFERENCES

1. O'Gorman M, Lake AM: Chronic inflammatory bowel disease in childhood. Pediatr Rev 1993;14:475–480.
2. Statter MB, Hirschl RB, Coran AC: Inflammatory bowel disease. Pediatr Clin North Am 1993;40:1213–1231.

PERITONITIS

MARK S. PASTERNACK, M.D.

Peritonitis most commonly is due to bacterial infection of the abdominal cavity but may be the result of mycobacterial or fungal infection or, occasionally, noninfectious inflammatory causes. Bacterial peritonitis occurs in two distinctive settings, known as primary, or spontaneous, bacterial peritonitis and secondary peritonitis. The former generally develops in patients with preexistent ascites following transient or sustained bacteremia or transmural migration of enteric bacteria into the peritoneal cavity. The latter, which is far more common, is a complication of a primary process involving an intraabdominal viscus, with secondary leakage of intraintestinal bacteria into the peritoneal cavity. The laboratory hallmark of spontaneous bacterial peritonitis is the recovery of a single pathogen from cultures of peritoneal fluid, whereas, in contrast, secondary peritonitis is associated with the recovery of multiple facultative and anaerobic pathogens. This classification system also has important therapeutic implications, since antibiotic therapy is the mainstay of treatment for spontaneous bacterial peritonitis but is only an adjunctive measure accompanying definitive surgical repair in the management of secondary peritonitis.

SPONTANEOUS BACTERIAL PERITONITIS

Spontaneous peritonitis is seen almost exclusively in children with underlying disease states, such as cirrhosis or nephrotic syndrome, that are associated with the development of ascites. Advances in treatment of the nephrotic syndrome, nutrition, and diuretic therapy have reduced the incidence of ascites in children and have led to a reduction in the incidence of spontaneous bacterial peritonitis. The pathogens responsible for this infection are encapsulated pathogens, such as *Streptococcus pneumoniae*, which commonly establish bacteremia in young children, and Enterobacteriaeceae, such as *Escherichia coli*. Children with advanced liver disease may be at increased risk of infection by such enteric bacteria as the result of impaired hepatic filtration of portal blood, by splenic dysfunction complicating portal hypertension, or by both.

The diagnosis of spontaneous bacterial peritonitis must be strongly considered when fever, abdominal pain, and tenderness accompanied by increased ascites develop in a child with preexistent ascites. Classic peritoneal signs of rigidity, guarding, and rebound tenderness are variably present. Occasionally, most local abdominal findings may be absent, and the diagnosis must be pursued with appropriate diagnostic studies in a child with ascites and fever. Laboratory studies should include a white blood cell count and differential, as well as blood cultures. In children with cirrhosis, the development of bacterial peritonitis may be accompanied by deterioration in previously stable liver function. The diagnosis of peritonitis should be ascertained directly by abdominal paracentesis. A small-volume midline paracentesis performed in the infraumbilical region using a small-guage (e.g., 22-gauge) needle carries a minimal risk of bleeding or bowel puncture but provides important data. Aspirated fluid should be analyzed for cell count, differential, albumin, lactate dehydrogenase (LDH), and amylase, as well as gram stain and culture (routine and anaerobic). In addition to routine cultures, direct inoculation of ascites fluid into a blood culture bottle may enhance the recovery of a pathogen. If a child with hepatic failure and coagulopathy requires paracentesis, suitable plasma factor or platelet replacement or both can be administered before diagnostic paracentesis.

Empiric intravenous antibiotic therapy should be effective against gram-positive cocci as well as gram-negative bacilli. Beta-lactam agents combined with beta-lactamase inhibitors (e.g., ampicillin-sulbactam or ticarcillin-clavulanate) provide suitable initial coverage, although in children with severe toxicity, dual coverage with one of these agents together with gentamicin should be used. A third generation cephalosporin agent, such as ceftriaxone or cefotaxime, may be considered, although such therapy does not provide optimal coverage for enterococci or *Staphylococcus aureus*, two occasionally encountered pathogens. Imipenem provides another choice for a single broad-spectrum agent. Children with immediate hypersensitivity to beta-lactam antibiotics should receive vancomycin and gentamicin. The initial empiric regimen should be revised as suitable identification and sensitivity data become available. In uncomplicated cases of spontaneous bacterial peritonitis, 2 weeks of intravenous therapy should be administered. Children who have persistent fever or other complications should be considered for repeat paracentesis to assess sterilization of ascites fluid and improvement in laboratory parameters.

Long-term complications of spontaneous bacterial peritonitis, such as late intraabdominal abscess, are rare, and the overall prognosis is more closely linked to the child's underlying disease.

SECONDARY PERITONITIS

Polymicrobial peritonitis is virtually always a complication of transmural bowel injury or disease, and its recognition is crucial to coordinate life-saving surgical intervention. The causes of the underlying bowel pathology responsible for secondary peritonitis vary as a function of age. Small bowel atresia, necrotizing enterocolitis, Hirschsprung's disease, volvulus, intussusception, strangulated hernia, appendicitis with perforation, perforated Meckel diverticulum or peptic ulcer, inflammatory bowel disease, and blunt as well as penetrating abdominal trauma all may be complicated by the development of peritonitis. In general, neonates and infants with peritonitis have a paucity of local findings and may manifest distention or ileus or both, together with systemic signs of sepsis with acidosis, hypotension, and oliguria. Older children generally demonstrate the more classic peritoneal signs of (initially localized) tenderness, rigidity of the abdominal musculature, local rebound, and ileus.

Routine laboratory evaluation is generally nonspecific. Leukocytosis is usually present, and coagulopathy accompanied by thrombocytopenia may be present if disseminated intravascular coagulation develops. Blood cultures are sometimes helpful in recovering pathogens. Radiologic assessment with an abdominal flat plate (kidney, ureter, and bladder) and upright may demonstrate obstruction, ileus, or free intraperitoneal air, the pathognomonic finding of visceral perforation. Close consultation with an experienced pediatric or general surgeon is crucial for the proper timing of exploratory laparotomy. When surgical exploration is imminent, direct intraoperative cultures may be obtained. Fluid should be collected by syringe, and the capped syringe should be transported directly to the bacteriology laboratory for direct culturing of routine facultative, anaerobic, and fungal pathogens. A gram stain will confirm the presence of polymicrobial sepsis. Occasionally, a diagnostic paracentesis may be considered, since a negative tap will support continued observation, but a positive tap will mandate urgent laporotomy.

Empiric antibiotic therapy should be administered promptly once the diagnosis of perforated viscus and secondary peritonitis is made. It is necessary to select agents that are efficacious against facultative gram-positive cocci and gram-negative enteric bacilli, as well as beta-lactamase-producing anaerobic gram-negative bacilli, such as *Bacteroids* sp. Enterococci sometimes are recovered from peritoneal cultures in this situation, and synergistic therapy (ampicillin and gentamicin) to cover these pathogens specifically should be given if there is moderate or abundant growth. A small quantity of *Candida* in peritoneal cultures does not mandate amphotericin B treatment routinely. Three-drug regimens that treat enterococci as well as facultative and anaerobic pathogens include ampicillin and gentamicin together with an agent, such as metronidazole or clindamycin, that is effective against anaerobes. Two-drug regimens with comparable coverage include the use of gentamicin together with a beta-lactam agent possessing anaerobic activity, such as ampicillin-sulbactam or ticarcillin-clavulanate. Clindamycin combined with gentamicin is a traditional two-drug combination but does not treat enterococcal infections. Monotherapy with broad-spectrum antibiotics possessing anaerobic activity, such as cefoxitin, is sometimes used after early surgical exploration or in patients with mild disease, particularly in patients with unstable renal function. Children who develop peritonitis during a prolonged hospitalization or in association with neutropenia caused by malignancy or chemotherapy should receive tobramycin or amikacin and an antipseudomonal beta-lactam to cover possible resistant nosocomial pathogens. Appropriate life support measures, including vigorous volume repletion, hemodynamic support, and correction of coagulopathy and acidosis are often required in cases of advanced peritonitis and mandate intensive care.

A patient with generalized peritonitis complicating visceral perforation may have a stormy postoperative course despite optimal surgical and medical care. Acute complications may include septic shock, respiratory failure (adult respiratory distress syndrome), and renal failure. Slow resolution of fever is common and can be associated with the development of late intraabdominal abscesses. Cross-sectional images using abdominal CT scanning or ultrasound or both should be obtained in attempts to identify such collections and place percutaneous drainage catheters.

PERITONITIS COMPLICATING PERITONEAL DIALYSIS

Peritonitis is the major complication of chronic ambulatory peritoneal dialysis. Dialysis-associated peritonitis has a distinctive spectrum of etiologic agents. Gram-positive skin flora, specifically staphylococci (coagulase-negative and coagulase-positive, e.g., *S. aureus*), streptococci, and diphtheroids *(Corynebacterium)* predominate, with gram-negative bacilli, including *Pseudomonas aeruginosa,* occurring less frequently, and fungi, specifically *Candida,* occurring occasionally. The diagnosis should be considered when peritoneal dialysis patients complain of abdominal pain and tenderness, with or without nausea, vomiting, and diarrhea. Fever is only variably present.

Cloudy dialysis drainage, even without symptoms, should be considered peritonitis until proven otherwise by negative cell counts and cultures. Analysis of dialysis fluid usually confirms leukocytosis (often $>500/mm^3$), although cultures may be negative in about one tenth of cases. Blood cultures generally are not helpful in this setting. Antibiotics frequently can be administered in the peritoneal dialysis fluid via the existing dialysis catheter, obviating the need for additional intravenous therapy. Initial empiric treatment with vancomycin and gentamicin may be modified once a pathogen is identified and sensitivity data become available. If initial cultures are negative and the child is improving, empiric therapy should be continued. Therapy should be continued for 2 weeks. If symptoms persist despite initial therapy, cultures for fungi and mycobacteria should be obtained. Removal of the percutaneous dialysis catheter must be considered if there is significant tunnel or exit site infection, fungal or mycobacterial infection, or medical failure, with relapsing bacterial infection despite appropriate therapy.

PERITONITIS COMPLICATING VENTRICULOPERITONEAL SHUNTS

Children with ventriculoperitoneal (VP) shunt infections usually come to medical attention because of headache, fever, or alterations in mental status due either to meningitis or increased intracranial pressure caused by shunt dysfunction. A minority of patients with VP shunt infections present instead with abdominal symptoms, such as localized abdominal pain, nausea, and vomiting, and findings of localized tenderness, distention, or even frank peritoneal signs. The differential diagnosis must include a coincidental process, such as appendicitis, catheter-induced intestinal perforation, and VP shunt infection with associated peritonitis.

Cross-sectional abdominal imaging may define a localized collection of infected cerebrospinal fluid or a localized intestinal perforation, which can be helpful in confirming a specific diagnosis. A shunt tap usually confirms VP shunt infection, with evidence of cerebrospinal fluid pleocytosis, hypoglycorrhachia, and elevated protein. Gram stain of the cerebrospinal fluid is positive in only a minority of cases. Culture usually recovers skin flora (coagulase-negative staphylococci and corynebacteria) or, occasionally, polymicrobial enteric flora if intestinal perforation has occurred.

Combined surgical and medical therapy involving removal of the infected shunt system, placement of a ventricular drain to control intracranial pressure, and parenteral antibiotic therapy is required. Vancomycin and gentamicin are administered empirically until a pathogen is identified and its sensitivities are known. Ventricular fluid can be monitored serially for cell count, chemistries, and culture to document sterilization. A new complete internal drainage system can be inserted 5 to 7 days after sterilization of cerebrospinal fluid. Intestinal perforation by a VP catheter does not generally require intestinal resection, but drainage of a localized abscess may be necessary.

MALABSORPTIVE DISORDERS

Eric S. Maller, M.D.
John B. Watkins, M.D.

The clinical presentation of malabsorptive disorders is extremely varied and may include generalized disturbances in growth and loss of weight or may be more limited to the absorption of a specific substrate, such as vitamin B_{12} or lactose. Adequate treatment requires establishment of the proper diagnosis, for example, identification of the child with cystic fibrosis who presents with poor weight gain and large, foul-smelling stools or identification of excessive sorbitol ingestion in the child who presents with normal growth and intermittent abdominal pain and watery diarrhea.

Classically, a discussion of the treatment of malabsorptive conditions has focused on the malabsorption of specific classes of nutrients (e.g., carbohydrates, proteins, and fats). However, because many disorders affect the absorption of more than one nutrient, an alternative approach is to consider the treatment of malabsorptive disorders in terms of their pathophysiology. In this fashion, one can determine whether they arise from abnormalities of the intestinal intraluminal processes (i.e., maldigestion), from intestinal mucosal function due to injury or loss of absorptive surface area following surgical resection, or, finally, from defects in the transport of absorbed nutrients from the enterocyte into the blood or lymphatics.

CARBOHYDRATE INTOLERANCE (TABLE 1)

Carbohydrate intolerance is a common presentation for malabsorptive disorders in children and may be due to the ingestion of poorly absorbed sugars or to disorders of both the intraluminal and the mucosal phase of digestion. Transient mucosal injury following a viral gastroenteritis or *Giardia* infestation commonly results in an acquired lactose intolerance. Symptoms may be short-lived, resolving over several days, or they may persist for several weeks or even months in the case of a resolving gluten-sensitive enteropathy *(celiac disease)*, depending on the extent of mucosal injury.

Treatment includes the short-term exclusion or decrease in the intake of lactose-containing foods. Alternatively, this may be achieved through the use of several newly developed formulations that contain glucose polymers derived from either corn or rice. These polymers have proved to be well tolerated in oral rehydration solutions and in infant formulas, providing both a reduced osmotic load and effective absorption. Late-onset lactase deficiency is the rule in most of the world's adult population, occurring in childhood typically after 5 to 6 years of age in white children and after 3 to 5 years of age in other selected populations, including black and Asian children. A commercial lactase enzyme preparation may be added to milk or sprinkled on food, and this will typically result in a 70% to 90% reduction in the lactose content. A prehydrolyzed, lactose-reduced milk is commercially available. Individuals with lactose intolerance often are able to tolerate yogurt with active cultures without symptoms, as the bacteria in the yogurt produce an enzyme that survives passage through the stomach to remain active in the intestine.

TABLE 1. Treatment of Malabsorptive Disorders

DISORDER	TREATMENT
Carbohydrate Intolerance	
Monosaccharide intolerance	
Congenital glucose-galactose malabsorption	Remove glucose and galactose from diet; substitute fructose
Sorbitol- and fructose-induced diarrhea	Remove offending carbohydrate from diet or substitute juices with lower sorbitol content
Disaccharide intolerance	
Lactase deficiency	Remove lactose from diet; add commercial lactase to milk; take commercial lactase tablets with meals containing lactose
Sucrase-isomaltase deficiency	Avoid sucrose in diet
Polysaccharide	
Amylase deficiency (congenital or secondary to pancreatic damage)	Avoid starch in diet
Fat Malabsorption	
Bile salt insufficiency (e.g., cholestasis, terminal ileal resection or dysfunction; primary bile acid malabsorption)	Low-fat diet; medium-chain triglyceride and fat-soluble vitamins A, D, E, K supplementation
Exocrine pancreatic insufficiency (e.g., cystic fibrosis, Shwachman syndrome, chronic pancreatitis)	Pancreatic enzyme replacement (enteric-coated or high lipase preparation or both) with H_2-blocker therapy; fat-soluble vitamin supplements; protein-calorie supplements
Intestinal lymphangiectasia	Medium-chain triglyceride and fat-soluble vitamin supplementation; low-fat diet
Abetalipoproteinemia	Treatment as for lymphangiectasia; vitamin E supplementation, parenterally or as oral alpha-tocopherol polyethylene glycol succinate—1000
Congenital lipase deficiency	Treatment as for exocrine pancreatic insufficiency
Selected Common Disorders Causing Mucosal Injury or Insufficient Absorptive Surface	
Celiac disease	Gluten-free diet; lactose-free diet until mucosal healing
Inflammatory bowel disease	Anti-inflammatory/immunosuppressive therapy; elemental enteral or possibly parenteral caloric supplementation
Short-bowel syndrome	Treat bacterial overgrowth with antibiotics; medium-chain triglycerides if extensive ileal resection; enteral or parenteral caloric supplementation
Bacterial overgrowth	Treat with appropriate antibiotics (e.g., trimethoprim-sulfamethoxazole, neomycin)
Parasitic infestation (e.g., *Giardia*)	Treat with metronidazole or other antiprotozoal drug; lactose-free diet if symptomatic
Specific Micronutrient Malabsorption	
Acrodermatitis enteropathica (zinc)	Zinc supplementation
Vitamin B_{12} malabsorption	Vitamin B_{12} supplementation usually parenteral; diagnose and treat any vitamin B_{12}-ingesting tapeworm (e.g., *Diphyllobothrium latum*)

Sucrase-isomaltase deficiency is present at birth, and mucosal function is otherwise normal. It may become apparent clinically later in infancy, coinciding with the introduction of sucrose-containing foods, such as fruits and fruit juices. Restriction of sucrose results in an amelioration of symptoms, which also occurs with increasing age probably as a result of adaptation of the colonic bacterial flora and changes in colonic function.

In infancy and with toddlers who are growing well, the most common cause of carbohydrate intolerance is the ingestion of large amounts of the poorly absorbed or nonmetabolizable carbohydrates fructose, and sorbitol. Symptoms result from an osmotic diarrhea. These sugars are commonly used to sweeten many foods and soft drinks. They are commonly found in fruit juices, purees, and sugar-free gum. Treatment focuses on decreasing the intake of carbohydrate-containing beverages or substituting foods with lower quantities of the offending sugar. Table 2 lists some common juices and their sorbitol and other carbohydrate content.

Glucose-galactose malabsorption and primary lactase deficiency are rare conditions but are of interest because they are due to congenital defects in specific transport and hydrolysis systems. These conditions are treated by removal of the specific sugar. Carbohydrate-free formulas are available for infants with profound carbohydrate intolerance and should never be used without providing a carbohydrate source, either orally or intravenously.

FAT MALABSORPTION (TABLE 1)

Fat malabsorption may occur in a wide variety of conditions, as fat digestion involves all phases of the digestive process: intraluminal, mucosal, and transport events. Intraluminal causes of fat malabsorption characteristically affect lipolysis and the micellar solubilization of nutrient lipids. Examples of this type of abnormality include pancreatic insufficiency due to cystic fibrosis or, less commonly, recurrent pancreatitis and the Shwachman syndrome.

These disorders may be treated effectively with pancreatic enzyme replacement therapy. The efficacy of treatment may be improved by the use of enteric-coated microspheres and, occasionally, reduction of gastric acid secretion with H_2-receptor blockers. Decreased intraluminal bile acid concentration occurs with cholestatic liver disease and ileal resection. Loss of the ileocecal valve compounds the problem by often leading to bacterial overgrowth of the small bowel and deconjugation of the bile salts. These disorders often result in selective deficiencies of the lipid-soluble vitamins, A, D, E, and K. Children with these disorders and all others with significant fat malabsorption should receive fat-soluble vitamin supplementation.

Vitamin E replacement is often the most difficult and, when inadequate, leads to a syndrome of progressive neuromuscular dysfunction. Adequate vitamin E replacement therapy may be achieved by the use of a water-soluble preparation of vitamin E, alpha-tocopheral polyethylene glycol succinate—1000 (TPGS), 25 IU/kg/d.

The liquid preparation of *vitamin D₂* (ergocalciferol) (1000 to 2000 U/d) is usually effective. If signs of vitamin D deficiency persist, the more potent 25- and 1,25-hydroxyvitamin D_3 products (calcifediol and calcitriol, respectively) also may be used.

Menadiol, a water-soluble preparation of vitamin K, is available in 5-mg tablets, and one-half tablet every other day with feeding is usually sufficient. Measurement of the prothrombin time can be used as an indicator of the adequacy of vitamin K replacement.

Vitamin A deficiency is the most difficult to recognize clinically, but it can be confirmed through the use of serum levels. Deficiencies are treated with replacement doses of 5000 to 10,000 U/d. To avoid toxicity, the adequacy of therapy should be evaluated by obtaining serum levels.

An abnormal intraluminal environment due to bacterial overgrowth results in low bile acid concentrations caused by the deconjugation of bile acids, which also may produce a secondary intestinal mucosal injury. Treatment is aimed at identification of the bacterial etiologies

TABLE 2. Carbohydrate Content and Osmolality of Fruit Juices

JUICE	CARBOHYDRATE (g/dl)				OSM/kg OF WATER
	FRUCTOSE	GLUCOSE	SUCROSE	SORBITOL	
Apple	6.2	2.7	1.2	0.5	638
Grape	7.5	7.1			1030
Pear	6.4	2.3	0.9	2.0	764
2% Sorbitol				2.0	142

From Hyams JS, Etienne NL, Leichtner AM, Theuer RC: Carbohydrate malabsorption following fruit juice ingestion in young children. Pediatrics 1988; 82:64–68.

and correction of any underlying motility disturbance or obstructed blind loop, which may have contributed to the overgrowth.

NET PROTEIN MALABSORPTION (TABLE 1)

Net protein malabsorption rarely, if ever, occurs in isolation. It may occur with fat malabsorption and disorders of pancreatic insufficiency. More commonly, it occurs in the setting of protein-losing enteropathy due to primary intestinal lymphangiectasia, small intestinal mucosal injury secondary to a variety of causes, including celiac disease, extensive Crohn's disease, eosinophilic gastroenteropathy, or severe infectious enteritis, especially in the infant. Additionally, any disorder that increases vascular back pressure into the hepatic venous and, hence, the portal venous system draining the intestine (e.g., constrictive pericarditis, congestive heart failure [especially right-sided], or hepatic venous or inferior vena cava obstruction due to a congenital web or malignancy) can result in secondary intestinal lymphangiectasia and protein malabsorption and loss into the stool.

Therapy centers on treating and correcting the underlying heart disease or vascular obstructive lesion, if possible, or healing the mucosal injury by using anti-inflammatory or immunosuppressive therapy (or both) in Crohn's disease and a gluten-free diet in celiac disease. Supplementation of calories with use of a medium-chain triglyceride supplement and a diet low in long-chain fat in the case of primary or secondary lymphangiectasia bypasses the need for intact lacteal and lymphatic function and results in improved nutrition and immune function.

MALABSORPTION SECONDARY TO DECREASE IN INTESTINAL SURFACE AREA (TABLE 1)

Finally, the malabsorptive processes that arise from a decrease in intestinal surface area and injury to the mucosa, such as celiac disease, small bowel resection, or extensive small bowel involvement secondary to inflammatory processes (e.g., Crohn's disease), may result in insufficient intestinal surface area to permit effective nutrient absorption or the maintenance of adequate fluid and electrolyte homeostasis. Celiac disease, or gluten-sensitive enteropathy, is a condition resulting from an immune-mediated injury in response to the presence in the diet of the gliadin fraction of gluten. This fraction is found in grains, such as wheat, barley, oats, and rye, and the disease is a specific diagnosis that requires a lifelong gluten-free diet. Many commercial substitutes for gluten-containing foods are available, as are cookbooks containing gluten-free recipes. Considerable knowledge and useful information may be obtained through national and local celiac disease organizations.

Inflammatory bowel disease, specifically Crohn's disease, requires targeted therapies to suppress the inflammatory response. These include immunosuppressant medications, such as prednisone, azathioprine, or cyclosporine, and other agents, including sulfasalazine and the newer 5-aminosalicylate derivatives. Nutritional rehabilitation of the patient is an important adjunct to these medications and often is necessary to ensure adequate growth and to ameliorate the inflammatory process.

In some malabsorptive conditions, particularly when adequate oral intake cannot be maintained, or in patients with severe mucosal injury or reduced surface area as the result of small bowel resection, enteral feeding administered by a nasogastric or a gastrostomy tube is an important adjunct to therapy. The selection of an appropriate formulation for the infant or child is based in part on the etiology of the malabsorptive condition. The normal progression is from blenderized to polymeric and then chemically defined or modular specialized formulas.

When normal growth is unable to be maintained by enteral feeding, total parenteral nutrition (TPN) may be necessary. Home parenteral nutrition is now an established form of treatment. A permanent central venous catheter can be surgically inserted and then used safely at home after a formal education and training program. The most effective care for children in home programs is achieved in conjunction with an experienced center able to provide adequate support services, including trained physicians, nurses, pharmacists, and nutritionists. The distribution of formulas, TPN solutions, and other supplies has been simplified by the emergence of a number of excellent national and regional companies. These companies may be able to provide home evaluation and nursing support so that a number of children can receive their nutritional therapy at night and continue their regular activities during the day.

It should be noted that it is often possible to use enteral feeding administered continuously at night either by nasogastric or gastrostomy feeding. This method is recommended over parenteral feeding because it is associated with a lower risk of complications, is simpler to administer, and is less expensive.

REFERENCES

1. Gaskin KJ, Waters DJ: Nutritional management of infants with cystic fibrosis. J Pediatr Child Health 1994;1:1–2.
2. Marotta RB, Floch MH: Dietary therapy of steatorrhea. Gastroenterol Clin 1989;18:485–512.
3. Roberts IM: Update on malabsorption. Comp Ther 1994;20(1):10–15.
4. Shmitz J: Malabsorption. In Walker WA, Durie PR, Hamilton JR, Walker-Smith JA, Watkins JB (eds): Pediatric Gastrointestinal Disease: Pathophysiology, Diagnosis and Management. Philadelphia, BC Decker, 1991;1:79–89.

PANCREATIC DISEASES

AUDREY H. BIRNBAUM, M.D.
NEAL S. LELEIKO, M.D., Ph.D.

ACUTE PANCREATITIS

Acute pancreatitis in childhood is relatively rare. The etiologies in children include blunt trauma, drug toxicity, and systemic multiorgan disease (usually a vasculitis). Viral illnesses, congenital anomalies of the pancreas, and metabolic disturbances, such as hyperlipidemia, also may cause acute pancreatitis, but up to 25% of cases may be idiopathic.

The management of acute pancreatitis has not changed much over the past few decades, with treatment aimed primarily at supporting the patient. Mild to moderate cases, with abdominal pain, epigastric tenderness, and ileus, may be managed in a ward setting. More severe cases associated with hypovolemia and shock or hemorrhagic pancreatitis, which may be accompanied by a bluish discoloration of the flanks (Grey Turner's sign) or umbilicus (Cullen's sign), require treatment in an intensive care unit. In these cases, central line placement for administration of fluids and assessment of volume status is essential. The objective of treatment is to expand the intravascular compartment by vigorous fluid and colloid administration. Administration of 20 ml/kg of normal saline (NS) or 5% albumin may be done initially. Since excessive administration of fluids may lead to pulmonary edema in these patients, central venous pressure should be monitored continuously. Electrolytes also must be monitored carefully, especially ionized calcium, which can saponify because of fat necrosis. Calcium gluconate 0.1 to 0.2 g/kg per dose (maximum 2 g) as a 10% solution should be administered slowly should hypocalcemia be present. Bradycardia may complicate calcium infusion, so bolus treatment is reserved for patients with tetany.

Nasogastric (NG) tube drainage is useful in providing patient comfort if vomiting is persistent. It is not required in the nonvomiting patient. NG tube drainage must be replaced milliliter for milliliter with appropriate replacement fluid. One-half NS with 10 mEq KCl/L is appropriate to replace gastric losses, but bicarbonate may be required if the drainage is bilious. Potassium should be added to intravenous fluid *after* urine output is adequately established, since acute tubular necrosis may occur in association with hypovolemic shock. Blood glucose must be monitored closely as hyperglycemia can occur. Hypomagnesemia also can occur in these patients and should be monitored.

Pain control is essential in patients with acute pancreatitis. Many opioid analgesics cause spasm of the sphincter of Oddi, potentially increasing obstruction to the flow of pancreatic secretions. We use fentanyl citrate 1 to 2 μg/kg intravenously every 1 to 2 hours or as a continuous infusion. Fentanyl minimizes sphincter spasm and may have less emetic properties than meperidine.

Once initial fluid and electrolyte replacement is given and the patient is hemodynamically stable, focus can be turned to futher treatment of the pancreatitis. In general, removal of the offending agent is key. Any drug known to cause pancreatitis should be discontinued. If duct stones are seen on ultrasonography, these will need to be removed via endoscopic retrograde cholangiopancreatography (ERCP). In patients with systemic vasculitis, it may be difficult to determine if the pancreatitis is due to medications (such as steroids or other immunosuppressives) or to flareup of the underlying disease with pancreatic involvement (which may require more intensive use of medication). Usually, a systemic disease that extends to involve the pancreas will show evidence of intensification in other organs.

Keeping the patient NPO is crucial. Total parenteral nutrition (TPN) is given to support the patient during this period. Since TPN decreases pancreatic secretions, it should be considered primary as well as supportive therapy in severe pancreatitis. Intravenous lipids have not been shown to worsen the pancreatitis and should be used to provide substantial calories. For lengthy courses, a feeding jejunostomy through which an elemental diet may be infused may be required. The objective of the elemental diet is to provide nutritional support with minimal stimulation of pancreatic enzymes.

Because the morbidity and mortality of acute pancreatitis remain high despite supportive care, various attempts have been made to ameliorate the course with pharmacotherapy. The most promising agent has been the somatostatin analog octreotide. Animal studies have demonstrated improved survival and decreased elevations in serum amylase and lipase. In humans, octreotide inhibits secretin secretion, cholecystokinin (CCK) release, and CCK-stimulated pancreatic enzyme secretion. It also slows gallbladder and gastric emptying rates and decreases sphincter of Oddi basal pressure. Despite these promising findings, clinical experience with somatostatin has been equivocal. Small randomized studies in adults have failed to show significant differences in outcome between treatment and control groups, but a metaanalysis of various controlled trials has demonstrated a significant decrease in mortality in the treatment groups. Doses of up to 1.35 μg/kg/h as a continuous infusion have been used in these studies. At this time, however, treatment with somatostatin analog should be reserved for the most refractory cases. Other drugs that have been used in the attempt to decrease pancreatic secretions include H_2-receptor antagonists, anticholinergic agents, calcitonin, glucagon, 5-fluorouracil, and aprotinin. None of these has had a significant effect on outcome in human studies.

PANCREATIC PSEUDOCYST

Pancreatic pseudocyst may develop as a complication of either acute or chronic pancreatitis. The pseudocyst contains high concentrations of pancreatic enzymes. It may be palpable on physical examination if large, or it may be noted incidentally on radiologic evaluation after an episode of pancreatitis. Clinical signs may include abdominal pain, back pain, nausea or vomiting, a palpable mass, fever, or jaundice. Pseudocyst usually develops 2 to 3 weeks after the initial pancreatitis. CT scanning is the diagnostic procedure of choice for evaluating the pseudocyst initially. Differentiating a pseudocyst from an infected phlegmon is important, as the latter may lead to generalized sepsis, with a high mortality rate.

Pancreatic pseudocysts usually resolve spontaneously with conservative management, especially if they are associated with acute pancreatitis. Pseudocysts > 5 cm that are present for more than 6 weeks usually require drainage. Percutaneous, CT-guided drainage is effective, but recurrences may occur in up to 60% of patients. CT or ultrasound studies should be followed every 2 to 4 weeks until resolution. Surgery with internal drainage (cystogastrostomy, cystoduodenostomy, or cystojejunostomy) and laparotomy with external drainage are effective surgical options. Internal drainage of infected cysts has a high rate of mortality and morbidity and therefore, should be avoided if possible. Laparotomy with external drainage may be complicated by recurrences for the development of wound infections or fistulas. Nonoperative internal drainage also may be performed if a skilled endoscopist is available. This can be accomplished by the endoscopic creation of a cystogastrostomy using blunt cautery that penetrates the lesser curvature of the stomach, providing a communication to the cyst. The use of an echoendoscope provides direct visual guidance during this procedure. Since this represents a fairly new therapeutic modality, its true role remains to be established.

The role of preoperative ERCP in pancreatic pseudocyst is controversial. If an ERCP demonstrates pseudocyst communication with the pancreatic duct, nonoperative drainage is preferred. If pancreatic duct obstruction is identified, operative management is required. Antibiotic prophylaxis before ERCP is recommended.

The patient should remain NPO if he or she has a persistent draining pseudocyst. Nutritional support must be provided to the patient in the form of TPN and intravenous lipids. In chronic cases, a feeding jejunostomy may need to be created, and a defined formula diet may be used. Somatostatin analog has a more defined role in the treatment of a persistent draining pseudocyst or pancreatic fistula than in the treatment of uncomplicated pancreatitis. A dose of 50 μg subcutaneously b.i.d. or t.i.d. may be used initially and titrated until secretions are effectively diminished. Somatostatin analog also may be given as a continuous infusion at 25 μg/h. Pediatric doses of 0.7 to 2 μg/kg per dose have been given by the subcutaneous route t.i.d.

Pancreatic phlegma, collections of infected necrotic pancreatic tissue, also may occur as a complication of acute pancreatitis and must be distinguished from a pseudocyst. A phlegmon usually is solid-appearing on CT scan and, even if fluid is present, does not contain the clearly demarcated borders of a pseudocyst. Pancreatic infection can occur in up to 9% of cases of acute pancreatitis. Most infected lesions contain gram-negative rods, although many are polymicrobial. The treatment of choice is needle aspiration of the lesion, with placement of a drain, or surgical debridement. Antibiotic coverage should be broad-spectrum and directed at enteric flora initially and then refined based on results of cultures and gram stain.

CHRONIC PANCREATITIS

Chronic pancreatitis and recurrent acute episodes of pancreatitis are rare disorders in childhood and suggest a specific underlying cause. An ERCP should be done to exclude congenital pancreatic anomalies, such as pancreas divisum, or duct abnormalities, such as stones or strictures. The presence of pancreas divisum, however, does not necessarily establish this anomaly as the cause of chronic pancreatitis. Other causes include drugs, hyperlipidemia, and hereditary pancre-

atitis. Pain management may be aided by the use of pancreatic enzyme supplementation, which may reduce endogenous pancreatic excretion via a negative feedback mechanism. This has the further advantage of alleviating any pancreatic insufficiency that may ensue from the chronic pancreatic inflammation. Severe, refractory pain may be an indication for surgical treatment of this condition.

PANCREATIC TRAUMA

Pancreatic trauma caused by blunt injury from motor vehicle accidents or bicycle handlebars is a common cause of acute pancreatitis in children. The diagnosis of serious pancreatic injuries, such as laceration or transection of the pancreas, after abdominal trauma may be difficult to make, and elevations in serum amylase are not always reliable indicators. Peritoneal lavage is of little diagnostic value. CT scanning, especially if done acutely, may miss serious pancreatic injury in 40% of cases. A high index of suspicion is, therefore, required, and cholangiography will detect the lesion, allowing directed intraoperative evaluation. If the main duct is intact, simple drainage may be all that is required. Injuries to the main duct in the body or tail of the pancreas require distal pancreatectomy and drainage. Injuries to the duct in the head of the pancreas require more extensive diverting procedures.

PANCREATIC INSUFFICIENCY STATES

Inherited pancreatic insufficiency may result from cystic fibrosis, the Shwachman-Diamond syndrome, or the Johansen-Blizzard syndrome. It may result also from chronic pancreatitis. Treatment is directed toward replacement of pancreatic enzymes with exogenous supplements. Fifteen grams of dietary fat are digested by roughly 8000 lipase National Formulary (NF) units. The number of pills or capsules to be taken, therefore, is titrated to the size of the meal. The effectiveness of enzyme supplementation can be assessed by measurements of 72-hour fecal fat, with the dose of enzyme adjusted accordingly. Gastric acid hypersecretion may reduce enzyme activity, so most products are now enterically coated. H_2-receptor antagonists may aid efficacy as well.

Not uncommonly, a patient with cystic fibrosis who apparently is getting sufficient enzyme extract will still have profound failure to thrive. This may be due to a combination of increased metabolic demands caused by respiratory disease or fever and decreased oral intake. Supplementary enteral feedings via NG or gastric tube may profoundly improve the longevity of these patients and aid their ability to tolerate procedures that otherwise might be impossible, such as lung transplantation. Any high-calorie formula diet may be used. Pancreatic supplements are given before the feed and are dosed according to the amount of fat in the formula. If feeds are given continuously overnight, a medium-chain triglyceride, protein hydrolysate formula is recommended, since exogenous enzymes cannot be given throughout the feed.

Fat-soluble vitamin deficiencies can occur with pancreatic insufficiency states. Water-miscible vitamins (Aquasol A and E) are more readily absorbed than their fat-soluble counterparts. Vitamin K is usually reserved for patients with prolonged prothrombin times (PT), and the oral dose ranges from 2 to 20 mg/d and is titrated to the PT.

PANCREATIC NEOPLASMS

Pancreatic tumors are rare in children. Nesidioblastosis in infants, caused by hyperplasia of islet cell precursor cells, may cause hypoglycemia because of excessive insulin release. Treatment is 95% pancreatectomy, which provides excellent results if no severe neurologic damage has resulted from the hypoglycemia. Insulinoma, a more common lesion in children than nesidioblastosis, also may cause hypoglycemia and also is treated effectively with surgical removal of the lesion. A gastrinoma may produce the Zollinger-Ellison syndrome, with hypersecretion of acid and debilitating and refractory peptic ulcer disease. The gastrinoma itself may be difficult to locate, so surgical removal is not always possible. Chronic treatment with H_2-receptor antagonists or omeprazole, a proton-pump inhibitor, may reduce the symptoms of this disease. Surgical treatment of acid hypersecretion, using methods such as antrectomy, may be indicated. Vasoactive intestinal polypeptide (VIP)-secreting tumors, usually of neurogenic origin, rarely may be found in the pancreas, producing secretory diarrhea. Salt and water replacement, sometimes with several liters per day of NS, often is required. Somatostatin analog effectively inhibits secretion, but identification of the lesion for removal should be the goal.

CONGENITAL MALFORMATIONS OF THE PANCREAS

Pancreas divisum (failure of embryonic fusion of the dorsal and ventral buds of the pancreas) is a common congenital lesion, occurring in 3% to 10% of the population. It is controversial whether this lesion predisposes to pancreatitis. Therefore, demonstration of this lesion on ERCP in a patient with recurrent pancreatitis is not necessarily an indication for surgical intervention. Annular pancreas, a far less common congenital lesion, usually shows evidence of intestinal obstruction. Duodenal stenosis may be present with this lesion, in addition to other congenital anomalies. Treatment is surgical creation of a duodenoduodeonostomy or duodenojejunostomy if obstructive signs are present.

REFERENCES

1. Jones DR, Vaughan RA, Timberlake GA: Pancreatic pseudocyst: Diagnosis and management. South Med J 1992;85:729–734.
2. Steinberg WM, Schlesselman SE: Treatment of acute pancreatitis: Comparison of animal and human studies. Gastoenterology 1987;93:1420–1427.
3. Wilson RH, Moorhead RJ: Current management of trauma to the pancreas. Br J Surg 1991;78:1196–1202.

NONHEMOLYTIC UNCONJUGATED HYPERBILIRUBINEMIA

HASSAN HESHAM A-KADER, M.D.
WILLIAM F. BALISTRERI, M.D.

Although unconjugated bilirubinemia is a common finding in neonates, the level of serum unconjugated bilirubin below which one can safely conclude that *kernicterus* will not develop is yet to be defined. Therefore, an understanding of the physiologic alterations and pathologic conditions that lead to unconjugated hyperbilirubinemia in the newborn is needed. Early recognition, careful monitoring, and prompt management are essential to prevent long-term complications.

PHYSIOLOGIC JAUNDICE

The elevated levels of *unconjugated* hyperbilirubinemia noted during the neonatal period are related to dynamic perinatal changes in hepatic physiology. The term *physiologic jaundice* is applied. However, other pathologic causes of an elevation in the unconjugated bilirubin fraction, such as excessive hemolysis, certain drugs, and specific diseases, must be excluded before the diagnosis of physiologic jaundice is made. Typically, the serum unconjugated bilirubin level peaks at the third day of life and declines within a few days, reaching a normal level at the age of 7 to 10 days. Levels above 12 mg/dl in the term infant and 15 mg/dl in premature infants are atypical and may warrant further investigation. If jaundice persists beyond 14 days of age, the urine should be tested for bilirubin, and serum total and *conjugated* bilirubin levels should be measured to rule out liver disease (*conjugated* hyperbilirubinemia). (See following discussion on cholestasis.) Treatment of unconjugated hyperbilirubinemia is rarely required.

MANAGEMENT

Phototherapy is an established and effective method that is widely used to control elevated serum levels of unconjugated bilirubin of any cause. Phototherapy usually is initiated in full-term infants at serum levels of unconjugated bilirubin higher than 15 mg/dl but at lower levels in the premature infant and in the presence of risk factors for kernicterus, such as hypoxia, acidosis, hemolysis, and infection. The resultant bilirubin photoisomers are less toxic and more readily excreted in bile. The use of phototherapy is not without risk. Therefore, phototherapy should be used conservatively. The most common side effect is increased insensible water loss, leading to dehydration. For this reason, fluid intake should be increased in patients under phototherapy. Loose stools also may result. The possibility of retinal damage necessitates protecting the eyes during phototherapy. Phototherapy should not be used in patients with conjugated hyperbilirubinemia because it may lead to hemolysis and skin bronzing.

Exchange transfusion has been used effectively to reduce markedly elevated levels of unconjugated hyperbilirubinemia unresponsive to phototherapy. Exchange is indicated when the serum bilirubin level exceeds 20 mg/dl in babies weighing more than 2000 g, when the bilirubin exceeds 10 to 20 mg/dl in those weighing between 1000 and 2000 g, or when the rise of bilirubin exceeds 0.5 mg/dl/h.

BREAST MILK JAUNDICE

Breast milk feeding may be associated with unconjugated hyperbilirubinemia. The mechanism has been postulated to be either an increased enterohepatic circulation of unconjugated bilirubin or inhibition of hepatic glucuronyl transferase. Bilirubin levels increase after the fourth day of life, peak at the age of 2 weeks, and gradually decrease. Less commonly, jaundice associated with breast milk may appear during the first 3 days of life. Although serum bilirubin levels may reach as high as 30 mg/dl, kernicterus has not been reported in association with breast feeding alone. Interruption of breast feeding results in a rapid decline of serum bilirubin, with either minimal or no increase following resumption. The condition is benign, and there is no need for phototherapy in treatment.

SPECIFIC DISEASES CAUSING UNCONJUGATED HYPERBILIRUBINEMIA

Crigler-Najjar Syndrome

Crigler and Najjar described a severe form of unconjugated hyperbilirubinemia occurring in the absence of hemolysis and in patients with no liver disease. There are at least two phenotypes. *Type I Crigler-Najjar syndrome*, transmitted in an autosomal dominant pattern, typically occurs soon after birth. The serum unconjugated bilirubin levels are markedly elevated (usually above 20 mg/dl). Kernicterus of some degree develops universally, and, therefore, early recognition and treatment are required. The marked hyperbilirubinemia is due to the complete absence of the enzyme bilirubin uridine diphosphate glucuronyl transferase in the liver. The diagnosis may be made by the combined clinical and biochemical findings. The absence of bilirubin diglucuronide from bile is characteristic. Patients should be treated aggressively from early life. At a minimum, phototherapy and exchange transfusion will be needed to control the hyperbilirubinemia. As the patient matures, phototherapy becomes less effective. The use of heme oxygenase inhibitors has been suggested recently. Short-term treatment with a heme oxygenase inhibitor has been shown to reduce the requirement for phototherapy and decrease serum bilirubin levels in patients with Crigler-Najjar syndrome. However, this needs to be studied further. Liver transplantation should be an early consideration in these patients. In the future, gene therapy or hepatocyte transfer may be used to supply the missing enzyme to affected patients.

Type II Crigler-Najjar syndrome, usually a less severe clinical condition, is transmitted in an autosomal recessive pattern. Lower serum levels of unconjugated hyperbilirubinemia (usually between 6 and 20 mg/dl) are found. Phenobarbital decreases serum bilirubin levels in these patients through induction of hepatic glucuronyl transferase activity.

Gilbert Syndrome

Gilbert syndrome is a mild, benign form of familial unconjugated hyperbilirubinemia (possibly autosomal dominant), affecting approximately 5% of the population. Unconjugated hyperbilirubinemia is noted after the neonatal period. The onset is usually after puberty. The total serum bilirubin level is typically less than 3 mg/dl, although levels up to 6 mg/dl may be seen during periods of illness or stress. Patients with Gilbert syndrome excrete bilirubin monoglucuronide in bile. There is reduced hepatic bilirubin glucuronyl transferase activity and a decreased amount of bilirubin diglucuronide in bile and serum. There is no risk for the development of kernicterus, since the disorder appears after the neonatal period and the serum bilirubin levels rarely reach extreme levels.

Although phenobarbital decreases serum bilirubin levels in patients with Gilbert syndrome, there is no need for treatment. Patients and families should be alerted to the fact that visible icterus may be noted during intercurrent infections and prolonged periods of fasting, and they should be reassured about the benign nature of this finding.

REFERENCE

1. Gourley GR: Disorders of bilirubin metabolism. *In* Suchy FJ (ed): Liver Disease in Children. St Louis, Mosby-Year Book, 1994:401–413.

CHOLESTASIS (CONJUGATED HYPERBILIRUBINEMIA)

L. GLEN LEWIS, M.D.
WILLIAM F. BALISTRERI, M.D.

The presence of conjugated hyperbilirubinemia (defined as a direct bilirubin fraction greater than or equal to 2 mg/dl or greater than 20% of the total bilirubin value) signals any one of a heterogeneous group of disorders. Appropriate therapy is dependent on identifying the underlying disease process. Novel therapies have emerged in recent years, expanding the list of treatable causes of cholestasis (Table 1). This review focuses on specific therapies available for disorders associated with conjugated hyperbilirubinemia. Management of the complications of cholestasis are discussed elsewhere. A detailed review of cholestatic disorders and an exhaustive patient evaluation are beyond the scope of this text.

DIFFERENTIAL DIAGNOSIS

The etiology of cholestasis and, therefore, the approach to the cholestatic patient vary with age. The neonate with a conjugated hyperbilirubinemia must be evaluated expeditiously, as early intervention may be lifesaving. Appropriate initial tests may include cultures of blood and urine, viral titers (if clinically indicated), urine clinitest for reducing substances (positive in galactosemia), thyroid hormone levels, sweat chloride determination, and alpha₁-antitrypsin phenotype. Positive findings should prompt confirmatory studies and the institution of therapy when available. In the majority of infants, initial screening studies will fail to yield a diagnosis. The patency of the bile ducts must then be determined. The absence of bile excretion into the gut, as demonstrated by acholic (colorless) stools, duodenal fluid aspiration, or biliary scintigraphy, suggests the diagnosis of biliary atresia. A liver biopsy may confirm the diagnosis of biliary

TABLE 1. Treatable Causes of Cholestasis

DISORDER	TREATMENT
Hepatitis	
Neonatal Infections	
Bacterial sepsis	Age-appropriate antibiotics
Congenital syphilis	Penicillin G
Congenital toxoplasmosis	Sulfadoxine and pyrimethamine
Congenital herpesvirus	Acyclovir 30 mg/kg/d divided t.i.d.
Autoimmune Hepatitis	Prednisone 2 mg/kg/d (max: 40 mg/d); azathioprine, 1 mg/kg/d (max: 50 mg/d)
Metabolic Disorders	
Hypopituitarism/hypothyroidism	Hormone replacement
Galactosemia	Galactose-free diet
Hereditary fructose intolerance	Sucrose and fructose-free diet
Tyrosinemia	NTBC*† 0.1–0.6 mg/kg/d
Wilson's disease	Penicillamine 20 mg/kg/d or trientine 20 mg/kg/d; zinc 100 mg t.i.d.
Neonatal iron storage disease	Deferoxamine 20–40 mg/kg/d; alpha-tocopherol*; N-acetyl-cysteine*; selenium*; prostaglandin E₁*
Inborn errors of bile acid metabolism	Ursodeoxycholic acid 100 mg/d; cholic acid 100 mg/d
Disorders of Biliary Tree	
Choledochal cyst	Cystectomy or Roux-en-Y
Spontaneous perforation of bile duct	Surgical closure or Roux-en-Y
Bile duct stenosis	Surgical resection
Obstruction (gallstone, bile or mucus plug, mass lesion)	Cholecystectomy; surgical drainage; mass resection
Biliary atresia	Kasai procedure

*Experimental: dosage for this disorder is not established.
†NTBC, 2-(2-nitro-4-trifluoromethylbenzoyl)-1,3-cyclohexanedione.

atresia or may suggest an alternative diagnosis, such as idiopathic neonatal hepatitis.

The differential diagnosis of cholestasis in children and adolescents varies somewhat from that in the neonate. A careful history, including the use of drugs or exposure to other potential toxins, should be obtained. Initial studies should include serologic tests for the known causes of viral hepatitis, autoimmune markers, and a serum ceruloplasmin determination as screening for Wilson's disease. Ultrasound can be helpful in demonstrating dilatation or obstruction of the biliary tree. A liver biopsy may be necessary to complete the investigation. Appropriate therapy for cholestasis is dependent on identifying the underlying cause at any age.

INFECTIOUS HEPATITIS

A myriad of infectious agents may be associated with conjugated hyperbilirubinemia. In infants with a conjugated hyperbilirubinemia, specific antimicrobial therapy must be initiated promptly in the clinical setting of bacterial sepsis or congenital infections, including syphilis, toxoplasmosis, and herpesvirus, to prevent additional morbidity or mortality.

Viral hepatitis can be associated with a conjugated hyperbilirubinemia in all age groups. No effective antiviral agents are available for acute disease. Therapy with alpha interferon has shown efficacy in adult patients with chronic hepatitis B infection in the setting of active viral replication. Alpha interferon therapy for chronic hepatitis C infection in adult patients has not resulted in viral eradication, and a sustained biochemical remission occurs only in a minority of patients.

AUTOIMMUNE HEPATITIS

Autoimmune hepatitis, frequently associated with antismooth muscle antibodies, antinuclear antibodies, or antiliver-kidney microsome antibodies, may present with conjugated hyperbilirubinemia in the pediatric population. Immunosuppressive therapy consisting of prednisone, frequently in combination with azathioprine, can be of benefit. Relapse is common following the withdrawal of immunosuppressive therapy. The minimal doses required to maintain biochemical remission are administered as long-term therapy.

METABOLIC DISORDERS

A vast number of metabolic disorders may present with conjugated hyperbilirubinemia. Correctly identifying the metabolic disturbance is imperative, as specific therapy is available for several potentially life-threatening entities.

Congenital hypopituitarism or hypothyroidism may present as neonatal cholestasis. The hepatic dysfunction typically resolves with appropriate hormonal therapy.

Neonatal iron storage disease is a familial disorder characterized by massive iron accumulation in multiple nonreticuloendothelial tissues and postnatal, progressive hepatic failure. Although it was previously considered uniformly fatal without orthotopic liver transplantation, preliminary results of successful experimental therapy using combined iron chelation (deferoxamine) and antioxidants (alpha-tocopherol, N-acetylcysteine, and selenium) plus prostaglandin E_1 have been reported recently.

Two treatable defects of bile acid synthesis have been described: 3beta-hydroxy-delta^5-C$_{27}$ steroid dehydrogenase/isomerase deficiency and delta^4-3-oxosteroid 5beta-reductase deficiency. The diagnosis can be made by fast atom bombardment-mass spectrometry analysis of urine from the cholestatic patient. Lifesaving replacement therapy with oral bile acids can prevent the formation of hepatotoxic bile acid intermediates and provide choleresis.

Focal biliary cirrhosis is a relatively common complication of cystic fibrosis. Microscopic changes of bile duct obstruction have been seen in 50% of autopsy cases. Cirrhosis and portal hypertension develop in 3% to 5% of children and adolescents with cystic fibrosis. Although not curative, ursodeoxycholate may slow disease progression.

Galactosemia and hereditary fructose intolerance are disorders of carbohydrate metabolism. Presentation is that of an acutely ill infant or child with a conjugated hyperbilirubinemia caused by the accumulation of hepatotoxic metabolites following ingestion of the offending sugar. Galactosemia due to absent galactose-1-phosphate uridyl transferase activity presents in early infancy and will remit on a galactose-free diet. Similarly, infants and children with hereditary fructose intolerance (fructose-1-phosphate aldolase deficiency) have symptoms after the introduction of fructose into the diet (typically at 4 to 6 months of age). The removal of all sources of fructose and sucrose from the diet is curative.

Tyrosinemia is a disorder of the degradation pathway for the amino acids tyrosine and phenylalanine. The deficient enzyme is fumarylacetoacetate hydrolase, the terminal enzyme of the pathway. Conjugated hyperbilirubinemia is accompanied by marked hepatic synthetic dysfunction. Experimental therapy using 2-(2-nitro-4-trifluoromethylbenzoyl)-1,3-cyclohexanedione (NTBC), a potent inhibitor of a more proximal enzyme in the tyrosine pathway, appears to prevent the formation of toxic intermediates. Although more data are needed, this therapy may obviate the need for liver transplantation for certain patients with tyrosinemia.

Wilson's disease is an autosomal recessive disorder of copper metabolism that leads to copper deposition in the liver, central nervous system, and other organs. Typically occurring in adolescence, cirrhosis and progressive neurological degeneration ensue in the absence of therapy. Chelation therapy with D-penicillamine (20 mg/kg/d up to 1 g/d in 4 divided doses) can be curative. Pyridoxine supplementation is appropriate because of the antipyridoxine effects of penicillamine. Significant side effects of penicillamine therapy have been reported, including bone marrow suppression, a variety of dermatologic manifestations, a lupuslike syndrome, and nephrotoxicity. Should cessation of penicillamine therapy be required, alternative therapy with triethylene tetramine dihydrochloride (trientine) has proven efficacious. Zinc, which inhibits the intestinal absorption of copper, may be useful as an adjunct, but its efficacy when used alone has not been fully established. Dietary restriction of copper is indicated as well.

BILIARY TREE DISORDERS AMENABLE TO SURGERY

When promptly and precisely recognized, a number of extrahepatic disorders presenting as conjugated hyperbilirubinemia are amenable to surgical therapy. These include choledochal cysts, spontaneous perforation of the bile duct, bile duct stenosis, and obstruction of the biliary tree secondary to gallstones or a mass lesion (see Disorders of the Biliary Tree). The goal of surgery is to restore biliary flow. A Kasai procedure (hepatoportoenterostomy) may be curative for some patients with extrahepatic biliary atresia or may reestablish bile flow, allowing a period of growth before the development of end-stage liver disease (and the need for hepatic transplantation). It is imperative to make the diagnosis of biliary atresia before 2 months of age, as the success rate of the Kasai procedure falls dramatically (under 20%) when performed on infants greater than 2 months of age.

SUMMARY

The number of treatable or potentially treatable disorders associated with conjugated hyperbilirubinemia continues to expand. In the future, definitive therapies consisting of targeted enzyme replacement or gene therapy may be available for certain metabolic diseases, offering a cure at the molecular level. However, until these novel therapies reach clinical practice, management of the complications of cholestasis and portal hypertension, including transplantation for end-stage liver disease, will remain necessary in treating these disorders.

CIRRHOSIS

MANOOCHEHR KARJOO, M.D.
PHILIP G. HOLTZAPPLE, M.D.

Cirrhosis is a chronic liver disease characterized by architectural changes of the liver associated with collagen accumulation, widespread fibrosis, and regenerative nodule formation. These changes are irreversible and can alter hepatic hemodynamics, nutrition, protein synthesis, and drug metabolism.

The most common causes of cirrhosis in children include metabolic and genetic diseases such as galactosemia, fructosemia, tyrosinemia, cystic fibrosis, alpha$_1$-antitrypsin deficiency, and Wilson's disease; infections such as chronic viral hepatitis B, C, and D and cytomegalovirus (CMV) infection; and other conditions such as total parenteral nutrition (TPN) with prolonged cholestasis, malnutrition, toxins, bile duct malformations, primary biliary cirrhosis, cardiac cirrhosis, autoimmune-induced chronic active hepatitis, and Indian childhood cirrhosis.

Patients with cirrhosis may present with fatigue, with signs of portal hypertension, such as gastrointestinal bleeding and ascites, with hepatic encephalopathy, and with nutritional or vitamin deficiencies. Investigations should include studies for metabolic disorders, viral etiology, structural bile duct abnormalities, and autoimmune-induced liver cirrhosis. A diagnosis often can be confirmed by liver biopsy.

The treatment of cirrhosis begins with recognition of the cause and elimination of possible offending agents in the diet. In individuals with metabolic disorders it is critical to eliminate galactose, fructose, tyrosine, phenylalanine, and methionine, depending on the problem. Prevention of cirrhosis in Wilson's disease includes reduction of dietary copper and D-penicillamine treatment. Excess administration of lipids, protein, and sugar beyond the liver's metabolic capacity during TPN therapy must be avoided. The control of nutrition is especially important in case of protein deficiencies. Beyond dietary changes, certain disorders require other action. For example, surgical correction of bile duct obstruction and biliary atresia must be accomplished in the early stage. Control of heart failure for prevention of cardiac cirrhosis is important. Finally, hepatitis B vaccination in infants and children should be considered.

NUTRITIONAL SUPPORT

Most patients with cirrhosis have evidence of significant malnutrition manifested by signs of protein-calorie malnutrition, steatorrhea, fat-soluble vitamin deficiency, and mineral deficiency. Long-term nutritional management with appropriate diet regimens is directed toward promoting growth and development, as well as the prevention of potential bleeding and ascites. Patients with advanced liver disease may have a high fecal fat loss. Their steatorrhea is due to insufficient intraluminal long-chain triglyceride lipolysis, secondary to decreased bile acid secretion. In such patients, medium-chain triglycerides that do not require bile salt solubilization before absorption can provide needed calories.

Fat-soluble vitamin supplementation may eliminate significant morbidity in cirrhosis. Vitamin A supplementation (10,000 to 15,000 IU/d) will prevent xerophthalmia, night blindness, and thickened skin. Vitamin D supplementation (5000 to 8000 IU/d) or as 25-hydroxycholecalciferol (3 to 5 μg/kg/d) should also be provided. This prevents metabolic bone disease, including rickets, and pathologic fractures. In patients with kidney disease, 1,25-hydroxycholecalciferol 0.25 μg/d should be considered. Vitamin E deficiency results in areflexia ophthalmoplegia, cerebellar ataxia, peripheral neuropathy, and posterior column dysfunction. A large dose (up to 50 to 400 IU/d, usually with 150 IU/kg/d as oral alpha-tocopherol A) may be required. If a patient fails to respond to a large dose of vitamin E orally, intramuscular dl-alpha-tocopherol (50 mg/d) could be considered. Vitamin K supplementation in an oral water-soluble form may be started at a dosage of 2.5 to 5 mg every other day and increased up to 5 mg/d. Patients with coagulopathy and bleeding unresponsive to oral therapy require intramuscular injections of vitamin K. Correction of coagulopathy may still be impaired as a result of markedly diminished platelet count over inadequate hepatic reserve.

The patient's serum calcium, phosphorus, and magnesium levels should be measured and supplemented as needed.

In the absence of liver failure, a protein-rich (1.5 to 2 g/kg/d), low-fat, and high-carbohydrate diet is recommended. In case of liver failure, protein intake is limited to 0.5 g/kg/d. A positive nitrogen balance can be achieved and encephalopathy can be avoided in patients with cirrhosis by the use of branched-chained amino acids as an oral supplement.

ASCITES

Treatment of ascites starts with a low sodium diet of 1 to 2 mEq/kg/d (or 250 to 500 mg/d) and fluid restriction to 1000 ml/m²/d. It is usually not necessary to restrict fluid intake in patients with adequate renal output (urine output >500 ml/m²/d). About 25% of patients will spontaneously diurese with sodium restriction alone. If this regimen is not sufficient, the aldosterone antagonist spironolactone 3 to 5 mg/kg/d in 3 or 4 divided doses can be started. The half-life of spironolactone is 12 hours. About 50% of patients will diurese on this dose. For the rest, the dose may be increased up to 10 to 12 mg/kg/d 72 hours after initial therapy. Patients unresponsive to this regimen may require hydrochlorothiazide 2 to 3 mg/kg/d or furosemide 1 to 2 mg/kg every other day up to twice daily. Serum sodium, potassium, urea, and creatine and urinary sodium and potassium should be measured regularly as long as the patient is on diuretics. While on diuretics, patients are prone to develop prerenal azotemia, hypokalemia, hyponatremia, hypotension, metabolic alkalosis, hepatic encephalopathy, and hepatorenal syndrome. Patients with ascites significant enough to compromise the respiratory status may respond to albumin infusion 1 g/kg, with close medical supervision. Slow diuresis will decrease the potential of renal failure. Therapeutic paracentesis with a slow albumin infusion equal in volume to that removed in the paracentesis will also decrease the chance of hepatorenal syndrome. There are few studies supporting therapeutic paracentesis treatment in children, but it is a relatively safe and effective treatment in adults. Complications of paracentesis include intravascular protein and volume loss, renal failure, and infection.

Ascites is a poor prognostic sign in patients with chronic liver disease. There is no evidence that the treatment of ascites alters the natural history of the underlying disease. The transjugular intrahepatic portosystemic stent (TIPS) shunt has been shown to be an effective treatment of refractory ascites and hepatorenal syndrome and has a positive effect on the nutritional status in adult patients. There is little experience with stent shunts in children, but this technique may become a future consideration for treatment of refractory ascites in children.

PORTAL HYPERTENSION AND GASTROINTESTINAL BLEEDING

Gastrointestinal bleeding in cirrhosis usually results from esophageal varices caused by increasing pressure within the portal vein. However, not all gastrointestinal bleeding is from variceal rupture. Bleeding may be due to esophagitis, gastritis, or peptic ulcer disease. A nasogastric tube with saline lavage will help in the assessment of active bleeding. Patients should be evaluated by upper endoscopy to localize the site of bleeding. Sclerotherapy or band ligation of esophageal varices can be performed at the time of endoscopy. Endoscopic control of bleeding actually controls 90% of variceal hemorrhage. However, bleeding may recur during long-term follow-up, especially from gastric varices. Blood replacement should be considered, but overinfusion must be avoided. If bleeding is controlled, the patient should receive H₂-blockers, sucralfate, or antacids to control coexisting acute mucosal inflammation. If the bleeding continues, vasopressin 0.3 U/kg (maximum 20 U) diluted in 2 ml/kg 5% dextrose should be administered over 20 minutes, followed by 0.3 U/1.73 m²/min for 12 to 24 hours, then tapered. If bleeding is persistent, placement of a Sengstaken-Blakemore tube should be considered. Long-term management includes chronic sclerotherapy and shunting. A variety of shunt procedures is available for patients with extrahepatic portal hypertension. Success varies depending on the procedure.

ENCEPHALOPATHY

Precipitating factors leading to hepatic encephalopathy or coma include gastrointestinal bleeding, large dietary protein load, infection, azotemia, vomiting, diarrhea, paracentesis, and severe constipation. Metabolic and electrolyte causes include hypokalemia, hyponatremia, hypomagnesemia, and hypocalcemia, and metabolic alkalosis may also contribute. The use of drugs such as diuretics or sedatives can precipitate encephalopathy. A comatose patient should be investigated for any of these precipitating conditions. Cultures of blood, ascitic fluid, and urine should be obtained. A nasogastric tube should be inserted with gastric lavage to investigate for upper gastrointestinal bleeding. Patients initially should be kept on no protein intake to reduce ammonia production. A nonabsorbable antibiotic, such as oral neomycin in a dosage of 100 mg/kg/d, should be started. Lactulose, a nonabsorbable sugar, produces short-chain fatty acids in the colon, leading to a drop in pH, thereby reducing ammonia reabsorption. For patients with end-stage liver disease and recurring hepatic encephalopathy, liver transplantation should be considered.

INFECTIONS

Bacterial peritonitis may occur as a consequence of contamination of the ascitic fluid with pneumococci, *Escherichia coli,* and other enteric organisms. Patients experience sudden onset of fever, anorexia, diarrhea, abdominal pain, distention, chills, and leukocytosis. Asymptomatic peritonitis is seen in a few patients. If peritonitis is suspected, a diagnostic peritoneal tap should be performed. A combination of ampicillin and gentamicin should be started in asymptomatic patients if the polymorphonuclear leukocyte count is >500/mm² in peritoneal fluid or >250/mm² with signs of peritonitis. Antibiotic therapy should be started before sensitivity is known.

LIVER TRANSPLANTATION

Liver transplantation should be considered in patients with cirrhosis who develop end-stage liver disease. Once a patient is accepted as a candidate, he or she is listed for transplantation on a candidate list when one or a combination of the following conditions is present: hepatic encephalopathy, recurrent and massive variceal hemorrhage, hepatorenal syndrome, recurrent episodes of cholangitis, spontaneous bacterial peritonitis or septicemia, poorly controlled ascites, hepatocellular carcinoma, and growth failure in children. Biochemical abnormalities, such as persistent indirect hyperbilirubinemia (more than 10 mg/dl), hypoalbuminemia (less than 2.5 g/dl), hypoprothrombinemia unresponsive to vitamin K, and hyperammonemia, are other conditions under which transplant is a consideration. The outcome of liver transplantation depends on the nutritional status of the patient, coagulation factors, and infection. Fortunately, survival has improved with the introduction of cyclosporine and FK 506 as immunosuppressive drug therapy in posttransplant patients. In infants, a segment of the left lobe of the liver from a living related donor has been used with good results.

REFERENCES

1. Suchy FJ, Shneider BL: Neonatal jaundice and cholestasis. *In* Liver and Biliary Disease. Baltimore, Williams & Wilkins, 1992:442–455.
2. Zetterman RK: Cirrhosis of the liver. *In* Diseases of the Liver and Biliary Tract. St. Louis, Mosby-Year Book, 1992:447–466.
3. Zetterman RK: Complications of cirrhosis. *In* Diseases of the Liver and Biliary Tract. St. Louis, Mosby-Year Book, 1992:467–488.

PORTAL HYPERTENSION

John T. Boyle, M.D.

Portal hypertension in childhood may be classified as *intrahepatic* or *extrahepatic*. Intrahepatic portal hypertension results from cirrhosis, which in the United States is most commonly caused by biliary atresia, chronic viral or autoimmune hepatitis, or alpha₁-antitrypsin deficiency. Extrahepatic portal hypertension is most commonly caused by portal vein thrombosis (cavernous transformation of the portal vein) or by hepatic venous or inferior vena caval obstruction (Budd-Chiari syndrome). The etiology in individual patients is usually suggested by real-time ultrasonography and Doppler flowmetry. Although the anatomy of the portal circulation is best defined by angiography, information, such as site of portal vein obstruction, distribution of collaterals, and dynamics of portal flow, is of therapeutic importance only when shunt surgery is being contemplated.

Portal hypertension results in splenomegaly and esophageal varices. Clinical presentations include asymptomatic splenomegaly (with or without laboratory evidence of thrombocytopenia, anemia, or neutropenia), upper gastrointestinal bleeding from ruptured esophageal or gastric varices, or, rarely, ascites or bleeding hemorrhoids. In patients who present for the first time with upper gastrointestinal bleeding, the possibility of bleeding esophageal varices is suggested primarily by a past history of jaundice, hepatitis, blood transfusion, sepsis, shock, chronic right-sided heart failure, pulmonary hypertension, exchange transfusion, omphalitis, or umbilical vein catheterization.

Because there are few reports in the pediatric literature regarding the management of variceal bleeding, therapy is based primarily on the adult experience. It is important to emphasize that there is no consensus on management policy in pediatric patients before, during, or after variceal bleeding.

TREATMENT

Management of Splenomegaly in Patients with Portal Hypertension

Every effort should be made to ensure that a child with portal hypertension leads as normal a life as possible. Normal school activity should be allowed, with the exception of contact sports and physical education activities involving prolonged running or jumping. Often, education of school officials is required to explain signs and symptoms of bleeding.

Although hypersplenism is a common complication of splenomegaly in patients with portal hypertension, bleeding and infection related to thrombocytopenia and neutropenia are rare. Hypersplenism is not an indication for splenectomy in such patients. Nevertheless, the presence of fever in a patient with portal hypertension demands immediate and careful evaluation to identify a source of infection. It is my practice to recommend pneumococcal immunization to patients with cirrhosis and hypersplenism.

Prophylactic Management To Prevent the First Variceal Bleed

Patients should avoid nonsteroidal anti-inflammatory agents, which may cause gastrointestinal inflammation or ulceration. Coughing associated with upper respiratory infections should be treated with antitussive agents.

The risk of first-time variceal bleeding in children with known portal hypertension is unknown. In adults, only 25% to 30% of patients with esophageal varices will experience variceal hemorrhage. Therefore, the risk-benefit ratio is widely believed to be against the use of repeated sclerotherapy and shunt surgery as prophylactic therapy before the first variceal bleed. In adults, a number of randomized, double-blind trials have reported a statistically significant reduction in the frequency of variceal bleeding for patients while on chronic beta-blocker therapy. Results have been best in patients with Child Class A or B (an index of liver dysfunction based on serum albumin, serum bilirubin, prothrombin time, and the presence of ascites and encephalopathy).

The main argument for prophylactic use of beta-blockade therapy is that there is little to lose. In the absence of cardiac decompensation, heart block, and reactive airway disease, propranolol appears to have a wide margin of safety in pediatric patients. It is imperative to remember that during acute bleeds, propranolol may mask compensatory hemodynamic changes, a fact that must be taken into account during resuscitative efforts.

Patients with documented portal hypertension should undergo endoscopy at least every 2 years. In patients judged likely to be compliant, a decision to use prophylactic propranolol should be based on the etiology of the portal hypertension and the appearance of the esophageal varices and overlying esophageal mucosa at the time of diagnostic upper endoscopy. High-risk patients include those with cirrhosis, especially associated with bile duct damage, or those with tense varices that bulge into the esophageal lumen and have small cherry-red spots, dilated blood vessels, or telangiectasia on top of the varices. The French have reported that approximately 80% of such patients will go on to have bleeding episodes. In addition, gastric varices are more frequent in children who bleed. I begin propranolol at a dose of 1 mg/kg/d three times a day orally and increase the dose by 0.5 mg/kg/d up to 3 mg/kg/d to achieve a 20% to 25% reduction in baseline heart rate. Side effects of weakness, lethargy, or depression may limit the ability to increase dosage to achieve a targeted reduction in heart rate.

Emergency Management of Acute Variceal Hemorrhage

Variceal hemorrhage usually results in hematemesis. Occasionally, however, a significant esophageal hemorrhage can present as melena without associated hematemesis. Any patient who presents with evidence of significant gastrointestinal hemorrhage (hematemesis, hematochezia, or melena) should have a nasogastric tube passed and the stomach aspirated. Suspicion of bleeding esophageal varices is not a contraindication to pass a nasogastric tube. Not only is the presence of blood diagnostic of an upper gastrointestinal bleed, but the color of the aspirate and response to lavage allows one to estimate the size of the bleed. Coffee-ground material in the lavage suggests a slow rate of bleeding that would not require immediate invasive measures to stop. Gastric lavage should be performed with normal saline at room temperature. The recommended volume for each infusion depends on age: 50 ml for infants, 100 to 200 ml for older children. There is no benefit to continuous lavage beyond 15 minutes if the return is not clearing. The tube can be left to gravity or low suction and irrigated every 15 minutes to assess the activity of bleeding.

The initial management of esophageal variceal hemorrhage is identical to that of massive upper gastrointestinal bleeding from any source. The first priorities are to reestablish hemodynamic stability and protect the airway. Effective placement of an endotracheal tube is indicated in any patient with massive upper gastrointestinal bleeding. Immediate resuscitation should be undertaken with crystalloid solutions (normal saline or Ringer's lactate) given as 20 ml/kg boluses until evidence of restoration of intravascular volume is observed, such as a rise in blood pressure or disappearance of physical signs of peripheral vasoconstriction. Colloid solutions, such as albumin or fresh frozen plasma, are used only when blood loss is massive and continuous and there is concern for a precipitous drop in plasma oncotic pressure (a risk factor for development of shock lung). Only rarely is low oxygen-carrying capacity of enough concern to require emergency transfusion of blood without complete crossmatch methods. Patients with significant hemorrhage should be given nasal oxygen. Overexpansion of the intravascular volume is to be avoided because it may contribute to rebleeding. Following initial resuscitation, further intravenous volume replacement should be titrated to match continuing blood loss. The decision to begin transfusion at this point depends on the hematocrit value taken at the time of restoration of blood volume. Remember that the initial complete blood count drawn at the time of presentation does not reflect the severity of the gastrointestinal bleed because of a delay in hemodilution. The volume of transfused packed red blood cells should be calculated to correct the hematocrit to 30%. In patients with suspected variceal bleeds, it is important to pay attention to the initial platelet count and prothrombin time, which may reflect the degree of hypersplenism or liver dysfunction. Platelet transfusion may be necessary for severe thrombocytopenia. Patients with increased prothrombin time should be given intravenous vitamin K and fresh frozen plasma. It is also important to look for precipitating factors in patients with suspected variceal bleeding. Because bleeding varices may be the presenting sign of sepsis in a patient with cirrhosis, any patient with fever should be started on broad-spectrum antibiotics pending result of blood cultures.

Emergency flexible endoscopy should be performed once the patient's vital signs have been stabilized. Actively bleeding esophageal varices or observation of a varix with an overlying clot confirms the site of variceal bleeding. Endoscopic detection of bleeding gastric varices or bleeding sites unrelated to portal hypertension (i.e., acute gastric erosions, peptic ulcer) will alter subsequent management. If active esophageal variceal bleeding is confirmed, the endoscopist has the option of performing emergency sclerotherapy to stop the hemorrhage. I prefer, however, to delay sclerotherapy until after the hemorrhaging has been controlled by pharmacologic agents or balloon

tamponade if there is difficulty obtaining a clear field of vision. Sclerotherapy should not be considered a therapeutic option to control bleeding gastric varices.

Pharmacologic therapy of acute variceal hemorrhage employs the splanchnic arterial vasoconstrictor *vasopressin* to reduce portal blood flow and pressure. Vasopressin infusion may be initiated before diagnostic endoscopy if there is evidence of massive continuing hemorrhage (after initial nasogastric lavage) or recurrent bleeding. Vasopressin is given by continuous intravenous infusion through a large-bore peripheral catheter. I empirically begin by infusing 0.1 U/min and increase the dose by 0.05 U/min every 30 minutes up to a maximum of 0.2 U/min in children younger than 5 years of age, 0.3 U/min in children younger than 10 years, and 0.4 U/min in patients older than 10 years of age. The vasopressin is given in 5% dextrose in water, the exact dilution being based on overall volumes of fluids being infused. Side effects, including myocardial ischemia, arrhythmia, cerebral and mesenteric ischemia, local tissue necrosis, activation of fibrinolysis, and water retention and hyponatremia, are potentially serious.

The concept that drugs that constrict the lower esophageal sphincter may decrease gastroesophageal collateral blood flow recently was suggested by an adult study describing control of acute variceal bleeding following intravenous infusion of metoclopramide. Metoclopramide 0.1 mg/kg IV every 4 hours may be given in conjunction with vasopressin. Once bleeding has been temporarily controlled, vasopressin infusion should be continued at the dose that controls the bleeding for a minimum of 12 hours, preferably until elective sclerotherapy can be performed. Most patients with variceal bleeding are started on intravenous cimetidine or ranitidine following initial resuscitative efforts to decrease gastric acidity and secretions.

Balloon tamponade is reserved for patients in whom pharmacologic therapy has failed and the rate of bleeding precludes safe sclerotherapy. A four-lumen modified Sengstaken-Blakemore tube should be inserted only by a physician skilled in its use. A pediatric tube is used in children younger than 10 years; the adult tube is used in adolescents. In all patients, the airway must be protected by an endotracheal tube. Passage through the nose is facilitated by pretreatment with oxymetazoline hydrochloride (Afrin) nose drops and generous lubrication of the tube. Once the tube is in the stomach, 50 to 100 ml of air is infused into the gastric balloon, and the tube is pulled back until resistance is encountered at the gastroesophageal junction. An emergency radiograph is obtained to ensure correct position. Additional air is infused into the gastric balloon (up to 150 ml in the pediatric balloon, 250 ml in the adult balloon), and the tube is pulled taut and taped to a support structure outside the body (i.e., an orthopedic support bar or a face guard of a football helmet slipped over the child's head). In the vast majority of cases, only the gastric balloon needs to be inflated to control bleeding. Only if esophageal bleeding continues should the esophageal balloon be inflated. The volume of air in the esophageal balloon is determined by pressure in the balloon (measured by connecting the inflow tube to a sphygmomanometer), which should not exceed 40 mm Hg. If bleeding is controlled, balloon tamponade should be maintained for 12 to 24 hours, at which time elective sclerotherapy should be performed. Complications associated with Sengstaken-Blakemore tubes include rupture or erosion of the esophageal or fundic mucosa, occlusion of the airway by the balloon, or aspiration around the endotracheal tube because of inadequate drainage of oral secretions from the esophageal body.

If endoscopic sclerotherapy is not performed at the initial diagnostic endoscopy, it should be done on an elective basis within 6 to 24 hours after active bleeding has been controlled temporarily by pharmacologic therapy or balloon tamponade. Direct obliteration of large varices at the gastroesophageal junction is best achieved by intravariceal injections of a variety of sclerosing agents. The procedure may be repeated every 2 to 4 weeks until all varices at the location are obliterated. Major complications of sclerotherapy include sepsis, bleeding, mediastinitis, esophageal stricture, esophageal perforation, pleural effusion, and pericardial effusion. Minor complications include transient dysphagia, transient retrosternal discomfort, low-grade fever (<38.5° C for less than 24 hours), and esophageal mucosal ulcer. I prescribe sucralfate slurry (0.5 to 1 g in 1 ounce of water) for 5 days following sclerotherapy.

Emergency shunt surgery is indicated only if two attempts at sclerotherapy fail to control active bleeding. The exact type of shunt performed depends on the experience and individual preference of the surgeon. Emergency shunt should be considered the last resort because of the high operative mortality and unpredictable occurrence of postoperative encephalopathy. An alternative to emergency shunt surgery in patients with cirrhotic portal hypertension is esophageal transsection with or without devascularization.

Therapeutic Management After an Episode of Variceal Bleeding

In patients who have had variceal bleeding, the aim is to prevent recurrent bleeding. The treatment options in pediatrics are repeated injection sclerotherapy, long-term pharmacologic therapy with beta-blocking agents, portosystemic shunt surgery, and liver transplantation.

In patients with known untreatable progressive liver disease (particularly patients with biliary atresia with progressive biliary cirrhosis or patients with alpha₁-antitrypsin deficiency that is progressing to cirrhosis), a significant variceal hemorrhage is an indication to list the patient for liver transplantation. Repeated sclerotherapy is the most widely practiced therapy before transplant in such patients. Experience with chronic pharmacologic therapy is limited. Every effort is made to avoid shunt surgery before transplantation, although shunt surgery is no longer considered an absolute contraindication to transplantation.

In patients with liver disorders without cirrhosis, such as congenital hepatic fibrosis, or with disorders amenable to specific medical therapy, such as chronic active hepatitis or Wilson's disease, repeated sclerotherapy should be the first-line treatment for prevention of subsequent bleeding episodes. In carefully selected patients with quiescent disease who experience recurrent bleeding despite sclerotherapy, shunt surgery is indicated.

There is no consensus on treatment to prevent further bleeding in patients with extrahepatic portal hypertension. Although long-term follow-up is limited, early reports indicate that the incidence of subsequent bleeding episodes is significantly reduced following repeated sclerotherapy. The rationale for repeated sclerotherapy is the natural history of childhood extrahepatic portal hypertension in which bleeding frequency dramatically decreases after adolescence, presumably because of the development of natural shunts. Even if shunt surgery is eventually required because of rebleeding from esophageal or gastric varices, sclerotherapy may serve as a temporizing measure until the patient is old enough to be a better candidate for shunt success. Long-term complications of sclerotherapy, described previously, vary with the injection technique, the sclerosing solution used and the length of follow-up. In reports to date, overall complication rates in the pediatric population have been acceptably low.

A number of difficulties have been reported following portosystemic shunts in children with extrahepatic portal hypertension, including a high incidence of rebleeding secondary to shunt thrombosis and development of mild hepatic encephalopathy. Most surgeons agree with Clatworthy's observation that shunts have a higher rate of long-term patency if they are constructed of veins larger than 1 cm in diameter. Angiographic evaluation or splenoportography is essential immediately before a shunting procedure to determine the size of available portal tributaries. Theoretically, the selective distal splenorenal shunt of Warren and Zeppa, which preserves portal flow to the liver while shunting varices into the systemic venous circulation via the spleen and its distal vein, is the shunt procedure of choice to prevent encephalopathy. Although some studies have reported that other types of shunt surgery may result in minor developmental or learning disabilities or both in patients with extrahepatic portal hypertension and normal liver function, more recent studies have refuted these findings. Because of the young age of patients requiring shunt surgery and the variability of the anatomy and pathology of the portal

tree in patients with extrahepatic portal hypertension, the first priority of surgery in this patient population must be long-term patency of the shunt. The surgeon, therefore, must decide which of a variety of shunt procedures is best for an individual patient.

CHRONIC ACTIVE HEPATITIS

IAN D. D'AGATA, M.D.
RONALD E. KLEINMAN, M.D.

Chronic active hepatitis (CAH) is a necroinflammatory process of the liver persisting for longer than 6 months. It encompasses a wide spectrum of disorders that share common histopathologic features but differ in etiology, pathogenesis, and response to therapy. In some patients, the only evidence of disease is biochemical abnormalities, whereas in others, disease may progress to overt liver failure and death. The histologic features of CAH include expansion of portal tracts by mononuclear inflammatory cells and piecemeal necrosis. Bridging necrosis occurs when hepatocellular necrosis is followed by fibrosis, which may progress to macronodular cirrhosis. Because it has become apparent that irreversible liver damage can occur in under 6 months and may, in fact, be present at the time of diagnosis (even in children with subclinical disease), CAH should be considered in any child with transaminase levels elevated to greater than three times normal values for more than 10 weeks. CAH may be caused by viral agents, drugs, metabolic disorders, and autoimmune processes. Prompt diagnosis is imperative to remove the offending drug or to suppress the inflammatory process in an effort to limit hepatocellular necrosis.

CHRONIC AUTOIMMUNE HEPATITIS

First described by Kunkel in 1951 and later termed *lupoid hepatitis* by Mackay when it was thought to be associated with systemic lupus erythematosus (SLE), chronic autoimmune hepatitis (CAIH) is a fairly common cause of CAH in children. It is diagnosed after excluding other possible metabolic, viral, or drug-related causes. Presenting symptoms may include jaundice, fatigue, rashes, and joint pains, and patients may have antinuclear and antismooth muscle or antiliver-kidney microsomal antibodies in the serum. Some patients only show a marked polyclonal elevation of gamma globulin.

Thus far, randomized prospective therapeutic trials have been conducted mainly in adults, with the resulting conclusions of such studies adapted for children. Prednisone is initiated at 2 mg/kg/d (total daily maximum [tdm] of 60 mg), and this dose is decreased by 5 to 10 mg every 2 to 4 weeks once the alanine aminotransferase (ALT) level is less than 2.5 times greater than normal. The goal is to attain the lowest possible dose capable of ensuring remission. In patients who respond poorly, develop severe side effects, or cannot be maintained on a low dose of steroids, azathioprine is added (1 to 1.5 mg/kg/d, tdm 75 mg), with frequent monitoring of CBC and platelets. Azathioprine potentiates the immunosuppressive effect of corticosteroids, but its side effects include renal, bone marrow, and pancreatic toxicity that may be significant and life threatening. Some studies suggest that liver biopsy should be performed early in the course of therapy and again 4 to 6 weeks after its discontinuation to confirm remission, but this is controversial. A repeat biopsy following the initial diagnostic biopsy, performed 6 to 12 months from the start of therapy, is appropriate if symptoms and biochemical signs of active inflammation persist. A rise in serum cholylglycine and ALT levels correlates well with histologic relapse. It is important to discriminate between chronic viral hepatitis and autoimmune CAH, as the use of interferon therapy for chronic viral hepatitis may exacerbate the autoimmune injury of CAH. Overall, 75% of patients will respond to immunosuppressive therapy for CAH. Half of these will relapse, and half can be weaned off steroids completely. Children with cirrhosis and advanced liver disease have a poorer prognosis, and orthotopic liver transplantation may be their only therapeutic option.

HEPATITIS B, C, AND D

Chronic hepatitis B (HBV) and hepatitis C (HCV) infection can progress to cirrhosis and hepatocellular carcinoma. Superinfection of chronic HBV disease with delta agent (HDV) may cause unusually severe liver disease. Hence, there exists an absolute need for efficacious therapy in chronic infectious hepatitis. Standard immunosuppressive agents, such as corticosteroids, are not routinely recommended, as they may enhance viral replication and even increase mortality. However, interest in corticosteroids and other agents, such as cyclosporine and muromonab-CD3 (Orthoclone OKT3), remains high, since the hepatocellular injury that results from HBV replication is, in large part, immune mediated.

Earlier trials of immunomodulating therapeutic agents in pediatric patients were not promising, perhaps because of inadequate dosing regimens, duration of therapy, and inappropriate patient selection. More recent trials have been encouraging. Alpha interferon (IFN-α) has been shown to be effective in treating children with both HBV and HCV-induced CAH. It is most useful when the infection is acquired after the neonatal period or when patients have very high titers of HBV DNA. In both HBV and HCV-affected patients (especially in the latter), there is an unfortunately high rate of relapse almost as soon as the IFN is stopped. The optimal dose of IFN-α therapy remains controversial, with a recommended range of 3 to 5 million units 3 times a week for 6 weeks. Recent trials with interferon gamma (IFN-γ) have failed to show a beneficial effect, although patients seem to tolerate it better than IFN-α, which is associated with flu-like symptoms, hair loss, fatigue, myelosuppression, and autoimmune thyroid dysfunction. Antivirals, such as ribavirin, are being examined in pilot studies, and initial results are mildly encouraging.

METABOLIC CAH

Wilson's disease is an autosomal recessive, inherited disorder of hepatic copper accumulation characterized by neurologic deterioration and progressive liver damage. Penicillamine therapy has proven extremely effective (10 to 20 mg/kg divided b.i.d. or t.i.d.) and must be instituted promptly to avoid irreversible damage. Neonatal or congenital hemochromatosis is a rare disease characterized by excessive iron stores in the liver and other organs, especially the heart and thyroid. Liver synthetic function progressively deteriorates, and liver transplantation often is required as the disorder progresses to complete hepatic failure. Supportive chelation may be beneficial until transplantation can be performed, although this remains controversial.

Alpha1-antitrypsin deficiency is the most common metabolic disorder leading to the need for liver transplantation in children. It is an autosomal recessive disorder associated with a reduction in serum concentrations of alpha1-antitrypsin. Among affected patients, those who are homozygous PiZZ have the lowest values, approximately 10% to 15% of normal. In such patients, an abnormal glycoprotein (due to two point mutations) is elaborated, which accumulates in the endoplasmic reticulum and cannot be secreted. Liver involvement is usually noticed in the first 2 months of life because of persistent jaundice. The liver may be enlarged, and the transaminases may be elevated. Ten percent of these infants have moderate to severe disease, with hepatic synthetic dysfunction and cholestasis. As many as 65% of PiZZ infants will have only biochemical evidence of abnormality, yet no overt liver disease, although it is not completely understood why. Fulminant hepatic failure is rare but may happen in the first year of life. Infants who present with cholestatic syndrome that resolves may then have cryptogenic cirrhosis in childhood.

The diagnosis of alpha1-antitrypsin deficiency is confirmed by serum alpha1-antitrypsin phenotype determination by isoelectric focusing or agarose electrophoresis at an acid pH. Serum concentrations can be misleading, since alpha1-antitrypsin is an acute phase reactant that will increase in inflammatory states, even in PiZZ individuals. Therapy for alpha1-antitrypsin-associated liver disease is supportive. If liver disease progresses to cirrhosis with portal hypertension and ultimately hepatic failure, liver transplantation is the treatment of choice. It is, however, important to remember that even individuals with moderate to severe liver dysfunction may have relatively slow rates of progression of liver disease.

The administration of synthetic androgens (e.g., danazol), useful in hereditary angioedema (where there exists a deficiency of a homologous protease inhibitor [C1 inhibitor]), increases alpha1-antitrypsin levels in only 50% of patients, and the increment is small. Weekly infusions of purified plasma-derived alpha1-antitrypsin over a 6-month period increase serum alpha1-antitrypsin concentrations. However, it is unclear how this may be of benefit to patients with liver disease where low levels of alpha1-antitrypsin are not the cause of hepatocellular necrosis. Gene replacement therapy is also being discussed. However, the ethical concerns are considerable; it is difficult to obtain stable levels of expression, and the continued presence of the abnormal gene has greatly limited this approach.

PHARMACOLOGIC CAH

A large number of drugs have been shown to cause CAH in children, including isoniazid, phenytoin, nitrofurantoin, methyldopa, and sulfonamides. Treatment consists in eliminating the offending drug, as well as supportive measures if synthetic function remains compromised. Orthotopic liver transplantation may be necessary if hepatic injury is irreversible and accompanied by hepatic failure.

REFERENCE

1. Mieli-Vergani G, et al: Different immune mechanisms leading to autoimmunity in primary sclerosing cholangitis and autoimmune chronic active hepatitis of childhood. Hepatology 1989;9:198–203.

DISORDERS OF THE BILIARY TREE

IAN D. D'AGATA, M.D.
RONALD E. KLEINMAN, M.D.

BILIARY ATRESIA

Extrahepatic biliary atresia (EHBA) is responsible for about one third of all cases of prolonged cholestasis in the neonatal period, with an incidence ranging between 1:8000 and 1:15,000 live births. It is characterized by the absence of all or portions of the extrahepatic biliary system, with obstruction to bile flow, resulting in secondary biliary cirrhosis when the obstruction is not relieved. The term *biliary atresia* was first coined by Holmes in 1916. He also devised the terms *correctable* and *noncorrectable* biliary atresia, which are still used today. The latter term describes a condition that was thought to preclude a satisfactory operative result. However, in 1959, Kasai introduced the hepatoportoenterostomy procedure, which, with modifications, remains the primary treatment for EHBA. Mortality, which in untreated infants is 100%, has been greatly reduced, and with the advent of orthotopic liver transplantation (OLT), the prognosis for long-term survival is excellent.

Fewer than 10% of infants have the correctable form of EHBA, in which there is either atresia of the common bile duct or hepatic duct and patent proximal extrahepatic and intrahepatic ducts. Operative correction may be achieved by anastomosis of the patent extrahepatic duct or gallbladder to a Roux-en-Y jejunostomy. In a hepatoportoenterostomy, all the extrahepatic structures are excised, and the porta hepatis is then anastomosed to a Roux-en-Y jejunal limb. This procedure has been used for both the correctable and noncorrectable forms of the disease because EHBA is a progressive disorder in which orginally patent extrahepatic ducts may undergo fibroobliteration.

Successful reestablishment of bile flow following a hepatoportoenterostomy is as high as 80% to 90%, and in all reported series, long-term success is always highest when the operation is performed before 2 months of age, with 90% survival at 10 years of age in children free of jaundice, infection, and cirrhosis. In contrast, the outcome is uniformly poor when the operation is delayed beyond 3 months of age, probably a result of progressive biliary cirrhosis and its complications. In view of this, OLT is probably the procedure of choice for those infants first diagnosed after 3 months of age. For most others, regardless of the extent of fibrosis and cholestasis, portoenterostomy should be performed. A decrease in serum bilirubin will occur in the majority of patients (50% to 75%), although long-term survival for this group is only 25% to 35%. The results of OLT after a failed Kasai procedure are equal to those after primary transplant, although it is technically more difficult to perform the transplant in the setting of a previous operation. Nevertheless, success is high enough with the portoenterostomy and the risks of immunosuppression and transplantation are great enough that the former procedure should be considered before OLT in very young infants.

If cholestasis redevelops within the first or second postoperative month, reoperation and reexcision at the hilus may prove successful. A similar approach may be useful in patients in whom the initial operation was unsuccessful, but results in both cases are poor. After the third postoperative month, reoperation is not helpful. Steroids and choleretics have been employed to increase bile flow, with mixed results. The most common and serious complication of a portoenterostomy is recurrent cholangitis, which occurs in 30% to 50% of all patients within the first postoperative year, with an average of one to three episodes per year. Cholangitis is heralded by fever, leukocytosis, and cholestasis. Anorexia, right upper quadrant tenderness, jaundice, and irritability also may be present. An infant with a portoenterostomy and longer than 24 hours of an unexplained fever requires hospital admission and IV antibiotics. Peripheral blood cultures may not yield the causative microorganisms, and if there are ongoing symptoms, culture of a liver biopsy specimen may be helpful. Broad-spectrum antibiotics, such as gentamicin or tobramycin (7.5 mg/kg/d divided t.i.d.), and a cephalosporin often are used. Antibiotics have varying degrees of penetration into the biliary system, and care must be taken to choose those that will ensure adequate concentrations in the bile. The use of prophylactic amoxicillin 40 mg/kg/d divided t.i.d. or trimethoprim-sulfamethoxazole 5 ml/10 kg b.i.d. PO for the first postoperative year is controversial.

In an effort to reduce the incidence of cholangitis, several variants of the original Kasai portoenterostomy have been devised. There are more than 20 of these, and, in general, they involve decompressing the Roux-en-Y limb and either lengthening or interrupting the intestinal conduit. Most of these procedures have failed to decrease the prevalance of cholangitis, and most actually are associated with a higher rate of infection, obstruction, and reoperation. A more recently devised intussuscepted antireflux segment, created in the Roux-en-Y jejunostomy, is more promising. Severe and sometimes intractable pruritus is another common consequence of persistent cholestasis. Different therapeutic regimens have been tried, with mixed results. In the face of obstruction, phenobarbital 5 mg/kg/d divided b.i.d., which promotes the bile salt independent component of bile flow, and binding resins, such as colestipol and cholestyramine 0.5 mg/kg/d, are not useful and may even be harmful. Emollients, nail clipping, and antihistamines are of some benefit. Plasmapheresis or biliary diversion may be helpful in the most severe cases. Infants with intermittent cholestasis following portoenterostomy often benefit from ursodeoxycholic acid (UDCA), a hydrophilic bile salt and potent choleretic. Recently, a new class of benzodiazepine antagonist with significant antipruritic properties, nalmefene, has been described. It is hoped that these agents may help to control this debilitating problem.

Portal hypertension with attendant ascites, hypersplenism, and esophageal, gastric, and intestinal varices is a life-threatening complication of uncorrected biliary atresia. Sclerotherapy or variceal banding may be necessary, along with other supportive measures, including diuretic therapy, until a liver transplant can be performed. The nutritional support of patients with biliary atresia and persistent cholestasis is critical to optimal growth and development until OLT. Since lipid malabsorption is universal, infants are placed on formulas containing medium-chain triglycerides and essential fatty acids and receive supplements of fat-soluble vitamins. These include vitamin A 10,000 to 25,000 IU/d, vitamin D 5000 to 8000 IU/d (ergocalciferol) or 3 to 5 μg/kg/d of 25-OH cholecalciferol, vitamin E 50 to 400 IU/kg/d or 15 to 25 μg/kg/d of tocopheryl polyethylene glycol succinate (TPGS), and vitamin K 2 to 5 mg/d. Water-soluble vitamins are administered at twice the RDA, and serum levels of minerals, such as calcium and zinc, should be monitored carefully.

CHOLEDOCHAL CYST

Choledochal cyst, a congenital biliary tract abnormality, is present in about 1:15,000 live births, affecting females three times as often as males. The cysts may involve either the intrahepatic or extrahepatic ducts or both. In the classic form, or type I, only the extrahepatic ducts show cystic dilatation. Less common forms include a choledochal diverticulum (type II), a choledochocele associated with ampullary obstruction (type III), extrahepatic bile duct cystic dilatation plus cylindrical or cystic intrahepatic biliary dilatation (type IV), and intrahepatic multiple cystic dilatation of Caroli (type V). The last usually is a diffuse disease not amenable to surgical treatment, but when it is unilateral, a lobectomy may be curative.

Treatment of the classic form of choledochal cyst is complete excision of the cyst. Choledochocystojejunostomy and simple cyst needle aspiration are no longer advocated, as there is more than a 5% increased risk of cholangiocarcinoma development in the residual cystic structures. Other complications of untreated choledochal cysts include cholangitis, stone formation, biliary cirrhosis, and pancreatitis.

CHOLELITHIASIS AND CHOLECYSTITIS

Cholesterol-predominant stones are most common in the older pediatric age population. These are the result of cholesterol supersaturation of bile, either through cholesterol overproduction or bile salt deficiency, but supersaturation alone is not a sufficient cause. Biliary phospholipid composition affects the capacity of bile to solubilize cholesterol, especially when it contains less hydrophobic W-3 fatty acids. Pigment stones in infants and children occur in the setting of chronic hemolytic disease or bacterial infection of bile. Other factors, such as anatomic abnormalities of the bile ducts and a dysfunctional gallbladder, predispose to stone formation because of bile stasis and possible secondary infection. Total parenteral nutrition, ileal resection (which decreases the enterohepatic recirculation of bile salts), diuretic use, and prematurity also have been associated with an increased incidence of gallstones. The treatment of asymptomatic cholelithiasis is controversial. Either no therapy or, in the case of small noncalcified cholesterol stones, UDCA 5 mg/kg b.i.d. may be given. This and chenodeoxycholic acid have proved useful in adults, but definitive studies in children are lacking.

Any patient with cholecystitis, acalculous or not, requires antibiotics and, ultimately, a cholecystectomy. Cholecystitis in the absence of stones is rare but has been described with *Salmonella*, *Shigella*, and viral infections and as a consequence of Henoch-Schoenlein purpura. Of note is that the incidence of gallbladder and biliary parasitic disease is increasing worldwide and in the United States particularly. *Giardia lamblia*, *Ascaris lumbricoides*, and *Opisthorchis viverrini* infections all have been associated with an increased risk of cholangiocarcinoma in endemic areas, and, hence, treatment may be more aggressive in such cases. Hydrops of the gallbladder, which may occur as a result of *Streptococcus*, *Salmonella*, *Leptospira*, and *Pseudomonas* infections, as well as in patients with Kawasaki's disease, may cause cholecystitis-like symptoms. Such cases are treated with appropriate antibiotics, and cholecystectomy may be necessary if the gallbladder fails to reduce in size.

PRIMARY SCLEROSING CHOLANGITIS

Primary sclerosing cholangitis (PSC) is a chronic disorder of the larger bile ducts. It may involve any portion of the intrahepatic or extrahepatic biliary system and results in strictures, stone formation, bile stasis, and decreased liver synthetic function. Its etiology is unknown, and there is a higher frequency of HLA DR3 and B8 in these patients than in healthy individuals. The characteristic lesion of PSC is fibroobliterative bile duct destruction, but this is present in only 10% to 50% of patients undergoing liver biopsy. Thus, histologic diagnosis can be difficult. The primary role of liver biopsy, therefore, is to both exclude other diseases and confirm that the pathologic changes present are consistent with PSC. Endoscopic retrograde cholangiopancreatography (ERCP) is a highly sensitive test for demonstrating PSC. This disease occurs predominantly in males and is often associated with both ulcerative colitis and immunodeficiency states. It may be caused by an immune-mediated process, as portal infiltrates consist mainly of T cells, and there are circulating autoantibodies, of which those directed against neutrophils have sparked the most interest. These perinuclear antineutrophil cytoplasmic antibodies (pANCA) have been found also in a significant number of patients with ulcerative colitis. UDCA and immunosuppressive agents such as methotrexate are the principal agents used to achieve remission. Once complete obstruction occurs, therapeutic ERCP may permit dilatation of stenotic areas of the affected bile ducts. With disease that progresses despite maximal medical therapy, patients become candidates for OLT.

REFERENCES

1. Balistrieri WF: Neonatal cholestasis. J Pediatr 1985;106:171–184.
2. Lopez RR, et al: Variation in management based on type of choledochal cyst. Am J Surg 1991;161:612–615.
3. Schreiber RA, Kleinman RE: Genetics, immunology and biliary atresia: An opening or diversion? J Pediatr Gastroenterol Nutr 1993;16:111–113.

TUMORS OF THE LIVER

SHUNZABURO IWATSUKI, M.D. Ph.D
THOMAS E. STARZL, M.D., Ph.D.

Increasing numbers of hepatic mass lesions are found incidentally by advanced imaging technology. Although most of these incidental tumors are histologically benign and do not require any therapy, they must be thoroughly investigated. Modern imaging technology is quite efficient in detecting small lesions but is not effective in producing pathognomonic findings of many hepatic lesions other than hemangiomas and cysts. Percutaneous needle biopsy often fails to establish a definitive diagnosis because of its limited sampling, and it can cause serious hemorrhage when unwisely performed for vascular lesions.

Major hepatic resections can now be performed with minimum operative risk (less than 5%), but no surgeon should explore a hepatic mass without having the competence to perform all of the major resections, including a right and left trisegmentectomy.

BENIGN TUMORS

Most of the benign tumors of the liver are asymptomatic and are found incidentally during studies for other disorders or during abdominal operations. The general approach to a small incidental tumor (less than 3 cm in diameter) that is considered benign is close observation after thorough investigation. When the tumor changes its imaging characteristics or increases in size during close observation, it must be excised immediately. Larger incidental tumors, other than

asymptomatic cavernous hemangiomas, deserve excisional therapy unless unequivocal benignity is confirmed.

Hemangiomas are the most common benign tumors of the liver. Giant cavernous hemangiomas should be treated by surgical excision, particularly when they are symptomatic (e.g., pain, mass-related complaints) or are found to have a necrotic center inside. The majority of giant cavernous hemangiomas require lobectomies or trisegmentectomies of the liver, but some located on the surface of the liver or pedunculated can be enucleated along pseudocapsular margins without significant loss of normal liver tissue. Ligation or embolization of the feeding hepatic artery and radiation therapy may be hazardous and do not have long-standing effects on the course of giant cavernous hemangiomas.

Infantile hemangioendotheliomas are seen most often in infants during the first 6 months of life and are distinct from cavernous hemangiomas. The lesions should be excised by anatomic hepatic resection whenever possible. Treatment with prednisone, diuretics, and digoxin can be used initially when the patient's condition prohibits surgery or the lesion is too extensive for resection. Response to prednisone may allow surgery to be performed safely in a few weeks. In extensive lesions, radiation to the liver may be used after pathologic diagnosis is confirmed. Favorable responses to steroids, radiation, and hepatic artery ligation or embolization have been reported. The treatment should be vigorous because complete regression and cure are possible.

Other benign tumors include liver cell adenoma, focal nodular hyperplasia, hematoma, mesenchymoma, teratoma, and fibroma. Radiologic differentiation of these benign tumors from malignant tumors is unreliable. Pathologic confirmation of benign tumors is mandatory for each lesion. Large benign tumors should be treated by surgical excision, particularly when they are symptomatic. Adenoma has a tendency to rupture and cause life-threatening hemorrhage. Some adenomas cannot be easily differentiated from low-grade hepatocellular carcinoma by needle biopsies. If the diagnosis is uncertain, the lesion should be excised with an adequate margin without delay.

Congenital hepatic cysts are usually asymptomatic and do not require any therapy. Although aspiration, internal drainage, marsupialization, fenestration, and sclerotherapy have all been recommended for symptomatic congenital cysts, these approaches are no longer justifiable for the treatment of single or localized multiple cysts because hepatic resections can be performed quite safely now.

MALIGNANT TUMORS

The most common primary malignant tumor of the liver in children is hepatoblastoma. Hepatocellular carcinoma is the second most common and usually occurs in older children. Sarcomas of the liver, such as rhabdomyosarcoma and angiosarcoma, are rare. None of these has a favorable outlook, but fibrolamellar hepatocellular carcinoma, which is common in older children and young adults, has a better prognosis than other types of malignancy.

The treatment for all malignant liver tumors is complete surgical excision by anatomic hepatic resection. Hepatic resection of more than the right or left lobe of the liver can be performed quite safely. For example, a large tumor occupying the right lobe of the liver and the medial segment of the left lobe can be resected by right hepatic trisegmentectomy, leaving only the left lateral segment of the left lobe (to the left of the falciform ligament), or a large tumor occupying the left lobe and the anterior segment of the right lobe can be resected by left hepatic trisegmentectomy, leaving only the posterior segment of the right lobe (posterior to the right hepatic vein). These major hepatic resections can now be performed by experienced surgeons with less than a 5% operative mortality.

We have found that computed tomography scan or magnetic resonance imaging is most useful in assessing the extent of the tumor, but findings can be misleading, particularly when a large tumor distorts normal anatomic boundaries. If the resectability is uncertain after extensive preoperative investigation, the patient should be referred to a surgeon who is experienced in major hepatic resection rather than undergo exploratory celiotomy by someone who is unprepared to undertake a definitive procedure.

After curative hepatic resection, we usually recommend that patients receive adjuvant chemotherapy for at least 1 year. We have been using combination chemotherapy with doxorubicin, dactinomycin, vincristine, and cyclophosphamide, and often mitomycin or cisplatin. The value of this approach has not been validated in randomized trials, but the patients who have received adjuvant chemotherapy after curative resections of large tumors have seemed to have longer tumor-free survival.

In general, liver transplantation (total hepatectomy and liver replacement) cannot offer good long-term results when applied to large malignant tumors that cannot be removed by subtotal hepatectomy. However, liver transplantation can result in a cure (more than 5-year survival) on more than isolated occasions. The most favorable lesions for transplantation, just as with resection, are the fibrolamellar hepatoma and epithelioid hemagioendothelial sarcoma. On the other hand, most of the patients who have received liver transplantation for other end-stage liver diseases, such as tyrosinemia and alpha₁-antitrypsin deficiency disease, and whose malignant tumors were small and incidental survived tumor free for several years.

The most common metastatic liver tumors in children are neuroblastoma and Wilms' tumor. Although chemotherapy and radiation therapy may be helpful in treating these metastatic tumors, the lesion should be excised whenever possible, particularly if it is localized to part of the liver. Hepatic resections for metastatic tumors are much safer than those for primary malignancy.

INTESTINAL TRANSPLANTATION

JORGE REYES, M.D.
ANDREAS TZAKIS, M.D.
SATORU TODO, M.D.

The clinical entity of intestinal failure includes an extremely varied array of causative diseases, associated anomalies, and complicating factors, with one common denominator: they all rely on total parenteral nutrition (TPN) for their survival. The introduction of TPN has improved the outcome of many patients and is the accepted therapeutic modality today. However, some patients suffer complications of this therapy, principally liver dysfunction and venous access complications, that limit its long-term use. Also, the frequent morbidity and need for specialized care and hospitalizations place a significant drain on the health care system. Finally, the social awkwardness and emotional demands on the family can hinder tremendously the normal developmental and behavioral maturity of children. There is an urgent need for achieving success with intestinal transplantation.

INDICATIONS

The inability to maintain a normal nutritional status by the use of the gastrointestinal tract alone constitutes intestinal failure (IF). Children with IF usually have had major bowel resections because of catastrophic gastrointestinal disease or suffer functional abnormalities as a result of motility or secretory/absorptive disorders.

The following are **major indications for intestinal transplantation** in children:

- Congenital malformations
- Gastroschisis
- Hirschsprung's disease
- Necrotizing enterocolitis
- Pseudoobstruction
- Volvulus

The composition of the allograft type focuses on the integrity of the remaining gut and other abdominal organs. Those patients with IF and cholestatic liver disease secondary to TPN are candidates for combined liver intestinal transplant (LITX). Guidelines used in assessing the need for a concomitant liver transplant include biochemical parameters, histology, and the presence of portal hypertension. Patients with functional disorders may require replacement of the entire gastrointestinal tract. Candidates for isolated intestinal transplant (ITX) are those who present incipient signs of TPN injury to the liver, although without significant damage, and those who have suffered multiple septic episodes from line infection, with consequent thrombosis, and are limited in the availability of access sites. These patients are in danger of progressively depleting these sites and should be considered for ITX.[3]

A potential small bowel transplant recipient should have a thorough assessment of nutritional history and present nutritional status, as well as an outline of the abdominal anatomy. This should allow for planning of the optimum time for transplantation, as well as for accurate planning of graft type.

THE OPERATION

A history of normal intestinal function in a patient referred for potential liver donation is considered adequate for possible intestinal donation. The donor should be hemodynamically stable, without a need for vasopressor support. There should be no history of cardiac arrest. The adequacy of the intestine is assessed by the donor team at the time of surgery. We select a donor of similar or smaller size than the recipient. The ABO blood groups should be identical, and there is no HLA matching.

The procurement of multiple visceral organs (en-bloc or as separate components) focuses on the isolation and cooling of the organs, preserving their vascular and parenchymal anatomy. The complete multivisceral retrieval includes the stomach, duodenum, pancreas, liver, and small and large intestine. After encirclement of the proximal aorta near the diaphragm and the distal aorta below the origin of the inferior mesenteric artery, the organs are flushed with chilled University of Wisconsin (UW) solution via a catheter inserted into the lower abdominal aorta. In situations where the liver is not required in the graft, it may be separated in situ after perfusion or at the back table. Back table irrigation of the intestinal lumen is required only when the colon is included in the graft. Manipulation of the graft lymphoreticular tissue (using polyclonal or monoclonal antilymphocyte antibody preparations or radiation) is not performed.

The recipient operation focuses on preservation of the remaining bowel and the status of the native liver. The final judgment as to graft type is made at this time. The liver is usually excised, preserving the retrohepatic vena cava as for a piggyback transplant. A portacaval shunt is used when the liver is removed, and the proximal gut is preserved (stomach, duodenum, pancreas, spleen), thus allowing decompression of these organs. This is not required in recipients of a complete multivisceral transplant (MVTX) or ITX graft.

Revascularization in the MVTX or LITX graft uses a Carrel patch containing the celiac and superior mesenteric arteries, which is anastomosed to the recipient infrarenal aorta (with or without an interposition graft of donor thoracic or abdominal aorta). The venous drainage of the graft is into the hepatic veins of the recipient. After reperfusion, the portacaval shunt may be taken down, and a recipient portal vein-to-donor portal vein anastomosis may be performed. In the ITX graft, the superior mesenteric artery is anastomosed into the infrarenal aorta. The venous drainage of this type graft can be into the native superior mesenteric vein, the portal vein at the level of the hepatic hilus, or the inferior vena cava. The graft is reperfused after unclamping of the arterial inflow, allowing bleeding to occur from the venous outflow anastomotic lines. This allows for drainage of the potassium-rich UW solution. The venous drainage clamps are then removed. The gastrointestinal tract is reconstructed in a standard fashion, anastomosing to native intestine proximally and distally. Biliary reconstruction is required only in recipients of an LITX graft and is performed to the most proximal end of the transplanted bowel. A proximal tube gastrostomy or jejunostomy or both complete the procedure.

POSTOPERATIVE MANAGEMENT

Immunosuppression is begun immediately after graft reperfusion using a combination of FK 506, steroids, and prostaglandin E_1 (Prostin). FK 506 0.1 to 0.15 mg/kd/d is administered initially by continuous IV infusion, targeting levels at between 2 and 3 ng/ml. FK 506 0.3 mg/kg/d PO is initiated once intestinal motility is present. A steroid taper of methylprednisolone is started at a dose of 100 mg and reduced over a period of 5 days to 10 mg. Prostaglandin E_1 is administered at 0.003 to 0.009 μg/kg/min intraoperatively, then continued for 5 days. We have observed a beneficial effect on FK 506 nephrotoxicity. The use of azathioprine to supplement baseline immunosuppression is considered in cases of recurrent rejection or FK 506 nephrotoxicity. The long-term management usually entails reduction of FK 506 and withdrawal of steroids. Most pediatric patients can be managed eventually by monotherapy with FK 506.[1]

POSTOPERATIVE CARE AND RESULTS

Postoperatively, recipients of MVTX and LITX receive the same level of intensive care as liver transplant recipients, since commonly these patients are in liver failure. However, they often require prolonged ventilatory support and have frequent fluid and electrolyte shifts. Recipients of ITX who generally do not have life-threatening complications immediately preoperatively recover faster after transplantation and are discharged from intensive care earlier. Although there may be renal dysfunction early secondary to the extensive procedure, blood product requirements, hemodynamic instabilities, and drug toxicities, only one patient has required kidney transplantation.

Infection

All patients receive prophylactic broad-spectrum IV antimicrobials. Appropriate specific antibiotics should be used with any history of recent preoperative nosocomial infections. Intestinal decontamination using a cocktail of oral antibiotics (amphotericin B, gentamicin, and colistin sulfate) is given for a period of 6 weeks and during episodes of rejection. Surveillance quantitative stool cultures are performed weekly. Translocation of bacterial organisms may occur during episodes of acute rejection when the mucosal barrier of the allograft has been damaged. A 2-week routine prophylaxis with ganciclovir focuses on the prevention of cytomegalovirus infection. *Pneumocystis carinii* pneumonia prophylaxis is with lifetime oral trimethoprim-sulfa-methoxazole.

Infections have been responsible for significant morbidity and mortality after intestinal transplantation and have been caused by bacterial, fungal, and viral organisms. They have presented as primary lung, peritoneal, and venous catheter infections or as systemic sepsis accompanying translocation phenomena in a graft damaged by rejection. The most frequent bacterial infections involve gram-positive cocci (staphylococci and enterococci). The viral pathogens include adenovirus, cytomegalovirus, parainfluenza, influenza B, and respiratory syncytial virus (RSV). Epstein-Barr virus (EBV) infection and posttransplant lymphoproliferative disease (PTLD) have occurred in six children and resulted in two fatalities. The disease has invariably involved the graft, and treatment by withholding of immunosuppression and antiviral therapy has resulted in limited control and cure of the disease. The intestinal graft may be rejected during the recovery phase, and although treatment with steroids and reinstitution of FK 506 immunosuppression has controlled most rejection episodes, some patients have had uncontrollable rejection and death.

Nutritional Support

In the immediate postoperative period, standard TPN solutions are used. After the first postoperative week, oral or enteral feedings can be initiated and advanced as tolerated. Voluntary eating has been difficult early, particularly in pediatric recipients. Therefore, enteral supplementation is critical. Functional assessment of the small bowel has been through the use of absorption studies of D-xylose and FK 506 and the quantitation of fat in the stool. A satisfactory absorption curve for D-xylose is the rule, and abnormal results should prompt a search for rejection. Maintenance of satisfactory FK 506 blood trough levels off of IV therapy has occurred at a mean of 28 days after transplant. Although excretion of fat in the stool is abnormal in most patients (because of the interruption of lymphatics at the time of harvesting), this does not have any clinical implications. The intestine is routinely evaluated by standard barium gastrointestinal series. Significant changes can be observed in cases of severe rejection, which can produce ablation of the normal mucosal pattern and a tubelike image, with strictures and dysmotility.[2]

Immunologic Monitoring

Evaluation of the anatomic and functional integrity of the graft relies on multiple clinical evaluations, supplemented by endoscopic examinations (both routine and when clinically indicated) and the histopathology of multiple endoscopically guided biopsies. Examination of the stoma and the enteral output is helpful, as is the presence or absence of blood in the stools. The differential diagnosis in these patients includes preservation injury, rejection, enteritis, and systemic sepsis.

Intestinal allograft rejection rarely may be asymptomatic but generally occurs with a combination of fever, abdominal pain and distention, nausea or vomiting, and a sudden increase in stomal output followed by its cessation. The presence of blood in the stool (secondary to mucosal sloughing) is an ominous sign that must be assumed to be rejection until proven otherwise. Sepsis can be associated with rejection of the intestinal allograft, since bacteria can translocate through the injured epithelium.

Endoscopically early rejection may show mucosal edema, erythema, and friability. If the rejection process is not controlled, the mucosa will become ischemic or dusty and present focal or defuse ulcerations. Sloughing of large areas of mucosa and complete loss of peristalsis may accompany severe rejection. Histologically, there is edema of the lamina propria, with mononuclear cell infiltrates, villous blunting, and cryptitis. Depending on the severity of rejection, there may be varying degrees of epithelial cell necrosis and regeneration. Complete mucosal and crypt loss with replacement by granulation tissue and pseudomembranes can be seen in the final phases.

The overall incidence of acute intestinal allograft rejection during the first 90 days after transplantation is reported to be 80% in ITX recipients and 77% in LITX recipients. The incidence of acute liver allograft rejection in the LITX recipients is 55%. The risk of rejection diminishes significantly after the third month. However, if there is an episode of infection with opportunistic organisms such as EBV, in which overall reduction of immunosuppression may be required, this risk may increase.

Graft rejection is treated initially with bolus steroid therapy (IV hydrocortisone or methylprednisolone) in cases of mild rejection and with a steroid taper in cases of moderate to severe rejection. The FK 506 trough levels should reach 3 to 5 ng/ml by either the oral or intravenous route. Muromonab-CD3 (Orthoclone OKT3) is used when rejection has progressed on a steroid taper but should be considered as the initial therapeutic agent in cases of severe mucosal injury and crypt damage.

COMPLICATIONS

Postoperative Bleeding

A combination of coagulopathy secondary to end-stage liver disease and multiple previous surgeries with significant vascularized adhesions and portal hypertension makes these patients susceptible to postoperative bleeding. Usually, bleeding can be found from a vascular anastomosis or extensive raw peritoneal surfaces. Preoperative coagulopathy is related to the liver failure, platelet defects, and fibrinolysis. Temporary graft reperfusion coagulopathy also may occur. Early exploration is the rule.

Biliary Complications

Biliary leaks occur in recipients of the LITX graft and present within the first 2 weeks of transplantation. Sepsis and the presence of biliary drainage through the abdominal wound or drains are the presenting signs. Immediate exploration with revision of the biliary anastomosis is required.

Vascular Complications

In our series, thrombosis of the hepatic artery occurred in 1 patient with an LITX, with consequent hepatic gangrene. This required retransplantation of the liver component of the graft, although a full LITX graft was desirable. The patient died of influenza B 3 weeks later.

Gastrointestinal Complications

The most common intestinal complication after intestinal transplantation has been bleeding, which usually reflects severe rejection and requires prompt enteroscopic assessment and biopsy. Leakage of either a proximal or distal gastrointestinal anastomosis, as well as native duodenal and colonic stumps and gastrostomy sites, has occurred. Presentation may be dramatic, with florid sepsis. Surgical revision of these leaks, antibiotic therapy, and frequent reexplorations may be required. Gastrointestinal motility disorders may occur in both native (gastric atony/pylorospasm) and transplanted bowel. Hypermotility should induce a search for rejection or bacterial overgrowth.

REFERENCES

1. Reyes J, Tzakis AG, Todo S, et al: Small bowel and liver/small bowel transplantation in children. Semin Pediatr Surg 1993;2:289–300.
2. Reyes J, Tzakis AG, Todo S, et al: Nutritional management of intestinal transplant recipients. Transplant Proc 1993;25:1200–1201.
3. Todo S, Tzakis A, Abu-Elmagd K, et al: Intestinal transplantation in composite visceral graft or alone. Ann Surg 1992;216(3):223–234.

ORGAN TRANSPLANTS: PANCREAS AND ISLET CELLS

MATHIAS D. BRENDEL, M.D.
CAMILLO RICORDI, M.D.

With few exceptions, insulin-dependent diabetes mellitus in patients of pediatric age is a result of the destruction of the pancreatic beta cells. The disease is caused by a combination of genetic predisposition and a postulated environmental factor, leading to an autoimmune reaction.

Insulin replacement, in combination with drug therapy for diabetes-related disease and diet, has been the gold standard of treatment for the last seven decades, greatly reducing acute morbidity and death. Yet the limitations of insulin administration are evident from the magnitude of late complications of the disease. These result mainly from microangiopathy and macroangiopathy because of the impaired carbohydrate metabolism. In consequence, diabetes represents the third leading cause of death by disease, is the leading cause of legal blindness (age group 45 to 64 years) and end-stage renal disease, forces 40% of amputations in patients (age group >45 years), and contributes largely to heart disease, stroke, and peripheral neuropathy.

As recently shown by the diabetes control and complications trial (DCCT), a synergistic effort of intensified insulin therapy, either by multiple daily injections or pump therapy, in combination with thorough glucose monitoring is capable of significantly reducing late complications. However, at best, even intensified insulin therapy mimics a gross approximation of the glucose homeostasis as compared with

physiologic control by the pancreatic islets. In addition, near normal glucose profiles under insulin therapy in association with inefficient counterregulation carry increased risks of hypoglycemic events

An alternative to exogenous insulin therapy, biophysiologic replacement of the pancreatic islet apparatus, offers normal glucose control by providing both a natural glucose-sensing system and appropriate (on-demand) insulin secretion. This type of biologic replacement can be achieved clinically by pancreas organ transplantation or by transplantation of pancreatic endocrine cells (islets of Langerhans). However, both procedures require continuous immunosuppression of the recipients, severely limiting the indications for transplantation in pediatric patients.

PANCREAS TRANSPLANTATION

Classification and Technique

Transplantation of whole or segmental pancreas can be defined as solitary (pancreas transplant alone, PTA) or combined transplant, in most cases following (pancreas after kidney, PAK) or simultaneous with a kidney transplant (simultaneous pancreas-kidney, SPK) or in combination with other organs, such as liver. Usually, organs from cadaveric donors are used as graft tissue. Recent advances in harvesting and organ preservation techniques (hypothermia and preservation solutions) allows organ storage up to 30 hours with preserved function. Most centers in the United States and in Europe perform transplantation of the whole pancreas and a duodenal segment adjacent to the papilla of Vater. Since maintaining the exocrine function of the pancreas requires drainage, the duodenal portion is anastomosed to either the bladder (pancreaticoduodenocystotomy) or the jejunum (pancreaticoduodenojejunostomy) via a Roux-en-Y limb or directly side-to-side. Pancreatic duct obliteration by synthetic polymers (neoprene, prolamine) represents a third alternative for pancreatic duct management.

Immunosuppression

Allogeneic transplantation of whole or segmental pancreas generally requires systemic immunosuppressive therapy. Currently, most centers use a multiple-drug combination of cyclosporine, azathioprine, and prednisone in conjunction with inductive functional depletion of lymphocytes in the recipient by polyclonal (anti-lymphocyte globulin, ALG) or monoclonal (muromonab-CD3 [Orthoclone OKT3]) antibodies. Rejection episodes usually are treated by high-dose corticosteroids, antilymphocyte antibodies, or a combination thereof.

Immune Monitoring

For simultaneous pancreas-kidney transplantation (SPK), evaluation of rejection episodes is facilitated by determination of serum creatinine levels, since kidney rejection precedes or parallels pancreas rejection in the great majority of cases. Single pancreas transplantation (SP) with bladder drainage allows functional surveillance through urine amylase levels. In the case of enteric drainage or duct obliteration, diagnosis proves more difficult and depends on indirect signs, such as fever and leukocytosis.

Patient and Graft Survival

The International Pancreas Transplant Registry (IPTR), recording cases worldwide, reported more than 4166 pancreas transplantations between 1986 and September 1993.[2] The 1-year patient survival rate within the last 6 years was 91%, and the 1-year pancreas graft survival rate, as defined by the patient's independence from exogenous insulin administration, was 74% for combined pancreas-kidney transplants worldwide and 49% for pancreas transplant alone. Favorable results for combined organ transplants are associated with more sensitive diagnostic criteria of rejection episodes and earlier immunosuppressive intervention therapy. In addition, graft survival appears to correlate positively with the number of HLA-A, B, and DR matches between donor and recipient, multiple immunosuppressive therapy, and the experience of the transplant center. In consequence, dramatic improvements in both patient and graft survival have been achieved within recent years.

Functional Outcome

Extending the analysis of survival statistics, the key criterion of the success of functional pancreatic endocrine replacement is the efficacy of the graft to restore normal glucose metabolism. Functional pancreas transplants lead to normal fasting glucose and hemoglobin A_{1c} (HbA_{1c}) values. Recipients may have delayed postprandial insulin secretion peaks and an abnormal glucose tolerance. This does not reflect an absolute insulin deficiency, since the majority of recipients have hyperinsulinemia, a phenomenon that is ascribed to the delivery of insulin from the graft into the systemic circulation, thereby circumventing the intrahepatic first-pass clearance. In addition, both impaired glucose tolerance and hyperinsulinemia are linked to increased insulin resistance and direct impairment of pancreatic beta cells as a consequence of the immmunosuppressive therapy. The long-term effects of elevated systemic insulin levels remain to be investigated.

Evaluation of the influence of pancreas transplantation on late complications is confounded by the limited number of functional pancreas grafts and the fact that the majority of recipients suffer from end-stage kidney disease. Thus, the effect is aggravated by uremia. It has been clearly demonstrated that cotransplanted kidneys are protected from diabetic nephropathy by simultaneous pancreas transplantation. Similar benefits from single pancreas transplantation on the native kidneys can, therefore, be expected. Clinical data on the beneficial effects on other diabetic late complications (retinopathy, neuropathy, vasculopathy) are still scarce but are substantiated by laboratory animal experiments.

Risk Analysis

Evaluation of the benefits versus the risks of pancreas transplantation must address (1) patient morbidity, (2) functional outcome, (3) the effects of additional drug therapy (immunosuppression), and (4) quality of life. Continuous improvements in patient morbidity and graft survival is to be expected but is limited by the fact of major abdominal surgery and the period of hospitalization. At present, the degree of metabolic control by functional pancreas grafts cannot be attained by any other treatment method. However, there are very limited data on long-term graft survival and function available. In addition, besides the adverse acute effects, the long-term consequences of the mandatory immunosuppressive therapy are not well understood. Pancreas transplantation, therefore, appears suitable for insulin-dependent patients with end-stage renal disease who are awaiting kidney transplantation and for patients with diabetes who require chronic immunosuppressive therapy because of replacement of other organs.

Considering the lack of ability to predict late complications of diabetes and the side effects of chronic immunosuppression, pancreas transplantation in pediatric patients at the first signs of other disease does not appear to be justified.

ISLET CELL TRANSPLANTATION

As compared with clinical transplantation of the vascularized pancreas, experience with clinical islet cell transplantation is very limited and is, therefore, considered an experimental procedure. Although single attempts at islet transplantation into human patients were made between 1970 and 1988, they remain anecdotal and largely unsuccessful. Recent advances in the isolation procedures allowed several centers to assess the value of islet transplantation over the last 4 years. Since only the pancreatic endocrine cells (comprising 1% to 2% of the pancreas mass) are needed to control carbohydrate metabolism, transplantation of these islet cells isolated from a whole pancreas offers advantages over whole organ transplantation. Islet transplantation is a simple and safe procedure that requires no surgery. In addition, complications related to persistent pancreatic exocrine secretion are

circumvented. It was demonstrated in animal experiments that islets can be subjected to manipulations that reduce immunogenicity, thus avoiding the need for chronic immunosuppression in the recipient. Alternatively, islet cells can be protected from immune rejection by semipermeable membranes. Isolated islet cells can be stored to facilitate functional matching procedures and allow accumulation of a critical mass required to reverse diabetes.

Classification and Technique

Islet cell transplantation can be separated into procedures involving islet transplant only (islet transplant alone, ITA) or in combination with kidney transplant (islet after kidney, IAK; simultaneous islet-kidney, SIK) or other organ transplants. Isolation of islet cells is performed mainly from cadaveric donors by enzymatic digestion (collagenase) in combination with mechanical disruptions.[3] The endocrine cell components are then separated from the exocrine tissue by density gradient centrifugation. In some cases, islets have been infused into the portal system of the liver by gravity drainage either through percutaneous transhepatic catheterization or through a patent umbilical vein.

Immunosuppressive Therapy

The initial trials to establish islet allograft function in human patients have been performed on patients who underwent simultaneous or preceding replacement of solid organs and, therefore, required medication to suppress immune rejection. Immunosuppressive therapy for the islet graft usually compromises induction by monoclonal (muromonab-CD3) or polyclonal (ALG) antibodies and maintenance therapy with prednisone, cyclosporine, or azathioprine (or a combination of these). In one center, FK 506 was used in combination with corticosteroids. In addition, in several cases, islet cells were placed in immunoprotective devices (diffusion chamber, microcapsules), with no further immunosuppressive therapy.

Immune Monitoring

In cotransplantation of solid organs (such as kidney, liver, heart-lung), functional markers for these organs in blood or urine may facilitate diagnosis of rejection episodes. Functional monitoring of islets by assessment of serum glucose, insulin, and C peptide is not sensitive enough to determinate rejection at a point where it would be still possible to salvage the islet graft by intervention therapy. To date, there is no early rejection marker available.

Patient and Graft Survival

The short period of use and the limited number of clinical islet cell transplantations do not provide a sufficient base for rigorous statistical analysis. To date, there has been no report of any fatal complications as a result of transplantation of purified islets. Because of the early phase of the islet transplantation trials, preserved C peptide secretion (≥ 1 ng/ml for ≥ 1 month) has been used as a more sensitive marker of graft survival than independence from exogenous insulin (the criterion used for vascularized pancreas grafts). Graft survival between 1974 and 1989 was 9 of 90 cases (5 patients achieved temporary independence from exogenous insulin). In contrast, 52 of 85 patients between 1990 and 1992 had prolonged periods of C peptide secretion (exogenous insulin independence in 18 of these subjects[1]). As of June 1993, 4 patients remain insulin independent from >127 to >326 days. The longest period of insulin independence was 2 years. Beneficial factors for functional graft survival appear to be the liver as transplant site, immunosuppressive induction therapy with antilymphocyte antibodies, and an islet transplant volume exceeding 8000 islets (average diameter 150 µm per kilogram body weight of the recipient.

Preliminary results favor functional islet allograft survival for simultaneous islet-kidney (SIK), islet after kidney (IAK), and islet-liver (SIL) transplantation. Similar to vascularized pancreas grafts, improved survival of SIK might result from earlier diagnosis of rejection episodes and intervention therapy. The SIL transplantations were performed in patients who had become insulin-dependent because of removal of their original pancreas for treatment of other disease, mostly carcinoma. Whereas islets usually are infused into the recipient's native liver, in these cases, the islets were placed into a co-transplanted liver and possibly encountered a microenvironment beneficial for engraftment. Furthermore, reversal of diabetes by islet transplantation appears to be largely facilitated in cases of nonautoimmune origin, possibly because of a smaller degree of insulin resistance and improved neovascularization of the transplanted islets. The limited data available have not revealed a significant influence of HLA (A, B, DR) antigen mismatches in islet graft survival.

Functional Outcome

Functional islet grafts are those that secrete enough insulin to allow discontinuation from exogenous insulin administration and normalize fasting serum glucose and HbA_{1c} levels. A similar degree of metabolic control can be reached by patients with lower levels of insulin secretion by islet grafts, who require supplementary administration of exogenous insulin. Similar to the case with vascularized pancreas grafts, postprandial insulin peak secretion may be delayed and glucose tolerance test profiles may be abnormal. In contrast to whole organ transplantation, no hyperinsulinemia is observed in the normoglycemic patients, indicating an effective hepatic insulin clearance. The limited number of patients and the short period of islet graft survival do not allow an evaluation of the impact on diabetic late complications.

Risk Analysis

Islet transplantation is safer than vascularized organ transplantation, as it is not associated with complications from general anesthesia, abdominal surgery, or management of exocrine pancreatic secretion. In addition, a possible rejection of an islet graft is not harmful to the patient. Islet transplantation is able to effectively control carbohydrate metabolism in the recipient, although the number of cases and duration of insulin independence still are very limited. The current requirements of chronic immunosuppression impose similar restrictions on the recipient population as described for the vascularized graft. In contrast to whole organ transplantation, it is evident from animal experiments that alteration of islet immunogenicity can circumvent the need for long-term immunosuppression. These approaches hold great promise for clinical transplantation. As they become reality, islet transplantation can be performed successfully in the very early stage of insulin-dependent (type I) diabetes.

REFERENCES

1. Hering BJ, Browatzki CC, Shultz A, Bretzel RG, Federlin KF: Clinical islet transplantation—Registry report, accomplishments in the past and future research needs. Cell Transplant 1993;2:269–282.
2. Moudry-Munns KC, Gruessner A, Sutherland DER: International Pancreas Transplant Registry report. Transplant Proc (in press)
3. Ricordi C (ed): Pancreatic Islet Cell Transplantation, 1892–1992—One Century of Transplantation for Diabetes. Austin, TX, R.G. Landes Company, 1992.

NAUSEA AND VOMITING

LEWIS R. FIRST, M.D.

Vomiting, one of the most common symptoms in pediatrics, represents the forceful expulsion of gastric contents through the mouth. It is a complex, coordinated process that is under control of the central nervous system. Nausea, frequently associated with vomiting, is a physical sensation that can be induced by visceral, vestibular, or emotional stimuli and may not necessarily progress to full emesis. It is characterized by a desire to vomit, as well as by other autonomic symptoms, such as salivation, pallor, diaphoresis, tachycardia, and anorexia.

MECHANISM AND SIGNIFICANCE

One cannot begin to consider the treatment of nausea and vomiting without an understanding of the mechanism by which vomiting occurs, as well as the realization of the broad spectrum of diseases that can cause vomiting. Vomiting itself is controlled by two medullary areas in the midbrain. A variety of chemical agents and mediators send signals (primarily dopamine and serotonin) into the vomiting center (located in the region of the nucleus solitarius or adjacent portion of the lateral reticular formation) and the chemoreceptor trigger zone (in the area postrema of the floor of the left ventricle), resulting in emesis. Therefore, to control the act of vomiting, one therapeutic approach is to suppress medullary activity and, in turn, gain motor control of vomiting.

Afferent stimuli to the medulla can arise from the posterior pharynx, abdomen, and other visceral organs, including the pleura, heart, and urogenital and biliary tracts, in response to obstruction or infection. Metabolic factors, vestibular abnormalities, and certain medications (particularly morphine derivatives) may all affect the vomiting center as well, acting either directly or indirectly through the chemoreceptor trigger zone. In addition, impulses can be submitted either by vagal or sympathetic afferents to the vomiting center.

One might think of the clinical significance of vomiting as being a defense system that acts to identify and remove any accidentally ingested toxins before they can progress further into the gastrointestinal tract and result in worsening gastrointestinal symptoms. Nausea in itself may be a protective reflex, in that anorexia helps to prevent further ingestion of potentially toxic materials, and the unpleasant sensations associated with nausea may create almost a behavioral aversion to an offending food or stimulus that would otherwise result in vomiting. The fact that vomiting can occur with some medications, such as chemotherapy, may again represent an appropriate physiologic protective response to the sensation of a toxin. Even the vomiting associated with gastrointestinal reflux may represent a defense system, in that the act of vomiting helps to remove refluxed gastric acid from inflaming the esophageal mucosa.

TREATMENT

An approach to the treatment of vomiting really begins with an assessment of whether the vomiting is acute or chronic, in combination with the age of the child. When vomiting is the principal symptom, the history should focus on a description of the vomitus, its relationship to meals, and whether it is projectile or simply represents spitting or rumination. Associated symptoms and signs may be useful, such as headache, visual symptoms, or vertigo, or other gastrointestinal symptoms, such as diarrhea, constipation, or jaundice. The assessment of anorexia also can be important in sorting out an etiology. Family histories for migraine or ulcer disease can be extremely useful. Vomiting without nausea may be a clue to a problem involving elevated intracranial pressure or mechanical obstruction within the gastrointestinal tract or other viscera, since this vomiting often is very sudden and not preceded by nausea. If the child does not appear acutely ill, psychosocial issues should be pursued that might contribute to poor feeding techniques. An inability to gain weight in the setting of vomiting may suggest a more chronic underlying process.

VOMITING IN INFANCY

Vomiting in the newborn that is associated with abdominal distention, is projectile, or contains blood or bile is more worrisome and warrants immediate investigation, including the use of appropriate radiologic studies (described elsewhere in this text). Bilious vomiting should be considered a surgical emergency until proven otherwise. It is worthwhile to consider sepsis, head trauma, narcotic withdrawal, peptic ulcer disease, and inborn errors of metabolism should vomiting be persistent in early infancy.

In the postneonatal period, feeding problems, as well as pyloric stenosis and viral and bacterial infectious disorders, are most common.

It is possible that an infant with cow's milk protein allergy can have vomiting.

VOMITING IN OLDER CHILDREN

In older children, acute vomiting is usually associated with abdominal pain and can represent obstruction or inflammation of an abdominal viscus. On the other hand, it may also be associated with congestion from upper respiratory infections, hepatitis, ingestions, pneumonia, or metabolic disorders, such as diabetes. Persistent vomiting in an older age group makes one more concerned about elevated intracranial pressure, migraines, peptic ulcer disease, and, in adolescents, anorexia nervosa and bulimia.

Once life-threatening obstructive or surgical disorders have been eliminated, most vomiting, particularly in older children, usually results from some very common etiologies, such as a viral gastroenteritis or food poisoning. In these cases, the vomiting usually resolves within 24 to 48 hours. Should the vomiting be persistent or be associated with the use of chemotherapy or other medication, some pharmacologic attention to its treatment appears warranted. A psychogenic etiology for the vomiting often is attributed to stress, which elevates epinephrine levels and, in turn, influences the chemoreceptive trigger zone. In the psychogenic setting, pharmacologic treatment may be warranted.

The cessation of vomiting is important in ensuring adequate hydration, as well as avoiding Mallory-Weiss tears in the gastric mucosa, which can result in hematemesis. Vomiting occasionally will result in episodes of aspiration and, in younger infants, failure to thrive. Dehydration and electrolyte abnormalities are the most worrisome aspects of persistent vomiting that warrant therapeutic attention. The entity of cyclic vomiting in older children (in which episodes of vomiting last a few hours to a few days) often is associated with

TABLE 1. Drugs Useful for Control of Nausea and Vomiting

DRUG	HOW SUPPLIED	PRINCIPAL SIDE EFFECTS
Antihistamines		
Promethazine (Phenergan)	Syrup: 6.25 mg/5 ml or 25 mg/5 ml	Headache
Child: 0.5 mg/kg per dose PO, IM, or IV q4–6h	Tablets: 12.5, 25, 50 mg	Abdominal pain
Adult: 25 mg PO or IM q4h	Suppository: 12.5, 25, 50 mg	Urinary urgency
	Injection: 25 mg/ml	Blood pressure changes
		Extrapyramidal and anticholinergic side effects
Dimenhydrinate (Dramamine)	Injection: 50 mg/ml	Drowsiness
Child: 1.25 mg/kg per dose PO or IM q.i.d.	Liquid: 12.5 mg/4 ml	Atropinelike effects
Adult: 50–100 mg per dose PO or IM q.i.d., 100 mg PR q.i.d.	Tablets: 50 mg	
	Suppository: 100 mg	
Dopamine Antagonists		
Metoclopramide (Reglan)	Injection: 5 mg/ml	Extrapyramidal restlessness, sedation, lowered threshold to seizure
Child and adult: 0.5–2 mg/kg per dose IV 30 min before chemotherapy and q2h for 2 doses, then q3h for 3 doses		
Thiethylperazine (Torecan)	Injection: 10 mg/2 ml	Extrapyramidal and anticholinergic effects
Child: 5 mg PO q.i.d. if <50 kg, 10 mg if >50 kg	Tablet: 10 mg	
Adult: 10–30 mg PO q.i.d.	Suppository: 10 mg	
10 mg IM t.i.d.		
Perphenazine (Trilafon)	Tablets: 2, 4, 8, 16 mg	Extrapyramidal and anticholinergic effects
Child: 2–5 mg IV with maintenance of 2–4 mg IV or PO q4h or 0.5 mg/h as continuous infusion	Injection: 5 mg/ml	
Adult: 8–16 mg PO b.i.d.–q.i.d. 8–10 mg IV or IM q6h or as continuous infusion		
Prochlorperazine (Compazine)	Injection: 5 mg/ml	Extrapyramidal, anticholinergic, sedation, dysphoria, orthostatic hypotension, lowered seizure threshold
Child: (>10 kg): 0.05 mg/kg IM q6h or 0.1 mg/kg PR or PO q6h	Syrup: 5 mg/5 ml	
Adult: 5–10 mg per dose IM or PO q6h or 25 mg PR b.i.d.	Oral concentrate: 10 mg/ml	
	Suppository: 2.5, 5, 25 mg	
Serotonin Antagonists		
Ondansetron (Zofran)	Tablets: 4, 8 mg	Headaches
Child: >3 y to adult: 0.15 mg/kg per dose IV 30 min before chemotherapy and then 4 and 8 h after first dose	Injection: 2 mg/ml	Constipation
		Diarrhea
		Transient elevation in liver function tests
		Seizures (rare)
Miscellaneous		
Phosphated carbohydrate solution (Emetrol)	Liquid: 1.87 g dextrose	Nontoxic
Child: 1–2 tsp q15min until nausea subsides	1.87 g fructose	
Adult: 1–2 Tbsp q15min until nausea subsides	21.5 mg phosphoric acid/5 ml	
For Psychogenic Vomiting		
Lorazepam (Ativan)	Tablets: 0.5, 1, 2 mg	
Usual dose: 2–3 mg/d in divided doses		
Diazepam (Valium)	Tablets: 2, 5, 10 mg	
Child: 1–2.5 mg t.i.d. or q.i.d.		
Adult: 2–10 mg t.i.d. or q.i.d.		

dehydration, as well as with migraines or stressful events or both. A therapeutic approach to this type of vomiting is certainly indicated, although often not very helpful.

ANTIEMETIC PHARMACOTHERAPY

For nausea and vomiting associated with a viral illness or an acute ingestion (assuming that the toxin has been appropriately dealt with), treatment is essentially supportive and consists of sips of clear fluids and a bland diet until the feelings of nausea and vomiting pass (usually within 24 to 48 hours). If the vomiting persists and dehydration becomes a potential concern, antiemetic pharmacotherapy may be indicated, particularly in older children, in whom the benefits of such therapy will outweigh the side effects. Unfortunately, most antiemetics are oral agents, and these may not be useful if acute vomiting is occurring unless they can be absorbed rapidly from the mouth or stomach before emesis recurs. Oral antiemetics may be more useful in the setting of anticipated vomiting, such as with chemotherapy or radiation therapy, or in the setting of persistent vomiting from hepatitis or psychogenic etiologies.

Most antiemetics work through the midbrain to influence central control of the sensations of nausea and vomiting. A complete list of antiemetics and their dosages appears in Table 1. The most common of these is metoclopramide, which blocks dopamine receptors in the chemoreceptor trigger zone and thus influences central control of vomiting. Unfortunately, it is associated with significant dystonic and dyskinetic reactions, including oculogyric crises, and, therefore, is not recommended for young children.

Phenothiazines are the drugs of choice for control of vomiting secondary to chemotherapy, with the most useful being thiethylperazine (Torecan), which can be given orally, intravenously, intramuscularly, or rectally. The dose is 10 mg for children 12 years of age or greater than 50 kg, and 5 mg is used in smaller children. It provides prophylactic protection if given on a regular basis around the clock (beginning with a dose administered before chemotherapy). The dosage frequency should be tapered to an individual's own need rather than given on a fixed, every 6 hour schedule. Other alternatives include perphenazine (Trilafon), which is available for intravenous or oral administration and can be given as a continuous infusion.

Prochlorperazine (Compazine) can be very useful in younger children for sedation and treatment of nausea but has less antiemetic effect than the two agents noted previously. It is given at 0.5 mg/kg PO, PR, or IM. Promethazine (Phenergan) works similarly to reduce the sensation of nausea and enhance sedation rather than significantly decreasing vomiting. Any child receiving a phenothiazine derivative should be alerted to the possibility of extrapyramidal side effects that can continue to occur for 48 hours after the drug is discontinued. They can be treated easily, however, with the use of diphenhydramine or another antihistamine.

A new addition to the chemotherapeutic antiemetic regimen is ondansetron (Zofran), a selective serotonin receptor antagonist. It is given intravenously 30 minutes before chemotherapy and then every 4 hours for two additional doses. The dose is 0.15 mg/kg per dose and is recommended for children 3 years of age or older.

Cannabinoid derivatives, although certainly not first-line agents, may be effective in controlling chemotherapy-induced emesis as well. Delta-9-tetrahydrocannabinol is available as a schedule 2 substance (Marinol) and can be given at a dose of 5 mg/m² to children every 4 hours up to a maximum of 15 mg/d starting 5 hours before chemotherapy. The side effects of cannabinoid derivatives are rare but may involve drowsiness, agitation, or general dysphoria.

Antihistamines, such as dimenhydrinate (Dramamine), may be useful as prophylaxis against nausea and vomiting resulting from motion sickness. It is not useful once the nausea and vomiting have started, however. Emetrol (a phosphated carbohydrate solution) also may be useful in children for relief of nausea associated with an upset stomach. It is not as efficacious in the cessation of vomiting once it occurs.

If a psychogenic etiology is determined, where the precipitation of vomiting is more of a factor than the actual effect, lorazepam or diazepam may be indicated. In the small infant in whom phenothiazines may be contraindicated because their side effects outweigh their benefits, promethazine (Phenergan) might be tried first, with the addition of diphenhydramine for poor response or if toxicity occurs. In situations of cyclic vomiting or episodes of psychogenic etiology, such techniques as biofeedback and other behavior modification and psychotherapy methodologies have been used successfully to decrease anticipatory nausea and vomiting cycles.

REFERENCES

1. Billet AL, Sallen SE: Management of nausea and vomiting. *In* Pizzo PA, Poplack DG (eds): Principles and Practices of Pediatric Oncology. Philadelphia, JP Lippincott, 1993:1051–1055.
2. Dodge JA: Vomiting and regurgitation. *In* Walker WA, Durie PR, Hamilton JR, Walker-Smith JA, Watkin JB (eds): Pediatric Gastrointestinal Disease. Philadelphia, BC Decker, 1991:32–41.
3. Roberts JT, Priestman TJ: A review of ondansetron in the management of radiotherapy-induced emesis. Oncology 1993;50:173–179.

RECURRENT ABDOMINAL PAIN

J. CARLTON GARTNER, JR., M.D.

Recurrent abdominal pain (RAP) is a common and, at times, vexing complaint for the pediatrician. The prevalence of the problem is approximately 10% in childhood, with a peak incidence in 9 to 10-year-old girls of about 25%. Apley's definition of RAP is still used: a child more than 3 years of age, more than three episodes over at least a 3-month period, and episodes severe enough to interfere with daily activity.[1] Although numerous organic disorders have been suggested as the primary etiology, true medical or surgical causes are found in less than 5% of children.

The pain in a child with RAP is located in the central abdomen, usually in the periumbilical area (60%) or lower abdomen (30%). It is usually either crampy (50%) or a dull ache (30%).[4] Most patients experience pain that lasts for minutes to several hours and recurs several times per week or per month. Rarely do patients experience daily pain. Associated symptoms described by children or their families are usually nonspecific: pallor, tiredness, mild anorexia, dizziness, and headache. Emesis, diarrhea, and constipation are reported less frequently. Despite careful questioning, it is usually difficult to relate episodes to meals or other possible triggering mechanisms.

PATIENT AND FAMILY CHARACTERISTICS

Most physicians recognize a typical personality type for children with RAP: perfectionist and overachieving. Several controlled studies have modified this profile. Anxiety, fearfulness, dependency, and poor self-esteem are found more frequently in children with RAP. There are significantly more stressful life events during the period of pain. Unfortunately, at least one study has demonstrated that patients with inflammatory bowel disease and RAP are different from a control population but not from each other when standard psychologic tests are administered.

Apley found that family members of children with RAP had an increased incidence not only of abdominal pain but also of several medical disorders: migraine, peptic ulcer disease, appendectomy, and "nervous breakdown."[1] Controlled studies have demonstrated that marital discord, maternal depression, and maternal health problems are more prevalent in families of children with RAP. Furthermore, somatization disorders occur in other family members at a higher than expected rate.

ETIOLOGY

Numerous theories for the cause(s) of childhood abdominal pain of a recurrent and chronic nature have been advanced. Older theories (conditioned learning, intestinal dyskinesia, carbohydrate malabsorption) explain symptoms in some patients. Abnormal intestinal motility and permeability have been described in separate studies. The most helpful approach clinically is multifactorial, and the physician should assume that patients with RAP have a genetic or gastrointestinal predisposition that is aggravated by personality, life events, or lifestyle.

Purely organic causes of RAP are rare, as demonstrated by long-term studies, such as those from the Mayo Clinic. In a series of 161 children with at least a 5-year follow-up (often far longer), Stickler and Murphy found 3 (1.9%) who developed definite organic disorders—Crohn's disease in each case.[5] Additionally, 20% had undergone laparotomy. A few other conditions causing abdominal pain deserve mention: urinary tract disorders, peptic ulcer disease, carbohydrate malabsorption, pancreatitis, and recurrent volvulus. Clues to these organic disorders may include peripheral abdominal pain, nocturnal pain, protracted emesis, growth deceleration or weight loss, and the absence of personality, or family factors that are typical for RAP. Abnormalities of physical examination or laboratory screening tests are more likely. In contrast, other vague complaints (e.g., headache, dizziness, limb pains) frequently accompany typical RAP.

TREATMENT

The therapy of RAP actually begins with a carefully done history and physical examination. A comprehensive and sensitive evaluation at this point will help prevent the random use of diagnostic tests and will also establish a solid relationship with the patient and family. Specific clues to organic disorders must be sought, as well as nuances of family functioning and life stresses. The possibility of child abuse must be considered as well. At the end of the evaluation, if specific organic disorders remain in the differential diagnosis, individualized specific testing must be completed, for example, endoscopy if peptic ulcer disease is a consideration. Most patients will not require extensive testing, and the performance of a few screening tests is the only necessity. These include complete blood count, sedimentation rate, urinalysis and urine culture, serum albumin and amylase/lipase, and stool testing for occult blood. Suggesting that further tests may be done later if symptoms worsen almost universally ensures that the problem will progress! The physician must be reassured before the family can be managed.[2]

Patients who have a typical history, normal physical examination, and negative screening tests usually can be managed by the pediatrician, with frequent follow-up. The first priority is to accept the pain as real but not secondary to defined medical or surgical conditions. Many families are helped by review of the frequency of the problem and the extremely low incidence of missed organic disorders in long-term follow-up studies. Factors that may aggravate the problem should be addressed, for example, hurried meals, constipation, hectic lifestyle, family discord, and stress. It must be emphasized that the child should remain in (or return to) school as treatment proceeds. Routine use of sedatives, antispasmodic agents, antacids, and elimination diets should not be part of the treatment plan. Most patients will improve with reassurance and careful, supportive follow-up. Rare patients with extremely chaotic family life and symptoms suggestive of major behavioral or psychiatric disturbance may require referral to a colleague in child psychiatry.

REFERENCES

1. Apley J: The Child with Abdominal Pains. Oxford, England, Blackwell Scientific Publications, 1975.
2. Gartner JC: Recurrent abdominal pain: Who needs a workup? Contemp Pediatr 1989;6:62–82.
3. Levine M, Rappaport LA: Recurrent abdominal pain in school children: The loneliness of the long distance physician. Pediatr Clin North Am 1984;31:969–991.
4. Liebman WM: Recurrent abdominal pain in children. A retrospective survey of 119 patients. Clin Pediatr 1978;17:149–153.
5. Stickler GB, Murphy DB: Recurrent abdominal pain. Am J Dis Child 1979;133:486–489.

CONSTIPATION AND ENCOPRESIS

Michael J. Pettei, m.d., Ph.D.

Constipation is a poorly defined problem that occurs commonly in the pediatric age group. Although only rarely associated with serious underlying disorders, it can be accompanied by significant functional disability and family discord. Constipation often is easily treated when it first occurs, but the individual commonly seeks medical help long after the initial symptoms, when its resolution is more difficult. The tendency to constipation often seems familial. Firm, infrequent stools may develop in infants and children with this tendency, producing pain. This may lead to voluntary withholding, with eventual onset of *encopresis* (involuntary stool passage), which constitutes a greater problem than the original constipation.

Since constipation is a symptom and not a disease, it is associated with many disorders. It is during the first few months of life that organic causes most commonly occur. Some of the disorders that can give rise to constipation include hypothyroidism, hypercalcemia, hypokalemia, lead ingestion, infant botulism, dehydration, and abnormalities in abdominal musculature or neuromuscular innervation. Structural problems, such as abdominal or pelvic masses, intestinal stenoses and strictures, and anorectal problems (e.g., anal fissures), may also occur with constipation. A number of medications, including anticholinergics, hematinics, and opiates, may cause constipation. The most frequently considered organic etiology in constipated infants is Hirschsprung's disease (congenital aganglionosis). Nevertheless, infants with functional constipation may pass less than one bowel movement daily. In the vast majority of children, no underlying abnormality is found, and the term *chronic functional (idiopathic) constipation* can be applied.

The diagnosis of chronic functional constipation rests principally on a detailed history and physical examination, with knowledge of the natural history of functional constipation. In the history, special attention should be paid to stool frequency and size, the age of onset, dietary intake, family history, withholding behavior, presence of soiling, and response to prior therapy. Vomiting, localized abdominal pain, inordinate abdominal distention, and failure to thrive or weight loss could indicate an organic cause. Physical examination must take particular note of the abdominal contents, anal tone and placement, sacral appearance, and rectal contents, as well as abdominal wall strength and neurologic status. When the patient with chronic constipation does not fit the usual developmental pattern, does not present the appropriate physical findings, or does not respond to therapy, further evaluation should be considered.

Although it seems likely that the mechanism underlying functional constipation may vary in patients of different ages and sex, the clinical presentation of chronic retentive constipation is usually quite similar in children, and therapy for constipation should take into account the particular developmental stage of the disorder. Therapy may need to be directed to (1) Symptomatic constipation, (2) Stool withholding, or (3) Eventual encopresis.

CONSTIPATION

Symptomatic Constipation

For children with acute constipation, dietary manipulation should be the mainstay of therapy. Newborns may have bowel movements with each feeding but on average have four bowel movements per day. Those who eliminate only one to two times per day during the first month may be demonstrating a tendency to develop constipation. Between 4 and 6 months of age, infants commonly have two to three movements per day, whereas the infant with a tendency to constipate often begins to skip days. Although many babies get through this period without difficulty, others experience painful defecation and develop anal fissures.

Dietary therapy forestalls later problems in the infant younger than 6 months of age with a tendency to constipation. Laxative fruits, such as apricots, prunes, and pears, and the nonstarchy vegetables should be encouraged, as should an occasional water or juice bottle. For those with persistently firm stools, stool softness can be increased via colonic fermentation. Carbohydrate preparations, such as dark corn syrup or malt soup extract (dark Karo syrup or Maltsupex 1 to 2 teaspoons one to three times per day) may be tried. Although the resulting colonic fermentative process softens stools, it also increases gas in the intestinal tract. Occasionally, this induces or worsens colicky behavior in the first few months of life. For this situation, glycerin suppositories or rectal stimulation with a lubricated cotton swab may be used for a short time to induce a daily bowel movement. For many young infants, defecation is accompanied by considerable grimacing and grunting. Parents should be reassured that as long as stools are of average frequency and consistency, no intervention is necessary.

In the latter part of the first year or in the second year of life, manifestations of constipation (anal fissures with streaks of blood on the stool, small hard scybala, infrequent defecation) should not be approached with reassurances that the child will outgrow the problem. Although this is true in some instances, other children experience increasing difficulties. Benign neglect at this age can result in a pattern of chronic constipation and stool-withholding behavior with eventual megarectum and encopresis. In the toddler, particular emphasis should be placed on the avoidance of excessive dairy products, especially to the exclusion of water or juice intake. Maltsupex may be useful, laxative fruit snacks (prunes, apricots, or raisins) may be substituted for sweets, and a number of different bran products (e.g., bran cereals and bran muffins) may be tolerated by older toddlers. In some instances, limited amounts of a stimulant, such as senna (Senokot or Castoria 1 or 2 teaspoons daily), or a lubricant (mineral oil 1 or 2 tablespoons daily) may be necessary for a short time. The medications should not be forced on an unwilling child but can be mixed with food products. For example, senna can be placed in juices and mineral oil in milk.

Voluntary Stool Withholding

Beginning as early as late infancy, but more commonly in the middle or latter part of the second year of life, children may begin to withhold stools voluntarily to avoid painful defecation. Another critical time for the development of stool withholding is during toilet training. Many toddlers develop an aversion to the toilet, resulting in withholding. When this is significant, training should be abandoned until regular, voluntary bowel movements have been reestablished. Parents often mistake stool withholding for exaggerated attempts at defecation. It is often useful in explaining this behavior to compare the stiff, erect posturing of withholding to the natural squat position of defecation. In the toddler who shows stool withholding behavior of short duration and in whom significant fecal retention or megarectum has not occurred, short-term therapy may suffice. One to two enemas (3 ml/kg 12 hours apart), followed by forced daily evacuation for 2 to 3 weeks with laxative therapy (Senokot or milk of magnesia 1 to 3 teaspoons per day usually q.h.s.), is usually sufficient. If withholding behavior is abolished, a daily bowel habit may be achieved by dietary therapy and bowel training. If necessary, low-dose mineral oil (1 to 2 tablespoons per day) or laxative therapy may be added, depending on the age of the child.

ENCOPRESIS

With chronic stool withholding, the lower colonic segment gradually becomes distended with accumulated stool. The urge to defecate then becomes irregular, since a stretched wall seems to decrease rectal sensation. A vicious cycle is thus set up. The retained material is difficult to pass, the patient refuses to try and holds back, the rectum and sigmoid are distended, their walls gradually overstretch, and the urge is appreciated less frequently. When the rectum has become sufficiently distended, any additional stool that arrives from the more proximal colon cannot be accommodated, resulting in involuntary stool passage (encopresis).

For children with chronic constipation who have progressed to an enlarged rectum and encopresis, treatment with a regimented program is useful. It is based on the assumption that maintaining a relatively empty rectum devoid of retained stool over time results in a decrease in rectal size and an increase of rectal sensitivity to distention. Encopresis (overflow soiling) will not occur if feces are not permitted to accumulate in the rectum. Thus, encouragement should be given to both the parents and the child that the most anxiety-provoking symptom, soiling, usually can be resolved quickly.

Treatment of Encopresis and Megarectum

The management of functional encopresis and megarectum can be divided into several steps. Before therapy is outlined, the parents and patient should be educated about the usual natural history of encopresis. After an explanation of stool retention and development of the megarectum, it should be pointed out that most soiling occurs involuntarily through an overflow-type mechanism, without the control of the child. Parental attempts to place blame are, therefore, inappropriate.

Disimpaction

The *initial* phase of therapy involves disimpaction. The most effective, yet acceptable method of achieving this is through the administration of hypertonic phosphate enemas (3 ml/kg up to 13.5 dl [4.5 oz.]) in most cases each morning and evening until the effluent is free of solid stool. On average, this entails two to four enemas (1 to 2 days). *Since these enemas in overdosage can result in hyperphosphatemia or electrolyte abnormalities, they should not be used in those with significant medical problems (e.g., cardiac or renal failure) or in the very young child.* No more than two enemas per day for 3 days should be advised without reexamination, which may include serum chemistries and an abdominal film. Other cleanout regimens may use medicated suppositories, oral laxatives, such as bisacodyl (Dulcolax) or senna, or polyethylene glycol-electrolyte solutions. Occasionally, the child presents with a fecaloma, a hard, inspissated stool concretion, and may require multiple mineral oil enemas between phosphate enemas to achieve cleanout.

Preventing Reaccumulation of Stool and Stopping Stool-withholding Behavior

The *second* phase of therapy is aimed at preventing the reaccumulation of retained feces and overcoming stool-withholding behavior, if present. Encopresis should not recur if rectal impactions are not permitted to accumulate. However, if therapy is not initiated to prevent retention, the child will simply return to the former state after time. To force one or two stools daily, a sufficient dose of stimulant or osmotic laxative (senna, milk of magnesia, or lactulose) should be prescribed (e.g., Dulcolax or Senokot 1 to 3 tablets usually q.h.s.). In those in whom impressive megarectum has developed over years, this regimen may need to be continued on a prolonged basis. (An alternative solution to this problem, the Davidson method, used high-dose mineral oil therapy [5 to 15 ml/kg divided b.i.d.] to achieve four to six bowel movements per day. However, this rigorous regimen is difficult for most children and has largely been abandoned.)

Establishing Regular Bowel Patterns

The *final* stage of treatment is directed at establishing a regular bowel pattern. Conditioning to at least daily stools ensures softer stools and is reasonable in children old enough to cooperate (3 to 4 years old). The child must be encouraged to sit on the commode for 5 to

15 minutes at least once a day, usually after a meal (particularly breakfast). Young children should be encouraged to rest their feet on a stool or other solid support to maintain mechanical leverage. For those on laxatives, the dosage should be decreased gradually over a few months while a regular bowel habit is formed. Low-dose mineral oil therapy (30 to 60 ml) may be added on laxative withdrawal to help maintain the bowel training.

For those who do not voluntarily comply with the bowel training program, more formalized behavior modification therapy may be of benefit. Manometric biofeedback may be useful for nonresponders. The family should be cautioned that interruption of the normal routine (e.g., vacation, periods of illness) may give rise to acute constipation, which should be addressed promptly with enemas or laxatives to avoid the recurrence of chronic problems. The rare child with *voluntary fecal soiling* without impaction or megarectum represents a significant behavioral problem and should have psychiatric evaluation.

SUMMARY

Constipation and encopresis are common and often functionally disabling problems in childhood. Diagnosis rests almost completely on a thorough history and physical examination. Therapy is usually effective, although sometimes prolonged. Early recognition and anticipatory guidance with preventive dietary measures can help avoid the establishment of chronic constipation and stool withholding. Attention to these disorders is important, as measured by the amount of functional disability that can be promptly relieved by therapy.

REFERENCES

1. Christophersen ER: Toileting problems in children. Pediatr Annu 1991;20:240–244.
2. Loening-Baucke V: Management of chronic constipation in infants and toddlers. Am Fam Physician 1994;49:397–400, 403–406, 411–413.
3. Nolan T, Oberklaid F: New concepts in the management of encopresis. Pediatr Rev 1993;14:447–451.

INFANT COLIC SYNDROME

BRUCE TAUBMAN, M.D.

Infant colic is a syndrome in which healthy infants, usually less than 3 months of age, have episodes of excessive, seemingly inconsolable crying. Most studies on infant colic include only infants whose parents report them to be crying more than 3 hours a day or to have more than 2 hours of crying a day on detailed behavior diaries. The etiology of this syndrome remains controversial, and, consequently, so does its treatment.

Some investigators have hypothesized that infants with colic have milk protein intolerance and recommend treatment with protein hydrolysate formula or milk protein-free diets for nursing mothers. There are studies which show that 20% to 30% of colicky infants improve with such treatments. However, these studies include infants with vomiting or diarrhea or both. Other studies, which appropriately exclude any infant with these symptoms, have failed to show any long-term improvement with this approach.

Many infants with colic will pass a great deal of flatus while crying and appear as if they are having abdominal pain. As a result, excessive gas has been suggested as a cause of the infant colic syndrome, and simethicone has been recommended as a treatment. However, no one has been able to document excessive gas production in these infants. There is only one well-designed double-blind crossover study on the use of simethicone as a treatment for colic.[1] It failed to show any significant therapeutic effect.

Since infants with colic often draw their legs up, harden their abdomens, and turn red in the face while crying, it has been assumed that their problem is abdominal pain per se. Antispasmodics, therefore, have been used as a treatment. Unfortunately, dicyclomine hydrochloride (Bentyl) is the only antispasmodic shown to be effective in some colicky infants, and it has serious side effects in that it can cause lethargy and sedation, an action that may explain its effectiveness. Furthermore, it has been reported to cause apnea, seizures, and even death when used in infants. Consequently the manufacturer (Marion Merrell Dow) has warned against its use in this age group.

An alternative to such treatments is based on the hypothesis that colicky infants are not crying because of pain. In support of this hypothesis, it is pointed out that the manner in which colicky infants cry is nonspecific, and a careful history and physical examination have failed to reveal any condition that would cause pain. It has been proposed that these infants begin crying to communicate their needs and wants.[2,3] If the cause of the crying is misinterpreted by the parents and responded to incorrectly, the colicky infant's temperament is such that he or she will continue to cry. After a while, the baby becomes so agitated and distraught as to be truly inconsolable. The key to treating infant colic syndrome is to interpret the meaning of the infant's crying before this occurs.

Treatment based on this hypothesis of the etiology of the infant colic syndrome includes several steps. First, the physician must take a careful history and do a careful physical examination to rule out any medical condition in the baby that may be causing pain. Having done this, the physician then has the difficult task of convincing the parents that their infant is healthy and not in pain. It must be explained that one cannot know why a baby is crying by observation.

Next, the physician must discern exactly how the parents are misinterpreting the infant's cries. This is difficult to do by the traditional approach of taking a careful history. Most parents with a colicky infant are emotionally distraught and sleep deprived. They often have difficulty recalling details needed to determine the context of their infant's crying and the sequence of their responses to the cries. It is, therefore, helpful, and often necessary, to have parents complete a behavior diary. Figure 1 is an example of one such diary used effectively in treating colicky infants. In addition to allowing the physician to observe the effectiveness of specific parental responses to their crying infant, it can be used to quantitate baseline crying and to monitor the effectiveness of counseling.

An examination of the diary may reveal that the parents are not truly demand feeding their infant. Despite being instructed to do so and believing they are complying, the parents may never consider feeding the baby more often then every 2 or 3 hours. This may be because of concern about overfeeding the baby, leading to abdominal pain or obesity or both. The diary may demonstrate that the parents are trying to bring order into their newly hectic lives by attempting to get their infant on a regular eating and sleeping schedule. Rather than responding to the infant's signals, the parents arbitrarily put the baby into the crib to sleep when he is not tired, do not feed the infant when he is hungry because it is too soon, or do not pick up the crying infant because they feel that he has not slept enough.

Parents may never offer an infant a pacifier because they believe it is harmful or they find it esthetically unpleasing. The diary may show that the parents never put their baby in the crib until he has fallen asleep in their arms, even though this may require hours of walking and rocking. By reviewing the diary, the pediatrician may discover that the parents are picking up their sleeping infant in response to nonspecific noises the infant is making, inadvertently waking the baby. This usually occurs when the infant is sleeping in the parents' room.

Occasionally, by the time the parents have consulted the physician, they are convinced that most of their infant's crying is as a result of pain. When this occurs, the diary will show that the parents only respond to the crying infant by walking and rocking the baby.

After reviewing the behavior diary and having some ideas of how and why the parents are misinterpreting their infant's cries, the pediatrician counsels them to treat infant crying as communication. It is explained that misinterpreting infant cries in some infants, such as

Daily Diary Page

Name _____

Day/Date: _____

A.M. P.M. (circle one)

Activity Code

S	=	Sleeping alone (not held)
SH	=	Sleeping held
F	=	Feeding
AAH	=	Awake, alone, and happy (in crib, infant seat, swing, etc., but not held)
AAC	=	Awake, alone, crying
AHH	=	Awake, held, and happy
AHC	=	Awake, held, and crying
(W)	=	Being walked
(R)	=	Being rocked
B	=	Being bathed
(P)	=	Pacifier

Hour	Start Time	Activity	Minutes of Crying
12			
1			
2			
3			
4			
5			
6			
7			
8			
9			
10			
11			

Total Minutes Crying: _____

FIGURE 1. Parents are instructed to note the time one behavior starts and a second begins, using the activity code shown.

theirs, results in continual and inconsolable crying and agitation. The five basic parental responses to infant crying are explained and reviewed: feeding, holding the infant (not walking with the baby), giving a pacifier, stimulating the infant visually and aurally, putting the infant to sleep. Parents are instructed to try each response in any order they feel appropriate until the infant stops crying. They are urged to try each response for only a minute or so so that they can try all responses within 5 to 7 minutes, before the infant becomes agitated and inconsolable. The baseline diary is reviewed with the parents, and the problems of that specific family are discussed.

It is important to stress to parents that the infant colic syndrome from which their baby is suffering is not their fault. Interpreting the meaning of the cry of any infant can be difficult. Without help, it can be close to impossible in infants who are irregular in their sleeping and feeding patterns and who require little sleep. It is certainly not the parents' fault that their infant has a temperament that causes him to become agitated and inconsolable when crying is misunderstood. It is also not their fault that much of their response to their crying infant has been based on inappropriate advice from family, friends, and even doctors.

After counseling of the parents, continued follow-up is usually needed. This can best be done by having the parents continue the behavior diaries, receiving feedback from the pediatrician until the crying is reduced to less then 1½ hours per day.

REFERENCES

1. Danielsson B, Hwang CP: Treatment of infant colic with surface active substance (simethicone). Acta Paediatr Scand 1985;74:445–450.
2. Taubman B: A randomized trial comparing parental counseling with elimination of cow's milk or soy milk protein for the treatment of infant colic syndrome. Pediatrics 1988;81:756–761.
3. Taubman B: Why Is My Baby Crying? New York, Simon & Schuster, 1993.

FOREIGN BODIES IN THE GASTROINTESTINAL TRACT

Lewis R. First, M.D.

The gastrointestinal tract can be a frequent location for the ingestion, aspiration, or insertion of a nonedible object by a child. Although the vast majority of foreign bodies in the gastrointestinal tract pass within 7 to 10 days without complication, it is important to be aware of the potential problems that can occur with such an event. It is also important to consider the possibility of a foreign body in the gastrointestinal tract even if the symptomatic child or family does not give a history of such an ingestion. The child who frequently puts objects in the mouth, is easily distractable, is fed inappropriate-for-age foods, or is given inappropriate-for-age toys runs a risk of foreign body aspiration or ingestion. Knowledge of what has been ingested, as well as where the object is located within the gastrointestinal tract, can help the practitioner decide on the most beneficial therapeutic approach.

If examination of the nasopharynx does not reveal an ingested object, a reasonable approach is to obtain plain radiographs that display the entire gastrointestinal tract from nasopharynx to rectum, since most foreign bodies made of glass or metal will appear radiopaque. Even if the object is not radiopaque, plain films may show air trapping suggestive of obstruction. Recently, metal detectors have been employed in some emergency rooms as another means of confirming the presence of a metallic foreign body and have been found to be as sensitive as the radiograph for detecting such an object. If the ingested metal object is sharp, however, a confirmatory radiograph is still needed to determine its nature and location.

A radiolucent foreign body that does not appear identifiable by plain film should be looked for with a barium swallow and upper gastrointestinal series to ensure that there is no obstruction at the gastric outlet or elsewhere. If esophageal perforation is a concern, a small amount of Gastrografin might be used instead of barium as the contrast agent in the esophagogram. If the object is suspected to be in the nasopharynx, a CT scan of this area is an alternative way to image for wooden objects or objects lodged in the deep soft tissues.

ESOPHAGEAL FOREIGN BODIES

The esophagus is a worrisome area should a foreign body lodge there, since edema, ulceration, perforation, or subsequent aspiration and pneumonia can result. Coins are the most frequent foreign bodies

to lodge in the esophagus of children. There are three common locations where obstruction or lack of forward movement can occur:

1. The cervical esophagus at the thoracic inlet (at the lower border of the cricopharyngeus muscle) (60% to 80%)
2. The cardioesophageal level (where the esophagus crosses the aorta) (5% to 20%)
3. The area of the gastroesophageal junction (10% to 20%)

Symptoms suggestive of an esophageal foreign body include refusal to eat solids, drooling, vomiting, dysphagia, cough exacerbated by feeds, and, rarely, no symptoms whatsoever except a good history for such an event. Symptoms of respiratory distress, such as stridor or tachypnea, can occur as a result of pressure on the airway from an impacted esophagus. In addition, mediastinitis, lung abscess, pneumothorax, or pleural effusion can result from an esophageal perforation secondary to a sharp object or from pressure necrosis from a lodged large object. If the object is lodged above the level of the cricopharyngeus muscle, a patient is able to localize it. Below this level, however, patient-guided localization is no longer reliable.

Fewer than 20% of children with an esophageal foreign body will have an abnormal physical examination. The most common signs include respiratory distress, fever, or palatal abrasions. Lungs should be listened to for decreased breath sounds or wheezes. Stool should be checked for blood.

Confirmation of an esophageal foreign body often can be made radiographically. An AP view of the chest will show an esophageal radiopaque foreign body en face (coronal view), whereas a tracheal object will appear in a sagittal anterior-posterior plane. A child who has had prior esophageal surgery who has symptoms suggestive of an esophageal foreign body after eating should proceed directly to an esophagogram or endoscopy, since many obstructive or hung-up foodstuffs are radiolucent and will not appear on plain film. If radiographs reveal such an object and the child is symptomatic, endoscopy should be performed as soon as possible. If clinical suspicion is high, even if the child is asymptomatic, with an object that has not moved from the esophagus in 24 hours, endoscopy should be done for exploration and removal of the object, since mucosa can grow around the object and make it even more difficult to remove over time.

If an ingested button disc battery lodges in the esophagus, the child should undergo rapid removal even if asymptomatic, since tissue injuries have been reported as early as 4 hours after ingestion. Glucagon has been reported to relax esophageal smooth muscle and attenuate lower esophageal sphincter (LES) tone and has been reported to be useful in moving foreign bodies from the lower third of the esophagus into the stomach. The initial dose is 0.05 mg/kg IV and can be repeated after 10 to 20 minutes. The impact of administering this in the pediatric population remains anecdotal at present.

Most esophageal complications occur after 24 hours or more of impaction. Recently, considerable success has been achieved by trained gastroenterologists using flexible endoscopy accompanied by conscious sedation (e.g., IV diazepam and meperidine), although endoscopy with general anesthesia has long been the gold standard reported in the literature.

The use of a 12–16F Foley catheter has been reported to be a successful method of removing rounded foreign objects lodged in the esophagus, but this method carries with it a host of potential complications that make this a less than desirable option. This technique involves the insertion, under fluoroscopic guidance, of a Foley catheter through the nose and past the object in the esophagus. The balloon is then inflated with contrast material, and the catheter is withdrawn into the oropharynx as the object is either coughed out or grasped for removal. The Foley technique does not allow direct visualization of the object and provides no airway protection. This technique may result in less than optimal control of where an object goes as it is brought up by the inflated catheter, allowing it to lodge in the hypopharynx or even to go down the trachea. It requires a prolonged radiation dose during the fluoroscopy as well. This method does not allow one to see if there is associated esophageal disease from pressure impaction of the foreign body or if there might be more than one foreign body left behind. Incorrect technique might result in perforation of the esophagus itself from the catheter. Endoscopy, as well as general surgery, should be available to the provider who attempts this technique.

If a large piece of meat lodges in the distal esophagus and the child is handling the secretions, 12 hours of observation can be in order while waiting for passage into the stomach. If the child is not handling secretions well or if symptoms suggestive of an obstructive food bolus in the esophagus persist, endoscopy should be used to either remove the bolus or push it into the stomach. The use of an enzyme, such as papain, to enhance digestion of meat lodged in the esophagus is not recommended, since such enzymatic preparations frequently result in complications. Papain can simultaneously perforate or digest the esophagus while working on the meat. Furthermore, papain will not digest bone fragments that may be present in the meat.

FOREIGN BODIES IN THE STOMACH AND INTESTINES

Once the esophagus has been cleared, other points of potential obstruction include the pylorus, duodenal C loop, duodenal-jejunal junction, ileocecal valve (the most common site for perforation from a long sharp object), and rectum. An object less than 15 mm in diameter detected in the stomach should not raise significant concern unless it remains there for at least 7 to 10 days without moving forward. Although sharp objects (e.g., bones, toothpicks, needles) suggest an increased risk of perforation, less than 1% do result in perforation with clinical symptoms, and almost all pass. Nonetheless, if such an object is detected in the stomach, especially if the object is greater than 5 cm long, endoscopy should be considered to avoid peritonitis and hemorrhage secondary to a perforation, although the data are unconvincing relative to just waiting.

The intestines, although being a site for perforation from a sharp object, rarely cause trouble, and almost all objects that clear the pylorus move easily through the intestines. The most frequently reported intestinal complications result from long narrow objects (greater than 5 cm) that have difficulty passing through areas of angulation, such as the duodenal sweep and the ileocecal valve, or that lodge in such locations as a Meckel's diverticulum or an inguinal hernia. Serial films every 3 to 5 days to monitor the course of such an object can be helpful to ensure that lodgment and, in turn, associated increased risk for complications is not occurring. Parental monitoring of the stool for passage of the object often is suggested, but it is unpleasant for parents, and compliance is questionable. Nonetheless, if an object has not progressed for 2 to 3 weeks in the intestine or if there is evidence of obstruction, hemorrhage, or perforation, a surgical approach must be considered.

Objects that have been inserted up the rectum that cause pain and discomfort usually can be removed manually with the help of a vaginal speculum for visualization. If it cannot be accessed manually, a sig-moidoscope may be necessary for adequate visualization and removal. If the object is fragile and may fragment with removal, general anesthesia is recommended before attempting such removal.

DISC BUTTON BATTERY INGESTIONS

One of the objects tht a child can swallow that causes great concern is the disc button battery found in many small computer toys and games, as well as in hearing aids and calculators. More than 500 such ingestions are reported per year. These batteries contain potassium hydroxide, manganese dioxide, and either mercuric or silver oxide and can cause significant injury throughout the proximal part of the gastrointestinal tract. The mechanism of this injury may be

1. Electrolyte leakage from the battery, with subsequent liquefaction necrosis and tissue destruction
2. Corrosive effects of mercuric oxide after leakage
3. Electrical current that can be generated, creating an electrical burn
4. Simply pressure necrosis from the impacted battery

All patients ingesting a battery must have at least one roentgenogram to determine its location. Induced emesis should never be attempted with these batteries, since the batteries may move retrograde and lodge in the esophagus, causing significant damage to surrounding tissue.

Since damage to the esophagus can occur quickly once a battery is lodged there (because the moist environment helps to generate a low voltage current), immediate removal via endoscopy is necessary. Neither battery diameter nor symptoms are predictive of battery position or damage in the esophagus, although batteries larger than 15 mm stand a higher risk of getting stuck. Any battery less than 15 mm that is detected in the stomach of a child under 6 years of age should be given 24 hours to pass before attempts are made to remove it endoscopically. The use of cathartics, such as magnesium citrate, or motility agents, such as metoclopramide, to enhance the propulsion of these batteries out of the stomach is largely anecdotal in the literature but may bring some success with little risk in these patients.

SUMMARY

The best therapeutic approach to foreign bodies in the gastrointestinal tract is to advocate prevention. Parents need to be made aware of the potential dangers of the small parts and objects their toddlers handle, as well as the damage that can result from such an apparently innocent object as the button battery. Better childproof battery compartments and a clearly written package warning regarding possible toddler ingestion of such batteries hopefully will reduce the incidence of related injuries.

REFERENCES

1. Crysdale WS, Sendi KS, Yoo J: Esophageal foreign bodies in children: 15-year review of 484 cases. Ann Otolaryngol Rhinol Laryngol 1991;100:320–324.
2. Litovitz T, Schmitz BF: Ingestion of cylindrical and button batteries: An analysis of 2382 cases. Pediatrics 1992:747–757.

7

Hematology

ANEMIA OF IRON DEFICIENCY

STEVEN ARKIN, M.D.

Iron deficiency arises when the iron requirement for daily needs and for growth exceeds the available iron supply (the sum of the iron endowment at birth plus absorbed iron). Early iron deficiency is evidenced by depletion of body iron stores, with a decrease in both serum ferritin and stainable iron in the bone marrow. With progression, serum iron levels fall and serum transferrin (total iron binding capacity) increases, resulting in a decreased percent saturation of transferrin ($<15\%$). As iron deficiency becomes more profound, supplies of iron become inadequate for optimal production of hemoglobin, myoglobin, and a variety of iron-containing enzymes, including catalase and the cytochromes, resulting in a microcytic anemia with elevation of the free erythrocyte protoporphyrin (FEP). Clinical symptoms may include irritability, listlessness, anorexia, reduced spontaneous activity, and dulled interest in the environment, as well as those signs and symptoms related to potentially severe anemia.

Treatment of iron deficiency includes iron replacement therapy and determination of the etiology of the iron deficit. This includes an evaluation for unusual or excessive iron losses and an assessment of the adequacy of dietary iron intake.

REPLACEMENT THERAPY WITH IRON

Oral therapy with iron salt preparations is the preferred mode of treatment because of efficacy, ease of administration, and cost. Available iron salt preparations include reduced iron (Fe) complexed to sulfate, fumarate, or gluconate (sulfate salt is preferred because of its cost advantage). Ferrous sulfate is available in drop (15 mg elemental Fe per 0.6 ml), syrup (30 mg elemental Fe per 5 ml), elixir (30 or 45 mg elemental Fe per 5 ml), and tablet form (40 or 60 mg elemental Fe per tablet) (Table 1). Drops are most appropriate for infants, syrup or elixir for toddlers, and tablets for older children. Although doses as high as 6 mg/kg/d of elemental iron have been recommended, the mathematics of blood turnover indicate that absorption of 1.5 mg/kg/d of elemental iron will allow for a maximal reticulocyte response (Table 2). With the increased efficiency of iron absorption in the setting of iron deficiency anemia, 2 to 3 mg/kg/d of elemental iron given orally, a dose associated with a minimum of side effects, is adequate to permit this level of absorption.

Absorption of iron given with meals can be decreased by 50% to 60%. Therefore, oral iron therapy should be divided into two or three daily doses given between meals. Food products, such as tea, coffee, and milk, contain compounds (tannic acid, polyphenols, oxalates, and phosphates) that can complex to iron, reducing its absorption by up to 75%, and should not be ingested concurrently with iron replacement therapy. Simultaneous ingestion of large amounts of vitamin C helps

to lower the redox state of ingested iron, increasing its absorption. However, vitamin C administration is usually not necessary for successful treatment of iron deficiency. To avoid temporary staining of the teeth, liquid iron preparations are best administered to the back of the tongue. Side effects of oral iron therapy are rare. They include gastrointestinal irritation, diarrhea, and constipation. When observed, such side effects often can be eliminated by giving the iron concurrently with meals.

Parenteral iron is usually not indicated in the treatment of iron deficiency. Exceptions include lack of compliance or the inability to absorb orally administered iron. All preparations of parenteral iron are high molecular weight compounds, with iron bound to a substance stabilizing the iron in the form of a complex. Iron dextran (Imferon, 50 mg of elemental Fe per milliliter) is the parenteral compound used most commonly in the United States. Required dosing with Imferon (in milliliters) can be calculated using the following formula.

$$
\begin{aligned}
\text{Dose of Imferon in milliliters} = \ & \text{wt (kg)} \\
& \times \text{desired rise in Hb (g/dl)} \\
& \times 0.75 \text{ dl/kg} \\
& \times 3.5 \text{ mg Fe/g Hb} \\
& \times 1 \text{ ml Imferon per 50 mg Fe} \\
& \times 1.5 \text{ (up to 50\% allowance} \\
& \quad \text{to replenish iron stores)} \\
or \\
= \ & \text{wt (kg)} \\
& \times \text{desired rise in Hb (g/dl)} \\
& \times 0.075
\end{aligned}
$$

TABLE 1. Ferrous Sulfate Formulary Information

PREPARATIONS	FeSO$_4$ CONTENT	IRON CONTENT	DOSAGE
Ferrous sulfate drops	75 mg/0.6 ml	15 mg/0.6 ml	2–3 mg/kg/d of elemental iron using the appropriate oral preparation divided × 3 between meals
Ferrous sulfate syrup	150 mg/5 ml	30 mg/5 ml	
Ferrous sulfate elixir	150 mg/5 ml	30 mg/5 ml	
Ferrous sulfate tablet	200 mg/tablet	40 mg/tablet	
	300 mg/tablet	60 mg/tablet	

Parenteral Iron Therapy for Correction of Anemia plus Replenishing Iron Stores

Iron dextran (Imferon) 50 mg Fe/ml	Total dose in ml = wt (kg) × desired rise in Hb (g/dl) × 0.075
	Maximum daily dose for child weighing <5 kg = 0.5 ml; <9 kg = 1 ml; for other patients = 2 ml
	If given IM, administer by Z track.

TABLE 2. Basis for Dosage in Iron Replacement Therapy

Assumptions
1. With treatment of iron deficiency, RBC production can increase fivefold over normal basal levels.
2. Blood volume in the pediatric patient is 0.8 dl (80 ml)/kg of body weight.
3. Normal hemoglobin is 12 g/dl.
4. Average lifespan of a red blood cell is 120 days.

Calculated Dosage
Daily turnover of Hb is [12 g/dl/120 d] × 0.8 dl/kg = 0.08 g/kg
Molecular weight of Hb = 64,373
Molecular weight of Fe = 55.85 (there are 4 Fe atoms per molecule of Hb)
Hb = 223.4/64,373 = 0.35% iron
Daily turnover of Fe = 0.35% Fe × 0.08 g Hb/kg = 0.28 mg Fe/kg/d
Maximal response to Fe therapy requires 5 × 0.28 mg Fe/kg/d = 1.4 mg Fe/kg/d

The maximum daily dose by weight is <4 to 5 kg, 0.5 ml; <9 kg, 1 ml; >9 kg, 2 ml. It may, therefore, be necessary to dose Imferon over multiple days. If given by the intramuscular route, Imferon should be injected into the buttock using a Z track to avoid skin staining. If given intravenously, it should be initiated with a 0.5 ml test dose. Toxicity of Imferon includes not only staining of the skin and pain at the injection site but also potential asthma and potential anaphylactic reactions. It has been associated with headache, nausea, vomiting, chills, fever, myalgia, arthralgias, dizziness, and urticaria.

Blood transfusion for iron deficiency anemia is rarely warranted but may be indicated in the setting of severe iron deficiency anemia with Hb <4 to 5 g/dl and impending cardiovascular decompensation. In this setting, transfusion of packed red blood cells either should be initiated as a partial exchange transfusion with repeated small aliquots of 10 to 20 ml each so that the patient remains isovolemic or should be given in small aliquots at a very slow rate (5 ml/kg over 3 to 4 hours), with administration of diuretics considered part way through the transfusion.

RESPONSE TO THERAPY

Clinical symptoms of iron deficiency rapidly respond to iron replacement therapy. Laboratory responses to iron replacement take longer. For moderate to severe iron deficiency anemia, an increased reticulocyte count should be detected within 2 to 3 days of beginning iron therapy, with the peak response at 7 to 10 days. In mild iron deficiency anemia, this reticulocyte response may be too small to detect. A Hb checked 2 to 4 weeks after initiation of iron therapy should have increased, with a rise proportional to the degree of anemia. In general, two thirds of the anticipated response should be apparent after 1 month, with an additional 2 to 4 months of iron therapy required to replenish iron stores. Following 3 months of iron therapy, the Hb, mean corpuscular volume (MCV), and FEP should be completely corrected in a pure iron deficiency anemia. Extension of iron therapy beyond 5 months offers no advantage and risks iron overload.

The reasons for treatment failure can include poor compliance, improper administration, incorrect dosage, ongoing blood losses, malabsorption, mixed nutritional deficiency, and poor iron utilization. Compliance with an oral iron regimen can be assessed by potassium ferricyanide testing of the stool, with a positive result confirming iron administration. Malabsorption of iron in nutritionally iron-deficient children can be assessed by administering an oral dose of 6 mg/kg of elemental iron. In the absence of malabsorption, a peak serum iron level >350 μg/dl should be detected 1 to 2 hours after the dose.

EVALUATION FOR BLOOD LOSSES

The iron-deficient child should be evaluated for ongoing blood loss. Gastrointestinal bleeding can be detected by guaiac testing of the stool. Causes of gastrointestinal blood loss include feeding unprocessed cow's milk during infancy, such anatomic causes as Meckel's diverticulum, infectious entities (bacterial or parasitic), and inflammatory bowel disease. Pulmonary blood loss (e.g., idiopathic pulmonary hemosiderosis, Goodpasture's syndrome) usually will result in transient infiltrates on chest x-ray. Confirmation may be provided by staining a morning gastric aspirate for iron and finding hemosiderin-laden macrophages. Congenital bleeding disorders, such as hemophilia and von Willebrand's disease, can result in significant blood losses through hemorrhage into the skin or joints or via mucous membranes (epistaxis, menorrhagia). A thorough history and, if necessary, screening coagulation tests can effectively confirm or exclude these entities. In the adolescent female, menstrual losses (40 ml of blood per month) and pregnancy (fetus, placenta, perinatal blood loss) may cause iron deficiency.

PREVENTION OF IRON DEFICIENCY

Dietary iron should be adequate both to replace iron losses and to maintain growth. The term newborn has an iron endowment of approximately 75 mg/kg and will require an additional 135 to 200 mg of iron in the first year of life. If fetal stores are reduced (preterm infant, fetal blood loss), this endowment is less, and more dietary iron will be required. To prevent the onset of iron deficiency, the Nutritional Committee of the American Academy of Pediatrics recommends iron supplementation of term infants with 1 mg/kg of iron per day (maximum 15 mg/d) to begin no later than 4 months and continue until 3 years of age. For preterm infants the recommendation is 2 mg/kg/d. For very low birthweight infants (1000 to 1500 g) 3 mg/kg/d and for infants <1000 g 4 mg/kg/d (maximum 15 mg/d) may be appropriate. For the infant receiving iron-supplemental foods (FeSO$_4$ or reduced Fe), the amount absorbed is inversely proportional to the iron concentration (Table 3). Despite this phenomenon, the additional iron content in the iron-fortified formulas more than offsets the reduced percentage of iron absorbed, resulting in increased net iron absorption. During the first 12 months of life, whole cow's milk should be avoided because it may cause occult enteric blood loss, which may contribute to iron deficiency anemia.

Since the introduction of solid food to the breast-fed baby's diet will reduce the efficiency of iron absorption (by as much as 80%), solid foods should be rich in iron. Iron-enriched dry cereals represent a good source of supplemental iron, providing 0.45 mg of iron per gram of dry cereal (or 7 mg of Fe per 100 g of cereal as fed; a 1 tablespoon portion provides 15 g of cereal); 12 tablespoons/d should be adequate to prevent the onset of iron deficiency. For the older child, iron in food is mostly present as nonheme irons, with a smaller amount as heme proteins. Nonheme iron (approximately 5% absorption), usually present in the form of ferric complexes, is more readily absorbed when reduced to the ferrous form (facilitated by the acidic environment in the stomach) and when complexed to readily absorbed components of the diet, such as fructose, ascorbic acid, citrate, and certain amino acids. The iron present in the heme proteins is more readily absorbed and less readily affected by other dietary components (up to 40% absorption). For children ages 4 to 10 years, the recommended daily iron intake is 10 mg/d. This should be increased to 18 mg/d at age 11 to allow for accelerated growth in adolescence.

ANEMIA OF CHRONIC DISEASE

Anemias of chronic, often inflammatory, disease states are associated with adequate total body iron stores but a lack of *bioavailable*

TABLE 3. Iron Content and Absorption of Various Milk Sources

MILK SOURCE	IRON ABSORPTION (%)	IRON CONTENT (mg/L)
Breast	50	0.5–1
Cow's milk	10	0.5–1
Iron-fortified formula	4	12

iron. The pathophysiology of these anemias is a result of impaired release of iron from the tissues, causing reduced serum iron and transferrin saturation. These disorders usually are characterized by a reduced or normal total iron-binding capacity and a normal to increased ferritin, the latter often elevated as an acute phase reactant. The resulting mild to moderate anemia ranges from normocytic to slightly microcytic. Treatment should be directed at the underlying chronic disorder. If there is a coexisting iron deficiency, a trial of iron replacement therapy may have a salutary effect.

MEGALOBLASTIC ANEMIA

PHILIP LANZKOWSKY, M.D., Sc.D., F.R.C.P., D.C.H.

ETIOLOGY

Megaloblastic anemias in children are relatively uncommon and usually are due to folate or, more rarely, vitamin B_{12} deficiency. The causes of folate deficiency include (1) inadequate diet, (2) malabsorption (which may be congenital or acquired, e.g., gluten-induced enteropathy, sprue, pancreatic insufficiency, short-gut syndrome), (3) drug-induced inhibition of dietary folate absorption (phenytoin, phenobarbital), (4) increased folate utilization (growth, increased metabolic rate, e.g., fever, thyrotoxicosis, malignant disease, hemolytic anemias), and (5) drug-induced inhibition of folate metabolism (methotrexate, pyrimethamine, trimethoprim).

The causes of vitamin B_{12} deficiency include (1) dietary insufficiency (rare), (2) absence or abnormality of gastric intrinsic factor, (3) abnormal absorption of the vitamin B_{12} intrinsic factor complex as a result of previous small intestinal surgery or lack of intestinal receptors (rare), and (4) inherited abnormalities of vitamin B_{12} transport protein.

Rarer metabolic causes of a macrocytic anemia (e.g., thiamine deficiency) have occurred in offspring of consanguineous marriages who had presented with neurologic abnormalities. The anemia was responsive to 25 mg of thiamine daily.

The metabolism of folic acid and vitamin B_{12} is interrelated, and this must be considered when therapy is instituted. Large doses of vitamin B_{12} may correct the hematologic problems caused by folate deficiency. Conversely, large doses of folate may correct the hematologic disturbances caused by lack of vitamin B_{12}. Folate, however, does not correct the neurologic problems associated with vitamin B_{12} deficiency, and large doses of folate should not be given until vitamin B_{12} deficiency has been excluded.

TREATMENT

Folic Acid Deficiency

Successful treatment of patients with folate deficiency involves (1) correction of the folate deficiency, (2) amelioration of the underlying disorder, if possible, (3) improvement of the diet by increased folate intake, and (4) follow-up evaluations at intervals to monitor the patient's clinical status.

The most recent recommended daily allowance (RDA) of folic acid for men and women aged 25 to 50 years is 200 µg/d and 180 µg/d, respectively, reflecting an allowance of 3 µg/kg/d. For infants from birth to age 1 year, it is 3.6 µg/kg/day. During pregnancy, the RDA is 400 µg/d. For lactating women, the RDA is 280 µg/d the first 6 months and 260 µg/d for the second 6 months. Rich sources of folate include liver, kidney, wheat bran, yeast, spinach, asparagus, black-eyed peas, lentils, and lima and navy beans. Green leafy vegetables, most whole grains, beef, almonds and peanuts, corn, beets, potatoes, turnip greens, and broccoli contain good amounts of folic acid. The vitamin is ubiquitous in foods.

In cases of a suspected folate deficiency, a therapeutic trial can be instituted with 50 to 100 µg of folate per day orally. This dose produces a prompt reticulocytosis in cases of folate deficiency but is without effect in patients with vitamin B_{12} deficiency. An optimal response occurs in most patients with 100 to 200 µg folic acid daily. Nevertheless, it is usual to treat deficient patients with 0.5 to 1.0 mg daily orally. Commercially available preparations include tablets (0.25, 0.4, 0.8, 1 mg) and an elixir (1 mg/ml). To reduce the folate content would not significantly reduce the cost, and because pteroylmonoglutamic acid does not produce side effects except in patients with vitamin B_{12} deficiency, there is little reason to reduce the dose. Further, a smaller oral dose might not always be effective in patients with folate malabsorption. In most patients, 5 mg of folic acid given orally daily for 7 to 14 days induces a maximal hematologic response and significant replenishment of body stores. This may be given orally because, even in those with severe malabsorption, sufficient folate is absorbed from this dose to replenish stores. Before folic acid is given (in these large doses), it is always necessary to ensure that vitamin B_{12} deficiency is not present.

In the rare case of isolated congenital folate malabsorption, maintenance IM doses of folic acid are required every 3 to 4 weeks.

Response to Treatment

The clinical and hematologic response to folic acid is prompt. Within 1 to 2 days, the patient's appetite improves (often becoming voracious) and a sense of well-being returns, with increased energy and interest in surroundings. There is a fall in serum iron (often to low levels) in 24 to 48 hours and a rise in reticulocytes in 2 to 4 days that reaches a peak at 4 to 7 days. Hemoglobin levels return to normal in 2 to 6 weeks. The leukocytes and platelets increase with the reticulocytes, and the megaloblastic changes in the marrow diminish within 24 to 48 hours. However, large myelocytes, metamyelocytes, and band forms may be present for several days.

Duration of Therapy

The duration of therapy depends on the underlying pathology, but usually folic acid is given for several months until a new population of red blood cells has been formed. It is often possible to correct the cause of the deficiency and prevent its recurrence (e.g., by an improved diet, a gluten-free diet in celiac disease, or treatment of an inflammatory disease, such as tuberculosis or Crohn's disease). In these cases, there is no need to continue folic acid for life. In other situations, however, it is advisable to give folic acid continually to prevent recurrence of the deficiency (e.g., chronic hemolytic anemia, such as thalassemia) or in patients with malabsorption who do not respond to a gluten-free diet.

Megaloblastic anemia occasionally develops in patients receiving drugs that are folic acid antagonists (methotrexate, pyrimethamine, trimethoprim). These drugs inhibit the enzyme that reduces dihydrofolate to tetrahydrofolate. In some cases, folate deficiency can be severe, especially in patients with marginal or depleted folate stores. In these cases, the antagonism can be overcome by folinic acid, one 5-mg tablet daily.

In cases of a functional deficiency of folate or cobalamin, such as in an inborn error of metabolism or transport, only massive doses of vitamin may be helpful. Diagnosis is made only by appropriate biochemical tests, often on cultured fibroblasts obtained by skin biopsy. Inborn errors are rare, and patients often show mental deficiency, aminoacidemia, and growth failure rather than presenting as simple cases of anemia.

Vitamin B_{12} Deficiency

In conditions in which a patient is at risk for vitamin B_{12} deficiency (e.g., total gastrectomy or ileal resection), prophylactic administration of vitamin B_{12} should be prescribed.

Patients with suspected vitamin B_{12} deficiency are given a therapeutic trial with 25 to 100 µg of vitamin B_{12}. This dose corrects the hematologic problem caused by this vitamin deficiency but does not correct the defect in folate-deficient patients. The reticulocyte response to this therapy is similar to that noted in folate deficiency.

Optimal doses for children are not as well defined as those for adults. When the diagnosis is firmly established, several daily doses of 25 to 100 μg may be used to initiate therapy. Alternatively, in view of the ability of the body to store vitamin B$_{12}$ for long periods, maintenance therapy can be started with monthly intramuscular injections of doses between 200 and 1000 μg. Most patients with vitamin B$_{12}$ deficiency require treatment throughout life.

Patients with defects affecting the intestinal absorption of vitamin B$_{12}$, because of abnormalities of either intrinsic factor or ileal uptake, respond to parenteral vitamin B$_{12}$. Such a therapeutic maneuver completely bypasses the defective step and is the chief means by which these two groups of patients are managed currently.

Patients with complete transcobalamin II deficiency respond only to large amounts of vitamin B$_{12}$ (1 mg IM twice or three times weekly). The exact mechanism of this response remains to be defined.

Patients with methylmalonic aciduria with defects in the synthesis of vitamin B$_{12}$ coenzymes are likely to be benefited by massive doses of vitamin B$_{12}$ (1 to 2 mg vitamin B$_{12}$ parenterally daily). However, not all patients in this group are benefited by vitamin B$_{12}$.

The very rare case of defective use of 5-methyltetrahydrofolate by intact cells with normal activity of methylmalonyl-CoA mutase characterized clinically by severe developmental delay, megaloblastic anemia, and homocystinuria responds to hydroxycobalamin and not cyanocobalamin and folic acid.

In vitamin B$_{12}$-responsive megaloblastic anemia, the reticulocytes begin to increase on the third to fourth day, rise to a maximum on the sixth to eighth day, and fall gradually to normal on about the twentieth day. The height of the reticulocyte count is inversely proportional to the degree of anemia. Beginning bone marrow reversal from megaloblastic to normoblastic cells is obvious within 6 hours and is completely normoblastic in 72 hours.

Prompt hematologic responses are also obtained with the use of oral folic acid. Folic acid, however, is contraindicated because it has no effect on neurologic manifestations and has been known to precipitate or accelerate their development. Indeed, megaloblastic anemia should never be treated before a serum folic acid or vitamin B$_{12}$ assay has determined the precise cause so that correct treatment can be administered. Iron occasionally is required when a generally inadequate diet has been given that is deficient in this mineral.

REFERENCE

1. Lanzkowsky P: Megaloblastic anemia. In Manual of Pediatric Hematology and Oncology, 2nd ed. New York, Churchill Livingstone, 1995.

HEMOLYTIC ANEMIA

LAWRENCE WOLFE, M.D.

Hemolytic anemia in childhood is related either to congenital errors in the structure or function of red cells, leading to short red cell survival, or to acquired immune system mechanical or oxidative injuries to red cells. Most congenital hemolytic anemias follow similar patterns, with the exception of sickle cell disease and thalassemia, which are discussed in different sections of this book. Acquired hemolytic anemias require therapies directed at reversing the process that is toxic to red cell lifespan.

In general, hemolytic anemias are characterized by lower than normal hemoglobins, elevated reticulocyte counts, elevated bilirubin, abnormal red cell morphology (approximately 80% of the time), and elevated lactic acid dehydrogenase. When red cells are hemolyzed in the intravascular space, hemoglobinemia and hemoglobinuria also are seen. Folic acid supplementation (1 mg) should be offered to all patients with the diagnosis of hemolytic anemia.

CONGENITAL HEMOLYTIC ANEMIA

The problems likely to be encountered by the pediatrician in dealing with congenital hemolytic anemia include neonatal hyperbilirubinemia (covered extensively in Chapter 21), chronic anemia, hyperplastic crisis of anemia, hypoplastic crisis of anemia, intermittent jaundice, cholelithiasis and cholecystitis, and the problems of subsequent splenectomy.

Chronic Anemia

It is unusual for patients with congenital hemolytic anemia to suffer chronic anemia serious enough to require ongoing transfusion. Most patients with hereditary spherocytosis have a hematocrit in the 25 to 35 range. Some of the extremely rare hereditary hemolytic anemias, such as hereditary pyropoikilocytosis, spheroelliptocytosis, stomatocytosis, or unstable hemoglobins (chronic Heinz body hemolytic anemia), may require ongoing transfusion. Decisions about whether to begin a transfusion program should relate not only to arbitrary hematocrit number but also to the child's individual capability to adapt and the manifestation of cardiopulmonary symptomatology. It is unusual for patients to be symptomatic with hematocrits of 25 or above. Hematocrits consistently below 25 may be tolerated on an individual basis. Care must be taken to ascertain formal diagnosis before transfusion to avoid problems of the mixing of donor with recipient red cells in subsequent diagnostic testing.

Once begun, there is always the question of how long to continue a transfusion program. With the exception of infantile hemolytic elliptocytosis, which may improve dramatically over the course of the first year of life, most patients with congenital hemolytic anemias will not have a trend toward improvement of their resting hematocrit and reticulocyte counts over time. Once a transfusion program is initiated, it is unlikely that at its cessation the hematocrit will be any higher than at its beginning. Hence, the decision in many cases relates to the age at which splenectomy can be performed safely, the known probable response of the patient's hemoglobin and hematocrit to splenectomy, the specific hemolytic anemia involved, and issues of iron overload. Our practice in these situations has been to follow the biochemical parameters of iron overload (iron/iron-binding capacity ratio greater than 75%, ferritin greater than 1000) and to conduct a provocative chelation (see section on thalassemia and iron overload) to determine how significant the iron overload might be. Consideration of early splenectomy to avoid the life disruption of a chronic transfusion program and the problems of transfusional iron overload may arise, but except in extraordinary circumstances, it has been our practice to try to avoid early splenectomy.

Hyperplastic Crisis

In hyperplastic crisis, the hematocrit decreases while the reticulocyte count increases, and the patient usually becomes jaundiced. This is the most common situation with which the pediatrician will deal, and it usually will occur around times of minor infection. In general, hyperplastic crisis usually does not lead to a diminution of hematocrit sufficient to warrant transfusion. Nonetheless, the pediatrician may wish to monitor the hematocrit if symptoms of anemia occur along with jaundice during a minor infection or if the child is beginning hyperplastic crisis from a relatively low hematocrit (around 25). Hyperplastic crisis tends to become most severe in viral infections that lead to significant reticuloendothelial hyperplasia and splenomegaly. As an example, the adolescent with hereditary spherocytosis who has escaped splenectomy because of mild disease can be transformed by infectious mononucleosis into a patient with a much lower hematocrit and a much higher reticulocyte count. Rarely, this hypertrophy remains after the viral infection has cleared and leads to a change in the pattern of the disease.

Hypoplastic Crisis

Hypoplastic crisis occurs when bone marrow erythroid production is suppressed, usually following viral infection. Because of the shortened red cell lifespan of hereditary hemolytic anemia, brief periods of red cell suppression will lead to drops in hematocrit. This phenomenon has been shown most consistently with parvovirus infection. However, there have been reports in the literature of other viruses causing this as well. The patient who has a lower hematocrit and higher reticulocyte count is obviously at greater risk for the effects of hypoplastic crisis. Decisions about transfusion in hypoplastic crisis relate to several factors: the actual drop in hematocrit, the length of time of the suppression, the expectation of return of reticulocyte function, and the patient's cardiopulmonary response to worsening anemia. Patients with extremely low hematocrits and early symptomatology should be transfused if there is no evidence of any reticulocyte response. On the other hand, patients with very low hematocrits yet stable cardiopulmonary adaptation, who have initial evidence of reticulocyte response, may be observed closely in hopes that they will begin to stabilize and then raise their hematocrits within a short period of time. If transfusion is required, it is best to avoid multiple donor exposure, especially in small children. In general, most patients will respond to the hypoplastic crisis within 5 to 10 days. Rarely, hypoplastic crisis expands to include other bone marrow lines, including white count and platelet count. This is the so-called aplastic crisis of hereditary hemolytic anemia. It is rarely seen and most likely reflects marrow injury secondary to parvovirus infection. It is important to supplement all patients who have hypoplastic or aplastic crisis with folate (1 mg/d) to make sure that there will be no blunting of recovery because of a lack of cofactors.

Intermittent Jaundice, Cholelithiasis, and Cholecystitis

In congenital chronic hemolytic anemia, a constant turnover of bilirubin pigment leads to a variety of syndromes. Any patient may have scleral or overt jaundice. Jaundice usually is seen either as a steady state or in association with hyperplastic crisis. Patients who have mild to moderate chronic jaundice or a history of gallstones or even those patients who appear to have mild syndromes with reticulocyte counts in the 5% range are at risk for gallbladder disease. The presence of hemolytic anemia enhances the risk of gallbladder disease in children dramatically. Children or adolescents with chronic hemolytic anemia who have symptoms at all suggestive of gallbladder disease should be evaluated with a gallbladder ultrasound and analysis of biochemical parameters. The natural history of gallstones picked up on surveillance ultrasound in young patients with hemolytic anemia is not known, although the presence of stones or a strong family history of gallbladder disease might tip the scales toward splenectomy. If a patient requires cholecystectomy for cholelithiasis, decision making about splenectomy should be made separately, considering the anemia and quality of life. Recurrent stone formation after cholecystectomy is rare.

Splenectomy

Formerly, patients with hereditary spherocytosis would likely be automatically scheduled for splenectomy. Splenectomies were performed in the neonatal or infant periods until data demonstrating a developmental time course for overwhelming postsplenectomy infection became available, with the timing for splenectomy rising to 5 years of age.

It seems clear now that not all patients with congenital hemolytic anemia require splenectomy. Hereditary spherocytosis improves most reliably with splenectomy. Other congenital hemolytic anemias may vary in their response to splenectomy, especially the more severe ones and the more unusual ones. Even in these latter cases, however, splenectomy usually will raise the hematocrit, leading to a better quality of life or the loss of a transfusion requirement. Added to the elective nature of splenectomy must be changing concerns about overwhelming postsplenectomy infection. At the same time that penicillin prophylaxis and appropriate vaccination with pneumococcal vaccine, *Haemophilus influenzae* vaccine, and meningococcal vaccine have diminished the threat of overwhelming postsplenectomy infection, concerns about penicillin-resistant strains of the pneumococcus and

lack of understanding about which patients are most at risk make a careful, conservative decision about splenectomy most appropriate.

Our current recommendations for splenectomy in hereditary sphenocytosis include the following.

1. Hematocrit consistently less than 30%
2. Reticulocyte count greater than 5%
3. Significant family history of gallbladder disease at a young age
4. Hypoplastic episode requiring transfusion

Since splenectomy generally is elective, the most stringent criteria should be used in making the decision for surgery in hereditary sphenocytosis. For other chronic hemolytic anemias, decision making usually will be based on the hope of ending the need for multiple transfusions or an attempt to raise the hematocrit to improve quality of life.

Enzyme Deficiencies

Decrease in the functional capacity of red cell glucose-6-phosphate dehydrogenase (G6PD) can result in an acute bout of hemolysis, especially after an oxidant stress, such as infection or drug administration. Drugs most commonly associated with such bouts of hemolysis include antimalarials, sulfonamides, aspirin, ascorbic acid, certain antibiotics, naphthalene, and benzene. Food exposure to fava beans also can cause hemolysis. The hemolysis occurs a short time after exposure to the inciting agent and will differ depending on the type of G6PD deficiency the patient has. The African American patient may develop a moderate anemia, although usually the hemoglobin stays greater than 6 g/dl. The Caucasian patient with the Mediterranean form of G6PD deficiency has virtually no levels in the red cells at any time and, thus, is at much greater risk for hemolysis. Some of these patients have an ongoing hemolytic anemia, with hemoglobinuria and jaundice. The most important approach for all patients with G6PD deficiency is the avoidance of oxidant stress. Certain stresses, however, such as infection, cannot be avoided, and hence some patients will have acute or chronic hemolysis, occasionally requiring transfusion. We have seen some amelioration of symptoms with use of daily oral vitamin E in Caucasian patients with the Mediterranean form of the disease and chronic hemolysis.

Pyruvate kinase deficiency is another red cell enzyme deficiency that leads to nonspherocytic hemolytic anemia. Problems with hyperbilirubinemia may begin at birth, and these patients seem at great risk for gallstones. Transfusion may be necessary. The response of this disease to splenectomy is variable, but it may be tried to end transfusion requirements or to enhance the quality of life. High doses of salicylates should be avoided in patients with pyruvate kinase deficiency.

ACQUIRED HEMOLYTIC ANEMIAS

Neonatal Hemolytic Anemia

Perhaps the trickiest neonatal hemolytic anemia to diagnose is oxidant hemolysis of the newborn. Most newborns have red cells with a temporary developmental sensitivity to oxidant stress. This can lead to a failure to protect hemoglobin from denaturation and a temporary Heinz body hemolytic anemia, which appears as a sudden bout of hemolysis with jaundice and a mild to moderate drop in hematocrit associated with the appearance of so-called bite cells in the peripheral blood. More commonly, the jaundice from oxidant hemolysis is a more significant problem than the anemia itself. In general, oxidant hemolysis of the newborn, if unassociated with an inborn enzymopathy such as G6PD deficiency, is self-limited, and the hematocrit begins to rise again within 5 to 7 days. Given a high suspicion of this phenomenon, the greatest challenge is to avoid excessive phlebotomy in the baby. As long as transfusion appears unnecessary, it is useful to watch these newborns carefully in the hope that this will be a self-limited disease. Red cell enzymes sent under these circumstances can be misleading because the population of red cells is very young and because oxidant injury selects for those red cells with the lowest capacity to protect themselves.

Immune Hemolytic Anemia

Immune hemolytic anemia is relatively rare in children (incidence of less than 0.2/100,000). It occurs when an antibody against a blood group antigen is generated that breaks immune tolerance. This occurs most commonly in an idiopathic manner (although often called post-infectious), or it can occur in response to an underlying disease or a secondary sensitization with specific drugs. The idiopathic, or post-infectious, type usually appears before the age of 4 years. Starting in late adolescence, the pattern of immune hemolytic anemia begins to resemble that of the adult, with fewer idiopathic cases and more cases related to underlying diseases, such as rheumatic or lymphomatous diseases.

There are basically two types of immune hemolytic anemia, and they respond differently to different therapies. We first discuss *warm or IgG* immune hemolytic anemia, which presents with spherocytosis and a positive direct antiglobulin test and is mediated by an abnormally produced IgG (usually in the Rh blood group system). The second type of immune hemolytic anemia is *IgM induced*, is often postinfectious (especially related to *Mycoplasma* infection or infectious mononucleosis), may be associated with a direct antiglobulin test positive for the third component of complement, and usually can be detected by testing the patient's blood for a high-titer cold agglutinin.

Warm IgG Immune Hemolytic Anemia

In general, children younger than 2 years of age and young adults older than 20 are more likely to suffer a chronic course, as well as a less explosive presentation. Most children will be over this illness by about 6 months. However, patients with chronic disease may require long-term therapies. The coexistence of anti-red cell antibodies with antiplatelet antibodies augurs for a more chronic course.

Patients with idiopathic warm immune hemolytic anemia usually are treated first with steroid therapy. Our practice is to begin with 4 mg/kg of prednisone daily for 2 to 4 days, with a taper to 2 mg/kg once there is evidence of improvement in hematocrit or reticulocyte count. High doses of steroids may interfere with macrophage receptors to the extent that there is immediate improvement in the rate of red cell destruction. Over a period of approximately 2 weeks after that, there may be a decrease in the actual production of antibody, leading to a more stable state with even less reticulocytosis. Hence, patients are usually on a dose of 2 mg/kg/d for at least 10 to 14 days. Once reticulocyte counts have fallen to 5% or less, the hematocrit is 25 or greater, and 10 to 14 days of steroid therapy have elapsed, one can begin to consider a taper of steroid therapy. Patients should be monitored carefully for exacerbations of hemolysis during the steroid taper.

In patients who are not responsive to steroids, intravenous gamma globulin may be tried. The success of intravenous gamma globulin in warm IgG autoimmune hemolytic anemia is far less consistent than it is in idiopathic thrombocytopenic purpura. In addition, higher doses are required (1 g/kg/d for up to 5 days). When giving intravenous gamma globulin, one may continue with steroid therapy in the hope of acquiring the delayed effect of diminished autoantibody production.

Usually, the practitioner has the option to attempt these therapies because most patients with autoimmune hemolytic anemia do not have life-threatening levels of anemia or have fallen to very low levels of anemia over a long enough time to provide physiologic compensation. It is important to remember that if a patient with autoimmune hemolytic anemia requires transfusion to avoid overt heart failure, it is unlikely that the blood bank will be able to find a fully compatible unit. For this reason, the blood bank usually follows the practice of administering the "least incompatible" unit. This usually can be transfused safely, although the red cells from the transfused unit will have a shortened lifespan because they usually will be coated with the autoantibody. Nonetheless, in life-threatening situations, one generally sees an improvement in anemia and cardiac function without transfusion reactionlike effects.

Those patients who do not respond to steroids or gamma globulin therapy and who demonstrate a serious transfusion requirement in an acute setting over 4 to 6 days may require urgent splenectomy. Because of concerns about postsplenectomy sepsis, especially in children under the age of 4 years, this procedure should be considered a last resort. Patients who fail to respond to splenectomy and still have active severe anemia may respond to plasmapheresis. In plasma exchange, a large amount of the autoantibody may be removed. In our experience, however, plasma exchange works only transiently unless significant immunosuppression occurs simultaneously. The use of immunosuppressive agents in autoimmune hemolytic anemia usually occurs after splenectomy has been attempted. Drugs that have been used include azathioprine, 6-mercaptopurine, and cyclophosphamide. For this author, cyclophosphamide is the drug that has worked most consistently when given in oral, daily, low doses. Concerns about long-term side effects are real. Therefore, immunosuppressive drugs should be used primarily for patients who have a clinically unacceptable degree of anemia that has not responded to corticosteroid, immunoglobulin, or splenectomy treatment or for those patients who cannot tolerate steroids or are too sick to have splenectomy. If cyclophosphamide therapy or immunosuppressive therapy is initiated, it generally takes 1 to 2 weeks before the effect can be noted. We usually switch from one drug to another if no dramatic change in the hemolysis has occurred after 1 to 2 months.

Cold Agglutinin Disease

Cold agglutinin disease is treated differently from warm autoimmune hemolytic anemia, although usually the anemia is more moderate. In general, patients with IgM anti-red cell antibodies or IgG antibodies that have a cold thermal (24° to 30° C) amplitude (meaning that they bind to red cells in the cold as opposed to the usual IgG property, which is to bind to red cells in the warm [approximately 37° C]) do not respond well to corticosteroids. The usual approach to such patients in childhood is to have them avoid exposure to the cold and to wait for the postinfectious time period to end (e.g., in *Mycoplasma* pneumonia and mononucleosis). If an attempt is made to transfuse such patients, it is important that blood be administered through a blood warmer to try to diminish binding of the cold-reacting antibody to the transfused red cells as they enter the circulation. Patients who have moderate to severe anemia and a demonstrable cold agglutinin may respond well to plasmapheresis. Because these abnormal IgMs tend not to bind directly to the red cells in the circulation (because of the higher temperatures) and because they are found predominantly within the intravascular space, plasmapheresis is more efficient in removal of this autoantibody than the abnormal IgG seen in autoimmune hemolytic anemia. Although this is a short-term effect, it usually can create enough time either for the patient to get over the postinfectious syndrome or to detect an underlying disease that can be treated.

Splenectomy is not effective in patients with cold agglutinin disease, and, hence, patients who have unacceptable anemia, no recognizable underlying illness, and a long time period from onset of disease (suggesting a lack of spontaneous resolution) should be considered for immunosuppressive agents. Once again, cyclophosphamide is the drug of choice and has a high rate of success, at least in adult patients with idiopathic IgM-induced disease.

Other Acquired Hemolytic Anemias

In general, other acquired hemolytic anemias are treated either by alleviating associated conditions or by transfusion. It is important to realize, however, that transfused red cells suffer the same fate as the patient's own.

The specific red cell morphology is often a clue to the cause, and such causes are varied. When fragmentation is seen, one should consider disseminated intravascular coagulation (DIC), cardiac valve dysfunction, hemolytic uremic syndrome, and giant hemangiomas. When spherocytes occur, one should consider thermal injury, toxins *(Clos-*

tridium), or venoms; with echinocytes, hypophosphatemia or uremia; with acanthocytes, severe liver disease, abetalipoproteinemia, anorexia nervosa, or neonatal vitamin E deficiency. Subsequent evaluation and therapy will be guided by the diagnosis.

REFERENCES

1. Becher P, Lux S: Disorders of the red-cell membrane. *In* Nathan DG, Oski FA (eds): Hematology of Infancy and Childhood, 4th ed. Philadelphia, WB Saunders Co, 1993.
2. Mentza WC: Pyruvate kinase and related disorders of glycolysis. *In* Nathan DG, Oski FA (eds): Hematology of Infancy and Childhood, 4th ed. Philadelphia, WB Saunders Co, 1993.
3. Schreiber A, Gill F, Manno C: Autoimmune hemolytic anemia. *In* Nathan DG, Oski FA (eds): Hematology of Infancy and Childhood, 4th ed. Philadelphia, WB Saunders Co, 1993.
4. Wolfe L: Neonatal anemias. *In* Hanoin RI, Lux SE, Stossel TP (eds): Blood—Principles and Practice of Hematology. Philadelphia, JB Lippincott Co, 1993.

ANEMIA OF CHRONIC DISEASE

James A. Stockman III, m.d.

The anemia of chronic disease is that anemia characterized by a decreased plasma iron, decreased total iron-binding capacity of the plasma, decreased saturation of transferrin by iron, decreased numbers of bone marrow sideroblasts, normal or increased levels of reticuloendothelial iron, and a normal or increased plasma ferritin level. It is seen in association with a wide variety of clinical disorders, including cancer, lymphoma, collagen vascular disease, severe tissue injuries, renal failure, and many infectious processes. It is important to recognize that each of these disorders may be associated with multiple sources of anemia, including blood loss, hemolysis, and drug suppression. Only when other possible causes of anemia have been excluded should a diagnosis of the anemia of chronic disease be made.

The anemia of chronic disease develops slowly, usually over the period of a month. The anemia is most often mild and less commonly mild to moderate. More severe degrees of anemia are not consistent with the anemia of chronic disease as the only diagnosis. The hematocrit concentration rarely falls below 30% in adults and the low 20% range in children. The anemia most commonly is normocytic and normochromic. The patients are reticulocytopenic. In approximately 15% of cases, it is associated with a low red cell mean corpuscular volume (MCV). Should a low MCV be found, concomitant iron deficiency should be looked for. In contrast to simple iron deficiency, the infrequent microcytosis of chronic disease is rarely proportional to the degree of anemia associated with these disorders.

The pathophysiology underlying the anemia of chronic disease is complex. In most instances, there is a slight shortening of red cell survival, an impaired marrow response to anemia, and an impaired flow of iron from reticuloendothelial cells to the bone marrow. The last accounts for the iron-deficient type of erythropoiesis seen in these disorders. Iron absorption may be either normal or diminished. The diagnosis of anemia of chronic disease can be made based on the clinical findings and the typical laboratory results noted. A bone marrow examination is not necessary in most instances.

Therapy for the anemia of chronic disease varies with the individual disorder. In most situations, there will be no specific therapy. Iron therapy, except when necessitated by the concurrent use of human recombinant erythropoietin, is of no value, since when given either orally or by intramuscular injection, it must first be cleared by the reticuloendothelial system. Occasionally, a patient with the anemia of chronic disease is also iron deficient. This is particularly common in children with rheumatoid arthritis, in whom gastrointestinal bleeding secondary to aspirin or nonsteroidal anti-inflammatory drug use occurs. Such patients may partially respond to iron.

ANEMIA WITH CHRONIC RENAL DISEASE

In renal disease, there can be many causes of anemia, including blood loss, aluminum toxicity, depletion of folate or iron, and a significantly shortened red cell survival. The predominant etiology, however, is diminished red cell production because of the decreased production of erythropoietin. Before the availability of human recombinant erythropoietin (EP), transfusional therapy was the only effective treatment for the anemia, although some patients responded to androgens. EP, however, is the therapy of choice. Children receiving 50 to 100 U/kg of EP two to three times a week in conjunction with dialysis should be expected to reach a hematocrit of 35% by 8 to 12 weeks, providing iron stores are adequate. At this level of hematocrit there should be no signs or symptoms of anemia. Once such a hematocrit is achieved, lesser amounts of EP (15 to 75 U/kg two to three times a week) are needed. EP usually is administered intravenously to achieve these results, but subcutaneous administration is equally effective. Even in iron-sufficient individuals, the tremendous stimulation of erythropoiesis by EP causes mobilization of considerable iron stores. An absolute or relative iron deficiency results, blunting the response to EP. For this reason, most patients require the oral administration of iron or the parenteral administration of iron dextran. EP usually eliminates the need for transfusional support.

EP therapy should produce improvements in energy, appetite, and sleep patterns. EP may cause a slight increase in platelet counts. The only significant side effect is hypertension, which is a relatively uncommon sequela of EP therapy in children. This can usually be managed with antihypertensive drugs while continuing the EP.

ANEMIA WITH CANCER

Children with hematologic and solid tumor malignancies frequently develop anemia. This can result from bone marrow infiltration, blood loss associated with thrombocytopenia, and the effects of chemotherapy. Disseminated intravascular coagulation, radiation, and infection also can result in anemia. Even without these causes, some patients with malignancy will have defective red cell production consistent with the type seen in the anemia of chronic disease. EP may be helpful for selected patients, but the usual management involves transfusional support.

ANEMIA OF CHRONIC INFECTION

During active infection producing systemic illness, the hemoglobin concentration declines approximately 15%, often within 1 week. Some infections are associated with a hemolytic anemia (*Haemophilus influenzae,* Epstein-Barr virus, *Clostridium perfringens*). When these are excluded, the anemia is most like that seen in other chronic disorders. Although anemia of chronic infection once was common in subjects with chronic osteomyelitis, subacute bacterial endocarditis, and tuberculosis, effective antimicrobial therapy has virtually eliminated it except for that seen in association with active HIV infection.

HIV infection causes ineffective hematopoiesis. As with other anemias of chronic disorders, it is normocytic and normochromic. A macrocytic anemia may be a consequence of treatment with zidovudine (AZT). Any child with HIV infection should have nutritional causes of anemia excluded. The anemia resulting from HIV infection may require transfusional support. In most instances, the degree of anemia is sufficiently mild that correction of the anemia is unnecessary. EP has been effective in adult clinic trials for HIV-related anemia, and it may be useful in children. Initial dosing would be the same as for patients with renal disease, although higher or lower doses may be needed.

ANEMIA OF CHRONIC INFLAMMATION

The most frequent noninfectious cause of chronic inflammation is collagen vascular disease, of which rheumatoid arthritis is predominant in the pediatric age group. Anemia in association with rheumatoid arthritis can be related to the anemia of chronic disease or to iron deficiency. Occasionally, patients will develop a macrocytic anemia because of abnormal folate metabolism.

The anemia of chronic inflammation seen in association with rheumatoid arthritis in childhood usually requires no specific therapy. It is important to exclude the presence of iron deficiency. Since the laboratory features of iron deficiency and the anemia of chronic disease overlap, a trial of iron therapy (elemental iron 2 mg/kg PO t.i.d.) is both diagnostic and therapeutic. There are insufficient data to warrant the use of EP, especially in view of the fact that the mild anemia seen in affected children is not likely to cause clinically apparent signs or symptoms.

THALASSEMIA

HELEN S. JOHNSTONE, M.D.

The thalassemias are hereditary anemias resulting from reduced or absent synthesis of the alpha- or beta-globin chains. In severe beta-thalassemia, the erythroid precursors are destroyed in the bone marrow, contributing to a transfusion-dependent anemia. Treatment consists of a regular blood transfusion program and chelation therapy to prevent iron overload.

TRANSFUSION THERAPY

Regular blood transfusions are given to maintain the hemoglobin level between 10 and 14 g/dl. The purpose is twofold, to suppress endogenous ineffective erythropoiesis and to prevent complications of chronic hypoxia. In general, 10 to 15 ml/kg of leukocyte-poor, packed red blood cells are infused at a rate of 5 ml/kg/h every 3 to 5 weeks. Removal of the leukocytes by a simple bedside filter can minimize fever and the urticarial reactions resulting from alloimmunization to leukocyte antigens. For patients who have had reactions in the past, pretreatment with acetaminophen and diphenhydramine hydrochloride can prevent recurrence of symptoms. Transfusion therapy is initiated in infancy based on the patient's symptoms. Indications for transfusion include poor appetite, a decrease in growth rate, and a decreased activity level despite the hemoglobin level. If the hemoglobin drops below 8 g/dl and is associated with increasing spleen size, transfusions are initiated. On an adequate transfusion program, one can expect the growth rate to be normal until the patient is 8 to 10 years of age. Maintaining the hemoglobin level above 10 g/dl prevents expansion of the bone marrow, with the associated cosmetic deformities and pathologic fractures that were seen in thalassemia patients in the past. Hypersplenism from splenomegaly secondary to extramedullary hematopoiesis can be delayed and sometimes prevented by early appropriate transfusion therapy. Dietary iron absorption from the gastrointestinal tract is reduced when the hemoglobin levels are normal or near normal.

One of the most common serious complications of transfusion therapy is the possibility of transmission of viral infections. Currently, blood is tested routinely for hepatitis A, B, and C virus and human immunodeficiency virus (HIV). Hepatitis B vaccine is given to all nonimmune patients before instituting transfusion therapy. Since most non-A, non-B transfusion-related hepatitis is believed to be caused by hepatitis C, we believe that the incidence of cirrhosis should decrease now that adequate testing for hepatitis C is done routinely.

MANAGEMENT OF CHRONIC IRON OVERLOAD

Repeated transfusions lead to a large quantity of iron accumulation and result in dysfunction of the liver, heart, and endocrine organs. Currently, the most effective available method to remove excess iron is daily subcutaneous infusions of deferoxamine. The goal of this therapy is to maintain iron balance without causing serious toxicity.

A regular chelation program begins at about 3 years of age, when the serum ferritin level is between 1000 and 1500 ng/ml. Growth failure, bone dysplasia, sensineural hearing loss, and retinal damage are associated with high-dose chelation therapy administered to young patients with minimal iron burdens. Ideally, deferoxamine should begin well before the development of irreversible organ damage. When one begins chelation at age 3 years and monitors the patient carefully for toxicity, serious complications usually can be avoided. The deferoxamine is given at 25 to 50 mg/kg diluted in sterile water to a concentration of 200 mg/ml. A 27-gauge butterfly needle is inserted into the subcutaneous tissue of the abdomen or thigh. The medication is infused slowly over 10 to 12 hours by means of a portable, battery-operated syringe infusion pump. The pump is strapped to the leg or secured with a belt around the waist. Skin irritation can be lessened by adding 5 to 10 mg of hydrocortisone to the medication and by rotating the infusion sites daily. One of the common problems with this management is poor compliance in adolescents and young adults. To maintain iron balance, chelation must be done for a minimum of 10 hours a night for at least 5 days per week. Experience has shown that compliance is better when the patients are instructed to treat themselves 7 days per week.

Patients who are severely iron overloaded and did not receive chelation therapy in early childhood may benefit from high-dose deferoxamine IV infusions at a maximum concentration of 15 mg/kg/h at the time of the blood transfusion and, if possible, for 48 hours or longer each month.

A low-iron diet, with limited red meats and drinking tea with meals, may assist in reducing iron absorption from food sources.

SPLENECTOMY

Some patients with thalassemia major will develop hypersplenism, with increased blood transfusion requirements. When the packed red blood cell requirement exceeds 250 ml/kg/y, most patients cannot maintain iron balance with the usual deferoxamine chelation program. Splenectomy will reduce the blood transfusion requirement and restore iron balance. Before splenectomy, the patient should receive pneumococcal vaccine. After splenectomy, penicillin 250 mg twice daily should be administered to reduce the incidence of pneumococcal sepsis. Splenectomy is not recommended for children less than 2 years of age because of the increased risk of overwhelming sepsis in these patients. On an intensive transfusion regimen, hypersplenism usually does not develop until later in childhood or early adolescence.

COMPLICATIONS OF IRON OVERLOAD

Cardiac Complications

The primary cause of death in patients with thalassemia is chronic congestive heart failure or cardiac arrhythmias. Studies have shown that such complications are largely prevented by a consistent chelation program instituted before 10 years of age. Cardiac death occurs primarily in noncompliant adolescents and young adults.

Endocrine Abnormalities

Growth Retardation

With a good transfusion program, children grow normally until 8 to 10 years of age, and then the growth rate begins to slow. This occurs even in children who began iron chelation at 3 years of age and have maintained iron balance with serum ferritin levels below 1000 ng/ml.

Abnormal Pubertal Development

Delayed onset of puberty is still common in children who began chelation therapy at 6 to 7 years of age. Hormone replacement can be administered to allow development of normal secondary sex characteristics.

Diabetes Mellitus

Diabetes mellitus is now seen in older patients who are noncompliant with chelation therapy. They are insulin dependent, and the diabetes is often difficult to control.

Hypoparathyroidism

Hypoparathyroidism usually occurs with symptoms of hypocalcemia. Treatment consists of calcium supplements and vitamin D.

BONE MARROW TRANSPLANTATION

Thalassemia can be cured with a successful bone marrow transplant using an HLA-matched sibling donor. The 2-year event-free survival after bone marrow transplantation is approximately 85% in large treatment centers in Italy and Greece. Thalassemia has been eradicated in 80% of the patients. Graft rejection may occur as long as 3 to 5 years after transplantation. The prognosis is best in children less than 16 years of age without significant hepatomegaly or hepatic fibrosis. Because of the 15% early mortality and the concern about possible malignancies in long-term survivors, bone marrow transplantation is less commonly recommended in centers in the United States.

ORAL IRON CHELATORS

Considerable research effort is being directed toward developing safe, effective oral iron chelating agents. One compound that is now in clinical trials and shows early promise is 1,2-dimethyl, 3-hydroxypyrid, 4-one(L-1). Urinary iron excretion is similar to that seen when subcutaneous deferoxamine is used, but stool iron is considerably less. Serum ferritin levels fell significantly in patients during the initial 24 months of a therapeutic trial. Longer trials will be needed before the safety and efficacy of this agent can be determined.

PREVENTION

The use of genetic counseling and antenatal diagnosis has reduced the number of new cases of thalassemia to fewer than 10% of the number expected in some regions of Cyprus and Italy. By the use of chorionic villous biopsy specimens or fetal blood sampling, an accurate diagnosis can be made at 8 to 14 weeks of gestation in many cases.

THALASSEMIA INTERMEDIA

Patients with thalassemia intermedia are those with homozygous or heterozygous beta-thalassemia who are able to maintain a hemoglobin of 6 to 9 g/dl without regular transfusions. Symptoms of chronic hypoxia or skeletal changes caused by marrow expansion may be indications for using a transfusion program in such individuals. Because of chronic anemia, iron absorption from the gastrointestinal tract may be increased. Low-iron diets should be prescribed, and serum ferritin levels should be monitored in all patients. Even those patients not requiring regular transfusions may need intermittent deferoxamine chelation therapy to maintain iron balance.

THALASSEMIA MINOR

Thalassemia minor, or thalassemia trait, may result in a mild, hypochromic microcytic anemia. The patients are usually asymptomatic and require no specific therapy. However, an accurate diagnosis is still important to provide genetic counseling to prospective parents. In addition, thalassemia trait must be distinguished from iron deficiency anemia. Toxicity from iron overload has been reported in patients with thalassemia trait as a result of chronic iron administration. Thus, individuals with thalassemia trait should not receive iron.

REFERENCES

1. Fosberg MT, Nathan DG: Treatment of Cooley's anemia. Blood 1990;76:435–444.
2. Lucarelli G, Galimberti M, Polchi P, et al.: Bone marrow transplantation in patients with thalassemia. N Engl J Med 1990;322:417–421.

SICKLE CELL DISEASE

Kwaku Ohene-Frempong, m.d.

Sickle cell disease (SCD) is a generic term for a group of disorders in which red blood cells can become sickled under physiologic conditions because of the presence of sickle hemoglobin (Hb S). The common types of these disorders are

- Hemoglobin SS disease (β^s/β^s)
- Hemoglobin SC disease (β^s/β^c)
- Hemoglobin S/beta-plus thalassemia $(\beta^s/\beta^+$ thal)
- Hemoglobin S/beta-zero thalassemia $(\beta^s/\beta^0$ thal)

Sickle cell trait (AS), the heterozygous condition, is not included among the sickle cell diseases because it is generally asymptomatic.

MOLECULAR GENETICS

Hb S results from a single base mutation in the 6th codon, GAG, of the beta-globin gene to GTG, resulting in a substitution of valine for glutamic acid as the 6th amino acid in beta-globin. The condition is inherited as an autosomal codominant trait. The β^s mutation is known to have at least five separate origins, four in Africa and one in the Arabian-Indian region.

PATHOPHYSIOLOGY

Oxygenated Hb S is soluble, allowing the red cell to be soft and deformable. However, when Hb S is deoxygenated, the β^6-valine causes the Hb S molecules to polymerize into long fibers that are insoluble and force the red cell to become rigid and distorted into sickle or other shapes. Sickle cells have a shortened lifespan (16 to 20 days) compared with normal red cells (120 days). They cause microvascular occlusion, leading to tissue ischemia, infarcts, and chronic organ damage. Sickle cells also cause endothelial damage to larger vessels, leading to thickened walls, severe stenosis, and occlusion or serving as nidi for thrombus formation. Involvement of larger vessels is responsible for acute events, such as stroke and probably other recurrent vasoocclusive events.

The clinical course of SCD is extremely variable. Much of this variability can be explained by the genotype of the common sickling disorders, with the following decreasing order of severity.

$$SS = S\beta^0 \text{ thal} > SC > S\beta^+ \text{ thal}$$

Fetal hemoglobin inhibits the polymerization of deoxy-Hb S. Patients with higher levels of Hb F have a milder clinical course than those with lower levels. Other genetic factors, such as alpha-thalassemia and the β^s-haplotype, also affect the clinical expression of SCD.

DIAGNOSIS

Historically, the leading cause of death in children with SCD has been bacterial septicemia, primarily caused by the pneumococcus. Twice-daily penicillin prophylaxis has been shown to decrease the incidence of pneumococcal septicemia in these children greatly. It is important to establish the diagnosis as soon after birth as possible so that penicillin prophylaxis can begin as early as 2 months of age. Testing for SCD is included in the newborn screening program of 43 states in the United States.

The best laboratory methods for establishing the diagnosis of SCD are those, such as electrophoresis, isoelectric focusing, and chromatography, that attempt to identify all the hemoglobin present in a blood sample. The simple tests that seek to establish the presence or absence of Hb S alone are not adequate for the diagnosis of

SCD. These simple tests may be negative in the presence of Hb S and high levels of Hb F and should not be used in infants. In all clinical settings, the SCD status of children, particularly those in groups with a high prevalence of the disease, needs to be established or documented.

CLINICAL COMPLICATIONS AND MANAGEMENT

Infection

In early childhood, the prevention and treatment of infection are the predominant clinical goals of managing SCD. Primarily because of splenic dysfunction, invasive bacterial infection with encapsulated organisms, particularly the pneumococcus, can have a rapidly progressive and fatal course in children with SCD. Children with SCD should be on antibiotic prophylaxis, twice-daily penicillin (125 mg for the first 2 to 3 years and 250 mg thereafter). Erythromycin may be used in those allergic to penicillin. Children with SCD should receive pneumococcal vaccine at 2 years of age and boosters every 4 to 5 years until the late teens. In addition, all children with SCD who exhibit signs and symptoms of infection should be managed as if they have pneumococcal sepsis until proven otherwise. Children under 6 years of age with fever or other signs of infection should be evaluated as quickly as possible in the emergency room, doctor's office, or clinic, should have blood and other specimens obtained for appropriate cultures, and immediately should be given a parenteral dose of broad-spectrum antibiotic, such as ampicillin, cefuroxime, or ceftriaxone, which has excellent coverage for the pneumococcus and *Haemophilus influenzae*. The choice and dose of antibiotic should be governed by the local prevailing conditions regarding antibiotic susceptibility of pneumococcal and *H. influenzae* strains. Traditionally, such patients have been admitted to the hospital for continued parenteral antibiotic therapy until cultures have proven negative for bacterial infection after 48 to 72 hours. Recently, outpatient management of children with SCD who have fever and do not appear ill has been adopted by several institutions. Ceftriaxone, a long-acting cephalosporin, has been given IV after obtaining cultures, and patients have been monitored subsequently at home. The long-term clinical efficacy of this less costly outpatient approach is under evaluation.

Painful (Vasoocclusive) Events

Episodic attacks of pain are the lifelong hallmark of SCD. Unfortunately, pain may be the least well managed complication of SCD. Medical staff, ill-prepared to deal with chronic/recurrent acute complications of any disease, too often become resistant to the needs of the SCD patient in pain and do not provide treatment that will lead to adequate pain relief. Unjustified concern over drug addiction often has led to inappropriate underdosing and scheduling of analgesics.

Uncomplicated pain in SCD is managed most appropriately at home with oral analgesics, such as acetaminophen, aspirin, ibuprofen, and other anti-inflammatory medication, alone or in addition to oral opioids, such as codeine, hydromorphone, and others. When home management of pain is deemed inadequate by the parent or patient, institution-based management may become necessary. Outpatient administration of parenteral analgesics, such as morphine or hydromorphone with or without an oral or parenteral nonsteroidal anti-inflammatory agent, is standard practice. The intravenous route is preferable to intramuscular injections because such injections are painful and lead to muscle fibrosis over the years. The use of parenteral meperidine is falling out of favor because of the toxic side effects, including seizures, caused by the metabolite, normeperidine. Patients can be managed in the outpatient setting (emergency room or day hospital) for several hours before a decision to admit or discharge is made. Inpatient management of pain should have the same goal, adequate pain relief, as home management. While on parenteral opioid analgesics, patients should have aggressive pulmonary care and be monitored carefully to prevent the development of pulmonary complications. Attempts to introduce contracts or to test different philosophies and protocols of pain management should not be made while the patient is in the hospital in pain. Such programs should be planned and adopted in outpatient comprehensive management programs.

Stroke (Cerebrovascular Accident)

Strokes may occur in children with SCD from as early as the second year of life. They are commonly due to cerebrovascular disease, leading to thrombotic infarcts or hemorrhage. Children with stroke usually present with hemiparesis, monoparesis, aphasia, seizures, or even coma. Often, the presentation is as subtle as a painless limp. Recognition of such subtle signs by parents and medical staff, especially in the younger children, is a challenge. Children suspected of a stroke should be evaluated as quickly as possible with thorough neurologic examination and an imaging study of the brain. The goal of the initial evaluation is to rule out intracranial hemorrhage, which may require surgical intervention. It is important to remember that the lesion of a new infarct may take several days to appear on computed tomography (CT). Magnetic resonance imaging (MRI) may be a more sensitive test for the detection of infarcts, especially in the early stages. However, stroke is a clinical diagnosis.

Management should begin soon after the initial evaluation. Stabilization of vital signs as necessary for comatose patients and early intravenous hydration for others are important. Simple or exchange transfusion with normal blood to reduce the level of Hb S–containing cells to less than 30% should be performed as quickly as possible, particularly in patients still exhibiting neurologic changes. In patients with seizures and other clinical problems at presentation, appropriate evaluation to rule out other causes should be included. Further management includes physical and occupational therapy as needed and chronic transfusion therapy to maintain Hb S at less than 30% to prevent the recurrence of stroke. Long-term transfusion should be performed by the exchange method, if possible, to reduce the rate of iron accumulation. Therapy for iron overload should be started when the ferritin level reaches about 2000 ng/ml.

Acute Chest Syndrome

Involvement of the lungs may be due to infection from a wide range of agents, infarction resulting from vasoocclusive events, or atelectasis due to involuntary splinting because of pain caused by infarcts of adjacent ribs. The common signs at onset include chest pain, mild to moderate dyspnea, and varying degrees of respiratory distress. Acute chest syndrome has the potential for rapid progression to involvement of several lobes or the entire lung. It is a major cause of death in SCD.

Management is oriented toward the maintenance of adequate oxygenation and treatment of underlying or associated infection. The use of simple or partial exchange transfusion to increase the oxygen-carrying capacity and reduce the percentage of Hb S cells often leads to faster resolution of acute chest syndrome. Broad-spectrum antibiotics with good coverage for pneumococci and *Mycoplasma* are used even in the absence of proven infection. Hydration should be managed carefully to avoid pulmonary edema.

Acute Anemia Caused by Acute Splenic Sequestration

The sudden pooling of blood from the general circulation into an enlarged spleen occurs typically in children under 5 years of age with SS and Sβ^0 thalassemia but may occur at older ages in patients with milder forms of SCD. The cause of this vascular event is unknown but is usually associated with signs and symptoms of infection. No organisms have been found consistently to be associated with acute splenic sequestration. In areas where it is common, malaria may precipitate acute splenic sequestration (as it does also in children who do not have SCD).

In a known SCD patient, diagnosis is established by the presence of a spleen much larger than at previous examination, severe anemia with reticulocytosis, left shift of granulocytes, and, often, thrombocytopenia. Clinically, the child shows signs of anemia and shock depending on the degree of hypovolemia. Hypovolemia associated with acute splenic sequestration can lead to death if not corrected in time.

The danger associated with acute splenic sequestration comes from hypovolemia, not anemia. Management starts with quick assessment and diagnosis, intravenous hydration to restore circulatory blood volume, and transfusion of red cells later to improve anemia. Transfusions should be performed cautiously, using small aliquots with periodic assessment of blood counts, since the usual response of the enlarged spleen to transfusion is to contract, thereby releasing more blood into circulation. Fatal *hyper*volemic shock has occurred as a result of overly aggressive transfusion aimed at rapid normalization of the anemia. Splenectomy has been performed in children with recurrent severe splenic sequestration. In children less than 4 years old, chronic transfusion therapy may be used to delay splenectomy until a later age, if necessary.

Acute Anemia Due to Erythroblastopenia

Erroneously termed *aplastic crisis,* the transient cessation of red cell production, often due to infection, is not unique to sickle cell disease. B19 parvovirus, which invades and destroys developing red cells (erythroblasts), is the most common cause of this complication in SCD as well as in other chronic hemolytic diseases.

Acute anemia due to erythroblastopenia is distinguishable from other causes of acute anemia by the reticulocyte count, which is typically much lower than expected. Occasionally, other cell lines may be affected, together with the red cells. Because it is gradual in development, the severe anemia of erythroblastopenia is generally well tolerated. Management involves investigation to rule out treatable bacterial infection in the febrile patient and transfusion of red cells. The decision to give red cells should be based on clinical evidence of compromise from severe anemia and not on the blood count alone. Transfusion should be performed cautiously in small aliquots with long intervals (4 hours) to allow for volume equilibration and avoidance of hypervolemia. Spontaneous recovery within 2 weeks or so of the onset of severe anemia is the rule.

Priapism

The incidence of acute priapism in the SCD patient is not well documented because the complication is often not recognized as such by the patient and not reported. The medical treatment of acute priapism includes hydration, pain management, and blood transfusion. Surgical management includes early aspiration of the corpora cavernosa to remove stagnated blood and allow the inflow of fresh well-oxygenated blood, followed by injection of alpha-adrenergic agents to restrict the flow of more blood. A combination of these medical and surgical regimens is carried out until the penis detumesces. Early intervention is advised to avoid the development of penile fibrosis and eventual impotence.

Right Upper Quadrant Syndrome

Recurrent pain in the right upper quadrant or epigastric region is a common feature of SCD. This often is caused by cholecystitis secondary to gallstones. When acute right upper quadrant pain is accompanied by fever or suspected infection, cholecystitis should be treated parenterally with appropriate antibiotics. Investigation for the presence of gallstones is usually performed with abdominal ultrasonography. Elective cholecystectomy is indicated when a patient with stones has frequent episodes of right upper quadrant syndrome.

PREPARATION FOR GENERAL ANESTHESIA AND SURGERY

Sickle cell disease patients often require surgery, and cholecystectomy is the most common procedure used. Conflicting data suggest that SCD patients have higher than expected perioperative complications. The most common complication is postoperative acute chest syndrome. To prevent sickling-related complications, standard preoperative care has included serial or exchange transfusion to reduce the percentage of Hb S cells to less than 30%. Postoperative care

should include aggressive respiratory therapy aimed at preventing acute chest syndrome.

CHRONIC ORGAN DAMAGE

The combined effects of chronic severe anemia and infarcts caused by microvascular occlusion lead gradually to deterioration in the functioning of most organs as patients age. The spleen often is the first organ to fail. In adults, renal, hepatic, cardiac, and pulmonary dysfunction is common. There is no treatment to prevent chronic organ damage at this time.

SPECIFIC TREATMENT

Experimental therapy for the treatment or cure of SCD is in progress. Hydroxyurea, the most widely evaluated agent in SCD, causes increases in the number of cells containing fetal hemoglobin (F cells) and in the level of fetal hemoglobin. The clinical efficacy of hydroxyurea therapy in SCD is under evaluation. Butyrates, another class of agents reported to increase fetal hemoglobin production, also are being tested. Bone marrow transplantation is slowly gaining application in SCD. Because of the perception of attendant danger and expense, clinicians have been slow in recommending and referring patients for bone marrow transplantation.

HEALTH MAINTENANCE

Sickle cell disease should be diagnosed as early as possible, preferably at birth, so that preventive care can begin before the development of complications. Children with SCD should receive all the regular immunizations, including hepatitis B, pneumococcal, and perhaps meningococcal vaccines. Penicillin prophylaxis should begin as early as 2 months of age and continue for at least 5 years. In areas where malaria is common, prophylaxis with the appropriate antimalarial agent is recommended. In the early years, patients should be examined every 3 to 4 months to evaluate changes in spleen size, degree of anemia, and growth. Education of parents regarding signs and symptoms of infection, splenic sequestration, severe anemia, respiratory distress, and the management of painful events is an important part of the care of children with SCD. Because SCD is a disease of acute complications, the health care team must be organized to recognize and respond appropriately to those complications. A multidisciplinary team of physicians, nurses, social workers, health educators, and genetic counselors is necessary to provide comprehensive health care to SCD patients.

CONGENITAL AND ACQUIRED DISORDERS OF COAGULATION

GERALD S. GILCHRIST, M.D.

INHERITED DISORDERS

General Principles of Management

The hemophilias and other inherited disorders of blood coagulation are characterized by an inherited inability to produce one of the plasma factors needed for normal hemostasis or by the inheritance of an abnormal coagulation factor with reduced functional activity.* The tendency to "spontaneously" bleed into joints and muscles, particu-

---

*With the exception of fibrinogen, which is usually measured in milligrams per deciliter of plasma, standard assay systems for other coagulation factors are based on the ability of the patient's plasma to correct the clotting time of factor-deficient plasma. The value is then expressed as a percentage of the correction produced by plasma from a normal pool of donors. Thus, the usual range of normal values is from 50% to 150% of normal but is sometimes expressed as 50 to 100 U/dl of activity.

larly in those with severe deficiencies (<1% of normal), can produce serious physical, economic, and psychosocial problems. Thus, the treatment of patients with hemophilia requires a multidisciplinary team approach, of which only one component is replacement of the missing factor by intravenous transfusion or in vivo stimulation of production or release of the deficient protein.

Awareness of the fact that blood products have been responsible for transmission of a variety of viruses, including HIV and hepatitis, has led to the development of increasingly more purified products derived from human plasma and production of various coagulation factors in vitro using recombinant DNA technology. These highly purified products can still stimulate the development of inhibitors to the missing factor but seem less likely to produce nonspecific changes in immune function related to the repeated infusion of plasma proteins from large pools of blood donors. Another approach to elevating factor VIII levels is to exploit the ability of desmopressin (DDAVP) to stimulate the release of preformed factor VIII from endothelial cells. This is effective only in patients with relatively mild hemophilia A or type I von Willebrand disease.

Comprehensive Care

The interdisciplinary approach to the management of patients with hemophilia and other inherited disorders of blood coagulation has resulted in the designation of comprehensive hemophilia diagnostic and treatment centers in the United States and Canada. These centers have the resources and expertise to provide a complete range of services to the affected patient and the family. In larger metropolitan areas, patients may receive their primary and ongoing care at the center, but in rural and less densely populated areas, it is essential that primary care physicians outside the center participate actively in the development and execution of appropriate management programs designed to meet individual needs. Periodic in-depth evaluations at a center are essential to monitor the appropriateness of the replacement therapy program, to detect significant complications of the disease or its treatment, and to ensure that the patient is given every opportunity to participate appropriately in the mainstream of society. At these sessions, patients are evaluated by a pediatric hematologist, orthopedic surgeon, specialist in physical medicine, dental surgeon, geneticist, and social worker. Laboratory studies include screening tests for the presence of an inhibitor, for evidence of liver and kidney disease, and for evidence of impairment of immune function.

After this multidisciplinary evaluation, the program for the upcoming year is reviewed with the patient, and, if necessary, appropriate modifications are made. This includes a replacement therapy plan, exercise programs to maintain or restore joint function, and communication with primary physicians, schools, employers, and appropriate community, regional, and state agencies. Plans are developed for surgical or medical consultation or treatment of other problems identified during the evaluation. More frequent evaluations may be necessary. It is now recommended that asymptomatic patients with evidence of exposure to HIV be evaluated at least every 6 months. Between visits to the center, patients are expected to submit monthly reports documenting the site and frequency of bleeds, their nature, and their response to therapy. This is of particular importance for patients on home treatment programs. These records are reviewed by the center personnel, and appropriate contacts are made with the patient, family, and primary physician regarding any recommended changes in treatment. This type of contact is greatly facilitated by hemophilia nurse specialists and social workers experienced in dealing with hemophilia patients and their problems. All patients and potentially affected family members should be made aware of the availability of cDNA probing techniques for carrier detection and prenatal testing.

Participation in most normal peer group activities should be encouraged, and this often requires providing in-service education for school personnel. Children should be permitted to participate in physical education programs to the extent that they are able. Contact sports should be avoided. Early entry in a competitive swimming program is recommended and provides an excellent physical, social, and psychologic outlet for the patient. Table 1 lists sports in which the physical, social, and psychologic benefits often outweigh the risks. For each individual the risk/benefit ratio must be evaluated. Attempting to isolate or overprotect the hemophiliac from all types of potentially dangerous activity can produce psychologic maladjustment that ultimately may prove more devastating than the physical crippling. The physician has the ultimate responsibility for advising appropriate restrictions for individual patients, taking all these factors into consideration.

Replacement Therapy

The prevention and treatment of hemorrhage and musculoskeletal deformities rank high in the list of priorities for the patient with hemophilia. At present, most material for replacement therapy is extracted from normal human plasma. There is limited indication for the use of single donor products, such as fresh frozen plasma (FFP) or cryoprecipitate, since neither product can be subjected to viral inactivation by heat or other means. In situations where no concentrated product is available, FFP remains the only means of supplying the missing procoagulant. Cryoprecipitate remains an important source of fibrinogen and is also useful in supplying the factor VIII needs of infants and young children, where a stockpile of units can be obtained by repeated pheresis of a single donor. Highly purified concentrates of factors VIII and IX are produced by immunoaffinity chromatography using monoclonal antibodies. Now that the genes have been cloned for a variety of clotting factors, products containing pure human factor VIII have been produced using recombinant DNA technology. Two such products are licensed in the United States and appear to be free of blood-borne infectious agents, although they are stabilized in human albumin. All blood-derived factor concentrates marketed in the United States are subjected to various procedures aimed at viral inactivation. Heat treatment or solvent-detergent treatment of concentrates has effectively eliminated HIV as a contaminant. Pasteurization, solvent-detergents, and monoclonal antibody purification seem to be effective in removing the hepatitis B and C viruses.

TABLE 1. Sports Participation

Recommended Sports
Golf
Swimming

Benefits Can Outweigh Risks
Baseball
Basketball
Bicycling
Bowling
Frisbee
Gymnastics
Horseback riding
Ice skating
Roller skating
Running and jogging
Skiing
Soccer
Tennis
Volleyball
Waterskiing
Weightlifting

Risks Outweigh Benefits
Boxing
Football
Hockey
Motorcycling
Racquetball
Skateboarding
Wrestling

Adapted from *Hemophilia and Sports,* American Red Cross and the National Hemophilia Foundation, New York, NY, 1984.

TABLE 2. Plasma-Derived Coagulation Factor Concentrates

PRODUCT NAME	MANUFACTURER	METHOD OF VIRAL INACTIVATION	HEPATITIS SAFETY	CLINICAL USE
Immunoaffinity Purified Factor VIII Products				
Monoclate-P	Armour	Pasteurized (60°C, 10 h)	Yes	Hemophilia A
Hemofil M	Baxter-Hyland	Solvent-detergent (TNBP/Triton X-100) 25°C, ≥10 h	Yes	Hemophilia A
Coagulation FVIII, method M	(Manufactured by Baxter-Hyland for American Red Cross from ARC collected plasma)	Solvent-detergent (TNBP/Triton X-100) 25°C, ≥10 h	Yes*	Hemophilia A
Intermediate Purity and High Purity Factor VIII Products				
Profilate OSD	Alpha	Affinity chromatography and solvent-detergent [tri(n-butyl) phosphate (TNBP) and polysorbate 80] 27°C, 6 h	Yes*	Hemophilia A
NY Blood Center FVIII-SD	NY Blood Center Melville Biologics	Solvent-detergent (TNBP and cholate) ≥24°C, 6 h	Yes	Hemophilia A
Koate HP	Miles	Solvent-detergent (TNBP and polysorbate 80), ≥24°C, 6 h	Yes*	Hemophilia A and VWD
Humate-P	Behringwerke (distributed by Armour)	Heated in solution (pasteurized), 60°C, 10 h	Yes	VWD
Koate-HS	Miles	Heated in solution (pasteurized) 60°C, 10 h	Yes*	VWD
Melate SD	NY Blood Center Melville Biologics	Solvent-detergent (TNBP and polysorbate 80) ≥24°C 6 h	Yes*	VWD
Coagulation Factor IX Products				
AlphaNine	Alpha	Heated in N-heptane solution, 60°C, 20 h	Yes*	Hemophilia B
AlphaNine SD	Alpha	TNBP and polysorbate 80 24°–30°C, > 24 h, and affinity chromatography	Yes*	Hemophilia B
Mononine 7M	Armour	Sodium thiocyanate, ultrafiltration	Yes	Hemophilia B
Factor IX Complex Concentrates				
Konyne 80	Miles	Dry heat, 80°C, 72 h	Yes*	Factor II, VII, IX, X deficiency Factor VIII inhibitor
Proplex T	Baxter-Hyland	Dry heat, 68°C, 144 h	No	Factor II, VII, IX, X deficiency
Profilnine HT	Alpha	Heated in N-heptane solution 60°C, 20 h	Yes*	Factor II, VII, IX, X deficiency
Bebulin VH	Immuno	Vapor heated (10 h, 60°C, 1190 mbar pressure plus 1 h, 80°C, 1375 mbar)	Yes	Factor II, VII, IX, X deficiency
Activated Factor IX Complex Concentrates				
Autoplex T	Baxter-Hyland	Dry heat, 68°C, 144 h	No	Factor VIII inhibitors
FEIBA VH	Immuno	Vapor heated (10 h, 60°C, 1190 mbar plus 1 h, 80°C, 1375 mbar)	Yes*	Factor VIII inhibitors

*Hepatitis safety established in another product prepared using similar methodology.
Some data from National Hemophilia Foundation's Medical and Scientific Advisory Council's recommendations, April 1995, Medical Bulletin No 226, the Foundation, New York, NY.

In developing a rational replacement therapy program, one must have (1) a knowledge of the potency of the various therapeutic products available for replacement therapy, (2) an awareness of the levels of the missing factor needed for hemostasis in the particular clinical situation, and (3) a knowledge of the approximate infusion half-life of the missing factor.

Tables 2 and 3 list the various products available in the United States for treatment of coagulation deficiencies. The potency of the lyophilized concentrates varies considerably, but each vial has the number of units of activity listed on the product label. Table 4 lists the equivalent volumes of products containing factor VIII or factor IX that contain 100 factor VIII or factor IX units, respectively. Table 5 lists the approximate half-disappearance times of various coagulation factors following infusion. The decay patterns are complex, but for practical purposes, these figures reflect the approximate time for the initial peak increments to decrease by 50%.

The in vivo recovery of the missing factor depends on its molecular weight and whether or not it is retained within the intravascular space. For example, after infusion of a given quantity of factor VIII, almost all of it is measurable in the circulation, and approximately 1 U of factor VIII per kilogram of body weight will elevate the in vivo factor VIII level by approximately 2%. On the other hand, when compared with factor VIII, factor IX is a smaller molecule and, since it is distributed extravascularly, will produce only 25% to 50% of the increment after infusion. These figures are approximations but are of practical value in day-to-day patient management.

TABLE 3. Recombinant Factor VIII Products

PRODUCT NAME	MANUFACTURER	METHOD OF VIRAL DEPLETION/INACTIVATION	HEPATITIS SAFETY
Recombinate Helixate	Baxter-Hyland Armour	Immunoaffinity chromatography, virucidal solutions, pasteurization	Yes
KoGENate Bioclate	Miles Armour	Anion and immunoaffinity chromatography, heat	Yes

TABLE 4. Equivalent Volume Containing 100 U* of Activity

| | FACTOR | |
PRODUCT	IX (ml)	VIII (ml)
Reference plasma	100	100
Fresh frozen plasma	125	110
Cryoprecipitate†	—	15–25
Factor VIII concentrate	—	0.5–2.0
Prothrombin complex concentrate	4	—
Factor IX concentrate	0.5–2.0	—

* 1 U is defined as the amount of coagulant activity present in 1 ml of plasma having 100% activity.

† The factor VIII content of individual bags is variable. The average bag of cryoprecipitate contains 100 factor VIII units, with a range of 50–200 U.

Prophylactic Replacement Therapy

With the availability of highly purified factor concentrates, it is now possible to provide satisfactory prophylaxis by changing the status of severely affected patients to mild or moderate, a significant change in terms of modifying the potential for long-term orthopedic complications. Reports from Sweden document completely normal joint function and x-ray appearance in a cohort of 15 patients who began prophylaxis at 1 to 2 years of age between 1979 and 1988.[1] This was achieved by preventing the factors VIII and IX levels from dropping below 1% to 5% of normal using 25 to 40 U of factor VIII per kilogram body weight three times a week. The same dose of factor IX was given twice weekly. This has required insertion of venous access devices in smaller children. The results were less impressive in a cohort of 20 boys who had begun prophylaxis at an older age or used lower doses, but even in this group, 50% had completely normal joint scores. This experience suggests that prophylaxis should be considered in younger children *before* they experience significant hemarthrosis. Although initially the cost of treatment will be higher, additional expenses will be offset by maintaining function and avoiding the need for much higher doses of concentrate to treat bleeds in damaged joints and major orthopedic reconstruction in adolescence and adulthood. Prophylaxis might also be considered in patients who have had CNS hemorrhage or recurrent hemarthroses in a single target joint or during periods of intensive rehabilitation.

Pharmacologic Approaches

A number of naturally occurring and synthetic hormones can elevate plasma levels of factor VIII and von Willebrand factor (VWF). These include estrogen, which stimulates increased synthesis, and l-deamino-8-D-arginine vasopressin (desmopressin, DDAVP), which causes release of factor VIII and VWF from endothelial cells and has been widely used to treat patients with relatively mild hemophilia A (factor VIII >5% of normal) and with mild to moderately severe type I von Willebrand disease. Following an IV infusion of 0.3 μg/kg of DDAVP, peak levels are seen within 15 to 30 minutes with the expected half-life of about 12 hours. The increment in factor VIII/VWF levels is variable but reasonably consistent within families. Since the baseline level may increase anywhere from 1.5- to 6-fold, each patient should have a trial dose, and factor VIII/VWF levels should be assayed to document the magnitude of the rise. If the peak level is considered suboptimal, supplemental replacement therapy will be necessary. It should also be appreciated that in most (but not all) patients, tachyphylaxis occurs, resulting in decreasing responsiveness if the drug is given more frequently than every 24 to 48 hours. Side effects of DDAVP, such as flushing, changes in blood pressure, tachycardia, and water retention, can be avoided by diluting the dose in 50 ml normal saline and administering over 30 minutes.

Subcutaneous injection of DDAVP appears to be at least as effective as the intravenous route and has obvious advantages for self-administration. Although DDAVP is approved by the FDA for subcutaneous administration for treatment of diabetes insipidus, it has not been licensed for this form of administration in factor VIII deficiency. The current intravenous formulation (4 μg/ml) makes it difficult to administer large doses in a single subcutaneous injection. A more concentrated version (10 μg/ml) is being developed and should obviate this problem. An intranasal formulation of DDAVP has been developed in Sweden and has recently been approved by the FDA. This product (Stimate) delivers 150 μg per activation. The effective dose is 150 μg in children weighing less than 50 kg and 300 μg in those over 50 kg. DDAVP can be used alone to control bleeding episodes and to cover dental extractions and even major surgery if the deficiency is relatively mild and hemostatic levels of factor VIII can be achieved and maintained.

Factor VIII Deficiency (Hemophilia A, Classic Hemophilia)

One factor VIII U/kg will elevate the plasma level by 2%. To achieve a 50% level in a 20 kg child, 500 U of factor VIII are given by rapid infusion. This would require approximately 5 bags of cryoprecipitate, ± 700 ml of plasma, or 2.5 to 10 ml of concentrate. After about 12 hours, the level will have dropped to 25%, and to maintain levels above 25% over a period of time, infusions will have to be repeated every 12 hours, using approximately 12.5 U/kg, a dose calculated to produce a 25% increment in plasma factor VIII level. The potency, in vivo recovery, and half-life are quite variable, so that levels of factor VIII may have to be monitored by specific assay. Factor level assays are not usually necessary in the treatment of isolated joint or muscle hemorrhage but are critical in the management of intracranial hemorrhage or in patients undergoing major surgery. This is most effectively done by measuring factor VIII before and 30 minutes after an infusion and repeating it 8 to 12 hours later. This provides an indication of the lowest level before infusion, the increment following infusion, and the decay rate. This information allows the dose to be adjusted when it is essential that minimum plasma levels be maintained. For patients undergoing major surgery, continuous infusion of factor VIII avoids the wide variations in plasma levels and reduces the number of assays needed to monitor therapy. A protocol for continuous infusion of factor VIII is outlined in Table 6.

In deciding which factor VIII product to prescribe, the treating physician must consider cost (which can vary from 30¢ to 90¢ per factor VIII unit) and purity (which ranges from crude cryoprecipitate to highly purified, rDNA-derived material) in relation to the patient's age and clinical situation, including prior HIV and hepatitis exposure. DDAVP is particularly useful in more mildly affected patients (>5% factor VIII) to cover acute bleeding episodes or minor and even major surgery.

Factor IX Deficiency (Hemophilia B, Christmas Disease)

The in vivo recovery of factor IX is less than that of factor VIII. One factor IX U/kg elevates the circulating plasma level by only about 1%. Thus, to achieve a peak postinfusion increment of 50%, 50 U/kg would have to be administered. A 20 kg child would require 1000 to 2000 ml of FFP. Concentrates contain 500 to 1500 U of factor IX in as little as 10 ml, so that 1000 U of activity can be administered in a volume of 20 ml. Because of the longer biologic half-life of

TABLE 5. Approximate Biologic Half-Life of Coagulation Factors After Infusion

FACTOR	HALF-LIFE
VII	4–6 h
VIII	12 h
V	20 h
IX	24 h
X	30 h
XI	48 h
Fibrinogen	72 h
II	72 h
XIII	10+ d

TABLE 6. Continuous Infusion of Factor VIII Concentrates

1. Bolus infusion to increase to desired level (1 U/kg elevates level by 2%)
2. To maintain
     25%: 1 U/kg/h
     50%: 2 U/kg/h
     75%: 3 U/kg/h
3. Factor VIII is dispensed in batches for 12 h infusions mixed in 500 or 1000 ml of normal saline
4. Assay factor VIII levels once daily to ensure that appropriate level is maintained

factor IX, the infusions can be given less frequently. However, it should be appreciated that the first phase of factor IX disappearance is rapid, and if high hemostatic levels are needed over a prolonged period of time, the frequency of infusions may approach that used in factor VIII replacement. In potentially life-threatening situations or to cover surgical procedures, laboratory monitoring of plasma factor levels is critical.

Although many centers believe that lower levels of factor IX may be adequate to produce hemostasis in various clinical situations, most tend to use the same general guidelines as are used for factor VIII-deficient patients. This means that most hemophilia B patients should be treated with concentrates. In the past, FFP was used to control minor bleeding in mildly affected patients with hemophilia B. However, the new, more purified factor IX preparations are less thrombogenic, have a reduced hepatitis risk, and are now considered to be the products of choice for treating hemophilia B (Table 2). DDAVP has no effect on factor IX levels.

von Willebrand Disease (VWD)

VWD is characterized by a deficiency of a plasma factor (VWF) that is necessary for the promotion of normal platelet-vessel interaction and the synthesis of factor VIII coagulant activity. A number of subtypes have been recognized. Some (e.g., type I) are characterized by reduced production of normal VWF, whereas in others (e.g., type II), there is production of an abnormal molecule. Type III refers to almost complete absence of VWF in plasma. Both sexes are equally affected. Bleeding tends to be mucosal and cutaneous, although hemarthroses can occur in patients with extremely low factor VIII levels. Epistaxis is common in childhood and is often aggravated by local lesions in the nose and, during the winter months, by reduced humidity. Thrombin-soaked nasal packs and cauterization are sometimes needed, and replacement therapy may be required. Menorrhagia can be severe but can usually be controlled with cyclic oral contraceptive therapy, in part because exogenously administered estrogen also stimulates increased synthesis of VWF and factor VIII in mildly to moderately affected females. DDAVP is very effective in shortening the bleeding time and elevating blood levels of factor VIII and VWF in those with mildly to moderately severe type I VWD. DDAVP can also improve hemostasis in those with type IIA VWD but is contraindicated in type IIB VWD because it produces in vivo platelet aggregation and thrombocytopenia.

A number of virus-inactivated factor VIII concentrates contain VWF and are generally preferable to random donor cryoprecipitate (Table 2). To prepare a patient for elective surgery, an infusion of plasma (10 to 15 ml/kg) cryoprecipitate (1 bag per 10 kg), or one of the wet heat-treated concentrates (Humate P, Koate HP, or Profilate HP) (Table 2) is given 8 to 24 hours earlier. In an emergency, enough material should be given to produce an immediate rise in factor VIII coagulant activity to 50%. This will provide adequate coverage during the period of in vivo synthesis. The decision to provide further therapy is determined by monitoring the plasma VWF and factor VIII levels, which should be maintained at 25% to 50% for 10 days after a major operation.

The bleeding time is often shortened 2 to 4 hours after infusion but rarely to normal. Hemostasis is usually satisfactory in spite of failure to correct the bleeding time.

Factor XI Deficiency (Hemophilia C, PTA Deficiency)

Very little factor XI enters the extravascular space, so that one can apply the same dosage calculations as for factor VIII. No concentrations are available, but satisfactory hemostasis can be maintained because the biologic half-life is from 40 to 48 hours. A series of three plasma transfusions in a dose of 10 ml/kg every 6 to 8 hours will produce a peak rise in factor XI of about 50%, and levels above 25% can be maintained easily with daily transfusions of 10 ml/kg or less. A monoclonal antibody-purified factor XI concentrate is being developed. In an emergency, partial exchange transfusion may be necessary if circulatory overload is a concern.

Factor XII Deficiency (Hageman Disease)

Deficiency of factor XII is not associated with abnormal hemostasis. No particular precautions or replacement therapy is needed in spite of the markedly prolonged in vitro coagulation times.

Factor XIII Deficiency

Deficiency of fibrin-stabilizing factor is easily treated. A single infusion of 2 to 3 ml of plasma per kilogram is sufficient to obtain normal hemostasis and correct the abnormal in vitro clot solubility. To reduce exposure to plasma from multiple donors, a single, healthy compatible donor can be identified for periodic plasmapheresis, since most patients will only require 250 to 500 ml of plasma every 2 to 4 weeks.

Congenital Afibrinogenemia, Hypofibrinogenemia, and Dysfibrinogenemia

Normal hemostasis requires plasma levels of 80 to 100 mg/dl and can be achieved readily with single donor cryoprecipitate, which contains about 250 mg per bag. After infusion, fibrinogen enters the extravascular space. Two to four bags of cryoprecipitate per 10 kg body weight will elevate plasma fibrinogen by 50 to 100 mg/dl. This can be administered over an 8- to 12-hour period to minimize volume overload, depending on the volume of cryoprecipitate in each bag. Adequate circulating levels can be maintained by daily infusion of 0.6 to 1 bag of cryoprecipitate per 10 kg body weight. Lyophilized factor concentrates are virtually fibrinogen free. A purified fibrinogen concentrate is entering clinical trials in the United States.

Deficiencies of Factors II, VII, and X

These rare inherited disorders do not respond to vitamin K therapy. Their in vivo recovery is similar to that of factor IX, although their biologic half-lives vary (Table 4). The same principles for the use of plasma or prothrombin complex concentrates apply. Even moderately severe deficiency of factor VII may result in very little bleeding. Successful operations have been performed on patients with as little as 20% of normal factor VII without factor replacement.

Factor V Deficiency

Factor V is extremely labile, and only fresh plasma or FFP should be used for replacement therapy. The in vivo recovery and biologic half-life are similar to those of factor IX, and the same general principles apply. Factor V is not a vitamin K-dependent factor and is not present in cryoprecipitate or other concentrates.

Special Treatment Situations
Musculoskeletal Hemorrhage

Prompt treatment is essential to control hemarthrosis or intramuscular bleeds, particularly those involving the gastrocnemius or if nerve compression is suspected. All patients and parents should be made aware of the early signs and symptoms of hemarthrosis and the need for prompt treatment, which should be made readily available on an outpatient basis if the patient is not on a home treatment program. If treatment is given in an emergency room, clinic, or doctor's office, an outline of the patient's treatment program should be kept on file as an ongoing prescription for replacement therapy. Physician evaluation is not necessary for patients who are known to the facility and have demonstrated a working knowledge of hemophilia and its treatment. Naturally, if the well-informed patient or parent requests it, evaluation by a physician is indicated.

A smooth-flowing system is essential to the success of an outpatient treatment program. Traditionally, when the need for replacement therapy had to be evaluated with each bleed, treatment was inevitably delayed because the average physician in an emergency room is usually less well informed about hemophilia than is the patient.

A copy of the patient's treatment program should be readily available in the emergency room, blood bank, or any other treatment facility. In addition, the patient should carry a copy of the program at all times. At the earliest sign of bleeding into an area that would require replacement therapy, a phone call is made to the treatment facility with a request that the appropriate number of vials or bags of materials be prepared for infusion at the time the patient anticipates arriving there. Occasionally, less responsible patients fail to keep these appointments, to the chagrin of hospital personnel, but this is a rare occurrence and should alert one to reevaluate whether that patient's outpatient treatment program is appropriate. Table 7 lists the principles for outpatient or home therapy for the treatment of musculoskeletal bleeding. Joint aspiration is rarely indicated and then only to relieve pressure symptoms in a markedly swollen joint.

Specific factor assays need not be monitored unless the clinical response is considered unsatisfactory. If assay is indicated and the increment in factor level is not consistent with the dose infused, the possibility of an inhibitor or some deterioration in the potency of the infusion material has to be considered.

The presence of synovitis with hypervascular friable synovium should be suspected in patients who have repeated bleeds into a single joint in spite of satisfactory increments in plasma procoagulant levels. The inflamed synovium sets the stage for recurrent hemorrhage. To break this vicious cycle, short, 4 to 5 day courses of prednisone (40 mg/m^2/d in three divided doses) are prescribed in conjunction with replacement therapy. If this fails to have the desired effect after 6 to 8 weeks of observation, a longer course of prednisone (3 to 4 weeks) should be considered. Alternatively, a prophylactic infusion program aimed at maintaining factor VIII or IX levels above 5% can be effective and should be continued for at least 3 months. In selected instances, surgical synovectomy should be considered in a joint that is the site of recurrent hemorrhage with synovial thickening but before radiographic evidence of hemophilic arthropathy has developed. Nonsurgical synovectomy using colloidal ^{32}P chromic phosphate has been employed successfully but must still be considered investigational. In older patients, joint replacement has successfully eliminated painful, crippling deformities in weightbearing and upper extremity joints.

Dental Management

Preventive dental care should be part of the hemophiliac's overall treatment plan. Most routine dental procedures can be performed without replacement therapy, particularly if regional anesthesia is avoided. Local infiltration of the affected tooth often can suffice. Loss of deciduous teeth is not usually associated with significant bleeding. If bleeding is persistent, however, oozing usually can be controlled with thrombin-soaked gauze.

Extraction of permanent teeth requires appropriate replacement therapy or DDAVP, with the aim of achieving a 50% level of the missing factor immediately before the procedure. Epsilon-aminocaproic acid (EACA, Amicar) or tranexamic acid (Cyklokapron) is given to inhibit fibrinolytic activity in the oral cavity. This prevents the fibrin clot in the tooth socket from dissolving. Clot formation is also enhanced by packing the socket with thrombin-soaked oxidized cellulose (Oxycel or Surgicel saturated with a solution of powdered thrombin dissolved in 0.5% sodium bicarbonate). The dose of EACA is 100 mg/kg PO or IV immediately before the procedure and every 6 hours for 7 to 10 days thereafter. It is administered most easily as a 25% syrup, which contains 1.25 g in each 5 ml, but is also available in tablet form. Tranexamic acid also is an effective antifibrinolytic agent

TABLE 7. Guidelines for Replacement Therapy of Joint or Muscle Hemorrhage

Treat at *earliest* sign of hemarthrosis or intramuscular bleed
Increase factor VIII or IX level to ± 40% of normal*
Repeat dose at 24 h if no response
Physician evaluation if still symptomatic at 48 h
Maintain mobility unless pain or swelling is severe

*It is often possible to produce hemostasis with lower levels if the treatment is instituted very early.

in a dose of 25 mg/kg PO or IV every 6 to 8 hours. These drugs should not be used in the presence of hematuria or if there is evidence of active intravascular coagulation. With a single infusion of replacement therapy or DDAVP and adequate consolidation of the clot, no further replacement therapy usually is necessary unless the clot is dislodged from the tooth socket.

Epistaxis and Intraoral Hemorrhage

Epistaxis is more common in patients with VWD than in those with hemophilia. Packing with thrombin-soaked oxidized cellulose (see Dental Management) is helpful if other local measures fail. Replacement therapy or DDAVP may be necessary, particularly if the oozing is generalized without an identifiable bleeding point to cauterize.

The toddler with hemophilia tends to have problems with intraoral bleeding as a result of trauma to the tongue, lips, frenum, or oral mucosa. Because it is impossible to immobilize these areas, the clot is easily dislodged, leading to recurrent bleeding and the need for repeated doses of replacement therapy. This series of events can be modified by prompt replacement therapy aimed at elevating factor levels to 50%, local application of thrombin-soaked oxidized cellulose, and oral EACA or tranexamic acid as recommended for dental procedures.

Pain Control

One of the goals of early control of bleeding is to reduce the need for analgesia. Particularly in older patients with established hemophilic arthropathy, drug abuse and addiction can be serious problems. In addition, aspirin and aspirin-containing drugs should not be used because of their action on platelet function and their ability to aggravate the preexisting hemostatic defect. A list of aspirin-containing drugs is available from the National Hemophilia Foundation. Although other nonsteroidal anti-inflammatory drugs, such as ibuprofen (Motrin), affect platelet function, the effect is rapidly reversed when treatment is discontinued. In contrast, the effect of aspirin persists for the lifespan of the exposed platelet. Thus nonsteroidal anti-inflammatory drugs deserve a trial in patients with symptoms suggestive of arthritis in joints that have been the site of recurrent hemorrhage in the past. Nonacetylated salicylates in the form of choline magnesium trisalicylate (Trilisate) or salicysalicylic acid (Disalcid) 500 to 1000 mg b.i.d. do not affect platelet function but do exert an anti-inflammatory effect. Although their effects on platelet function are less well defined, phenylbutazone, phenothiazides, and phenacetin should be avoided in patients with bleeding disorders.

Hematuria

Hematuria is often unresponsive to replacement therapy in spite of hemostatic blood levels being attained. Bedrest for 24 to 48 hours seems to be advantageous in some patients. Prednisone, 40 to 60 mg/m^2/24 h in divided doses usually causes the hematuria to subside in 48 hours, after which the dose should be tapered and stopped over the next 3 days. EACA or other antifibrinolytic therapy is contraindicated in the management of hematuria and can result in clot formation in the urinary tract.

Inhibitors

Approximately 10% of those with severe hemophilia A develop inhibitors that are capable of neutralizing infused factor VIII. The frequency of inhibitor formation is much lower in hemophilia B. Some patients have low titers of inhibitor (<5 Bethesda units) and do not have an anamnestic rise in inhibitor level after an infusion. These inhibitors often can be overcome by treating with larger and more frequent doses of the missing factor. In patients with more potent inhibitors, a number of therapeutic approaches have been tried. Some investigators have recommended withholding replacement therapy, hoping that the inhibitor titer will drop, but this rarely happens and usually leads to increasing disability from untreated musculoskeletal hemorrhages. Various trials of immunosuppressive therapy have not met with success in hemophiliacs with inhibitors. In life-threatening situations, exchange transfusion using the continuous-flow centrifuge has been effective in replacing the patient's inhibitor-containing plasma with normal plasma. The beneficial effect is temporary, since the antigenic stimulus invariably produces an anamnestic antibody response and even higher levels of inhibitor within 5 to 7 days.

A number of other approaches have been developed for management of high responders. These include the use of activated and nonactivated prothrombin complexes to bypass the need for factor VIII, highly purified porcine factor VIII, induction of immune tolerance using varying doses and schedules of factor VIII, and immunoabsorbance of IgG antibodies during plasmapheresis. Two newly developed rDNA products, factor VIIa and tissue factor, are currently being evaluated.

The high-responding patient must be managed by a center having all the resources to treat and monitor bleeding episodes.

Head Injury

Any significant injury to the head in a patient with an inherited disorder of blood coagulation deserves immediate replacement therapy before proceeding with careful neurologic evaluation. Any patient with hemophilia and a headache lasting more than 6 to 8 hours should receive replacement therapy, with immediate infusion of sufficient material to elevate the factor level to 100%. Surgical evacuation of intracranial accumulations of blood should be undertaken in a hemophilia center where facilities are available for careful monitoring of blood levels.

Nerve Compression

Compression of peripheral nerves can occur whenever there is bleeding in a closed fibromuscular compartment. Hemorrhage into the iliopsoas sheath can lead to permanent femoral nerve palsy. Early recognition and prompt replacement therapy are essential. On occasion, surgical decompression is necessary if there is danger of permanent loss of neuromuscular function.

Major Surgery

Elective surgical procedures should be undertaken only in hospitals with facilities to monitor coagulation factor levels and only after it has been established that the patient has no evidence of an inhibitor. Factor levels above 30% have to be maintained for 7 to 10 days after major procedures by either intermittent or continuous infusion of the missing factor.

Emergency surgical procedures should be performed after administering enough of the missing factor to produce a blood level of 100%. If specific factor assays cannot be done, normalization of the partial thromboplastin time can be accepted as reasonable indirect evidence of satisfactory response, but the patient should be transferred to a hemophilia center as soon as possible if the patient's condition permits.

Immunizations

All children should receive routine immunizations, all of which can be given subcutaneously. In addition, hepatitis B vaccine should be given to all patients who are likely to be exposed to blood products. The child who is HIV positive or lives in a household with an HIV-infected parent or sibling should receive killed polio vaccine (Salk) to prevent passage of live virus in the household.

Home Infusion Therapy

Home therapy should be considered if the patient requires reasonably frequent factor infusions or DDAVP and after careful psychosocial evaluation of the patient and the family. Formal training in infusion procedures and intravenous technique is mandatory, and it is the responsibility of the supervising physician and the hemophilia center team to ensure that the patient and family are completely familiar with the indications for treatment and the signs and symptoms that would mandate physician evaluation.

Home treatment has obvious psychologic and economic advantages for both the patient and the family. In addition to making early treatment more available, home therapy also means that, for the first time, many of the patients have some control over their lives and the management of their disease. Home infusion is not without hazards, however. These include lack of medical supervision, increased danger of hepatitis in relatives, poor intravenous technique, overuse of material, product deterioration, and illegal use of intravenous equipment. The patient and family should keep detailed records, and, as with the outpatient treatment program, they are advised to check with the physician if more than two successive daily infusions are needed for control of a single bleeding episode. Furthermore, each patient on the home infusion program must return at least once a year for evaluation of the total management program. A number of studies have shown that there is increased use of replacement therapy initially, but this eventually levels off. However, even if replacement therapy use remains high, this is usually balanced by the reduced cost of treatment and the improvement in school and work attendance. To guard against product deterioration, it is essential that the patient have adequate instructions and facilities for storage. To ensure that patients who are traveling in other areas receive prompt and appropriate therapy, each patient is provided with a card outlining the diagnosis and the dose of replacement therapy. This is also useful in protecting patients who have to account to law enforcement authorities for venipuncture marks and the possession of venipuncture equipment.

The institution dispensing the infusion material has an obligation to guard against abuse and sale of venipuncture equipment through illegal channels. To monitor this, we insist that all materials are appropriately disposed of after use. Patients are encouraged to restock their supply when they have enough material left for only one infusion. Ordinarily, we supply enough for four infusions at a time, and this can be done through the mail. A number of home care companies arrange for shipment of therapeutic materials, arrange to bill third party payers, and keep the hemophilia center updated on each patient's product use. However, this does lead to additional costs.

Educational Resources

A wide variety of educational materials is available from the National Hemophilia Foundation, The SoHo Building, 110 Greene Street, Suite 303, New York, NY 10012. These include informative brochures suitable for patients, physicians, teachers, nurses, and other individuals who deal with the hemophilic patient and family. The brochures cover such subjects as pain control, dental care, physical therapy, financial counseling, teaching home therapy, sports, and so on. In addition, the Foundation publishes a *Directory of Hemophilia Treatment Centers* and descriptions of state and federal programs for assisting the hemophiliac and the family. The World Federation of Hemophilia, 4616 St. Catherine Street West, Montreal, Quebec, Canada H3Z, 1S3, publishes a *Guide for Traveling Hemophiliacs,* which lists hemophilia centers located in 72 countries.

ACQUIRED DISORDERS

Vitamin K Deficiency

Hemorrhagic Disease of the Newborn

Prevention. In healthy full-term infants, the problem of hemorrhagic disease of the newborn has been virtually eliminated by the administration of vitamin K at or soon after delivery. The naturally occurring compound, vitamin K_1 oxide (phytonadione), is the preferred form because synthetic vitamin K analogs can produce hemolysis. Neonatal hemolysis and the risk of kernicterus are particular problems in the presence of a deficiency of red cell glucose-6-phosphate dehydrogenase (G6PD). It has been well established that as little as 0.025 mg of vitamin K_1 can prevent the deficiencies of the vitamin K-dependent factors in a neonate with reasonably mature liver function. Thus, the recommended dose of 0.5 to 1.0 mg IM or SC or 1 to 2 mg PO is far in excess of the neonate's physiologic needs, and higher doses have no added beneficial effect. Particularly with the water-soluble analogs, higher doses increase the risk of kernicterus. Infants of mothers being treated with phenytoin (Dilantin) or phenobarbital occasionally are found immediately after birth to have hemorrhage secondary to depletion of vitamin K-dependent factors. This is in contrast to the usual case of hemorrhagic disease of the newborn, where the various clotting factors are transferred transplacentally and symptoms become manifest only beyond the first 24 hours of age. Some recommend the administration of vitamin K during labor to the mother who is on anticonvulsant therapy to prevent bleeding secondary to the trauma of delivery.

Treatment. Premature infants, particularly those with such complications as hypoxia, acidosis, or infections, do not respond to the administration of vitamin K as well as healthy term infants. When hemorrhagic manifestations are proved to be due exclusively or in large part to a deficiency of vitamin K-dependent factors, the clinician has to resort to the use of replacement therapy with fresh plasma or FFP if the patient is not responsive to vitamin K. The amount of procoagulant that can be safely administered to the newborn in this fashion is limited by the relatively low concentrations of procoagulants in whole plasma. On an average, plasma contains 1 U of procoagulant activity in each milliliter, and an infusion of 10 mg/kg will produce an elevation of only about 10% in the circulating level of factor IX and the other vitamin K-dependent factors. Because of concern for volume overload, central venous pressure should be monitored constantly, particularly if an umbilical vein catheter is already in place for other reasons. As a practical approach, 10 ml of FFP/kg body weight can be administered every 12 hours, and this should provide hemostatic levels of the missing factors, although the levels of each procoagulant will vary because of variations in in vivo recovery and intravascular biologic half-life. For example, factor VII, although stable in stored plasma, has a short in vivo half-life of 4 to 6 hours. In contrast, 50% of infused prothrombin (factor II) is still present 72 hours later.

Prothrombin complex concentrates are commercially available (Table 2). In these concentrations, the vitamin K-dependent factors are concentrated in approximately 1/25 the volume, compared with plasma. However, because of the increased risk of hepatitis and thrombosis, these concentrates should not be used unless it has been impossible to provide satisfactory hemostatic levels with single donor plasma.

High-risk neonates should continue to receive supplemental parenteral or oral vitamin K, particularly if they are receiving broad-spectrum antibiotics or total parenteral nutrition.

Impaired Intestinal Absorption

Vitamin K deficiency can develop as a result of fat malabsorption and after prolonged administration of broad-spectrum antibiotics. Thus, patients with conditions in which vitamin K deficiency might

be anticipated should receive the water-soluble form of the vitamin prophylactically. For treatment of bleeding in these situations, intramuscular or intravenous vitamin K_1 should be given. Replacement therapy with blood products is rarely necessary.

Liver Disease

In advanced liver disease, there is defective synthesis of the vitamin K-dependent clotting factors, and treatment with vitamin K often is ineffective. If there is overt bleeding or if the patient is being prepared for surgery, plasma infusions may be necessary. If possible, prothrombin complex concentrates should be avoided because of the added risk of hepatitis in the face of preexisting liver dysfunction. Thrombosis risk hazard may be increased in the patient with liver disease who is unable to clear activated coagulation factors from the circulation.

Coumarin Anticoagulants

The coumarin anticoagulants are rarely used therapeutically in pediatric practice, but they can cross the placenta, producing neonatal bleeding. More commonly, accidental ingestion of medication or rat poison can produce severe depletion of vitamin K-dependent factors. Intravenous administration of 50 mg of vitamin K_1 will normalize the prothrombin time within 6 to 12 hours, regardless of how much dicumarol is taken. A prolonged coumarin effect lasting up to 3 weeks occurs after ingestion of brodifacoum, one of the second-generation anticoagulant rodenticides. Compared with warfarin, which has a plasma half-life of 14 hours, the in vivo half-life of brodifacoum is closer to a week. Repeated daily doses of vitamin K are necessary to bypass the prolonged inhibition of gamma-carboxyglutamation. The synthetic water-soluble analogs are less effective than the naturally occurring compound.

Circulating Anticoagulants

Circulating inhibitors of coagulation can develop in children without preexisting coagulation factor deficiency. They may be directed against specific coagulation factors but usually are nonspecific and appear to be directed against the prothrombinase complex. They are rarely associated with abnormal hemostasis in spite of significant in vitro abnormalities. Treatment is directed at the underlying disease, for example, systemic lupus erythematosus. Problems have not been encountered at renal biopsy, even when significant in vitro inhibition is present. Many of these inhibitors, particularly those detected during preoperative screening, seem to be related to viral infections and gradually disappear over weeks or months without specific therapy.

REFERENCE

1. Nilsson IM, Berntorp E, Lofqvist T, Pettersson H.: Twenty-five years of experience of prophylactic treatment in severe hemophilia A and B. J Intern Med 232:25–32, 1992.

PLATELET DISORDERS

DIANA S. BEARDSLEY, M.D., Ph.D.

THROMBOCYTOPENIA

Therapy for thrombocytopenia depends on the etiology for the decrease in platelet count. There are two basic mechanisms to be considered: decreased platelet production and increased platelet destruction. Differentiating between these two states usually can be accomplished by an assessment of the patient's clinical history and an examination of the bone marrow for the presence of megakaryocytes. The platelet equivalent of the erythrocyte reticulocyte count has not yet achieved clinical use. However, a flow cytometric assay of young, reticulated patients is undergoing evaluation and holds promise for evaluating platelet destruction without examination of the bone marrow. Recently, a cytokine that stimulates platelet production, thrombopoietin, has been identified, but it is not yet possible to assay this growth factor clinically. It is hoped that induction of platelet production eventually will be possible using appropriate cytokine therapy.

Thrombocytopenia Due to Decreased Platelet Production

Aplastic anemia, whether congenital or acquired, causes a decrease in all circulating blood cells because of production failure. A common cause for decreased platelet production is the use of myelosuppressive chemotherapeutic agents. Therapy for childhood leukemia and solid tumors has become more intensive, and bone marrow transplantation has been available to more patients in recent years. The addition of radiotherapy as part of such aggressive treatment regimens further increases the effect on bone marrow production. The duration of neutropenia can now be moderated by the use of growth factors, but thrombocytopenia remains a serious consequence of intensive chemotherapy and bone marrow transplantation.

Transfusion of Platelet Concentrates

The current treatment for patients who have defective platelet production as a result of primary bone marrow failure or secondary to myelosuppressive chemotherapy and radiotherapy relies on replacement therapy in the form of transfusion with platelet concentrates. Transfusion is indicated for the patient with clinical hemorrhage regardless of the platelet count. Prophylactic platelet transfusion is considered appropriate for the patient with severe thrombocytopenia. Early studies showed that spontaneous hemorrhage rarely occurs at a platelet count over 20,000/mm³. Recently, this threshold has been lowered to 10,000 or even 5000/mm³.

Random donor platelets are the standard transfusion product used by most blood centers. These concentrates are prepared by differential centrifugation of individual units of donated whole blood, each of which contains approximately 5.5 to 7.5 × 10¹⁰ platelets. Multiple units are pooled to prepare an individual patient's therapeutic dose. The platelet dose may be determined by estimating that 1 unit of platelets per square meter of body surface area will increase the recipient's platelet count by 10,000 to 20,000/mm³ in an afebrile, uninfected, nonalloimmunized recipient with a normal spleen.

Assessment of the effectiveness of platelet transfusion can be documented by determining the immediate posttransfusion platelet count, a measure of *platelet recovery*. Traditionally, this platelet count was measured 1 hour after completion of the platelet transfusion, although the platelet concentration 5 minutes after transfusion is equal to the 1-hour measure. *Platelet survival* is determined by the platelet count 24 hours after transfusion. In general, immune platelet destruction leads to poor platelet recovery, whereas nonimmune factors are more likely to affect platelet survival. Platelet recovery and survival can be assessed accurately by calculating the corrected count increment (CCI) either within the first hour (recovery) or 24 hours (survival) after the platelet transfusion.

$$CCI = \frac{[\text{Posttransfusion count} - \text{pretransfusion count} (/\mu l)] \times BSA \ (m^2)}{\text{No. of platelets infused} \ (\times \ 10^{-11})}$$

Platelet concentrates contain both erythrocytes and leukocytes. The leukocyte contamination presents several potential complications. Graft-versus-host (GVH) disease can occur in the severely immunocompromised patient. The problem is alleviated by gamma-radiation. Radiation of directed donor units is standard practice to avoid GVH disease in even an immunocompetent recipient who might receive a transfusion from an HLA homozygous family member. Cytomegalovirus (CMV) infection also can result from transfusion with leukocyte-containing blood products. As CMV infection is an adverse risk factor for bone marrow transplantation, patients who may become candidates for transplantation should receive only blood products free from CMV. These include donations from CMV-seronegative donors as well as frozen, washed erythrocytes. Filtration with leukocyte filters

may be an alternative approach to elimination of CMV, although this modality continues to be investigated. Platelets for transfusion to newborn infants also should be chosen to reduce the risk for CMV and GVH disease.

All platelet concentrates should be administered through a standard 170 μm blood filter to remove aggregates. To maintain platelet function, platelets are stored at 25° C with constant motion on a rocker. Because of the risk of bacterial growth at this storage temperature, platelets cannot be stored for more than 5 days.

The patient who requires multiple platelet transfusions is at risk for becoming alloimmunized against platelet antigens and refractory to platelet transfusion. The frequency is higher for immunocompetent recipients, such as patients with aplastic anemia, than it is for immunosuppressed patients, such as those undergoing intensive chemotherapy. Alloimmunization to HLA antigens is responsible for most cases of immune refractoriness, although alloimmunization against platelet-specific antigens or the formation of autoantibodies also can occur. Anti-HLA alloimmunization results from the presence of lymphocytes in platelet concentrates. Platelets lack class II HLA antigens and, therefore, are not capable of stimulating an alloimmune response. However, platelets can be destroyed by the resulting HLA alloantibodies.

Special leukocyte filters may reduce HLA alloimmunization, and ultraviolet B (UV-B) radiation is under investigation as another approach to this problem. Alloimmunization can be assessed by documenting a posttransfusion corrected platelet count increment of <5000 in the absence of nonimmune factors that might cause platelet destruction. Further support for HLA alloimmunization may include a test for anti-HLA antibodies against a panel of cells of known HLA type. Platelet transfusion support for the alloimmunized patient should use platelets from a donor matched as closely as possible for the HLA class I antigens. Although single donor (apheresis) platelet concentrates are used routinely for all platelet transfusions at some centers, this process is more often employed to prepare allotype-specific platelets for patients who have become alloimmunized against HLA antigens. Platelets from a donor of the best available HLA-A and HLA-B allotype are appropriate for the patient who repeatedly has poor platelet count increments after transfusion with random donor platelets, particularly if anti-HLA serum antibodies have been detected. Directed donations from family members are contraindicated for the child who may be a candidate from allogeneic bone marrow transplantation, to avoid unnecessary sensitization. Erythrocyte ABO blood group antigens are found on platelets to varying degrees. Therefore, platelets of a compatible ABO type are preferred at some blood centers. Rhesus antigens are not found on platelets; however, Rh-negative recipients could become alloimmunized by Rh-positive erythrocytes in platelet concentrations.

Thrombocytopenia Due to Increased Platelet Destruction: Immune Thrombocytopenic Purpura

Thrombocytopenia can result from immune or nonimmune platelet destruction. Specific therapy depends on the precise etiology of the platelet destruction. Platelet transfusion is usually not effective in correcting thrombocytopenia of this type. Therefore, transfusion is generally reserved for the patient with life-threatening hemorrhage. In some situations (e.g., thrombotic thrombocytopenic purpura), platelet transfusion is contraindicated.

Immune thrombocytopenic purpura (ITP), a relatively common cause of thrombocytopenia in childhood, is discussed first and in greatest detail. Some of the therapeutic modalities were found empirically to be effective in this syndrome, whereas others were chosen to modulate the humoral autoimmune response causing the platelet destruction. Initial management of ITP includes one of three options: close observation with or without corticosteroids or IV immunoglobulin.

Whether or not pharmacologic therapy is prescribed for ITP, an important aspect of management is close observation and careful monitoring. Aspirin, other nonsteroidal anti-inflammatory drugs, and any anticoagulant therapy should be discontinued. Immunizations and allergic desensitization programs should be interrupted temporarily, as these stimulants for the immune system can exacerbate immune thrombocytopenia. Activity should be modified commensurate with the risk for hemorrhage. For the child with clinical evidence of active bleeding, especially mucosal or internal hemorrhage, hospitalization is appropriate. If thrombocytopenia is not severe and the signs of bleeding are minimal, altered activity under observation at home may be reasonable as long as the parents and caretaker(s) are educated about the signs and symptoms of serious hemorrhage and a plan for safe activities is made. Contact sports, bicycling, and unsupervised play usually are unwise for the thrombocytopenic child, but more restrictive recommendations must be made on an individual basis.

Corticosteroid therapy for autoimmune thrombocytopenia has been employed for nearly 50 years. Although this approach does not affect the eventual outcome of ITP, steroid treatment may decrease the period of thrombocytopenia. Oral prednisone in a dose of 2 mg/kg/d (maximum 60 to 80 mg/d) is a common treatment given for 1 to 2 weeks and then tapered to stop by 1 month of treatment. There may be some merit to giving a higher oral dose (3 to 5 mg/kg/d) for the first few days of treatment. Some investigators favor a brief intravenous course of very high dose steroids (methylprednisolone 30 mg/kg/d, maximum 1 g, for 3 days), which yields a rapid rise in platelet count. It is important to ascertain that the child does not have acute leukemia as a cause of thrombocytopenia before initiation of steroid therapy, since the long-term prognosis could be adversely affected.

Purified immunoglobulin administered intravenously at high doses (IV-IgG 400 mg/kg/d for 5 days *or* 1 g/kg/d for 2 days) has been documented to be effective in the vast majority of children with ITP. The mechanism by which IV IgG affects platelet concentration in ITP is not well understood.

The rare child who experiences life-threatening hemorrhage will be best served by institution of multiple therapeutic modalities: high-dose steroids, intravenous immunoglobulin, splenectomy, and other surgical intervention as indicated. Platelet transfusions at frequent intervals may be of some benefit in decreasing catastrophic bleeding even if the platelet count does not rise.

Splenectomy results in remission of ITP in about 70% of cases. Since 90% of children with ITP will remit within 6 to 12 months with or without therapy (i.e., acute ITP), splenectomy is generally reserved for the child with chronic ITP or with serious bleeding. The most significant complication of splenectomy is sepsis with encapsulated bacteria. This risk can be minimized by educating the patient and family regarding the need for prompt medical attention, immunizing the patient against *Streptococcus pneumoniae, Haemophilus influenzae* B, and *Neisseria meningitidis,* and prescribing prophylactic antibiotic (penicillin or substitute) treatment for at least the first year postoperatively.

For the child with ITP who requires treatment beyond the approaches discussed, a number of options are available, all of which carry greater side effects or risks than do first-line therapies. Possible approaches include immunosuppressive agents, such as low-dose cyclophosphamide, azathioprine, and vinca alkaloids. Purified anti-Rh(D) immunoglobulin can cause a rise in platelet count in the Rh_o(D)-positive patient with ITP. This form of therapy has been reported to be most effective *before* splenectomy.

Neonatal Thrombocytopenia

Thrombocytopenia is common among newborns who have other medical problems. Viral infections, bacterial sepsis, and birth asphyxia may lead to increased platelet utilization or to underproduction of platelets. Affected newborns are usually transfused with platelet concentrates to maintain a platelet count judged to be hemostatically adequate (e.g., 20,000/mm^3 to 100,000/mm^3) based on the assessment of an individual infant's hemorrhagic risk.

Neonatal Alloimmune Thrombocytopenia

When a mother and fetus have platelets bearing different allelic forms of antigenic platelet glycoproteins (Pl^A, Bak, or other antigen systems), alloimmunization may occur during pregnancy. Alloimmunization does not occur in all incompatible pregnancies, but may affect the first infant of a mother who is immunoresponsive. Platelet alloantibodies that cross the placenta destroy fetal platelets, leading to perinatal or antenatal intracranial hemorrhage in 10% to 20% of cases. The first affected infant in a family usually presents as an otherwise healthy, full-term newborn with severe thrombocytopenia unresponsive to transfusion of random donor platelets. The baby's mother has a normal platelet count and negative history for thrombocytopenia. This condition differs from maternal ITP or drug-induced thrombocytopenia in that there is a greater risk for severe bleeding but a shorter postnatal duration of neonatal alloimmune thrombocytopenia (NATP). Therapeutic options for the infant with severe thrombocytopenia or evidence of clinical hemorrhage include intravenous immunoglobulin, exchange transfusion, or transfusion of antigen-negative platelets. Platelets from the mother are usually used; these platelets can be assumed to be negative for the pertinent antigen even before specific allotyping. The maternal platelets need to have excess plasma removed and may also be gently washed to further minimize the transfusion of maternal antiplatelet antibody. As with other directed donor transfusions, these platelets need to be irradiated to protect against GVH disease.

After the first recognized case in a family, subsequent infants are known to be at risk for NATP. Maternal platelets can be available before a planned cesarean section delivery. Although this approach to management reduces the risk of perinatal bleeding, it offers no protection from antenatal hemorrhage. Identification of the precise alloantigen incompatibility and determination of paternal zygosity for that antigen can establish the probability (50% or 100%) of recurrence. Percutaneous blood sampling has been used to type the fetal platelets and to determine the fetal platelet count in utero. There is a risk of fetal exsanguination unless platelets are also transfused to the affected fetus. Some centers have reported correction of fetal thrombocytopenia after administration of intravenous immunoglobulin weekly to the mother, although this therapy is not effective in all cases. Pregnancies at risk for NATP should be managed in consultation with a platelet immunologist and a high-risk perinatal center skilled in fetal blood sampling and familiar with current recommendations in this rapidly changing field.

FUNCTIONAL PLATELET DISORDERS

Some patients who have a normal platelet count are at risk for excessive bleeding because those platelets do not function normally. Table 1 lists some congenital and acquired qualitative platelet disorders for which therapy may be needed at times of hemorrhagic stress. Appropriate therapies for these conditions vary according to the severity and cause of the hemorrhagic episode.

Congenital Platelet Disorders

Correction of intrinsic platelet disorders may require transfusion with normal platelet concentrates. For adhesion and aggregation defects, platelets are transfused to supply a hemostatically adequate number of normal platelets (see discussion on platelet transfusion). Signaling and storage pool defects require only a small transfused

TABLE 1. Disorders of Platelet Function

Congenital Platelet Disorders
Glanzmann's thrombasthenia
Bernard-Soulier syndrome
Collagen receptor disorder

Acquired Platelet Disorders
Uremia
Aspirin or NSAID secretion defect
Other drug-induced platelet dysfunction
Antibody-induced platelet dysfunction

dose of normal platelets for correction, since the patient's platelets are capable of participating in aggregation once a stimulus is provided. Isoimmunization may occur after transfusion of normal platelets to individuals who have platelets lacking surface glycoproteins (e.g., Glanzmann's thrombasthenia or Bernard-Soulier syndrome). Since isoantibodies may preclude adequate therapy in the future, transfusions should be reserved for severe bleeding episodes. Ancillary approaches to treatment include local measures to halt bleeding and pharmacologically induced increases in circulating von Willebrand's factor and inhibition of fibrinolysis.

Acquired Platelet Disorders

Uremia

Whenever feasible, it is best to treat acquired platelet dysfunction by removing the underlying cause. The primary hemostatic defect associated with uremia usually responds to aggressive dialysis. Additional or alternative therapies aimed at increasing von Willebrand's factor levels are also often effective. Although cryoprecipitate was once used for this purpose, desmopressin acetate (Stimate 0.3 μg/kg) is preferred for short-term therapy. The greatest experience has been with intravenous desmopressin, although an intranasal preparation has recently been licensed for this use. For patients with oral hemorrhage, inhibition of fibrinolysis with epsilon aminocaproic acid or tranexamic acid is recommended.

Drug-induced Platelet Dysfunction

Aspirin and most other nonsteroidal antiinflammatory drugs (NSAIDs) inhibit the cyclooxygenase enzyme of platelets and cause defective activation and granule secretion. Aspirin can bind covalently to the active site of cyclooxygenase; the platelet dysfunction resulting from a single dose of aspirin lasts for the lifespan of affected platelets (7 to 10 days). Most other NSAIDs bind reversibly to cyclooxygenase; therefore the platelet defect resolves after the drug is cleared from the circulation. Trilisate, one NSAID that does not affect platelet function, is an appropriate antiinflammatory agent for patients with underlying coagulopathies. The optimum therapy for drug-induced platelet disorders is to withhold the responsible medication. For emergency treatment of severe bleeding, transfusion with a single unit of normal platelets should correct the clinical defect.

Other medications have been less predictable as a cause of platelet dysfunction. Before a surgical procedure or at the time of hemorrhage, it is wise to determine the patient's bleeding time. Appropriate management depends on the hemorrhagic risk and the severity of the platelet defect.

Antibody-mediated Platelet Dysfunction

Some platelet antibodies interfere with normal platelet function. Acquired Glanzmann's thrombasthenia and Bernard-Soulier syndrome have been reported; milder platelet dysfunction can also be caused by autoantibodies. ITP therapy for affected patients must be individualized based on the available options.

DISSEMINATED INTRAVASCULAR COAGULATION

HARVEY J. COHEN, M.D., Ph.D.

Disseminated intravascular coagulation (DIC) is a syndrome and not a disease. It is the result of an acquired failure of hemostasis characterized by poorly controlled protease activity in the blood, resulting in an increase in fibrin formation and fibrinolysis. It is always triggered by an underlying disease process. DIC can be caused by tissue injury, obstetric complications, cancer, overwhelming infections, cardiovascular disease, immunologic phenomena, liver disease,

pancreatitis, pulmonary disease, neurologic disease, and certain toxins, such as snake venoms. The term *purpura fulminans* is used to describe DIC associated with widespread arterial and venous thrombosis. The most common clinical manifestations of purpura fulminans include skin necrosis, gangrene of the digits, and hemorrhagic adrenal infarction. Purpura fulminans is seen most commonly in children following streptococcal or meningococcal infections.

PATHOGENESIS

DIC is manifested by a decrease in clotting factors, an increase in fibrin split products, and a decrease in platelet count. A microangiopathic hemolytic anemia may also be part of this syndrome. It is important to keep in mind that DIC is not an exaggerated version of normal clot formation and clot lysis. Rather, it occurs when the intricately balanced interplay among clotting factors and inhibitors is overcome. DIC may be initiated by exposure of blood to tissue factor or to any of a wide variety of proteolytic enzymes. This may lead to destruction of clotting factors, fibrinolysis, or a neutralization of natural anticoagulants, such as antithrombin III or antiplasmin. Most patients with acute DIC have no pathologic evidence of stable fibrin clot formation despite having greatly increased fibrin activity and soluble fibrin in their blood. Thus, thrombosis, although sometimes seen in DIC, often is not a problem. Solid fibrin clot formation also may be limited by rapid fibrinolysis, depletion of fibrinogen, and inhibition of fibrin polymerization by circulating fibrin split products.

DIAGNOSIS

The diagnosis of clinically significant DIC is not usually difficult. If a patient with an underlying disorder has an elevated prothrombin time (PT) or partial thromboplastin time (PTT) associated with a decrease in fibrinogen and an increase in fibrin split products together with thrombocytopenia, the diagnosis can be made with reasonable certainty. *The presence of liver failure causes the most difficulty in diagnosing DIC, since it can produce similar abnormalities.* Determining factor VIII activity may be helpful in distinguishing the two phenomena, since factor VIII is consumed in DIC but is made normally in liver failure. The PT provides a rough indication of the degree to which components of the extrinsic pathway have been depleted, whereas the PTT provides a rough indication of the degree to which components of the intrinsic pathway have been depleted.

THERAPY

Success in the treatment of DIC is dependent on the ability to both diagnose and treat adequately the underlying disease. High-grade DIC that persists once such treatment has been given is an ominous sign. The mortality rate in severe DIC is high, exceeding 80% in some series. Death, however, usually results from progression of the underlying disease rather than the DIC itself. Because it is not possible to accomplish the reversal of the underlying disease process rapidly enough in some instances, it is important to attempt to reverse the coagulopathy of patients with DIC. Such steps may be lifesaving.

Treatment Options

Two treatment options are available for the reversal of DIC: replacement of clotting factors and platelets and the use of pharmacologic inhibitors of coagulation or fibrinolysis. It must be kept in mind that the treatment is designed not to reverse or correct clotting abnormalities but to correct and prevent bleeding or, rarely, excessive clot formation.

Replacement Therapy

Clotting factors and coagulation inhibitors may be replaced by giving fresh frozen plasma (FFP). Although theoretically the use of FFP might be construed as adding fuel to the fire and exacerbating the DIC, this does not occur. This may be because FFP contains not only coagulation factors but also regulators of coagulation that are deficient in DIC. In patients with DIC, there is also increased fibrinolysis, and, therefore, a disproportionate consumption of fibrinogen may be occurring. This can be detected and followed by the quantitative fibrinogen assay. If this occurs, cryoprecipitate, which contains 5 to 10 times more fibrinogen than whole plasma, can also be used. Thrombocytopenia in DIC is often not severe unless accompanied by other disorders associated with decreased platelet production. When needed, however, platelets can be given as part of the therapeutic regimen. The potential for volume overload and transmission of blood-borne viral infections must be kept in mind whenever blood products are given.

General guidelines for replacement therapy are to give FFP (approximately 10 to 15 ml/kg) to achieve a PT within 2 to 3 seconds of the control value. Cryoprecipitate (approximately 1 bag per 5 kg) is given for a fibrinogen level of less than 100 mg/dl, and platelet transfusions (1 to 3 U/10 kg) are given for a platelet count of less than 20,000/ml or, if there is major bleeding, with a platelet count of less than 50,000/ml.

Antithrombin III concentrates have been shown to affect experimental DIC, but clinical experience with this product is limited. It is important to keep in mind that patients with DIC are at risk for vitamin K and folate deficiency. Thus, if DIC is prolonged, the use of vitamin K (5 to 10 mg/d) and folic acid (1 mg/d) should be considered.

Inhibitors of Coagulation and Fibrinolysis

The use of heparin and antifibrinolytic agents in DIC is still controversial. Treatment with these agents has never been shown conclusively to improve survival in DIC and is associated with the risk of either exaggerating bleeding (heparin) or increasing thrombosis (antifibrinolytic agents). Nonetheless, these agents need to be considered on an individual basis.

Heparin is particularly likely to help patients with DIC associated with certain cancers, especially acute promyelocytic leukemia, and chronic DIC disorders, such as those due to vascular diseases and retained dead fetus. It is also rational to give heparin to patients with evidence of purpura fulminans. If heparin is used, a dose of 5 to 10 U/kg/h, significantly lower than that normally used for anticoagulation, is recommended. Heparin should be given by continuous intravenous infusion whenever possible. When heparin is used in the treatment of DIC, the dose should be sufficient to prolong the partial thromboplastin time to approximately 1.5 times control, similar to what is done in patients with deep venous thrombosis. ε-Aminocaproic acid and tranexamic acid are lysine analogs that inhibit fibrinolysis. These drugs may reduce bleeding and fibrinogen consumption in patients with increased fibrinolysis. However, they run the risk of converting a bleeding disorder into a thrombotic condition. They should, therefore, be used with great caution. When used to treat DIC, these antifibrinolytic drugs usually are given in conjunction with heparin to minimize the potential for thrombosis. Antifibrinolytic agents, together with heparin, have been useful in treating the coagulopathy associated with acute promyelocytic leukemia, and antifibrinolytic agents alone have been beneficial in patients with the Kasabach-Merritt syndrome. If ε-aminocaproic acid is used, it should be given at a dose of 3 g/m² over 1 hour as a loading dose, followed by 1 g/m² every hour by continuous infusion.

Other Therapies

Other therapeutic modalities that have been used in the treatment of DIC include antiplatelet agents, dextrans, alpha-adrenergic blocking agents, and protease inhibitors. A genetically engineered protease inhibitor, alpha₁-antitrypsin Pittsburgh, has been shown to inhibit thrombin and other clotting factor protease activities and has attenuated DIC and improved survival in experimental DIC. These and other experimental agents have not been approved for therapeutic use. It is hoped that the development of specific coagulation factors may offer promise in the future.

LANGERHANS CELL HISTIOCYTOSIS

JEFFREY M. LIPTON, M.D., Ph.D.

Langerhans cell histiocytosis (LCH), previously referred to as histiocytosis X, was originally categorized by many as a malignant neoplasm and, as such, had been treated with aggressive chemotherapy and radiation therapy. Although these modalities are still used, significant differences between LCH and true malignant disease suggest conservative management for many patients. The clinical course of malignant neoplasia is relentlessly progressive, with virtually no survival in untreated patients (stage IV-S neuroblastoma being a notable exception). LCH is characterized by frequent spontaneous remissions and exacerbations. Morbidity and survival in untreated patients vary depending on the extent of disease. Pathologically, the lesions of LCH appear as reactive infiltrates, possessing little of the cellular atypicality and homogeneity characteristic of malignancy. However, clonality has been demonstrated in lesions from patients with local as well as systemic disease. Although the etiology of the phenomena that comprise LCH is unknown, LCH appears to represent an immune regulatory disorder triggered by unknown stimuli, resulting in the proliferation of a family of Langerhans-like cells not under the control of the local tissue-specific microenvironment.

Historically, LCH comprises eosinophilic granuloma, localized lesion(s) confined to bone, Hand-Schüller-Christian syndrome (protracted multiple site involvement with the classic but rare triad of skull defects, diabetes insipidus, and exophthalmos), and Letterer-Siwe syndrome (visceral lesions involving skin, liver, lungs, bone marrow, lymph nodes, spleen, and other reticuloendothelial organs). Since there is a continuum of disease that frequently does not fit these rigid and arbitrary criteria, it is important, before considering therapy, to group each patient prognostically using known demographic and

TABLE 1. Grouping System for Histiocytosis

Factor	Points
Age (y)	
≥2	0
<2	1
Extent of disease	
≤4 organs	0
>4 organs	1
Dysfunction* (1, 2, or 3 systems)	
No	0
Yes	1

Group 1†	Total Points
0	Monostotic eosinophilic granuloma
I	0
II	1
III	2
IV	3

*(1) Hepatic dysfunction: One or more of the following: hypoproteinemia (total protein <5.5 g/dl or albumin <2.5 g/dl), hyperbilirubinemia (>1.5 mg/dl), edema ascites. (2) Pulmonary dysfunction: One or more of the following: tachypnea, dyspnea, cyanosis, cough, pneumothorax, pleural effusion. (3) Hemopoietic dysfunction: One or more of the following: anemia in the absence of iron deficiency or significant infection (10 g/dl hemoglobin), leukopenia (<4000/dl), thrombocytopenia (<100,000/dl).

†By arbitrarily assigning either 0 or 1 point for the absence or presence of one of the three important prognostic variables, a number of total points is obtained and a patient is assigned a group.

From Lipton JM: Histiocytic syndromes. *In* Hoffman R, Benz EJ Jr, Shattil SJ, Furie B, Cohen HJ (eds): Hematology: Basic Principles and Practice. New York, Churchill Livingstone, 1991:604. Adapted from Osband ME, et al: Histiocytosis-X: Demonstration of abnormal immunity. N Engl J Med 304:147, 1981. Copyright 1994. Massachusetts Medical Society. All rights reserved.

clinical variables. The initial evaluation of patients with LCH should determine the site and extent of disease to identify cosmetically and functionally significant lesions. Of note, precise pathologic criteria for the diagnosis of LCH have been established by the Histiocyte Society.*

Once the extent of the disease is determined, the patient is grouped according to the criteria outlined in Table 1. The grouping helps determine both therapy and prognosis. Patients in groups 0 and I and some in group II do quite well, with little morbidity and no mortality. They frequently need little or no systemic therapy. Patients in group III (and many in group II) require systemic therapy and generally do well, whereas significant morbidity and even mortality are encountered in group IV patients. One of the main goals of therapy is to minimize loss of function and prevent cosmetic deformity. The agents used should be thought of as immunosuppressive rather than antineoplastic. Patients are treated to obtain disease control, followed by tapering of drug doses to achieve the lowest dose that maintains control. Eventually, almost all patients who respond will be able to discontinue treatment completely. However, systemic treatment lasting from 1 year to occasionally as long as 5 years is not uncommon, and late recurrences do occur.

SUPPORTIVE CARE

The primary caretaker coordinates the care of these patients. Subspecialty consultation is sought from dermatologists, dentists, orthopedists, otolaryngologists, endocrinologists, and others experienced in managing LCH.

Severely ill patients are hospitalized and given maximal antibiotic, ventilatory, nutritional (including hyperalimentation), blood product, skin care, physical therapy, medical, and nursing support as required. Scrupulous hygiene is quite effective in limiting auditory canal, cutaneous, and dental lesions. Debridement, and even resection of severely affected gingival tissue, is used to limit oral involvement. The seborrhea-like dermatitis of the scalp may improve with the use of a selenium-based shampoo twice a week. If shampooing is not effective, topical steroids are used sparingly for short-term control of small areas. We do not advocate the use of topical nitrogen mustard lotion. Many patients require hormone replacement for diabetes insipidus or other manifestations of hypopituitarism.

LOCAL THERAPY (SURGERY AND RADIATION THERAPY)

After complete evaluation, those patients with disease involving a single bone and, in some instances, patients with disease involving

*The Histiocyte Society is dedicated to the advancement of knowledge regarding the clinical syndromes that constitute the disorders including Langerhans cell histiocytosis known as *the histiocytoses*. For further information, phone (609) 881-4911.

multiple lesions and multiple bones are managed with local therapy. This involves surgical curettage for patients whose lesions are in easily accessible, noncritical locations. Surgical restraint must be exercised to prevent drastic cosmetic and orthopedic deformities and loss of function. Localized radiation therapy (usually 600 to 900 cGy, with 450 cGy for small lesions and up to 1500 cGy for large lesions) in 200-cGy fractions, using only megavoltage equipment, is employed. Older patients may require slightly higher doses (2000 cGy for large lesions). Care is taken to prevent radiating potentially sensitive normal structures, such as the lens and thyroid, if possible. Patients at risk for skeletal deformity, visual loss secondary to exophthalmos, pathologic fractures, vertebral collapse, and spinal cord injury or those suffering from severe pain or symptomatic adenopathy, even when multiple lesions exist, may receive radiation therapy to those areas. Lesions in poorly accessible sites, such as the orbit, and those with recurrence after curettage are also radiated. Diabetes insipidus (DI) may occur at any time during the course of LCH. Patients and their families are instructed to report signs of DI as soon as they develop. If they are identified within 48 hours of the onset of symptoms, these patients receive local radiation to the hypothalamus and pituitary. This approach is controversial, however, and the response rate is not optimal. Since individual lesions in patients with unifocal disease have a higher rate of response than those in patients with multifocal disease, patients who appear to have an isolated lesion and fail to respond to appropriate radiotherapy should be carefully reevaluated for additional sites of disease.

CHEMOTHERAPY

Patients in group I and some in group II can be observed for signs of spontaneous improvement. If symptomatic lesions or failure to thrive is evident, treatment should be pursued. Falling off the growth curve or a persistently elevated erythrocyte sedimentation rate may indicate significant systemic disease. Patients in groups II and III will benefit dramatically from chemotherapy, whereas those in group IV frequently will die despite chemotherapy. Experimental modalities, such as bone marrow transplantation, are being pursued at specialized centers for group IV patients who are nonresponsive to conventional chemotherapy.

The basic principle of systemic therapy is to begin with the most benign treatment and then add increasingly toxic agents, never making the treatment worse than the disease while trying to prevent permanent disability. Table 2 outlines our current chemotherapeutic treatment program. Other agents, including particularly etoposide and cyclosporine, are in use in ongoing clinical studies. We currently individualize therapy in those patients failing programs I and II.

Careful monitoring of blood counts and clinical status is maintained, since chemotherapeutic toxicity can cause severe complica-

---

TABLE 2. Current Mount Sinai School of Medicine Chemotherapeutic Treatment Program for Treatment of Langerhans Cell Histiocytosis

Program I

1. Vinblastine 0.15 mg/kg/wk IV as a single weekly dose. If the patient is not improved after 2 weeks, increase the dose by 0.025 to 0.05 mg/kg/wk. The highest nonmyelosuppressive, nonneurotoxic dose is used. In addition, if there is no or slow improvement or a more rapid response is required, *add*

2. Prednisone 2 mg/kg/d PO. With improvement, taper to smallest effective dose on an alternate-day schedule. With continued improvement or satisfactory control, a slow taper of prednisone is undertaken, but prednisone should be discontinued before the vinblastine taper. Vinblastine is tapered from weekly to every other week to every 3 or 4 weeks, and then the dosage is reduced to 0.15 mg/kg/every 4 weeks before discontinuation. Reinstate lowest effective dose for disease rebound.

Program II *(if program I fails)*

1. Methotrexate 10 mg/m²/wk IM, IV, or PO
   and
2. 6-mercaptopurine (6-MP) 20 mg/m²/d PO for 14 days of 21-day cycle

The highest nontoxic dose is used (toxicity: myelosuppression, mouth sores, hepatotoxicity). On improvement, both drugs are slowly tapered. Methotrexate is tapered from weekly to every other week to every 3 weeks. PO therapy may be instituted. The 6-MP schedule is maintained while the dose is reduced 10%–15% per cycle. Reinstitute lowest effective dose for disease rebound.

tions in these already compromised patients. We recommend treatment by physicians experienced in the administration of these agents. Alkylating agents, chlorambucil in particular, should be avoided because of the substantial risk of chemotherapy-induced malignancy. Trimethoprim-sulfamethoxazole (Bactrim) prophylaxis should be instituted in patients for whom long-term immunosuppressive therapy is anticipated.

LONG-TERM FOLLOW-UP

All patients with systemic LCH receive long-term follow-up. Patients are monitored for potential chronic disabilities, such as cosmetic or functional orthopedic and cutaneous disorders, as well as emotional problems that may arise from the disease or the treatment. Patients having or at risk for hearing impairment, loss of permanent dentition, pulmonary fibrosis, cor pulmonale, portal hypertension, cirrhosis, diabetes insipidus, growth failure, and other endocrinologic disorders are followed closely by appropriate subspecialists.

REFERENCES

1. Komp DM: Concepts in staging and clinical studies for treatment of Langerhans cell histiocytosis. Semin Oncol 18:18–23, 1991.
2. Lipton JM: Histiocytic syndromes. *In* Hoffman R, Benz EJ Jr, Shattil SJ, Furie B, Cohen HJ (eds): Hematology: Basic Principles and Practice. New York, Churchill Livingstone, 1991:604.
3. Malone M: The histiocytoses of childhood. Histopathology 19:105–119, 1991.

APLASTIC ANEMIA

WAYNE R. RACKOFF, M.D.
DAVID A. WILLIAMS, M.D.

Aplastic anemia is the result of absent or defective production of terminally differentiated blood cells. The resultant pancytopenia leads to bleeding, infections, and complications of anemia. The term *aplastic anemia* describes a number of conditions in which there is some degree of failure in all cell lines produced in the bone marrow. These conditions usually are acquired during life, but a number of inherited bone marrow syndromes also exist (Table 1). Acquired aplastic anemia is associated with exposure to chemicals (e.g., benzene derivatives), viruses (e.g., hepatitis B), and drugs (e.g., chloramphenicol). However, no causative factor is found in as many as 50% of patients.

DEFINITION

Severe acquired aplastic anemia is defined by the presence of moderate to severe hypocellularity on examination of a bone marrow biopsy and two of the following: neutrophil count less than 500/mm³, platelet count less than 20,000/mm³, and reticulocyte count less than 1% (corrected for hematocrit). Untreated, severe acquired aplastic anemia has a high mortality rate. Patients with severe pancytopenia require specific treatment to reverse their bone marrow failure and supportive care to treat anemia, thrombocytopenia, and infections related to prolonged neutropenia. Currently, approximately 60% to 80% of patients who have bone marrow transplantation may be expected to survive, and approximately 60% of patients who are treated with immunotherapy may be expected to survive.

BONE MARROW TRANSPLANTATION

The current treatment of choice for a patient whose peripheral blood counts fulfill the definition of severe aplastic anemia is bone marrow transplantation from an HLA-matched sibling. Umbilical cord blood from an HLA-matched sibling also has been used as a marrow source. Siblings of the patients should have HLA typing performed as soon as possible after the patient is diagnosed with severe aplastic anemia, and bone marrow transplantation should be carried out as

TABLE 1. Inherited Bone Marrow Failure Syndromes

Fanconi's anemia
Shwachman-Diamond syndrome
Dyskeratosis congenita
Amegakaryocytic thrombocytopenia
Reticular dysgenesis
Familial aplastic anemia

soon as possible after a donor is identified. The initial typing usually can be completed in less than 1 week. Immunosuppressive therapy is not given before transplantation if a suitable donor is available. Blood product use should be minimized to avoid alloimmunization of the patient. Patients who have an HLA-compatible bone marrow donor in their family should not receive blood products from family members because alloimmunization may increase the risk of bone marrow graft rejection. A recognized pediatric bone marrow transplantation center should be contacted to assist in the HLA typing of siblings and to make arrangements for transplantation if a donor is identified.

In some centers, the cure rate for severe acquired aplastic anemia exceeds 80% for patients who receive bone marrow from an HLA-matched sibling. The results of bone marrow transplantation using alternative donors, for example, HLA-matched unrelated donors and partially matched family members, are less encouraging, with survival rates of 30% to 60% depending on the type of donor. Better measures to prevent graft-versus-host (GVH) disease, with T cell depletion of the donor marrow and immunosuppression of the recipient, may improve these rates. At this time, bone marrow transplant from alternative donors should be considered only after a patient has failed immunosuppressive therapy.

IMMUNOSUPPRESSIVE THERAPY

If an HLA-matched family member is not identified, immunosuppressive therapy should be given. The immunosuppressive therapy should include cyclosporine, corticosteroid, and antithymocyte globulin (ATG) given in combination or sequentially. A promising new protocol currently under evaluation uses cyclosporine concomitant with ATG. In this protocol, ATG is given at a dose of 40 mg/kg/d for 4 days with cyclosporine (12 mg/kg/d for adults, 15 mg/kg/d for children). Methylprednisolone (1 mg/kg/d) is given during the first 10 days of treatment to prevent serum sickness associated with the use of ATG. The dose of cyclosporine is adjusted to maintain a therapeutic level for 6 months. ATG should not be given to a patient with known hypersensitivity to horse serum, and a skin test should be administered before the first dose. The combination of cyclosporine, ATG, and corticosteroid is effective in 50% to 60% of patients.

ANDROGEN THERAPY

Androgen therapy is not usually effective for patients with severe acquired aplastic anemia but is the treatment of choice for some inherited bone marrow failure syndromes and may be tried if other treatment fails in acquired aplastic anemia. A 2 to 4 month trial of oral oxymetholone (dihydrotestosterone) 2 to 5 mg/kg/d is a reasonable starting point. If a patient does not respond to an androgen preparation, a trial with a different preparation will sometimes result in a response. It appears that patients with hepatic disease may be treated safely with parenteral androgen preparations (e.g., nandrolone 5 mg/kg/wk).

HEMATOPOIETIC GROWTH FACTORS

The administration of recombinant human granulocyte macrophage–colony-stimulating factor (GM-CSF) to patients with severe acquired aplastic anemia results in increased neutrophil counts in most patients. Unfortunately, only a small minority of patients will have increases in red blood cell or platelet production. The advent of hematopoietic growth factors with the potential to stimulate multiple lineages or treatment with combinations of growth factors offers hope of more efficacious treatment in the future.

SUPPORTIVE CARE

All patients with severe aplastic anemia will require supportive care for anemia, thrombocytopenia, and infection. Transfusions of red blood cells and platelets should be minimized to reduce the risk of alloimmunization, especially in patients who are bone marrow transplant candidates. All blood products should be negative for cytomegalovirus, radiated to 1500 cGy, and given through a leukocyte depletion filter. Our approach is to transfuse based on symptoms (bleeding, tachycardia, fatigue) rather than on specific peripheral blood count levels. In some centers, platelet transfusion is given if the platelet count is less than 20,000/mm³, and packed red blood cells are given to maintain a hemoglobin of 7 g/dl.

In a patient with a neutrophil count of less than 1000/mm³, fever or other signs of infection should prompt a thorough evaluation to identify the source of infection. Empiric treatment with broad-spectrum antibiotics should begin while awaiting the results of blood cultures and other diagnostic tests. Early consideration should be given to the use of antifungal medications because many patients with prolonged neutropenia will become infected with opportunistic fungi. The role of granulocyte transfusion in the supportive care of children with acquired aplastic anemia remains controversial. If granulocyte transfusion is considered, it should be used for the neutropenic patient with life-threatening sepsis that is unresponsive to initial treatment with antimicrobials.

Aplastic anemia is a rare disease of childhood, leaving families with little support from other families who have experienced the disease. The Aplastic Anemia Foundation of America [(301)-955-2803] may be helpful to these families in coping with the disease.

REFERENCES

1. Camitta BM, Doney K: Immunosuppressive therapy for aplastic anemia: Indications, mechanisms, and results. Am J Pediatr Hematol Oncol 12:411–424, 1990.
2. Smith DH: Use of hematopoietic growth factors for treatment of aplastic anemia. Am J Pediatr Hematol Oncol 12:33, 1990.
3. Storb R, Champlin RE: Bone marrow transplantation for severe aplastic anemia. Bone Marrow Transplant 8:69–72, 1991.

NEUTROPENIA

LAWRENCE WOLFE, M.D.

TYPES OF NEUTROPENIA

Establishing the diagnosis of acute or chronic neutropenia does not in and of itself assess the patient's risk of infection. Neutropenia is often stratified as mild (1000 to 1500 granulocytes per microliter), moderate (500 to 1000 granulocytes per microliter), or severe or intense (0 to 500 granulocytes per microliter). Patients whose neutropenia is their only risk factor for infection (postinfectious or viral neutropenia, immune neutropenia) appear to be at less risk than other patients whose neutropenia is more intense (Kostmann's syndrome) or who have other immune system or nutritional problems (e.g., chemotherapy, aplastic anemia, leukemia, Shwachman-Diamond syndrome). Ultimately, the experience of each patient is the best guide to the problems that neutropenia may cause. An attempt is made to distinguish different characteristics of certain groups of neutropenic patients.

RAISING THE NEUTROPHIL COUNT

The first principle in treating neutropenia of any source is to consider a plan to try to raise the granulocyte count. In the case of acute viral granulocytopenia, this plan simply consists of expectant treatment—awaiting a rise in the granulocyte count within 5 to 10 days. In the case of neutropenia secondary to bone marrow failure, planning to ameliorate the situation would depend on the nature of the bone marrow failure. Iatrogenic bone marrow failure from chemotherapy, as well as certain congenital neutropenias (e.g., Kostmann's syndrome, Shwachman-Diamond syndrome) may respond to humoral factors, such as granulocyte-colony stimulating factor (G-CSF) or granulocyte macrophage-colony stimulating factor (GM-CSF). The use of these factors in chemotherapy-induced neutropenia is well established, but their use in congenital bone marrow failure neutropenia is less well documented at this time. Some temporary results have been seen, but no long-term remissions on the basis of short courses of these growth factors have been achieved. When bone marrow failure is a result of infiltrative disease or severe bone marrow injury, such as aplastic anemia, the specific condition requires treatment before the neutropenia will resolve.

Postinfectious neutropenia, or so-called immune neutropenia, usually occurs in a child who previously had a normal granulocyte count but does not bring the granulocyte count back up after what appears to be a postinfectious syndrome. These patients can have granulocyte percentages less than 2% to 5%. Such patients are clearly at risk for infection. However, bacteremia is rare. Prednisone at a dose of 2 to 4 mg/kg/d will raise the white count in a large percentage of such cases after approximately 5 to 7 days. There is a paradox in the use of prednisone to raise the white count, as part of the immunodeficiency of steroids probably relates to a diminution of neutrophil and reticuloendothelial function. It is, therefore, not surprising that the use of intravenous gamma globulin has been investigated in this condition, analogous to its use for immune thrombocytopenic purpura (ITP). In doses of 1 g/kg for 1 to 5 days, many patients with immune neutropenia will achieve a temporary rise in their white count. When does one consider the use of these drugs in immune neutropenia, especially when the patient is asymptomatic? We do not use these drugs prophylactically except in the case where elective surgery or some other immune system challenge is about to occur. In general, we reserve the use of these therapies for situations where actual infection exists. If a patient with immune neutropenia has been shown in the past to respond to gamma globulin, this should be the first alternative in patients with febrile illness or infection.

PRINCIPLES OF TREATING THE NEUTROPENIC PATIENT

When approaching the neutropenic patient for the first time, there are basically two scenarios. The first is in the patient who, despite the presence of intense neutropenia, is currently suffering no symptoms or signs of ongoing infection. The second is in the situation where the patient is neutropenic and also has fever or illness.

The Neutropenic Patient Without Signs of Fever or Illness

In the patient with neutropenia who does not appear actively infected, questions of therapy, beyond raising the white count, include (1) What else can be done to maximize the patient's immune system function? (2) What is the role of antibiotic prophylaxis? (3) What is the role of prophylactic environments?

Gamma globulin levels should be determined in patients with neutropenia in order to ensure that adequate humoral immunity is available. Attention should be paid to the nutritional status of the patient, as malnourished patients have immune system dysfunction related to both protein-calorie malnutrition and vitamin and trace element deficiency. In patients in whom complement deficiency is suspected (e.g., active systemic lupus erythematosus), an effort should be made to correct the underlying condition to aid recovery from complement deficiency.

Antibiotic prophylaxis would seem to be appropriate in the situation where symptomatic neutropenia exists. Patients with congenital neutropenia, such as Kostmann's syndrome, do seem to benefit from antibiotic prophylaxis. In the time before antibiotic prophylaxis, these patients often suffered from deep pulmonary infections, as well as severe skin infections. In the patient with so-called immune neutropenia and in patients with severe neutropenia from other causes (e.g., Shwachman-Diamond syndrome or idiopathic), the use of antibiotic prophylaxis is considered more controversial. Many of these children go through life with few infections beyond typical nuisance viral infections in which there is an increase in susceptibility to secondary infection. In such circumstances, it seems prudent to follow the patient for a period of time to determine whether multiple episodes of infection will occur. If the child develops frequent episodes of otitis media or difficult or unusual skin infections, prophylactic antibiotics may be considered. Otherwise, to balance side effects versus benefits, it would seem reasonable to withhold antibiotic prophylaxis in patients who have long periods when they are asymptomatic.

Prophylactic antibiotics (with the exception of *Pneumocystis carinii* pneumonia prophylaxis) usually are not used in neutropenic patients with either iatrogenic neutropenia and immune system dysfunction (chemotherapy) or noniatrogenic immune system dysfunction (aplastic anemia and acquired immunodeficiency syndrome). This is to avoid creating multiply resistant organisms that would represent a greater threat to the patient.

Isolation of the patient with neutropenia is indicated primarily for patients who are expected to have sustained neutropenia in concert with immune dysfunction for long periods of time. Patients with neutropenia alone without concomitant immune system dysfunction should not be strictly isolated. Patients who have concomitant neutropenia and immune system dysfunction are at risk for secondary superinfection after viral infection and may be encouraged to avoid situations where they might come in contact unknowingly with someone who is sick. We reserve true isolation for those patients who are admitted to the hospital with neutropenia expected to last longer than 7 to 10 days and who are at risk for nosocomial infection.

Neutropenia in Association with an Infected Area or Fever

The major concern in observing an obvious infection in a patient with neutropenia is that the signs and symptoms of inflammation usually engendered by a given infection may be masked by the lack of white blood cells to create the inflammatory response or that fever as the only sign of bacteremia may be missed. All patients with neutropenia and fever should have blood cultures, urine culture, and specific cultures associated with any potential source of infection.

Bacteremia

Bacteremia represents 10% to 20% of infectious complications in neutropenic patients. Bacteremia can occur in association with recognizable sources (e.g., catheter-related infections, urosepsis, or pneumonia) or may be occult. If catheter-related sepsis is a possibility, vancomycin may be added expectantly to treat potential *Staphylococcus epidermidis* infection.

In patients with bacteremia from other known sources or occult sources, specific treatment for the organism detected, as well as broad-spectrum antibiotic coverage (often including a semisynthetic penicillin and an aminoglycoside), should continue for 14 days and longer for patients who remain neutropenic. In patients in whom there is no expectation of granulocyte return, therapy may end at 14 afebrile days, but patients should be observed carefully, as the incidence of return of fever or bacteremia is significant.

SPECIFIC EXAMINATION OF THE NEUTROPENIC PATIENT AND REGIONAL APPROACH TO THERAPY OF INFECTIONS

Examination of the neutropenic patient begins with careful noting of vital signs and observation for toxicity. Examination of the skin for evidence of cellulitis or septic emboli is important. The presence of either should lead to consideration of treatment of gram-positive and gram-negative infections and also inclusion of anti-*Pseudomonas* therapy with a semisynthetic penicillin (e.g., Timentin) and an aminoglycoside. Areas of cellulitis or septic emboli may be aspirated or biopsied and cultured in an attempt to determine a specific bacteriologic diagnosis. The skin should be examined closely for other diagnostic rashes, such as varicella zoster, especially in immunosuppressed patients.

The head and neck examination should include meticulous inspection of the tympanic membrane, including mobility analysis (because of the lack of pus formation behind the eardrum in neutropenia), and funduscopic examination for abnormalities that might create a suspicion of opportunistic infection. The nose should be examined carefully for excoriation or infected sores, and rapid parenteral treatment should begin if cellulitis or invasive bacterial infection is suspected.

Mouth lesions occur commonly in neutropenic patients, and aphthous stomatitis can be a problem. Such aphthous sores may come and go, especially in patients with cyclic forms of neutropenia. Oral doses of tetracycline timed with the patient's cycle in cyclic neutropenia occasionally can diminish aphthous stomatitis. Mouth rinse solutions containing tetracycline also have been helpful. Other than these approaches, most treatments relate to controlling pain. When aphthous stomatitis or chemotherapy-induced stomatitis becomes severe, these sores may act as a potential source of secondary infection within the mouth or can be potential sources of bacteremia. When there is evidence of mouth infection or dental infection, our practice has been to use high doses of penicillin or clindamycin parenterally. In chronically neutropenic patients, patients with cyclic neutropenia, and patients on chemotherapy with intermittent severe neutropenia, colonization with *Candida*, as well as herpes simplex stomatitis, can occur. We routinely put our patients with chronic neutropenia on a mouth care regimen involving the use of soft toothbrushes, thrice-daily rinses with peroxide and water, and prophylactic use of oral nystatin or clotrimazole (Mycelex) troches. For patients with neutropenia associated with either congenital or iatrogenic (chemotherapy) immune deficiency, we use fluconazole orally when *Candida* infection appears truly established in the mouth. If there is severe Candidiasis in the mouth, especially if it is associated with signs or symptoms of concomitant esophagitis and unresponsive to oral fluconazole, we often use a short course of amphotericin B. Intravenous acyclovir is the treatment of choice for herpetic gingivostomatitis and usually works promptly. Patients on chemotherapy may have recurrent bouts of herpetic infection, and these episodes may be prevented by oral prophylactic acyclovir.

Patients with chemotherapy-induced stomatitis should always be suspected of having ulcerations at any level of the gastrointestinal tract, making bacteremia, especially gram-negative bacteremia, more likely in the febrile patient with neutropenia and mouth sores.

Sinus tenderness or headaches suggestive of sinus involvement should be considered carefully. Evidence of severe sinus infection or rapidly progressive sinus infection requires an approach more aggressive than simple oral antibiotic treatment, as spread of bacterial or fungal infection into the CNS may occur. The sinuses should be examined radiologically (often with CT scan) or directly for biopsy. There should be serious concern over the possibility of fungal infection (*Aspergillus* or *Mucor*), and if such infection is suspected, appropriate therapy with aggressive antifungal treatment and possibly surgery should be instituted promptly.

The neck should be examined for adenopathy and swelling, but suppleness of the neck may not be helpful in evaluation of the presence or absence of meningitis.

The upper and lower respiratory tracts are extremely common portals of infection in the neutropenic patient, making the chest examination extremely important. Analogous to the difficulty of seeing infiltrates on chest x-rays because of the lack of neutrophils, it may be difficult to hear rales or adventitious sounds in the chest of patients who have neutropenia. When examination reveals even a suspicion of chest disease, many issues arise. As physical signs and x-ray appearance may be diminished, the progression of chest disease in the intensely neutropenic patient may be difficult to monitor. Shallow tachypnea or evidence of hypoxia in the absence of prolonged expiration should raise the possibility of *P. carinii* pneumonia. Careful attention should be paid to the inspiratory/expiratory ratio for signs of obstruction and to respiratory rate and depth, looking for any physical examination evidence of pneumonia or pneumonitis.

In some situations, bacterial or opportunistic infection may be progressing without much in the way of respiratory compromise until the return of granulocyte function, with its accompanying inflammation. Since chest symptoms in neutropenic patients are very common and can progress so rapidly, patients with neutropenia and chest disease should be monitored in the hospital with frequent examinations, nursing observation, serial chest x-rays, and continuous oxygen saturation monitoring, if appropriate. Broad-spectrum antibiotics are administered unless the physical examination or radiologic pattern of illness suggests *P. carinii* pneumonia (diffuse interstitial infiltrate and hypoxemia) or fungal disease. The use of bronchoscopy or open lung biopsy for diagnosis usually is reserved for patients who do not respond to appropriate antibiotic therapy in the first 48 to 72 hours, patients with rapidly progressive loss of pulmonary function, or patients with nodular or unusual patterns of lung disease suggestive of nonbacterial origin. Antibiotic therapy should consist of drugs aimed at both gram-positive and gram-negative infection, especially in the patient with neutropenia and immune compromise, as well as a consideration of *Mycoplasma, Legionella,* or *P. carinii* pneumonia.

We have been discussing the patient who has chest disease along with neutropenia. Another potential situation is the neutropenic patient already under treatment with antibiotics who experiences the new onset of a pulmonary infection while on antibiotics and still neutropenic. The appearance of pulmonary infiltrates and pulmonary signs and symptoms in patients who have already been on antibiotics for several days is worrisome. Clinical experience has suggested that if this occurs in concert with a rise in the white count, it may simply represent an inflammatory response. Most such patients will recover without major changes in therapy. However, when this pattern occurs in the presence of continuing intense neutropenia, fungal infection should be considered, and more invasive approaches to diagnosis, including broncoscopy or lung biopsy, should be entertained. In patients with a sudden, rapid deterioration of pulmonary function, precluding invasive procedures, switching to a different pair of broad-spectrum antibiotics and adding amphotericin B has been our practice.

The appearance of a new cardiac murmur as a result of endocarditis is an unusual finding. Patients with chemotherapy-induced neutropenia often have concomitant anemia, and new flow murmurs frequently appear. Our experience is that most patients with fever and bacteremia are unlikely to have endocarditis but rather may have indwelling line infections without true cardiac infection.

In patients who have received chemotherapy, there is a particularly significant chance of gastrointestinal ulceration and surface mucosal ulceration. Hence, examination of the abdomen is important. Bowel sounds should be carefully ausculated and documented. As true peritoneal signs may be absent in the presence of neutropenia, changes in bowel sounds are important, as is the presence of distention. The cecum often is a sensitive place in patients with prolonged neutropenia. Careful examination of the right lower quadrant is important, and any evidence of pathology within the abdomen on physical examination should lead the physician to order a kidney ureter, and bladder (KUB) examination to look for free air or changes in the bowel wall (pneumatosis cystoides intestinalis).

Patients with substernal or midepigastric pain in association with other symptoms of esophagitis may have simple hyperacidity. In the neutropenic patient, however, this symptom may represent localized infection of the esophagus by *Candida* or herpes simplex. In nontoxic or ambulatory patients, we have employed endoscopy primarily for specific diagnosis and treatment. Information on sicker patients might be obtained by barium swallow. However, our tendency in very sick patients has been to begin oral fluconazole and acyclovir along with an antacid regimen, maintaining an expectant approach to improvement.

Patients with neutropenia should *not* be subjected to rectal examination or to the placement of anything in the rectum, except under the most unusual circumstances where examination of the rectum seems appropriate. This prohibition helps to avoid both bacteremia and perirectal abscess. In the event that perirectal tenderness develops in a patient who is neutropenic, concern about the formation of a diffuse perirectal abscess leads us to initiate antibiotics that cover anaerobic and gram-negative organisms. If, in fact, there is concern about appendicitis or typhlitis (inflammation of the cecum) or if there is a true need to do a formal rectal examination, it is best to allow the most experienced physician as a single examiner as opposed to subjecting the patient to multiple rectal examinations. If there is a suggestion of typhlitis, it is critical that patients be given antibiotics with aerobic and anaerobic coverage, as the incidence of bacteremia is quite high. We usually use clindamycin in addition to a semisynthetic penicillin and an aminoglycoside in patients with suspected typhlitis. Such patients can have pain mimicking an acute abdomen or a perforated appendix, and they may also have associated significant gastrointestinal bleeding. It has been our approach to attempt simply to maintain these patients on antibiotics with supportive care and bowel rest. When severe gastrointestinal bleeding occurs, consideration of surgical intervention may be necessary.

Diarrhea in the neutropenic patient is common and may be a side effect of chemotherapy (chemotherapy-induced colitis). In patients who have been on antibiotics for a long period of time, the diarrhea may represent overgrowth of *Clostridium difficile* (pseudomembranous colitis). Once the toxin of *C. difficile* is recognized through standard laboratory procedures, patients can be treated with oral vancomycin or metronidazole. Diarrhea, especially bloody diarrhea, can also indicate the onset of typhlitis.

The neurologic examination should be performed carefully, with the understanding that symptoms are more common than formal signs when neutropenic patients develop infections in the central nervous system. CNS contamination should be suspected in the presence of the most mild meningeal signs, neck or back pain, lethargy, or any change in the level of consciousness. Although meningitis is uncommon in these patients, if there is any doubt, a spinal tap should be part of the septic workup.

FEVER AND NO SOURCE OF INFECTION

As a general rule, patients with immune neutropenia or acute postviral neutropenia may be less prone to bacteremia, opportunistic infection, or rapid spread of localized infection. Nonetheless, in the presence of fever or evidence of toxicity, it is our practice to treat these patients aggressively after appropriate cultures are taken with broad-spectrum antibiotics, at least for the first 48 to 72 hours to preclude the remote possibility of bacteremia or infection with an unusual bacterial agent. Antibiotic choices may vary dramatically by physician practice and known hospital and community flora, but they should include broad coverage with such choices as single-agent ceftriaxone, a semisynthetic penicillin and an aminoglycoside, or vancomycin and ceftazidime.

Patients who have neutropenia and fever and no source and who are immunocompromised should be admitted to the hospital and placed on broad-spectrum antibiotics, including anti-*Pseudomonas* coverage and coverage specific to the bacterial profile of the institution. In the course of the patient's hospitalization, if the fever should go away and cultures remain negative, broad-spectrum antibiotics should be continued until such time as the neutropenia has resolved. This practice is based on extensive studies demonstrating that breakthrough bacteremia will occur if there is early withdrawal of antibiotics before resolution of neutropenia. If a specific source or infection with a specific organism becomes known during this time, that organism should be aggressively treated, but broad-spectrum antibiotics should continue until neutropenia resolves. If the patient continues to be febrile despite broad-spectrum antibiotics and still has no obvious source, culturing on a daily basis should continue. Such cultures should include both fungal and bacterial cultures of blood, culture of urine and any wound or skin involvement, and CSF culture if appropriate. If the patient remains febrile on broad-spectrum antibiotics over 5 days and there is evidence of toxicity by clinical judgment or by actual vital sign changes, consideration should be given to the use of antifungal therapy, specifically amphotericin B. This drug should not be added to a regimen without due consideration, as it is associated with renal problems, severe potassium wasting, and perhaps prolonged neutropenia. Unfortunately, testing for fungal infection still has not approached our capacity to detect bacteremia. Hence, it is important to consider fungal infection early in patients who have not responded appropriately to antibiotics and in patients who seem at higher risk because of the degree of their immunosuppression. Clues to fungal infection may include unexplained pulmonary infiltrates or budding yeast in the urine.

If the patient rapidly becomes afebrile on antibiotics and is not expected to have a return of granulocytes, treatment may be stopped at 14 afebrile days, although careful observation should follow, since there is still a risk of breakthrough bacteremia at this time.

REFERENCES

1. Curnutte J: Disorders of granulocyte function and granulopoiesis. *In* Nathan DG, Oski F (eds): Hematology of Infancy and Childhood. Philadelphia, WB Saunders, 1993:904–977.
2. Freifeld A, Hathorn J, Pizzo P: Infectious complications in the pediatric patient. *In* Pizzo P, Poplack D (eds): Principles and Practice of Pediatric Oncology. Philadelphia, JB Lippincott, 1993:987–1020.

POLYCYTHEMIA

SHELLY C. BERNSTEIN, M.D., Ph.D.

During the first week of life, hemoglobin values above 22 g/dl or hematocrit values of more than 65% should be considered evidence of polycythemia. In childhood and adolescence, hemoglobin values above 17 g/dl or hematocrit values of more than 50% are significant. The diagnosis should be verified by venipuncture. Capillary blood samples should not be used. Hemoconcentration due to dehydration must be excluded as a cause.

NEONATAL POLYCYTHEMIA

Polycythemia in the neonate may be due to twin-to-twin transfusion, maternal-fetal transfusion, delayed cord clamping, placental insufficiency, cogenital adrenal hyperplasia, maternal diabetes mellitus, Down syndrome, or Beckwith's syndrome. The signs and symptoms may consist of lethargy, plethora, cyanosis, jaundice, respiratory distress, congestive heart failure, seizures, priapism, thrombocytopenia, renal vein thrombosis, necrotizing enterocolitis, hypoglycemia, and hypocalcemia. Many infants with polycythemia are, however, asymptomatic. Prophylactic treatment is not recommended. However, all infants with polycythemia should be monitored carefully, and at the first sign of symptoms, treatment should be instituted. Treatment should be designed to reduce the venous hematocrit value to approximately 60%, accomplished by partial exchange transfusion, using 5% albumin to reduce the hematocrit value while maintaining the blood volume. The volume of exchange may be estimated from the following formula.

Volume of exchange (ml) =

$$\frac{\text{Blood volume} \times (\text{observed Hct} - \text{desired Hct})}{\text{Observed Hct}}$$

The infant's blood should be removed in volumes of 10 ml for full-term (and smaller volumes for low birth weight) infants and replaced with an equal volume of 5% albumin. A blood volume of 80 ml/kg may be estimated for newborn infants. The procedure is usually performed through an umbilical venous line. Simple phlebotomy should not be performed unless the infant is hypervolemic.

CHILDHOOD POLYCYTHEMIA

Primary Polycythemia

Polycythemia Vera

This disorder, rarely seen in childhood, consists of an increase in red cell mass of unknown etiology, often accompanied by thrombocytosis. The Polycythemia Vera Study Group recommends phlebotomy for patients under the age of 40 years. Erythrocytapheresis with isovolemic exchange of saline or 5% albumin, rather than simple phlebotomy, should be performed to maintain the hematocrit between 40% and 45%. Patients with complications (such as massive splenomegaly, vascular obstruction, or symptoms associated with hypermetabolism) or with extreme thrombocytosis (platelet counts greater than $1.0 \times 10^{12}/L$) should be treated with myelosuppressive agents. Hydroxyurea at a dose of 30 mg/kg PO in three divided doses per day is given until the platelet count falls to $1.0 \times 10^{11}/L$. At that time, busulfan at a dose of 0.12 mg/kg (maximum dose of 6 mg) PO per day for 7 days is given. This dose may be repeated for another 7 days if significant myelosuppression does not occur. Periodic pulses of busulfan may be required to control thrombocytosis and may need to be performed on a regular basis. Repeated erythrocytapheresis will lead to iron deficiency, causing an increase in whole blood viscosity related to decreased erythrocyte deformability, as well as thrombocytosis. Therefore, iron deficiency should be avoided by oral iron supplementation.

Benign Familial Polycythemia

This term is used to describe familial cases with increased red cell mass that are otherwise normal, with no other recognizable etiology. Therapy is warranted only when the patient has symptoms related to hyperviscosity. Erythrocytapheresis or phlebotomy may then afford symptomatic relief.

Secondary Polycythemia

These conditions refer to an increase in red cell mass secondary to recognizable cause. This may result either from tissue hypoxia, leading to a compensatory increase in production of erythropoietin, or from a pathologically increased production of erythropoietin despite normal tissue oxygenation.

Cyanotic Congenital Heart Disease

Children with cyanotic congenital heart disease develop polycythemia in response to chronic systemic arterial desaturation. Symptoms are headaches, irritability, anorexia, and dyspnea. In addition, polycythemia, when accompanied by iron deficiency, may be associated with an increased incidence of intravascular thrombosis and a consumptive coagulopathy. Arterial desaturation should be surgically corrected, if possible. If the patient is symptomatic, reduction of hematocrit values should be attempted by partial exchange transfusion or erythrocytapheresis. Since acute phlebotomy in these patients may result in vascular collapse, cyanotic spells, cerebrovascular accidents, or seizures, sudden hemodynamic alterations should be avoided. Hence, erythrocytapheresis is the preferred method in most cases. The red blood cells removed are replaced continuously by infusion of equal volumes of saline or 5% albumin. The hematocrit should be reduced to 60% to 65% over about 1 hour. How much can be removed is a function of patient tolerance. Typically, one cannot reduce by more than 10% to 15% at a single sitting. On average, automated hematocrits are 3% to 5% lower than spun hematocrits in patients with cyanotic congenital heart disease. Thus, the degree of polycythemia must be defined by which method is used. Because of the complications associated with iron deficiency and polycythemia, iron deficiency should always be corrected. These measures have led to reduced coagulation abnormalities, decreased operative mortality, and symptomatic improvement in polycythemic patients with cyanotic congenital heart disease.

Abnormal Hemoglobins

A number of rare hemoglobin variants have been described with a marked increase in oxygen affinity and compensatory polycythemia via increased production of erythropoietin. Other than erythrocytosis, affected individuals have minimal clinical manifestations, with the exception of one reported family with Hb Malmö, the children of which were reported to have cardiovascular symptoms. Hematocrit values rarely are high enough to necessitate treatment.

Congenital methemoglobinemia due to NADH-diaphorase I deficiency and acquired methemoglobinemia due to exposure to various agents capable of oxidizing heme iron to the ferric state may produce cyanosis and polycythemia. Treatment of methemoglobinemia, regardless of the etiology, is dictated by the severity of the hypoxia. Most patients with hereditary disease require no therapy. Severe methemoglobinemia can be treated initially by methylene blue in a dose of 1 to 2 mg/kg administered intravenously as a 1% solution. Further treatment is accomplished with daily oral doses of methylene blue 1 to 2 mg/kg.

Inappropriate Erythrocytosis

Polycythemia has been associated with a number of tumors in which erythropoietin secretion is elevated, such as Wilms' tumor, hepatoma, cerebellar hemangioblastoma, and benign lesions of the kidney, such as cysts and hydronephrosis. Endocrine disorders, such as pheochromocytomas, aldosterone-producing adenomas, and Cushing's syndrome, as well as exogenous administration of testosterone or growth hormone, also may cause increased red cell mass. Correction of the underlying condition results in elimination of the polycythemia.

The availability of the red cell cytokine erythropoietin has led to its use and possible overuse. Anecdotal reports of athletes trying to "blood dope" in an undetectable fashion may have resulted in fatalities. Hence, inappropriate use of erythropoietin needs to be investigated in an adolescent athlete who has a very high hematocrit.

REFERENCES

1. Berk PD, Goldberg JD, Donovan PB, Fruchtman SM, et al: Therapeutic recommendations in polycythemia vera based on polycythemia vera study group protocols, Semin Hematol 23:132–143, 1986.
2. Hocking WG, Golde DW: Polycythemia: Evaluation and management. Blood Rev 3:59–65, 1989.
3. Landaw SA: Polycythemia vera and other polycythemic states. Clin Lab Med 10:857–871, 1990.

ACUTE LEUKEMIA

PHILIP P. BREITFELD, M.D.

The treatment of leukemia in children is truly one of the therapeutic successes in medicine over the last three decades. There are approximately 2500 to 3000 new cases of acute leukemia in children each year in the United States, and with modern therapy, about 65% of these children will be cured and live to old age. This is a dramatic change from the 1960s, when only 20% of children were curable. Two factors have contributed significantly to this progress. First, basic as well as clinical research in leukemia has translated into better therapy. Second, better supportive care has lessened the chance of death from side effects of therapy, especially infection.

Both acute lymphoblastic leukemia (ALL) and acute myelogenous leukemia (AML) occur in childhood. Seventy-five percent of children with leukemia present with ALL, and the remaining 25% with AML. In general, the chance of surviving ALL (65% to 70%) is greater than that of surviving AML (35% to 40%). In addition, the therapeutic approach to ALL significantly differs from the approach to AML. Nonetheless, the future promises to bring improved treatment for both forms of leukemia in childhood.

CLINICAL PRESENTATION OF ACUTE LEUKEMIA

Children of any age can present with leukemia, although the peak incidence occurs in young schoolage children. The presenting symptoms and signs can range from the subtle to the dramatic. Most children have a several week history of malaise, with or without fever. Bone pain, loss of appetite, and weight loss are not uncommon. There may be pallor, epistaxis, bruising, lymphadenopathy, and hepatosplenomegaly. A chest x-ray may reveal an anterior mediastinal mass. The hemogram can be normal but often shows anemia and thrombocytopenia. The child may have leukopenia or leukocytosis, with blast cells noted in the differential. Because the presentation may be subtle and because there are no specific presenting symptoms or signs, the differential diagnosis of a child with possible leukemia might include an undefined viral syndrome, mononucleosis, immune thrombocytopenic purpura (ITP), rheumatoid arthritis, and aplastic anemia. Once a diagnosis of acute leukemia is seriously entertained, a prompt referral to a tertiary care center with a pediatric hematology-oncology specialist is recommended.

POTENTIAL EMERGENCIES AT PRESENTATION

Many children with newly diagnosed leukemia need prompt medical attention to prevent certain life-threatening complications of the disease. Severe anemia (Hb < 7 g/dl) and severe thrombocytopenia (< 15,000/mm³) require prompt transfusion. A child with an anterior mediastinal mass may have compression of the trachea that could threaten the airway. Small doses of radiation directed toward the area of compression may be required, especially before any sedation of the child is considered. Leukocytosis (WBC >100,000/mm³) can cause stasis in blood vessels, leading to CNS stroke or pulmonary infiltrates and hypoxia, especially in AML. Urgent exchange transfusion or leukophoresis is indicated for this complication. Rapid proliferation and death of leukemia cells can cause the acute tumor lysis syndrome, with renal failure secondary to hyperuricemia, hypocalcemia, hyperkalemia, and hypophosphatemia. Treatment includes allopurinol (250 mg/m²/d) and intravenous hydration at twice the maintenance rate, with added sodium bicarbonate to achieve a urine pH of 7.5. No potassium should be added to this fluid. Occasionally, renal dialysis is required if urine output is inadequate or if life-threatening electrolyte imbalance occurs. Finally, when a child presents with leukemia and fever, he or she may be at risk for severe sepsis, especially if the absolute neutrophil count is below 500/mm³. Prompt administration of broad-spectrum antibiotics, such as piperacillin and gentamicin, is indicated. In summary, once a diagnosis of leukemia is seriously suspected, a CBC with differential and platelet count, chemistry panel, a bioximeter reading, and a chest x-ray are necessary to determine if the child requires emergency care at a referral center.

SUPPORTIVE CARE

Improvements in the supportive care of children with acute leukemia have contributed to better survival rates, as well as enhancing the quality of life. We believe that adherence to the principles outlined here makes the delivery of chemotherapy safer and adds to the comfort of the child undergoing therapy.

For symptomatic control of vomiting associated with chemotherapy, ondansetron is the drug of choice, especially for moderate to severe emesis seen mainly with chemotherapy for AML. Ondansetron has replaced the phenothiazines, since it does not cause extrapyramidal side effects and effectively controls emesis without sedation. Constipation is a frequent side effect from vincristine, especially in ALL induction, and we recommend the administration of stool softeners before development of symptomatic constipation.

Transfusion Support

Blood component therapy is essential for children with acute leukemia. In ALL, most transfusions of red cells and platelets are given in induction and are relatively infrequent after this time. Children with AML are generally red cell and platelet transfusion dependent during each cycle of therapy. We recommend using radiated and filtered blood components for all patients. For those children who are cytomegalovirus (CMV) antibody negative, we use CMV-negative blood components. We routinely transfuse 10 to 15 ml/kg of packed red blood cells for Hb less than 8.0 g/dl and 5 U/m² of random donor platelets when the platelet count is less than 15,000/mm³. If a patient is septic or experiencing intravascular coagulation (DIC), we maintain higher levels of Hb and platelets.

Infection

Since infection is the second most common cause of death in children with leukemia, close attention to fever in this setting is essential. The most life-threatening infections in children with acute leukemia are bacteremias that occur as a consequence of neutropenia. Thus, if a child is neutropenic and has a temperature exceeding 38.5°C, we recommend that the child be seen urgently for a septic workup, which includes a comprehensive physical examination, cultures of blood and urine, and chest x-ray. This must be followed by the prompt administration of broad-spectrum antibiotics in the hospital. The most likely organisms are *Escherichia coli, Klebsiella, Pseudomonas,* and *Staphylococcus aureus.* We use piperacillin and gentamicin as initial empiric therapy and continue this until the neutrophil count exceeds 500/mm³. The risk of fungal infection increases as the length of neutropenia increases. Therefore, for prolonged neutropenia and fever (more than 5 to 7 days), we empirically add amphotericin B as antifungal therapy. The frequent use of central venous catheters (CVLs) has made certain bacterial infections more common. *Staphylococcus epidermidis* and enterococcus are common at our institution, and we commonly use vancomycin, especially in the febrile, nonneutropenic child who has a CVL in place.

Pneumocystis carinii pneumonia also is common, especially in children with ALL. For this reason, all children with acute leukemia are placed on prophylactic doses of trimethoprim-sulfamethoxazole three times a week. We occasionally must withhold this therapy secondary to neutropenia. Any child on chemotherapy who has a cough, elevated respiratory rate, and evidence of hypoxia should be assumed to have *Pneumocystis* and should be treated in the hospital with therapeutic doses of trimethoprim-sulfamethoxazole and followed carefully.

Varicella is the viral infection of most concern in acute leukemia. The immune suppression of chemotherapy places the nonimmune child at risk for disseminated varicella on exposure to the virus. If a nonimmune child is exposed to varicella, varicella immune globulin (VZIG) should be administered within 72 hours of exposure. If the child develops chickenpox, acyclovir should be administered until symptoms have disappeared. The use of VZIG and acyclovir has greatly reduced the mortality of varicella in acute leukemia.

The use of growth factors or colony-stimulating factors (CSFs) to shorten the duration of neutropenia has increased greatly over the last 5 years. The most commonly prescribed growth factor in children is granulocyte-colony stimulating factor (G-CSF). Since its role in childhood leukemia is yet to be established, we do not recommend the routine use of G-CSF in childhood leukemia. Several national studies are assessing its role in high-risk ALL and AML induction.

Psychosocial Support

All children with acute leukemia and their families require close attention to psychologic needs. The stresses of diagnosis and treatment often bring old issues to the surface, as well as create new ones. Continuity is needed for the assessment and management of such problems. This often can be provided by the primary oncologist and nurse but also requires a social worker or a psychologist (or both) who is familiar with leukemia in childhood.

ACUTE LYMPHOBLASTIC LEUKEMIA

ALL is the most common form of acute leukemia in childhood. The peak incidence is between 3 and 6 years of age. No specific cause of ALL in children has been established. However, ionizing and electromagnetic radiation have received considerable attention. Because there is still much to learn about the biology and treatment of ALL in children and because this is a relatively rare disorder, we recommend that all children with ALL be referred to a pediatric hematology-oncology specialist. These children can then be placed on a clinical research treatment program designed to offer the latest therapy, which will contribute to our further understanding and therapy of this disease.

The diagnosis of ALL can be established only by obtaining a diagnostic bone marrow aspiration. Except for rare exceptions, this should be performed by the treating pediatric hematologist-oncologist. In addition to morphologic analysis of the specimen, cytochemical staining, flow cytometric analysis, and cytogenetics are now standard tests performed on the marrow sample. Many centers perform additional scientific and biologic tests in the leukemic marrow at diagnosis. Today, the flow cytometric analysis and cytogenetic analysis are critical, since the results of these tests can alter therapy and prognosis. For example, the presence of the Philadelphia chromosome (t[9,22]) in leukemic blast cells is a very poor prognostic feature, and children with T cell ALL require more aggressive therapy to achieve good results. Thus, the first step beyond establishing the diagnosis of ALL is the full and accurate characterization of the lymphoid blasts.

With this information, the child is placed into one of several prognostic groups. The definition of these groups varies somewhat depending on therapy and the choice of the investigator designing the clinical research program. Nonetheless, general categories of risk can be described. These are designated as low risk (of relapse), intermediate risk, high risk, and very high risk (Table 1). Specific therapy is determined by the risk group. In general, chemotherapy rather than bone marrow transplantation is recommended for children with ALL. Bone marrow transplantation in first remission is reserved for those few children with very high risk ALL who have less than a 40% chance of cure with even the most aggressive modern chemotherapy programs.

Induction Therapy

Certain general components or phases of therapy are recommended for all children. Once the diagnosis of ALL is established, all children

TABLE 1. Childhood Acute Lymphoblastic Leukemia: Risk Groups

	LOW	INTERMEDIATE	HIGH	VERY HIGH
Age (yr)	2–10	>1	>1	Any
WBC	<10,000	10,000–50,000	50,000–100,000	>100,000
Massive LN*	−	−	+	±
HSM*	−	−	+	±
T cell	−	−	+	±
t(9,22)	−	−	−	+

*LN, nodes >5 cm; HSM, hepatosplenomegaly.

TABLE 2. Commonly Used Agents in Acute Leukemia

AGENT	DOSE	ROUTE	FREQUENT SIDE EFFECTS
Vincristine	$1.5-2.0$ mg/m^2 q1-4wk	IV	Constipation, peripheral neuropathy, alopecia
Prednisone	$40-120$ mg/m^2 q.d. $\times$ 5	PO	Salt or water retention, hyperglycemia, hypertension, behavioral changes
Asparaginase	6000 U/m^2 MWF, 25,000 U/m^2 q.wk.	IM	Allergic reactions, hyperglycemia, pancreatitis, hepatitis
Doxorubicin	$30-60$ mg/m^2 q3wk	IV	Myelosuppression, heart failure, mucositis, emesis
Methotrexate	$20-40$ mg/m^2 q.wk.	PO IV IM	Mucositis, hepatitis, myelosuppression
6-Mercaptopurine	50 mg/m^2 q.d. 1 g/m^2 q.wk.	PO IV	Myelosuppression, hepatitis
Cytarabine	100 mg/m^2/d $\times$ 7 $1-3$ g/m^2 q12h for $2-4$ d	IV	Myelosuppression, emesis, conjunctivitis, cerebellar dysfunction
Daunomycin	45 mg/m^2 q.d. $\times$ $2-3$	IV	Myelosuppression, heart failure, mucositis, emesis
Etoposide	150 mg/m^2/d $\times$ 3	IV	Myelosuppression, hypotension, alopecia
5-Azacytidine	100 mg/m^2/d $\times$ 3	IV	Myelosuppression (prolonged), emesis
6-Thioguanine	$75-100$ mg/m^2/d $\times$ 4	PO	Myelosuppression, hepatitis

undergo induction therapy. This involves a month of therapy and is designed to achieve remission. Remission is determined by demonstrating that there is no evidence of leukemia in the blood, bone marrow, and spinal fluid. Agents commonly employed to achieve remission in ALL include vincristine, prednisone, asparaginase, doxorubicin, and intrathecal methotrexate (Table 2). Remission occurs in approximately 95% to 97% of children with ALL, and failure to achieve remission is generally an ominous sign. Up to 50% of children will require 1 to 2 weeks of hospitalization during induction for treatment of possible infection or other complications of treatment. Up to 2% of children will die from complications of therapy during this period.

CNS Leukemia and its Prevention

Only 2% to 3% of children with ALL will present with leukemia in the central nervous system defined as detectable lymphoblasts in the spinal fluid. However, it is likely that all children at diagnosis have subclinical evidence of CNS leukemia and, thus, are at risk for the future development of overt CNS leukemia unless specific therapy is given that addresses this issue. Many of the medications given systemically for leukemia do not penetrate the CNS at the doses administered. Thus, historically, both intrathecal chemotherapy, generally methotrexate, and whole brain radiation have been employed to treat this sanctuary site. With this combination, only 5% or less of children with ALL will suffer a CNS relapse. However, because whole brain radiation places the child (especially the child less than 3 years) at risk for neuropsychologic complications, such as learning disabilities, whole brain radiation is now reserved for those children with high and very high risk leukemia. Early results suggest that for low and intermediate risk patients, intrathecal chemotherapy is sufficient to prevent the development of CNS leukemia.

Intensification-Consolidation

Most treatment programs for ALL include a 1 to 2 month phase of treatment after induction designed to further reduce the leukemic cell burden, which, although undetectable by standard means, is still substantial. Additional systemic agents, such as cytarabine and cyclophosphamide, often are employed in this phase. During this phase, CNS prophylaxis is emphasized. This often includes weekly intrathecal chemotherapy and whole brain radiation. A similar phase without the CNS prophylaxis is often administered 6 months into therapy and is called *delayed intensification*. This phase interrupts maintenance therapy.

Maintenance Therapy

This phase of therapy consists of 3 to 4 week cycles of medications, including vincristine, prednisone, methotrexate, and 6-mercaptopu-

rine. The goal of therapy is to eliminate any undetectable residual leukemia, referred to as minimal residual disease. This therapy is delivered on an outpatient basis, and the risks of serious complications are low, since the goal of treatment is to minimize the myelosuppressive effects of therapy by maintaining an absolute neutrophil count above 750/mm^3 and a platelet count above 100,000/mm^3. These cycles are repeated until approximately 2 full years of therapy are completed. Some centers treat boys for 3 years. At the end of treatment, a diagnostic bone marrow and spinal tap are performed to document continued remission.

Relapse

Although modern therapy is effective for childhood ALL, approximately 25% of children still suffer a relapse. Thus, relapse remains the most likely cause of death from leukemia. The timing of the relapse has a substantial effect on the probability of cure. If a bone marrow relapse occurs while the patient is still receiving treatment, the chance of long-term survival, even with the most intensive chemotherapy, is less than 25%. Thus, an allogeneic bone marrow transplant from an HLA-identical sibling is recommended once a second remission has been achieved. Unfortunately, only 20% of children will have a sibling donor, and only 75% of relapsed patients will achieve a second remission. Currently, the efficacy and safety of autologous bone marrow transplantation and unrelated donor allogeneic transplants for children who relapse on therapy are being studied. Such transplants would be used if a matched sibling bone marrow donor is not available. If relapse occurs after the elective cessation of therapy, the outlook is more favorable. If the intensity of prior therapy was moderate and the duration of the first remission was long, retreatment with aggressive chemotherapy may cure up to 35% of these children. However, up to 50% of children are curable with an allogeneic marrow transplant from an HLA-matched sibling donor. Thus, if available, an allogeneic bone marrow transplant is recommended even if the relapse occurs late. Some centers have reported a 50% event-free survival for children who relapse off therapy and who have undergone a purged autologous bone marrow transplant. The role of an unrelated matched-donor transplant is still controversial, especially for a child suffering from a late bone marrow relapse.

If an isolated CNS relapse occurs, many investigators consider that this event is heralding a more widespread systemic (bone marrow) relapse. This is demonstrated by the observation that approximately 35% of patients with an isolated CNS relapse are curable with retreatment with chemotherapy. For this reason, especially if the CNS relapse occurs on treatment, some investigators will consider bone marrow transplantation for these children. This area remains controversial, however.

ACUTE MYELOGENOUS LEUKEMIA

The therapy for and chance of cure with AML in childhood is substantially different from that of ALL. For the last two decades, extremely intensive and relatively short chemotherapy programs have been used to treat children with AML and have resulted in curing about 35% of such children. Although this represents a substantial improvement in survival from the 1960s, there has been little progress in outcome since the 1980s. Thus, there is intense interest in developing new programs that might offer even better chances for survival in childhood AML.

Induction Therapy

As with ALL, induction therapy is designed to eradicate all detectable disease. However, the therapy is much more myelosuppressive and often causes prolonged neutropenia, leading to a substantial risk for infection, both bacterial and fungal. In addition, induction in AML often lasts 2 months. Most children will require hospitalization during induction for AML, as they frequently require multiple antibiotics and transfusions. Almost all centers use cytarabine, either as a continuous infusion or at high doses with bolus therapy, and daunomycin (Table 2). Some investigators will add etoposide during induction. Substitutes for daunomycin, such as idarubicin and mitoxantrone, are being investigated. The chance of achieving remission is about 80% to 85%. As many as 5% to 10% of children will die from a serious infection during induction.

For those children who present with a subtype of AML, called acute promyelocytic leukemia (APML), there are several special considerations during induction. When given standard chemotherapy programs, these children have a substantial risk for hemorrhage secondary to DIC. Frequent platelet and plasma infusions are required, and some investigators use low-dose continuous infusion heparin. Finally, a national randomized trial is underway in children to determine if retinoic acid as a single agent will be as effective as standard induction chemotherapy in obtaining remission in APML.

Continuation Therapy

Once remission is achieved, if an HLA-identical sibling is identified, an allogeneic bone marrow transplant is recommended. These children have a 60% chance of survival but may suffer from graft-versus-host (GVH) disease. The remaining 80% of children without a sibling donor have a 40% to 50% chance of cure with further intensive chemotherapy. Continuation therapy usually consists of high-dose cytarabine, etoposide, 5-azacytidine, and 6-thioguanine. The duration of treatment is controversial, but most centers stop treatment after a total of 6 to 8 months from diagnosis. We are currently testing in a randomized fashion whether continued chemotherapy or a purged autologous bone marrow transplant is better once remission is achieved in children without a matched sibling donor.

Relapse/Refractory AML

The remission rate for children with either relapsed or refractory AML has been disappointing and is in the range of 50%. Newer programs employing mitoxantrone may improve this, however. Even if achieved, the duration of a second remission in AML tends to be quite short. Thus, allogeneic bone marrow transplantation from a matched sibling donor is recommended for such children. If available, this approach offers a 30% to 40% chance of survival. The efficacy of autologous and unrelated donor bone marrow transplantation is being studied.

REFERENCES

1. Cassano WF, Eskenazi AE, Frantz CN: Therapy for childhood acute lymphoblastic leukemia. Curr Opin Oncol 5:42–52, 1993.
2. Hoelzer D: Acute lymphoblastic leukemia—Progress in children, less in adults. N Engl J Med 329:1343–1344, 1993.
3. Klingebiel T, et al: Role and perspectives of BMT in AML: The BFM experience. Bone Marrow Transplant 7(Suppl 3):66–70, 1991.
4. Rivera GK, Pinkel D, Simone JV, Hancock ML, Crist WM: Treatment of acute lymphoblastic leukemia. N Engl J Med 329:1289–1295, 1993.

THE CHILD CURED OF CANCER

MOLLY R. SCHWENN, M.D.

By the year 2000, an estimated 1 of every 900 young adults will be a survivor of childhood cancer. Because of the increasing number of children surviving cancer, the prevention of and surveillance for long-term sequelae of treatment continually grow in importance.

BACKGROUND

In the history of treatment of childhood malignancy, the initial focus was on increasing the number of survivors. As effective treatments emerged, the pediatric, surgical, and radiation oncologists who design and carry out treatment protocols began to modify therapy to minimize late toxicity. Such efforts have required courage on the part of parents, patients, and investigators, since reduction of therapy can, at best, produce a cure rate equal to the standard treatment and risks lowering the number of children cured of their cancer. Finding the appropriate balance between therapy aggressive enough to cure the maximal number of children and therapy that will have acceptable long-term sequelae is an ongoing process. In general, the higher the likelihood of survival for a given malignancy, the more intense are the efforts to find less toxic treatment. The elimination of prophylactic CNS radiation for some children with acute lymphoblastic leukemia (ALL) and the use of chemotherapy to avoid mutilating surgery for certain children with pelvic rhabdomyosarcoma were among the pioneering efforts in this attempt. Just as the enrollment of children with cancer in multiinstitutional studies was vital to producing curative therapies, ongoing enrollment in large, national group studies is critical to answering randomized treatment reduction questions.

THERAPEUTIC MODALITIES

The treatment of cancer in children involves the use of surgery, radiation therapy, and chemotherapy alone and in combination. Each has recognized sequelae.

Surgery for tumor resection may involve the removal of or injury to organs and surrounding structures. Such procedures range from unilateral nephrectomy for Wilms' tumor to mutilating procedures, such as amputation or hemipelvectomy, for bone tumors. The introduction of limb-sparing procedures to avoid amputation has been a dramatic orthopedic surgical innovation, lessening the consequences of cancer treatment for some survivors.

Radiation affects normal tissue both in the field of radiation and outside the field via scatter and other mechanisms, such as immunosuppression. This damage is generally dose dependent and exaggerated in the infant and young child. For example, cranial radiation for brain tumors at doses ranging from 4000 to 6000 cGy causes more profound sequelae than the lower doses (1800 to 2800 cGY) used for treating or preventing CNS leukemia, and the sequelae are most pronounced in children under 3 years of age. Other organs or tissues that are particularly sensitive to radiation include the spinal cord, thyroid, kidney, heart, and the growing end of long bones. For example, approximately 50% of survivors of Hodgkin's disease who have received radiation to the neck or mediastinum will develop thyroid dysfunction (usually chemical hypothyroidism) 6 months to 20 years after therapy. Daily thyroid replacement hormone frequently is prescribed. Before this decade, most patients with Wilms' tumor received whole abdomen radiation to a dose of 2000 cGy, which caused ovarian dysfunction and sterility in the majority of females treated. In recent years, the dose of radiation, the field, and the number of children who receive radiation all have been reduced.

Radiation can also cause or contribute to the development of secondary malignancies. For example, osteogenic sarcoma may develop in bones treated for Ewing's sarcoma, and breast cancer may develop in individuals treated for Hodgkin's disease. There may be a long latency period before secondary solid tumors occur. This provides an example of why physician and patient education is a very important component of long-term care.

In addition to the better known acute side effects of chemotherapeutic agents, such as nausea and hair loss, these drugs can cause a variety of late toxicities, often dependent on total cumulative dose or dose schedule. Alkylating agents (e.g., nitrogen mustard, cyclophosphamide) can cause or contribute to secondary malignancy and to sterility. Anthracyclines (e.g., doxorubicin, daunorubicin) may cause left ventricular dysfunction and congestive heart failure. Cisplatin can lead to hearing loss, bleomycin to pulmonary fibrosis, and the epipodophyllotoxins (etoposide [VP-16] and teniposide [VM-26]) to secondary leukemia (AML). This last association is an example of a toxicity that was not suspected until 1990, when the drugs had been in use for more than 10 years. It should be recognized that there is frequently an interaction between or additive effect of radiation and chemotherapeutic drugs in producing organ toxicity and secondary malignancy.

PSYCHOSOCIAL DIFFICULTIES

More difficult to identify and measure are psychosocial difficulties, which may be subtle yet lead to profound consequences for the child cured of cancer. Discussion of school function, peer relationships, and, for the older survivor, job performance, sexual function, marriage, and childbearing is of critical importance. Referral for detailed neuropsychologic testing may reveal specific deficits that can be addressed in the school setting and improve educational performance and satisfaction. Groups where adolescents and young adults can share their experiences with regard to the special issues they face in dating, obtaining employment, and obtaining insurance are valuable.

PRACTICAL ISSUES

In evaluating the child or adolescent who is a survivor of childhood cancer, each visit should be sufficiently long to permit time for discussion, education, and counseling, as well as a comprehensive physical examination. The physician evaluating a childhood cancer survivor must have or must obtain the following baseline information: the original diagnosis and tumor location, the treatment modalities (and doses) used, and the age when treatments were given. Since there is a latency period for certain side effects, time since treatment can be an important factor.

Measurements of blood pressure, weight, and height with plotting of growth velocity, evaluation of Tanner stage (pubertal development may be delayed, absent, or precocious), and skeletal examination (looking for spinal deformity, leg length discrepancy) are particularly important. Laboratory tests can be useful following certain treatments—for example, urinalysis for survivors with missing or damaged kidneys, thyroid studies for those who received brain, neck, or chest radiation—but generally are not the major focus of follow-up visits.

Echocardiograms are performed for survivors who have had significant doses (>300 mg/m^2) of anthracyclines and for those who exhibit any signs or symptoms of congestive heart failure. Evaluation of symptoms suggestive of arrhythmia (such as syncope) should include 24-hour Holter monitoring. Pulmonary function tests may aid in the evaluation of symptoms following chest radiation and such drugs as bleomycin.

Decreased growth velocity or short stature should be evaluated with a wrist film for bone age and thyroid function tests, and referral to a pediatric endocrinologist for possible growth hormone testing and replacement therapy should follow. Pediatric endocrinologists or gynecologists can be important for the evaluation and treatment of estrogen deficiency. Semen analysis can be predictive of infertility, as long as sufficient time has passed to allow for the possibility of recovery.

Audiology evaluation should be done for any child who has received cisplatin, has school problems, or has any hearing complaints, such as tinnitus. The administration of aminoglycosides and vancomycin for fever and neutropenia and infections associated with treatment also may contribute to ototoxicity. Preferential seating in the classroom and other locations may be helpful. However, hearing aids may be necessary to improve function and adjustment.

Most pediatric cancer centers have developed special clinical settings to follow survivors on an annual basis. Visits should include discussion of cancer prevention and early detection. Survivors should be given sufficient information about their treatment so they will be able to advocate for themselves. Additional details on evaluation and treatment of late effects in survivors, including guidance for the primary physician, are available from various sources.[1-4]

REFERENCES

1. Blatt J, Copeland DR, Bleyer WA: Late effects of childhood cancer and its treatment. *In* Pizzo PA, Poplack DG (eds): Principles and Practice of Pediatric Oncology, 2nd ed. Philadelphia, JB Lippincott, 1993:1091–1114.
2. Carter MC, Thompson EI, Simone JV: The survivors of childhood solid tumors. Pediatr Clin North Am 38:505–526, 1991.
3. Copeland DR: Neuropsychological and psychosocial effects of childhood leukemia and its treatment. CA 42:283–295, 1992.
4. DeLaat CA, Lampkin BC: Long-term survivors of childhood cancer: Evaluation and identification of sequelae of treatment. CA 42:263–282, 1992.

ANEMIA AND WHEN TO TRANSFUSE

CYNTHIA F. NORRIS, M.D.
STEVEN E. MCKENZIE, M.D., Ph.D.

The need for a red blood cell (RBC) transfusion depends on the clinical presentation, laboratory parameters, and suspected diagnosis. Questions that need to be answered before an RBC transfusion is given include

- What is the hemoglobin level? Is it accurate?
- Is the patient symptomatic, or has he compensated for the degree of anemia?
- Is there ongoing blood loss?
- Are laboratory values consistent with RBC destruction or decreased bone marrow production?
- Is the disease process one in which *giving* an RBC transfusion could make things worse?

INDICATIONS

The most important factor to consider when deciding whether to give an RBC transfusion is the clinical appearance of the child. Signs or symptoms of hypovolemia or circulatory failure indicate a need for prompt intervention. The child may complain of dizziness or fatigue. Ominous physical findings include hypotension, tachycardia, pale, cool, or mottled skin, prolonged capillary refill, decreased or absent peripheral pulses, and a cardiac gallop. The neonate may have difficulty feeding or be sleeping excessively. These signs and symptoms tend to develop in the child who has experienced a *rapid* drop in hemoglobin. Since the body has not had time to compensate, prompt restoration of the hemoglobin or blood volume or both is essential to maintain tissue oxygenation and perfusion.

Sometimes anemia is discovered before the patient becomes symptomatic. If the anemia is moderate to severe and the hemoglobin is continuing to fall (secondary to ongoing blood loss, decreased bone marrow production, or continued RBC destruction), an RBC transfusion should be considered, as the patient's red cell reserve is low. The decision to transfuse will depend on the child's baseline hemoglobin (which varies with age) and how rapidly the hemoglobin is continuing to fall. *In an asymptomatic child there is no absolute hemoglobin level at which an RBC transfusion is always indicated.*

Blood loss may result from an obvious injury or trauma or may be subtle, as in occult gastrointestinal bleeding. Stool should be checked for the presence of blood as part of the overall evaluation of anemia if the etiology is unclear. The reticulocyte count is typically elevated if the blood loss is chronic and iron stores are sufficient but may not be affected in the acute setting.

Anemia resulting from decreased bone marrow production may be isolated to the RBC line (Diamond-Blackfan syndrome or transient erythroblastopenia of childhood) or may be a component of pancytopenia (aplastic anemia or leukemia). The reticulocyte count is inappropriately decreased for the degree of anemia, and bone marrow examination may reveal an erythroid maturational arrest.

Anemia resulting from hemolysis (RBC destruction resulting in increased RBC production by the bone marrow) may also require transfusion. The hemolysis can be caused by a problem intrinsic or extrinsic to the RBC. Intrinsic causes of hemolysis include RBC membrane, enzyme, or hemoglobin disorders. Extrinsic causes of hemolysis include immune-mediated hemolytic anemia (HA), microangiopathic HA, and drug-induced or infection-induced HA. The patient may be jaundiced, and laboratory evaluation reveals an elevation in the unconjugated bilirubin level. Other byproducts of RBC destruction (urobilinogen) also can be found in the urine.

Although RBC transfusions may be indicated for many symptomatic hemolytic anemias, there is one exception: the child suspected of having an undefined antibody-mediated hemolytic anemia. Giving an RBC transfusion to such individuals may cause further RBC destruction, resulting in worsening of the anemia and precipitation of renal failure. Direct and indirect Coombs testing will help with this diagnosis.

In summary, the *symptomatic* child with anemia requires prompt treatment with an RBC transfusion to prevent heart failure and restore adequate tissue oxygenation. Asymptomatic children with a low hemoglobin who have evidence of ongoing blood loss, continued RBC destruction, or decreased to absent bone marrow production are also at high risk and should be followed closely. If there is no indication that the primary process is resolving, an RBC transfusion should be seriously considered, since the red cell reserve is low. In both instances, there is usually time to talk to a hematologist or the blood bank. Both can help guide the decision about the need for an RBC transfusion.

Certain diseases are commonly associated with the need for an RBC transfusion. Patients with aplastic anemia or leukemia are followed by a hematologist or oncologist. Others who have severe iron deficiency anemia are followed by a primary care physician. In almost all instances, however, the initial presentation is to the primary care physician. Table 1 lists some common conditions that require RBC transfusion.

Iron Deficiency Anemia

Iron deficiency anemia is best managed with oral iron replacement therapy. Current treatment guidelines recommend 6 mg/kg/d of elemental iron to be given in three divided doses. Intravenous iron is available (although rarely used primarily because of the risk of anaphylaxis) for the child unable to comply with oral therapy. Intramuscular iron is available but not recommended. Patients who are clinically symptomatic from their iron deficiency are the exception to this rule. These individuals should receive an RBC transfusion in addition to iron supplementation. (See also earlier discussion of iron deficiency anemia in this chapter.)

Sickle Cell Disease

Sickle cell disease (SCD) has many associated complications that require RBC transfusion. In the acute setting of a cerebral vascular accident (CVA) or severe acute chest syndrome (ACS), prompt intervention with an RBC transfusion is necessary to decrease the percentage of sickle hemoglobin, thus slowing the process of infarction and improving oxygenation to ischemic tissue. Splenic sequestration crisis can cause a rapid drop in hemoglobin in an individual whose baseline hemoglobin is only 8 or 9 g/dl. Aplastic crisis secondary to human parvovirus B19 infection can also quickly result in severe anemia, given the shortened RBC lifespan in sickle cell patients. Both scenarios may dictate intervention with an RBC transfusion if the

---

TABLE 1. Conditions That May Require RBC Transfusions

1. Severe iron deficiency anemia
2. Sickle cell anemia
   a. In acute setting of stroke, severe acute chest syndrome, severe splenic sequestration, aplastic crisis, or priapism
   b. In chronic setting for patients with a history of stroke, recurrent severe vasoocclusive crisis, recurrent acute chest syndrome, recurrent splenic sequestration, or recurrent priapism
   c. Before elective surgery
3. Thalassemia (Cooley's anemia)
4. Hereditary spherocytosis, hereditary elliptocytosis, and other RBC membrane disorders in the setting of aplastic crisis secondary to human parvovirus B19 infection
5. Bone marrow failure syndromes (aplastic anemia, Fanconi's anemia)
6. Bone marrow infiltration syndromes (leukemia)
7. Chemotherapy-related anemia
8. Neonatal anemia
   a. Symptomatic anemia from blood loss (phlebotomy, abruptio placentae), decreased RBC production, or increased RBC destruction (ABO or Rh disease)
   b. Anemia with respiratory disease (especially if on O_2 or ventilator)
   c. Growth failure (controversial)
9. Acute hemorrhage due to
   a. Trauma
   b. Gastrointestinal bleeding
   c. Underlying bleeding disorder
   d. Surgery (intraoperative or postoperative)
   e. Pulmonary hemosiderosis

---

patient is symptomatic from anemia. (See also earlier discussion of sickle cell disease in this chapter.)

Certain individuals with severe or recurrent complications of SCD benefit from a chronic transfusion program aimed at reducing their percentage of hemoglobin S. A list of these complications can be found in Table 1. Data on the duration of transfusion therapy indicated for these conditions are sparse. A hematologist should be involved in the care of these individuals.

A final indication for RBC transfusion in the child with SCD is before elective surgery. The aim is to reduce the percentage of sickle hemoglobin to <30% to decrease ACS and other postoperative complications. How to do this best is under investigation.

Thalassemia

Children with beta-thalassemia major (Cooley's anemia) require a chronic transfusion regimen to improve tissue oxygenation and suppress erythropoiesis. The benefits include improved growth and development, decreased stress on the heart, decreased hepatosplenomegaly, fewer bony deformities, and decreased gastrointestinal absorption of iron. Most centers aim to maintain a minimum hemoglobin level of 10 to 12 g/dl during childhood but will accept lower levels (9 to 10 g/dl) after the pubertal growth spurt is complete. Without chronic transfusion therapy, these children will die early of heart failure or inanition. (See also earlier discussion of thalassemia in this chapter.)

RBC Membrane Disorders

Children with RBC membrane disorders have a hemolytic anemia that frequently results in a baseline hemoglobin level of 8 to 11 g/dl. When these children contract parvovirus B19, which infects RBC progenitors, RBC production can cease. The resulting aplastic crisis can cause significant anemia. If the child is symptomatic or signs of bone marrow recovery are absent (reticulocyte count of zero or absence of nucleated RBCs on the peripheral smear), an RBC transfusion should be considered.

Bone Marrow Failure or Infiltration Syndromes

Bone marrow failure syndromes (aplastic anemia, Fanconi's anemia) and syndromes in which the bone marrow is infiltrated (leukemia) result in varying degrees of anemia. RBC transfusion will not correct the underlying process but is indicated for supportive care. Transfusions enable individuals with such syndromes to have a relatively normal activity level and help to prevent cardiac failure. RBC transfusions are also useful in the individual whose bone marrow is suppressed from chronic or intensive chemotherapy.

Neonates

Neonates comprise another group of individuals who sometimes require RBC transfusions. Neonates primarily develop anemia as a consequence of

- Acute perinatal blood loss (abruptio placentae)
- Hemolytic anemia (ABO or Rh incompatibility)
- Phlebotomy-related blood loss
- Rare congenital anemias

All these etiologies may result in a symptomatic anemia that requires RBC transfusion. Anemic neonates with respiratory disease also benefit from RBC transfusions to improve tissue perfusion and oxygen delivery. A target hematocrit of >40% is recommended. A more controversial indication for RBC transfusion in the anemic neonate is growth failure. Some studies report improved growth with RBC transfusion therapy, whereas other studies report no benefit.

Acute Blood Loss

Individuals with acute blood loss need RBC transfusions to correct their anemia and hypovolemia. The cause of the bleeding needs to be identified promptly and corrected. If blood loss is severe, a coagulopathy may develop secondary to loss of platelets and other clotting factors. Plasma concentrate (fresh frozen plasma and cryoprecipitate) and platelet transfusion should be considered if bleeding persists and laboratory values measuring hemostasis (PT, PTT, fibrinogen, and platelet counts) are abnormal.

Occasionally, a child will have signs and symptoms of circulatory collapse secondary to massive ongoing blood loss. There may not be time to obtain a type and crossmatch. In this situation, transfusion of an O-negative unit of whole blood or packed red blood cells (PRBC) is appropriate. *In all other circumstances, ABO and Rh-compatible blood should be given to avoid the possibility of an alloantibody-mediated transfusion reaction.* Following this practice avoids significant patient morbidity and mortality.

BLOOD PRODUCTS AVAILABLE

Whole Blood

Whole blood may be used in cases of acute blood loss where signs of hypovolemia exist, especially if more appropriate products are not available. Fresh whole blood is recommended for exchange transfusion and following open heart surgery with cardiopulmonary bypass in infants.

Packed Red Blood Cells

PRBC are prepared by centrifuging a unit of whole blood and retaining the cellular layer. Consequently, varying numbers of white blood cells (WBC) and platelets also may be found in a unit of PRBC. PRBCs are the component of choice for treatment of most pediatric anemia, especially in cases of RBC underproduction or nonimmune-mediated destruction.

Frozen Deglycerolized Packed Red Blood Cells

Fresh RBC can be frozen using the cryoprotectant glycerol. When ready for use, they are thawed and deglycerolized by washing, which removes 92% to 95% of the WBCs. Freezing red cells is useful for patients who have been multiply transfused and have developed several alloantibodies, making the selection of red cells difficult. A reserve can be maintained by freezing. Frozen deglycerolized packed cells are also used in some centers for neonatal transfusion, since small

alliquots of a single unit can be frozen, limiting donor exposure. In addition, freezing eliminates the risk of CMV transmission.

Washed Red Blood Cells

RBCs can be washed to remove plasma proteins that cause allergic transfusion reactions. Any child with a history of an *allergic transfusion reaction* should receive washed RBCs. An allergic transfusion reaction is characterized by hives and wheezing. It should not be confused with a *febrile transfusion reaction*, which is caused by the body's response to WBC by-products.

Cytomegalovirus (CMV)-Negative Products

Transfusion of CMV-negative products will decrease the risk of CMV disease in the susceptible host. CMV status is determined by screening the donor unit for CMV antibody. CMV-negative products are indicated for use in low birth weight infants (<1200 g) and in all CMV-negative immunocompromised patients.

Irradiated Products

Irradiation of any blood product with >2500 cGy will inactivate donor lymphocytes and prevent them from proliferating once transfused into the recipient. Irradiation is necessary to prevent the development of graft-versus-host (GVH) disease in a recipient with a deficiency in cell-mediated immunity. Absolute indications for the use of an irradiated product include

- Bone marrow transplant recipients
- Low birth weight (<1200 g) infants
- Children with known or suspected T cell deficiency syndromes (DiGeorge syndrome, severe combined immunodeficiency syndrome, Wiskott-Aldrich syndrome)
- Patients receiving directed donor blood from a biologic relative.

Relative indications include

- Cancer patients receiving chemotherapy or radiation therapy
- Neonates receiving intrauterine transfusion or subsequent transfusion after birth (regardless of birth weight)
- HIV-positive individuals

Leukofiltered Products

Leukocyte depletion filters used at the time of infusion of RBC will remove >99% of donor leukocytes. Indications for the use of a WBC filter include

- Patients who have a history of febrile nonhemolytic transfusion reactions
- Patients on chronic transfusion protocols as prophylaxis against alloimmunization
- Patients who require frequent RBC transfusions to prevent HLA sensitization (thereby decreasing the risk of platelet refractoriness)
- Patients awaiting organ transplantation for whom HLA sensitization should be avoided.

TECHNIQUE OF RBC TRANSFUSION

How much blood to give is always the first question. As a guideline, 3 ml/kg of PRBC should raise the hemoglobin level 1 g/dl. Children whose hemoglobin level is >5 g/dl and who are not symptomatic can tolerate 10 ml/kg of PRBC over 3 to 4 hours. If the hemoglobin level is <5 g/dl or the child has symptoms of heart failure, PRBC volumes of 3 to 5 ml/kg over 4 hours would be more appropriate.

Children whose anemia developed gradually need to be monitored for signs of fluid overload during and after receiving their PRBC transfusion. A diuretic, such as furosemide at 0.5 to 1 mg/kg IV up to 10 mg, may be necessary. A repeat CBC performed at least 1 hour after the transfusion has finished will help guide the decision about the need for additional transfusion therapy. If the expected rise in hemoglobin has not occurred, evidence of ongoing blood loss or RBC destruction should be sought. If the patient is still symptomatic at the current hemoglobin level, additional transfusion should be considered.

ALTERNATIVES AND ADJUNCTS TO TRANSFUSION THERAPY

Recombinant Human Erythropoietin (rHu-EPO)

Erythropoietin is a glycoprotein hormone that stimulates erythropoiesis. It is produced by recombinant DNA technology. Erythropoietin therapy has proven beneficial in patients with anemia of prematurity and anemia resulting from chronic renal disease. Other forms of chronic anemia may also benefit from EPO therapy. Current clinical trials are addressing this issue. There is no role for EPO in the management of acute symptomatic anemia. Patients receiving erythropoietin should be given iron supplements to prevent the development of iron deficiency anemia.

Steroids, Intravenous Gamma Globulin (IVIG), Splenectomy, and Immunosuppressive Agents

Steroids, IVIG, splenectomy, and immunosuppressive agents are all treatment strategies to consider in the child who presents with an autoimmune hemolytic anemia. A hematologist can help guide the management of these children's anemia.

Iron Therapy

Iron replacement is necessary for an individual with iron deficiency anemia. There are two main reasons for the development of iron deficiency anemia—decreased iron intake (nutritional) and increased iron loss secondary to blood loss. Anemia resulting from either etiology will benefit from iron therapy.

EXCHANGE TRANSFUSION

Exchange transfusion is a process whereby whole blood is removed from a patient and replaced with either donor whole blood or components. The exchange can be full (involving the entire blood volume) or partial. The process functions to remove a substance (antibodies or nondialyzable poison) or to replace RBCs. Anemia-related conditions that may require an RBC exchange transfusion include

- Severe anemia with heart failure and euvolemia (enables one to bring up the hemoglobin level quickly)
- Severe hyperbilirubinemia of the newborn (especially secondary to Rh incompatibility)
- Sickle cell patients with CVA or severe ACS or before emergent surgery
- Sickle cell patients on chronic transfusion therapy who have problems with iron overload (who cannot or will not chelate)
- Polycythemia and hyperviscosity (phlebotomy is another alternative)

The procedure can be performed manually or automatically. The first pass through an automated pheresis machine is 78% efficient at removing antibody and replacing RBCs. A second pass increases the efficiency to 90%. Additional passes do not substantially alter the outcome. A hematologist should guide the pheresis procedures.

ADVERSE REACTIONS TO BLOOD TRANSFUSION

MARTIN T. FOSBURG, M.D.

Although concern about AIDS has raised fears about the safety of blood transfusion to unprecedented levels, transfusion therapy is measurably safer now than at any time in the past. The development of tests to identify blood donors carrying hepatitis C, the major cause of non-A, non-B hepatitis, the increasing sensitivity of screening tests

for other transfusion-borne infections, the refinement of donor selection procedures to achieve an ever healthier donor pool, and the development of filters to allow widespread use of leukocyte-depleted blood products have all contributed to this progress. Despite these advances, transfusion therapy will never be risk free.

The best way to prevent side effects of transfusion therapy is to avoid or minimize transfusion. Over the past decade, indications for transfusion of red blood cell, plasma, and platelet products have been critically reviewed and, in many instances, made more stringent. Automatic transfusion at a given hemoglobin concentration or platelet count is no longer acceptable medical or surgical practice. Transfusion should never be used to correct a laboratory value but instead to prevent or reverse specific clinical problems resulting from lack of one or more elements of blood. Since each component of banked blood (red blood cells, granulocytes, lymphocytes, platelets, plasma, and citrate anticoagulant) has potential side effects, patients should be transfused with the minimal necessary amount of the required component(s).

It is, perhaps, a sign of the times that confrontation with a frightened patient or irate parent is often the first adverse consequence of ordering a blood product. It behooves the physician to educate himself or herself sufficiently to anticipate and answer the concerns likely to be raised by patients and their families.

TRANSFUSION REACTIONS

About 5% of transfusions are associated with some form of reaction. These are separated into three broad categories: hemolytic, febrile nonhemolytic, and urticarial, although there is considerable overlap among them in etiology, symptoms, and therapy.

Hemolytic Reactions

Hemolysis results from the interaction between antibodies in the recipient plasma and antigens on the surface of transfused red blood cells. These antibodies have two sources. Naturally occurring antibodies, such as those to blood groups A and B, are developed in response to exposure to bacterial antigens. After infancy, immunocompetent individuals will have sufficient titers of anti-A or anti-B to provoke intravascular hemolysis with transfusion of ABO-incompatible blood. Alternatively, antibodies may develop in response to transfusion of red blood cells with antigens not found in the recipient. Up to 15% of chronically transfused patients may develop antibodies to minor (neither ABO nor Rh) blood group antigens.

Pretransfusion testing to prevent hemolytic transfusion reactions includes ABO and Rh typing of donor and recipient red blood cells, screening donor and recipient plasma for red cell antibodies, and performing a crossmatch, that is, mixing recipient serum and donor red blood cells. These tests are sufficiently sensitive that when hemolytic reactions do occur, they almost invariably result from clerical errors: either improperly labeling patient or donor specimens or giving a blood product to the wrong patient. Such errors are very rare because of the rigid rules regarding handling specimens in the blood bank and patient identification before blood administration. Most instances of blood going to the wrong patient happen in such settings as the operating or emergency suites, where the rules may be broken in crisis situations.

The clinical signs of an acute hemolytic reaction may include fever, chills, nausea, emesis, dyspnea, anxiety, chest/abdominal/back pain, tachycardia, hypotension, shock, and anuria. In anesthetized or critically ill patients, the initial symptoms may be bleeding and shock. The symptoms are due to antibody-antigen interaction, with consequent complement activation. Since the diagnosis of hemolysis usually is not immediately apparent from the clinical symptoms, laboratory confirmation is essential. The differential diagnosis includes another type of transfusion reaction, coincident sepsis, and transfusion of blood contaminated with bacteria. Laboratory findings confirming hemolysis include anemia, spherocytosis, hemoglobinemia, hemoglobinuria, a positive Coombs' test and, in some cases, hypofibrinogenemia (DIC).

Therapy is aimed at preventing/reversing shock and establishing urine flow. Consumption coagulopathy is first treated by stopping the transfusion, thereby removing the precipitating factor. Fresh frozen plasma, cryoprecipitate (for fibrinogen), and platelet concentrates are administered as needed to correct coagulation abnormalities. The use of heparin (bolus of 100 U/kg, followed by an infusion of 10 to 15 U/kg/h) in patients with DIC should be reserved for those with persistent bleeding despite blood product support or those who otherwise deteriorate with supportive care alone.

Delayed Hemolytic Reactions

These relatively rare reactions are seen in multiply transfused and multiparous patients. A patient previously sensitized to minor red cell antigens may have antibody titers below the level necessary for detection if there has been a sufficient interval since the transfusion. Following a subsequent transfusion, an anamnestic response occurs. In about a week (3 to 14 days), sufficient antibody is produced to cause hemolysis. The clinical signs and symptoms associated with an immediate reaction are generally absent. The usual presenting symptom is unexplained anemia, which may be profound, sometimes accompanied by fever and elevated bilirubin. The diagnosis is confirmed by a positive Coombs' test and identification of a new red cell antibody. The only way to make the diagnosis is to be aware of this entity and order a repeat Coombs' test when a multiply transfused or multiparous patient develops unexplained anemia following transfusion. Frequently, delayed hemolytic reactions occur in patients with concurrent bacterial or viral infection.

Febrile Nonhemolytic Reactions

The occurrence of fever (>2° F over baseline), chills, and diaphoresis within minutes to hours following onset of transfusion is most often caused by a reaction between antibodies in the host and leukocyte (and, less often, platelet or plasma protein) alloantigens in the blood product. Since formation of these antibodies requires prior exposure, only multiply transfused (and multiparous) patients are at risk. Such reactions are common with platelet transfusion and almost universal with granulocyte transfusion. Many patients chronically transfused with packed red blood cells will also develop febrile reactions. *Febrile, nonhemolytic reactions can be entirely prevented or lessened in severity by administering white blood cell-depleted red cell products and platelet concentrates. Since the vast majority of nonhemolytic reactions to blood transfusion are associated with leukocytes, the use of leukocyte-poor blood products is highly desirable, even in patients likely to need even relatively short-term transfusion therapy.*

Washing red cells dilutes the plasma 1:600 but leaves 10% of the original white cells. Frozen, deglycerolized red cells retain only 1/ 1×10^6 of the original plasma and <1% of the white cells. Third generation red blood cell and platelet leukofilters, which can be used in the blood bank or at the bedside, produce a 3 to 4 log reduction in total white blood cells, granulocytes, and lymphocytes. Platelets may be leukocyte depleted also by differential centrifugation. Of the available methods for leukocyte removal, filtration is the simplest, least expensive, and most effective.

Although the cause of most febrile, nonhemolytic transfusion reactions has been assumed to be due to reactions between leukocytes in blood products and antileukocyte antibodies in recipients, recent data (1993–1994) suggest that some proportion of these reactions is due to cytokines (in particular interleukin 6, tumor necrosis factor alpha, interleukin 1 beta) contained in the plasma of stored blood products. These cytokines, some of which are known pyrogens, are synthesized and released by leukocytes during storage. The evidence implicating cytokines in febrile nonhemolytic reactions includes the correlation between high blood product cytokine levels and a febrile reaction, the fact that both cytokine levels and the incidence of febrile reactions increase with time of blood product in storage, and the failure of leukocyte removal to prevent all episodes of febrile transfusion reactions. Leukocyte depletion remains highly effective for preventing

febrile reactions. However, the use of blood products with short storage times as well as methods to remove plasma from blood products (by utilizing washed platelet concentrates or either washed or frozen deglycerolized blood cells) may prove beneficial in those patients who continue to have reactions despite leukocyte depletion and premedication.

The symptoms of febrile reactions range from a minor elevation in temperature to a syndrome of high fever, rigors, pain, dyspnea, and hypotension. Transfusion-associated acute lung injury (TRALI) is a rare but serious problem caused by a reaction between white blood cells and granulocyte antibodies. The antibodies are usually, but not always, of donor origin. The resulting circulating immune complexes lead to complement activation, granulocyte deposition and degranulation in the pulmonary circulation, and endothelial damage, with increased capillary permeability eventuating in a clinical syndrome similar to adult respiratory distress syndrome (ARDS). Clinical symptoms, including dyspnea, chest pain, hypoxemia, hypovolemia, hypotension, and pulmonary infiltrates on x-ray, usually arise within 6 hours of transfusion. The diagnosis is confirmed by the presence of granulocyte antibodies.

The likelihood and, to a certain extent, severity of febrile reactions are related to the number of white cells in the transfused product and the rate of transfusion. Granulocyte transfusions have such a high incidence of moderate to severe febrile reactions that pretreatment with narcotics, acetaminophen, and steroids is routine in many centers. The problem is magnified by the fact that recipients of granulocytes are often critically ill before transfusion. Granulocyte transfusions must be given slowly, and patients must be very closely monitored.

Urticarial Reactions

Urticaria can be seen with the first transfusion a patient receives. Allergy to a protein in the donor plasma is often suspected but rarely proven. Reactions are seen with fresh frozen plasma, intravenous gamma globulin (IV IgG), less often with cryoprecipitate, and rarely with factor concentrates. Reactions to albumin are extraordinarily rare. These reactions vary in severity from a single small wheal to life-threatening urticaria with upper airway obstruction or anaphylaxis. Where possible (i.e., with red cell transfusion), such reactions can be prevented by the use of plasma-poor products.

Patients with anaphylactic reactions to plasma or plasma products should be tested for IgA deficiency and receive IgA-depleted plasma products. About 1 in 650 persons either lack IgA or have antibody of limited specificity and thus form anti-IgA when exposed to plasma or IgA-containing plasma products, such as some types of IV IgG.

The distinction between allergic and febrile reactions is not absolute. Patients with allergic reactions may have fever and chills, whereas those with febrile reactions may have manifestations of urticaria.

TREATMENT OF TRANSFUSION REACTIONS

The initial treatment of all transfusion reactions is symptomatic and directed to the specific symptoms present and their severity. In all cases, the transfusion should be stopped immediately. In patients with minimal symptoms (e.g., a slight fever or appearance of one wheal), the transfusion may be resumed after the physician has examined the patient, reviewed the situation (including the patient's previous transfusion history), determined that a serious reaction is not occurring, and administered appropriate therapy. Even then, the patient should be observed carefully, and the transfusion should be restarted at a slow rate. If the symptoms are moderate or severe, the transfusion is stopped, and the remaining blood product, along with freshly drawn patient blood and urine specimens and a written description of the incident, is returned to the blood bank. (If facilities are available at the bedside, the urine is dipsticked for blood, a spun hematocrit is obtained, and the supernatant plasma is examined for evidence of hemolysis.) With these samples, the blood bank can quickly determine (1) that this was the correct unit for the patient,

(2) whether hemolysis has occurred, and (3) if there is a new antibody in the patient's serum or coating the red blood cells. Thereby, both hemolytic reactions and clerical errors may be identified.

Mild febrile reactions may require no treatment or respond to oral or rectal acetaminophen. Moderate or severe reactions with fever, rigors, and pain respond to a combination of acetaminophen and opiates. Morphine 0.1 mg/kg IV over 3 to 5 minutes (or other parenteral opiate) is the treatment of choice to reverse or prevent rigors. Opiates should not be used if there are severe urticarial symptoms or hypotension. Pulmonary reactions to leukoagglutinins may be lessened in severity or prevented by pretreatment with low-dose steroids, for example, hydrocortisone 1 mg/kg IV. Patients with established TRALI generally require ventilation and aggressive fluid therapy, with close monitoring of central venous and pulmonary wedge pressures. High-dose methylprednisolone (25 to 50 mg/kg IV, followed by 2 to 4 mg/kg/d divided q6h until recovery) may accelerate recovery.

Mild to moderate urticarial symptoms are best treated with oral or intravenous diphenhydramine (Benadryl) 1.25 mg/kg (or other H$_1$-blocker) given slowly through a large-bore IV. It can cause considerable pain and burning if pushed rapidly into a small peripheral vein. If symptoms are more severe, methylprednisolone 2 mg/kg IV is added. Patients with persistent symptoms 1 hour or more after treatment with parenteral H$_1$-blockers and steroids may benefit from the addition of an H$_2$-blocker, such as ranitidine 1 mg/kg given by slow (5 min) IV infusion. Patients with recurrent urticaria with transfusion can be pretreated with these agents. Since steroids have a delayed onset of action, premedication should be given 45 to 60 minutes before transfusion.

Life-threatening urticarial and anaphylactic reactions with upper airway obstruction, bronchospasm, or shock require emergency treatment. Aqueous epinephrine 1:1000 0.01 ml/kg (max: 0.5 ml) IM is given immediately and may be repeated 5 to 10 minutes later. Methylprednisolone 2 mg/kg IV push should be given immediately after the first dose of epinephrine. If there is good response, epinephrine hydrochloride (SusPhrine) 0.005 ml/kg SC (max: 0.3 ml) is then given. If bronchospasm persists, aminophylline 6 mg/kg IV is given over 15 minutes, followed by an infusion of 1 mg/kg/h. In life-threatening allergic reactions, antihistamines play a subsidiary role and may be administered only after epinephrine, steroids, and aminophylline for persistent urticarial symptoms. Early treatment with epinephrine is the key to stopping these reactions before refractory complications develop.

Severe reactions characterized by hypotension and some combination of fever, rigors, urticaria, pain, nausea, and emesis may be due to intravascular hemolysis, severe allergic reactions, or sepsis from transfusion of contaminated blood. The initial treatment is aimed at restoring the circulation, preventing shock, and maintaining urine output. If there is any symptom suggesting urticaria or anaphylaxis, epinephrine should be administered as described. Normal saline 20 ml/kg over 3 to 5 minutes is given for hypotension and may be repeated once if there is an inadequate response. Methylprednisolone 2 mg/kg IV is administered simultaneously. If hypotension persists, a central venous catheter is essential for guiding further therapy. If the central venous pressure (CVP) is <4 to 6 mm Hg, further volume repletion with crystalloid, colloid, or red cells is necessary before administration of pressors or diuretics. When venous pressure is restored, dopamine 5 µg/kg/min (or other pressor) can be started. If the arterial pressure and CVP are adequate but the patient has not voided, a single dose of mannitol 200 mg/kg IV over 3 to 5 minutes or furosemide 1 mg/kg IV push may be used to induce diuresis. (Renal failure in this setting is due to shock or complement activation, both resulting in decreased renal perfusion.) If anuria persists despite restoration of the circulation and diuretic therapy, dialysis may be needed.

Patients who spike high fevers with rigors with transfusion should have blood cultures drawn and broad-spectrum antibiotics administered (e.g., vancomycin 50 mg/kg and ceftazidime 50 mg/kg, both IV) within a maximum of 15 minutes, unless there is a compelling reason not to do so (such as a history of similar reactions). Delay in initiating administration of antibiotics can make the difference between an uneventful recovery and shock, multiple organ failure, and death in patients with bacterial sepsis from contaminated blood or other causes.

All settings where transfusions are administered should have the indicated medications and materials immediately at hand (including antibiotics) and personnel trained so that drugs can be located, drawn up, and administered without delay. A chart listing medications and dosages, kept near to hand, can prove invaluable in an emergency.

BACTERIAL CONTAMINATION

Blood products may be contaminated by bacteria introduced at the time of collection. The most common pathogens in platelet concentrates, which are stored at room temperature, are skin flora. Enteric organisms, such as *Pseudomonas cepacia* and *Yersinia enterocolitica*, which can grow in the cold and use citrate as a carbon source, are found in red blood cell products. Although as many as 0.4% of red blood cell or platelet units test positive by culture, the risk of bacterial contamination resulting in clinical sepsis is considerably lower, about 1/15,000 units of platelets in one study. Time in storage is an important risk factor, and maximal storage time for platelets was reduced from 7 to 5 days because of the excessive risk of bacterial infection in units stored longer than 5 days. The symptoms (which include pallor, fever, rigors, pain, emesis, and hypotension) usually appear after a latent period of about 30 minutes. If the organism produces endotoxin, however, the symptoms are almost immediate. Transfusion of blood through an infected indwelling central venous catheter, particularly if it has been capped before the transfusion, produces symptoms identical to those found with transfusion of an infected blood product. Treatment is described previously. The diagnosis is confirmed by gram stain of a centrifuged specimen from the suspected unit and cultures of the unit, patient and access device.

CITRATE TOXICITY

Blood products are anticoagulated by the addition of citrate, which prevents clotting by binding calcium. When infused rapidly, citrate may cause acute hypocalcemia. Those products containing the most plasma (whole blood, fresh frozen plasma, and platelet concentrates) have the highest risk of producing toxicity. Citrate toxicity is seen most often in patients already prone to hypocalcemia because of small size (neonates), shock, or hepatic or renal failure who receive large amounts of citrate-containing blood products. Examples are exchange transfusion in neonates and massive transfusion of whole blood or plasma or both for acute blood loss.

The symptom complex of citrate intoxication in children is pallor, abdominal pain, and emesis, followed by hypotension and bradycardia. In anesthetized and critically ill children, hypotension and bradycardia may be the initial symptoms. The diagnosis is made by finding an ionized calcium level depressed by >25%. (Total calcium, in contrast, will be normal or elevated.) Treatment is a slow (3 to 5 min) infusion of calcium chloride 100 mg/ml (10%), 0.3 ml/kg, or calcium gluconate 100 mg/ml (10%), 1.0 ml/kg, with close monitoring of pulse and blood pressure. Too rapid administration of calcium can cause abdominal pain, hypertension, and reflex bradycardia. The calcium must be administered through a separate or well-flushed, secure intravenous setup. Patients receiving large amounts of citrate-containing blood products, particularly those who are prone to hypocalcemia, should be carefully followed by serial determinations of ionized calcium.

VOLUME OVERLOAD

Circulatory overload and congestive heart failure may result from rapid administration of blood products, particularly in patients with volume intolerance from cardiac or renal compromise. Common settings include patients with profound anemia (e.g., sickle cell patients during an aplastic crisis) and critically ill patients with cardiomyopathy and consumption coagulopathy. Such patients can receive packed red blood cells slowly (1 to 2 ml/kg/h) with close monitoring, including measurements of CVP. A diuretic (e.g., furosemide 1 mg/kg) may be administered if signs of congestive failure, such as tachypnea, respiratory distress, and hypoxemia, develop. This method is not appropriate for plasma products where more rapid transfusion is necessary. An alternative is to give plasma products or red cells by exchange transfusion. A partial exchange, replacing aliquots of patient blood with packed red cells, can rapidly raise the hematocrit. Plasmapheresis allows for the delivery of a virtually unlimited amount of red cell or plasma products rapidly without risk of volume overload.

ALLOIMMUNIZATION

Multiply transfused patients may become sensitized to HLA and other antigens found on leukocytes and platelets. HLA sensitization may preclude solid organ or bone marrow transplantation. In addition, sensitization may make patients refractory to platelet transfusions. This may lead to lethal bleeding complications in patients requiring prolonged platelet support for intensive chemotherapy or bone marrow transplantation. All such patients should receive leukocyte-depleted blood products from the time of diagnosis.

TRANSFUSION-ASSOCIATED GRAFT-VERSUS-HOST DISEASE

Transfusion of $>1 \times 10^7/kg$ lymphocytes to an immunodeficient patient can cause graft-versus-host disease (GVHD). Susceptible patients include fetuses receiving intrauterine transfusions, premature infants, those with inherited immunodeficiency, patients undergoing intensive chemotherapy or total nodal radiation, some patients with AIDS, those undergoing solid organ transplantation, and bone marrow transplantation candidates. Immunocompetent patients can get GVHD if they receive a sufficient dose of lymphocytes from HLA *identical or closely matched donors,* such as parents or siblings. All cellular blood products can cause GVHD. Once acquired, it is >90% fatal. There is no therapy. GVHD can be prevented by radiating blood products at a dose of 1500 to 5000 cGy.

PROBLEMS ASSOCIATED WITH MASSIVE TRANSFUSION

Rapid replacement of more than one blood volume is associated with several potential problems.

Citrate Toxicity

This has been discussed previously.

Alkalosis and Hypokalemia

During massive transfusion, patients may develop alkalosis from metabolism of citrate to bicarbonate. Each unit of whole blood generates 22.8 mEq of bicarbonate. In response to alkalosis, potassium moves into cells in exchange for hydrogen. It may be difficult to correct hypokalemia while the patient is alkalotic.

Dilutional Coagulopathy

A moderate drop in the platelet count frequently is associated with massive transfusion. Platelet transfusion may be indicated if the count falls to <50,000 mm³ in patients at high risk for bleeding. Stored whole blood is deficient in factors V, VIII, and XI. Massive transfusion with such blood may cause depletion of these factors.

Pulmonary Dysfunction

Microaggregates composed of leukocyte and platelet debris accumulate during storage of whole blood. Depending on the age and type of blood product transfused, a variable number of microaggregates are administered. These settle in the pulmonary capillary bed and may cause hypoxemia via alterations in pulmonary blood flow. This is avoided by transfusing through a microaggregate filter.

Hyperkalemia

The plasma potassium level of whole blood increases to >20 mEq/L by day 28 of storage. Massive transfusion of aged blood may produce acute hyperkalemia sufficient to cause cardiac arrest. Use of whole blood stored less than 7 days or packed red cells and fresh frozen plasma instead of whole blood can prevent this problem.

Hypernatremia

Fresh frozen plasma obtained from whole blood anticoagulated with citrate phosphate dextrose (CPD) has a sodium concentration of about 165 mEq/L. Acid citric dextrose (ACD) plasma, obtained via apheresis, has a sodium concentration of about 150 mEq/L. Massive transfusion with CPD plasma can cause hypernatremia. The label on the plasma bag will indicate the type of anticoagulant in use. Provision of an adequate amount of free water will ameliorate this problem.

Hypothermia

Massive transfusion of inadequately warmed blood products can cause hypothermia, particularly in neonates and other patients with temperature instability. Symptoms include chills, bradycardia, and hypotension. The use of a calibrated blood warmer will prevent this problem. Warming blood in hot water is not recommended, as it can easily overheat or underheat the blood.

AIR EMBOLUS

This problem has been rare since collapsible plastic bags were substituted for glass bottles. In a seriously ill patient, as little as 10 ml of air can cause symptoms of acute chest pain and dyspnea. Treatment consists of clamping the intravenous tube and placing the patient in a head-down, feet-up position on the left side. Careful attention to intravenous apparatus and the use of infusion pumps with pressure-sensitive alarms and automatic shutoffs can prevent accidental infusion of air.

INFECTION

Transmission of viral infection remains the most common lethal side effect of transfusion therapy. Posttransfusion hepatitis, AIDS, and cytomegalovirus (CMV) infection are responsible for most serious transfusion-related infections in developed countries.

Testing

All blood collected in the United States undergoes the following tests: hepatitis B surface antigen, hepatitis B core antibody, ALT, antibodies to HIV-1, HIV-2, HTLV-I, Hepatitis C virus, and syphilis. CMV testing is available but not legally mandated.

Posttransfusion Hepatitis
Hepatitis B

Until a generation ago, up to 30% of transfusions led to hepatitis B. The elimination of paid donors and the introduction of screening tests for hepatitis B viral antigens reduced the incidence to about 1 in 10,000 transfusions. The present risk of acquiring hepatitis B by transfusion is about 1 in 200,000. It is still possible to transmit hepatitis B if an infected person donates early in the incubation phase. Of infected persons, 10% to 15% develop chronic active or persistent hepatitis that may end in cirrhosis and liver failure. Chronic infection with hepatitis B increases the risk of hepatocellular carcinoma. Because of these serious sequelae, all patients scheduled to receive chronic transfusions should receive hepatitis B vaccine.

Hepatitis C

Previously known as transfusion-associated non-A, non-B hepatitis, hepatitis C has had an incidence of 10%. Initially asymptomatic in 70% of cases, 50% progress to chronic hepatitis and 25% to cirrhosis, portal hypertension, and liver failure. Hepatitis C has been a major cause of chronic liver disease in the United States and by far the most serious adverse consequence of blood transfusion. The virus responsible for hepatitis C was isolated in 1989, and an effective screening test was introduced soon after. All blood for transfusion has been screened for antibodies to hepatitis C since 1990. Studies have shown that the incidence of hepatitis C transmission was decreased by >90% by screening with this first-generation test. The risk in the period 1990–1992 was about 1 in 3300 units. As a second-generation test was introduced in 1992 and a third, even more sensitive, test has since been developed, the risk at present and in the near future should be even lower. Since the risk of acquiring this serious chronic illness was 1 in 10 less then 10 years ago, this represents a triumph of preventive medicine.

Acquired Immunodeficiency Syndrome

HIV-1, the human immunodeficiency virus, can be transmitted by any blood product except for certain plasma products processed by heat treatment. The risk of acquiring AIDS via transfusion peaked between 1976 and 1983. Two major strategies were developed to deal with this problem. Comprehensive donor screening was introduced in 1984 to eliminate those at high risk for the disease from the donor population. This reduced the risk by about 80%. In 1985, a screening test for antibodies to HIV was introduced nationwide. AIDS can still be transmitted by blood that has tested negative for HIV antibody if it is donated during the incubation phase of the disease. The risk of acquiring HIV by screened blood in the United States was estimated to be between 1 in 80,000 and 1 in 200,000 in the period 1989–1992. Since that time, both donor screening techniques and the antibody tests have been improved. The current risk is close to 1 in 200,000. The future is uncertain. The introduction of more sensitive tests for HIV antibody and antigen will no doubt decrease the number of infected units in the donor pool. However, if the disease spreads widely into the general heterosexual population, current donor screening procedures that focus on high-risk groups may not be as effective. HIV-2 has not been implicated in transmission by blood products. To date, it has been isolated in only 40 patients in the United States. Despite this, all blood has been tested for HIV-2 since mid-1992.

Directed donation, in which recipients bring in friends and family members to serve as their donors, was accepted with reluctance by the blood bank community in response to pressure from a public understandably alarmed by this lethal illness. A number of anecdotal reports recently supplemented by the results of a large multiinstitution study have shown the incidence of positive HIV antibody tests in directed donors to be equivalent to or higher than that of the general donor population. Further, directed donor blood has a higher incidence of positive results for each of the other donor screening tests. There is no doubt that using directed donor blood does patients a disservice. Sadly, it is unlikely that these facts will persuade many parents and patients to forego directed donation. In contrast, such programs as advance donation before elective surgery, hemodilution, and intraoperative red cell salvage actually decrease the risk of acquiring AIDS and other infections and should be encouraged.

Human T Cell Lymphotrophic Virus Type I

This retrovirus causes T cell lymphoma and leukemia, as well as tropical spastic paresis (TSP) and HTLV-I associated myelopathy (HAM). The risk of viral transmission in 1990–1992 was roughly 1 in 70,000 transfusions. A screening test for antibodies to HTLV-I has been used since 1988. Actual instances of acquiring HTLV-I-associated diseases as a result of transfusion are extremely rare and not yet documented in the United States.

HTLV Type II

Since the HTLV-I test picks up the majority of units containing HTLV-II and it was not certain that HTLV-II was associated with human disease, testing for HTLV-II has not been mandated. Recent data have revealed HTLV-II to be associated with a neuromuscular disease similar to TSP/HAM. Since nearly half of the units positive for HTLV-II are not picked up by the HTLV-I test, it is possible that HTLV-II testing will be added in the future.

Cytomegalovirus

CMV does not pose a significant threat to immunocompetent individuals. However, it can lead to lethal systemic infections in immunodeficient patients, such as low birth weight neonates and CMV antibody-negative bone marrow and solid organ transplant candidates and recipients. CMV is carried in and transmitted by leukocytes. Leukofiltration with third-generation filters prevents CMV transmission by red blood cells obtained from CMV-positive donors. It is likely that leukofiltration is similarly effective for platelet concentrates, but the final data are not yet in. Blood products from CMV antibody-negative donors do not transmit the virus. All at-risk patients should receive leukofiltered blood products or products from CMV antibody-negative donors.

Malaria

As malaria is readily transmitted by red cells from infected individuals, blood banks do not accept donors who have resided in or traveled to areas where malaria is endemic. Isolated outbreaks of malaria from transfused blood result from using the blood of donors who are unaware that they are carrying the disease. The presenting symptom usually is fever of unknown origin. The illness may be difficult to diagnose, since it is rarely considered in the differential diagnosis in areas where malaria is not endemic.

Parvovirus

This DNA virus, the causative agent of fifth disease (erythema infectiosum) in children, is transmissible via blood products. As the virus multiplies in and destroys erythroid precursors, infection poses a risk of aplastic crisis in patients with chronic hemolytic anemia who require rapid red cell production to maintian a safe hemoglobin level. There is no screening test for this agent, so the risk to transfusion recipients is not known. Parvovirus B19 should be suspected in patients who show suppressed erythropoiesis following transfusion.

Chagas Disease

An illness endemic to large areas in Central and South America, Chagas disease, due to *Trypanosoma cruzi,* inevitably will become a problem as more persons from endemic areas migrate to the United States. Both testing for *T. cruzi* and questions to identify donors likely to carry the disease may need to be added to current testing and screening procedures.

Other Infections

Epstein-Barr (EB) virus, syphilis, filariasis, brucellosis, and babesiosis are potentially transmissible via transfusion.

PROBLEMS ASSOCIATED WITH CHRONIC RED BLOOD CELL TRANSFUSIONS

Iron Overload

Iron causes dose-related damage to the skin, liver, various endocrine organs, and the heart. Each milliliter of packed red blood cells contains 1 mg of iron. Chronically transfused patients develop signs of organ damage (skin darkening, liver damage) at iron accumulations of 400 to 600 mg/kg. This is followed by insulin-dependent diabetes, pubertal failure, and growth failure. Patients die from congestive heart failure/arrhythmias at iron accumulations of greater than 1000 mg/kg. Laboratory signs of iron overload are elevated serum ferritin and fully saturated transferrin. Chelation therapy with daily 12 hour infusions of deferoxamine can prevent serious organ damage if initiated early and may partially reverse organ damage in affected patients. Since this therapy is cumbersome and expensive, alternatives to chronic red cell transfusion (erythropoietin, renal transplant, bone marrow transplant) should be pursued.

Hypersplenism

Chronic red cell transfusions will lead to hypersplenism in some proportion of patients. The mechanism is not fully defined. Hypersplenism may lead to a shortened survival of transfused red cells, thus increasing transfusion requirements, as well as causing leukopenia and thrombocytopenia. Splenectomy may be needed to normalize transfusion requirements or, rarely, to correct symptomatic cytopenias.

MEASURES TO AVOID REACTIONS

With currently available technology, many transfusion-related adverse effects can be prevented or minimized. Transfusion should be avoided or minimized, but if it is necessary, autotransfusion via predonation, intraoperative salvage, or hemodilution should be used where possible. When banked blood is needed, the patient should receive only the needed component(s). Medical and nursing staff should be educated in the diagnosis and treatment of transfusion reactions. Patients receiving blood products should be observed closely, and the transfusion should be stopped and appropriate therapy administered at the first sign of a reaction. Leukocyte-depleted blood products should be used for all chronically transfused patients and those with a history of previous adverse reactions. Appropriate precautions as outlined here should be taken when giving blood products to immunosuppressed patients and during massive transfusion.

BONE MARROW TRANSPLANTATION

CHARLES S. AUGUST, M.D.

The first successful bone marrow transplants (BMTs) were reported simultaneously in 1968 in a child with severe combined immunodeficiency disease (SCID) and a second with Wiskott-Aldrich syndrome. Since then, allogeneic BMTs with histocompatible sibling donors have been carried out in increasing numbers of congenital disorders of blood cell number and function, congenital and acquired marrow aplasia, lysosomal storage diseases, acute and chronic leukemias, myelodysplasia, and many solid tumors. Table 1 lists those diagnoses about which there is a consensus in recommending BMT and those diagnoses for which BMT is frequently carried out but for which the indications are less clearly defined. The latter transplants are best undertaken in the setting of clinical research.

From the genetic standpoint, three types of marrow transplants are performed. *Allogeneic* BMT is transplantation of marrow from a genetically dissimilar donor of the same species. Until recently, this usually has been an HLA-identical sibling. Because of a desire to offer BMT to a larger number of patients who might benefit from it, BMTs with HLA-identical unrelated donors, as well as partially mismatched related and unrelated donors, have been attempted. *Autologous* BMT is the transplantation (reinfusion) of a patient's own previously harvested marrow. *Syngeneic* BMT is transplantation of marrow from an identical twin.

HISTOCOMPATIBILITY REQUIREMENTS

At first, BMT was restricted to siblings who were histocompatible, defined as donor and recipient possessing identical HLA-A and B (class I) antigens, and unreactive in the mixed lymphoycte culture (MLC) test. Now, serologic testing for DR and DQ (class II) antigens and molecular biologic tests (DNA typing using oligonucleotide probes) have almost replaced the MLC. At present, related donors identical at all but one HLA antigen may be used in BMT for the leukemias. Parent-to-child transplants (haplotype mismatched) are performed routinely for children with SCID after removing T-lymphocytes from the marrow to prevent lethal graft-versus-host disease (GVHD).

The existence of computerized registries of volunteer marrow donors whose HLA types are known offers another alternative for needy patients who lack HLA-identical family members. Such registries exist in many countries of the world, and information about the

TABLE 1. Indications for Allogeneic Bone Marrow Transplantation with HLA-Identical Sibling Donors

Consensus Indications
Severe combined immunodeficiency disease*
Wiskott-Aldrich syndrome
Malignant infantile osteopetrosis
Growth factor-resistant congenital cytopenias
Therapy-resistant leukocyte function defects
Severe acquired aplastic anemia
Fanconi's anemia (constitutional aplastic anemia)
Myelodysplastic syndromes, preleukemia (monosomy 7)
Chronic myelogenous leukemia: juvenile and adult-types
Familial hemophagocytic lymphohistiocytosis
Beta-thalassemia when chelation is not possible

Frequent Indications
Acute lymphoblastic leukemia†
   First remission with Philadelphia chromosome, 4;11, and 8;14 translocation
   Second remission and beyond
Acute nonlymphoblastic leukemia (myelogenous, myelomonocytic, megakaryoblastic, erythroblastic)
   First remission and beyond†
Neuroblastoma, metastatic with poor prognosis
Non-Hodgkin's lymphoma, recurrent or refractory
Hodgkin's disease, recurrent after 2 treatment modalities

*Also parent to child.
†Most, but not all, pediatric oncologists favor BMT in first remission for patients with ANLL and in second and subsequent remissions for children with ALL. See references.

existence of matched unrelated donors (MUD's) may be obtained rapidly from most marrow transplant centers. *As of April 1994, the U. S. National Marrow Donor Program had registered 1.2 million volunteer donors.*

Matched unrelated donor transplants are being performed by experienced transplant teams for all of the common indications for BMT. The results of these transplants are somewhat poorer than the results of BMTs from related donors because of a higher incidence of graft rejection and GVHD. Another disadvantage is the long time required for identifying an appropriate donor (average 5 to 6 months). *Thus, when a BMT is indicated and no related donor is available, a search for an unrelated donor should begin early.* Such transplants are best performed in a research setting.

ABO-mismatched transplants may be carried out simply by removing red cells or plasma from the nucleated marrow cells depending on the direction of the mismatch. The ultimate hematopoietic stem cell does not have enough A or B substance on its surface to be destroyed by anti-A or anti-B isohemagglutinins.

PREPARATION FOR BMT

Children with SCID accept allogeneic grafts because of their congenital immunoincompetence. All other BMT recipients require preparative treatment. This treatment is intended (1) to assure acceptance of the graft, that is, to establish immunologic tolerance, (2) to cure the underlying disease, for example, acute leukemia, and (3) to create space in the recipient's marrow for the donor marrow cells to reside. *Achieving durable engraftment becomes more difficult if recipients have been multiply transfused with blood products before BMT. This is especially so if family members have been used as donors.* It is thought that such transfusions expose future BMT recipients to transplantation antigens—especially the so-called minor histocompatibility antigens—that may be shared by their eventual marrow donors. *Thus, it is recommended that family members not be used as donors of blood products* and that, once the indication for BMT has been established, the transplant be carried out as soon as possible. Of the three tasks, the second is the most difficult, especially when the underlying disease is neoplastic.

In general, preparative treatments for BMT may be divided into three levels of intensity. The preparation for patients with aplastic anemia is least intense. This usually consists of a near lethal dose of cyclophosphamide, combined with cyclosporine or antithymocyte globulin (ATG). Preparation for patients with leukemia in remission is intermediate. It may consist of near lethal chemotherapy added to a lethal dose of total body radiation (TBI) or two drugs both given in near lethal doses, for example, busulfan and cyclophosphamide. The most intensive treatment in pediatric BMT is given to children with relapsed leukemia, progressive solid tumors, or leukemia where the donors are other than HLA-identical siblings. This may involve multiple drugs, at least one of which will be given in a near lethal amount, and TBI. An example of this is a treatment for advanced neuroblastoma consisting of cisplatin, teniposide, high-dose melphalan, and TBI. The short-term and long-term toxicities of each class of preparative regimens differ. Some commonly used preparative treatments are summarized in Table 2.

AUTOLOGOUS BMT

Autologous BMT is primarily a rescue technique enabling oncologists to increase the doses of anticancer drugs or radiation or both to levels that are lethal to the hematopoietic and lymphoid systems. Marrow is obtained from patients before or after recovery from chemotherapy and is stored frozen. After patients have been treated with supralethal courses of chemotherapy, the marrow cells are thawed, then reinfused. Hematopoietic stem cells obtained from peripheral blood are also used effectively for hematopoietic rescue both alone and together with marrow cells. Although developed primarily for use in adults, this therapy is now beginning to be applied to small children.

In children, autologous BMT has been studied mostly in metastatic neuroblastoma and less often in lymphomas and Hodgkin's disease, Ewing's sarcoma, rhabdomyosarcoma, and brain tumors that have relapsed or are otherwise resistant to conventional therapy. In general, a requirement for attempting BMT in these patients is that the tumors respond to alkylating agents or radiation. Recently, several techniques have been developed for removing leukemia cells from marrow, thus permitting autologous BMT to be extended to the acute leukemias.

The advantages of autologous BMT over allogeneic BMT include freedom from the requirement for a histocompatible donor and the absence of graft rejection and GVHD. The disadvantages of autologous BMT include the possibility that the marrow contains tumor cells and the necessity of removing (or purging) them and the absence

TABLE 2. Commonly Used Preparative Regimens for Bone Marrow Transplantation

Acquired Aplastic Anemia (Newly Diagnosed, Minimally Transfused)
Cyclophosphamide 50 mg/kg/d × 4 d

Acquired Aplastic Anemia (Multiply Transfused)
Cyclophosphamide 50 mg/kg/d × 4 d
Antithymocyte globulin 30 mg/kg/d × 3 d *or* TBI 300 cGy *or* total lymphoid radiation 750 cGy

Acute Leukemia/Chronic Leukemia/Myelodysplasia
Cyclophosphamide 60 mg/kg/d × 2 d
Fractionated TBI 1200–1400 cGy (200 cGy b.i.d. × 6 or 7 d)
or
Cytosine arabinoside 3 g/m² per dose q12h × 12 doses
Fractionated TBI 1200–1400 cGy (200 cGy b.i.d. × 6 or 7 d)
or
Cyclophosphamide 50 mg/kg/d × 4 d
Busulfan 1 mg/kg q6h × 4 d

Neuroblastoma
Melphalan 140 and 70 mg/kg/d
Cisplatin 30 mg/m²/d × 4 d
Etoposide 100 mg/m²/d × 4 d
Fractionated TBI 333 cGy/d × 3 d

TABLE 3. Preventive Measures To Reduce the Incidence of Complications of Bone Marrow Transplants

EVENT	PREVENTIVE MEASURE
Malnutrition	Intravenous hyperalimentation
Acute radiation toxicity	Fractionate TBI, shield lungs or other organ if necessary
Early infection	Oral, nonabsorbable antibiotics, antifungals, ± laminar air flow unit and sterile environment
Aspergillus infection	HEPA filtration of air supply
GVHD	Low-dose methotrexate × 100 d *or* low-dose methotrexate × 11 d + cyclosporine × 6 months *or* cyclosporine ± prednisone × 6 months
Transfusion-associated GVHD	Radiate all transfused blood products to 2000–3000 cGy
Pneumocystis carinii pneumonia	Trimethoprim-sulfamethoxazole 20 mg/kg/d* × 10–14 d before BMT, 5 mg/kg/d thrice weekly starting 10 weeks posttransplant
Herpes simplex reactivation	For seropositive patients, acyclovir 250 mg/m² q8h daily day +3 to day +21
Cytomegalovirus disease	Seronegative blood products, leukocyte-depletion filters, IV IgG 400–500 mg/kg weekly for 4 months if donor or recipient is seropositive

*Dose of trimethoprim.

of a graft-versus-tumor effect. In addition, some techniques for removing tumor cells from marrow appear to prolong the time required for full hematopoietic reconstitution.

Whether autologous BMT is experimental or not often depends on the stage of the disease being treated. It is well established that supralethal chemoradiotherapy followed by autologous BMT has salvaged *some* children with recurrent or progressing solid tumors who otherwise would have died. Thus, its use in that setting is not experimental. Whether autologous BMT is the best treatment for children with poor prognosis tumors who have achieved complete remissions is not clear. Protocols testing this approach are being studied in children with a variety of tumors, including metastatic neuroblastoma, Ewing's sarcoma, rhabdomyosarcoma, non-Hodgkin's lymphoma, and some brain tumors.

COMPLICATIONS

Historically, the outcome of BMTs has been determined by whether or not a number of potentially fatal complications have occurred. These include early infections, the acute toxic effects of the preparative regimen, graft rejection, acute or chronic GVHD, interstitial pneumonia—especially that caused by *Pneumocystis carinii* and cytomegalovirus (CMV)—and recurrence of the original disease.

Children, particularly very young children, tolerate chemoradiotherapy well, seldom reject their marrows, and infrequently develop severe GVHD. The administration of TBI in fractions rather than as a single dose has markedly reduced regimen-related acute toxicity. Prophylactic measures and transfusing blood products from donors who are uninfected by CMV have minimized mortality from CMV disease. A number of these strategies are listed in Table 3. At present, the survival of children who have undergone BMT is determined largely by whether or not the underlying disease has been cured. The quality of that survival is determined primarily by whether the children have chronic GVHD and secondarily by the cumulative toxicities of all the therapies received in the course of the disease.

Graft-Versus-Host Disease

GVHD may be defined as an attack by immunologically competent T lymphocytes directed against foreign transplantation antigens expressed on the cells of an immunologically incompetent host. *GVHD occurs most frequently in the context of clinical BMT but has also occurred following transfusions containing live lymphocytes to immunologically immature premature infants, to patients receiving immunosuppressive chemotherapy or x-ray therapy, to patients with congenital or acquired immunodeficiencies (e.g., SCID and AIDS), and very rarely to a normal person.* In the last instance, it is believed that, by chance, a critical matching of HLA antigens has occurred such that the recipient (host) has not recognized the donor lymphocytes as foreign, thus allowing them to survive and cause GVHD.

GVHD may be acute, defined as developing within the first 100 days, or chronic, developing thereafter. Acute GVHD is an acute mononuclear cell inflammatory reaction that targets skin, gastrointestinal tract, liver, and, when intact, the bone marrow. Severity is graded by the extent of damage to the skin, liver, and gastrointestinal tract (Table 4). Grade II–IV GVHD occurs in approximately 10% to 25% of transplants in children under 10 years of age and 25% to 40% of transplants in children ages 11 to 21 years. In BMTs using alternate donors, these percentages approach 60% to 90%. Grade IV GVHD is usually fatal.

Patients with acute GVHD greater than grade II require treatment. Prednisone or intravenous methylprednisolone may be given in divided doses of 2 to 4 mg/kg/d for 5 to 7 days and subsequently tapered when the patient responds. If there is no response or the patient worsens during treatment, high-dose bolus prednisolone may be given in doses of 750 to 1000 mg/m²/d for 5 days. ATG in doses of 10 to 15 mg/kg/d may be given daily or every other day for 7 doses if necessary. *Caution should be exercised if the patient has received a previous course, since ATG is horse protein, and serum sickness or other severe allergic reaction may result from a second exposure.*

Chronic GVHD most often occurs in patients who have survived acute GVHD, but it also may occur de novo. Its features include both focal and generalized scleroderma, sicca syndrome involving salivary and lacrimal glands and other mucous membranes, malabsorption, hepatic fibrosis, and many laboratory features of autoimmunity. Muscles, serosal surfaces, lungs, and esophagus are less frequently involved. Overwhelming infection with pyogenic bacteria occurs, and both hypogammaglobulinemia and functional hyposplenism have been observed. The pathogenetic mechanism common to most all of the involved organs is chronic mononuclear cell inflammation that progresses to fibrosis.

Treatment for chronic GVHD is reserved for patients with extensive disease. Prednisone and cyclosporine are given together or on alternate days in the lowest doses required to control the disease. Azathioprine, cyclophosphamide, or procarbazine (all at 1.5 mg/kg/d) may be added if necessary. Prophylactic therapy with trimethoprim-sulfamethoxazole, oral nystatin, vigorous oral hygiene, artificial tears and saliva if necessary, and sun-blocking agents also are essential elements of therapy. In spite of aggressive treatment, long-term survival of children with extensive disease is only 20% to 30%.

RESULTS OF BMT IN CHILDREN

Accurate outcome data are by no means available for all of the BMTs that are currently being undertaken in children. However, when an HLA-identical family member is used as donor, the 3-year disease-free survival may be expected to be 70% to 80% in children with aplastic anemia, 55% to 65% in children with acute lymphoblastic leukemia (ALL) in second remission and acute nonlymphoblastic leukemia (ANLL) in first remission, and 95% in SCID. In SCID, survival with T lymphocyte-depleted HLA-nonidentical marrow (usually from a parent) is approximately 60%.

The results of autologous BMT for leukemia are as yet immature, but for ANLL in first remission and ALL in second remission, the 3-year disease-free survival will probably be in the range of 30% to 50%. Whether this is better than that achieved with conventional therapy is being addressed in a series of studies sponsored both by the Pediatric Oncology Group and the Children's Cancer Group.

Results of allogeneic BMT from alternate donors (matched unrelated, partly mismatched related, and unrelated) are just beginning to be reported. In general, the outcomes are complicated by an increased incidence of graft rejection and late graft loss, as well as more frequent and more severe GVHD.

LATE EFFECTS AND QUALITY OF LIFE

There are now a growing number of children who have survived hitherto fatal illnesses because they have had BMTs. Some information about the late effects of BMT on such children has begun to appear.

Growth appears to change minimally after BMT for aplastic anemia (the least intensive preparative therapy employed) except in children with chronic GVHD undergoing prolonged treatment with steroids. After BMT for leukemia, there is a modest decrease in growth that is exaggerated in those children who develop chronic GVHD. Children cured with the most intensive preparative therapies grow very slowly and after a few years can usually be differentiated from their peers by virtue of their small size. Growth hormone deficiency has occurred in a substantial percentage of children with leukemia who received cranial radiation in addition to their transplant-associated TBI. Thyroid dysfunction is common in children who have received local radiation to the neck in addition to or as part of their pretransplant treatment.

CNS function may be adversely affected in patients who have BMT after cranial radiation. Leukoencephalopathy has been observed in 7% of such patients. In a pilot study evaluating school performance, children transplanted without additional CNS radiation performed as well as their siblings. Cataracts occur in about 80% of patients prepared for BMT with single-dose TBI. Only 20% of patients receiving either fractionated TBI or no TBI develop cataracts. Chronic steroid therapy accelerates cataract development.

Exercise tolerance is reduced in the survivors of BMT and appears to be more related to cardiac than to pulmonary dysfunction. Resting heart and lung functions tend to be normal. However, chronic GVHD or the development of interstitial pneumonitis significantly impairs lung function thereafter.

Gonadal damage occurs in almost all patients prepared for BMT with busulfan and cyclophosphamide, as well as with TBI-containing regimens. Virtually all patients who survive BMT for leukemia are destined to be sterilized. By contrast, retention of fertility is common after BMT for aplastic anemia. The late effects of BMT on the gonadal

TABLE 4. Clinical Grading of Acute Graft-Versus-Host Disease

GRADE	SKIN	LIVER	GASTROINTESTINAL TRACT	PERFORMANCE
I (mild)	Maculopapular rash <50% BSA*	0	0	100%
II (moderate)	Rash or erythroderma 50%–100% BSA	Bilirubin <3 mg/dl	Diarrhea <600 ml/m²/d	80%–100%
III (moderately severe)	Generalized erythroderma	Bilirubin 3–15 mg/dl	Diarrhea >600 ml/m²/d	<80%
IV (severe)	Erythroderma and desquamation	Bilirubin >15 mg/dl	Diarrhea >600 ml/m²/d + pain, ileus	↓ BP and shock

Modified from the Seattle grading criteria for use in children. In Glucksberg H, Storb R, Fefer A et al: Clinical manifestations of graft-versus-host disease in human recipients of marrow from HLA-matched sibling donors. Transplantation 18:295–304, 1974.
*BSA, body surface area.

development of children who have been transplanted early in life have yet to be reported.

Because patients undergoing BMT are exposed to mutagenic drugs and radiation, endure long periods of immunosuppression, and develop GVHD and viral infections, it is not surprising that they develop second tumors. In addition, some individuals who may be genetically predisposed to develop cancer or leukemia in the first place may develop a second malignancy if they are cured of the first. Three types of secondary malignancies have been reported: (1) leukemic relapses in donor cells, (2) viral-associated tumors, for example, Epstein-Barr virus-associated lymphomas, and (3) solid tumors and leukemias. The risk of developing second tumors after BMT is greater than that after conventional therapy and much greater than in the general population. Reliable estimates of these risks are just now beginning to emerge.

Finally, one must realize that late effects are cumulative and that children undergoing BMT for cancer and leukemia late in the course of their diseases will experience a summation of the late effects of both the conventional and BMT-related therapies they have received. This fact provides a strong rationale for performing BMT early in the course of a patient's illness. Moreover, late effects may be related not just to the antineoplastic therapies but to antimicrobial and immunosuppressive treatment as well. Such late adversities, as well as the inherent risks of the transplant itself, emphasize the importance of unbiased, comprehensive discussions of benefits and risks that lead to informed consent.

REFERENCES

1. D'Angio GJ, Sinniah D, Meadows AT, Evans AE, Pritchard J (eds): Practical Pediatric Oncology. London, Edward Arnold, 1992.
2. Green DM, D'Angio GJ (eds): Late Effects of Treatment for Childhood Cancer. New York, Wiley-Liss, 1992.
3. Johnson FL, Pochedly C (eds): Bone Marrow Transplantation in Children. New York, Raven Press, 1990.
4. Pinkel D: Bone marrow transplantation in children. J Pediatr 122:331–341, 1993.
5. Whedon MB (ed): Bone Marrow Transplantation: Principles, Practice, and Nursing Insights. Boston, Jones & Bartlett, 1991.
6. Weinstein HJ, Rappeport JM, Ferrara JLM: Bone marrow transplantation. *In* Nathan DG, Oski FA (eds): Hematology of Infancy and Childhood, 4th. ed. Philadelphia, WB Saunders Co, 1993.

Spleen and Lymphatic System

INDICATIONS FOR SPLENECTOMY

FOUAD M. HAJJAR, M.D.
HOWARD A. PEARSON, M.D.

There are a number of indications for splenectomy. However, because of the recognition of the syndrome of overwhelming post-splenectomy infection (PSI), patients should be evaluated individually regarding the necessity and timing of the operation. Because the incidence of PSI is highest in infancy and early childhood, whenever possible, the operation should be deferred until the child is at least 6 years of age.

The indications for splenectomy can be divided into medical and surgical categories.

MEDICAL INDICATIONS

Congenital Hemolytic Anemias

Hereditary spherocytosis and hemolytic elliptocytosis are related to abnormalities of spectrin, an important constituent of the red blood cell membrane. These diseases are manifested as chronic hemolytic anemias, and many patients with well-compensated hemolysis are totally asymptomatic. Removal of the spleen completely corrects the hemolysis, although the membrane defect persists. Early splenectomy (before age 6 years) should be considered only in children with severe anemia that affects growth and activity. Splenectomy may prevent cholelithiasis and the rare aplastic crises.

Certain severe, nonspherocytic hemolytic anemias (pyruvate kinase deficiency) are improved—although not usually cured—by splenectomy.

Immunohematologic Disorders

Splenectomy may be indicated for children with very severe or chronic immunohematologic disorders, notably idiopathic thrombocytopenic purpura (ITP) and autoimmune hemolytic anemia (AIHA).

In childhood, ITP is usually self-limited, more than 90% of patients recovering within 9 to 12 months. Chronic (> 1 year duration) cases are usually cured or substantially improved by splenectomy. However, rare causes of chronic thrombocytopenia, especially the Wiskott-Aldrich syndrome, must be considered and excluded before one recommends the operation in young males.

Most cases of AIHA are very acute but self-limited. Chronic cases may benefit from splenectomy. In multiply transfused patients (e.g., those with refractory anemias, Cooley's anemia), a state of accelerated destruction of transfused red blood cells often develops. Splenectomy usually corrects this, even when the spleen is not greatly enlarged.

Staging for Hodgkin's Disease

Staging laparotomy and splenectomy are still advised for patients with stage I and II Hodgkin's disease, for whom radiation therapy is the treatment of choice. Partial splenectomy is not advocated. More extensive disease (stage III and IV) is treated primarily with systemic chemotherapy, and staging laparotomy and splenectomy are not generally employed.

Hypersplenism

The term hypersplenism is used when four elements are present: (1) peripheral cytopenia, (2) normal or increased marrow production of the affected cell line, (3) significant splenomegaly, and (4) cure after splenectomy. Obviously, a diagnosis of hypersplenism is often entertained even when all of these criteria are not met.

Patients with massive splenomegaly, as in lipidoses, especially Gaucher disease, often have low white blood cell and platelet counts. Such cytopenias may reflect increased dilution in an enlarged splenic pool rather than accelerated destruction. Therefore, splenectomy may not be indicated unless infection or bleeding is occurring. However, in massive splenomegaly, splenectomy may be indicated to relieve the considerable mechanical burden of a greatly enlarged organ.

SURGICAL INDICATIONS

Splenic Cysts

Splenic pseudocysts result from liquefaction of intrasplenic hemorrhage and most often are a result of splenic trauma. Splenic pseudocysts and rare true cysts may necessitate splenectomy because of their large size. Ultrasonography is diagnostic. Splenic malignancies other than those of reticuloendothelial origin are very rare.

Traumatic Rupture of the Spleen

Long considered an absolute indication for emergency splenectomy, traumatic injury of the spleen is now approached more selectively. Most instances of acute splenic injury can be managed nonoperatively if the patient and the hematocrit value are stable. Serial imaging studies show spontaneous repair of the lacerated spleen within 1 to 2 months. If the patient is hemodynamically unstable, splenorrhaphy or other techniques to surgically repair the spleen may obviate the need for total excision.

The risk of PSI after removal of the spleen because of trauma is low, especially in children older than 6 years of age. Splenosis subseqently develops in about 50% of children undergoing splenectomy for trauma, but the protective effect of splenosis is uncertain.

REFERENCES

1. Pearson HA, Johnston D, Smith KA, Touloukian RJ: The born again spleen. Return of splenic function after splenectomy for trauma. N Engl J Med 298:1389–1392, 1978.
2. Touloukian RJ: Splenic preservation in childhood. World J Surg 9:214–221, 1985.

POSTSPLENECTOMY SEPSIS

FOUAD M. HAJJAR, M.D.
HOWARD A. PEARSON, M.D.

Among its many functions, the spleen plays a major role in protection of the host against bacteria when the blood is infected. This role has been well documented since the first report on postsplenectomy sepsis in 1952 by King and Shumacker.

The anatomy of the spleen is unique. The spleen facilitates filtering foreign elements, such as bacteria, from the blood by phagocytosis. It also initiates the production of opsonic antibody by splenic lymphocytes.

Both the liver and spleen participate in filtration and phagocytosis. Efficient hepatic phagocytosis is opsonin dependent and requires the presence of preformed specific antibodies (IgM or IgG) and complement. The spleen, in contrast, can clear organisms effectively in the absence of specific antibody. In the nonimmune host, therefore, the spleen performs most of the filtration and phagocytic activity. In its absence, bacteria cannot be cleared effectively from the blood. As a result, overwhelming bacteremia ensues.

Severe or fatal sepsis with disseminated intravascular coagulation (DIC) in patients with functional or anatomic asplenia (postsplenectomy infection, PSI) is a well-recognized phenomenon. Although the risk of PSI is lifelong, risk is greatest in young children in the first year following surgery, probably as a result of the paucity of naturally acquired antibodies. The reason for splenectomy is another important determinant of risk. The incidence of infection is greater in patients splenectomized for an underlying hematologic or oncologic disease than in patients splenectomized for trauma. The increased risk is especially high if there is a concomitant immunologic abnormality.

The organisms responsible for PSI are, in most cases, encapsulated bacteria. *Streptococcus pneumoniae,* irrespective of serotype, causes more than half of such infections. Implicated next most often are *Haemophilus influenzae* type b (HIB) and *Neisseria meningitidis. Escherichia coli, Pseudomonas aeruginosa. Staphylococcus aureus,* and group B streptococci have caused PSI in small numbers of patients. Increased severity of malaria and of babesiosis has been described also in splenectomized patients.

IMMUNIZATION

Since *S. pneumoniae* and *H. influenzae* type b cause the majority of cases of PSI and because polysaccharide vaccines are available, immunization against infection with these organisms should be performed before elective splenectomy or immediately thereafter in cases of emergency splenectomy. These polysaccharide antigens stimulate the formation of circulating antibodies in the immunologically mature asplenic patient, although their immunogenicity in unconjugated form in infants and young children may be sharply limited. A polyvalent pneumococcal vaccine composed of the unconjugated capsular polysaccharides of the 23 capsular types responsible for approximately 90% of invasive pneumococcal infections is available. Children under 2 years of age may respond poorly to this vaccine. If a child is vaccinated before 2 to 3 years of age, revaccination may be desirable at age 6 to 8 years, although definitive evidence supporting this practice is lacking. Rarely, severe local reaction may follow revaccination of adults, but such reactions do not appear to be a problem in children.

The newly available conjugate HIB vaccine to prevent infection with *H. influenzae* type b is immunogenic in infants as young as 2 to 3 months of age. It is especially important that it be administered to asplenic children younger than 2 years of age. A booster dose of vaccine should be given at age 5.

A tetravalent meningococcal polysaccharide vaccine to prevent infection with organisms of serogroups A, C, Y, and W-135 is available (in the United States). Most of these polysaccharides are not predictably immunogenic in children younger than 2 years of age. The vaccine is recommended for asplenic patients 2 years of age and older.

It should be emphasized that there are no studies demonstrating conclusively the efficacy of these vaccines in preventing PSI. However, vaccination against the encapsulated bacteria is recommended because the vaccines are safe and the infections they are designed to prevent are often fatal.

PROPHYLACTIC ANTIBIOTICS

Prophylactic penicillin, used in patients younger than 4 years of age with the functional hyposplenism from sickle cell disease, decreases the incidence of pneumococcal sepsis by 85%. Penicillin prophylaxis is indicated for all young asplenic patients. The recommended dosage for infants younger than 6 months is 62.5 mg PO of penicillin VK, twice daily, 125 mg PO twice daily for those between 6 months and 2 years, and for those over the age of 2 years, 250 mg PO twice daily. Erythromycin may be substituted for penicillin in allergic patients.

Some authorities recommend indefinite penicillin prophylaxis in all asplenic patients. Others do not use it in children older than 6 years of age. A study in progress should determine whether prophylactic penicillin can be stopped safely in children with sickle cell disease at 6 years of age.

It is very important to apprise asplenic patients and their families about the role of the spleen and to instruct them to seek immediate medical attention for any significant febrile illnesses (temperature >102°F). Health care providers should also be aware of the possible serious significance of fever in asplenic patients.

TREATMENT OF SUSPECTED SEPSIS

Any significant febrile illness (temperature >102°F) or lower grades of fever if the patient has chills in a splenectomized patient should be taken seriously. Blood culture specimens should be obtained. *Appropriate intravenous antibiotic therapy should be instituted immediately, even before culture reports are available.* Antibiotics should be selected based on the most common pathogens and certainly should be active against pneumococci and *H. influenzae.* We recommend cefuroxime 150 mg/kg/d divided in three doses IV or ceftriaxone 50 mg/kg/d in a single dose IV.

When the patient appears ill, hospitalization is indicated. Even if not admitted, febrile patients should be closely observed for several hours after the institution of antibiotic therapy.

SPLENECTOMY, CONSERVATIVE MANAGEMENT

Splenectomies should be performed only when absolutely indicated, and, when possible, an attempt should be made to defer splenectomy in infants and younger children until a later age (older than 6 years). Pediatric surgeons have become more conservative in the management of splenic trauma and splenic rupture. It is often possible to manage these patients nonoperatively. Splenic repair, partial splenectomy, and peritoneal implantation (induction of splenosis) also have been advocated.

REFERENCE

1. Gaston MH, Verter JI, et al: Prophylaxis with oral penicillin in children with sickle cell anemia. A randomized trial. N Engl J Med 314:1593–1599, 1986.

LYMPH NODE INFECTIONS

SHELDON L. KAPLAN, M.D.

Lymphadenitis, especially in the cervical and axillary regions is encountered frequently in young children. The empiric management of lymphadenitis is dependent on the history, physical findings, and the degree and duration of illness. Acute cervical lymph node enlargement is usually related to viral upper respiratory infections that resolve spontaneously.

Staphylococcus aureus and group A streptococcus are by far the most common bacteria associated with acute suppurative cervical lymphadenitis in young children. Thus, in the absence of any clues from the history or physical examination to suggest other etiologies, treatment of acute suppurative lymphadenitis is directed against *S. aureus* and group A streptococcus. If the child is not ill, has only low-grade fever, and has only mild to moderate lymph node enlargement, an oral agent, such as dicloxacillin 25 to 50 mg/kg/d in four divided doses or cephalexin 25 to 50 mg/kg/d in four divided doses, can be initiated. Amoxicillin-clavulanate (40 mg/kg/d of amoxicillin component in three divided doses) may be more convenient to use but may be associated with more diarrhea than the other two agents. For the penicillin-allergic child, erythromycin 40 mg/kg/d in four divided doses and clindamycin 30 mg/kg/d in three divided doses are alternative agents. If the child's lymphadenitis improves within 36 to 48 hours of initiating treatment, the oral agent can be continued for a duration of 10 days.

If the child is moderately or severely ill appearing or has marked lymph node enlargement, a parenteral antibiotic should be administered. An aspirate of the lymph node for culture is optimal before starting the parenteral agent. I prefer nafcillin or oxacillin 150 mg/kg/d in four divided doses for IV therapy. Cefazolin 100 mg/kg/d in four divided doses and clindamycin 30 to 40 mg/kg/d in three divided doses are alternative parenteral agents for the penicillin-allergic child. Once the child has improved with regard to overall condition as well as lymph node size and tenderness, one of the oral agents suggested can be used to complete therapy.

Anaerobic bacteria may be associated with inflamed lymph nodes draining infections of the teeth or gingiva. In this instance, penicillin V 50 mg/kg/d in four divided doses, clindamycin, or amoxicillin-clavulanate can be administered.

Axillary lymphadenitis and inguinal lymphadenitis also usually are caused by *S. aureus* and group A streptococcus, in association with cellulitis, an insect bite, an abrasion, or some other injury to the skin. An approach similar to that outlined for routine cervical lymphadenitis can be taken for these regions.

In the neonate and young infant, group B streptococcus is an important cause of cervical lymphadenitis. A penicillinase-resistant penicillin (methicillin, nafcillin) will be appropriate for group B streptococcus as well as for *S. aureus* in this age group.

Lymph nodes from which material can be repeatedly aspirated or that develop fluctuance should be drained surgically. Moist warm dressings applied intermittently may promote localization of the infection before drainage.

In a child who has received two or more *Haemophilus influenzae* type b conjugate vaccines, *H. influenzae* type b would be a very unusual cause of cervical lymphadenitis. *Francisella tularensis* should be considered in the differential diagnosis of cervical lymphadenitis when a history of a tick bite in an endemic area is elicited. Treatment of lymphadenitis accompanying tularemia is streptomycin 30 to 40 mg/kg/d IM divided every 12 hours for 3 days, followed by 15 to 20 mg/kg/d IM divided every 12 hours for 4 days. If streptomycin cannot be obtained, gentamicin 7.5 mg/kg/d in divided doses every 8 hours is an alternative agent. Doxycycline 2 to 4 mg/kg/d PO divided every 12 hours is an alternative for older children. Therapy is provided for 10 days.

Several viruses can be associated with impressive cervical lymphadenopathy, as well as generalized lymph node enlargement. Epstein-Barr virus, cytomegalovirus, varicella, and herpes simplex are among the most common viral agents associated with lymph node hyperplasia.

Subacute or chronic lymphadenitis is more likely to be caused by agents other than group A streptococcus, although *S. aureus* may be implicated in such patients. Atypical mycobacteria most frequently associated with cervical lymphadenitis are *Mycobacterium avium-intracellulare* complex, *Mycobacterium kansasii, Mycobacterium fortuitum,* and *Mycobacterium scrofulaceum.* Medical therapy usually is not recommended in treating infections caused by these atypical mycobacteria because the standard chemotherapeutic agents generally are not active against them. Lymph nodes that are smaller than 3 cm and soft usually resolve with time. The decision to excise the infected lymph node frequently is based on the appearance of the child and the desire to avoid the development of a chronic draining sinus. Excisional biopsy of lymph nodes larger than 3 cm or associated with overlying skin changes (thinning, discoloration) is the management of choice when definitive treatment is desired. Lymphadenitis caused by *Mycobacterium tuberculosis* is treated with the routine regimens using multiple drugs (isoniazid, rifampin, and pyrazinamide).

Cat-scratch disease is another important cause of lymphadenitis and should be considered in the proper setting. *Bartonella henselae,* the etiologic agent of cat-scratch disease, is susceptible to a number of antibiotics in vitro, but it is unclear if antimicrobial therapy affects the course of lymphadenitis in this illness. Aspiration of the lymph node one or more times and warm compresses may help reduce the pain and discomfort and hasten resolution. Some patients may require surgical excision.

Most normal children with acute toxoplasmosis and cervical adenitis do not require specific therapy.

REFERENCE

1. Margileth AM: Cervical adenitis. Pediatr Rev 7:13–24, 1985.

LYMPHEDEMA

JAMES M. LEWIS, M.D.

Lymphedema is defined as chronic swelling of a body part due to the accumulation of lymph in interstitial tissues. This imbalance in lymph formation and transport may be due to maldevelopment or dysfunction of lymphatic vessels, lymph node obstuction, or chronic venous stasis.

Lymphedema is broadly classified as either primary (idiopathic) or secondary. *Secondary lymphedemas* are caused by processes that destroy or obstruct the lymphatic vessels and nodes: neoplasm (primary or metastatic), recurrent lymphangitis or cellulitis, parasitic infestation, excisional surgery, trauma, and radiation. Although the etiology of *primary lymphedema* is unknown, evidence points to an underlying developmental insufficiency that may be triggered by environmental factors. The continuum of primary lymphedemas is subdivided further by age of onset into congenital, praecox (3 months to 35 years), and tarda (greater than 35 years). *Milroy's disease* is strictly defined as familial congenital lymphedema, whereas *Meige's disease* represents familial lymphedema praecox. Primary lymphedema may be present in several genetic disorders, including Turner's syndrome, Noonan's syndrome, distichiasis-lymphedema syndrome, intestinal lymphangiectasis, and yellow nail syndrome.

DIAGNOSIS

The diagnosis of lymphedema is made clinically by careful history and physical examination. Lymphedema praecox most commonly presents as insidious, painless swelling in the lower extremity of an adolescent girl. Lymphoscintigraphy with technetium-99m (^{99m}Tc)-labeled antimony-sulfur colloid may be helpful in questionable cases to both diagnose lymphedema and differentiate primary from secondary causes. *Lymphangiograms, venograms, and biopsies are not indicated.*

TREATMENT

The treatment of secondary lymphedemas is directed toward the underlying etiologic agent. *Filariasis,* a common cause of lymphedema in tropical countries, may be treated early with diethylcarbamazine to decrease lymphangitis and prevent fibrosis. In later stages, lymph nodovenous shunting procedures may be performed to create alternate pathways for lymphatic drainage. Severe lymphedema or elephantiasis with extreme disfigurement, decreased mobility, and recurrent lymphangitis may require subcutaneous excisional procedures, such as the Charles operation.

The treatment of idiopathic primary lymphedema consists primarily of supportive measures to decrease tissue fluid, improve existing lymphatic flow, and prevent further subcutaneous fibrosis. Lymphedema, however, is a chronic disease with no therapeutic regimen available to completely restore the extremity to a normal appearance. Although diuretics have been effective in reducing edema in adults, they are not recommended for pediatric patients. The affected lower extremity should be elevated by raising the top of the bed 15 to 30 cm (6 to 12 in) at night and maintaining as often as is possible a horizontal position during the day. Exercise may improve lymphatic flow by the extrinsic compression of lymph vessels by muscle contractions and arterial pulsations. The external support of a carefully fitted high-pressure elastic stocking (Jobst) will augment this effect and prevent further accumulation of fluid. Intermittent, sequential compression of the limb by programmable pneumatic pump (Jobst, Wright Linear, Lympha-Press) in a daily regimen (used at night), combined with elastic hose, has provided dramatic improvement in selected patients. Progressive injury to lymphatics causing worsening of the edema may be prevented by the avoidance of trauma, careful hygiene of the skin and nails, and prophylaxis or vigorous treatment of bacterial or fungal infections.

There is experimental evidence that benzo-[α]-pyrene therapy reduces lymphedema and decreases secondary inflammation. This medication provides an alternative mechanism for removal of excess protein by increasing tissue macrophage proteolysis. 5,6-Benzo-[α]-pyrene, however, is not yet available for general use in North America.

Cellulitis and lymphangitis secondary to group A streptococci or coagulase-positive staphylococci are frequent complications of lymphedema. Typically, chills and fever occur, and patients may appear toxic with lethargy, headache, nausea, and vomiting. Local signs include erythema, induration, tenderness, enlargement of the extremity or lymph nodes, and red streaking. Therapy should include intravenous antibiotics, bedrest, moist heat, and analgesics. Lymphangiosarcoma is a rare, late but dreaded complication of lymphedema. The development of a violaceous lesion, especially if accompanied by ulceration or necrosis, requires prompt diagnosis by multiple deep biopsies followed by aggressive medical and surgical therapy.

Surgical treatment of lymphedema is reserved for patients with severe, progressive disease with complications who do not respond to intensive medical therapy. Because of the unpredictable course of primary lymphedema, surgery should be postponed until the full extent of the swelling is apparent or the child is older than 2 years. Procedures to debulk genital lymphedema, however, may be the exception to this rule. All surgical options have a low success rate, with frequent complications, persistent disproportion, and residual scarring.

The chronic, progressive nature of lymphedema often causes considerable family, social, and emotional problems, particularly for adolescents. Patients and parents can benefit from thorough explanations, genetic counseling if appropriate, and opportunities to express feelings and participate in therapeutic decisions.

REFERENCES

1. Casley-Smith JR, Morgan RG, Piller NB: Treatment of lymphedema of arms and legs with 5,6-benzo-[α]-pyrene. N Engl J Med 329:1158–1163, 1993.
2. Klein MJ, Alexander MA, Wright JM, et al: Treatment of adult lower extremity lymphedema with the Wright linear pump: Statistical analysis of a clinical trial. Arch Phys Med Rehabil 69:202–206, 1988.
3. Smeltzer DM, Stickler GB, Schirger A: Primary lymphedema in children and adolescents: A follow-up study and review. Pediatrics 76:206–218, 1985.

MALIGNANT LYMPHOMAS

LINDA GRANOWETTER, M.D.

Childhood lymphomas are cancers of lymphoid tissue that are classified as non-Hodgkin's lymphoma (NHL) and Hodgkin's disease. Taken together, the lymphomas are the third most common group of pediatric neoplasms, accounting for approximately 10% of all cancers diagnosed in children. NHL are tumors of lymphocyte progenitor origin and may be classified as developing from B cell or T cell origin, much like pediatric acute lymphoblastic leukemia. The cell of origin of Hodgkin's disease is still controversial. These tumors are linked by a common presentation, an enlarging mass of lymphoid tissue. They differ in that NHL, even when apparently localized, is a systemic disease at presentation as it originates from lymphoid cells destined to circulate. Usually, the clinical onset is rapid. Hodgkin's disease more often presents, as in adults, with orderly progression from one group of lymph nodes to the next contiguous group. The onset is usually more indolent. These differences in clinical presentation underlie some differences in the philosophy of treatment of these tumors.

HODGKIN'S DISEASE

Appropriate application of current treatment modalities has made successful treatment of Hodgkin's disease in children the rule; 10-year relapse-free survival rates are close to 90%. Excellent survival rates give treating physicians the luxury to design and select treatment programs for Hodgkin's disease that result in the least complications and late effects. Thus, many appropriate treatment programs exist, and there are many differing treatment philosophies. Some treatment plans require only radiation therapy (in full doses, see later), more include radiation therapy and chemotherapy (combined modality therapy), and some plans use only chemotherapy. The choice among the options is based on the patient's age and stage. For example, an adult with early stage disease is most often treated with radiation therapy alone. However, a growing child with the same stage disease is most often treated with combined modality (chemotherapy and reduced dose radiation) to avoid adverse effects on growth. This difference in treatment strategy is central and informs even the pediatric oncologist's approach to staging. In general, pediatric Hodgkin's disease patients are best treated at centers that treat children with cancer routinely and are thus sensitive to the special treatment requirements of children. Further, most such centers are associated with national treatment study consortiums. Thus, patients are offered the most up-to-date treatment programs.

Staging

The universally accepted staging system for Hodgkin's disease is shown in Table 1. Anatomic staging is denoted by stages I through IV. Letters denote the absence or presence of systemic symptoms or clarifications of the extent of disease. The first step in appropriate staging is an accurate history that emphasizes the presence or absence of systemic signs, such as weight loss > 10% in the 6 months preceding diagnosis (without dieting), fevers greater than 38°C for 3 days, or drenching night sweats. The presence of any one of these

TABLE 1. Staging Classification for Hodgkin's Disease

STAGE	DEFINITION
I	Involvement of a single lymph node region (I) or of a single extra-lymphatic organ or site (I$_E$)
II	Involvement of two or more lymph node regions on the same side of the diaphragm (II) or localized involvement of an extralymphatic organ or site and one or more lymph node regions on the same side of the diaphragm (II$_E$)
III	Involvement of lymph node regions on both sides of the diaphragm (III), which may be accompanied by spleen (III$_s$) or by localized involvement of an extralymphatic site or organ (III$_E$) or both (III$_{SE}$) III$_1$ ± splenic, hilar, celiac, portal nodes III$_2$ + paraaortic, iliac, mesenteric nodes
IV	Diffuse or disseminated involvement of one or more extralymphatic organs or tissues with or without associated lymph node involvement

No systemic symptoms = A
One or more of the following symptoms = B
  Presence of fever > 38°C for 3 consecutive days
  Drenching night sweats
  Unexplained loss of >10% of body weight in the 6 months before diagnosis

symptoms is a condition to consider a patient stage B. The absence of symptoms denotes stage A. Patients may also have pruritus or alcohol intolerance, but these symptoms do not result in the designation of stage B status. The physical examination must completely define the areas of clinical involvement, with accurate assessment of all abnormal lymph nodes and hepatosplenomegaly.

Accurate imaging is the next step in appropriate staging. Basic imaging should include chest radiograph, computed tomography (CT) of the chest, abdomen, and pelvis, and gallium and bone scanning. Magnetic resonance imaging (MRI) may be a complementary modality, particularly for delineation of abdominal and pelvic nodal areas. Gallium scanning, particularly of the chest, if positive at diagnosis, may be used to accurately follow disease. Whereas chest CT scans may remain abnormal after successful therapy, gallium scans generally become negative. Bipedal lymphangiography may be used to evaluate the presence of disease in iliac and lower paraaortic lymph nodes. However, lymphangiography is technically difficult in children, and there is a risk of reaction to the dye. Thus, this procedure is only warranted if the results will clearly influence the choice and specifics of therapy. Bone marrow aspirate and biopsy are required and may be done as part of a staging laparotomy.

Staging laparotomy that includes complete splenectomy, liver biopsy, and subdiaphragmatic lymph node sampling provides the most accurate staging. As many as one third of patients will be upstaged on the basis of surgical staging. However, the necessity of staging laparotomy is controversial because of the risks of postsplenectomy sepsis and postsurgery adhesions, which must be weighed against the benefits of such surgery. Patients with advanced disease at diagnosis will clearly require treatment with systemic chemotherapy. Thus, the usefulness of staging laparotomy is limited to patients whose protocols require radiation of all involved fields (who have equivocal imaging studies) or patients whose protocols require surgical staging. Many oncologists believe that patients who receive adequate systemic chemotherapy do not require the accuracy of surgical staging. Young children who will be treated primarily with chemotherapy and limited, if any, radiation therapy despite early stage disease most likely should not undergo staging laparotomy. Most pediatric oncologists would reserve staging laparotomy for fully grown adolescents who have clinical stage I (and occasionally stage II nonbulky) disease, who might appropriately be treated with radiation alone. In these patients, anatomic staging remains important to guide the treatment decision. If staging laparotomy is required in a female and pelvic radiation is

likely to be part of the treatment regimen, oophoropexy to move the ovaries out of the radiation field may be considered to decrease the risk of infertility. However, there is a risk of infertility after oophoropexy itself.

Treatment Programs

Radiation Therapy

Extended field radiation is therapy to all areas of known disease plus the adjacent nodal areas, involved field radiation is radiation only to areas of known disease, and total nodal radiation encompasses all nodal areas. Full-dose radiation is generally 35 to 44 Gy, and low-dose radiation is generally 15 to 25 Gy. Fully grown patients with stage I disease may be treated with extended field radiation. Some would treat patients with stage I disease confined to the upper cervical nodes with 35 to 40 Gy to the involved field alone. These patients generally have been surgically staged. Some institutions, however, will treat fully grown patients with disease confined to the high neck by clinical staging with full-dose radiation alone, as the risk of relapse is very low, and those who relapse still have high cure rates with chemotherapy used after relapse. Patients with massive mediastinal disease (I$_x$ or II$_x$)* generally benefit from radiation therapy in a program that includes chemotherapy. In children, the extensive use of full-dose radiation is limited because of the negative effects of radiation on growth of bone and soft tissue and the risk of radiation-induced late malignancies.

Combined Therapy

Combined modality therapy refers to chemotherapy plus radiation therapy. In general, the radiation dose employed when chemotherapy used is lower (15 to 25 Gy). Thus, the risk of growth disturbance and second malignancy due to radiation is decreased. Radiation programs used as part of combined modality programs usually treat the involved field only, although some regimens call for extended field or total nodal radiation. Most regimens call for radiation therapy after chemotherapy is complete, but equally successful regimens call for sandwich therapy, that is, chemotherapy followed by radiation and then completion of chemotherapy.

Chemotherapy

The classic chemotherapy regimen is MOPP: mechlorethamine (nitrogen mustard), Oncovin (vincristine), procarbazine, and prednisone. Variations of this protocol, such as COPP (substitution of cyclophosphamide for nitrogen mustard) or CVPP (cyclophosphamide, vinblastine, procarbazine, and prednisone), are also useful and may be less toxic. The primary long-term toxicities of these regimens are infertility and a risk of second malignancies due to the akylating agents employed. A newer and equally successful regimen, ABVD [Adriamycin (doxorubicin), bleomycin, vinblastine, and dacarbazine] decreases the risk of infertility and second malignancy but is associated with the risk of cardiomyopathy caused by doxorubicin and pulmonary restrictive disease caused by bleomycin. Variants of ABVD, such as ABV (deletion of dacarbazine) and ABVE (substitution of etoposide for dacarabazine), also have proven useful. Many investigators choose to limit the risk of toxicity by alternating MOPP and ABVD, thus using half as much of each regimen. Because the risk of late effects is related to cumulative dose, limiting the total dose of each agent is likely to decrease the risk of late effects. Newer regimens are being developed to further reduce exposure to agents with the risk of significant late effects. An example of such a regimen under investigation is OPPA: vincristine, prednisone, procarbazine, and doxorubicin. Combined modality used for a limited number of cycles (3 to 4 months) is appropriate for early stage disease. Advanced disease is generally treated with 6 to 12 months of chemotherapy. Several useful chemotherapy regimens are detailed in Table 2.

---

*x = bulky mediastinal disease, that is, mediastinum is more than one third of the cardiothoracic diameter.

TABLE 2. Treatment Regimens for Hodgkin's Disease

NAME	DRUGS	DOSE (mg/m²)	ROUTE	DAYS
MOPP*	Mechlorethamine (nitrogen mustard)	6	IV	1,8
	Oncovin (vincristine)	1.4 (max: 2)	IV	1,8
	Prednisone	40	PO	1–14
	Procarbazine	100	PO	1–14
COPP*	Cyclophosphamide in place of nitrogen mustard in MOPP			
	Cyclophosphamide	500	IV	1,8
ABVD*	Adriamycin (doxorubicin)	25	IV	1,15
	Bleomycin	10	IV/SC	1,15
	Vinblastine	6	IV	1,15
	Dacarbazine	375	IV	1,15
ABVE*	Etoposide in place of dacarbazine in ABVD			
	Etoposide	100	IV	1–5
OPPA*	Oncovin (vincristine)	1.5 (max: 2)	IV	1,8,15
	Adriamycin (doxorubicin)	40	IV	1,15
	Prednisone	60	PO	1–14
	Procarbazine	100	PO	1–14
MOPP/ABV	Mechlorethamine (nitrogen mustard)	6	IV	1
	Oncovin (vincristine)	1.4 (max: 2)	IV	1
	Prednisone	40	PO	1–7
	Procarbazine	100	PO	1–14
	Doxorubicin	35	IV	8
	Bleomycin	10	IV/SC	8
	Vinblastine	6	IV	8
	Dacarbazine	375	IV	1,15

*Each cycle = 1 month, repeat every 28 days.

Chemotherapy regimens given without radiation therapy have been used successfully in two settings. Patients with advanced disease have been successfully treated on 6 to 12 month programs. Patients with early stage disease have been successfully treated with 3 to 4 month chemotherapy regimens. For the rare patient under 5 years of age, chemotherapy without radiation may well be the most appropriate treatment regimen.

Relapse Therapy

Relapse in patients treated initially with radiation therapy alone has an excellent outlook when treated with chemotherapy. However, relapse after treatment with chemotherapy is more difficult to cure, particularly if relapse occurs on chemotherapy or shortly after the end of therapy. Although many patients will achieve second durable remissions on noncross-resistant chemotherapy regimens with or without radiation and some patients are salvaged with radiation therapy alone, the chance for long-term cure is diminished. New drug regimens show promise, but very high dose chemotherapy followed by autologous bone marrow rescue may be the most appropriate treatment regimen for patients in second or later remission of Hodgkin's disease.

Late Effects

Patients successfully treated for Hodgkin's disease must be monitored carefully for late effects. The risk of a second malignancy may be as high as 10% at 15 years. Myeloid leukemia in patients treated with combined modality therapy (particularly when the chemotherapy included a high cumulative dose of alkylating agents, such as nitrogen mustard, cyclophosphamide, and procarbazine) is about 4%. The highest time period of risk for secondary leukemia is 5 to 10 years after therapy is complete, and the risk of a secondary solid tumor increases over time.

Infertility is a significant late effect of therapy. Females who have received pelvic radiation are at risk for infertility as well as early

ovarian failure. Thus, women so treated should be counseled to consider relatively early childbearing if children are desired. Chemotherapy alone is less likely to cause infertility in women. Male infertility is a common late effect of chemotherapy, with the majority of males developing infertility after six cycles of MOPP, and as many as a third after ABVD. A small number of male patients will recover fertility years after therapy, but the option of sperm banking should be offered to pubertal males who are to receive chemotherapy.

Other late effects for which patients must be monitored include thyroid dysfunction after radiation therapy involving the neck, cardiac dysfunction after doxorubicin, and pulmonary disease after bleomycin. Knowledge of these late effects continues to spur interest in developing successful but less toxic treatment regimens.

NON-HODGKIN'S LYMPHOMA

An understanding of treatment strategies for non-Hodgkin's lymphoma requires the understanding that pediatric non-Hodgkin's lymphomas are similar to the childhood lymphoid leukemias. Indeed, in certain settings, the distinction between lymphoma and leukemia may be blurred. The childhood non-Hodgkin's lymphomas differ from adult lymphomas in that virtually all are considered *diffuse* according to the commonly used Rappaport classification schema. There is general concordance between histologic subtype and the cell of derivation. The large cell tumors are generally of B cell origin, lymphoblastic lymphomas are generally of T cell origin, and the undifferentiated lymphomas (including Burkitt's lymphoma) are generally of B cell origin (Table 3). Specific clinical syndromes are associated with each subtype. For example, the lymphoblastic lymphomas (T cell lymphoma) characteristically present with a rapidly enlarging mediastinal mass, bulky adenopathy, and often with massive hepatosplenomegaly. Bone marrow involvement is not uncommon. The classic presentation of an American Burkitt's lymphoma of B cell origin is a rapidly enlarging abdominal mass with ascites. Other characteristic presentations of Burkitt's lymphoma include presentation with a jaw mass, involvement of Waldeyer's ring (tonsillar lymphoma), and intussusception.

Staging and Diagnosis

The clinical staging system of childhood NHL (Table 4) considers the anatomic extent of disease and also the overall tumor burden. Initial evaluation includes history, physical examination, blood count, and chest radiograph. In some patients with rapidly enlarging mediastinal or abdominal masses, delay in diagnosis may be dangerous because of the onset of respiratory compromise and increased risk of metabolic complications. For these patients, bone marrow aspirate, spinal fluid examination, and cytologic examination of pleural, ascitic, or rarely pericardial fluid may yield a rapid diagnosis, avoiding surgical biopsy. The cells obtained may be examined for evidence of tumor chromosome and immune marker studies. If these sites do not yield a diagnosis, lymph node sampling generally is required. However, the risk of general anesthesia in a patient with a rapidly enlarging mediastinal mass is considerable, and this risk must be weighed heavily, and if possible, the tissue should be obtained under local anesthesia. If general anesthesia is used, flow-volume loops to predict the degree of airway obstruction and CT imaging to assess the caliber

TABLE 3. Histology and Immunophenotype in Childhood Non-Hodgkin's Lymphoma

HISTOLOGY	IMMUNE MARKERS
Lymphoblastic	Majority T cell may be pre-B cell (common ALL phenotype)
Undifferentiated Burkitt's lymphoma, non-Burkitt's (pleomorphic)	B cell
Large cell	May be B cell, T cell

TABLE 4. Staging System for Childhood Non-Hodgkin's Lymphoma (Murphy Staging System)

STAGE	DEFINITION
I	Single extranodal tumor, *or* a single anatomic (nodal) area with the exclusion of the mediastinum or abdomen
II	Single tumor (extranodal) with regional node involvement, *or* two or more nodal areas on the same side of the diaphragm, *or* primary gastrointestinal tract tumor (often ileocecal), with or without associated mesenteric nodes
III	Two single extranodal tumors on opposite sides of the diaphragm, *or* two or more nodal areas above and below the diaphragm, *or* any primary intrathoracic tumor (mediastinum, pleura, thymic), *or* extensive primary intraabdominal disease Any paraspinal or epidural tumor (regardless of other site[s])
IV	Any of the above with CNS or bone marrow involvement (bone marrow blasts >5% and <25%); marrow involvement >25% denotes leukemia

of the trachea are mandatory. More careful imaging studies may be deferred if it is clear that the disease is initially advanced.

Further staging studies in a stable patient should include abdominal and pelvic CT or ultrasound or both, CT of the chest if the mediastinum is involved, and bone scan. Serum chemistries, including electrolytes (particularly calcium, phosphorus, and potassium), uric acid, and creatinine, are essential, since perturbations of these indicators are evidence of high tumor burden. In addition, the serum lactate dehydrogenase is an excellent indicator of overall tumor burden and prognosis. As the NHL are generally considered systemic diseases at diagnosis, there is no need for staging laparotomy or surgery to remove tumor beyond a simple biopsy.

Initial Management

Initial management of the NHL patient must include careful attention to the metabolic status of the patient because acute tumor lysis may occur spontaneously and is hastened by the initiation of therapy. Rapid tumor lysis results in a syndrome characterized by elevated uric acid, potentially resulting in uric acid nephropathy, hyperkalemia, and hyperphosphatemia, with associated hypocalcemia. Occasionally, hypercalcemia is seen. In addition, the kidneys may be infiltrated with tumor, or large nodal masses may cause renal obstruction, contributing to the risk of renal failure. Meticulous attention to electrolyte and renal status is required before and during therapy. In some patients dialysis is required.

Initially, patients should be vigorously hydrated with twice maintenance fluids, using sufficient sodium bicarbonate to raise the urine pH to greater than 7. Potassium must not be in the hydrating solution unless severe hypokalemia is documented. If potassium is added, the serum potassium must be monitored carefully. Should the phosphorus/calcium product exceed 70, increasing the risk of calcium-phosphorus deposition in the kidney, or if symptomatic hypocalcemia occurs, it may be necessary to stop alkalinization but continue vigorous hydration. Hyperkalemia may be life threatening, and the patient must be carefully monitored by using serum chemistries and electrocardiogram to determine if the laboratory value correlates with the clinical risk. Initially, alkalinization and oral sodium polystyrene may be used to treat hyperkalemia, and glucose-insulin infusions or even dialysis may be required in extreme cases. Allopurinol in the dose of 300 to 500 mg/m²/d must be given (as one daily dose or divided b.i.d. or t.i.d.) to all patients. Oral aluminum hydroxide antacids should be used to help control elevated phosphorus levels.

Bulky disease may interfere with organ function, and this must also be critically monitored. Mediastinal masses may be associated with pleural and even pericardial effusions. Patients may present with stridor, wheezing, superior vena cava obstruction, and even cardiac tamponade. Temporary relief may be obtained by thoracentesis, which also may yield a diagnosis. Very rarely, pericardiocentesis is required

for alleviation of cardiac tamponade. Most importantly, prompt initiation of chemotherapy generally reverses these symptoms rapidly and dramatically. Thus, any patient with a significant mediastinal mass should be managed in an institution that can rapidly reach a diagnosis and initiate therapy.

In very rare instances, radiotherapy to the mediastinal mass may be required to alleviate symptoms. This is not ideal, however, as T cell lymphoma may be completely cured with chemotherapy alone. A rapidly growing abdominal mass, particularly like that occurring in Burkitt's lymphoma, may cause respiratory distress because of massive ascites, often with associated pleural effusion. Thoracentesis or paracentesis gives temporary relief and may yield the most rapid diagnosis. Chemotherapy generally gives rapid resolution of symptoms, but the patient must be fastidiously monitored and treated for metabolic derangements associated with rapid tumor lysis.

Treatment Programs

Successful treatment for childhood NHL has been accomplished by the understanding of the systemic nature of these entities and the predilection for marrow and central nervous system dissemination, as in the childhood leukemias. Treatment programs are based primarily on extent of disease and on histologic subtype. Examples of a few of the many successful treatment programs are found in Table 5.

Localized Disease

Even localized tumors, that is, stage I or II tumors, have the potential for systemic spread. Thus, they are treated with systemic chemotherapy. In the past, successful regimens generally were 6 to 8 months in duration. Recently, excellent prognosis for patients with nonlymphoblastic lymphoma treated with regimens as short as 12 weeks has been demonstrated. Radiation therapy is not indicated in patients with localized disease, and CNS prophylaxis by intrathecal medication is generally reserved for patients who have head and neck primary lesions and are thus at increased risk for CNS relapse.

Nonlocalized Disease

Patients with stage III or IV disease generally are treated with multiagent chemotherapy regimens that include intrathecal CNS prophylaxis. Treatment regimens are specific to the tumor histology, as previous studies have shown differing outcomes for histologic subtypes depending on the chemotherapy regimens employed (Table 5). Radiation therapy is not required, with the exception of craniospinal radiation for patients with CNS disease at the time of diagnosis or with overt testicular disease.

Lymphoblastic lymphoma patients respond to intensive chemotherapy regimens similar to programs devised for the treatment of high-risk acute lymphoblastic leukemia. Virtually all of these regimens include an induction period of about 4 to 6 weeks, a consolidation period of 4 to 6 weeks, and maintenance therapy to complete 18 months to 2 years. These regimens always include multiple chemotherapy agents, generally on a rotating basis. All successful regimens include intrathecal medication to decrease the risk of CNS dissemination, and craniospinal radiation is required for treatment of those patients with CNS disease at presentation. Successful regimens for the treatment of lymphoblastic lymphoma are listed in Table 5. The LSA_2L_2 regimen was one of the first successfully employed, and other simplified regimens also have proven successful. Overall, about 75% of children with lymphoblastic lymphoma will be free of disease 2 years after diagnosis, with few late relapses.

Undifferentiated Lymphoma (Burkitt's and non-Burkitt's)

Early success in the treatment of nonlymphoblastic lymphoma was achieved with the COMP regimen (Table 5), with about 60% long-term survival. Current regimens for nonlymphoblastic or undifferentiated lymphomas generally use the elements of COMP, often with the addition of doxorubicin or the addition of alkylating agents, such as ifosfamide (with etoposide) and cytarabine. All successful regimens incorporate aggressive intrathecal chemoprophylaxis against CNS dis-

TABLE 5. Childhood Non-Hodgkin's Lymphoma: Examples of Treatment Regimens

REGIMEN	INDUCTION	CONSOLIDATION	MAINTENANCE	CNS (IT) PROPHYLAXIS	DURATION	APPLICATIONS
A-COP+	Vincristine Prednisone Doxorubicin Cyclophosphamide	Vincristine Prednisone Doxorubicin Cyclophosphamide	Methotrexate 6-Mercaptopurine	Methotrexate Cytarabine Hydrocortisone	2 months / 7 months	Localized, nonlymphoblastic / Localized, lymphoblastic
LSA₂L₂	Cyclophosphamide Vincristine Methotrexate Doxorubicin	Cytarabine 6-Thioguanine L-Asparaginase Camustine	6-Thioguanine/cyclophosphamide Hydroxyurea/doxorubicin/methotrexate Cytarabine/vincristine	Methotrexate	18 months	Nonlocalized, lymphoblastic
COMP	Cyclophosphamide Vincristine Methotrexate Prednisone		Cyclophosphamide Vincristine Methotrexate Prednisone	Methotrexate	18 months (6 localized)	Nonlymphoblastic Large cell
LMB84	Cyclophosphamide* Prednisone* Vincristine* Vincristine HD methotrexate + LV Doxorubicin Cyclophosphamide Prednisone Cytarabine	HD methotrexate Cytarabine	Vincristine HD methotrexate + LV Prednisone Cyclophosphamide Doxorubicin	Methotrexate Hydrocortisone	4 months	B cell leukemia and lymphoma, excluding CNS disease at diagnosis
APO	Doxorubicin Prednisone Vincristine	Doxorubicin Prednisone Vincristine Mercaptopurine Asparaginase ±RT	Doxorubicin Prednisone Vincristine Mercaptopurine Methotrexate	Methotrexate	24 months	Large cell Lymphoblastic

*Prephase.
HD, high dose.
LV, leucovorin rescue.

ease. Current treatment regimens offer 60% to 80% long-term survival. Patients with advanced stage Burkitt's lymphoma, once believed to have a dismal prognosis, are now achieving 60% to 80% survival rates on very intensive, short (3 to 6 months) regimens. Radiation therapy is used only for overt CNS system disease or testicular disease.

Large Cell Lymphoma

Large cell lymphoma may be treated successfully with the APO regimen (Table 5), with cure rates of close to 75%. Ongoing research is designed to further improve survival by incorporating additional agents into this successful regimen. Radiation therapy is not generally used, with the exception of biopsy-proven residual tumors after chemotherapy induction.

Supportive Care

All of the chemotherapy regimens for advanced lymphoma are intensive, and patients experience periods of profound immunosuppression and myelosuppression. Transfusion support with radiated blood products is generally required. Aggressive management of fever and infectious complications is critical. Many of the aggressive treatment programs now are investigating the use of the cytokines, G-CSF or GM-CSF, to decrease the duration of myelosuppression, with the hope of decreasing infectious complications and prolonged hospitalizations. All pediatric patients undergoing lymphoma therapy should be managed at centers where there is expertise in the management of pediatric cancer and its complications.

Late Effects

Two of the potential effects on long-term survivors of non-Hodgkin's lymphoma include infertility due to the use of alkylating agents and cardiac dysfunction in patients who received doxorubicin. These are similar to those effects seen in patients successfully treated for Hodgkin's disease. In addition, second malignant tumors have been related to the alkylating agents, and secondary myeloid leukemia has

been associated with the use of epidophylotoxins (such as etoposide). As patients with NHL require CNS prophylaxis or treatment for overt disease, there is the potential of learning disabilities and other neuropsychologic sequelae. This is particularly true in young children (less than 5 years of age) who have received cranial radiation. Brain tumors as a second malignancy are a rare consequence of cranial radiation. Thus, children who have survived NHL must be monitored carefully, with particular attention to neuropsychologic sequelae.

AIDS AND LYMPHOMA

AIDS has been shown to be associated with an increased risk of NHL, particularly B cell lymphomas (undifferentiated, Burkitt's lymphoma). In addition, Hodgkin's disease may be increased in incidence in patients who have positive HIV serology or AIDS. Ongoing research is designed to determine how such patients fare on standard chemotherapy regimens. Early data indicate that pediatric patients who are HIV positive and have lymphoma may respond well to standard regimens. However, their management obviously is complicated by the incorporation of antiretroviral medication, when appropriate, and an even heightened risk of infectious complications. It is recommended that treatment centers test all newly diagnosed lymphoma patients for HIV infection so that we can learn the true incidence and course of lymphoma in HIV-infected patients.

BURKITT'S LYMPHOMA

JOHN T. SANDLUND, M.D.
WILLIAM M. CRIST, M.D.

Burkitt's lymphoma (BL), as defined by the National Cancer Institute Working Formulation, is a high-grade, small, noncleaved cell non-Hodgkin's lymphoma (NHL). It represents approximately one third of the NHLs of childhood, with large cell and lymphoblastic subtypes accounting for the other two thirds. Most patients with BL present with advanced stage disease involving the abdomen, with tumor arising from Peyer's patches in the ileocecal area. The clinical presentation often resembles appendicitis or intussusception. Extranodal primaries in the head and neck region are common.

BL is one of the most rapidly growing tumors, requiring immediate confirmation of diagnosis, staging workup, and initiation of histology-specific and stage-specific therapy.

DIAGNOSTIC WORKUP

The diagnosis of BL is made pathologically. Examination of the resected or biopsied tumor mass reveals a diffuse pattern of cells with medium-sized, round to ovoid nuclei, approximately the size of interspersed benign histiocyte nuclei (starry-sky appearance). The nuclei have prominent nuclear membranes and contain two to five prominent basophilic nucleoli, with an irregular distribution of coarse reticulated chromatin. A distinct rim of basophilic cytoplasm with prominent vacuolization is observed on cytologic preparations of ascites, pleural fluid, bone marrow, or spinal fluid. Cytogenetic analysis reveals either the characteristic [t(8;14)] or a variant [t(2;8), t(8;22)] translocation in the lymphoma cells. BL has the phenotype of a relatively mature B cell, typically with expression of B4 (CD19), B1 (CD20), B3 (CD22), and surface immunoglobulin.

STAGING WORKUP

Therapy is determined by the stage of disease at presentation, necessitating an accurate staging workup preferably performed rapidly so that treatment can commence. This should include a complete physical examination, with computed tomography (CT) scan of the abdomen and pelvis, CT of the head and neck (if involvement is detected on physical examination), bone scan, and gallium scan. A spinal tap should be performed for cytologic examination, including cell count and differential. Bilateral bone marrow aspirates and biopsies also should be performed to determine whether there is lymphomatous infiltration. If greater than 25% lymphoma cells are present in the bone marrow, the patient is considered to have Burkitt's leukemia (i.e., B cell ALL). The staging workup should be completed within 24 to 48 hours of presentation, with classification according to the St. Jude NHL system as previously described.

INITIAL MANAGEMENT

BL may be associated with life-threatening metabolic complications. Therefore, in addition to a complete blood count, serum chemistries including electrolytes, uric acid, calcium, phosphorous, and lactic dehydrogenase (LDH) should be measured as soon as possible at presentation. Uric acid-associated nephropathy is a fairly common problem, particularly in patients with a large tumor burden (LDH > 500 U/L). This condition may be exacerbated by the administration of chemotherapy, when the rapid lysis of large numbers of tumor cells results in the release of potassium, phosphate, and uric acid (tumor lysis syndrome). Thus, before chemotherapy is administered and simultaneous with the staging workup, vigorous hydration (3 to 4 L/m²/d), allopurinol administration, alkalinization of urine with NaHCO₃ (urine pH to 7), and diuresis (mannitol and furosemide) are indicated. A nephrologist should be consulted at presentation in cases of large tumor burden, in the event that dialysis is required.

TREATMENT

Role of Surgery

Surgery has a limited role in the management of BL. The only indication for surgery, other than a diagnostic biopsy, is in the case of an abdominal (ileocecal) primary tumor with or without involvement of mesenteric nodes only. If the mass can be completely resected, the patient is downstaged from a III to a II and is a candidate for less intensive therapy.

Role of Radiation

Radiation is not used routinely in the initial management of BL. It has been shown to add only toxicity. It may be considered in cases of spinal cord compression by a tumor mass. However, chemotherapy alone usually results in rapid tumor reduction. Cranial radiation has been used in the very successful French regimen for children with involvement of the central nervous system (CNS) at diagnosis. However, its use with intrathecal chemotherapy in preference to intrathecal chemotherapy alone for overt CNS involvement remains controversial.

Role of Chemotherapy

Chemotherapy is the primary therapeutic modality in the treatment of BL. It has been shown that for patients with limited stage disease, the intensity of therapy can be safely reduced without compromising cure. The most recent clinical trial by the Pediatric Oncology Group demonstrated that with three cycles of CHOP [cyclophosphamide, Adriamycin (doxorubicin), vincristine, prednisone] and weekly vincristine (7 doses), a 5-year event-free survival of greater than 90% could be achieved.

Improvement in the treatment outcome for patients with advanced stage disease has been achieved by the development of shorter (2 to 12 months) but more intensive treatment regimens. Initial strategies included the incorporation of fractionated high-dose cyclophosphamide, high-dose methotrexate with leucovorin rescue, and high dose cytarabine. Some recent protocols have included etoposide or ifosfamide or both. CNS prophylaxis and treatment with intrathecal methotrexate and cytarabine is another important component of successful treatment regimens. The French Pediatric Oncology Society has reported among the best results to date with an event-free survival (EFS) of over 90% for stages I–IV NHL and 87% (median follow-up 20 months) for patients with B cell (Burkitt's) leukemia. In the same study, they also reported a 70% EFS for those presenting with CNS disease, a group that formerly had a particularly poor prognosis.

FUTURE DIRECTIONS

Patients with BL and CNS involvement remain the worst risk group and require improvement in therapeutic approach, which may include the routine use of Ommaya reservoirs or the incorporation of new agents that can be administered intrathecally. The dramatically improved treatment outcome for patients without CNS involvement creates the challenge of reducing morbidity of therapy without compromising cure.

Patients with recurrent disease have a dismal prognosis requiring a more intensive or novel approach, which may include growth factor support or bone marrow transplantation or both.

REFERENCES

1. Magrath IT. Malignant non-Hodgkin's lymphoma. In Pizzo PA, Poplack DG (eds): Principles and Practice of Pediatric Oncology. Philadelphia, 1988.
2. Patte C, Leuerger G, Richie H, Bertrand Y, Cage C, Méchinaud F, Lutz P, Michon J, Baruchel A, Courbon B: High cure rate in B-cell (Burkitt's) leukemia in the LMB89 protocol of the SFOP (French Pediatric Oncology Society). Proc ASCO 12:317, 1993.
3. Sandlund JT, Hutchison RE, Crist WM: The non-Hodgkin's lymphomas. In Vietti T, Fernbach D (eds): Clinical Pediatric Oncology, 7th ed. St. Louis, Mosby, 1991.

9

Endocrine System

HYPOPITUITARISM AND GROWTH HORMONE THERAPY

DENNIS M. STYNE, M.D.

Growth hormone (GH) was originally extracted and purified from human pituitary glands donated postmortem. For more than 25 years, this limited source of GH was used solely to treat classic GH-deficient patients. In 1983, the use of human pituitary-derived GH was linked with Creutzfeldt-Jakob disease, which occurred more frequently in young patients previously treated with human GH. Because recombinant DNA–derived GH was in clinical trials at that time, the use of human pituitary–derived GH was eliminated and all patients in the United States were switched to recombinant DNA–derived GH. Recombinant DNA–derived GH supplies theoretically are unlimited, and new pressures arose to treat children with disorders other than GH deficiency.

DIAGNOSIS

Despite decades of study, it remains difficult to determine who is GH deficient. The classic patient demonstrating poor growth rate (below the 5th percentile on growth velocity charts or under 4 cm per year between ages 5 and 10 years), cherubic appearance, proportionate short stature, increased subcutaneous adiposity, low serum GH on secretagogue testing, and low spontaneous secretion of GH is not difficult to diagnose. However, many patients vary from this classic description, including those with late-onset growth failure because of a tumor or central nervous system radiation. This section considers only evaluation of GH secretion and not diagnosis of such neurologic disease.

Deciding which patient has inadequate GH secretion is difficult for several reasons. Random GH determinations are useless because serum GH concentrations are low much of the day in normal as well as in GH-deficient patients. Thus, stimulated GH concentrations must be considered to determine maximal GH secretion. However, standards are questionable because normal GH secretion reported in most clinical studies is based on analysis of children who are statistically short, the subjects who are most likely to undergo testing for GH deficiency. The radioimmunoassay employed to determine GH concentrations has significant influence. For example, a GH level of slightly higher than 10 µg/L, which would be considered normal in most laboratories, may be reported as a value of 7 µg/L or less by a different laboratory because of differences in assay techniques. Nonetheless, most authorities accept stimulated GH concentrations of less than 10 µg/L as abnormal.

Two tests of GH secretion are necessary to determine sufficiency or deficiency because any normal child has a 10% to 20% chance of failing to respond to one secretagogue during one test. Peak GH concentrations are measured 10 minutes after 10 minutes of vigorous exercise, and 30, 60, and 90 minutes after the start of a 30-minute IV infusion of 0.5 g/kg of arginine (maximum of 20 g), an oral dose of L-dopa (125 mg for body weight up to 15 kg, 250 mg up to 35 kg, and 500 mg over 35 kg; L-dopa usually causes nausea), or a PO dose of clonidine (0.1 to 0.15 mg/m²; clonidine causes drowsiness and possibly hypotension or bradycardia). Insulin-induced hypoglycemia by the IV infusion of a bolus of 0.075 to 0.1 U/kg push is effective but dangerous as a test of GH. This insulin tolerance test requires confirmation of a normal basal glucose before the infusion of insulin and maintenance of an available intravenous line for emergency infusion of 25% dextrose infusion if the blood glucose drops too far and causes coma or seizure. GH-releasing hormone is available for testing but, although theoretically preferable, has not demonstrated improved results over the use of the older agents above.

Alternative methods of testing for GH deficiency are proposed but not all add much to diagnostic possibilities. For example, integrated GH concentration over a 24-hour period is obtained by frequent blood sampling through an indwelling catheter without administration of a secretagogue. Alternatively, some investigators believe that frequent sampling over only the 12 hour nighttime sleep period is equally informative. In fact, such determinations of integrated concentrations of GH do not appear preferable to stimulated GH values for the diagnosis of GH deficiency.

Serum insulin-like growth factor 1 (IGF-1) concentrations are related to GH secretory status and also to age and nutritional status. Thus, whereas IGF-1 levels are diagnostically low in an older child with classic GH deficiency, they may be misleadingly low in a young normal subject or a malnourished patient. The combination of serum IGF-1 and IGF-2 determinations increases the accuracy of diagnosis, but there are patients with normal values of both factors who may still benefit from GH therapy. The measurement of IGF-binding protein-3 (IGFBP-3), a high-molecular weight protein that varies directly with GH secretory status, is a new addition to the diagnostic armamentarium. IGFBP-3 is said to differentiate GH deficiency better in the newborn and in infancy than does IGF-1, but IGFBP-3 also is sensitive to nutritional status. The measurement of GH-binding protein (GHBP), a circulating protein that has the identical sequence of the extracellular domain of the GH receptor, may offer clinical insight. Patients with GH resistance (Laron dwarfism) have low GHBP and low growth hormone cellular receptor concentration, suggesting that the serum concentration of GHBP reflects the prevalence of GH receptors. GHBP is higher in obesity whereas GH is lower, and GHBP is lower in starvation, when GH is elevated. GHBP is inversely related to body mass index (BMI). Subtle abnormalities of GHBP as related to GH secretion may indicate the etiology of the short stature of some patients according to some studies.

Thus, the diagnosis of patients with conditions other than classic GH deficiency still remains problematic. Studies of children who are significantly short (height >3.5 SD below the mean for age), with a significantly delayed bone age but normal GH secretion, show no more than a 50% chance of response to GH therapy with an increase in growth velocity. Most short children are not as severely affected and stand a lesser chance to respond to GH.

It appears that one way to determine whether a severely short child with no endocrine, systemic, nutritional, or psychosocial condition to explain decreased growth could benefit from GH is to attempt a 3- to 6-month trial period of the medication, with exacting measurements for 3 to 6 months before therapy and during treatment. Unfortunately, short-term observation of such patients does not answer the question of whether such therapy will increase their final height.

TREATMENT

GH is administered almost solely by pediatric endocrinologists. Possible side effects must be discussed with the family before therapy is initiated. Elevation of blood glucose with GH therapy is more theoretical than demonstrable, and potential local infection at the injection site is possible. Slipped capital epiphysis occurs with increased frequency in patients receiving GH, and these patients usually are thinner than the customary subject with slipped capital epiphysis. A few children and young adults previously treated with GH have developed leukemia without any predisposing cause (such as chromosomal breakage syndromes, previous tumors, or prior radiation). The incidence of such cases was so low that it could not be determined whether they were due to GH therapy, but it now appears that there is no relationship to GH therapy. GH therapy does not increase the incidence of recurrence of tumors. Most recently, two cases of pseudotumor cerebri accompanied by papilledema and headache occurred in patients taking GH. Limited evidence indicates that the condition is reversible after discontinuation of GH.

Recombinant DNA-derived GH is administered by injection with various possible doses and regimens. Subcutaneous injection has proved to be efficacious and easier and is, therefore, preferable to the older intramuscular injection technique. Dosing daily or six times per week improves growth rate over the previous three per week regimen when the total weekly dose is maintained constant. Initially, a weekly dose of 0.3 mg/kg of methionyl GH and 0.18 mg/kg of recombinant DNA-derived GH was recommended. However, doses of up to double this amount are now used in some cases of GH deficiency. The percentage gain in growth rate is less than the percentage increase in dose, and higher doses are, therefore, considerably more expensive for height achieved.

GH therapy in GH deficiency exerts greater effects in patients with younger bone ages. Thus, in the first decade of life, doubling the growth rate is often seen (e.g., 4 cm/y pretreatment, increasing to 8 to 9 cm/y after therapy), whereas during the teenage years, therapy may add only 2 cm/y to the pretherapy rate. Furthermore, growth is greater in the first year of therapy compared with that in the later periods. Long-term studies of patients treated in past decades demonstrate final heights below that expected for genetic potential, probably as a result of several factors—the combination of the limited supply of GH and mandatory periods without therapy, together with older patient ages at the time of diagnosis and onset of therapy in previous decades. Nonetheless, it appears that if GH therapy is started in the first years after birth and is administered consistently, the GH-deficient patient is likely to reach a height close to the genetic potential.

GH is being used in diagnosable conditions other than GH deficiency with some success. Patients with Turner's syndrome who received 25% increased doses of GH and showed increased growth rate and girls with Turner's syndrome receiving GH had taller final heights on the average than untreated girls with Turner's syndrome. Despite these findings, treatment of Turner's syndrome with GH is not yet routine. In several studies, patients with severe renal disease had increased growth rate when treated with GH, and GH treatment in renal disease is now officially approved by the FDA.

Other Therapy for Growth Hormone Deficiency

Other agents are used in the treatment of GH deficiency and allied conditions. Administration of growth hormone-releasing factor (GHRF) by injection, infusion, or nasal insufflation is under clinical study at several sites. GHRF will increase the growth of patients who have a responsive pituitary gland, as do most patients with idiopathic GH deficiency (idiopathic GH deficiency is considered in most cases to be the result of a deficiency of the production or release of GHRF). Patients increase their growth rate with GHRF therapy, but this form of therapy usually requires several doses a day of a medication, in contrast to GH treatment, which is given once a day. This technical difficulty, unless solved through clinical trials, might limit the ultimate utility of GHRF.

Insulin-like growth factor 1 (IGF-1) is considered to be responsible for the actual linear growth in patients who are treated with GH. Recently, IGF-1 was sequenced and cloned, and now therapeutic amounts of IGF-1 are available. Clinical studies suggest that IGF-1 will increase the growth rate of patients with Laron dwarfism who lack GH receptors and thus cannot respond to GH therapy. IGF-1 might prove ultimately to be a useful therapeutic agent in more classic types of GH deficiency as well. Patients with GH deficiency, however, lack GH-responsive IGFBPs, and the half-life of IGF-1 may be too short to allow it to be used in a convenient therapeutic manner. Thus, IGFBPs might themselves be used as therapeutic agents in the future.

It is clear that future therapy of GH disorders will be dynamic, and many new modes of therapy will be developed over the next years.

REFERENCES

1. Brown P: Human growth hormone therapy and Creutzfeldt-Jakob disease: A drama in three acts. Pediatrics 81:85, 1988.
2. Fine RN, et al: Recombinant human growth hormone treatment of children with chronic renal failure: Long-term (1- to 3-year) outcome. Pediatr Nephrol 5:477, 1991.
3. Laron Z, et al: Effects of insulin-like growth factor on linear growth, head circumference, and body fat in patients with Laron-type dwarfism. Lancet 339:1258, 1992.
4. Rosenfeld RG, Hintz FL: Growth hormone therapy in Turner syndrome. *In* Rosenfeld RG, Grumbach MM (eds): Turner Syndrome. New York, Marcel Dekker, 1990:393–404.
5. Styne DM: Normal growth and pubertal development. *In* Sanfilippo JS (ed): Pediatric and Adolescent Gynecology. Philadelphia, W.B. Saunders, 1994:20–33.
6. Styne DM: Growth. *In* Greenspan FS, Baxter JD (eds): Basic and Clinical Endocrinology. Norwalk, Conn, Appleton and Lange, 1994:128–159.
7. Underwood LE, Van Wyk JJ: Normal and aberrant growth. *In* Wilson JD, Foster DW (eds): Williams' Textbook of Endocrinology, 8th ed. Philadelphia, W.B. Saunders, 1992:1079–1138.

SHORT STATURE

Thomas Moshang, Jr., M.D.

An individual who is more than 2 standard deviations (SD) shorter than the mean for an age, sex, and ethnically matched population of normal individuals is defined as being short. Short stature is not a disease or a symptom or a sign. However, short stature is a finding that may be indicative of disease. Therapy of short stature should, therefore, be directed at the primary illness manifested by poor linear growth. It is not within the scope of this therapeutically oriented textbook to discuss the diagnostic evaluation of short stature. Rather, this section focuses on hormonal therapy of some of the more common causes of short stature.

GROWTH HORMONE THERAPY

Growth Hormone Deficiency

The classic and incontestable indication for growth hormone (GH) therapy is GH deficiency. Complete GH deficiency is not difficult to diagnose, as it is manifested by extremely slow growth, markedly delayed bone age, low levels of insulin-like growth factors (IGF), and an inadequate rise in GH levels following administration of pharmacologic GH secretagogues. However, it may be reasonably argued that, similar to other systemic disorders, GH hormone deficiency may be partial or incomplete, and human GH (hGH) treatment is, therefore, also indicated for such disorders. The definition of partial or incomplete GH deficiency includes those children who are phenotypically similar to those with complete GH deficiency but whose provocative GH tests are more marginal or whose overnight spontaneous GH levels are abnormally low. In the United States, there is general agreement that GH levels less than 10 µg/L following pharmacologic stimuli constitute inadequate responses, in view of the fact that children with incomplete GH deficiency may have a marginal rise in GH levels following pharmacologic GH secretagogues. An inadequate level of GH as determined by frequent (every 20 minutes) sampling during sleep or over a 24-hour period is recognized as GH neurosecretory dysfunction. This latter form of incomplete GH deficiency has been clearly documented in children surviving cranial radiation for cancer. It is important to remember that a child with the clinical features of complete GH deficiency with low levels of IGFs and low GH levels during frequent blood sampling is likely to be GH insufficient, even if GH concentrations following pharmacologic testing are significantly increased (i.e., >10 µg/L). The rationale for this judgment is that all factors, including physiologic tests, are consistent with GH deficiency and are more relevant than normal GH responses to pharmacologic stimuli.

GH treatment regimens for children with GH deficiency during the era of treatment with cadaveric pituitary-derived hGH were based on availability and short-term dose-response studies. In 1985, the advent and availability of recombinant GH provided uninterrupted treatment, but the use of older dosing regimens, 0.18 to 0.3 U/kg/wk, administered intramuscularly three times weekly, persisted. A number of subsequent studies evaluating dosing regimens suggested that higher doses administered more frequently were more efficacious. In the United States, the present standard doses of hGH being administered are 0.15 mg to 0.3 mg/kg/wk (equivalent to 0.39 to 0.78 U/kg/wk). There are ongoing dose-response studies in Europe and the United States evaluating the safety and efficacy of even higher dosing regimens. The present doses of hGH, however, have caused such side effects as pseudotumor cerebri not seen with older administration protocols. Further contemplated increases in hGH doses raise the possibility of inducing acromegalic changes and other side effects.

The manner and frequency of administration of hGH have evolved over the past several years. Administration by intramuscular injection was recommended to decrease the sensitization of the patient and to lessen the potential development of anti-GH antibodies. Not only is the incidence of antibodies with recombinant hGH low, but also, more importantly, growth failure due to antibodies blocking the biologic activity in GH is virtually nonexistent. This knowledge has permitted the administration of hGH routinely by subcutaneous injections, which is less painful. However, the benefit provided by this change in route of injection may have been negated by more frequent injections. Several studies indicate that the same weekly dose of hGH administered daily as compared with thrice weekly results in better growth velocity for the first several years of treatment. This differential in terms of growth velocity is less by the third year of hGH treatment. Whether final height is enhanced by more frequent or higher doses of hGH is not yet established. There is no doubt that the availability of recombinant hGH, providing uninterrupted treatment, has resulted in GH-deficient children achieving more normal final heights as compared with the era when cadaveric pituitary-derived hGH was limited and treatment was interrupted frequently because of the scarcity of hGH.

Based on such studies, the recommendations at present for hGH treatment are daily doses of 0.02 to 0.04 mg/kg SC. The patients are monitored at 3-month intervals during the first year, and the dose is adjusted according to weight gain. Bone age determinations should be monitored yearly and more frequently with signs of adolescence.

Some patients have experienced accelerated puberty and rapid skeletal maturation during adolescence, essentially negating some of the benefits of hGH treatment. Investigators are considering both increasing the dose of hGH during adolescence (a period of development during which GH levels are normally highest) and using gonadotropin-releasing hormone agonists to delay or slow puberty when undue acceleration of bone age occurs.

Although hGH therapy is relatively free of side effects, there are both minor and major concerns perhaps related to the higher dosing regimens. Occasional patients develop peripheral edema during hGH therapy, which generally will subside without therapy and without discontinuation of hGH therapy. Some endocrinologists do lower the dose or discontinue hGH temporarily. Another noted effect is an increase in nevi formation for a variable period of time, although there have been no reported cases of malignant change with proliferation of nevi. Recently, a small number of cases of pseudotumor cerebri, manifested by headache and papilledema, have occurred during hGH treatment. One patient at Children's Hospital of Philadelphia was noted to have papilledema during a routine ophthalmologic examination without any other symptoms or changes in the brain based on magnetic resonance imaging (MRI). The pseudotumor cerebri generally subsides spontaneously, although many endocrinologists will discontinue treatment temporarily. There is concern that slipped capital femoral epiphysis (SCFE) may be related to hGH treatment in some patients. SCFE seems to occur in children receiving hGH at ages younger than expected, but the association may be due to the rapid growth generally seen in the first several years of hGH treatment rather than to hGH itself.

Insulin resistance can be induced by hGH treatment. Although glucose concentrations generally remain normal, increased insulin levels have been documented. Generally, after a period of time, despite continuing hGH treatment, insulin levels decrease to normal levels. However, in several patients with insulin resistance, clinical diabetes mellitus was precipitated by continuous hGH treatment.

The most serious concern about using hGH treatment is related to the possible mitogenic properties of hGH. In 1988, Japanese investigators reported a small but significant number of hGH-treated patients who developed leukemia. An international survey of the worldwide experience of hGH-treated children revealed a higher than anticipated number (32 cases have now been reported). Statistical analyses based on patient years of hGH treatment suggest that the risk factor is increased approximately three-fold if all the cases are included. However, the largest number of leukemia cases were clustered in Japan or included children with previous malignancies or radiation or both. Several meetings, including international committees, reviewing this problem have concluded that although the risk factor for leukemia with hGH treatment may be slightly increased, the actual risk is probably minimal.

Normal Variant Short Stature

Normal variant short stature (NVSS) refers to children who are short but who are, by all indications including GH testing, normal and healthy. There are a number of ongoing trials, both in single institutions and in large multicenter studies, evaluating hGH treatment of NVSS. One such trial being conducted at the National Institute of Child Health and Development includes control subjects who are receiving placebo injections. Although all studies show initial growth response to hGH by NVSS children, final height has not been proven to be increased. In fact, studies of relatively small numbers of patients indicate that final height is not improved. The results of all of the studies taken together are still controversial, and treatment of such children should be reserved for the ongoing clinical trials still in progress.

Turner's Syndrome

Clinical trials, including a large multicenter study being conducted for more than 10 years, indicate that hGH treatment improves the stature of Turner's syndrome patients. Before hGH treatment, the data from Europe and the United States (over several generations) consistently indicated that the mean final height in Turner's syndrome is 143 cm, despite either low-dose anabolic steroids or late (after age 14 years) treatment with estrogens or both. The hGH treatment trials demonstrate an improvement in final height of approximately 8 cm as compared with historic controls. Although some of the hGH trials suggest that the combination of low-dose anabolic steroid and hGH provides better initial growth, it is not clear that there is any additional advantage in terms of final height when compared with hGH therapy alone. The dose of hGH used for treatment of Turner's syndrome is 0.055 mg/kg/d, slightly higher than the dose used for GH deficiency. There are no data to indicate the appropriate age for initiation of therapy, but the youngest girls with Turner's syndrome in the largest US multicenter study were 8 years of age. Until such data are available, waiting until age 5 or 6 years (or when growth has clearly decelerated) before initiation of hGH treatment is appropriate.

Other Conditions Associated with Growth Failure

Because of the unlimited quantities available for treatment, recombinant hGH has been used in a number of genetic and systemic disorders associated with short stature. These conditions include chondrodystrophies, Down syndrome, intrauterine growth retardation, Diamond-Blackfan syndrome, and chronic renal failure (CRF). Most of these trials have been uncontrolled and of short duration, except in CRF. In general, similar to children with normal variant short stature, children with any of these conditions seem to respond to hGH with an increase in growth velocity over the short term. However, the growth response seems to be of limited duration.

The largest trials and the best controlled studies have been the studies in children with CRF. The growth retardation associated with CRF is particularly severe and emotionally devastating. The growth response to hGH has been significant, and 5-year data show continued significant growth. There is some concern that hGH treatment has accelerated renal failure in some patients. Although final height outcome in CRF is not yet established, the emotional improvement in many of these children supports continued study of hGH treatment in CRF.

GROWTH HORMONE–RELEASING HORMONE (GHRH) AND GROWTH HORMONE–RELEASING PEPTIDES (GHRPs)

GHRH

Pituitary GH production and release are regulated by GHRH and somatostatin. Hypothalamic dysfunction is the basis of GH deficiency for many GH-deficient children, especially those who received cranial radiation and also those with idiopathic and genetic variants of GH deficiency. Several trials with GHRH have shown improved growth in those children with hypothalamic GH deficiency. At present, GHRH still must be administered by subcutaneous injection and has the additional disadvantage of requiring multiple doses per day. Because GHRH is a much smaller molecule than GH, the potential possibility is that other routes of administration (oral or intranasal) would permit multiple dosing without injections and provide a more physiologic form of treatment.

GHRP

Several peptides, not known to be physiologically natural, have demonstrated GH-releasing properties similar to GHRH. These are called growth hormone-releasing peptides (GHRP). The intriguing aspect of these small molecules is their potential clinical use via other routes of administration. One such GHRP has been demonstrated via intranasal administration to cause GH release similar to levels achieved by intravenous administration in human adult volunteers. The safety and efficacy of these peptides over the long term have not yet been completely evaluated. The use of GH-releasing substances, including GHRH, must still be considered experimental.

INSULIN-LIKE GROWTH FACTOR 1 (IGF-1)

Growth Hormone Resistance Syndromes

Since the original description by Laron, a number of families with inherited GH resistance have been observed. These patients are phenotypically similar to those with GH deficiency but have normal to elevated basal and stimulated GH levels. The defect resides in the GH receptor, and biochemically, these patients are diagnosed by the low levels of GHBP (which is identical to the extracellular domain of the GH receptor) and low levels of IGF-1. Because of this defective or absent GH receptor, these patients are clinically and biochemically unresponsive to exogenously administered hGH. Several patients with this syndrome have been treated with IGF-1 and have demonstrated improved growth and anabolic biochemical changes similar to those achieved with hGH treatment. The use of IGF-1 is still in the earliest phases of clinical trials, and some of the side effects have included hypoglycemia and, in one adult, an unexplained shocklike condition that responded to fluid therapy.

ANDROGEN THERAPY

Constitutional Delay of Growth and Development (CDGD)

CDGD refers to normal children proceeding through growth and adolescent development at a tempo slower than average. Although these children, by definition, are not hormonally deficient and do not have evidence of systemic illness resulting in growth failure, their growth rate may be slow enough to cause concern and adversely affect their self-image. During childhood, when the children are smaller than one would expect from their families, the height differential as compared with peers is maintained. Even during childhood, there is clinical evidence of delay (delayed bone age, delayed dental age), reflecting the slower process of physical maturation. It is during the early teenage years, when their peers begin to accelerate growth, that anxiety related to short stature increases in children (especially boys) with CDGD.

The use of low-dose androgens to treat CDGD in boys has been standard therapy for over 30 years. Although there was concern in the 1960s that even low doses of androgens would cause premature closure of epiphyses, a number of reports over the last 20 years agree that low-dose androgens prescribed appropriately do not cause premature closure of epiphyses and do not result in shorter adult stature. However, it should be made clear to parents and to the child with CDGD that low-dose androgen treatment will increase growth velocity (and only modestly) but will not improve final height. Unrealistic expectations by the child will further compound the psychosocial difficulties, which are the only indication for intervention in an otherwise normal child.

Both oral and parenteral forms of androgens have been used to treat CDGD. In the past, oral alkylated androgens and mucosally absorbed (buccal or sublingual) methyltestosterone were popular. Most of these preparations are no longer marketed because of abuse. Fluoxymesterone, oxandrolone, and methyltestosterone Linguets are still available, but the major form of androgen treatment is depot testosterone. Parenteral testosterone affords several advantages, including more consistent blood levels and decreased toxicity. Oral alkylated androgens have been associated with cholestatic jaundice and liver toxicity, including hepatic tumors.

The treatment regimen for males with CDGD must consider both dose appropriateness and age appropriateness. To minimize the likelihood of premature closure of epiphyses, it is suggested that androgens be used to stimulate growth when the bone age is at least 11 years. A recommendation is that treatment be delayed until the boy with CDGD is 13 or 14 years old and the bone age is >11 years. Further, the patient's serum testosterone concentrations should still be in the prepubertal or very early pubertal range, indicating that growth velocity is not likely to increase in the next year or so. There are a number of recommended treatment protocols. A dose of 50 to 100 mg of depot testosterone per month intramuscularly for several months (three or four monthly injections) and no treatment for a subsequent several months is one standard treatment program. It occasionally is necessary to repeat the cycle of treatment, but more than two such cycles generally are not necessary. All patients should be monitored closely, that is, followed at 3-month intervals with bone ages every 6 months. Testosterone levels and other laboratory studies based on clinical findings should be repeated at intervals. A serum testosterone concentration in the midadolescent range off treatment indicates impending spontaneous growth and is an appropriate indicator to withhold further treatment. Obviously, a marked advancement in bone age also is an indication to discontinue treatment.

ESTROGEN THERAPY

Constitutional Delay of Growth and Development

In general, girls are not as concerned about delay in growth and sexual development. If diagnostic studies indicate that final height will be normal, most girls are tolerant of this delay and are not anxious for therapeutic maneuvers. This is especially true because epiphyseal fusion appears to be mediated by estrogen action. Low doses of estrogen (100 ng/kg/d) used for treatment of growth in Turner's syndrome can stimulate growth without excessive skeletal maturation. However, there are no commercial preparations of these very low doses of estrogen that were used for clinical trials. In those occasional female patients who are unable to tolerate delay in growth and sexual maturation, conjugated estrogen at 0.3 mg/d PO for 3 months can be prescribed. There should be reassessment after an additional 3 months without estrogen treatment. This dose of estrogen has stimulated short-term growth in both Turner's syndrome and hypogonadal female patients. Prolonged continuous treatment will result in premature epiphyseal fusion.

REFERENCES

1. August GP, Lippe BM, Blethen SL, et al: Growth hormone treatment in the United States: Demographic and diagnostic features of 2332 children. J Pediatr 116:899–903, 1990.
2. Cara JF, Johanson AJ: Growth hormone for short stature not due to classic growth hormone deficiency. Pediatr Clin North Am 37:1229–1254, 1990.
3. Richman RA, Kirsch LR: Testosterone treatment in adolescent boys with constitutional delay in growth and development. N Engl J Med 319:1563–1567, 1988.
4. Rosenfield RG: Nonconventional growth hormone therapy in Turner syndrome: The United States experience. Horm Res 33:137–143, 1990.

TALL STATURE

MARY M. LEE, M.D.
LYNNE L. LEVITSKY, M.D.

In recent years, referrals for the evaluation and treatment of the healthy child or adolescent with tall stature have become less common because social standards for acceptable heights have changed. Treatment with supraphysiologic doses of sex steroids to promote rapid epiphyseal fusion has proved to be the most effective therapy. Although this therapy was pioneered initially in the United States, European pediatric endocrinologists have been the most forceful advocates of the use of pharmacologic measures to limit statural growth. Overall, many more adolescent females than males have been referred and treated for tall stature. With the growing involvement of young women in competitive athletic activities, however, taller height is often perceived as advantageous rather than as socially handicapping, and fewer families are seeking medical intervention.

DIAGNOSIS

In the prepubertal child, rapid growth with crossing of height percentiles may herald the onset of early adrenarche or puberty or both or may be associated with thyrotoxicosis or exogenous obesity. These growth patterns cause early epiphyseal fusion and will not result in unusually tall adult stature. Other pathologic causes of excessive linear growth, such as Marfan syndrome, Klinefelter's syndrome, Sotos' syndrome, pituitary gigantism, or homocystinuria, have phenotypic features and growth patterns that usually are readily distinguishable from benign familial or constitutional tall stature. In familial tall stature, the typical pattern of accelerated linear growth during infancy and early childhood causes height to deviate upward across growth channels at an early age without undue skeletal maturation. Height during childhood is greater than 2 SD above the mean (greater than the 97th percentile), and growth velocity is often above the 50th percentile for age. The predicted adult height is also 2 SD above the mean but is consistent with the midparental height and genetic potential. Although the criteria for initiating treatment for tall stature vary among individual pediatric endocrinologists and depend on societal norms in different countries, the general consensus in western society is that treatment is not warranted unless the predicted adult height is greater than 183 cm (6 feet) for women and greater than 200 cm (6 feet 6 inches) for men. Even then, the majority of pediatric endocrinologists in the United States are concerned about the immediate and long-term risks of high-dose sex steroids and hesitate to intervene. Others will treat only for overriding medical or psychologic indications, such as severe progressive scoliosis and kyphosis or significant emotional stress and social dysfunction secondary to the tall stature.

THERAPY

Currently, high-dose estrogen therapy is the most effective treatment for tall stature in girls. Estrogen is thought to reduce final height by two mechanisms. High-dose estrogen therapy inhibits growth hormone-stimulated insulin-like growth factor 1 (IGF-1) synthesis and also causes discordant osseous maturation, with bone age advancing more rapidly than linear growth for chronologic age. Although a greater height reduction is achieved when therapy is started at a younger age, treatment usually is deferred until the onset of spontaneous pubertal changes to avoid inappropriately early pubertal maturation. Initiation of treatment at a bone age of 10 to 12 years is believed to be optimal for maximizing height reduction without inducing early puberty. In practice, the age at which treatment commences usually is predetermined by the age at referral. High-dose estrogens are continued until the bone age reaches 15 years or until the growth rate has declined to less than 2 cm/y. The recommended doses have decreased over the years from 0.5 to 1 mg ethinyl estradiol (or 5 to 20 mg conjugated estrogens) daily to 0.1 mg ethinyl estradiol daily (current recommendation). A recent study showed that three different doses of ethinyl estradiol (0.1, 0.2, and 0.5 mg) were all equally efficacious and caused similar reductions of final height by 3 cm/y of treatment. A progestational agent, such as medroxyprogesterone acetate (5 to 10 mg) is added for the first 10 days of each calendar month. This permits regular withdrawal bleeding and avoids endometrial hyperplasia with erratic breakthrough bleeding. It may also protect against future endometrial malignancy. Most studies have shown that adult height is reduced by about 40% of the remaining height potential at the start of therapy, with final heights varying from 2 to 9 cm below the initial predicted height.

The reluctance to treat healthy girls with high-dose estrogens stems from concern about the immediate risk of thromboembolic phenomena and uncertainty about the long-term effects on the cardiovascular system and on carcinogenesis of estrogen-responsive organs. Decreased antithrombin III and protein S levels can be found in adolescents treated with estrogens for tall stature, and several cases of deep vein thrombosis have been reported. We have seen one episode of clinically significant pulmonary emboli as a result of such thrombosis. Posttreatment amenorrhea and anovulatory cycles from suppression of the hypothalamic-pituitary axis seem to resolve within 6 to 12 months. Minor short-term side effects of high-dose estrogen therapy include nausea, headaches, weight gain, galactorrhea, and leg cramps.

Supraphysiologic doses of testosterone have been used similarly to limit growth in the few males with tall stature who seek treatment. In contrast to estrogens, high-dose testosterone increases growth velocity while disproportionately advancing osseous maturation. The younger the age at which treatment is started, the greater is the reduction in final height. Treatment started at a bone age of 12 to 14 years will reduce the final height by 5 to 7 cm (50% of remaining height) without causing unusually early pubertal maturation. The previously recommended regimen was testosterone enanthate or cypionate 500 mg IM given every 2 to 4 weeks until a bone age of 17 years is reached. However, a recent study showed that the acceleration in osseous maturation induced by 6 months of testosterone enanthate therapy (500 mg every 2 weeks) persisted for another 6 months after therapy was discontinued. Thus, a short-term course of testosterone may be sufficient to diminish final height potential significantly. A 6-month treatment period with reevaluation of the remaining growth potential periodically has been recommended as an optimal regimen for reducing adult height while minimizing the risks of high-dose testosterone therapy. Posttreatment gonadal suppression seems to be more of a concern with prolonged high-dose testosterone than with estrogen therapy. In an early study, although most of the patients (21 of 24) had normalization of testicular size for chronologic age within 18 months after treatment, 3 had prolonged abnormalities in testicular volume and sperm count. Other side effects of treatment include weight gain, edema, and severe acne.

Several other treatment modalities with potentially less toxicity than high-dose sex steroids have been tried for the treatment of familial tall stature, with limited success. These include the use of bromocriptine to oppose the dopaminergic stimulation of GH release, pirenzepine to block cholinergic effects on GH secretion, and long-acting somatostatin analogs. Despite promising preliminary results of somatostatin analog therapy, final height data are not available to judge its efficacy.

CONCLUSION

The decision to treat healthy individuals with familial tall stature is a difficult one. The potential side effects and risks of high-dose sex steroid therapy must be weighed against the limited height reduction and poorly documented psychologic benefits of prolonged estrogen or testosterone treatment to limit linear growth.

REFERENCES

1. Bramsig JH, Lengerke HJ von, Schmidt H, Schellong G: The results of short-term (6 months) high-dose testosterone treatment on bone age and adult height in boys of excessively tall stature. Eur J Pediatr 148:104–106, 1988.
2. Conte FA, Grumbach MM: Estrogen use in children and adolescents: A survey. Pediatrics 62:1091–1097, 1978.
3. Crawford JD: Treatment of tall girls with estrogen. Pediatrics 62:1189–1195, 1978.
4. Ignatius A, Lenko HL, Perheentupa J: Oestrogen treatment of tall girls: Effect decreases with age. Acta Paediatr Scand 80:712–717, 1991.
5. Norman EK, Trygstad O, Larsen S, Dahl-Jorgensen K: Height reduction in 539 tall girls treated with three different dosages of ethinyloestradiol. Arch Dis Child 66:1275–1278, 1991.
6. Zachmann M, Ferrandez A, Murset G, Gnehm HE, Prader A: Testosterone treatment of excessively tall boys. J Pediatr 88:116–123, 1976.

THYROID DISORDERS

ROSALIND S. BROWN, M.D., F.R.C.P.(C.)

Disorders of the thyroid gland often are subtle in presentation, but the deleterious consequences of late or inappropriate diagnosis and treatment may be irreversible, especially in the newborn infant. Deficient or excessive function may be due to an intrinsic thyroid abnormality (primary) or may result from pituitary (secondary) or hypothalamic (tertiary) disease. In some cases, thyroid function is af-

fected by circulating immunoglobulins with stimulating or blocking properties. In general, severe congenital abnormalities of the thyroid present in infancy, whereas acquired abnormalities, such as autoimmune thyroid disease, develop later in childhood and adolescence. Infants may be affected passively, however, because of the transplacental passage of maternal immunoglobulins.

THYROID DISEASE IN INFANCY

Congenital Hypothyroidism

Congenital hypothyroidism (CH) occurs in 1 in 4000 live births and is one of the more frequent treatable causes of mental retardation. Since optimal results depend on early diagnosis and adequate treatment and since the early signs and symptoms are subtle, neonatal screening programs have been developed that test dried blood spots obtained in the first few days of life. In North America, thyroxine (T_4) is tested initially, and thyrotropin (TSH) is measured secondarily if the T_4 is low. (It should be recalled that the normal range for serum T_4 concentration in neonates, 6.6 to 16.3 μg/dl, is much higher than the adult reference values provided by most laboratories.)

Any infant with a low T_4 and elevated TSH concentration (>20 mU/L) is presumed to have primary congenital hypothyroidism until proven otherwise and should be assessed without delay. However, infants tested before 2 or 3 days of age may have a falsely elevated TSH value because of the postnatal TSH surge. Potential causes of *transient* hypothyroidism (e.g., maternal iodine exposure, antithyroid medication, or autoimmune disease) should be excluded, and the diagnosis should be confirmed by repeat measurement of free T_4 index and TSH in serum. If adequate facilities are available, all infants with confirmed CH should have a radionuclide scan (preferably ^{123}I) to verify that a permanent thyroid abnormality is present and to distinguish thyroid agenesis, dysgenesis, or ectopia, sporadic conditions, from thyroid dyshormonogenesis, which is genetically determined (autosomal recessive). This should be performed within 5 days of diagnosis but need not delay initiation of therapy, since TSH values remain increased for several weeks. Babies of mothers with autoimmune thyroid disease should be checked for TSH receptor blocking antibodies, since maternal blocking antibody-induced CH is indistinguishable clinically from thyroid agenesis/dysgenesis and may be associated with absent uptake on radionuclide scan. Unlike the latter, however, it is transient and familial. Assessment of skeletal maturation (bone age) may be helpful in estimating the degree of in utero hypothyroidism. Consultation with a pediatric endocrinologist is recommended because of the possible complexities in diagnosis and therapy in some cases, the importance of family education and counseling, and the irreversible consequences if therapy is delayed or suboptimal. Parental education and genetic counseling by trained personnel should be provided once a definitive diagnosis has been established.

Treatment with levothyroxine sodium should be initiated as soon as the diagnosis is confirmed. There is no advantage to using the more biologically active isomer, triiodothyronine (T_3), since most brain T_3 is derived by the intracellular conversion of T_4 (derived from serum) to T_3. Similarly, desiccated thyroid or thyroid extract should be avoided because of variable potency. Thyroxine tablets can be crushed and mixed with a small amount of fluid or food. Alternately, we have found that most babies have no difficulty swallowing the small tablet whole if it is placed on the tongue. A high initial dose of 10 to 15 μg/kg is recommended, particularly in infants whose initial T_4 is low (<5 μg/dl), so as to normalize the T_4 as soon as possible, preferably within 2 weeks. Small infants can be started on 25 μg/d. Subsequent adjustments are made according to the clinical response and the results of thyroid function tests (T_4 and TSH). Parents should be instructed to double the dose of medication for 1 day in the event that a tablet is missed. One aims to normalize linear growth and intellectual development by maintaining the serum T_4 in the upper half of the normal range (10 to 16 μg/dl; 130 to 206 nmol/L). Serum TSH should be suppressed into the normal range (<10 mU/L), although this may take several weeks to occur. Infants should be monitored closely (every few months) particularly in the first 3 years of life when the brain is undergoing growth and maturation and less often thereafter. Although this is still controversial, many experts believe that early, appropriate postnatal treatment will normalize mental development even in babies with in utero hypothyroidism, as evidenced by a delayed bone age at birth, and that treatment failures are most likely to be due to noncompliance or inadequate therapy.

Some infants will have an elevated TSH (10 to 20 mU/L) even after apparently appropriate treatment despite T_4 levels in the upper half of the normal range. This may be due to relative pituitary insensitivity or to noncompliance. In babies in whom noncompliance is not suspected, an attempt should be made to increase the replacement dosage judiciously as tolerated. Clinical thyrotoxicosis (fussiness, difficulty falling asleep, poor weight gain, jitteriness) should be avoided, however, because of the possible deleterious consequences of persistent hyperthyroxinemia on brain maturation and the possible development of premature cranial synostosis. In babies with CH in whom an organic basis was not established at birth and in whom transient disease is suspected, a trial off replacement therapy can be initiated after the age of 3 years, by which time most thyroxine-dependent brain maturation has occurred.

Occasionally, a low T_4 is found in association with a normal TSH. This may occur in babies with thyroxine-binding globulin (TBG) deficiency (approximate incidence 1 in 5000 to 10,000 live births), congenital hypopituitarism (1 in 50,000), in premature or low birthweight newborns, or in sick euthyroid syndrome. No treatment is indicated in TBG deficiency, since the free T_4 (and thus the metabolically active fraction) is normal. Babies with secondary hypothyroidism due to congenital hypopituitarism may be recognized clinically because of evidence of other pituitary hormone deficiencies (e.g., hypoglycemia, microphallus in males) and should be suspected in infants with midline facial defects. Urgent diagnosis and hormonal replacement are important and may be life saving. These infants tend to require lower doses of levothyroxine (25 μg/d) than do those with primary hypothyroidism. Thyroid replacement should be initiated concurrent with hydrocortisone to avoid the possible development of acute adrenal insufficiency. Treatment is not indicated in premature, low birthweight, or sick newborns whose T_4 is low, but thyroid function testing should be repeated every 2 weeks until it normalizes because of the rare occurrence of delayed onset of CH. Similarly, any baby suspected clinically of having hypothyroidism should have repeat thyroid function testing because of rare errors in the screening programs.

Neonatal Goiter

Goiter in the newborn is rare but may be large enough to cause respiratory embarrassment. It is associated most frequently with maternal treatment with high-dose thioamides (propylthiouracil, PTU, or methimazole) for Graves' disease and is self-limited. Other causes include neonatal Graves' disease or thyroid dyshormonogenesis, although goiter is rarely prominent at birth in the latter condition. Treatment with levothyroxine is indicated only if the TSH is elevated. In rare cases of large fetal goiter, intrauterine therapy with weekly intraamniotic injections of 250 μg levothyroxine (in addition to reduction of the maternal PTU dose) has been effective.

Neonatal Graves' Disease

Neonatal hyperthyroidism is almost always due to the transplacental passage of maternal TSH receptor-stimulating antibodies that mimic the action of TSH. Although transient, neonatal hyperthyroidism may persist for several months, depending on antibody potency and titer. Rarely, it is longer lasting. Infants with neonatal Graves' disease frequently are small for gestational age and become symptomatic at the end of the first week of life, when maternal antithyroid medication (e.g., PTU) has been cleared from their circulation. Diagnosis is confirmed by demonstration of a significantly elevated serum concentration of T_4 (and total T_3) associated with a suppressed

TSH. Measurement of TSH receptor-stimulating antibodies will verify the etiology of the hyperthyroidism.

Specific therapy is dependent on the severity of disease. In mildly affected infants, observation and serial monitoring of thyroid function may be sufficient. In severely afflicted neonates, on the other hand, urgent intervention may be necessary. In addition to supportive measures (including the provision of adequate fluids, calories, and temperature control), conventional therapy includes short-term thioamide administration (PTU 5 to 10 mg/kg/d or methimazole 0.5 to 1 mg/kg/d) in three or four divided doses and a beta-adrenergic agent to reverse the hyperadrenergic state (propranolol 2 mg/kg/d in two or three divided doses) if the cardiac effects are significant. An iodide salt that blocks thyroid hormone secretion acutely (e.g., Lugol's solution, which contains 5% iodine and 10% potassium iodide with 126 mg of iodine per milliliter), 8 mg every 8, hours is added frequently for more immediate thyroid suppression. Treatment with digitalis may be necessary if high-output heart failure develops despite these measures. In severe cases, glucocorticoids (e.g., prednisone 2 mg/kg/d in three divided doses for up to 10 to 14 days) have been used because of their acute effect of blocking thyroid hormone secretion. Recently, treatment with the iodine-containing radiocontrast agent sodium ipodate alone 0.5 g PO every 3 days has been shown to result in prompt and sustained control of the hyperthyroidism. In rare cases, intrauterine therapy of affected fetuses has been advocated because of the adverse effects of prolonged fetal and neonatal hyperthyroidism.

Gradual tapering and discontinuation of medication are based on close monitoring of thyroid function tests (T_4 and T_3). Conversely, the dose of thioamides and iodide can be increased if a significant therapeutic effect is not seen within a few days. Careful follow-up both during therapy and after treatment has been discontinued is necessary to avoid the development of hypothyroidism or hyperthyroidism and to detect the occurrence of relapse.

THYROID DISEASE DURING CHILDHOOD AND ADOLESCENCE

Goiter

Thyroid disease is much more common in the child and adolescent than in the neonate and has a striking predilection for females. The most common presentation is goiter, which occurs in 2% to 3% of schoolchildren in North America, a noniodine-deficient population. Goiter may be asymptomatic or may be associated with hypothyroidism or hyperthyroidism. The most frequent cause of asymptomatic goiter in North America is chronic lymphocytic (Hashimoto) thyroiditis (CLT), an autoimmune disorder, which should be distinguished from colloid goiter because CLT carries a risk of hypothyroidism and colloid goiter does not. Less often, children with mild, undiagnosed dyshormonogenesis may present because of a goiter. CLT is distinguished from other causes of goiter by the firmness of the gland clinically, the occasional finding of a delphian node in the midline of the neck just superior to the thyroid, the frequent family history of autoimmune thyroid disease, and demonstration of significant titers of antithyroid antibodies (antithyroid peroxidase, TPO, formerly known as antimicrosomal and antithyroglobulin, Tg), which are markers of underlying thyroid immune damage. Serum concentration of TSH should be measured to detect unrecognized primary hypothyroidism.

Thyroid suppression is indicated in all children with goiters who have an elevated TSH whether or not their serum thyroxine is decreased. Treatment of children whose TSH is normal is controversial. Measurement of TSH should be repeated in a few months before treatment is initiated in those in whom it is minimally elevated (e.g., 10 to 15 mU/L), since there is some evidence that the disease may be reversible in milder cases.

Acquired Hypothyroidism

Children with hypothyroidism are recognized most frequently because of poor linear growth, the height being more affected than the weight. The classic signs and symptoms of hypothyroidism (e.g., lethargy, cold intolerance, constipation, dry skin or hair texture), if present, are often minimized or ignored by the patient and family and must be questioned about carefully. The most common cause is CLT. Nongoitrous CLT (primary myxedema) or a previously undiagnosed dysgenetic/ectopic thyroid should be suspected in hypothyroid children with a small or nonpalpable thyroid gland. The bone age is usually significantly delayed. There is an increased incidence of CLT in patients with insulin-dependent diabetes mellitus, Down syndrome, and Turner's syndrome. Rarely, CLT may be part of an autoimmune polyglandular syndrome, including hypoadrenalism, hypoparathyroidism, and diabetes mellitus.

Laboratory diagnosis of primary hypothyroidism is based on the demonstration of an elevated TSH. If the T_4 is normal, the child is said to have compensated hypothyroidism. The presence of elevated titers of anti-TPO (and anti-Tg) antibodies supports an autoimmune etiology. TSH receptor-blocking antibodies, found in some children and adults with nongoitrous CLT, may block TSH-induced stimulation of thyroid function and growth, as a result of which hypothyroidism is worsened and a goiter fails to develop. In some adults, disappearance of these blocking antibodies has been associated with normalization of thyroid function.

In contrast to neonatal hypothyroidism, where urgent normalization of thyroid function is important to minimize the deleterious effects of hypothyroidism on the developing brain, rapid replacement is not essential in the older child. On the contrary, rapid normalization may result in unwanted side effects (e.g., deterioration in school performance because of short attention span, hyperactivity, insomnia, irritability, and behavior difficulties), particularly in those with long-standing, severe thyroid underactivity. In these children, it is preferable to increase the replacement dose slowly. Typical initial replacement doses of levothyroxine are 6 μg/kg for children 1 to 5 years of age, 4 μg/kg for those ages 6 to 10 years, and 3 μg/kg for those 11 years of age and older. We generally start with 25 μg/d for 2 weeks and increase by that amount every 2 weeks as tolerated until the desired amount is reached. It is wise to counsel both parents and teachers that side effects of medication may occur, that they are due to the medication rather than the child deliberately misbehaving, and that, in general, they tend to be self-limited. In the rare child in whom the signs and symptoms are longer lasting, even slower replacement may be necessary. In contrast, in children with mild hypothyroidism, full replacement usually can be initiated at once without much risk of adverse consequences. T_4 and TSH should be measured after the child has received the recommended dosage for at least 6 to 8 weeks. Once a euthyroid state has been achieved, patients should be monitored every 6 to 12 months. Close attention is paid to interval growth as well as to the presence of clinical evidence of hypothyroidism or hyperthyroidism.

In patients with a goiter, one tends to use a somewhat higher T_4 dose than for simple replacement so as to keep the TSH in the low normal (0.3 to 1.0 mU/L in an ultrasensitive or third-generation assay) rather than normal range. In this way, one attempts to suppress the goitrogenic effect of TSH. Therapy in CLT tends to be most effective initially but may not always reduce gland size, particularly in individuals whose glands have extensive lymphocytic infiltration. Overtreatment should be avoided both because of the adverse effects of clinical thyrotoxicosis and because of the potential danger of osteoporosis that has been demonstrated in adults with prolonged hyperthyroxinemia. Goiter size should be monitored in 3 to 4 months initially and every 6 to 12 months thereafter. Serum TSH should be estimated to ensure compliance and adequacy of the dose of medication. Treatment is continued indefinitely.

Hyperthyroidism

Over 95% of cases of hyperthyroidism in children and adolescents are due to Graves' disease. The clinical diagnosis is confirmed by the finding of increased concentrations of circulating thyroid hormones, with elevation of total T_3 frequently being more striking than that of T_4. Demonstration of a suppressed TSH by an ultrasensitive RIA

method excludes much rarer causes of hyperthyroxinemia, such as TSH-induced hyperthyroidism (e.g., due to a pituitary adenoma) and thyroid hormone resistance. If an elevated T_4 is found in a clinically euthyroid patient, an abnormality of thyroxine-binding globulin (either familial or acquired, for example, a result of administration of oral contraceptives in an adolescent female) or rarer binding protein abnormalities (e.g., familial dysalbuminemic hyperthyroxinemia) should be considered. Demonstration of TSH receptor-stimulating antibodies by either radioreceptor assay (usually referred to as TSH binding inhibitory IgGs, TBII) or bioassay (often called thyroid-stimulating antibodies, or TSAbs) will distinguish Graves' disease from CLT, which rarely may present with a hyperthyroid phase. In the latter case, thyrotoxicosis is due to the release of preformed hormone from an inflamed, damaged gland rather than to gland overactivity. Antithyroid treatment, therefore, is contraindicated. In contrast to adults, because of the desire to minimize unnecessary radiation in children, radioactive iodine uptake and scan are used to confirm the diagnosis only in atypical cases or if measurement of TSH receptor-stimulating antibodies is negative.

Medical therapy with one of the thiouracil derivatives (PTU or methimazole) usually is the first approach to therapy. In severe cases, beta-adrenergic blockers (e.g., propranolol 10 mg t.i.d.) can be added to control the adrenergic hyperresponsiveness for the first 2 or 3 weeks. PTU and methimazole are well absorbed after oral administration and actively concentrate in the thyroid gland. Both agents block synthesis of T_4 and T_3 by interfering with the organification of iodine and the coupling of iodinated tyrosines into thyroglobulin. Although PTU has the theoretical additional advantage of interfering with the conversion of T_4 to the more active isomer T_3, this effect is not significant in vivo. We usually prefer methimazole because of its longer half-life, an advantage in adolescents in whom compliance frequently is an issue. The initial dosage of PTU is 5 to 7 mg/kg/d in three divided doses, and that of methimazole is 0.5 to 0.7 mg/kg/d given twice daily. Patients should be followed every 4 to 6 weeks until the serum concentration of T_4 (and total T_3) normalizes. At this point, one can either decrease the dosage of thioamide drug by 30% to 50% or, alternatively, wait until the TSH begins to rise and add a small, supplementary dose of levothyroxine (1 μg/kg/d).

Maintenance doses of PTU may be given twice daily. Methimazole may be administered once daily. The optimum duration of therapy is unknown. We usually treat for at least 2 years following attainment of a euthyroid state. In patients treated with antithyroid drugs alone, a small drug requirement to maintain euthyroidism, diminution in goiter size, lack of orbitopathy, and lower initial degree of hyperthyroxinemia (T_4 <20 μg/dl; T_3:T_4 ratio <20) is a favorable indicator that drug therapy can be gradually tapered and withdrawn. Persistence of TSH receptor-stimulating antibodies, on the other hand, indicates a high likelihood of relapse. Approximately 50% of patients will go into long-term remission within 4 years, with a continuing remission rate of 25% every 2 years for up to 6 years of treatment. There is some evidence that combined therapy might be associated with an improved rate of remission, although this remains controversial.

In addition to the need for long-term therapy and the significant risk of relapse once therapy is discontinued, the disadvantages of the thiouracil derivatives include toxic drug reactions, which occur in 5% to 14% of children. These include erythematous rashes, urticaria, and arthralgias. Rarely, more severe sequelae, such as hepatitis, a lupuslike syndrome, thrombocytopenia, and agranulocytosis, occur. Most reactions are mild and do not contraindicate continued use. In more severe cases, switching to the other thioamide frequently is effective. The risk of the exceedingly rare life-threatening complications, hepatitis and agranulocytosis, appears to be greater within the first 3 months of therapy, when a higher dosage of medication (particularly PTU) is used, and in older individuals. Since the onset is precipitous and idiosyncratic, routine monitoring of the white blood cell count or liver function tests is not generally recommended. It is important to caution all patients, however, to immediately stop their medication and consult their physician should they develop unexplained high fever, gingival sores, or jaundice.

Definitive therapy with either medical (radioactive iodine) or surgical thyroid ablation usually is reserved for patients who have failed medical management, developed a toxic drug reaction, or are noncompliant. In recent years, however, radioactive iodine is being favored increasingly, even as the initial approach to therapy. This is particularly so in adolescents with behavior problems, in children who are mentally retarded, and in those about to leave home (e.g., to go to college). The advantages are the relative ease of administration and the reduced need for medical follow-up. An ablative dose of radioactive iodine usually is used, since this is not associated with an increased risk of subsequent thyroid neoplasia. However, a majority of patients become hypothyroid and require lifelong thyroid replacement therapy. Despite widespread concerns about the use of this form of treatment in the young, the gonadal exposure has been estimated to be similar to that when standard roentgenographic studies are performed, and there has been no evidence of increased congenital malformations in offspring, extrathyroidal malignancies, or of any other untoward complications in several long-term follow-up studies.

Subtotal thyroidectomy, the third therapeutic modality, is performed less frequently now than in the past. This form of therapy is usually reserved for patients who have failed medical management. It is indicated in the rare patient with significant ophthalmopathy in whom radioactive iodine therapy is contraindicated and in those who refuse radioactive iodine therapy. Because of the associated complications of recurrent laryngeal nerve paralysis, hypoparathyroidism, and, rarely, death, this therapy should be performed only by an experienced pediatric thyroid surgeon. Following surgery, most patients become hypothyroid and require lifelong thyroid replacement therapy. If inadequate tissue is removed, hyperthyroidism may recur. Rarely, unsightly keloid formation may occur at the site of the scar.

Thyroid Nodules

Thyroid nodules are rare in childhood, but there is some evidence that they are more likely to be carcinomatous than are similar masses in adults. A history of prior head and neck radiation (e.g., for treatment of head or neck cancer) increases the risk of malignancy. The possibility of a rare medullary thyroid carcinoma should be considered if there is a family history of thyroid cancer or pheochromocytoma or if the child has multiple mucosal neuromas and a marfanoid habitus.

Clinically, a malignancy is suspected if the mass is solitary (i.e., unassociated with a goiter or other evidence of thyroid nodular disease), fixed to the surrounding soft tissue, and associated with regional cervical adenopathy or hoarseness. These signs need not be present in all cases, however. Children with clinical and biochemical (elevated titers of anti-TPO and anti-Tg antibodies) evidence of underlying CLT in whom malignancy is less likely may be carefully watched initially without therapy (if TSH is normal) or treated with suppressive doses of levothyroxine (if TSH is elevated). Further evaluation is not indicated unless there is evidence of nodular enlargement. If medullary thyroid carcinoma is suspected, measurement of calcitonin either in the basal state or after calcium/pentagastrin stimulation (elemental calcium 2 mg/kg IV over 50 to 60 seconds; pentagastrin 0.5 μg/kg given by bolus IV injection over 5 to 10 seconds) should be performed.

The optimal diagnostic and therapeutic approach to the solitary nodule is controversial. Needle biopsy is the diagnostic method of choice in older children and adolescents but requires an experienced clinician and cytologist. If the nodule is cystic, needle biopsy and aspiration of the cyst may be curative. Although the finding of a cyst lessens the likelihood of malignancy, carcinomas have been found in the walls of cysts. Therefore, cysts that recur after repeated aspirations probably should be treated by excision biopsy.

If an experienced cytologist is not available, open surgical biopsy is indicated in a young patient or when malignancy is suspected. Additional procedures that may be helpful include radionuclide (^{123}I) thyroid scan and ultrasound. The former is employed frequently to assess nodular function, since there is an increased risk of malignancy

in cold or nonfunctioning nodules. Ultrasonography may be useful in determining whether a nodule is cystic. Benign lesions are treated by lobectomy. There is no evidence that such patients benefit from thyroid suppression to prevent recurrences. Carcinoma is usually treated with near-total thyroidectomy and dissection of adjacent involved areas. This frequently is followed by radioablation. Because malignant tumor remnants often are sensitive to TSH, suppressive doses of levothyroxine are indicated postoperatively.

In cases where malignancy is not suspected, suppressive doses of levothyroxine can be tried.

Painful Thyroid Glands

Tenderness of the thyroid gland may be due to an acute (bacterial) or subacute (viral) inflammation, both of which are exceedingly rare in childhood. Acute suppurative thyroiditis is characterized by severe pain, redness and swelling in the region of the thyroid gland, cervical adenopathy, and fever. Recurrent attacks and involvement of the left lobe suggest a pyriform sinus fistula as the route of infection. The affected area should be aspirated and cultured in both aerobic and anaerobic media for diagnosis and determination of antimicrobial sensitivity. Ultrasonography can be used to evaluate the possibility of abscess formation, and therapy with high-dose parenteral antibiotics should be initiated as soon as possible to prevent abscess formation. Surgical drainage or lobectomy or both are necessary if abscess formation occurs. Barium swallow should be performed if a pyriform sinus is suspected, and if one is found, complete extirpation of the fistula is necessary to prevent recurrence.

Subacute thyroiditis is characterized by low-grade fever, malaise, mild thyromegaly, pain, and tenderness in the region of the thyroid gland. Characteristically, an initial thyrotoxic phase lasting several weeks to months is followed by a mild hypothyroid period of several months duration. In contrast to Graves' disease, the thyrotoxicosis is associated with a low radioactive iodine uptake. Complete recovery is the rule, although rarely, repeat exacerbations may occur. Analgesics, such as acetaminophen or aspirin, usually are sufficient for pain relief. In more severe cases, glucocorticoids may be tried, although they do not alter the course of the disease. PTU is contraindicated.

PARATHYROID DISEASE

HARALD JÜPPNER, M.D.

Parathyroid hormone (PTH), a peptide with 84 amino acids, is the major regulator of calcium-phosphate homeostasis through its actions on bone and kidney. PTH shares significant structural and functional homology with the PTH-related peptide (PTHrP) that is the major cause of the syndrome of humoral hypercalcemia of malignancy. Both peptides bind to and activate the same, widely expressed PTH-PTHrP receptor that belongs to the superfamily of G-protein-coupled receptors. Unlike PTH, which is synthesized and secreted only by the parathyroid glands, PTHrP is expressed in a large variety of fetal and adult tissues. Recent gene ablation experiments have shown that PTHrP is of vital importance for normal embryonic development, indicating that PTHrP and the PTH-PTHrP receptor serve yet unknown autocrine/paracrine functions.

The therapy of parathyroid diseases involves recognition of states of underactivity and overactivity, both primary and secondary (Table 1; see also Chapter 10). Increased PTH secretion may be associated with hypercalcemia (primary or tertiary hyperparathyroidism) or with frank or relative hypocalcemia (pseudohypoparathyroidism [PHP] or uncompensated secondary hyperparathyroidism). Decreased PTH secretion as in hypoparathyroidism is usually associated with hypocalcemia.

TABLE 1. Drug Therapy of Parathyroid Disease

Hypocalcemia

Acute Treatment

Elementary calcium at 10–20 mg/kg BW slowly over 10–20 min, i.e., 1–2 ml/kg BW of 10% Ca-gluconate, which contains 9 mg/ml of elementary calcium

Repeat q4–6h or institute continuous infusion (check compatibility with other IV solutions); maximal recommended dose of elementary calcium: 60 mg/kg BW/24 h

Cardiac monitoring required: bradycardia, QRS changes

Note that hypocalcemia may be secondary to magnesium deficiency

Chronic Treatment of Hypoparathyroid States

(Individual dose adjustment required)

Vitamin D_3: 50 µg/kg/d as single dose (10 µg of cholecalciferol = 400 U)

1.25 $(OH_2D_3$: 0.01–0.05 µg/kg/d as single dose

Calcium carbonate or calcium citrate: 50–100 mg/kg BW per day given in 3–4 doses

Hypercalcemia

Acute Treatment of Life-Threatening Hypercalcemia

Forced diuresis with normal saline and appropriately added potassium at 1.5 times of maintenance; after achieving adequate hydration, furosemide may be given at 1 mg/kg BW IV q6h if necessary

Calcitonin: 2–8 U/kg BW IV, SC, or IM; repeat q6–12h

Bisphosphonates:

Plicamycin (Mithracin): 15–25 µg/kg BW per day IV over 4–8 h

Etidronate (EHDP, Didronel): 5–10 mg/kg BW per day IV over 3 consecutive days

Pamidronate (APD, Aredia): 60–90 mg/d (in adults, a single IV dose normalizes serum calcium levels in 80%–100% of patients)

Peritoneal dialysis or hemodialysis with low-calcium dialysate

Supportive Therapy

Glucocorticoids to decrease intestinal calcium absorption (prednisone: 2 mg/kg BW per day)

Cellulose sodium phosphate to reduce intestinal calcium absorption (Calcibind given PO in 3–4 doses)

Reduction of dietary calcium and vitamin D_3

HYPOCALCEMIA

In comparison to maternal blood calcium levels, fetal concentrations are maintained considerably higher through an active, fetus-directed calcium transport mechanism in the placenta. Because of this relative hypercalcemia and an increased set point of the parathyroid calcium sensor, the intrauterine secretion of PTH is limited. After delivery, the cessation of maternal calcium supplies results in a rapid decrease in neonatal blood calcium concentrations. This leads to increased PTH secretion, which then mobilizes calcium from bone, enhances the reabsorption of calcium in the maturing kidney, and stimulates the renal 1 α-hydroxylase to synthesize the biologically active 1,25$(OH)_2$ vitamin D_3.

Early neonatal hypocalcemia with total calcium concentrations below 7 mg/dl usually occurs during the first 3 days of life and is associated with increased concentrations of plasma PTH. The incidence is considerably higher in premature infants and in newborns of mothers with diabetes mellitus or hyperparathyroidism. Symptomatic hypocalcemia requires immediate treatment with intravenous calcium (Table 1), and prolonged intravenous or oral therapy may be necessary until the mechanisms for renal tubular calcium reabsorption and intestinal absorption are fully adapted.

Hypocalcemia that develops after several weeks or months of life may have a wide variety of causes, including phosphate loading, magnesium or vitamin D deficiency, parathyroid hypoplasia or aplasia with associated immunologic deficiencies (DiGeorge syndrome), polyglandular autoimmune disease, thyroid or parathyroid surgery, renal tubular disease (i.e., cystinosis), or renal failure. Splicing defects of the PTH pre-mRNA or mutations in the preprosequence of PTH have been described for familial forms of hypoparathyroidism. Furthermore, recent studies indicate that some forms of hypoparathyroidism are caused by activating mutations in the parathyroid calcium sensor. Mutations in the secreted PTH(1-84) have not been identified.

Pseudohypoparathyroidism (PHP) as the cause of hypocalcemia usually becomes clinically apparent in older children but may not develop until adulthood. PHP comprises several groups of only partially understood disorders characterized by hypocalcemia and hyperphosphatemia despite elevated concentrations of circulating PTH. Because of an end-organ resistance, the infusion of PTH usually fails to increase urinary cAMP and phosphate excretion (types Ia and Ib) or reveals a defective urinary elimination phosphate yet normal cAMP excretion (type II). PHP type Ia is the classic form of end-organ resistance toward PTH, which is characterized by the typical laboratory findings and several clinical features, including short stature, round face, varying degrees of intellectual impairment, and multiple bony abnormalities (short metacarpals and metatarsals), collectively termed Albright's hereditary osteodystrophy (AHO). PHP type Ia is thought to be caused by an abnormality or deficiency in Gsα, which also explains the high frequency of associated endocrine deficiencies (e.g., hypothyroidism). Clinically, pseudo-pseudohypoparathyroidism (pseudoPHP) is often indistinguishable from PHP type Ia, and both disease entities have been described in kindreds of the same family. However, patients with pseudoPHP show no abnormality in the control of calcium homeostasis, despite an equivalent deficiency in Gsα. Patients with PHP type Ib are phenotypically normal, have no associated endocrine diseases, and show laboratory findings that are indistinguishable from those of patients with PHP type Ia. PHP type Ib is thought to be caused by a defect in the PTH-PTHrP receptor or in the regulation of its cell surface expression. PHP type Ia or Ib may present with hyperparathyroid bone disease as a result of selective renal resistance toward PTH.

Treatment of acute, symptomatic hypocalcemia should be carried out with great care, with cardiac monitoring. The usual doses of elemental calcium are listed in Table 1 and discussed at greater length in Chapter 10 in Hypocalcemia and Tetany.

Vitamin D therapy usually is an important part of treating chronic hypocalcemia as seen in hypoparathyroidism or the different forms of PHP. The active form of vitamin D, calcitriol (Rocaltrol) [1,25 $(OH)_2D_3$] is relatively costly but very effective. Its advantage is its relatively short half-life, which permits a more rapid correction of toxicity than other forms. Calcitriol is available in 0.25 and 0.5 µg capsules, which contain a viscous oil. For very small children, an 18-gauge needle may be used to withdraw the oil into a 1-ml syringe, so that small doses may be given. Vitamin D_3 and calcifediol (25-OHD) have longer half-lives. Vitamin D_3 is available in tablets or solution and must be metabolized successively in liver and kidney. Large doses (usually 50,000 to 100,000 U/d, occasionally 150,000 units) may be needed, and toxic effects persist for a long time. Calcifediol has to be 1α-hydroxylated in the kidney and offers no particular advantage for the therapy of parathyroid disorders (the compound comes in 20 and 50 µg capsules and is given in a dose of 3 to 6 µg/kg/d).

Dihydrotachysterol (DHT), a synthetic vitamin D metabolite, does not need renal 1α-hydroxylation. It was often the treatment of choice before the availability of calcitriol and is available in tablets of 0.125, 0.2, and 0.4 mg. A solution of 0.2 mg/ml, once easily available, is now very hard to obtain. In addition to vitamin D or its analogs, oral calcium supplementation may be helpful in chronic hypoparathyroid states (Table 1).

Monitoring of serum calcium is important for proper management. After initiation of therapy, serum calcium should be checked twice weekly for several weeks and then at least every 3 months. If hypercalcemia occurs, all forms of vitamin D and calcium supplements must be stopped until levels of calcium normalize. Additionally, monitoring urinary calcium/creatinine ratios is useful, as hypercalciuria may precede hypercalcemia. (This ratio is normally 0.05 to 0.19; a value of >0.35 constitutes significant hypercalciuria and is likely to lead to nephrocalcinosis). It is important to note that hypoparathyroid individuals tend not to have an intact calcium reabsorptive mechanism and so may become hypercalciuric at relatively low levels of serum calcium. Therefore, aiming for a low-normal serum calcium (8 to 9 mg/dl) is ideal. The use of thiazide diuretics to enhance urinary calcium resorption has been considered at a dose of 0.5 mg/kg/d, not to exceed 100 mg in any individual.

HYPERCALCEMIA

Synthesis and secretion of PTH by the parathyroid glands is tightly regulated by calcium and is mediated by a cell surface, calcium-sensing protein that belongs to a novel class of G-protein-coupled receptors (its gene is located on chromosome 3q). Other important regulators of PTH secretion include 1.25 $(OH)_2$ vitamin D_3 and Mg^{2+}. Primary hyperparathyroidism (HPT) as the cause of hypercalcemia is very rare in young children and adolescents. However, the infantile form of HPT is an acutely life-threatening disease that usually requires immediate parathyroid surgery. Recent findings indicate that this severe neonatal disorder is caused by homozygotic mutations in the calcium-sensing receptor of the parathyroid cell. Most cases of benign familial hypocalciuric hypercalcemia (FHH) are also caused by these mutations, and this abnormality represents the heterozygotic form of infantile HPT. A second, less frequent form of FHH has been mapped to chromosome 19, and linkage to either chromosome 3 or 19 has been excluded for a third form of the disease. Other causes of hypercalcemia include treatment with or accidental ingestion of vitamin D preparations (accidental fortification of milk with exceedingly high concentrations of vitamin D has been described), tumor-associated hypercalcemia secondary to humoral or osteolytic mechanisms, multiple endocrine neoplasia (MEN), Williams-Beuren syndrome, type Jansen metaphyseal chondrodysplasia, sarcoidosis, immobilization, or autonomous hyperparathyroidism caused by prolonged renal failure. Another recently described form of mild, familial hypercalcemia is associated with elevated circulating concentrations of PTHrP.

The steps for therapy of hypercalcemia are outlined in Table 1. The acute management generally consists of generous (>1.5 times maintenance) fluid administration, with loop diuretics. The addition of bisphosponates and calcitonin may be helpful. However, if the situation does not reverse, it may be important to consider dialytic therapy with low-calcium dialysate as a temporizing measure. Utlimately, uncontrollable hypercalcemia as a result of hyperparathyroidism may require parathyroidectomy.

REFERENCES

1. Broadus AE, Stewart AF: Parathyroid hormone-related protein. Structure, processing, and physiological action. In Bilezikian JP, Levine MA, Marcus R (eds): The Parathyroids. Basic and Clinical Concepts. New York, Raven Press, 1994, 259–294.
2. Kronenberg HM, Bringhurst FR, Nussbaum S, Jüppner H, Abou-Samra AB, Segre GV, Potts JT, Jr: Parathyroid hormone: Biosynthesis, secretion, chemistry, and action. In Mundy GR, Martin JT (eds): Handbook of Experimental Pharmacology: Physiology and Pharmacology of Bone. Heidelberg, Germany, Springer-Verlag, 1993, 185–201.

DISORDERS OF THE ADRENAL GLAND

PETER A. LEE, M.D., Ph.D.
SELMA SIEGEL WITCHEL, M.D.

HYPOADRENALISM (ADDISON'S DISEASE)

Adrenal insufficiency refers to inadequate glucocorticoid or mineralocorticoid secretion. Malaise, weight loss, anorexia, vomiting, and fatigue are typical symptoms of adrenal insufficiency. Hypoglycemia, hyperkalemia, hyponatremia, and hypotension also may occur. Pathophysiologic mechanisms resulting in adrenal insufficiency are primary adrenal failure, impaired hypothalamic-pituitary signaling,

or iatrogenic adrenal suppression with pharmacologic glucocorticoid therapy. Etiologies of primary adrenal failure can be congenital (adrenal hypoplasia, ACTH unresponsiveness) or acquired (autoimmune, tuberculosis, toxins). Hypothalamic-pituitary dysfunction can impede ACTH secretion, leading to adrenal insufficiency, often with more subtle clinical features, since mineralocorticoid secretion is generally preserved. Causes of decreased ACTH secretion can be congenital (panhypopituitarism, central nervous system development anomalies) or acquired (tumors, infiltrative lesions, postradiation therapy). Corticotropin-releasing hormone (CRH) stimulation may help distinguish hypothalamic and pituitary causes of hypoadrenalism.

Rationale for Therapy

Acquired or congenital adrenal insufficiency necessitates the physiologic replacement of the significant hormones that the adrenal gland cannot synthesize and secrete. When the adrenal gland is inadequately developed (hypoplasia or aplasia) or has been destroyed, as by tuberculosis or toxins (Addison's disease), glucocorticoid and mineralocorticoid therapy is essential. For ACTH-deficient or unresponsive states, usually only glucocorticoid therapy is needed, since ACTH stimulation is generally not obligatory for adequate mineralocorticoid (aldosterone) secretion.

Routine therapy involves physiologic doses of glucocorticoid drugs given orally (Table 1). The usual dose may be doubled or tripled during stress or for initial therapy. During illness or surgery when the patient is unable to tolerate oral medication, the parental route is necessary. The intravenous route provides the most prompt delivery, the subcutaneous route is the next quickest, and the intramuscular route is the slowest. Mineralocorticoid therapy does not require an increased dose during stress. However, since hydrocortisone has significant mineralocorticoid effect, stress doses of this glucocorticoid may provide adequate coverage for initial therapy or stress coverage.

Acute Treatment

The patient with untreated Addison's disease (primary adrenal insufficiency) or with Addison's disease and major stress without greater than physiologic replacement therapy faces a life-threatening situation. The primary threat in the previously undiagnosed patient relates to mineralocorticoid deficiency (hyperkalemia, hyponatremia, and dehydration). Therefore, *initial therapy is rehydration* and *correction of the electrolyte abnormality*. Once appropriate blood samples for determination of glucose (including rapid measurement), electrolytes, urea nitrogen, cortisol, ACTH, and plasma renin activity have been obtained, therapy can be initiated. Fluid therapy should begin with normal saline (10 to 20 ml/kg/h for the first 1 to 2 hours). If the child is hypoglycemic, 2 to 4 ml of $D_{25}W$ can be added (50% dextrose 1 to 2 ml diluted 1:1 with sterile water).

Hydrocortisone (because it has a mineralocorticoid as well as a glucocorticoid effect in these doses) is the recommended drug, using an initial bolus of 50 mg in infancy, 100 mg during childhood, and 200 mg once body mass approximates adult size. The bolus should be followed by one-half the initial dosage given by intravenous infusion (not bolus) every 6 hours. Once the patient is stabilized and

TABLE 1. Glucocorticoid Therapy

	EQUIVALENT DOSE (GLUCOCORTICOID EFFECT)	REPLACEMENT DOSE (mg/m²/24 h)
Oral		
Hydrocortisone	100	15–18
Prednisone	20	4–5
Methylprednisolone	12.5	3–4
Dexamethasone	1.25	0.23–0.27
Parenteral		
Cortisone acetate	75	12.5–15
Hydrocortisone	62.5	7–12

recovery has begun, the dose can be decreased by one half at 1 to 3 day intervals until *physiologic replacement dose (7 to 12 mg/m²/24 h)* is reached. Because the significant mineralocorticoid effect of large doses of hydrocortisone wanes, fludrocortisone (Florinef) should be added during tapering of the hydrocortisone dose. To change glucocorticoid to oral replacement therapy, see Chronic Therapy.

At times of major physical stress, such as febrile (>37.5°C) illness, major trauma, or surgery, stress doses (approximately three times physiologic replacement) should be given. If one considers the upper range of production rates per day of 12 mg, tripling this dose would be 36 mg/m²/d of hydrocortisone. If the child is clinically stable and can tolerate oral medication, the usual daily dose can be given orally in tripled quantities until the stress has subsided. If this duration has been 5 days or less, the dose can be dropped back to the physiologic range. If longer, the dose can be tapered to double replacement for 3 to 5 days before being dropped back to the physiologic range.

If the patient is vomiting or too ill to take oral medications, parenteral glucocorticoid must be used. Parents or caretakers should be prepared for such an emergency situation by having *available at home hydrocortisone sodium succinate* in a ready-to-mix vial, with syringes and needles. Caretakers should be instructed to give this medication either subcutaneously or intramuscularly. The dose is 50 mg for a child less than 2 years of age and 100 mg for the older child. Whenever such an emergency situation arises, the injection should be given. Immediate medical attention then should be sought for further assessment, determination of underlying causes of the stress, need for specific therapy for the precipitating illness, and continuing need for increased glucocorticoid therapy. The need for fluid and electrolyte therapy should be ascertained by clinical evidence of dehydration and determination of glucose and electrolyte levels.

Intramuscular cortisone acetate does not provide an acute effect but can be used for continuing coverage during illness or surgery. Because significant circulating levels are not attained until 24 hours after injection, coverage can be provided only for subsequent days. An injection of 45 mg/m²/d can be given to provide the stress dose for the next 2 to 3 days. Such a regimen can be used the day before elective surgery to provide on board stress glucocorticoid levels and backup coverage should the infusion fail during anesthesia.

Chronic Therapy

Although daily physiologic replacement using parenteral glucocorticoid therapy falls within the range of daily production rates of 7 to 12 mg/m²/d, 1.5 to 2 times this amount is required for therapy orally. Daily *oral replacement doses* usually range from *12 to 18 mg/m²*. During childhood, hydrocortisone usually is used. It is available as a *liquid (2 mg/ml)* and as *tablets (5 and 10 mg)*. Because of the relatively short half-life of hydrocortisone, the most physiologic replacement *regimen* is *three times a day*. Dose calculations are based on body surface area. For example, a child who weighs 15 kg and is 99 cm tall has a surface area of 0.6 m². To begin treatment and ensure adequate therapy initially, she could be started on about 18 mg/m²/d, or 10 mg. The dose can be divided to mimic the diurnal variation pattern and provide the greatest coverage when the child is most active. For instance, the patient could be given 5 mg on arising in the morning, 2.5 mg in midafternoon after school, and the final 2.5 mg at bedtime.

The daily dose should be adjusted if there is clinical evidence of glucocorticoid excess or deficiency. Weight gain, poor growth rates, and other signs consistent with Cushing's syndrome suggest overtreatment, whereas weight loss, fatigue, and hyperpigmentation (in primary adrenal insufficiency) imply inadequate treatment. Laboratory monitoring is of limited usefulness in the determination of appropriate therapy in adrenal insufficiency. Twenty-four hour urinary free cortisol levels within the normal range suggest appropriate dosage if hydrocortisone is used. However, plasma ACTH levels are generally not helpful, since with appropriate therapy for primary adrenal insufficiency, levels often will be above the usual normal range. Because a continuous feedback system is not operative when periodic medication is given and appropriate therapy does not result in persistent ACTH

suppression, ACTH levels are useful only when they are extremely elevated or persistently suppressed. An extremely elevated level suggests inadequate dosing or noncompliance, and a persistently low level indicates overtreatment (or ACTH deficiency).

The mineralocorticoid *fludrocortisone (Florinef)* is available as *scored 0.1 mg tablets,* and the usual dose is 0.1 mg/d, ranging from 0.05 to 0.15 mg, except in early infancy, when the requirement is greater and 0.2 to 0.3 mg may be needed for the first few months of life. Plasma renin levels are useful to assess the adequacy of mineralocorticoid therapy. Generally, if the patient appears well, electrolytes will be compensated and within the normal range, perhaps at the cost of excessive salt intake and renin secretion. Excessive mineralocorticoid effect may cause hypertension. Therefore, treatment with mineralocorticoid, as with glucocorticoid, should be adjusted based on clinical findings.

CONGENITAL ADRENAL HYPERPLASIA

The congenital adrenal hyperplasias are a group of disorders that impair conversion of cholesterol to steroid hormones, principally cortisol, occurring secondary to blocks at any step in the biosynthetic pathways. Decreased cortisol levels lead to increased ACTH secretion such that certain steroid hormones are excessively secreted. The signs and symptoms of each specific type of congenital adrenal hyperplasia are related to which steroid hormones are overproduced in addition to those of glucocorticoid deficiency. In 21-hydroxylase deficiency, the most common form of congenital adrenal hyperplasia, decreased cortisol synthesis leads to increased adrenal androgen production. Aldosterone biosynthesis also may be impaired. Virilization and decreased mineralocorticoid production can occur in 3β-hydroxysteroid dehydrogenase deficiency. Since deoxycorticosterone has mineralocorticoid activity, 11β-hydroxylase deficiency is characterized by glucocorticoid deficiency, virilization, and hypertension. Two separate catalytic sites on P450c17 perform 17α-hydroxylase activity and 17,20-lyase activity. The signs and symptoms of decreased P450c17 activity include glucocorticoid deficiency, hypertension, and decreased sex steroid synthesis. However, the clinical features may vary depending how each enzyme activity is affected.

Principles of Treatment

Except for rare forms of adrenal hyperplasia, these enzyme deficiencies (most commonly 21-hydroxylase deficiency) result in compromised ability to produce cortisol, which in turn results in excessive ACTH stimulation, with the production of excessive amounts of steroids not affected by the enzyme block. Decreased activities of 21α-hydroxylase or 11β-hydroxylase result in excessive production of adrenal androgens. This causes virilization of the female fetus, premature pubarche, peripheral precocious puberty in males, excessive growth and bone maturation during childhood, and hirsutism and oligomenorrhea and amenorrhea at and after puberty. Decreased activity of 3β-hydroxysteroid dehydrogenase can cause ambiguous genitalia in the neonate because of excessive androgen levels in the female fetus and inadequate testosterone levels in the male fetus. After birth, principal manifestations are similar to those of 21α-hydroxylase deficiency.

Appropriate treatment of these disorders is the *replacement of physiologic amounts* of glucocorticoid, which not only provides for the patient's needs but also provides sufficient feedback to *suppress the excessive ACTH secretion*. When ACTH levels decrease, adrenal androgen production decreases to age-appropriate levels. If the enzyme blockade involves the production of aldosterone as well (such as in severe cases of 21-hydroxylase deficiency), oral mineralocorticoid may be necessary.

With 21α-hydroxylase deficiency or 3β-hydroxysteroid dehydrogenase deficiency, mineralocorticoid synthesis may be impaired, and replacement therapy with fludrocortisone is necessary. Mineralocorticoid therapy is generally not necessary with 11β-hydroxylase or 17α-hydroxylase/17,20-lyase deficiencies in which deoxycorticosterone is secreted. However, with 11β-hydroxylase deficiency, the neonate or older treated patients with intercurrent gastroenteritis may have salt loss.

Acute Treatment, Initial Therapy

The initial therapy for enzyme deficiencies is the same as described for adrenal insufficiency. If this condition is severe enough to present in infancy, adrenal insufficiency usually develops between day 5 and day 10 of life. In males, the presenting findings are excessive weight loss and vomiting. Among infant females, virilized genitalia provide the clue to suspect this diagnosis. When the patient presents with evidence of an acute adrenal crisis, *initial treatment* should be directed *toward fluid and electrolyte needs* while *concomitantly giving stress doses of glucocorticoid*. Before initiation of steroid therapy, a blood sample should be obtained for determinations of 17-hydroxyprogesterone, 17-hydroxypregnenolone, progesterone, androstenedione, dehydroepiandrosterone, deoxycortisol, electrolytes, and plasma renin activity. Hyponatremia and hyperkalemia indicate the need for mineralocorticoid, which is provided by large doses of hydrocortisone. Fludrocortisone should be added as soon as oral medication can be given. Until adequate sodium has been retained, and sometime during infancy, supplemental salt (1 to 2 g/d) may be required.

If the newborn is not stressed, *oral liquid hydrocortisone*, supplied 2 mg/ml, can be begun at *18 mg/m²/d divided into three doses*. Subsequent adjustments are made based on the guidelines discussed under Chronic Therapy.

Chronic Therapy

Although the guidelines for doses with glucocorticoids are similar to those for adrenal insufficiency, monitoring therapy is more complex with congenital adrenal hyperplasia. The goal is to give adequate amounts of glucocorticoid to suppress excessive ACTH and adrenal androgen secretion. If the dose completely suppresses ACTH secretion, however, the amount of glucocorticoid will be excessive and will suppress growth. Therefore, glucocorticoid must be adjusted so that growth is not stimulated by excessive adrenal androgens or suppressed by excessive glucocorticoid. Therapy is monitored by assessing growth rate and physical evidence of androgen and glucocorticoid excess, skeletal age x-rays at 6 to 24 month intervals, and a plasma or urinary index of androgen secretion (androstenedione, testosterone in females or prepubertal males, and urinary 17-ketosteroid excretion). Plasma 17-hydroxyprogesterone levels are a difficult index for monitoring therapy for 21-hydroxylase deficiency, since levels are not expected to be within the usual normal range and must be obtained 2 to 3 hours after the previous glucocorticoid dose. Similar difficulties may be present when attempting to monitor therapy for 11β-hydroxylase deficiency using deoxycortisol and for dehydroepiandrosterone for 3β-hydroxysteroid dehydrogenase deficiency.

DISORDERS OF MINERALOCORTICOID SECRETION

Adrenal Cortical Hypertension

Elevated mineralocorticoid levels lead to sodium retention, with subsequent hypertension, increased potassium excretion, and suppressed plasma renin activity. Although rare, elevated mineralocorticoid levels may occur during childhood in two types of congenital adrenal hyperplasia, 11β-hydroxylase deficiency and 17α-hydroxylase/17,20-lyase deficiency, in idiopathic hyperaldosteronism, and in aldosterone-secreting adenomas.

Dexamethasone-suppressible hyperaldosteronism is an inherited disorder in which the hyperaldosteronism and hypokalemia improve with glucocorticoid therapy. The pathophysiology is explained by a mutation involving the 11β-hydroxylase gene usually expressed in the zona fasciculata and the gene encoding aldosterone synthetase expressed in the glomerulosa. This intergenic recombination event places the promoter region of the gene usually expressed in the fasciculata in the aldosterone synthetase gene, making its action responsive to ACTH rather than to angiotensin II. This explains why

treatment with dexamethasone to suppress ACTH is effective in this disorder.

Apparent mineralocorticoid excess is characterized by hypertension, hypokalemia, and suppression of the renin-angiotensin axis. A deficiency of 11-hydroxysteroid dehydrogenase results in decreased conversion of cortisol to its inactive metabolite, cortisone. Urinary free cortisol excretion is elevated, although patients do not have other stigmata of Cushing's syndrome. The excessive cortisol acts as a mineralocorticoid.

Corticosterone methyloxidase I and II deficiency, defects of mineralocorticoid synthesis, results in aldosterone deficiency. During childhood, the clinical features include hyponatremia, hyperkalemia, and failure to thrive.

Hypercortisolism

Cushing's syndrome signifies excessive cortisol levels. Clinical features include obesity, decreased muscle mass, fatigue, and increased bruisability. Growth failure occurs in childhood. Premature sexual hair, altered carbohydrate tolerance, and decreased bone mineral density may be present. The most common form of Cushing's syndrome is iatrogenic, caused by pharmacologic glucocorticoid therapy. Excessive adrenal cortisol secretion can be primary because of adrenal tumors or secondary to excessive ACTH secretion. The term, Cushing's disease, refers to excessive pituitary ACTH secretion.

Pituitary Surgery

Transphenoidal pituitary surgery is the treatment of choice among children with Cushing's disease in whom pituitary adenomas can be identified. However, hypophysectomy generally is avoided among children without obvious adenomas but with pituitary ACTH excess to avoid hypopituitarism. Therefore, such children can be treated with either bilateral adrenalectomy or radiation therapy. Radiation therapy does not produce an effect for several months. During the interim, medical therapy may be used to treat glucocorticoid excess.

When pituitary adenomas can be identified and removed, the patient may become immediately cortisol deficient, since secretion by the remaining ACTH-secreting cells is suppressed. Therefore, not only should these *patients be covered during surgery with stress doses of cortisol,* but also replacement levels of cortisol should be maintained after surgery until adequate endogenous secretory capacity can be demonstrated. If the patient experiences evidence of withdrawal from the excessive cortisol (including arthralgias, edema, fatigue, hypotension), the dose should be tapered gradually over weeks or months.

Pituitary Radiation

Radiation therapy has a relatively *low remission rate* and a delay before remission among patients who do respond. There is also a risk of developing *other pituitary hormone dysfunction*. Therefore, such therapy should be used with caution during childhood.

Medical Therapy

Medical therapy for Cushing's syndrome is inadequate and should be used only while awaiting results of radiation therapy, in preparation for adrenal surgery, or in patients unable to tolerate surgery. Ketoconazole has produced the best results.

Adrenal Surgery

Bilateral adrenalectomy is appropriate therapy for patients with Cushing's disease without detectable adenomas and for those in whom pituitary surgery or radiation has failed to produce remission. The result is primary adrenal insufficiency, and therapy is as outlined previously. Consequences may include regrowth of adrenal remnants or adrenal rest tissue or the development of Nelson's syndrome (hyperpigmentation and growth or development of pituitary adenomas).

Surgical resection is the initial treatment for adrenal tumors, whether adenomas or carcinomas. During childhood, adenomas may secrete primarily cortisol or primarily androgens. Carcinomas, although rare, are relatively more common in childhood and account for up to one half of cases of noniatrogenic Cushing's syndrome, especially among the very young. Such carcinomas often produce not only excessive cortisol but also other adrenal steroids. They are rapid growing and may have metastasized by the time they are diagnosed. Initial treatment is surgical, but medical therapy also may be needed in an attempt to control steroid excess and growth of metastases.

Patients with bilateral adrenal nodular hyperplasia require bilateral adrenalectomy. In this, as in any situation in which the adrenal glands are removed, patients must be treated for adrenal insufficiency.

Withdrawal of Exogenous Glucocorticoids

Cushing's syndrome is most commonly iatrogenic, the result of administration of supraphysiologic doses of glucocorticoids. The withdrawal of such pharmacologic therapy may be limited by the underlying condition. The following guidelines are provided for the situations in which withdrawal is possible. The dose can be *reduced by one half* at *intervals of 3 days until physiologic replacement levels* are attained (Table 1). From this point on, the dose should be tapered more slowly and with caution, remembering that increased doses are indicated during times of stress until one can be confident of full recovery of the adrenal axis. Generally, the dose can be *lowered every 7 to 10 days by increments of about 25% of the replacement dose.* After one-fourth replacement, the taper can be dropped to only the morning dose and then to the morning dose every other day. Thereafter, the dose can be stopped. Major illness or stress or exacerbation of the underlying condition may cause resumption of steroid therapy. If so, guidelines as outlined can be used to stop therapy again. If the drug is given for 5 days or less, it can be stopped abruptly.

The tapering schedule described should be used if the pharmacologic doses have been given for more than 2 months. If treatment has been for less than 1 month, the taper can be very abbreviated; if less than 1 week, no taper is required. Stress coverage may be required for up to a year after a period of prolonged suppression.

ADRENAL TUMORS

Adrenal tumors may secrete excessive quantities of glucocorticoids, mineralocorticoids, and adrenal androgens. Those that secrete excessive glucocorticoids present as Cushing's syndrome. Virilizing tumors can cause premature pubarche, accelerated growth velocity, hypertension, clitoromegaly in girls, and peripheral precocious puberty in boys. Histologic differentiation of adrenal carcinomas from adenomas may be difficult, but generally tumors that have invaded the capsule or are metastatic at the time of surgery have a poorer prognosis. Rarely, adrenal tumors secrete estrogens, leading to gynecomastia in boys and premature thelarche in girls.

Pheochromocytoma

Pheochromocytomas are rare biogenic amine-secreting tumors arising from chromaffin tissue. The clinical manifestations, headache, diaphoresis, palpitations, and hypertension, are due to the effects of the biogenic amines. Paroxysmal symptoms may occur. Although most occur within the adrenal medulla, they can develop anywhere along the sympathetic chain from the brain to the pelvis. Malignant tumors are uncommon. Pheochromocytomas comprise one feature of multiple endocrine neoplasia syndrome type IIA. Definitive diagnosis depends on demonstration of excessive endogenous catecholamine levels: 24-hour urinary excretion of vanillylmandelic acid (VMA), normetanephrine-metanephrine, and free catecholamines. Ultrasound, CT scan, and MRI scan may help localize the tumor(s).

Neuroblastoma

Neuroblastomas, tumors derived from primitive neuroblasts, may be located wherever sympathetic nervous tissue is found. Presenting clinical features include abdominal mass, weight loss, and fever. Urinary catecholamine secretion is elevated in 85% to 90% of patients. The finding of multiple copies of the N-*myc* oncogene is associated with more rapid progression of disease. Ganglioneuromas, benign

tumors detected incidentally, may present spontaneous maturation of neuroblastomas.

Treatment

Treatment is surgical after proper preparation with *adrenergic blockade.* Phenoxybenzamine may be used in doses from 0.25 to 1.0 mg/kg/d. Because the effect is cumulative, the dose should be begun low, with increases if needed after several days. Treatment generally can be accomplished with removing the adrenal cortex. Severe hypertension or hypotension may occur postoperatively.

REFERENCES

1. Miller JW, Crapo L: The medical treatment of Cushing's syndrome. Endocr Rev 14:443–458, 1993.
2. Morel Y, Miller WL: Clinical and molecular genetics of congenital adrenal hyperplasia due to 21-hydroxylase deficiency. Adv Hum Genet 20:1–68, 1991.
3. Sheps SG, Jiang NS, Klee GG, et al: Recent developments in the diagnosis and treatment of pheochromocytoma. Mayo Clin Proc 65:88–95, 1990.

ENDOCRINE DISORDERS OF THE TESTIS

MICHAEL A. WOOD, M.D.
JOSEPH I. WOLFSDORF, M.B., B.Ch.

Endocrine disorders of the testis impair secretion of testosterone. Unresponsiveness of target tissues to androgens can cause similar clinical appearances. There is a wide spectrum of abnormalities in children with hypogonadal states. A complete diagnosis is critical before starting therapy.

MANAGEMENT DURING INFANCY

Male genital development in utero requires normal production of testosterone, its conversion to dihydrotestosterone, and a normal response to androgens in target tissues.

Micropenis or Ambiguous Genitalia

The most important initial step in management is proper measurement of the phallus size and comparison to normal standards for age. At term, the third percentile for stretched length of the penis is 2.8 cm (2.5 cm is 2.5 SD below the mean and is used as the lower limit of normal) and width is 0.9 cm. Not infrequently, a normal phallus is buried in suprapubic fat.

True micropenis results either from defective testosterone secretion or action in utero or from a field defect in perineal development that usually is accompanied by other major anomalies of the urogenital tract. Early testosterone deficiency causes severe hypospadias or ambiguous or female-appearing genitalia. Later or less severe testosterone deficiency typically causes micropenis without other genital abnormalities. The karyotype is important in guiding management decisions.

The association of *isolated micropenis* with prolonged neonatal jaundice or hypoglycemia suggests congenital hypopituitarism. Vanishing testes is suggested by high serum levels of gonadotropins. Testosterone is given to demonstrate responsiveness of the phallus.

Therapy of *micropenis with perineoscrotal hypospadias* is dictated by the specific diagnosis, which must be established before treatment is started. Etiologies include 46,XY gonadal dysgenesis, vanishing testes, congenital adrenal hyperplasia (deficiency of sidechain cleavage enzyme, 17α-hydroxylase, 17,20-lyase, 3β-hydroxysteroid dehydrogenase), 5α-reductase deficiency, and partial androgen insensitivity. Treatment of congenital adrenal hyperplasia is discussed in the section on adrenal disorders. After measuring serum levels of testosterone, dihydrotestosterone, and gonadotropins, a trial of human chorionic gonadotropin (hCG) is performed to assess the ability of testicular tissue (if present) to produce testosterone and to measure its conversion to dihydrotestosterone. If these mechanisms are normal, phallus size increases modestly. If testosterone production is inadequate, testosterone enanthate is used to evaluate androgen responsiveness. If testosterone and dihydrotestosterone levels are normal, the diagnosis may be androgen insensitivity, and a trial of high-dose testosterone may be indicated.

Severe microphallus, despite a 46,XY karyotype, is an indication for assigning a female gender and rearing the child as a girl (see section on Ambiguous Genitalia). If the level of serum testosterone is normal but dihydrotestosterone is markedly reduced, the child has 5α-reductase deficiency, and topical dihydrotestosterone 2% in a cream base can be applied twice daily to the penis before surgical correction. Therapy may be repeated throughout childhood to promote growth of the phallus and maintain an average size for age. Testosterone is ineffective in this condition.

Gender assignment with *mixed gonadal dysgenesis (45,XO/46,XY)* depends on the appearance of the external genitalia. Patients are at high risk of developing gonadoblastomas, and gonadectomy should be performed before puberty. Testicular prostheses are implanted in the scrotum before school age to obviate any ambiguity about sexual identity or body image. These are replaced with adult-sized prostheses in midadolescence.

Diagnostic and Therapeutic Protocols

Human chorionic gonadotropin (hCG) stimulation with 500 IU or 3000 IU/m² of hCG is given SC or IM three times a week (Monday, Wednesday, and Friday). If the level of testosterone is inadequate 24 to 48 hours after the third dose or if the initial testosterone and dihydrotestosterone values are normal or high-normal and partial androgen insensitivity is the likely diagnosis, treatment with testosterone is indicated (Table 1).

Testosterone enanthate 25 mg is given IM every 3 to 4 weeks for 3 months. After three doses of testosterone, a measurable increase (>0.5 cm) should occur in the stretched length of the penis. No growth suggests androgen insensitivity, and a course of high-dose testosterone (50 to 100 mg IM every 2 to 3 weeks) may be given for 2 to 3 months. Linear growth and bone age must be carefully monitored. If the infant responds adequately, IM testosterone 75 mg/m²/y can be given intermittently during childhood until the phallus reaches the average length for age. *Topical testosterone* 1% in a cream base gives less uniform results than parenteral testosterone. Close follow-up in conjunction with a urologist experienced in treating ambiguous genitalia is essential.

Cryptorchidism

In the neonate with bilateral cryptorchidism, severe virilizing congenital adrenal hyperplasia of a 46,XX infant must be urgently ruled out. Such infants can present with a normal appearing phallus and apparently undescended testes. Cryptorchidism may occur in infants with hypogonadism, as part of a syndrome (more than 40 have been described), or as an isolated phenomenon.

The earlier the testes are brought into the scrotum, the greater the likelihood of fertility and avoidance of testicular pathology. Testes,

ideally, should be brought into the scrotum before 2 years of age. In recent placebo-controlled studies (retractile testes excluded), hCG was ineffective in the treatment of undescended testes. Spontaneous testicular descent often occurs in the first 6 months of life. Therefore, we recommend surgical correction for undescended testes at about 1 year of age. hCG may be given to assess the ability of undescended testes to secrete testosterone. If the undescended testis really is a retractile testis, hCG may cause its descent.

MANAGEMENT AT PUBERTY

Minimal change in genital size occurs from birth until the onset of puberty. Secondary sexual development at puberty is caused by increased production of testosterone and, to a lesser extent, dihydrotestosterone. An important developmental task for boys during puberty is to develop a healthy body image. Regardless of the diagnosis, the boy must be reassured that, with therapy, he will lead a normal male adult life. Fertility usually becomes a concern for the patient only on reaching adulthood but often is a major concern of the parents of the infant or young child with testicular dysfunction.

Constitutional Delay of Puberty

At age 14 to 15 years, with a bone age ≥12.5 years, a diagnostic and therapeutic trial of testosterone enanthate is given 50 to 100 mg IM monthly for three to six doses. This increases penis size and promotes growth of pubic hair in most boys and does not affect final adult height. A second course may be given if the results of a single course of therapy are not satisfactory.

Primary or Secondary Hypogonadism

Treatment to induce sexual maturation should commence when the bone age is ≥11 years. In normal puberty, gradually escalating testosterone production occurs over 2 to 3 years until adult levels (production rate 4 to 7 mg/d) are achieved at Tanner stage IV. Treatment should attempt to mimic the natural course.

Parenteral Testosterone

Testosterone, esterified at the 17β-hydroxyl position (enanthate or cypionate), is commonly prescribed for hypogonadism. The enanthate and cypionate sidechains make the esters less polar and more fat soluble and retard their absorption. They are available in 100 to 200 mg/ml vials in sesame and cottonseed oil, respectively. The starting dose is 50 mg IM monthly for 6 months. The monthly dose is increased by 50 mg every 6 months. After reaching a dose of 100 mg/mo, we decrease the dosing interval to every 2 weeks because serum testosterone levels tend to fall below normal 2 weeks after a single monthly dose. Measurement of trough levels of testosterone can be used to guide further increases in dose. A typical adult dose is 200 mg at 2-week intervals and is reached in 36 months. A higher dose can be used less frequently (e.g., 300 mg at 3-week intervals) but causes unduly high peak values in the first few days after each injection. Injections less often than every 3 weeks result in symptoms of hypoandrogenism. Complaints with this form of therapy are minimal

TABLE 1. Medications Used for Endocrine Disorders of the Testis

DRUG	BRAND NAME (COMPANY)	VEHICLE	CONTENTS PER VIAL
Testosterone enanthate	Delatestryl (Gynex)	Sesame oil	100–200 mg/ml 1 ml syringe; 5 ml vial
Testosterone cypionate	Depo-Testosterone (Upjohn)	Cottonseed oil	100–200 mg/ml
	Virilon IM (Star)	Cottonseed oil	200 mg/ml (10 ml vial)
Methyltestosterone	Android (ICN)	Tablets	10, 25 mg
	Virilon (Star)	Capsules	10 mg
	Testred (ICN)	Capsules	10 mg
Fluoxymesterone	Halotestin (Upjohn)	Tablets	2, 5, 10 mg
Human chorionic gonadotropin (hCG)	Profasi (Serono)	Water	5000–10,000 IU/vial

and primarily relate to discomfort from intramuscular injection. If therapy is begun after the age of 18 years, the schedule can be compressed into 24 months. More rapid increases can cause excessive libido and priapism. Supraphysiologic serum testosterone levels occur for the first few days after each injection and may have a transient deleterious effect on plasma lipoproteins (decreased HDL, apo A-I, and increased LDL) and suppress gonadotropins in those with partial deficiencies. The normal diurnal variation of testosterone levels cannot be reproduced with this method of treatment.

Other delivery systems are being developed, including trocar-inserted crystalline testosterone pellets, testosterone microcapsules, and testosterone patches for either scrotal or truncal skin absorption. The patches are replaced daily and mimic the diurnal variation of testosterone. These systems are not widely accepted and have not been tried in children.

Side effects that may occur with any testosterone preparation include acne, fluid retention, worsening of sleep apnea, breast tenderness or gynecomastia, and weight gain.

Although achievement of fertility is not usually an important therapeutic issue for pediatricians seeing adolescent males, it is important to inform patients with secondary forms of hypogonadism caused by hypothalamic-pituitary dysfunction that spermatogenesis can be induced and fertility achieved by pharmacologic means. Such therapies are complex and expensive, and patients should be referred to endocrinologists with expertise in the treatment of these disorders.

Oral Androgens

The 17α-alkylated testosterone compounds were used in the past to maintain secondary sexual characteristics in boys in whom initial virilization was accomplished with testosterone esters. Oral therapy was better tolerated than intramuscular injection. Because these compounds may cause cholestasis, aminotransferase elevation, peliosis hepatis, and hepatocellular carcinoma, their use is not recommended in children. High levels in the liver on first pass have adverse effects on lipoproteins, a drop in HDL and an increase in LDL. In rare circumstances, when parenteral use of testosterone is impossible or potentially harmful (e.g., hemostatic disorders), oral androgens may be used. The dose of methyltestosterone (17α-methyltestosterone, half-life 2.5 hours) to maintain secondary sexual characteristics is 5 to 20 mg twice a day. It is available in 10 and 25 mg tablets and capsules. The longer acting preparation, fluoxymesterone (9α-fluoro-11β-hydroxy-17α-methyltestosterone, Halotestin, half-life 10 hours), is given once daily. It is available in 2, 5, and 10 mg tablets, and the usual dose is 10 to 20 mg.

GYNECOMASTIA

JOSEPH I. WOLFSDORF, M.B., B.Ch.

Gynecomastia refers to benign enlargement of the male breast, and in pediatric medicine, it occurs in three age groups: newborn, prepuberty, and puberty.

NEWBORN

Sixty to ninety percent of newborn infants of both sexes have palpable breast tissue that increases in size in the first few days of life. Neonatal gynecomastia results from transplacental passage of maternal estrogen to the fetus and can be expected to resolve spontaneously within a few weeks or, in occasional cases, a few months. No investigation or therapy is required. Gynecomastia may be accompanied by galactorrhea (witch's milk), and it is important to instruct parents not to manipulate the baby's breasts in an attempt to discharge the milk because this can lead to infection.

PREPUBERTY

Gynecomastia before puberty is rare and warrants a thorough search for a possible source of exogenous estrogens, such as ingestion of contraceptive pills, use of an estrogen-containing cream, or consumption of milk, meat, or poultry that contains estrogens. The breast is exquisitely sensitive to estrogen. Consequently, gynecomastia can develop in boys exposed to trace amounts of estrogens in foods. This makes it difficult or impossible to identify the source in many instances. Furthermore, gynecomastia may persist after the exposure to estrogen has ceased. Thus, at the time of evaluation, the causative pharmacologic or environmental factor may no longer be present. Other causes of prepubertal gynecomastia should be assiduously sought by endocrinologic investigation and appropriate imaging techniques. Ultrasonography of the testes may help to identify an impalpable testicular tumor, and computed tomography (CT) and magnetic resonance imaging (MRI) of the abdomen are useful to search for adrenal tumors. These include estrogen-secreting adrenal or testicular tumors, congenital adrenal hyperplasia (especially 11β-hydroxylase deficiency), and trophoblastic (human chorionic gonadotropin or hCG-secreting) tumors. The virilization of sexual precocity may be associated with gynecomastia, as it would in normal adolescent development. Treatment of the underlying disorder will stop progression of the gynecomastia. If the workup is negative, the patient may be said to have idiopathic prepubertal gynecomastia, for which there is no specific therapy, and the gynecomastia can be expected to resolve spontaneously within a few years.

PUBERTY

A firm disc of subareolar breast tissue, often slightly tender, which may be accompanied by elevation of the areola, is common in healthy adolescent boys. The prevalence varies depending on the ages of the subjects and the criterion used to define gynecomastia but has been found to be as high as 69%. The diameter of the breast usually does not exceed 4 cm. Pubertal gynecomastia is usually most evident at 13 to 14 years of age, corresponding to Tanner stages III–IV pubertal development. The breasts are typically unequal in size, and the discrepancy can be marked. The patient and his parents should be reassured that this is a normal developmental phenomenon related to the production of sex hormones and does not signify a pathologic state. It can be expected to regress spontaneously within 24 months and does not require treatment.

Extremely prominent breast enlargement can occur as an expression of pubertal gynecomastia (pubertal macromastia), but before one ascribes it to this cause, it is appropriate to undertake a thorough search to rule out an estrogen-secreting tumor of the adrenal gland or testis or a trophoblastic (hCG-secreting) tumor. Other pathologic causes of gynecomastia are drug exposure, liver disease, Graves' disease, and disorders characterized by testicular deficiency (e.g., Klinefelter's syndrome or other cause of primary hypogonadism). Drugs that may cause gynecomastia are shown in Table 1. The presence of galactorrhea warrants testing for a prolactinoma. The testes should be examined carefully for the presence of a tumor, and their size should be determined as accurately as possible. A testicular volume exceeding 4 ml or a length greater than 2.5 cm excludes Klinefelter's syndrome from further consideration. Differentiation of mammary tissue from adipose tissue by palpation may be difficult in obese youths in whom the appearance of gynecomastia (pseudogynecomastia) usually is principally the result of accumulation of adipose tissue in the area of the breast. True gynecomastia can be differentiated from pseudogynecomastia by examination of the patient in the supine position. The breast is grasped between the thumb and forefinger, which are moved gently toward the nipple. If gynecomastia is present, a firm or rubbery, mobile, disclike mound of tissue will be felt arising from beneath the nipple and the areolar region. If the enlargement is caused by adipose tissue, no such disc of tissue will be palpable. Weight loss will reduce the size of breasts largely composed of adipose tissue. Gynecomastia must be differentiated from rare tumors, such

TABLE 1. Drugs That May Cause Gynecomastia

Hormones Androgens and anabolic steroids Chorionic gonadotropin Estrogens and estrogen agonists **Antiandrogens or Inhibitors of Androgen Synthesis** Cyproterone Flutamide **Antibiotics** Isoniazid Ketoconazole Metronidazole **Histamine H$_2$-receptor Antagonists** Cimetidine Ranitidine	**Cardiovascular Drugs** Amiodarone Captopril Digitoxin Enalapril Methyldopa Nifedipine Reserpine Verapamil **Psychotropic Agents** Diazepam Haloperidol Phenothiazines Tricyclic antidepressants **Recreational Drugs** Alcohol Amphetamines Heroin Marijuana

as lipoma, neurofibroma, and breast cancer, that may present as breast enlargement.

Testosterone therapy is contraindicated in adolescent gynecomastia and will actually increase the size of the breasts. It may be indicated, however, in patients with Klinefelter's syndrome with subnormal testosterone levels, but its effect on gynecomastia is not consistently beneficial.

Severe physiologic gynecomastia with more than 5 cm breast tissue and pronounced areolar changes will seldom resolve spontaneously or, if it does, will take several years to occur. Because pronounced gynecomastia is difficult to conceal and is a source of extreme embarrassment to the afflicted youth, treatment to reduce the volume of breast tissue is warranted. Various drug regimens have been reported to be effective for the treatment of gynecomastia. However, the studies have not all been well controlled, nor have the beneficial effects of these medications been widely confirmed.[1] Dihydrotestosterone heptanoate, which cannot be aromatized to estrogen, has been used to treat patients with prolonged pubertal gynecomastia. A reduction in breast volume occurred in the majority of subjects, but only one fourth had a complete response. Testolactone, an aromatase inhibitor, has been used in an uncontrolled trial in a small number of patients with pubertal gynecomastia. Patients received 450 mg/d for up to 6 months, and breast size decreased without side effects when the drug was taken for at least 2 months. A placebo-controlled, double-blind study of the use of this drug for treatment of pubertal gynecomastia has not been performed. Both clomiphene citrate and tamoxifen have been used for their antiestrogenic effects. Clomiphene, in a relatively large dose of 100 mg/d for 6 months, was associated with a complete reduction in breast volume in two thirds of patients, without side effects. Tamoxifen cannot be recommended for use until its efficacy and safety are clearly demonstrated in controlled clinical trials.

If a trial of medical therapy is unsuccessful or if the gynecomastia has been present for several years, the glandular tissue of the breast should be removed surgically. A reduction mammoplasty through a circumareolar incision is recommended sooner rather than later to spare the boy further embarrassment and any possibility of confusion about his sexual identity. Modern surgical techniques can be expected to result in a barely noticeable hairline scar.

REFERENCES

1. Braunstein GD: Gynecomastia. N Engl J Med 328:490–495, 1993.
2. LeRoith D, Sobel R, Glick SM: The effect of clomiphene citrate on pubertal gynaecomastia. Acta Endocrinol (Copenh) 95:177–180, 1980.
3. Zachmann M, Eiholzer U, Muritano M, Werder EA, Manella B: Treatment of pubertal gynaecomastia with testolactone. Acta Endocrinol (Copenh) (Suppl) 279:218–226, 1986.

AMBIGUOUS GENITALIA

SELVA S. SCHENKMAN, M.D.
EDNA H. SOBEL, M.D.

The assignment of gender usually occurs in the delivery room. The case of a newborn with ambiguous genitalia represents a medical and social emergency. Designation of sex must await expeditious and rational investigation to establish the sex of rearing. *During this period, the infant must be monitored for the emergence of a metabolic problem: hypoglycemia or hyponatremia.* The family will require support. Explanation that the sex structures of the child developed incompletely during fetal life is needed. Diagrams of fetal sexual differentiation will be helpful to show the similarities of external genital appearance of boys and girls at the third month of gestation.

A good history is required to differentiate exogenous (maternal) from endogenous (fetal) causes of ambiguity. A family history of unexpected neonatal death will direct attention to the possibility of an adrenal enzyme defect.

Useful details in physical examination include the presence of palpable gonads and perineal malformations. Rectal examination is helpful because the cervix of an infant girl often is palpable. The presence of internal feminine structure may be revealed by pressure on the uterus, which may cause mucus to be extruded from a urogenital sinus. Ultrasonography is usually not definitive because there is little fat to provide contrast.

Laboratory procedures should be chosen on the basis of probable etiology. Those usually selected are karyotype, which is much more reliable than a buccal smear, and 17-OH progesterone, 11-deoxycortisol, and testosterone.

Spot urine checks for sodium (Na$^+$) and potassium (K$^+$) ratio can be useful because abnormal salt balance will become evident in the urine before it is reflected in the plasma. By the fifth day of life, plasma renin, Na$^+$, and K$^+$ will identify the infant with salt-wasting congenital adrenal hyperplasia (CAH). Other procedures, such as adrenocorticotropic hormone (ACTH) stimulation and gonadotropin stimulation, will come later, if needed.

It is useful to design the investigation in accordance with knowledge of normal sex differentiation. Sex differentiation is sequential and involves several phases from the moment of conception. The genetic sex is determined at fertilization. The gonadal sex is determined by the chromosomes. The function of the gonadal axis determines the internal and external phenotype. Finally, gender identity is acquired postnatally by the individual through lived experiences, environment, and personal hormonal milieu.

The fetal ovary does not secrete testosterone or müllerian inhibiting factor (MIF). The normal female is born without male differentiation of the external genitalia and without mullerian repression (with uterus and fallopian tubes). The fetal testis does secrete testosterone and MIF. Fetal androgens cause stimulation of the wolffian ducts, posterior migration of the labioscrotal folds so that the phallus lies anterior to the scrotum, elongation of the genital tubercle, midline fusion of the genital folds, and swellings to form the penis and scrotal sacs. In the male, the source of androgen is the fetal testis. In a female fetus, any source of androgen will cause complete or partial male differentiation of external genitalia. Failure to secrete enough androgen results in various degrees of male pseudohermaphroditism.

There are four pathophysiologic categories of sexual ambiguity.

1. Virilization of an ovary-bearing 46,XX female *(female pseudohermaphroditism)*. Such a child has normal internal müllerian structures and is potentially fertile. The etiology is fetal or transplacental. In the fetus, increased androgen production occurs because of an enzyme block that interferes with cortisol production and leads to increased ACTH secretion. In 90%, the error is 21-OH deficiency, and in 10% it is 11-OH or 3-BOH dehydrogenase deficiency. All are inherited as autosomal recessive traits.

Leydig cell tissue in a 46,XX fetus with dysgenetic testes produces androgen, which masculinizes the genitalia. Such testes usually do not produce MIF, so the mullerian structures are preserved.

Androgen may reach the fetus in the first trimester from a maternal virilizing disorder or because of androgen treatment of the mother. One must remember that androgens can be ingested by accident (e.g., use of geriatric vitamin preparations).

2. Gonads palpable and incomplete masculinization of the testis-bearing 46,XY male *(male pseudohermaphroditism)*. The etiology includes hypothalamic-hypophyseal abnormality, whereby the fetal testis does not receive stimulation to produce testosterone. Such infants may become hypoglycemic because of insufficient growth hormone or ACTH. Androgen synthesis may be defective in adrenal and testis 20,22-desmolase deficiency, 17,20-desmolase deficiency, or 17-OH dehydrogenase deficiency. A human chorionic gonadotropin (hCG) stimulation test may be useful during infancy to clarify the testicular capacity to produce androgen.

Abnormalities in testosterone metabolism are another possible cause: 5α-reductase deficiency, abnormality of testosterone receptors, or a postreceptor defect. If one testis is defective, müllerian structures may persist on that side.

Androgen insensitivity comes into question only if a normal-appearing girl has an inguinal hernia. The sex of rearing must be feminine in such a child.

3. *True hermaphroditism.* In this case, the infant has both ovarian and testicular tissues, with abnormal internal and external genital structures. In 80%, karyotype is 46,XX; in 10%, 46,XY; in 10%, mosaicism (5% have female genitalia and 45,X/XY).

The gonad distribution encountered most frequently is ovary/testis or ovatestis/ovary. In the management of patients with no palpable gonads, exploratory laparotomy is almost always included. If the gonad is dysgenetic or streak, it should be removed. If there are functional ovaries and female external appearance, the testicular tissue should be removed. If there is a testis in an abnormal position and male gender can be assigned, the testis should be exteriorized, and any müllerian remnants or streak gonad should be removed. hCG stimulation and accurate hormonal evaluation should be carried out before laparotomy.

4. Anatomic disruption of normal female or male structures. In these disorders, defects of embryogenesis are included. The mechanism is neither hormonal nor chromosomal. The endocrinologist as a subspecialist should be involved for the clarification and management of sex reversal or for hormone replacement therapy in the case of gonadal reversal.

Sex assignment in infants with sexual ambiguity must involve all

these points but will be dictated mainly by the external genital appearance and the capacity of potential full function at the time of puberty and adulthood. In virilized female infants with CAH, the female gender should always be assigned, as these patients have normal internal mullerian structures and fertile ovaries.

Reconstructive surgery should be performed before age 3 years, when the toddler is first aware of his or her sex identity. Newborn males with microphallus and hypogonadism should be closely monitored for the possible appearance of hypoglycemia. Hypopituitarism should be ruled out, and hormone replacement therapy should be started when indicated. Dysgenetic tissue (gonads) should be resected, as the potential for malignancy increases with age. In cases of complete androgen insensitivity (testicular feminization), the testes should remain in place until after puberty, as they allow feminization at puberty and their potential for malignancy is very low.

Genetic workup and counseling may be indicated, since many of these conditions are inherited as autosomal recessive or X-linked traits, and other family members may have heterogeneous clinical expressions.

Once an infant is given a sex of rearing, the family should have a clear understanding and no doubts in their minds. Psychologic support and therapy should be made available when necessary for the family and child.

REFERENCES

1. Drucker S, New MI: Disorders of adrenal steroidogenesis. Pediatr Clin North Am 34:1055–1066, 1987.
2. Lippe M: Ambiguous genitalia. *In* Lavin N (ed): Manual of Endocrinology and Metabolism. Boston, Little, Brown and Company, 1994:189–198.
3. Money J: Psychologic counseling: Hermaphroditism. *In* Gardner LI (ed): Endocrine and Genetic Diseases in Childhood and Adolescence, 2nd ed. Philadelphia, WB Saunders Co, 1975:609–618.
4. Saenger P: Abnormal sexual differentiation. J Pediatr 104:1–17, 1984.
5. Styne DM: Ambiguous genitalia. *In* Fitzgerald PA (ed): Handbook of Clinical Endocrinology. Greenbrae, CA, Jones Medical Publications, 1986:65–79.

PRECOCIOUS AND DELAYED PUBERTY

DENNIS M. STYNE, M.D.

The appearance of secondary sexual characteristics begins between 9 and 14 years of age in approximately 95% of boys and between 8 and 13 years of age in approximately 95% of girls (± 2 SD). Thus, the appearance of puberty before the lower limit is precocious, and lack of pubertal appearance after the upper limit is delayed. Although psychologic effects of disorders of puberty can be significant if the patient is considerably outside the normal limits, this chapter deals solely with pharmacologic therapy of these disorders.

PRECOCIOUS PUBERTY

Isosexual precocity indicates feminization in girls (possibly with normal pubertal virilization) or virilization in boys at an age below the normal limits. True or central precocious puberty (CPP) is a premature reawakening of the hypothalamic-pituitary-gonadal axis, leading to the normal sequence of secondary sexual development at an age below the normal limits. Endocrine testing reveals hypothalamic-pituitary and gonadal function to be the same as found in normal puberty. Thus, serum pituitary gonadotropin concentrations are in the pubertal range for the given laboratory, and the luteinizing hormone (LH) response to the administration of gonadotropin-releasing hormone (GnRH) is completely pubertal (in most laboratories, more than 15.7 mIU/ml rise in LH after 100 μg of GnRH by IV administration). Serum gonadal sex steroid concentrations are likewise in the normal pubertal range (usually more than 20 ng/dl of testosterone in boys and 10 pg/ml of estradiol in girls in most laboratories). Physical development progresses rapidly, slowly, or in a waxing and waning course, depending on the individual patient, and menses occur in many girls well before the normal range. In boys, normal pubertal enlargement of the testes to a size greater than 2.5 cm in length or more than 4 ml in volume is characteristic of CPP. Height velocity increases, and skeletal development, reflected in bone age determinations, advances rapidly. Thus, the patient will be tall, but growth will cease early because of premature epiphyseal fushion, and a short adult stature results.

CPP may occur from a variety of causes. Idiopathic precocious puberty becomes a diagnosis of exclusion after all other etiologies for CPP are eliminated. Familial precocious puberty (except for premature Leydig cell and germ cell maturation) usually is apparent from family history. In this entity, early development is more borderline (usually not earlier than 6 years of age) than significantly out of the normal limits (such as 1 to 4 years of age). CPP may follow the treatment of a long-standing virilizing disorder, such as congenital adrenal hyperplasia, which was not treated with glucorticoids for several years, or a virilizing adrenal tumor removed after exerting its androgenic effects for a significant time. A hamartoma of the tuber cinereum is ectopic hypothalamic tissue that precipitates the entire endocrine course of puberty well before the lower normal age limits. Usually, hamartomas of the tuber cinereum are diagnosed on MRI or CT scan and do not require biopsy. There are conflicting views concerning the treatment of these hamartomas, but as hamartomas do not enlarge or produce further neurologic complications and as their endocrine effects are treatable with GnRH agonist, we do not recommend surgical therapy. All types of CPP may be treated with long-acting GnRH agonists.

However, CPP may result from a CNS neoplasm that will require its own primary therapy before treatment of CPP is invoked. A brain tumor must be in the differential diagnosis of any case of CPP, and an MRI or CT scan is a mandatory step in evaluation. Treatment for CNS neoplasms is beyond the scope of this section.

The most mild cases of CPP without significant advancement of bone age or elevation of pubertal hormones may not require therapy, since final height may not be affected. Cases of CPP with rapid advancement of secondary sexual characteristics, height velocity, and bone age, accompanied by testosterone greater than 20 ng/dl in boys less than 8 years of age and menarche before 9 years of age in girls, may require treatment. If therapy is offered for CPP, GnRH agonists are the agents of choice. GnRH agonist molecules are altered native GnRH molecules with increased affinity for GnRH receptors and with prolonged half lives and increased resistance to enzymatic degradation. Native GnRH is released from the hypothalamus in episodic pulses. If a constant infusion of GnRH is administered, pituitary gonadotropes reduce their response to GnRH by a decrease in cellular GnRH receptor numbers and an uncoupling of the receptors from their intracellular processes (downregulation), leading to a cessation of gonadotropin secretion. Each individual dose of GnRH agonist acts as a constant infusion of GnRH and decreases gonadotropin secretion, leading, in turn, to absence of gonadal sex steroid secretion and, ultimately, cessation or regression of pubertal progression.

GnRH agonists originally were administered daily by subcutaneous injection or several times per day by intranasal insufflation. Now, depot preparations are given once per month, leading to improved compliance and more consistent effect. Various chemical structures lead to similar effects, but only three preparations are commercially available in the United States. Histrelin acetate is given as a daily SC dose of 10 μg/kg; nafarelin acetate is given as a nasal spray in a daily dose of 1600 μg/d divided into two 800 μg/d doses; and leuprolide acetate is given as an every 4 week IM dose of 0.3 mg/kg.

GnRH is first administered in the lower dose range, and 3 weeks after a dose, serum LH, follicle-stimulating hormone (FSH), and sex steroid determinations indicate whether complete suppression is achieved. The dose is increased as indicated while monitoring of LH, FSH, and estradiol continues. Bone age determinations at 6-month intervals indicate whether control of skeletal growth is achieved.

Appropriate therapy leads to suppression of all pubertal hormones and a decrease in bone age advancement to the normal ratio of 1 year advance in bone age to the equivalent of 1 year advance in height. Menses, if started, will cease, and an increase in final height prediction over predictions made at the start of therapy occurs over several years of therapy. Cessation of therapy allows resumption of pubertal development. Initial studies demonstrated an increase in adult height in treated patients compared with untreated patients. The worst effect of a course of therapy would be incomplete suppression of gonadal sex steroids, leading to continued progression of bone age and ultimate short stature while the treating physician is lulled into complacency by observing a cessation of the rapid pubertal development over the untreated state.

Incomplete Sexual Precocity

If secondary sexual characteristics occur through a pathway different from the normal process of puberty, incomplete sexual precocity (ISP) occurs. Thus, autonomous secretion of ovarian estrogens, testicular androgens, or, in boys, human chorionic gonadotropin (hCG) from a liver or CNS tumor leads to ISP. Testicular, ovarian, or adrenal tumors must be treated primarily to suppress ISP. Enzymatic defects in adrenal steroidogenesis leading to congenital adrenal hyperplasia are treated with glucocorticoids in a dose appropriate to suppress ACTH without suppressing growth.

Familial germ cell and Leydig cell maturation (called testotoxicosis) is an X-linked disorder leading to autonomous testicular function with suppression of hypothalamic-pituitary gonadotrope function. GnRH agonists are not effective initially, but ketoconazole, an antifungal agent that interrupts steroidogenesis as a side effect, testolactone, an aromatase inhibitor, and spironolactone or flutamide, antiandrogens, have been used to good effect to suppress the process. After suppression of the autonomous process, CPP occurs as a result of the virilizing effect of increased testosterone secretion on the hypothalamic-pituitary-axis. GnRH then becomes useful for this secondary CPP.

The McCune-Albright syndrome consists of the triad of café-au-lait spots, polyostotic fibrous dysplasia, and precocious puberty, although other endocrine conditions with hyperfunction (such as pituitary gigantism and hyperthyroidism) are described. This condition, which affects so many systems, appears to be caused by abnormalities in the G-protein system leading to constant stimulation of multiple organs. The antiaromatase agents testolactone and fadrozole are reported to treat the pubertal manifestations of McCune-Albright syndrome successfully. Recurrent, idiopathic, autonomous ovarian cysts that appear in McCune-Albright syndrome do not necessarily require surgical removal, since medroxyprogesterone acetate, an inhibitor of ovarian steroidogenesis, is effective therapy. Medroxyprogesterone acetate is also an inhibitor of testicular steroidogenesis and was used in familial germ cell and Leydig cell maturation.

DELAYED PUBERTY

Delay in pubertal development to an age above the upper limits of normal or cessation of development after the initial appearance of secondary sexual characteristics can be a danger sign indicating a serious illness. However, because approximately 2.5% of all normal children will enter puberty after the accepted upper limits of normal, delay in pubertal development need not always trigger an expensive workup. It is the examining physician's duty to determine which patient needs serious evaluation and which patient requires only reassurance. Usually, constitutional delay in puberty resolves into spontaneous pubertal development by 18 years of age.

Constitutional delay in puberty occurs in a patient with a significantly delayed bone age (>2 SD from the mean) who has a height and height velocity appropriate for bone age but all through life is short for chronologic age. There frequently is a family history of constitutional delay in puberty in a parent or sibling. When teenagers have constitutional delay in puberty, their social life and school work may suffer, sometimes to the point of depression. Although we do not treat all subjects with constitutional delay in puberty with sex steroids, if there appears to be a significant problem with body image, low-dose sex steroid replacement for a few months may improve the patient's outlook while awaiting spontaneous pubertal development. However, excessive therapy will advance bone age, prematurely close epiphyses, and cause a loss of final adult height.

Girls with delayed puberty may receive oral ethinyl estradiol in a dose of 10 μg or conjugated estrogens 0.3 mg daily for 3 months to cause some breast development. Treatment is followed by a 3-month period of observation for continued pubertal development. If no spontaneous development occurs, another course of therapy is appropriate if the subject continues to evidence distress.

Boys with delayed puberty may receive injections of testosterone enanthate every 4 weeks in a dose of 50 to 200 mg (I recommend 100 mg) for three injections. If no pubertal development is appreciated over the next 3 months, another course of therapy may be administered. Daily oral testosterone is usually less effective and more complicated to administer, and methylated testosterone preparations carry the risk of hepatic toxicity.

Permanent absence of pubertal development may originate from a lack of gonadotropin secretion (hypogonadotropic hypogonadism) or an absence of gonadal function (hypergonadotropic hypogonadism). Hypogonadotropic hypogonadism may be isolated and idiopathic, may occur with other congenital hypothalamic-pituitary deficiencies, and may be associated with congenital midline defects ranging from cleft palate to holoprosencephaly. Kallmann's syndrome combines hypogonadotropic hypogonadism and anosmia or hyposmia. Acquired hypogonadotropic hypogonadism may be caused by a CNS tumor, infection, trauma, or post-CNS radiation therapy for various conditions. Hypergonadotropic hypogonadism occurs in the presence of testicular or ovarian failure. This may be idiopathic, autoimmune, or postradiation or may be due to a karyotypic abnormality, such as Klinefelter's or Turner's syndrome.

Boys with either hypogonadotropic or hypergonadotropic hypogonadism may receive testosterone replacement at an appropriate age to start puberty. The dose should be started low to avoid priapism in a patient never previously experiencing testosterone. Every 4 weeks, a dose of 100 mg is administered and raised in 3- to 6-month or longer intervals to 200 to 300 mg every 4 weeks. Since a change in energy level may be noted with every-4-week dosage, every-2-week dosage of one-half the total monthly dose may be tried to smooth the testosterone effects over the whole month. If the patient has growth

hormone deficiency and has not been treated with growth hormone to the stage of near adult height, the sex steroid dose should start in the lower range to avoid rapid advancement of skeletal development. Combined growth hormone and testosterone in appropriate doses will better approximate the normal pubertal environment than will growth hormone alone and is preferable in a patient well treated with growth hormone through the prepubertal years. The amount of pubic hair that develops on testosterone therapy may not be acceptable to the subject. Intramuscular hCG was administered in studies of subjects with hypogonadotropic hypogonadism to successfully increase pubic and axillary hair growth.

Girls with hypogonadotropic or hypergonadotropic hypogonadism should receive ovarian steroids in a regimen appropriate to support secondary sexual development and menstrual flow. Estrogen is administered as ethinyl estradiol initially in doses from 5 to 10 μg, gradually increasing to 20 to 30 μg/d by adding 5 to 10 μg at 6-monthly intervals. Initially, ethinyl estradiol is given daily, but as breakthrough bleeding is noted or 6 months pass, the dose is given on days 1 to 21 of the month according to the calendar. Conjugated estrogen in equivalent, appropriate doses may be used in place of ethinyl estradiol. After cycling begins, progesterone in the form of medroxyprogesterone acetate is given in 5 to 10 mg doses on days 12 to 21 of the month. Menstrual flow should follow this schedule of therapy. Growth hormone was used to increase the growth of girls with Turner's syndrome in several national studies and now is being used more frequently in girls not enrolled in clinical trials.

Boys and girls with hypogonadotropic hypogonadism due to hypothalamic conditions may receive GnRH by programmable pump to advance puberty, but the therapy is so cumbersome that it is usually reserved for subjects desiring fertility. Women have had ovulation and men have had sperm formation with this regimen.

REFERENCES

1. Grumbach MM, Styne DM: Puberty: ontogeny, neuroendocrinology, physiology. *In* Wilson JD, Foster DW (eds): Williams' Textbook of Endocrinology, 8th ed. Philadelphia, W.B. Saunders, 1992:1139–1222.
2. Styne DM: Growth. *In* Greenspan FS, Baxter JD (eds): Basic and Clinical Endocrinology. Norwalk, Conn, Appleton and Lange, 1994:501–524.
3. Styne DM: Puberty and its disorders. *In* Kohler PO (ed): Current Science: Current Opinions in Endocrinology and Diabetes. Philadelphia, 1994:46–51.
4. Styne DM, Grumbach MM. Puberty in the male and female: its physiology and disorders. *In* Yen JCC, Jaffe RB (eds): Reproductive Endocrinology, 2nd ed. Philadelphia, W.B. Saunders, 1991:511–554.

10

Diabetes and Metabolic Disorders

INSULIN-DEPENDENT DIABETES MELLITUS

Nejib Raboudi, M.D.
Lynne L. Levitsky, M.D.

DIAGNOSIS

The diagnosis of insulin-dependent diabetes mellitus (IDDM) is usually obvious. If initial symptoms of polydipsia, polyuria, and polyphagia with weight loss over a period of days to weeks are ignored, early IDDM may progress to frank diabetic ketoacidosis, requiring aggressive management with intravenous fluids and insulin. Often, in children with adequate access to medical care, IDDM is suspected because of minimal symptomatology associated with glycosuria and slight hyperglycemia (blood glucose 150 to 200 mg/dl). When these children are free from intercurrent illness, a fasting plasma glucose greater than 140 mg/dl and a 2-hour postprandial blood glucose of greater than 200 mg/dl (a glucose tolerance test is rarely indicated) will be diagnostic of diabetes. Rapid confirmation that the diabetes is IDDM requires measurement of elevated anti-islet or anti-insulin antibodies. Eventually, the evolution of the disorder to true insulin deficiency (lack of C-peptide response to meals, development of ketosis-prone state) permits this distinction without immunologic data. Therapeutic intervention is recommended even in very early diabetes because insulin therapy may postpone complete loss of insulin secretory capacity.

GENERAL GOALS OF THERAPY

The outcome of the NIH-sponsored Diabetes Control and Complications Trial (DCCT) fully supports the goal of maintaining near-normal blood glucose levels to reduce substantially the risk of long-term complications in patients with diabetes. Although only patients between the ages of 13 and 39 years were enrolled in this study, implementation of rigorous blood sugar control in the younger population should be considered and tailored on an individual basis. The challenge is to achieve these goals and avoid serious hypoglycemic episodes that put the young child at risk of brain injury. The intensity of diabetes management for each patient is, therefore, guided by glycemic control, as measured by glycosylated hemoglobin, and by concern about hypoglycemia. In general, children under the age of 5 are managed to prevent hypoglycemia, and this often leads to higher blood sugars than are accepted in older children and adolescents.

INITIAL MANAGEMENT OF CHILDREN WITH IDDM

All newly diagnosed children with ketoacidosis require a short-term hospitalization for therapy of ketoacidosis. Children with blood sugars greater than 800 mg/dl often are admitted for therapy because of the small risk of central nervous system (CNS) complications during oral rehydration.

The decision to hospitalize a hyperglycemic child who does not have ketoacidosis should be predicated on the clinical stability of the child at the time of diagnosis, the emotional, intellectual, and economic resources of the family, and the availability of adequate clinical support for the initiation of outpatient education and therapy. If the patient is stable (normal vital signs, able to maintain oral hydration, without nausea or vomiting, and with normal sensorium) and the family is capable of rapidly absorbing diabetes survival skills, outpatient management by a team consisting of a pediatric endocrinologist or other physician trained in diabetes management, diabetes nurse educator, and dietitian can be provided. Psychologic support staff (psychologist, social worker) must be available as is felt indicated by the management team.

Survival education must include instruction in insulin administration and blood sugar testing, information about the symptoms, signs and treatment of hypoglycemia, hyperglycemia, and ketoacidosis, and initial nutritional education. Mastery of these skills should be assessed at intervals.

The family should have complete instructions as to how to reach a designated clinician-member of the diabetes management team and should receive an algorithm for insulin administration based on preceding blood sugars. It is our practice to have the family call before insulin injections for at least the first 48 hours and to call us for blood sugars beyond established guidelines (usually less than 80 or greater than 250 mg/dl in the first week). The family and child should return in 5 to 7 days to recheck skills and deal with new questions and problems. They should be seen again in 2 weeks, at 1 month, and then at 2 to 3 month intervals, with telephone consultation as necessary between visits. A checklist of management skills and information to be covered and assessed is found in Table 1.

Initiation of insulin therapy with hands-on teaching of insulin injection to the family (and to the child as is age-appropriate) is essential as a first management step to free family members from fears of this aspect of therapy and allow them to learn other survival skills. It is our custom to begin outpatient insulin therapy by planning a split-mixed (NPH or Lente, with regular), b.i.d. insulin regimen with supplemental regular insulin (0.05 to 0.1 U/kg) to be administered based on telephoned blood glucose reports, and gradual prospective increments in planned insulin dose as needed. The starting total daily dose of insulin is less than we anticipate will be required to achieve euglycemia. We begin with 0.3 to 0.5 U/kg body weight, with two thirds given before breakfast and one third given before the evening meal. The smaller calculated total dose is reserved for children under the age of 5 and for children discovered to have incidental modest hyperglycemia without ketosis. The larger calculated total dose would be used for teenagers, individuals with slight ketosis, and those with higher postprandial blood sugars. Two thirds of the insulin dose in the morning is given as NPH or Lente, and one third is given as regular insulin. At the evening meal, the insulin is usually split equally between regular insulin and NPH or Lente.

TABLE 1. Checklist of Management Skills and Information for the Child with Diabetes

1. Materials should be provided
   a. Resources for diabetes education (books, pamphlets, videos). Suggested sources include:
      (1) Travis LB: An Instructional Aid on Insulin-Dependent Diabetes Mellitus, 9th ed., 1993. Century Business Communications, Inc., P.O. Box 200633, Austin, TX 78720-0633. Telephone (512) 832-0611 (available in English and Spanish).
      (2) Chase HP. Understanding Insulin-Dependent Diabetes, 7th ed. Denver, CO, Hirschfeld Press, 1992.
      (3) Franz M, Etzwiller DD, Joynes JO, Hollander PM: Learning To Live Well with Diabetes. 1991. Chronimed Publishing, 13911 Ridgedale, Minnetonka, MN 55305. Telephone 1 (800) 848-2793, Ext. 765.
      (4) Betschart J: It's Time To Learn About Diabetes, A Workbook on Diabetes for Children. 1991. Chronimed Publishing, 13911 Ridgedale, Minnetonka, MN 55305. Telephone 1 (800) 848-2793, Ext. 765 (available with a video).
   b. Prescriptions for insulin (2 vials of each type to be used), syringes, glucagon emergency kit, glucose meter and strips, lancets and lancet device, ketone testing strips, alcohol wipes, and a MedicAlert application. Ensure that prescriptions are filled before discharge, materials are checked, and use is rehearsed with the family.
2. Essential information about diabetes should be taught and recall assessed
   a. Function/location of pancreas
   b. Normal glucose metabolism and insulin effects
   c. Difference between insulin-dependent and noninsulin-dependent diabetes. Emphasize continuing need for insulin
   d. Need for blood testing for glucose and urine testing for ketones
   e. Hypoglycemia: Signs and symptoms, causes, management at different levels of severity, importance of glucagon emergency kit with demonstration of kit, MedicAlert information
   f. Hyperglycemia and ketoacidosis: Signs and symptoms, causes, and management
   g. Nutrition and diabetes: Ensure nutritional consultation, stress importance of consistency of timing and carbohydrate content of meals, interaction of diet, insulin, and exercise
   h. Adaptation to daily living: Managing problems in school, travel, treatment when the child is ill, and social management issues
3. Skills necessary for diabetes management should be demonstrated and observed
   a. Blood glucose testing and recording
   b. Urine ketone testing and recording
   c. Drawing up and administering insulin: Types of syringes, mixing of two insulins, site rotation, insulin storage, disposal of insulin syringes
   d. Adjustment of insulin and food based on blood glucose results
4. Emotional needs should be assessed and support provided
   a. Provide information about diabetes support groups, diabetes organizations, and camping programs
   b. Arrange referrals to social service, visiting nurse as necessary
5. Follow-up
   a. Provide telephone numbers for emergency assistance
   b. Provide guidelines for telephone consultation
   c. Provide follow-up appointments with clinicians (physician, nurse, dietician as appropriate)
   d. Discuss plans for follow-up laboratory studies

If the patient is admitted to the hospital, a split-mixed insulin regimen as described for outpatient management can be initiated, and supplemental regular insulin (0.05 to 0.1 U/kg) can be administered before meals for blood glucose values greater than 300 mg/dl. The prospective split-mixed insulin regimen can then be adjusted upward as indicated by the need for regular insulin supplementation. Alternatively, multiple regular insulin injections before each meal and at bedtime can be instituted. This latter approach offers a greater opportunity for the patient and family to practice insulin injection technique. Distribution of the total planned insulin dose as 40% before breakfast, 20% before lunch, 30% before dinner, and 10% at bedtime usually matches the carbohydrate intake of these meals and the insulin requirement at those times. At bedtime, the insulin can be given as NPH or Lente to control blood sugar during the night. After a day or two on a multiple-insulin dose regimen, the daily total insulin requirement may be calculated from the previous insulin requirement and divided appropriately, as outlined previously, to manage the patient with only two injections of combined insulins a day. If euglycemia has been achieved, the estimate of the insulin requirement in a hospital setting should be reduced by 10% to 20% on discharge from the hospital to avoid hypoglycemia when the patient resumes normal activity. The goal during hospitalization is not to achieve a target range of glucose but rather to ensure that the patient and parents are skilled enough to be able to do insulin injections and to recognize and promptly correct hypoglycemic events. Follow-up visits and telephone contacts as described for outpatient management are used to bring blood glucose levels to near normal. This process usually takes several weeks and is aided by the onset of the *remission* phase.

Appropriate attention to nutrition goes hand-in-hand with insulin therapy. The nutritionist must work closely with the clinician, suggesting insulin dose adjustment, so that both diet and insulin are tailored to the changing needs of the child.

LONG-TERM MANAGEMENT OF IDDM

The components of long-term management include adjustment of insulin therapy based on glycemic control, nutritional counseling based on caloric need and glycemic control, and attention to the developmental psychosocial needs of child and family. Prospective planning for anticipated maturational changes in insulin need and food intake based on activity level and pubertal stage permit smooth management. Changes in therapeutic regimen must be timely, logical, and concordant with the functional capacity of the family of the child with diabetes. Twenty-four hour access to advice and support must be available.

Insulin Therapy

Patients with IDDM have very limited endogenous insulin secretion at diagnosis and no insulin secretory capacity after a few years of diabetes. The use of oral hypoglycemic drugs is contraindicated because stimulation of residual beta-cell function early in the course of IDDM could theoretically lead to more rapid onset of complete insulin deficiency. The goal of insulin therapy is to reduce the blood glucose level to as near normal as possible without causing hypoglycemia.

Insulin Preparations

Insulin preparations are listed in Table 2. Premixed combinations of human regular and NPH insulins are available but are not often used in childhood because they lack flexibility of dosage. Diluent may be obtained from the insulin manufacturer to prepare diluted insulin for small children requiring adjustments of 0.5 U of insulin

TABLE 2. Insulin Preparations

INSULIN TYPE	SOURCE	PREPARATION	ONSET (h)	PEAK ACTION (h)	DURATION (h)
Regular	Human, beef, pork, beef-pork	Crystalline zinc	0.5	2–4	4–6
NPH	Human, beef, pork, beef-pork	Neutral protamine Hagedorn-protamine-zinc insulin suspension	2–4	6–8	16–24
Lente	Human, beef, pork, beef-pork	Amorphous and crystalline zinc suspension	2–4	6–8	16–24
Ultralente	Beef	Crystalline zinc suspension	2–4	None	28–36
Ultralente	Human	Crystalline zinc suspension	2–4	Variable 8–12	20–28

Insulin vials should be refrigerated, not frozen. Vials should not be used for longer than 2 months, and the last 10% of insulin suspensions (NPH, Lente, Ultralente) should be discarded. Insulin-zinc preparations are naturally bacteriostatic but can become contaminated with time and poor technique. Insulin loses up to 10% of potency per month at room temperature. Dispersed insulins should be checked for homogeneity after gentle mixing (rolling of vial between the palms) before use and discarded if aggregates are noted. Differences in timing between human and animal NPH and Lente insulins are discussed in the text.

or less. Families using diluted insulin must be instructed carefully so that they do not make errors based on insulin syringe calibrations. All routinely available insulin preparations in the United States contain 100 U of insulin per milliliter (U100). More concentrated U500 regular insulin can be obtained for special uses. In other countries, U40 and U80 (40 and 80 U/ml, respectively) insulin is still available. Patients contemplating foreign travel should be aware of this so that they do not introduce dosage errors through the use of incompatible syringes and insulin. Maintenance insulin is normally administered subcutaneously. Only regular insulin should be administered intravenously or intramuscularly for the treatment of acute metabolic decompensation (diabetic ketoacidosis). There is variability in subcutaneously administered insulin action and duration depending on the patient, the injection site, and the means of administration. Peak concentrations are reached more rapidly with abdominal than with thigh injections, and onset is more rapid with the use of jet injection devices compared with needles and syringes. Exercise of an injected limb will increase the rate of release of insulin, as will hyperthermia (hot tubs, fever) or rubbing of the area.

Methods of Insulin Administration

Insulin is usually administered using a disposable syringe and needle calibrated in units. Twenty-five, 30, 50, and 100 U syringes can be obtained. Alternative insulin administration devices include jet injectors. These devices disperse an ultrafine spray subcutaneously and speed the kinetics of insulin absorption. They are expensive and cumbersome, require cleaning, and take some effort to change insulin mixtures. Jet injectors have been found useful by exceedingly needlephobic children, but it is usually possible to deal with the phobic behavior rather than to offer a mechanical solution. Pen injectors supplied with an insulin-containing cartridge and disposable needles can be useful for dialing up doses of extra regular insulin before meals for teenagers taking multiple daily injections. However, pen injectors have not improved diabetes control in adolescents. External insulin

pumps are rarely useful in the childhood population. Because the infused insulin is relatively short-acting, discontinuation of subcutaneous infusion can rapidly lead to ketoacidosis. Only individuals committed to blood glucose testing four or more times a day should consider using an insulin pump. Pumps should never be used to resolve problems of poor control and poor adherence to regimen.

Design of the Insulin Regimen

The daily replacement dose of insulin is usually 0.7 to 1 U/kg. The amount of insulin needed is not necessarily an indicator of difficulty of control. Adolescents are insulin resistant and may require up to 1.3 U/kg/d. Young children (less than 5 years of age) may be quite insulin sensitive and require as little as 0.5 U/kg/d. Insulin requirement changes with age, duration of diabetes, and activity level. The honeymoon or remission phase of diabetes is the postdiagnosis period of residual insulin release capacity and may last a few weeks to several years. Insulin requirements are often less than 0.5 U/kg/ d during this time. Although during the remission phase of diabetes, it may be feasible to maintain children on a single-dose regimen of intermediate and regular insulin or even to discontinue insulin, this is in general inadvisable. Prolonged maintenance of endogenous insulin release seems dependent on excellent glycemic control because of exogenous insulin therapy. It is believed that residual beta-cells are less accessible to immunologic attack when at rest.

The insulin regimen should be designed around the patient snack and meal pattern to avoid postprandial glycemic excursions. Commonly used regimens are described in Table 3.

A stepped approach to insulin administration often is useful. Our initial management in the child is a b.i.d. split-mixed intermediate and regular insulin regimen as described in the section on Initial Management of Children with IDDM. However, adequate glycemic control between dinner and breakfast may not be possible with predinner intermediate insulin. Human intermediate insulins in particular have a somewhat earlier peak (6 hours compared with 7 to 8 hours)

TABLE 3. Insulin Administration Regimens

REGIMEN*	INSULINS AND ADMINISTRATION
Split-mixed b.i.d.	Intermediate insulin (NPH or Lente) is mixed with regular insulin and administered before breakfast and dinner.
Split-mixed t.i.d.	Morning insulin is distributed as in split-mixed b.i.d., but evening insulin is given as regular before dinner, and Lente or NPH (with extra regular as indicated by blood glucose) is given at bedtime.
Regular-Ultralente	Beef-pork Ultralente is used as basal insulin (approximately 20% of total requirement), and regular insulin is given separately before each meal to match carbohydrate content of meal and planned activity.
Split-mixed b.i.d. human Ultralente	Human Ultralente may be used as an intermediate-acting insulin, given with regular insulin before breakfast and before dinner. Sometimes, the extra peak engendered by the mix of the two insulins works to the benefit of the patient, providing lunch or afternoon insulin coverage. However, changes in the amount of regular insulin may alter the timing and intensity of insulin action (see text). To avoid this, the Ultralente and regular can be administered separately. This regimen can be used for only the morning or evening insulin in combination with an intermediate and regular mix to cover the other time period.

*Only the regular-Ultralente regimen covers carbohydrate intake at lunch. However, any of these regimens can be modified to include additional regular insulin administered before lunch. Moreover, supplementation with regular insulin before high-carbohydrate snacks allows flexibility of daily meal planning for older children.

and shorter duration (16 to 20 hours compared with 24 hours) than do animal insulins and may not provide full insulin coverage between dinner and the next morning. If morning glycemic control is inadequate or nocturnal hypoglycemia becomes a problem, we take one of two approaches. The preferred approach is to move the evening intermediate insulin to the parental bedtime (10 to 11 PM). This then peaks in the early morning hours, protecting the child from nocturnal hypoglycemia and resolving morning hyperglycemia. An alternative approach is to administer human Ultralente insulin before dinner. Ultralente preparations contain some excess zinc for stability. If Ultralente is given mixed with regular insulin, a variable additional insulin peak, depending on the ratio of human Ultralente and regular insulin, will be noted 4 to 8 hours after administration. This may be avoided if the parents are willing to administer human Ultralente in a syringe separate from regular insulin.

Two to three injections of insulin a day usually will prevent major glycemic excursions related to breakfast and dinner. Regular insulin should be administered at least 45 minutes before meals. In very young children with capricious appetites, it rarely may be necessary to give insulin during or after meals to ensure that intake will be sufficient. Some older children and families are willing to take on the additional management responsibility of checking blood glucose before lunch and supplementing with regular insulin at that time as necessary. Insulin adjustment is based on previous blood glucose records, knowledge of the peak and duration of action of administered insulins, and anticipated food intake or level of physical activity. No tailoring of insulin dose will retrospectively deal with unplanned carbohydrate intake and other departures from a prescribed regimen.

Local Effects of Insulin Therapy

Lipohypertrophy (insulin hypertrophy) is due to the local lipogenic effect of insulin and can be avoided by rotating insulin injection sites. However, because insulin absorption varies so much from site to site, patients should be advised to inject insulin in the same regions (arms, legs, abdomen, buttocks) at the same time each day to avoid variability of onset and peak insulin effect. Lipoatrophy is rarely seen with pure human or porcine insulin. This local loss of fat tissue is secondary to an immune response to impure insulins.

Blood Glucose Self-Monitoring

Rationale and Suggested Patterns for Blood Glucose Testing

The best measure of chronic diabetes control is the glycosylated hemoglobin determination (see Monitoring Long-Term Glycemic Control). However, frequent blood glucose determinations permit intelligent adjustment of the insulin dose. We recommend at least three times daily blood glucose testing but are delighted when families agree to test even more frequently to solve problems related to glycemia. We currently employ the following guidelines for blood glucose testing.

1. Test routinely at least before insulin administration at breakfast and dinner so that adjustments can be made in regular insulin dose and at bedtime so that decisions can be made as to whether extra food is necessary to prevent nocturnal hypoglycemia. In general, a prebed blood glucose of less than 120 mg/dl would be an indication for increasing the size of the bedtime snack (1½ times for glucose of 90 to 120 mg/dl, double the usual snack if blood sugar is less than 90 mg/dl).
2. Test before treating hypoglycemic reactions, or if the reaction is too severe to permit this relatively leisurely approach, test immediately after treatment, to document that the feelings of hypoglycemia are associated with low blood sugar.
3. Test blood glucose at specific problem times, as indicated in these common examples.
   a. Many children have high blood glucoses before dinner but eat after-school snacks 1 to 2 hours before dinner. A blood glucose test before the afternoon snack will help to determine when morning intermediate-acting insulin has been raised sufficiently

to produce euglycemia before the snack. Further increases in morning Lente or NPH insulin might lead to hypoglycemia at the end of the school day.
   b. If attempts to lower morning blood sugars by increasing evening insulin seem likely to produce nocturnal hypoglycemia, we request testing at 2 AM for several days. Values at 2 AM should not be less than 80 mg/dl.

Equipment for Blood Glucose Self-Monitoring

The new generation of glucose meters, although still requiring finger puncture to obtain a drop of blood, supply a blood glucose value in less than 1 minute, and in the best of them, timing is started by placement of a drop of blood on a strip inserted into the meter. Moreover, they are very sensitive to improper use so that it is difficult to produce artifactually low readings. Many have a date, time, and memory function to permit review of data directly from the meter and also perform a mean glucose calculation based on previous timed readings. These characteristics encourage accurate recordkeeping and integration of the data into diabetes management decisions. Some meters can download glucose values into computers. This capacity is of variable use because judgments as to necessary acute changes in insulin regimen probably should be based on only the previous 7 to 10 days of readings, numbers easily encompassed without a computer printout.

A variety of springloaded lancets can be purchased that make repeat blood glucose tests essentially pain-free. In contrast to the rotational regimen for insulin administration, all blood glucose tests may be performed using small regions on the side of one or more chosen fingers. These areas rapidly become callused, and the perceived discomfort of blood sugar testing is further minimized. A major difficulty of blood glucose testing is that the strips are expensive. Blood glucose testing supplies for a 30-day period of four-times-daily testing will cost over $60.00, and few health insurance plans cover this cost. On the other hand, if the information obtained from blood glucose testing is used intelligently, glycemic control can be improved and hypoglycemic risk can be diminished.

Diet

Nutritional counseling is begun within the first day or two of insulin therapy. The initial prescription by the physician may be an age-based estimate of caloric need.

Caloric intake = 1000 + 100 × Age (in years up to 12 years)

However, further adjustment must be based on an assessment of the eating habits, cultural practices, and special needs of the patient and family. The meal plan should be kept as close as possible to previous patterns, modifying only components judged inappropriate to meet the child's need for normal growth and development. A diet that is balanced in carbohydrate will facilitate a strategy in which insulin dosage and timing are determined according to food intake and lifestyle. A reevaluation of these nutritional needs should be made every 3 to 6 months.

We attempt to provide 10% to 20% of energy from protein and less than 30% from fat. Monounsaturated fat intake is encouraged. In children less than 2 years old, fat intake should not be limited. Complex carbohydrate intake is advised. Other modifications of nutritional intake may be individualized based on specific needs (obesity, undernutrition). The distribution of the total caloric intake depends on the age and cultural needs of the child. Most children taking in a standard United States diet will receive three meals, as well as a late afternoon and prebedtime snack. Young children usually also take a snack in the midmorning, as do their friends without diabetes.

The approach to nutritional management of the child with diabetes depends to a large extent on parental sophistication.

Exchange Lists

American Diabetes Association exchange lists divide foods into six categories (free foods, milk, fruit, vegetable, bread, and meat, with meats considered either high fat or low fat). Foods can be exchanged within each group to promote consistency of meal content. Picture books of food exchanges and food exchange lists for various ethnic foods in English and other languages may be obtained from the American Diabetes Association.

Carbohydrate Counting

Carbohydrate counting is a more sophisticated method of introducing consistency into the meal plan. Since the major determinant of the postprandial glucose rise is the glucose load in the meal, stability from day to day in the amount of carbohydrate in each meal will facilitate adjustment of the premeal insulin dose. However, high sugar drinks (soft drinks and juices) should be discouraged because they are a readily absorbed source of carbohydrate and raise the blood sugar level very quickly if ingested alone. When incorporated into a meal plan, sucrose-containing food has no adverse effect on the blood sugar level provided insulin doses are adjusted accordingly.

Development of Effective Management Plan

Anticipatory guidance must be employed to assist families and children in coping with potential pitfalls in the management of diabetes. Parenting the child with diabetes is made easier if specific guidelines are offered.

Target Glucose Levels

Parents should be given age-related target guidelines for glycemic control. Our goal of therapy in children over the age of 5 years is to achieve preprandial blood glucose levels between 70 and 130 mg/dl and 1 hour postprandial levels no higher than 180 mg/dl in 70% or more of blood tests. This goal is modified depending on the age of the patient and the level of concern about severe consequences of hypoglycemic episodes on brain development. In children less than 5 years of age, we aim for preprandial values between 100 and 200 mg/dl without hypoglycemia (blood sugars of 50 mg/dl or less). Infants and toddlers often have such frequent daytime food intake that all blood glucose determinations after the morning value are postprandial. We use the glycosylated hemoglobin as an aid in interpreting the quality of glycemic control and defining individual goals. Target glucose goals are relatively easy to reach during the initial remission phase of diabetes and become progressively harder to achieve.

Insulin Adjustment

We instruct families to make adjustments in intermediate or long-acting insulins only every 2 to 3 days based on general patterns of hypoglycemia or hyperglycemia or specific episodes of hypoglycemia or hyperglycemia at the times of the peak of the insulin. Daily changes in these insulins may be necessary in unusual circumstances. For instance, children receiving every-other-day glucocorticoid therapy for another condition may need to increase their NPH the evening of the glucocorticoid day to deal with glucocorticoid-stimulated gluconeogenesis. Children who have rigorous sports schedules requiring prolonged bursts of exercise on a random basis through the week (swimmers, long-distance runners) may need to decrease their morning or evening intermediate or long-acting insulin on the high activity days.

Regular insulin can be changed at each dose based on blood glucose and anticipated food intake. We develop an algorithm with each family to permit adjustment of regular insulin depending on blood sugar and anticipated intake. Usually, an adjustment of 1 to 5 U of regular insulin is sufficient to cope with glycemic swings and increased intake.

Particular attention should be paid to persistently elevated before-breakfast blood sugar values because high levels may indicate increased nocturnal fasting gluconeogenesis and interfere with glycemic control during the rest of the day. The Somogyi phenomenon (posthypoglycemic hyperglycemia) is still invoked to explain morning hyperglycemia in children. All studies suggest that the posthypoglycemic counterregulatory hormone response has only a limited effect on morning blood glucose values. Instead, morning hyperglycemia is usually secondary to both insufficient insulin at that time (waning of intermediate-acting insulin) and the insulin resistance of the morning hours probably induced by endogenous nocturnal pulses of growth hormone (dawn phenomenon).

Insulin Need

During the initial education period after diagnosis, the remission phase of diabetes should be discussed. Families should be encouraged to recognize that a period of improved control and diminished insulin requirement after initial therapy is not a sign that the diabetes has improved or that it will disappear. Families should be taught to recognize that higher blood glucose levels and increased insulin needs are the earliest signs of increasing insulin deficiency. Too often, young adolescents with diabetes are given complete control of this disorder and look on the loss of the remission phase as a "failure," best not communicated to parents or medical personnel. Parents should be encouraged to review blood glucose values in the memory of the child's glucose meter nonjudgmentally and to bring the meter to each office visit for review with medical caregivers.

The insulin resistance of puberty should be discussed so that parents and children recognize that adolescent behaviors are not the only reasons for diminished glycemic control during puberty.

Components of Anticipatory Guidance and Management

At the time of diagnosis, the main focus is to provide an overview of the physiopathologic basis of diabetes and to teach the basic skills. This is also a critical time to assess the patient's family setting and needs and to develop an individualized strategy of achievable goals. Because of the vigilance and ongoing decision making required to care for a child with diabetes properly, this disorder can unmask latent family disorganization or difficulty. Intact, organized families usually manage children with diabetes well. The clinicians and educators involved in diabetes management should provide continuing and responsive psychologic support and be prompt in helping to resolve management problems.

Positive Parenting Behaviors. The parent should present diabetes management to the child as a positive force for a healthy life. The parent of the child with diabetes should recognize and support the child's individuality as distinct from the child's chronic illness. Other children and family members should not be neglected. The parent's vital role in maintaining diabetes control during adolescence should be stressed. Children should not be permitted autonomy of diabetes care until the late teens.

Parents, if smokers, should be encouraged to discontinue smoking because smoking is an important risk factor in diabetes complications, and children are likely to imitate parental behaviors.

Advice for the Overburdened Parent. Parents are often overwhelmed by the burden of daily management in a child with diabetes. The vigilance necessary to manage a child with this disorder may exhaust the major caretaker in a marriage and deprive other siblings of attention. Too often, parents of young children with diabetes are sleep-deprived and feel that they cannot leave their children for fear of untoward events. Some minor electronic aids can allow the parents of children with diabetes to deal more easily with their management tasks. Parents of children who have had nocturnal hypoglycemia may wish to keep an auditory baby monitor in their child's room so that they will waken if there are changes in breathing patterns. Parents may feel more comfortable leaving their child if they have a means for rapid contact. We occasionally recommend pagers to parents who are particularly concerned about these issues.

It is important that both parents be involved in this difficult task. If possible, single parents should call on other family members to assist them. Diabetes camps and support groups provide additional opportunities for both respite and support for families and children. Many local diabetes support groups organize babysitter lists of experienced individuals.

Changes in Management of Children with Diabetes at Different Developmental Ages. School-age children should learn, with their parents, how to deal with new supervision at school. During these early years, it is important for children with diabetes to develop mastery of diabetes-related skills as an extension of the other developmental tasks of childhood and learn to participate progressively in their own care under continued parental supervision. Preadolescents may be able to do blood sugar testing and insulin injection and to discuss insulin dose adjustment with parents, but they should never be unsupervised. Maintenance of control of diabetes during adolescence requires a vigilant parent with high self-esteem and a strong sense of mission. Parental abdication inevitably leads to major problems in diabetes control.

Physician's Role in Managing the Adolescent to Adult Transition

The adolescent years are particularly stressful for patient and family because of physiologic pubertal changes that interfere with blood sugar control. In addition, the usual autonomy issues of adolescence are new challenges in caring for young people with diabetes. The transition to early adulthood can be eased if the clinicians responsible for diabetes care subtly shift interactions away from the parents and toward a direct relationship with the adolescent. Continuous support and respect of confidentiality are key elements in establishing a relationship of trust between the health care provider and the adolescent with diabetes. Family and individual counseling should be initiated if necessary. Common adolescent issues are complicated by the presence of diabetes. Such issues should be discussed prospectively with the teenager and the parent, as is appropriate. Adolescents who attempt to improve control may experience weight gain as a complication of the improved control. Such weight gain may be managed by clandestine omission or reduction in insulin. Issues of sexual activity, contraception, and pregnancy should be discussed at patient visits. Smoking and the use of alcohol and other drugs may become manifestations of adolescent dysfunction and also should be discussed at intervals. If the adolescent is guided appropriately toward full responsibility for diabetes management, the family will be able to relinquish its role successfully at the appropriate time.

Monitoring Long-Term Glycemic Control

Measurement of glycosylated (glycated) hemoglobins (GHb) provides an integrated assessment of blood glucose values over the preceding 2 to 3 months. The different glycohemoglobins are formed by a nonenzymatic reaction of sugars with the free amino groups of the hemoglobin molecule (glycation). For example HbA_{1C} is the β-chain N-terminal glycosylated glycohemoglobin. The higher the glucose level, the greater the formation of these glycosylated hemoglobins.

Several techniques have been developed to separate glycated and nonglycated hemoglobin and to measure the hemoglobin components: HbA_{1C}, HbA_1, or total GHb. There is no established standard and no universally accepted reference method. It is very important for health professionals caring for diabetic children to be aware of what these different assays mean and how they correlate with mean glucose values. It is also important to recognize pitfalls of the different methods. Measures of glycosylation of HbA will give aberrantly low readings in patients with sickle cell trait and aberrantly high readings if there is persistence of fetal hemoglobin. Other abnormal hemoglobins also may interfere with this assay. Only the total glycohemoglobin method can be used to assess long-term control in the presence of abnormal hemoglobins. Abnormal red cell turnover can affect the accuracy of all methods. Correlations in individuals with normal hemoglobins for three different commonly used methods are presented in Figure 1.

We measure HbA_{1C} every 2 to 3 months. In children less than 5 years of age, our goals are limited. To avoid hypoglycemia, we try to maintain the HbA_{1C} (HPLC) below 10% (mean blood glucose of 250 mg/dl). In children of school age, we aim to maintain HbA_{1C} within the range of the well-controlled group of subjects in the Diabetes Control and Complications Trial (mean HbA_{1C} 7.2%, mean

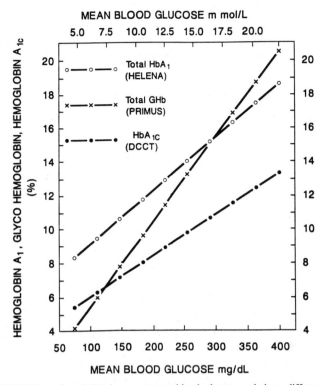

FIGURE 1. Correlation between mean blood glucose and three different commonly used assays for glycated hemoglobin. (Modified from Santiago JV: Lessons from the diabetes control and complications trial. Diabetes 42:1549–1554, 1993. © American Diabetes Association; reprinted with permission.)

blood glucose of 155 ± 30 mg/dl). This is not often feasible without severe hypoglycemia. We are very pleased when children maintain values less than 8% (mean blood glucose of 180 mg/dl).

MANAGEMENT OF INTERCURRENT EVENTS

Parents and children should be instructed as to management of extremes of blood sugar, strenuous exercise, and intercurrent illness.

Treatment of Hypoglycemia

Although blood glucose levels of 60 mg/dl may be seen commonly in normal children after an overnight fast, we define hypoglycemia for the purpose of diabetes management as a blood glucose of 60 mg/dl or less. Counterregulatory responses to a decreasing blood glucose can be detected at 70 mg/dl in normal children. Children with poorly controlled diabetes may develop hypoglycemic symptoms with blood glucose levels in the normal range. In contrast, children who have had recurrent hypoglycemia may fail to manifest autonomic symptoms of hypoglycemia yet may develop decreased mentation without warning. All children should be taught to carry sugar with them to treat sudden hypoglycemia. Approximately 40 kcal (10 g) of carbohydrate (two large sugar cubes, two glucose tablets, four small hard candies, or 4 ounces [120 ml] of juice, regular soft drink, or milk if available) are sufficient to raise blood glucose levels within 15 minutes and reverse most hypoglycemic reactions. If a meal is anticipated within the next hour, no further treatment usually is necessary. If there will be a longer time before a meal, carbohydrate-containing food with a longer action should also be consumed (100 kcal of crackers and cheese or peanut butter, 8 ounces [240 ml] of milk, or similar foods). Overtreatment will lead to hyperglycemia and can be avoided by retesting blood glucose in 15 to 30 minutes to confirm that it is in the normal range. Hypoglycemia of great enough severity to cause clouding of mentation may require the use of double the amount of carbohydrate as sugar-containing syrups or pastes (instant glucose, cake frosting in a tube, maple syrup, or honey), administered orally by a responsible caretaker. Glucose is not absorbed through the buccal mucosa. Only sugar that is swallowed will be absorbed into the bloodstream. Severe hypoglycemia associated with loss of consciousness or seizure can be treated by the family with subcutaneous glucagon. Glucagon is available as a 1 mg emergency kit containing powdered glucagon in a lactose carrier and packaged with a glass syringe containing diluent. The family should tape an insulin syringe to the kit. Glucagon should be administered by injecting diluent into the powdered glucagon vial and then using the insulin syringe to administer the dissolved glucagon. The diluent syringe cannot be used easily to administer the glucagon preparation. A full syringe of the size used by the child (0.3 [30 U] to 1 mg [100 U]) will be sufficient to raise the blood glucose within 15 minutes. The child should be fed immediately because transient nausea with vomiting often develops 30 minutes to 1 hour after glucagon administration. Severe hypoglycemia with recovery may nonetheless lead to mentation changes that persist for up to 8 hours or may produce a hemiparesis that persists for 8 to 24 hours.

Prevention of Hypoglycemia

One to two minor episodes of hypoglycemia every week may be unavoidable in well-controlled children. More frequent or severe hypoglycemia calls for a reexamination of the insulin therapy regimen, as well as a search for an obvious cause for hypoglycemia, such as omission of a meal/snack, increased exercise, or inappropriate insulin administration.

Treatment of Hyperglycemia and Impending Ketoacidosis

If blood glucose is elevated above 300 mg/dl and there are associated signs of illness, urine ketones should be tested promptly. If there is no ketonuria, a search for a cause of hyperglycemia (recent food intake, decreased exercise, inappropriate insulin dose) should be made. Exercise should not be used routinely to treat hyperglycemia. If hyperglycemia is the result of insulin deficiency, exercise may worsen high blood sugars and predispose the child to ketosis. Hyperglycemia may be treated with additional regular insulin (0.05 to 0.1 U/kg per dose) given every 4 to 6 hours until blood sugar returns to the normal range. Hyperglycemia associated with ketonuria without evidence of severe ketoacidosis (alteration of consciousness, uncontrollable vomiting) also may often be handled with oral rehydration and supplemental insulin. Incipient diabetic ketoacidosis of this type should be treated with subcutaneous regular insulin (0.1 U/kg per dose) every 4 to 6 hours until blood glucose is in the normal range and symptoms of ketoacidosis clear. Blood sugars and urine ketones should be tested every 2 hours. Oral rehydration should be with sips of fluid containing electrolyte and some glucose. Aspartame-containing diet soft drinks are not appropriate for complete oral rehydration because they are very low in sodium. Iced diet soft drinks can be alternated with canned broth or bouillon. Replacement of 2 to 3 ounces (60 to 90 ml) an hour in the preschooler, 3 to 5 ounces (90 to 150 ml) in the schoolage child, and 5 to 7 ounces (150 to 210 ml) an hour in the adolescent, as tolerated, usually will be sufficient. Sugar-containing drinks should be added when the blood sugar is less than 300 mg/dl. Telephone management of impending ketoacidosis should be attempted only if the family is very reliable.

Strenuous Exercise

Exercise, like insulin, increases muscle glucose uptake and can lead to hypoglycemia in well-insulinized individuals during physical activity or several hours later. When exercise is anticipated, it can be managed by reducing the insulin dose that will peak during the exercise by 10% to 20% or more. Alternatively, the child can be given an extra snack before or during physical activity. In children who are very sensitive to the prolonged effects of exercise, an extra snack at bedtime can reduce the risk of nocturnal hypoglycemia.

Intercurrent Illness

Febrile episodes are usually associated with modest insulin resistance. It is often necessary to provide additional insulin in excess of 10% of the total daily dose at each meal and at bedtime. However, when children are intolerant of oral intake (vomiting and nausea), it may be necessary to decrease the usual dose of insulin by 30% in anticipation of poor oral intake and judiciously to withhold regular insulin. When the child is able to tolerate small meals, we may then suggest small doses of regular insulin before each meal. To avoid both dehydration and hypoglycemia, children should be encouraged to take small quantities (1 to 3 teaspoons) of a sugar-containing soft drink every 15 to 20 minutes. Instructions for a carbohydrate-containing liquid regimen should be supplied to the parent by the dietitian so that carbohydrate calories can be maintained during illness. If the child is having diarrhea, electrolyte-containing oral rehydration solutions should be taken. Mixing these over-the-counter solutions with clear juices (1 volume of juice for 7 volumes of rehydration solution, for example) makes them more palatable to older children. Blood glucose and urine ketones should be monitored every 4 hours until the symptoms subside. The development of ketonuria usually is related to persistent dehydration and may be inhibited by more aggressive rehydration. Such hydration should be carried out with a combination of sugar-containing drinks and broths or bouillon drinks so that sodium depletion does not occur (see Treatment of Hyperglycemia and Impending Ketoacidosis). In rare instances, a short course of intravenous fluid therapy will be required. Telephone management is sufficient for most episodes of intercurrent illness, but the child should be evaluated by the physician if ketonuria or hyperglycemia is unremitting for 6 to 8 hours, the child is deteriorating clinically, or oral hydration is not possible.

Perioperative Management

For minor surgical procedures, the patient can be scheduled as the first patient of the day, and insulin should be withheld until after surgery. For longer procedures, 30% to 50% of the usual intermediate insulin dose can be given subcutaneously on the morning of surgery, and the child can then be supplemented with regular insulin every 4 to 6 hours (0.05 to 0.1 U/kg) as necessary until oral intake is possible. The normal evening insulin dose is then given. Alternatively, combined intravenous infusion of dextrose and insulin perioperatively and postoperatively may be employed. In a patient receiving a 5% dextrose infusion, 0.05 to 0.1 U/kg/h of infused regular insulin usually is required to maintain blood sugar in the 120 mg/dl to 180 mg/dl range. These insulin requirements can be higher in a setting of severe infection or steroid use. Blood sugar levels should be monitored at 1 to 2 hour intervals during intravenous insulin therapy.

Travel Across Time Zones

Patients taking two or more injections of insulin a day who are prepared to check blood sugar and take extra regular insulin as needed have a rather easy adjustment to changes in time zones. For changes of 2 hours or less, no compensation is necessary. Advance or loss of time by 12 hours requires only substituting the appropriate insulin for the time of day at the arrival point. A 6 hour backward time shift might call for a small supplement of regular insulin (10% or 20% of total daily dose) before the first meal on arrival, with intermediate-acting insulin and regular insulin administered at the next appropriate time for the arrival zone. A 6 hour advance in time would call for a reduction of 20% to 30% in the first dose of intermediate-acting insulin in the new time zone.

Inappropriate Insulin Doses

Inadvertent Missed Insulin Doses

If recognition of a missed dose occurs within 2 hours of the normal time of administration, the intermediate insulin may be given late, with regular insulin added depending on the blood sugar. If insulin administration is delayed by 3 to 6 hours, it is often better to give one half of the intermediate insulin dose and supplement with regular insulin at discovery and before meals until the next dose of intermediate insulin. Regular insulin alone can tide the patient over until the next intermediate insulin dose if discovery is even later.

Inadvertent Overinsulinization

Most minor insulin overdoses can be treated at home. A child who has received two or three times the appropriate dose should be fed frequently (every 2 to 4 hours) and have blood glucoses checked before feedings for the anticipated duration of the overdose. Larger amounts of insulin may require judicious observation in a hospital setting, with intravenous glucose available as necessary.

Diabetic Ketoacidosis

Presentation and Pathophysiology

Typically, new-onset patients present with a history of a few days to weeks of polyuria, polydipsia, weight loss, and abdominal pain with or without vomiting. In a previously diagnosed patient with diabetes, omission of insulin injections for more than 24 hours will lead to diabetic ketoacidosis (DKA), as can intercurrent illness with poor oral intake, vomiting, or insulin resistance. DKA in patients with known diabetes is always preventable with appropriate intervention. On physical examination, Kussmaul respirations, dehydration with increased pulse and hypotension, acetone odor on the breath, and altered consciousness may be apparent. However, even in the presence of infection, many patients are afebrile. Stretching of the liver capsule resulting from increased hepatic lipid production can cause tender hepatomegaly.

DKA is the metabolic consequence of insulin deficiency. This results in hyperglycemia, ketoacidosis, and increased release of counterregulatory hormones, such as glucagon, catecholamines, cortisol, and growth hormone. Counterregulatory hormones play an important role in the pathogenesis of DKA. Glucagon enhances gluconeogenesis, glycogenolysis, lipolysis, ketogenesis, and renal natriuresis. Epinephrine stimulates hepatic gluconeogenesis, glycogenolysis, and lipolysis. Cortisol decreases peripheral uptake of glucose and enhances lipolysis, gluconeogenesis, and proteolysis. Finally, growth hormone increases hepatic glucose production, decreases peripheral glucose uptake, and has a peripheral lipolytic effect, enhancing ketogenesis.

Decreased peripheral glucose uptake and enhanced hepatic and renal gluconeogenesis are the major contributors to hyperglycemia. Renal losses of water, sodium, potassium, calcium, magnesium, phosphate, and bicarbonate are in part the result of hyperglycemia-induced osmotic diuresis. Dehydration results in a decrease in glomerular filtration and impairment of the acid-base buffering capacity of the renal tubule.

Because insulin deficiency facilitates the activation of lipase, lipolysis is enhanced, and there are increased plasma levels of free fatty acids (FFA). Circulating FFA are transported to the liver and other peripheral tissues. During ketoacidosis, levels of malonyl CoA (a critical intermediate in the synthesis of long-chain fatty acids) decrease because the excess of glucagon interrupts the transformation of glucose-6-phosphate to malonyl CoA. This results in a shunting of FFA from lipogenesis to ketogenesis, with accumulation of acetoacetic and beta-hydroxybutyric acid, creating an anion gap acidosis. In addition, DKA reduces renal and muscle metabolism of ketoacids.

Laboratory Studies

When DKA is suspected, a rapid determination of blood glucose level and ketones in the urine using test strips should always be confirmed by the chemistry laboratory. Plasma glucose concentration is usually greater than 250 mg/dl, bicarbonate is less than 15 mEq/ L, and there is ketonemia and ketonuria. The acidosis is enhanced by lactic acidosis induced by dehydration. The nitroprusside method commonly used to measure ketones measures acetoacetate and acetone

but does not measure beta-hydroxybutyrate. Because beta-hydroxybutyrate is in excess in severely acidotic and dehydrated individuals, the magnitude of ketonemia can be underestimated. As the acidosis is corrected, the ratio of acetoacetate/beta-hydroxybutyrate returns to normal, and the patient may exhibit increased ketonuria.

Serum electrolyte levels vary according to the degree of urinary losses and duration of symptoms before presentation. Urine losses of sodium during DKA average 70 mEq/L. Hyperglycemia and hyperlipemia contribute to factitious hyponatremia. For each 100 mg of glucose over the normal value of 100 mg/dl, the serum sodium value is decreased by approximately 1.6 mEq/L.

Potassium concentration is also variable depending on renal losses and fluid shifts between body fluid compartments. However, total body potassium stores are invariably low. Initial phosphate levels are also variable, but body stores are depleted. Although calcium is lost in the urine, serum values usually are normal. Blood urea nitrogen can be elevated from dehydration. Creatinine may be spuriously elevated when measured by the Jaffe reaction because acetoacetate is a nonspecific chromogen in this assay.

Amylase levels may be elevated and, with coexisting abdominal pain, may suggest surgical abdomen. Although the amylase has been found to be of nonpancreatic origin, persistent abdominal pain should be fully evaluated because DKA can be precipitated by a surgical emergency. Elevated white blood cell (WBC) count with a polymorphonuclear leukocytosis is most commonly a stress response. However, a marked elevation of the WBC count might indicate that occult infection precipitated DKA. Hemoglobin and hematocrit values are elevated if dehydration is severe.

Therapy

Therapy of DKA involves not only insulin administration but also correction of fluid and electrolyte losses.

Fluid and Electrolyte Therapy. The first priority in treating DKA is to restore intravascular volume. Ten to twenty milliliters per kilogram of 0.9% saline should be administered over 1 to 2 hours for initial volume expansion. If the patient is in shock, additional 0.9% saline (10 to 20 ml/kg) may be necessary to restore volume. Fluid (0.45% saline) should then be infused as maintenance and deficit to correct estimated losses over 24 to 36 hours. Urine losses during rehydration should be discounted and not replaced. If serum potassium values are normal or low, potassium (40 mEq/L provided as half potassium chloride and half potassium phosphate) should be added to the infusate as soon as the patient voids. Very rare patients will require greater (60 to 80 mEq/L) potassium supplementation. If initial serum potassium is elevated, potassium should be measured again in 2 to 4 hours, and potassium should be replaced only after serum potassium has normalized. Phosphate replacement (as potassium phosphate) is prudent. Phosphate levels fall as treatment begins, and hypophosphatemia can occur but usually is asymptomatic. With phosphate deficiency the 2,3-diphosphoglycerate levels may fall, and the oxygen-dissociation curve will shift to the left. Therefore, there is a potential risk of tissue hypoxia because hemoglobin will not readily release oxygen to the tissues. There is little evidence that sodium bicarbonate is useful in the routine treatment of diabetic ketoacidosis. However, when the arterial pH is less than 7, the respiratory center may be depressed, worsening the acidosis because of loss of respiratory compensation. Therefore, sodium bicarbonate can be administered as 0.2 × base excess × body weight over 20 to 30 minutes if the arterial pH is less than 7.1 and the patient is clinically unstable. Appropriate insulin and fluid therapy will ensure full correction of the acidosis.

Restoration of fluid volume often leads to a decrease in blood glucose of 100 mg/dl or more. Acidosis also may improve, but insulin therapy is necessary to continue correction. When the glucose value is less than 300 mg/dl, 5% dextrose is added to the 0.45% saline solution to avoid hypoglycemia. If serum sodium decreases or remains

132 mEq or less during therapy, the sodium concentration of the infusate can be increased to 0.9%. If the patient is still acidotic but blood glucose is 200 mg/dl or less, the glucose concentration of the infusate can be increased to 10%.

Insulin Therapy. Subcutaneous, intramuscular, and intravenous routes of insulin therapy are effective in treating diabetic ketoacidosis. For most purposes, intravenous insulin infusion is the most effective route, correcting the hyperglycemia smoothly and allowing flexible adjustment of the insulin dose. Insulin infusion is given at a rate of 0.1 U/kg/h. Regular insulin can be piggybacked into the infusion as a solution of 1 U/kg in 100 ml of 0.9% saline, infused as 10 ml/h. To retain potency, insulin infusates should be discarded every 6 hours. An initial loading dose of insulin is not necessary. When the blood glucose reaches 250 mg/dl and the patient is no longer acidotic, the insulin infusion rate should be decreased to 0.05 U/kg/h. A decrease of blood glucose of 75 to 100 mg/dl/h is anticipated using this regimen. If blood glucose does not decrease, the insulin infusion rate may be increased. If blood glucose decreases too quickly, additional glucose should be added to the infusion. When continuous intravenous insulin infusion is not possible, intramuscular insulin administered as 0.1 to 0.2 U/kg every 2 hours has been shown to be effective. The insulin dose must be calculated carefully and administered using a tuberculin or other syringe calibrated in milliliters rather than units because the short needles of swaged insulin syringes can be used for intramuscular therapy in only the smallest of children. Because subcutaneous insulin absorption is slow and variable if perfusion is poor, we usually reserve subcutaneous insulin therapy for the telephone management of incipient DKA.

Other Interventions. Occasionally, other interventions are necessary. Intubation will secure the airway in a patient with vomiting and altered level of consciousness. A nasogastric tube will decompress abdominal distention in case of acute gastric dilatation. Urinary catheterization may be necessary if there is concern about anuria. Concomitant infection should be treated aggressively with the appropriate antibiotic therapy.

Clinical and Laboratory Monitoring. Close monitoring of the patient is essential to prevent or abort untoward events. Vital signs and neurologic status should be recorded hourly, as should blood glucose. If monitoring of glucose is a bedside procedure, both instrument and operator must be accurate. An initial electrocardiogram and a follow-up electrocardiogram at 6 to 8 hours will monitor potassium repletion. Electrolyte and pH determination should be repeated every 2 to 4 hours as needed, depending on the clinical severity, and all urine samples should be tested for ketones. Such careful assessment is required for at least the first 12 hours of therapy, until the patient is awake, responsive, and able to take sustenance orally. Phosphate and calcium levels should be rechecked at 6 to 8 hours and then before discontinuation of intravenous therapy. Urine output should be monitored.

Transition to Subcutaneous Insulin. Because the half-life of intravenous regular insulin is only 4 to 6 minutes, subcutaneous insulin must be administered before the intravenous infusion is discontinued. When the child is ready to eat and has a venous blood pH greater than 7.3 and a blood glucose less than 300 mg/dl, subcutaneous insulin may be given, and the insulin infusion can be discontinued. Subcutaneous insulin therapy in newly diagnosed patients should follow the general guidelines suggested in Initial Management of Children with IDDM. Initial daily insulin requirements of 0.5 to 1 U/kg should be anticipated after DKA. Children with known IDDM usually can resume their customary insulin regimen unless the onset of DKA has been related to insufficient insulin therapy. An etiology for the DKA should be determined. If an acute illness has led to decompensation, the necessity for closer monitoring and follow-up should be stressed to the parents. If no etiology can be determined, it is likely that failure to administer insulin is the problem. When supervision of insulin administration is delegated to a responsible adult, no further recurrences of DKA need be anticipated.

Complications

The development of cerebral edema is a concern during management of DKA. Although rare, cerebral edema is a major cause of diabetes-related death and disability in children. Children at greatest risk are younger at diagnosis, have a more prolonged period of ketoacidosis before diagnosis, and remain persistently hyponatremic during therapy. The pathogenesis of symptomatic cerebral swelling is not well understood. Overhydration with dilute fluids has been etiologic in some instances. Asymptomatic cerebral swelling may be found in children with DKA before initiation of therapy and during therapy. A rapid drop of glucose and sodium concentration leading to discordant changes in osmolality between the CNS and the periphery has been implicated in causing cerebral edema. Underlying tissue hypoxia, inappropriate ADH release, and CNS intravascular thrombotic events may also play a role. Symptomatic patients should be diagnosed quickly and treated aggressively. Typically, after improvement of the state of consciousness and during recovery from ketoacidosis, the patient develops symptoms of headache, irritability, decreased level of consciousness, and even seizures. Decreased pulse rate and a widened pulse pressure are signs of impending brain herniation. Focal neurologic signs and brainstem dysfunction with decerebrate posturing may be followed by brain death. Children who remain comatose and never have transient CNS recovery from DKA are more likely to have had intracranial vascular thrombotic events before therapeutic intervention rather than the development of cerebral edema during therapy.

If increased intracranial pressure is suspected, fluid intake should be reduced to low maintenance (1000 ml/m²/d), and 1 to 2 g/kg IV of mannitol should be administered and repeated every 4 to 6 hours. Intubation and hyperventilation may improve outcome. A CT scan or other imaging study should be obtained, but therapy should not await confirmation of cerebral edema because brain herniation may occur rapidly. Neurosurgical involvement should be requested to monitor intracranial pressure and ultimately to consider surgical decompression of the cerebral swelling.

IDENTIFICATION AND TREATMENT OF CHRONIC COMPLICATIONS OF IDDM IN CHILDREN

Children and adolescents with diabetes can develop other associated disorders. Chronic lymphocytic thyroiditis develops in up to 10% of children with IDDM. At each visit, the thyroid gland should be examined, and thyroid enlargement should be an indication to obtain thyroid function studies. TSH and antithyroid antibodies should be checked yearly after the first decade of life. Other endocrinopathies (adrenal insufficiency, for example) are decidedly less common. Serum lipids should be assessed yearly. Although hyperlipidemia can be the result of poor control of diabetes, hyperlipidemia separate from hyperglycemia should be treated appropriately.

The onset of degenerative complications of diabetes correlates with diabetes duration and control as assessed by glycohemoglobin. The prepubertal years appear to be less critical for the development of complications. However, the habits learned during those years are important for the maintenance of diabetes control during puberty and adulthood. Early complications may be seen in pubertal children.

Sclerodactyly (finger contractures) is associated with poor control and diabetes duration. This is a clinical marker of enhanced glycosylation and is associated with a higher frequency of retinopathy, cardiomyopathy, and diminished pulmonary compliance. Improved glycemic control can reverse sclerodactyly. Nephropathy can begin in puberty. Adolescents should have yearly measures of microalbumin in 12 hour overnight urine samples. If microalbuminuria is detected and is persistent on repeat testing, treatment is strongly encouraged. Hypertension should be treated vigorously because it is a risk factor for nephropathy. ACE inhibitors are the drugs of choice in IDDM for both microalbuminuria and hypertension. Early retinopathy may be detected, and pubertal and postpubertal patients should have yearly retinal examinations.

Peripheral neuropathy should be assessed clinically (vibration sense, deep tendon reflexes) in pubertal and postpubertal patients. Persistent gastrointestinal symptoms may reflect autonomic neuropathy and might require further evaluation and therapy.

FUTURE PROSPECTS FOR DIABETES MANAGEMENT

Attention to glycemic control, even in the imperfect manner currently available, has changed the life prospect for children with diabetes. In the near future, we may expect the marketing of an external glucose sensor that will determine glucose levels without blood sampling, a rapidly acting insulin now in clinical trials that could resolve many insulin-food mismatch issues, and the development and testing of drugs that may ameliorate or prevent complications related to nonenzymatic glycosylation.

Attempts to cure diabetes have focused on transplantation and mechanical devices. Pancreatic transplantation has been successful in alleviating insulin dependency in a number of patients with IDDM. Islet transplantation also has been successful occasionally. Unfortunately, the required immunosuppressive therapy is associated with major risks and long-term complications. It is not clear that either quality of life or outcome is remarkably improved by pancreas transplantation, although management needs are obviously altered. Pancreas or islet transplantation will become a therapeutic option in childhood if immunologic barriers to rejection can be managed specifically. Similarly, implanted mechanical devices to administer insulin will offer hope for children when they are matched with glucose sensors. We speculate that a better understanding of the glucose sensor and the insulin release mechanism of the beta-cell might permit a biologic approach to the cure of diabetes.

Families are often concerned about the potential for prevention of diabetes in siblings of the affected child. Immunosuppressive therapies (cyclosporine, azathioprine) have been successful in ameliorating the severity of newly diagnosed IDDM for variable periods in uncontrolled and a few controlled trials. However, the complications of immunotherapy are substantial, and these agents are not suggested for routine use as prophylactic or adjunctive therapies. Siblings and other family members of a child with diabetes can be screened for diabetes susceptibility using a combination of predictive antibodies and specific measures of glucose tolerance. Families wishing to become involved in prospective controlled trials to inhibit the development of diabetes should be encouraged to make contact with a major diabetes center to learn about available studies. Individuals who are identified to have high levels of predictive antibodies and deteriorating glucose tolerance may be eligible for these studies.

REFERENCES

1. American Diabetes Association: Position statement. Nutrition recommendations and principles for people with diabetes mellitus. Diabetes Care 17:519–522, 1994.
2. American Diabetes Association: Position statement. Standards of medical care for patients with diabetes mellitus. Diabetes Care 17:616–623, 1994.
3. Diabetes Control and Complications Research Group: Effect of intensive diabetes treatment on the development and progression of long-term complications in adolescents with insulin-dependent diabetes mellitus: Diabetes Control and Complications Trial. J Pediatr 125:177–188, 1994.
4. Franz MJ, Horton ES Sr, Bantle JP, et al: Nutrition principles for the management of diabetes and related complications. Diabetes Care 17:490–518, 1994.
5. Levitsky LL, Edidin DV: Diabetic ketoacidosis. *In* Vidyasagar D, Sarnaik AP (eds): Neonatal and Pediatric Intensive Care. Littleton, MA, PSG Publishing, 1985:175–188.
6. Rother KI, Levitsky LL: Diabetes mellitus during adolescence. Endocrinol Metab Clin North Am 22:553–571, 1993.

HYPOGLYCEMIA AND GLYCOGEN STORAGE DISEASES

LAWRENCE G. LEICHTMAN, M.D.

Hypoglycemia, defined as an abnormally low level of blood glucose, is not a disease but a symptom of an abnormal process involving metabolic or endocrine systems or increased glucose use. Hypoglycemia is said to exist when plasma glucose levels are less than 35 mg/dl in a full-term infant, below 25 mg/dl in a premature infant, or below 40 mg/dl in older infants and children. Hypoglycemia in the newborn may be asymptomatic, mild, severe, or persistent and intractable. In older infants, poor feeding, weak or high-pitched cry, limpness, cyanosis, and vomiting may occur. In children, symptoms are primarily neurologic and may include confusion, irritability, listlessness, eye-rolling, jitteriness, headache, and frank encephalopathy with seizures and coma. Ultimately, significant long-standing hypoglycemia may produce irreversible nervous system damage. *In the absence of a definitive diagnosis, it is important to obtain the necessary studies rapidly, before the initiation of therapy.* These studies should include urine ketones, serum lactic acid, insulin, cortisol, and growth hormone levels. An aliquot of plasma should be frozen for additional studies to be determined by the patient's future course.

IMMEDIATE THERAPY

Rapid restoration of the normoglycemic state is the key to treatment. Intravenous glucose at 0.5 to 1 g/kg or 2 to 4 ml/kg/min of a 25 g/dl (25%) dextrose solution should be administered at a rate of 1 ml/min. Following this initial bolus, the infusion should continue at 8 to 10 mg/kg/min, with frequent monitoring of the blood glucose concentration. If hypoglycemia persists despite adequate therapy, hyperinsulinemia should be considered. If hyperinsulinemia has been documented, diazoxide given PO at a dose of 5 to 30 mg/kg/d in three doses may prove useful. Even after glucose levels have stabilized and adequate feeding has been reinstated, intravenous glucose should be continued at a slower rate. The infusion of intravenous glucose should never be terminated abruptly, as this may provoke a rebound phenomenon. If the child is a known type I diabetic, treatment can be given with oral glucose or with the intramuscular administration of glucagon (a dose of 1 mg is usually sufficient).

LONG-TERM THERAPY

Long-term therapy is entirely dependent on the etiology of hypoglycemia. The etiologies can be divided into disorders of utilization, metabolic processes that interfere with glucose release, and endocrine disorders. Immediate disorders that can cause hypoglycemia must be first ruled out. These include sepsis, congenital heart disease, insulin-dependent diabetes mellitus (IDDM), drug and alcohol ingestion, and ketotic and functional hypoglycemia.

Decreased Release of Glucose from the Liver

Glycogenosis Types Ia and Ib

This disorder usually presents in the first year of life with seizures secondary to hypoglycemia or with abdominal enlargement because of massive hepatomegaly. Recurrent hypoglycemia is a major problem and may cause mental retardation. There is eventual stunting of growth yet moderate obesity due to treatment regimens. The disorder is due to severe deficiency of specific hepatic enzymes, glucose-6-phosphatase in type Ia and translocase in type Ib. Both cause an inability to release glucose from glycogen breakdown in the liver. A negligible amount of glucose is produced by an alternate pathway of lactate to glycogen, which then releases glucose through the action of amylo-1,6-glucosidase.

Treatment protocols aim to prevent hypoglycemia and to suppress hyperlacticacidemia by dietary therapy. After the glucose requirement is calculated (as milligrams per kilogram body weight per minute), therapy can be initiated. In general, the glucose requirement is 8 to 9 mg/kg/min for infants and 5 to 7 mg/kg/min for older children. Taking the patient's glucose requirement into account, three elements of the diet need special consideration: formula feeding, nasogastric drip feeding at night, and the use of uncooked cornstarch. A milk-based formula with a low lactose content should be used if breast milk is not available. Maltose may be added to allow increased nighttime feeding intervals to 3 to 4 hours. Gastric drip nighttime feedings may consist of a milk-based formula, lactose restricted and without sucrose. Dextrimaltose may be added to cover the glucose requirement. After infancy, uncooked cornstarch has been found to prolong euglycemia from 4 to 6 hours. The recommended dose is 1.75 to 2.5 g/kg per feeding in cool, chilled diet soda, Kool-Aid, or water. Fructose, galactose, and their polymers are to be avoided. Continued frequent monitoring of serum glucose and lactate levels is required to maintain adequate growth and development. Liver transplantation has been used for patients with intractable hypoglycemia, but the risk of a severe bleeding diathesis during the surgical procedure plus the risk of rejection and long-term immunosuppression precludes transplantation for all but the most severe cases. Long-term observations of adults with type Ia glycogenosis have noted an increased risk of liver neoplasm. Most of the tumors are benign hepatomas, but occasional carcinomatous transformation has occurred.

Glycogenosis Type III, Amylo-1,6-Glucosidase Inactivity

Type III glycogenosis patients manifest symptoms similar to those of type I but in a much milder form. Thus, patients are not as seriously affected by minor infections. Hepatomegaly and hypoglycemia are usually present later in childhood. Disease symptoms seem to abate during adolescence. Management is directed toward maintenance of normoglycemia and prevention of hepatic enlargement. A diet rich in proteins and containing starch as the primary carbohydrate source is recommended. Raw cornstarch is as beneficial as in type I disease. Avoidance of prolonged periods of starvation is mandatory.

Glycogen Synthetase Defect

This disease results from a defect in glycogen synthesis. Though rare, it has been reported in several families. Patients have hypoglycemia, hepatomegaly, and doll-like facies. There may be secondary inhibition of gluconeogenesis, as well as inability to synthesize glycogen. Dietary control with high-protein feeding, as well as the use of cornstarch and corticosteroids, has proven successful to minimize the inflammatory response.

Hepatic Fructose-1,6-Diphosphatase Deficiency

This disorder manifests as hypoglycemia with concomitant ketosis and lactic acidosis. The major event is total failure of gluconeogenesis. Substrate loading with fructose, glycerol, alanine, sorbitol, or dihydroxyacetone may result in hypoglycemia and lactic acidosis. In the neonatal period and infancy, breast milk may be protective because of its lack of fructose. Treatment consists of a low-protein diet free of sucrose, fructose, and sorbitol. Management must aim to prevent catabolism, as this may rapidly provoke hypoglycemia and lactic acidosis.

Fructose-1-Phosphate Aldolase B Deficiency and Galactose-1-Phosphate Uridyl Transferase Deficiency

Each of these diseases causes hypoglycemia because of the inability to metabolize either fructose or galactose. Treatment of either one consists primarily of restricting the offending sugar. In each case, however, dietary management requires careful consultation with dietitians, since both sugars are present in numerous prepared products. Parents are urged to read the ingredients of all prepared foods.

Primary Defects in Gluconeogenesis

Pyruvate Carboxylase Deficiency

This enzyme controls the first step of gluconeogenesis and is activated by acetyl CoA. The release of glucose from lactate recycling is, therefore, impaired. Resuscitation of the hypoglycemic, acidotic infant requires immediate glucose and bicarbonate replacement. Maintenance of carbohydrate intake in the presence of lactic acidemia is necessary. Uncooked cornstarch has proven beneficial in some of these patients.

Secondary Defects in Gluconeogenesis

This is a rapidly enlarging group of diseases that can affect fatty acid oxidation pathways by direct loss of enzymes. Defects include medium-chain, long-chain, or short-chain acyl CoA dehydrogenase deficiency, holocarboxylase synthetase deficiency, 3-hydroxy,3-methyl glutaryl CoA lyase deficiency, primary carnitine deficiency, or carnitine palmitoyl CoA transferase deficiency. Organic acidurias, such as methylmalonic aciduria and propionic aciduria, can produce similar symptoms. All produce hypoglycemia by essentially the same pathway: the lack of acyl CoA shuttling into the mitochondria for beta-oxidation of fatty acids. Under periods of stress, the body uses lactate and beta-hydroxybutyrate to produce glucose. The body first depletes liver glycogen resources and then proceeds to metabolize fatty acids. Therefore, when these infants become stressed by infection or starvation, severe hypoglycemia may occur along with hepatomegaly, Reye-like symptoms, and, occasionally, sudden infant death.

Treatment of defects of fatty acid oxidation consists primarily of glucose resuscitation at high rates (6 to 8 mg/kg/min). Sodium bicarbonate therapy at 2 to 4 mEq/kg over the first 4 to 6 hours usually is necessary to stabilize acidosis. Protein and fats should be initially withheld and started back slowly. High blood glucose levels may help spur lipolysis and decrease shunting through the defective fatty acid pathways. Carnitine at a rate of 100 to 150 mg/kg/d divided in three doses is supportive. Long-term therapy primarily centers around avoidance of prolonged periods of starvation (greater than 6 to 8 hours) and careful monitoring of blood glucose levels during infectious illnesses. Organic acidurias may benefit from long-term therapy with carnitine.

Beta-ketothiolase and succinyl CoA transferase deficiencies affect the ability to use ketones. Hypoglycemia may occur in these diseases during periods of stress or infection. Prevention of carbohydrate starvation, especially during intercurrent illness, is necessary. Carnitine at 100 mg/kg/d in three divided doses is also beneficial.

HYPERINSULINEMIA

Hyperinsulinemia results in hypoglycemia by suppressing hepatic release of glucose as well as by increasing glucose use. The two major forms of hyperinsulinemia in children are the hyperinsulinemia occurring in type I diabetes mellitus and the hypoglycemia of nesidioblastosis.

Hypoglycemia in children with diabetes mellitus following the injection of insulin without eating is a medical emergency. Oral glucose may be beneficial, but one must be cautious, as obtunded patients may aspirate liquids. If the child is not conscious, glucagon 0.03 to 0.3 mg/kg IM up to a maximum dose of 1 mg may be given. Parents of insulin-requiring diabetics should be familiar and comfortable with the use of glucagon, which should also be available in school for the school nurse to use. Tightly regulated diabetic patients are always at risk for hypoglycemic episodes, but the risk may be ameliorated by the child's taking high carbohydrate snacks just before intense physical activity.

The most difficult patients to manage are those with hyperinsulinism secondary to nesidioblastosis. These patients, if not treated rapidly, may suffer irreversible CNS damage or death. Placement of a central venous catheter for maintenance glucose (15% to 25%) administration at 10 to 12 mg/kg/min is the first step. In the event that high dextrose infusion rates are necessary (16 to 24 mg/kg/min), a course of intravenous synthetic cyclic somatostatin may be effective in suppressing insulin release. This may be combined with glucagon therapy. Such therapy is recommended only as a short-term strategy.

In the mildly affected patient, diazoxide, a nondiuretic benzothiazide, is an effective agent in controlling hypoglycemia by suppressing further insulin release. Patients who respond to diazoxide usually will be maintained without intravenous glucose support. The usual dose is 5 to 20 mg/kg/24 h PO in two divided doses. Side effects of diazoxide include water retention, hypertrichosis, and hyperuricemia.

Patients who have not responded within 2 weeks of initiation of therapy with high-dose glucose, glucagon, and somatostatin are candidates for subtotal or total pancreatectomy. Some patients will not respond even if only 10% of pancreatic tissue remains. Almost all such patients become either temporarily or permanently diabetic. Immediately postoperatively, glucose levels may be erratic because of secondary diabetes mellitus but should respond to the principles of management of type I diabetes mellitus.

HORMONAL DEFICIENCIES

An isolated deficiency of almost every endocrine secretion directly involved in carbohydrate homeostasis or energy metabolism has been associated with or implicated in hypoglycemia. Most such patients present in the newborn period. In most cases, the hypoglycemia is mild or transient, providing a clue for endocrinologic evaluation. Congenital glucagon deficiency may be associated with more severe and recurring hypoglycemia. Once the hormonal deficiency(ies) are identified, replacement therapy is given. In the case of growth hormone deficiency, conventional therapy consists of growth hormone injections three times a week. Hypoglycemia has been reported in some cases so treated and responds to daily injections instead. Cortisol replacement therapy consists of 10 to 15 mg/m² of hydrocortisone in two divided doses.

Finally, it is important to note that young children as a group are prone to become hypoglycemic when fasted (ketotic hypoglycemia) or if caloric intake is severely compromised during illness. Because of this vulnerability, it is always prudent to prevent prolonged interruption of nutritional needs of the child.

REFERENCES

1. Fernandes J, Leonard JV, Moses SW, et al: Glycogen storage disease: Recommendations for treatment. Review. Eur J Pediatr 147:226–228, 1988.
2. Greene HL, Slonim AE, Burr IM: Type I glycogen storage disease: Five years of management with nocturnal feedings. J Pediatr 96:590–595, 1980.
3. Robinson BH: The lacticacidemias. In: Lloyd JK, Scriver CR (eds): Genetic and Metabolic Diseases in Pediatrics. London, Butterworths, 1985.

CARBOHYDRATE DISORDERS

Mira Irons, M.D.

THE GALACTOSEMIAS

Three inborn errors of galactose metabolism have been identified. Each of these is due to an inherited deficiency of one of the three enzymes of the galactose metabolic pathway whereby galactose, which is derived from the galactose-containing disaccharide lactose, is ultimately converted to glucose-1-phosphate.

Classic galactosemia, the most common of these disorders, is due to a deficiency of the enzyme galactose-1-phosphate uridyltransferase. Lack of this enzyme results in the accumulation of both galactose-1-phosphate and galactose. Since the sugar of milk is lactose, neonates with classic galactosemia who are fed either breast milk or a milk-based formula may develop the symptoms of lethargy, feeding intolerance, vomiting, weight loss, renal tubular dysfunction, hyperbili-

rubinemia, and liver dysfunction with coagulopathy. Approximately 25% of affected infants also develop bacterial sepsis, most commonly due to gram-negative organisms, presenting by the end of the first or second week of life. The accumulation of galactose-1-phosphate is believed to be the cause of many of these clinical symptoms. Cataracts, which are noted on physical examination, result from the accumulation of galactitol, a galactose metabolic product, in the lens. If milk is not withdrawn and the infant survives this neonatal illness, the disease produces mental retardation, cirrhosis, and cataracts.

Several variant transferase deficiency states in which affected individuals have 10% to 35% of normal transferase activity are also known. The most frequent of these is the Duarte variant. Individuals with one gene for classic galactosemia and one gene for the Duarte variant have 25% of normal transferase activity. Patients with these variant forms of the disorder are generally asymptomatic but may present with clinical symptoms depending on the degree of enzyme deficiency present.

A deficiency of galactokinase, the first enzyme in the pathway, results in accumulation of galactose in blood and urine and galactitol in urine and ocular lenses. The only clinical manifestation of this disorder is the development of cataracts.

A deficiency of the enzyme UDP-galactose-4-epimerase, the third enzyme in the pathway, results in accumulation of not only galactose and galactose-1-phosphate but also UDP-galactose. Since this inborn error has been described only recently, less is known about this disorder. However, it appears that those in whom the enzyme deficiency is limited to erythrocytes are asymptomatic, whereas those with a more generalized deficiency may have a phenotype similar to that seen in untreated classic galactosemia.

Diagnosis

Since newborn screening for galactosemia is performed in most states of the United States and in many other countries around the world, many affected infants are identified before they become clinically ill. Screening methods in use identify the presence of either galactose and galactose-1-phosphate or transferase activity (by a specific spot enzyme assay) in the newborn filter paper blood specimen. In the absence of newborn screening, the suspicion of galactosemia is based on clinical presentation. In this instance, a urine test for reducing substances (Clinitest) will be positive, whereas the urine test for glucose (Clinistix) will be negative. The diagnosis can then be confirmed by the identification of galactose or galactose-1-phosphate in the blood and measurement of the appropriate enzyme in erythrocytes, cultured fibroblasts, or liver.

Therapy

The mainstay of therapy for affected individuals is the elimination of lactose by removing milk and milk products from the diet. In infancy, this is accomplished by the use of soybean-based formulas or a casein hydrolysate, such as Nutramigen or Alimentum. Older children and adults should remain on milk-free diets. The appropriate amount of calcium and vitamins must be added to the diet. Since lactose and milk solids are common additives to many foods and medications, close attention to product labels is required. Nutritional guidance by a dietitian is helpful to ensure that the diet contains sufficient amounts of calories, vitamins, protein, and minerals and is appropriate for growth and development. Education of the parents (and ultimately the child) will be required as the child grows to ensure that foods or medications that contain lactose are not ingested.

In addition to elimination of lactose from the diet, affected neonates may also require hospitalization and treatment for dehydration, sepsis, or coagulopathy. Resolution of clinical symptoms begins within several days of initiation of therapy.

Compliance with the diet is monitored by measuring erythrocyte or whole blood galactose-1-phosphate and urinary galactose. Even well-treated patients may have detectable erythrocyte galactose-1-

phosphate levels. This galactose-1-phosphate is believed to be produced endogenously from UDP-glucose.

Patients with galactokinase deficiency are also treated with a milk-free diet. This results in elimination of galactose and prevents the development of cataracts.

Patients with epimerase deficiency who are symptomatic should be treated in the same way as those with classic galactosemia. These patients may require a small amount of galactose to promote the synthesis of galactoproteins and galactolipids.

Patients with galactosemia have been found to have lower levels of UDP-galactose, and newer forms of therapy are being investigated that may increase UDP-galactose levels in affected patients. One such treatment regimen involves the administration of uridine. However, the use of uridine in the treatment of galactosemia is still experimental and should be given only in the setting of a controlled clinical trial.

When treatment is begun early in life, affected individuals do not develop the triad of mental retardation, cirrhosis, and cataracts. However, even well-treated individuals have been noted to develop learning disabilities, speech and language disorders, neurologic disease, and behavioral problems. Girls with galactosemia may develop premature ovarian failure, resulting in amenorrhea or oligomenorrhea, infertility, and osteoporosis because of estrogen deficiency.

Genetics

All of the galactosemias are inherited in an autosomal recessive manner, so that couples with one affected child have a 1 in 4, or 25%, risk of having another affected child in each subsequent pregnancy. Prenatal diagnosis is available by either measurement of enzyme activity or specific DNA testing in fetal tissue obtained by either amniocentesis or chorionic villus biopsy.

Mothers at risk for having a child with galactosemia often are placed on lactose-restricted diets during pregnancy, with calcium supplementation, on the premise that this will decrease the galactose load to the fetus and eliminate some of the complications of the disorder. However, galactose-1-phosphate has been noted in the cord blood of infants born to mothers who strictly eliminated lactose from their diets during pregnancy, which raises the possibility that even the galactosemic fetus may produce galactose-1-phosphate endogenously.

OTHER DISORDERS OF CARBOHYDRATE METABOLISM

Hereditary Fructose Intolerance

Hereditary fructose intolerance is due to a deficiency of fructose-1-phosphate aldolase B, one of the enzymes of the fructose catabolic pathway. The ingestion of fructose or sucrose (which contains fructose) results in the accumulation of fructose-1-phosphate and subsequent hypoglycemia because of inhibition of gluconeogenesis and glycogenolysis. Symptoms are first noted in breast-fed infants when they are weaned to solids, and fruits and vegetables are introduced. Neonates may present with symptoms if fed with soybean-based formulas that contain sucrose.

Symptoms usually include feeding intolerance, failure to thrive, and vomiting but may also include hypoglycemia, metabolic acidosis, hepatomegaly, renal tubular dysfunction, alterations of consciousness, and seizures. The diagnosis may remain unknown unless a careful dietary history reveals that exacerbations of illness occur after the ingestion of fructose- or sucrose-containing foods. Some patients may learn to restrict their diets and avoid the foods that make them ill.

Treatment of acute illness requires elimination of all fructose- and sucrose-containing foods and administration of intravenous fluids with glucose. Long-term therapy consists of strict avoidance of all dietary sucrose and fructose. Patients should inform all physicians caring for them of their condition or wear medical alert bracelets indicating this diagnosis, since many intravenous fluids contain fructose or sorbitol, which may be life-threatening to affected individuals.

Disorders of Gluconeogenesis

Disorders of gluconeogenesis are extremely rare and are caused by deficiency of enzymes, such as pyruvate carboxylase, phosphoenolpyruvate carboxykinase, or fructose-1,6-diphosphatase. Affected patients present with hypoglycemia, lactic acidosis, seizures, hepatomegaly, hypotonia, failure to thrive, lethargy, and rarely coma and death. These symptoms are precipitated by prolonged fasting, febrile illness, or ingestion of fructose, sorbitol, or glycerol.

Treatment of acute episodes includes administration of large quantities of intravenous glucose to treat the hypoglycemia and sodium bicarbonate to correct the acidosis. Long-term therapy includes the avoidance of fasting and frequent or continuous feedings with a diet high in carbohydrates. See section on Hypoglycemia and Glycogen Storage Diseases.

REFERENCES

1. Gitzelmann R, Steinmann B, Van Den Berghe G: Disorders of fructose metabolism. *In* Scriver CR et al (eds): The Metabolic Basis of Inherited Disease. New York, McGraw-Hill, 1989:407–413.
2. Holton JB, de la Cruz F, Levy HL: Galactosemia: The uridine diphosphate galactose deficiency-uridine treatment controversy. J Pediatr 123:1009–1013, 1993.
3. Korson M, Irons M, Levy HL: Hereditary metabolic diseases. *In* Avery ME, First LR (eds): Pediatric Medicine. Baltimore, Williams & Wilkins, 1994:1025–1038.
4. Segal S: Disorders of galactose metabolism. *In* Scriver CR et al (eds): The Metabolic Basis of Inherited Disease. New York, McGraw-Hill, 1989:453–480.

DIABETES INSIPIDUS

LOUIS J. MUGLIA, M.D., Ph.D.
JOSEPH A. MAJZOUB, M.D.

ETIOLOGY

Diabetes insipidus (DI) exists when, in the presence of plasma hyperosmolality, an appropriately concentrated urine is not formed. This defect stems from either insufficient secretion of vasopressin *(hypothalamic or central DI)* or renal unresponsiveness to vasopressin *(nephrogenic DI)*.

Hypothalamic Diabetes Insipidus

Hypothalamic DI occurs most frequently in association with tumors involving the hypothalamus or following their resection (craniopharyngioma, germinoma). Because the magnocellular neurons of the hypothalamic paraventricular and supraoptic nuclei, which synthesize vasopressin destined for release from the posterior pituitary, are distant from the pituitary, substantial suprasellar extension of anterior pituitary tumors must develop before the occurrence of DI. DI, however, develops in approximately 20% of patients following the surgical removal of anterior pituitary tumors, particularly when associated with high transection of the pituitary stalk. Infiltrative malignancies (leukemia, lymphoma) and systemic diseases (histiocytosis, sarcoidosis, Whipple's disease) may cause substantial destruction of vasopressin-containing neurons with little mass effect. Nonsurgical trauma, vascular lesions, infection, and pituitary infarction associated with parturition are less common causes.

Idiopathic hypothalamic DI comprises a relatively common subgroup of patients. Pedigrees exhibiting an autosomal dominant mode of inheritance have been described, but the majority of these cases are not familial. Recently, several groups have reported point mutations in the vasopressin gene that result in DI. In familial hypothalamic DI, screening DNA from children for vasopressin mutations will allow identification of susceptible individuals before development of symptoms, since in the majority of pedigrees, polyuria does not occur until after the first year of life.

Nephrogenic Diabetes Insipidus

Nephrogenic DI most commonly results from acquired defects, such as chronic tubulointerstitial renal disease, obstructive uropathy, hypercalcemia, hypokalemia, or drug effects (e.g., lithium). A congenital X-linked recessive form has also been defined.

CLINICAL FEATURES

Thirst, polyuria, and polydipsia are the hallmarks of DI. Urine output in general exceeds 3 L/m^2/d, with nocturia (and sometimes enuresis) a common feature. The urine is often colorless, even on the first morning voiding. A marked preference for cold liquids is expressed by most patients, with drinking occurring through the night. In infants, failure to thrive or recurrent fever of unknown origin may be the primary complaints.

To screen for DI, it is useful to obtain a serum sample and second-voided urine sample after a defined fast. The duration of the fast should be determined by the usual length the patient can abstain from fluids to avoid excessive dehydration. A serum osmolality of greater than 295 mOsm/kg of water (H$_2$O) with a urine osmolality less than 295 mOsm/kg H$_2$O establishes the diagnosis. If the serum osmolality is less than 295 mOsm/kg H$_2$O and the urine osmolality is less than 600 mOsm/kg H$_2$O, a water deprivation test is needed to establish the diagnosis. Hourly serum and urine electrolytes and osmolality, as well as weight, are measured beginning at 4 hours of fasting until the serum osmolality rises above 295 mOsm/kg H$_2$O or the urine osmolality exceeds 600 mOsm/kg H$_2$O. Blood pressure and pulse should be monitored hourly to guard against the development of clinically important hypovolemia.

THERAPY

Postoperative Management

Water balance is normally regulated by vasopressin and thirst. The potential for significant problems arises when both of these components are compromised, as in postoperative situations in which intravenous fluids are used and damage to the hypothalamus or posterior pituitary has occurred. Patients in this setting should be monitored and stabilized in an intensive care unit. During the postoperative period, DI can develop in many patients undergoing craniotomy and manipulation of the hypothalamic-pituitary region. The classic triphasic response may develop in cases of pituitary stalk transection, in which, after an initial 1 to 3 days of DI, inappropriate vasopressin secretion develops that may last for several days before the subsequent return of DI.

Because of this lability in neuroendocrine function, it is often best to manage acute postoperative DI *in children,* especially infants and toddlers, with fluids alone, avoiding the use of vasopressin therapy. This method consists of matching input and output hourly within the range of 1 to 3 L/m^2/d (40 to 120 ml/m^2/h). These limits are derived assuming an obligate daily solute excretion of approximately 500 mOsm/m^2 and normal renal function without an excess of extrarenal water loss (due to vomiting, diarrhea, diaphoresis, and so on). When intravenous fluids are used, the basal 40 ml/m^2/h should be given as D$_5$ ¼ normal saline (NS) and the rest, depending on the urine output, as 5% dextrose in water (D$_5$W). Potassium chloride (40 mEq/L) may be added if oral intake is to be delayed for several days. For hourly urine volumes under 40 ml/m^2/h, no additional fluid should be administered. For hourly urine volumes in excess of 40 ml/m^2/h, the excess volume should be replaced with D$_5$W up to a total maximum replacement of 120 ml/m^2/h. For example, in a child with a surface area of 1 m^2 (approximately 30 kg), the mimimal infusion rate would be 1 m^2 times 40 ml/m^2/h = 40 ml/h of D$_5$ ¼ NS. If an hourly urine output was 60 ml, an additional 20 ml/h D$_5$W would be given, for a total infusion rate of 60 ml/h. This may result in a serum sodium in the 150 mEq/L range and a mildly volume contracted state, should DI be present. Patients may also become mildly hyperglycemic on this regimen, particularly if they are also receiving postoperative glu-

cocorticoid therapy. This fluid management protocol, because it does not employ vasopressin administration, prevents any chance of hyponatremia.

In children of school age and older or in patients experiencing excessive hyperglycemia on the fluid replacement regimen described, a vasopressin infusion (Pitressin) provides an effective means of antidiuresis when the appropriate safeguards are taken. Vasopressin infusions are instituted at 1.5 mU/kg/h, which results in maximal antidiuresis. To avoid water intoxication, fluids are restricted to 1 L/m^2/d once a reduction in urine output is observed. Whenever exogenous vasopressin is administered along with intravenous fluids, thirst and vasopressin regulatory mechanisms are bypassed, providing a setting in which serious complications associated with water intoxication may occur. When this protocol is used, great care must be taken to avoid iatrogenic hyponatremia. With either protocol, patients may be switched from intravenous to oral fluids as soon as possible to facilitate their management.

Chronic Diabetes Insipidus

Therapy for patients with chronic DI must be individualized. In infants with continued DI, formula is continued at 3 L/m^2/d without vasopressin replacement. Institution of exogenous vasopressin therapy in this age group would require fluid restriction to a degree that would jeopardize adequate growth. For children and adolescents with an intact thirst mechanism, intranasal desamino-D-arginine vasopressin (DDAVP) is begun as a single nighttime dose of 2.5 to 10 μg, with a usual duration of action of 12 to 24 hours. A second dose may be given in the morning if adequate antidiuresis is not maintained. Patients are instructed to alternate nares to minimize mucosal edema and irritation, which can reduce absorption, as can rhinorrhea and congestion. Excessive doses may cause mild abdominal cramping or diarrhea. All patients should be allowed a period of at least 1 to 2 hours daily when escape from the effects of DDAVP occurs so that any excess water accumulated may be excreted. This minimizes the chance of water intoxication.

Partial Vasopressin Deficiency

In patients with partial vasopressin deficiency states, chlorpropamide (4 mg/kg/d) has been found to augment residual vasopressin action. Hypoglycemia is the primary complication of this therapy.

REFERENCES

1. Bartter FJ, Detea CS: Diabetes insipidus, its nature and diagnosis. Lab Management 20:23, 1982.
2. Coggins CH, Leaf A: Diabetes insipidus. Am J Med 42:807, 1967.
3. Harris AS: Clinical experience with desmopressin: Efficiency and safety in central diabetes insipidus and other conditions. J Pediatr 114:711–718, 1989.
4. Knoers M, Monnens LA: Amiloride-hydrochlorothiazide vs indomethacin-hydrochlorothiazide in the treatment of nephrogenic diabetes insipidus. J Pediatr 117:499–502, 1990.

HYPOCALCEMIA AND TETANY

Rita D. Swinford, m.d.
John T. Herrin, m.b.b.s.

Tetany is a condition of neuromuscular irritability resulting from hypocalcemia or hypomagnesemia. This hyperexcitable state of the peripheral and central nervous system is manifest as a sustained contracture, or paralytic, state in which the muscles of the feet assume a characteristic position of toes down and increased arch, and the hand shows extension of the fingers with the thumb tightly adducted into the palm and wrist flexion (Trousseau's sign). Hyperexcitability of facial muscles results in a positive Chvostek's sign. An occasional patient will demonstrate grand mal seizures or focal seizure activity. These characteristic changes are common outside the neonatal period and, in fact, may be provoked in an infant by handling or during the elicitation of muscle reflexes.

Tetany-associated laryngospasm and even laryngeal closure with respiratory difficulty may be seen spontaneously in some patients, whereas tight vocal cord adduction may be precipitated by attempted endotracheal intubation. Additionally, patients may exhibit severe apprehension, loss of deep tendon reflexes, hypotension, and ECGs showing prolonged ST segment and Q-T interval with ventricular arrhythmias. An older patient may not reveal the full-blown typical tetanic pattern but rather a history of cramping and stiffness. The laryngospasm may be described by family members as "honking" during breathing.

Calcium and magnesium ions are important in the regulation of vascular tone and the maintenance of membrane potentials. Changes in their homeostasis in disease states and acid-base disturbances can produce painful and uncontrolled muscular contraction, cardiac arrhythmias, and respiratory or locomotor difficulties. Acute empiric management aims to provide sufficient control to allow investigation and institution of rational long-term therapy. Table 1 provides guidelines to further investigation following measures for symptomatic relief. Stabilization and repletion are performed concurrently.

Although rational or chronic treatment necessitates correction of the underlying cause as well as provision of calcium or magnesium and acid-base correction, empiric therapy may be required in the acute setting of tetany. Hypocalcemia and hypomagnesemia are the result of a number of underlying disease processes. Knowledge of potential causes can allow rapid clinical evaluation of the tetanic state and permit correction, with adjustments depending on the clinical response and chemical monitoring. Symptoms are related not only to the rate of calcium decline but also to the absolute level of ionized calcium.

THERAPY

Hypocalcemia

Serum calcium is predominantly an intracellular ion, existing mainly in bone (99%). Intravascularly, 40% of available calcium is bound to plasma albumin, with the remaining 60% freely ionizable and a small amount complexing with serum citrates, phosphates, and bicarbonate ions. Three biologic processes regulate calcium homeostasis: gastrointestinal absorption of calcium, turnover of bone, and renal calcium reabsorption mediated by parathyroid hormone (PTH) and vitamin D_3. Alterations in any of these mechanisms can result in decreased availability of circulating ionized calcium. An ionized calcium below 3.5 mg/dl (0.88 mmol/L) represents hypocalcemia and is likely to result in symptomatic tetany.

Acid-base status influences serum calcium levels. Acidosis decreases calcium binding to serum proteins, thereby increasing the amount of filtered and excreted calcium. Acidosis also increases the amount of calcium released from bone and inhibits PTH-mediated calcium reabsorption in the distal tubule. Alkalosis, on the other hand, increases the fraction of calcium bound to serum proteins and stimulates PTH secretion, which promotes calcium reabsorption.

Emergency therapy consists of returning the serum ionized calcium level to normal, if possible, by correction of the pathophysiologic process (Table 2). For example, in hyperventilation tetany, rebreathing into a paper bag adjusts the acid-base deficit by elevating the partial pressure of carbon dioxide and normalizing serum pH with correction of tetany. In a symptomatic patient with tetany and observed seizure activity, elemental calcium at 10 mg/kg (0.5 mEq/kg) should be provided slowly IV over 10 to 20 minutes. The ECG should be monitored during this infusion, since bradycardia and QRS changes can be seen. Following the initial bolus, 10 mg/kg of elemental calcium should be infused IV every 4 to 6 hours. Plasma ionized calcium levels should be monitored before each infusion. The aim should be to restore total serum calcium to 7 mg/dl in the premature neonate or 8 mg/dl in the full-term infant (Table 2). In the older child, the calcium requirement remains elevated. Thus, either sup-

TABLE 1. Etiology of Hypocalcemia and Hypomagnesemia

Hypocalcemia
Neonatal Period
Early (onset within first 3–4 days of life)
1. Postnatal calcitonin surge (prematurity)
2. Delayed PTH response, mother with IDDM
3. Perinatal anoxia and preeclampsia
4. Infant of mother with hyperparathyroidism
Late (5–10 days of age)
1. Maternal vitamin D deficiency
2. Elevated serum phosphate, dietary phosphate loading
3. Hypomagnesemia
4. Parathyroid agenesis

Beyond the Neonatal Period (several weeks to months)
Vitamin D deficiency
Hyperphosphatemia and aggressive treatment of hypophosphatemia
Prematurity: "Late-late" hypocalcemia at 2–4 months
Parathyroid hypoplasia (DiGeorge syndrome)
Transient hypoparathyroidism, infant of mother with hyperparathyroidism
Acquired idiopathic hypoparathyroidism
Polyglandular autoimmune disease
Surgical (thyroidectomy, parathyroidectomy)
Renal tubular disease (galactosemia, cystinosis)
Transient hypocalcemia (citrated products, albumin infusion)
Hyperventilation syndrome with tetany
Chronic renal failure
Anticonvulsant therapy: phenytoin and phenobarbital

Hypomagnesemia
Factors Associated with Increased Renal Magnesium Excretion
Extracellular volume expansion
Loop diuretics, furosemide and ethacrynic acid
Osmotic diuretics, mannitol/diuresis, urea and glucose
Metabolic acidosis
Cisplatin administration
Amphotericin treatment
Aminoglycoside nephrotoxicity
Cyclosporine treatment
Fanconi's syndrome
Chronic interstitial nephritis/renal disease

Factors Associated with Decreased Intestinal Absorption
Vitamin D deficiency
Selective malabsorption (intestinal and biliary fistulas)
Inadequate intake
Prolonged intravenous therapy
Generalized malabsorption (nontropical sprue)
Severe diarrhea, ulcerative colitis, gastroenteritis
Prolonged nasogastric suction
PTH deficiency (hypoparathyroidism)

Factors Associated with Endocrine Disorders
Diabetes mellitus
Primary hyperparathyroidism and primary aldosteronism

plemental intravenous infusion providing 20 to 40 mg/kg/d or oral supplements of 60 to 100 mg/kg/d of elemental calcium should be given. Vitamin D as 1,25-dihydroxycholecalciferol intravenously as Calcijex (0.01 μg/kg) or orally as Rocaltrol (0.125 to 0.25 μg) can be used to increase calcium gastrointestinal absorption, particularly in patients with longer-term calcium losses (e.g., chronic renal failure, pseudohypoparathyroidism, Fanconi's syndrome).

Hypomagnesemia

Not unlike calcium, magnesium is also contained predominantly in bone (two thirds of the total reserve). Magnesium plays an essential role in intracellular metabolism, including the production and use of energy. Magnesium's regulation and control are less well understood, however. Cellular availability is closely linked to mobilization from the gastrointestinal tract (vitamin D and PTH mediated), kidney, and bone. Magnesium is highly bound to plasma proteins and other serum

TABLE 2. Treatment of Hypocalcemia

Calcium Supplementation

Oral Calcium
Neonates: 50–150 mg/kg elemental calcium per day
Children: 45–65 mg/kg of elemental calcium per day
Adults: 1–2 g of elemental calcium per day

Calcium carbonate	
Os-Cal	500 mg (25 mEq) per tablet
Os-Cal with vitamin D	250 mg (12.5 mEq) per tablet
Calci-Chew	500 mg (25 mEq) per flavored packet
Calci-Mix	500 mg (25 mEq) per dissolvable capsule
Nephro-Calci	600 mg (30 mEq) per tablet
Calcium citrate	
Citracal	200 mg (10 mEq) per tablet
Calcium glubionate	
Neocalglucon syrup	115 mg (5.6 mEq)/5 ml

Parenteral Calcium
Calcium chloride
  135 mg (7 mEq) per 5 ml or 10 ml injection
Calcium gluconate
  90 mg (4.5 mEq) per 10 ml injection (ampoule)

Acute Hypocalcemia

Level: Ionized Calcium <0.88 mmol/L and <3.5 mg/dl or Symptoms
1. Determine clinical impact
2. Check ionized calcium and rate of decline
3. Development of symptoms depends on serum pH, concomitant hypomagnesemia, hypokalemia, hyponatremia, sedatives, and anticonvulsant drugs
4. Slowly give 10 mg/kg (0.5 mEq/kg) IV over 10–20 min to reverse tetany
   Repeat with 10 mg/kg infusion q4–6h
   Begin oral therapy if possible 60–100 mg/kg/d elementary calcium
   Begin vitamin D therapy: Calcijex (IV) or Rocaltrol (PO)
5. Treat associated electrolyte abnormalities if present

Neonatal Hypocalcemia

Premature infant: Treat with serum level of 0.62–0.72 mmol/L
Term infant: Treat with serum level of 1.50–1.75 mmol/L

Treatment
1. IV calcium gluconate (10% solution) 1–3 ml slowly (<1 ml/min); not to exceed 2 mg/kg body weight; may be repeated up to four times in one 24 hour period
2. Maintenance: IV 20–50 mg/kg of elemental calcium per day by use of calcium gluconate or calcium glubionate
3. Formula should be changed to low-phosphate formula with Ca:PO$_4$ ratio of 4:1 (e.g., Similac PM 60/40)
4. Correct hypomagnesemia if present. Short-term treatment using 50% magnesium sulfate 0.1–0.2 ml/kg one or two doses and possibly 1 more in the next 12 to 24 hours. Long-term treatment should be oral

buffers. Classically, patients with chronic severe hypomagnesemia (less than 1 mEq/L) are hypocalcemic as well. This is thought to be secondary to the permissive magnesium effect on PTH.

Hypocalcemia can be difficult to correct unless magnesium deficits are corrected concurrently. Although magnesium can be given intravenously in an emergency, slow adjustment of magnesium is preferred because (1) bolus correction of magnesium typically is followed by enhanced renal excretion, and (2) rapid changes in extracellular magnesium can produce toxicity (somnolence, hypotension, and sedation with or without respiratory compromise). Therapy can be divided into several categories: (1) prevention of magnesium depletion in high-risk groups, (2) replenishment of an established depletion, and (3) emergency therapy of symptomatic depletion.

Hypomagnesemia occurs most frequently in patients who have chronic diarrheal disorders with intestinal magnesium wasting. Intestinal fluids are rich in magnesium. The upper intestinal tract fluids contain about 1 mEq/L magnesium, and diarrheal fluids and fistulous drainage contain 15 mEq/L magnesium. Additional causes include

TABLE 3. Magnesium Supplementation

Oral Magnesium	Children: 3–6 mg/kg of elemental magnesium divided t.i.d. or q.i.d. (400 mg max)
	Adults: 200–400 mg elemental magnesium divided t.i.d. or q.i.d.
Magnesium gluconate	
Magonate 500	27 mg (2.4 mEq) per tablet
Magonate suspension	54 mg (4.5 mEq)/5 ml
Magnesium oxide	
Mag-Ox 400	241 mg (19.86 mEq) per tablet
Antacids	
Maalox suspension	83 mg (7 mEq)/5 ml
Laxatives	
Milk of Magnesia	500 mg (42 mEq)/15 ml
Parenteral Magnesium	25–50 mg/kg per dose q4–6h, max 1 g in 1 h
Magnesium sulfate	
24 mg (2 mEq)/ml	
48 mg (4 mEq)/ml	

renal tubular magnesium wasting either from iatrogenic causes, such as diuretic therapy, chemotherapy (particularly cisplatin), aminoglycoside treatment, or cyclosporine administration. Patients with inherent tubular dysfunction or those on prolonged parenteral nutrition, particularly if rapid restoration of protein and caloric balance is attempted, may also develop hypomagnesemia.

In emergencies, such as hypomagnesemic seizures, magnesium sulfate 20% (4 mEq/ml) at a dose of 0.4 to 0.8 mEq/kg (50 to 100 mg/kg) of elemental magnesium per dose IV or IM should be administered. With marked asymptomatic depletion, parenteral replacement will be necessary. Magnesium sulfate 25 to 50 mg/kg (0.2 to 0.4 mEq/kg/d) can be added to IV fluids or given IM every 6 hours for several doses unless thrombocytopenia is present. Oral supplements can be started early in the form of elemental magnesium (3 to 6 mg/kg/d) divided into 6- to 8-hour supplements. With oral magnesium supplements, frequent dosing is preferred, as magnesium also has cathartic and laxative properties that will further exacerbate magnesium losses. Magnesium gluconate is better tolerated than magnesium sulfate, resulting in less diarrhea and less abdominal cramping. It can be given in tablet or suspension form. Magnesium oxide can be used as an alternative oral supplement in patients with severe losses secondary to long-term cancer therapy, cisplatin and amphotericin treatment, or congenital magnesium-wasting syndromes (Table 3).

REFERENCE

1. Ichikawa I: Pediatric Textbook of Fluids and Electrolytes. Baltimore, Williams & Wilkins, 1990.

RICKETS

Thomas O. Carpenter, M.D.

The term *rickets* refers to the gross skeletal abnormalities resulting from unorganized proliferation of cartilage in the growth plates of long bones. *Osteomalacia,* or the inadequate mineralization of true bone tissue, usually accompanies the growth plate abnormality in children. Adults subjected to similar pathophysiologic events are said to have osteomalacia, in contrast to rickets, as their epiphyseal growth plates are mineralized. In active rickets, radiographs of epiphyseal areas of rapidly growing long bones reveal characteristic fraying, flaring, and cupping of the epiphyses. The bone may be generally demineralized, and a coarse trabecular appearance sometimes indicated by a ground-glass appearance to the shaft of the bone often is present. The characteristic epiphyseal signs may be less prominent in

TABLE 1. Causes of Rickets

	CALCIOPENIC	PHOSPHOPENIC
Nutritional	Vitamin D deprivation Calcium deprivation	Phosphate deprivation
Transport	Intestinal malabsorption of vitamin D or calcium	Renal tubular defects in phosphate reabsorption
Metabolic	Increased clearance of vitamin D metabolites Impaired 25- and 1-hydroxylase Tissue resistance to 1,25D and receptor mutation	

a child who is not growing well. The progress of healing of the active abnormality can be monitored by sequential radiographs at a selective site. The predominant long-term complication of the lesion is severe malalignment of the lower extremities. *The immediate goal of medical treatment is to heal the active epiphyseal lesions, thereby preventing progression of the longer-term bow or knock-knee deformities, which in untreated disease may become irreversible and require corrective orthopedic intervention.*

The pathophysiologic events resulting in rickets or osteomalacia can be generally attributed to the reduced availability of mineral to the skeleton. It is convenient to classify these disorders as predominantly resulting from either a reduced availability of calcium to the mineralizing tissue or a reduced availability of phosphate (Table 1). These groups of disorders have some distinguishing clinical characteristics, although diagnoses should always be confirmed biochemically, as treatment strategies for these forms of rickets differ. In general, the calciopenic forms of rickets have a greater extent of upper body involvement, including rachitic rosary, bossing of the frontal bone, and craniotabes in small children, whereas the phosphopenic forms have predominantly lower extremity disease. Alkaline phosphatase values tend to be lower in the renal phosphate wasting forms than in other forms of the disease. It is important to determine the precise type of rickets in order to implement the most effective therapy.

CALCIOPENIC RICKETS

These disorders can result from a primary deficiency of calcium, a primary defect in the availability or activity of vitamin D, or some combination of these mechanisms. Vitamin D is a compound that is metabolized to a steroidlike hormone and plays a major role in intestinal calcium absorption. Vitamin D either is ingested from foodstuffs and absorbed as a fat-soluble substance or is synthesized in the skin via an ultraviolet light-dependent pathway. Vitamin D from either source circulates, and in liver cells, it is hydroxylated to 25-hydroxyvitamin D (25-OHD), the most abundant circulating metabolite. Since circulating 25-OHD is the best available index of body stores of the vitamin, this compound is most appropriately measured when confirming a diagnosis of vitamin D deficiency or intoxication. 25-OHD is further hydroxylated in the kidney to 1,25-dihydroxyvitamin D [1,25(OH)$_2$D], the potent metabolite well characterized with respect to effecting intestinal calcium absorption.

Vitamin D Deprivation

This form of rickets is still seen in certain at-risk populations. A typical presentation is that of a black child less than 18 months of age presenting in the late winter or early spring. The baby is usually fed breast milk only, with no vitamin supplementation. Often, the mother's vitamin D status is marginal. The child may have rachitic abnormalities in the skull, ribs, and both upper and lower extremities. Hypocalcemia and tetany may be present, but not necessarily. The diagnosis is established by the low levels of circulating 25-OHD in the circulation. Effective treatment is provided by daily supplementation with 1000 to 2000 U or oral vitamin D (Table 2). Treatment is continued for up to 4 months or until correction of the elevated serum alkaline phosphatase activity. In the event that calcium intake is limited, a minimum dietary intake of 30 mg of elemental calcium per kilogram of body weight must be provided, using calcium supplements if necessary. This will protect against severe decreases in serum calcium, due to the hungry bone syndrome, seen with vitamin D therapy. The movement of calcium from the intravascular compartment to the skeletal compartment can exceed the replenishment of circulating calcium in the early stages of vitamin D therapy. After healing of the bones, vitamin D supplementation should be continued indefinitely at recommended daily allowance (RDA) amounts, usually found in most multivitamin preparations (400 U/d). An alternative form of therapy can be applied when there is concern about compliance. This form of therapy employs a large oral or intramuscular dose of vitamin D. Either 600,000 units of vitamin D is given once, or two doses of 300,000 units are given within a 24-hour period. Tetany may occur with treatment if dietary calcium is inadequate. Vitamin D and its related therapeutic metabolites are listed in Table 2.

Calcium Deficiency

If calcium intake is less than 250 mg/d for long periods, a clinical syndrome of calcium-deficiency rickets may occur. Calcium-deficiency rickets presents in similar fashion to vitamin D deficiency, with the exception of a normal circulating 25-OHD level. The cir-

TABLE 2. Vitamin D and Related Therapeutic Agents

VITAMIN	FORMULATION		TYPICAL DAILY DOSE*	APPROXIMATE COST FOR 1 MONTH OF TREATMENT†
Vitamin D (calciferol)	Solution:	8,000 IU/ml	2,000 IU	$10
Drisdol	Tablet:	25,000 IU	25,000 IU	$ 8
		50,000 IU	50,000 IU	$12
25-OH Vitamin D (Calcifediol)	Tablet:	20 µg	20 µg	$32
Calderol		50 µg	50 µg	$52
Dihydrotachysterol	Solution:	0.2 mg/5 ml	0.5 mg	$35
Hytakerol, DHT	Tablet:	0.125 mg	0.5 mg	$88
		0.2 mg	0.5 mg	$78
		0.4 mg	0.5 mg	$50
1,25(OH)$_2$ vitamin D (calcitriol)	Tablet:	0.25 µg	0.5 µg	$58
Rocaltrol		0.50 µg	0.5 µg	$65
Calcijex	IV solution:	1 µg/ml	0.01 µg/kg per dose	$14 for 10 kg child
		2 µg/ml	3 times/wk	$12 for 10 kg child

Note: 1 µg vitamin D$_2$ = 40 IU.
* May vary significantly, depending on condition.
† These are average wholesale prices. Retail prices vary slightly.

TABLE 3. Oral Calcium Preparations

PREPARATION	CALCIUM CONTENT	COST/100 g Ca
Calcium glubionate		
Neocalglucon	115 mg/5 ml	$180
Calcium gluconate		
500 mg tablet	45 mg/tablet	$143
Calcium carbonate		
Tums/Equilet	200 mg/tablet	$ 16
Tums-EX	300 mg/tablet	$ 15
Calci-Chew/Os-Cal 500	500 mg/tablet	$ 18
Calci-Mix	500 mg capsule for sprinkling on food	$ 20
Nephro-Calci/Caltrate	600 mg/tablet	$ 15
Titralac tablet	168 mg/tablet	$ 22
Titralac Plus suspension	200 mg/5 ml	$ 26
Rolaids-Ca Rich	220 mg/tablet	$ 16
Alka-Mint	340 mg/tablet	$ 17
Calcium lactate		
325 mg tablet	42 mg/tablet	$ 62
650 mg tablet	84 mg/tablet	$ 38

culating $1,25(OH)_2D$ is usually elevated. This syndrome is rare in the United States. It responds to adequate calcium supplementation, and selected oral calcium preparations useful in pediatrics are listed in Table 3.

Defects in Metabolism or Action of Vitamin D

These disorders have been named vitamin D-dependent rickets, relating to early reports of favorable clinical responses to therapeutic vitamin D, followed by relapsing rickets on reduction to RDA level supplementation of the vitamin. Such patients were said to be "dependent" on pharmacologic doses of vitamin D. More recently, these disorders have been identified as defects in the metabolism of 25-OHD to $1,25(OH)_2D$ (vitamin D-dependent rickets, type I, or VDDR-I) or in the action of $1,25(OH)_2D$ (vitamin D-dependent rickets, type II, or VDDR-II). The latter of these disorders, although rare, has been well characterized in a number of families and can be shown to result from various mutations in the $1,25(OH)_2D$ receptor (VDR). Mutations have been found in the DNA and hormone-binding regions of the receptor. A nonfunctional truncated protein results from another mutation.

Treatment of VDDR-I is best accomplished with $1,25(OH)_2D_3$. Initially, doses of up to 3 μg/d may be required, but after correction of hypocalcemia, maintenance doses of 0.25 to 1 μg/d are more common. It has been recommended to administer the medication in two divided daily doses. VDDR-II has been treated with variable success with very high dose regimens of $1,25(OH)_2D_3$ (up to 35 μg/

d). More recently, it has been demonstrated that long-term intravenous calcium infusions, with follow-up nocturnal calcium administration, can effectively heal the bone disease in this condition. Obviously, treatment of this rare condition should involve a specialist in bone and mineral metabolism.

Gastrointestinal and Hepatobiliary Disease

Disorders affecting vitamin D absorption in the proximal small intestine may result in vitamin D deficiency despite normal dietary intake. Cystic fibrosis is a typical cause of this phenomenon, but this form of rickets is seen also in other disorders of fat malabsorption, including inflammatory bowel disease, celiac disease, and short bowel syndromes. Treatment with 5000 to 10,000 IU of vitamin D daily has been recommended, with monthly follow-up of mineral and vitamin levels, so that appropriate adjustments in dosing can be made. Others have suggested the use of the more polar $1,25(OH)_2D_3$, which is, in part, absorbed in water-soluble form and, therefore, is less dependent on intact fat absorption. Dosages of 0.1 to 0.2 μg/kg body weight per day have been suggested as initial doses.

Severe hepatobiliary disease may impair 25-hydroxylation of vitamin D, although this is not a commonly encountered syndrome. Presumably, imminent liver failure must be present to lead to a significant clinical defect. High doses of vitamin D (up to 50,000 IU/d) or 25-OHD (1 to 3 μg/kg body weight per day) are recommended.

PHOSPHOPENIC RICKETS

Nutritional Phosphorus Deprivation

Although phosphorus is ubiquitous in western diets, nutritional phosphorus deprivation occurs in our society in a pediatric setting. Breast milk phosphorus content is generally inadequate to meet the needs of the rapidly mineralizing skeleton of the premature infant. It has been suggested that oral supplementation with 20 to 25 mg of elemental phosphorus per kilogram of body weight per day will treat this form of rickets. Recently, breast milk fortifier products (Table 4) have been developed to provide calories as well as other nutrients to breast milk. The use of fortifier provides sufficient phosphorus to limit the risk of the development of rickets while allowing the child to benefit from breast feeding. The preventive use of breast milk fortifier (one to two packets per ounce [30 ml] of breast milk) is recommended for all premature infants for whom breast milk is the sole source of nutrition. In babies receiving 150 ml of breast milk per kilogram per day, the fortifier provides approximately 35 to 65 mg of supplemental phosphorus per kilogram per day. (Calcium is also provided in the fortifier, and reductions in alkaline phosphatase levels have been demonstrated with its use.) Many nurseries use fortifier routinely until a premature infant is discharged from the hospital (at about 1800 g body

TABLE 4. Recommended Phosphate Salts for Treatment of Hypophosphatemic Rickets

FORMULATION	ELEMENTAL PHOSPHORUS CONTENT	COMMENTS	APPROXIMATE MONTHLY COST (1 g P per day)
Neutra-Phos capsule	250 mg	Dissolved in water	$34
packet	250 mg	Dissolved in water	$31
Neutra-Phos K capsule	250 mg	Dissolved in water	$41
packet	250 mg	Dissolved in water	$37
K-Phos-Neutral tablet	250 mg		$12
Phospho-soda solution	1 g/8 ml	Used only in small quantities when neutral preparations are not tolerated; cathartic	$2.70
Enfamil Human Milk fortifier	45 mg per 4 packets	Prevention of phosphate-deficiency rickets of prematurity	$2–4/d for infants receiving 4 oz breast milk per day, providing 27–54 mg of supplemental P per day

weight). It is not clear whether continuation of fortifier beyond hospital discharge is warranted. It can be argued that fortification until term gestational age is reached would benefit the skeleton.

Phosphate deprivation, however, may be only one of several components of rickets in the premature infant. To provide adequate vitamin D, it has been recommended that premature infants be supplemented with 800 IU daily of vitamin D. Furthermore, the bone disease in prematures may not always be attributable to rickets. Osteoporosis also may be present.

Primary Hypophosphatemic Rickets

Several syndromes of renal tubular phosphate wasting result in phosphopenic rickets. The prototype of these disorders is X-linked hypophosphatemic rickets, which is characterized by hypophosphatemia, a low renal tubular threshold for phosphate reabsorption, and normal circulating levels of $1,25(OH)_2D$, which is inappropriate for hypophosphatemia. Circulating calcium usually is normal or slightly depressed. The therapeutic strategy is to increase the available phosphate with oral phosphate supplements. However, this strategy as the only treatment generates secondary hyperparathyroidism. To maintain adequate calcium levels with phosphate supplementation and to protect against the development of secondary hyperparathyroidism, $1,25(OH)_2D_3$ is added in combination with phosphate salts. We tend to use modest doses of these compounds and repeatedly reinforce motivation for compliance. We generally initiate treatment in small children with low doses of both compounds: up to 0.5 g of elemental phosphorus per day with 0.5 μg of $1,25(OH)_2D_3$ per day. Phosphate salts are ideally administered 3 to 5 times per day, and $1,25(OH)_2D_3$ is given in two divided daily doses. Nevertheless, it appears that even with these modest doses, secondary hyperparathyroidism and nephrocalcinosis may ensue, although the clinical significance of these complications is not clear. Because of the necessity for both frequent follow-up and access to specialized laboratory tests, a specialist in pediatric bone disease should be consulted regarding management issues. Patients with this disorder may have significant bone pain in adulthood despite the absence of epiphyseal disease. Such patients may also benefit from modest phosphate and $1,25(OH)_2D_3$ treatment. Various recommended phosphate preparations are listed in Table 4. Neutral phosphate salts are generally preferable so that patients are not obliged to ingest an acid load.

Another form of hypophosphatemic rickets that presents with similar biochemical findings and may have quite low circulating levels of $1,25(OH)_2D$ is related to the presence of small benign tumors that secrete a substance acting on the kidney. This disorder, oncogenic osteomalacia, has been reported in association with linear nevus syndrome in children but is more common in adult age groups. Surgical removal of the tumor results in amelioration of skeletal and biochemical abnormalities.

Hereditary hypophosphatemic rickets with hypercalciuria is a rare autosomal recessive disorder in which the hypophosphatemia-vitamin D axis remains intact. Elevated $1,25(OH)_2D$ is seen. Hyperabsorption of calcium and hypercalciuria occur. Treatment consists of phosphate supplementation without additional vitamin D metabolites.

MISCELLANEOUS BONE DISEASES

Certain forms of bone disease manifest rachitic elements as components of more complex pathophysiology. In many cases, there is no specific treatment option, and each patient must be evaluated on an individual basis. For instance, metabolic bone disease may be encountered during the course of total parenteral nutrition. Other than ensuring a normal vitamin and mineral status of these patients, no specific therapy has been useful.

Patients on anticonvulsant therapy may have a variety of histologic bone abnormalities. The isolated occurrence of rickets is not the usual scenario. Earlier reports indicated that circulating 25-OHD may be decreased in patients taking phenobarbital or phenytoin. We recommend that individuals taking these medications receive the RDA of

vitamin D (400 IU) from the usual sources but no pharmacologic supplementation unless overt disease develops.

Chronic renal failure can result in a complex bone disorder called *renal osteodystrophy*. This mixed skeletal lesion can consist of osteomalacia as well as osteopenia and aluminum-induced mineralization defects if aluminum-containing medication has been used as a phosphate binder. Hyperparathyroidism and low circulating levels of $1,25(OH)_2D$ are often present, as is chronic metabolic acidosis. Treatment with $1,25(OH)_2D_3$ (in oral dosages of up to 1.5 μg/d) can be used to suppress PTH levels, and dietary phosphate intake should be restricted. Hyperphosphatemia should be treated with calcium carbonate rather than aluminum hydroxide. Intravenous $1,25(OH)_2D_3$ (0.01 μg/kg per dose) given three times weekly has been suggested as a PTH suppressant, but experience in children is limited. Newer vitamin D metabolites that have PTH-suppressive effects but limited hypercalcemic effects offer promise in the future approach to this complicated problem.

Rachitic disease may occur in other renal diseases, such as tubulopathies, including renal tubular acidosis and the Fanconi's syndrome. These disorders may occur as isolated renal defects or as part of a renal or systemic disease that may require specific diagnosis and treatment. Specific treatment of these disorders is addressed elsewhere.

COMPLICATIONS OF TREATMENT

The use of vitamin D metabolites in an unmonitored fashion can create severe complications. Most commonly, sequelae from vitamin D intoxication are related to hypercalcemia and hypercalciuria, which can have long-term effects on renal function. Therefore, after initial dosing with these compounds, serum and urinary calcium and creatinine determinations are performed within 2 weeks of the initial dosing and after adjustments in dose. On stable doses with long-term treatments, these tests are performed every 3 to 4 months. If serum calcium becomes greater than 11 mg/dl or the urinary calcium/creatine is greater than 0.35 (mg/mg), adjustments in dose are warranted. If severe hypercalcemia is present, vitamin D administration should be discontinued, and specific measures for the treatment of hypercalcemia should be instituted.

The use of phosphate salts in X-linked hypophosphatemia has been associated with development of secondary hyperparathyroidism. Therefore, circulating PTH levels are useful in monitoring these patients every 6 months. If rise in PTH occur, either the phosphate dose should be decreased, or if serum and urinary calcium parameters permit, the dose of $1,25(OH)_2D_3$ should be increased.

The use of both vitamin D metabolites and phosphate (particularly in combination) has been associated with the development of nephrocalcinosis of the renal pyramids. The long-term significance of this finding is not entirely clear, but renal function should be monitored closely in all patients who develop this complication. Cessation of chronic treatment may be indicated if detectable changes in renal function occur.

IDIOPATHIC HYPERCALCEMIA

BARBARA R. POBER, M.D.
THOMAS O. CARPENTER, M.D.

Idiopathic hypercalcemia is defined as an elevation in total serum calcium above 11 mg/dl, diagnosed after the exclusion of other known causes of hypercalcemia. Hypercalcemia may be mild (11 to 13 mg/dl) with little symptomatology or more severe (>13 mg/dl), generally accompanied by failure to thrive, abdominal pain, vomiting, constipation, muscle weakness, polydipsia, and polyuria. A complication of long-standing hypercalcemia can be nephrocalcinosis.

One of the most common causes of hypercalcemia in childhood is *Williams syndrome*. This syndrome is a rare (1 in 20,000) genetic condition that can include transient hypercalcemia and hypercalciuria, cardiovascular abnormalities (most commonly supravalvar aortic stenosis), extreme irritability during infancy, slow physical growth, characteristic facial appearance, learning difficulties, and mental retardation.

Williams syndrome has recently been shown to be caused by deletion of the gene elastin. However, the cause, true frequency, and natural history of the hypercalcemia of Williams syndrome remains unknown. The hypercalcemia may be secondary to excess absorption from the gastrointestinal tract. There have been no consistent abnormalities detected in levels of parathyroid hormone, calcitonin, and vitamin D.

THERAPY

Treatment of persistent mild hypercalcemia consists of dietary restriction of calcium (to <400 mg/d which is less than half the recommended daily allowance [RDA]), elimination of vitamin D supplementation, and avoidance of excess sunlight. Corticosteroids (prednisone, 1 to 2 mg/kg/d) will also gradually reverse hypercalcemia as a result of increased intestinal absorption of calcium, but long-term steroid treatment is not indicated because of possible adverse effects. Given the fact that hypercalcemia is typically transient, long-term therapy of any modality is generally not indicated, and attempts to discontinue therapy should be made on a regular basis. Individuals with Williams syndrome, even those who are normocalcemic, should avoid markedly excess dietary calcium, as hypercalcemia has recurred under such circumstances.

Extremely severe hypercalcemia (>15.0 mg/dl) should be treated with intravenous fluids and furosemide (1 mg/kg every 6 hours), as needed. Hypercalcemia secondary to excess bone resorption can be treated with calcitonin (salmon calcitonin, 4 IU/kg every 12 hours IM or SC) or bisphosphonate preparations, although there is minimal experience in children with this class of drugs.

Familial hypocalciuric hypercalcemia occurs secondary to decreased calcium clearance in the kidneys and appears to be secondary to a mutation in the extracellular calcium receptor. This is a benign autosomal dominant disorder, and no treatment is required. However, in rare instances of homozygosity, severe neonatal hyperparathyroidism may ensue. This condition usually requires emergency surgery to correct the severe hypercalcemia.

HEPATOLENTICULAR DEGENERATION (WILSON DISEASE)

LAWRENCE G. LEICHTMAN, M.D.

Wilson disease rarely presents in the pediatric patient with the classic clinical triad of Kayser-Fleischer corneal rings, hepatic cirrhosis, and neurologic dysfunction. Despite this, it is necessary to diagnose Wilson disease early, before the onset of irreversible organ damage and disease progression. Symptoms in children rarely begin earlier than 5 years of age, and the most common presentations are between 10 and 20 years old. Manifestations of Wilson disease are protean, but the hepatic form is most common in childhood. About half of the patients who present with neurologic symptoms either give a history of unexplained hepatitis or hemolytic anemia from which there has been a full recovery or are found to have hepatosplenomegaly on physical examination. Initial neurologic symptoms consist of dystonia, dysarthria, akinesia, a behavior disorder, or psychiatric illness. The neurologic features are of two forms. The most severe, and least common, is lenticular degeneration (dystonic form) that predominantly occurs in young adults and is refractory to therapy. The more

common form, pseudosclerosis, can occur at any age and is more amenable to therapy. Without treatment, the pseudosclerosis form can progress to the severe form.

Wilson disease has a wide variability of presentations in terms of age of onset, mode of presentation, and response to therapy. There is, however, often a familial similarity of presentation. Although the hepatic and neurologic manifestations are best known, Fanconi syndrome (with or without progressive renal failure), osteoarthritis, hematologic crises, cardiomyopathy, and endocrinopathies, such as parathyroidism, may occur. The hepatic and neurologic manifestations usually precede other symptoms. Psychiatric disturbances may range from subtle changes in personality, falling off of school performance, difficulty in writing, hysteria, development of speech defect to schizophrenia.

The liver is the *central* homeostatic organ for copper metabolism. Genetically determined deficiency of ceruloplasmin does not cause liver or brain disease. The two most fundamental disturbances of copper metabolism in Wilson disease are a reduction in the rate of incorporation of copper into ceruloplasmin and a reduction in biliary excretion of copper. The first effect is the progressive accumulation of copper in the liver. In some patients, there are only minor effects for years. In other patients, the accumulation of copper leads to severe liver damage and death because of liver failure. In older patients, spillage of copper into the general circulation leads to its deposition in various extrahepatic tissues, producing the distinctive clinical manifestations. Acute liver crises and hematologic crises can cause extreme spillage of copper into the general circulation.

THERAPEUTIC RATIONALE

Excessive storage of copper in viscera leads to organ system failure because the patient is unable to mobilize, use, and detoxify this trace metal. The principles of therapy are based on enhancing the mobilization and excretion of copper, limiting copper intake, and monitoring the function of copper-toxic target organs. Successful therapy requires early recognition and diagnosis of Wilson disease.

Pharmacotherapy is the central approach for achieving negative copper balance in patients. D-Penicillamine is the most effective agent used in the treatment of these patients.

THERAPY

D-Penicillamine in a starting dose of about 250 mg/d (20 mg/kg/d) is increased progressively over a few weeks, to 750 to 1000 mg/d. *Treatment is pursued indefinitely,* since the copper balance becomes positive every time it is stopped. D-Penicillamine therapy should be individually adapted, depending on the patient's tolerance to the drug and its efficacy. The initial dose may be calculated as 20 mg/kg/d divided into two to four doses per day. In all patients, 24-hour urinary copper excretion should be monitored, with adjustment of dose to achieve losses of over 2 g/d of copper in the early stages of treatment. After a year or two of therapy, the amount of copper available to mobilize from viscera decreases, and excretion of over 1 g/d is satisfactory. Because D-penicillamine inhibits pyridoxine-dependent enzymes, patients should be given daily supplements of 12.5 to 25 mg/d of vitamin B_6. In patients with far advanced neurologic disease L-dopa has proven a variably successful treatment.

Oral zinc sulfate can be used as an adjunctive treatment or, in cases of intractable complications to D-penicillamine, can be used as the primary treatment of Wilson disease. The dose is 50 to 100 mg/kg given three times a day. Zinc has an antagonistic action against copper in many metabolic processes. Its inhibitory effect on copper absorption has been used to maintain a negative copper balance and to reverse abnormal biochemical and pathologic abnormalities in patients already treated with D-penicillamine. Since zinc therapy also competes with iron absorption, patients treated with zinc sulfate should be monitored for iron deficiency.

Ongoing patient evaluation should include regular assessment of renal and hepatic function; 24-hour urine copper excretion should be followed periodically at a yearly interval after the initial year of D-penicillamine therapy. Clinical confirmation of successful therapy can be confirmed by slitlamp examination for Kayser-Fleischer corneal rings that should disappear over 1 to 2 years from the institution of chelation therapy.

Hematologic manifestations may occur either as a direct effect of Wilson disease or as a complication of D-penicillamine therapy. During hemolytic crises, the patient may manifest significant cupriuria and elevated serum copper levels. Thrombocytopenia and leukopenia may occur secondary to hypersplenism.

Skin rashes, thrombocytopenia, nephrotic syndrome, and acute arthritis are the most frequently encountered side effects of D-penicillamine therapy. Cessation of therapy generally leads to resolution of these problems, and slow reintroduction often is tolerated without recurrence. Reduction of the dose to 50 mg/d for 7 days is usually sufficient. Twenty milligrams per day of prednisone can be given for 2 weeks while the D-penicillamine dose is being increased. Elastosis perforans is a more persistent and usually irreversible complication.

The outcome of treatment is determined mainly by the amount of organ damage incurred before the onset of therapy. A normal life span with normal health is likely for patients diagnosed before the onset of hepatic cirrhosis or serious neurologic damage. Treatment stops active liver damage, and the degree of hepatic fibrosis may decrease markedly. The reduction of neurologic symptoms is variable and may not respond to D-penicillamine therapy alone. Movement disorders may be treated with L-dopa or trihexylphenidyl or both. Psychotic symptoms may respond to standard antipsychotic medications. Patients on active therapy may become so complacent about their good health that they may discontinue therapy. Serious symptoms not readily reversed by resumption of therapy may occur within 6 to 18 months, with rapidly fatal outcome.

As an alternative therapy, *triethylene tetramine dihydrochloride* (Trientine) may be used. This drug induces cupriuresis as great as or greater than that produced by D-penicillamine, and can be given for a long duration without any side effects. The usual dose is 600 mg three times a day or 900 mg twice a day. Its use has been restricted by its limited availability, though it is no longer an investigational drug. Trientine is available as an orphan drug, and therapy tends to be costly.

OTHER CONSIDERATIONS

To minimize copper deposition, dietary restriction of copper should be advocated during the first 2 months of chelation therapy. Foods high in copper that should be limited or excluded include liver, nuts, dried fruits, chocolate, cocoa, mushrooms, brain, shellfish, and broccoli. The average American diet includes 3.5 to 5 mg of copper per day. The patient with Wilson disease should be limited to 1.5 mg/d.

Patients with advanced liver failure with fulminant Wilson disease can still ultimately receive D-penicillamine therapy, but they must be stabilized for 6 months before initiating therapy. In such patients, copper levels can be as high as 30 μmol/L, and these levels set up a vicious cycle of cell damage. Peritoneal dialysis and plasmapheresis are the most effective of the established measures for initial stabilization. Addition of albumin to the peritoneal dialysate and maintenance of plasma albumin levels by infusion have helped in binding the copper.

Some Wilson disease patients may require liver transplantation. Criteria for liver transplantation have been established in three groups of patients: (1) patients with fulminant hepatitis, (2) severely decompensated cirrhotic children who have failed to improve after 2 to 3 months of adequate chelation therapy, and (3) effectively treated patients in whom severe hepatic insufficiency and hemolysis develop following noncompliance with chelation therapy. These last candidates are less than ideal, as it is unlikely that they will comply with lifelong immunosuppression.

Two reports have described babies with unusual connective tissue changes born to women on D-penicillamine therapy for cystinuria and rheumatoid arthritis, respectively. Interference with collagen cross-linking by D-penicillamine was blamed. None of the 11 babies born to mothers taking Trientine for Wilson disease has had any abnormality. Animal studies have shown that the teratogenic effects of D-penicillamine and of trientine can be prevented by copper supplementation. Excessive copper stores in patients may be protective for the fetus. For the present, it is possible to continue D-penicillamine therapy during the pregnancy if the maternal disease has been treated for a relatively short time. In long-treated patients, no clinical effects are seen during rests from therapy of 6 to 9 months, and cessation or reduction of dose during pregnancy might be considered.

Siblings of a patient with Wilson disease have a 1 in 4 risk of developing the disease. These siblings should be examined for liver or neurologic disease and for Kayser-Fleischer rings and be measured for serum copper, serum ceruloplasmin, and urinary copper. Linkage studies may be of some benefit in genetic counseling, but because they are only 80% to 90% reliable, they may not be sufficient for discovering heterozygotes. With more effective linkage studies, prenatal diagnosis would be possible but is of questionable benefit for a late-onset disease that is treatable. Newborn screening is possible but difficult because of low levels of ceruloplasmin in newborns. Early symptomatic diagnosis through constant awareness should be sufficient.

REFERENCES

1. Brewer GJ, Yuzbasian-Gurkan V: Wilson disease. Medicine 71:139–164, 1992.
2. Sternlieb I: The outlook for the diagnosis of Wilson's disease. J Hepatol 17:263–264, 1993.

PHENYLKETONURIA AND RELATED DISORDERS

MARY G. AMPOLA, M.D.

Hyperphenylalaninemia occurs because of inability to convert the essential amino acid phenylalanine to tyrosine. This may be secondary to a primary defect in the apoenzyme itself, namely, phenylalanine hydroxylase, or in the production of the necessary cofactor for the reaction, tetrahydrobiopterin. The biopterin defects are discussed in a separate section. Defects of the apoenzyme can involve a wide variety of mutations, over 150 at latest count. Most patients have compound mutations, that is, different gene mutations on each of the two number 12 chromosomes, which carry the gene (location 12q24.1). The large number of possible mutation combinations explains the wide range of enzyme activity, ranging from no residual activity to almost normal function. The result is great variability in clinical severity.

PHENYLKETONURIA

Phenylketonuria (PKU) results when the enzyme defect is significant enough to elevate phenylalanine levels into a clinically detrimental range. The classification of the hyperphenylalaninemias is detailed in Table 1. The incidence of abnormalities severe enough to require treatment ranges from 1:10,000 to 15,000 individuals in the United States. Benign elevations account for about one and one-half times this number. Generally, phenylalanine levels above 6 mg/dl require treatment. Clinically significant hyperphenylalaninemias are more common than average in individuals of Irish, Scotch, Belgian, German, and Yemenite Jewish origin, as well as in French Canadians. Blacks appear to have a lower than average incidence.

The hallmark of classic PKU is progressive neurologic dysfunction with psychomotor retardation, which can be severe to profound. Hypopigmentation results in fair skin, blue eyes, and light hair. In addition, seizures, eczema, and a musty odor may be present.

TABLE 1. Classification of Hyperphenylalaninemias

	PLASMA PHENYLALANINE LEVEL (mg/dl)	MENTAL RETARDATION	NEED FOR TREATMENT
Classic PKU	>20	Virtually all	All
Atypical (variant) PKU	6–20	Mild to moderate	Most
Benign persistent hyperphenylalaninemia	<6	None	None*
Biopterin defects	4–40	Normal to severe	All

*Affected women should be treated during pregnancy if blood phenylalanine is over 6 mg/dl.

TABLE 2. Medical Foods Used in Treatment of Phenylketonuria in the United States

MEDICAL FOOD	INTENDED AGE FOR USE	ENERGY-YIELDING NUTRIENTS (% OF TOTAL CALORIES)
Analog XP*	Infancy	L-Amino acids (11%), fat (39%), carbohydrate (50%)
Lofenalac†	Infancy, childhood	Casein hydrolysate (13%), fat (35%), carbohydrate (52%)
PKU-1†	Infancy	L-Amino acids (28%), carbohydrate (72%)
Phenex 1‡	Infants, toddlers	L-Amino acids (17%), fat (45%), carbohydrate (38%)
Periflex*	Over 1 y	L-Amino acids (23%), fat (37%), carbohydrate (40%)
Maxamaid XP*	1–8 y	L-Amino acids (71%), carbohydrate (29%)
Maxamum XP*	8 + y, pregnancy	L-Amino acids (46%), carbohydrate (54%)
Phenyl-Free†	2 + y, pregnancy	L-Amino acids (20%), fat (15%), carbohydrate (65%)
PKU-2†	Childhood	L-Amino acids (90%), carbohydrate (10%)
Phenex 2‡	Childhood, adults	L-Amino acids (23%), fat (37%), carbohydrate (40%)
PKU-3†	Adolescence, pregnancy	L-Amino acids (95%), carbohydrate (5%)

*Scientific Hospital Supplies, Gaithersburg, Maryland.
†Mead-Johnson, Evansville, Indiana.
‡Ross Laboratories, Columbus, Ohio.

Basic Treatment Principle

The basic treatment principle for PKU involves lowering the intake of phenylalanine and providing extra tyrosine to compensate for that which is not being generated. The sequelae of PKU are the result of accumulation of phenylalanine. Phenylalanine is an essential part of all proteins, comprising 3% to 5% of natural protein. The phenylalanine intake must be lowered to that needed to meet the minimum growth requirement. This requirement cannot be met with natural foods without exceeding the limit of phenylalanine tolerance. Thus, a significant portion of the patient's protein is given in the form of a medical food product. Such formulas contain little or no phenylalanine but all of the other necessary amino acids, vitamins, minerals, and fats. Additional calories are provided as carbohydrate.

Nutritional needs other than phenylalanine are the same for children with PKU as for normal children. A carefully monitored diet that includes a medical food product plus a carefully controlled intake of low-protein foods will result in normal growth. At present, there is no practical alternative to the diet, although extensive research continues in such areas as gene therapy.

Diagnosis

The Guthrie bacterial inhibition assay test has become the standard diagnostic procedure, using blood collected as spots on filter paper. The test is done in the newborn period before discharge from the hospital. It is clear that even testing at 24 hours of age will show some elevation in most babies who later prove to have clinically significant hyperphenylalaninemia. The normal phenylalanine level is up to 2 mg/dl, and the Guthrie test will detect any levels 4 mg/dl or greater and permit an estimate of the degree of phenylalanine elevation. All babies with elevations of any degree should be retested for confirmation using fluorimetric or high-pressure liquid chromatography (HPLC) amino acid analysis. Urine testing using ferric chloride reagent for urinary phenylketones is unreliable, as there are many false negatives for up to several weeks after birth. Once the elevation has been confirmed, the baby should be screened for defects in pterin metabolism (see section on Biopterin Defects).

Initial Treatment

To prevent permanent neurologic damage, PKU treatment should begin within the first 2 to 3 weeks of life. Referral should be made to an experienced treatment center. The blood phenylalanine should be lowered into a therapeutically safe range (under 6 mg/dl) as soon as possible. This is accomplished by giving the medical food product alone at first, which usually requires 2 to 4 days and can be done easily on an outpatient basis, minimizing the impact of the diagnosis on the family. Although it is possible to breast feed a PKU baby, this must involve careful monitoring of the number of feedings and the time allotted at the breast. This requires significant supplementation with medical food products.

There are various types of medical foods, all of which provide 80% to 90% of the daily requirement of protein, as well as most vitamins and minerals (Table 2). Such preparations contain a variable amount of energy, ranging from an insignificant amount of carbo-

hydrate and fat to up to 70% of the daily energy requirements, provided by such sources as dextrose, dextrimaltose, cornstarch, polycose, and corn or other oils.

Ongoing Treatment

Once the phenylalanine level has been brought to the desired therapeutic range, that is, 3 to 6 mg/dl, a small amount of natural protein must be provided to meet the child's ongoing growth needs. Standard infant formula or evaporated milk is used. Alternatively, breast feedings in limited amounts can be used, which is estimated by weighing the baby before and after feedings and taking into account the changing protein content of breast milk over time.

At 4 to 6 months, solids are begun as usual. Cereals and fruits are usually introduced first and vegetables thereafter. Generally, foods very high in protein, such as meat, cheese, fish, eggs, nuts, and legumes, are not tolerated. All the natural foods are given in measured or weighed amounts, which includes virtually all foods except pure fats and sugars. No vegetables or fruits are truly free foods, and all need to be counted in the total phenylalanine intake. Generally, the phenylalanine from natural foods is provided in parallel with the medical food, and both are distributed through the day. This allows full use of both the phenylalanine in food and the amino acids and other major nutrients in the formula.

The child will need to be seen twice a week initially, with visit intervals increased gradually as the phenylalanine level stabilizes. In general, intervals between blood level measurements approximate 2 to 3 weeks by 6 months of age, 4 weeks by 1 year of age, and 4 to 6 weeks thereafter, depending on the degree of overall control. At each visit, a full 3-day food intake diary is brought. The interval since the last visit is reviewed in terms of intake of medical food, health, and the family's and child's adjustment and compliance with the diet. A physical examination is performed at appropriate intervals, and growth is followed carefully. Ongoing support and counseling are provided. The blood phenylalanine level is measured, ideally using quantitative methods, such as HPLC or fluorimetric methods. Analysis of the approximate levels using Guthrie bacterial inhibition assays is not precise enough for optimal control. More frequent measurement of the phenylalanine level is unnecessary and, indeed, of little use unless the analysis method is accurate and results are communicated within a matter of days after the sample is taken.

As noted, solids are begun at 4 to 6 months of age. As the phenylalanine intake in solid foods increases, the amount of phenylalanine in normal infant formula, evaporated milk, or breast milk is decreased until all of the phenylalanine is provided in the form of natural foods. Because the medical foods are very strong tasting and generally better accepted by nipple than by cup, we have found it useful to introduce small amounts of formula directly into the mouth daily via a teaspoon or a small glass, beginning at about 6 months of age. Weaning is carried out as early as possible to a spout cup and then a regular cup. The medical food becomes the permanent milk substitute and continues to supply up to 90% of the protein, vitamins, and minerals. As noted, the treatment goal in the early years is a phenylalanine level of 3 to 6 mg/dl.

Although the medical foods are designed to provide sufficient tyrosine to compensate for that not being produced from phenylalanine, it has become clear that this goal is not always achieved. Blood tyrosine levels should be measured periodically. Since it is difficult to measure blood tyrosine levels under 1 mg/dl accurately, we have found it desirable to aim to maintain the levels between 1 and 2 mg/dl. This ensures that there is sufficient tyrosine for all needs, including pigmentation and neurotransmitter production. Tyrosine supplementation using pure powder, either mixed into the formula or given in applesauce or other foods, may be needed at times to reach this goal.

Phenylalanine requirements vary with the degree of residual enzyme activity, with classic PKU patients, who have essentially no residual enzyme function, tolerating the least phenylalanine. In addition, the phenylalanine requirement varies with age, generally being highest in early infancy, when most PKU patients will tolerate 60 to 90 mg/kg/d of phenylalanine. As growth rate slows, this tolerance decreases to about 20 mg/kg by 1 year and to 10 mg/kg in late childhood in classic PKU patients. These tolerances are less than one-tenth the normal tolerance to phenylalanine.

After each blood test, the clinic prescribes a certain amount of phenylalanine as exchanges or equivalents to be given each day. Each exchange contains 15 mg of phenylalanine. Foods are chosen and menus are planned using food lists indicating portion size and the corresponding number of exchanges or equivalents.

It is not necessary at any time to perform formal loading studies with high-protein foods in large amounts to document the ongoing need for limitation. The general principle should be to treat each patient "to tolerance" at every age. Should the child at any point begin to tolerate normal or close to normal amounts, this will become obvious as the phenylalanine intake is gradually increased in response to dropping blood phenylalanine levels. Patients with atypical PKU certainly tolerate more phenylalanine than do patients with classic PKU.

Hunger is a significant problem in the treatment of PKU patients, although the medical food is quite filling and satisfying. Specialty low-protein products are available to prevent hunger and help meet energy needs. Pastas, cookies, gelatin, and flour for baking are available, although very expensive. It is best to introduce these products as early as possible, since acceptance when they are introduced later is problematic. It is important to note that aspartame, also available as Equal or Nutrasweet, contains a significant amount of phenylalanine, and foods containing this sweetener should be avoided. All foods, including fruits and fruit juices (which have sometimes been considered phenylalanine-free foods), must be counted in the total phenylalanine intake. Finally, there are a number of foods that have no phenylalanine or only trace amounts. These are designated free foods and include pure carbohydrates or fats, such as sugar candies, nondiet soft drinks, margarine, and butter. These free foods provide extra calories.

Patients are followed closely for protein, calorie, fat, vitamin, and mineral intake. It generally is not necessary to supply extra vitamins or minerals if the intake of medical food is adequate. In the past, some shortages of trace elements have been reported, but newer formations have addressed these issues. Growth is closely followed, with frequent height, weight, and head circumference measurements. Periodically, amino acid profiles, iron indices, and albumin determinations are made. If supplementation is needed, such as extra iron during adolescence, this is provided separately.

One of the major problems in PKU management is medical food refusal because of taste. Chronic refusal certainly can result in weight loss, lethargy, and other nutritional and developmental sequelae. This is often a problem at weaning, and toddlers may lower their intake as they enter their normal negative period. Schoolage children often refuse to take the formula to school for ingestion at lunch time because of its unpleasant smell. In this instance, the amount of phenylalanine given at lunch is kept as low as possible and that formula portion is given with a snack after school. Adolescents often refuse the formula as part of an antiauthority rebellion pattern. A change in formula brand or addition of flavoring to the formula is sometimes helpful. Occasionally, behavioral or psychologic intervention is indicated and should be provided without delay at any age.

Phenylalanine intake over the amount prescribed can certainly elevate blood phenylalanine levels. Medical food refusal also results in elevated levels because of endogenous protein breakdown. Similarly, the catabolic state associated with illnesses can result in hyperphenylalaninemia, and it is notable that the elevated levels can precede the clinical symptoms by 1 or 2 days. Although no firm evidence exists that the intermittent elevations during illnesses cause permanent damage, we have found it prudent to recommend that from the very first sign of any illness (e.g., fever, coryza), the phenylalanine intake from food should be lowered to at least half the baseline amount. This helps moderate the phenylalanine spikes during illness.

It is very important to avoid overlimitation of phenylalanine, which may result in insufficient amounts for optimal protein synthesis. If severe, the deficit can result in growth deficiency, dermatitis, brain damage, or even death.

In addition to the medical care these patients require, it is important to carry out ongoing education. The family, including the extended family, must be supported and taught about PKU, including genetic and reproductive issues. Repeated explanations about the disorder and the importance of the diet, as well as encouragement for the child to take responsibility as early as possible, are critical. The patient should be encouraged to be open about his diet with friends and to downplay but not hide the importance and difficulty of maintaining the diet. The child should be taught the phenylalanine values of various foods, how to make the formula, and the meal-to-meal tracking of what has been eaten. By the preteen or early teen years, the patient should be self-motivated and within the next few years should be largely independent in terms of diet.

Results of Treatment

With careful dietary management, these patients generally achieve normal IQ levels, that is, IQs commensurate with those of the rest of the family. Minor specific deficits, including visual-motor, visuospatial, and executive function defects, have been described. In addition, a larger proportion of these patients than in the general population develop some or all of the features of disorders of attention. Their response to such medications as methylphenidate (Ritalin) often is dramatic.

Duration of Treatment

There is no known age at which the low phenylalanine diet can be terminated safely. Although older patients may tolerate blood phenylalanine levels up to 12 to 15 mg/dl without obvious short-term adverse effects, long-term elevations above 20 mg/dl have been shown to result in cognitive losses and emotional difficulties. The latter include depression, anxiety, thought disorders, agoraphobia, irritability, and personality changes. EEG abnormalities may be found, and eczema may appear. Extreme cases have manifested frank psychosis. Even mild elevations are described by patients as resulting in a sense of "fogginess," inability to concentrate, distractibility, and sleep dysfunction.

Reinstituting the diet once the patient has been off treatment for any length of time is extremely difficult, since it means resuming medical food ingestion and strict adherence to the low-protein diet. However, restarting the diet at any time certainly helps prevent further damage and may improve concentration, learning ability, and behavior, as well as decreasing seizures in some patients.

Genetic Analysis/Prenatal Diagnosis

It is now possible to detect many of the phenylalanine hydroxylase enzyme mutations or other changes using mutation-specific oligonucleotide probes. In families where both gene defects are defined and detectable, prenatal diagnosis in subsequent pregnancies is possible.

Maternal PKU

It has been amply documented that fetuses of women with elevated blood phenylalanine levels are at risk. This is because the excess phenylalanine from the mother readily crosses the placenta and may result in a fetal level up to two times as high as in the maternal circulation. Maternal PKU may be associated with intrauterine growth retardation, microcephaly, mental retardation, and congenital heart disease in the fetus. The risk is greatest for women with classic PKU, over 90% of whose fetuses are mentally retarded. Generally, the risk and severity of the maternal PKU syndrome in the fetus are related to the degree of elevation of the maternal blood phenylalanine level. It is important to note that these risks occur despite the fact that most of these fetuses are heterozygotes and would otherwise have been unaffected. Thus, it is extremely important to educate all hyperphenylalaninemic females about the risk of the maternal PKU syndrome.

The National Maternal PKU Collaborative Study has been under way for a number of years. It has revealed that even if the woman starts the diet immediately on learning she is pregnant, significant damage may already have occurred. Prevention of the fetal effects of maternal PKU requires regulation of the blood phenylalanine level beginning before conception. It has become clear with time that the critical maternal level is 6 mg/dl. The fetus of any woman whose level is higher during pregnancy is at risk. Even women who have not themselves received treatment for PKU (i.e., benign hyperphenylalaninemics with levels between 6 and 10 mg/dl) require treatment during pregnancy.

Although results must be considered preliminary because of the limited number of pregnancies thus far fully studied, it appears that mothers whose blood phenylalanine levels remain below 6 mg/dl beginning before conception and throughout pregnancy deliver fetuses who are essentially normal. It is obvious that maintenance of the low-phenylalanine diet requires monitoring by an experienced center to ensure that all the nutritional needs of both the mother and fetus are maintained throughout the pregnancy.

BIOPTERIN DEFECTS

In addition to a primary defect of phenylalanine hydroxylase, as described for PKU, elevated phenylalanine levels may result from deficiency of the enzyme's essential cofactor, tetrahydrobiopterin (BH_4). As a group, the three enzyme defects that can lead to BH_4 deficiency are called the pterin defects.

Two other critical hydroxylases in addition to phenylalanine hydroxylase require BH_4 as a cofactor. Activities of tyrosine hydroxylase, responsible for the production of dopamine and norepinephrine, and tryptophan hydroxylase, crucial for serotonin synthesis, are also seriously reduced. Production of these three neurotransmitters is, thus, inadequate. These deficiencies, together with hyperphenylalaninemia, lead to neurologic deficits. The enzymes guanosine triphosphate cyclohydrolase (GTPC) and 6-pyruvoyltetrahydropterin synthase (PTS) are responsible for synthesis of BH_4, and dihydropteridine reductase (DHPR) regenerates the biologically active BH_4 from its dihydro form.

Diagnosis

Only a small percentage of infants found to have elevated phenylalanine levels in newborn screening (less than 3%) have one of these rare disorders. If the hyperphenylalaninemia is confirmed, each infant should be tested to rule out biopterin defects, since the standard PKU diet alone is insufficient to control the features of these disorders.

Urine neopterin and biopterin are determined, and the neopterin/biopterin ratio is calculated. In GTPC deficiency, both neopterin and biopterin are decreased. In PTS deficiency, the neopterin is increased and the biopterin is decreased, so the ratio that normally is about 1:1 is greatly increased. In contrast, DHPR is best tested in blood by enzyme assay in RBC or cultured skin fibroblasts. These urine and blood tests are readily collected and sent on the same filter papers as are used for standard newborn PKU screening. Enzyme studies to confirm the GTPC and PTS deficiencies can be carried out in cultured fibroblasts. In addition, the assay for PTS can be done in RBCs.

It is notable that PTS deficiency has been reported to occur in a benign form, involving only peripheral tissues and not the brain. Thus, in this disorder, it is essential to measure CNS neurotransmitter metabolite levels to differentiate the benign form from that requiring treatment.

Prenatal diagnosis for DHPR deficiency may be carried out using amniocytes, chorionic villus biopsy tissue, or fetal RBCs. For PTS deficiency, pterin metabolites may be measured in amniotic fluid, and the enzyme may be assayed in fetal RBCs. Finally, quantitation of pterin metabolites in amniotic fluid and enzyme assay in fetal WBCs or liver are available.

Clinical Features

Symptoms become obvious by about 4 months of age, and they include feeding and swallowing problems, with failure to thrive and repeated respiratory infections, including pneumonia. Lethargy, hypotonia, and hyperreflexia are present, and there is slow motor development. Fairness of skin and hair and dermatitis are similar to those in PKU patients. Hyperthermia and sleep disorders also are common. Choreiform movements and seizures, including myoclonus, appear. Eventually, mental retardation and progressive neurologic deterioration follow unless the child is treated.

Treatment

All patients should be treated with a standard phenylalanine-restricted diet if the blood phenylalanine level exceeds 6 mg/dl. Direct BH_4 treatment in a dose of 20 to 40 mg/kg/d has been used in a limited number of patients, largely because of its cost. L-Dihydroxyphenylalanine (L-dopa), a precursor of dopamine, is given in doses of 5 to 15 mg/kg/d. L-5-Dihydroxytryptophan (L-5-HTP) is a precursor of serotonin, and the dose used is 5 to 20 mg/kg/d. Carbidopa is a decarboxylase inhibitor that lessens conversion of L-dopa to dopamine and L-5-HTP to serotonin in the bloodstream before they reach the target organ, the brain. Carbidopa is given in doses of 1 to 4 mg/kg/d. Folate depletion has been reported in DHPR deficiency, requiring folinic acid in doses of 12.5 to 37.5 mg/d.

The efficacy of therapy is determined by frequent monitoring of clinical status and, ideally, also by monitoring CSF neurotransmitter metabolite levels. Medication doses are adjusted accordingly.

Early in their course of treatment, most patients have experienced mild choreoathetosis, dystonia, and diarrhea. These findings have generally disappeared within 1 to 2 months. Higher doses have caused vomiting and Parkinson-like dyskinesia.

Results of Treatment

There have been indications of improvement in neurologic status, but the long-term prognosis is unclear and probably will be variable. To minimize the potential for irreversible CNS damage, the diagnosis should be made and treatment should be initiated as early in life as possible.

AMINO ACID DISORDERS

PAIGE KAPLAN, M.B.B.Ch.

Amino acid and organic acid disorders are rare but always should be considered in the diagnosis of the sick neonate or infant with nonspecific signs, such as poor feeding, recurrent vomiting, lethargy, and seizures, and in older infants and children with developmental delay, cerebral palsy, seizures, behavior disorders, or obtundation with intercurrent illnesses. Early diagnosis and treatment may prevent toxic brain damage, with normal or near normal neurologic function. Organic acidoses such as maple syrup urine disease (MSUD), urea cycle defects (UCD), and nonketotic hyperglycinemia usually present in the neonatal period. Phenylketonuria (PKU) and some urea cycle defects and organic acidopathies may present in late infancy and childhood. Newborn screening programs may detect PKU (universal), homocystinuria, and MSUD (some programs). Enzyme deficiencies, specific for each disease, result in accumulation of toxic metabolites proximal to the enzyme block and deficiency of metabolites required for growth and energy distal to the block. Amino acid disorders are inherited as autosomal recessive traits, except for ornithine transcarbamylase (OTC) deficiency, an X-linked recessive trait. There may be a history of siblings or, in the case of OTC deficiency maternal cousins and uncles too, with unexplained infant or childhood death, retardation, or cerebral palsy.

DIAGNOSTIC TESTS

Bedside screening. In MSUD, equal parts of 2,4-dinitrophenylhydrazine (2,4-DNPH) and urine will produce a cloudy, yellowish solution. This test is pathognomonic for MSUD. Urine with sodium cyanide-nitroprusside becomes deep red in homocystinuria (false negatives occur).

Initial tests in the undiagnosed infant should include blood gases, ammonium, and glucose. In organic acid disorders, there will be acidosis, sometimes with moderately increased ammonium. In UCD, there is about a 20-fold elevation of ammonium, with normal or alkaline pH. Other tests include plasma amino acids, blood lactate and pyruvate, urine amino, organic, and orotic acids. Diagnosis of both amino acid disorders and organic acid disorders can be made with these tests.

PRINCIPLES OF TREATMENT

The cornerstones of therapy are removal of toxic metabolites and provision of essential amino acids for growth and energy.

In the acutely ill neonate, protein feeds should be discontinued even before the diagnosis is confirmed. High-caloric intake must be maintained with glucose infusions (10% to 12.5% solution via peripheral catheter; in MSUD it may require a 20% solution via central catheter). A one and one-half to twofold increase in fluid volume can be given as well as the necessary appropriate amounts of bicarbonate and electrolytes. In MSUD, when the diagnosis has been established, an intravenous amino acid solution devoid of the nonmetabolizable amino acids should be added with intravenous carbohydrate and lipid to promote anabolism. Hyperglycemia (>150 mg/dl) requires small doses of insulin (0.01 U/kg per dose). Toxic levels of ammonium or branched-chain amino and keto acids may require lowering by dialysis (continuous arteriovenous hemofiltration, peritoneal dialysis, or hemodialysis).

Chronic therapy of amino acid disorders centers around diet. The diet is essentially vegetarian. The amount of protein given is that of the required daily allowance according to age. There are proprietary infant formulas devoid of the amino acids that cannot be metabolized and fortified with vitamins and trace elements. However, small quantities of these (essential) amino acids must be given, in the form of limited amounts of a regular protein-containing formula or individual

amino acid solutions. The amounts are titrated to give an amino acid level slightly above the normal plasma concentration.

After infancy, solid foods are introduced. A varied diet is permitted by the development of food exchanges based on the protein content of each food. Additional vitamin, trace element, and amino acid supplements also may be needed and will vary with each individual. In a small percentage of cases, the disease may be due to a deficiency of the cofactor of the enzyme. At the time of diagnosis, it is prudent to administer pharmacologic doses of the appropriate vitamin cofactor, pyridoxine (vitamin B_6) in homocystinuria, thiamine (vitamin B_1) in MSUD. A trial of such cofactors should be given for several weeks. It is controversial whether carnitine administration for organic acid or amino acid disorders is beneficial.

For optimal care, intensive continuous instruction of all caretakers (parents, other family members, and child care workers) is crucial. Before the patient is discharged from the hospital, the parents must demonstrate ability to administer the treatment regimen and must have a sufficient understanding of the disorder to treat the child. They must be adept at weighing the protein formula powder and mixing it in a blender with appropriate quantities of water, recording the daily diet, and interpreting the daily urine test for ketones (a sign of decompensation). Metabolic and neurologic decompensation can occur during intercurrent illnesses (even trivial), fevers, stress, or excessive intake of whole protein. Dehydration and acidosis need prompt therapy. At the start of the illness, all protein should be withheld, and alternative sources of high calories should be given. A 50% increase in calories should be given, if feasible, by oral or nasogastric feeds. If these measures fail, hospitalization is needed for the modified parenteral nutrition described previously.

Routine interim evaluations by specialists in metabolic diseases are recommended. Although early diagnosis and good chronic control will optimize the intellectual and growth outcome, specific deficits in growth and development have been the usual outcome in most inborn errors of metabolism. Liver transplantation has been performed in tyrosinemia type I and ornithine transcarbamylase deficiency. There is potential for gene therapy in amino acid disorders. Support groups for families are helpful, and genetic counseling is very important, as in *each* pregnancy the carrier parents conceive *together,* there is a 25% recurrence risk. Availability and reliability of prenatal diagnosis vary for each disease. Homozygote and heterozygote (carrier) detection is available by enzyme assay or DNA analysis for some diseases.

THERAPY OF SPECIFIC AMINO ACID DISORDERS

Maple Syrup Urine Disease

Deficient activity of the branched-chain keto acid dehydrogenase results in marked increases of the branched-chain amino acids (BCAA) (leucine, isoleucine, valine) and their keto acids (BCKA). Affected neonates become symptomatic after 3 to 7 days, with nonspecific signs of poor feeding, increasing lethargy, obtundation, and dehydration, mimicking sepsis. The characteristic maple syrup odor and a history of previously affected siblings aid in diagnosis. The infants have ketoacidosis, 20-fold increases in plasma BCAA, and elevated urine BCKA. *Crucial factors for a better outcome are early institution of treatment (optimally by 5 days of age) and good chronic control.* Affected children can have intellectual abilities in the same range as their parents. Children treated presymptomatically have much higher IQs than their symptomatic siblings. Inadequately treated children may develop spasticity, seizures, and mild to severe retardation.

Principles of treatment were described previously. Home monitoring may be done by checking urine ketones and a 2,4-DNPH test (variable reliability) daily and by impregnating filter paper with blood from a fingerprick every 2 to 4 weeks and mailing it to a reference laboratory where the BCAA levels can be measured quantitatively within a few days. Dietary changes can be made accordingly. During periods of decompensation requiring hospitalization, plasma amino acids should be measured approximately every 12 hours. The isoleucine and valine levels decrease more rapidly than the leucine level and should be supplemented when they have fallen to approximately twofold above normal. If this is not done, the leucine levels will not decrease into the therapeutically acceptable range. Enteral feedings should be started gradually when there is no further vomiting or diarrhea and the leucine levels are falling. During a period of decompensation, cerebral edema may develop, with cerebellar herniation and death in some cases and permanent neurologic damage in others. Dialysis and surgical decompression of increased intracranial pressure may be required.

Urea Cycle Defects

Carbamyl-phosphate synthetase (CPS) deficiency, ornithine transcarbamylase (OTC) deficiency, citrullinemia (CIT), and argininosuccinic aciduria (ASA) may manifest catastrophically in the newborn period. These diseases may present later in life if there is a milder enzyme deficiency. Arginase deficiency has a different clinical presentation: spasticity and choreoathetotic movements become apparent after 1 year of life. Ammonium levels are more than 20-fold elevated in patients with UCD. The plasma amino acid citrulline is very low or absent in CPS and OTC deficiencies and markedly elevated in the others, particularly citrullinemia. Urine orotic acid will be absent in CPS deficiency and elevated in OTC deficiency. In CPS, OTC, CIT, and ASA, the initial emergency treatment described earlier is implemented. In addition, large amounts of the ammonium can be removed by using sodium benzoate intravenously (loading dose 250 mg/kg, followed by 250 mg/kg/d in four divided doses) and sodium phenylacetate enterally. Ucephan, a combination of these two drugs, can be given enterally. Trials with sodium phenylbutyrate (as another method of removing nitrogen) are being conducted. Dialysis may be needed to lower excessively high ammonium levels. Chronic treatment involves protein restriction, the use of special formula, and Ucephan (or sodium benzoate) orally. The prognosis for morbidity and mortality in neonatal UCD is poor but is somewhat better for those presenting at later ages. Prenatal diagnosis is available, but first, the enzyme or molecular defect in the proband has to be delineated.

Homocystinuria

Homocystinuria, an inborn error of sulfur metabolism, is caused mainly by cystathionine β-synthase deficiency. About 50% of patients will respond to very high doses (250 to 500 mg/d) of pyridoxine (pyridoxine responders, PR).

Four main systems are involved: brain, eyes, skeleton, and blood vessels. Mental retardation occurs frequently, but IQ ranges from 10 to 138 (median 78 for PR, 56 for pyridoxine-nonresponsive, PNR, patients). Seizures (20%), dystonia (uncommon), and psychiatric disorders (50%) occur. Ocular findings may occur, including dislocated lenses with associated myopia (usually after 2 years) and glaucoma. A marfanoid habitus, osteoporosis, and scoliosis are common. A major cause of morbidity and mortality is thromboembolism in the cerebral, peripheral, and coronary arteries (50%), and venous occlusion also may occur.

Homocystine and methionine accumulate in plasma and urine. For accurate testing in blood, plasma must be separated immediately after venipuncture. False negative results occur in screening tests (cyanide-nitroprusside and chromatography) or if the patient is taking folate or vitamin B_6.

At the time of diagnosis, a trial of high-dose pyridoxine (500 to 1000 mg/d) and folic acid 0.5 mg is given for several weeks. If the methionine and homocystine levels normalize in plasma and disappear from urine, the patient is considered pyridoxine responsive. Therapy with approximately 150 mg pyridoxine per day is given initially. The dose may be increased or decreased according to the amounts of homocystine and methionine measured. Some methionine restriction in the diet may be helpful in PR. Newborn screening is done in some states but may not detect all the vitamin B_6-responsive homocystinuric patients.

Diet therapy, the main form of management in homocystinuria, is aimed at lowering homocystine, the toxin responsible for most pathology. Methionine is the only source of homocystine. A methionine-restricted diet is difficult to implement after infancy but delays lens dislocation and prevents seizures and retardation (mean IQ is 35 points higher than that of late-treated patients). Betaine, a methyl donor, increases conversion of homocystine to methionine, and a betaine dose of 6 to 9 g/d lowers homocystine levels substantially. There are anecdotal reports that betaine improves behavior, decreases seizure frequency, and may retard or prevent thromboembolism. The high methionine level does not appear to be harmful. Daily acetylsalicylic acid and dipyridamole may prevent thromboembolism.

At 30 years of age, more than 75% NPR and more than 95% PR will be alive. Two thirds of the deaths are attributed to thromboembolic events. Surgery has resulted in thromboembolism in 4% of 586 procedures. Maintenance of treatment and good hydration perioperatively and intraoperatively may be important factors.

Pregnancy has occurred, mainly in PR, with a high rate of fetal loss but no increased incidence of abnormalities in the liveborn. Prenatal diagnosis is possible using cultured amniocytes or cultured chorionic villi. Heterozygotes are reported to have an increased incidence of peripheral and cerebral occlusive arterial and venous disease and myocardial infarction.

Tyrosinemia

Hereditary tyrosinemia type I is caused by fumarylacetoacetate hydrolase deficiency. It affects the liver and kidneys, resulting in high tyrosine and methionine, succinylacetone (urine), δ-aminolevulinic acid, and α-fetoprotein. The disease manifests soon after birth with vomiting, diarrhea, failure to thrive, and jaundice. The liver disease may be fulminating or chronic with cirrhosis and eventual hepatocellular cancer in the first two decades. Renal disease manifests with aminoaciduria, glucosuria, and rickets. Acute porphyric episodes cause great pain. Enzyme assay can be done on erythrocytes (although a recent blood transfusion may give a false negative result).

Treatment with a diet restricted in tyrosine and phenylalanine improves the renal aspects but does not prevent liver failure or development of hepatoma. Liver transplantation cures the liver disease but does not affect the kidney. There is innovative therapy[3] using an inhibitor of the enzyme 2-nitro-4-trifluoromethylbenzoyl-1,3-cyclohexanedione (NTBC). In a small group of patients treated with NTBC, the formation of the toxin succinylacetone and hepatotoxic and nephrotoxic compounds decreased, liver function improved, α-fetoprotein decreased, and liver nodules regressed (except in 1 patient). Increased physical activity, alertness, and improved appetite were noted. No side effects have been noted so far.

Prenatal diagnosis by measurement of the enzyme in CVS or cultured amniotic cells and measurement of increased succinylacetone in amniotic fluid is reliable.

REFERENCES

1. Berry GT, Heidenreich R, Kaplan P, Levin F, Mazur A, Palmieri M, Yudkoff M, Segal S: Branched-chain amino acid-free parenteral nutrition in the treatment of acute metabolic decompensation in patients with maple syrup urine disease. N Engl J Med 324:175–199, 1991.
2. Kaplan P, Mazur A, Field M, Berlin JA, Berry GT, Heidenreich R, Yudkoff M, Segal S: Intellectual outcome in children with maple syrup urine disease. J Pediatr 119:46–50, 1991.
3. Lindstedt S, Holme E, Locke EA, Hjalmarson O, Strandvik B: Treatment of hereditary tyrosinemia type I by inhibition of 4-hydroxyphenyl pyruvate dioxygenase. Lancet 340:813–817, 1992.
4. Scriver CR, Beaudet AL, Sly WS, Valle D (eds): The Metabolic Basis of Inherited Disease, 6th ed. New York, McGraw-Hill, 1989.

DISORDERS OF PORPHYRIN, PURINE, AND PYRIMIDINE METABOLISM

LAURIE S. SADLER, M.D.
F. BRUDER STAPLETON, M.D.

The porphyrias are a group of heritable disorders, each due to deficiency of an enzyme involved in the heme biosynthetic pathway. Heme biosynthesis involves eight enzymatic steps. With the exception of the first enzyme of the pathway, δ-aminolevulinic acid (ALA) synthase, partial deficiency of each enzyme results in a specific form of porphyria. The erythropoietic porphyrias are associated with hemolytic crises and cutaneous manifestations. In contrast, the hepatic porphyrias may manifest as abdominal, autonomic, or central nervous system (CNS) symptoms with or without cutaneous manifestations.

In the first step of heme synthesis, the enzyme ALA synthase catalyzes the condensation of succinylcoenzyme A with glycine to form ALA. ALA synthase is subject to feedback inhibition by heme. As a result, deficiency of any enzyme distal to ALA synthase will result in an increased activity of ALA synthase, resulting in the accumulation of precursors. ALA dehydrase condenses two molecules of ALA to form monopyrrole porphobilinogen (PBG). PBG deaminase catalyzes the condensation of four molecules of PBG to form hydroxymethylbilane, which may either spontaneously form uroporphyrinogen I or be converted to uroporphyrinogen III by the enzyme uroporphyrinogen III synthase. Uroporphyrinogen decarboxylase converts uroporphyrinogen III to coproporphyrinogen III, which undergoes oxidative decarboxylation using corproporphyrinogen oxidase with conversion to protoporphyrinogen IX. The latter is oxidized to porphyrin IX by protoporphyrinogen oxidase. In the final step, ferrochelatase catalyzes the insertion of ferrous iron into protoporphyrin.

Heme is involved in numerous critical biologic functions, including oxygen binding and transport as hemoglobin and myoglobin, electron transport as cytochromes, the degradation of hydrogen peroxide in peroxisomes, and mixed function oxidation as cytochrome P450. Drugs that are metabolized by the hepatic cytochrome P450 system may precipitate acute crises of the hepatic porphyrias. Examples include barbiturates, sulfonamides, griseofulvin, and anticonvulsants, such as carbamazepine, phenytoin, primidone, and valproic acid. Other potentially unsafe drugs include clonidine, erythromycin, rifampin, and theophylline. Menstruation and exogenous estrogens also may exacerbate porphyria.

ALA DEHYDRATASE DEFICIENCY

ALA dehydratase deficiency porphyria (ALADP) is an autosomal recessively inherited disorder and the least frequent of the porphyrias. Patients present with symptoms indistinguishable from those of acute intermittent porphyria. Diagnosis is based on elevated urinary ALA excretion without elevation of PBG. The rare occurrence of this disorder limits information regarding treatment. Intravenous glucose infusion and the avoidance of recognized exacerbating factors, such as stress, fasting, and alcohol, have diminished symptoms in some cases.

ACUTE INTERMITTENT PORPHYRIA

Acute intermittent porphyria (AIP), the most common of the heritable porphyrias, is an autosomal dominantly inherited disorder that results from a partial deficiency of PBG deaminase. The vast majority of heterozygotes remain symptomatic throughout life. Endogenous and exogenous environmental factors most often precipitate acute exacerbations of disease.

Clinical expression of AIP is extremely rare before puberty. Abdominal pain is the most common initial symptom and may be so severe as to warrant surgical intervention. Other gastrointestinal symptoms include nausea, vomiting, diarrhea, and ileus. Autonomic symptoms also may include tachycardia, hypertension, fever, diaphoresis,

and tremor. Neuropathy represents another common feature of AIP, with motor neuropathies occurring more frequently than sensory neuropathies. Seizures, paresis, and even respiratory paralysis may occur. Psychiatric manifestations may include anxiety, insomnia, paranoia, and depression.

Diagnosis of AIP is based on elevated urinary excretion of ALA and PGB, as well as demonstration of diminished erythrocyte PBG deaminase activity. The red urine seen in severe cases is due to urinary porphyrins or the conversion of PBG to porphobilin by light, heat, or acid. Recent localization of the PBG deaminase gene to the long arm of chromosome 11 has allowed for the use of haplotype analysis for carrier detection.

Prevention of acute exacerbations includes adequate nutrition, avoidance or drugs known to precipitate attacks, and the treatment of intermittent crises. Treatment of acute attacks involves the administration of large amounts of carbohydrate, with careful fluid and electrolyte management, since hyponatremia secondary to inappropriate ADH secretion has been observed. Appropriate pharmacologic treatment of pain, gastrointestinal symptoms, and hypertension also is warranted. Treatment with intravenous hematin, a heme compound containing ferric iron, in doses of up to 4 mg/kg b.i.d. may reduce the overproduction of porphyrins and their precursors by feedback inhibition of ALA synthase and diminish neurologic symptoms. Potential complications of this therapy include thrombophlebitis, coagulopathy, and hemolysis. Haem-arginate, which acts to repress ALA synthase, and Sn-protoporphyrin, which inhibits hepatic heme oxygenase and reduces the rate of degradation of hepatic heme, are promising new therapies with fewer serious complications. In addition, luteinizing hormone–releasing hormone agonists, which inhibit ovulation, may reduce the incidence of AIP associated with menstruation.

CONGENITAL ERYTHROPOIETIC PORPHYRIA

Congenital erythropoietic porphyria (CEP) is a rare, autosomal recessive disorder in which homozygotes show decreased activity of uroporphyrinogen III synthase (URO III synthase). Infants may present with pink to red-brown staining of diapers because of urinary porphyrin excretion. Mutilating cutaneous photosensitivity exacerbated by sunlight is characteristic and may result in marked scarring, atrophy, pseudoscleroderma, and joint contractures. Additional features include alopecia, hypertrichosis, and erythrodontia. Hemolytic anemia and splenomegaly also occur.

Diagnosis is based on clinical symptoms and the demonstration of elevated amount of urinary, fecal, and erthrocytic porphyrins. Diminished URO III synthase has been documented in both fibroblasts and aminocytes. Treatment is primarily preventive, with avoidance of sun exposure, trauma, and infection. Red blood cell transfusions for treatment of hemolysis may suppress bone marrow activity and decrease porphyrin production. Splenectomy has resulted in the short-term reduction of hemolysis, porphyrin excretion, and cutaneous photosensitivity. Orally administered activated charcoal has been shown to lower porphyrin levels in skin and plasma.

PORPHYRIA CUTANEA TARDA

Porphyria cutanea tarda (PCT) is a common, heterogeneous, often sporadic disorder. Familial cases are inherited in an autosomal dominant manner. URO decarboxylase activity is reduced by about 50% in affected individuals. Sporadic PCT usually appears in adulthood, whereas childhood manifestations are more typical of familial PCT. Clinical features include cutaneous photosensitivity, skin fragility with poor wound healing following even minor trauma, hyperpigmentation, hypertrichosis, and pseudoscleroderma. Environmental factors, such as alcohol, estrogens, iron, and polychlorinated cyclic hydrocarbons, may precipitate or exacerbate sporadic PCT.

Diagnosis is based on clinical findings and the presence of elevated levels of urinary uroporphyrin and, to a lesser extent, coproporphyrin. The presence of fecal isocoproporphyrin is essentially diagnostic. Measurement of erythrocyte URO decarboxylase is diagnostic in familial cases. Avoidance of precipitating factors remains an important aspect of overall treatment. Intermittent phlebotomy may reduce urinary porphyrins and improve clinical status by reducing hepatic iron stores. Low-dose chloroquine therapy also been used with some success.

CONGENITAL HEPATOERYTHROPOIETIC PORPHYRIA

Congenital hepatoerythropoietic porphyria (HEP) is a rare autosomal recessively inherited disorder resulting from homozygous URO decarboxylase deficiency and is clinically indistinguishable from CEP. Diagnosis is based on elevated levels of urinary uroporphyrins and erythrocyte zinc protoporphyrin. Less than 10% of normal erythrocyte URO decarboxylase activity is also diagnostic. Avoidance of sun exposure is the current mainstay of treatment, as other therapies have proved ineffective.

HEREDITARY COPROPORPHYRIA

Hereditary coproporphyria (HCP) is a rare autosomal dominantly inherited disorder caused by a partial deficiency of coproporpyrinogen oxidase, with resultant accumulation of coproporphyrins, and is clinically similar to AIP, although symptoms are often milder. In addition, cutaneous photosensitivity has been observed in approximately 30% of cases. Diagnosis is based on clinical findings suggestive of AIP, with normal PBG deaminase activity. Increased urinary and fecal coproporphyrins, with predominance of the latter, aid in diagnosis. Avoidance of precipitating factors remains an essential aspect of treatment. Acute exacerbations are treated as in patients with AIP.

VARIEGATE PORPHYRIA

Variegate porphyria (VP) is an autosomal dominantly inherited disorder resulting from a partial deficiency of protoporphyrinogen oxidase. It is common in South Africa, and clinical manifestations are indistinguishable from those observed in AIP and HCP, although cutaneous photosensitivity tends to be more frequent and chronic. As in HCP, the diagnosis of VP should be considered when clinical findings suggest AIP, particularly with documentation of normal PBG deaminase activity. Diagnosis is based on the demonstration of elevated urinary and fecal porphyrins, although these substances may not be significantly elevated in prepubertal or elderly heterozygotes. Quantitation of lymphocyte or fibroblast protoporphyrinogen oxidase activity is diagnostic. Treatment is similar to that for AIP, with avoidance of known precipitating factors and management of acute attacks. In addition, photoprotective measures are essential. Beta-carotene and analogs have been used with partial success.

ERYTHROPOIETIC PROTOPORPHYRIA

Erythropoietic protoporphyria (EPP) is an autosomal dominantly inherited disorder resulting from partial deficiency of ferrochelatase. EEP usually begins with cutaneous manifestations in childhood. Short-term exposure to sunlight or, in some cases, artificial light results in burning, erythema, and edema. Skin fragility and severe scarring, as may be observed in CEP, are infrequent findings. Hepatobiliary dysfunction, although rare, may also occur with the development of gallstones or the deposition of protoporphyrin crystals in hepatocytes, with resultant hepatic failure. There are no recognized precipitating factors.

Diagnosis is based on cutaneous photosensitivity and documentation of elevated levels of free protoporphyrin in plasma, erythrocytes, and stool. Urinary porphyrins remain normal. Treatment involves the use of photoprotective measures. Oral administration of beta-carotene to maintain serum levels at 600 to 800 µg/dl has been partially effective in improving light tolerance, the mechanism of which probably involves the binding of oxygen free radicals. In addition, cholestyramine has been shown to diminish both photosensitivity and hepatic protoporphyrin accumulation.

HEREDITARY OROTIC ACIDURIA

Orotic aciduria (OA) is the most frequent disorder of pyrimidine metabolism. An autosomal recessive disorder, OA results from deficiencies of orotate phosphoribosyltransferase and orotidine 5'-monophosphate decarboxylase. These two enzymes, coded for by a single gene, catalyze the synthesis of uridine 5'-monophosphate synthetase (UMPS). All affected individuals develop a megaloblastic anemia unresponsive to folate, ascorbic acid, and vitamin B_{12} during childhood. The urinary excretion of large amounts of orotic acid results in precipitation of crystals within the urinary tract. Other clinical findings include failure to thrive, developmental delay, an increased frequency of congenital cardiac defects, leukopenia, and impaired cell-mediated immunity.

Diagnosis is based on elevated levels of urinary orotic acid. Treatment of OA involves pyrimidine replacement with oral uridine, which has proven effective in the amelioration of megaloblastic anemia, decreased urinary orotic acid excretion, and improved strength and level of alertness. A high fluid intake is recommended to reduce crystal formation. Adrenal corticosteroids have been used with limited effectiveness in the treatment of anemia.

URIC ACID DISORDERS

Uric acid is the end product of purine metabolism in humans and is poorly soluble in biologic fluids. This weak organic acid is over 10 times more soluble at pH 7.0 than at pH 5.0. In children, mean serum uric acid values slowly increase from 3 mg/dl at 2 years of age to 4.5 mg/dl at age 15 years. Approximately two thirds of the daily uric acid production is eliminated by the kidneys, and the rest is eliminated through the gastrointestinal tract. Urinary uric acid excretion is substantially greater in children than it is in adults. Disorders of uric acid produce gouty arthritis and acute renal failure from hyperuricemia and urinary stones from hyperuricosuria.

Hyperuricemia

Hyperuricemia may be the result of increased uric acid production or impaired urinary urate excretion or both. Idiopathic hyperuricemia or gout is an uncommon affliction of children and has a strong predilection for boys. Acute gouty arthritis may be managed effectively with allopurinol at doses of 5 to 10 mg/kg/d and colchicine at 0.5 to 1 mg/kg/d. Allopurinol inhibits xanthine oxidase and reduces uric acid production and urinary acid excretion. Secondary hyperuricemia is most often the result of neoplasia, although hyperuricemia is also common in hemolytic anemias, polycythemia, and thrombocytosis. Acute hyperuricemia is a prominent component of the tumor lysis syndrome that occurs during induction therapy of children with large tumor burdens. Prevention of acute renal failure in the face of acute and severe hyperuricemia requires a large volume of fluids, given orally or intravenously, to ensure a high urine volume. In children with tumor lysis syndrome, 3000 to 5000 ml/m²/d is provided intravenously. Intermittent administration of mannitol at a dose of 0.5 to 1 g/kg per dose, followed by furosemide 1 to 2 mg/kg per dose, may be helpful if urine volume declines. Urine pH is maintained above 6.5 with either sodium bicarbonate or potassium citrate given every 4 to 6 hours to promote urinary urate solubility. Children with chronic hyperuricemia should avoid purine-rich foods, such as organ meats.

Lesch-Nyhan Syndrome

Deficiency of the enzyme hypoxanthine guanine phosphoribosyltransferase (HGPRT) is an X-linked recessive disorder. Young men with Lesch-Nyhan syndrome have hyperuricemia, gout, nephrolithiasis, mental retardation, and self-mutilating behavior. This condition may present as acute renal failure in the newborn period. Partial deficiency of HGPRT may not be detected until gouty arthritis develops during the second decade of life. Therapy includes allopurinol, a low purine diet, a large fluid intake, and urinary alkalinization.

Adenine Phosphoribosyl Transferase

A deficiency of adenine phosphoribosyl transferase (APRT) is associated with urolithiasis. Other manifestations include hematuria and dysuria. Occasionally, acute renal failure occurs. This enzyme deficiency is inherited as an autosomal recessive trait. Urinary stones are composed of 2,8-dehydroxyadenine and are radiopaque. Stone analysis by isotachoporesis or high-performance liquid chromotography (HPLC) is required to distinguish calculi from uric acid stones. Therapy includes a high fluid intake, a low-purine diet, and allopurinol. Unlike uric acid, the solubility of 2,8-dehydroxyadenine is *reduced* in alkaline urine.

Xanthinuria

When hypouricemia (serum uric acid <2 mg/dl) is associated with decreased urinary uric acid excretion and radiolucent nephrolithiasis, xanthinuria should be suspected. Xanthinuria, an autosomal recessive condition, has a markedly increased urinary excretion of xanthine because of a deficiency of the enzyme xanthine oxidase. Therapy includes a high fluid intake and urinary alkalinization with either sodium bicarbonate or citrate therapy. Secondary xanthinuria and xanthine lithiasis are unusual complications of allopurinol therapy, especially in patients with Lesch-Nyhan syndrome.

REFERENCES

1. Baldree LA, Stapleton FB: Uric acid metabolism in children. Pediatr Clin North Am 37:391–418, 1990.
2. Kauppinen R, Mustajoki P: Prognosis of acute porphyria: Occurrence of acute attacks, precipitating factors, and associated diseases. Medicine 71:1–13, 1992.
3. Straka JG, Rank JM, Bloomer JR: Porphyria and porphyrin metabolism. Annu Rev Med 41:457–469, 1990.

LYSOSOMAL STORAGE DISEASE

WILLIAM A. GAHL, M.D., Ph.D.

Lysosomal storage disorders are rare inborn errors of metabolism resulting from the accumulation of molecules within cellular lysosomes. They can be divided into two groups based on the type of defect causing the storage. In lysosomal transport defects, such as cystinosis and infantile free sialic acid storage disease, the basic defect is failure to transport a small molecule, that is, cystine or sialic acid, out of the lysosome and into the cytoplasm. In lysosomal enzyme defects, which comprise the vast majority of lysosomal storage disorders (Table 1), the basic defect is deficiency of an enzyme that degrades macromolecules, such as glycosaminoglycans, glycolipids, gangliosides, or glycoproteins. Patients with lysosomal storage disorders are generally normal at birth but progressively develop symptoms within the first year of life. The severity, rapidity of progression, and age at onset vary widely. The specific organ systems affected by lysosomal storage diseases depend on the tissues in which the storage material accumulates. Diagnosis is based on clinical suspicion occasioned by the presence of hepatosplenomegaly, bony abnormalities, coarse facial features, developmental delay, or renal disease and is confirmed by a biopsy showing storage material in lysosomes or by demonstration of the deficiency of a specific enzyme. Several disorders defined by the presence of storage material in cellular lysosomes have no known etiology. Most lysosomal storage disorders have an incidence between 1 in 10,000 and 1 in 200,000 and are inherited in an autosomal recessive fashion. Hunter disease and Fabry disease are X-linked.

SYMPTOMATIC THERAPY

For most lysosomal storage diseases, there is no specific therapy directed toward the primary defect, and treatment is symptomatic. Nevertheless, a few general principles follow from the physical and

TABLE 1. Lysosomal Storage Diseases

Transport Defects
Cystinosis
Infantile free sialic acid storage disease
   (Salla disease)*

Enzyme Defects
Mucopolysaccharidoses (MPS)
Hurler disease, MPS I H
   (Scheie, MPS I S)*
Hunter disease, MPS II†
Sanfilippo A, B, C, D, MPS III A, B, C, D
Morquio disease, MPS IV
Maroteaux-Lamy disease, MPS VI
β-Glucuronidase deficiency, MPS VII

Mucolipidoses (ML)
I-cell, ML II
   (ML-III)*
ML-IV

Lipidoses
Wolman disease, acid lipase deficiency
   (cholesteryl ester storage disease)*
Farber lipogranulomatosis
Niemann-Pick disease
Gaucher disease
Krabbe disease
Fabry disease†
Metachromatic leukodystrophy

Gangliosidoses
GM-1 gangliosidosis
GM-2 gangliosidosis, Tay-Sachs disease
GM-2 gangliosidosis, Sandhoff disease

Glycoproteinoses
Fucosidosis
Mannosidosis
Sialidosis
Aspartylglycosaminuria

Miscellaneous
Pompe disease, glycogenosis type II
Acid phosphatase deficiency

*Diseases in parentheses are milder, probably allelic, forms of the prototype disease.
†X-linked; all others are autosomal recessive.

developmental impairment common to many of the disorders. Personal and dental hygiene must often be provided by caretakers, and seizure control should be managed with the use of conventional anticonvulsants. Patients with mental retardation can benefit from educational and training programs attuned to the level of their performance. The resources of local social service agencies should be tapped, and institutional care may be required. It should not be assumed that all individuals with lysosomal storage diseases exhibit intellectual impairment. In general, patients with cystinosis are mentally intact, as are those with Morquio disease, Maroteaux-Lamy disease, Gaucher disease, Pompe disease, Hunter disease, and certain other storage disorders. Intelligence may be normal despite dysmorphic facial features. Hydrocephalus occurs in patients with mucopolysaccharidoses, and ventriculoperitoneal shunts often are indicated. Patients with Sanfilippo disease often have major behavioral problems and require aggressive pharmacotherapy. An occasional patient will have a paradoxical response to sedatives, with exacerbation of agitation.

Bone and joint problems afflict patients with several different lysosomal storage diseases, especially the mucopolysaccharidoses, and should be addressed via orthopedic consultation and aggressive physical therapy. Instability of the atlantoaxial joint, caused by odontoid hypoplasia in Morquio disease or in glucuronidase deficiency, may require prophylactic cervical fusion. The acroparesthesias of Fabry disease usually can be alleviated with carbamazepine or diphenylhydantoin.

Obstructive airway disease can often be palliated by tonsillectomy and adenoidectomy, but affected patients remain at increased risk for general anesthesia. Many children with mucopolysaccharidoses and mucolipidoses have recurrent ear infections and require myringotomy and methylene ventilation tube placement.

Periodic ophthalmologic examinations are useful in several lysosomal storage diseases. The corneal clouding of mucopolysaccharidoses and the corneal whorls of Fabry disease are diagnostically helpful. Cystine crystals in the corneas of patients with cystinosis may be seen on slitlamp examination.

Cardiac care is essential for patients with mucolipidoses, as well as those with Pompe disease. Pneumonias are often a terminal event for bedridden or inactive patients with various lysosomal storage diseases, and the family and caretakers must jointly consider the extent to which lifesaving efforts will be pursued.

In institutionalized or developmentally delayed patients, constipation is often a problem and can be treated with stool softeners, laxatives, and enemas. Feeding may be difficult and can be managed by tube feeding or a gastrostomy.

Patients with cystinosis and with Fabry disease may develop renal insufficiency. Specific symptomatic therapy can include renal transplantation for untreated cystonisis (at approximately 10 years of age) or Fabry disease (in the third to fifth decades of life). Patients with Gaucher disease or Niemann-Pick disease may require splenectomy for symptomatic hypersplenism.

TREATMENTS DIRECTED TOWARD BASIC DEFECTS

Recently, inroads have been made into treatments directed toward the basic defect in specific lysosomal storage diseases. One example involves *cysteamine therapy* in nephropathic cystinosis. Cysteamine, which has been approved by the U.S. Food and Drug Administration, chemically converts lysosomal cystine into two compounds, cysteine and cysteine-cysteamine mixed disulfide, both of which freely leave lysosomes. The consequent cystine depletion, if initiated in infancy, allows for preservation of renal function and a normal growth rate. In addition, cysteamine eyedrops can dissolve corneal crystals.

Enzyme replacement has shown remarkable efficacy for patients with Gaucher disease. Alglucerase (glucocerebrosidase, Ceredase) has proven beneficial with respect to hematologic parameters and overall well-being in Gaucher patients. Candidates for this therapy should be prepared for the $300,000 per year cost of the drug at the present time. Enzyme replacement for other diseases, such as Fabry disease (alpha-galactosidase deficiency), and the GM-2 gangliosidoses has been attempted in a few individuals, but the short half-life of the infused enzyme has made this therapy less useful. More stable enzyme is being developed for future studies. The existence of animal models for MPS I, MPS VI, MPS VII, fucosidosis, and certain gangliosidoses means that enzyme replacement can be attempted in these diseases after appropriate trials in nonprimates.

Bone marrow transplantation has been attempted in a variety of mucopolysaccharidoses, including MPS I, II, and VI, and in metachromatic leukodystrophy, Gaucher disease, and a few other lysosomal storage diseases. In general, improvements in parenchymal organ storage levels and enzyme activities have been observed; corneal clearing, joint mobility, and reduced hepatosplenomegaly have occurred. However, the key issue for most of the storage diseases is the prevention or amelioration of central nervous system (CNS) disease. Targeting of enzymes or enzyme-containing cells to the CNS by physical or biochemical means is essential. To date, clinical efficacy with respect to the CNS has not been demonstrated unequivocally, and further studies with longer follow-up are critical. Optimism regarding bone marrow transplantation in lysosomal storage disease must be tempered by this realization, and complete discussions with the patient and family are essential. Amnion implants have not proven helpful.

The prospect of using gene therapy for selected lysosomal storage diseases now appears on the horizon. Genes have been cloned for many of the pertinent enzymes, including iduronidase (MPS I), alpha-

galactosidase (Fabry disease), and glucocerebrosidase (Gaucher disease). These genes can readily be placed into retroviral or adenoviral vectors. At least two issues require concerted attention. First, the vectors must be targeted to the tissues of interest. This appears feasible for some tissues, such as the liver, but targeting to the CNS will prove more challenging. A second issue is how to achieve long-term, high-level expression in the targeted cells. Although retroviruses are integrated into the host genome of dividing cells and offer prolonged expression, adenoviruses express transiently and require repeated administrations. Determination of the optimal vehicle for gene therapy also depends in part on how much enzyme is needed to achieve normal function and how safe the vehicle is. Only somatic gene therapy, not germline therapy, is being considered at this time.

GENETIC COUNSELING AND PRENATAL DIAGNOSIS

One of the most important pursuits in the management of lysosomal storage diseases involves genetic counseling, an endeavor that is heavily influenced by the severity of the disease. For autosomal recessive disorders, the main concern is for future pregnancies, whereas for X-linked disorders, the mother's family should be investigated. Several autosomal recessive and X-linked diseases can be detected in the heterozygote state, provided that the laboratory has wide experience in performing the assays and studies obligate heterozygotes at the same time. The screening of Ashkenazi Jews for Tay-Sachs heterozygosity has had a significant impact on the occurrence of this disorder, but such widespread screening has not occurred for other disorders. Many lysosomal storage diseases can be diagnosed prenatally, either through chorionic villus sampling from the sixth to eighth week of gestation or through amniocentesis in the thirteenth to sixteenth weeks of gestation. These diagnoses rely either on deficiency of the pertinent enzyme activity in the chorionic villi or cultured amniocytes or on molecular genetic techniques involving restriction fragment length polymorphisms or direct hybridization assays of the mutant portion of the gene. Not all at-risk families are suitable for prenatal diagnosis using molecular genetic technology. In utero therapy has not been attempted for lysosomal storage diseases.

With a few exceptions, the prognosis for patients with classic lysosomal storage disorders is poor. Therapy for these diseases can be advanced only by participation of both patients and physicians in clinical trials.

REFERENCE

1. Scriver CR, Beaudet AL, Sly WS, Valle D (eds): The Metabolic Basis of Inherited Disease, 7th ed. New York, McGraw-Hill, 1995:2427–2879.

HYPERLIPOPROTEINEMIA

JOSEPH LOSCALZO, M.D., Ph.D.

CLASSIFICATION OF DYSLIPIDEMIAS

Childhood dyslipidemias may be operationally categorized by plasma or serum lipid measurements as hypertriglyceridemia, elevated low-density lipoprotein (LDL) cholesterol, low high-density lipoprotein (HDL) cholesterol (hypoalphalipoproteinemia), or a combination of these abnormalities (Table 1). Dyslipidemias in childhood affect

TABLE 1. Operational Diagnostic Categories of Pediatric Dyslipidemias

I.	Hypertriglyceridemia
II.	Elevated low-density lipoprotein cholesterol
III.	Decreased high-density lipoprotein cholesterol
IV.	Combinations of these disorders

TABLE 2. Range of Lipid Values in Children and Adolescents

AGE (y)	TOTAL CHOLESTEROL (mg/dl)			LDL CHOLESTEROL (mg/dl)			HDL CHOLESTEROL (mg/dl)			TRIGLYCERIDES (mg/dl)		
	5TH PERCENTILE	MEAN	95TH PERCENTILE	5TH PERCENTILE	MEAN	95TH PERCENTILE	5TH PERCENTILE	MEAN	95TH PERCENTILE	5TH PERCENTILE	MEAN	95TH PERCENTILE
0–4												
Males	114	155	203							29	56	99
Females	112	156	200							34	64	112
5–9												
Males	121	160	203	63	93	129	38	56	75	30	56	101
Females	126	164	205	68	100	140	36	53	73	32	60	105
10–14												
Males	119	158	202	64	97	133	37	55	74	32	66	125
Females	124	160	201	68	97	136	37	52	70	37	75	131
15–19												
Males	113	150	197	62	94	130	30	46	63	37	78	148
Females	120	158	203	59	96	137	35	52	64	39	75	132

Data from Lipid Research Clinics Population Studies Data Book.

principally two organ systems, the pancreas and the vasculature. Markedly elevated levels of triglycerides (>400 mg/dl) are associated with an increased risk of acute pancreatitis. Elevated total or LDL cholesterol or both (as reflected in an elevated total/HDL cholesterol ratio) are associated with an increased risk of atherosclerosis. Population values for total cholesterol, LDL and HDL cholesterol, triglycerides, and the total/HDL cholesterol ratio are given in Tables 2 and 3.

Atherosclerotic vascular disease is a process that begins in childhood, continues throughout life, and becomes clinically apparent (with rare exception, such as in homozygous familial hypercholesterolemia or type IIA hyperlipoproteinemia) only in middle age or later. The decision to treat dyslipidemic disorders in children or adolescents that are manifested by atherogenic lipoprotein profiles must be predicated on evidence supporting the views that these disorders (1) are associated with (preclinical) atherosclerotic disease in childhood, (2) track from childhood into adulthood, and (3) when diagnosed in childhood, predict the development of clinical atherosclerotic disease in adulthood.

Recent epidemiologic evidence supports the first two views.[2,3] In the Bogalusa Heart Trial, serum total cholesterol and LDL cholesterol levels were associated with the size and number of aortic fatty streaks. Longitudinal clinical tracking studies (Muscatine study) indicate that approximately one half of those children with total or LDL cholesterols above the 75th percentile had elevated levels 12 years later (Bogalusa) and that two thirds of children with total cholesterol above the 90th percentile had levels above the 75th percentile in adulthood (Muscatine). Inferential evidence exists in support of the view that children with a genetically determined atherogenic lipoprotein profile develop atherosclerotic coronary heart disease in adulthood.

TABLE 3. Range of Total/HDL Cholesterol in Children and Adolescents

AGE (y)	5TH PERCENTILE	MEAN	95TH PERCENTILE
5–9			
Males	2.1	2.8	4.2
Females	2.2	3.5	4.8
10–14			
Males	2.2	2.9	4.3
Females	2.3	3.0	4.2
15–19			
Males	2.2	3.4	5.2
Females	2.1	3.0	4.7

POPULATION SCREENING

The decision about which population of children to screen for atherogenic lipid profiles is controversial. Recent recommendations by the National Cholesterol Education Program[1] suggest screening children and adolescents if a parent or grandparent has had premature cardiovascular disease or if a parent has an elevated total cholesterol level (≥240 mg/dl). Acceptable, borderline, and high levels of total and LDL cholesterol in this at-risk population are shown in Table 4. *If these recommendations were to be routinely adopted, approximately 25% of children in the United States would be screened, and approximately 50% of these (or 14 million) would be candidates for therapy (Table 5), which, in the majority, would involve changes in diet.*

TREATMENT

Dietary Management

Dietary modification remains the first approach and mainstay of therapy for children with dyslipidemias. As a general principle of dietary management, the physician should seek to achieve the ideal body weight with normal growth velocities in all cases. In those children or adolescents with elevated total or LDL cholesterol, dietary therapy should commence with the institution of an American Heart Association Step-one diet designed to reduce total fat intake to less than 30% of total calories and to reduce cholesterol intake to less than 100 mg/4200 kJ/d. Of the less than 30% of dietary calories as fat, less than 10% should be derived from saturated fats, 10% from monounsaturates, and 10% from polyunsaturates. If careful adherence to this diet fails to achieve the treatment goals, the Step-two diet should be implemented. In this diet, total cholesterol should be reduced to less than 75 mg/4200 kJ/d, and saturated fat should be reduced to less than 7% of total calories. Both diets should also contain the recommended dietary allowances of total calories, protein, minerals,

TABLE 4. Ranges of Total and LDL Cholesterol in Children and Adolescents from Families with Premature Cardiovascular Disease or Hypercholesterolemia

CATEGORY	TOTAL CHOLESTEROL (mg/dl)	LDL CHOLESTEROL (mg/dl)
Acceptable	<170	<110
Borderline	170–199	110–129
High	≥200	≥130

TABLE 5. General Therapeutic Options in Pediatric Dyslipidemias

TREATMENT	LIPID ABNORMALITY*		
	↑ TG	↑ LDL-C	↓ HDL-C
Dietary modification	+	+	+
Bile acid sequestrants	−	+	−
Nicotinic acid†	+	+	+
HMG CoA reductase inhibitors†	−	+	±
Fibric acid derivatives†	+	±	+

*TG, triglycerides; LDL-C, low-density lipoprotein cholesterol; HDL-C, high-density lipoprotein cholesterol; HMG, hydroxymethylglutaryl.
†Use only in selected cases as discussed in text.

and vitamins. Children 2 years of age and younger should be excluded from these dietary modifications because of the importance of dietary fat in neural growth and development.

The goal of dietary therapy should be to reduce LDL cholesterol below 130 mg/dl minimally or below 110 mg/dl ideally. Pharmacologic therapy should be considered in children 10 years of age or older who, despite aggressive diet therapy, maintain an LDL serum cholesterol ≥190 mg/dl or who have a positive family history of premature atherosclerotic vascular disease or two or more other cardiovascular risk factors and who maintain an LDL serum cholesterol ≥160 mg/dl (Table 6).

Pharmacotherapy

Among the lipid-lowering agents currently available, the bile acid sequestrants or binding resins are the best studied and most commonly used in children. Resins administered at 0.3 to 0.4 g/kg/d will lead to an additional 10% to 30% reduction in total and LDL cholesterol beyond the effect of diet alone. Notwithstanding the potential these agents have to produce fat malabsorption, no changes in levels of vitamins A, D, E, or K have been detected with their use. *Folate levels are, however, significantly reduced, for which reason children treated with resins should receive folate supplementation 1 hour before or 2 hours after treatment.*

Nicotinic acid also effects a further reduction in total and LDL cholesterol beyond that produced by diet and bile acid sequestrants, with the additional benefit of an increase in HDL cholesterol. Hydroxymethylglutaryl CoA reductase inhibitors (lovastatin, pravastatin, simvastatin) are very effective in lowering total and LDL cholesterol as well, but their long-term safety has yet to be determined. The unknown safety features of these agents with long-term use and their potentially adverse effects on cholesterol synthesis in the CNS, adrenal glands, and gonads preclude the general application of their use in children and adolescents—with the exception of those rare individuals with homozygous familial hypercholesterolemia. Fibric acid derivatives (gemfibrozil, clofibrate) may also prove useful in selected cases, but, again, their safety with long-term administration has not been determined in the pediatric population.

Other General Therapeutic Considerations

In addition to these general pharmacotherapeutic principles, individuals with atherogenic lipid profiles should be instructed in other

TABLE 6. Characteristics of High-Risk Patients in Whom Pharmacologic Therapy May Be Considered

1. LDL cholesterol ≥190 mg/dl or ≥95th percentile for age
2. LDL cholesterol ≥160 mg/dl and
   a. A family history of premature atherosclerotic vascular disease
   or
   b. Two other cardiovascular risk factors

aspects of risk factor modification. Appropriate attention should be paid to nonlipid factors that may have an indirect impact on lipid metabolism, including physical activity, smoking cessation, and blood pressure control. Other secondary causes for dyslipidemias should be considered and treated when appropriate, including hypothyroidism, diabetes mellitus, nephrotic syndrome, autoimmune diseases (especially systemic lupus erythematosus), and renal failure.

Specific Treatment of Selected Dyslipidemias

Selected disorders that may necessitate special therapeutic considerations include marked hypertriglyceridemia, particularly hyperchylomicronemia, and familial hypercholesterolemia.

Hyperchylomicronemia

Hyperchylomicronemia (Fredrickson type I hyperlipoproteinemia) is a consequence of deficient lipoprotein lipase activity that is a rare (<1 in 100,000) autosomal recessive disorder, the hallmarks of which are marked elevations in triglycerides (>1000 mg/dl), eruptive xanthomas, and, most importantly, recurrent pancreatitis. Two types of molecular abnormalities have been found to produce this phenotype, apoprotein CII deficiency and circulating inhibitor(s) of lipoprotein lipase. Treatment is best effected with a very low dietary fat intake and the use of medium-chain triglycerides in cooking to improve dietary palatability. Severely symptomatic individuals with apoprotein CII deficiency may benefit from plasma transfusion. Avoidance of alcohol use in adolescence should be advised.

Secondary Hypertriglyceridemia

Secondary severe hypertriglyceridemia from hypothyroidism, diabetes mellitus, systemic lupus erythematosus, nephrotic syndrome, and renal failure is generally associated with levels less than 1000 mg/dl. Treating the underlying condition is of paramount importance as an initial approach, with additional benefit derived from fat restriction and weight reduction. Rarely, nicotinic acid or fibric acid derivatives (e.g., gemfibrozil) may be required for optimal treatment, but the use of these agents should be restricted to those individuals with triglycerides between 400 and 1000 mg/dl who fail to respond to alternate conservative measures and continue to suffer episodes of pancreatitis.

Familial Hypercholesterolemia

Familial hypercholesterolemia is a rare disorder (1 in 1,000,000) caused by an abnormality in the function or a true absence of the LDL (apo B/E) receptor. This disorder is marked by the development of accelerated atherosclerosis and consequent myocardial infarction or stroke in the first two decades of life. For this reason, aggressive treatment directed toward reducing LDL cholesterol should be prescribed early. Hydroxymethylglutaryl CoA reductase inhibitors, at the very least, should be considered in all such patients, and in selected cases, more aggressive therapeutic options may be required, including plasmapheresis, LDL-apheresis, portacaval anastomosis, partial ileal bypass, and liver transplantation.

Heterozygous familial hypercholesterolemia is much more prevalent than the homozygous form (1 in 500) and is a milder disorder, the hallmarks of which are tendinous xanthomas, LDL cholesterol higher than the 99th percentile and usually at twice the mean value for any given age range, and a family history suggesting monogenic transmission (three generations affected with xanthomas, premature atherosclerotic coronary heart disease, or isolated LDL cholesterol elevations with normal triglycerides levels). Treatment with hydroxymethylglutaryl CoA reductase inhibitors may be required in late adolescence in affected individuals.

Hypoalphalipoproteinemia

The treatment of severely depressed HDL cholesterol (marked hypoalphalipoproteinemia) is generally more difficult than that for the disorders discussed thus far. Aerobic exercise, avoidance of tobacco use, and achievement of ideal body weight may lead to a 5 to 10 mg/dl increase in HDL cholesterol in selected individuals. Treatment with nicotinic acid or fibric acid derivatives may be required in high-risk adolescents.

REFERENCES

1. American Academy of Pediatrics National Cholesterol Education Program: Report of the Expert Panel on Blood Cholesterol Levels in Children and Adolescents. Pediatrics 89:525–584, 1992.
2. Lauer RM, Lee J, Clarke WR: Factors affecting the relationship between childhood and adult cholesterol levels: The Muscatine Study. Pediatrics 82:309–318, 1988.
3. Webber LS, Srinivasan SR, Wattigney WA, Berenson GS: Tracking serum lipids and lipoproteins from childhood to adulthood—The Bogalusa Heart Study. Am J Epidemiol 133:884–899, 1991.

UREA CYCLE DISORDERS

Mark L. Batshaw, M.D.

Congenital deficiencies of each of the five enzymes in the urea cycle and one of its activators (N-acetylglutamate synthetase) have been described.[2] These disorders include deficiencies of carbamylphosphate synthetase (CPS), ornithine transcarbamylase (OTC), argininosuccinate synthetase (AS or citrullinemia), argininosuccinate lyase (AL or argininosuccinic acidemia), and arginase. In the classic presentation, the infant with a complete defect (other than arginase) develops hyperammonemic coma during the first week of life. Individuals having partial defects can first manifest symptoms as early as infancy or as late as adulthood. In these patients with partial deficiencies, symptoms can mimic a number of common neuropsychiatric disorders, including cyclical vomiting, migraine, psychosis, and stroke. Prognosis is influenced by the site of the enzyme defect, its severity, the age at presentation, and the rapidity of making a diagnosis and instituting therapy.[1]

Long-term treatment of urea cycle disorders relies on the principles of restricting nitrogen intake and stimulating alternate pathways of waste nitrogen excretion. Attempts at enzyme replacement through liver transplantation have been attempted recently, and the future prospects of gene therapy look promising.

NITROGEN RESTRICTION THERAPY

In infants, nitrogen restriction involves the use of a high-calorie, low-protein diet supplemented with essential amino acids. This is accomplished most readily by using small amounts of natural protein, an essential amino acid formula (UCD Formula, Mead-Johnson), and supplemental calories provided by a nonprotein-containing formula (Formula 80056, Mead-Johnson) (Table 1). In older children, nitrogen restriction can be accomplished by using a protein-restricted diet similar to that used in chronic renal failure. Complete OTC and CPS deficiencies require more severe nitrogen restriction than do other defects.

ALTERNATE PATHWAY THERAPY

Approaches to stimulating alternate pathways of waste nitrogen excretion vary with the site of the enzymatic block (Fig. 1). In CPS and OTC deficiencies, sodium benzoate and sodium phenylacetate (or its conjugate phenylbutyrate) have been used. Sodium benzoate is conjugated with glycine to form hippurate, which is cleared by the kidney at fivefold the glomerular filtration rate (GFR). One mole of waste nitrogen is synthesized and excreted as hippurate for each mole of benzoate ingested. The hippurate synthetic mechanism rests primarily in hepatic mitochondria. Sodium phenylacetate conjugates with glutamine to form phenylacetylglutamine, which is excreted by the kidney. Glutamine contains two nitrogen atoms, whereas glycine contains one. Thus, 2 moles of waste nitrogen are removed for each mole of phenylacetate administered. Over 40% of total waste nitrogen can be excreted as phenylacetylglutamine. Commonly used therapeutic doses are either 250 mg/kg/d each of benzoate and phenylacetate (given as Ucephan) or 500 mg/kg/d alone of phenylbutyrate.

These drugs, although effective for long-term therapy, may not be well tolerated by the child or family. Sodium phenylacetate has an acid aftertaste and a clinging unpleasant odor. Sodium phenylbutyrate tastes and smells better. Toxicity of benzoate and phenylacetate has been rare, but severe overdoses (4 to 10 times normal) lead to symptoms that mimic hyperammonemic episodes, including lethargy, hyperventilation, metabolic acidosis, and cardipulmonary collapse. Plasma levels of benzoate and phenylacetate should be measured periodically and in the event of hyperammonemic crisis or clinical signs of toxicity. Plasma levels of benzoate should be kept at <5 mg/dl, and phenylacetate should be kept in the range of 0 to 15 mg/dl.

ARGININE AND CITRULLINE SUPPLEMENTS

In the case of AS and AL deficiencies, arginine can stimulate waste nitrogen excretion through enhanced production and excretion of citrulline and argininosuccinic acid. Argininosuccinic acid contains both waste nitrogen atoms destined for excretion as urea. Furthermore, it has a renal clearance rate equal to the GFR. Thus, provided it is continuously synthesized and excreted, it should serve as an

TABLE 1. Long-Term Treatment of Urea Cycle Disorders (g/kg/d)

DISORDER	NATURAL PROTEIN	ESSENTIAL AMINO ACID (UCD FORMULA)	CITRULLINE	ARGININE	SODIUM BENZOATE	SODIUM PHENYLBUTYRATE*
CPS/OTC deficiency	0.6	0.6	0.17	—	0–0.25	0.25–0.5
OTC-deficient females	0.6–1.2	—	0.17	—	0–0.25	0.25–0.5
AS deficiency	1.2–1.5	—	—	0.4–0.7	0–0.25	0.25–0.5
AL deficiency†	1.5–2	—	—	0.4–0.7	—	—
Arginase deficiency‡	0.5–1.5	—	—	—	0–0.25	0.25–0.5
NAGS§	1.2–1.5	—	—	0.18	0–0.25	0.25

Calories supplemented with Mead Johnson Product 80056

*If used without benzoate, 0.50; if used with benzoate, 0.25.
†Citric acid can be given as Bicitra at a dose of 2 mmol/kg/d.
‡Ornithine or lysine can also be given at a dose of 0.1–0.25 g/kg/d.
§N-Carbamylglutamate is also given at a dose of 0.38 g/kg/d.

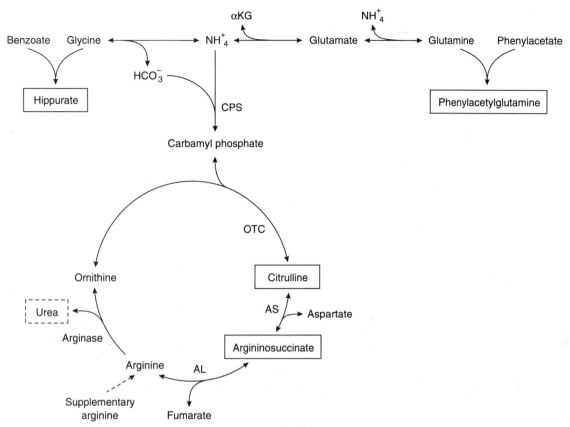

FIGURE 1. Alternative pathways of waste nitrogen excretion in urea cycle disorders. Supplemental arginine stimulates the synthesis and excretion of citrulline in patients with AS deficiency (citrullinemia) and of argininosuccinic acid in patients with AL deficiency (argininosuccinic acidemia). Sodium benzoate acylates glycine, forming hippurate, and sodium phenylacetate (or phenylbutyrate) acetylates glutamine, forming phenylacetylglutamine, both of which can be readily excreted. (From Msall M, Batshaw ML, Suss R, Brusilow SW, Mellits ED: Neurologic outcome in children with inborn errors of urea synthesis. N Engl J Med. 1984;310:1500–1505. Reprinted by permission of the *New England Journal of Medicine*.)

effective substitute for urea as a waste nitrogen product. Like argininosuccinic acid, citrulline can be a means of waste nitrogen excretion, although it contains only the one nitrogen atom from ammonium and has a more limited urinary excretory capacity than argininosuccinic acid.

In AL deficiency, the efficacy of arginine supplementation may be limited by a deficiency in aspartate, which normally combines with citrulline to form argininosuccinic acid. There is some evidence that with arginine supplementation, aspartate levels are depleted, leading to citrulline accumulation and decreased urinary argininosuccinic acid excretion. It has been suggested that a supplement of citrate may prevent this from occurring by repleting aspartate stores through the production of oxaloacetate.[3]

In CPS and OTC deficiencies, arginine (or citrulline) must be provided as an essential amino acid, but it does not stimulate an alternate waste nitrogen pathway. Arginine deficiency in these children results in an erythematous scaling and weeping rash. The lack of availability of an alternate pathway in complete CPS and OTC deficiencies may explain their more severe course compared with AS and AL deficiencies.

For *N*-acetylglutamate synthetase deficiency, effective treatment has involved protein restriction combined with supplements of arginine and treatment with *N*-carbamylglutamate. Arginine is an activator of residual *N*-acetylglutamate synthetase activity, and *N*-carbamylglutamate is an analog of the deficient *N*-acetylglutamate. Therapy has resulted in an increase in serum urea nitrogen, a decrease in plasma ammonium levels, and clinical improvement.

Arginase deficiency has been treated with an arginine-restricted diet supplemented with benzoate and phenylacetate.

ENZYME REPLACEMENT VIA LIVER TRANSPLANTATION

A number of patients with various urea cycle disorders have received orthotopic liver transplants to provide enzyme replacement therapy. In the majority of cases, this procedure has improved the metabolic abnormalities and permitted a normal protein intake. However, its effectiveness is hampered by expense, limited availability of donor organs, and high morbidity and mortality.

MANAGING INTERCURRENT HYPERAMMONEMIC CRISES

Early identification and treatment of intercurrent hyperammonemic episodes is essential both because treatment is more effective at lower ammonium levels and because neurologic outcome appears to be a function of duration of severe hyperammonemia.

Anticipatory management of hyperammonemia is often feasible in a previously diagnosed case. Increases in ammonium levels have been found to lag by days to weeks behind elevations in glutamine, which serves as a storage form of nitrogen. Therefore, periodic measurement of plasma amino acids (which include glutamine) and ammonium may permit adjustment of therapy before clinical symptoms appear. When asymptomatic biochemical abnormalities are detected, the patient usually responds to lowering nitrogen intake or increasing the doses of arginine, benzoate, or phenylacetate (phenylbutyrate) or any combination of these.

If symptoms of vomiting and lethargy become evident and ammonium levels are more than threefold to fivefold elevated, more aggressive treatment is needed (Fig. 2). This involves hospitalization, with complete elimination of protein and the beginning of intravenous treatment with arginine, benzoate, and phenylacetate. There is some

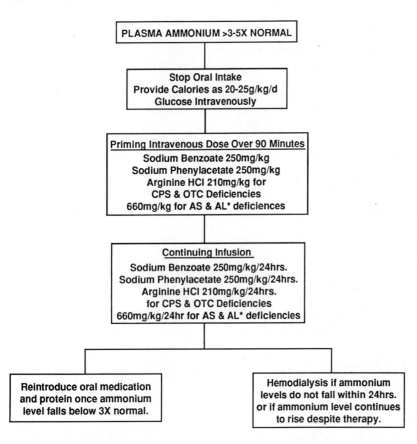

FIGURE 2. Algorithm for treatment of symptomatic hyperammonemic episode. *For AL deficiency, arginine treatment alone should be sufficient.

evidence that carnitine supplements (50 to 100 mg/kg/d) may be helpful during hyperammonemic crises. Neomycin and lactulose have been suggested as a means of decreasing nitrogen production by intestinal bacteria in hepatic encephalopathy, but their role in the treatment of urea cycle disorders is unclear.

In the event that ammonium levels do not respond to this conservative management and biochemical or clinical symptoms worsen, hemodialysis should be initiated. There has been controversy about the relative effectiveness of peritoneal dialysis, exchange transfusion, hemodialysis, and continuous arteriovenous hemofiltration (CAVH). Yet nitrogen balance studies clearly show the advantage of hemodialysis, with CAVH being second best if hemodialysis is unavailable. Hemodialysis should be continued until ammonium levels fall to less than fivefold normal.

MANAGING THE NEONATE WITH A UREA CYCLE DISORDER

In the newborn period, treatment of hyperammonemia may be anticipatory or reactive. In families who have had a previously affected child or in OTC-deficient kindreds, the birth of an at-risk or prenatally diagnosed infant provides the opportunity for prospective management. Within hours of birth, the child can be placed on oral therapy with arginine, benzoate, and phenylacetate (phenylbutyrate).

For infants who have been diagnosed during hyperammonemic coma, hemodialysis should be started immediately. In addition, arginine, benzoate, and phenylacetate should be given intravenously at the same doses used to treat intercurrent hyperammonemia. There is a clear correlation between duration of neonatal hyperammonemic coma and outcome. Infants in coma for more than 4 days are likely to have severe developmental disabilities, including mental retardation and cerebral palsy.[4]

THE FUTURE: GENE THERAPY

Although there have been significant advances in treatment, mortality and morbidity remain unacceptably high. Gene therapy holds the promise for improving this outcome. The OTC gene carried on an adenovirus vector has resulted in transduction and enhancement of OTC activity seen after injection in the OTC-deficient sparse fur mouse.[5] This offers hope for improved treatment of hyperammonemic coma, although immunologic response to the adenovirus may limit its repeated use. For long-term correction ex vivo, hepatocyte retrovirus transfer may be undertaken. A defective recombinant retrovirus has been used to transduce primary hepatocytes derived from sparse fur mice. Transduction was highly effective, and enzymatic assays demonstrated that a partial biochemical correction of the OTC defect was achieved.

REFERENCES

1. Batshaw ML, Robinson MB, Hyland K, Djali S, Heyes MP: Quinolinic acid in children with congenital hyperammonemia. Ann Neurol 34:678–681, 1993.
2. Brusilow SW, Horwich AL: Urea cycle enzymes. *In* Scriver CR, Beaudet AL, Sly WS, Valle D (eds): The Metabolic Basis of Inherited Disease, 7th ed. New York, McGraw-Hill, 1994.
3. Iafolla AK, Gale DS, Roe CR: Citrate therapy in argininosuccinate lyase deficiency. J Pediatr 117:102–105, 1990.
4. Msall M, Batshaw ML, Suss R, Brusilow SW, Mellits ED: Neurologic outcome in children with inborn errors of urea synthesis. N Engl J Med 310:1500–1505, 1984.
5. Stratford-Perricaudet LD, Levrero M, Chasse J-F, et al: Evaluation of the transfer and expression in mice of an enzyme-encoding gene using a human adenovirus vector. Hum Gene Ther 1:241–256, 1990.

11

Connective Tissue

JUVENILE RHEUMATOID ARTHRITIS AND SPONDYLOARTHROPATHY SYNDROMES

Ilona S. Szer, M.D.

The chronic arthritis syndromes are a diverse group of conditions characterized by inflammation of the connective tissues. Manifestations of this chronic inflammation may include arthritis, fever, and rash, as well as evidence of specific extraarticular organ inflammation, such as nephritis, carditis, and uveitis. To control the often crippling and sometimes fatal sequelae of inflammation, the management of rheumatic diseases in children calls for a coordinated, interdisciplinary approach to care that not only addresses the specific disease manifestations but also ensures normal function for both the child and the family at home, at school, and in the local community.

A high level of expertise is required from professionals experienced in caring for children and skilled in pediatric rheumatology, nursing, physical and occupational therapy, nutrition, social services, ophthalmology, and orthopedics. Ideally, this team of experts should be available each and every time the child is seen at the tertiary pediatric rheumatology center to avoid fragmentation of care, miscommunication, and multiple visits. At the level of the local community, a similar team of consistent providers led by the pediatrician should be identified. All of the health providers must have knowledge of the federal and state education laws regarding special services for chronically ill children. Through education, the parents become child advocates and, as such, members of the management team. Yearly school meetings should be encouraged and, whenever possible, should be attended by a member of the health care team to outline the specific individual education plan (IEP) for the child and ensure optimal function in the classroom.

JUVENILE RHEUMATOID ARTHRITIS

The principles of therapy for children with juvenile rheumatoid arthritis (JRA) are largely the same whether the onset of the disease was pauciarticular (four or less joints involved), systemic (hectic fever, anemia, rash, lymphadenopathy, polyserositis), or polyarticular (five or more joints involved), even though these onset subtypes represent distinct clinical entities with the common feature of chronic joint inflammation. The overall prognosis for children with JRA is good. Children with pauciarticular onset JRA carry a more favorable prognosis regarding long-term joint function than do those children who have multiple joint involvement. Because rapid bony destruction is not as common in children as it is in adults with chronic arthritis, maintenance of proper joint function and strength is critical. This is accomplished by anti-inflammatory drugs and physical and occupational therapy. Nonetheless, up to a third of children with polyarticular

and systemic JRA are at risk for permanent disability and require aggressive medical intervention.

The short-term goal of drug therapy is to reduce the inflammation, which produces pain, swelling, warmth, and tenderness. Once pain control is achieved, children are able to tolerate an individualized exercise program aimed at maintaining normal ambulation, joint range of motion, muscle strength, and both reducing and preventing flexion contractures and muscle atrophy. With daily physical and occupational therapy, many children with arthritis are able to participate in normal recreation and play and are independent in activities of daily living, including unassisted ambulation. The use of wheelchairs, buggies, and crutches should never be encouraged. These and other assistive devices should be deferred for as long as possible. Above all, a positive attitude toward an independent and productive future should be encouraged and practiced.

Drug Therapy

Control of inflammation is the goal of the medical therapy for children with chronic arthritis. In general, the milder the disease, the less medicine will be required to achieve control. Approximately 5% of children with JRA may not require drug treatment as they do not experience pain, stiffness, or limitation of motion. Painless swelling that does not interfere with function may be left untreated unless there is muscle atrophy from even minimal favoring or documented leg length discrepancy resulting from accelerated local growth.

Nonsteroidal Anti-inflammatory Drugs

Salicylates. Until recently, salicylates were the mainstay of treatment for children with JRA. During the past several years, salicylates have been replaced by other nonsteroidal anti-inflammatory drugs (NSAIDs) because of the ease of administration, fewer side effects, and no need for frequent monitoring of laboratory studies. Salicylates are, nonetheless, effective anti-inflammatory agents. Salicylates come in a variety of sizes and preparations requiring different dosing regimens (Table 1). In general, an anti-inflammatory serum level of approximately 20 mg/dl or 200 mg/L can be achieved within 10 days of initiating salicylates at 70 to 100 mg/kg/d for children weighing less than 25 kg and 50 to 70 mg/kg/d for children whose weight exceeds 25 kg. The dose for all patients should be titrated to the desired clinical response, as some children respond to a lower dose and others may require a much higher amount. For example, children with systemic onset JRA may not benefit from salicylates until the dose exceeds 120 mg/kg/d before the required anti-inflammatory level and subsequent control of symptoms are achieved. Unfortunately, the rate of intolerance rises when the salicylate level approaches 25 to 30 mg/dl. The most commonly encountered side effects in young children are irritability and personality changes, with a concomitant rise in hepatic transaminase levels. These abnormalities are usually dose related and resolve when the drug is reduced or stopped. Nausea, vomiting, and rapid, heavy breathing indicating metabolic acidosis

TABLE 1. Drug Therapy for Chronic Childhood Arthritis

	SIZE (mg/tablet)	SCHEDULE	DOSE (mg/kg/d)	MAXIMUM AMOUNT (mg/d)
Nonsteroidal Antiinflammatory Drugs (NSAIDs, First-Line Agents)				
Salicylates				
Acetylsalicylate (A.S.A.)	81, 325	t.i.d. or q.i.d.	60–100	2500
Choline magnesium (Trilisate)	500,* 750, 1000	b.i.d.	50	2250
Choline salicylate (Arthropan)	650*	t.i.d.	50	2250
Salsalate (Disalcid)	500, 750	b.i.d.	50	2250
Acetylsalicylate (Zorpin)	800	b.i.d.	50	3200
Nonsalicylated NSAIDs Approved for Children				
Naproxen (Naprosyn)	250, 375, 500	b.i.d. or t.i.d.	10–15	750
Naproxen liquid (Naprosyn)	125*	b.i.d. or t.i.d.	10–15	750
Tolmetin sodium (Tolectin)	200, 400	t.i.d. or q.i.d.	15–30	2000
Ibuprofen (Advil, Motrin)	200, 300, 400	t.i.d. or q.i.d.	30–70	2400
Ibuprofen liquid (Pediaprofen)	100*	t.i.d. or q.i.d.	30–70	2400
NSAIDs Not Approved for Children				
Indomethacin (Indocin)	25, 50	t.i.d. or b.i.d.	1–3	150
Indocin SR	75	b.i.d.	1–3	150
Sulindac (Clinoril)	150, 200	b.i.d.	4–6	400
Piroxicam (Feldene)	20	q.d.	0.5	20
Diclofenac (Voltaren)	25, 50, 75	b.i.d.	2–3	200
Fenoprofen (Nalfon)	200, 300, 600	q.i.d.	40–50	3200
Slow-Acting Antirheumatic Drugs (SAARDs) (Second-Line Agents)				
Sulfasalazine (Azulfidine)	500	b.i.d.	40–60	3000–4000
Gold salts				
Myochrysine, Solganal,		q.wk.†	0.5–1	25 (<12 y), 50
Auranofin (Ridaura)	3	q.d.	0.1	6
Hydroxychloroquine (Plaquenil)	200	q.d.	3–6	400
Penicillamine (Cuprimine)	125, 250	q.d.	5–10	500
Immunosuppressive Drugs (Third-Line Agents)				
Methotrexate (oral)	2.5	q.wk.	5–10‡	20–25
Methotrexate IM		q.wk.†	5–10‡	20–25
Cyclosporine (Sandimmune)	50, 100	q.d.	2–5	200
Azathioprine (Imuran)	50	q.d.	1–2	150

*mg/5ml.
†Intramuscular.
‡mg/m².

are clear indicators of salicylism and call for prompt discontinuation of the drug. The risk of Reye syndrome associated with salicylate intake has been emphasized recently. Fortunately, only a handful of case reports describe an association of high-dose, chronic salicylate use with Reye syndrome. In our clinic, we recommend stopping aspirin temporarily for children with chickenpox and flu-like syndrome with vomiting, although very few if any of our patients are currently receiving salicylates. In addition, we recommend flu vaccines for children receiving NSAIDs.

Nonsalicylated Nonsteroidal Anti-inflammatory Drugs. Naproxen (Naprosyn) and tolmetin sodium (Tolectin) are the only other NSAIDs labeled by the FDA for use in children with chronic arthritis. Ibuprofen has recently become available to control fever and pain and, therefore, is often used to treat arthritis as well (Table 1).

At a dose of 10 to 15 mg/kg/d, naproxen has become the initial drug of choice for children with arthritis. This drug is preferred because of its easy, twice-daily dosing schedule. It is available in liquid form appropriate for young children. It may be given to the child at breakfast and dinner, avoiding administration at school. Similar to other NSAIDs, a trial of at least 1 month is required before changing to another medication because of lack of response. Naproxen is generally well tolerated and safe. Rarely, gastrointestinal intolerance, headache, and drowsiness necessitate discontinuation. Several recent studies reported an association between naproxen and a distinctive

photodermatitis, termed naproxen-induced pseudoporphyria. This complication appears to affect children who are blond and have fair skin. Naproxen should be stopped in children who develop scarring after minor trauma on sun-exposed areas, such as the face and hands.

At a dose of 15 to 30 mg/kg/d, tolmetin is a useful agent to treat arthritis in children who either do not respond to naproxen or cannot tolerate it. Tolmetin is usually well tolerated, but its effectiveness may not be as high as that of naproxen. A 1-month trial is probably sufficient, although 3 months may be needed, before changing to another agent. Similar to naproxen, gastrointestinal irritation and headache may limit its use, but photodermatitis has not been reported.

Ibuprofen recently has been approved for treating fever and minor aches and pain in children. Although the indication for arthritis is still pending, ibuprofen is often used to treat arthritis. The recommended dose that achieves an anti-inflammatory effect is 30 to 70 mg/kg/d.

Over the last decade, many additional NSAIDs have become available for adults with arthritis, and some of these have been tested in children through collaborative multicenter trials. Dosing, efficacy, and side effects are known, but the FDA has not approved their use in children. These NSAIDs include indomethacin, fenoprofen, meclofenamate sodium, sulindac, piroxicam, and diclofenac (Table 1). I usually start treatment with naproxen, followed by tolmetin or ibuprofen. During the past 2 to 3 years, I have not prescribed salicylates or combinations of NSAIDs, although others have done both successfully. If any of the approved agents fail to sufficiently control inflammation, an NSAID not approved for children—but one that has been studied for both safety and efficacy in a pediatric setting—may be tried. All anti-inflammatory medications should be taken either with milk or after a meal. It may be appropriate to prescribe antacids, such as Tums. Sucralfate at 0.5 or 1 g to be taken 30 minutes before the anti-inflammatory medication can be used to minimize gastrointestinal intolerance.

The total length of treatment varies for each patient. Generally, anti-inflammatory therapy is required for as long as there is active inflammation. For most children with pauciarticular onset JRA, therapy is continued for 1 to 2 years, using as parameters the clinical signs and symptoms and weaning the medicine 3 to 4 months after the signs of inflammation have resolved completely. Blood tests may not be of value in assessing the activity of the disease but may be used for those patients who had abnormal tests at the onset of their arthritis. The antinuclear antibody, often positive in children with arthritis particularly if it is complicated by iritis, may remain in their serum for many years and does not serve as a guide to drug management.

Children with polyarticular and systemic onset JRA require treatment for many years, often marked by periods of lesser disease activity, during which lower doses or no medicine may be given. The principle of the least medicine sufficient to control inflammation that interferes with normal function applies at all times.

Second-Line Agents

The slow-acting antirheumatic drugs (SAARDs), also known as disease-modifying or remittive agents, are reserved for those children with multijoint disease who are at risk for crippling and disability. These children are adversely affected despite proper use of NSAIDs and are threatened with poor function, such as nonambulation and dependence on others for activities of daily living, such as dressing, feeding, and toileting. SAARDs, which include gold salts, penicillamine, hydroxychloroquine, and sulfasalazine, must be given by the pediatric rheumatologist because of the high risk of side effects and the absolute need for close follow-up. Gold salts, currently available both as intramuscular injection (Myochrysine or Salgenol) and in pill form (auranofin) may be useful for children with polyarticular JRA, particularly older girls who have rheumatoid factor-positive rheumatoid arthritis. Both preparations have been studied in children and were shown to be only mildly effective but quite toxic. Up to 30% of children do not tolerate intramuscular gold, necessitating withdrawal. The incidence of side effects, as well as efficacy, is somewhat less with the oral preparation. Reasons for discontinuation include allergic rashes and itching, mouth sores, diarrhea, proteinuria, and eosinophilia. Children with systemic onset JRA are at serious, albeit small, additional risk for the development of life-threatening disseminated intravascular coagulation (DIC), reported after the second injection of intramuscular gold. This complication has not been observed following adminstration of auranofin, although it has been seen in children with systemic onset JRA who did not receive gold. Although the potential for inducing remission exists with gold therapy, this event is exceedingly rare. More commonly, there seems to be a modification of disease activity resulting in improved function, less pain and stiffness, and more endurance. It may take up to 6 months for clinically appreciable changes to occur, but a positive effect may be noted after the second month. A 6-month trial of one or the other form of gold may be attempted for selected patients.

Hydroxychloroquine (Plaquenil) is commonly used to treat adults with arthritis. This agent, whose mechanism of action is not understood, has been studied in children and found no more effective than placebo. However, because of its relative short-term safety, it may be tried for 3 to 6 months if the disease is not too aggressive and time is of no issue. Long-term toxicity of hydroxychloroquine is limited to the eyes and is secondary to accumulation of the drug in the macula. We recommend yearly ophthalmologic evaluations and discontinuance of the drug if there is interference with color or peripheral vision.

D-Penicillamine, often helpful in adult rheumatoid arthritis, has not been found effective in children when compared with placebo. The rate of side effects is high, making this agent of limited, if any, use in the pediatric rheumatology setting.

Sulfasalazine (Azulfidine), a combination of salicylate and sulfa that is effective in controlling symptoms of inflammatory bowel disease, has been studied in adults with arthritis and is used increasingly in children. It appears to be both safe and efficacious in treating arthritis, especially in older children with spondyloarthropathy syndromes. Controlled studies in children with arthritis are needed.

Corticosteroids

Systemic and local steroids have a limited but important role in the treatment of JRA. The use of steroids should be restricted to the pediatric rheumatology clinic and should be avoided at all costs. There are, however, several specific criteria for the use of steroids. First, daily steroids are often necessary to control the extraarticular manifestations of systemic onset JRA, such as hectic fever, anemia, and pericarditis. Steroids should be weaned gradually and discontinued as soon as control of these signs and symptoms is achieved. Although the initial indication for corticosteroids is not arthritis, joint inflammation responds exceedingly well to steroids, and tapering may result in worsening of joint symptoms.

For selected patients with polyarticular JRA, small doses of approximately 5 mg of prednisone daily or every other day may enable an otherwise bedridden child to function more independently. Second, a local steroid injection into an inflamed or contracted joint may significantly improve the function of a child with monoarticular disease unresponsive to medical and physical therapy. Some pediatric rheumatologists advocate repeated injections and have shown that many children thus treated remit and do not require further intervention.

Although steroids are potent anti-inflammatory agents and offer rapid relief of symptoms, the many risks associated with their administration, in addition to osteoporosis, avascular necrosis of bone, and muscle atrophy, should absolutely discourage their use in children with chronic joint inflammation.

Third-Line Agents

Immunosuppressive drugs, including methotrexate, cyclophosphamide (Cytoxan), azathioprine (Imuran), chlorambucil, and cyclosporine (Sandimmune), are reserved for those children whose disease is crippling and unresponsive to conventional therapies.

Methotrexate has been used widely during the last few years and should be considered separately from the other immunosuppressive agents. A multicenter trial of methotrexate versus placebo was completed several years ago and documented significant improvement in children who received the drug. There were no serious side effects noted during a 6-month trial. Long-term continuation of the study documents sustained benefit without serious side effects. Thus, this agent is effective while not posing a high risk of side effects over many years of administration. Similar to adult trials, methotrexate was effective in 70% of children compared with 20% receiving placebo. Most patients who respond, however, may not enter a true remission. Recent data from studies of adult patients and anecdotal reports from pediatric rheumatologists suggest that the dose may need to be increased with time and that discontinuation of the drug may result in severe, difficult to control exacerbations. These considerations in children are all the more potent, as we may be committing our young patients to a lifetime of immunosuppressive therapy. Side effects may include bone marrow, liver, gonadal, and, rarely, renal toxicity.

Cyclosporine has been reported as a helpful agent to treat adults with severe arthritis. We recently reported a successful pilot study of 12 children who received cyclosporine to treat severe JRA and dermatomyositis. Although only several children with JRA have been treated thus far and more studies are needed to support these findings, cyclosporine may offer benefit to children with severe unresponsive arthropathy.

Azathioprine, cyclophosphamide, and chlorambucil have not been studied in children with arthritis and are used anecdotally with appropriate caution.

Physical Management

Physical and occupational therapy form a cornerstone in the management of chronic childhood arthritis. Since the potential for remission exists for many children, it is imperative to preserve joint integrity. Tendon and ligament shortening and muscle atrophy are common in JRA.

The goal of a physical therapy program, including passive, active, and resistive exercises, is to preserve a full range of motion, muscle strength, independent ambulation, and gross motor activity. This is accomplished by a daily exercise program carried out at home by the parent, at school by the school therapist, or in a hospital or health club setting. Normal play and recreation are always encouraged.

The goal of occupational therapy is to preserve independence in activities of daily living and age-appropriate function, often curtailed by arthritis of the small joints of the hands and wrists. Daily exercise in addition to specific training in various tasks is prescribed and monitored by the occupational therapist.

Nighttime use of splinting devices and braces should be limited to persistent contractures only. The most frequent use of splinting is in wrist arthritis to arrest progressive loss of dorsiflexion (extension) and to prevent ulnar deviation and hand weakness. Splints are fabricated to encourage as much dorsiflexion as possible and to maintain the position of function. I do not prescribe resting or day splints unless children report pain or fatigue while writing or are threatened with impending fusion in a dysfunctional position. Air splints may sometimes be used, at night only, for children with elbow flexion contractures or small children with knee contractures. Bivalved knee braces are prescribed for children with persistent flexion contractures and are worn during sleep. Frequently, small lifts are placed inside shoes or over the soles of shoes for children with leg length discrepancy. This is particularly common in youngsters with pauciarticular onset JRA who have inflammation of one knee or ankle. Leg lengths must be monitored regularly because, with time, the discrepancy diminishes and the lift should be removed.

Serial casting, particularly for persistent knee flexion contractures that prove unresponsive to physical therapy and nighttime splinting, may be tried and is successful when performed by experienced therapists under the supervision of a pediatric rheumatologist. Attention to the risk of posterior tibial subluxation, quadriceps weakness, and loss of flexion cannot be overemphasized.

Iridocyclitis

One of the most important and potentially devastating extraarticular complications of JRA is inflammation of the anterior uveal tract. Iritis or iridocyclitis is asymptomatic but can be diagnosed easily by a slitlamp examination, which reveals cells and flare in the anterior chamber of the eye. Children with pauciarticular onset JRA are at the highest risk for the development of this complication, which may result in blindness if unrecognized and left untreated. Ophthalmologic evaluations must be performed quarterly for children with pauciarticular onset JRA and once or twice per year for all other children with chronic arthritis. The need for slitlamp examination continues for several years after the arthritis has remitted. Treatment is highly successful if initiated early and before scarring has occurred. Management consists of local steroid eyedrops, often given in conjunction with mydriatic drops. Unfortunately, long-term side effects of local steroid application include cataract formation and, rarely, glaucoma and must be balanced against the risk of iritis. Rarely, children with iritis will require systemic steroids to control inflammation.

Systemic Onset JRA

Extraarticular manifestations of this disease often overshadow the arthritis and require special management. Control of fever and pain may sometimes be accomplished with NSAIDs alone. However, cau-

tion must be taken when these medications are given to children with active systemic manifestations because of the risk of DIC associated with systemic JRA, particularly when the level of serum albumin is low. A rise in liver enzymes and the presence of fibrin degradation products and prolonged PTT necessitate immediate discontinuation of the NSAID and initiation of high-dose steroids.

When systemic JRA is complicated by severe anemia or pericarditis, oral steroids usually are required for control. The dose of 1 to 2 mg/kg/d or 3 to 4 mg/kg every other day achieves response in virtually all children. Pericarditis, if present, is often complicated by a pericardial effusion, which rarely requires surgical drainage. The procedure can be done in the cardiac catheterization laboratory, and the drain can be left in place for 24 to 48 hours. By this time, systemic steroids usually take effect, and drains may be removed. Once control is achieved, steroids are weaned to an alternate-day regimen and slowly discontinued while NSAIDs are maintained. Since systemic manifestations abate in the majority of children within 6 to 12 months, long-term management focuses on chronic arthritis and is identical to that discussed previously.

SPONDYLOARTHROPATHY SYNDROMES

Adolescents with spondyloarthritis are treated similarly to youngsters with other forms of chronic arthritis, with additional attention to lumbosacral spine flexibility and chest expansion. The physical therapy program focuses on both range of motion and strengthening of low back and respiratory muscles. Spondyloarthritis responds well to tolmetin and naproxen. If control is not achieved with NSAID alone, sulfasalazine has been shown to benefit adult patients with spondyloarthropathies, and we and others have used it successfully in many adolescents (Table 1). The starting dose of sulfasalazine is approximately 25% of the therapeutic amount. We increase the dose of sulfasalazine by doubling the daily amount every week until the recommended daily dose is reached. This caution often avoids gastrointestinal intolerance, such as diarrhea and abdominal cramping. Liver function should be monitored monthly.

Methotrexate may also be tried, but gold, hydroxychloroquine, and penicillamine are not usually beneficial. Eye involvement in spondyloarthritis is acute and symptomatic and responds well to local steroid drops.

DERMATOMYOSITIS AND POLYMYOSITIS

LAURIE C. MILLER, M.D.
LORI B. TUCKER, M.D.
JANE G. SCHALLER, M.D.

Dermatomyositis and polymyositis are inflammatory myopathies occurring uncommonly in childhood. Both are characterized by inflammatory infiltrates in muscle tissue in association with muscle weakness. The muscle weakness may begin acutely and severely or may develop insidiously over many months. Dermatomyositis is further characterized by cutaneous findings, including Gottron's papules (a papulosquamous eruption on the extensor surfaces of the metacarpal phalangeal joints and occasionally on the extensor surfaces of the elbows and knees) and a periorbital heliotrope hue. Typical periungual capillary dilatation often may be seen by capillaroscopy. Criteria for diagnosis include the presence of symmetric proximal muscle weakness, characteristic rash, elevated muscle enzymes [aldolase, creatine phosphokinase (CPK), alanine aminotransferase, aspartate aminotransferase, lactate dehydrogenase (LDH)], myopathic findings on electromyogram (EMG), and typical muscle biopsy findings. Pathologically, muscle biopsies show fiber necrosis, variation in fiber size, endothelial swelling and varying degrees of occlusion of small blood vessels, and perivascular inflammatory infiltrates. Vasculitis also may be seen in other involved tissues. In patients without typical rash, EMG and biopsy are mandatory. With typical rash, these are sometimes deferred by experienced examiners.

Polymyositis (myositis in the absence of rash) is unusual in childhood. Therefore, the rest of this discussion refers to dermatomyositis. Inclusion body myositis is also a rare myopathy in childhood, and typically, these patients respond poorly to corticosteroids. Diagnosis is based on demonstration of abnormal tubular filaments in myofibrils. Atypical forms of muscular dystrophy and other rare conditions, such as mitochondrial myopathy, may mimic dermatomyositis.

TREATMENT

Initial treatment with corticosteroids has become standard care for patients with dermatomyositis or polymyositis, despite the lack of controlled trials in either adults or children. Dosage and treatment regimens differ among pediatric rheumatologists, but the most common recommended treatment is 2 mg/kg/d of prednisone in divided doses for at least 1 month, followed by consolidation and then very gradual tapering. Changes in medication are guided by muscle strength testing and levels of serum muscle enzymes (CPK and aldolase). Medication is not tapered until muscle enzymes return to normal and muscle strength is improving. Dosage is reduced by no more than 10% at each change. We prefer daily rather than every other day steroids. Corticosteroid treatment should continue for a minimum of 2 years. Most patients seen early in the course of disease can be tapered to 5 mg/d prednisone after about 12 to 18 months. Considerable evidence has accumulated suggesting that early, high-dose treatment improves the outcome of dermatomyositis and may decrease the incidence or severity of long-term complications, such as calcinosis. Large intravenous doses of pulse doses of steroids are used in some centers, particularly in children with palatal or respiratory muscle involvement. Techniques to determine bioavailability of oral prednisone may some day permit improved individualization of therapy, as there is some evidence of impaired gastrointestinal absorption during the active phase of the disease.

Most patients seen early in the course of disease do well with the standard steroid regimen. However, adjunctive therapy is necessary for some patients, including those with severe onset disease (extreme muscle weakness, severe systemic involvement), those with a relapsing course, or those with chronic persistent disease. Adjunctive therapy may also provide significant steroid-sparing effect. Azathioprine, methotrexate, and cyclosporine have all been reported to have beneficial effects in the treatment of recalcitrant dermatomyositis in children. In addition, chlorambucil has been used in adults. We have used methotrexate as a first choice among these drugs: of 16 children with recalcitrant dermatomyositis, the 12 treated at least 8 months with oral methotrexate (20 mg/m²/wk) regained normal muscle strength. Baseline chest x-ray and pulmonary function tests are obtained before initiation of therapy. No experience with intramuscular methotrexate has been reported, and there are theoretical reasons to avoid intramuscular injections in patients with myopathy.

Some investigators prefer cyclosporine as an adjunct to prednisone therapy. A number of case reports indicate that some children may respond well to this drug. A group of 14 children with recalcitrant dermatomyositis treated with cyclosporine in London all responded well to cyclosporine at doses of 2 to 8 mg/kg/d, with minimal renal compromise.

Intravenous immunoglobulin has been reported to improve muscle strength in some patients, although this has not been demonstrated in controlled trials. Five children treated in Toronto with IVIg (1 g/kg/d for 2 days each month for 6 months) all showed improved muscle strength and rash. Prednisone was decreased or stopped in all patients. In Florida, 6 children with persistent dermatomyositis treated with IVIg (400 mg/kg/d for 4 days, then the same dose monthly for 6 months) maintained or improved muscle strength, and prednisone could be decreased in 5 of the 6 children. In another study, 15 of 20 adults with refractory dermatomyositis had significant clinical improvement after IVIg.

For patients who do not respond to these agents, the use of chlorambucil, cyclophosphamide, plasmapheresis, leukapheresis, phototherapy, and lymphoid radiation has been proposed. Data to support the use of these agents, particularly in children, are lacking. A recent controlled trial of leukapheresis and plasma exchange in 39 adult patients with dermatomyositis or polymyositis found no difference between these treatments and sham pheresis.

Physical therapy is an important component of treatment for children with dermatomyositis. Initially, gentle range of motion exercises can prevent contractures that can develop surprisingly quickly in immobile patients. After the acute phase of inflammation, physical therapy becomes critical to maintain range of motion and to improve endurance and muscle strength.

The skin manifestations of dermatomyositis may be quite troublesome cosmetically. In most children, the skin manifestations improve concurrent with muscle strength, but in some patients (usually with chronic persistent disease), the rash may remain prominent out of proportion to the degree of muscle weakness. In some children, the rash, as well as the muscle weakness, may respond to hydroxychloroquine. Rarely, hydroxychloroquine use exacerbates the rash. Sunscreens are useful, since in some patients the rash is photosensitive.

Treatment of Complications of Dermatomyositis

In most patients, disease manifestations are limited to muscle and skin, although gastrointestinal involvement is not uncommon. All patients should be assessed for palatal, esophageal, and respiratory function and should be hospitalized if significant problems are detected. Severe weakness of the muscles of speech and swallowing may increase the risk of aspiration. Aside from drug treatment of the underlying disease, evaluation by a speech pathologist and observation of the patient while he or she is eating may be useful. Offering purees, liquid dietary supplements, or a soft diet may aid in maintaining nutritional support. Hard, particulate foods, such as nuts, should be avoided.

Serious gastrointestinal complications are seen infrequently in the present era of treatment. Formerly, intestinal perforations resulting from small vessel vasculitis in the intestinal wall were a common cause of death. Radiologically, the occasional patient may be found to have pneumatosis intestinalis. Gastrointestinal symptoms should be evaluated carefully in all patients. Many gastrointestinal manifestations of dermatomyositis respond to prednisone treatment, but occasionally a patient will develop an acute abdomen, requiring surgery.

Cardiac abnormalities are rarely reported in childhood dermatomyositis. Arrhythmias may occur but generally do not require specific treatment. Pericarditis, tamponade, and myocarditis have been described. Children with pronounced weakness have restrictive pulmonary disease, and in contrast to adults, interstitial lung disease is uncommon. The presence of specific autoantibodies to a variety of aminoacyl transfer RNA synthetases identify patients with an increased risk for interstitial pneumonitis. Some of these individuals also have Raynaud syndrome or arthropathy. The existence of such autoantibodies in pediatric patients has not been documented, and the incidence is thought to be low. Pulmonary disease related to dermatomyositis must be distinguished from opportunistic infections in an immunocompromised host and from possible methotrexate toxicity.

Calcinosis occurs in 20% to 30% of patients, although this proportion seems to be decreasing as patients are recognized earlier and treatment improves. A long list of treatments for calcinosis has been reported, including diphosphonates, aluminum hydroxide, colchicine, probenecid, and warfarin, but no reliable treatment for this difficult complication has been identified. In one study, children who had or subsequently developed calcinosis had an increased incidence of staphylococcal skin infections. The immunologic basis for the apparent increased susceptibility to staphylococcal infections in these patients remains unknown.

EOSINOPHILIC FASCIITIS

Eosinophilic fasciitis is an extremely rare disorder characterized by painful induration of the fascia and soft tissues, especially of the extremities, and peripheral blood or tissue eosinophilia. Deep tissue biopsy (skin to muscle) is necessary to demonstrate the characteristic eosinophilic and mononuclear cell infiltrates that are found in subcutaneous tissue and fascia. Eosinophilic fasciitis must be differentiated from the recently described eosinophilia-myalgia syndrome related to tryptophan ingestion. Responsiveness to corticosteroid treatment is usual, although some patients have gradual development of cutaneous fibrosis. Complications can include progressive flexion contractures, especially of the hands, localized morphea, or carpal tunnel syndrome. Children with more extensive disease and a younger age of onset appear to have increased risk of development of residual cutaneous fibrosis resembling localized scleroderma. In some children with this complication, penicillamine has been used as an adjunctive measure. Cimetidine, colchicine, cyclosporine, and chloroquine have been reported to be effective anecdotally, with variable results. We have tried methotrexate, with limited success.

Physical and occupational therapy should be initiated to maintain strength, range of motion, and flexibility. Splinting occasionally may be beneficial, and surgical procedures may improve hand function in some children.

SYSTEMIC LUPUS ERYTHEMATOSUS

BALU H. ATHREYA, M.D.

Systemic lupus erythematosus (SLE) is a multisystem disease with protean manifestations. The natural history of the disease is characterized by exacerbations and remissions, and the variability of manifestations between individuals makes it difficult to conduct controlled clinical trials of available forms of therapy. There are also differences of approach in defining what constitutes activity of the disease and what constitutes a flare. Consequently, treatment of SLE is largely empirical and should be managed in conjunction with a pediatric rheumatologist experienced in the care of these patients.

GENERAL MANAGEMENT PRINCIPLES

General principles of management of SLE in children should include the following.

1. Individualizing treatment according to the organ system(s) involved and the severity of the involvement
2. Preventing major flares to the extent possible by avoidance of precipitating factors, such as sun exposure, certain drugs, and emotional stress
3. Detecting and managing flares early
4. Minimizing the toxicity related to therapeutic modalities
5. Recognizing and treating secondary problems, such as infections and hypertension, promptly
6. Planning for the child's growth and psychosocial development—not just for the disease

Careful attention should be paid to the following general measures: (1) education of the child and the family, (2) counseling on nutrition, exercise, and precipitating factors such as exposure to sun and medications, (3) stress reduction, (4) discussions concerning sex education, including use of birth control methods and risks of pregnancy, (5) discussions about the effects of disease and drugs on growth and development, and (6) discussions that involve educational and vocational counseling.

PHARMACOLOGIC THERAPY

The rash of SLE with or without mild systemic symptoms, such as fever, malaise, and arthralgia, is best treated with an antimalarial drug. Hydroxychloroquine is the preferred drug, starting at 7 mg/kg/d for 2 months, then reduced to 5 mg/kg/d, with the maximum daily dose not to exceed 400 mg. Topical steroids may also be used for limited cutaneous involvement, with care taken not to induce cutaneous atrophy (especially facial).

For more resistant dermatitis (e.g., lupus profundus), dapsone may be tried in an experimental protocol. It is important to test for glucose-6-phosphate dehydrogenase (G-6-PD) deficiency before using hydroxychloroquine and dapsone.

Nonsteroidal anti-inflammatory drugs (NSAIDs), for example, salicylates, tolmetin, indomethacin, and naproxen, may be beneficial for children with low-grade fever, arthritis, and mild pleuropericarditis with or without the addition of small doses of prednisone (0.25 mg/kg/d). However, NSAIDs are known to cause hepatotoxicity (particularly with salicylates) and, infrequently, serious nephrotoxicity. Therefore, careful monitoring is indicated. *Because ibuprofen has been associated with an aseptic meningitis syndrome in SLE, this is not a preferred NSAID for patients with SLE.* Salicylsalicylic acid, choline magnesium salicylate, and sulindac may be safer nonsteroidal drugs for use in patients with SLE, although they have not been approved for use in children.

Prednisone 0.5 to 1 mg/kg/d in divided doses is indicated for moderate systemic disease, including high fever, myositis, mild pleuropericarditis, arthritis, weight loss, and lymphadenopathy. For more severe disease characterized by high fever, pleuropericarditis or myocarditis, hemolytic anemia, thrombocytopenia, most neurologic problems, and glomerulonephritis, high-dose oral prednisone (2 mg/kg/d in divided doses) is used for 4 to 6 weeks, followed by gradual tapering after stabilization of the activity of the disease. Although the benefits of intravenous bolus methylprednisolone (pulse steroid therapy) are not well established in conditions other than rapidly progressive renal disease, one may use this form of therapy in acutely ill children with rapidly progressive multisystem disease. Caution is indicated in the use of pulse steroid therapy in the presence of an infection, hypertension, electrolyte abnormalities, or myocarditis. The dose is usually given as 30 mg/kg of methylprednisolone (maximum dose 1000 mg) suspended in 50 to 100 ml of 5% dextrose in water (D_5W) over 45 to 60 minutes, with careful, frequent monitoring of cardiac status and blood pressure. In children with hypertension, it may be safer to administer the calculated dose slowly over 1 to 2 hours.

Recent studies have established the value of intravenous cyclophosphamide for severe renal disease in adults. In a recent multicenter trial involving children and adolescents with SLE, intravenous cyclophosphamide was used only in children who had failed to establish a satisfactory response to optimal steroid treatment. In the presence of rapidly progressive renal disease (particularly diffuse proliferative glomerulonephritis), one may elect to use intravenous cyclophosphamide as follows after informed parental consent: 750 to 1000 mg/m² body surface once a month for 6 months. Some centers continue this therapy once every 2 to 3 months for 1 to 2 more years. A nadir white blood cell (WBC) count should be checked 10 to 14 days after each dose and the dose adjusted to maintain the WBC count in the 3000 to 4000/mm³ range. Recent reports indicate that this therapy is not curative; indeed, the disease tends to flare when the treatment is stopped. One hopes, however, to achieve a satisfactory delay in the progression of the renal lesion. Newer protocols of intravenous cyclophosphamide therapy include the use of ondansetron to reduce emesis and mesna to reduce bladder toxicity. However, the increased incidence of herpes zoster and the long-term effects on fertility and oncogenicity are of concern.

Once the disease is brought under control, the aim of further therapy should be to reduce the dose of prednisone to the lowest possible level, preferably given every other day, consistent with control of activity. Azathioprine, methotrexate, and hydroxychloroquine may be used as steroid-sparing agents to achieve this goal, depending on the organ system involved and the severity of the disease.

One other treatment of value is intravenous human gamma immunoglobulin (IVIg). This is particularly useful for the treatment of thrombocytopenia in SLE and, to a lesser extent, for the treatment of hemolytic anemia. The dose is 1 g/kg to be given on consecutive days. For severe, rapidly progressive disease with multisystem involvement, the use of plasmapheresis in combination with intravenous cyclophosphamide is justifiable.

FOLLOW-UP

Serologic abnormalities (anti-ds DNA antibodies, complement) alone without evidence of increasing disease activity do not necessitate treatment. In children already taking steroids or immunosuppressive agents for established organ system involvement, some authorities believe that serologic abnormalities should be normalized as nearly as possible to avoid irreversible renal disease. However, such a goal of therapy may lead to the use of unacceptable doses of steroids for prolonged periods, subjecting the child to the other drug-related morbidities of SLE—opportunistic infections, aseptic necrosis, premature atherosclerosis, and early myocardial infarction. Therefore, I do not try to normalize serology—if the patient is clinically well. However, I use serologic tests to help decide how rapidly to withdraw steroids.

The prognosis for childhood SLE has improved considerably, with a 10-year survival rate of over 95%. However, data on long-term effects of the disease (chronic renal failure, organic brain disease) and treatment (growth failure, sterility, atherosclerosis, myocardial infarction, and malignancy) are not available or only now are becoming recognized. Future studies on these very important clinical issues and on the use of biologic or pharmacologic agents with more precise immunomodulatory effects are expected to improve the treatment and outcome of children with SLE.

12

Nephrology Issues and Genitourinary Tract

PENIS, SPERMATIC CORD, AND TESTES

James Mandell, M.D.

PENIS

Circumcision

Circumcision of the normal penis has been a focus of concern and controversy for some time. The uncircumcised penis is covered by a relatively adherent foreskin for the first few years of life. Thereafter, it may or may not be easily retracted for proper hygiene. The only consensus is that good hygiene is important for health commencing with puberty. The possible problems associated with the intact foreskin are phimosis, paraphimosis, balanoposthitis, and urinary tract infection. Phimosis is the inability to retract the foreskin, and paraphimosis is the inability to pull the foreskin back over the glans after first retracting it. Balanoposthitis is infection or inflammation of the prepuce or shaft skin due to trauma or poor hygiene. Removal of the material produced by the subcoronal glands (smegma) is the main hygienic issue. Urinary tract infections in otherwise normal male infants are much more common in those who are uncircumcised. However, the rate of urinary tract infection in infants, circumcised or not, is quite low. The problems with the circumcised phallus are the cost of the procedure, the potential surgical complications, and the longer-term risk of meatal stenosis.

Epispadias

Epispadias can occur as an isolated finding without bladder exstrophy but is much less common than hypospadias. It also can range in severity from distal (glanular) to very proximal (penopubic). Dorsal chordee is common. With the severest forms, urinary incontinence also may be present because of deficient formation of the bladder neck and urethral sphincter. Repair of epispadias is approached in a similar time frame to repair of hypospadias unless incontinence is present. If it is, primary attention is directed at bladder neck reconstruction, with many more potential complications and deviations from a straightforward course.

Other Anomalies

Several other congenital anomalies are seen that may require surgical intervention. Chordee without hypospadias may create potential future problems with sexual function. Penile web or torsion may be unsightly or functionally significant. Micropenis is a very difficult problem to address. If the phallus is less than 2 cm in stretched length, that child probably will not function well in an adult male sexual role. Exogenous testosterone may be given to determine end-organ responsiveness. Megalourethra, which is represented by an elongated, tortuous phallus with outpouching of the urethra, may be an isolated finding, but one should look for the other stigmata of prune-belly syndrome (absent or hypoplastic abdominal musculature, cryptorchidism, renal anomalies).

Acquired problems include priapism, which is a persistent erection, not physiologic in nature. In children, it can be associated with hematologic abnormalities, such as sickle cell disease or leukemia. Treatment is variable, and effectiveness is debatable. Injection of the corporal bodies with dilute epinephrine may be effective in achieving detumesence.

Meatal stenosis is a narrowing of the urethral meatus due to chronic irritation. This is found almost exclusively in circumcised males.

SPERMATIC CORD AND TESTES

The *acute scrotum* is one of the most common and potentially significant genital problems in childhood. The differential diagnosis includes torsion of the testicle, torsion of the appendages of the testicle or epididymis, incarcerated hernia, epididymitis, orchitis, allergic reaction, and trauma. Torsion is certainly the most common of these entities and one of the most important to recognize because of its potential for testicular loss. Torsion of the testicle occurs in a bimodal age pattern, the first in the immediate postnatal period and the other near puberty. Neonatal torsion has been thought to have a different anatomic and clinical presentation than the childhood form. This, however, may not be entirely true, as we have seen at least 6 cases of bilateral neonatal torsion, both synchronous and asynchronous. This implies that the risk of acquired anorchia exists in both groups. The childhood presentation may be more easily confused with an inflammatory condition, but the rule is that the presentation of an acutely painful swollen hemiscrotum is torsion of the testicle until proven otherwise. The treatment if the condition is seen early enough (<8 hours) is immediate surgical exploration, detorsion of the affected side if salvageable, or if not, orchiectomy. Septopexy (fixation to the scrotal septum) of the other testicle is mandatory.

Torsion of the appendix testis or epididymis is also very common but carries none of the same risks. The problem is that it is not always possible to differentiate between the two. The use of radionuclide flow scans or Doppler ultrasound may be helpful. In terms of other differential diagnostic possibilities, a careful examination usually will be able to distinguish between them. Although viral epididymoorchitis is seen in childhood, the diagnosis of epididymitis due to bacterial source is one of exclusion. If the latter is definitively diagnosed, urologic evaluation is indicated.

Tumors of the testis are relatively rare in childhood but can be quite aggressive, especially postpubertally. The diagnosis is usually made on the basis of the physical finding of a painless, firm mass in the testicle. Laboratory studies should include determination of alpha-fetoprotein and the beta unit of human chorionic gonadotropin (hCG). An inguinal approach with radical orchiectomy is standard. Depending on the age at presentation and the histology, the need for retroperitoneal lymphadenectomy or chemotherapy or both is decided. In early childhood, the teratomas or granulosa cell tumors are more likely to behave benignly if they are completely excised. Postpubertally, however, most tumors are managed as in the adult.

Varicocele of the scrotum is a collection of dilated veins draining the testis. It is much more common to the left side and may occur in as many as 10% of adolescent males. The importance of this finding is related to the fact that males presenting with infertility have a high incidence of varicoceles, and ligation of the varicocele has been said to improve the sperm count and fertility. It has been shown that the testicle associated with moderate-size to large varicocele is often smaller and softer than its corresponding mate. Whether this means that spermatic vein ligation ultimately will change the incidence of infertility in these adolescents is unknown.

Other lesions of the spermatic cord include spermatocele and hydrocele. Spermatocele is unusual, is unlikely to be symptomatic, and rarely requires surgical intervention. Hydrocele of the cord is sometimes difficult to differentiate from a communicating hydrocele and often comes to surgical intervention. If the hydrocele is seen in the neonatal period and is not extremely tense, it can be followed during the first year of life to see if it resolves.

Undescended testes (cryptorchidism) are one of the most common genital abnormalities seen in early childhood. The incidence is between 3% and 4% in neonates and declines to around 1% at 1 year of age. The cause is multifactorial and may be influenced by hormonal and mechanical factors. The long-term risks associated with cryptorchidism include testicular injury, loss of fertility potential, and malignant neoplasms of the testicle. The diagnosis of nondescent is made by careful physical examination. The differentiation between retractile and true undescended testis is difficult in some cases and has led to bias in outcome studies. Retractile testes do not require surgery in most cases. It is best to examine the child froglegged and as relaxed as possible. Nonpalpable testes present diagnostic dilemmas, especially if bilateral. If neither testicle can be felt on repeated examinations, an endocrine evaluation for anorchia should be instituted. This involves obtaining baseline serum follicle-stimulating hormone (FSH), luteinizing hormone (LH), and testosterone levels. Repeat levels are drawn after performing an hCG study by giving three to five injections of hCG at a dose of 1000 to 2000 IU. If the baseline gonadotropins (FSH, LH) are elevated and the poststimulation testosterone level does not rise, the absence of any functioning testicular tissue must be considered. Many studies, including ultrasonography, computed tomography (CT), magnetic resonance imaging (MRI), and gonadal venography, have been advocated for the evaluation of nonpalpable testes. Currently we use laparoscopy to locate possible intraabdominal testes and proceed with repair under the same anesthesia.

The treatment of undescended testes remains controversial. Early intervention (around 1 year of age) is the current consensus, but conflicting data about hormonal treatment with and without surgery are reported. Surgical treatment remains the standard in the United States. The technique usually involves a groin incision, with mobilization of the adjacent hernia sac, if present, and a separate scrotal incision to make a pouch for the testicle. In the small number of cases where the testicle is intraabdominal, surgical options include laparoscopic orchidopexy (the latter term implies surgical fixation), open orchidopexy, or orchiectomy if the other testicle is descended and the intraabdominal testicle is too high to bring down or is very dysmorphic. The laparoscopic and open techniques include one-stage and two-stage procedures, with the first stage in the latter using clipping of the gonadal vessels in an attempt to promote collateral vessel growth along the vas deferens. Another option is autotransplantation of the gonadal vessels to the groin. In the rare cases where the undescended testis is associated with a chromosomal mosaicism, biopsy and removal of the nondescended testis should be entertained.

None of the surgical treatments, even if performed early, have been proven to enhance fertility potential, decrease the very low risk of later carcinogenesis, or influence hormonal production from the testicle that is preserved, even in the intraabdominal gonad. Historical

series do suggest, however, that waiting until near puberty to bring the testicle down does not allow for fertility potential. The additional benefit of orchidopexy is to allow for later easy examination of the previously cryptorchid testes to look for the development of masses.

INGUINAL HERNIAS AND HYDROCELES

STEPHEN E. DOLGIN, M.D.

ELECTIVE INGUINAL HERNIA REPAIR

Death from incarcerated inguinal hernias was not uncommon in the nineteenth century. Now, it is, in part because elective repair is advocated and can be accomplished safely when the diagnosis is made. Some of the advantages of an elective operation are that it is, by definition, cancelled if the child is sick with an intercurrent illness and performed only if appropriate time has been allowed for the stomach to empty before induction of anesthesia. These intentions are explained to the parents preoperatively.

Standard preoperative measures include a visit with the surgeon and a documented recent history and physical examination. Psychologic preparation should be directed toward the child and the parents. The child can be guided through the process with minimal stress only if the parents' anxiety can be contained. The truth is a useful guide in preparing the child old enough to understand. A well-trained pediatric anesthesiologist offers an important safety factor, which should help contain the parents' fears. While waiting for elective repair, parents should be informed about incarceration—how it presents and what to do.

The Young Premature Baby

The risk of incarceration is greatest in the youngest babies, so elective repair is advocated even in the small premature baby before discharge home from the neonatal intensive care unit. In this setting, 24 hours of cardiorespiratory monitoring in the hospital will be necessary after administration of the anesthetic because of the risk of postoperative apnea. Although general anesthesia is standard, there is a role for a spinal anesthetic in an occasional small baby.

Locating the Testes

Locating the testes is a critical step before hernia repair. Cryptorchidism is common and is associated with hernias. The undescended testis is not expected to complete spontaneous descent after hernia repair because of scarring. Therefore, orchidopexy is necessary even in the youngest baby undergoing hernia repair if the testis is not descended.

Inguinal Hernias in Girls

Although inguinal hernias are much more common in boys, inguinal hernias in girls present specific problems. The ovary often enters the hernia as a smooth movable lump in the inguinal area. When an ovary is incarcerated, repair should be scheduled without delay because there is some risk of ischemia.

The possibility of androgen insensitivity (the most common form of male pseudohermaphroditism) arises in any premenarchal girl with an inguinal hernia unless a female karyotype has excluded this possibility. Suspicion is increased with bilateral, prolapsed (inguinal) gonads or any sign of virilization (although patients with classic testicular feminization have a normal female phenotype). Since testes produce mullerian inhibiting substance, mullerian structures are not present in patients with androgen insensitivity. Androgen insensitivity can be excluded by karyotype, sonography confirming mullerian structures, measurement of a normal vagina, or, intraoperatively, by demonstrating a normal fallopian tube.

Operative Repair

The operation on a boy with an inguinal hernia includes reducing the contents of the hernia sac into the peritoneal cavity and ligating the sac at the internal ring, protecting the vas deferens and the testicular vessels. I usually approximate the muscles deep to the cord laterally, which buttresses the internal ring, to help prevent recurrence. In a girl, I confirm a normal fallopian tube, do a comfortable ligation of the sac, reduce the ligated sac, and close the internal ring. Bupivacaine is injected into the wound and around the ilioinguinal nerve to help with postoperative analgesia. Some pediatric anesthesiologists employ a caudal block, which is a satisfactory alternative to supplement postoperative pain management.

Contralateral Repair

Although often done, it is not obligatory to explore a clinically negative contralateral side. I do not promise to do so, since the decision depends on there being no problems in repairing the known hernia. I usually do explore the contralateral side in boys less than 2 years old and in girls less than 6.

Postoperative Course

The operation is done on an ambulatory surgery basis except for those at risk of postoperative apnea, who will spend 24 hours in the hospital for monitoring after the anesthetic. Such individuals include the young premature and the extremely young term baby. There is minimal restriction of activities after the procedure. Infants are back to themselves in 24 to 72 hours. Occasional acetaminophen is usually the only medication needed by young children. Adolescents generally will require oral narcotics.

The usual hernia repairs leave no long-term consequences except a memory for the parents and a small, cosmetically favorable scar in the child's lower abdominal skin crease. Uncommon complications include wound infections, recurrences, and rare injuries to the vas or testicular vessels. A very large hernia, especially in a small baby, may leave considerable swelling that can take months to resorb. Parental anxieties are much better managed if these possibilities have been reviewed before the repair.

HYDROCELES

Distinguishing a hydrocele from a hernia is usually easy. This distinction should not be blurred, since only the hernia always requires an operation. Unless abdominal or pelvic viscera enter the groin, the scrotal mass should not be called a hernia. A hernia always has an inguinal component, and a hydrocele usually does not. A loop of intestine gives a characteristic squelch, like the feeling of stepping in mud, when it is reduced. Transillumination is a useful maneuver to reassure everyone that a scrotal swelling is not a solid tumor. Transillumination does not, however, prove that the swelling is a hydrocele, since there may be fluid in a loop of intestine that will transilluminate.

Although some texts advocate hydrocele repair if it is still present at age 1, I do not hold to this practice. Hydroceles may still resolve after this age and will not necessarily eventuate in a hernia. In the absence of a hernia, a hydrocele should be repaired if it is readily reducible by examination, progressively enlarging, or persisting as years pass.

Inguinal Hydroceles

When hydroceles extend up into the inguinal area, they can be misconstrued as incarcerated hernias, since they are not usually reducible. A loculated hydrocele of the cord may confuse the pediatrician. It appears to a parent as a third testis. It is a discrete movable cystic mass in the groin or upper scrotum, and it cannot be reduced into the peritoneal cavity. It can, however, be moved around easily. The patient with a hydrocele will have no symptoms and a soft abdomen.

The inguinoscrotal hydrocele, especially with a retroperitoneal component, can provide a formidable challenge to the surgeon. Sub-

stantial swelling is expected after the repair, and occasionally, there is persistence of fluid, which usually will respond to aspiration. Aspiration is useless, however, in managing hydroceles that have not been repaired.

Hydrocele Repair

A hydrocele repair is done through an inguinal incision. The processus vaginalis is ligated at the internal ring, and distal fluid is drained. In the case of an enormous hydrocele, resection of part of the distal sac is appropriate.

REFERENCE

1. Rescorla FJ, Grosfeld JL: Inguinal hernia repair in the perinatal period and early infancy: clinical conditions. J Pediatr Surg 19:832–837, 1984.

VULVA AND VAGINA

ANDREA M. VANDEVEN, M.D., M.P.H.
S. JEAN EMANS, M.D.

CONGENITAL ANOMALIES AND DEVELOPMENTAL DISORDERS

Ambiguous Genitalia

All instances of abnormal appearance of male and female genitalia in the newborn should be promptly investigated (see Chapter 9). These entities, which are characterized by varying degrees of virilization, include congenital adrenocortical hyperplasia, bilateral cryptorchidism, and unilateral cryptochidism with incomplete scrotal fusion or hypospadias. The spectrum of virilization seen is determined by the extent of fetal androgen exposure. With clitoromegaly, the clitoris is enlarged, but other genital and ureteral structures are intact. In extensive virilization, the labia are fused in the midline, creating an apparent scrotum, obliterating the vaginal opening.

Congenital adrenocortical hyperplasia (CAH) represents the most common cause of ambiguous genitalia in the 46,XX newborn. Because of the variability in enzymatic block, ambiguity may range from labial fusion with or without slight clitoromegaly to an apparent male phallus with labial fusion and rugae on the labioscrotal folds. The diagnosis of CAH should be made as soon as possible after birth because of the need to institute mineralcorticoid and glucocorticoid replacement to prevent dehydration, hyponatremia, and hyperkalemia. Surgical genital reconstruction may be necessary for recession of the clitoris, creation of an adequate vagina, and division of the labioscrotal folds.

Genotypic females without evidence of CAH either have been exposed to virilizing hormones (maternally derived or exogenous) or may have pure hermaphroditism or idiopathic female pseudohermaphroditism. Patients with mixed gonadal dysgenesis have a mixture of mullerian and wolffian structures and often asymmetry of internal and external genitalia. The gonads are dysgenetic, and, generally, the testis does not virilize the external genitalia completely. Genotypic males with ambiguous genitalia may suffer from hypogonadotropic hypogonadism (Kallmann's syndrome), true hermaphroditism, or male pseudohermaphroditism (including androgen insensitivity). In all these situations, gender assignment depends on the external genitalia, the response to hormones (chosen on the basis of the particular enzymatic deficiency), and the possibility of future fertility and coital adequacy. All organs of the opposite sex should be removed, including intraabdominal testes in patients with male pseudohermaphroditism and mixed gonadal dysgenesis, because of the risk of future malignancy. Finally, all patients with genital abnormalities should have a careful search for associated anomalies of the urinary tract.

Precocious Puberty

Although usually benign, isolated premature pubic hair development (adrenarche) may be secondary to a mild adrenocortical enzyme deficiency (e.g., 21-hydroxylase or 3-beta-hydroxysteroid dehydroxygenase deficiency) or may be the first sign of a true precocious puberty. Clitoromegaly may be the result of excess androgens of either ovarian or adrenal origin and can be caused by adrenal and ovarian tumors, as well as congenital adrenal hyperplasia and Cushing's syndrome. Premature pubertal development is most often idiopathic, but central nervous system (CNS) lesions, CAH, primary hypothyroidism, tumors, and McCune-Albright syndrome are among the causes. True isosexual precocity must be differentiated from pseudoprecocious puberty (where estogren is produced independently of hypothalamic-pituitary regulation). Rarely, exogenous estrogen sources, such as ingested birth control pills or estrogen creams, are to blame.

Treatment is focused on the underlying disorder. For idiopathic precocious puberty, treatment with GnRH analogs can shut down the pubertal process temporarily and allow a delay in further development, menses, and epiphyseal fusion until a later age.

Agenesis of the Vagina

Vaginal agenesis is usually associated with uterine agenesis. However, on rare occasions, there may be a uterus with agenesis of the cervix or vagina. A vagina can be surgically created or fashioned by using graduated dilators during adolescence. However, if there is functional uterine tissue, menstrual flow obstruction must be alleviated early in life surgically. GnRH analogs can be used to delay onset of menses.

Imperforate Hymen and Transverse Vaginal Septum

Although the diagnosis of imperforate hymen usually is made in the newborn nursery or during early childhood by routine genital examination, it occasionally is made in adolescence. Patients can be asymptomatic or can have a history of cyclic abdominal pain and amenorrhea associated with a bluish, bulging hymen (hematocolpos). Excision of the hymen is recommended. Puncture alone without definitive surgical repair will not allow complete drainage of menstrual flow and may predispose the patient to infection.

A complete transverse vaginal septum is a rare cause of hematocolpos or mucocolpos in children and adolescents and may result in endometriosis if untreated. The external genital examination is normal, but the vagina appears shortened. There is a palpable midline mass on rectovaginal or vaginal examination. Surgical repair is indicated, with the approach dictated to some degree by the thickness of the septum.

Labial Adhesion

Agglutination of the labia minora is seen primarily in young girls between age 3 months and 6 years. It is generally thought that agglutination results after the healing of irritated labia. The condition is usually of no consequence and will spontaneously resolve either during childhood or at puberty because of estrogen effect.

For adhesions that impair vaginal or urinary drainage, the most effective treatment is application of an estrogen-containing cream, such as Premarin, twice daily for 2 to 3 weeks and then at bedtime for another 2 to 3 weeks. The parent should be instructed specifically on where to apply the cream. When separation has been achieved, application of a bland ointment, such as petrolatum (Vaseline) or A and D ointment, should be continued at bedtime to prevent recurrence, and good hygiene should be emphasized to avoid vulvitis. In the event that separation does not occur despite good compliance with the estrogen cream, lidocaine 5% (Xylocaine) ointment may be applied to the adhesion, and the labia may be gently teased apart with a Calgiswab. In rare cases, it may be necessary to separate the adhesions in an operation.

VULVOVAGINITIS

Presenting symptoms of vulvovaginitis can include genital irritation, dysuria, and vaginal discharge, which sometimes can be mixed with blood. Although the infection or irritation may have been localized at onset, by the time of presentation it may have become generalized. The etiology of vulvovaginitis is closely linked to the age of the patient, which determines the microenvironment of the genital tract and the patient's likely exposure to various infectious agents. In contrast, the physiologic leukorrhea associated with maternal estrogens in the newborn period and also with rising estrogen levels in early puberty may be labeled as abnormal and require reassurance from the physician. Nonspecific vulvovaginitis related to poor hygiene accounts for the majority of symptoms in prepubertal children, whereas vulvovaginitis in adolescents is often related to a sexually transmitted disease (STD).

Nonspecific Vulvovaginitis

The vulvar skin of the prepubertal girl is susceptible to irritation and is easily traumatized because of the absence of protective hair and labial fat pads and the lack of estrogenization in the presence of poor hygiene related to the proximity of the vagina and anus. Obesity and the wearing of tight clothing or noncotton underwear may contribute by causing occlusion and maceration of the vulva. If cultured, normal flora (lactobacilli, diphtheroids, *Staphylococcus epidermidis*, alpha streptococci) or gram-negative enteric organisms (usually *Escherichia coli*) are usually identified.

The emphasis of treatment is on hygienic measures, including the use of cotton underpants, the avoidance of nylon tights or tightly fitting clothing or other irritants (harsh soaps or bubble baths), front-to-back wiping after using the toilet, and handwashing. Sitz baths and protective ointments, such as petrolatum or A and D ointment, may be used to relieve the discomfort. Persistent nonspecific vaginitis not responding to 3 to 4 weeks of hygienic measures often resolves with a 10-day course of oral antibiotics, such as amoxicillin. In persistent cases of nonspecific vulvovaginitis, topical treatment with an estrogen-containing cream or several months of a low-dose antibiotic at bedtime can be considered.

Specific Infections and Infestations

Specific infections in prepubertal girls usually are caused by respiratory, enteric, or sexually transmitted organisms. The respiratory pathogens include group A beta-hemolytic streptococci (*Streptococcus pyogenes*), *Streptococcus pneumoniae*, and *Neisseria meningitidis*. *Staphylococcus aureus*, *Moraxella catarrhalis*, and *Haemophilus influenzae* can occur as normal flora but also have been linked to some cases of vaginitis. *Shigella* is the most common enteric pathogen, causing a mucopurulent, occasionally bloody discharge that is associated with diarrhea in only a quarter of affected girls. *Yersinia* also has been reported as a cause of vaginitis. Pinworms (*Enterobius vermicularis*) may be suspected in young girls who have perineal pruritus and can be diagnosed either by using a piece of tape touched to the perianal area to examine for the eggs or by inspection by parents with a flashlight at night when the child is asleep, looking for the fine, ½-inch (1.5 cm) long, white, threadlike worm. Recommendations for the treatment of vulvovaginitis due to specific organisms in the prepubertal child are listed in Table 1.

Both adolescents and prepubertal children can develop *Candida* vaginitis, but it is far more common in the postmenarchal patient. The diagnosis of *Candida* (by KOH preparation, revealing pseudohyphae and budding yeast, or positive Biggy agar culture) in the toilet-trained prepubertal child who has not had a recent course of antibiotics should prompt evaluation for possible diabetes mellitus. In children, topical antifungal creams are usually sufficient, but in persistent cases, a small urethral catheter attached to a syringe filled with an antifungal cream can be used as an intravaginal applicator. Treatment options are listed in Table 1. Persistent and recurrent *Candida* infections in the adolescent may be secondary to diabetes, obesity, antibiotic use, or HIV infection.

Pediculosis pubis (crabs) is generally transmitted by sexual contact. Adolescents may present with severe itching, and on inspection of the genital area, small, moving adult lice or tiny (1 to 2 mm), firmly attached flakes (nits) are visible on the pubic hair. Treatment with 1% lindane (Kwell) shampoo lathered on and left for 5 minutes is effec-

TABLE 1. Treatment of Vulvovaginitis and Cervicitis

ETIOLOGY	TREATMENT
Prepubertal Child*	
Group A β-streptococcus (*Streptococcus pyogenes*) *Streptococcus pneumoniae*	Penicillin V potassium 125–250 mg q.i.d. PO × 10 d
Chlamydia trachomatis	Erythromycin 50 mg/kg/d PO × 10 d
	Children ≥ 8 y of age, doxycycline, 100 mg b.i.d. PO × 7 d
Neisseria gonorrhoeae	Ceftriaxone 125 mg IM. Patients who cannot tolerate ceftriaxone may be treated with spectinomycin, 40 mg/kg IM once
	Children ≥ 8 y of age should also be given doxycycline, 100 mg b.i.d. PO × 7 d
	Children > 45 kg are treated with adult regimens
Candida	Topical nystatin, miconazole, or clotrimazole cream
Shigella	Trimethoprim-sulfamethoxazole 8 mg 40 mg/kg/d PO × 7 d
Staphylococcus aureus	Cephalexin 25–50 mg/kg/d PO × 7–10 d
	Dicloxacillin 25 mg/kg/d PO × 7–10 d
	Amoxicillin-clavulanate 20–40 mg/kg/d (of the amoxicillin) PO × 7–10 days
Haemophilus influenzae	Amoxicillin 20–40 mg/kg/d PO × 7 d
Trichomonas	Metronidazole 125 mg (15 mg/kg/d) t.i.d. × 7–10 d
Pinworms (*Enterobius vermicularis*)	Mebendazole 1 chewable 100-mg tablet, repeated in 2 wk
Adolescent†	
Bacterial vaginosis	Metronidazole 500 mg PO b.i.d. × 7 d *or* 2-g single dose
	Metronidazole gel 0.75% b.i.d. vaginally × 5 d
	Clindamycin 300 mg PO b.i.d. × 7 d
	Clindamycin vaginal cream 2% q.h.s. × 7 nights
Candida	Clotrimazole‡ 1% cream, 1 applicatorful vaginally q.h.s. × 7 nights
	Clotrimazole‡ 100 mg vaginal tablets vaginally q.h.s. × 7 nights
	Miconazole‡ 100 mg suppository vaginally q.h.s. × 7 nights
	Miconazole 2% cream‡ 1 applicatorful vaginally q.h.s. × 7 nights
	Butoconazole 2% cream, 1 applicatorful vaginally q.h.s. × 3 nights
	Terconazole 0.4% cream, 1 applicatorful vaginally q.h.s. × 7 nights
	Terconazole 0.8% cream or vaginal suppository q.h.s. × 3 nights
	Fluconazole 150 mg PO single dose
Chlamydia trachomatis§	Doxycycline 100 mg PO b.i.d. × 7 d
	Azithromycin 1 g PO
	Erythromycin 500 mg q.i.d. × 7 d or 250 mg q.i.d. × 14 d (if pregnant)
	Ofloxacin 300 mg b.i.d. × 7 d (> 18 y, not pregnant)
Neisseria gonorrhoeae§‖	Ceftriaxone 125 mg IM
	Cefixime 400 mg PO
Trichomonas	Metronidazole 2 g PO single dose

*Reprinted with permission from Emans SJ, Goldstein DP: *Pediatric and Adolescent Gynecology,* 3rd ed, Boston, Little, Brown & Co, 1990:78.
†From Vandeven AM, Emans SJ: Vulvovaginitis in the child and adolescent. Pediatr Rev 14(4):147, 1993.
‡Available over the counter.
§Refer to Centers for Disease Control guidelines for other treatment options.
‖Patients diagnosed with *N. gonorrhoeae* should receive a course of treatment for *Chlamydia* as well.

tive, as is 1% permethrin cream rinse (Nix) left on for 10 minutes. After rinsing, the hair should be cleaned with a fine-tooth comb to remove the nits. Repeat treatment in 1 week will lessen recurrences. Clothing and blankets should be laundered, since these can transmit the lice.

Sexually transmitted infections are a comon cause of specific vulvovaginitis in the adolescent (see Chapter 22). Adolescents may also present with vaginal discharge secondary to cervicitis. It should be kept in mind that if the patient is diagnosed with one sexually transmitted infection, she is at higher risk for others. For that reason, there should be consideration of screening for other sexually transmitted infections (such as syphilis and HIV) and thoughtful evaluation of persistent symptoms despite adequate treatment and good compliance. Treatment of the young woman's sexual partner is also necessary. Because of changing resistance patterns, as well as the development of new treatment regimens, the physician is advised to keep abreast of the Centers for Disease Control guidelines, which are updated regularly. The recommendations given are current as of September 1993.

Sexually transmitted infections can be seen in prepubertal children as well and, when diagnosed, should prompt a thorough evaluation for possible sexual abuse. In situations where the child appears to have a nonspecific vulvovaginitis with a scant mucoid discharge and accompanying vulvar erythema, it is often unnecessary to do specific cultures for sexually transmitted infections. However, if the discharge is persistent, purulent, or recurrent despite good hygiene measures or if there is a suspicion of sexual abuse, the physician is obligated to evaluate the symptoms more carefully with appropriate microscopic examination and culture.

Gonorrhea

Adolescents can present with gonococcal cervicitis, urethritis, pelvic inflammatory disease (PID), pharyngitis, and arthritis, although many infections are asymptomatic. In prepubertal girls, *Neisseria gonorrhoeae* infections result from sexual abuse, and all contacts and siblings should be cultured. The Gram stain of the discharge may reveal gram-negative, intracellular diplococci, which is suggestive but not conclusive of infection in females. Therefore, particularly in children, culture confirmation is necessary. In teens there is a high rate of coinfection with *Chlamydia trachomatis,* and so treatment for both infections is indicated. Treatment options are listed in Table 1. Treatment should be followed by rescreening 1 month later because of the high chance of reinfection.

Chlamydia

Chlamydia trachomatis infection is associated with mucopurulent cervicitis, salpingitis, and urethritis in adolescent females. In prepubertal children, *Chlamydia* contracted at birth can persist until the child is 2 years of age, but in older children, especially those with a history of antibiotic therapy in infancy, sexual abuse is the usual mode of transmission. For that reason, although rapid tests using immunoassays and slide tests are acceptable for screening high-risk populations, such as sexually active adolescents, they are inappropriate for use in children because of unacceptably high false positive and false negative rates. Only *Chlamydia* culture should be used in children or in adolescent rape victims. Treatment options are listed in Table 1. After treatment the patient should be rescreened because of reinfection.

Trichomonas Vaginitis

Trichomonas vaginalis is a flagellated parasite that causes a frothy, malodorous, yellow-green or gray discharge in adolescents. It is sometimes detected on culture or found in a routine Pap smear or urinalysis. Although usually considered a sexually transmitted infection, the organism can survive in wet towels, so that a nonsexual mode of transmission is theoretically possible but highly unlikely. The treatment recommendations are given in Table 1.

Bacterial Vaginosis

Bacterial vaginosis, formerly known as "nonspecific vaginitis," results from the complex alteration of microbial flora of the vagina with overgrowth of anaerobic organisms and *Mycoplasma hominis,* with an absence of normal hydrogen peroxide-producing lactobacilli. Although *Gardnerella vaginalis* is typically found in patients with this diagnosis, this organism is also found in many asymptomatic patients, including those who are virginal. Three of four criteria must be met for the diagnosis: (1) homogeneous discharge, (2) pH over 4.5, (3) positive "whiff" test (mixing 1 drop of the discharge with 1 drop of 10% KOH to see if an amine odor is liberated), and (4) the presence of at least 20% clue cells. Cultures for *G. vaginalis* are not helpful and alone should not be diagnostic of this condition. Currently, asymptomatic patients are not treated. Current recommendations are in Table 1.

Genital Herpes

Herpes simplex type 2 (HSV 2) generally is associated with genital infections, although between 5% and 15% of first episodes are actually due to HSV 1. Patients may have vulvar, cervical, urethral, or rectal infections, manifested by vesicles that rupture in 1 to 3 days, producing painful ulcers. There may be systemic symptoms consistent with a viral illness (malaise, fever, headache). Patients may have asymptomatic viral shedding, although symptomatic patients are most infectious. In simultaneous oral and genital infections, HSV 1 is more likely to be associated with labial recurrences and HSV 2 with genital recurrences. Although both HSV 1 and HSV 2 can be transmitted via sexual abuse, HSV 2 is more likely to be sexually acquired. A positive Tzanck preparation is highly specific for HSV but not very sensitive. The diagnosis can be confirmed by culture.

In mild cases, symptomatic treatment with good local hygiene, sitz baths, dry heat (cool setting on a hair dryer), topical application of 2% lidocaine jelly, and analgesics may be used. In primary outbreaks, oral acyclovir 200 mg 5 times a day for 10 days can shorten the duration of symptoms and viral shedding and reduce the number of new lesions. However, it has no effect on recurrence rates. Oral acyclovir is less effective in recurrent infection, although it may help to suppress frequent recurrences (200 mg 2 to 5 times a day or 400 mg twice a day for 6 months). Topical acyclovir offers no advantages over the oral preparation, and there is no indication for the simultaneous use of both oral and topical medication.

Condyloma Acuminatum

Human papillomavirus (HPV) is a DNA virus with more than 50 subtypes that can cause, depending on subtype, both exophytic cauliflower genital warts and flat condyloma. HPV has become the most prevalent cause of sexually transmitted viral infection, and it is associated with the development of genital neoplasia. Infections with the genital types may be apparent clinically or may be detected on the basis of an abnormal Pap smear or biopsy. Application of 3% to 5% acetic acid to vulvar, vaginal, and cervical tissue often will demonstrate subclinical HPV infection in what appears to be normal tissue.

Detailed discussion of treatment options is beyond the scope of this article. However, most patients with condyloma deserve careful evaluation by a gynecologist, often including biopsy before the lesions are removed. Especially in cases of possible sexual abuse, it is often useful to obtain biopsy material for subtyping. Without treatment, exophytic warts usually regress over 3 to 5 years. Although podophyllin traditionally has been recommended, it must be applied frequently and is contraindicated in well-vascularized perianal and vaginal tissues because of absorption. Many physicians have turned to 25% to 85% strength trichloroacetic acid (TCA), which is applied directly to the lesion, followed immediately by normal saline or aloe vera gel to ease the burning sensation. TCA is reapplied weekly. In extensive or unresponsive cases, laser or cryocautery may be indicated.

Miscellaneous Causes of Vaginal Discharge

Discharge with or without accompanying vulvovaginitis can be caused by a variety of entities. Vaginal foreign bodies can cause a foul-smelling, occasionally blood-tinged discharge. In adolescents, it is most likely a retained tampon, and in young children, bits of toilet paper. In young children, small foreign material can often be flushed out with gentle vaginal irrigation using a small-diameter urinary catheter attached to a syringe. Allergic or irritative vulvovaginitis can be caused by contraceptive creams, soaps, douches, latex products, and occasionally, sperm. Rectovaginal fistulas (Crohn's disease) and mullerian anomalies with obstruction also can cause chronic vaginal discharge. Finally, psychosomatic vulvovaginitis, with constant scratching of the vulva, can cause genital irritation and discharge.

VULVAR MANIFESTATIONS OF SKIN DISEASES

Seborrhea, psoriasis, and atopic dermatitis can affect the genital area and are usually associated with characteristic skin lesions on the rest of the body. Burow's solution may be helpful in weepy lesions, and superinfections should be treated with appropriate oral or topical antibiotics. The prolonged use of potent steroid creams in the genital area is to be avoided because of the risk of absorption in this highly vascularized area.

Diaper Rash

Diaper dermatitis is the most common rash in infancy. This dermatitis is classified as an irritant dermatitis secondary to prolonged contact with ammonia or, less commonly, to residual detergents in diapers. Secondary infection with *Candida* is common, characterized by satellite, beefy red papules scattered beyond the borders of the dermatitis. The parents are advised to keep the area as dry as possible, and 1% hydrocortisone cream can be used alone if there is no candidal infection. Otherwise, nystatin or clotrimazole (Lotrimin) cream should be used twice daily, alternating with 1% hydrocortisone cream after each diaper change.

Lichen Sclerosus

This poorly understood vulvar dystrophy is being diagnosed more often in children, primarily because of physician awareness. It is seen most frequently in prepubertal girls and postmenopausal women, and for that reason, a hormonal abnormality has been questioned as a possible cause. There can be extragenital lesions. Classically, the lesions are symmetric, ivory-white macules that coalesce to form a figure-of-eight around the vulva and anus. The atrophic skin is easily damaged, and patients may present with hemorrhagic bullae or "blood blisters." Because of the genital location and the association with easy injury, these children frequently are brought to a physician by a parent concerned about possible sexual abuse.

Since the cause is unknown, definitive recommendations for treatment are difficult. In mild cases, good hygiene is stressed, and the guidelines for the care of nonspecific vulvovaginitis are followed. If necessary, a 1- to 3-month course of a low-potency topical steroid cream, such as 1% or 2.5% hydrocortisone, or a shorter course of a more potent steroid, such as fluocinolone acetonide or betamethasone valerate, is indicated. Rarely, it may be necessary to try 2% topical testosterone propionate cream, although this treatment may be less acceptable because of androgen absorption, causing pubic hair growth or clitoral enlargement.

CYSTS, MASSES, AND TUMORS

Cysts may be developmental or epidermoid or may develop as a result of a blockage of the various gland ducts. The position and the histology of the cyst allow categorization. Bartholin cysts cause acute pain and swelling, and their location is diagnostic. They are associated with infections caused by *N. gonorrhoeae, Chlamydia,* or other organisms and should be treated with incision and drainage, with culture of the drained material. Paraurethral duct cysts may compress the urethra because of their location and may need to be removed for that reason. They are often seen in newborns and often disappear without treatment.

Before surgery is done, urologic or gynecologic malformations, such as urethral diverticulum, ectopic ureterocele, hymenal or vaginal cyst, or obstructed hemivagina, should be excluded by examination and ultrasound and the use of intraoperative radiopaque dye injected into the cyst. Labial abscesses can sometimes be treated conservatively with oral antibiotics and sitz baths, although surgical drainage may be necessary. Urethral prolapse is characterized by an annular doughnutlike friable mass that may be bleeding. Prolapse usually resolves in 1 to 4 weeks with nonsurgical treatment, including sitz baths, topical estrogen cream or antibiotic ointment, and oral antibiotics.

The most common benign tumors in children are nevi and cavernous hemangiomas. Nevi in the vulva should be treated as would nevi elsewhere on the body: changes should be monitored and excision considered if necessary. Vulvar nevi in adolescents should be electively excised. Hemangiomas will resolve and should be left untreated unless they are rapidly growing or prone to trauma. They can be removed surgically or by laser excision. Malignant tumors, usually sarcomas, are rare and more often of vaginal than of vulvar origin. The malignant tumor that involves the vagina, uterus, bladder, and urethra of very young girls most frequently is sarcoma botryoides, also known as embryonal rhabdomyosarcoma. The tumor usually starts within the vagina, and as it grows, it appears as a prolapse of grapelike masses through the urethra or hymen. The tumor grows quickly, and the prognosis is poor unless the diagnosis is made early. Treatment is with a combination of chemotherapy and aggressive surgery, along with radiation therapy for some patients.

Diethylstilbestrol (DES) was used to prevent miscarriages from the mid-1940s to the early 1970s. In utero exposure to DES and the related nonsteroidal estrogens hexestrol and dienestrol is associated with the development of vaginal adenosis and clear cell adenocarcinoma of the cervix and vagina. Vaginal adenosis consists of alteration of the columnar epithelium in the vagina and squamous metaplasia. DES exposure is also associated with structural abnormalities of the vagina and cervix, including fibrous ridges, hoods (a circular fold that partially covers the cervix), large ectropions, hypoplasia of the cervix, and pseudopolyp. Clear cell adenocarcinoma may involve any portion of the vagina or cervix or both. Most are polypoid nodules, but some are flat or ulcerated with a granular surface. The primary mode of therapy is with radical surgery, with adjunctive chemotherapy and radiation therapy indicated depending on staging.

TRAUMA

Trauma to the genital area can result from accidental straddle falls and from sexual assault. A straddle injury typically causes ecchymoses in the vulva and periclitoral folds, and lacerations of the labia minora and periurethral tissues are sometimes seen. It is extremely unusual for a child to have a tear of the hymen without a penetrating injury, such as from a direct fall onto a nail or stick. Thus, sexual abuse

should be carefully considered when hymenal trauma is seen, especially if a credible explanation is lacking. In children with fresh genital trauma and bleeding, it is often necessary to anesthetize the child to be able to carefully examine the vagina for deep trauma that may penetrate to the bladder, rectum, or peritoneum. In situations of sexual assault, specimens should be collected for forensic investigation (rape kit).

Minor injuries of the labia will heal without scarring, but even small hymenal tears often will heal in such a way that the hymenal rim will be irregular with clefts or demonstrate focal scarring or thickening. In other instances, the hymen will be found to be attenuated or diffusely thickened. Synechiae are sometimes seen. It must be kept in mind that most girls who have been sexually abused have either nonspecific (irritation, friability) or normal findings on physical examination.

UTERUS, FALLOPIAN TUBES, AND OVARIES

Margaret Polaneczky, M.D.

Many common gynecologic disorders in the adolescent can be evaluated and treated completely by the pediatrician. Whenever possible, a thorough pelvic examination should precede the institution of any therapy. If performed in a sensitive manner by an experienced clinician, the examination need not be a traumatic experience for the patient. In the patient deemed unsuitable for speculum examination, a careful bimanual and rectal examination, supplemented by ultrasonography if necessary, can often provide enough information to allow further evaluation and treatment to proceed.

COMMON MENSTRUAL DISORDERS

The average age of menarche in the United States is 12.8 years, with a range of 9 to 16 years. Menarche usually occurs within 2 to 2.5 years after breast budding and 1 year after the growth spurt. Up to 50% of young women do not ovulate during their first few menstrual cycles. As a result, menses in the young adolescent may be irregular and are often prolonged or heavy.

Normally, young women should begin to have regular, ovulatory cycles by 1 to 2 years after menarche. Normal cycle length ranges from 21 to 45 days, with menstrual flow lasting 2 to 7 days. The average blood loss during a normal menstrual period is 30 to 40 ml, or up to four well-soaked pads or tampons per day. On the first and second days, flow may be slightly heavier.

Primary Amenorrhea

Primary amenorrhea is defined as any one of the following: (1) the absence of menarche by age 16 years in the otherwise normal pubertal female, (2) the absence of menarche by age 14 years in the young woman who lacks breast and pubic hair development, or (3) the failure of menarche to appear within 2 years of completed sexual maturation.

The diagnostic evaluation of primary amenorrhea is summarized in Figure 1. The workup begins with a complete history and physical examination, after which the patient may be classified into one of four diagnostic groups based on the presence or absence of breast development and internal female genitalia. Follicle-stimulating hormone (FSH) levels, testosterone levels, and karyotype are then performed selectively to arrive at a final diagnosis. Treatment is best undertaken in conjunction with an endocrinologist or adolescent gynecologist. Although prognosis will vary according to diagnosis, treatment should be designed to achieve, whenever possible, the following goals.

1. Successful gender identification
2. Normal height and breast development

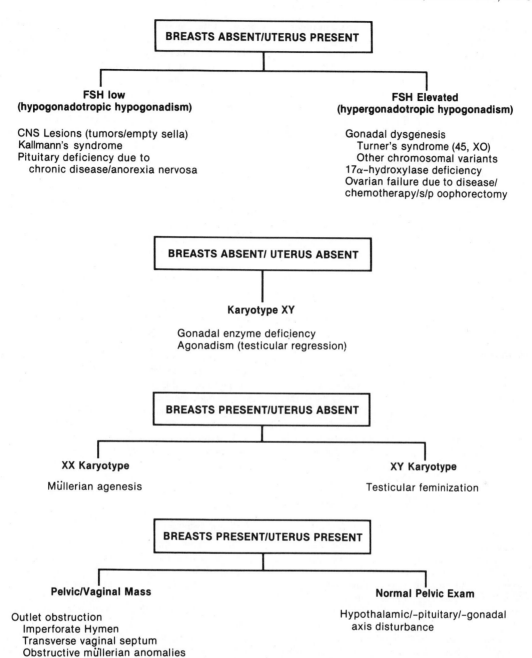

FIGURE 1. Diagnostic approach to patients with primary amenorrhea. FSH, follicle-stimulating hormone; CNS, central nervous system. (Adapted from Maschak CA, et al: Clinical and laboratory evaluation of patients with primary amenorrhea. Obstet Gynecol 57:719, 1981. Reprinted with permission from the American College of Obstetricians and Gynecologists.)

3. Normal sexual function
4. Cyclic menstrual bleeding
5. Preservation of reproductive function
6. Protection from bone and cardiovascular consequences of estrogen deficiency
7. Prevention of future malignancy

Hypogonadotropic Hypogonadism

These individuals have primary amenorrhea accompanied by sexual immaturity. Pelvic examination reveals the presence of a normal vagina and uterus. FSH levels are low, indicating that the primary defect lies in either the pituitary or the hypothalamus. Careful central nervous system (CNS) evaluation should be performed to rule out the presence of a cranioparyngioma or other CNS lesion.

A typical individual in this category is the young woman who has permanent deficits of pituitary hormones as a result of radiation ther-

apy or surgery for a brain tumor. Others include those with the empty sella syndrome or Kallmann's syndrome. In addition, individuals with severe early-onset anorexia nervosa or certain chronic diseases, such as thalassemia major, often experience hypogonadotropic primary amenorrhea as a result of hypothalamic-pituitary dysfunction.

All of these patients require estrogen replacement therapy to induce sexual maturation, prevent bone loss, and allow for normal menstrual function and vaginal lubrication. In patients with pituitary insufficiency, therapy may also include growth hormone, thyroid hormone, and adrenal replacement.

Estrogen replacement typically begins with low-dose conjugated estrogens (Premarin, 0.3 to 0.625 mg daily on days 1 to 25), with medroxyprogesterone acetate (Provera, 5 to 10 mg added on days 14 to 25). An alternative regimen for the younger adolescent is to begin with estrogen alone to induce breast development, adding cyclic progestin once menses ensue. In either case, it is usually necessary to increase the estrogen dose to 1.25 mg over 1 to 2 years in order to complete breast development.

Suggested long-term estrogen replacement regimens are summarized in Table 1. Because recent evidence suggests that the duration of progestin is more important than the dose in preventing the development of uterine malignancy due to unopposed estrogen, 12 days of progestin therapy is now recommended rather than the traditional 10 days of therapy. Micronized 17β-estradiol (Estrace), in doses of 1 to 2 mg, is an alternative to conjugated estrogens. Another long-term treatment option is to use an oral contraceptive. This is often easier for the patient than taking two different medications. Because oral contraceptive therapy will be continued indefinitely, pills containing high doses of the more atherogenic progestin, levonorgestrel, should be avoided. Oral contraceptive therapy should not be used until breast development is complete because there has been some concern that their use before then may lead to tubular breast formation. The estrogen patch (0.05 to 0.1 mg/d), is a good alternative for younger adolescents who may have problems with daily oral compliance.

It is important to remember that the ovaries and internal genitalia of these patients, although unstimulated, are otherwise normal. The patient and her parents should be advised that future pregnancy is possible. This is usually accomplished by combining estrogen replacement with induction of ovulation using human menopausal gonadotropins (hMG).

Hypergonadotropic Hypogonadism

Patients with hypergonadotropic hypogonadism present with sexual immaturity and amenorrhea. Pelvic examination reveals the presence of a vagina and uterus. FSH levels are elevated, revealing the primary defect to be in the gonad. Blood karyotype should be performed, and at least 20 cells should be counted to increase the detection rate of mosaic abnormalities. The most common chromosomal abnormality associated with hypogonadotropic hypogonadism is Turner's syndrome (XO karyotype) and its mosaic variants. Less common are other X chromosomal variants. Even rarer are primary defects in ovarian steroid production due to 17α-hydroxylase deficiency or ovarian failure secondary to ataxia-telangiectasia, galactosemia, or myotonic dystrophy.

If karyotype reveals the presence of any portion of a Y chromosome, surgical removal of the gonadal streak must be performed to avoid malignant degeneration. Gonadectomy is usually performed before puberty because the gonad is nonfunctional.

The short stature associated with Turner's syndrome and its variants is due to the absence of growth-regulating genes usually present on the X chromosome. Estrogen replacement therapy alone is usually insufficient for achieving the dual goals of increased height and normal pubertal development in these patients. Both recombinant growth hormone and anabolic steroids have been used as adjuncts to estrogen replacement in young women with Turner's syndrome. The relative timing of growth hormone therapy and estrogen replacement will depend on the age at which the diagnosis of Turner's syndrome is

made. If the diagnosis is made during early childhood and growth is found to be abnormal, growth hormone therapy may be begun first, with estrogen replacement begun in early adolescence (around age 10) to achieve normal pubertal development. However, if the diagnosis of Turner's syndrome is made in adolescence, concurrent growth hormone and estrogen therapy may be begun. Concurrent androgen therapy also has been used in maximizing final height in Turner's syndrome patients. Incremental growth may be greater when androgens are used in conjunction with growth hormone. However, the possibility of accelerated bone maturation with androgen therapy requires close monitoring of skeletal age. Because neither recombinant growth hormone nor androgen therapy has been approved by the U.S. Food and Drug Administration for treatment of short stature in Turner's patients, experts recommend that treatment with these agents only be undertaken in association with physicians conducting approved research protocols.

When estrogen replacement is given to Turner's syndrome patients, low doses (i.e., 0.3 mg conjugated estrogen or 5 μg ethinyl estradiol) are used initially to begin breast development without accelerating epiphyseal closure. The rate of further estrogen dose increase will depend on the patient's age and skeletal status, as indicated by bone age, which should be determined annually once therapy is begun. Younger adolescents (those under age 13) may be maintained on 0.3 mg conjugated estrogens for up to 2 years before increasing to 0.625 mg conjugated estrogens. At this point, menses usually ensue, and progestin is added. Because higher doses of estrogen usually will be necessary to complete breast development, the dose of estrogen is increased after this point every 6 months to a year to the equivalent of 1.25 mg conjugated estrogens daily, always accompanied by cyclic progestin. Once final height is achieved, estrogen treatment regimens are the same as those discussed earlier (Table 1).

Rare pregnancies have been reported in Turner's patients, usually those with mosaic karyotypes. In general, however, Turner's patients are incapable of producing genetic offspring. The patient and her parents should be advised that because of recent advances in reproductive technology, future childbearing may be possible using oocyte donation.

Testicular Regression and Testicular Enzyme Deficiencies

Individuals with this rare form of hypergonadotropic hypogonadism are genetic males who lack testosterone because of a gonadal enzyme deficiency or early gonadal regression (vanishing testes). They appear female and present with sexual immaturity and primary amenorrhea. However, pelvic examination reveals a blind vaginal pouch and absent uterus. FSH levels are elevated, and XY karotype confirms the diagnosis.

Treatment includes surgical removal of the intraabdominal gonads and estrogen replacement therapy as outlined previously. Obviously, one needs to be judicious in counseling these patients in order to avoid gender confusion. Classic practice has been to tell the patient that her reproductive organs never developed and to avoid discussion of genetic sex. However, this may not be appropriate for all patients, and discussion must be tailored to the individual.

Testicular Feminization (Androgen Insensitivity)

Individuals with this disorder are chromosomal males who have normal internal male gonads but lack normal androgen receptor function. Despite circulating male levels of testosterone, the wolffian ducts fail to develop and the external genitalia develop as female. Because there is normal gonadal production of müllerian-inhibiting factor (MIF), the müllerian system regresses during development, leaving only fibrous remnants of internal genitalia.

At puberty, a normal growth spurt occurs and breasts develop as a result of low levels of estrogens, which are produced directly by the gonad and made peripherally from androgen conversion. Because puberty appears to be progressing normally, these individuals do not usually present until late in adolescence, when the expected menses never arrive. The patient at presentation appears to be a normally

---

TABLE 1. Suggested Estrogen Replacement Regimens

- Conjugated estrogens (Premarin) 0.625–1.25 mg on days 1–25
  plus
  Medroxyprogesterone acetate (Provera) 5–10 mg on days 14–25

- 17β-estradiol (Estrace) 1–2 mg on days 1–25
  plus
  Medroxyprogesterone acetate (Provera) 5–10 mg on days 14–25

- Oral contraceptive (30–35 μg estrogen with nonandrogenic progestin)

- Estraderm patch (0.05–1 mg/d) twice weekly for days 1–25
  plus
  Medroxyprogesterone acetate (Provera) 5–10 mg on days 14–25

developed female of normal height but with absent or sparse axillary and pubic hair. Pelvic examination reveals an absent or shortened vagina. Confirmatory laboratory studies include XY karyotype and male testosterone levels.

Consultation with a gynecologist should be made at this point to plan for gonadectomy and long-term estrogen replacement. The male gonads, which may be either intraabdominal or inguinal, carry a 20% risk of malignant degeneration and should be removed. Classic teaching has been that gonadectomy be deferred until after full height and breast development have occurred (usually 16 to 18 years of age). However, a number of patients have now been described with incomplete forms of testicular feminization who become virilized during puberty. For this reason, some experts recommend gonadectomy at the time of diagnosis, regardless of the pubertal status of the patient. Once the gonads have been removed, long-term estrogen replacement should begin. Typical treatment regimens are 0.625 to 1.25 mg conjugated estrogens or 1 to 2 mg 17β-estradiol daily. (Lower initial doses may be used to induce breast development in individuals whose gonads were removed before puberty.) Because no uterus is present, cyclic progestin need not be added. Patients should be counseled that future pregnancy will not be possible. The decision to discuss genetic sex is best made on an individual basis and is usually deferred until after adolescence.

Mullerian Agenesis (Rokitansky-Kuster-Hauser Syndrome)

This is a fairly common disorder, found in 15% of patients presenting with primary amenorrhea. Affected individuals are genetic females who have normal functioning ovaries but lack a vagina and uterus as a result of anomalous development of the müllerian system. They classically present either in late adolescence with primary amenorrhea or in early adulthood after unsuccessfully attempting intercourse. On examination, these young women are of normal height and exhibit normal breast and axillary hair development. Although the external genitalia are normal, the vagina either is absent or forms a blind pouch of variable length. Karyotype confirms a normal XX chromosomal complement, and excludes rare forms of incomplete androgen insensitivity or pseudohermaphroditism.

Once the diagnosis is made, intravenous pyelography should be performed because of the 15% to 40% incidence of associated renal abnormalities in this disorder. Cardiac and skeletal examination detects associated disorders in as many as 12% of patients.

Careful counseling is the key to helping these young women maintain self-esteem and a healthy body image. Rather than being told they were "born without a vagina," they should be told that their vagina is "not completely developed." A gynecologic specialist should be consulted early in the course of the evaluation to plan for the creation of a functioning vagina once the patient has achieved full growth and is psychologically prepared. The classic operation has been the *McIndoe split-thickness graft*. However, the *Williams procedure*, which combines a very simple surgical procedure with postoperative dilators, is now the usual first-line surgical approach. The nonsurgical *Frank procedure* involves the use of progressively larger surgical dilators to create a functioning vagina. A racing bicycle seat with attached dilators works well for many patients. The long-term success of either method depends on patient involvement in learning how to maintain the created vagina. Other operative approaches are used more often outside the United States and include vaginoplasty using either intestine *(Baldwin method)* or peritoneum *(Rothman method)* and abdominal suspension of the vaginal pouch combined with dilatation *(Veschetti method)*. Although combined perineal and laparoscopic approaches to vaginoplasty may gain popularity in the future, they are not widely used at present.

Because these patients have normally functioning ovaries, hormonal replacement is not necessary. Although individuals with müllerian agenesis cannot carry a pregnancy or give birth, they should be counseled that genetic offspring may be possible through ovum retrieval, in vitro fertilization, and embryo transfer to the uterus of a volunteer surrogate.

Outlet Obstruction

This category includes young women with imperforate hymen, transverse vaginal septum, or other genital tract anomalies that lead to obstruction of menstrual effluent. These patients often present with a history of normal Tanner development, amenorrhea, and cyclic pelvic pain. Pelvic examination or ultrasonography reveals a pelvic mass, usually a distended vagina or hematocolpos.

Treatment of a transverse vaginal septum or imperforate hymen involves simple surgical excision of the obstructing membrane. If the obstruction occurs as a result of cervical agenesis or other anomalies, such as bicornuate uterus with a blind horn, repair is more complicated. The surgery should be performed by a gynecologist or surgeon with expertise in the repair of congenital genital anomalies.

The coexistence of renal and müllerian anomalies should prompt a thorough evaluation of the urinary tract in patients with obstruction due to anomalous genital tract development. Future pregnancy rates vary, depending on the nature of the obstruction and repair, ranging from 25% to 100%. Patients presenting with obstruction due to imperforate hymen can be reassured that associated abnormalities are rare and that reproductive function is expected to be normal.

Abnormalities of the Hypothalamic-Pituitary Axis

When pubertal development and pelvic anatomy are normal yet menses has not occurred, there is usually a disturbance in the hypothalamic-pituitary axis. Possible causes include systemic disease, pituitary adenomas, constitutional delay, exercise-induced amenorrhea, and anorexia nervosa. The management of these patients is identical to that of patients with secondary amenorrhea.

Secondary Amenorrhea and Oligomenorrhea

Secondary amenorrhea is defined as the absence of menstruation for at least three cycles or at least 6 months in females who have already experienced regular menstruation. Oligomenorrhea is defined as four or fewer menses per year. Although menses are often irregular in young adolescents, they should stabilize within 1 to 2 years from the time of menarche. Amenorrhea or oligomenorrhea occurring more than 2 years after menarche should be considered abnormal and warrants investigation and treatment. Oligomenorrhea or amenorrhea accompanied by galactorrhea or hirsutism should be investigated regardless of how much time has passed since menarche.

The diagnostic evaluation of secondary amenorrhea is summarized in Figure 2. After one excludes pregnancy, a thyroid-stimulating hormone (TSH) and prolactin level should be obtained to rule out thryoid disease and pituitary adenoma. Androgen level determinations are also indicated if the patient is hirsute. If the initial TSH level is elevated, the patient should be referred for thyroid replacement therapy. Normal menses should resume once the patient becomes euthyroid. Hirsute patients with elevated dehydroepiandrosterone sulfate (DHEAS) or testosterone levels need further evaluation to rule out ovarian or adrenal tumors, congenital adrenal hyperplasia, and Cushing's syndrome. Consultation with a pediatric endocrinologist or gynecologist is recommended at this point.

If TSH and prolactin levels are normal, a progestational challenge is performed to evaluate estrogen status. One frequently used regimen for this test is medroxyprogesterone acetate (Provera, 5 to 10 mg for 10 days). This regimen results in a withdrawal bleeding in the patient with an estrogen-primed uterus, establishing the diagnosis of anovulation, usually due to *polycystic ovarian syndrome* (PCOS). Absence of a withdrawal bleed mandates determining an FSH level to distinguish patients with hypothalamic dysfunction from those with ovarian failure. If withdrawal bleeding does not occur and there is a history of previous uterine curettage, a combined estrogen-progestin regimen should be given (conjugated estrogens, 2.5 mg daily for 25 days, with medroxyprogesterone acetate, 5 to 10 mg, on days 14 to 25). Failure to bleed after this is indicative of Asherman syndrome, and the patient should be referred to a gynecologist for further evaluation and therapy.

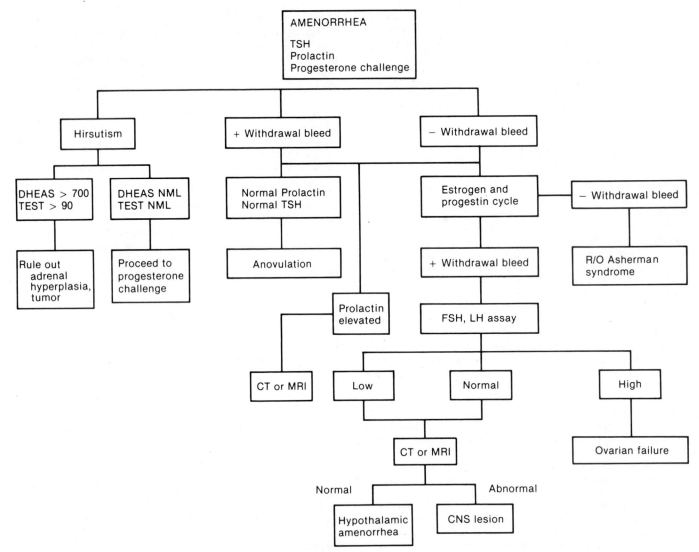

FIGURE 2. Evaluation of secondary amenorrhea. TSH, thyroid-stimulating hormone; DHEAS, dehydroepiandrosterone sulfate; FSH, follicle-stimulating hormone; LH, luteinizing hormone; R/O, rule out; CT, computed tomography; MRI, magnetic resonance imaging; CNS, central nervous system; NML, normal. (Modified from Speroff L, et al: Clinical Gynecologic Endocrinology and Infertility, 4th ed. Baltimore, Williams & Wilkins, 1989:178. Copyright 1989 Leon Speroff, MD)

Pregnancy

The young woman who presents with amenorrhea must be considered pregnant until proven otherwise. It is best to have a low threshold of suspicion for ordering pregnancy testing because the menstrual history may be unreliable in the adolescent patient. The possibility of an ectopic gestation should be considered in any pregnant patient who gives a history of spotting or pelvic pain, however minimal, or if examination of the pregnant patient reveals a normal-sized uterus, adnexal mass, or adnexal tenderness. If an ectopic pregnancy is suspected, immediate referral to a gynecologist or emergency room can be lifesaving.

If pregnancy is diagnosed, sensitive, nondirective counseling should take place immediately, and appropriate referrals should be made. The teenager should be encouraged, when possible, to inform her parents. For many reasons, teenagers frequently delay obtaining prenatal care or do not obtain care at all. Those who desire pregnancy termination often delay until it is too late. Judicious and persistent follow-up is important in ensuring that the teenager actually keeps her referral appointments.

Polycystic Ovarian Syndrome

The most common cause of anovulation in the postmenarchal adolescent is polycystic ovarian syndrome (PCOS). PCOS is a term applied to a heterogeneous group of disorders distinguished by anovulation due to asynchronous production of gonadotropins and ovarian hormones. In its classic presentation, PCOS is characterized by oligoamenorrhea, hirsutism, obesity, and infertility. The ultrasonographic ovarian appearance is that of multiple thick-walled cysts, and endocrinologic evaluation reveals elevated levels of ovarian androgens, hyperinsulinemia, and increased LH/FSH ratio. However, there is significant individual variation in the clinical expression of PCOS. A small but important subset of individuals with PCOS has the constellation of hyperandrogenism, insulin resistance, and acanthosis nigricans, the so-called Hair-AN syndrome.

The etiology of PCOS remains unclear, although any explanation as to its origins must account for the basic aberrations seen in LH and FSH levels. Because PCOS typically presents at menarche, it has been theorized that the disorder may be the result of what has been termed an "exaggerated adrenarche." According to this theory, peripheral conversion of excess adrenal androgens at puberty leads to elevated estrogen levels, which in turn institute an elevated LH production by the pituitary that is characteristic of PCOS. Other theories focus on the action of insulin growth factors as the primary initiators of elevated ovarian production. Whatever the initial event, local ovarian androgens inhibit follicular development and ovulation. Conversion of ovarian androgens leads to elevated peripheral estrogen levels, which perpetuates the abnormal LH secretion characteristic of the disorder. Persistent anovulation results in prolonged periods of unopposed stimulation of the uterine endometrium, leading to breakthrough bleeding, prolonged and heavy menses, and long-term risk for endometrial hyperplasia and malignancy.

Adolescents with PCOS generally come to the attention of the clinician when they present with dysfunctional uterine bleeding (DUB). The clinical picture is one of amenorrhea interrupted by periods of heavy, often prolonged menses. Obesity is fairly common in these young women. Hirsutism is less frequent but, when present, must be evaluated thoroughly to rule out adrenal or ovarian hormone-producing neoplasms before attributing it to PCOS. Although FSH and LH levels may confirm the clinical diagnosis, they are not necessary. Neither is an ultrasound, since the polycystic appearance typically occurs only in those with long-standing anovulation and may not be present in younger adolescents with PCOS.

Oral contraceptives are the mainstay of treatment for PCOS and act in several ways in treating the manifestations of the disorder. By suppressing pituitary gonadotropins, they render the ovary quiescent, thus decreasing production of ovarian androgens. In addition, the progestin component of the oral contraceptive acts on the uterine endometrium to counteract the effects of prolonged endogenous estrogen and, over time, will result in lighter, shorter, more regular menses. Finally, the elevated levels of sex hormone-binding globulin induced by action of the oral contraceptive further decrease serum and tissue levels of free androgens and estrogens. A low-dose (30 to 35 μg) oral contraceptive is preferred. In patients with DUB, a higher-dose 50 μg pill with a strong progestin, such as Ovral or Demulen 1/50, can be very useful in gaining initial control over abnormal bleeding. (See later discussion of Dysfunctional Uterine Bleeding.)

The newer oral contraceptive formulations containing the synthetic progestins desogestrel and norgestimate have a theoretical advantage over older pill formulations. In vitro studies of these progestins show less binding to androgen receptors and increased progestin activity compared with levonorgestrel and norethindrone. However, there are at present no controlled clinical trials in the United States that demonstrate superior efficacy of the new progestins over the older preparations in treating either the hirsutism or menorrhaghia associated with PCOS.

More severe cases of hirsutism due to PCOS that do not respond to oral contraceptive therapy alone can be treated with antiandrogens, such as spironolactone 50 to 100 mg PO b.i.d. Oral contraceptive therapy should be continued in this case, both for continued androgen suppression and because spironolactone can be teratogenic to the developing male genital system. Gonadotropin-releasing hormone (GnRH) agonists, such as nafarelin, leuprolide, and buserelin, are an alternative to oral contraceptive therapy for ovarian suppression. However, the hypoestrogenic effects of these medications make them generally unsuitable for use in all but the most refractory cases of hirsutism.

Teenagers with PCOS who are not sexually active or who prefer not to take an oral contraceptive can be treated with cyclic progestin to induce menses and protect against the long-term risk of endometrial hyperplasia. This can be done one of two ways. For the first 10 days of each month, 10 mg of medroxyprogesterone acetate can be administered to induce regular menses. Alternatively, 10 days of medroxyprogesterone acetate can be administered every 3 months in the absence of spontaneous menses. This latter regimen has the advantage of allowing for the return of normal menses, which will occur in 60%

to 70% of patients who present in early adolescence with amenorrhea due to immaturity of the hypothalamic-pituitary-ovarian axis.

Although patients with PCOS may experience infertility, the overall prognosis for a future successful pregnancy is good. A small but significant percentage will conceive spontaneously. Approximately 75% of remaining patients will ovulate after treatment with clomiphene citrate (Clomid).

Hyperprolactinemia

It is estimated that 5% to 10% of patients with both amenorrhea and elevated serum prolactin and 25% of those with amenorrhea, galactorrhea, and high prolactin levels have pituitary adenomas. Therefore, all patients with elevated prolactin should undergo CNS imaging of the pituitary either by computed tomography (CT) scan or magnetic resonance imaging (MRI). Prolactinomas are classified as either microadenomas (<1 cm) or macroadenomas (>1 cm). Less than 5% of microadenomas progress to macroadenomas. Other causes of hyperprolactinemia include medications, stress, breast stimulation, hypothyroidism, and renal failure. Psychotropic medications, in particular, are a common cause of drug-induced hyperprolactinemia and galactorrhea.

Hyperprolactinemia from any cause results in hypoestrogenemia, and these patients are at real risk for osteoporosis if not treated. Treatment has several goals: normalization of prolactin levels, return of normal estrogen levels, resumption of normal menses, and preservation of fertility.

Primary treatment of pituitary adenomas used to be surgical, namely, transsphenoidal resection. Rates of response were as high as 80%. However, *cure rates* were only 10% to 40% because tumor regrowth and recurrence of hyperprolactinemia were common. As a result, medical therapy with bromocriptine (Parlodel) is generally recommended for all microadenomas. Recent evidence suggests that bromocriptine therapy alone is probably appropriate for most macroadenomas and should be attempted for at least 6 months before consideration of surgical resection.

Bromocriptine is a dopamine agonist that inhibits prolactin release by the pituitary, resulting in the shrinkage of pituitary lactotrophs. Approximately 80% to 90% of patients with microadenomas respond to bromocriptine therapy. Since effects of this therapy include nausea, headache, and orthostatic hypotension. Therefore, therapy is begun with low doses (1.25 mg), which are taken only at bedtime. If this is tolerated, the dose is gradually increased over several weeks until appropriate reduction in prolactin levels occurs. Final therapeutic doses range from 2.5 to 15 mg daily, usually taken in two divided doses. Prolactin levels should be measured frequently, and the patient should be maintained on the lowest dose that will produce normal prolactin levels. Menses usually resume in 6 to 8 weeks; suppression of galactorrhea may not occur for several months.

Administration of bromocriptine via the vagina can provide higher sustained levels of circulating drug at lower doses because of increased absorption and avoidance of first-pass enterohepatic circulation. For patients unable to tolerate the side effects of bromocriptine, vaginal administration may allow for normalization of prolactin levels at lower drug dosages, thus reducing potential gastrointestinal side effects associated with higher oral doses. The initial dose is 1.25 mg inserted at bedtime into the posterior vaginal fornix. As with oral therapy, prolactin levels are monitored frequently, and the dose is increased gradually until euprolactinemia is attained.

Some patients require estrogen replacement therapy along with bromocriptine for menses to occur. It should be remembered that once prolactin levels normalize, ovulation will usually return and contraception will be necessary. The decision whether and when to stop therapy is individualized and controversial. Tumor regrowth will occur in the majority of cases.

There is a subgroup of patients with hyperprolactinemia and amenorrhea who have no visible tumor on CT scan or MRI. These young women with functional hyperprolactinemia are still at risk for osteoporosis secondary to hypoestrogenemia. Treatment is either bromocriptine, as detailed previously, or estrogen replacement therapy if bromocriptine is not used. Most of these patients respond to very low doses of bromocriptine, such as 1.25 mg daily. If the patient elects not to take any medication, close observation with periodic bone mass measurements and calcium supplementation is indicated.

Prognosis for future pregnancy in patients with hyperprolactinemia is good. Bromocriptine therapy usually results in ovulation. The decision to continue bromocriptine therapy during pregnancy depends on the size of the adenoma, visual field measurements, and the presence or absence of associated symptoms, such as headache.

Ovarian Failure (Hypergonadotropic Amenorrhea)

A typical patient in this category is the young woman who has had her ovaries removed as the result of malignancy or who has experienced ovarian failure secondary to cancer chemotherapy or radiation therapy for Hodgkin's disease. In the absence of such a history, patients with premature ovarian failure should have a karyotype determined, since premature ovarian failure in adolescence may be due to variants of gonadal dysgenesis or Turner's mosaicism. If any portion of a Y chromosome is present, gonadectomy should be performed. Patients with normal chromosomes should be referred for further evaluation to rule out autoimmune and multiple endocrine disorders.

Treatment consists of lifelong estrogen replacement. A typical regimen is 0.625 to 1.25 mg conjugated estrogens on days 1 to 25, with 5 to 10 mg medroxyprogesterone acetate added on days 12 to 25. Note that 12 days a month of progestin therapy is now being recommended rather than the traditional 10 days as a result of recent evidence that longer duration of progestin offers better protection against endometrial cancer. An oral contraceptive is an alternative estrogen replacement regimen and, for many teenagers, is simpler to take. Periodic bone density measurements taken during the first several years of therapy ensure the adequacy of estrogen replacement.

Because pregnancy may occur in as many as 10% of patients with premature ovarian failure, contraception is advised for those not taking an oral contraceptive. Prognosis for future fertility is poor, but pregnancy may be accomplished in patients who elect to undergo oocyte donation with embryo transfer to their intact uterus. Rare pregnancies have been reported after high-dose estrogen in combination with exogenous gonadotropins has been given to patients with ovarian failure and intact ovaries.

Exercise-Induced Amenorrhea

As many as 50% of teens involved in competitive athletics experience hypothalamic amenorrhea. Ballet dancers also commonly experience this form of amenorrhea. Although the etiology of this disorder is not well understood, it may result from a complex interplay of low body fat percentage and psychologic stress. Elevated prolactin levels are often found in these individuals and may contribute as well. Whatever the cause, young women with this disorder are estrogen-deficient and should, therefore, be treated.

The simplest way to treat exercise-induced amenorrhea is to decrease the amount of exercise. If amenorrhea persists or if the patient is unwilling to curtail her training, estrogen replacement therapy should be begun because these women are hypoestrogenic and at risk for osteoporosis. Compliance with estrogen replacement therapy can be a problem in the serious athlete, and fractures in such individuals have been reported. Periodic bone density measurements documenting bone loss may help to persuade such individuals to comply with treatment. All patients with exercise-induced amenorrhea should be encouraged to increase their calcium intake, either by diet or by supplements, to 1500 mg daily. However, one must emphasize to the patient that unless estrogen therapy is added, the use of calcium alone probably does nothing to help maintain bone mass.

Anorexia Nervosa

Anorexia nervosa is a potentially life-threatening disorder characterized by abnormal eating habits, severe weight loss, and distorted body image. Although the exact nature of the hypothalamic amenorrhea that occurs in most patients with anorexia nervosa is unclear, these patients are almost always estrogen deficient.

The complex medical and psychologic problems associated with anorexia nervosa mandate a team approach to management of patients with this disorder, employing psychiatric counseling, close medical supervision, nutritional consultation, and estrogen replacement therapy. Estrogen replacement can be given as conjugated estrogens (0.625 to 1.25 mg on days 1 to 25, with the addition of 10 mg medroxyprogesterone acetate on days 12 to 25). Alternatively, an oral contraceptive can be used. Menses will usually return spontaneously once normal weight is achieved. Chronic estrogen replacement, calcium supplementation, and periodic bone density measurements are indicated for the young woman whose anorexia persists for more than a year.

Dysmenorrhea

Dysmenorrhea, or painful menstruation, is the most common gynecologic problem in the adolescent female and the leading cause of school absenteeism in this population. *Primary dysmenorrhea* is defined as painful menses with no identifiable pelvic pathology. *Secondary dysmenorrhea* refers to painful menses resulting from a pelvic abnormality, such as endometriosis or pelvic inflammatory disease (PID). A careful pelvic examination, including rectovaginal examination, should be performed in the adolescent presenting with dysmenorrhea to exlude pelvic pathology before initiating therapy for primary dysmenorrhea. Failure of treatment for presumed primary dysmenorrhea warrants repeated evaluation for pelvic pathology and referral to a gynecologist.

Most dysmenorrhea during adolescence is primary. Because it occurs almost exclusively in ovulatory cycles, it typically begins several months after menarche and may worsen gradually as ovulatory cycles become established. Although the etiology of dysmenorrhea is not completely understood, almost all of the symptoms of primary dysmenorrhea can be explained by the action of uterine prostaglandins. For this reason, therapy of primary dysmenorrhea aims to decrease prostaglandin production by the endometrium.

Prostaglandin synthetase inhibitors (PGIs) are the first-line treatment for mild dysmenorrhea in the adolescent who is not sexually active. These medications work by blocking the production of prostaglandins within the endometrium. A wide range of PGIs is available, although not all classes are suitable for treatment of dysmenorrhea. Most patients experience significant relief with the fenamate and propionic acid derivatives without untoward side effects. Some of the more commonly used regimens are outlined in Table 2. Because of side effects, indomethacin, phenylbutazone, and oxyphenylbutazone should be avoided. Aspirin has been shown to be no more effective than placebo in relieving dysmenorrhea.

Treatment with a PGI should be initiated at the onset of the menstrual flow and continued for the duration of symptoms. Because most of the newer PGIs have a rapid onset of action, there is no need to begin treatment before the onset of menses. If there is no response,

TABLE 2. Prostaglandin Synthetase Inhibitors Effective in the Treatment of Primary Dysmenorrhea

DRUG	DOSE
Fenamates	
Meclofenamate sodium (Meclomen)	100 mg t.i.d.
Mefenamic acid (Ponstel)	500 mg initially, then 250 mg t.i.d.
Propionic Acid Derivatives	
Ibuprofen (Advil, Motrin)	400 mg q.i.d.
Naproxen sodium (Anaprox DS)	550 mg t.i.d.
Naproxen (Naprosyn)	500 mg initially, then 250 mg q.i.d.
Ketoprofen (Orudis)	25–50 mg q.i.d.

the initial dose can be increased. Switching to a different class of PGI may also be effective. If this fails, the oral contraceptive should be considered.

The oral contraceptive is effective in more than 90% of patients with primary dysmenorrhea and is the treatment of choice for the sexually active teenager. It acts by preventing ovarian stimulation of endometrial prostaglandins and by decreasing the total amount of endometrium available for prostaglandin production. Any low-dose (30 to 35 μg) pill can be used. Because the reduction in prostaglandin production is cumulative over time, the maximal effect of the oral contraceptive may not be seen for several months. If symptoms persist after several months, a PGI can be added. Failure of medical treatment at this point warrants referral to a gynecologist for further evaluation and possible laparoscopy. Consideration should also be given to the possibility that psychologic factors may be involved in the etiology of the patient's pain.

Transcutaneous electrical nerve stimulation (TENS) is undergoing investigation as a treatment for dysmenorrhea. TENS most likely works as a pure analgesic without directly affecting the activity or production of endometrial prostaglandins. Although still experimental, TENS has few reported side effects and may be an alternative therapy for those patients with dysmenorrhea who for some reason are unable or unwilling to take oral contraceptives or PGIs.

Dysfunctional Uterine Bleeding

DUB is defined as abnormal endometrial bleeding occurring in the absence of structural pelvic pathology. In the adolescent, DUB is usually the result of anovulation secondary to immaturity of the hypothalamic-pituitary-ovarian axis. Prolonged periods of anovulation lead to an overestrogenized endometrium lacking the progesterone-induced stability and control of sloughing that normally occurs with ovulatory menses. The clinical presentation is that of prolonged periods of amenorrhea interspersed with prolonged heavy menses. Over time, bleeding may begin to occur every 1 to 2 weeks and can be life threatening.

DUB is a diagnosis of exclusion. Therefore, all patients presenting with abnormal vaginal bleeding should have a careful history and thorough pelvic examination (including a Papanicolaou smear, wet mount, and screening for *Neisseria gonorrhoeae* and *Chlamydia*) to rule out pelvic pathology, such as trauma, genital tract malignancy, vaginitis, cervicitis, and pelvic inflammatory disease. Pregnancy should always be considered in the differential diagnosis of abnormal vaginal bleeding. Bleeding disorders (e.g., von Willebrand disease and idiopathic thrombocytopenic purpura) should be ruled out when DUB presents at menarche or is associated with significant hemorrhage or anemia.

The management of the patient with DUB depends on the severity of the bleeding and the level of anemia and is summarized in Table 3.

Mild DUB

DUB presenting without acute hemorrhage or anemia may be managed with observation and reassurance only. However, most adolescents and their parents would prefer some form of treatment, given the inconvenience and anxiety accompanying unpredictable menses. These patients can be offered the regimen described next for patients with moderate DUB.

Moderate DUB

This category includes patients presenting with mild anemia (hemogloblin >10 g/dl) but no acute bleeding. If the patient is sexually active, an oral contraceptive is the treatment of choice and should be prescribed in the routine fashion. Any monophasic low-dose pill can be used.

An alternative to oral contraceptive therapy is the use of cyclic progestin in the teenager who is not sexually active. Medroxyprogesterone acetate (10 mg) is given for 5 to 7 days every 35 to 40 days in the absence of spontaneous menses. This regimen allows for the

TABLE 3. Management of Dysfunctional Uterine Bleeding (DUB)

Mild DUB: inconvenient, unpredictable bleeding/Hb > 12 g/dl
Reassurance
Fe supplementation
Consider oral contraceptive
Reevaluate every 3–6 mo

Moderate DUB: irregular, prolonged, heavy bleeding/Hb > 10 g/dl
Hormonal therapy:
    Medroxyprogesterone acetate (Provera) (10 mg/d for 5–7 d q35–40d)
       or
    Oral contraceptives
Fe supplementation
Menstrual calendar
Reevaluate in 1–2 mo

Severe DUB: irregular, heavy prolonged bleeding/Hb < 10 g/dl
Not actively bleeding
    Oral contraceptive
    Fe supplementation
    Reevaluate in 1–3 mo
Active mild to moderate bleeding
    Ovral, 1 tablet q6h for 24–48 h, tapered over the following week to 1 tablet daily
    Fe supplementation
    Reevaluate in 1 wk, then in 1–3 mo
Active heavy bleeding
    Hospitalize
    Transfuse if necessary
    Hormonal therapy:
        Ovral, 1 tablet q6h for 24–48 h, tapered over the week to 1 tablet daily *or* conjugated estrogens (Premarin), 20–25 mg IV q4h for maximum 6 doses with concurrent Ovral, 1 tablet q6h, tapered over the following week to 1 tablet daily
            followed by
        Oral contraceptive for 6–12 mo (consider continuous regimen, i.e., without placebos, until Hb normalizes)
    D & C if hormonal therapy fails
    Reevaluate 1–2 wk and 1 mo after discharge, then in 1–3 mo until menstrual pattern and Hb stable

Adapted from Muram D: Vaginal bleeding in childhood and adolescence. *In:* Menstrual Cycle Disorders. Obstet Gynecol Clin North Am 17:405, 1990.
Hb, hemoglobin; D & C, dilatation and curettage.

recognition of the return of ovulatory menses. However, progestin alone may not halt DUB if it has been prolonged. Estrogen often is needed as well to restore endometrial tissue where severe desquamation has occurred. An oral contraceptive, therefore, provides the best treatment in such situations. Iron therapy should be added to either regimen, and the patient should be reevaluated frequently.

Severe DUB

Patients who present with Hb levels lower than 10 g/dl but who are1 not actively bleeding should be placed on an oral contraceptive and given iron supplementation. Because prolonged bleeding may result in little residual endometrial tissue on which progestin may exert its organizational effect, a high-estrogen, high-progestin oral contraceptive (e.g., Ovral, Demulen 1/50) should be used. The patient should be reevaluated frequently to ensure the efficacy of treatment.

Patients presenting with mild to moderate bleeding and anemia can usually be managed as outpatients with intensive oral contraceptive therapy. A high-estrogen, high-progestin oral contraceptive can be given (one tablet every 6 hours for 24 to 48 hours). Bleeding should diminish or stop within 12 to 24 hours on this regimen. The patient should be warned that this regimen may cause nausea, and appropriate antiemetics should be prescribed when necessary. Over the next week, the dose can be gradually tapered to one tablet daily for the next several months, followed by a monophasic low-dose (30 to 35 μg) pill for another 3 to 6 months. At this point, if the patient does not require contraception, the oral contraceptive can be discontinued, and bleeding can be reassessed.

Patients presenting with life-threatening bleeding or severe anemia require hospitalization, possible transfusion, and high-dose estrogen therapy. Premarin (20 to 25 mg) can be given intravenously ever 4 hours for a maximum of six doses. Because the endometrium resulting from such therapy is inherently fragile, concurrent progestin must be given. This can be in the form of an oral contraceptive (e.g., Ovral one tablet every 6 hours for 24 to 48 hours), which is then tapered gradually to once a day dosage. Alternatively, medroxyprogesterone acetate (10 mg every 12 hours) can be used initially and replaced with an oral contraceptive in 24 to 48 hours, which is then tapered gradually to once a day. Bleeding that does not respond to intravenous estrogen requires immediate dilatation and curettage (D & C).

The first menses following hormonal therapy for DUB is usually heavy and may worsen a preexisting anemia. In the patient with a low hemoglobin level whose bleeding has stopped, the oral contraceptive can be given in a continuous fashion (i.e., without placebos) to prevent withdrawal bleeding. Once the hemoglobin level is increased, the patient can be allowed to cycle regularly on the oral contraceptive.

DUB persists for up to 2 years in 60% of patients, 4 years in 50%, and 10 years in 30%. Most patients with a prolonged history of DUB have PCOS and should be maintained on either cyclic progestin or an oral contraceptive.

GONORRHEA, CHLAMYDIAL INFECTION, AND PELVIC INFLAMMATORY DISEASE

Gonorrhea and chlamydial infections are occurring in epidemic proportions in adolescents, most likely as a result of increasing sexual activity in this population. The serious sequelae of these infections, if untreated, include pelvic inflammatory disease, infertility, Fitz-Hugh-Curtis syndrome, ectopic pregnancy, and pelvic adhesions.

Gonorrhea

The majority of reported cases of infection with *Neisseria gonorrhoeae* occur in adolescent females. Overall, 3% to 7% of teenage females attending family planning clinics test positive for gonorrhea. Rates may be higher in certain populations, such as indigent teens.

Symptoms suggestive of gonorrheal infection include vaginal discharge, dysuria, and vaginal burning or irritation. However, the majority of gonorrheal infections in the adolescent female are asymptomatic, and, therefore, screening for gonorrhea is recommended on a twice-yearly basis for all sexually active teenagers. Suggestive physical findings include mucopurulent cervical discharge, cervical friability, and inflammation of the endocervical glands. Specimens for screening should be taken from the endocervix. The addition of a rectal culture increases the yield of detection by 5%. Pharyngeal cultures probably do not add significantly to the detection rate but should be performed if the history or physical examination is suggestive.

Although culture remains the gold standard for gonorrhea testing, difficulties in specimen handling can significantly decrease its sensitivity in some settings, and results are generally not available for 48 hours. DNA hybridization (e.g., Gen-Probe) is a rapid screening alternative to gonorrhea culture. The sensitivity and specificity of the Gen-Probe assay are approximately 90% to 98%, respectively. Other rapid screening tests for gonorrhea include monoclonal antibody tests (e.g., Phade bact GC [Omni]) fluorescent antibody tests (e.g., Syva [MicroTrak]), and rapid enzyme assay (e.g., Neisstrip, Gonochek II). All are useful as initial rapid screening tests in settings where culture is unavailable. Culture confirmation of positive screening tests in low-prevalence populations is recommended. It should also be noted that none of the nonculture techniques tests for antibiotic resistance.

Treatment for uncomplicated gonorrheal infection should be given to any adolescent female with a positive screening culture. Patients with a history or physical findings suggestive of gonorrheal infection,

or who report sexual contact with an individual with suspected urethritis, should be cultured *and* treated at the same visit. Patients who present with PID should be cultured and hospitalized for intravenous antibiotic therapy. All cases of gonorrhea must be reported to the state for contact tracking and notification.

Table 4 summarizes the current Centers for Disease Control (CDC) recommendations for the treatment of uncomplicated gonorrheal infection. These recommendations have undergone major changes in the past decade as a result of the emergence of antibiotic-resistant organisms. Most large urban centers now report endemic levels of penicillinase-producing *N. gonorrhoeae* (PPNG), tetracycline-resistant *N. gonorrhoeae* (TRNG), and organisms with chromosomally mediated resistance to multiple antibiotics (CMRNG). For this reason, the CDC recommends ceftriaxone as first-line therapy for uncomplicated gonorrheal cervicitis. To date, no ceftriaxone-resistant gonococcus has been isolated, and ceftriaxone has the added advantage of being effective against incubating syphilis. Because recent research has shown that 125 mg ceftriaxone is equally effective to the previously recommended 250 mg dose, current CDC recommendations are to use the lower dose as first-line therapy for uncomplicated gonorrhea infection. It should be noted, however, that ceftriaxone is currently available only in 250 mg dose units.

Cefixime (Suprax) 400 mg orally in a single dose is a new and welcome option for treatment of gonorrhea infections in adolescents. Although cefixime is similar to ceftriaxone in its antimicrobial spectrum, bactericidal levels are not as high. However, the oral mode of administration provides a distinct advantage over ceftriaxone; administration under direct supervision will guarantee compliance. It is not known whether cefixime can cure incubating syphilis.

Spectinomycin is a second-line regimen reserved for patients allergic to cephalosporins. Spectinomycin resistance has been reported in some areas, so it is best used in conjunction with culture and sensitivity testing. Additional cephalosporins that have shown activity against the gonococcus are listed in Table 4.

The quinolones, although recommended for treatment of both gonorrhea and *Chlamydia* infections, have been associated with arthropathy and are contraindicated in adolescents age 17 and under. The two recommended quinolone regimens for treatment of uncomplicated gonorrheal cervicitis in adolescents over age 17 are (1) ciprofloxacin

---

TABLE 4. Treatment of Uncomplicated Gonorrhea Cervicitis in Adolescents

Recommended Regimens
Ceftriaxone 125 mg IM in a single dose
or
Cefixime (Suprax) 400 mg PO in a single dose
plus
Treatment for coinfection with *Chlamydia* (see Table 5)

Alternative IM Regimens
Spectinomycin 2 g IM in a single dose
or
Ceftizoxime 500 mg IM in a single dose
plus
Treatment for coinfection with *Chlamydia* (see Table 5)
or

Alternative Oral Regimens
Cefuroxime axetil 1 g PO in a single dose
or
Cefpodoxime proxetil 200 mg PO in a single dose
plus
Treatment for coinfection with *Chlamydia* (see Table 5)
Note: Only ceftriaxone has been shown to be effective against incubating syphillis. Other approved cephalosporins include cefotaxime 500 mg IM, cefotetan 1 g IM, and cefoxitan 2 g IM. Resistance to spectinomycin exists in certain geographic areas.

500 mg orally in a single dose and (2) ofloxacin 400 mg orally in a single dose.

Depending on the geographic location, the incidence of concomitant infection with *Chlamydia* can be as high as 60%. *For this reason, all patients undergoing treatment for gonorrhea must receive treatment for chlamydial infection as well, even when only gonorrhea is isolated.*

All adolescents receiving treatment for gonorrhea should be screened for syphilis and counseled regarding human immunodeficiency virus (HIV) risks, HIV testing, and condom use. Hepatitis B vaccination is recommended in all adolescents and should be instituted at this time if it has not already been accomplished. Screening for hepatitis B antibody before vaccination may be useful in those adolescents who are at risk for having already acquired the infection. Although the diagnosis of gonorrhea mandates a report to the state for contact tracing and notification, attempt should be made by the provider to assist the patient in having her partner(s) treated. The patient should be advised to refrain from sexual activity until both she and her partner have been treated. If CDC recommended regimens are used for treatment, a test of cure is not necessary. However, retesting 2 weeks to 1 month after treatment is recommended in order to detect reinfection from an untreated partner.

Chlamydia

Chlamydia trachomatis is the most common sexually transmitted organism in the United States. Among sexually active adolescent females, the incidence of chlamydial cervicitis ranges from 8% to 33% and is highest among inner-city teens attending family planning clinics. Any sexually active adolescent is at risk for chlamydial infection, although risk is highest in those who have multiple sexual partners, a history of gonorrhea, or a history of a partner with urethritis and in those who do not use barrier contraceptives. In addition, the finding of purulent cervical discharge associated with cervical friability—so-called mucopurulent cervicitis—is highly predictive of a positive culture for *C. trachomatis*. Most infections with *Chlamydia* in the female are asymptomatic, including *Chlamydia*-associated PID, which is notorious in this regard.

All sexually active adolecent females should be screened for chlamydial cervicitis twice yearly, and treatment should be given to any teenager with a positive screening test or hisory of possible exposure to an infected partner. Available screening tests for *Chlamydia* include *Chlamydia* culture, direct fluorescent antibody (DFA) tests (e.g., MicroTrak), enzyme immunoassay (e.g., Chlamydiazyme), DNA hybridization (e.g., Gen-Probe), and more recently, polymerase chain reaction (PCR) (e.g., Amplicor). *Chlamydia* culture, although still the gold standard for *Chlamydia* testing, is both timely and costly and has in many institutions been replaced by the more rapid and less expensive nonculture techniques. Although DFA tests have an advantage over other techniques by reporting the presence or absence of endocervical cells in the specimen, they are generally less sensitive than culture and the newer DNA techniques. Gen-Probe provides a highly sensitive, rapid, and inexpensive screening method for gonorrhea and *Chlamydia* using a single swab. Its sensitivity and specificity in sexually active adolescent populations are close to that of *Chlamydia* culture. However, the test can be problematic in screening low prevalence populations, where its positive predictive value can be as low as 50%. For this reason, culture is sometimes used to confirm positive results before treatment. In initial testing, PCR has equaled or exceeded culture in its sensitivity, with close to 100% specificity, and may eventually replace *Chlamydia* culture as the gold standard. PCR testing of urine holds promise for diagnosing chlamydial urethritis in both men and women.

September 1993 CDC recommendations for the treatment of *Chlamydia* cervicitis are outlined in Table 5. These differ from previous recommendations primarily in the addition of a single-dose, long-acting oral azolide antibiotic, azithromycin, to the list of preferred regimens. (Tetracycline is no longer recommended because of low compliance with its four times a day regimen.) Azithromycin appears

TABLE 5. Treatment of Uncomplicated Chlamydial Cervicitis in Adolescents

Recommended Regimens
Doxycycline 100 mg PO b.i.d. for 7 d
or
Azithromycin 1 g PO in a single dose

Alternative Regimens
Erythromycin base 500 mg PO q.i.d. for 7 d
or
Erythromycin ethylsuccinate 800 mg PO q.i.d. for 7 d
or
Sulfisoxazole 500 mg PO q.i.d. for 10 d
Note: Safety and efficacy of azithromycin in pregnancy and in adolescents under age 16 has not been established. Sulfisoxazole is the least desirable regimen because of its inferior efficacy.

to be similar to doxycycline in both efficacy and toxicity and has a distinct advantage in being single-dose therapy. It is considerably more expensive than both doxycycline and erythromycin and has not been approved for use in pregnancy or in adolescents under age 16. Despite its expense, it is the preferred treatment for adolescents age 16 and older because of its guaranteed compliance. Ofloxacin, a quinolone antibiotic, is approved for treatment of *Chlamydia* infection but is contraindicated in adolescents age 17 or under and in pregnancy. It is also expensive, and provides no advantage over doxycycline. For this reason, it has been omitted from Table 4. If used in adolescents over age 17, the dose is ofloxacin 300 mg PO b.i.d. for 7 days.

Because of concerns about antibiotic potential for teratogenicity, some practitioners routinely obtain a negative pregnancy test before treating *Chlamydia* in the adolescent. This practice may delay treatment in settings where on-site urine pregnancy testing is unavailable and is not routinely recommended unless the menstrual history or pelvic examination suggest pregnancy. Erythromycin is the preferred therapy in pregnant or suspected-pregnant adolescents. If gastrointestinal side effects lead to noncompliance, a liquid preparation may be better tolerated. If this fails, amoxicillin 500 mg PO t.i.d. for 7 to 10 days can be used, although there are only minimal data concerning its effectiveness. The use of oral and intravaginal clindamycin preparations is under investigation and may provide a future alternative treatment of *Chlamydia* in pregnant adolescents.

All adolescents receiving treatment for *Chlamydia* infection should be screened for gonorrhea and syphilis and counseled regarding HIV risks, HIV testing, and condom use. Their partners should receive prompt evaluation and treatment for exposure to *Chlamydia*. Some states now mandate reporting of *Chlamydia* infection for contact tracing and notification. The patient should be advised to refrain from intercourse until both she and her partner have completed treatment. Of all the treatment regimens for *Chlamydia*, only azithromycin, when administered on-site, has guaranteed patient compliance. Because all nonculture *Chlamydia* screening techniques have the potential for false positive results due to detection of nonviable organisms, nonculture test of cure for *Chlamydia* should be delayed at least 3 weeks after completion of treatment to allow for excretion of all dead organisms. However, a brief follow-up visit at 1 to 2 weeks can be useful in assuring both compliance and partner notification. This visit is also a good time to reinforce condom use and contraception. *Chlamydia* retesting is not performed until approximately 4 weeks after completion of therapy and will detect both treatment failures and reinfection from an untreated partner.

About 15% of patients with *Chlamydia* are infected only in the urethra and not the cervix. These patients may present with the so-called acute urethral syndrome, defined as dysuria and urinary frequency accompanied by sterile pyuria. Because specimens of *Chlamydia* from the urethra are often of low yield, these patients should receive presumptive treatment for *Chlamydia*, using the same treatment regimens as for chlamydial cervicitis.

Pelvic Inflammatory Disease (PID)

PID refers to ascending infection of the uterus, fallopian tubes, and ovaries, most often as a consequence of gonorrheal or chlamydial cervicitis. It is one of the most serious gynecologic disorders of adolescence. Long-term sequelae of PID include infertility, ectopic pregnancy, pelvic adhesions, and chronic pelvic pain.

Risk factors for PID include multiple sexual partners, young age at first intercourse, prior history of *N. gonorrhoeae* or *Chlamydia* infection, and lack of any contraceptive use. The risk of acquiring PID for the sexually active 15-year-old female is estimated to be as high as 1 in 8.

Because the signs and symptoms of PID may be subtle or nonspecific, clinical diagnosis often is difficult and has been shown to be inaccurate as often as 35% of the time when compared with laparoscopy. Laparoscopy, though more specific, is generally reserved for patients with more severe clinical signs who fail empiric therapy or in whom the diagnosis is unclear. When tubal infection is mild or when endometritis alone is present, laparoscopy may in fact be negative. Endometrial biopsy can be useful in detecting endometritis but is probably not appropriate for routine use in adolescents with suspected PID.

In recognizing both the serious public health consequences of PID and the often subtle presentation of the disease, the CDC in 1993 liberalized the criteria for PID, essentially eliminating fever and leukocytosis as essential elements in the diagnosis. This is extremely important information for adolescent practitioners, who are particularly urged to have a low threshold for making the diagnosis in their sexually active patients. Empiric therapy has little morbidity when compared with the long-term consequences of undiagnosed or untreated tubal infection in the adolescent.

Empiric treatment for PID should be begun in any adolescent who presents with the following *minimum criteria* for PID, and in whom another cause cannot be found.

Minimum Criteria for Diagnosis of PID
- Lower abdominal tenderness
  plus
- Adnexal tenderness
  plus
- Cervical motion tenderness

Complaints of dysuria, dyspareunia, abnormal bleeding, new onset breakthrough bleeding on oral contraceptives or other long-acting hormonal contraceptives, and dysmenorrhea may be the only presenting symptom in the adolescent with PID and should prompt further investiation and consideration of treatment. The practitioner is reminded that a negative pregnancy test is another essential in ruling out ectopic gestation before instituting treatment for PID in the adolescent.

In sicker adolescents, use of the following additional *routine criteria* and *elaborate criteria* for PID will assist in differentiating teens with uncomplicated PID from those with other conditions, such as appendicitis or tuboovarian abscess, in whom delays or errors in diagnosis can carry significant morbidity.

Routine Criteria for Diagnosis of PID
- Oral temperature >38°C
- Abnormal cervical or vaginal discharge
- Elevated erythrocyte sedimentation rate
- Elevated C-reactive protein
- Laboratory documentation of cervical infection with *N. gonorrhoeae* or *C. trachomatis*

Elaborate Criteria for Diagnosis of PID
- Histopathologic evidence of endometritis on endometrial biopsy
- Laparoscopic abnormalities consistent with PID

Approximately 20% of adolescents with acute PID have concomitant tuboovarian abscesses. Because as many as 70% of these may be missed on initial examination by the pediatrician, *use of pelvic ultrasonography should be routine whenever an adolescent female is diagnosed with acute PID in the pediatric setting.*

Treatment of PID in the adolescent female mandates hospitalization for intravenous antibiotic therapy. There is no place for ambulatory treatment in this population, for a number of reasons. Teenagers typically present later in the course of infection than older patients with PID and thus tend to have more serious infection. In addition, adolescents have high rates of noncompliance with outpatient regimens, as well as with timely follow-up. Finally, earlier, aggressive management may be associated with lower rates of serious sequelae, such as ectopic pregnancy and infertility.

Antibiotic therapy should include broad-spectrum coverage aimed at eradicating *N. gonorrhoeae* and *Chlamydia,* as well as gram-negative bacilli, aerobic streptococci, and anaerobes. The 1993 CDC recomendations for the treatment of PID are given in Table 6. Intravenous antibiotic therapy should be continued for at least 48 hours after the patient shows significant clinical improvement. Because oral doxycycline has similar bioavailability to the intravenous form, oral doxycycline may be used if normal gastrointestinal function is present. Although intravenous clindamycin now appears to be effective against chlamydial infection, the oral formulation has not been proven in this regard. For this reason, it is probably best to use the doxycycline-containing regimen if chlamydial infection is strongly suspected. Failure of the patient to improve clinically within 24 to 48 hours of hospitalization mandates consultation with a gynecologist and consideration of laparoscopy to ensure definitive diagnosis and treatment.

The presence of right upper quadrant pain in the setting of acute PID suggests perihepatic involvement, the so-called FitzHugh-Curtis syndrome. These patients are treated in a similar fashion to those with uncomplicated PID. However, failure of clinical improvement mandates right upper quadrant ultrasonographic examination to rule out the presence of a perihepatic abscess. If significant right upper quadrant findings persist after resolution of PID, consideration should be given to other reasons for the pain, such as hepatitis or gallbladder disease.

While the patient is in the hospital, she should be well hydrated with intravenous fluids and given appropriate pain medication. Bedrest in the semi-Fowler position is recommended because it is the most comfortable for the patient with abdominal pain and because it will facilitate drainage of purulent material into the cul-de-sac. Screening for syphilis should be performed, and testing for HIV should be done with the patient's consent after appropriate pretest counseling. HIV testing is especially important because recent studies have suggested that the prevalence of HIV infection in patients presenting with PID is higher than in similar control populations. Adolescents with PID who have not yet completed a course of hepatitis B vaccine should be screened for this infection and vaccinated if they are antibody negative. The time in the hospital should be used to educate the patient about sexually transmitted diseases and birth control. If the patient is not using birth control, she can be offered contraception at this time. Condom use should be reinforced. The patient's sexual partner(s)

TABLE 6. Recommended Antibiotic Regimens for Treatment of Pelvic Inflammatory Disease (PID)

- Cefoxitin 2 g IV q6h *or* cefotetan 2 g IV q12h
    plus
  Doxycycline 100 mg IV or PO q12h

- Clindamycin 900 mg IV q8h
    plus
  Gentamicin 2 mg/kg loading dose IV, then 1.5 mg/kg IV q8h

Note: Continue treatment for a total of 4 days *and* until the patient is afebrile for at least 48 h; the patient is then discharged on either clindamycin 450 mg PO q.i.d. or doxycycline 100 mg PO b.i.d. to complete 10–14 d of therapy

should be contacted and treated. When possible, parental involvement should be sought and encouraged, especially in the very young adolescent.

At discharge, the patient is given a prescription for either oral doxycycline or clindamycin to complete 14 days of therapy. She can be seen for follow-up in 1 week, at which time a pelvic examination should be performed. Rescreening for gonorrhea and *Chlamydia* should be delayed until 3 to 4 weeks after discharge.

When pelvic abscess is suspected based on physical or ultrasonographic examination, the clindamycin-containing treatment regimen will provide broader anaerobic coverage. Alternatively, clindamycin or metronidazole can be added to the doxycycline-containing regimen if chlamydial coverage is of chief concern. The duration of antibiotic therapy in this situation is controversial. Intravenous antibiotic coverage should be continued, at minimum, for 5 to 7 days and until the patient has been afebrile for at least 48 to 72 hours, the white blood cell count has normalized, and the patient's abdominal examination is completely benign. At this time, follow-up and ultrasonographic examination should show the abscess to be either stable or decreased in size. If this has not occurred, a gynecologist should be consulted.

If ultrasound shows the abscess to be resolving, the patient may be discharged on oral antibiotics. Although either oral doxycycline or clindamycin may be used, clindamycin provides more effective anaerobic coverage and may be more appropriate. Alternatively, some clinicians will use oral doxycycline plus metronidazole to ensure optimal coverage for both *Chlamydia* and anaerobes. The patient should be seen in an outpatient setting at 1 week, 4 weeks, and 8 weeks after discharge. Failure to note either complete or near-complete resolution of the pelvic abscess by ultrasonography at 6 to 8 weeks after discharge mandates referral to a gynecologist for appropriate surgical management. Occasionally, pelvic masses, such as endometriomas or ovarian neoplasms, may be misdiagnosed as tuboovarian abscesses in the setting of acute PID.

Brief mention should be made of the use of other antibiotic regimens for the treatment of PID. Recent studies have been done evaluating the effectiveness of some of the newer penicillins, multigeneration cephalosporins, and quinolones, either alone or in combination with other drugs, in the treatment of PID. Until further data are available on these regimens, it is recommended that the CDC guidelines be followed in treating the adolescent female with PID.

Gonorrhea and Chlamydial Infections in Children

Gonorrhea and chlamydial infections can occur in prepubertal females as a result of sexual abuse, although the prevalence is low. *Chlamydia* is seen more often than *N. gonorrhoeae* in these circumstances. Upper genital tract infection in children is rare, and most infections with *Chlamydia* and *N. gonorrhoeae* are confined to the vagina or extragenital sites. Vaginal, rectal, and pharyngeal specimens must be obtained for culture in all children in whom sexual abuse is suspected, since their history of assault may be incomplete. Treatment is given only if infection has been documented and is similar to that of adults with uncomplicated infection, although doses may need to be adjusted for children weighing under 45 kg.

CERVICAL CYTOLOGY

Regular cervical Pap smears should be obtained in all females beginning at age 18 years or at the onset of sexual activity. From 10% to 14% of sexually active teenagers have abnormal Pap smear findings on routine screening. The sexually active young adolescent, given her young age at first intercourse and likelihood of multiple partners over her lifetime, is at high risk for cervical cancer and should be advised to have at least yearly Pap smears for the rest of her life.

HPV disease, sometimes manifested as venereal warts, accounts for the majority of abnormal Pap smears in the adolescent population. HPV disease is occurring in epidemic proportions in young, sexually active women. As many as 50% of university students show evidence of HPV infection by DNA analysis of cervical and vulvar smears.

TABLE 7. Management of Papanicolaou Smear Abnormalities as Reported Under the 1988 Bethesda System

REPORT	RECOMMENDED ACTION
Specimen adequacy	
Satisfactory	No further action
Unsatisfactory or less than satisfactory	Repeat smear
Descriptive diagnoses	
Inflammation	Rule out vaginitis, cervicitis; otherwise, follow Pap routinely
Cervical cytology	
Within normal limits	No further action
Atypical squamous cells of undetermined significance	Evaluate for vaginitis or cervicitis; treat if present and repeat smear in 4–6 wk; if no evidence of vaginitis or cervicitis, refer to gynecologist for further evaluation
Low-Grade Squamous Intraepithelial Lesion (SIL)	
Cellular changes associated with HPV	If no history or clinical evidence of condyloma, or prior history of abnormal Pap smear, repeat Pap smear in 3 mo; if second Pap smear shows persistent HPV changes, refer to gynecologist for evaluation; if history of condyloma or visible condyloma present, refer to gynecologist for evaluation or treatment
Mild dysplasia or CIN	Referral for colposcopy and biopsy
High-Grade Squamous Intraepithelial Lesion (SIL)	
Moderate dysplasia, CIN 2	Referral to gynecologist for colposcopy and biopsy
Severe dysplasia, CIN 3	
Carcinoma in situ, CIN 3	
Squamous cell carcinoma	

HPV, human papillomavirus; CIN, cervical intraepithelial neoplasia.

Young women with external genital warts are 3.8 times more likely to develop cervical carcinoma in situ than young women without warts. They, therefore, constitute a particularly high-risk subgroup of teenagers.

Pap smear classification was changed in 1988 in an attempt to make the diagnostic categories more meaningful in terms of malignancy risk and treatment. The numerical class system has been replaced by a system based on the presence of squamous intraepithelial lesions (SIL) of low malignant potential (HPV changes and mild dysplasia), high malignant potential (moderate dysplasia, severe dysplasia, and carcinoma in situ), or invasive carcinoma. The suggested management of these Pap smear categories is summarized in Table 7. Referral to a gynecologist for any abnormal Pap test is appropriate if the practitioner has any question regarding management.

Mention should be made about the management of those patients with grossly visible lesions on the cervix. These patients should be referred immediately to a gynecologist for colposcopy and cervical biopsy. It is not appropriate merely to perform a Pap smear and manage on the basis of the Pap smear alone.

OVARIAN MASSES

Ovarian masses in the pediatric population may present with abdominal pain, mass, or distention. Hirsutism or precocious puberty may be the only symptom of hormonally active tumors. Nausea and vomiting, when present, may indicate ovarian torsion or associated gastrointestinal involvement, such as a bowel obstruction. The differential diagnosis and management of ovarian masses in the pediatric population vary considerably with age and pubertal status. For this reason, our discussion focuses on three distinct age groups: the fetus/neonate, prepubertal child, and adolescent.

The use of ultrasound has led to increased detection of ovarian cysts in the fetus and neonate. These cysts are usually diagnosed in the third trimester of pregnancy or during the immediate neonatal period. The overwhelming majority are benign and follicular in origin, and most will resolve spontaneously. In reported series, ovarian torsion occurs in up to 20% to 30% of cases. Whereas some series report increased torsion rates in larger cysts (5 cm or larger), others have found no association between ovarian size and risk of torsion.

Almost all cases of antenatal ovarian cysts can be managed expectantly during pregnancy. In utero aspiration is reserved for cases where compression of pulmonary or abdominal viscera is present. Treatment after delivery will depend on the appearance of the cyst and its evolution over time. In general, serial sonograms during the third trimester and early neonatal period will document resolution of the cyst. Change in sonographic appearance from simple to complex has been reported to occur after delivery. This may be due to hemorrhage within the cyst and often will resolve. Indications for immediate surgery in the neonatal period include large space-occupying lesions and ultrasonographic evidence of torsion. Both complex and simple cysts that do not decrease in size during follow-up should be managed surgically. Surgical management will depend on the appearance of the ovary and the amount of viable ovarian tissue remaining. In general, most cysts can be excised, allowing preservation of the ovary, although torsion may mandate removal of the entire adnexa.

Most abdominopelvic masses in the prepubertal female are ovarian in origin. The most frequent cause of ovarian enlargement before 3 years of age is a physiologic ovarian cyst. Two to five percent of females between ages 2 and 8 can be found to have small (2 to 3 mm), functional ovarian cysts on ultrasound. Although large cysts in general are rare after age 2, they may be found in conjunction with precocious puberty at any age.

After 5 years of age, most ovarian masses in the prepubertal female are neoplasms of germ cell origin, the most common of which is the benign teratoma. Malignancy rates in ovarian neoplasms in this age group have been reported to be as high as 30%. Although germ cell tumors, such as immature teratomas, dysgerminomas, endodermal sinus tumors, embryonal carcinoma, and gonadoblastomas, predominate, tumors of epithelial origin also occur. Ovarian metastases of neuroblastoma and rhabdomyosarcoma have been reported and may be difficult to distinguish clinically from primary ovarian neoplasms.

Ultrasound is the primary diagnostic tool for evaluating pelvic masses in children. It is highly accurate in determining the location of the tumor and in differentiating masses of ovarian origin from other pelvic lesions, such as lymphomas, appendicitis, or mesenteric cysts. The ultrasonographic appearance of ovarian torsion is highly specific and mandates immediate surgery. Other indications for immediate surgical evaluation and treatment include symptomatic masses, solid or complex masses, and masses associated with calcification or ascites. When possible, conservative surgery with preservation of the adnexa is performed. Chemotherapy for ovarian malignancies will depend on histologic type.

Simple ovarian cysts in the prepubertal female may present symptomatically or can be an incidental finding on ultrasound performed for other indications. The overall rate of malignancy in ovarian cysts diagnosed on ultrasound ranges from 5% to 10%. Although the management of simple ovarian cysts remains somewhat controversial, cysts greater than 5 cm in diameter are usually managed surgically because of the potential risk of ovarian torsion. Asymptomatic simple cysts less than 5 cm in diameter may be observed with serial sonograms, provided they are decreasing in size. Simple cysts that do not resolve should be excised.

After puberty, the most common pelvic mass is an enlarged pregnant uterus. The possibility of an ectopic pregnancy must always be considered as well, especially if there is pain or a prior history of PID. The association of pain, primary amenorrhea, and a pelvic mass in the absence of pregnancy suggests obstruction of menstrual effluent caused by mullerian abnormalities. However, most ovarian masses in the adolescent age group are either follicular or hemorrhagic cysts.

The incidence of malignancy ranges from 6% to 10%, and the malignancy is almost always of germ cell origin. Benign cystadenomas will be diagnosed in 10% to 20% of adolescents with ovarian masses.

Pelvic masses in the adolescent that present with fever, abdominal pain, nausea and vomiting, or evidence of acute abdomen should be managed aggressively. The differential diagnosis in these instances can be wide and includes tuboovarian abscess, ovarian torsion, appendicitis, bowel obstruction, and other gastrointestinal lesions. Ultrasound can be extremely helpful in establishing the diagnosis. Ovarian torsion frequently presents with a history of intermittent pain associated with nausea and vomiting. The patient's pain, which can be severe, may seem out of proportion to the findings on abdominal examination. Classic surgical management of ovarian torsion has been to excise the affected ovary because of the perceived risk of embolism from the involved ovarian vessels. However, this risk has never been substantiated clinically. Timely intervention with untwisting of the involved pedicle is, therefore, indicated if the ovary appears viable.

In the adolescent patient, asymptomatic ovarian enlargement of less than 5 cm noted on routine examination can be followed clinically. If ovarian enlargement persists over two menstrual cycles, ultrasonography is indicated. If a sonogram shows the cyst to be clear and unilocular, the most likely diagnosis is a functional cyst, which can be managed conservatively with observation alone. Oral contraceptive suppression is not necessary, since controlled randomized study has shown similar rates of cyst resolution with observation versus suppression. The patient may be reassessed by either pelvic examination or ultrasound after 4 to 6 weeks. At this point, most functional cysts will have resolved or decreased significantly in size. If the cyst is the same size or larger, surgical evaluation, usually by laparoscopy, is indicated.

If the initial sonogram shows the cyst to be complex in nature, the possibility of pregnancy or a tuboovarian abscess should be ruled out. If there is a history of dysmenorrhea or findings on examination suggestive of endometriosis, adnexal enlargement may be due to an endometrioma. Referral for possible laparoscopy or excision should be made. Occasionally, ultrasonographic findings may suggest a dermoid cyst. MRI at this point can be diagnostic, and referral to a gynecologist is appropriate. The possibility of ovarian malignancy must always be considered in the differential diagnosis of a complex ovarian mass. However, most complex ovarian cysts in the adolescent age group are hemorrhagic corpus luteal cysts that usually resolve spontaneously. These patients can be managed expectantly with reevaluation in 6 to 8 weeks, at which point the cyst should be either resolved or significantly decreased in size. Depending on the size of the cyst, physical activity should be limited in the interval to minimize the risk of rupture or torsion. Mild analgesics can be given if necessary, although the presence of anything other than minimal discomfort warrants referral to rule out torsion or rupture. Persistence or enlargement of the cyst after 6 to 8 weeks warrants referral for surgical management.

If the sonogram shows the mass to be larger than 5 cm, a gynecologist should be consulted. Depending on the patient's symptoms and medical status and the radiographic appearance of the ovary, larger masses occasionally may be managed expectantly but only in consultation with a gynecologist. If the sonogram shows the ovary to contain a solid mass or to be suspicious of malignancy, immediate referral for surgical management should be made.

PREMENSTRUAL SYNDROME

Premenstrual syndrome (PMS) refers to a constellation of symptoms, such as bloating, mood swings, depression, headache, and cramps, that occur 7 to 14 days before the menses and usually resolve at some point after menstrual flow has begun. Studies have shown a consistently high prevalence of premenstrual symptomatology in adolescent females, ranging from 73% to 96% of young women studied.

The cause of PMS is unknown, although numerous theories exist. Most presume that the symptoms are hormonally mediated, but no consistent hormonal abnormalities have been found in patients with

PMS. A variety of medications have been used to treat PMS, including oral contraceptives, diuretics, vitamin supplements, and progesterone suppositories. No single treatment has withstood the test of a well-controlled, double-blind placebo trial, although in a given patient, any one of these therapies may provide symptomatic relief.

For the adolescent patient with premenstrual symptoms, first-line therapy includes education, reassurance, a well-balanced diet, and restriction of salt, sugar, and caffeine. Regular aerobic exercise may increase well-being and alleviate mild depressive symptoms. If dysmenorrhea is significant, PGIs or an oral contraceptive can be used. Caution should be used in prescribing diuretics in the adolescent patient, particularly those with eating disorders. However, a trial of a mild diuretic (such as spironolactone 25 mg daily during the week preceding the menses) may alleviate breast tenderness and bloating in some individuals. Progesterone suppositories should be reserved for severe cases and prescribed in consultation with a gynecologist. The use of GnRH agonists is under study and holds promise for the older female with severe PMS. It is probably not suitable therapy for the adolescent patient. Antidepressants appear to be promising treatment for patients with debilitative PMS. They should, however, be used only in adolescents who have psychiatric depression and then only in consultation with a psychiatrist.

CHRONIC PELVIC PAIN

The management of chronic or recurrent pelvic pain in the adolescent depends on the history and nature of the pain and the extent of the prior diagnostic evaluation. Many times, a careful history reveals the pain to be cyclic in nature, suggesting the diagnosis of dysmenorrhea. A trial of PGIs or oral contraceptives may offer significant relief, in addition to confirming the diagnosis. Pain that is cyclic and related to ovulation (*Mittelschmerz*) may also respond to oral contraceptive therapy.

The evaluation of noncyclic pain includes a thorough pelvic examination, with screening for pregnancy, urinary tract infection, sexually transmitted diseases, and occult blood. Associated gastrointestinal symptoms suggest pathology of the gastrointestinal tract, and radiologic or endoscopic evaluation may be indicated. Thickening or nodularity of the uterosacral ligaments in association with dysmenorrhea suggests a diagnosis of endometriosis. A history of sexually transmitted disease, PID, or abdominal surgery suggests either subclinical PID or pain from pelvic adhesions. Psychologic factors may play a role in some adolescents with chronic pelvic pain and should be considered early in the diagnostic workup. Recent studies have shown that an approach that combines psychologic evaluation with medical diagnostic evaluation and therapy has the most success in resolving chronic pelvic pain.

Laparoscopy should be reserved for those adolescents with abnormal findings on pelvic examination or whose diagnosis remains elusive despite persistent symptoms that compromise normal activity. Approximately 30% of young women undergoing laparoscopy for chronic pelvic pain have normal findings at surgery. Of the rest, PID and endometriosis are the most frequent pathologic diagnoses.

RENAL HYPOPLASIA AND DYSPLASIA

GHALEB H. DAOUK, M.D., S.M.
JULIE R. INGELFINGER, M.D.

RENAL MALFORMATIONS

Developmental defects of the kidney are common, affecting 10% of all births, and are divided into a number of categories (Table 1). Renal hypoplasia is characterized by a reduced number of complete nephrons caused by failure of normal inductive interaction of the ureteric bud and metanephric blastema. Renal dysplasia, characterized by abnormal parenchymal differentiation, appears to result from abnormal interaction of renal anlage at any time during gestation. Hypoplasia and dysplasia are histologically distinct, yet may coexist in the same kidney. Furthermore, both hypoplasia and dysplasia may be unilateral or bilateral.

This section does not discuss detailed anatomy and pathophysiology of each entity shown in Table 1, but major features and clinical presentations are summarized there. Table 1 also outlines the various categories of renal dysplasia. From the clinical perspective, however, there are common concerns in managing this group of patients that need to be addressed.

EVALUATION

General considerations involve assessment of anatomy, renal function, and general physiologic status. Adequate anatomic delineation of the renal malformation is essential. Visualization by ultrasound constitutes a good noninvasive screening modality. Subsequently, voiding cystourethrography may be indicated to rule out associated problems, such as posterior urethral valves, reflux, and bladder abnormalities. CT scans and MRI examinations are rarely needed. Intravenous pyelography (IVP) is required infrequently, although characteristic patterns may be confirmatory. In contrast, radionuclide scanning may provide an index of both renal function and anatomy. As the child with hypoplasia or dysplasia grows, serial measurements of renal growth using ultrasound may prove helpful for predicting the child's course. Periodic imaging of the kidneys may be warranted to observe for potential tumorigenesis in dysplastic tissues, although whether such kidneys actually have oncogenic potential is debated (and the potential now is thought by many nephrologists to be negligible).

APPROACH TO UNILATERAL HYPOPLASIA OR DYSPLASIA

Long-term management is strongly influenced by whether the renal abnormalities are unilateral or bilateral. Unilaterally small kidneys are most often found in asymptomatic children. Such kidneys frequently have both hypoplastic and dysplastic elements and may have ipsilateral reflux or obstruction, either of which requires follow-up. Since there is a small but definite chance that an affected child will develop hypertension, blood pressure should be monitored.

Children with a unilateral, multicystic, dysplastic kidney present with an enlarged, cystic abdominal mass of renal tissue associated with ureteral atresia. Contralateral abnormalities are present in approximately 30% of cases, so renal function and anatomy of the normal kidney must be followed over time. Until recently, removal of a unilateral, multicystic, dysplastic kidney has been performed traditionally to confirm the diagnosis and avert the potential development of hypertension, infection, and, possibly, malignant degeneration. However, the basis for removal has been challenged, given critical review of the data. Thus, we suggest noninvasive imaging techniques for monitoring rather than removal. We recommend that a multicystic, dysplastic kidney be removed only if the kidney fails to involute, is associated with infection, or is associated with hypertension.

The entity of unilateral, segmental renal hypoplasia, the so-called Ask-Upmark kidney, is important to mention, as it is associated with hypertension. This malformation is characterized by a unilaterally small kidney with a unique configuration: segmental decreased lobulation and deep cortical transverse grooves. Whereas it was once thought that this was a form of aberrant nephrogenesis in a renal segment, it now seems more likely that the anomaly is caused by acquired infection in the presence of reflux. The hypertension associated with this lesion should be treated medically. If the hypertension proves intractable, a partial nephrectomy should be considered.

Unilateral renal lesions that compromise the involved kidney invariably lead to contralateral hypertrophy. Whether the uninvolved kidney is able to keep up with renal functional demands depends on whether it is truly normal and also on metabolic demand. Because of this, long-term follow-up is essential. Although there are substantial

TABLE 1. Congenital Malformations of Kidney and Associated Organs*

DISEASE CATEGORY	PATHOLOGY	CLINICAL COURSE
Renal agenesis		
Unilateral	(a) Associated ipsilateral genitourinary anomalies	(a) Less severe on the clinical spectrum
	(b) Hypertrophied contralateral kidney	(b) Solitary kidney's function needs monitoring
Bilateral	(a) Twice as common in males	Incompatible with life
	(b) Associated severe malformations, such as pulmonary hypoplasia, Potter syndrome	
Hereditary aplasia and dysplasia	(a) Familial and bilateral aplasia	Incompatible with life
	(b) Recurrence risk 8%; 12.5% associated malformations present	
Renal hypoplasia	Congenital small kidney not associated with parenchymal maldifferentiation or secondary to other disease	
	(a) Bilaterally kidneys <50% of expected weight	Proteinuria, polyuria, polydipsia, urine
Oligonephronia	(b) Few and hypertrophied glomeruli	Concentrating defect and salt wasting in the first 2 y; dehydration, vomiting, growth retardation
Simple	Same as above but without nephronic hypertrophy	Same features
Renal dysplasia		
Bilateral aplasia	Kidneys fail to develop	Potter syndrome; incompatible with life
Multicystic, dysplastic kidney	Enlarged kidney with large peripheral cysts and atretic pelvicaliceal system and ureter; VUR* may be present contralaterally	Infection and tumors are rare complications; when bilateral, results in Potter syndrome; VCUG indicated to rule out contralateral VUR
Hypoplastic dysplasia (hypoplasia)	Associated with variety of ureteral anomalies; variable degree of dysplasia	May retain initial functionality; VUR with infection, stone formation, hypertension, and renal failure are all possible complications
Dysplasia in duplex systems		
Ectopic ureterocele	Common, more frequent in girls (6:1); ectopic ureterocele with duplicated pelvicaliceal system most common; cystic upper ureter with abnormal insertion site; upper pelvis and calyceal system often rudimentary	Amenable to surgical correction with good prognosis
Lower pole dysplasia	Less common; lower pole often nonfunctional; associated VUR and hydronephrosis	Surgically correctable, with good prognosis
Prune-belly and megacystis-megaureter syndromes	Multiple congenital anomalies affecting abdominal wall musculature, dilated cystic ureters with severe VUR	Amenable to complex surgical correction
Diffuse cystic dysplasia	Bilateral, enlarged kidneys with diffusely cystic parenchyma; thin but patent ureter with hypoplastic bladder; needs to be differentiated from multicystic and polycystic kidney disease	Clinical course depends on severity of dysplasia and associated anomalies in its hereditary variants
Hereditary and multiple anomaly syndromes; sporadic	Associations with Meckel syndrome, Zellweger, Jeune, oral-facial-digital, and trisomy D	
Hereditary renal aplasia or dysplasia with VUR	VUR associated with different anomalies	
Congenital nephromegaly	Unilateral: In association with contralateral renal hypoplasia	Associated nephroblastomatosis is a potential for nephroblastoma
	Bilateral: Beckwith-Wiedemann, Perlman syndrome	Increased risk for other malformations
Congenital hydronephrosis	Mostly due to UP junction obstruction	Abdominal mass felt with severe hydronephrosis
	More commonly unilateral with a predilection to the left side; bilateral in 20% of patients, mostly in very young males	Abdominal pain and hematuria in older children
Renal ectopia and malrotation	Seen in 1 in 800 radiologic kidney examinations; often dysplastic with hydronephrosis, and in 25% calculi are present; pelvic kidneys can be associated with rectal or vaginal malformations	Asymptomatic unless affected contralateral kidney, or hypertension from associated renal artery stenosis
Renal fusion	Horseshoe kidney seen in 1 in 600 radiologic examinations; male/female = 2:1; associated with Turner's syndrome	Higher predisposition to calculus formation and renal infection if hydronephrosis is present
Renal duplication	Occurs in 5% of all autopsies; complete duplication is rare	Mostly asymptomatic
Supernumerary kidney	Extremely rare	Asymptomatic
Renal tubular dysgenesis	Similar to bilateral agenesis with Potter facies, oligohydramnios, pulmonary hypoplasia; hereditary, ?X-linked	Incompatible with life

*Unilateral renal agenesis, hypoplasia, and dysplasia account for the greatest majority of these malformations.
†VUR, vesicourethral reflux.

data that hyperfiltration is associated with this situation, no long-term data concerning therapy with low-protein diet or medications in children are available.

Renal function needs to be assesssed for each child presenting with evidence of renal hypoplasia or dysplasia. Serum urea nitrogen and creatinine levels roughly reflect function but are insufficient alone. An estimated clearance may be obtained using the Schwartz formula:

$$\text{Patient's length in cm} \times \frac{\text{constant*}}{\text{serum creatinine}}$$
$$= \text{glomerular filtration rate (GFR) in ml/min/1.73 m}^2$$

*Constant = 0.45 for premature infants, 0.5 for infants and young children, and 0.55 for older children.

A formal creatinine clearance using blood and timed urine collections (or exogenous clearances using inulin or iothalamate) may also prove useful. Electrolyte balance, calcium regulation, renal tubular function, and hematopoiesis must be assessed, as renal contribution to homeostasis in these areas may be aberrant. Thus, serum pH, bicarbonate, sodium, potassium, and chloride levels should be measured at intervals, as should calcium and vitamin D regulation, renal tubular function (urinary concentrating and diluting ability, phosphate reabsorption, amino acid handling, acidification ability), and hematopoiesis. The presence or absence of proteinuria should be established. All of these parameters should be followed at intervals determined by the initial presentation.

APPROACH TO BILATERAL HYPOPLASIA OR DYSPLASIA

The child with bilateral hypoplasia or dysplasia may have associated abnormalities (Table 1). The outlook for a child with bilateral renal disease depends on the amount of functioning renal parenchyma. Severely affected infants may present with oligohydramnios and the pulmonany hypoplasia seen with this finding and may not survive the neonatal period. However, more often, such infants do survive but have tenuous renal function, possibly requiring end-stage renal disease (ESRD) care within the first year of life. More often, such children present with small kidneys, decreased renal function, and a renal concentrating defect.

There is a strong association of renal dysplasia with vesicoureteral reflux (VUR), megaureter, or obstructive uropathy. For this reason, early evaluation of the lower urinary tract is essential.

MANAGEMENT OF DECREASING RENAL FUNCTION

Children with renal hypoplasia or dysplasia syndromes, even unilateral, should be followed by a pediatric nephrologist. Prevention of progression of renal failure is the optimal aim of management. However, little is known about how best to accomplish this aim. Recent studies in adult patients indicate that the use of converting enzyme inhibitors, relatively low-protein diets, and control of hypertension forestall progression in glomerulopathies, but no analogous studies are available in children with any form of renal disease. However, it is important to control hypertension (BP within the normal centiles for age), ensure adequate nutrition, control metabolic bone disease, and treat anemia (with recombinant erythropoietin and adequate iron and folate for the former to be effective). The management of chronic renal failure is discussed near the end of this chapter.

The question as to whether agents, such as angiotensin-converting enzyme inhibitors (ACEI), prevent hyperfiltration (increased GFR per nephron with glomerular hypertension) in children is unresolved. At the present time, there are no data in children to support the use of such medications routinely, although the concept is appealing. Our recommendation is to consider the use of ACEI in the presence of proteinuria or hypertension, remembering that caution is advised, especially as hyperkalemia may ensue in patients with chronic renal failure.

Hypertension in the context of renal hypoplasia or dysplasia may be associated with renovascular malformations and requires complete evaluation, with concomitant hypotensive therapy and subsequent correction if a vascular lesion is found.

Growth failure may result from both inadequate nutrition and insufficient response to growth hormone. Ensuring adequate calorie intake, as well as adequate nutrients, is important. Additionally, therapy with recombinant human growth hormone may enhance linear growth.

GENETIC COUNSELING

Table 1 displays the known hereditary and genetic factors affecting several renal malformations. With rapidly advancing molecular genetic research into the human genome, an exponential increase in our knowledge of the genetic basis of many diseases is expected. It is appropriate, therefore, for the physician caring for children with renal malformations of known hereditary or genetic nature to advise or refer the family for specialized genetic counseling. In addition, antenatal diagnosis should be encouraged for the mother's subsequent pregnancies when studies may be expected to be revealing.

Antenatal ultrasonography often can reveal severe cases of renal malformations early in pregnancy, since kidneys form early in gestation. As in utero surgical intervention techniques improve, correction of certain renal malformations, especially those involving obstruction of urinary flow, will be amenable to such fetal surgery.

Amniotic fluid sampling for fetal cell DNA analysis looking for direct evidence of genetic mutation or indirectly using techniques such as DNA restriction fragment length polymorphism (RFLP) is now feasible. DNA analysis is generally done using direct DNA amplification through the polymerase chain reaction (PCR) technique and nucleotide base sequencing, whereas RFLP involves DNA amplification by PCR, then cutting by specific restriction enzymes that generate a pattern of DNA fragments (bands on gel electrophoresis) of different lengths depending on the sites of cutting for the restriction enzyme. Then, a comparison is made between a normal DNA pattern (usually unaffected members of that family) versus the pattern of DNA fragments from the propositus. However, there are few syndromes resulting in hypoplasia or dysplasia that can be diagnosed definitively in this manner.

FOLLOW-UP AND SPECIALTY REFERRALS

After confirming the initial diagnosis and establishing the degree of severity of renal hypoplasia or dysplasia, follow-up of the child's overall health, as well as renal function, must be monitored, with the primary physician having the coordinating role. Renal function and metabolic control as described are usually followed by the pediatric nephrologist at a frequency that depends on the degree of renal failure and the presence of hypertension.

REFERENCES

1. DeKlerk PP, Marshal FF, Jeffs RD: Multicystic dysplastic kidney. J Urol 118:306, 1977.
2. Risdon AR: Development, developmental defects, and cystic diseases of the kidney. *In* Heptinstall RH (ed): Pathology of the Kidney. Boston, Little, Brown & Co, 1993:124.
3. Roodhooft AM, Birnholz JC, Holmes LB: Familial nature of congenital absence and severe dysgenesis of both kidneys. N Engl J Med 310:1341, 1984.
4. Zerin JM, Ritchey MI, Chang ACH: Incidental vesicoureteral reflux in neonates with antenatally detected hydronephrosis and other renal abnormalities. Radiology 187:157–160, 1993.

HYDRONEPHROSIS

BOYD H. WINSLOW, M.D.
RAYMOND D. ADELMAN, M.D.

Before the advent of modern techniques for sonographic detection of fetal hydronephrosis, the management of hydronephrosis in neonates, infants, and toddlers was very simple. Generally, patients presented with obvious symptoms or signs leading to the detection of an anatomic abnormality in the urinary tract. The spectrum of presenting signs and symptoms included urinary tract infection and urosepsis, hematuria, polyuria, flank masses, colicky abdominal pain, and finally, failure to thrive, with poor appetite and general malaise. It was not difficult in this setting to move directly on to surgical therapy after appropriate radiographic testing had confirmed and defined the urinary tract anomaly precipitating the illness.

Routine antenatal ultrasonography with consequent detection of hydronephrosis in the fetus has rendered the workup and management of hydronephrosis in the infant far more complex. Now the pediatrician, the pediatric nephrologist, and the pediatric urologist, working in concert, carry the added burden of having to determine which child is at risk for deterioration of renal function and which child will continue to do well without surgical therapy. The debate surrounding this issue is ongoing, and its participants range from those who advocate watchful waiting to those who advocate early surgery to support the developing kidney even when there is the slightest suspicion of obstruction. Since the pivotal question is the presence or absence of true obstruction, the real debate has to do with the way we test children rather than the way we treat children. A number of factors pertaining to fetal and neonatal renal function and the nature of currently available imaging techniques make the definition of obstruction exceedingly difficult. Ultrasonography itself is well known to be highly operator-dependent, and, further, its delineation of hydronephrosis is related to degree of hydration. Since the developing kidney has limited concentrating ability, it is generally believed that the neonatal kidney produces copious dilute urine and, in essence, is in a state of diuresis. In this state, the ultrasound examination would likely yield a large number of false positive evaluations in which the infant has a physiologic hydronephrosis. Further, the radionuclide diuretic renogram, a study frequently used to confirm the presence of true obstruction, may be difficult to interpret if the subject is already in a state of diuresis and cannot respond with further diuresis to the administration of furosemide (Lasix). Renal insufficiency or a baggy, markedly distended collecting system, or both, may further limit an adequate response to furosemide. The application of Doppler ultrasound techniques enables us to determine the resistive index of a hydronephrotic kidney. Again, the lack of standards for the neonatal kidney hampers the use of these diagnostic modalities in defining the presence of obstruction.

Finally, it must be understood that the neonatal kidney is indeed in a state of transition. With maturation, the neonatal kidney gains in glomerular filtration rate (GFR) and in concentrating ability. Since these functional parameters have a profound effect on the results gleaned from imaging techniques, it becomes very difficult to use absolute values as a guide to selection of surgical versus nonsurgical treatment. Furthermore, it may be difficult to determine whether improvement in renal function reflects a response to relief of obstruction or a normal maturational improvement in renal function over time.

In addition to the entity of physiologic hydronephrosis already mentioned, the differential diagnosis of fetal and neonatal hydronephrosis includes ureteropelvic junction obstruction, ureterovesical junction obstruction, vesicoureteral reflux (VUR), intravesical obstruction (which is usually caused by posterior urethral valves in boys), and neurogenic bladder dysfunction related to spinal dysraphism or sacrococcygeal teratoma. In addition, a number of conditions can be present that lead erroneously to the diagnosis of hydronephrosis. These include multicystic dysplasia, megacalycosis, and the hypoechoic pyramids found normally in the fetal and neonatal kidney.[3] Nonobstructive dilatation also may be seen with diabetes insipidus, prune-belly syndrome, or acute urinary tract infection, especially in infants. Since some of these conditions have the potential to interfere with renal development, the management team must have a plan for surveillance and intervention founded on valid physiologic principles.

Keeping in mind the uncertainties implicit in the diagnosis and management of hydronephrosis in the neonate and small infant, the management of fetal hydronephrosis becomes even more difficult. In our maternal fetal medicine program, we believe that in utero intervention is justifiable only when fetal survival is challenged by the presence of bilateral or infravesical obstruction, with resultant fetal oliguria and oligohydramnios. Currently, researchers in fetal physiology are investigating the value of serial fetal bladder aspirations to determine when renal function is in jeopardy.[1] Sadly, the salvage rate of vesicoamniotic shunting procedures in infants at risk has been extremely low. At this time, antenatal intervention should be seen as experimental and indicated rarely, if at all, in the therapy of hydronephrosis.

The neonate with hydronephrosis should undergo, when fitness permits, studies including serum creatinine and electrolytes, postnatal ultrasound with Doppler flow determination of resistive indexes, and voiding cystourethrography. These studies should be obtained as early as possible, if only for baseline parameters. One should not be deceived by a diminution in degree of hydronephrosis in the earliest postnatal ultrasound. Some neonates may be mildly volume depleted in the first few days of life, leading to an underestimate of the degree of hydronephrosis. Rarely does the neonate in the first few days of life require surgical intervention for obstruction. When possible, we start the neonate on prophylactic antibiotics while we await maturation and then obtain a second set of parameters to help us define the presence of obstruction. The selection of antibiotics is an important one. We avoid using trimethoprim-sulfamethoxazole (Bactrim, Septra) because of hepatic immaturity and nitrofurantoin (Macrodantin) because of our inability to detect G6PD deficiencies in the neonatal population. Amoxicillin seems to be the best choice, given at one-third to one-half the therapeutic dose. Usually, when the child is about 6 weeks of age, we can move on to the more typical use of trimethaprim-sulfamethoxazole as the prophylactic antibiotic of choice.

The male neonate with obstructive posterior urethral valves should undergo surgical therapy as soon as possible. With today's excellent neonatal resectoscopes, even the smallest neonate is a candidate for primary transurethral valve ablation. Of course, the neonate with valves can be so ill as to require prolonged catheter placement or diversion of the urinary tract by vesicostomy or supravesical diversions in rare situations. Because of changes in the detrusor musculature of the infant with valves, these young boys must undergo surveillance for upper tract deterioration much the same as the other infants with ureteropelvic junction (UPJ) obstructions or ureterovesical obstructions.

At about 1 month of age, the infant with hydronephrosis is restudied with ultrasonography and diuretic radionuclide renography. The magnitude of pelvic calyceal dilatation by ultrasonography or radiography cannot predict the presence or severity of obstruction reliably. If obstruction is believed to be clearly evident, surgical intervention can be undertaken safely. In our center, pediatric urologists and nephrologists meet on a regular basis to discuss the ongoing surveillance of such cases. In the absence of compelling information to the contrary, we recommend surgery for those infants who have progressive dilatation, poor washout of radionuclide on a well-tempered furosemide renogram, or diminished or diminishing renal function as compared with its normal counterpart and when urinary tract infection or failure to thrive seems attributable to urinary tract obstruction. In many cases, nonoperative management is indicated. The majority of mild to moderate lesions improve. Even kidneys with severe hydronephrosis and poor isotope washout may improve or normalize.

After the 1-month milestone, we think it necessary to maintain prophylactic antibiotics and imaging surveillance every 3 months. Although some use the pressure perfusion study described by Whittaker, we do not use this test routinely (antegrade perfusion of the renal pelvis with monitoring of pressure as a function of increasing flow) as a serial diagnostic test. We believe that if our index of suspicion is high enough to justify such an invasive test, surgical correction should be undertaken.

Parents of infants in this follow-up study are counseled regarding the changes in imaging or performance that would lead us to recommend surgery. We are candid with each family in presenting our goal as preservation of renal function. We maintain an aggressive posture with regard to treatment of obstruction despite reports that delayed pyeloplasty can return renal function to predeterioration levels in many cases.[2]

The infant with stable hydronephrosis and stable renal function must be followed for a long period of time. One needs only to look back at data accumulated before fetal ultrasonography to find that UPJ obstructions may remain quiescent for many years before the sentinel urinary infection, bleed, or episode of pain mandates surgical intervention. One must assume that, over time, continued expansion of the renal pelvis or changes in urinary flow characteristics may cause the previously asymptomatic obstruction to become clinically significant. Whatever the case, we prefer to use the advance notice provided by antenatal ultrasonography and serial postnatal imaging to help us avoid such clinical crises. All too often, we have seen children in whom surgery was withheld under the guise of conservative, careful management when, in fact, prompt surgery would have removed risk and eliminated years of worry for the family and child in question. Long-term follow-up is indicated for these patients, since some may show progressive deterioration in renal function, with hypertension, proteinuria, and development of focal glomerulosclerosis, many years after successful surgery and after a long period of stable renal function.

REFERENCES

1. Johnson MP, Bukowski TP, Reitleman C, Isada NB, Pryde PG, Evans MI: In utero surgical treatment of fetal obstructive uropathy: A new comprehensive approach to identify appropriate candidates for vesicoamniotic shunt therapy. Am J Obstet Gynecol 170:1770–1779, 1994.
2. Koff SA, Campbell KD: The nonoperative management of unilateral neonatal hydronephrosis: Natural history of poorly functioning kidneys. J Urol 152:593–595, 1994.
3. Stark JE, Weinberger E: Ultrasonography of the neonatal genitourinary tract. Appl Radiol 22:50–53, 1993.

THE NEUROGENIC BLADDER

ANDREW S. BREM, M.D.

IDENTIFICATION OF NEUROGENIC BLADDER

Identification of a neurogenic bladder, with its associated renal risk factors, is the key to appropriate management. Although a neurogenic bladder can be an acquired defect that follows a spinal tumor or injury, it most often results from a congenital deformity of the lower spine, such as meningomyelocele or sacral agenesis. Children with neurogenic bladder frequently provide clinical clues that lead to the proper diagnosis. Continual dribbling, recurrent urinary tract infections, and constipation often can be elicited in the history, even in infants. The constipation arises from altered rectal sphincter tone. Physical findings in these patients with disrupted lower spinal nerve roots include abnormalities of the lower spine, poor anal sphincter tone, and diminished lower extremity reflexes, sensation, and muscle tone.

The bladder appears to have a fairly simple task. It stores previously produced urine and then selectively and efficiently empties that urine. Any defect in these processes will eventually affect renal structure

and function. During gestation, the fetal kidney (metanephros) produces urine from about the 10th week of development. Since nephron formation continues through the 34th week of gestation, abnormal bladder drainage during those early weeks can lead to renal dysplasia. Poor bladder drainage and urinary obstruction after birth, when the kidneys grow but do not form additional nephrons, also may adversely influence renal function. Reflux of stagnant urine from a dysfunctional neurogenic bladder to the kidneys can occur and be a risk factor for recurrent urinary tract infections. Moreover, a neurogenic bladder often exhibits a high resting intravesicular hydrostatic pressure, which can be transmitted directly to a growing kidney via a refluxing ureter. A high resting bladder pressure is observed in patients who display poor bladder compliance as the bladder fills. These noncompliant bladders are frequently small and trabeculated. Vesicoureteral reflux, urinary infections, and a high resting intravesicular pressure together have been shown to alter renal growth and produce scarring in affected kidneys, especially during the first 5 to 6 years of life, when the bulk of renal growth occurs.

MANAGEMENT OF THE CHILD WITH NEUROGENIC BLADDER

Management of the child with neurogenic bladder is both exacting and time consuming. Once the diagnosis is suspected on clinical grounds, a radiographic assessment of both the upper and lower urinary tracts is required. The renal parenchyma can be initially evaluated by ultrasound, looking specifically for the degree of hydronephrosis and renal size. Ultrasound, however, does not provide information about relative renal function. A renal technetium-99m-diethylenetriaminepentaacetic acid (^{99m}Tc-DTPA) or MAG 3 scan does supply a qualitative assessment of each kidney's function. Both ultrasound and radionuclide scans provide a significant degree of information with a minimal amount of patient discomfort. A voiding cystourethrogram (VCUG) must be done to assess the lower urinary tract, specifically the bladder and urethra. By introducing dye directly into the bladder and following its course fluoroscopically, an appraisal of bladder size, emptying capability, and reflux can be made. Although a radionuclide VCUG can give similar information on reflux and bladder emptying with less radiation, it does not provide the anatomic detail of a standard VCUG. After the initial evaluation, the radionuclide VCUG can be used to follow the course of patients over time.

Urodynamic studies supply additional complementary information, measuring bladder hydrostatic pressures during filling and voiding. Electromyographic studies of the external sphincter also can be coupled to the urodynamic testing, looking specifically at external urinary sphincter activity during bladder filling and emptying. The urodynamic studies as a group are more difficult to perform in the newborn and may be difficult to interpret when there is a significant degree of reflux. Using some or all of these studies, one can classify children with neurogenic bladder into a high pressure trabeculated bladder group or a low pressure compliant bladder group. Children with a high pressure bladder appear at greater risk for the development of significant renal insufficiency over time.

DEFINITIVE THERAPY

Relief of urinary obstruction with appropriate urinary drainage, maintaining a low intravesicular pressure, and providing urinary continence are the goals of treatment. In the newborn or very young infant with a neurogenic bladder, a vesicostomy may provide a low pressure urinary outlet, since urinary continence is less of an issue with a child in diapers. If the ureters are significantly dilated, diversion of both ureters may be done as a temporary drainage procedure. The Credé maneuver is not recommended, as it only transmits the increased bladder hydrostatic pressure directly to both kidneys. Older children often can be treated with clean intermittent urinary catheterization four or five times per day. This technique is effective in maintaining urinary continence and lowering bladder hydrostatic pressure. When combined with clean intermittent catheterization, the artificial bladder sphincter has been useful for patients who continue to demonstrate

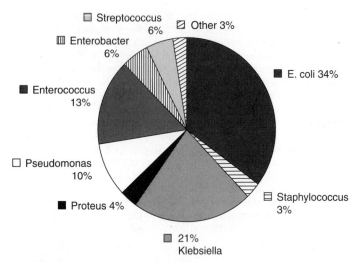

FIGURE 1. Common bacterial organisms recovered in patients with myelomeningocele maintained on clean intermittent catheterization. (Data from Ehrlich O, Brem AS: A prospective comparison of urinary tract infections in patients treated with either clean intermittent catheterization or urinary diversion. Pediatrics 70:665–669, 1982.)

urinary incontinence with catheterization alone. Patient compliance with a regular catheterization program is essential if the sphincter is to be used. In some patients, the intravesicular pressure is so high that a bladder augmentation may be required to improve bladder compliance. At times, anticholinergic medications, such as oxybutynin chloride (Ditropan), can be prescribed to decrease bladder tone and hydrostatic pressure. These agents have limited usefulness because of their side effects, including aggravating preexisting constipation. Urinary diversion, either with an ileal or colon conduit, is now generally believed to be an intervention of last resort.

In patients with a neurogenic bladder, the presence of a stagnant pool of urine provides a culture medium allowing for the development of urinary tract infections as a comorbid process. In young children, reflux coupled with a high pressure bladder can force infected urine directly into renal parenchyma, setting the stage for eventual scarring. Providing good bladder drainage clearly lowers the risk of infection by removing the culture medium. The most common organism encountered in children with urinary tract infections and a neurogenic bladder is *Escherichia coli,* although other organisms are frequently found (Fig. 1). When using antibiotics prophylactically to maintain a sterile urine, the objective should be to use a drug of low cost, with minimal side effects, and with a slow urinary excretion rate. Such agents as sulfamethoxazole nitrofurantoin (Furadantin) are reasonable initial choices in patients with normal renal function. Amoxicillin also can be used safely, even in patients with a significant degree of renal impairment. These drugs are generally administered at bedtime, once a day, or at most on a twice-daily basis at one-third to one-half the usual daily dose. Since asymptomatic bacteriuria will occur in at least a third of children maintained on clean intermittent catheterization, only clinically evident urinary tract infections should be treated with specific changes in antibiotic selection and dose. Synthetic penicillins and cephalosporins in conventional doses often are used to treat acute symptomatic infections. Symptoms of an acute urinary tract infection might include any or all of the following: fever, abdominal pain, flank pain, and worsening renal function.

Children with neurogenic bladder and persistent obstructive uropathy may experience a decrease in glomerular filtration rate (GFR) and a rising serum creatinine even in the absence of recurrent urinary tract infections. Efforts must be directed toward identifying the locale and degree of obstruction so that appropriate urinary drainage procedures can be instituted. More subtle forms of renal dysfunction may also occur in the renal distal tubule and collecting duct. These alterations in function include an acquired hyperchloremic distal renal tubular acidosis (RTA), a defect in potassium secretion leading to

hyperkalemia, or an inability to excrete a concentrated urine. Children with this form of RTA may demonstrate significant growth delay. The acidosis is generally treated with sodium bicarbonate 1 to 2 mEq/kg/d or an equivalent dose of sodium citrate (Bicitra) 1 mEq/ml. The hyperkalemia is resistant to mineralocorticoids but usually is not clinically troublesome. Dietary modifications restricting the intake of potassium usually will suffice as treatment. The urinary concentrating defect, which is resistant to vasopressin, also can account for growth delay. The large intake of water leads to a sense of fullness and a decreased ingestion of food (calories). Such a child will maintain a low urine specific gravity or osmolality in the face of obvious dehydration.

In summary, the care of the child with neurogenic bladder involves a team approach. The goals of management are to ensure proper urinary drainage and prevent the progression of renal failure, if possible. The pediatrician, pediatric nephrologist, and pediatric urologist all have important roles to play in ensuring normal growth and development in children afflicted with this condition.

REFERENCES

1. Bauer S, Hallett M, Khoshbin S, Lebowitz RL, Winston KR, Gibson S, Colodny AH, Retik AB: Predictive value of urodynamic evaluation in newborns with myelodysplasia. JAMA 252:650–652, 1984.
2. Brem AS, Martin D, Callaghan J, Maynard J: Long-term renal risk factors in children with meningomyelocele. J Pediatr 110:51–55, 1987.
3. Ehrlich O, Brem AS: A prospective comparison of urinary tract infections in patients treated with either clean intermittent catheterization or urinary diversion. Pediatrics 70:665–669, 1982.
4. Lapides J, Diokno AC, Silber SJ, Lowe BS: Clean intermittent self-catheterization in the treatment of urinary tract disease. J Urol 107:458–461, 1972.
5. McLorie GA, Perez-Marero R, Csima A, Churchill BM: Determinants of hydronephrosis and renal injury in patients with myelomeningocele. J Urol 140:1289–1292, 1988.
6. Uehling DT, Smith J, Meyer J, Bruskewitz R: Impact of an intermittent catheterization program on children with myelomeningocele. Pediatrics 76:892–895, 1985.

EXSTROPHY OF THE BLADDER

JAMES MANDELL, M.D.

Bladder exstrophy is characterized by a defect in the anterior abdominal wall, with the inner lining of the bladder and urethra exposed. On close inspection, one can see the ureteral orifices at the bladder trigone and the posterior aspect of the bladder neck. The rectus muscle and fascia and the symphysis pubis are widely separated. The rectum is anteriorly placed, and inguinal hernias are commonly present. In males, there is a spadelike glans and a dorsal urethral groove, and one can see the prostate, verumontanum, and ejaculatory ducts. In females, there is a bifid clitoris and anteriorly placed vagina. The bladder varies in size and compliance. In some cases, it can be indented easily with the examiner's finger, and in others, there is a fibrotic plate.

The functional problems associated with bladder exstrophy include urinary incontinence and a foreshortened, dorsally curved phallus with complete epispadias. The difficulties underlying achieving continence involve decreased bladder capacity and the lack of a continence mechanism. The bladder capacity may not be sufficiently large to accommodate socially acceptable voiding intervals because of either anatomic or functional deficiencies. There is also complete absence of a continence mechanism at both the bladder neck and urogenital diaphragm. The presence of the dorsally curved, short phallus (chordee) is caused by the attachment of the corporal bodies to the inferior aspect of the widely separated pubic ramus. Although the upper urinary tracts are invariably normal at birth in infants with exstrophy, the ureters enter the bladder nonobliquely, leading to reflux once the bladder is closed. There is little or no functional defect in gait associated with the widened pubis or rotated pelvic bones.

Management of the child with bladder exstrophy is neither simple, consistent, nor universally successful. Currently, if a newborn is recognized with this defect, emergent referral to a pediatric institution is recommended. Before transfer and surgery, the bladder should be covered with a cellophane (Saran) wrap. Petrolatum (Vaseline) gauze should be avoided. An initial ultrasound is performed and is almost always normal. We favor an immediate (within 72 hours) closure of the bladder. The surgical technique involves mobilization of the bladder and closure of the bladder, the bladder neck, and the posterior urethra. No attempt is made to tighten the bladder neck to achieve continence. The closure may also include dissection of the prostate gland off the urethral plate, creation of short paraexstrophic skin flaps, and penile lengthening by mobilization of the corpora cavernosa. The pubis is approximated with sutures and held in place for 3 weeks postoperatively with lower extremity traction and internal rotation of the hips. During this initial postoperative period, ureteral stents and a suprapubic bladder catheter are left in place. Complications commonly seen following this initial procedure include wound dehiscence and bladder prolapse through the newly created bladder neck. Helpful surgical hints include using a complete lower body skin preparation and draping to enable good manual approximation of the symphysis, the use of a posterior or anterior pelvic osteotomy if the child is out of the immediate neonatal period, anchoring of the closed bladder to the abdominal or retroperitoneal fascia, and the use of absorbable sutures to approximate the pubis.

If the bladder is too small to close primarily, delayed closure is recommended, either along with an initial urinary diversion or with a simultaneous bladder augmentation. Pelvic osteotomy is mandatory in this setting. Correction of the episadias is usually performed between 2 and 4 years of age. In the female, repair of the bifid clitoris is also done. If the bladder capacity is less than 60 ml, the urethral repair is carried out first. If the bladder is of good size, it can be done simultaneously with the bladder neck reconstruction and ureteral reimplants. The last is done using the crossed trigonal technique. Techniques for achieving continence include bladder neck reconstruction using part of the native bladder and surrounding tissues or, failing this, insertion of an artificial sphincter. Ureterosigmoidostomy has been used for many years with some success, but we no longer consider this a satisfactory primary form of treatment because of later development of carcinomas at the ureteral-rectal anastomosis.

Long-term issues involving continence and sexual and psychologic health and performance cannot be overlooked. These children will need surgical input well into adult life, and perfection is never achieved.

PATENT URACHUS AND URACHAL CYSTS

ANTHONY ATALA, M.D.
ALAN B. RETIK, M.D.

The allantois appears around day 16 of gestation as an outpouching from the caudal wall of the yolk sac. As the bladder enlarges, the allantois involutes to form a thick tube called the urachus. The urachus allows free communication between the urinary bladder and the umbilicus in the abdominal wall. After birth, the urachus becomes a fibrous cord called the median umbilical ligament. The lumen in the inferior portion of the urachus remains patent approximately one third of the time during gestation. The abnormalities associated with the umbilicus are usually due to embryologic abnormalities of the urachus. The treatment of such abnormalities is surgical.

PATENT URACHUS

Failure of the urachus to regress completely results in a patent urachus, a communication between the bladder and umbilicus. The usual presenting sign is a discharge of fluid from the umbilicus, which

increases with voiding. Urethral obstruction may be present. Umbilical swelling due to an associated umbilical hernia or urachal vascular engorgement and skin discoloration may be present.

A voiding cystourethrogram may demonstrate the patent urachus and may also rule out the presence of a lower urinary tract obstruction. Fluid analysis for blood urea nitrogen and creatinine may be helpful. Injection of methylene blue transurethrally may confirm the communication. Treatment consists of identification and extraperitoneal excision of the urachal tract with a bladder cuff.

EXTERNAL URACHAL SINUS

Persistence of the distal urachus with an opening at the umbilicus results in an external urachal sinus. This may become symptomatic at any age but usually occurs during childhood. Drainage, fever, paraumbilical tenderness, and inflammation may be present. A voiding cystourethrogram should be done to rule out a patent urachus and the presence of lower urinary tract obstruction. Sinography may aid in the diagnosis. Treatment consists of excision of the sinus. Concomitant removal of any attached intraperitoneal structure is necessary if omphalomesenteric duct remnants are present.

URACHAL CYSTS

A urachal cyst occurs when both ends of the urachus are closed and only the central portion of the canal remains patent. The central lumen may enlarge from epithelial desquamation and degeneration. Such cysts are usually asymptomatic until they attain a considerable size or become infected. Lower abdominal pain is the most frequent presenting complaint and may be associated with fever, voiding symptoms, gastrointestinal upset, or a palpable mass or a combination of these features. Peritoneal irritation may give rise to symptoms that mimic an acute abdomen. Rupture of the cyst into the bladder, umbilicus, or peritoneal cavity may occur. Diagnostic studies should include a voiding cystourethrogram in the lateral position to demonstrate the compressive effect on the bladder and an ultrasound study. Treatment consists of removal of the cyst if it is uninfected and drainage and marsupialization if an abscess is present. Another alternative is first to drain the cyst percutaneously with ultrasound guidance and subsequently to perform a surgical excision.

REFERENCES

1. Avni EF, Matos C, Van Regemorter G, Goolaerts JP, Diard F: Symptomatic patent urachus in children: The contribution of ultrasound. Ann Radiol 30:482–485, 1987.
2. Persutte WH, Lenke RR, Kropp K, Ghareeb C: Antenatal diagnosis of fetal patent urachus. J Ultrasound Med 7:399–403, 1988.
3. Rich RH, Hardy BE, Filler RM: Surgery for anomalies of the urachus. J Pediatr Surg 18:370–372, 1983.

DISORDERS OF THE BLADDER AND URETHRA

ANTHONY ATALA, M.D.
ALAN B. RETIK, M.D.

DISORDERS OF THE BLADDER

Malignant Tumors

Epithelial Tumors

Epithelial tumors of the bladder are extremely rare in children. Transurethral resection of the bladder lesion is necessary to confirm the diagnosis and to establish if any muscle invasiveness is present. Most commonly, the lesions are noninvasive and do not require further surgical treatment. These children are followed with periodic cystoscopy and bladder washing for cytology and flow cytometry. If the lesion is consistent with carcinoma in situ, a cycle of intravesical chemotherapy is administered. If the lesion is muscle invasive, radical cystectomy may be indicated.

Rhabdomyosarcomas

A more common malignant tumor of the urinary tract in children is rhabdomyosarcoma (RMS). Rhabdomyosarcoma is the most common soft tissue sarcoma in children, comprising about 10% of childhood cancers. Approximately 20% to 30% of all RMS occur in genitourinary sites. Genitourinary RMS occurs more frequently in infants and young children, with 75% of cases occurring in children under 4 years of age. The major sites are bladder and prostate, paratesticular regions, female reproductive organs, and retroperitoneal/pelvic regions. Embryonal histology is present in over 90% of children with genitourinary RMS. Approximately one third of such tumors have a botryoid appearance. The alveolar and pleomorphic types are rare in children.

The clinical presentation usually includes urinary frequency, urgency, or retention, hematuria, lower abdominal discomfort, or constipation. An abdominal mass is usually palpable during physical examination. Radiographic studies, including ultrasound, CT, or MRI, are helpful in evaluating the extent of the tumor.

After adequate biopsy tissue has been obtained, chemotherapy is initiated, followed by restaging with CT or MRI, cystoscopy, and biopsy. A decision is then made regarding further surgery. Radiation treatment is used in patients with positive margins on permanent sections or residual disease. Overall, with chemotherapy, radiation treatment, and surgery, the tumor-free survival rate for RMS exceeds 70%. Approximately 60% of survivors have functional bladders after 5 years, which is a considerable improvement over a decade ago.

Benign Tumors

Benign bladder tumors in children are extremely rare. Bladder hemangiomas are benign vascular lesions that usually present with gross hematuria. Usually, children have similar lesions elsewhere in the body. Visualization of the lesion during cystoscopic examination confirms the diagnosis. Fulguration is generally effective for small lesions. The more common larger lesions are usually managed with a partial cystectomy.

Neurofibromas may also occur in the bladder. Although most of these lesions are benign, they can cause obstruction if they grow to a substantial size. Malignant degeneration has been reported in approximately 10% of cases. Wide excision is the treatment of choice. Other benign bladder tumors include fibroma, leiomyoma, nephrogenic adenoma, and dermoid cyst. These lesions usually present with hematuria and tend to be treated with simple excision.

Bladder Diverticula

Bladder diverticula are herniations of bladder mucosa between the detrusor muscle. The majority of diverticula are congenital, although a few are acquired because of outlet obstruction or infection. The most common location is lateral and cephalad to the ureteral orifice. Congenital bladder diverticula may cause vesicoureteral reflux due to the paucity of smooth muscle present in the periureteral region. Bladder diverticula can also cause obstruction at either the bladder neck or urethral region. Generally, however, they are entirely asymptomatic and are found incidentally. Bladder diverticula are best demonstrated by voiding cystourethrography at the time the postvoid film is obtained. Surgical excision is indicated if the diverticulum is obstructive, is a locus for infection, or is associated with high degrees of vesicoureteral reflux.

DISORDERS OF THE URETHRA

Benign Tumors

Urethral benign tumors are extremely rare. Urethral hemangiomas occur infrequently, causing hematuria or bloody discharge. Small lesions are treated with fulguration, and larger lesions may need radical excision, with subsequent urethral reconstruction. Other uncommon benign tumors of the urethra include neurofibroma and leiomyoma, both amenable to local excision either transurethrally or with open surgery.

Meatal Stenosis

Meatal stenosis in boys occasionally may be associated with another urologic anomaly. However, it is most often an acquired lesion following circumcision, usually secondary to meatitis or trauma. A diagnosis can be established only after a careful physical examination that includes observation of voiding. If the meatus has a pinpoint opening, with a narrow urine stream, if deflection of the urinary stream is evident, and if the child is straining to empty his bladder, a diagnosis of meatal stenosis can be ascertained. A meatotomy, which involves a ventral incision in the thin fused area, should alleviate the stenosis.

Hypospadias

Hypospadias is a congenital defect of the penis wherein there is incomplete development of the anterior urethra. The urethral opening is proximal to its usual location at the center of the glans. The abnormal urethral opening may be anywhere along the ventral aspect of the penis, the scrotum, or perineum. Approximately 60% of hypospadias are distal, involving either the proximal glanular, coronal, or distal penile shaft regions. Approximately 20% of hypospadias occur in the midpenile region along the midshaft. Another 20% occur proximally, either in the penile, penoscrotal, scrotal, or perineal region.

The incidence of hypospadias in studies of large populations has been reported to be from 1 to 8/1000 male births. The diagnosis is made during physical examination. The physical examination determines the severity of the hypospadias and is also aimed at identifying any associated anomalies. These include meatal stenosis, penile torsion, urethrocutaneous fistula, chordee (a ventral curvature of the penis), and penoscrotal transposition. A neonatal circumcision should not be performed in a patient with hypospadias. The prepuce is routinely used during the repair, and the cosmetic results may be compromised if there is a shortage of preputial tissue. Thus, such patients should not be circumcised.

Approximately one fourth of patients with hypospadias and undescended testes have an intersex anomaly. Therefore, all such patients should be evaluated for intersex with determination of karyotype, serum analysis for FSH, LH, and testosterone, and urinary 17-ketosteroids and 17-hydroxycorticosteroids. If a phallus is small, its size may be enlarged preoperatively by the use of topical testosterone or dihydrotestosterone cream or parenteral testosterone.

Surgical treatment is performed between 6 and 18 months of age. Regardless of the severity of hypospadias, the goals are the same. These include creating a straight penis, positioning of the meatus on the penile tip, normalization of the direction of voiding, creating a urethra of adequate and uniform caliber, and symmetry in appearance of the glans and shaft. Although most hypospadias are amenable to a single-stage surgical repair, a few more complex defects require two separate surgical procedures. The glanular hypospadias can be repaired with a meatal advancement procedure. The more proximal subglanular and penile shaft defect usually can be corrected with penile shaft skin or preputial flaps. Grafts from other donor sites, such as nonpenile skin, bladder, or buccal mucosa, can also be used for the more complex repairs.

Even in the hands of the most experienced surgeons, hypospadias repair may be associated with a complication rate of as high as 25% for the more complex repairs. Complications include urethrocutaneous fistula, stricture, diverticula, and persistent chordee. A careful preoperative evaluation, precise surgical technique, and appropriate postoperative care are required to minimize the complication rate and achieve the desired objectives of hypospadias surgery.

Posterior Urethral Valves

Posterior urethral valves represent the most common cause of bladder outlet obstruction in the male newborn. Although initially described as three types of valves in 1919, with a fourth type described in 1983, only type one and type three valves are clinically significant. Type one valves arise from either side of the verumontanum as leaflets that extend distally to the anterior urethral wall at the level of the urogenital diaphragm. Type two valves represent membranous valves that run outward from the verumontanum to the bladder neck. Type three valves consist of a diaphragm usually located at the verumontanum with a small central perforation. Type four valves are seen in patients with prune-belly syndrome, when the prostate folds on itself, causing a partial obstruction. Overall, type one valves make up more than 95% of those seen, and type three valves make up over 4%. Even though different embryologic defects are present, there is no difference in the clinical presentation, pathophysiology, or management of children with either type one or type three valves.

A large number of babies with posterior urethral valves are now being diagnosed prenatally with ultrasonography. The prenatal ultrasound may show a large, thickened bladder with a dilated prostatic urethra and bilateral hydroureteronephrosis. Valves cause varying degrees of urinary tract obstructive changes, ranging from severe hydronephrosis with renal dysplasia to a relatively normal upper urinary tract. Severe obstructive uropathy due to posterior urethral valves may lead to the development of oligohydramnios, with subsequent pulmonary hypoplasia. Survival in these instances is markedly decreased. Prenatal intervention for the severe forms of this condition was first performed in the early 1980s. This type of intervention, however, has slowed considerably because of poor results in terms of survival and associated infant morbidity.

The prenatal findings of posterior urethral valves should be confirmed at birth with a voiding cystourethrogram. The classic appearance is that of a dilated and elongated posterior urethra, a cutoff of urethral caliber just proximal to the membranous urethra, often bladder neck hypertrophy, and occasionally the leaflets are visible as filling defects. A baseline renal and bladder ultrasound should be obtained. Newborns with posterior urethral valves who are not diagnosed prenatally usually present with an abdominal mass, failure to thrive, urinary ascites, azotemia, or urosepsis. When the newborn or infant is acutely ill, prompt management of acidosis, sepsis, and fluid and electrolyte abnormalities is essential. The serum creatinine is monitored, with the realization that it reflects the mother's levels for the first week of life. An increase in the serum creatinine levels with serial measurements during the first week of life, however, is indicative of worsening renal function in the neonate.

Once the diagnosis of posterior urethral valves is made, the bladder is drained transurethrally with a catheter or small caliber feeding tube. A Foley balloon catheter is not recommended because of its tendency to occlude the ureteral orifices. Broad-spectrum antibiotics are administered. When the patient is stable, valve ablation is performed cystoscopically. Valve ablation by either a perineal urethrostomy or transvesically may be necessary in the small infant whose penile urethra cannot accommodate the cystoscope. In certain situations, a vesicostomy may be performed. If the valves are ablated and there is continued obstruction or increase in creatinine, a higher diversion may be indicated, using either a cutaneous pyelostomy or loop ureterostomy. If valve ablation results in adequate urinary emptying, close observation is still imperative.

Although the radiographic appearance of the urethra after valve ablation returns to normal almost immediately, the trabeculation and hypertrophy of the bladder will take much longer to resolve. Vesicoureteral reflux, if present, may improve or cease entirely. In a subset of patients, there is a continued impairment in bladder compliance that may be associated with a decreased bladder capacity or high voiding pressures. These patients may require long-term management with intermittent catheterization alone or in conjunction with anticholinergic or alpha-sympathomimetic agents. Failure of these methods of treatment may lead to the need for bladder augmentation with urinary reconstruction.

Older boys with valves may present at any age depending in part on the severity of obstruction. Voiding dysfunction, hematuria, and urinary tract infections are frequent reasons for older boys with posterior urethral valves to come to medical attention. A full urodynamic and radiographic evaluation is necessary before proceeding with valve ablation. Careful follow-up is essential because of the common sequelae of impaired bladder function.

Anterior Urethral Valves

An anterior urethral diverticulum may arise due to a segmental defect of the corpus spongiosum. The diverticulum may enlarge, extending beyond the anterior margin, producing an obstructing valvular mechanism. Children usually present with some symptoms of urinary obstruction or infection. On physical examination, there may be a swelling present just proximal to the penoscrotal junction that will produce urinary drainage if pressure is applied. A voiding cystourethrogram is diagnostic. Small diverticula may be managed with endoscopic resection, whereas larger ones may require open excision with urethroplasty.

Urethral Polyps

Urethral polyps are congenital lesions that are always benign. They arise in the area of the verumontanum and usually have a long stalk. Children present with urinary infection, hematuria, or intermittent obstruction. A voiding cystourethrogram usually shows a filling defect, which may vary in location. Although less reliable, an ultrasound may also show a polyp. Removal of the polyp usually can be performed cystoscopically. Incomplete removal may lead to a later recurrence.

Urethral Prolapse

Urethral prolapse occurs most commonly in young black girls. The presenting symptoms are bloody spotting and dysuria. The diagnosis is made on physical examination, when an inflamed everted mucosa is seen surrounding the urethral meatus. These patients can usually be managed with estrogen cream applications two or three times daily for 2 weeks. If a prolapsed urethra persists for several months, formal excision may be necessary.

Urethral Duplication

Duplication of the uretha is a rare anomaly. Three major varieties may occur. In type one, there is complete duplication of the urethra. Urine will flow from both urethras. In type two, there is a bifid urethra that may or may not have two external openings. Type three indicates that the ventral meatus is in a perineal location. In all of these categories, the ventral urethra is the most normal. Presenting symptoms include voiding with two urinary streams, infection, or purulent discharge. A voiding cystourethrogram is helpful in delineating the anatomy and confirming the diagnosis. Treatment depends on the anatomy of the duplication and its clinical manifestations. Surgery should be considered for disturbing symptoms, such as a divergent double stream, incontinence, or a cosmetic deformity, such as an epispadiac meatus. Surgical treatment may involve complete excision of the accessory urethra, transurethral excision of the intraurethral system, or formal urethroplasty.

Megalourethra

Megalourethra is a rare entity associated with developmental abnormalities of two types: fusiform (complete type) and scaphoid (incomplete type). A fusiform megalourethra has a deficiency of both the corpora cavernosa and the corpus spongiosum. The penis is flaccid and markedly distended. This type is usually associated with severe forms of the prune-belly syndrome. If the patients survive, treatment of this defect is usually unsatisfactory, and sex conversion may be necessary. The scaphoid variety has an abnormal corpus spongiosum. Treatment usually involves trimming of the uretha.

Urethral Gland Abnormalities

There are two groups of periurethral glands, the diaphragmatic glands and the bulbar glands. These glands empty their secretions through their appropriate ducts into the urethra. Any obstruction within the ducts may cause retention cysts, abscess formation, or a dilated duct. In addition, urine may reflux into a dilated duct. Any of these conditions may lead to symptoms of obstruction or infection. If symptomatic, transurethral fulguration of the retention cysts may be performed. Most children are asymptomatic and do not require any treatment.

REFERENCES

1. Colodny A: Urethral lesions in infants and children. *In* Gillenwater JY (ed): Adult and Pediatric Urology. St. Louis, Mosby Year Book, 1993:1995.
2. Hays DM: Bladder/prostate rhabdomyosarcoma: Results of the multi-institutional trials of the Intergroup Rhabdomyosarcoma Study. Semin Surg Oncol 9:520–523, 1993.
3. Retik AB, Casale A: Hypospadias. *In* Libertino J (ed): Pediatric and Adult Reconstructive Urology. Baltimore, Williams & Wilkins, 1990:501.
4. Rimon U, Hertz M, Jonas P: Diverticula of the male uretha: A review of 61 cases. Urol Radiol 14:49–55, 1992.
5. Rosenfeld B, Greenfield SP, Springate JE, Feld LG: Type III posterior urethral valves: Presentation and management. J Pediatr Surg 29:81–85, 1994.

VESICOURETERAL REFLUX

RONALD J. HOGG, M.D.

Vesicoureteral reflux (VUR) refers to retrograde passage of urine from the bladder into one or both ureters. This may occur spontaneously or only during voiding. The severity of the disorder is defined by the level of the collecting system reached by refluxing urine, as shown by dye or radioisotope during a voiding cystogram, and the extent to which there is dilatation of the pelviureteral system. Most authorities have adopted the International Classification of VUR, which subdivides the disorder into five grades of severity, with grade I being the least severe (nondilating reflux into the ureter only) and grade V being the most severe (reflux causing significant blunting of the majority of the calyceal fornices associated with gross dilatation and tortuosity of the ureters).[6]

Although the VUR classification questions appear to have been resolved, the importance of VUR as the marker of possible renal scarring from ascending urinary tract infection (UTI) (reflux nephropathy, RN) has come under increased scrutiny in recent years. It has been well established that VUR occurs in approximately 30% to 40% of children under 5 years of age with UTIs. However, the assumption that children without VUR are safe from renal parenchymal injury has been shown to be erroneous.[4,5] For example, in a recent study of 150 children with their first UTI, Ditchfield et al.[4] reported that whereas 88 of 300 kidneys (almost 30%) had at least one cortical defect shown by renal cortical scanning, over half of the scarred kidneys (54/88, 61%) had no evidence of VUR by voiding cystourethrogram (VCUG). However, cortical defects were noted in 47% of the 72 kidneys in which VUR was found. The authors noted that the specificity of VCUG in predicting a renal cortical defect was 82.1%, whereas the sensitivity was only 38.6%. They raised the possibility that demonstrating VUR by VCUG may be less important than showing renal scars by cortical scanning when defining which patients are at risk for RN and should, therefore, be treated.[4]

MANAGEMENT

Medical Management

The optimal management of VUR varies according to the severity of the disorder and the presence or absence of associated abnormalities. There is good agreement that the initial—and often the only—treatment necessary for mild to moderate grades of VUR involves measures to keep the urine free of infection while waiting for the VUR to resolve spontaneously. Sterility of the urine is usually achieved by (1) limiting the exposure of the urethra to fecal bacteria by encouraging the patient and parent to practice good hygiene, (2) maintaining a high urine flow rate via high fluid intake, and (3) placing the patient on a low prophylactic dose (1 to 2 mg/kg/d) of an appropriate antibiotic, such as trimethoprim-sulfamethoxazole or nitrofurantoin. In addition, constipation should be avoided in patients with VUR, since this can interfere with normal bladder emptying and further increase the risk of ascending bladder infections. Having done all these things, it is important to ensure that the patient's urine remains sterile by obtaining serial urine cultures every 1 to 2 months.

A relatively new aspect of the medical management of VUR concerns the treatment of this disorder when it is diagnosed or suspected in utero by a prenatal sonogram.[6] This diagnosis needs confirmation by a postnatal study before long-term treatment is undertaken, but it is appropriate to begin prophylactic treatment immediately after birth to avoid a UTI in the postnatal period before obtaining a VCUG. The prophylactic antibiotic most frequently prescribed during the first 2 months of life is amoxicillin. After 2 months, it is reasonable to change to the standard prophylaxis described previously. By starting therapy in anticipation of a diagnosis of VUR, it is to be hoped that renal injury from the first UTI may be avoided. This may reduce the number of patients in whom renal scarring has already occurred when the diagnosis of VUR is made. However, the recent incorporation of neonatal antibiotic prophylaxis has not completely abolished the finding of abnormal renal cortical scans when VUR is first identified, thus providing evidence that some of the RN scars may represent areas of maldevelopment or dysplasia that are not related to renal parenchymal infection.

Another series of observations has drawn attention to the fact that a diagnostic workup for VUR may be necessary for symptom-free siblings of children with VUR, of whom approximately one third may have VUR.[5] Furthermore, Buonomo et al.[3] recently reported that 6 of 16 siblings in whom this diagnosis was made had scintigraphic evidence of renal damage. Not surprisingly, based on their results, Buonomo et al.[3] recommended that screening radionuclide VCUGs and cortical scanning when appropriate should be undertaken early in life in the siblings of all children known to have VUR.

Results of Medical Management of Mild VUR

In a prospective study by the Southwest Pediatric Nephrology Study Group (SPNSG) reported by Arant,[2] 59 patients with VUR grades I to III but no significant radiologic signs of renal injury were treated medically for 5 years and followed with annual VCUGs and serial annual intravenous pyelograms (IVPs). At the end of the 5 years, 17% of the previously normal kidneys had decreased growth—based on their planimetric surface area—and 12 of the kidneys (in 11 patients) showed renal scarring. Whether these scars were the results of renal parenchymal damage sustained before the institution of medical treatment could not be ascertained by this study. It is noteworthy that VUR was never demonstrated in 4 of the kidneys in which scars developed during the period of study. Another unexpected, but important, finding was that VUR was demonstrated at the first or second year follow-up VCUG in 9 of 34 (27%) kidneys in which VUR was *not* seen in the baseline study. These two observations raise additional questions regarding the relevance of radiologic evidence of VUR to renal injury in children with recurrent UTIs and the failure to exclude VUR with a single VCUG in such children.

Surprisingly, the incidence of renal parenchymal injury in the SPNSG study was approximately 10% in ureters with *no* VUR and in those with VUR grades I and II but occurred in 28% of the ureters with grade III VUR. Overall, the rate of resolution of mild degrees of VUR observed in the SPNSG studies was excellent. At the end of 5 years, over 80% of the ureters with grade I and II VUR had no evidence of VUR (based on two consecutive negative VCUGs), and a higher or unchanged grade of VUR was seen in only 3 of 51 ureters. In addition, VUR had resolved in 46% and improved in 40% of the 33 ureters with grade III VUR. None of the ureters with grade III VUR had more severe reflux at the end of the follow-up. The SPNSG study thus demonstrated that a high rate of resolution of mild VUR can be anticipated following medical treatment of VUR but that monitoring for renal scarring and other signs of renal injury should be continued, since these abnormalities may occur occasionally in mild cases of VUR and even when VUR is not demonstrable. Whether the outcome would be improved by surgical reimplantation has not been studied in patients with mild to moderate degrees of VUR.

Surgical Management of Moderate to Severe VUR (Grades III to V)

A number of studies have been done to assess the effect of ureteral reimplantation procedures on the clinical course of patients with more severe degrees of VUR. Such studies have shown that the frequency of UTIs is somewhat higher in the surgical group, who do not receive long-term antibiotics, but the number of episodes of pyelonephritis is less. Contrary to previous assumptions, there has been no significant decrease in the frequency of new scarring in patients in whom the VUR has been corrected surgically. It should be noted, however, that many of the patients already had scarred kidneys at the time they entered into the study.

In a randomized clinical trial of medical versus surgical management of infants and children with grades III and IV primary VUR, Weiss et al., reporting for the International Reflux Study, found that new renal scarring developed in 22% of medical and 31% of surgical patients ($p < 0.04$).[7] Pyelonephritis occurred in 15 medical patients versus 5 surgical patients ($p < 0.05$). There was no significant change in glomerular filtration rate within or between groups. The rate of resolution in patients with grade IV reflux was approximately 8% per year in the medical patients, and 75% still had reflux after 3 years of observation.

SUMMARY

The current uncertainty regarding optimal treatment for infants and children with VUR makes it difficult to provide concise, generalized recommendations. The overall goal has not changed, however, that is, to prevent or limit the degree of renal parenchymal damage that may result from VUR and its associated complications. It seems clear that attempts to maintain the urine sterile should remain the cardinal feature. Also important should be attempts to facilitate complete bladder emptying and a high urine flow rate. The extent to which surgical intervention will complement these approaches will hopefully become clearer in future years. For the present time, it would appear prudent to rely mainly on aggressive medical measures for most patients, especially those with mild to moderate degrees of VUR. It is important to reiterate that even patients with mild VUR must be considered at risk for renal damage—no matter what treatment is used.

REFERENCES

1. Andrich MP, Majd M: Diagnostic imaging in the evaluation of the first urinary tract infection in infants and young children. Pediatrics 90:436–441, 1992.
2. Arant BS Jr: Medical management of mild and moderate vesicoureteral reflux: Follow-up studies of infants and young children. A preliminary report of the Southwest Pediatric Nephrology Study Group. J Urol 148:1683–1687, 1992.
3. Buonomo C, Treves ST, Jones B, Summerville D, Bauer S, Retik A: Silent renal damage in symptom-free siblings of children with vesicoureteral reflux: Assessment with technetium Tc-99m dimercaptosuccinic acid scintigraphy. J Pediatr 122:721–723, 1993.
4. Ditchfield MR, DeCampo JF, Cook DJ, Nolan TM, Powell HR, Sloane R, Grimwood K, Cahill S: Vesicoureteral reflux: An accurate predictor of acute pyelonephritis in childhood urinary tract infections? Radiology 190:413–415, 1994.
5. Noe HN: The long-term results of prospective sibling reflux screening. J Urol 148:1739–1742, 1992.
6. Weiss RA: Vesico-ureteral reflux (VUR) in children. Kidney 25:1–6, 1993.
7. Weiss R, Duckett J, Spitzer A, for the International Reflux Study in Children: Results of a randomized clinical trial of medical versus surgical management of infants and children with grades III and IV primary vesicoureteral reflux (United States). J Urol 148:1667–1673, 1992.

INFECTIONS OF THE URINARY TRACT

EUGENE D. SHAPIRO, M.D.

Although seemingly a straightforward problem, the diagnosis and management of bacterial infections of the urinary tract in children require clinicians to make a number of relatively complex decisions. How should the diagnosis be made? Should the patient be hospitalized? What antimicrobials should be used? Which radiographic studies should be obtained? There are many options available, and there is no single correct approach to these issues.

DIAGNOSIS

There are many potential problems in establishing the diagnosis of a urinary tract infection (UTI) in a child. The classic gold standard definition of a bacterial infection of the urinary tract, the isolation of $\geq$100,000 colony-forming units (CFU) of bacteria from a midstream, clean-catch sample of urine, is based on old studies conducted in adult women. Recent studies have indicated that among adult women with dysuria, of those with bacteria isolated from specimens obtained by suprapubic aspiration, nearly half had counts less than 100,000 CFU/ml of urine (some had as few as 100 CFU/ml). No comparable studies have been conducted in children. However, the isolation of a pure culture of a uropathogen in concentrations between 5000 and 100,000 CFU/ml of urine in two or more different clean-catch samples from a *symptomatic* child should also be considered evidence of a UTI.

In young children, the diagnosis of a UTI is complicated by the difficulty of obtaining uncontaminated specimens of urine and by the sometimes nonspecific nature of their symptoms. Indeed, fever may be the only symptom of pyelonephritis in an infant. Because, especially in infants, the urinalysis is imperfect as a screening test for a UTI, cultures of the urine should be obtained in all infants in whom a UTI is suspected. Specimens of urine obtained by the bag collection method have an unacceptably high rate of contamination. Consequently, if a child who may have a UTI is unable to provide a midstream, clean-catch specimen of urine, a specimen of urine for culture should be obtained by either suprapubic aspiration or urethral catheterization before antimicrobial therapy is initiated. Any growth of bacteria in a sample obtained by suprapubic aspiration and counts $\geq$1,000 CFU/ml in a sample obtained by urethral catheterization generally are considered to be indicative of a UTI.

Whatever criteria are used for defining a UTI, the diagnosis depends on the concentration of bacteria in the urine, which may be influenced by the rate of production of urine, how long the urine has been in the bladder, and how the specimen is stored after it is collected. Since bacteria may multiply in urine that is at room temperature, it is important promptly either to inoculate the culture media or to refrigerate the specimen until the media can be inoculated. The interpretation of the significance of bacteriuria is complicated further by the entity of covert or asymptomatic bacteriuria. When asymptomatic children are screened, some (up to 2.5% of boys and 1% of girls under 6 months of age and 1% to 3% of girls older than 6 months) will have significant ($\geq$100,000 CFU/ml) concentrations of bacteria in multiple samples of urine. Although still somewhat controversial, most studies have indicated that the vast majority of children with asymptomatic bacteriuria, left untreated, have an excellent prognosis, and impairment of their renal function will not occur. Consequently, most experts do not recommend routine screening of asymptomatic children for bacteriuria.

TREATMENT

The goals of treatment are (1) to alleviate the acute symptoms, (2) to prevent or to minimize damage to the renal parenchyma, and (3) to prevent recurrent infections and their attendant morbidity. Infections that are limited to the lower urinary tract (e.g., cystitis) generally are not associated with significant sequelae. On the other hand, bacterial infections that involve the renal parenchyma, especially those that occur during infancy or early childhood and those that are associated with either vesicoureteral reflux or obstruction (e.g., posterior urethral valves), may result in scarring and permanent loss of functional renal tissue.

The microorganisms most often responsible for infections of the urinary tract are shown in Table 1. Once the diagnosis is established, the physician must decide whether a child should be hospitalized, which antimicrobial to use, how to administer it (i.e., orally or parenterally), and which radiographic studies of the urinary tract to obtain.

The risk of permanent renal damage as a consequence of infection is inversely related to the age of the child. Most infection-associated scarring of the kidney (and the consequent loss of functional renal tissue) occurs during the first and second years of life. Scarring occurs only rarely in children older than 5 years. Consequently, aggressive treatment is justified in younger children. In addition, pyelonephritis is sometimes associated with bacteremia in young infants. I do not routinely obtain blood cultures in children suspected of having pyelonephritis unless they are young infants, are immunocompromised, appear toxic, or have a type of heart disease that puts them at risk of endocarditis.

Fortunately, many antimicrobial agents are effective against the bacteria that commonly are responsible for infections of the urinary tract. The choice of an antimicrobial to treat a patient with a UTI should be guided by tests of the antimicrobial susceptibility of the bacteria that are isolated. Patients with uncomplicated infections limited to the lower urinary tract (e.g., cystitis) can be treated effectively as outpatients with orally administered antimicrobial agents. Pending the identification of the responsible bacteria and the results of the antimicrobial susceptibility tests, amoxicillin, trimethoprim-sulfamethoxazole, and a cephalosporin all are reasonable agents to use for empiric therapy in a patient in whom cystitis is suspected (doses are shown in Table 2). There is uncertainty about how long to treat patients with cystitis. I usually treat for 5 to 7 days. Because concentrations in the urine of most antimicrobials used to treat UTIs far exceed concentrations in the serum (often by a factor of 100 or more), even so-called resistant strains of bacteria may be eradicated. A single large dose of an antimicrobial may be effective for treating cystitis. However, because both the rate of failure of treatment and the frequency of recurrent infections are somewhat higher after single-dose treatment, such therapy generally should be reserved for older children and adolescents in whom the benefits of assured compliance (when the single dose is administered before the child leaves the office) outweigh these disadvantages. Many of the newer, orally administered cephalosporins (e.g., cefprozil, cefpodoxime, loracarbef, and cefixime) are effective for treating most UTIs, since the bacteria that commonly cause UTIs in children usually are susceptible to these agents. However, there is no evidence that these drugs are superior

TABLE 1. Organisms that Cause Urinary Tract Infections

*Escherichia coli**
Klebsiella sp.
Enterobacter sp.
Proteus sp.
Enterococci
Group B streptococci†
Staphylococcus saprophyticus‡
Pseudomonas sp
Fungi§

*Causes approximately 85% of first episodes of UTI.
†Occurs primarily in newborns.
‡Occurs primarily in female adolescents.
§Occurs primarily in patients who recently have had urologic surgery, who have indwelling catheters, who are taking antimicrobials chronically, or who are immunocompromised.

TABLE 2. Empiric Antimicrobial Treatment of Cystitis*

DRUG	DOSE
Amoxicillin	50 mg/kg/d divided t.i.d. (max: 2–3 g/d)
Trimethoprim-sulfamethoxazole	6 mg/kg/d of trimethoprim divided b.i.d. (max: 0.5–1 g/d)
Cephalexin	50 mg/kg/d divided q.i.d. (max: 2–3 g/d)

*Treat for 5–7 days.

to the older, less expensive, and more widely used antimicrobials for treating children with a UTI. Consequently, the decision about which drug to use should be based on cost, convenience, and adverse side effects (as well as the antimicrobial susceptibility of the bacteria isolated from the culture of the urine).

It may be difficult to distinguish between infections of the upper and of the lower urinary tract on clinical grounds alone (particularly in infants and young children). Factors that should be considered in deciding how to manage patients with possible infection of the upper urinary tract (pyelonephritis) include (1) the patient's clinical appearance and the need for supportive care (patients who are moderately or severely dehydrated, who are in shock, or who appear toxic should be hospitalized and treated with fluids and antimicrobials administered intravenously), (2) the age of the patient, (3) the expected compliance with treatment, and (4) the reliability of follow-up.

Table 3 shows antimicrobials that are recommended for parenterally administered empirical treatment of pyelonephritis. Before the organism that is causing the infection is identified and its antimicrobial susceptibility determined, the clinician may be able to ascertain the morphologic characteristics of the organism (e.g., gram-positive diplococci or gram-negative rods) to help guide the choice of antimicrobials by examining a gram-stained smear of the urinary sediment. The decision of whether to hospitalize the patient and to treat parenterally should be based on factors that were outlined previously. Hospitalization generally is warranted for a child with pyelonephritis who is under 3 months of age, as well as for most who are 6 months of age or younger. *To consider managing a child with pyelonephritis as an outpatient, it is critical that there be good compliance with the prescribed treatment regimen and that absolute reliability of follow-up be assured.*

Although there are many antimicrobials that are effective for treating pyelonephritis when administered orally, they can work only if they are administered appropriately. Furthermore, even if the caretaker does administer the antimicrobial reliably, if the child is vomiting (a common symptom of pyelonephritis), the drug may not be absorbed and treatment may be ineffective. One attractive option to ensure that a patient with pyelonephritis who will not be hospitalized receives adequate antimicrobial treatment is initially to administer parenterally a dose of ceftriaxone (50 mg/kg). This will result in concentrations in the kidney and in the urine for at least 24 hours that far exceed the minimal inhibitory concentration of most of the common bacterial pathogens (one exception is the enterococcus). Subsequent treatment with an orally administered agent may be guided by the antimicrobial susceptibility of the bacteria that are isolated. Although orally administered amoxicillin is usually effective, many experts prefer trimethoprim-sulfamethoxazole to treat pyelonephritis orally because of the higher concentrations that are achieved in renal tissue by this combination.

Once the antimicrobial susceptibility of the bacterium that caused the infection is known, antimicrobial therapy may be modified so that treatment is directed more specifically against the responsible organism. For hospitalized patients who are allergic to penicillins and cephalosporins, aztreonam (90 to 120 mg/kg/d administered q8h; maximum 6 to 8 g/d) may be a suitable alternative agent. Antimicrobial

TABLE 3. Empiric Antimicrobial Treatment of Pyelonephritis

Hospitalized Patients (Antimicrobials Administered IV)

Ampicillin *and*	100–150 mg/kg/d divided q6h (max: 12 g/d)
Gentamicin	5–7.5 mg/kg/d divided q8h* (max: 300 mg/d)
Alternatives are ampicillin and	
Cefotaxime *or*	100–150 mg/kg/d divided q8h (max: 12 g/d)
Ceftriaxone *or*	50–75 mg/kg/d in a single dose (max: 2–4 g/d)
Ceftazidime	100–150 mg/kg/d divided q8h (max: 6–8 g/d)

Outpatients

Trimethoprim-sulfamethoxazole *or*	6 mg/kg/d of trimethoprim administered PO b.i.d.
Ceftriaxone†	50 mg/kg/d (max: 2 g/d) administered IM or IV in a single dose

*The higher dose is for neonates and young infants. If renal function is impaired or treatment is to be continued for several days or longer, concentrations of gentamicin in serum should be monitored and the dosage altered as appropriate.

†Switch to trimethoprim-sulfamethoxazole or another suitable orally administered agent after 24–48 h.

treatment usually is continued for 10 to 14 days, although patients who initially were treated parenterally may be switched to an orally administered antimicrobial once they have stopped vomiting and are improving clinically. A culture of the urine 24 to 48 hours after the initiation of treatment is useful to document that the urine has been sterilized. Even after appropriate antimicrobial treatment has been initiated in patients with uncomplicated pyelonephritis, it may take up to 48 to 72 hours for the inflammation to subside and for symptoms, such as fever and vomiting, to resolve. If after this time the patient has not had a favorable clinical response to treatment or if obstruction of urinary flow is suspected (e.g., because of a history of renal stones or a known anatomic abnormality), appropriate radiographic studies, such as ultrasound, IVP, or CT scan, should be undertaken to determine whether surgical intervention may be necessary.

After treatment for pyelonephritis has been completed, it is advisable to administer to infants and young children with first-time infectons low-dose prophylactic antimicrobials to prevent recurrent infections until the anatomy of the urinary tract has been evaluated with a voiding cystourethrogram and a renal ultrasound. If significant vesicoureteral reflux or certain other abnormalities are found, long-term antimicrobial prophylaxis may be indicated. For prophylaxis, I usually use trimethoprim-sulfamethoxazole (1 to 2 mg/kg of trimethoprim) in a single daily dose at night. Nitrofurantoin (1 to 2 mg/kg dose) is a suitable alternative agent.

IMAGING OF THE URINARY TRACT

Investigation of the functional anatomy of the urinary tract is an important aspect of managing the patient with a UTI. The goal of imaging is to detect anatomic or functional abnormalities, such as posterior urethral valves, vesicoureteral reflux, or obstruction of the ureteropelvic junction, intervention for which may prevent either recurrent infections or obstructive uropathy and associated renal damage. Radiographic studies may be helpful in defining the extent of any renal damage and in assessing the prognosis of the patient. In children with pyelonephritis, vesicoureteral reflux is a particularly common problem that is important to detect, since at least in young children, prevention of infection can minimize renal scarring and may help to avoid the need for surgical intervention.

I believe that all children with pyelonephritis, regardless of their age, should undergo a renal ultrasound. The ultrasound may be obtained anytime during or after the acute infection. As long as the patient has responded appropriately to treatment, I usually wait several weeks so that edema of the kidney has resolved. If the ultrasound

demonstrates normal kidneys and the child is 5 years of age or older, additional studies usually are not necessary unless a second episode occurs. Although the ultrasound may fail to detect mild to moderate degrees of vesicoureteral reflux, even if such reflux is present, scarring of the kidney is rare in children older than 5 years. Because younger children have a relatively high frequency of treatable anatomic abnormalities or vesicoureteral reflux and because they are at risk of permanent renal damage from some of these conditions, I believe that all such children younger than 5 years should also be evaluated with a voiding cystourethrogram. There is controversy about whether infection can itself cause vesicoureteral reflux. Nevertheless, I usually wait 4 to 5 weeks before I obtain the voiding cystourethrogram. Although radionuclide renography provides sensitive data about renal function, in most patients who have had an ultrasound and a voiding cystourethrogram, the results will not change how the patient is managed. Consequently, I do not routinely order this test. Such tests may be useful in some patients with advanced or complicated disease and when surgical intervention is being considered.

REFERENCES

1. Hoberman A, Chao H-P, Keller DM, Hickey R, Davis HW, Ellis D: Prevalence of urinary tract infection in febrile infants. J Pediatr 123:17–23, 1993.
2. Lohr JA: Use of routine urinalysis in making a presumptive diagnosis of urinary tract infection in children. Pediatr Infect Dis J 10:646–650, 1991.
3. McCracken GH Jr: Diagnosis and management of acute urinary tract infections in infants and children. Pediatr Infect Dis J 6:107–112, 1987.

PERINEPHRIC AND INTRANEPHRIC ABSCESS

RAYMOND D. ADELMAN, M.D.
STEPHEN R. SHAPIRO, M.D.

Perinephric and intranephric abscess formation in children is rare. In most cases, early antibiotic therapy probably aborts the process. When suppuration and necrosis have occurred, an abscess is formed. A renal carbuncle represents coalescence of multiple abscesses into a multiloculated cavity. A perirenal abscess occurs when the infection extends beyond the renal capsule but is confined by Gerota's fascia. A pararenal abscess is present if the infection extends beyond Gerota's fascia. *Staphylococcus* and *Escherichia coli* are the most common causes of renal abscesses. Other organisms include *Proteus, Pseudomonas, Salmonella,* and anaerobic organisms, especially *Bacteroides. Candida* and *Torulopsis* also may be seen, especially in immunocompromised patients or those with diabetes or a history of multiple courses of antibiotic therapy.

Recent abdominal or urologic surgery is a common antecedant in children with perinephric abscess. Renal abscesses can also occur in healthy children from a minor, remote cutaneous, respiratory, or dental site. With gram-negative infection, an underlying urinary tract abnormality may exist, such as vesicoureteral reflux, obstructive uropathy, renal vein thrombosis, renal calculi, or renal trauma. Abscesses involving *Staphylococcus* or hemolytic streptococci have been associated with congenital heart disease. Children with an abnormal host response to infection, such as those with chronic granulomatous disease, diabetes mellitus, or leukemia, or those under treatment with immunosuppressive drugs, such as transplant recipients, are predisposed to renal abscesses. Recent or concomitant infections may be found in such children, including endocarditis, carbuncle, psoas abscess, and necrotizing enterocolitis. After confirmation of the diagnosis by ultrasonography or computerized tomography (CT), blood and urine cultures should be obtained. Blood cultures are usually negative, whereas urine cultures predict the perinephric abscess organism in up to 20% of cases. However, pathogens isolated from the urine often correlate poorly with those cultured from the abscess, especially in abscess infection with multiple organisms. In this instance and with persistent signs and symptoms, aspirate cultures may guide the clinician in the adjustment of antibiotic therapy. Because urine and blood cultures are often not helpful and because it may be difficult to distinguish an abscess radiographically from other lesions (Wilms' tumor in the infant and child, renal cell carcinoma in the teenager, as well as renal hamartoma and lymphoma), we recommend fine-needle aspiration and percutaneous drainage of the abscess unless contraindications exist. The aspirated material should be cultured aerobically and anaerobically, and fungal cultures should be performed. A gram stain should be made, and, if indicated, stains for fungi and acid-fast bacilli should be done. Negative cultures are obtained in 5% to 10% of cases.

If the condition of the child permits, a trial of intensive antibiotic treatment may be warranted before percutaneous aspiration or surgical drainage and is successful in about 25% of patients. Currently, percutaneous catheter drainage offers an attractive alternative to open surgical drainage for patients with a perinephric or intranephric abscess. After needle aspiration of the purulent material, a catheter or multiple catheters can be inserted into the abscess cavity or cavities. Percutaneous drainage of the urine from the kidney can be accomplished simultaneously if indicated for obstructive uropathy (ureteropelvic junction obstruction, ureteral calculi). The abscess cavity can be irrigated with antibiotic solution, or in some cases, the catheter may be left indwelling, without irrigation, in combination with antibiotic therapy. Resolution of the abscess occurs in several days to 4 to 6 weeks. Percutaneous abscess drainage duplicates surgical treatment in providing decompression, continual drainage, and evacuation. In most reported cases, adequate drainage of the abscess cavity has been accomplished with a catheter size as small as 8.3 French using a pigtail variety of catheter.

Indications for removal of the catheter include resolution of fever, cessation of drainage, return of the white blood cell count to normal, and a sinogram showing nearly complete closure of the abscess cavity. Following removal of the catheter, the drainage tract will close rapidly if infected material has been adequately removed.

Percutaneous drainage of the abscess will fail if the cavity is inadequately drained, if multiple pockets of pus are not recognized, or if there is continuous drainage despite adequate catheter placement (suggesting an enteric fistula). Percutaneous techniques have now proved suitable even for the small infant or neonate, in whom renal abscesses are, fortunately, extremely rare.

Although percutaneous drainage is successful in the vast majority of patients, some patients may require operation instead of percutaneous drainage or following it. The decision to perform surgery should be based on the patient's general condition, associated pathologic findings, and the condition of the involved kidney. For example, poorly functioning or nonfunctioning kidneys, particularly those with multiple abscesses, may indicate a need for surgical treatment, such as nephrectomy and drainage. The clinical response is also critical. Failure of percutaneous drainage to result in defervescence of signs and symptoms within 48 to 72 hours may suggest inadequate drainage.

Initial antibiotic therapy must include gram-negative coverage for *E. coli*, *Proteus*, and *Pseudomonas* and coverage for *Staphylococcus*. An aminoglycoside and an antistaphylococcal agent in combination may be necessary. Tobramycin 6 to 7.5 mg/kg/d is recommended. Ceftazidime 100 to 150 mg/kg/d may be substituted for tobramycin. Intravenous doses of cefazolin 100 mg/kg/d or nafcillin 100 to 150 mg/kg/d continue to provide the best coverage for *Staphylococcus*. In patients allergic to penicillin, vancomycin 45 to 60 mg/kg/d should be substituted. Antibiotic doses should be lowered appropriately for neonates. *Candida* infections will require amphotericin B or fluconazole or both. Anaerobic coverage also may be indicated. Although documentation in the literatue does not exist, it is assumed that parenteral therapy should be continued for 1 to 2 weeks, followed by oral therapy for an additional 2 to 4 weeks, as indicated by the clinical condition.

HEMOLYTIC-UREMIC SYNDROME

JERRY M. BERGSTEIN, M.D.

The hemolytic-uremic syndrome (HUS) is a common cause of acute renal failure in children. The disease is characterized by a microangiopathic hemolytic anemia, thrombocytopenia, and acute renal failure.

PATHOGENESIS

The causes of HUS are listed in Table 1. The disease most commonly follows a gastroenteritis produced by an enteropathogenic strain of *Escherichia coli* (ATCC No. 0157:H7). The reservoir of this organism is the intestinal tract of domestic animals. It is usually transmitted by undercooked meat or unpasteurized milk. The organism elaborates a toxin called verotoxin (a similar toxin is produced by *Shigella* sp.), which apparently is absorbed from the gut, leading to HUS.

Recent studies suggest that the pathogenic feature common to all causes of HUS is the capacity to injure endothelial cells. Direct (cytotoxins, endotoxin) or indirect (through the activation of neutrophils or the production of antiendothelial cell antibodies) endothelial cell injury results in the generation of factors that promote clotting (tissue factor, tumor necrosis factor, interleukin 1, platelet-activating factor, large multimers of Von Willebrand factor) and inhibit fibrinolysis (plasminogen activator inhibitor 1), leading to microvascular thrombosis in the kidneys and other organs.

In HUS, fibrin thrombi in the glomerular capillaries and arterioles lead to renal insufficiency. The anemia results from mechanical damage to the erythrocytes as they attempt to pass through the fibrin thrombi. Thrombocytopenia is due to adhesion of platelets to the microthrombi and to removal of damaged platelets from the circulation by the reticuloendothelial system.

CLINICAL MANIFESTATIONS

HUS is most common in children under age 4 years. It is usually preceded by diarrhea, which is frequently bloody. The prodrome phase is followed in 5 to 10 days by the sudden onset of pallor, irritability, oliguria, and, occasionally, petechiae, edema, jaundice, and hepatosplenomegaly. Extrarenal involvement may include the central ner-

TABLE 1. Etiology of Hemolytic-Uremic Syndrome (HUS)

Infection
Enteropathogenic *Escherichia coli* (ATCC No. 0157:H7)
Shigella
Campylobacter jejuni
Yersinia enterocolitica
Streptococcus pneumoniae
Bartonella sp.
Viruses

Systemic Disorders
Transplantation
Systemic lupus erythematosus
Pregnancy (preeclampsia, postpartum)
Malignancies
Severe hypertension
Kawasaki disease

Toxins
Cisplatin
Mitomycin
Cyclosporine
Estrogen-containing oral contraceptives
Radiation

vous system (irritability, seizures, coma), colitis (melena, perforation), diabetes mellitus, and rhabdomyolysis.

DIAGNOSIS

The diagnosis is supported by detection of a microangiopathic hemolytic anemia, characterized by fragmented erythrocytes on the blood film and evidence of intravascular hemolysis (elevated plasma hemoglobin and reticulocyte count, decreased plasma haptoglobin) in association with thrombocytopenia and a variable degree of renal insufficiency. Evidence for disseminated intravascular coagulation (DIC) is absent, but vitamin K deficiency may occur. Findings on urinalysis are surprisingly mild. Appropriate studies should be obtained to seek known causes of the syndrome (blood and stool cultures, antinuclear antibody titer) and to exclude other causes of acute renal failure, especially those associated with microangiopathic hemolytic anemia (bilateral renal vein thrombosis, malignant hypertension, systemic lupus erythematosus, and thrombotic thrombocytopenic purpura).

TREATMENT

Complications of the disease are primarily related to the microangiopathic state (anemia) and the degree of renal insufficiency (acidosis, hyperkalemia, fluid overload, congestive heart failure, hypertension, uremia). Each time the hemoglobin falls below 7 g/dl, the patient is transfused with 10 ml/kg of packed red blood cells. The management of acute renal failure is summarized in a later section of this chapter.

Presumably, recovery of renal function depends on removal of glomerular thrombi. If endogenous fibrinolytic mechanisms (mediated by the elaboration of tissue plasminogen activator and urokinase) remove glomerular thrombi before the development of ischemic necrosis, glomerular function will be restored. Although several forms of therapy (corticosteroids, anticoagulants, platelet inhibitors, fibrinolytic agents, fresh-frozen plasma with or without plasmapheresis) pointed toward resolving glomerular thrombi have been proposed, none are of proven benefit, and all have potential risks. Peritoneal dialysis was previously looked on as supportive therapy only, but recent studies indicate that in addition to controlling the uremic state, early peritoneal dialysis promotes recovery by removing an inhibitor (plasminogen activator inhibitor 1) of glomerular fibrinolytic activity from the circulation. Plasma levels of this inhibitor at presentation correlate with the degree of renal failure, and normalization of plasma inhibitor levels by dialysis or by spontaneous recovery within 16 days after presentation is associated with recovery of renal function.

Thus, peritoneal dialysis is initiated as soon as it is clear that the patient is progressing to renal failure. A Tenckhoff catheter is inserted into the peritoneal cavity, and dialysis is initiated with a dialysate volume of 30 to 50 ml/kg. Dialysate is exchanged on hourly cycles (inflow 10 minutes, dwell 35 minutes, drain 15 minutes) for up to 16 days. If the patient has not recovered renal function after 16 days of hourly exchanges, continuous ambulatory peritoneal dialysis is initiated.

With aggressive management of the acute renal failure, more than 90% of patients will survive the acute phase, with most recovering normal renal function.

REFERENCES

1. Bergstein JM, Riley M, Bang NU: Role of plasminogen-activator inhibitor type 1 in the pathogenesis and outcome of the hemolytic-uremic syndrome. N Engl J Med 327:755–759, 1992.
2. Kaplan BS, Trompeter RS, Moake JL (eds): Hemolytic-Uremic Syndrome and Thrombotic Thrombocytopenic Purpura. New York, Marcel Dekker, 1992.
3. Kelles A, Van Dyck M, Proesmans W: Childhood haemolytic uremic syndrome: Long-term outcome and prognostic features. Eur J Pediatr 153:38–42, 1994.
4. Robson WL, Leung AK, Brant R: Relationship of the recovery in the glomerular filtration rate to the duration of anuria in diarrhea-associated hemolytic-uremic syndrome. Am J Nephrol 13:194–197, 1993.
5. Stewart CL, Tina LU: Hemolytic-uremic syndrome. Pediatr Rev 14:218–224, 1993.

UROLITHIASIS

F. BRUDER STAPLETON, M.D.

Urolithiasis is being recognized with increasing frequency in children, particularly in high-risk groups with neurogenic bladder, bronchopulmonary dysplasia, corticosteroid therapy, hyperalimentation, steatorrhea, or antineoplastic chemotherapy. Pediatricians must have a high sensitivity to the possibility of urolithiasis because the classic symptom of incapacitating renal colic is unusual in children. Abdominal or flank pain occurs in approximately 50% of children with urolithiasis. Either microscopic or macroscopic hematuria heralds urinary stones in greater than 90% of such patients. Urinary infection is a common complication.

DIAGNOSIS

Preventive medical therapies should be directed toward specific etiologies of urolithiasis. Whenever possible, evaluation of urolithiasis should begin with analysis of the stone mineral composition. In the case of struvite (infection-related), cystine, or urate stones, specific diagnoses may be determined through stone analysis, and the diagnostic evaluation can be narrowly directed. In the majority of patients, however, the stone will be composed of calcium oxalate, and further extensive metabolic studies are warranted. Further diagnostic studies should be deferred until the stone episode has resolved and urinary infection has been eradicated. For patients with calcium oxalate or calcium phosphate stones or in whom a stone is not recovered, a 24-hour urine is collected while the patient is eating a customary diet. The urine is analyzed for calcium, oxalate, uric acid, citrate, and cystine. Normal values following infancy are given in Table 1. Urinary excretory values during infancy may be significantly different from those in older children. An abnormal value should be confirmed with a second collection. When hypercalciuria is discovered, serum concentrations of parathyroid hormone, calcium, phosphorus, and bicarbonate should be determined. Urinary tract infection always should be excluded in children with urolithiasis.

Further characterization of the pathogenesis of confirmed hypercalciuria is warranted. Twenty-four-hour urine calcium excretion is measured after 2 weeks of dietary calcium and sodium restriction. Persistent hypercalciuria without hypercalcemia suggests a renal tubular defect, primary hypercalciuria, or renal tubular acidosis. When dietary calcium and sodium restriction result in normalization of urinary calcium excretion, the diagnosis of absorptive idiopathic hypercalciuria is assigned.

MEDICAL THERAPY

Therapies for urolithiasis consist of preventive medical management and acute intervention of obstructive calculi. General management includes hypotonic diuresis with water loading and, when appropriate, antibiotic therapy for urinary infection or analgesics or both.

Hypercalciuria accounts for approximately 40% of all children with urolithiasis. In addition to an increased water intake, a no-added salt and low-oxalate diet is recommended. In some children, dietary sodium restriction alone may normalize urinary calcium excretion. For children with absorptive hypercalciuria that fails to correct with salt

TABLE 1. Normal Values for Urinary Excretion

Calcium	<4 mg/kg/d
Uric acid	<0.57 mg/dl GFR
Oxalate	<50 mg/1.73 m^2 BSA
Citrate	>400 mg/g creatinine
Cystine	<60 mg/1.73 m^2 BSA

restriction, a reduction in dietary calcium intake (400 to 600 mg/d) is recommended. If urinary calcium excretion does not decline to the normal range with such dietary management, hydrochlorothiazide 1 to 2 mg/kg/d is used as an additional anticalciuric measure. Thus, for children with hypercalciuria unresponsive to dietary calcium and sodium restriction, hydrochlorothiazide is prescribed. All children receiving diuretic therapy should be advised to ingest a diet rich in potassium and should have serum potassium concentrations monitored. Alkali therapy 2 to 4 mEq/kg is given to patients with renal tubular acidosis. Citrate therapy (potassium citrate) is helpful in patients with reduced urinary citrate excretion and hypercalciuria.

Primary hyperoxaluria requires aggressive medical therapy and dietary oxalate restriction. Urinary calcium excretion is reduced by hydrochlorothiazide diuretic therapy (2 mg/kg/d) and large doses of inorganic phosphates. Pyridoxine is administered in an attempt to reduce oxalate production in patients with type I hyperoxaluria. The starting dose is 10 mg/kg/d and may be increased gradually to a total dose of 500 mg/d. Magnesium hydroxide is given to increase the solubility of calcium oxalate. Sodium citrate, given at a dose of 100 mg/kg/d, may reduce calcium oxalate crystal formation. Hyperoxaluria secondary to gastrointestinal disease requires therapy for the primary malabsorptive disorder.

Therapy for uric acid stones includes efforts to alkalinize the urine and to maintain a high urine flow rate. Diagnostic studies should determine whether a treatable cause of hyperproduction of uric acid is present. When uric acid production is increased, as in Lesch-Nyhan syndrome, allopurinol therapy 5 to 10 mg/kg is warranted. Therapy with potassium citrate is useful in decreasing the risk of urinary urate crystallization by alkalinization of the urine.

Cystinuria also requires aggressive urinary alkalinization and a large fluid intake to produce a hypotonic diuresis. When recurrent stones persist despite these measures, D-penicillamine is helpful in reducing the risk of urolithiasis. Penicillamine combines with cystine to form a more soluble cysteine-disulfide complex. Unfortunately, D-penicillamine has a large number of adverse effects, including gastrointestinal discomfort, loss of taste perception, bone marrow depression, proteinuria, membranous glomerulopathy, optic neuritis, myasthenia gravis, and trace metal deficiencies. Potentially less toxic agents, mercaptopropionylglycine (MPG) and captopril, have been suggested as alteratives to D-penicillamine, although neither drug has been approved as therapy for cystinuria in children.

SURGICAL THERAPY

Approximately 40% of urinary stones in children will be passed spontaneously. A number of surgical procedures are available for the removal of calculi within the urinary tract. Surgical management of urinary stones in children ranges from surgical lithotomy to extracorporeal shockwave lithotripsy. Traditional surgical lithotomies are often required when nephrolithiasis is associated with congenital obstruction that can be corrected simultaneously. Because many stones in children are discovered in the lower ureter, cystoscopic manipulation and basket extraction is a common procedure. The success of cystoscopic extraction depends on the size of the calculus. This technique of stone removal is indicated only for urinary stones in the lower third of the ureter.

Percutaneous nephrolithotomy has been used in children with upper tract stones. The advantage of this technique is the ability to avoid general anesthesia and major surgical trauma. Unfortunately, small children require general anesthesia during the procedure, and the large size of the surgical instruments relative to the smaller pediatric renal mass has limited the widespread application of this surgical approach. As smaller instruments are developed and greater experience with this technique is gained, percutaneous treatments may be applied in greater numbers of children.

Extracorporeal shockwave lithotripsy has been used effectively for the dissolution of upper tract calculi in children. This therapy is difficult to apply to infants because of the requirement for immersion.

Children are positioned in a large immersion tank while seated in a harness platform. Styrofoam padding is used to position the child and shield the lung fields from pulmonary contusion. General anesthesia is required to ensure immobility and to provide adequate analgesia. Upper tract stones less than 2 cm in diameter are particularly amenable to shockwave lithotripsy. Lower tract stones and staghorn calculi are not suitable. Cystine stones often respond poorly to shockwave lithotripsy.

A major problem with the use of extracorporeal shockwave lithotripsy in children is that of adjusting the port and gantry to fit small pediatric patients. Complications of lithotripsy include entry site ecchymosis, pain, ureteral obstruction, subcapsular renal hematuria, branchial nerve palsy, cardiac arrhythmia, and pancreatitis. Shockwave lithotripsy is contraindicated in children with hemorrhagic diatheses. Recently, a new piezoelectric lithotriptor has been developed. This method localizes the stone with ultrasound and does not require either immersion or, in most cases, anesthesia. Hematuria following the procedure is less common than with shockwave lithotripsy, and no radiation exposure is required.

REFERENCES

1. El-Damenhoury H, Bürger R, Hohenfellner R: Surgical aspects of urolithiasis in children. Pediatr Nephrol 5:339–347, 1991.
2. Millner DS, Murphy ME: Urolithiasis in pediatric patients. Mayo Clin Proc 68:241–248, 1993.
3. Stapleton FB: Nephrolithiasis in children. Pediatr Rev 11:21–30, 1989.

FLUID AND ELECTROLYTE THERAPY IN CHILDREN

SHERMINE DABBAGH, M.D.
BASSAM ATIYEH, M.D.
LARRY E. FLEISCHMANN, M.D.
ALAN B. GRUSKIN, M.D.

A well-recognized characteristic of the kidneys is their ability to adapt to a wide range of dietary intake, metabolic requirements, and extrarenal losses so as to maintain homeostatic balance during periods of acute change. This equilibrium is possible because of participation of multiple organ systems, including the lungs, the endocrine system, the central nervous system (CNS), and various membrane transport systems in the gastrointestinal and renal systems. In this chapter, we consider fluid and electrolyte therapy during health and disease.

NORMAL PHYSIOLOGY

Body Fluid Compartments

The internal milieu of the body is largely water contained within compartments. It accounts for 50% to 60% of the total body weight in adults and older children but can be as high as 70% to 85% in newborn infants and premature babies, respectively. Total body water decreases with age and is dependent on body habitus. Obese patients have less total body water than muscular lean individuals, since adipose tissue contains only 10% water, whereas muscle is 75% water.

Generally, water and solutes move from one compartment to another down a concentration gradient using diffusion or carrier-facilitated diffusion. The extent of this movement is dependent on the degree of membrane permeability, hydrostatic or oncotic pressure differences, and the orientation of the electric domain if the solute diffusing has an electric charge. In addition, solutes traverse through membranes using active transport, particularly when moving from a compartment of lower concentration to one of higher concentration. An example of such a process is the Na^+-K^+-activated adenosine triphosphatase pump, which is driven by energy derived from the hydrolysis of adenosine triphosphate. This pump maintains an intracellular high concentration of K^+ and an extracellular high concentration of Na^+, thus maintaining a negative intracellular potential difference.

The *extracellular fluid (ECF)* constitutes one third of the total body water and is distributed in two compartments: plasma and interstitial fluid. It is characterized by high concentrations of Na^+ and Cl^- and by the ability of small molecular weight solutes to freely diffuse throughout the compartments. Plasma is 4% to 5% of the total body weight, and interstitial fluids (ISF) are 15% to 20%. Starling forces govern the circulation between the capillaries and the ISF. The principal cation in the ECF is sodium. Chloride and bicarbonate are the principal anions. There are small differences in the concentrations of these ions between ISF and plasma as dictated by the Gibbs-Donnan equilibrium.

An integral part of the ECF is transcellular fluid, which accounts for 1% to 3% of the body weight. It is separated from blood by endothelium and epithelium and is in constant interchange with the other fluids. It represents such collections as cerebrospinal, peritoneal, pleural, and synovial fluids, aqueous and vitreous humors of the eye, and intraluminal, hepatic, pancreatic, and biliary tree fluids.

The *intracellular fluid (ICF)* represents two thirds of the body weight. The cellular membrane allows the passive diffusion of water, and active transport mechanisms maintain a high intracellular K^+ concentration (and hence a negative transmembrane potential difference). The tonicity (or osmolality) in most cells is equal to that of ECF. Thus, the addition or removal of solute or water or both from either side of the membrane results in a rapid flow of water across the membrane to attain osmolal equilibrium.

The anatomy of these body fluid compartments changes from fetal life to adulthood. Whereas the full-term newborn infant is 79% water with an ECF/ICF water ratio of 1.25, the water content drops to 60% by 1 year of age, which is maintained as a constant throughout life. The ECF/ICF ratio continues to decline throughout the first and second decades, reaching 0.77 at 1 to 2 years and 0.48 by 16 years by decreasing the ECF volume. Because of the higher ECF volume in infants, more sodium and chloride per kilogram of body weight and less potassium are found.

Energy Requirements

During steady state, caloric intake and heat production balance caloric expenditure and heat losses. Basal energy expenditure encompasses requirements for baseline activity (basal metabolic rate), physical activity, and thermal stress. The energy requirement for food to be assimilated and metabolized is in the order of 10 kcal/kg/d, and fecal losses account for 5 to 10 kcal/kg/d. In the growing child (a unique situation in pediatrics), 25 kcal/kg/d are required for the biosynthesis of new lipids, carbohydrates, proteins, and nucleic acids. In addition, fever increases and hypothermia decreases daily energy requirements by 12% per degree Celsius, provided that the temperatue change is sustained. Clinical situations characterized by increases in the metabolic rate, such as sepsis and hyperthyroidism, may increase energy requirements by as much as 50%, and myxedema may decrease these requirements by as much as 25%.

Thus, a relationship exists between the weight and the daily caloric requirements, as described by Holliday and Segar[2] and as depicted by the following.

Weight (kg)	Caloric Requirement
3–10	100 kcal/kg/d
10–20	1000 kcal + 50 kcal/kg for each kg >10
>20	1500 kcal + 20 kcal/kg for each kg >20

One observes that an infant expends (and hence requires) more energy per unit weight than does an adolescent or an adult, which is related to the higher surface area/body weight ratio and growth requirements.

Ideally, parenteral maintenance therapy should provide an equal number of calories for those expended. In short-term parenteral therapy, enough glucose should be provided to prevent ketosis and severe tissue catabolism. This is achieved in the form of 5% dextrose to provide 20% of the total calories expended. Generally, severe catabolism could be avoided for 24 to 48 hours.

FLUID AND ELECTROLYTE REQUIREMENTS (Table 1)

Water Requirements

Maintenance fluid requirements can be regarded to replace water losses through the skin and gastrointestinal, respiratory, and urinary systems. These losses average 100 ml/100 kcal expended per day. *Insensible water losses* occur via the skin (which accounts for two thirds of the losses) and the pulmonary system. Generally, these losses are affected by the ambient humidity, clothing, body temperature, respiratory rate, and age of the child. The volume of the insensible water loss can be related to energy expenditure. Losses through the skin and lungs are electrolyte free and account for 30 and 15 ml/100 kcal expended per day, respectively.

Losses from the gastrointestinal tract during health account for 5 to 10 ml/100 kcal/d. However, during episodes of diarrhea, which promotes gastrointestinal water loss and, in most instances, inhibit its absorption, water losses can be as high as 100 ml/100 kcal/d and may constitute up to 10% or more of the total body weight.

Urine volume is determined by the solute load presented to the kidneys. The final urine osmolality depends on this solute load and the ability of the kidneys to concentrate and dilute. Compared with adults, infants have a limited ability to dilute and concentrate their urine. Whereas the minimum and maximum urine osmolality in adults can reach 80 and 1200 mOsm, respectively, urine osmolalities of an infant usually range between 200 and 800 mOsm/kg H_2O. Thus, an infant is prone to readily develop dehydration in the presence of diarrhea or vomiting and limited access to fluids.

The *urinary loss of water* is proportional to the renal solute load (and hence total caloric expenditure). In normal infants and children, it is equal to 50 to 75 ml/100 kcal/d. Water excretion can be excessive in the presence of tubulointerstitial diseases (e.g., acute interstitial nephritis), central or nephrogenic diabetes insipidus, or immature tubular function (e.g., prematurity). Under these circumstances, water losses can reach 300 ml/100 kcal/d.

In calculating fluid replacement, a physician should be aware of several factors that will determine the patient's response:

1. Endogenous sources of water may contribute as much as 20 ml of water/100 kcal metabolized per day (oxidation of fat and carbohydrates generates 12 to 17 ml/100 kcal metabolized, and tissue catabolism during periods of stress generates 3 ml/100 kcal).
2. Traditional maintenance fluids in an oliguric or anuric patient will result in fluid overload because of the inability to eliminate 50 to 75 ml of water per 100 kcal/d. Thus, these patients need to have their urinary outputs closely monitored and fluid prescriptions promptly adjusted during these clinical situations.
3. It is imperative that all persistent fluid losses from the gastroin-

TABLE 1. Daily Fluid and Electrolyte Requirements

CONSTITUENT	WATER (ml/100 kcal/d)	SODIUM (mEq/100 kcal/d)	POTASSIUM (mEq/100 kcal/d)
Normal maintenance	100	1–3	1–2
Normal output			
Urine	50–75	0.5–5	0.1–2
Sweat	0–5	0–1	0.1–0.2
Gastrointestinal tract	5–10	0.2–0.5	0.1–0.2
Growth	0–15	0–0.75	0–0.75
Intake			
Ingestion	Variable	Variable	Variable
Oxidation	12–17		
Tissue catabolism	3		

testinal tract (e.g., stool losses or nasogastric losses) are promptly replaced in addition to the patient's maintenance fluid therapy.

Sodium Requirements

During steady state, the total body sodium content is approximately 40 to 45 mEq/kg. The bulk of it resides in the extracellular fluid and bone. Typically, sodium requirements range between 1 and 3 mEq/100 kcal/d. Urine is the major source of sodium loss in normal children, and it varies between 0.5 and 5 mEq/100 kcal/d (or 0.1% to 10% of the daily sodium load filtered by the kidneys). These losses are modified by clinical disease. In the presence of osmotic diuresis or tubulointerstitial disease or prematurity, the urinary Na^+ losses exceed 5 mEq/100 kcal/d, and hence these patients are at risk of developing hyponatremia. On the other hand, dehydrated children (who have renal function) can decrease urine Na^+ concentrations to below 10 mEq/L. Losses via sweating or the gastrointestinal tract during health account for 0.5 mEq/100 kcal/d each. In addition, growing children expend up to 0.75 mEq Na^+/100 kcal for growth.

As with water replacement, a physician should be aware of the Na^+ losses via the gastrointestinal tract or urine during periods of disease when prescribing Na^+ replacement to avoid hyponatremia or hypernatremia.

Potassium Requirements

During steady state, total body potassium stores approximate 50 to 55 mEq/kg body weight and exist in muscle and other intracellular compartments. Although it is primarily an intracellular ion, K^+ is easily exchangeable, a property that maintains serum K^+ concentration between 3.6 and 5.5 mEq/L. The normal requirements for potassium are 1 to 2 mEq/100 kcal/d. Potassium requirements for growth are highest in the newborn period and can be as high as 0.75 mEq/100 kcal/d to maintain appropriate intracellular potassium concentrations.

Potassium is excreted via many routes. Losses through the colon account for 0.1 to 0.2 mEq K^+/100 kcal/d and are regulated by aldosterone. This route of excretion assumes an important role in oliguric renal failure, when K^+ excretion through the gut could triple. Losses through sweat amount to 0.1 to 0.2 mEq/100 kcal/d, which increase during periods of strenuous exercise or in cystic fibrosis. Normal urinary excretion of K^+ ranges between 0.1 and 2 mEq/100 kcal/d and is influenced by numerous factors, such as insulin, $beta_2$-adrenergic stimulation, aldosterone, acid-base status, and delivery of sodium to the distal tubule of the kidney.

Disturbances in K^+ homeostasis may involve transcellular shifts from the intracellular compartment, as in metabolic acidosis or tissue necrosis, or increased losses via the kidneys, as in congenital or acquired renal diseases (e.g., Bartter's syndrome or diuretic therapy) or increased losses via the gastrointestinal tract, such as diarrhea or vomiting.

Alkali Requirements

The primary challenge to the kidneys in acid-base homeostasis is to reclaim filtered bicarbonate (primarily in the proximal tubule) and to excrete hydrogen in the distal tubule in the form of titratable acids (e.g., phosphates) or ammonium salts. It is estimated that 320 mmol of CO_2 (volatile acid) are produced per kilogram of body weight per day from the metabolism of carbohydrates, protein, and fat. These are in equilibrium with a normal Pco_2 of 40 to 45 mm Hg. The oxidation of amino acids results in the production of fixed acids at a rate of 1 to 3 mEq/kg/d. In perturbations of acid-base balance, respiratory compensation occurs within 12 to 24 hours to maintain blood pH within the normal range. The addition of acid to the body invokes the participation of several extracellular and intracellular buffering mechanisms, which include the bicarbonate-carbonic acid system, albumin, hemoglobin, and bone.

There are no alkali requirements in the absence of metabolic acidosis. However, in a child with renal failure, 1 to 2 mEq of alkali/kg/d need to be provided to neutralize the fixed acid load produced from the metabolism of amino acids. This can be provided in the form of $NaHCO_3$ or sodium acetate.

DEFINITIONS

Before we consider replacement therapy during disease, a few definitions need to be clarified. *Hypertonicity* results from an increase in the concentration of solutes that do not cross the cell membrane. Examples of such solutes include mannitol, glucose (in the absence of insulin), and hypernatremia. With an increase in the tonicity of the extracellular fluids, there is a shift in fluids from the intracellular to the extracellular space, resulting in reduction of cell size. On the other hand, *hyperosmolality* is caused by increased concentration of solutes that may or may not cross the cell membrane. Such solutes include urea or alcohol, which are permeant with respect to the membrane, and sodium, which does not cross the membrane. Hence, there is no change in the size of the intracellular and extracellular spaces. Thus, an increase in serum urea concentration results in hyperosmolality without hypertonicity, whereas hypernatremia causes hypertonicity and hyperosmolality.

REPLACEMENT THERAPY DURING DISEASE

Dehydration

Neonates and young infants are more prone to develop dehydration than older children and adults, and dehydration may result from either a decrease in fluid intake due to such causes as coma or lethargy or increased losses via the gastrointestinal tract (vomiting, diarrhea), the kidneys (osmotic diuresis, salt-losing nephropathy, diuretics, diabetes insipidus), and the skin (burns, cystic fibrosis, heat prostration).

The degree of dehydration is estimated by the amount of weight loss, which frequently is not known. A quick estimate of body weight, knowing the age, could be made using the following formula.

$$Weight (kg) = [Age (years) \times 2] + 10$$

Alternatively, the physical examination may provide clues to determine the degree of dehydration (Table 2). Older children tend to develop symptoms at lower degrees of dehydration compared with infants because older children have lower total body water content and extracellular volume.

During intravascular volume depletion, renal function is preserved for long periods of time. Although there is a tendency for the intrarenal vascular resistance to increase during dehydration, this vasoconstricting effect is attenuated by the vasodilating effect of prostaglandins on the afferent arteriole, along with the intrinsic autoregulation property of these arterioles. There is increased vasoconstriction of the efferent arterioles in the presence of low-dose angiotensin II, which results in preservation of glomerular pressure. In addition, numerous neural and hormonal factors affect tubular function to increase fractional reabsorption of sodium and other solutes. Any breakdown in these compensatory mechanisms results in severe afferent arteriolar vasoconstriction and prerenal failure. Since creatinine is unabsorbable, the increase in the serum concentration of creatinine is modest. The reabsorption of urea is enhanced by the slow tubular urine flow and results in BUN/creatinine ratios of 40:1 or more. There is a decrease in the urine output, accompanied by an increase in the specific gravity and osmolality (because of an increase in the concentration of antidiuretic hormone). Frequently, urine sodium concentration falls below 20 mEq/L. Metabolic acidosis is common due to loss of bicarbonate through the gastrointestinal tract and increased acid production because of increased catabolism.

Dehydration is classified according to the observed serum sodium concentration. Hyponatremic dehydration is defined as occurring when the serum Na^+ is less than 130 mEq/L. Hypernatremic dehydration is defined as occurring when serum Na^+ is more than 150 mEq/L, and isonatremic dehydration occurs when the serum Na^+ is between 130 and 150 mEq/L.

Isonatremic Dehydration

Isonatremic dehydration is the most common form of dehydration and accounts for 80% of all cases of dehydration. It results from a proportional loss of water and solute. Since net water loss is isotonic,

TABLE 2. Clinical Assessment of the Severity of Dehydration

CLINICAL SIGNS	MILD (4%–5%)	MODERATE (6%–10%)	SEVERE (>10%)
Vital signs			
Pulse	Normal	Increased	Increased and weak
Blood pressure	Normal	Normal to low	Very low, orthostatic, shock
Respiratory rate	Normal	Normal to deep	Rapid and deep
General appearance			
Infants	Fussy, thirsty, alert	Fussy, restless, thirsty, lethargic but arousable	Drowsy to comatose, not arousable, gray color, limp, cold, and sweaty
Older children	Thirsty, restless, alert	Thirsty, restless, postural hypotension	Apprehensive, comatose, cold, mottled skin, cyanotic
Mucous membranes	Normal to slightly dry	Dry	Parched
Anterior fontanel	Normal	Sunken	Markedly depressed
Eyes	Normal	Sunken	Markedly sunken
Capillary refill	< 3 s	3–5 s	> 5 s
Skin turgor	Normal	Decreased (may have a doughy feel in hypernatremic dehydration)	Markedly decreased (may have a doughy feel in hypernatremic dehydration)
Urine output	Mildly decreased, diaper may be dry	Decreased, diaper is dry, concentrated urine with specific gravity of 1.02–1.03	Decreased, diaper is dry, decrease in the number of diapers changed during the day, concentrated urine with specific gravity > 1.03

there is no change in the tonicity of the remaining fluids, and there is no redistribution between the intracellular and extracellular compartments. All the losses occur from the ECF, and hence there is a decrease in the blood volume. Gastrointestinal losses with or without decreased intake and increased urinary losses are the most common causes of isonatremic dehydration. The severity of dehydration can be assessed using the signs summarized in Table 2.

It is important to answer a number of questions before proceeding with a rehydration regimen.

Is there significant volume reduction with cardiovascular compromise? Although some studies have shown that the clinical estimate of the severity of dehydration could be inexact, it serves as a starting point to approximate body fluid deficits.

Is there a potassium disturbance? It is not unusual for patients with diarrheal isotonic dehydration to accumulate a potassium deficit of 8 to 10 mEq/kg. Remembering that potassium is an intracellular ion, we conclude that serum potassium concentrations may not reflect the body potassium stores. In addition, serum potassium levels are influenced by the acid-base status of the patient. For example, metabolic acidosis may obscure a frank hypokalemia due to transcellular shifts.

Is there a perturbation in acid-base status? Generally, bicarbonate loss in the stools results in a hyperchloremic metabolic acidosis with a normal anion gap. If the patient has decreased oral intake and is in a catabolic state, there may be an increase in the anion gap because of protein and fat breakdown, with resultant acid generation. Most patients develop a pure metabolic acidosis. However, patients need to be assessed for combined disorders by plotting the blood pH, P_{CO_2}, and bicarbonate concentration on an acid-base nomogram that depicts the Henderson-Hasselbalch equation. A few rules of thumb may apply in the absence of the nomogram: (1) In a compensated metabolic acidosis, the last two digits of the pH are equal to the P_{CO_2}. (2) Use of the regression formula (Winter's formula) may assist to verify the existence of a pure metabolic acidosis.

Winter's formula: P_{CO_2} (mm Hg) = 1.5 × [HCO_3^-] + (8 ± 2)

(HCO_3^- concentration is determined using blood chemistry and not the Henderson-Hasselbalch nomogram.)

Is there compromise of renal function? Typically, infants present with history of decreased urine output at the time of the emergency room visit. Thus, it is important to assess whether the patient is in prerenal failure or acute renal failure.

During the rapid or initial phase of deficit therapy, the integrity of the circulation is restored and vital signs are stabilized. If shock

is present, 5% plasmanate or albumin should be administered at 10 to 20 ml/kg over 30 to 60 minutes. In the absence of shock, 20 ml/kg of normal saline or Ringer's lactate can be administered over 1 hour. Therapy is continued until circulation is restored and the patient voids.

During the repletion phase, it is customary to replace half of the deficit over the first 8 hours and the rest over the ensuing 16 hours. The amount of fluids and sodium given over the initial phase is subtracted from the total amount required to replace the deficit. The sodium and potassium losses in isonatremic dehydration are estimated to be 8 to 10 mEq/kg each. To replace the sodium deficit, a solution containing 5% dextrose and 0.3 normal saline is sufficient. Generally, potassium chloride is added to the intravenous solution at a concentration of only 20 to 30 mEq/L and should be added only after the patient voids. It is important to remember that the maintenance fluid calculations are based on a urine output approximating two thirds of the administered volume. All ongoing losses (eg., diarrhea) are replaced with an appropriate concentration of sodium.

Hyponatremic Dehydration

Hyponatremic dehydration accounts for around 5% of all cases of dehydration and occurs when the net losses are hypertonic. The most prevalent case scenario is a young child with gastrointestinal losses that are counterbalanced by the intake of hypotonic solutions, such as sugar water, flat ginger ale or 7-UP. Thus, ECF fluid shifts into the intracellular compartment (which is less hypotonic), making the symptoms of hyponatremic dehydration more profound than other forms of dehydration for the same degree of fluid depletion. This form of hyponatremia should be distinguished from other forms of hyponatremia not associated with volume deficit, such as the syndrome of inappropriate antidiuretic hormone (ADH) secretion, nephrotic syndrome, liver cirrhosis, and congestive heart failure, since the treatment for such conditions is different from that associated with dehydration.

The treatment of hyponatremic dehydration is similar, in principle, to isonatremic dehydration, except for the need to account for the extra Na^+ needed to correct the hyponatremia. The extra Na^+ is calculated using the following formula.

Extra Na^+ = (135 mEq/L − measured Na^+) × total body water
(Total body water = 0.6 × body weight)

Again, half of the deficit is replaced over the first 8 hours, and the rest is administered over 16 hours. Typically, a solution containing 5% dextrose and 0.45 to 0.6 normal saline is administered. The use of hypertonic saline (3% saline) is reserved for patients with CNS symptoms (eg., seizures) caused by the hyponatremia or with a serum Na$^+$ concentration of less than 120 mEq/L. It is estimated that 5 ml of hypertonic saline per kilogram of body weight will raise the serum Na$^+$ concentration by 4 to 5 mEq/L.

Hypernatremic Dehydration

This type of dehydration results from the net loss of hypotonic fluid and accounts for around 15% of the cases of dehydration. It is seen commonly in infants with gastrointestinal losses who are given high sodium-containing fluids, such as concentrated formulas, bouillon soup, or chicken or beef broth. It may occur in a breast-fed neonate, in which case the sodium content of breast milk should be determined. If the sodium content is elevated, breast feeding should be discontinued, and commercial infant formulas should be started after correction of the hypernatremia. Other causes of hypernatremic dehydration include fever and diabetes insipidus.

Because of the hypertonicity of the extracellular fluid, the intracellular fluid shifts into the extracellular space, with resultant maintenance of circulatory integrity. Thus, the typical signs of dehydration, such as tachycardia, loss of skin integrity, and hypotension, are less pronounced than in other forms of dehydration. Shock is rare in hypernatremic dehydration. When the weight loss is above 10%, the skin starts to feel doughy. Generally, the child is irritable and lethargic and has a high-pitched cry. With the increase in the severity of the condition, coma, increased muscle tone, and seizures may be observed.

Acute CNS symptomatology correlates with the severity of the hypernatremia and, hence, the hypertonicity. Of interest is the observation that the serum sodium concentration and the severity of the acute CNS symptoms may not correlate with the degree of recovery. Permanent CNS sequelae have been reported in children with serum Na$^+$ concentrations of 160 mEq/L. The overall mortality rate is around 10%. In severe cases of hypernatremic dehydration, there may be tearing of the bridging vessels, followed by subarachnoid and subdural hemorrhage. Hyperglycemia, hypocalcemia, and hyperuricemia are frequent occurrences. The etiology of the hypocalcemia remains unknown. However, it is believed that there is reduced cellular uptake of glucose due to stress, which accounts for the hyperglycemia.

The treatment of hypernatremic dehydration requires gradual correction of the fluid deficit, usually over 48 to 72 hours. Rapid correction may lead to brain edema. When hypernatremia is persistent, brain cells accumulate idiogenic osmoles—which are amino acids, particularly taurine. These idiogenic osmoles restore brain cell volume to normal or near-normal levels. During the correction of hypernatremic dehydration, if water enters the brain cell rapidly and since it takes several hours to days for these osmoles to be depleted, the brain cell will swell, causing cerebral edema, herniation, and death.

To estimate the volume of free water required to correct the hypernatremia, one can use the following formula.

$$Na^+_{now} \times TBW_{now} = Na^+_{ideal} \times TBW_{ideal}$$
$$TBW \text{ (total body water)} = 0.6 \times body \ weight \ (kg)$$

Sodium should not be decreased by more than 10 to 15 mEq/L/d. The sodium to be given can be calculated as 80 to 100 mEq/L of the estimated loss. Because of the predilection of children to develop hyperglycemia, it may be necessary to use 2.5% dextrose solutions (instead of 5% dextrose). Generally, 0.2 normal saline solutions are used for hydration in these patients. Calcium gluconate may be added depending on serum calcium. Once the child has urinated, potassium chloride at a concentration of 30 to 40 mEq/L is added.

ELECTROLYTE DISORDERS

Hyponatremia

Hyponatremia, defined as a serum Na$^+$ concentration of less than 130 mEq/L, occurs in 1.5% of hospitalized children, excluding the newborn period. Central nervous system symptoms usually manifest when the serum Na$^+$ levels are 120 mEq/L or less. The acuity of the symptoms is related to the rapidity with which the hyponatremia developed.

The pathophysiology of CNS symptoms is related to the movement of water from the plasma into the brain with the development of hyponatremia, which results in cerebral overhydration. Associated with this water movement are the symptoms of apathy, lethargy, agitation, vomiting, altered consciousness, seizures, and even death. However, the brain swelling is generally less than one would predict for the magnitude of water movement across the blood-brain barrier as a result of two protective mechanisms. (1) With the movement of water into the brain, there is an increase in the interstitial fluid hydrostatic pressure, leading to loss of fluid into the cerebrospinal fluid, which is eventually returned to the systemic circulation via the arachnoid villi. (2) Cellular loss of intracellular potassium and organic osmoles (amino acids) renders the intracellular space less hypertonic and, hence, protects against brain swelling.

The cardiovascular response is dependent on the intravascular volume status. In cases of dehydration, hyponatremia causes further contraction of effective blood volume by shifts of fluid from the extracellular to the intracellular space. In addition, ADH secretion is stimulated by the hypovolemia, which overrides the suppressive effect of hypoosmolality (hyponatremia), thus compounding the hyponatremia. In the presence of ADH, the kidney elaborates concentrated urine with low urine concentrations of Na$^+$ in cases of hypovolemia not associated with renal disease or diuretic use.

Etiology

The treatment of hyponatremia is dependent on the etiology (Fig. 1). The evaluation of hyponatremia involves answering a number of questions based on the history, physical examination, and laboratory data. These include a determination of whether the low sodium reflects a true decrease, reflects a quirk in the way the laboratory assays the ion, or is a result of the presence of an impermeable solute. A number of causes deserve consideration.

Pseudohyponatremia occurs in nephrotic syndrome associated with hyperlipidemic (common in children) and hyperproteinemic states (rare in children). In these conditions, the hyponatremia as assayed by the laboratory is not real. Serum Na$^+$ concentrations are expressed in milliequivalents per liter of plasma, which normally is 93% water (proteins and lipids account for 70 ml). With an increase in plasma lipids or protein, the stated serum sodium is artificially low, as assayed by flame spectrophotometry. Newer methods that read direct potentiometry or delipidation of the plasma give accurate determinations of serum sodium in the presence of hyperlipidemia. If these methods are not available, one can determine the serum osmolality by freezing point depression. If this is normal, the serum sodium is more likely to be normal or close to normal, and the patient does not require supplementation with sodium chloride.

Factitious hyponatremia, on the other hand, occurs in the presence of an impermeant solute such as mannitol or glucose (in the absence of insulin). The plasma osmolality and tonicity are high, resulting in the shift of fluid from the intracellular to the extracellular space. Thus, the reported sodium concentration is low. Serum sodium concentration is lowered by 1.6 mEq/L for every 100 mg/dl increase in serum glucose or mannitol.

Hypovolemic Hyponatremia. This condition is characterized by a depletion of salt in excess of water through renal or extrarenal routes. Patients commonly present with the signs and symptoms of dehydration. Their total body sodium is also decreased. For more details, review preceding text.

Euvolemic Hyponatremia. This condition is characterized by hypo-osmolality associated with a normal or near-normal total body sodium. Thus, the signs and symptoms of intravascular volume depletion are absent. When present, they pertain to the CNS because of the hyponatremia. The prototype of euvolemic hyponatremia is the *syndrome of inappropriate antidiuretic hormone secretion (SIADH)*.

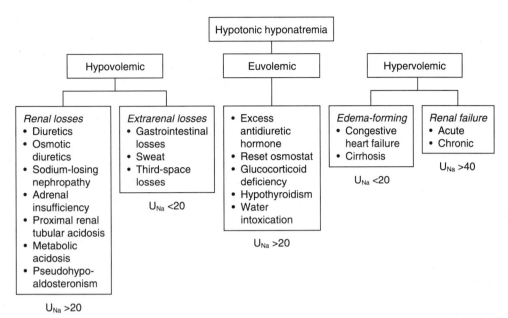

FIGURE 1. The differential diagnosis of hypotonic hyponatremia is shown, along with the typical urinary sodium concentrations. U_{Na} is expressed in milliequivalents per liter.

The syndrome is defined as the inappropriate concentration of the urine with respect to the serum in the presence of hypotonic hyponatremia and the absence of abnormal renal function, congestive heart failure, liver cirrhosis, glucocorticoid deficiency, hypothyroidism, and edema. SIADH is a problem of excessive water retention due to increased ADH secretion. Because of volume expansion, atrial natriuretic hormone levels are elevated and aldosterone concentrations are depressed, causing an increase in the urine sodium concentration.

Hypervolemic Hyponatremia. This category of diseases is characterized by an increase in the total body water and sodium. The pathophysiology of the hyponatremia in such conditions as congestive heart failure is related to a decrease in the effective circulating blood volume, which activates baroreceptors. This activation causes an increase in ADH secretion, water retention, dilution of the extracellular space, and resultant hyponatremia and avid urinary sodium retention.

Treatment

Irrespective of the etiology, if the patient is symptomatic or if the serum sodium concentration is less than 120 mEq/L, he should receive sufficient sodium to increase the Na^+ concentration to 125 mEq/L, a level at which symptoms are alleviated. Then, specific therapy is directed toward the underlying cause. Rehydration and volume expansion are the mainstay of therapy for hypovolemic dehydration, as discussed previously. Euvolemic patients require fluid restriction. For the severely hyponatremic and symptomatic patient, it may be necessary to administer furosemide, followed by replacement of the urinary sodium losses with normal or hypertonic saline. Similarly, the treatment for hypervolemic hyponatremia is fluid restriction.

Hypernatremia

Hypernatremia is defined as a serum sodium in excess of 150 mEq/L and is generally a disorder of water balance. Total body sodium content can be low, normal, or high, depending on the etiology of the hypernatremia. The hypernatremia causes hyperosmolality and hypertonicity. There is a shift of water from the intracellular to the extracellular compartments, which results in intracellular dehydration. For more details on the pathophysiology and symptomatology accompanying hypernatremia, refer to the section on Hypernatremic Dehydration.

The causes of hypernatremia are depicted in Table 3. The treatment of hypovolemic hypernatremia was discussed previously. In cases of

acute salt intoxication, the hypernatremia may be corrected by rapid fluid administration, since the idiogenic osmoles have not had the chance to accumulate. However, this may result in hypervolemia. In a child with severe salt intoxication and a serum sodium above 200 mEq/L, peritoneal dialysis must be performed, with frequent monitoring of electrolytes.

TABLE 3. Causes of Hypernatremia

Sodium Excess
Concentrated formula
Intravenous or oral administration of NaCl or $NaHCO_3$
Breast milk

Water Deficit
Diabetes insipidus
  A. Central
    1. Idiopathic
    2. Head trauma
    3. Suprasellar or infrasellar tumors
    4. Granulomatous diseases (tuberculosis, Wegener's granulomatosis, sarcoidosis)
    5. Infection
    6. Cerebral hemorrhage
  B. Nephrogenic
    1. Primary (congenital)
    2. Secondary
      a. Renal disease (obstructive uropathy, renal dysplasia, reflux nephropathy, polycystic kidney disease)
      b. Systemic disease with secondary renal involvement (amyloidosis, sickle cell disease)
      c. Drugs (amphotericin, lithium, aminoglycosides)
Excessive water loss via skin
  Burns
  Fever
  Exposure to high temperatures (e.g., radiant warmers)
Excessive water losses in excess of salt
  Gastrointestinal losses
  Osmotic diuretics
  Diabetes mellitus

Inadequate Intake
Adipsia
No access to free water

Hypokalemia

Normal serum concentrations of potassium (K^+) range between 3.6 and 5.5 mEq/L. Hypokalemia is defined as occurring when the serum potassium concentration is below the lower limits of normal. Serum K^+ concentrations are 0.4 mEq/L greater than plasma levels due to the release of intracellular K^+. A low or high K^+ concentration reflects the plasma concentration but not the total body K^+. Also, a normal serum K^+ level does not necessarily mean that the intracellular K^+ is normal.

Etiology

Most clinically significant hypokalemic states occur because of a net loss of potassium from the body. The causes of hypokalemia are listed in Table 4. Renal losses of potassium can be seen with transport systems in the proximal or distal tubules. Diseases such as renal tubular acidosis (types I and II), cystinosis, and interstitial nephritis secondary to toxins such as cisplatinum, are but a few examples of states causing hypokalemia. Diuretics are the most common iatrogenic cause for hypokalemia by increasing urine flow and sodium delivery to the distal tubule. On the other hand, vomiting and diarrhea are the most common causes of hypokalemia due to extrarenal losses in the pediatric age group.

TABLE 4. Causes of Hypokalemia

Hypokalemia Without Potassium Depletion
High white blood cell counts
In vivo insulin

Transcellular Shifts
Alkalosis
Insulin excess
Beta-adrenergic agonists
Theophylline toxicity
Barium intoxication
Hypokalemic periodic paralysis

Potassium Depletion
Nutritional
Inadequate intake (e.g., anorexia nervosa)

Extrarenal Causes
Copious perspiration
Gastrointestinal losses
Laxative abuse
Gastrointestinal fistulas
Geophagia
Rectal villous adenomas

Renal Causes
Renal tubular acidosis
Carbonic anhydrase inhibitors
Fanconi's syndrome
Diabetic ketoacidosis
Ureterosigmoidostomy
Chloride depletion
    Vomiting/gastric drainage
    Congenital chloride diarrhea
    Cystic fibrosis
    Diuretics
    Posthypercapnic alkalosis
Potassium wasting
    Bartter's syndrome and other hereditary K^+ wasting disorders
    Pyelonephritis and interstitial disease
    Magnesium wasting
    Postobstructive diuresis
    Diuretic phase of acute tubular necrosis
    Antibiotics

Endocrinopathies
Hyperaldosteronism
High glucocorticoid concentration
Cushing's syndrome
Licorice ingestion

Symptoms and Signs

The symptoms and signs of hypokalemia vary considerably among patients, depending on whether the potassium loss is acute or chronic. Mild to moderate degrees of hypokalemia are generally well tolerated by children. Severe hypokalemia results in manifestations that are independent of the underlying cause and relate to the neuromuscular system. Skeletal muscle weakness is the earliest manifestation of hypokalemia, occurring at concentrations of less than 3 mEq/L. With progressive decrease in potassium concentration, patients experience restless leg syndrome, fatigue, cramps, paralysis, and rhabdomyolysis. Frank muscle necrosis may occur at potassium levels of less than 2 mEq/L. The cardiac manifestations of hypokalemia include abnormalities in rhythm due to slowing of repolarization. The electrocardiographic abnormalities include depression of the ST wave, lower T wave voltage, and appearance of the U wave.

Chronic hypokalemia may lead to structural and functional abnormalities in the kidney, which include reduced renal blood flow and glomerular filtration rate, renal hypertrophy, tubuloepithelial dilatation, vacuolization, and sclerosis. Functionally, patients experience polyuria and develop acidification and concentration defects. Such patients may also develop glucose intolerance.

Diagnosis

The underlying cause for hypokalemia may not be readily apparent. Measurement of urinary potassium concentration may be helpful in determining the cause. A low urinary potassium of 10 mEq/L or less, in the absence of recent diuretic use, implies near maximal urinary potassium conservation and suggests an extrarenal etiology for the hypokalemia or inadequate intake.

Treatment

The choice for the treatment of hypokalemia depends on the severity of the potassium deficit and the symptoms and signs. Since the serum potassium concentration does not reflect the status of the body potassium stores, treatment of hypokalemia should be performed cautiously. Mild hypokalemia responds to oral supplementation using high potassium-containing foods, such as potatoes, bananas, oranges, and orange juice. Oral supplementation with potassium chloride or other related potassium compounds is necessary in moderate hypokalemia. Doses of 3 to 5 mEq/kg/d or more may be necessary. Most liquid preparations of potassium chloride are bad tasting, except for Kay Ciel, which provides 20 mEq/15 ml (10% solution). The side effects of oral potassium supplementation include gastrointestinal irritation (vomiting and ulceration) and potassium intoxication.

Intravenous supplementation should be reserved for severe hypokalemia (K < 2 mEq/L). Potassium chloride can be added to the intravenous solution at a concentration as high as 40 mEq/L (if administered peripherally) and 60 to 80 mEq/L (if administered centrally). Patients with neuromuscular and cardiac symptoms can be given 0.3 to 0.5 mEq/kg over 1 hour by slow IV infusion. This dose is repeated according to the assayed serum potassium. Adjunct therapeutic measures, such as potassium-sparing diuretics, may be necessary to achieve potassium balance.

Hyperkalemia

Hyperkalemia is defined as a serum potassium concentration above 6.0 mEq/L in the newborn period and above 5.5 mEq/L in older infants and children. Hyperkalemia does not always imply an increase in body potassium stores. Normally, the kidneys provide the primary defense against acute increases in serum potassium concentration. Thus, with a few exceptions, hyperkalemia occurs with great frequency in disease states characterized by decreased urine output and glomerular filtration rate.

Etiology

The causes of hyperkalemia are listed in Table 5. Pseudohypokalemia represents an in vitro elevation in serum potassium in the absence of any clinical manifestations related to the measured per-

TABLE 5. Causes of Hyperkalemia

Spurious or Pseudohyperkalemia
Hemolysis
Thrombocytosis
Leukocytosis
Ischemic blood drawing
Abnormal erythrocytes
    Acquired
    Familial pseudohyperkalemia

Transcellular Shifts
Acidosis
Hyperglycemia; insulin deficiency
Beta-adrenergic blockade
Arginine hydrochloride
Succinylcholine
Digitalis toxicity
Hyperkalemic periodic paralysis
Fluoride intoxication
Exercise

Increased Potassium Load
Oral or intravenous potassium supplementation
Use of aged bank blood
Geophagia
High doses of potassium-containing medications (e.g., penicillin)
Tissue release of potassium
    Burns
    Rhabdomyolysis
    Starvation

Decreased Renal Excretion of Potassium
Acute renal failure
Chronic renal failure
Mineralocorticoid deficiency
    Addison's disease
    Hereditary enzymatic defects
        Congenital adrenal hyperplasia
        Isolated aldosterone deficiency
    Hyporeninemic hypoaldosteronism
    Drugs
        Angiotensin-converting enzyme inhibitors
        Indomethacin
        Cyclosporine
        Heparin
Primary defects in potassium secretion
    Acquired disorders
        Renal transplantation
        Lupus nephritis
        Amyloidosis
        Obstructive uropathy
        Sickle cell nephropathy
    Hereditary
        Pseudohypoaldosteronism
    Drugs
        Amiloride
        Spironolactone
        Triamterene

turbation. Generally, serum potassium is higher than plasma potassium by 0.5 mEq/L because of release of the cation from cells during clotting. Thus, it is not surprising that patients with conditions characterized by elevated platelet or white blood cell counts may manifest hyperkalemia. To confirm the presence or absence of hyperkalemia, potassium should be assayed in plasma rather than in serum in cases of thrombocytosis or leukocytosis.

An oral intake of as little as 50 mEq of potassium by an adult may cause a transient increase in serum potassium of 0.5 to 1 mEq/L. Seventy to ninety percent of that load is sequestered intracellularly within 15 to 30 minutes and ultimately is excreted in the urine. Thus, when the kidneys are functioning normally, large amounts of oral potassium may be given without dangerous sequelae. However, if potassium is given at a rate greater than 0.5 mEq/kg/h, life-threatening hyperkalemia may result.

Manifestations of Hyperkalemia

The clinical manifestations of hyperkalemia relate to interference with the electrophysiologic activities of muscle, particularly the heart. Electrocardiographic changes include tenting or symmetric peaking of the T wave in the precordial leads and depression of the ST wave. With increasing severity, there is widening of the QRS complex, lengthening of the PR interval, first-degree or second-degree heart block, disappearance of the P wave, and finally atrial standstill. Ventricular fibrillation or asystole follows. In addition to the cardiac effects, hyperkalemia affects electrical activities in other muscles. Tingling, parasthesias, and flaccid paralysis may occur. There also is an increase in aldosterone synthesis and pancreatic insulin and glucagon release. Interestingly, hyperkalemia induces a decrease in systemic blood pressure in hypertensive patients, which may be related to inhibition of renin release and the natriuretic effect of hyperkalemia.

Diagnosis

The history and physical examination, with particular attention to the manifestations of chronic and acute renal failure (e.g., growth, nutrition, intake of food, presence or absence of hypertension, presence or absence of hematuria or proteinuria, ingestion of medications), may provide clues to the etiology of the hyperkalemia, in addition to the laboratory assessment. Information regarding renal potassium con-

servation can be obtained by assaying for urinary potassium. A fractional excretion of potassium of less than 30% despite progressive hyperkalemia may indicate the presence of aldosterone deficiency.

Treatment

The treatment of hyperkalemia (Table 6) depends on the plasma potassium concentration, renal function, and cardiac manifestations. The presence of electrocardiographic changes is an indication for emergency treatment of hyperkalemia. Calcium gluconate should be administered intravenously to reverse the cardiac effects of hyperkalemia by increasing the threshold potential, thus allowing the excitable cells to repolarize and fire a signal again. Potassium can be shifted into the intracellular compartment by the use of glucose and insulin or sodium bicarbonate (in the presence of metabolic acidosis). When adequate renal function is present, the excretion of potassium can be enhanced by the use of loop diuretics. Potassium could be eliminated via the gastrointestinal tract by using the cation exchange resin, Kayexalate (which exchanges 1 mEq of potassium for 1 mEq of sodium). It is usually administered with 30% to 70% sorbitol to prevent the resin from forming concretions. Its onset of action is dependent on the route of administration. Generally, 1 g/kg per dose lowers the serum potassium by 1 mEq/L. Dialysis remains the last therapeutic measure to be used. It is indicated in cases of hyperkalemia in the presence of renal failure to remove increased potassium loads. Because of the needed setup time, other measures are to be used to stabilize the patient.

ACID-BASE DISORDERS

The pH of the extracellular fluids is maintained in the narrow range of 7.35 to 7.45. When a disease state alters the pH, several compensatory mechanisms play a role to offset the perturbation. Chemical buffering is the primary defense against any change in blood pH. These buffers include bicarbonate (the major chemical buffer), protein, hemoglobin, phosphates, and sulfates. The relationship between pH, H_2CO_3, and HCO_3^- is expressed by the Henderson-Hasselbalch equation.

$$pH = pK + \log [HCO_3^-]/[H_2CO_3]$$

which is usually transformed to

$$pH = pK + \log [HCO_3^-]/(0.03 \times P_{CO_2})$$

where pK is the dissociation constant for carbonic acid-bicarbonate system, $[HCO_3^-]$ is the concentration of serum bicarbonate in mmole per liter, and P_{CO_2} is the partial pressure of CO_2 in millimeters of mercury.

When chemical buffering fails to offset a change in the blood pH, two secondary mechanisms play a pivotal role. Respiratory compensation for a metabolic disorder commences within minutes and is complete within 12 to 24 hours. Renal compensation from a respiratory disorder is slower, beginning within hours and requiring 2 to 5 days to be completed. It is important to remember that these compensatory mechanisms do not return the blood pH to normal, except in respiratory alkalosis.

Acid-base disorders can be classified into simple and mixed disorders. Thus, a patient may develop a simple metabolic acidosis or alkalosis or a simple respiratory acidosis or alkalosis or a combined respiratory/metabolic disorder, such as metabolic and a respiratory acidosis. We focus our discussion on the simple metabolic disorders of metabolic acidosis and metabolic alkalosis.

Metabolic Acidosis

Metabolic acidosis occurs when the blood pH falls below 7.35 and results because of the net loss of HCO_3^- or a net gain of acid. This disorder can be classified into two major categories: high anion gap and normal anion gap acidosis. The anion gap is determined as follows.

$$\text{Anion gap} = [Na^+] + [K^+] - [Cl^-] - [HCO_3^-]$$

and represents unmeasured anions and cations. Normally, the anion gap is 12 ± 2 mEq/L. In a compensated metabolic acidosis, there is an increase in the serum chloride to maintain a normal anion gap.

Etiology

The causes of metabolic acidosis based on the anion gap are depicted in Table 7. In the pediatric age group, the most common cause of normal anion gap metabolic acidosis is diarrhea, where considerable loss of bicarbonate and potassium may occur in the stools. The hypokalemia and acidosis stimulate ammoniagenesis and ammonium excretion to increase the urine pH in some patients above 5.3. Thus, it may be difficult to distinguish between renal tubular acidosis and metabolic acidosis due to diarrhea losses. Determining the urinary anion gap ($Na^+ + K^+ - Cl^-$) has been shown to reflect a rough estimate of urinary ammonium. Patients with metabolic acidosis due to diarrhea losses have a negative anion gap and urinary pH of 5.5 or less, whereas patients with renal tubular acidosis exhibit positive urinary anion gaps with urine pHs exceeding 6.

Diabetic ketoacidosis is a common cause of high anion gap acidosis and results from overproduction and underutilization of ketoacids. With treatment, these ketoacids are metabolized, with net acid excretion by the kidneys and generation of HCO_3^-. Lactic acidosis most commonly results from tissue hypoxia due to shock or sepsis. When severe, lactic acidosis has a high mortality rate.

Ethylene glycol ingestion occurs when infants and toddlers ingest antifreeze. Hence, it is more common to observe these ingestions during the winter months. Ethylene glycol is metabolized to glycolic acid, which results in elevated anion gaps. An important clue to the presence of ethylene glycol intoxication is the osmolal gap, which is the difference between the measured and the calculated osmolality (normal gap <10).

Diagnosis

Uncomplicated metabolic acidosis manifests with an increase in blood acidity, hypobicarbonatemia, and hypocapnia. Determination of the anion gap helps to distinguish between the two categories of metabolic acidosis (high anion gap versus normal anion gap acidosis). When fully compensated, several rules may apply. (1) For every 1 mEq/L decrease in the serum bicarbonate level, there is a 1 to 1.5 mm Hg decrease in P_{CO_2}. (2) The last two digits of the blood pH correspond to the P_{CO_2}. (3) Winter's formula (shown previously) calculates the expected P_{CO_2}, thus enabling us to compare it with the measured P_{CO_2} and to determine whether the patient has a simple metabolic acidosis or a combined disorder.

In the presence of a high anion gap acidosis, determination of renal function and serum phosphate is necessary to rule out renal failure as a cause of metabolic acidosis. On the other hand, determination of urinary anion gap may help to distinguish between metabolic acidosis secondary to diarrhea and distal renal tubular acidosis.

Manifestations

The pulmonary manifestations of metabolic acidosis are tachypnea and hypocapnia. Patients may present with Kussmaul or labored breathing. The cardiovascular effects include depression of myocardial contractility, resulting from decreased intracellular pH. The arterial vasodilatation of acidosis is counterbalanced by the vasoconstrictory effects of catecholamines. Generally, there is hyperkalemia due to transcellular shifts. There also is an increase in ionized calcium concentration because of the displacement of this divalent ion from albumin.

Other manifestations include fatigue, weakness, and malaise in chronic metabolic acidosis. Nausea, vomiting, and abdominal pain may accompany chronic and acute metabolic acidosis. When metabolic acidosis is severe, stupor and coma may occur, particularly when associated with toxin ingestion. In infants and toddlers, there may be growth retardation.

TABLE 6. Treatment of Hyperkalemia

Mild Hyperkalemia	**Transcellular Shifts**
Dietary restriction	Sodium bicarbonate
Discontinue oral potassium supplements	*Dose:* 1–2 mEq/kg per dose IV
Discontinue medications that are potassium-sparing or contain potassium	*Onset of action:* 15–30 min
Penicillin	Glucose and insulin
Angiotensin-converting enzyme inhibitors	*Dose:* 0.3–0.5 g/kg/h with 1 U insulin per 4–5 g glucose IV
Amiloride	*Onset of action:* 15–30 min
Spironolactone	
Triamterene	**Removal of Potassium**
Eliminate conditions that favor hyperkalemia	Kayexalate
Acidosis	*Dose:* 1 g/kg per dose PO or via retention enema
Sodium restriction	*Onset of action:* 60 min by enema; 120 min PO
Intravascular volume depletion	Furosemide
	Dose: 1 mg/kg per dose IV
Reversal of Membrane Effects	*Onset of action:* 15–30 min
Calcium gluconate	Dialysis
Dose: 100–200 mg/kg per dose IV	Hemodialysis
Onset of action: Few minutes	Peritoneal dialysis

TABLE 7. A Mnemonic Classification of High Anion Gap* and Normal Anion Gap† Metabolic Acidosis

High Anion Gap	Normal Anion Gap
Methanol	Ureteroenterostomy
Uremia	Small bowel fistula
Diabetic ketoacidosis	Extra chloride
Paraldehyde	Diarrhea
Inborn errors of metabolism (e.g., organic acidemia)	Carbonic anhydrase inhibitors
Lactic acidosis	Addison's disease
Ethylene glycol, ethanol	Renal tubular acidosis, rehydration
Salicylates	Pancreatic fistulas, posthypocapnia, parenteral alimentation

*The mnemonic for high anion gap acidosis is MUD PILES.
†The mnemonic for normal anion gap acidosis is USED CARP.

Treatment

Once a diagnosis is established, treatment is directed to correcting the underlying cause. Attention should be paid to correcting the intravascular volume and potassium depletion and removal of the toxin (if applicable). Sodium bicarbonate should be administered in cases of renal tubular acidosis, uremia, or other bicarbonate-losing causes. Doses as high as 8 to 10 mEq/kg PO may be necessary. In renal tubular acidosis, potassium supplementation is necessary. This can be provided by the use of sodium/potassium citrate (Polycitra), which provides 2 mEq of bicarbonate, 1 mEq of sodium, and 1 mEq of potassium per milliliter.

When the blood pH is less than 7.2, the patient is at risk of developing the complications of metabolic acidosis, and intravenous bicarbonate therapy should be considered. The dose of bicarbonate can be calculated from the following formula.

$$\text{NaHCO}_3 \text{ dose (mEq)} = (\text{desired HCO}_3^- - \text{observed HCO}_3^-) \times 0.5 \times \text{body weight}$$

The pH should not be raised above 7.25 to 7.3 to prevent overshoot metabolic alkalosis. This usually corresponds to a bicarbonate concentration of 12 to 15 mEq/L. In cases of hypernatremia associated with metabolic acidosis, *Tris*-hydroxymethylaminomethane (Tham) may be used. Consideration for hemodialysis using a bicarbonate-containing bath should be given when bicarbonate cannot be given.

Metabolic Alkalosis

Metabolic alkalosis is defined as a primary increase in serum bicarbonate concentration, with resultant alkalemia and secondary hypercapnia. There is a concomitant drop in serum chloride levels in association with hypokalemia. Metabolic alkalosis can be *generated* by either loss of H^+, gain of bicarbonate, or loss of extracellular fluid, with more chloride than bicarbonate being wasted. In order for alkalosis to be *maintained,* factors should exist to prevent the kidney from excreting the excess bicarbonate. The most commonly encountered factor is extracellular volume depletion, which decreases the glomerular filtration rate, stimulates proximal reabsorption of bicarbonate (and other solutes), and triggers the renin-angiotensin-aldosterone system, with resultant distal tubular sodium reabsorption and H^+ and K^+ excretion. Other factors include mineralocorticoid excess and chloride and potassium depletion. Hypokalemia stimulates bicarbonate reabsorption by the proximal tubule and enhances H^+ excretion (by the distal tubule) and ammoniagenesis.

Etiology

Metabolic alkalosis can be classified into two categories: (1) chloride responsive and (2) chloride resistant (Table 8). The most common causes of sodium chloride-responsive metabolic alkalosis are vomiting and nasogastric suctioning. During the generation phase of metabolic alkalosis in vomiting or nasogastric suctioning, there is a rise in serum bicarbonate and urine pH, a fall in net acid excretion, and an increase in urinary sodium and potassium. This results in intravascular volume and potassium depletion. The alkalosis is maintained because of the decrease in the glomerular filtration rate and increased aldosterone levels, with resultant avid sodium reabsorption and an increase in net

acid excretion. The extrarenal response to metabolic alkalosis involves buffering of excess bicarbonate by titration of noncarbonic acid buffers in the plasma and intracellular space and hypoventilation, resulting in a steady-state increase in Pco_2. Administration of sodium chloride effects expansion of the extracellular space, bicarbonaturia, and correction of the alkalosis.

Diagnosis

Determination of the urinary chloride concentration is helpful in classifying metabolic alkalosis and guiding therapy. A urinary chloride concentration of less than 10 mEq/L is indicative of chloride-responsive metabolic alkalosis, whereas a urinary chloride concentration of more than 20 mEq/L implies the existence of chloride-resistant alkalosis. In addition, the disorder is characterized by an elevated anion gap. Blood gas determination is helpful in assessing whether the patient has a simple or a mixed disorder. Generally, for every 1 mEq increase in the serum bicarbonate concentration, there is an equivalent 0.5 to 1 mm Hg increase in Pco_2. In addition, the expected rise in Pco_2 may be calculated as follows.

$$Pco_2 = 0.9 \times HCO_3^- \pm 2$$

Manifestations

Patients with metabolic alkalosis usually present with the signs and symptoms pertaining to the underlying etiology, dehydration, or hypokalemia. Perhaps the most significant complication of severe metabolic alkalosis is the development of refractory supraventricular and ventricular arrhythmias, mostly noted in the critically ill. Stupor, mental confusion, lethargy, muscle weakness, and cramping may

TABLE 8. Classification of Metabolic Alkalosis

Chloride Responsive
Gastric juice loss (vomiting, nasogastric suctioning)
Posthypercapnia
Congenital chloride diarrhea
Cystic fibrosis
Postdiuretic therapy
Ingestion of chloride-deficient formulas

Chloride Resistant
Primary hyperaldosteronism
Primary hyperreninism
Congenital adrenal syndrome
Cushing's disease
Exogenous steroid administration
Bartter's syndrome
Potassium depletion
Liddle's syndrome
Licorice ingestion
Hypercalcemia
Hyperparathyroidism
Milk-alkali syndrome
Refeeding alkalosis
Massive transfusions

develop. Oxygen delivery to tissues is diminished due to shift in the oxygen-hemoglobin dissociation curve to the left, which may be a contributory factor in the pathophysiology of the neuromuscular disturbances. In addition, there may be a decrease in serum ionized calcium concentration and increased lactate production. The latter contributes to the elevated anion gap commonly observed in metabolic alkalosis.

Treatment

Generally, the treatment of metabolic alkalosis is aimed at correcting the intravascular volume and potassium depletion. Patients are supplemented with sodium chloride orally or intravenously. In chloride-resistant metabolic alkalosis, attention should be paid to correcting the underlying cause. Acidifying agents may be needed when the blood pH is greater than 7.55. Hemodialysis or peritoneal dialysis with high chloride-containing and low bicarbonate-containing baths could be lifesaving in patients with renal failure and metabolic alkalosis.

REFERENCES

1. Holliday MA, Barratt TM, Avner ED: Pediatric Nephrology. Baltimore, Williams & Wilkins, 1994.
2. Holliday MA, Segar WE: Maintenance need for water in parenteral fluid therapy. Pediatrics 19:823, 1957.
3. Ichikawa I (ed): Pediatric Textbook of Fluids and Electrolytes. Baltimore, Williams & Wilkins, 1990.
4. Kokko JA, Tannen RL (eds): Fluids and Electrolytes. Philadelphia, WB Saunders Co, 1990.

MALIGNANT HYPERTHERMIA

MATTHEW J. STENZEL, M.D.
DAVID S. JARDINE, M.D.

Malignant hyperthermia (MH) is a pharmacogenetic myopathy manifested as a hypermetabolic disorder of intracellular movement of calcium in the sarcoplasmic reticulum (SR) of skeletal muscle, where Ca^{2+} accumulates in the cytosol. MH usually presents after administration of succinylcholine or a volatile anesthetic agent and results in severe lactic metabolic acidosis and hyperpyrexia. The temperature may rise as fast as 0.5° C to 1° C every 5 minutes and may exceed 43° C (109.4° F). A rise in Ca^{2+} may result in sustained muscle contracture, (contraction that is nonpropagated and prolonged), as well as masseter spasm (trismus), whole body rigidity, and hypertension initially, followed by hypotension and shock. In addition, hypercarbia, tachycardia, diaphoresis, and excessive heat production may ensue. Renal failure secondary to rhabdomyolysis and myoglobinuria may be seen along with hyperkalemia, increased creatinine phosphokinase (CPK), and disseminated intravascular coagulation. Cerebral edema is a late sign that may be followed by coma and death.

The incidence of MH is approximately 1 in 15,000 for children to 1 in 62,000 in adults with the use of potent inhalational anesthetics with or without succinylcholine. There appears to be a slight male predominance in the illness. Mortality from MH initially approached 70% but with earlier diagnosis decreased to 28%. Since dantrolene was introduced in 1979, mortality is now <10%.

The exact pathophysiology of MH is not known. However, MH is thought to be a myopathy in which there is an acute loss of intracellular control of calcium. Rigidity occurs when unbound myofibrillar calcium nears the contractile threshold. The wave of depolarization from end plate to transverse tubule (T tubule) is transferred to the SR. Sustained muscle contraction causes a large increase in heat production and hypercarbia. The energy for this contraction is derived initially from aerobic metabolism, glycolysis, neutralization of H^+ ions (acid), and hydrolysis of high-energy phosphate compounds. After readily available oxidative substrates are depleted, subsequent heat production is due to lactate formation. There is a 3-fold increase in O_2 consumption ($\dot{V}O_2$) and a 15 to 20-fold increase in blood lactate.

Muscle physiologists have not identified the abnormality that causes the excitation contraction coupling link between the transverse tubule of skeletal muscle and SR. In 1988, the ryanodine receptor (RYR1) gene, which codes for the skeletal muscle calcium release channel, was described. It is possible that one or more mutations in the gene result in altered structural and functional properties of the calcium release channel in response to depolarization from the neuromuscular junction (NMJ) and T tubule system. Inheritance of MH is probably autosomal dominant with variable penetrance in humans. The locus for halothane sensitivity in humans is the long arm of chromosome 19.

TRIGGERING OF MH

The most important known triggers of MH are the volatile anesthetic agents (halothane, isoflurane, enflurane, sevoflurane, desflurane, methoxyflurane) and the depolarizing muscle relaxants (succinylcholine). Other drugs considered unsafe include ether, chloroform, and decamethonium. Drugs for which there are insufficient or controversial data include curare, metocurine, calcium salts, ketamine, catecholamines, and phenothiazines. Drugs that are definitely safe include barbiturates, narcotics, antipyretics, antihistamines, antibiotics, local anesthetics (both esters and amides), althesin, pancuronium, atracurium, vecuronium, propranolol, and droperidol (although this dopamine antagonist may precipitate neuroleptic malignant syndrome).

The onset of MH may be explosive with succinylcholine. Fasciculation (temporary total body muscle contractions) is a normal response to succinylcholine and is qualitatively different from the contracture seen in MH. Hyperkalemia, myoglobinemia, myoglobinuria, rhabdomyolysis, acute tubular necrosis with renal failure, and bradycardia are all potential signs that succinylcholine is triggering MH via the depolarizing effect of this drug on the muscle end plate.

Barbiturates, tranquilizers, and nondepolarizing muscle relaxants (NDMR) may delay the onset of MH for several hours or block succinylcholine triggering MH (but not reliably). Many people who develop MH have previously tolerated anesthetics that included potent triggering agents without visible difficulty. Although MH usually occurs within 2 to 4 hours of administration of a triggering agent, delayed onset has been reported up to 25 hours after the initiation of an anesthetic.

DIAGNOSIS

Early signs of MH may not be apparent until emergence from anesthesia. The differential diagnosis includes hyperthyroidism, pheochromocytoma, neuroleptic malignant syndrome, and familial fever. MH should be suspected when the signs and symptoms listed previously occur during or after an anesthetic that includes a known triggering agent.

Laboratory studies should show an increase in $PaCO_2$ (>60 mm Hg with a base deficit −5 to −7 mEq/L) and decreased $P\bar{v}O_2$ (approximately 35 mm Hg with PaO_2 > 100 mm Hg) unless these values have been normalized with aggressive mechanical ventilation and increased FIO_2. Mixed venous oxygen ($P\bar{v}O_2$) will fall as muscle metabolic demand increases. Accurate diagnosis of mild cases may be difficult because the alterations in $PaCO_2$ and $P\bar{v}O_2$ may be subtle. The diagnosis of fulminant MH is established if (1) $PaCO_2$ > 60 mm Hg and increasing ($PaCO_2$ normal before trigger), (2) $P\bar{v}CO_2$ > 90 mm Hg and increasing, (3) base deficit more than −5 mEq/L and falling, (4) temperature increasing 1° C/5 min or faster, with (5) rigidity, masseter spasm, and contracture. Following the onset of MH, CPK may be elevated above 20,000 units.

TREATMENT

The onset of MH is usually recognized, and treatment is initiated in the operating room. However, because subtle signs of MH may be missed in the operating room or the onset of MH may not occur until after the patient has left the recovery room, it is important that all physicians who care for patients postoperatively be able to recognize and treat MH. Acute therapy for MH includes discontinuing all anesthetic agents and securing the airway with an endotracheal tube. The patient should be hyperventilated with 100% O_2 to remove excess CO_2 production. The physician should request prompt assistance. If the patient is in the operating room, the physician should change the ventilator breathing circuit. Dantrolene should be started immediately at 2.5 mg/kg IV q5–10min not to exceed 10 mg/kg. Dantrolene has a half-life of 10 to 15 hours and should be repeated as necessary. Sodium bicarbonate at 2 to 4 mEq/kg IV may be needed to neutralize ongoing lactic acidosis. The initiation of measures to control fever include iced IV fluids, iced gastric lavage, and surface cooling. Cooling should be halted at 38 to 39° C to prevent hypothermia.

Continuous hemodynamic monitoring is achieved with arterial, central venous, or pulmonary artery lines, as large fluid shifts may occur with resuscitation. The urinary output should be monitored with a Foley urinary catheter. Acute tubular necrosis may occur if hypotension follows the onset of MH. The urine should be examined for myoglobinuria as a sign of rhabdomyolysis. Mannitol may be used for decreased urine output.

Laboratory values should be monitored frequently, including arterial blood gases, electrolytes, liver function tests, BUN, creatinine, lactate, and glucose. Coagulation studies, platelet count, serum hemoglobin, and myoglobin also should be obtained. CPK in cases of MH will commonly rise to >1000 and is an important piece of diagnostic information. The monitoring of temperature, muscle tone, urine output, and response to ongoing therapy is also important. Hyperkalemia needs to be treated slowly unless the high potassium has precipitated ventricular tachycardia or fibrillation. Dantrolene is the most important agent to halt the progression of hyperkalemia. For severe hyperkalemia, regular insulin (0.1 to 0.2 U/kg IV) and glucose (0.5 to 1 g/kg IV) may be given. Calcium may exacerbate MH and should not be used to treat hyperkalemia. Arrhythmias may be treated with procainamide or lidocaine.

Dantrolene is the only known specific therapeutic drug for MH. It selectively blocks Ca^{2+} release from SR and rapidly halts the increase in metabolism. Dantrolene should be repeated 2.5 mg/kg IV up to 10 mg/kg (exceed this dose if necessary) q10–15h for at least several doses until there are no signs of recurrence of MH. Retriggering of MH can occur 10 to 15 hours later as dantrolene wears off because of redistribution, metabolism, and excretion. Dantrolene is absolutely necessary in acute or fulminant MH. Although control of symptoms may be achieved by the use of other means, such as external cooling and hyperventilation, the patient may still die secondary to hypermetabolism leading to irreversible cellular injury. Because dantrolene blocks Ca^{2+} release from the SR, it causes moderate muscle weakness. Side effects of dantrolene are rare if it is taken for less than 3 weeks but may include serious complications, such as pulmonary edema, thrombophlebitis, and elevated liver enzymes.

Ca^{2+} antagonists (such as nimodipine, verapamil, nifedipine, diltiazem), and sympathetic antagonists, such as beta-adrenergic blockers, e.g., propranolol, are ineffective in the treatment of MH. Ca^{2+} channel blockers may interfere with dantrolene and cause hyperkalemia or retrigger MH.

ANESTHESIA FOR MH-SUSCEPTIBLE PATIENTS

Anesthetic agents known to cause MH must not be used in MH-susceptible patients. Because there is a wide variety of anesthetic agents known *not* to trigger MH, MH-susceptible patients usually do not need prophylactic dantrolene. Preparation of the anesthesia machine is important and includes measures to eliminate residual halogenated anesthetic gases. Such measures include removal or sealing

of vaporizers, replacement of lines with fresh gas outlet hose and CO_2 absorbant, use of a disposable fresh breathing circuit, and a flush of 6 L/min of 100% O_2 for 5 minutes. When an agent that carries some risk of triggering MH must be used, prophylactic dantrolene should be given the night before surgery 2.5 to 4 mg/kg PO, as well as 2 mg/kg IV before induction. The disadvantages of this approach are that dantrolene may make the patient weak and may prolong nondepolarizing muscle relaxants.

EVALUATION OF SUSCEPTIBILITY

Evaluation of MH susceptibility (MHS) usually begins with a history of the patient or family. Noteworthy events include difficulty with previous anesthetics, unexpected family deaths, or masseter spasm. A genealogy going back two generations looking for information about anesthetic exposure and adverse reactions helps to estimate the likelihood of exposure to triggering agents. After the history, physical examination and measurement of CPK (especially CK MM fraction) may be helpful. CPK values must be interpreted from a resting, fasted patient without recent trauma. CPK is elevated in approximately 70% of MHS patients.

If the diagnosis is clearly established in a patient, close relatives may be considered susceptible without further testing. If the CPK is normal on several occasions but the patient has a positive history of hyperthermia associated with anesthesia, a muscle biopsy is necessary for contracture studies.

The only reliable test demonstrating MHS is the caffeine and halothane in vitro contracture test (IVCT). The IVCT is invasive, expensive, and time consuming and must be performed in a close enough location to a test center for rapid transit of the fresh specimen (5 to 6 hours). Contracture thresholds are about 95% reliable in evaluating MHS using halothane, caffeine, or both. Positive contracture in patients with myopathies that are not directly related to MH is inconclusive as to susceptibility. Patients must not be given dantrolene before muscle biopsy because it may mask identification of an MHS patient. The muscle specimen must be viable (i.e., twitch when electrically stimulated). The IVCT is very sensitive. Positive results correlate well with MH survivors determined by previous anesthetic challenge. The specificity of the IVCT is unknown.

For assistance in the management of patients with MH, call the MH hotline: (209) 634-4917; request index zero, MH consultant.

REFERENCES

1. Gronert GA, Schulman SR, Mott J: Malignant hyperthermia. *In* Miller RD (ed): Anesthesia, 3rd ed. New York, Churchill Livingstone, 1990: 935–956.
2. Larach MG, Landis JR, Schaeffer Bunn J, Diaz M: The North American malignant hyperthermia registry. Anesthesiology 76:16–27, 1992.
3. Rosenberg H, Seitman D: Pharmacogenetics. *In* Barash P, Cullen B, Stoelting R (eds): Clinical Anesthesia. Philadelphia, JB Lippincott, 1989:459–472.

HEAT-RELATED ILLNESSES INCLUDING HEMORRHAGIC SHOCK AND ENCEPHALOPATHY SYNDROME AND HEAT STROKE

DAVID S. JARDINE, M.D.
MATTHEW J. STENZEL, M.D.

HEMORRHAGIC SHOCK AND ENCEPHALOPATHY SYNDROME

Hemorrhagic shock and encephalopathy syndrome (HSES) is an illness that usually strikes children under 1 year of age. The cardinal aspects of this illness are shock, encephalopathy (usually including seizures), and coagulation abnormalities.[1] Despite the name, most patients do not have severe clinical hemorrhage. However, all patients with this illness have laboratory evidence of a coagulopathy. The outcome of patients with this illness is poor, with a high rate of mortality and frequent neurologic impairment among survivors.

HSES was first described in 1983 as a new disease "distinct from previously recognized disorders." Since the original account, more than 150 cases have been reported in the literature. The author of the original description of HSES has speculated that it might be caused by defective regulation of serum proteases. However, numerous authors have noted the striking similarity between HSES and heat stroke in infancy.[2] Although this issue has yet to be resolved, the preponderance of those who have published on the subject suggests that heat stroke is the most likely cause of this illness. Both mathematical and animal models have been put forward to explain how an infant may become severely hyperthermic while asleep in bed. These models indicate that the crucial determinant of heat transfer from the infant to the environment is the proportion of exposed (uncovered) skin. When this falls below a critical minimum, heat transfer to the environment is less than endogenous heat production, so the infant's temperature must rise. Many children who suffer HSES also have a minor viral illness. The fever engendered by the viral illness may serve to accelerate the temperature rise of an infant who has an inadequate quantity of exposed skin, and may increase the risk of HSES.

Diagnosis

Because there are no biologic markers for HSES (or for heat stroke), the diagnosis of HSES is based on a characteristic set of clinical and laboratory findings. The clinical presentation of HSES is so similar to that of bacterial sepsis that it is frequently mistaken for bacterial sepsis. HSES should be suspected in any child under 1 year of age who is admitted with the diagnosis of possible sepsis and who has shock requiring fluid resuscitation or vasopressors. HSES should also be suspected in any child who has had a temperature of ≥41.1° C (106° F). Temperatures of this magnitude are usually recorded in the child's home. By the time the child is admitted to the hospital, the temperature is usually unremarkable. Although HSES has been described in children over 1 year of age, it is much less frequent in this age group.

HSES usually strikes children who did not have a preexisting medical abnormality. Many, but not all, of those who suffer HSES have a minor viral infection before the onset of the illness. Characteristically, the patients are found in bed to be severely ill, usually after a period of sleeping unobserved. Morning is the most frequent time of presentation, when parents attempt to awaken the child. At the time of discovery, the child is usually pale, limp, and unresponsive. Seizures may be present at the time of discovery but often do not occur until shortly after the child is admitted to the hospital. *All children with HSES are in shock at the time of presentation and need fluid resuscitation. In our experience, approximately half of the children need vasopressor support to restore an adequate blood pressure.*

Patients with HSES have prerenal azotemia and metabolic acidosis at the time of presentation. Both of these abnormalities resolve with restoration of adequate blood pressure. Over the next several days, these patients show a characteristic progression of laboratory abnormalities. Creatine phosphokinase (CPK), alanine aminotransferase (ALT), and aspartate aminotransferase (AST) are normal or minimally elevated on admission but rise progressively after onset of HSES, usually reaching maximal levels within the first 72 hours of illness.

Anemia and thrombocytopenia, two other characteristics of HSES, may not be evident at the onset of illness, but within 24 hours hemoglobin and platelet concentrations have often fallen to dangerously low levels. Despite thrombocytopenia and elevation of prothrombin time (PT) and partial thromboplastin time (PTT), clinical bleeding, even after venipuncture, is usually not a severe problem and can be controlled with application of direct pressure. Almost always by the fourth or fifth day after onset of HSES, all laboratory abnormalities demonstrate a clear trend toward normal.

To facilitate the diagnosis of HSES, it is useful to collect the required laboratory data at the time of admission and on the morning following admission. If the ALT, AST, and CPK remain normal for the first 24 hours, HSES is eliminated as a possible diagnosis. If these values show a characteristic rise, the laboratory values noted should be collected daily for 4 more days to document the evolution of these abnormalities. Although the progression of these laboratory changes is useful as a diagnostic tool, the severity of derangement in laboratory values is not related to the prognosis in HSES. The risk of mortality and neurologic injury does not appear to be related to the peak values of CPK, ALT, and AST or to the degree of anemia and thrombocytopenia.

Treatment

Treatment of HSES is supportive. Because of the severity of the illness and the life-threatening nature of some of the abnormalities that occur, most patients with HSES will be cared for in a pediatric intensive care unit. Although this illness is probably caused by heat stroke, most victims of HSES have temperatures that are within the usual febrile range (<41° C) at the time of admission to a medical institution. Specific measures aimed at cooling the child other than removing blankets and clothing are not necessary.

Treatment of shock and control of seizures usually dominate the care of these children in the first few hours after onset. Isotonic fluids, such as lactated Ringer's solution, should be used for initial resuscitation. Fluids should be administered rapidly in increments of 10 ml/kg. After each increment of fluid, blood pressure should be determined, and peripheral perfusion should be observed. If adequate blood pressure and perfusion have not been obtained after the administration of 40 ml/kg of intravenous fluids, central venous access should be established to allow measurement of central venous pressures as a guide for further fluid therapy. If a double-lumen catheter is placed, it can be used for infusion of medication and fluids while allowing simultaneous measurement of central venous pressure.

Once central venous pressure has been restored (usually 8 to 15 mm Hg) a vasopressor infusion should be initiated if the patient remains hypotensive. We employ dopamine as the primary vasopressor in HSES. Although most patients respond adequately to dopamine, those who are most severely affected may need a second vasopressor. In this situation, we employ epinephrine. Characteristically, patients will not need vasopressor therapy for more than 24 hours. Most patients have no vasopressor requirements and normal fluid requirements beyond the first day of illness.

Many patients with HSES have a metabolic acidosis at the time of presentation. In mild cases of HSES, the acidosis is corrected by restoration of normal blood pressure, and no further intervention is necessary. In severe cases of HSES, the metabolic acidosis may be extreme (pH < 7.20). When confronted with this problem, we have administered $NaHCO_3$ to correct the acidosis partially. The metabolic acidosis usually is well controlled within 24 hours, and serum pH returns to normal. Nevertheless, serum lactate often remains elevated for several days despite a normal serum pH.

Seizures, which may not be present when a child is discovered to have HSES, often occur in the first hours of therapy. These usually can be controlled by administration of one or two anticonvulsants in doses sufficient to attain therapeutic levels. The anticonvulsant we use initially is phenobarbital. If the seizures are not controlled after administration of 20 mg/kg of phenobarbital, we obtain a serum level of phenobarbital and administer phenytoin while awaiting the results. Because of the potential for additional myocardial depression with the administration of phenytoin, we infuse the dose slowly (20 mg/kg over 40 to 60 minutes).

Respiratory depression occurs frequently in HSES. Management of this problem calls for endotracheal intubation and mechanical ventilation. Although respiratory depression may occur before the administration of anticonvulsants, it is observed most frequently after the treatment of seizures. Patients with HSES often will need mechanical ventilation for the first several days of the illness. The duration of mechanical ventilation is determined by the rate of neurologic improvement, as patients with HSES usually do not have intrinsic lung disease. Consequently, the ventilator settings necessary to maintain adequate arterial blood gases are usually low.

All patients with HSES have a coagulopathy, with prolongation of the PT and PTT, elevation of d-dimer (or fibrin split products), and thrombocytopenia. Even though the name of the illness derives from the hemorrhagic diathesis occasionally observed in the most severe cases, clinical hemorrhage in HSES is unusual. When bleeding becomes a problem, it usually can be managed by transfusion of platelets and fresh frozen plasma. Consumption of clotting factors and platelets in HSES is usually not so rapid that platelet and factor transfusions must be repeated more than once or twice.

It is difficult to distinguish between the clinical presentation of HSES and that of bacterial sepsis. Until blood cultures have been negative for 72 hours, children suspected of having HSES should be treated with antibiotics that would be used to treat bacterial sepsis of unknown etiology.

Outcome

Initial reports of HSES documented mortality rates of 70%, with similarly high rates of permanent neurologic injury among survivors. Subsequently, more than 150 cases of HSES have been reported, and the less severe manifestations of this illness have been appreciated. Although it is possible to survive HSES without residual neurologic injury, approximately 30% of those afflicted with this illness will die. It is more difficult to determine the frequency with which permanent neurologic damage occurs among the survivors, but it appears to occur in 30% to 50%. Other than the supportive measures discussed, there appear to be no therapeutic interventions that improve the outcome.

HEAT STROKE

Our survival depends on regulating our temperature within a very narrow range. When heat stress persists, the physiologic strain of preventing hyperthermia begins to take a toll, resulting in minor heat-related illnesses (heat cramps and heat exhaustion). If thermoregulation fails and the temperature rises to injurious levels, heat stroke occurs. Heat stroke is defined as tissue damage caused by excessive heat. It develops at body temperatures in excess of 41.6° C (106.9° F).[3] The extent of the injury depends on the height of the temperature *and* its duration. A child may tolerate a brief temperature of 42.5° C with little evidence of injury, but longer exposure to a temperature of 41.8° C may cause severe injury. Heat stroke takes two forms: nonexertional heat stroke (also called classic heat stroke) and exertional heat stroke.

Children who suffer heat stroke do not have primary thermoregulatory abnormalities. The neurophysiologic control of temperature regulation is intact but is overwhelmed by excess accumulation of heat. When a victim of heat stroke is removed from the offending circumstances, his temperature rapidly returns to normal. However, it is important to recognize that the injury caused by heat stroke lingers long after the temperature returns to normal. Hyperthermia at the time of presentation with heat stroke is not necessary to establish the diagnosis. Rather, the diagnosis is made by recognition that environmental circumstances and physical activity were sufficient to cause accumulation of injurious levels of heat and that the clinical and laboratory findings are consistent with heat stroke.

Heat Cramps

Heat cramps are muscle cramps that occur after work in a hot environment in muscle groups used extensively. Typically, the onset of cramping is after exertion has ceased and the individual is relaxing. Frequently, patients affected by this problem have attempted to maintain adequate hydration by intake of hypotonic fluids during exercise. Although heat cramps are not dangerous, they may cause substantial discomfort. Hyponatremia and hypochloremia frequently accompany heat cramps. The cause of heat cramps is not known, but the cramping rapidly concludes after the administration of salt, either orally or intravenously, in the form of electrolyte solution.

Heat Exhaustion

Heat exhaustion is characterized by thirst, fatigue, weakness, discomfort, and mental status alteration. It occurs in individuals who have been sweating copiously during physical exercise, usually in a hot environment. Both water and salt depletion are implicated in the pathogenesis of this illness. Treatment consists of rehydration and gradual correction of hypernatremia if this is present. If the patient is conscious, oral rehydration may be the preferred route if heat exhaustion is not severe. For unconscious or more severely affected patients, parenteral hydration is the route of choice. Correction of hypernatremia at an excessive rate can lead to serious neurologic problems, including seizures and cerebral edema. If hypotension occurs with heat exhaustion, the victim should be considered to be suffering from heat stroke.

Nonexertional Heat Stroke

This form of heat stroke (also called *classic heat stroke*) occurs in hot environments in the absence of physical exertion. Because the environment is so hot, the mechanisms used to transfer heat to the environment (primarily sweating and cutaneous vasodilatation) are insufficient to keep the body temperature at 37° C. When the temperature exceeds 41.6° C (106.9° F), tissue injury occurs. Victims of this illness frequently have had long periods of sustained sweat loss. If the physiologic production of sweat has become ineffective, the victim may have dry (anhydrotic) skin at the time of presentation.

Children are at special risk for this form of heat stroke because they are often unable to take measures to cool their environment. For example, deaths in children have occurred after they were left unattended in an automobile with the windows rolled up. The temperature in a dark-colored automobile with the windows rolled up has been reported to rise from 36° C to 67° C after 15 minutes in the sun. Heat stroke has also occurred in children who have been left unattended in excessively heated dwellings.

Because circulation of warm blood from the core to the skin and sweat losses are important to maintain thermal homeostasis, conditions that alter sweat production or reduce the ability to circulate blood to the skin increase the risk of heat stroke. Phenothiazines, anticholinergics, and tricyclic antidepressants reduce sweating and, thus, may increase the risk of heat stroke. Circulation of blood to the skin may be reduced by congestive heart failure, the use of diuretics, or the use of beta-blockers.

Exertional Heat Stroke

Exertional heat stroke affects those who have been working vigorously in warm environments. The heat produced by the body rises dramatically during muscular work. In adults, average work may increase heat production by fivefold compared with the basal state. Intense work can produce sustained heat production that is eight times greater than basal heat production. In the pediatric age group, exertional heat stroke is most likely to strike young athletes, especially those who perform strenuous activity for long periods of time (long distance runners and football players having strenuous practice sessions). Misdirected training regimens that include water deprivation and wearing of excessive clothing or clothing that reduces evaporation of sweat increase the risk of heat stroke.

Symptoms and Laboratory Abnormalities in Heat Stroke

At presentation, the patient may not be hyperthermic if sufficient time has passed between removal from the offending environment and arrival at a medical institution. Patients suffering from heat stroke are in shock and have neurologic abnormalities, including coma, constricted pupils, and seizures. Laboratory abnormalities usually include prerenal azotemia, progressive coagulopathy (elevation of PT, PTT, and d-dimer), anemia, and thrombocytopenia. Elevations of CPK, ALT, and AST are usually modest at the time of admission but reach a maximum at approximately 48 to 72 hours.

Treatment

Heat stroke is a medical emergency. If the victim of heat stroke is still hyperthermic on arrival in an emergency room, immediate steps must be taken to reduce the temperature. Although complicated regimens have been described to lower temperature rapidly, forced evaporation remains the most effective way to cool a patient. Forced evaporation is performed by removing the patient's clothing, spraying the victim with cool water, and using a large fan to augment evaporation. Because the heat of vaporization for water is great (2406 kJ/ kg H_2O), forced evaporation has been shown to be as effective as covering the body with cold packs.

Treatment of heat stroke is identical to treatment of HSES. Dantrolene has been used without success to ameliorate the injury that occurs in heat stroke. Dantrolene is effective for treatment of malignant hyperthermia because it relaxes skeletal muscle by preventing calcium ion release from the sarcoplasmic reticulum. Heat stroke is the result of tissue injury caused by recent hyperthermia, not by ongoing muscular contraction, as is the case with malignant hyperthermia.

Outcome

Much of the outcome of heat stroke is determined by the severity of the injury before the patient arrives at the hospital. Aggressive medical care is necessary to prevent additional injury to the patient from hypotension, seizures, or hypoxia. Although most patients will survive heat stroke with minimal sequelae, even with optimal medical care, some patients succumb to heat stroke or sustain permanent neurologic injury.

REFERENCES

1. Bacon CJ, Hall SM: Haemorrhagic shock encephalopathy syndrome in the British Isles. Arch Dis Child 67:985–993, 1992.
2. Caspe WB, Nucci AT, Cho S: Extreme hyperpyrexia in childhood: Presentation similar to hemorrhagic shock and encephalopathy. Clin Pediatr 28:76–80, 1989.
3. Knochel JP: Heat stroke and related heat stress disorders. Disease-A-Month 35:301–377, 1989.

HEMATURIA AND PROTEINURIA

BARBARA R. COLE, M.D.

Hematuria and proteinuria are signs of diseases of the urinary tract. Consequently, their therapeutic management is determined by elucidating their causes. Following are the major questions to be asked when one sees a patient with one or both of these signs.

1. What should I do to evaluate the patient?
2. How extensive should the evaluation be if the etiology is not readily apparent?
3. How should I follow and manage the patient if the cause cannot be determined?

GROSS HEMATURIA

The evaluation of gross hematuria differs from that of microscopic hematuria, for the etiologies of the two are likely different. *Gross red hematuria is often caused by an abnormality of the lower urinary tract.* Thus, as seen in Table 1, sources of such bleeding include trauma to any part of the urinary tract, infections (particularly cystitis), stones, sickle cell trait, and, much less commonly, bleeding from arteriovenous malformations, renal vein thrombosis, congenital or hereditary anomalies, or coagulopathies. *Gross brown or cola-colored urine indicates that the blood has been in the bladder long enough for the conversion of hemoglobin to acid hematin to produce the brown color.* Thus, bleeding from the upper urinary tract (including kidney) is the more likely source. Free hemoglobin and myoglobin also impart

TABLE 1. Etiologies of Hematuria

	MORE COMMON	LESS COMMON
Gross Red Hematuria		
	Infection	Sickle cell trait
	Trauma	Arteriovenous malformations
	Stones	Congenital or hereditary anomalies
		Coagulopathies
		Renal vein thrombosis
Gross Brown Hematuria		
	IgA nephropathy	Renal vein thrombosis
	Henoch-Schönlein purpura with nephritis	Other glomerulonephritides
	Postinfectious acute glomerulonephritis	
Microscopic Hematuria		
	Infection	Resolving acute glomerulonephritis
	Hypercalciuria	IgA nephropathy
	Trauma	Hereditary nephritis
	Undefined	Other nephritides
		Sickle cell disease
		AIDS nephropathy
		Benign familial hematuria

a brown color to urine, so the diagnosis of hematuria relies on seeing red cells in the urine.

Kidney diseases that may produce gross brown hematuria include IgA nephropathy, Henoch-Schönlein purpura with nephritis, postinfectious acute glomerulonephritis, and, much less commonly, crescentic glomerulonephritis and the nephritis of such systemic diseases as systemic lupus erythematosus.

The evaluation of gross red hematuria is first directed toward detection of a lower urinary tract abnormality. The urinalysis would be expected to show a full field of RBCs, small amounts of protein commensurate with the blood, and no casts. Infections usually produce pyuria as well. Historical information may suggest infections or trauma, although traumatic events may not have been witnessed by parents and not remembered by small children. A 5-year-old boy presented to our hospital last year with severe hypertension and only microscopic hematuria. Intravenous urography suggested a healing laceration of the kidney. With much thought, the parents found they had a videotape of their son's jumping on a bed that showed that he had fallen across the bedpost, striking his flank! He apparently, however, had no gross hematuria.

In addition to urinalysis and urine culture to detect infections, an important feature of evaluation is imaging. Ultrasound examination is usually performed first, but intravenous urography may be very helpful in the detection of blood that is extravasating into the retroperitoneal space. Ultrasound examination may reveal stones, obstruction from blood clots, or when the bladder is full, abnormalities of the lower urinary tract. Gross hematuria with trauma not uncommonly reveals the preexistence of hydronephrosis or hereditary abnormalities, such as autosomal dominant polycystic kidney disease. Their retroperitoneal placement protects normal kidneys from most blunt trauma, but the increased size associated with hydronephrosis or cysts makes those kidneys more vulnerable.

Therapy of Gross Red Hematuria

The treatment of gross hematuria due to trauma is usually supportive. Bedrest, high fluid intake (usually intravenous administration of 2.5 to 3 L/m² body surface area), and analgesia as necessary allow resolution of the gross hematuria in a few days. When the kidney is lacerated, however, surgical repair or nephrectomy may be necessary to prevent exsanguination. Urologic consultation must be sought early in these cases.

Specific and supportive treatment of urinary tract infections is discussed in a previous section in this chapter. Treatment of gross bleeding due to the presence and movement of stones is aimed at high fluid intake, with the purpose of aiding stone passage. Obstruction from the stones should also prompt urologic consultation. Treatment of gross hematuria from sickle cell trait is aimed at ensuring the absence of any complicating feature, such as infections, and then supplying large fluid intake. Approaches to hemostasis in the face of coagulopathies are directed to the specific coagulopathy. Bleeding from arteriovenous malformations is sometimes difficult to detect and may require angiography for diagnosis. This procedure is usually reserved for those who have sufficient bleeding to drop the hematocrit or for those with recurrent bleeding.

It should be appreciated that gross hematuria may be sufficient to cause obstruction from clots in the ureters or bladder. Thus, urine output should be monitored carefully and related to intake, and renal function, assessed by serum creatinine values, should be measured serially.

Therapy of Gross Brown Hematuria

A different approach to evaluation and management is required for those with gross brown hematuria, since it is usually renal in origin. Historical information and physical examination are of great benefit. Those with IgA nephropathy not infrequently have a coincident upper respiratory infection, and the gross hematuria resolves as the upper respiratory infection clears. Those with postinfectious glomerulonephritis may have a history of pharyngitis 7 to 14 days before the onset of the hematuria or may have or have had impetigo for several weeks. Those with Henoch-Schönlein nephritis develop rash, abdominal pain, or arthralgias. Those with hemolytic-uremic syndrome may have had prior diarrhea, sometimes bloody. Patients with the more rare nephritides generally are quite ill and may have symptoms secondary to renal insufficiency or volume retention. Urinalysis is helpfully revealing in glomerular disease. Proteinuria is quantitatively greater and may reach nephrotic range (>2 g/d). The red cells, having passed through the glomerular basement membrane, are small and dysmorphic. Microscopic inspection shows defects or outpouchings in the red cell membrane that are described as *blebs*. Casts are common, and red cell casts often can be detected with serial observation. The reader is referred to the section on Glomerulonephritis for evaluation and management of these entities.

MICROSCOPIC HEMATURIA

Etiologies of microscopic hematuria, defined as greater than 3 to 5 RBCs on two of three successive concentrated urine samples, are myriad. To perform an exhaustive evaluation that might be necessary to diagnose a specific but elusive abnormality would be traumatic to the patient and expensive. Furthermore, it would be to little avail, for many conditions do not require specific, or even supportive, therapy. The objective, then, should be to develop an evaluation scheme that will answer two questions. (1) Is this condition one that is likely to be progressive? (2) Does this condition require treatment?

The most common causes of microscopic hematuria (Table 1) are infections, hypercalciuria, lower urinary tract trauma (including perineal inflammation from bubble baths or masturbation and urethral trauma from catheterization or self-exploration), and undefined causes. Less commonly seen, but still relatively prevalent, is microscopic hematuria secondary to resolving acute glomerulonephritis and such nephritides as IgA nephropathy (which is often associated with microscopic hematuria between bouts of gross hematuria) and Henoch-Schönlein purpura. More uncommon still are membranoproliferative glomerulonephritis, hereditary nephritis, crescentic glomerulonephritis, and systemic diseases, such as systemic lupus erythematosus, sickle cell disease, and AIDS nephropathy. Other diseases, such as Wegener's granulomatosis, are rare in childhood. In addition, microscopic hematuria, incidentally found, may be the presentation

of congenital malformations, such as horseshoe kidney, and inherited ones, including autosomal dominant and autosomal recessive polycystic kidney disease, uremic medullary cystic kidney disease, and medullary sponge kidney.

Interstitial and tubular diseases may be the source of microscopic hematuria. Interstitial disease may be infectious or allergic in nature. The hematuria of tubular disease may well be coincident with infection or hypercalciuria. Finally, any of those entities noted to produce gross hematuria may occur with only microscopic findings.

The initial evaluation is directed toward answering the two questions about whether the disease is likely to progress and need intervention. A careful history is most important, and physical examination, particularly blood pressure measurement, growth, and presence of rash or edema, gives clues as to severity and duration of disease. Family history is particularly important, since benign familial hematuria and Alport's disease are not uncommon in some areas.

In addition to the history and physical examination, the urinalysis may be helpful in differentiating possible causes. Pyuria may indicate an infectious etiology. *It is important to relate the number of white cells per high power field to the degree of concentration of the urine.* The designation of 2 to 5 WBCs/hpf as "normal" is that for a concentrated urine. A more dilute urine might have only that number but represent an abnormal excretion. The presence of calcium oxalate crystals may direct the evaluation toward hypercalciuria or stones, and the presence of cystine crystals might indicate cystinuria. The presence of proteinuria suggests a more likely renal origin of the cells, particularly when it is 3+ or 4+ by dipstick or >500 mg/m²/d. Casts also direct attention toward the kidney and, depending on the type of cast, to glomerular or tubulointerstitial disease. An inappropriately dilute urine also suggests tubulointerstitial disease, and glucosuria raises the possibility of proximal tubular damage.

When history, physical examination, and urinalysis fail to provide direct leads to diagnosis, a few laboratory screening items are warranted. The answers to the two basic questions of progression and treatment are provided by their results. Those laboratory tests (Table 2) include assessment of blood urea nitrogen and serum creatinine, serum complement (C3), antinuclear antibody titer, quantitation of urinary protein by protein/creatinine ratio (<0.25) or 12 to 24-hour collection, urine calcium/creatinine ratio (substantiated by 24-hour urine collection if the value is in the suspicious range—<0.15), and urinary tract imaging, initially by ultrasonogram. If the hematuria is of recent onset, a urine culture and tests to detect recent streptococcal infection (such as antistreptolysin O and antihyaluronidase or streptozyme titers) may be warranted. Analysis of the parents' urines completes the initial evaluation. If the patient is African American, a sickle cell screen should be included.

The likelihood of a progressive disease or one that needs treatment is remote if all of these screening tests are within normal limits. Even so, there are a few chronic diseases that may be present and that will manifest themselves later. Two major diseases to be considered are IgA nephropathy and hypercalciuria. IgA nephropathy may begin as microscopic hematuria long before the presence of proteinuria or

---

TABLE 2. Initial Laboratory Evaluation of Microscopic Hematuria

Blood
Blood urea nitrogen and serum creatinine
Complement (C3), antinuclear antibody titer
Sickle cell screen (when appropriate)

Urine
Urinalysis of patient and parents
Urine protein/creatinine
Urine calcium/creatinine

Imaging
Renal ultrasound

recurrent bouts of gross hematuria are seen. The majority of pediatric patients with hypercalciuria have the absorptive type, so if the patient has avoided milk-containing foods for a day or two, the urine calcium/creatinine may be normal. All this leads to the practice of following patients with no specific diagnosis through time. Serial visits at 3 to 6 month intervals for 1 to 2 years, followed by yearly assessment thereafter, usually either establishes the disappearance of the hematuria or leads to the discovery of new findings, such as the appearance of proteinuria, that indicate the need for further evaluation.

In the meantime, there is no need for any therapeutic intervention. Limitation of activity or dietary modification is not needed, and every attempt should be made to assure parents and patient that there is no need for worry.

PROTEINURIA

The detection of small amounts of proteinuria by dipstick examination is exceedingly common. In fact, some 19% of 15-year-old males have been shown to have proteinuria on at least one of seven daily examinations.[4] Exercise and fever may be the two most common etiologies of trace to 2+ proteinuria seen in office and emergency room visits. However, the incidence of proteinuria in two or more urine samples collected at rest falls to <0.2% of subjects tested. Once again, the interpretation of the significance of positive dipstick proteinuria can be aided by noting the specific gravity. The appearance of 1+ proteinuria in a very concentrated specimen is representative of a quantitatively low protein excretion, whereas that reading in a very dilute specimen may represent a large excretion. The protein/creatinine ratio is even more helpful in interpretation.

Proteinuria has several designations. It may be *transient,* which is the case with exercise- or fever-induced proteinuria, *orthostatic* in which it is present only when the patient is in the upright position, or *fixed* or *persistent,* in which it is present in all urine specimens. Persistent proteinuria has four possible causes.

1. Increased glomerular permeability to plasma proteins, as is the case with any kind of glomerulonephritis
2. Decreased reabsorption of filtered proteins, which occurs with proximal tubular diseases, including lead intoxication
3. *Overflow,* in which excessive amounts of plasma proteins are produced (seen in multiple myeloma, for example) and filtered, exceeding the threshold for reabsorption
4. Conditions in which tissue proteins are produced by tubular or lower urinary tract structures

This *secretory proteinuria* may occur in pyelonephritis or cystitis, in analgesic nephropathy, or in diseases of the accessory sex glands. When proteinuria is persistent in children, it is likely associated with either increased glomerular permeability or decreased tubular reabsorption.

The first step when one sees a patient whose urine contains protein, particularly if the quantity is small (up to 2+), is to define whether it is persistent. A second urine specimen should be obtained when the patient is afebrile and has not just exercised. Should that one be positive as well, the next appropriate maneuver is to determine whether the proteinuria is orthostatic. One can approach this by having the patient dipstick the urine twice daily for a period of time. The first time should be immediately on arising in the morning, and the second time in the late afternoon or evening. A running account will show negative dipsticks in the morning and positive ones in the evening if the proteinuria is orthostatic in nature. Another approach is to have the patient collect two 12-hour urine specimens, one at bedrest and the other while ambulatory. If the proteinuria is orthostatic, it will be quantitatively normal (<30 mg/m²/12 h) in the recumbent specimen and greater in the ambulatory specimen.

Orthostatic proteinuria is seen in many adolescents, particularly male. There is no evidence that this is a progressive condition and no evidence that full activity does anything to harm the kidney. Thus, there should be assurance to the parents and patient that there is no cause for concern, and there should be no activity limitations imposed. It may be advisable to follow the patient for a few years to ensure that no new findings develop.

Persistent proteinuria, on the other hand, is a worrisome sign and warrants evaluation. It is fairly uncommon to have proteinuria as a sole finding when there is significant disease. Usually there are concomitant red blood cells or casts or both when glomerular diseases exist, and there may be pyuria with inflammatory diseases of any portion of the genitourinary tract. Three glomerular diseases in which proteinuria may be a sole finding are minimal change disease (in which case, the full-blown nephrotic syndrome may not be evident), focal sclerosing glomerulonephritis, and membranous glomerulonephritis. In children, membranous glomerulonephritis is uncommon, and when present, it is frequently associated with either hepatitis B infection or with systemic lupus erythematosus, and other signs or symptoms are present. Occasionally, proteinuria is seen as the first sign of smoldering chronic rejection in renal allograft recipients.

The evaluation for a patient with persistent proteinuria is like that of the patient with microscopic hematuria, with exceptions. First, history and physical examination may be very helpful in directing evaluation. The urinalysis, as noted previously, may give clues. Thereafter, it is important to quantitate the proteinuria, for larger amounts of protein are more common in glomerular diseases than in tubular diseases, and in some cases, it may be helpful to determine what kinds of protein are excreted. In minimal change disease, nearly all the protein excreted is albumin. In glomerulonephritides, the damage to the glomerular basement membrane allows both albumin and the larger globulins to filter. A urinary protein electropheresis discriminates the types of protein present in the urine. Should tissue proteins from the genitourinary tract or tumor-associated proteins (light chains, for example) be the culprits, the protein electrophoresis will detect them and allow more appropriate evaluation. An assessment of glomerular filtration rate, serum complement levels, antinuclear antibody titers, serum protein (total protein and albumin), serum cholesterol, and renal imaging completes the baseline evaluation. When silent infection is suspected, urine cultures are warranted. When tubulointerstitial disease is suspected, urine histology and tubular function studies may be helpful.

When should one perform a renal biopsy? If proteinuria is persistent, >500 mg/m²/d, and thought to be due to glomerular changes, a renal biopsy is necessary to determine both the diagnosis and the degree of injury. If proteinuria is persistent and accompanied by any of the following—hematuria, a decrease in glomerular filtration, or hypocomplementemia—a biopsy is helpful in making a diagnosis. If proteinuria is accompanied by the nephrotic syndrome and the patient is not in the typical age range for minimal change disease (18 months to 6 years) or is steroid resistant, a biopsy is warranted. The reader is referred to the section on nephrotic syndrome for further discussion of therapy. It should be underscored that persistent proteinuria is a more ominous sign than is persistent microscopic hematuria, and the presence of both is most ominous. Thus, exact diagnosis, insofar as is possible, is mandatory to provide the specific therapy required.

REFERENCES

1. Lieu TA, Grasmeder HM III, Kaplan BS: An approach to the evaluation and treatment of microscopic hematuria. Pediatr Clin North Am 38:579–592, 1991.
2. Schroder CH, Bontemps CM, Assmann KJM, et al: Renal biopsy and family studies in 65 children with isolated hematuria. Acta Paediatr Scand 79:630–636, 1990.
3. Stapleton FB: Morphology of urinary red blood cells: A simple guide to localizing the site of hematuria. Pediatr Clin North Am 34:561–569, 1987.
4. Vehaskari VA, Robson AM: Proteinuria. *In* Edelmann CM Jr (ed): Pediatric Kidney Disease, 2nd ed. Boston, Little, Brown and Co., 1992:542.

RENAL VEIN THROMBOSIS

Ann P. Guillot, M.D.

Renal vein thrombosis (RVT) in childhood occurs most often in the newborn but also may occur in a variety of settings, such as with nephrotic syndrome or after renal transplantation. The severity of clinical findings varies widely, with the most severe effects being seen in those patients who have sustained bilateral thrombosis.

Diagnosis of RVT is best made with the aid of ultrasonography with Doppler flow study of the renal veins. It may be helpful to determine split renal function by radionuclide scintiscan. The diagnosis can be confirmed by magnetic resonance imaging (MRI). Use of iodinated contrast, particularly of high osmolality, is contraindicated, since it may contribute to elevating the serum osmolality, sometimes one of the contributing factors in the genesis of RVT.

The first and perhaps most important part of therapy is to identify, and reverse if possible, any underlying factors contributing to the onset of RVT. These may include extracellular and intravascular volume contraction with decreased renal blood flow or sepsis with loss of vascular tone and consequent decreased renal blood flow. Hyperosmolar states should be corrected slowly and carefully to avoid cerebral edema. Other underlying factors may involve congenital or acquired deficiencies in antithrombin (AT) III, protein C, or protein S.

Restoration of normal intravascular volume and correction of metabolic acidosis and electrolyte abnormalities must be the first priority. Once the intravascular volume has been restored, dialysis should be instituted if there is absent or poor renal function. Hypertension may be managed by removal of excess fluid load and by the use of antihypertensives. It is advisable to use an antihypertensive drug that is easily titratable in the acute setting to avoid episodes of poor renal and cerebral perfusion. Nitroprusside should be used in the severely hypertensive child, and the child's blood pressure (BP) should be continuously monitored during its use. In the child whose hypertension is mild, more gradual control of BP may be achieved with oral or parenteral hydralazine or with nifedipine used sublingually.

Identification of AT III, protein C, and protein S deficiencies may be helpful in predicting the success of heparin therapy, as heparin acts in part to bind to AT III. In addition, acquired protein C deficiency recently has been identified as a concomitant of sepsis. In the future, replacement of missing protein C is a possibility (although it is not available commercially at this time).

As RVT is a progressive phenomenon, beginning in the renal parenchyma and progressing centrally toward the renal veins and then the inferior vena cava, the surgical approach (thrombectomy) usually has been found ineffective and is not recommended. The only situation in which thrombectomy should be considered is that in which there is occlusion of the inferior vena cava. Even then, thrombectomy would be expected to have a very high attendant morbidity and mortality risk. Early nephrectomy is not warranted and also bears a high operative risk.

Anticoagulant therapy has been recommended in adults with RVT, but its benefit has not been shown conclusively in children. If there is unilateral RVT with preservation of some renal function, there is a risk of progression. That risk may be decreased by careful anticoagulation with heparin (75 to 100 U/kg load, followed by an infusion of 22 to 25 U/kg/h). The activated PTT may be followed to adjust the heparin dose. Heparin should be continued for 5 to 7 days, after which the patient may be transferred to warfarin therapy. Warfarin can be started at a dose of 0.2 mg/kg/d in a single dose. Dosing has not been well studied in children with deep vein thrombosis (DVT) or RVT but may be adjusted to achieve an international normalized ratio of 2 to 3. Warfarin should be continued for about 3 months and may be expected to decrease the risk of thrombus extension and of pulmonary embolus.

Thrombolytic therapy has been described as successful in isolated cases of extensive RVT. The most dramatic successes have been those in which the thrombolytic agent was delivered to the affected renal vein directly via central venous catheter. Systemic thrombolysis has also been described. Streptokinase 2000 U/kg is given as a loading dose, with an infusion of 1000 U/kg/h for 6 to 12 hours. It should be noted that the reports of successful thrombolytic therapy have all been anecdotal, and such therapy should be considered only in those cases in which bilateral RVT is suspected, where there is concern about pulmonary embolus, or when massive, acute RVT has been confirmed.

Management of RVT in the long term may include management of hypertension in 20% of the survivors of the acute episode. Blood pressure management may include antihypertensive drugs. Angiotensin-converting enzyme (ACE) inhibitors should be used with caution, and the glomerular filtration rate (GFR) should be followed closely if they are used. Other agents may be used, including hydralazine and beta-blockers. A few children will benefit by late nephrectomy if a severely scarred affected kidney remains, is not contributing significantly to the overall GFR, and may be contributing to hypertension.

REFERENCES

1. Mocan H, Beattie TJ, Murphy AV: Renal venous thrombosis in infancy: Long-term follow-up. Pediatr Nephrol 5:45–49, 1991.
2. Oliver WJ: Renal vein thrombosis in infancy. Pediatr Rev 4:61–66, 1990.
3. Ricci MA, Lloyd DA: Renal vein thrombosis in infants and children. Arch Surg 125:1195–1199, 1990.

ACUTE AND CHRONIC GLOMERULONEPHRITIS

Sudesh P. Makker, M.D.

The term "acute glomerulonephritis" refers to a glomerular disease that has an acute onset and generally a short, self-limiting course. A classic example of acute glomerulonephritis is poststreptococcal glomerulonephritis. Chronic glomerulonephritis, on the other hand, refers to a glomerular disease that most probably has an insidious onset and follows a prolonged, protracted course, often leading to chronic renal failure, for example, membranoproliferative glomerulonephritis. However, it must be recognized that a chronic glomerulonephritis may come to attention with what appears to be an acute onset (sudden onset of swelling or gross hematuria). Whether, in such cases, the onset is truly acute or only represents an exacerbation of underlying asymptomatic microscopic hematuria or proteinuria secondary to a chronic glomerulonephritis is difficult to determine in most cases. Therefore, the main distinguishing feature between acute and chronic glomerulonephritis is the course.

ACUTE GLOMERULONEPHRITIS

Most cases of acute glomerulonephritis in children are due to poststreptococcal glomerulonephritis (PSGN). An occasional child may develop acute glomerulonephritis following other infections, for example, pneumococcal infection or mumps. Because an overwhelming majority of acute glomerulonephritis is poststreptococcal, the terms "acute glomerulonephritis" and "PSGN" often are used interchangeably. For the subsequent discussion, I use the term PSGN.

Diagnosis

PSGN may develop following an upper respiratory tract or a skin infection with nephritogenic strains of group A beta-streptococci. The latent period for pharyngitis-associated infection is usually 10 days and for impetigo-associated infection is about 21 days. Many children do not volunteer a history of pharyngitis or impetigo. Therefore, it is important to observe for healed or healing skin lesions on physical examination. Most children present with sudden onset of painless gross hematuria (tea-colored or Coke-colored urine) and, usually, some edema. The edema can be generalized and may result in pulmonary edema and congestive heart failure. Hypertension is very common, and patients may first present with symptoms of hypertensive encephalopathy, that is, headache, vomiting, lethargy, and seizures. Oliguria is frequent, and an occasional patient may present with anuria. The diagnosis of PSGN in most children can be made from the history, physical examination, and urinalysis, including examination of the urine sediment and a few simple laboratory tests. Urinalysis in most children shows proteinuria that may range from 1+ to 4+, hematuria, and abnormal urine sediment, which may include dysmorphic red blood cells, white blood cells, and various types of casts, including red blood cell casts. Other laboratory tests helpful in the diagnosis and management of PSGN are listed in Table 1. Renal biopsy generally is not required for the diagnosis, but if the course is not one of steady improvement, a renal biopsy should be performed. Such a course could occur in a child whose underlying disease is chronic membranoproliferative glomerulonephritis, which was exacerbated by a recent streptococcal infection. The child would present with an acute onset, would have laboratory evidence of a recent streptococcal infection, as well as low serum complement, and thus the disease could be confused with PSGN, but this child, as opposed to a child with PSGN, would not show a steady resolution.

Management

Because PSGN in most children is self-limited, the management is essentially supportive. However, such complications as hypertension and renal failure are frequent and require additional treatment.

Supportive Care

It is not necessary to put the child to bed unless the patient is extremely sick (hypertensive encephalopathy). Salt intake should be restricted. However, excessive salt restriction requires an unpalatable diet and is generally not necessary. Most patients can be managed by prescribing regular diet with no added salt and no salty foods. However, in patients with severe hypertension and fluid overload, sodium intake should be restricted to 1 to 2 mEq/kg/d. Fluids should be restricted to an amount equal to 24-hour urine volume plus insensible loss and any other losses. Blood pressure should be monitored every 4 hours, and a record of intake and output should be kept. A urinalysis should be performed daily at the bedside by dipstik, and blood chemistries should be monitored daily. However, if hyperkalemia is present, blood chemistries may need to be checked every 4 to 6 hours, and dietary potassium may be restricted. If the child's throat culture or skin cultures are positive for group A beta-streptococci, the child should be given a 10-day course of penicillin 400,000 units three times a day, or erythromycin 40 mg/kg/d in three divided doses if the child is allergic to penicillin, to prevent the spread of disease.

TABLE 1. Laboratory Tests for Diagnosis and Management of PSGN and Chronic Glomerulonephritis

Throat culture
Serum for antistreptococcal antibodies (streptozyme, antistreptolysin O [ASO], anti-DNAase B, antihyaluronidase)
Serum complement (CH50, C3, C4)
Serologic tests for antinuclear antibody, hepatitis B surface antigen, antineutrophil cytoplasmic autoantibodies (ANCA), and syphilis
Serum chemistries (electrolytes, blood urea nitrogen, creatinine, total proteins, albumin, cholesterol, calcium, phosphorus)
24-hour urine for protein and creatinine clearance or spot urine for protein/creatinine ratio
Chest x-ray, if evidence of heart failure
Renal biopsy

Similarly, family members should have throat or skin cultures taken, and those with positive results should be treated.

Hypertension

Hypertension is very common and can be life threatening (hypertensive encephalopathy). Asymptomatic moderate hypertension can be treated effectively in most patients with vasodilators with or without loop diuretics. Hydralazine 0.2 mg/kg per dose can be given IV or IM repeated every 30 minutes, if necessary. Most patients with PSGN respond promptly to a single dose. If the patient also has fluid overload and the response to the first dose is transient, the patient can be given furosemide 1 to 2 mg/kg per dose IV for better control of blood pressure. In the majority of cases of PSGN, the blood pressure can be controlled with this approach, but if life-threatening hypertension (hypertensive encephalopathy) is present, aggressive management is needed to lower the blood pressure immediately. This can be done by a rapid IV injection of diazoxide 3 to 5 mg/kg per dose. The patient should then be transferred to the intensive care unit, where the blood pressure can be controlled with closer supervision and the use of other potent drugs—nitroprusside, labetalol, nifedipine. In most cases of PSGN, hypertension can be managed easily with a few intravenous doses of hydralazine with or without furosemide, and chronic administration of oral antihypertensive drugs is generally not needed. Some patients may need a few days of oral therapy with hydralazine (1 to 3 mg/kg/d in three or four divided doses) or nifedipine (0.25 to 1 mg/kg/d in three or four divided doses) with or without furosemide (1 to 2 mg/kg/d).

Renal Failure

Renal failure, comprising fluid retention, azotemia, hyperkalemia, hyperphosphatemia, acidosis, and anemia, is mild to moderate in most children with PSGN and can be managed adequately with supportive care. Rapidly deteriorating renal failure with glomerular crescents on renal biopsy [rapidly progressive gomerulonephritis (RPGN)] may occasionally develop (in less than 5% of cases). Some of these patients may require dialysis for some time before the resolution of their disease begins. In general, the prognosis for RPGN associated with PSGN is much better than that of RPGN associated with other glomerular diseases.

Fluid Overload

If edema is mild to moderate and not accompanied by congestive heart failure or pulmonary edema, the patient can be observed and given supportive care, as outlined previously, and diuretics generally are not necessary. However, if congestive heart failure, pulmonary edema, and severe hypertension are present, the patient should be given diuretics. Furosemide 1 to 2 mg/kg given IV is sufficient in most cases and can be repeated as necessary. If the patient is anuric or there is no response to furosemide, dialysis should be started.

Hyperkalemia

Hyperkalemia is common in PSGN, and efforts should be made to maintain serum potassium between 4 and 5 mEq/L. If serum potassium rises above 5.5 mEq/L, the patient should be started on polystyrene sulfonate ion exchange resin (Kayexalate) at a dose of 1 to 2 g/kg/d PO in three or four divided doses to remove potassium from the gastrointestinal tract by exchanging sodium for potassium. Additionally, the patient can also be started on furosemide orally or intravenously to increase urinary losses of potassium. If serum potassium reaches 6 mEq/L, Kayexalate should be given rectally in 20% sorbitol in the same dose as used for retention enema, and the patient should be maintained on oral Kayexalate. Higher serum potassium levels, particularly if associated with electrocardiographic (ECG) evidence (peaked T waves, widening of QRS complex, flattening of P waves), are life threatening and deserve immediate attention. Treatment consists of intravenous administration of calcium gluconate, sodium bicarbonate, and dextrose with or without insulin. If ECG changes are absent, in addition to Kayexalate and furosemide, the patient should be started on intravenous glucose with or without insulin. We generally start with glucose alone 1 to 2 g/kg as 20% solution and rely on the endogenous insulin, but insulin can be added in an emergency. However, if ECG changes are present, all four agents can be used simultaneously, and the patient should be monitored by ECG. It must be recognized that all these measures are only temporary, and if no improvement in the underlying renal failure is apparent, the patient should be prepared for emergency hemodialysis or peritoneal dialysis.

Hyperphosphatemia

Mild to moderate hyperphosphatemia is common but rarely needs treatment because of the self-limiting nature of PSGN. If the course is of slow resolution, patients can be given calcium carbonate (40% elemental calcium) with meals at a dose equivalent to 600 to 1200 mg of elemental calcium per day.

Acidosis

Mild acidosis is common and usually does not require treatment. In fact, correction of acidosis may precipitate tetany because it further reduces ionized calcium in the serum. Ionized calcium may be borderline or low because of the presence of hyperphosphatemia associated with renal failure. Therefore, acidosis in PSGN is not treated unless it is severe (bicarbonate <12 mEq/L), and it is corrected slowly and not until hypocalcemia has been corrected first. The amount of sodium bicarbonate needed can be calculated as

$$mEq = body \quad wt \times 0.6 \times (desired \quad bicarbonate - observed \quad bicarbonate)$$

When NaHCO$_3$ is indicated, only half of this amount should be given over a 12-hour period. Intravenous bicarbonate infusion is used only in an emergency. Otherwise, it should be given orally in three or four divided doses per day.

Prognosis and Follow-Up

The prognosis of PSGN in children is excellent. Only a rare child may develop chronic disease. Renal failure and hypertension are transient and resolve in most cases within 1 to 2 weeks. Serum complement should be checked in every patient and should become normal in 10 to 12 weeks. If serum complement remains low, the diagnosis of PSGN is in doubt. In most cases, urine becomes normal within a few months, but it may take up to 2 years to resolve in a few patients.

CHRONIC GLOMERULONEPHRITIS

Chronic glomerulonephritis includes a large number of diseases that can be classified based on the etiology or the characteristic morphologic features detected on light, immunofluorescence, and electron microscopic study of renal biopsy tissue. The management of common, chronic glomerulonephritis encountered in children is discussed.

Management

The management of chronic glomerulonephritis may be divided into two categories: supportive and specific.

Supportive Management

The supportive management of chronic glomerulonephritis consists of provision of adequate nutrition, maintenance of fluid and electrolyte and cation balance, treatment of hypertension and complications of chronic renal failure, education of the patient and family, and provision of psychosocial support.

Nutrition and Fluids and Electrolytes. My approach is to provide 100% of the required daily allowance of calories for all patients. Protein is restricted to 1 g/kg/d if renal failure is present, and sodium is restricted to 1 to 2 mEq/kg/d if edema and hypertension are present. If the patient has nephrotic syndrome but no renal failure, protein is not restricted. Some restriction of potassium and phosphorus occurs

automatically when protein is restricted. Any additional restriction becomes difficult, since so many of the foods we eat have a fair amount of potassium and phosphorus. Further restriction of these in the diet makes it difficult to prepare a palatable diet, with the result that most children refuse to eat or eat little. This, added to the poor appetite associated with their disease, further compromises their nutrition. Therefore, I restrict potassium to 1 mEq/kg/d only if hyperkalemia is present and remains uncontrolled despite the addition of Kayexalate. Phosphorus is restricted when hyperphosphatemia cannot be managed with oral calcium carbonate supplementation. For the same reasons, I do not restrict fluids in most patients unless there is progressive fluid retention that cannot be managed with chronic diuretic therapy. Some fluid restriction automatically occurs when sodium is restricted.

Complications of Chronic Renal Failure. (See also Chronic Renal Failure later in this chapter.) **Hypertension** is a common problem and usually requires the use of one or more antihypertensive drugs (Table 2). Edematous patients generally will also require diuretics. With the availability of newer drugs, I generally start patients with nifedipine, gradually increasing to the maximum dose. If edema is present, furosemide is added. If blood pressure is not controlled with this regimen, angiotensin-converting enzyme inhibitors (ACE inhibitors), alpha-adrenergic antagonist, beta-adrenergic antagonist, vasodilators, alpha- and beta-adrenergic antagonist, and central sympatholytic agents (clonidine) are added one at a time in the order given. The principle is to use one drug at a time and increase the dose to the maximum tolerated dose before adding the next agent. However, when the next drug is added, it should be started at a lower dose. Diuretics need to be used in patients with edema but are also helpful in controlling blood pressure in nonedematous patients when used in conjunction with other antihypertensive drugs. In the past, a popular effective combination was hydrazaline (vasodilator), propranolol (beta-blocker), and furosemide (diuretic).

Fluid Retention. The mainstay of therapy for fluid retention associated with normal renal function or mild to moderate renal failure is the use of diuretics, particularly furosemide, which is sufficient in most patients to control edema. However, judicious fluid and sodium restrictions are needed in more difficult cases. Fluid retention associated with severe renal failure that is not controlled using such treatment should be treated with dialysis.

Hyperphosphatemia and Hypocalcemia. Some degree of hyperphosphatemia is common in chronic glomerulonephritis and should be managed by using calcium carbonate. The aim is to bind phosphorus in the gastrointestinal tract. Therefore, calcium carbonate should be given with meals. The dose is empiric and depends on the phosphorus content of the diet. The dose can be increased progressively every couple of days until the serum phosphorus becomes normal. At this stage, if there is evidence of secondary hyperparathyroidism, 1,25-dihydroxyvitamin D (Rocaltrol) can be started at a dose of 0.25 μg/d and progressively increased until the serum parathormone level becomes normal or hypercalcemia develops. Throughout the course, the serum Ca × P product should be kept below 70 to 75 mg/dl. Higher values can produce metastatic calcification in tissues, including the kidney, leading to further decline in renal function. If hypercalcemia develops, both calcium and vitamin D are discontinued temporarily but can be reinstituted once serum calcium returns to normal.

Acidosis. Chronic acidosis associated with chronic glomerulonephritis is managed by oral sodium bicarbonate or Shohl's solution or Bicitra 1 to 3 mEq/kg/d. However, it must be remembered that these medications add to the sodium load, which worsens fluid retention and hypertension.

Hyperkalemia. The treatment of acute hyperkalemia is discussed under acute glomerulonephritis. Chronic hyperkalemia is managed by using oral Kayexalate 1 to 2 g/kg/d in three or four divided doses and by dietary restriction of potassium to 1 to 2 mEq/kg/d if nec-

TABLE 2. Treatment of Hypertension in Chronic Glomerulonephritis

DRUG	INITIAL DAILY DOSE*	MAXIMUM DAILY DOSE*	COMMENTS
Calcium Channel Blocker			
Nifedipine	0.25 mg/kg	1–2 mg/kg (180 mg)	Use with caution in congestive heart failure, particularly in combination with beta-blockers
Angiotension-Converting Enzyme Inhibitors			
Captopril	0.05–0.1 mg/kg	4 mg/kg (200)	Use with caution with diuretics, may precipitate renal failure; watch for hyperkalemia
Enalapril	1.25–2.5 mg	40 mg	
Lisinopril	2.5 mg	20 mg	
Alpha-Adrenergic Antagonist			
Prazosin	1–2 mg	10 mg	
Beta-Adrenergic Antagonists			
Propranolol	1–2 mg/kg	8 mg/kg	Monitor for bradycardia; contraindicated in reactive airway disease, heart block, and congestive heart failure; use with caution in patients with diabetes mellitus, as it may mask symptoms of hypoglycemia
Atenolol	25 mg	100 mg	
Alpha- and Beta-Adrenergic Antagonists			
Labetalol	50 mg	300–600 mg	Same as beta-adrenergic antagonists
Vasodilator			
Hydralazine	0.2–1 mg/kg	2–8 mg (200 mg)	Reflex tachycardia; tachyphylaxis; as monotherapy, not very effective
Central Sympatholytic			
Clonidine	0.05–0.1 mg 0.1 mg patch	2 mg 0.6 mg patch	Rebound hypertension following sudden withdrawal
Diuretics			
Furosemide	1–2 mg/kg	320 mg	Hypokalemia, metabolic alkalosis, volume depletion, and deterioration of renal function
Hydrochlorothiazide	1–2 mg/kg	100 mg	Same as above; not effective if glomerular filtration rate <25 ml/min/1.73 m²

*The exact doses in children have not been determined.

essary. Chronic use of diuretics (furosemide or hydrochlorothiazide) also helps in the treatment of hyperkalemia.

Anemia. Mild anemia is not uncommon in chronic glomerulonephritis and may result from decreased erythropoietin production or nutritional deficiency due to poor intake. Hematocrit levels between 20% and 30% are acceptable and do not require aggressive measures, such as blood transfusions, to correct anemia. Blood transfusions in these patients are poorly tolerated and can lead to dangerous hypervolemia, including severe hypertension and pulmonary edema, and thus should be avoided. In some patients, iron deficiency may develop due to poor nutrition and can be treated with oral iron supplementation. If nutritional deficiencies of iron or vitamins have been corrected and the hematocrit falls between 15% and 20%, erythropoietin 25 to 50 U/kg SC may be given once or twice a week until the hematocrit increases to the 20% to 30% level. However, there is limited experience with erythropoietin in such situations, and care should be taken in its use. One should also be aware of potential complications, such as hypertension, seizures, and thrombosis.

Specific Management

Specific management of chronic glomerulonephritis consists of treatment of the underlying etiology in cases where the etiology is known, for example, congenital syphilis and nonspecific immunosuppression in those chronic glomerulonephritides that are immunologically mediated.

Glomerulonephritides with Known Etiology. Congenital syphilis-associated glomerulonephritis is treated with aqueous crystalline penicillin G 50,000 U/kg IV every 6 hours for 14 days. Treatment of shunt nephritis requires removal of the infected atrioventricular shunt and the use of appropriate antibiotics. Similarly, subacute bacterial endocarditis is treated with appropriate antibiotics. Treatment of glomerulonephritis associated with malaria or other parasitic infections requires appropriate antiparasitic therapy. Treatment of

chronic glomerulonephritis associated with chronic hepatitis B in the past has been only supportive, but recently recombinant human interferon-α 5 million U/m² on alternate days for 12 to 16 weeks has been used in some patients, with beneficial effects. The experience with this drug is limited, and the exact dose and duration of therapy are not yet established. Treatment of glomerulonephritides occuring following exposure to certain drugs involves discontinuation of the suspected drugs. In general, treatment of all these glomerulonephritides is based on removal or eradication of the inciting agent, following which resolution of the glomerular disease usually occurs.

Immunologically Mediated Glomerulonephritides of Unknown Etiology. Because these diseases are mediated by antibodies and the nature of the inciting agent (exogenous or autoantigens) is not known in most cases, they have been treated with immunosuppressive agents to control their progression. The aim is to reduce antibody production or remove antibodies from circulation. The former is achieved by nonspecific immunosuppressive drugs that affect not only the antibody production but also the entire immune response at various steps, as well as the inflammatory and repair processes. The latter is achieved by plasmapheresis. Common immunosuppressive drugs include corticosteroids and cytoxic drugs, such as cyclophosphamide, chlorambucil, and azathioprine and, recently, cyclosporine. These drugs have multiple and some serious side effects and should be used with caution and under close supervision, with the patient and family having full knowledge of the potential risks. Long-term use of corticosteroids, particularly if they are used daily, can lead to cushingoid obesity, growth retardation, osteoporosis, avascular necrosis of bones, posterior subcapsular cataracts, atrophic skin, striae, hypertension, infections, hirsutism, and diabetes mellitus, among other side effects. Cytoxic drugs can lead to bone marrow suppression, serious infections, and gonadal toxicity and can predispose to possible malignancies in the future. This is only a partial list of their side effects, and the reader should obtain a complete list of the side effects of each drug from appropriate sources.

A patient who is receiving high doses of daily corticosteroids is followed every week, particularly if there was hypertension before the start of therapy. Also, if immunosuppressive drugs are being used, the patient should be seen every week, and complete blood counts (CBC) should be obtained. In addition to monitoring the side effects of medications, laboratory tests assessing the activity and improvement of the disease should be obtained. These include examination of urine sediment, quantitative proteinuria (24-hour proteinuria or protein/creatinine ratio on a random urine sample), total serum protein and albumin if the nephrotic syndrome is present, renal function, erythrocyte sedimentation rate, and relevant serologic tests—serum complement (C3, C4, CH50), anti-DS DNA antibodies, antineutrophil cytoplasmic antibodies (ANCA), and antiglomerular basement membrane antibodies. The following glomerulonephritides may be treated with these immunosuppressive drugs.

MEMBRANOPROLIFERATIVE GLOMERULONEPHRITIS. Consensus is now developing that membranoproliferative glomerulonephritis (MPGN) is improved by corticosteroids. Patients with nephrotic syndrome or renal failure or both are generally given daily prednisone 2 mg/kg (60 mg maximum). After 4 to 6 weeks, the patient is switched to alternate-day prednisone at twice the daily dose (80 mg maximum), which then is slowly reduced to a maintenance dose of 20 to 40 mg (alternate-day therapy). The maintenance dose is continued for a long time, and the duration of therapy is individualized, depending on the response. Patients who are not nephrotic and have no renal failure can be started on alternate-day prednisone.

MEMBRANOUS GLOMERULONEPHROPATHY. Although there have been no controlled trials in children, based on results in adults and my own experience, it appears that membranous glomerulonephritis (MGN) also can be treated with corticosteroids. I start MGN patients on daily prednisone as discussed for MPGN, but the duration of maintenance therapy is generally 6 to 12 months.

LUPUS NEPHRITIS. Most cases of lupus nephritis can be controlled with daily prednisone 2 mg/kg/d (maximum 80 mg), following which the dose is slowly tapered to a maintenance dose of approximately 0.2 mg/kg/d. Depending on the duration of control, some patients can be switched to alternate-day prednisone (0.4 to 0.5 mg/kg) and maintained on alternate-day prednisone for a long time. The use of daily steroids often results in exacerbation of hypertension, but it can be managed effectively with the currently available antihypertensive agents, and one should not be hesitant to use daily steroids to control the disease. Patients whose disease is difficult to control on daily prednisone or who require large daily doses to maintain control are given *additional* immunosuppressive drugs. These drugs assist in maintaining control of the disease on lower doses of prednisone and, thus, help in reducing the side effects of steroids. Several approaches have been used. I generally add chlorambucil 0.2 mg/kg/d PO in two divided doses. Once further improvement is observed, the dose of prednisone is gradually reduced, and chlorambucil is withdrawn after 3 months. If at any time the WBC drops below 4000/mm³, chlorambucil is discontinued. Depending on the condition of the patient, chlorambucil may be restarted, and some patients will require more than one course of chlorambucil. Other approaches include the addition of azathioprine 2 mg/kg/d PO or cyclophosphamide 2 mg/kg/d PO, which can be given for a variable time (months), or cyclophosphamide 500 to 750 mg/m² IV every 1 to 3 months. With the latter, to prevent urinary bladder toxicity, sodium 2-mercaptoethane sulfonate (MESNA) is given as an intravenous bolus injection in a dose equal to 20% of the cyclophosphamide dose just before cyclophosphamide administration and then again at 4 and 8 hours after the dose of cyclophosphamide. Close supervision of patients is essential while using these drugs. Plasmapheresis has not been found to be effective in a controlled study in adults, and its role in children is uncertain. It must be emphasized that management of severe lupus nephritis is difficult and challenging, and one has to exercise great caution and sound clinical judgment to avoid overzealous immunosuppression, as it is the cause of death in many patients.

RAPIDLY PROGRESSIVE GLOMERULONEPHRITIS. RPGN consists of rapidly deteriorating renal function with extensive glomerular crescents seen on renal biopsy and may be seen with PSGN, MPGN, MGN, lupus nephritis, Henoch-Schönlein purpura, IgA nephropathy, vasculitis, or Goodpasture syndrome, or it may be idiopathic. Idiopathic RPGN is treated with pulses of IV methylprednisolone 15 to 30 mg/kg/d (maximum 1 g) on 3 or 4 consecutive days, followed by 2 mg/kg/d of daily prednisone for 4 to 6 weeks. The disease is uncommon in children, and no controlled studies have been performed. However, in my experience, the above approach has proven to be beneficial. Except for RPGN associated with PSGN, pulse steroid therapy can also be tried in RPGN. Some of these patients may also require other measures, such as plasmapheresis, anticoagulants, and the use of one of the three cytotoxic drugs, azathioprine 1 to 2 mg/kg/d, cyclophosphamide 1 to 2 mg/kg/d, or chlorambucil 0.1 to 0.2 mg/kg/d, for a variable duration of time depending on response. When using anticoagulants, we start with IV heparin 50 to 75 U/kg, sufficient to maintain partial thromboplastin time at twice the normal level. Patients can be started simultaneously on oral anticoagulants (4 to 8 mg of warfarin sodium as a loading dose). Heparin is discontinued once the prothrombin time becomes twice the normal level, and this is maintained on a maintenance dose of 1 to 2 mg/d of warfarin sodium. Depending on the response, the patient is gradually taken off anticoagulants and cytotoxic drugs but continued on variable doses of corticosteroids until recovery has occurred or the disease is considered refractory.

HENOCH-SCHÖNLEIN PURPURA. Most patients with Henoch-Schönlein purpura (HSP) only need supportive care and recover spontaneously. Patients with more severe involvement who have nephrotic syndrome, renal failure, or RPGN have a less favorable prognosis, and we treat such patients with corticosteroids in a similar manner to patients with MGN. Patients with RPGN have the worst prognosis and are treated more aggressively with intravenous pulses of methylprednisolone and other drugs, as described earlier.

WEGENER GRANULOMATOSIS AND OTHER VASCULITIDES. Patients with Wegener granulomatosis are treated with prednisone and cyclophosphamide. Prednisone is given at a dose of 1 mg/kg/d, and cyclophosphamide is given at 2 mg/kg/d. After 4 to 6 weeks, the patient is generally switched to alternate-day prednisone at twice the daily dose (maximum 80 mg), which is gradually reduced over several months, depending on the progress. Cyclophosphamide 1 to 2 mg/kg/d is continued for at least a year after remission of disease. Relapses are treated with daily prednisone and cyclophosphamide. Other vasculitides, for example, antineutrophil cytoplasmic autoantibody-associated vasculitis and polyarteritis, are treated similarly, but the duration of treatment with prednisone and cyclophosphamide is more variable and individualized.

GOODPASTURE SYNDROME. This rare disorder in children is treated with a combination of plasmapheresis and immunosuppressive drugs. Plasmapheresis (3 to 4 L of plasma exchange) is performed daily *or on alternate days,* and immunosuppression is started with prednisone 2 mg/kg/d (maximum 80 mg), cyclophosphamide 1 mg/kg/d, and azathioprine 1 mg/kg/d. Depending on the improvement in antiglomerular basement membrane antibodies, cyclophosphamide and azathioprine are generally discontinued after 8 weeks, and the dose of prednisone is gradually reduced. The response to therapy depends on the severity of disease when therapy is instituted. Patients with severe renal failure at onset are less likely to respond, whereas a great majority (70% to 80%) of patients with mild to moderate renal failure show improvement.

IgA NEPHROPATHY. Patients without nephrotic syndrome or renal failure are given supportive care and are followed every 3 to 6 months. Patients with RPGN, which is rare, are managed as are other patients with RPGN. The management of children with significant proteinuria and nephrotic syndrome is controversial, but they can be treated with prednisone 2 mg/kg/d (maximum 60 mg) for 4 to 8 weeks and then switched to alternate-day prednisone. Other immunosuppressives also may be used, but it is not clear whether they are beneficial.

Nonimmunologically Mediated Chronic Glomerulonephritides. Alport syndrome, nail patella syndrome, and associated glomerulonephritides are managed with supportive care.

REFERENCES

1. Makker SP: Glomerular diseases. *In* Kher K, Makker S (eds): Clinical Pediatric Nephrology. New York, McGraw-Hill, 1992:175–276.
2. Welch TR: Current management of selected childhood renal diseases. Curr Prob Pediatr November-December 1992.

THE NEPHROTIC SYNDROME

NORMAN D. ROSENBLUM, M.D.

The nephrotic syndrome is defined by the presence of the following features: proteinuria > 40 mg/m²/h or > 50 mg/kg/24 h, a serum albumin < 2.5 g/dl, hypercholesterolemia, and edema. In childhood, the incidence of the nephrotic syndrome is 2 to 3/100,000 children. In children 2 to 7 years of age, the male/female ratio is 2:1, whereas adolescent males and females are equally affected.

The etiology of the nephrotic syndrome may be considered as primary or secondary. The vast majority of primary cases in early childhood are due to minimal change disease. A minority of cases are caused by congenital nephrotic syndrome, idiopathic focal and segmental glomerulosclerosis, membranous nephropathy, and idiopathic membranoproliferative glomerulonephritis. Secondary causes include systemic lupus erythematosus, Henoch-Schönlein purpura, malaria, syphilis, and renal vein thrombosis. In children ≤ 10 years old, minimal change disease accounts for 93% of cases, whereas in the second decade of life, it accounts for far fewer cases (about 50%). During these years, other etiologies become more important and include systemic lupus erythematosus (18%), idiopathic membranoproliferative glomerulonephritis (14%), idiopathic focal and segmental glomerulosclerosis (5%), and membranous glomerulonephritis (5%).[3]

The clinical approach to the child with the nephrotic syndrome is guided by the recognition that an underlying diagnosis of minimal change disease can be predicted with a high degree of certainty on the basis of noninvasive clinical testing. A renal biopsy is generally not indicated in the 1 to 10-year age group, in which the prevalence of minimal change disease is very high. In contrast, a diagnostic renal biopsy is usually performed in children < 10 months and > 10 years old because of the higher incidence of other primary glomerulopathies.

The presence or absence of specific clinical characteristics is predictive of an underlying diagnosis of minimal change disease. A nephrotic child 10 months to 10 years of age with a normal glomerular filtration rate (GFR) has an 85% chance of having minimal change disease. In the absence of hematuria, diastolic hypertension, and hypocomplementemia, the chance increases to 92%. A urinary selective protein index (urinary clearance of IgG compared with that of transferrin) of < 0.1, that is less than 10%, increases the chances further to 96%. Finally, response to glucocorticoids, with a full remission in the nephrotic syndrome, increases the chances of minimal change disease to 98%. It is important to note that the presence of microscopic hematuria, diastolic hypertension, or an elevated blood urea nitrogen (BUN) does not rule out the diagnosis of minimal change disease. For example, 30% of children with minimal change disease present with microscopic hematuria. With these considerations in mind, the initial clinical approach to the nephrotic child is to perform a comprehensive clinical examination, examine the urinary sediment, and measure the serum third component of complement (C3), the BUN, and the serum creatinine. The selective protein index also may be measured. With this information, it is possible to make further decisions regarding specific treatment.

GENERAL TREATMENT MEASURES

It is extremely important that all efforts be made to help children with the nephrotic syndrome to lead as normal a life as possible. Since the nephrotic syndrome is often a chronic disorder, long-term strategies are needed to optimize the functioning of the child within the family, with friends, and at school.

Education

Education of the child, family, and school personnel and emotional support to relieve anxiety are essential components of therapy. At the time of diagnosis, the parents and child should be educated about the nature of the disorder, the implications of proteinuria, the usual response to steroids, the positive prognosis in steroid-responsive patients, and the effect of sodium and water intake on edema in the relapsing state. It is essential that the family understand that although proteinuria and edema are serious manifestations requiring treatment and that these manifestations may recur many times even in the face of treatment, the long-term prognosis in most patients is total resolution by the end of adolescence, without any evidence of residual renal dysfunction. Many families are better able to cope with the illness if they understand, in general terms, how proteinuria and edema occur. As well, every effort should be made to provide the family with the tools that enable them to manage the illness in collaboration with the physician and nurse. In this respect, it is essential that parents and children learn to use urinary dipsticks to measure protein, keep records of these measurements on a daily basis, learn to weigh the child at home, and attain a good understanding of the signs of infection.

Diet

For the most part, there is no need to restrict the diet. In fact, appetite is often markedly diminished when the patient is nephrotic. Diets that provide the recommended daily allowance of calories and protein are appropriate. To optimize nutritional intake, special attention should be paid to the food preferences of the child. There is no evidence that a sodium allowance more restrictive than a no-added-salt diet reduces anasarca, hastens the response to therapy, or alters the course of the disease. Water restriction is appropriate when the patient is nephrotic and should be equal to insensible losses (350 to 500 ml/m²/24 h). If the patient follows a low-salt diet, water intake will be automatically lowered as a result of diminished thirst. There is no indication that an excessive protein intake is efficacious.

Activity

Patients may lose weight by being supine, but there is no evidence that restriction of activity influences the course of the disease. Bedrest is rarely indicated. In general, children restrict their own level of activity according to how they feel. Attempts to forcibly restrict their level of activity rarely work and set up needless conflicts between the parent and child. In addition, there is great psychologic benefit to encouraging the child to take part in normal activities insofar as it is possible. Schoolage children should attend school unless they feel ill. Strenuous exercise in the nephrotic state is difficult to maintain and should be discouraged.

Hospitalization

As a general rule, hospitalization is not preferred, since it is disruptive to the child and family and dislodges a sense of control from the family. At the time of initial presentation, the tests needed to make the diagnosis, the education regarding the disorder, and the initial management can usually all be orchestrated in an ambulatory setting. However, in certain circumstances, this is not practical, and a short hospitalization is required. Subsequently, hospitalization should only be necessary for the treatment of edema unresponsive to the usual interventions or for the treatment of serious infections, such as peritonitis.

Immunizations

There are very few controlled data available regarding the need for, response to, or complications from various immunizations in nephrotic children. The child receiving steroids should not receive live virus vaccines. Other immunizations may be administered, but an appropriate immune response is not assured in patients who are being treated with corticosteroids. Although case reports have suggested that immunization may precipitate a relapse, no controlled studies have been performed to test whether this is, in fact, the case. Polyvalent pneumococcal vaccine administered to nephrotic patients will produce an increase in antibody titers. However, pneumococcal sepsis and peritonitis do occur in immunized patients. This is due, in part, to the fact that the vaccine contains only a subset of all the pathogenic serotypes.

Infection

The recognition and prompt treatment of intercurrent infections is a major goal of therapy. Common infections in the nephrotic syndrome include septicemia, peritonitis, pneumonia, cellulitis, urinary tract infection, and septic arthritis. Although *Streptococcus pneumoniae* is the most common organism producing sepsis and peritonitis, gram-negative infections with *Escherichia coli, Proteus,* and *Klebsiella* account for a sizable proportion of cases of peritonitis.

Varicella-zoster infections are of particular concern in patients treated with systemic high-dose corticosteroids. The risk of severe or fatal varicella infections is increased in these patients. Therefore, it is wise to determine the antibody titer against the varicella-zoster virus in these patients when they are in remission (i.e., in the absence of proteinuria and attendant hypogammaglobulinemia). In the relapse state, it is safest to assume inadequate circulating antibody against the virus. In a nonimmune patient or in an immune patient being treated with high-dose steroids, varicella-zoster immune globulin (VZIG) should be administered to the child within 72 hours of exposure to the virus. VZIG will either prevent or ameliorate the disease in the immunocompromised host. If VZIG is given, the incubation period for varicella is up to 28 days postexposure to the virus (versus 10 to 21 days in the normal host). In a nonimmune patient with a clear history of exposure, it is wise to taper the dose of corticosteroids quickly to less than 1 mg/kg/d until the incubation period has passed. In patients who develop varicella, such a steroid taper is also indicated, as is treatment with intravenous acyclovir.

Edema

Diuretic therapy is not necessary for the control of cosmetic edema alone. However, a moderate dose of a thiazide diuretic may be used. The restriction of salt intake is the most important intervention for minimizing the increase in extracellular fluid volume. The family should be instructed to avoid preprepared foods that contain large amounts of salt, hide the salt shaker at home to avoid the use of extra salt on foods, and substitute salt-free snack foods for those (e.g., potato chips) that contain large amounts of salt. These interventions are most effective if the family members make a joint decision not to bring salty foods into the house. Additional measures to control edema are important in the presence of respiratory symptoms, hyponatremia, skin breakdown, or severe elevation of the BUN. Intravenous salt-poor albumin 1 g/kg per dose administered over 2 hours every 12 hours with furosemide 1 mg/kg is an effective strategy for establishing negative salt and water balance. This regimen may be required for 4 to 5 days in patients with severe hypoalbuminemia. Additional diuretics in addition to furosemide do not increase the efficacy of treatment. During treatment, patients should be monitored carefully for hypertension during and immediately after the albumin infusion. After a vigorous diuresis has occurred, patients should be monitored carefully for the signs of plasma volume depletion, as indicated by hypotension, persistent tachycardia, and signs of poor peripheral perfusion. A depleted plasma volume can predispose the patient to venous thrombosis, renal failure, and a hyponatremic, hypokalemic metabolic alkalosis.

SPECIFIC THERAPY

Corticosteroids

Corticosteroids are the first line of therapy for children in whom the diagnosis of minimal change disease is clinically predicted or biopsy proven. There are several different published treatment protocols. None of these have been shown to offer any therapeutic advantage over the other (Table 1). One regimen consists of prednisone 60 mg/m^2/d (maximum 80 mg/d) PO divided in three or four doses for 28 days followed by 40 mg/m^2 PO every other morning for another 28 days. The prednisone is then discontinued. An alternative approach is prednisone 2 mg/kg/d divided t.i.d. (maximum dose 80 mg/d) until the urine is protein free for 7 days. The prednisone is then given at 2 mg/kg every other day and tapered by decreasing the dose steadily with a view toward discontinuing it at the end of 1 month. Ninety-two percent of children respond to prednisone with either a complete remission (protein-free urine and normal serum albumin) in 82% or a partial remission (proteinuria with a serum albumin > 2.5 g/dl) in 10%. Of prednisone-responsive patients, 73% respond with a complete remission in 3 weeks, 93% in 8 weeks, and 96% in 12 weeks. In view of the risks of steroid toxicity with prolonged daily therapy, many physicians do not extend treatment beyond 8 weeks. If the patient has not responded by this point, a diagnostic renal biopsy is indicated. Patients who are steroid resistant, that is, do not respond to a full course of therapy with a decrease in proteinuria, also require a renal biopsy. Their pathologic diagnosis is usually focal and segmental glomerulosclerosis (FSGS). A small minority of these patients have minimal change lesion. The therapy of these patients is not discussed further in this section.

Treatment of Relapses in Steroid-Responsive Patients

The nephrotic syndrome frequently recurs in those who have achieved a remission with steroid therapy. A relapse is defined by the occurrence of proteinuria on 7 consecutive days. The number of relapses in the first 6 months after diagnosis is predictive of the subsequent course. If no relapse occurs, there is a 93% chance that less than three relapses will occur in the next 18 months. The occurrence of three or more relapses in the first 6 months is indicative of many relapses subsequently. Relapses occur in 70% of patients with presumed or proven minimal change disease. Of these patients, 11% have a single relapse and then become disease free, 20% relapse infrequently (less than two relapses in the first 6 months), and 40% relapse frequently (more than two relapses in the first 6 months).[2] Within the frequently relapsing group of patients is a subgroup of patients who are classified as steroid dependent. This subgroup is defined by a relapse on two separate occasions as the steroid dose is being discontinued or a relapse that occurs within 2 weeks of steroids being discontinued.

TABLE 1. Recommended Regimens for Treatment of Patients with Minimal Change Nephrotic Syndrome

Corticosteroids
Prednisone
  Daily: 60 mg/m^2/d (maximum 80 mg/d) in 3 divided
    doses
  Alternate day: 40 mg/m^2/d every other morning
  or
  Daily: 2 mg/kg/d (maximum 80 mg/d) in 3 divided
    doses
  Alternate day: 2 mg/kg every other morning

Cytotoxic Drugs
Cyclophosphamide
  2–3 mg/kg/d × 8 weeks given with corticosteroids
Chlorambucil
  0.2 mg/kg/d × 8 weeks

Treatment of the first relapse after diagnosis and of subsequent infrequent relapses is similar to that for the initial episode of nephrosis, except that some physicians taper the steroids over a longer period (8 weeks) after a remission has occurred. Treatment of relapse in the patient with frequently relapsing nephrotic syndrome includes induction of remission with prednisone, followed by a prednisone taper over 8 to 12 weeks to 0.5 mg/kg q.o.d. for 6 months. For steroid-dependent patients, several strategies may be tried to maintain a remission:

• Tapering of steroids gradually from every day to every other day
• Tapering of steroids over a more extended time period
• Treatment with methylprednisolone instead of prednisone.

Some patients respond better to methylprednisolone than prednisone, suggesting that the variable pharmacokinetics of prednisone may be of therapeutic significance in these patients.

Cytotoxic Drugs in Relapsing Steroid-Treated Patients

Frequently relapsing and steroid-dependent patients are at risk of developing *growth failure as well as other toxic steroid side effects*. Two cytotoxic drugs, cyclophosphamide and chlorambucil,[1] have been used extensively, with the goal of inducing a lasting remission and, therefore, sparing the patient further exposure to corticosteroids. Cyclophosphamide reduces the frequency or eliminates relapses entirely in 80% to 90% of frequently relapsing or steroid-dependent patients. The duration of remission after treatment with cyclophosphamide is related to the duration of therapy. Patients who are treated concomitantly with steroids have a longer remission than patients treated with cyclophosphamide alone. In a cohort of frequently relapsing or steroid-dependent patients, treatment with cyclophosphamide 2 to 3 mg/kg/d along with corticosteroids 0.5 to 1 mg/kg/d for 8 weeks maintained a remission in 44% of the patients at 4 years. The response to cyclophosphamide was found to be better in patients who (1) were frequently relapsing versus those who were steroid dependent, (2) were > 9 years of age at the time of diagnosis, and (3) had a longer duration of disease at the time of treatment. If relapse occurs after therapy with cyclophosphamide, the frequency of subsequent relapses is the same as before treatment.

The acute side effects of cyclophosphamide include *leukopenia, intercurrent infection*, alopecia, nausea, gastrointestinal discomfort, and hemorrhagic cystitis. Concomitant corticosteroid therapy decreases the severity of leukopenia. To avoid hemorrhagic cystitis, it is best to treat patients with cyclophosphamide after achieving a remission with corticosteroids, since it is easier to achieve the desired levels of fluid intake and urine output in the patient who does not retain salt and water. Cyclophosphamide-treated patients are immunosuppressed. Intercurrent infections must be quickly recognized and treated. The long-term risks of treatment are the late occurrence of malignancies, *sterility*, ovarian fibrosis, and amenorrhea. The male gonad is at higher risk than that of the female. The dose threshold for azoospermia is not exactly known, but a total exposure of ≤ 168 mg/kg causes abnormalities of sperm morphology and motility but does not cause infertility. The dose-toxicity relationship for ovarian fibrosis is not well defined. Most females treated with the total amount of cyclophosphamide used in the nephrotic syndrome have been able to reproduce.

Chlorambucil is a well-studied and commonly used cytotoxic drug. In a dose of 0.15 to 0.2 mg/kg/d for 8 weeks (8.4 to 11 mg/kg total) chlorambucil induces a remission in 92% to 100% of steroid-dependent or frequently relapsing patients. These remissions tend to be longer lasting than those induced with cyclophosphamide. Remission rates of 87% and 78% have been reported at 30 months and 5 years, respectively.[4] Older children with disease of a longer duration are more likely to experience a prolonged remission. The acute side effects of chlorambucil seem to be less frequent than those observed with cyclophosphamide. They include *leukopenia*, gastrointestinal upset, and focal seizures. Leukopenia can be partially ameliorated by concomitant therapy with steroids. The seizures are not dose related and

are infrequent. Accompanying electroencephalographic abnormalities resolve after the drug is discontinued. Long-term risks include oligospermia or azoospermia, ovarian fibrosis, and leukemia. *Oligospermia and azoospermia* have been reported with cumulative doses of 9 and 11.6 mg/kg, respectively. The actual safe dose for spermatogenesis is unknown but is probably in the range of 7 to 10 mg/kg. The dosage threshold for toxicity in the female is not well defined. Leukemia has developed in chlorambucil-treated patients. However, the cumulative doses in these patients far exceeded those used in the treatment of the nephrotic syndrome.

Other Treatment Alternatives in the Steroid-Toxic Patient

Some patients do not sustain a lasting remission after treatment with corticosteroids and cytotoxic drugs. Cyclosporine has been reported to induce a sustained remission in about 50% of such patients. In these studies, the dose was 3 to 5 mg/kg/d, aiming for a trough serum level of 25 to 130 μg/ml (determined by radioimmunoassay). Sustained treatment with cyclosporine is required, since patients relapse when the drug is withdrawn. Several other drugs have received limited examination in patients with steroid-resistant nephrotic syndrome. These include levamisole, pulse intermittent intravenous methylprednisolone, and the angiotensin-converting enzyme inhibitors. At present, these drugs should be reserved for use when standard approaches have failed and in the context of treatment trials.

REFERENCES

1. Arbeitsgemeinschaft fur Padiatrische Nephrologie: Effect of cytotoxic drugs in frequently relapsing nephrotic syndrome with and without steroid dependence. N Engl J Med 306:451–454, 1982.
2. Grupe WE: Primary nephrotic syndrome in childhood. *In* Barness LA (ed): Advances in Pediatrics. Chicago, Year Book Publishers, Inc, 1979:163–207.
3. Ingelfinger JR: Nephrotic syndrome in the second decade of life. J Adoles Health Care 1:42–45, 1980.
4. Williams SA, Makker SP, Ingelfinger JR, Grupe WE: Long-term evaluation of chlorambucil plus prednisone in the idiopathic nephrotic syndrome of childhood. N Engl J Med 302:929–933, 1980.

RENAL TUBULAR DISORDERS

JUAN RODRIGUEZ SORIANO, M.D.

CYSTINURIA

Cystinuria is an autosomal recessive disease characterized by the excessive urinary excretion of cystine and dibasic amino acids (lysine, ornithine, and arginine). The basic abnormality is a transport defect present both in renal tubular epithelium and in intestinal mucosa. A mutation in the gene (rBAT) coding for the synthesis of a specific amino acid transporter has been identified recently. The increased cystine excretion leads to precipitation in the form of cystine stones. Treatment is indicated only in homozygous subjects and is directed toward the prevention of stone formation and the dissolution of stones that have already been formed.

Because crystallization of cystine depends mainly on the concentration of cystine in the urine (crystallization occurs when cystine concentration exceeds 300 mg/L at a urine pH between 4.5 and 7 and increases to about 500 mg/L at a urine pH of 7.5 or above), the most important therapeutic measure is the combined administration of large amounts of fluid and alkaline salts. Morning urine should be checked for pH, aiming to obtain values above 7.5. Unfortunately, this regimen has had limited success because, for many patients, especially children, it is often difficult to follow. An alternative therapy is to decrease urinary excretion of cystine to levels that are below the crystallization range. The safest way to obtain these levels is to restrict salt intake. In adults, the reduction of sodium intake to about 50 mmol/d, along with a high fluid intake, contributes to maintain a safe range of cystine excretion. Similar data are not available for children, but there is no reason to expect a different therapeutic effect.

If stone formation cannot be prevented by decreasing cystine excretion to below the crystallization range, the best option is to initiate treatment with D-Penicillamine (Cuprimine). D-Penicillamine in a divided dose of 30 mg/kg/d is a dimethylcysteine that reduces cystine excretion by reacting with cystine to form a more soluble mixed disulfide. Its success depends in great part on a careful monitoring of urinary cystine excretion, which should be kept below 200 or 300 mg/d/1.73 m². The main disadvantage of this therapy derives from the undesirable side effects of D-penicillamine administration, which can include fever and rash, leukopenia, proteinuria and nephrotic syndrome, systemic lupus erythematosus, collagen abnormalities, and loss of taste. D-Penicillamine is a powerful vitamin B₆ antagonist, and patients on long-term therapy should always receive a supplementary dose (100 mg/d) of pyridoxine.

Other therapies are of little value in children. A low-methionine diet also reduces cystine excretion, but its value is questioned because of poor patient compliance. Captopril, an angiotensin II-converting enzyme inhibitor, reduces cystine excretion by forming a more soluble mixed disulfide, but its use in children has not been successful.

FANCONI SYNDROME

Renal Fanconi syndrome represents a clinical entity characterized by a multiple dysfunction of the proximal tubule, which leads to glycosuria, generalized amino aciduria, hyperphosphaturia, and proximal renal tubular acidosis. Other abnormalities of renal tubular function (tubular proteinuria, hyperuricosuria, hypercalciuria, renal loss of sodium and potassium, and diminished concentrating capacity) also may be present. Glomerular filtration rate (GFR) is not affected initially but may decline secondarily. The main consequences of the tubular dysfunction are growth retardation, polyuria, hypophosphatemic rickets, hypokalemia, and metabolic acidosis. Fanconi syndrome may be either idiopathic or secondary to a variety of causes. Nephropathic cystinosis represents the most important cause of infantile Fanconi syndrome.

The clinical course and prognosis of the syndrome depend on the specific cause. In general, secondary forms may improve or disappear when the cause is avoided or some therapy is possible. In the primary forms, only supportive care may be offered, which aims to treat or prevent rickets, correct the acidosis and hypokalemia, and maintain a normal fluid balance. However, little effect on growth is to be expected.

Supportive Care

Bone lesions of *rickets* and *osteoporosis* are resistant to regular vitamin D therapy and are best treated with oral phosphate supplements and active metabolites of vitamin D. Hypophosphatemia can be partly compensated by oral administration of neutral phosphate (1 to 3 g/d in a divided dose to avoid vomiting, diarrhea, or abdominal discomfort). Various solutions are available. Joulie's solution contains 145 g Na₂HPO₄·H₂O and 18.2 g NaH₂PO₄·H₂O dissolved in 1 L of water with syrup base and provides 30.4 g of elemental phosphorus per milliliter. A marketed product is K-Phos-Neutral, which yields 250 mg of elemental phosphorus per tablet. Calcitriol or 1,25-(OH)₂D₃ (Rocaltrol) is given at the initial dose of 15 to 20 ng/kg/d and is increased over several months to a maintenance dose of 30 to 60 ng/kg/d. High doses of vitamin D (up to 2000 to 4000 U/kg/d) or dihydrotachysterol (up to 10 to 25 μg/kg/d) may also be used successfully. Frequent (as often as monthly) monitoring of serum calcium and urinary calcium/creatinine ratio is recommended. Repeat renal ultrasonography studies may provide early detection of nephrocalcinosis. It should be remembered that hypocalcemic tetany can be induced by acute alkalinization, especially if citrate or bicarbonate is administered at the same time as phosphate.

Patients with Fanconi syndrome waste bicarbonate and thus have proximal renal tubular acidosis (RTA). Chronic acidosis interferes with normal growth and contributes to the development of bone lesions. In proximal RTA, treatment must compensate for the urinary losses of bicarbonate and for the endogenous production of acid. Because patients with this disorder often excrete more than 10% of the filtered amount of bicarbonate when the serum level is brought within the normal range, the minimal starting dose of alkali is between 6 and 10 mmol/kg/d. However, larger doses are frequently needed. Alkali administration enhances the urinary loss of potassium, and the preparations used should include both sodium and potassium salts.

Because citrate excretion is not decreased, there is no special need to give the anion in the form of citrate. A mixture of sodium and potassium bicarbonate (1:1) can be given with excellent results. However, bicarbonate ingestion may cause bloating and flatulence, and citrate salts are often more palatable. A solution containing 2 g citric acid, 3 g sodium citrate, and 3.3 g potassium citrate per 30 ml in a nonalcoholic syrup base (Polycitra) provides 1 mmol of sodium and 1 mmol of potassium per milliliter of syrup base. It is better tolerated when diluted in juice, water, or formula. The aim of treatment is to maintain as normal a serum bicarbonate level as possible day and night. Thus, doses should be frequent, with the last one as late at night as possible.

In severe forms of proximal RTA, alkali alone may be ineffective because of the gastrointestinal intolerance to the enormous doses needed or because of rapid loss of the base into the urine. Also, progressive increases in the amount of sodium and potassium salts administered may expand the extracellular fluid volume and be paradoxically followed by a worsening of metabolic acidosis and hypokalemia. In these circumstances, hydrochlorothiazide may be useful because it improves renal bicarbonate reabsorption and allows the dose of alkali to be reduced. The initial dose of hydrochlorothiazide is about 1.5 to 2 mg/kg/d divided into two or three doses. However, after correction of the acidosis, a smaller dose may be sufficient. An additional benefit of hydrochlorothiazide in patients with Fanconi syndrome is diminution of urinary calcium and phosphate excretion, with subsequent improvement of rickets. However, hydrochlorothiazide administration enhances urinary potassium losses and may aggravate the hypokalemia.

Hypokalemia is a frequent finding in Fanconi syndrome and always requires correction. The aim of therapy is to keep the serum potassium level above 3.0 mmol/L, if possible. Although potassium is generally given (as potassium bicarbonate or potassium citrate) to correct the acidosis, an additional amount may be necessary. A solution of 2 g citric acid and 6.6 g potassium citrate per 30 ml nonalcoholic syrup base (Polycitra K) contains 2 mmol of potassium per 1 ml of syrup base. If acidosis is not present, potassium may be given as the gluconate, phosphate, or chloride salt.

When polyuria is present, fluid intake must be increased to avoid dehydration. A good practice, especially in infants, is to dissolve the required salts in the minimal amount of fluid required for the whole day. Additional water is also given, if necessary. It must be remembered that an excessive fluid intake may lead to overexpansion of extracellular fluid volume and aggravation of proximal tubular dysfunction. Acute management of fluid and electrolyte disturbances may be extraordinarily difficult in infants with Fanconi syndrome secondary to nephropathic cystinosis. In selected cases, it may be useful to administer indomethacin (Indocin 2 to 5 mg/kg/d). Indomethacin induces a marked improvement in proximal tubular function and reduces the abnormal urinary losses.

Carnitine deficiency may develop in patients with Fanconi syndrome and requires oral L-carnitine supplementation. L-Carnitine should be given at a starting dose of 50 to 100 mg/kg/d in divided doses every 6 hours and later titrated to maintain plasma free carnitine levels in the normal range without side effects. Muscle carnitine repletion requires prolonged therapy for many years. That muscle carnitine deficiency has been corrected can be assured only by muscle biopsy.

Specific Therapy

Nephropathic cystinosis is an autosomal recessive disorder characterized by the accumulation of cystine within body tissues due to a defect in cystine transport across lysosomal membranes. The increased content of cystine has a deleterious effect on many enzymatic systems and leads to cell death. Many organs are involved, including kidney, thyroid, eye, liver, pancreas, brain, and muscle. The child presents at a young age with Fanconi syndrome. Untreated, a progressive and unremitting glomerular failure develops, and renal death takes place before the patient reaches 10 years of age.

Although supportive care is also of paramount importance, there is strong evidence that cysteamine therapy, when started early, may slow down the progression to terminal renal failure. Cysteamine is a free thiol that depletes cystine stores from cells by reacting with cystine to form cystine-cysteamine mixed disulfide, which is able to egress from the cytosolic lysosomes by means of an intact lysine carrier system. Cysteamine is given every 6 hours as an oral cysteamine hydrochloride solution containing 50 mg of free base per milliliter. The starting dose of 10 mg/kg/d must be increased every 2 weeks to reach a dose of 50 to 60 mg/kg/d. Thereafter, the dose must be titrated to maintain leukocyte cystine levels below 1 nmol ½ cystine per 1 mg of protein. The dose should not exceed 90 mg/kg/d. This therapy ideally should be given shortly after birth, which is possible when cystinosis is diagnosed early because a sibling was affected. With early treatment, glomerular function is significantly preserved, and linear growth is clearly improved. When therapy is started later, especially when glomerular damage has already occurred, the benefit to the kidney is less apparent, although the therapy may contribute to preserve the function of other organs (eye, thyroid, pancreas, brain, and muscle).

The taste and smell of cysteamine are repulsive and may result in a high noncompliance rate. Therefore, the use of phosphocysteamine is a possible alternative. This drug has cystine-depleting effects similar to those of cysteamine but does not have its offensive odor because cysteamine is formed by intestinal hydrolysis and is quickly absorbed. Corneal crystal deposition may be improved by the use of cysteamine eyedrops.

Unfortunately, although early cysteamine therapy offers some hope for cystinotic patients, many still progress to end-stage renal failure at the end of their first decade. Renal transplantation has represented an important advance because transplanted kidneys do not accumulate cystine and do not suffer a progressive functional deterioration as a consequence of cystine deposits. In fact, the rate of rejection in patients with cystinosis appears to be significantly lower than in children with other chronic renal diseases. The success of renal transplantation has permitted children with cystinosis to live to adulthood, thus allowing the damage of many organs besides the kidney to become evident. The appearance of these complications (hypothyroidism, progressive blindness, diabetes mellitus, pancreatic exocrine dysfunction, myopathy, cerebral atrophy) mandates consideration of the use of cysteamine even after renal transplantation and, probably, for the lifetime of the patient.

RENAL TUBULAR ACIDOSIS

The term renal tubular acidosis is applied to a group of transport defects in the reabsorption of filtered bicarbonate or in the excretion of hydrogen ion. The RTA syndromes are characterized by a relatively normal GFR and a metabolic acidosis accompanied by a normal plasma anion gap. On clinical and pathophysiologic grounds, RTA can be classified as *proximal RTA* (type 2), which is caused by a primary defect in proximal tubular bicarbonate reabsorption, *distal RTA* (type 1), which is caused by an impaired distal hydrogen ion secretion, and *hyperkalemic RTA* (type 4), which is due to impaired ammoniagenesis and is associated with aldosterone deficiency or resistance.

Proximal RTA

Proximal RTA may occur in children as a primary and isolated entity or may be accompanied by other proximal tubular defects (Fanconi syndrome). Therapy of proximal RTA as observed in the Fanconi syndrome was discussed previously. When proximal RTA presents as an isolated entity, the correction does not specifically require potassium. Alkali can be given in the form of sodium bicarbonate or sodium citrate (a useful preparation is Shohl's solution, which contains 140 g citric acid and 98 g sodium citrate dissolved in water to a total volume of 1 L; 1 ml provides 1 mmol sodium). Primary proximal RTA manifests clinically with growth failure and persistent vomiting in early infancy. Alkali therapy induces a rapid increase in growth rate and can be discontinued after several years without reappearance of symptoms. The self-limited course of infantile proximal RTA contrasts with that of distal RTA, which appears to be persistent even when the clinical onset is in infancy.

Distal RTA

Treatment of distal RTA consists of giving enough alkali to maintain correction of the acidosis and normalization of urinary excretion of calcium and citrate. Potassium is also needed, regardless of the serum potassium value, and in cases of severe hypokalemia, it should be given before correcting the acidosis. Although the effects of sodium bicarbonate on acid-base homeostasis are indistinguishable from those of sodium citrate, the latter is preferred because it is more effective in increasing urinary excretion of citrate. The amount of sodium and potassium bicarbonate needed to correct the acidosis is often not enough to raise the low citrate excretion. Therefore, treatment is best accomplished by Polycitra. The total dose of citrate is determined mainly by the concomitant excretion of bicarbonate and is equal to the urinary excretion of bicarbonate plus about 2 mmol/kg/d to compensate for endogenous acid production. Therapeutic requirements may be as high as 10 to 15 mmol/kg/d during the first years of life, decreasing to about 3 mmol/kg/d in older children.

The aim of treatment is not only to correct the acidosis but also to normalize calcium excretion and, thus, prevent further development of nephrocalcinosis and nephrolithiasis. Unfortunately, parenchymal calcification already present is not reversible. The efficacy of treatment, when started early in infancy, is demonstrated by normal growth and complete arrest of further nephrocalcinosis. If excessive doses of alkali are used, the overexpansion of extracellular fluid volume leads to a paradoxical increase in urinary calcium excretion, which is rapidly corrected when doses are reduced.

Other therapeutic measures are of little or doubtful value. Vitamin D is generally not needed. Hydrochlorothiazide is not only of limited benefit but is also potentially dangerous because it may aggravate the hypokalemia. Patients treated for distal RTA are at risk of pseudoephedrine intoxication when this drug is used because its renal excretion is minimal in alkalinized urine.

Hyperkalemic RTA

The cause of hyperkalemic RTA should be found in order to manage this disorder adequately. Potassium-retaining drugs should be discontinued at once. If there is extracellular fluid volume contraction, it should be corrected. This is critical in patients with salt-losing aldosterone deficiency. In patients with chronic renal disease and hyporeninemic hypoaldosteronism, treatment decisions should be made from the symptoms and the severity of the hyperkalemia. Acidosis and hyperkalemia may be corrected by high doses of fludrocortisone. Prolonged treatment, however, may be complicated by excessive salt retention, with increased risk of cardiovascular compromise or arterial hypertension. Reduction of potassium intake, administration of potassium-binding resins or, preferably, periodic administration of furosemide will allow the dose of fludrocortisone to be reduced, thus preventing such complications. In many cases, sodium bicarbonate or citrate (~2 mmol/kg/d) also is necessary.

Therapy in patients with hyperkalemic RTA associated with states of mineralocorticoid resistance is detailed in the following section.

PSEUDOHYPOALDOSTERONISM

The term "pseudohypoaldosteronism" has been coined to describe disorders of electrolyte homeostasis characterized by an apparent state of renal tubular unresponsiveness to the action of aldosterone and manifested by hyperkalemia and metabolic acidosis.

Type 1 Pseudohypoaldosteronism

Primary type 1 pseudohypoaldosteronism is a hereditary condition characterized by salt wasting, hyperkalemia, and metabolic acidosis in the presence of markedly elevated plasma renin activity and aldosterone concentration. This name includes two clinically and genetically distinct entities with either exclusively renal or multiple target organ (kidney, sweat and salivary glands, colon) defects. The latter form is recognized by the severe salt wasting and by the elevated concentration of sweat and salivary electrolytes.

Renal type 1 pseudohypoaldosteronism is treated with sodium chloride supplementation (3 to 6 g/d), which is followed by marked clinical and biochemical improvement, that is, correction of volume contraction, hyperkalemia, and metabolic acidosis. The amount of sodium chloride required is deduced from the normalization of plasma potassium concentration and renin activity. Although the primary defect persists for life, improvement may occur beyond 1 or 2 years of age because of maturation of proximal tubular transport, development of salt appetite, and improvement in the renal tubular response to mineralocorticoids. Older children with renal type 1 pseudohypoaldosteronism are generally asymptomatic while eating a normal salt intake, but the plasma aldosterone concentration remains elevated. Exceptionally, subtle symptoms leading to growth failure or even overt salt wasting may persist to late childhood.

Multiple target organ type 1 pseudohypoaldosteronism is less frequent, more difficult to treat, and of worse prognosis. These patients manifest severe salt-wasting episodes early after birth, and death may ensue during the neonatal period. There is a poor response to sodium chloride supplementation alone, and rectal administration of ion exchange resins and dietary manipulation reducing the intake of potassium are also necessary. Improvement with age is less apparent, and therapy must be maintained throughout childhood and probably throughout life.

Some infants present an apparently primary unresponsiveness to aldosterone that is only manifested by hyperkalemia and metabolic acidosis, without overt salt wasting. This syndrome, called *early childhood hyperkalemia,* presents clinically with failure to thrive and frequent vomiting. Therapy is generally required during the first years of life in the form of sodium bicarbonate alone or associated with ion exchange resins. The disorder appears to be transient, and at about 5 years of age, therapy is no longer needed.

Secondary forms of type 1 pseudohypoaldosteronism have been documented frequently in young infants with urinary tract infection, associated with both obstructive and nonobstructive renal lesions. After medical or surgical therapy, all abnormalities quickly disappear. These observations indicate that renal ultrasonography and urine cultures should be performed in any infant presenting with salt wasting, hyperkalemia, and metabolic acidosis to exclude structural renal lesions or infection as the cause of the electrolyte disturbances.

Type 2 Pseudohypoaldosteronism

Type 2 pseudohypoaldosteronism, also called chloride-shunt syndrome or Gordon syndrome, is a familial condition presenting with arterial hypertension, hyperkalemia, metabolic acidosis, suppressed plasma renin activity, and normal glomerular function. It is also called Spitzer syndrome when arterial hypertension is absent. This disease represents an inherited tendency to hyperreabsorb the filtered sodium chloride, which leads to short stature and expansion of extracellular

fluid volume, with resultant hyporeninemic hypoaldosteronism. Hypertension is an important feature in adolescents and young adults but not in children.

Dietary salt restriction or diuretic therapy results in complete reversal of both clinical and biochemical abnormalities, with return of blood pressure to normal values (when it is elevated), rise in plasma renin activity and aldosterone concentration, and correction of hyperkalemia and metabolic acidosis. Furosemide administration is effective, but it aggravates the hypercalciuria frequently observed in this condition and, thus, increases the risk of urolithiasis. The ideal treatment is the administration of hydrochlorothiazide 1.5 to 2 mg/kg/d, which is as effective as furosemide in the reversal of hyperkalemia and metabolic acidosis but also corrects the hypercalciuria. However, long-term prognosis remains uncertain.

BARTTER'S SYNDROME

Bartter's syndrome, as observed in infants and children, is an autosomal recessive disorder characterized by hypokalemia, metabolic alkalosis, and normal blood pressure despite hyperplasia of juxtaglomerular apparatus, hyperreninemia, and hyperaldosteronism. The syndrome starts in infancy with failure to thrive, anorexia, vomiting, polyuria, polydipsia, tendency to dehydration, salt craving, and muscle wasting. Tetany is rare in children and is observed more frequently in adults. Short stature is common in children presenting with the symptoms early in life. More rarely, these children present with rickets, nephrocalcinosis, gout, or oligophrenia. An extremely severe neonatal form is characterized by oligohydramnios, prematurity, hypercalciuria, and nephrocalcinosis. Bartter's syndrome is associated with a chloride reabsorption defect in the distal nephron, which results in potassium wasting, hypokalemia, and increased secretion of prostaglandins. Concomitant elevations of plasma renin activity and angiotensin II stimulate aldosterone secretion but do not cause arterial hypertension because the vasoconstrictive effect of angiotensin II is opposed by the vasodilatory effect of prostacyclin.

Treatment

Treatment of Bartter's syndrome must include an attempt to correct the hypokalemia. Potassium chloride supplements 1 to 3 mmol/kg/d up to 500 mmol/d are always necessary. The amount needed will change according to the patient, and the supplements must balance the amount of potassium wasted through the kidney. Unfortunately, potassium supplements alone are almost completely ineffective in most cases because the administered potassium is quickly lost into the urine. Addition of spironolactone (Aldactone 10 to 15 mg/kg/d) or triamterene (Dyazide 10 mg/kg/d) may be initially effective in the control of hypokalemia, but this effect is often very transient. The administration of a beta-adrenergic inhibitor, such as propranolol 1 mg/kg/d, does not offer any additional advantage.

Therapy of Bartter's syndrome is best accomplished by the use of prostaglandin inhibitors: indomethacin (Indocin 2 to 5 mg/kg/d), acetylsalicylic acid (aspirin 100 mg/kg/d), ibuprofen (30 mg/kg/d), or ketoprofen (Orudis 20 mg/kg/d). Indomethacin is the drug most frequently used and is remarkably well tolerated by these patients, although attention should be paid to signs of intolerance or toxicity, such as nausea, vomiting, abdominal pain, peptic ulcer, hematopoietic toxicity, or liver damage. The possibility of developing pseudotumor cerebri should be considered because it has been reported to occur after both indomethacin and ketoprofen therapy. The early effect of prostaglandin inhibitors is spectacular, with improved well-being, strength, and activity, diminution of polyuria and polydipsia, and instigation of normal or even catchup growth. There is an immediate increase in serum potassium values. These, however, rarely rise above 3.5 mmol/L. Plasma renin activity and aldosterone concentration decrease to a normal range, and the vascular response to angiotensin II or norepinephrine also normalizes. The only renal tubular defect that remains unmodified after indomethacin therapy is the tubular impairment in sodium chloride reabsorption, which is, therefore, believed to constitute the primary metabolic event.

The efficacy of long-term use of prostaglandin synthesis inhibitors has been clearly established. With time, there is some recurrence of hypokalemia and hyperreninemia, but clinical improvement is generally maintained. If the symptoms reappear, the dose of indomethacin should be readjusted, or a combined therapy of indomethacin and spironolactone should be initiated. In adults, angiotensin II-converting enzyme inhibitors (captopril, enalapril) have been tried, with conflicting results. There are no data justifying the use of these drugs in children.

Addition of magnesium salts should always be considered when hypomagnesemia is present. Magnesium deficiency may be seen occasionally in Bartter's syndrome but is a cardinal feature of the syndrome of *familial hypokalemia-hypomagnesemia* or Gitelman syndrome, which is often confused with Bartter's syndrome. Patients with Gitelman syndrome present with recurrent episodes of tetany, without polyuria or growth retardation. Outstanding biochemical features include hypomagnesemia, hypokalemia, metabolic alkalosis, and hypocalciuria. These patients are best treated with magnesium salts alone, with no need to add either potassium salts or prostaglandin inhibitors. Although many magnesium salts have been used in the treatment of hypomagnesemic states, we prefer the use of magnesium chloride ($MgCl_2$) which also compensates for ongoing urinary chloride losses. Magnesium chloride has a high magnesium content, is very soluble, and is not dependent on gastric acidity for absorption. Also, its administration is less often followed by diarrhea, although this complication may still develop with increasing dose. We use a 5% solution that contains approximately 0.5 mEq (0.6 mg) magnesium ion per milliliter. The total dose should be individualized for each patient and given at 6- to 8-hour intervals. In our experience, continuous administration of $MgCl_2$ not only partly corrects the hypomagnesemia and prevents the appearance of tetanic episodes but also normalizes plasma potassium concentration, acid-base equilibrium, renin-aldosterone axis, and urinary calcium excretion.

NEPHROGENIC DIABETES INSIPIDUS

Nephrogenic diabetes insipidus (NDI) is an X-linked recessive disorder characterized by a resistance to the antidiuretic action of both endogenous and exogenous vasopressin. The basic molecular defect is a mutation in the gene coding for the synthesis of the renal receptors (V_2) for vasopressin, located in the long arm of chromosome X (Xq28). The vascular receptors (V_1) retain a normal response to the hormone.

Treatment

Therapy consists of lifetime administration of water in amount and frequency necessary to compensate for the obligatory urinary loss, thus avoiding chronic dehydration, hyperelectrolytemia, and secondary neurologic damage. This goal is easily attained in older children and adults, but great difficulties may be encountered in infants, especially when thirst is absent. Administration of solute-poor milk reduces urinary water requirements and helps to maintain an adequate water balance. Occasionally, it is necessary to give water around-the-clock through a gastric tube to allow the infant prolonged periods of rest. This procedure is extremely important to prevent subclinical nocturnal dehydration.

The discovery that hydrochlorothiazide decreases urinary output has enormously facilitated the management of NDI patients, especially during infancy. The decrease in urinary volume observed following administration of the diuretic is accompanied by an increased concentration of urinary solutes and decreased clearance of free water. It has been shown that the effect is mediated through sodium depletion, with increased proximal tubular reabsorption of sodium and decreased delivery of fluid to the distal nephron. Hydrochlorothiazide also increases the inner medullary osmolality and thus favors passive water reabsorption from the collecting duct. The recommended dose is 1.5

to 2 mg/kg/d divided into two or three doses and accompanied by a moderate restriction of salt intake (~1.2 mmol/kg/d). In infants, it may be given in a suspension form containing 10 mg/ml. Giving sodium chloride in excess interferes with the antidiuretic effect. However, prolonged thiazide therapy increases kaliuresis and may induce the development of profound hypokalemia. The simultaneous administration of potassium supplements is necessary in most cases.

As a result of the limited benefit and possible complications of thiazide administration, other drugs have been used, generally in association with thiazide therapy. Prostaglandin synthesis inhibitors, such as indomethacin 2 to 5 mg/kg/d, acetylsalicylic acid 100 mg/kg/d, ibuprofen 30 mg/kg/d, and ketoprofen 20 mg/kg/d, have also shown a beneficial effect on urinary output, additive to the antidiuretic effect of hydrochlorothiazide. Thiazide administration reduces urinary output by about 20% to 50%, and indomethacin reduces urinary output by another 20% to 30%. This combined therapy is especially useful in infants and young children. The mechanism by which prostaglandin inhibitors reduce urinary output in patients with NDI is not known but is probably related to a reduction in GFR, with a proportional increase in proximal reabsorption of water and sodium. As mentioned in the discussion of Bartter's syndrome, prolonged use of prostaglandin synthesis inhibitors may cause renal, gastrointestinal, hematopoietic, and central nervous system complications, and such therapy should be carefully followed.

The safest therapy that can be offered today to infants and children with DNI is the combined administration of hydrochlorothiazide and amiloride 0.2 to 0.3 mg/kg/d. This drug combination is marketed in tablets containing 50 mg of hydrochlorothiazide and 5 mg of amiloride hydrochloride, but in infants, it is better to use independent medications. Hydrochlorothiazide is given in suspension form containing 10 mg/ml, and amiloride is given as the calculated part of a 5 mg tablet crushed and mixed with food. With this therapy, along with moderate dietary salt restriction, urinary volume does not differ significantly from that obtained with combined hydrochlorothiazide-indomethacin therapy, but lesser side effects occur. Amiloride also has an additive antidiuretic effect, probably by further increasing sodium excretion, reducing extracellular fluid volume, and enhancing water and sodium reabsorption in the proximal tubule. Amiloride has antikaliuretic properties, and when it is given in association with hydrochlorothiazide, there is no need for potassium supplementation.

ACUTE RENAL FAILURE

JONATHAN D. HEILICZER, M.D.

Acute renal failure (ARF) is sudden, rapid impairment of kidney function, commonly associated with azotemia and oliguria. ARF in infants and children has varied etiologies, and specific therapy for some etiologies is discussed in other sections of this chapter. However, in general, therapy is symptomatic and supportive. The clinical approach to therapy can be divided into three areas:

1. Prevention of impending or potential ARF.
2. Management of established ARF.
3. Maximizing recovery of renal function.

This review focuses mainly on the second area, the symptomatic and supportive management of established ARF, with brief comments on the first and third areas.

IMPENDING ARF

Certain disease states or renal injuries, as well as iatrogenic procedures (i.e., cardiac surgery or cancer chemotherapy), can place children at risk for the development of ARF. Any state that potentially decreases blood flow or oxygenation to the kidneys can lead to ARF. Thus, dehydration due to gastroenteritis, peripheral vasodilation secondary to septic shock, and perinatal asphyxia can all precipitate ARF. As restoration of volume, vascular tone, and oxygen are obviously important in ensuring adequate renal blood flow and function, careful assessments of systemic blood pressure and intravascular volume are essential. In the most critical cases, insertion of a central venous catheter to measure central venous pressure (CVP) should be considered. Many critical care authorities advocate more advanced monitoring using a balloon-tipped Swan-Ganz catheter. However, this type of catheter carries added risk and requires considerable expertise in placement and use. It is rarely justified in children unless there is significant cardiac dysfunction. A percutaneously inserted end-hole venous catheter advanced into the right atrium (or superior vena cava) is usually sufficient. If the measured CVP is less than 5 mm H_2O or the patient is hypotensive, fluid resuscitation is mandatory. Isotonic fluid, normal saline being the fluid of choice, should be infused at a rate of at least 20 ml/kg/h until CVP is above 5 mm H_2O and systemic blood pressure is restored to normal. Hypovolemic shock states may require a more rapid rate of fluid delivery. Isotonic fluids other than normal saline should be reserved for specific types of hypovolemia (albumin for nephrotic children or whole blood for hemorrhage). Ringer's lactate, although isotonic, contains potassium, phosphate, and other electrolytes that the injured nephron might not adequately handle and is best avoided.

In these prerenal patients, renal function and urine output should improve once vascular tone and volume are restored. If the child remains oliguric despite adequate fluid replacement and lack of postrenal obstruction, a cautious challenge with a diuretic can be considered. Furosemide 1 to 2 mg/kg IV may be used in an attempt to improve urine output. However, one must bear in mind that diuretics do not enhance the glomerular filtration rate (GFR) but rather increase urine output by decreasing resorption of fluid from the tubule. If sufficient renal damage has occurred to markedly diminish GFR, diuretic use alone will not prevent the establishment of ARF and may cause potential harm. Ototoxicity can occur if furosemide is infused at a rate greater than 15 mg/min.

Dopamine, furosemide, and the osmotic diuretic mannitol have all been popularly advocated as being able to prevent or blunt ARF in children undergoing treatment for nonrenal problems (e.g., cardiac surgery). Studies indicate that such therapy can be of potential help only if used in a prophylactic manner before or immediately during an insult. Dopamine infused at a continuous rate of 1 to 3 μg/kg/min will enhance renal blood flow, increase GFR, and increase sodium excretion. Furosemide and mannitol increase solute excretion, theoretically preventing tubular collapse and blockage by cellular debris (i.e., casts).

MANAGEMENT OF ESTABLISHED RENAL FAILURE

Once ARF is established, conservative and symptomatic management can be employed successfully in the vast majority of patients. Only a few patients will require renal replacement therapy (hemodialysis, peritoneal dialysis, or hemofiltration). The technical aspects of these modalities are discussed elsewhere, but the indications for implementation when conservative therapy proves insufficient are discussed in subsequent paragraphs.

Children with established ARF, whether oliguric or nonoliguric, must have adequate monitoring, as outlined in Table 1. This will allow management to be individually tailored and discover abnormalities, correct complications, and prevent further deterioration in fluid, electrolyte, acid-base balance, blood pressure, and nutritional status.

Fluids

Monitoring of intravascular volume and attempting to maintain euvolemia is essential. In critically ill children, CVP monitoring is very helpful. Other children can be monitored with blood pressure and peripheral perfusion assessments alone. Strict accounting for all fluid intake and output is mandatory and allows for meticulous calculation of an individual's fluid requirements.

TABLE 1. Monitoring

Strict accounting and recording of all fluid intake and output
Blood pressure and central venous pressure (if available) recorded at least every 2–4 h
Daily weights, using exactly the same scale each day
Frequent laboratory data
  Daily CBC, differential and platelet count
  Daily full biochemistry—to include electrolytes, BUN, creatinine, Ca^+, PO_4^{2-}, albumin, and liver enzymes
  Venous blood gas (VBG)* with Na^+, K^+, Hct, and ionized Ca^+ q4–6h

*VBG is easier and less painful to obtain clinically. Unless there is concern about O_2, arterial blood is not needed.

All children with ARF should have intake restricted to insensible water loss and replacement of some percent of their fluid output (i.e., measured urine, nasogastric, or other losses). Insensible water loss can be estimated at 400 ml/m^2/d for children in an environment that is of normal temperature and humidity. Children on closed system ventilators breathing humidified gas will lose less water and, therefore, should have a lower estimate (300 ml/m^2/d). Insensible water loss contains no electrolytes and this intravenous replacement should theoretically contain no electrolytes, just glucose and water.

Replacement of output should be on a milliliter per milliliter basis, calculated hourly in very ill children. These replacement fluids do contain electrolytes. The most scientific method of calculating the concentrations is to obtain an aliquot of output fluid for laboratory measurement of electrolytes. However, in most situations, replacement with 0.45 normal saline is a reasonable estimate.

The CVP ideally should be maintained in a range between 5 and 10 cm H_2O. Values below 5 cm H_2O may require volume expansion. Values above 10 cm H_2O signify fluid overload and require further fluid restriction. If a child is fluid overloaded, restriction to insensible water losses or insensible water losses plus less than 100% of output should be considered. This more restricted regimen is continued until euvolemia is reestablished. Only then, a return to the original insensible water losses plus 100% of output should clinically maintain fluid balance.

Electrolyte Balance

Potassium

Other than the underlying primary illness, the major cause of morbidity and mortality associated with ARF is hyperkalemia. Potassium (K^+) levels greater than 6 mmol/L can cause direct cardiac toxicity by lowering the firing threshold of cardiac muscle. This is heralded by changes in the electrocardiogram (ECG)—initially manifested by peaked T waves, followed by ST wave depression, widening of the QRS complex, ventricular tachycardia, and asystole. The level of K^+ at which these changes occur varies in individual patients. However the rate of K^+ rise as opposed to a specific peak level is the major concern. Cardiac toxicity may be further aggravated by acidosis. Frequent review of the K^+ level (and serum pH), as well as accounting for all sources of exogenous K^+, is imperative. The necessity for penicillin therapy (which can add 1.7 mEq of K^+ per million units) or for packed red cell transfusions must be carefully evaluated.

All exogenous sources of intravenous K^+ should be withheld unless the serum K^+ is less than 3.5 mmol/L. If the child is stable and, therefore, able to take enteral nutrition, oral K^+ in the diet should be restricted to 1 g/d. However, enteral feeding should probably be withheld until the child is quite stable. In fact, one should consider prophylactic K^+ removal, an excellent method being continuous nasogastric suction (poor man's dialysis). An alternative is the use of Kayexalate.

If K^+ rises to greater than 6 mmol/L in an oliguric patient, manipulation of K^+ to blunt cardiac toxicity should be instituted as outlined in Table 2. Only urine output, nasogastric suction, polystyrene sulfonate ion exchange resins (Kayexalate), and dialysis actually

TABLE 2. Emergent Hyperkalemia Therapy

DRUG	DOSE	ROUTE	REMARKS
NaHCO$_3$*	1–2 mEq/kg	Slow IV over 5 min	Transfers K$^+$ intracellularly, can aggravate H$_2$O balance; effect lasts for several hours; USE WITH GREAT CAUTION IN NEONATES
D$_{25}$W	0.5 g/kg	IV infusion over 2 h	Transfers K$^+$ intracellularly; DO NOT USE 50% dextrose in children because of hypertonicity
Regular insulin	0.3 U/g glucose	IV infusion with D$_{25}$W	Transfers K$^+$ intracellularly
10% Ca^{2+} gluconate*	100 mg/kg	Slow IV over 5 min	Transfers K$^+$ intracellularly; monitor ECG for bradycardia; effect lasts for ~1 h
Kayexalate	1 g/kg	PO, NG, PR	Exchanges K$^+$ for Na; mix with 20% sorbitol for PR, 70% for PO/NG; can aggravate H$_2$O balance; USE WITH GREAT CAUTION IN NEONATES

*NaHCO$_3$ and calcium gluconate are incompatible. Clear IV between infusions.

remove K$^+$ from the body. The other methods change the extracellular K$^+$ concentration by either transferring K$^+$ intracellularly (NaHCO$_3$, glucose, and insulin) or increasing the cardiac muscle cell's firing threshold (calcium gluconate). Polystyrene sulfonate ion exchange resins must be used in combination with a cathartic, such as sorbitol, to prevent constipation. Resin exchange is more efficient in K$^+$ removal when given orally or via nasogastric tube, but the exchange occurs more rapidly when given rectally. Such resin exchange therapy should be avoided in premature infants who are at risk for necrotizing enterocolitis.

Sodium

Hyponatremia in oliguric ARF is almost always related to increases in total body water and is a sign of too liberal fluid intake. Rarely is any treatment required, other than fluid restriction to maintain the serum sodium (Na$^+$) greater than 130 mmol/L. However, should the serum Na$^+$ fall rapidly or fall below 120 mmol/L, central nervous system (CNS) complications ranging from seizures to coma can result. Hypertonic salt (3% NaCl), which has a concentration of ~0.5 mEq/ml, should be given in a quantity sufficient to raise the serum Na$^+$ to a level of at least 125 mmol/L. The Na$^+$ level should be raised slowly, at a rate of less than 1 mmol/L/h over several hours, to prevent a more permanent CNS catastrophe. This therapy carries the further risk of aggravating the fluid balance in an already overloaded patient.

Acid-Base Balance

Early in the course of ARF, pulmonary compensation maintains the serum pH at or close to a normal level. However, failure of the body's main outlet for hydrogen ions, the kidney, inevitably results in metabolic acidosis. The resulting acidosis is usually mild, with the serum pH staying above 7.25 and serum HCO$_3$ above 15 mEq/L. These levels are reasonably tolerated, and intervention is not necessary. Infusions of NaHCO$_3$ should be considered only if the serum pH falls below 7.2 and, even then, given only with caution. Such therapy is hypertonic and can result in fluid overload (water retained with NaHCO$_3$), tetany, or hypernatremia. In premature infants, using NaHCO$_3$ can pose the significant risk of intraventricular hemorrhage. Again employing nasogastric suction to remove acid (and K$^+$) can be helpful in mitigating the need for NaHCO$_3$. The addition of calcium carbonate (CaCO$_3$) as a phosphate binder can provide a source of base without Na$^+$ and, therefore, water. In children who must be mechanically ventilated for their underlying nonrenal condition, serum pH can often be maintained by manipulating ventilator settings. When managing pH with ventilator compensation, care should be exercised to maintain the Pco$_2$ above 30 mm Hg so as not to compromise cerebral blood flow.

Calcium and Phosphorus

Children with ARF may present with, or at some point develop, hyperphosphatemia and hypocalcemia. Patients with some types of renal disease may have low serum protein, thus lowering the mea-

surable total serum calcium. As illustrated in Table 1, the best measurement of calcium is the serum ionized calcium concentration. On occasion, the calcium level may be sufficiently low as to cause tetany or arrhythmias. An acute IV infusion of 10% calcium gluconate at a dose of 100 mg/kg can be given over 1 hour while continuously monitoring an ECG tracing.

In the nonsymptomatic patient, first lowering the serum phosphorus (PO$_4^{2-}$) and avoiding metastatic calcification syndrome is indicated. Hyperphosphatemia can be managed by dietary restriction and the addition of phosphate binders. However, the major route for PO$_4^{2-}$ removal is via the urine or dialysis. Phosphate binders prevent PO$_4^{2-}$ from being adequately absorbed from the gut. In children, binders containing aluminum or magnesium are contraindicated because of potential accumulation of heavy metal in brain and bone. Oral CaCO$_3$ is the binder of choice, not only helping to blunt hyperphosphatemia but also supplying a source of base and calcium. A dose of 300 to 400 mg/kg divided four times a day, preferably given with meals, is usually effective. Exogenous sources of PO$_4^{2-}$ should be limited. It is especially important to avoid enemas (e.g., Fleet) and cathartics that deliver large PO$_4^{2-}$ loads.

Hypertension

Two factors contribute to the rise in blood pressure in ARF patients: fluid overload and hyperreninemia. Volume-mediated hypertension is best treated with fluid retention. In worst case scenarios, fluid removal will be necessary. As noted previously, response to diuretics may be poor in ARF, and only a single trial is recommended. Dialysis or hemofiltration becomes necessary if restriction or diuresis is unsuccessful. While awaiting assembly of dialysis or hemofiltration, one can temporize severe volume-mediated hypertension (diastolic greater than 95th percentile for age) with a vasodilator, such as nifedipine (Table 3).

Renin-mediated hypertension is especially prominent in primary nephritis syndromes and collagen vascular disease. Such hypertension is treated pharmacologically. Chronic drugs of choice are angiotensin-converting enzyme (ACE) inhibitors, such as enalapril. Acutely, a vasodilator (nifedipine) is probably more efficacious. Nifedipine has a fairly rapid onset orally or sublingually and is advantageous in children with poor venous access. Should chronic as opposed to occasional treatment be required, the longer-lasting ACE inhibitors can be used.

Absolute control of blood pressure is not the goal of acute therapy. As hypertension in ARF is usually transient, parameters should be set up allowing for treatment of acute pressures above the 95th percentile and to maintain pressure below that range. Should blood pressure drop below an individualized level, antihypertensive medication should be withheld.

Nutrition

Children with ARF are extremely catabolic. This catabolism is aggravated by other metabolic disturbances, particularly acidosis. Additionally, these patients are at risk for calorie-protein malnutrition

TABLE 3. Hypertension Therapy

DRUG	DOSE	ROUTE	REMARKS
Nifedipine	0.5 mg/kg	Sublingual	Rapid vasodilator, very efficacious; for small doses, puncture 10-mg capsule and withdraw drug with syringe for titrated dose; max in adolescent: 80 mg/8 h; smaller children titrated accordingly
Diazoxide	1–3 mg/kg	IV bolus or slow push	DO NOT DELIVER bolus in central line; max: 3 doses in 15-min period; availability of nifedipine has diminished use
Labetalol	1–3 mg/kg	IV titrate to BP	A combined alpha- and beta-blocking agent; onset in 5 min; can cause urinary retention
Enalapril	Start with 1.25–2.5 mg/q12h per dose	PO	Converted to active form by liver; recommended as chronic therapy, not for acute use
Enalapril	0.625 mg q6h	IV	As above

because of both the need to restrict intake and their diminished appetite. Malnutrition can delay recovery and induce other complications, such as diminished immune function. Therefore, nutritional issues should be addressed early in the child's course to improve survival.

Oral/enteral feeding as opposed to total parenteral nutrition (TPN) is the preferred nutritional route. The oral/enteral method is able to provide more calories in a smaller fluid volume and with less risk than TPN. Enteral feeding is restricted to a total of 2 gNa$^+$ and 1 g K$^+$ per day, with similar limitation of PO$_4^=$. Intake in nondialyzed children should be limited to high-value dietary protein of 1 to 1.5 g/kg/d. The oral fluid amount must be restricted as outlined previously. Only fluids with a low sodium content should be offered, such as water, ginger ale, 7-Up, and Kool Aid.

In critically ill children, TPN should be started via a central venous catheter as soon as fluid, electrolyte, and acid-base balance is achieved. Hypertonic glucose solution with 0.5 g/kg/d of amino acids, at least 100 mg/kg/d of calcium gluconate, and multivitamins is mixed in sufficient sterile water to approximate insensible water losses. The glucose and protein concentrations can be increased on a daily basis to a maximum of 25% dextrose and 1.5 g/kg of protein. Once a better grasp of the child's output is gained or regular renal replacement therapy has begun, water content (and therefore calories) can be increased to include this added amount. Once this output replacement is added to the TPN, some amount of Na, with equal amounts of chloride and HCO$_3$, should be added as well. Patients on TPN can receive added calories and essential fatty acids in the form of 20% lipid infusions at a starting dose of 1 g/kg (maximum of 2 to 3 g/kg/d).

Essential amino acid solutions, in both oral (Amin-Ade) and intravenous forms (Nephramine, Ren Amin), have been advocated as the ideal protein source for renal failure therapy. Theoretically, they help recycle urea nitrogen and lessen uremia. These solutions carry some risks, including nephrotoxicity related to prolonged use. Thus, they can be considered for short-term acute uses in combination with some nonessential amino acids. The current recommended ratio of essential/nonessential amino acids in ARF is 2:1, with the major portion of the essential amino acids provided in branched-chain form.

Miscellaneous Therapy

The physician should carefully review all medications required by any child with ARF. The risk versus benefit of any drug normally excreted by the kidney should be evaluated. Serum levels of all potentially toxic drugs, such as aminoglycosides and digoxin, should be followed, and doses should be adjusted to maintain levels in a therapeutic range. Drugs metabolized and mainly excreted by the liver probably do not need any adjustment.

Specific Therapy

Beyond treatment of the child's underlying etiology, investigators have sought therapies that might affect the mechanisms that locally injure the nephron. At present, there are no clinically available medications proven to reverse or enhance recovery from ARF in humans. As previously noted, dopamine, furosemide, and mannitol are efficacious only before or close to the renal insult. The hormone thyroxine, adenine nucleotides (ATP, MgCl$_2$), and calcium antagonists (nifedipine, verapamil, and diltiazem) all have shown promise in the laboratory. Each of these agents appears to help with different aspects of cell repair. Protocols involving one or a combination of these and similar agents may arrive at the bedside in the near future.

Renal Replacement Therapy

Dialysis or hemofiltration is indicated when conservative therapy proves inadequate and to enable an expanded fluid allowance required for nutrition (Table 4). More than conservative therapy is required when metabolic acidosis or hyperkalemia or both are not sufficiently controlled. Fluid overload that may inevitably lead to cardiopulmonary compromise is also an indication for renal replacement therapy.

Elevations of BUN above an individualized level (probably 50 mg/dl in a neonate, 70 mg/dl in a child, and 90 mg/dl in an adolescent) are not absolute indications for additional therapy. However, such levels of azotemia are a harbinger that absolute criteria will occur in short order. Dialysis or hemofiltration can be considered when nutritional needs require expansion of the fluid allowance.

As with any invasive procedure, elective as opposed to emergent dialysis or hemofiltration has a higher success rate. Such therapy mandates the expertise of a pediatric nephrologist. The choice of which modality will depend on the size and condition of the individual patient and the judgment of the nephrologist.

RECOVERY FROM ARF

After some period of time, whether or not renal replacement therapy is required, most patients will begin to recover native renal function spontaneously. The initial indications will be a plateau of BUN and serum creatinine levels and, eventually, improved urine output. Careful monitoring during recovery remains an important therapeutic anchor. Polyuria, electrolyte washout, hypertension, and infection are all potential complications that can cause rapid swings in a child's status. Approximately a third of patients who succumb to ARF do so during this phase.

TABLE 4. Indications for Renal Replacement Therapy

Intractable hyperkalemia*
Persistent metabolic acidosis*
Fluid overload—impending cardiopulmonary compromise*
Advancing uremia
  BUN >50 mg/dl in neonate
       >70 mg/dl in child
       >90 mg/dl in adolescent
Deliver improved caloric intake

* Absolute indications.

Fluids

Glomerular function recovers before tubular function, leading to polyuria. This phase was previously known as "high-output ARF." Calculation of fluid requirements should continue to be based on insensible water losses ($400 \ ml/m^2/d$) plus 100% of output. Return of the nephron's ability to concentrate may lag behind GFR by several or more days. Thirst may be a useful guide in maintaining the fluid balance, especially in older children. In others, a careful trial titrating output replacement downward should be attempted. If polyuria persists, a return to the original 100% replacement is carried out, with a repeat challenge contemplated at a later time.

Electrolytes

The delay in tubular recovery prevents adequate reabsorption and secretion of electrolytes. Potassium, calcium, phosphorus, bicarbonate, and hydrogen ion are the major concerns. In this phase, hypokalemia can occur and is equally as dangerous as the hyperkalemia of the oliguric phase. Hypokalemia causes cardiac toxicity by lowering the muscle cell firing threshold and can lead to death. Once the serum K^+ falls below 3.5 mmol/L, K^+ should be added at a steady rate (not variable rate) intravenously, and the oral K^+ should be liberalized. If K^+ falls below 3.0 mmol/L, a supplemental intravenous infusion of KCl is recommended at a rate no faster than 0.25 mEq/kg in 1 hour while monitoring the ECG.

Calcium is usually well maintained by continuing intravenous calcium at the previously noted doses, in addition to calcitriol (1,25-vitamin D) at a starting dose of 0.01 to 0.05 $\mu g/kg/d$) PO.

Phosphorus is important for respiratory muscle action. Again, because of a lack of tubular reabsorption, hypophosphatemia can occur. When serum PO_4^{2-} falls below 5 mmol/L, phosphate binders should be discontinued. PO_4^{2-} levels of less than 1.5 mmol/L can lead to spontaneous respiratory arrest. PO_4^{2-} in either the Na^+ or K^+ form can be added at this point (the oral route is preferred).

Control of metabolic acidosis may be lost due to bicarbonate loss and poor hydrogen ion secretion by the tubule. In this phase, the addition of sufficient $NaHCO_3$ orally or intravenously is well tolerated.

PROGNOSIS

The availability of renal replacement therapy is the most significant reason for the relatively recent decrease in morbidity and mortality in children with ARF. The individual prognosis is tied not only to care of ARF but also to the underlying specific etiology. In many cases, a prognosis and a specific diagnosis cannot be elucidated without a renal biopsy. How much renal function is recovered and whether or not any sequelae occur is again a function of the underlying etiology.

The foregoing is intended as an outline of generalized ARF therapy in infants and children. The practitioner is cautioned that ARF is a complex, life-threatening syndrome that may range from mild and insidious to severe and explosive. Management in conjunction with a pediatric nephrologist is highly recommended.

REFERENCES

1. Bernstein JM, Erk SD: Choice of antibiotics, pharmacokinetics, and dose adjustments in acute and chronic renal failure. Med Clin North Am 74:1059–1076, 1990.
2. Cronin RE: Drug therapy in the management of acute renal failure. Am J Med Sci 292:112–119, 1986.
3. Feld LG, Cachero S, Springate JE: Fluid needs in acute renal failure. Pediatr Clin North Am 37:337–350, 1990.
4. Mandal AK, Visweswaran RK, Kaldas NR: Treatment considerations in acute renal failue. Drugs 44:567–577, 1992.
5. Wolfson M, Kopple JD: Nutritional management of acute renal failure. In Lazarus JM, Brenner BM (eds): Acute Renal Failure. New York, Churchill Livingstone, 1993:467–485.

CHRONIC RENAL FAILURE

KATHY JABS, M.D.
ELISABETH SIMON, M.D.

Chronic renal failure (CRF) is an uncommon problem in childhood with an estimated incidence of 1 to 3 per million population less than 16 years of age. Because its signs and symptoms may be nonspecific (e.g., growth retardation), detection often depends on the careful observation of the primary physician. Once recognized, the complications of CRF vary with the degree of renal insufficiency and the nature of the primary renal disease. Children with glomerular filtration rates (GFR) greater than 70% of normal for age have minimal signs and symptoms, as the remaining functioning nephrons adapt and compensate. When the GFR decreases to 25% to 50% of normal, treatment may be needed to maintain a normal metabolic status. In addition, stress or an intercurrent illness may result in dehydration, hyperkalemia, acidosis, and an acute decrease in renal function.

The goals of treatment for a child with CRF are to compensate for renal inability to maintain homeostasis by using dietary restrictions and supplementation of calories, vitamin D, and minerals as needed. In addition, the progression of renal failure may be slowed through treatment of infections, blood pressure control, and avoidance of nephrotoxins. Such an approach will decrease the long-term consequences of CRF. As CRF is a progressive condition, the ultimate treatment will be renal replacement therapy (dialysis or transplantation). The physiologic and psychologic outcome for children receiving renal replacement therapies can be enhanced by proper treatment before the development of end-stage renal disease (ESRD). The kidney plays an important role in maintaining homeostasis, so that renal dysfunction affects electrolyte and water balance, blood pressure, acid-base balance, calcium and phosphate metabolism, hemoglobin level (patients are anemic), and the clearance and accumulation of endogenous and exogenous toxins (Table 1). There are also long-term effects on growth and cognitive development from renal dysfunction. This chapter addresses approaches to compensate for renal dysfunction as CRF progresses. The approaches to the treatment of each disorder are summarized in Table 2.

MAINTENANCE OF SODIUM AND WATER BALANCE

A decrease in the kidney's filtering capacity usually does not lead to volume overload unless the GFR is less than 10% of normal for age. Thus, only a subset of children (including those with nephrosis) require fluid restriction. The need to restrict intake can complicate the care of those infants with renal dysplasia who have low, relatively fixed urine outputs. In such infants, it is necessary to increase the caloric density of formula to deliver sufficient calories while maintaining euvolemia. A child's fluid restriction would be the sum of insensible losses (300 to 400 ml/m^2 BSA), urine output, and any other losses. Patients and their parents need to be made aware of the fact that certain foods, such as fruits and vegetables, have a high water content that can substantially contribute to the child's daily fluid intake.

In contrast, a substantial proportion of CRF in children is due to renal dysplasia or obstructive uropathy associated with renal tubular dysfunction accompanied by an inability to concentrate the urine. These children may require chronic supplementation with free water. Chronic volume depletion in such children has been associated with poor growth. In addition, children with abnormal urinary concentrating ability are at increased risk for dehydration during gastrointestinal illnesses or periods when they have inadequate access to water. Careful attention to clinical indications of volume status, such as weight, skin turgor, and perfusion, are needed, since the usual signs, such as urinary specific gravity, cannot be used. The initial management of a child with CRF and dehydration is comparable to that of

TABLE 1. Disorders Associated with Chronic Renal Failure

> Salt and water overload
> Salt and water depletion
> Acidosis
> Hyperkalemia
> Bone mineral metabolism abnormalities
> Acidosis
> Anemia
> Growth retardation
> Cognitive dysfunction

a normal child and includes the rapid restoration of intravascular volume with a 10 to 20 ml/kg IV saline bolus. In determining the subsequent replacement for ongoing losses, it should be kept in mind that the kidneys will not appropriately conserve or excrete salt and water so that maintenance fluid protocols may not be appropriate.

A normally functioning kidney can adapt to a range of sodium intake from 40 to 200 mEq/d. However, changes in sodium intake are poorly tolerated in children with CRF. Sodium wasting can occur in children with renal dysplasia, medullary cystic disease, or obstructive uropathy. To compensate for sodium wasting, supplementation with 2 to 15 mEq/kg of sodium per day is needed. The amount needed can be quantitated by measuring the 24-hour urinary sodium excretion or estimated by the response to supplementation. Sodium losses in infants with fixed urine outputs and low sodium formulas may result in hyponatremia because of imbalances between sodium and water intake and urinary losses. In children with normal serum sodium levels, more subtle symptoms of sodium depletion, such as malaise, poor weight gain, and growth retardation, may occur. Acute illness can further decrease sodium intake, and the resultant negative sodium balance may significantly decrease intravascular volume. Conversely, sodium retention may occur if a child's intake is greater on average than his ability to excrete it. The result of the expanded extracellular fluid volume may be hypertension, peripheral edema, and pulmonary edema. Chronic treatment entails salt and water restriction and, in children with sufficient renal function, the addition of diuretics. In the case of pulmonary edema or severe hypertension, treatment includes antihypertensive medications, vigorous diuresis with furosemide, and, if necessary, ultrafiltration of fluid with continuous filtration or dialysis.

HYPERTENSION

As is the case for children with hypertension and normal renal function, children with CRF and blood pressure consistently >95% for age merit treatment. The goal of treatment is to decrease or avert the cardiovascular sequelae of chronic hypertension. In addition, well-controlled blood pressure may decrease the rate of CRF progression. The effect of blood pressure control on the progression of CRF may be maximal with a reduction of blood pressure to the 50th centile for age. In the case of severe hypertension, appropriate treatment is indicated in order to avoid sequelae such as hypertensive encephalopathy, stroke, and congestive heart failure. In choosing an antihypertensive medication, it is helpful to keep in mind that hypertension in CRF may be due to expanded vascular volume because of salt and water overload, activation of the renin-angiotensin system, or a combination of the two mechanisms. The treatment of chronic hypertension in children with CRF may include salt and water restriction or diuretics, weight control in the setting of obesity, and antihypertensive medications. Most children will require antihypertensive medications (Table 3). The optimum medication or combination of medications controls blood pressure and optimizes compliance through minimal side effects and infrequent dosing. As a general rule, a single agent should be initiated at less than the maximal dose and then increased to its maximum before adding a second drug. Careful monitoring is needed as the doses of the antihypertensive medications are adjusted, as a rapid decrease in blood pressure may compromise the GFR. A major part of the long-term monitoring of blood pressure rests with the patient or family and the teaching of blood pressure measurement with provision of a cuff for home use. Involvement of the school or visiting nurse may be helpful.

Renin-mediated hypertension is frequent in children with CRF due to pyelonephritic scarring, glomerulonephritis, hemolytic-uremic syndrome, polycystic kidney disease, and some forms of renal dysplasia. Although they are effective for the treatment of hypertension of various etiologies, converting enzyme inhibitors are particularly useful for patients with renin-mediated hypertension. The available agents vary in half-life and, therefore, the dosing interval is shortest with captopril (3 to 5 mg/kg/d two or three times a day) and longer with enalapril (staring dose 0.08 mg/kg per dose once or twice a day) or ramipril (once a day). The appropriate interval can be determined by the blood pressure pattern. If blood pressure is well controlled initially and the effect diminishes at the time for the next dose, the shorter of the recommended dosing intervals is indicated. Children should be

TABLE 2. Approaches to Treatment and Monitoring of Disordered Homeostasis in CRF

DISORDER	APPROACH TO TREATMENT	MONITORING
Renal sodium wasting	NaCl supplementation	Volume status, GFR, serum sodium
Urinary concentrating defect	Free water supplementation	Volume status, serum sodium
	Ready access to water	
Decreased sodium excretion	Dietary restriction, diuretics	Volume status, blood pressure
Hyperkalemia	Dietary restriction	Blood potassium level, electrocardiogram
	Exchange resin, dialysis	
Acidosis	Supplementation with bicarbonate, citrate, acetate	HCO_3 level, venous pH
Calcium-phosphate metabolism	Vitamin D supplementation	Blood levels of Ca, P, PTH
	Dietary phosphate restriction	Bone films
	Intestinal phosphate binders	
	Calcium supplementation	
Hypertension	Sodium restriction	Blood pressure, volume status
	Diuretics	
	Antihypertensive medications	
Anemia	Iron supplementation	Iron, total iron-binding capacity (TIBC), ferritin hemoglobin, hematocrit
	Recombinant erythropoietin	
Growth retardation	Caloric supplementation if needed	Height, growth velocity
	Maintain metabolic status	
	Recombinant growth hormone	

TABLE 3. Medications for Management of Hypertension in CRF

TYPE OF AGENT	MEDICATION	DOSE*	DOSING INTERVAL
Diuretic	Chlorothiazide	10–40	b.i.d.
	Hydrochlorothiazide	1–4	b.i.d.
	Furosemide	0.5–1	b.i.d. or q.d.
Vasodilator	Nifedipine	0.25–1	t.i.d. or q.i.d.
	(Procardia XL)		b.i.d. or q.i.d.
	Hydralazine	1–8	t.i.d. or q.i.d.
	Minoxidil	0.1–1	b.i.d. or q.d.
	Prazosin	0.030–0.3	t.i.d.
Beta-blocker	Atenolol	1–2	b.i.d. or q.d.
	Propranolol	0.5–4	q.i.d.
Converting enzyme inhibitor	Captopril	0.3–5	t.i.d.
	Enalapril	0.16	b.i.d. or q.d.

*Total dose per day in milligrams per kilogram of body weight.

carefully monitored after initiation of such agents as there is a risk of increased potassium levels in patients dependent on increased aldosterone to excrete a daily load of potassium. In this case, converting enzyme inhibitors would increase potassium. Beta-adrenergic blocking agents are also useful in children with CRF, as they may be dosed daily or twice a day, act by competitive inhibition of catecholamine action on the heart and at the kidney to decrease renin release, and have minimal side effects. There are a number of selective beta-blockers that have a greater effect on cardiac $beta_1$-receptors than bronchial $beta_2$-receptors. One such agent is atenolol, which is administered daily or twice a day (1 to 2 mg/kg/d). The nonselective agent, propranolol, is less desirable, as it has central nervous system effects on behavior and sleep and is usually dosed three or four times a day (1 to 10 mg/kg/d). These drugs may also contribute to hyperkalemia, as they decrease skeletal muscle uptake of a potassium load.

Vasodilators, such as calcium channel blockers, hydralazine, minoxidil, and prazosin, are used frequently. As these agents decrease blood pressure, vascular volume increases. Thus, a diuretic will be needed to maintain their effectiveness. In addition, the vasodilatation results in tachycardia, so that these agents are frequently used in association with beta-blockers. The choice of agents in this class varies with the size of the child, the severity of the hypertension, and the experience of the clinician. The long-acting preparations of nifedipine (Procardia XL) provide the best consistent blood pressure control and are dosed once or twice a day. The short-acting forms of nifedipine more frequently result in wide variations in blood pressure throughout the day. The total daily dose of the two formulations of nifedipine is the same (0.25 to 1 mg/kg). Hydralazine is a useful agent for small children who cannot swallow pills, despite the need for three or four times a day dosing (1 to 8 mg/kg/d). Minoxidil is a very potent agent that is usually effective in children with refractory hypertension (0.1 to 2 mg/kg/d once or twice a day). In addition to the risk of hypotension, the most significant adverse effect in a child is the resultant hirsutism. The potent alpha-adrenergic blocking agents, prazosin and labetalol, may also be used for blood pressure control. Prazosin is typically administered three times a day (10 to 100 μg/kg per dose). Labetalol (a combined alpha- and beta-blocker) is a better agent for hypertensive crises, as its short half-life necessitates dosing four times a day in chronic use, resulting in wide swings in blood pressure between doses.

Management of severe hypertension differs from chronic blood pressure management in that rapid reduction of blood pressure is attempted to avoid such sequelae as hypertensive encephalopathy (Table 4). In an emergency setting, sublingual nifedipine (0.25 to 0.5 mg/kg) is frequently effective. It can be repeated after 20 minutes if there has been an inadequate reduction in blood pressure. The dose is difficult to administer accurately to small children. However, the capsule can be punctured, the liquid aspirated into a tuberculin sy-

ringe, and the appropriate amount (0.035 ml corresponds to about 1 mg) administered. After administering the nifedipine, intravenous access should be obtained for further treatment. Hydralazine can be an effective agent administered intravenously or intramuscularly (0.1 to 0.2 mg/kg). The dose can be doubled and repeated every 20 minutes. A more effective agent is intravenous labetalol, which can be administered as a bolus (0.25 mg/kg) and repeated in escalating doses (0.5 to 1 mg/kg). Blood pressure control may be maintained by the constant infusion of labetalol at 1 to 3 mg/kg/h. A child who requires an infusion is typically cared for in the intensive care unit. If labetalol is inadequate, blood pressure can be controlled with infusion of nitroprusside (0.5 to 3 μg/kg/min). It should be kept in mind that the toxicity of this agent (thiocyanate) is increased in children with renal compromise.

MAINTENANCE OF POTASSIUM HOMEOSTASIS

Patients with renal insufficiency usually have a reduced capacity for excreting potassium when the GFR is less than 5% of normal. However, children with marked involvement of the renal interstitium (e.g., reflux nephropathy, obstructive uropathy, interstitial nephritis, or some renal cystic lesions) may have a tendency toward hyperkalemia at higher levels of renal function. Hyperkalemia may be exacerbated by use of angiotensin-converting enzyme inhibitors, such as captopril or enalapril, which decrease aldosterone secretion. The use of beta-adrenergic blockers may also contribute to hyperkalemia by decreasing the movement of extracellular potassium into skeletal muscle cells. The primary goal is prevention rather than treatment of hyperkalemia. This is achieved through limitation of foods rich in potassium, such as tomatoes, potatoes, and oranges. In addition, acidosis leads to a rise in the serum potassium level, and, hence, maintenance of acid-base equilibrium contributes to maintenance of potassium homeostasis. Some medications, such as penicillin VK, also contain potassium. However, these rarely lead to hyperkalemia.

A serum potassium level of >6 mEq/L must be carefully evaluated by ensuring its accuracy and looking for signs of cardiac toxicity. Inaccuracies in potassium measurement can be due to hemolysis of

TABLE 4. Treatment of Hypertensive Crises

MEDICATION	INITIAL DOSE*	ROUTE OF ADMINISTRATION
Nifedipine	0.25 mg/kg	Sublingual
Labetalol	0.25 mg/kg	IV bolus
	1 mg/kg/h	IV infusion
Hydralazine	0.1–0.2 mg/kg	IV or IM q4h
Nitroprusside	0.5 μg/kg/min	IV infusion

*Dose per administration. A dose for a single bolus and the infusion rate are given for labetalol.

the specimen or to local muscle release of potassium with prolonged tourniquet application. The latter may increase serum potassium by 1 to 2 mEq/L. While awaiting the results of a repeat potassium level, an ECG may be obtained to look for electrical evidence of hyperkalemia (e.g., peaked T waves, widening of the QRS complex, flattened P waves, and, more significantly, ectopic rhythms and intraventricular block). Since conduction abnormalities are due to changes in the membrane potential because of intracellular-extracellular electrolyte partitioning, acute increases in potassium levels are more likely to result in ECG changes at a lower serum level than chronic hyperkalemia. When in doubt, it is best to treat hyperkalemia while awaiting the results of repeat sampling, since reducing a normal potassium level rarely will have any adverse effects, whereas delaying treatment for hyperkalemia can be potentially fatal. In the absence of ECG changes, it is reasonable to treat any serum potassium level greater than 6.5 mEq/L. The potassium load may be decreased by the administration of the exchange resin sodium polystyrene sulfonate (Kayexalate), which is a resin that works by exchanging sodium for potassium via the colonic mucosa. Each gram of Kayexalate per kilogram of body weight can decrease the serum potassium level by about 1 mEq/L, and multiple doses may be administered. Kayexalate can be administered orally or rectally. It is coadministered with sorbitol (20% solution) to decrease the constipation that would result from administration of the resin and decrease its efficacy. Since contact with the colonic mucosa is necessary for its action, rectal administration can more rapidly decrease potassium levels. However, it may be more difficult to administer. To ensure prolonged contact between the gut and the drug, the Kayexalate enema must be retained. This can be accomplished by inserting a Foley catheter into the rectum and inflating the balloon to prevent expulsion of the resin. Since the potassium is exchanged with sodium, the administration of Kayexalate results in a significant sodium load to the patient—a fact that must be kept in mind in patients with hypertension or volume expansion.

In children, potassium levels above 7 mEq/L, especially in conjunction with ECG changes, may cause immediate changes in cardiac membrane polarization, requiring immediate action. Ventricular tachycardia or fibrillation due to hyperkalemia can be reversed with the IV administration of 10% calcium gluconate 0.2 to 0.5 ml/kg over 2 to 5 minutes. Potassium can be driven into the cells and the serum level decreased by administration of IV sodium bicarbonate 1 to 2 mEq/kg or intravenous glucose and insulin. These treatments will only alter the distribution of potassium or diminish cardiac sensitivity to hyperkalemia. They will not decrease the body's potassium content. These patients will, therefore, require a decrease in the potassium burden, which can be achieved through reduction of intake, administration of Kayexalate, and dialysis. The choice of approaches will vary with the setting and condition.

MAINTENANCE OF ACID-BASE BALANCE

There are several potential etiologies for acidosis in CRF, including proximal tubule bicarbonate wasting, inadequate distal tubule ammonia production, and (with severely depressed GFR) retention of sulfates, phosphates, and organic acids. Distal tubular dysfunction resulting in acidosis and hyperkalemia may develop in children with obstructive uropathy with only mild renal insufficiency. As the GFR decreases, all children with CRF will have a metabolic acidosis because of inability to excrete their daily acid load. Chronic acidosis may contribute to poor growth and metabolic bone disease as bone mineralization is diminished by bone buffering of acid.

To compensate for the body's daily acid generation, base supplementation of 2 to 4 mEq/kg is generally needed each day. The amount of acid generated is decreased somewhat by the decreased intake associated with intentional protein and phosphate restriction. Since acid is generated throughout the day, base is optimally supplemented three times a day. The choice of agent depends on the patient's age and preference. Sodium bicarbonate tablets contain 4 to 8 mEq of bicarbonate per tablet. A bicarbonate solution may be made up but

has a very short shelf life. Baking soda, which contains 44 mEq of bicarbonate per teaspoon, can be added to formula or food but is not very palatable. In contrast, citrate solutions are generally well tolerated. The available preparations include Polycitra (1 mEq potassium citrate and 1 mEq sodium citrate per milliliter), Polycitra K (2 mEq of potassium citrate per milliliter), and Bicitra (1 mEq sodium citrate per milliliter). The Polycitra forms are usually avoided because of the potassium load. One milliequivalent of citrate is equivalent to 1 mEq of bicarbonate. Treatment with sodium bicarbonate or citrate also provides a significant sodium load, which may be a particular problem in a child with hypertension or volume problems. An alternative is the provision of base via administration of calcium carbonate, citrate, or acetate.

MAINTENANCE OF CALCIUM AND PHOSPHORUS BALANCE

As the GFR decreases, children with CRF develop hyperphosphatemia as a result of decreased renal phosphate excretion. Hypocalcemia results from decreased intestinal calcium absorption due to decreased renal 1-alpha hydroxylation of 25-hydroxyvitamin D. The decrease in total calcium and increase in serum phosphate result in decreased ionized calcium. The decrease in ionized calcium levels and in 1,25-dihydroxyvitamin D both stimulate an increase in parathyroid hormone (PTH) level. The serum calcium level can initially be maintained by bone resorption. Therefore, a patient's calcium and phosphate balance must be assessed by measurement of calcium, phosphate, and PTH levels. A low normal calcium level accompanied by elevated PTH and alkaline phosphatase levels indicates that the blood calcium level is being maintained at the expense of bone mineralization. It is helpful to obtain a bone series at intervals to assess for the presence of renal osteodystrophy.

To treat the hypocalcemia of CRF appropriately, sufficient dietary calcium must be provided along with replacement of vitamin D to enhance intestinal absorption. The most physiologic approach to vitamin D supplementation is to provide the active vitamin D metabolite, calcitriol (Rocaltrol). It is available in 0.25 and 0.5 μg capsules and is dosed daily. An appropriate starting dose is 0.015 μg/kg/d. Although the half-life of calcitriol is short, is has prolonged biologic activity and can be given in an alternate-day schedule if the size of the smallest capsule prevents daily dosing. Infants or any child who cannot swallow tablets can be treated with dihydrotachysterol (Takerol), which is a synthetic form of vitamin D that requires hepatic hydroxylation. It is available in suspension (0.25 mg/ml) or a tablet (0.125 mg), and 0.01 mg/kg is a reasonable starting dose.

To maintain the ionized calcium level, phosphate restriction is needed. Since nutrients high in phosphate, such as dairy products, are also good sources of calcium, calcium supplementation is needed. This is discussed further later. It is difficult to avoid phosphorus in the diet, since it is contained in almost all foods. Thus, in addition to a phosphorus-restricted diet, patients need to take phosphorus binders with all their main meals and major snacks. In the past, aluminum hydroxide was the mainstay of therapy. However, the aluminum is absorbed and inadequately cleared by the kidneys, so its accumulation can lead to bone disease, anemia, and encephalopathy. Calcium-based binders are now used with the addition of aluminum hydroxide only in rare cases. The use of calcium-based phosphate binders has the added advantage of providing calcium and base, as well as binding dietary phosphate. Calcium carbonate is available in a number of generic preparations and in various flavors in Tums tablets, which are palatable and chewable. There are also liquid preparations. Calcium acetate is available in a number of preparations that may be swallowed intact. Acetate is a better binder of phosphate than carbonate, so that approximately half of the amount can be used. The optimum phosphate binder for an individual child is that preparation that is best tolerated by the patient resulting in improved compliance. As it is necessary to take the phosphate binder at least three times a day, the child's cooperation is necessary. The dose required varies with a child's food intake, so that it is empirical and based on carefully monitored laboratory studies. In addition to the diet, another potential source of phosphorus is a Fleet enema, and this agent should be avoided in children with CRF.

Careful monitoring of calcium and phosphate levels is necessary to determine the appropriate dosing of phosphate binders and vitamin D. The enhanced intestinal absorption of calcium with vitamin D supplementation in the face of inadequate phosphate restriction can lead to hypercalcemia and metastatic calcifications. To monitor a child's bone metabolism optimally, it is helpful to check a PTH level every 6 months in addition to checking the calcium and phosphate every 1 to 3 months.

ERYTHROPOIESIS

Most children with CRF will have a normochromic, normocytic anemia once the GFR is reduced to 20% of normal. Although the primary cause of anemia is deficient erythropoietin synthesis by the kidney, blood loss, decreased erythrocyte survival, and inhibition of erythropoiesis also contribute. Gastrointestinal blood losses, which are due to uremic platelet dysfunction, often result in iron deficiency. Children with CRF should have their iron stores regularly assessed by measurement of iron, total iron-binding capacity (TIBC), and ferritin. The serum ferritin is generally a good measure of iron stores. However, ferritin can be elevated as an acute phase reactant in renal failure. The transferrin saturation (iron/TIBC) is used to monitor the availability of iron for erythropoiesis. A transferrin saturation <15% is insufficient for optimum erythropoiesis, and saturations of 15% to 20% may reflect relative iron deficiency. The transferrin saturation becomes a less useful measure when there is a block of the reticuloendothelial release of iron and the ferritin more accurately reflects iron stores. Iron supplementation with 2 to 6 mg/kg is indicated in children with inadequate iron stores. The choice of iron preparation is primarily determined by the form that will aid in compliance. Ferrous sulfate is readily absorbed and causes the highest incidence of gastrointestinal complaints. Iron polysaccharide preparations are more easily tolerated but have decreased absorption.

Erythrocyte transfusions should be avoided in children with CRF, as they are a potential source of viral infection, as well as alloimmunization. Exposure to multiple HLA antigens may sensitize children so that it is difficult to find a suitable donor for kidney transplant, or if a kidney is found, the risk of graft loss due to rejection is increased. If a transfusion is necessary to treat acute symptoms, relatives who may be sources of living related allografts should not donate blood so that the risk of sensitization to a potential donor is avoided. Treatment with recombinant human erythropoietin should be considered in patients who require regular transfusions and in those who are symptomatic from their anemia. Recombinant erythropoietin must be used with care, in consultation with a physician experienced in its use. A typical initial dose is 50 U/kg (subcutaneously two to three times a week). The erythropoietin comes in single-use vials of 2000, 3000, 4000, and 10,000 U/ml, so the dose should be selected for ease of measurement, as well as optimum use of the product. It is necessary to monitor the hematocrit carefully every 1 to 2 weeks in order to maintain the desired target. The optimum hematocrit is not established, but a reasonable goal is the low end of the normal range for age. To maximize the erythropoietic response to erythropoietin, adequate iron stores are needed. Iron supplementation is reasonable when the transferrin saturation is less than 30%. The increased vascular volume and blood viscosity associated with an increase in hematocrit can exacerbate hypertension and contribute to pulmonary edema in a child who has an expanded vascular volume before treatment. Blood pressure and volume status must be monitored carefully, and hypertension must be treated promptly when correcting anemia with recombinant erythropoietin.

BLEEDING DISORDER

As the degree of uremia increases, children with CRF can develop a bleeding disorder. Most patients with CRF will have a mild to moderate decrease in their platelet number. More importantly, uremia inhibits platelet aggregation. Platelet transfusions are not typically helpful, as the transfused platelets will also be dysfunctional in a uremic environment. The extent of the platelet defect can be assessed by a determination of bleeding time. An abnormal bleeding time increases the risk of a closed procedure, such as renal biopsy, but is less frequently a problem in surgical procedures in which bleeding sites can be visualized and addressed. The platelet function can be temporarily improved by the IV administration of 0.3 μg/kg of 1 deamino-(8-D-arginine)-vasopressin (DDAVP) 30 to 60 minutes before a procedure. The dose can be repeated once after 24 hours. The platelet dysfunction can be exacerbated by the use of inhibitors of platelet aggregation, such as aspirin. The bleeding time has been shown to improve with correction of anemia with recombinant human erythropoietin.

GROWTH

One of the most significant problems for children with CRF is growth retardation. A number of factors may contribute to poor growth, including inadequate nutrition, acidosis, renal osteodystrophy, anemia, and endocrine abnormalities. The level of GFR at which growth is affected varies with the nature of the primary renal disease. Renal tubular defects resulting in acidosis and salt and water wasting may diminish growth at a mildly depressed GFR. Children with cystinosis are also at risk for hypothyroidism, which diminishes growth apart from the effects of renal insufficiency. Their thyroid function should be monitored, and thyroxine treatment should be instituted as appropriate. In addition to the effects of renal disease, treatment with corticosteroids may further diminish growth. The effects of any of these abnormalities on the adult height achieved by children with CRF are greatest in the periods of most rapid growth, that is, infancy and adolescence.

To optimize growth, it is important to make sure that nutrition is adequate. A dietary intake of less than 80% of the RDA has been associated with poor growth in children with CRF. Metabolic abnormalities, including acidosis, hypocalcemia, and hyperphosphatemia, should be adequately treated. In a euthyroid child with well-controlled metabolic status, abnormalities of growth hormone axis should be considered. Children with CRF have a decreased bioactivity of insulin-like growth factor I (IGF-I), which is the mediator of growth hormone activity. Treatment with recombinant human growth hormone can overcome this abnormality despite normal endogenous growth hormone levels. Therefore, it is reasonable to consider recombinant human growth hormone treatment (rhuGH) in a child with CRF who is growing at a subnormal rate (annualized growth velocity less than 4 to 5 cm/y) and has a height below the 5th percentile for age or is falling off the curve. Daily treatment with rhuGH (0.05 mg/kg SC) enhances the growth of children with CRF. The effect of this treatment should be reassessed every 3 to 6 months. If a child shows an inadequate response, his metabolic and nutritional status should be reviewed. If there is no apparent basis for an inadequate response, the dose may be increased. During rhuGH treatment, it is important to monitor calcium metabolism (including PTH levels) carefully, as accelerated growth can exacerbate hyperparathyroid bone disease and result in rickets or slipped epiphyses. Children who are obese or who are receiving corticosteroids should also have glucose metabolism monitored with glucose tolerance tests and glycosylated hemoglobin levels.

ELIMINATION OF DRUGS

The kidney is one of the principle organs involved in elimination of drugs. The physician treating children with CRF with any medication must ask several questions: "Is elimination of this drug impaired in renal insufficiency?" "Is this drug a nephrotoxin that may further diminish renal function?" "Is the availability of the drug altered in uremia?" It is beyond the scope of this section to present an exhaustive listing of drugs and their elimination characteristics. However, listings of those medications that have altered pharmacokinetics in renal failure are readily available in the *PDR* and most formularies. Dose adjustments in uremia can be achieved by decreasing the amount of the individual dose or increasing the interval between doses. The latter approach makes the most sense, as the distribution of the drug is rarely affected by renal failure. Therefore, the peak level attained is unaltered. The rate of metabolism varies, however, resulting in a longer half-life of those drugs that are excreted unchanged in the urine or metabolized by the kidney. Whenever drug levels are easily obtainable, they should be followed. In addition, such drugs as phenytoin, which are highly protein bound, have decreased protein binding in uremia. The free level of the drug is, therefore, increased, so that total as well as free levels should be followed, and the dose should be adjusted on the basis of the free drug levels.

Children with CRF may be more susceptible to the effects of potential nephrotoxins, such as aminoglycosides. Such medications should be used with care, and the drug levels should be closely monitored if such medications are clinically indicated. In addition to the risk for nephrotoxicity, children with CRF are at increased risk for ototoxicity due to repeated courses of aminoglycosides. This effect is cumulative and should be considered in choosing an antibiotic regimen. Nonsteroidal anti-inflammatory agents also should be avoided, since they can reduce renal perfusion and further diminish GFR. Medications that are secreted by the proximal tubule compete with creatinine secretion. As the GFR decreases, a greater proportion of creatinine excretion comes from tubular secretion. Competition for tubular secretion by administration of a medication, such as cimetidine, may increase the serum creatinine level without altering GFR. This should be kept in mind in the evaluation of an acute rise in serum creatinine.

DIET

As may be deduced from the preceding discussion, the nutritional management of the child with CRF must concurrently address two goals: decreasing the intake of foods that are high in substances that cannot be eliminated adequately by a diseased kidney and provision of adequate calories to optimize growth. Dietary intake is often inadequate in children with CRF because of anorexia, dysgeusia or alterations in taste, and dietary restrictions. It is necessary for a renal dietitian to consider a child's eating style and preferences in developing an individualized diet plan. Intake of adequate calories is important in order to maintain an anabolic state, which will both optimize growth and decrease urea generation from amino acids used for energy rather than protein synthesis. The typical diet for a child with CRF should provide at least the RDA for calories, with protein contributing 7% to 9% of the calories. Protein restriction to less than 0.8 g/kg is not recommended for children, as there is no evidence that it will affect the progression of CRF and it will hinder growth. Some children, such as those with nephrosis, will require increased protein intake to compensate for increased losses.

Infants with CRF present a particular nutritional challenge. Most of these infants will have inadequate spontaneous intake and will, therefore, require nasogastric feedings. In addition, many require fluid restriction, so that adequate caloric intake cannot be achieved with standard 20 kcal/oz formula. The formula must be altered by increasing the caloric density through the addition of glucose polymers, corn oil, and in some cases, protein. A caloric density of 40 kcal/oz is easily tolerated, and some infants require increased caloric density as high as 60 kcal/oz. In caring for an infant with CRF, it must be remembered that height lost during the rapid growth of infancy is not easily replaced. If a child has inadequate intake, aggressive measures must be taken to ensure adequate nutrition. This need for special feedings or nasogastric tubes is not readily accepted by some parents, but the clinician must not allow long periods of time to pass with inadequate intake.

RENAL REPLACEMENT THERAPY

Regardless of the primary renal disease responsible for CRF, the renal failure will inexorably progress, and the child will develop ESRD. ESRD is defined by the need for renal replacement therapy with dialysis or transplantation rather than an absolute level of GFR. There are a number of therapeutic decisions for the family to make, so it is important to begin preparations for renal replacement therapy early in the course of CRF. In general, the better informed the child and the family are, the more easily they will deal with ESRD. It is the responsibility of every physician caring for the child with CRF to ensure that the patient is introduced to a team experienced in pediatric dialysis and transplantation. Early discussions include a review of the types of dialysis and the pros and cons of hemodialysis and peritoneal dialysis. Both forms of dialysis are effective for children with CRF. However, peritoneal dialysis is often technically easier in infants and small children. In older children, the choice of dialysis modality is primarily based on the preferences of the child and family. Both hemodialysis and peritoneal dialysis are time consuming, but there are lifestyle differences with the two types of dialysis. Renal transplantation is considered the treatment of choice by pediatric nephrologists, since a well-functioning transplant allows a return to normal homeostasis. Furthermore, a child with a transplant that is functioning well is more likely to have normal cognitive and social development than a child on dialysis. In many cases, careful planning will allow preemptive transplant (transplantation without a prior course of dialysis). There is no absolute level of urea nitrogen or creatinine at which renal replacement is necessary. Treatment should be initiated when there are subtle symptoms of uremia, such as weight loss or increasing fatigue. In addition to medical preparations for dialysis and transplantation, a renal social worker can assist the child and family in dealing with the financial and emotional challenges of CRF. The opportunity to speak with other children and families who have dealt with the same issues is often very helpful.

SOCIAL AND PSYCHOSOCIAL ISSUES

The ultimate goal in the treatment of the child with CRF is to achieve physical and emotional well-being. Children should be encouraged to participate in school fully and to engage in other activities as much as possible. The primary physician can assist the family in interactions with the school. If academic assistance is indicated, it should be provided, but the child should not be kept from normal peer interactions or normal behavioral expectations. It is very rarely necessary for a child to have long-term home tutoring. The family should be assisted in maintaining as close to a normal life as possible. Attention to the home and school environments is important in the long-term social and behavioral development of the child with CRF.

IMMUNIZATIONS

The preventive health care of the child with CRF should not be overlooked. Primary responsiveness to immunizations diminishes with decreasing GFR, so it is important to have the child fully immunized according to current recommendations of the Advisory Committee on Immunization Practices. It may be helpful to follow a schedule for accelerated immunizations in some children. The only contraindications to immunization are the use of live virus vaccines (MMR, polio) in children who are immunocompromised by corticosteroids or other agents. Household contacts of immunocompromised children should not receive live poliovirus vaccine.

PERITONEAL DIALYSIS

Steven R. Alexander, m.d.

The peritoneal cavity has been used in the treatment of children's disorders for at least 70 years. In 1918, Blackfan and Maxcy described the successful treatment of severely dehydrated infants using intraperitoneal injections of saline solution, a technique that is still used today in rural areas of some developing countries. Peritoneal dialysis was first used to treat children with acute renal failure (ARF) more than 40 years ago, and since the 1960s, it has widely been considered to be the dialytic treatment of choice for ARF in infants and young children, primarily because the technique is intrinsically simple, safe, and easily adapted for use in patients of all ages and sizes. The technique has been adapted even for infants weighing as little as 350 g.

Renal replacement therapy for pediatric patients was once limited to peritoneal dialysis in all but the most highly specialized pediatric centers. Many more pediatric nephrology programs can now routinely offer hemodialysis and hemoperfusion in patients weighing as little as 5 kg, and the recent development of continuous hemofiltration [either continuous arteriovenous hemofiltration (CAVH) or continuous venovenous hemofiltration (CVVH)] has added another valuable renal replacement technique to the arsenal of the pediatric nephrologist. However, peritoneal dialysis remains the most frequently employed pediatric renal replacement therapy worldwide for both ARF and chronic renal failure (CRF).

INDICATIONS FOR DIALYSIS

Acute Renal Failure

In general, the indications for renal replacement therapy in children with ARF (see also section in this chapter on Acute Renal Failure) may be summarized as follows.

1. Circulatory overload, usually manifest by congestive heart failure, hypertension, or pulmonary edema
2. Intractable metabolic acidosis
3. Hyperkalemia
4. Severe hyponatremia or hypernatremia in the oligoanuric patient
5. Uremic encephalopathy, usually associated with very high or rapidly rising serum urea nitrogen concentrations
6. Bleeding, if due to uremia
7. The need to remove fluid so that optimal nutrition, transfusions, and other therapies can be given to the oligoanuric patient

For children with ARF, the choice among the available therapeutic modalities (hemodialysis, peritoneal dialysis, or continuous hemofiltration) should take into account the degree of expertise of the facility as well as the patient's size, clinical condition, and prognosis for recovery of renal function. Severe, life-threatening hyperkalemia or acidosis is most effectively treated with hemodialysis, although peritoneal dialysis may be preferred in some centers because of the rapidity with which it can be instituted. The hemodynamically unstable patient will tolerate hemodialysis poorly and should be treated with peritoneal dialysis or continuous hemofiltration. Hemodialysis or hemoperfusion is preferred for treatment of poisonings.

Chronic Renal Failure

Chronic maintenance dialysis is required when the creatinine clearance falls below 5 to 10 ml/min/1.73 m². Dialysis is often instituted at higher clearances in infants and young children when growth is poor, especially if head circumference growth rate falls below normal. The decision to begin chronic dialysis must always be individualized, but every effort must be made to begin dialysis soon enough to avoid any potentially severe or life-threatening consequences of renal failure, such as circulatory overload or hyperkalemia. Dialysis is often begun while the child is being prepared for renal transplantation, although nearly 25% of North American children now receive transplants without any prior dialysis.

Today, the chronic dialytic therapy of choice for most young pediatric patients (those younger than 15 years of age) in North America and parts of western Europe is continuous peritoneal dialysis (CPD), which can be performed in the home. CPD can be performed manually (i.e., continuous ambulatory peritoneal dialysis, CAPD) or with the aid of an automated cycler (i.e., continuous cycling peritoneal dialysis, CCPD, or nightly intermittent peritoneal dialysis, NIPD). These therapies may be used in children of any age, and all offer distinct advantages over hemodialysis as maintenance renal replacement ther-

apy: near steady-state biochemical and fluid control, no disequilibrium syndrome, greatly reduced dietary restrictions, freedom from repeated dialysis needle punctures, improved control of hypertension, and a reduced requirement for blood transfusions (which now is reflected in lower required doses of recombinant human erythropoietin). Most important, the simplicity and safety of CPD allow performance in the home by all but the most disrupted families, thereby returning the child with end-stage renal disease (ESRD) to regular school attendance and allowing family vacations and other normal childhood activities. During CAPD, the child (most children assume responsibility for some, if not all, of their own CPD home care after age 11 or 12 years) or the parent exchanges the dialysis solution four or five times in each 24 hours, using plastic containers commercially available in several different volumes and dextrose concentrations. In CCPD and NIPD, an automated cycler is employed to perform the fluid exchanges during the 8 to 12 hours that the infant or child is in bed each night. Cycler dialysis has several advantages over CAPD in convenience for the child and the family, making it the current favorite in many large pediatric dialysis centers in the United States.

Of the cycler techniques, NIPD is becoming increasingly popular. When the daytime exchange volume is <50% of the usual nighttime exchange volume, the treatment is, by convention, termed NIPD. There are children who do not tolerate the daytime exchange. Patients with a history of abdominal wall hernias, prune-belly syndrome, and continent urinary tract diversions do better with NIPD. In small children, the daytime exchange may contribute to anorexia. Adolescents frequently complain about the cosmetic effects of the daytime exchange, preferring a near-empty abdomen, which they believe allows them to wear more stylish clothing.

It is necessary to prescribe more nightly exchanges with NIPD to achieve solute clearances equal to those obtained with CAPD or CCPD. Middle molecule clearance with NIPD will always be inferior to that of CAPD or CCPD, resulting in as yet unknown long-term effects.

Another variant of peritoneal dialysis, tidal peritoneal dialysis (TPD), also is used in some children to decrease dialysis time or to improve dialysis tolerance. The technique is essentially a cycling technique in which the initial fill is large (40 to 50 ml/kg), and then subsequent relatively rapid partial drainage and refill (10 to 25 ml/kg) is performed without full emptying until all cycles are done.

CONTRAINDICATIONS TO PERITONEAL DIALYSIS

There are few absolute contraindications to peritoneal dialysis in pediatric patients. The absence of an adequate peritoneal cavity, as in infants with omphalocele, diaphragmatic hernia, or gastroschisis, is an obvious contraindication. Recent abdominal surgery is only a relative contraindication, as long as there are no draining abdominal wounds. Patients with urinary tract diversions, such as vesicostomies or ureterostomies, and with bilateral polycystic kidneys, colostomies, gastrostomies, and prune-belly syndrome have all been successfully treated with peritoneal dialysis. Following renal transplantation, peritoneal dialysis can be used to treat acute renal allograft dysfunction or severe rejection episodes when the allograft has been placed in an extraperitoneal location. Extensive intraabdominal adhesions may prevent successful peritoneal dialysis in some patients. The presence of a ventriculoperitoneal shunt in hydrocephalic children or the presence of a severe infection of the abdominal wall may also be a relative contraindication, although, again, the decision to begin peritoneal dialysis must be individualized, weighing risks against the availability of an alternative dialytic method.

PHYSIOLOGIC PRINCIPLES

The physiology of peritoneal dialysis has been studied extensively in adult subjects, but relatively few studies have been done in children. The peritoneum functions as a semipermeable membrane that permits the passage of water and solutes by the processes of diffusion and convection. Anatomic studies have shown that the surface area of the peritoneum is proportional to that of the body surface area in both children and adults. Thus, the peritoneal membrane in the child is larger, relative to body weight, than in the adult, and this property may be reflected by an increased ability to transfer solutes and water across the peritoneum of younger patients. Available data on this subject remain sparse and inconclusive, however. What is known is that the child's peritoneum allows passage of glucose into the blood from the dialysate and the transfer of proteins out of the blood into the dialysate more rapidly than is seen in adults. Removal of fluid (ultrafiltration) from children, especially infants, may be difficult using long-dwell exchanges (e.g., >2 hours) because the relatively rapid absorption of dextrose from the dialysate results in a more rapid decline in the osmolar gradient between blood and dialysate. Higher concentrations of dextrose in the dialysate and shorter dwell times are commonly employed in infants to offset these problems. Recent studies have suggested that the subdiaphragmatic lymphatic absorption of dialysate is greater in children than in adults, providing yet another reason why ultrafiltration may be difficult in some children.

CATHETER PLACEMENT

Access to the peritoneal cavity may be achieved readily using a temporary (percutaneous) catheter, although after about 72 hours, the incidence of peritonitis rises sharply when the same temporary catheter is used. Surgical placement of a chronic peritoneal catheter, even in the setting of ARF, has the obvious advantages of ensuring good immediate function and indefinite catheter life span. These advantages must be weighed in the individual patient against the risks and delays associated with an operative procedure that may require general anesthesia.

Percutaneous placement of a temporary peritoneal catheter in children is a simple procedure requiring great care and attention to detail. This procedure has been associated with all of the serious complications one might expect to see in cases of penetrating abdominal trauma, from massive hemorrhage to bowel perforation. Disposable catheters appropriate for use in children are widely available. Traditional techniques employ a trocar to perforate the peritoneum, which is distended at the time of catheter placement. This method has been replaced in some centers by the use of a modified Seldinger technique, which eliminates the trocar. The Seldinger technique requires puncture of the only mildly distended peritoneal cavity with an 18-gauge needle, through which a guidewire is inserted into the peritoneal cavity. The needle is then withdrawn. The hole in the abdominal wall and peritoneum is enlarged with dilators of increasing size inserted over the guidewire until the peritoneal catheter is itself inserted over the guidewire, and the guidewire is then withdrawn.

Although the Seldinger (guidewire) method is gaining popularity, the trocar technique is still widely used, and many of the technical pearls are common to both methods. The trocar technique is described in detail next.

Trocar Catheter Insertion

The catheter is inserted as follows.

1. Empty the bladder with a small sterile feeding tube (8 French). This tube is removed after successful placement of the peritoneal catheter to reduce the risk of urinary tract infection.
2. Ensure adequate sedation of older infants and children. Adults can be instructed to perform a Valsalva maneuver at the moment of trocar insertion, but children are rarely able to cooperate to this degree. Good sedation may increase the intraperitoneal priming volume required to safely perforate the now relaxed child's peritoneum. Careful attention must be given to cardiorespiratory status throughout the procedure to prevent respiratory embarrassment caused by a large priming volume.
3. Scrub the skin of the lower abdomen with a surgical skin cleaner, followed by the application of an appropriate antiseptic, such as povidone-iodine.

4. Inject a local anesthetic subcutaneously and carry down to the peritoneum at a point in the midline that is two-thirds the distance up from the symphysis to the umbilicus.
5. Use a 16-gauge polyethylene over-the-needle catheter (e.g., Intracath) to infuse dialysate to distend the abdomen. Smaller needles (18 to 21 gauge) may be used without polyethylene catheters, but inflow is slower and subcutaneous dialysate infusion may go unrecognized for some time. The Intracath (with needle in place) is attached to the dialysate inflow line and inserted below the skin surface. An assistant then opens the clamp on the inflow line. By watching the drip chamber in the inflow line, one can see dialysate pass drop by drop into the subcutaneous tissue. The Intracath is then advanced until a steady stream of dialysate is observed in the drip chamber, demonstrating free flow of dialysate into the peritoneal cavity. The needle catheter is advanced a bit farther, with the inflow line momentarily detached while the steel needle is withdrawn, the line reattached, and the remaining plastic catheter advanced until it is well within the peritoneal cavity. At least 30 ml/kg of warmed dailysate is infused while close attention is given to the vital signs of the child. Neonates may require additional ventilatory or circulatory support or both at this stage. When adequately filled, the abdomen will be fully distended, and the abdominal wall will be taut enough to provide firm resistance to insertion of the dialysis trocar catheter. Large priming volumes may be required. The absolute limit in each case is determined by the point at which the inflow stream begins to fluctuate with respiration.
6. After removing the Intracath, make a small stab wound with a No. 11 blade at the site of the puncture, with care taken not to enter the peritoneum proper.
7. Trim the dialysis catheter, if necessary, for smaller infants. Ideal intraperitoneal catheter length may be estimated as 1 cm less than the distance from xiphoid to umbilicus. This ensures that the first fenestrations of the catheter will reside at least 3 cm inside the peritoneal cavity. Generally, short catheters perform better than long ones. The cut edges of a trimmed catheter should be beveled with iris scissors to reduce the risk of injury to abdominal viscera.
8. Insert the catheter and trocar together (the catheter riding the trocar into the peritoneal cavity), using a rotating motion and steady pressure directed at right angles to the plane of the abdominal wall at the insertion site. Considerable force may be needed to puncture the peritoneum. If the abdominal wall can be depressed substantially without penetrating the peritoneum, additional distending fluid is needed. Once the peritoneum has been penetrated, the trocar and catheter are directed toward the right or left lower quadrant. The catheter is advanced as the trocar is withdrawn.
9. When good inflow and outflow of dialysate have been demonstrated, trim the extraabdominal portion of the catheter so that only 4 to 6 cm extends above the abdominal wall. The catheter is secured with a silk pursestring suture and water-resistant tape.
10. Should initial in-and-out exchanges yield cloudy or persistently bloody fluid or result in the appearance of diarrhea or polyuria (the high dextrose concentration of dialysate quickly resolves any question about the origin of the diarrhea or polyuria), remove the catheter immediately and replace it. Poor catheter drainage is a much more frequently encountered problem at this stage and is usually due to omental envelopment or obstruction of the temporary catheter. When this occurs, it is probably best to replace the temporary catheter with a surgically placed chronic catheter.
11. When a percutaneously placed catheter is used, initial exchange volumes are usually 20 to 30 ml/kg, with a gradual increase to 40 to 50 ml/kg over the first 24 hours of dialysis. When surgically placed catheters are used, a smaller exchange volume (20 ml/kg) is necessary during the initial 24 hours of dialysis to reduce the likelihood of dialysate leakage at the insertion site.
12. Warm the dialysate to body temperature to prevent hypothermia and enhance diffusion of small solutes.

TABLE 1. Peritoneal Dialysis Solution Containing Bicarbonate*

	ml	Na$^+$ (mEq)	Cl$^-$ (mEq)	Mg^{2+} (mEq)	SO$_4^{2-}$ (mEq)	HCO$_3^-$ (mEq)	HYDROUS DEXTROSE (g)
NaCl (0.45%)	896	69	69				
NaCl (2.5 mEq/ml)	12	30	30				
NaHCO$_3$ (1 mEq/ml)	40	40				40	
MgSO$_4$ (10%)	1.8			1.5	1.5		
D$_{50}$W	50						25
Total	998.8	139	99	1.5	1.5	40	25

Modified from Nash MA, Russo JC: Neonatal lactic acidosis and renal failure: The role of peritoneal dialysis. J Pediatr 91:101–105, 1977.
*Calculated osmolality = 423 mOsm/kg H$_2$O.

PRESCRIPTION IN ACUTE RENAL FAILURE

The initial peritoneal dialysis prescription for the child with acute renal failure should reflect the clinical status of the patient and the goals of dialytic therapy. In the severely uremic child with hyperkalemia and acidosis, frequent exchanges are used during the initial stabilization on dialysis. With dialysate that contains 2.5% dextrose, the exchange volume is infused over 5 to 10 minutes, allowed to dwell for 15 to 35 minutes, and allowed to drain for 5 to 15 minutes. More than two complete exchanges per hour can be accomplished but are rarely worthwhile. The amount of ultrafiltration required is determined by the fluid status of the child. Relatively euvolemic children may be dialyzed with 1.5% dextrose solutions, although adequate fluid removal to allow intravenous alimentation, transfusions, and other therapies often necessitates the use of 2.5% dextrose solutions. The most hypertonic solution (4.25% dextrose) is reserved for patients who are fluid overloaded. Hyperglycemia, hypernatremia, and hypovolemia are common complications associated with prolonged use of 4.25% dextrose solutions. Heparin (500 U/L) is routinely added to the dialysate during the first 24 hours of treatment and during episodes of peritonitis.

Some critically ill infants are unable to tolerate the lactate that is absorbed from commercially available dialysis solutions because absorbed lactate worsens the lactic acidosis in these patients. Dialysate can be reformulated to contain bicarbonate instead of lactate, as shown in Table 1. Note that calcium must be supplemented intravenously when bicarbonate-containing dialysate is used.

Initial stabilization on peritoneal dialysis often requires 24 to 48 hours of frequent exchanges (30 to 60 minutes each, depending on catheter function and nursing staff resources) to remove accumulated solutes and excess fluid and to correct acidosis and hypertension. Once the patient is stabilized, if a permanent catheter is in place, peritoneal dialysis may be continued indefinitely while the return of renal function is awaited. By gradual extension of dwell periods and increase in exchange volumes, a typical maintenance CAPD regimen (e.g., 35 to 40 ml/kg per exchange, four to six exchanges per 24 hours) may be reached in a few days. Continuous, prolonged-dwell peritoneal dialysis (either CAPD or CCPD) has become the standard approach to the treatment of ARF in our center, once the child has been stabilized with an appropriate period of frequent exchanges to correct fluid and electrolyte disturbances and to lower the blood urea nitrogen (BUN). The near steady-state biochemical and fluid control achievable with CAPD and CCPD may be of particular benefit to critically ill children with ARF whose cardiovascular status may be precarious.

PERITONITIS

The most common complication of both acute and chronic peritoneal dialysis is peritonitis. Sixty-five percent of children treated with CAPD or CCPD for ESRD have at least one episode of peritonitis before they have completed the first 12 months of therapy. The most frequently cultured pathogens are *Staphylococcus epidermidis* and *Staphylococcus aureus,* although gram-negative organisms and *Can-*

dida sp. account for 20% to 30% of peritonitis episodes. Antimicrobial agents should not be administered prophylactically but, rather, should be started empirically before culture results are available when patients show signs and symptoms of peritonitis. Peritonitis usually presents with cloudy peritoneal effluent in a mildly febrile child who may also have abdominal pain and tenderness. The peritoneal effluent will usually contain more than 100 white blood cells per cubic millimeter, more than 50% of which are polymorphonuclear neutrophils. Although gram stain of the centrifuged effluent demonstrates organisms in only 25% of cases that eventually show positive cultures, it is still a worthwhile test because gram stains provide the first evidence of fungal (usually *Candida*) infections, allowing early institution of antifungal therapy. When signs and symptoms of peritonitis are present, a sample for gram stain, cell count, and culture is obtained, and antibiotic therapy is begun immediately, using the intraperitoneal route.

Authorities now recommend beginning intraperitoneal therapy with either of the following combinations: a first-generation cephalosporin with an aminoglycoside or a third-generation cephalosporin with vancomycin. Empiric therapy continues until bacteriologic identification of the organism has been accomplished. Dosages for typical initial (empiric) intraperitoneal antibiotic therapy are shown in Table 2. Currently recommended doses and routes for many antimicrobials commonly used to treat peritonitis are shown in Table 3.

Although uncommon, fungal peritonitis remains a serious problem. Following an episode of fungal peritonitis, many children suffer peritoneal membrane failure and must be transferred to hemodialysis. Treatment is controversial. Amphotericin B, given intravenously, and catheter removal remain the mainstays of therapy for fungal peritonitis in most pediatric dialysis programs. The current approach begins with amphotericin B given at a dose of 1 mg/kg in a single daily IV infusion, after one daily dose at 0.25 mg/kg to observe for adverse reactions. After the third day of therapy, the dialysis catheter is removed, and the child is treated for a short period (3 to 7 days) with hemodialysis. At this point, a new permanent peritoneal dialysis catheter is surgically implanted, and treatment with amphotericin B is continued for a total of 21 days. The short period of hemodialysis is intended to allow sterilization of the peritoneal cavity in the absence

TABLE 2. Empiric Intraperitoneal Antibiotic Dosages for Suspected CPD Peritonitis

	LOADING DOSE*	MAINTENANCE DOSE
Cephalothin† *plus*	25 mg/kg (in a single exchange)	250 mg/L
tobramycin† *or*	1.7 mg/kg (in a single exchange)	6 mg/L
Vancomycin† *plus*	15 mg/kg (in a single exchange)	30 mg/L
ceftazidime†	25 mg/kg (in a single exchange)	125 mg/L

*Loading doses are not recommended in minimally symptomatic patients.
†May be mixed in dialysis fluid without affecting potency.

TABLE 3. Antibiotic Dosing Guidelines for Peritonitis in Children Receiving Continuous Peritoneal Dialysis

| | DOSE* | | |
| | INITIAL | | MAINTENANCE |
	mg/kg	mg/L of Dialysate	(mg/L of Dialysate)
Aminoglycosides†			
Amikacin‡	5–7.5 IV/IP	—	6–12
Gentamicin‡	1.5–1.7 IV/IP	—	4–8
Netilmicin‡	1.5–2 IV/IP	—	4–8
Tobramycin‡	1.5–1.7 IV/IP	—	4–8
Cephalosporins: First Generation			
Cefazolin	—	500	250
Cefonicid	—	125	25
Cephalothin	—	500	100
Cephradine	—	250	125
Cephalexin	12.5 PO		12.5–25 mg/kg per dose q8h PO
Cephalosporins: Second Generation			
Cefamandole	—	500	250
Cefmenoxine	—	1000	50
Cefoxitin	—	500	100
Cefuroxime	—	500	75–200
Cephalosporins: Third Generation			
Cefoperazone	—	1000	200–500
Cefotaxime	—	1000	250
Cefsulodin	—	500	25
Ceftazidime	—	500	125
Ceftizoxime	—	500	125
Ceftriaxone	—	500	125–250
Penicillins†			
Ampicillin	—	250	50
Azlocillin	—	250	250
Ticarcillin	—	500–1000	125
Miscellaneous			
Vancomycin	15 IV/IP	—	15–30
Clindamycin	—	150	150
Aztreonam	—	500	250
Imipenem	—	500	100
Cilastin	—	250–500	50–100
Trimethoprim	—	—	40
Sulfamethoxazole	—	—	200

*Current recommendations are adapted from the adult literature and are subject to change as new information on pediatric dosage becomes available.
† Aminoglycosides and penicillins cannot be mixed for intraperitoneal (IP) administration.
‡ Blood levels should be monitored to avoid toxicity.

of a foreign body (the catheter) while limiting the time off peritoneal dialysis and, thus, the opportunity for intraperitoneal adhesions to form. Some authorities advocate the addition of oral antifungal agents (e.g., fluconazole or ketoconazole) to the intravenous amphotericin B regimen, but this advice is controversial.

HEMODIALYSIS

ROBERT A. WEISS, M.D.

Although successful kidney transplantation provides the optimal mode of renal replacement therapy for the child with end-stage renal disease (ESRD), a kidney may not be available. Thus, dialytic therapy is the necessary bridge to sustain life until transplantation (or retransplantation). Absolute indications to initiate dialysis usually occur when the glomerular filtration rate (GFR) falls below 5 ml/min/1.73 m². Serum concentrations of BUN and creatinine are not very reliable as indicators of GFR, as BUN depends on dietary protein intake, which may decline with anorexia of uremia, and there may be loss of muscle mass (creatinine is generated from muscle creatine) as well. The mean of the urea and creatinine clearance is the best estimate of GFR under these circumstances. Biochemical indications to start dialysis include hyperkalemia (>6 mEq/L), hypocalcemia (<7 mg/dl) usually due to hyperphosphatemia, and acidosis (serum HCO_3 < 12 mEq/L). Clinical symptoms are vague: fatigue (most frequently attributed to the accompanying anemia of advanced chronic renal failure, CRF), malaise, anorexia, nausea, vomiting, and disturbances in sleep pattern and concentration. Clinical signs include drug-resistant hypertension, encephalopathy, pericarditis, neuropathy, and extracellular fluid (ECF) volume overload. Similar parameters indicate the need for emergency dialysis for acute renal failure (ARF).

Hemodialysis (HD) is a process by which accumulated solutes that are normally cleared by the kidneys via glomerular filtration leave the blood by diffusion across a semipermeable membrane. The concentration gradient is maintained by countercurrent flow of a crystalloid solution on the other side of the membrane. Regulation of ECF volume is accomplished by convective transport of isotonic fluid down a transmembrane pressure gradient generated by the positive hydrostatic pressure in the blood compartment and negative pressure in the dialysate compartment. This process is termed ultrafiltration (UF). Most HD patients undergo treatment thrice weekly for 3 to 4 hours per session. It is important to recognize that 9 to 12 hours of HD per week is only sufficient to ameliorate or prevent some, but not all, of the complications of uremia and that HD is quite unphysiologic by its intermittent nature.

Of the 130,000 adults who require maintenance dialysis therapy for ESRD, 85% receive HD, usually at a medical facility. In contrast, the proportion for children is closer to 50%, with the rest receiving peritoneal dialysis (PD), a home technique. However, as is frequently the case for pediatric patients with advanced CRF, a parental kidney donor is available, transplantation is undertaken just before the patient reaches ESRD, and thus dialysis is avoided. The majority of pediatric HD patients are those waiting for a cadaver donor (no live-related donor available) either for a first or a repeat transplant and those for whom PD has failed or is not chosen as the dialytic modality. Thus, only a small proportion of such pediatric ESRD patients require more than several years of dialytic support. In contrast, adults with ESRD frequently receive long-term maintenance HD because of medical contraindications to transplantation or lack of interest.

VASCULAR ACCESS

In general, the choice of dialysis modality is dictated by the ability to access the semipermeable membrane (artificial in the case of HD, natural in the case of PD). Since diffusive transport of solutes is dependent on the rate of blood flow delivered to the membrane, HD requires access to a high rate of flow venous system. For emergency HD, the femoral-iliac system can be accessed via a percutaneously placed double-lumen catheter (one for blood withdrawal, the other for blood return). HD catheter lumens are specifically designed with a large internal diameter to minimize resistance and, thus, maximize blood flow. This access site is amenable only for children >15 kg. Its location makes the risk of infection significant and confines the patient to the recumbent position. Generally, the catheter is inserted and removed for each HD treatment, which limits its use to the short term. In contrast, the right atrium catheter is typically inserted percutaneously in the operating room via the internal jugular system and tunneled to exit on the upper chest wall. Such devices are frequently used also for permanent vascular access in infants and small (<15 kg) children. Despite the potential complications of infection or thrombosis or both, catheter survival is typically measured in weeks to months. For older and larger children for whom permanent vascular access is required, an arteriovenous fistula is created. The radial or brachial artery is anastomosed to the cephalic vein to produce several high blood flow rate venous tributaries. The arterialization process requires several weeks, so that this form of vascular access is not practical for emergency or temporary HD. To access the fistula, any two veins are punctured with large-gauge (low-resistance) needles, one for blood withdrawal and one for blood return. As the success of fistula surgery is correlated to vessel size and fistula vein puncture is painful (two needles thrice weekly!), infants and young children generally receive HD via catheter, and older children and adolescents by fistula. An alternative to the fistula is the surgical interposition of either a prosthetic (polytetrafluoroethylene) or autologous (saphenous vein) blood vessel between a native artery and vein in either the upper or lower extremity. This conduit can be punctured in the same fashion as arterialized native veins for HD. However, the longevity of the prosthetic graft frequently is compromised by infection or thrombosis or both, similar to the right atrial catheter. An additional potential complication of such arteriovenous shunts is high-output congestive heart failure. Data are being accumulated in a national registry to assess technique survival, as vascular access difficulties frequently require switching either temporarily or permanently from HD to PD.

HEMODIALYSIS PRESCRIPTION

This term is defined as the dialyzer (plastic casing that contains the semipermeable membrane) selected, duration of individual treatment, number of treatments per week, blood flow rate, dialysate (crystalloid solution selected to flow countercurrent to blood in the dialyzer), and heparinization schedule. The goal is to provide sufficient clearance of small molecular weight solutes by diffusion and sufficient isotonic fluid removal to restore ECF volume to normal, so that the symptoms and signs of uremia are minimized. Quantitation of the adequacy of HD has been standardized for adults but not for children. The term

K_t/V = clearance of urea in ml/min by dialyzer × time in minutes/estimated volume of distribution of urea (total body water × weight in kg)

is thought to be the best reflection of HD efficiency. Because actual urea clearance, rather than the dialyzer manufacturer's data, and the actual volume of distribution of urea are difficult to measure under routine circumstances, most nephrologists use the urea reduction ratio

Urea reduction ratio = difference between pre- and post-HD BUN/pre-HD BUN

A value of >60% correlates well with a K_t/V of >1.2, which in turn is associated with adequate HD.

The extracorporeal circuit (dialyzer and blood tubing) should be no more than 10% of the estimated blood volume, lest hemorrhagic hypotension occur. Whereas a wide variety (size, diffusion, and ultrafiltration characteristics) of dialyzers is available for adults, this is not the case for the small dialyzers needed for infants and children. Dialyzer selection is usually first based on the priming volume, that is, the volume of blood contained in the dialyzer, then the urea clearance achievable at the blood flow rate that the vascular access can provide. Ideally, one aims for a urea clearance of 2 to 3 ml/min/kg. For example, a 10 kg infant has an estimated blood volume of 75 ml/kg = 750 ml. Neonatal tubing has a volume of 28 ml, and the smallest dialyzer, 0.41 m² surface area, has a priming volume of 40 ml. Thus, the extracorporeal circuit would contain 68 ml, less than 10% of the 750 ml blood volume of the patient. Selection of a larger dialyzer or blood tubing would be unwise. If HD is necessary for smaller infants, the extracorporeal circuit can be primed with blood (circuited through a warmer!) from the blood bank.

The blood flow rate selected is the highest that the vascular access can support, given the resistance in the system, without producing excessive pressure on the dialysis membrane, with the attendant risk of rupture and blood loss. A good fistula or graft can support 300 to 400 ml/min. Blood flow rates of 50 to 100 ml/min for an infant undergoing HD via right atrial double-lumen catheter are acceptable.

The duration of each treatment is generally 3 to 4 hours, adjusted according to the measures of HD efficiency mentioned previously. Lower blood flow rates translate into longer treatments to accomplish similar urea clearance. Three HD treatments per week are sufficient for most chronic or maintenance HD patients. However, those who are unwilling or unable to adhere to the dietary limitations required to limit interdialytic expansion of ECF volume (salt and water restriction) may require a fourth treatment per week. Selection of dialysate is usually limited to commercially available solutions. There is flexibility in the potassium concentration (most commonly 2 mEq/L to provide a steep enough concentration gradient for removal by diffusion), calcium (usually 3.5 mEq/L to produce net influx of Ca from dialysate bath to the patient's blood), and either acetate as a base precursor or bicarbonate. Systemic heparinization is required to prevent clotting as blood contacts the dialyzer membrane. Activated clotting time is used to regulate the degree of anticoagulation. If the patient is at high risk for bleeding, the heparin dose can be reduced or infused into the tubing just before the dialyzer with a protamine infusion as blood leaves the dialyzer (regional heparinization). Alternatively, citrate can be used as an anticoagulant. Finally, the patient's dry weight is estimated as that body weight for which ECF volume is normal. Generally, the patient's blood pressure is correlated with ECF volume, and ultrafiltration to below the dry weight produces hypotension because of excessive contraction of ECF volume. Since there is no or only limited excretion of salt and water during the hours between HD treatments, ECF volume expands from dietary intake of salt and water, with a rise in blood pressure. Each HD treatment must restore the ECF volume by ultrafiltration back to the patient's dry weight.

NUTRITION AND DIET

Studies in both adults and children have demonstrated the clinical and biochemical similarities between protein-calorie malnutrition and uremia. Thus, although adequate HD replaces a small proportion of normal excretory function, anorexia persists. In addition, the diet is restricted in sodium, potassium, and water, which makes it difficult to achieve even the RDA for protein and calories. The degree of restriction often depends on whether or not there is some residual GFR, as even 2 ml/min/1.73 m² generally means the patient will produce several hundred milliliters of urine daily, with substantial excretion of sodium and potassium, which, in turn, can permit the patient a more liberal diet. The nutritional goal for calories is 2000/m², for protein 3 to 4 g/kg for infants with linear reduction to 1g/kg for adolescents, and for fluids 400 ml/m² to replace insensible water losses plus urine output. Conventional restriction of dietary sodium and potassium is 40 mEq/m² and 30 mEq/m², respectively. As hyperphosphatemia is intimately involved in the pathogenesis of renal osteodystrophy, intake of phosphorus should also be restricted. However, since phosporous is ubiquitous in foodstuffs, this is not practical. Such agents as calcium carbonate, citrate, and acetate are used with meals to bind phosphorous into an insoluble calcium salt, which is then excreted in the stool. The doses of these preparations are adjusted according to the serum phosphorus concentration and the nature of the patient's food preferences. Finally, a daily multivitamin that includes folic acid (removed by HD) is recommended.

COMPLICATIONS OF HEMODIALYSIS

Anemia

The erythropoietin produced by normal kidney tissue, deficiency of which is the main cause of the anemia of ESRD, is now commercially available for replacement therapy. Most HD patients receive 50 to 150 U/kg IV into the dialysis tubing during each HD treatment. As long as iron stores are sufficient, HD patients can be maintained with a normal hemoglobin concentration. The only untoward effect of exogenous erythropoietin therapy is the rise in blood pressure associated with the increase in blood volume. At worst, this requires intensification of the patient's antihypertensive drug regimen. The success of exogenous erythropoietin in avoiding the need for blood transfusion has virtually eliminated transfusion-associated diseases, such as hepatitis B and C, which previously had been a major source of morbidity for HD patients. HD patients should undergo the hepatitis B vaccination series.

Blood Pressure

Most HD patients are chronically hypertensive due to inability to regulate ECF volume and a dysregulated renin-angiotensin system. The dietary salt restriction and ultrafiltration during HD frequently are sufficient to control ECF volume and, thus, blood pressure (BP). Those HD patients whose BP requires drug therapy can receive any antihypertensives, but some, such as the angiotensin-converting enzyme inhibitor class, require an extended dosing interval. In the rare circumstance that BP cannot be controlled by the combination of diet, ultrafiltration, and drugs, bilateral nephrectomy is indicated to remove the source of renin.

Hypotension can occur during HD, particularly when aggressive ultrafiltration is required to remove salt and water that has accumulated since the most recent HD treatment. The ultrafiltration process during HD removes salt and water from the plasma volume. If interstitial fluid fails to refill this space rapidly enough, *hypotension* may result, requiring saline infusion to restore BP. This can become a vicious cycle, with saline infused during HD to maintain BP resulting in an expanded ECF volume and *hypertension* after the HD treatment is terminated. Mannitol (0.5 to 1 g/kg) infusion during HD to produce an osmotic shift of interstitial salt and water into the plasma volume is often useful to counteract this sequence of events.

Cardiovascular Effects

Left ventricular hypertrophy, secondary to chronic hypertension, is a very strong predictor of mortality among adult HD patients. In addition, most HD patients have both hypercholesterolemia (with high LDL fraction) and hypertriglyceridemia. These conditions result in accelerated atherosclerosis (coronary artery/cerebrovascular disease) in adults and probably in children as well. Pediatric HD patients should undergo surveillance echocardiography, and every effort should be made to maintain normal BP. To date, there has been very little experience with long-term drug therapy for the hyperlipidemia of uremia for such patients.

Pericarditis is an uncommon manifestation of advanced uremia and occurs either around the time ESRD is reached or after months to years of maintenance HD. It is observed less frequently in PD patients, and the risk of hemorrhage into the pericardial sac is increased by the heparinization generally required for HD. The treatment usually is intensified HD for several weeks, although some nephrologists switch pericarditis patients to PD, not only to avoid heparinization but also because PD may clear as yet unknown toxins associated with the development of pericarditis. Surgical pericardiectomy and pericardial window, as well as intrapericardial steroids, have been used for more resistant cases. Cardiac tamponade and late constrictive pericarditis are the most serious complications of pericarditis in HD patients.

Osteodystrophy

Lack of the 1-alpha-hydroxylase normally found in healthy kidney tissue results in deficiency of 1,25-dihydroxycholecalciferol (calcitriol), which, in part through chronic hypocalcemia, produces hyperplasia of the parathyroid glands. This secondary hyperparathyroidism produces the osteitis fibrosa bone lesion of renal osteodystrophy, which can be very debilitating in infants and children. Fortunately, calcitriol is now available commercially and frequently is given intravenously during each HD treatment. However, careful attention must be paid to serum calcium and phosphorus. Hyperphosphatemia in ESRD is due to limited excretion of the daily burden of dietary phosphorus. Removal of phosphorus by HD is not sufficient to restore the serum phosphorus concentration to normal without the use of calcium salts to limit gastrointestinal absorption of dietary

phosphorus. The concentration of calcium in the dialysis bath (dialysate) is important in the regulation of serum calcium concentration, which, in turn, feeds back on parathyroid hormone secretion. Currently, the use of calcium salts as phosphorus binders, with exogenous calcitriol therapy, can result in *hypercalcemia*. This condition, when associated with the hyperphosphatemia of ESRD, may cause extraskeletal calcification, both vascular and soft tissue. Thus, low-calcium (2.5 or 3 mEq/L) dialysate is now prescribed for many HD patients. This maneuver allows intensive use of calcitriol, which is the most efficacious method to suppress parathyroid hyperplasia. Should this form of therapy fail to control the osteitis fibrosa of secondary hyperparathyroidism, surgical three and three-quarters parathyroidectomy, with or without implantation of the remaining fragments of parathyroid tissue into the subcutaneous tissue of the forearm for later retrieval, is necessary.

Seizures

Although urea is not an effective osmol, distributing itself throughout the total body water compartment, patients with very high BUN (>150 mg/dl) are at risk for the dialysis disequilibrium syndrome. It most frequently occurs during the first or second HD treatment. This is an encephalopathic state, typically associated with generalized seizure(s), which is thought to be due to rapid removal of osmoles from the brain. It can be prevented by slow reduction of urea by inefficient HD (low blood flow rate) and the use of intravenous mannitol or high-sodium dialysate to limit osmolar shift. Those pediatric HD patients with a preexisting seizure disorder are at even higher risk. Acute drug therapy for seizures in HD patients is similar to that for children with normal renal function, as all anticonvulsants are metabolized by the liver. However, there is a difference in protein binding of phenytoin in uremia.

Psychosocial Aspects

Above and beyond the nature and possible complications of HD treatments themselves is the associated technologic and staff dependency that HD requires. In contrast, PD is generally performed at home (during sleep if a cycler machine is used). Most pediatric HD patients miss school frequently, thus falling behind and suffering not only the social isolation and poor self-esteem of serious chronic illness but also difficulty in peer relationships related to subpar academic achievement. In addition, the stress of HD increases the divorce rate in the parents of such children. The goal for pediatric HD patients is to allow them as much responsibility for their care as is feasible and integrate them into their family, peer group, and school. An experienced pediatric ESRD social worker is invaluable in this regard.

REFERENCE

1. Harmon WE, Jabs K: Hemodialysis. *In* Holliday MA, Barratt TM, Avner ED (eds). Pediatric Nephrology, 3rd ed. Baltimore, Williams & Wilkins, 1994:1354–1372.

RENAL TRANSPLANTATION

ANUP SINGH, M.D.

AMIR TEJANI, M.D.

In the past decade, treatment choices for pediatric patients with end-stage renal disease (ESRD) have broadened. With the use of cyclosporine, graft survival and patient survival have improved significantly. Patients on renal replacement therapy (e.g., hemodialysis, peritoneal dialysis), in general, have a poorer quality of life, develop significant renal osteodystrophy, and exhibit severe growth retardation. These two modalities are, therefore, acceptable only as initial forms of replacement therapy pending transplantation. Currently, a quarter of all children in the U.S. transplant registry had preemptive transplantation without previous dialysis. Also, renal transplantation is more cost effective than dialysis.

The five most common causes of pediatric ESRD are hypoplastic, dysplastic kidneys, obstructive uropathy, focal segmental glomerulosclerosis, reflux nephropathy, and systemic immunologic disease.

IMMUNOBIOLOGY

The human immune response is an intricate array of mechanisms designed to eliminate a foreign body not recognized as self. This, however, proves a great hindrance to transplantation, wherein a foreign tissue is incorporated into the human body. The major components of the immune response include histocompatability antigens, T lymphocytes, B lymphocytes, and cytokines.

The major human histocompatibility complex (MHC), also known as the human lymphocytic antigen (HLA), is encoded in a series of genes on the short arm of chromosome 6. These are groups of cell surface antigens that define the nonself nature of transplanted organs. The particular allele combination one inherits from each parent is known as a haplotype. Introduction of an HLA profile from a donor organ that is not compatible with the recipient HLA initiates the immune response.

Lymphocytes act as the main arsenal of the immune system: B cells are responsible for the humoral response, and T cells are responsible for the cellular arm of the immune system and for delayed hypersensitivity. There are several cell types that process and present foreign protein to the T cell. These include monocytes, macrophages, B cells, and dendritic cells. In turn, such cells then secrete their own cytokines (monokines), which promote and direct the immune response. Interleukin 1 (IL-1), produced by macrophages and other presenting cells, stimulates T cells to release interleukins, leading to further proliferation and activation of T cells and finally resulting in graft loss.

Rejection is a process by which the body's immune system recognizes a tissue as foreign and attempts to destroy it. Rejection is categorized as hyperacute, accelerated acute, acute, and chronic. Hyperacute rejection occurs in the first 24 hours posttransplantation, often immediately on release of vascular clamps, and always leads to loss of the graft. This phenomenon is believed to be secondary to preformed antibodies to the graft. Accelerated acute rejection occurs within 24 to 72 hours and is believed to be due to the contribution of preformed antibodies and T cell mechanisms, since it can be reversed by antirejection therapies. Acute rejection is the most common form of rejection and is a cellular response that generally occurs after the tenth day of transplantation and is usually amenable to reversal. Chronic rejection is defined as the gradual loss of renal function due to mechanisms that have not been elucidated.

DONOR SELECTION

For patients on dialysis or reaching ESRD, two options for transplantation are available. A patient may receive a living related kidney from a close relative when possible, or the patient may await a cadaveric kidney by enrolling in the nationwide transplant waiting list. The demand for cadaveric organs has dramatically increased the waiting time for recipients. Transplantation with kidneys from living unrelated donors or distant relatives has been performed in small numbers of patients, with results comparable to or better than those for cadaveric donors. Such grafts constitute an underused resource that may help organ shortage.

Living Related Donors

In the latest report of the North American Pediatric Renal Transplant Cooperative Study (NAPRTCS), 45% of kidneys for transplantation came from living donors. The U.S. renal database shows a 20% living related donor (LRD) procurement rate for adults. The American experience is different from the European experience, where renal transplantation relies mostly on cadaveric sources, with pediatric

LRD patients accounting for 21%. The major benefit of a living donation is improved outcome.

The use of living donors is not without controversy. Opponents of living donation emphasize that the long-term impact of organ donation from young adults is not known. Risks to donors include perioperative morbidity and mortality and a long-term risk of living with one functioning kidney. Potential donors have to go through an exhaustive predonation workup that varies a little from one center to the other. Kidney donor exclusion criteria as followed by our center are listed in Table 1. Long-term follow-up of donors, looking at metabolic, endocrine, and hematologic change, showed only mild elevations of diastolic blood pressure and baseline serum creatinine.

Actuarial graft survivals for LRD kidney transplant are 89%, 83%, and 70% for 1, 2, and 5 years, respectively. Overall, the projected median graft half-life is 21 years. Black race, recipient age <2 years old, and ≥5 prior nonspecific transfusions are significant relative risk factors for a poor outcome.

Cadaveric Donors

There is a continuing increase in the number of pediatric patients in ESRD. However, the availability of organs remains low, and the increased demand has greatly prolonged the waiting time for cadaveric organ recipients. Different strategies have been employed to encourage organ donation, including educating the public to consider organ donation, teaching of housestaff and primary physicians to be alert to the possibility of organ donors, managing brain-dead patients to sustain organ viability, increasing the yield of donations by letting transplant coordinators speak to the family at the earliest possible time, and compensating the donating family to help in burial services.

The actuarial graft survival for cadaveric transplant is 75%, 69%, and 58% at 1, 2, and 5 years respectively. The projected median half-life of a cadaveric kidney is 14.4 years. Recipient age <2 years, donor age <2 years, and cold ischemia time >24 hours are significant risk factors for poor outcome.

IMMUNOSUPPRESSION

Azathioprine

Azathioprine is a thioether derivative of mercaptopurine that was first synthesized by Elion in 1961. It is metabolized in the liver to its active form. Its biochemical effects are complex and not fully understood. It inhibits both RNA and DNA synthesis by preventing synthesis of adenylic and guanylic acids from inosinic acid, and it causes a de novo suppression of purine synthesis by pseudofeedback inhibition.

The drug is usually given as a single daily dose of 1 to 2 mg/kg. Immunosuppression activity peaks 1 to 2 hours after intake and decreases to baseline within 12 to 24 hours. It inhibits promyelocytes in the bone marrow, resulting in a decrease in number of circulating monocytes capable of differentiating into macrophages.

TABLE 1. Exclusion Criteria for Living Donations

Age less than 18 or greater than 60 years*
Hypertension
Diabetes
Abnormal GFR
Significant proteinuria
Urologic abnormality that might increase risk to donor
Obesity*
Psychiatric disorders
HIV positivity
Positive crossmatch
Cardiac abnormalities
Abnormal liver enzymes

*Relative contraindication.

Monitoring of peripheral white count is recommended routinely for patients on azathioprine. Severe bone marrow depression may ensue, thus making the patient susceptible to infections. If necessary, the dose of azathioprine should be decreased by 25% to 50%, with frequent monitoring of peripheral white count. Azathioprine also has been reported to cause hepatotoxicity and cholestasis. Pancreatitis is a rare complication. Since it is converted to its inactive form, 6-thiouric acid, by xanthine oxidase, the drug should not be used in conjunction with allopurinol.

Corticosteroids

The immunosuppressive effects of steroids have been known since the 1920s. The first successful use of steroids for renal transplantation was in 1960 at Peter Bent Brigham Hospital, when cortisone was used for reversal of an acute rejection. Corticosteroid therapy was later added to azathioprine therapy as maintenance immunosuppression in most centers.

Corticosteroids exert their immunosuppressive action by inhibiting macrophage and mononuclear cell transcription of mRNA for both IL-1 and IL-6 and possibly for other lymphokines. Inhibition of IL-1 indirectly inhibits IL-2 production, which is responsible for T cell proliferation.

The side effects of prolonged steroid use are numerous. They include the development of cushingoid features, increased susceptibility to infection, poor wound healing, osteoporosis, cataracts, hyperglycemia, aseptic necrosis of bone, psychosis, peptic ulcer disease, obesity, and acne. In children, steroid-induced inhibition of linear growth, hyperlipidemia, and hypertension are particularly worrisome.

Cyclosporine

Cyclosporine consists of a cyclic structure of 11 amino acids. It was isolated from a fungus *Tolypocladium inflatum*. Since its introduction, it has improved graft survival significantly and currently is the primary drug for maintenance immunosuppression.

The cyclosporine molecule is hydrophobic but soluble in organic solvents and lipids. It has a selective inhibition of the immune response. Its main mechanism of action is through the inhibition of IL-2 synthesis, eventually blocking T cell proliferation. Cyclosporine binds to a binding protein, cyclophilin, in the cytoplasm. This complex inhibits the enzyme calcineurin, which is responsible for dephosphorylation and activation of a transcriptional factor called nuclear factor of activated T cells (NF-AT). NF-AT activates RNA polymerase, resulting in transcription of IL-2 and other lymphokine genes. Thus, cyclosporine inhibits this activation.

Cyclosporine is available in two oral forms, a liquid preparation and soft gelatin capsules. Absorption from the gastrointestinal tract is incomplete, with bioavailability of 30%. Within the blood, one third of the absorbed drug is bound to lipoproteins, and most of the drug is bound to erythrocytes. High concentrations are found in the liver and the pancreas. The drug is metabolized by the P450 liver microsome system, and, thus, great caution should be exercised when using concomitant drugs that either stimulate or suppress the enzyme system (Table 2).

Large doses of cyclosporine are used initially immediately post-transplantation, and the drug is tapered gradually according to center protocols down to about 5 to 6 mg/kg/d. Trough levels are monitored using whole blood assays with high-pressure liquid chromatography (HPLC) or radioimmunoassay, using monoclonal antibody.

Nephrotoxicity is the most worrisome side effect of cyclosporine. The drug causes a reversible constriction of the afferent arteriole, leading to a functional decrease in renal blood flow and filtration rate. Other toxicities include chronic interstitial fibrosis, hyperuricemia, hypertension, hepatotoxicity, hypertrichosis, gingival hyperplasia, and such CNS complications as coarse tremors and dysesthesias.

Monoclonal Antibody—OKT3

OKT3 has been in clinical use since 1987. It is produced by hybridization of a murine antibody-secreting B lymphocyte with a

TABLE 2. Known Drug Interaction with Cyclosporine

INCREASE CYCLOSPORINE LEVELS	DECREASE CYCLOSPORINE LEVELS
Ketoconazole	Phenytoin
Erythromycin	Phenobarbital
Danazol	Carbamazepine
Verapamil	Rifamycin
Diltiazem	
Metoclopramide	
Nicardipine	
Fluconazole	
Itraconazole	
Methylprednisolone	
Bromocriptine	
Nephrotoxic Synergy	
Gentamicin	Trimthoprim-sulfamethoxazole
Tobramycin	
Amphotericin	
Ketoconazole	
Melphalan	
Cimetidine	
Ranitidine	
Diclofenac	

nonsecreting myeloma cell line, the neoplastic potential of which permits perpetual secretion of the antibody. Its main action is directed against the CD3 complex, which is involved in antigen recognition and cell stimulation on the surface of T lymphocytes. It causes T cell receptors to undergo endocytosis and to be lost from the cell surface, thus making them ineffective. Such T cells later are opsonized and removed from the circulation by the reticuloendothelial system (RES).

For induction purposes, OKT3 is started immediately after transplant, given in the standard dose for 3 to 5 days. Cyclosporine is withheld until serum creatinine comes down to less than 3 mg/dl. Because of severe first-dose side effects, OKT3 is initially administered with close monitoring of vital signs, preferably in an intensive care unit. Most patients develop antibodies to the murine monoclonal antibodies, thus restricting future use.

Significant life-threatening adverse reactions with OKT3 may occur because of the release of T cell-derived cytokines, such as tumor necrosis factor (TNF), IL-2, and interferon gamma. Together these cytokines cause the cytokine release syndrome, which includes fever, chills, nausea, and vomiting, occurring a few hours after injection and usually abating after the third dose. Pulmonary edema may occur in hypervolemic patients. Transient deterioration in renal function as marked by a rise in serum creatinine is commonly seen. Neurologic complications are common, particularly a self-limited aseptic meningitis that resolves spontaneously on discontinuance of the drug.

Polyclonal Antibodies—ATG

Polyclonal antibodies are produced by immunization of rabbits or horses with human lymphoid tissue and then harvesting and purifying the sera to obtain the antibodies. At present, only one is available on the market, Upjohn ATG (ATGAM). ATG is used for rejection prophylaxis or induction therapy and treatment of steroid-resistant rejections.

ATG is usually given intravenously through a central line over 6 hours in 500 ml of 0.9 NaCl solution. The drug is highly sclerosing and will cause thrombosis and thrombophlebitis of small veins. The dose used is 10 to 20 mg/kg/d for 5 days for induction or rejection prophylaxis. Its mechanism of action is not clear. Total lymphocyte counts drop after its administration due to either lysis or clearance by the RES. Premedication with diphenhydramine HCl and methylprednisone is recommended to prevent or minimize allergic reactions. Careful monitoring of vital signs is recommended.

The first-dose reaction commonly seen with OKT3 does not occur with polyclonal antibody. Most of the reactions are due to the large amount of protein being infused. Fever, chills, and arthralgias are common, and serum sicknesslike reactions can occur after prolonged use. The potency of these preparations fluctuates from batch to batch. The presence of unwanted antiplatelet antibodies and antileukocyte antibodies may produce significant thrombocytopenia and leukopenia, warranting reduction or termination of therapy.

REJECTION

Rejection is a process by which the body recognizes transplanted tissue as foreign and mounts a response to it. Forty-five days posttransplantation, 39% of live donor transplant recipients and 54% of cadaver graft recipients have been treated for at least one rejection episode. By 2 years posttransplant, 59% of live donor recipients and 74% of cadaver donor recipients have experienced at least one rejection episode.

Patients with acute rejection will manifest one or all of the following: rise in serum urea and creatinine, decrease in urine output, graft tenderness, hypertension, and fever. Other causes of graft dysfunction should always be considered, such as cyclosporine toxicity, prerenal azotemia, obstructive uropathy, renal artery stenosis, and viral and bacterial infections.

Definitive diagnosis can be made only by tissue biopsy. Tissue evidence of acute cellular rejection includes edema and infiltration of the interstitium with numerous leukocytes predominantly of lymphocytic origin. Extension of lymphocytes and monocytes into the walls and lumina of tubules leads to degenerative changes of tubular epithelial cells, defined as tubulitis.

High-dose steroid therapy is the initial mainstay therapy for rejection, but 20% to 30% of acute rejection episodes do not respond to steroids. However, 90% of these do respond to OKT3 (monoclonal antibody). The standard dose is 5 mg given as a bolus IV through a Millipore filter for an average of 10 days. If the drug is well tolerated, patients may receive the remaining doses on an outpatient basis. The cyclosporine dose is reduced to half during the initial phase of treatment and increased to the prerejection level a few days before discontinuation of OKT3. ATG is used in the same manner as for induction for 10 to 14 days as a last resort for those patients who continue to reject post-OKT3 treatment.

Overall, 55% of acute rejection episodes are reversible (return to baseline serum creatinine), 38% are partially reversible, and about 7% end in graft failure or patient death.

COMPLICATIONS OF TRANSPLANTATION

Surgical complications posttransplantation include wound infections (10%), lymphocele (1% to 10%), postoperative bleeding, graft thrombosis (0.5% to 3.5%), renal artery stenosis (2% to 12%), urinary leaks, and ureteral obstruction.

With the continued use of T cell immunosuppressive agents, one of the major complications of transplantation is the lifelong risk of infection with viruses, protozoa, bacteria, and fungi. Special attention needs to be given to cytomegalovirus (CMV) disease, varicella exposure, and infection with *Mycobacterium tuberculosis* in the urban setting. Ideally, all children should be immunized before transplantation. After transplantation, live vaccines are not recommended (e.g., MMR, OPV). Another medical complication of transplantation is chronic rejection, which in some studies accounts for 25% of graft loss. The exact etiology of chronic rejection is unknown, but there is a significant relationship between the number of acute episodes of rejection, low cyclosporine dose (<5 mg/kg/d), number of infections, and the incidence of chronic rejection.

Hypertension after transplant is seen frequently and is usually multifactorial. Patients receiving steroids tend to be hypertensive compared with those not receiving steroids. Poor graft function, cyclosporine toxicity, and renal artery stenosis are other possible causes. Hyperlipidemia is seen frequently in children on steroids, and its long-term cardiovascular effect is worrisome. Progressive osteopenia has been reported in patients. Osteonecrosis of the femoral head is one of the most feared orthopedic complications. Glucose intolerance is commonly seen in patients who are somewhat obese and on high doses of steroids.

Recurrence of Original Disease

Recurrence of the original disease is more frequent in children than in adults. It has been reported to be the cause of graft failure in 2% to 5% of transplanted kidneys. In children, recurrence could be due to an inherent inborn error of metabolism or recurrence of a glomerular disease.

Oxalosis, an inborn error of metabolism due to deficiency of the hepatic enzyme peroxisomal alanine glyoxylate aminotransferase, has a high recurrence rate. Renal deposition of oxalate occurs during episodes of renal insufficiency and may lead to graft failure. The ideal management of this metabolic disorder is a combined liver-kidney transplant.

Focal glomerulosclerosis, a common cause of ESRD in children, is known to recur and cause graft failure. Higher doses of cyclosporine can control proteinuria and prolong graft survival. Other recurrent glomerular diseases include membranoproliferative disease (MPGN types I and II), Henoch-Schönlein purpura, IgA nephropathy, and hemolytic-uremia syndrome.

Growth

One of the main reasons to opt for early transplantation in children is premised on the notion that with normal renal function, catchup growth may be achieved. Data from NAPRTCS shows linear growth to be poor before and after transplantation. Linear growth was best among recipient less than 6 years of age at transplantation and all recipients who received alternate-day prednisone. Achieving steroid withdrawal shows positive correlation with catchup growth.

Malignancies

There is a growing concern about the increasing incidence of neoplasm posttransplantation. The incidence in adults has been reported to be between 2.5% and 3%. In children, 27 (1.36%) of 2053 registered patients in NAPRTCS have developed malignancies, the most common being lymphoproliferative disorders. The use of multiple immunosuppressive agents has been implicated.

REFERENCES

1. McEnery PT, Stablein DM, Arbus G, Tejani A: Renal transplantation in children. N Engl J Med 326:1727–1732, 1992.
2. Stablein D, Tejani A: Five-year patient and graft survival in North American children: A report of the North American Pediatric Renal Transplant Cooperative Study. Kidney Int 44:S16–21, 1993.
3. Tejani A, Butt KMH, Rajpoot D, et al: Strategies for optimizing growth in children with kidney transplants. Transplantation 47:229–233, 1989.
4. Tejani A, Stablein D, Fine R, Alexander S: Maintenance immunosuppression therapy and outcome of renal transplantation in North American children. A report of the North American Pediatric Transplant Cooperative Study. Pediatr Nephrol 7:132–137, 1993.

MALIGNANT TUMORS OF THE KIDNEY

JAMES S. MISER, M.D.

Malignant tumors of the kidney account for approximately 6% of all tumors that arise in children. Wilms' tumor, the most common malignant kidney tumor of childhood, occurs in about 1 in 10,000 children. Primitive neuroectodermal tumors, neuroblastomas, rhabdomyosarcomas, and primitive sarcomas also rarely arise in the kidney. Renal cell carcinoma, the most common malignant renal tumor in adults, is very rare in children. Mesoblastic nephroma is seen almost exclusively in infants and is almost always benign in behavior. Two additional tumors, rhabdoid tumor of the kidney and clear cell sarcoma of the kidney, have, in the past, been included in the National Wilms' Tumor Studies but must be clearly distinguished from Wilms' tumor because of their less favorable prognosis.

Malignant tumors of the kidney most commonly present with an asymptomatic abdominal mass; however, abdominal pain, hematuria, hypertension, and fever may be present at diagnosis. Common entities in the differential diagnosis of malignant tumors of the kidney include other abdominal malignancies, such as neuroblastoma, hepatoblastoma, lymphoma, primitive neuroectodermal tumor, desmoplastic small cell tumor of the abdomen, and rhabdomyosarcoma. Common benign kidney tumors include cysts, hamartomas, abscesses, and nephroblastomatosis. Hydronephrosis must also be included in the differential diagnosis.

WILMS' TUMOR

Wilms' tumor may present in association with congenital anomalies, most commonly hemihypertrophy, aniridia, and genitourinary anomalies. Moreover, patients with hemihypertrophy and aniridia have a high incidence of Wilms' tumor, and, as a result, they are often screened with renal ultrasonography.

Diagnostic Evaluation

Wilms' tumor spreads by direct extension through the renal capsule and renal sinus and by metastatic spread through blood vessels and lymphatics. The most common site of distant metastases is the lung; metastases to the liver, lymph node, brain, and bone also occur. The diagnostic evaluation of Wilms' tumor includes an abdominal computed tomogram (CT) with contrast, an abdominal ultrasound (specifically, to examine involvement of the blood vessels by tumor), a chest radiograph, a chest CT, complete blood count, and urinalysis. Evaluation of the bones by bone scan and skeletal survey should be included for patients with clear cell sarcoma of the kidney because of the propensity of this tumor to metastasize to bone. Evaluation of the brain by CT scan or magnetic resonance imaging (MRI) should be undertaken for clinical indications and in patients with rhabdoid tumors.

Prognostic Factors

The two most important factors that determine therapy for Wilms' tumors are the stage of the disease and histology. The staging system of the National Wilms' Tumor Study is shown in Table 1. The prognosis of patients with higher-stage tumors has improved greatly with advances in treatment, so that tumor stage now has a greater impact on treatment than on prognosis.

Histology is an extremely important factor in planning treatment for Wilms' tumor. Favorable histology Wilms' tumor is typically triphasic, with blastemal, epithelial, and stromal components, although one component may predominate. Unfavorable histology includes tumors with diffuse anaplasia, clear cell sarcomas, and rhabdoid tumors. The extent of the anaplasia in the tumor deposits in lymph nodes and metastases may also be of importance.

It can be anticipated that cytogenetic and molecular events will be correlated with the outcome of Wilms' tumor in the near future and, thus, will determine therapy in future studies.

Treatment

The current treatment of children with Wilms' tumor has evolved as the result of the first three multiinstitutional National Wilms' Tumor Studies. The most accepted initial approach to Wilms' tumor is surgical removal of the primary tumor. This approach allows careful surgical and pathologic staging and complete evaluation of the tumor for unfavorable histopathologic and biologic features. When very large tumors are encountered, preoperative therapy may avoid surgical complications. This approach, however, will result in incomplete characterization of the histology and stage of the tumor.

TABLE 1. National Wilms' Tumor Study: Staging Criteria

STAGE	CRITERIA
I	Tumor limited to the kidney and completely excised. The surface of the renal capsule is intact. The tumor was not ruptured before or during removal. There is no residual tumor apparent beyond the margins of excision.
II	Tumor extends beyond the kidney but is completely excised. There is regional extension of the tumor (i.e., penetration through the outer surface of the renal capsule into the perirenal soft tissue). Vessels outside the kidney substance are infiltrated or contain tumor thrombus. The tumor may have been biopsied, or there has been local spillage of tumor confined to the flank. There is no residual tumor apparent or beyond the margins of excision.
III	Residual nonhematogenous tumor confined to the abdomen. Any of the following may occur. a. Lymph nodes on biopsy are found to be involved in the hilus, the periaortic chains, or beyond. b. There has been diffuse peritoneal contamination by the tumor, such as by spillage of tumor beyond the flank before or during surgery or by tumor growth that has penetrated through the peritoneal surface. c. Implants are found on the peritoneal surfaces. d. The tumor extends beyond the surgical margins either microscopically or grossly. e. The tumor is not completely resectable because of local infiltration into vital structures.
IV	Hematogenous metastases. Deposits beyond stage III (e.g., lung, liver, bone, and brain).
V	Bilateral renal involvement at diagnosis. An attempt should be made to stage each side according to the above criteria on the basis of extent of disease before biopsy.

From D'Angio GJ, Breslow N, Beckwith JB, et al: Treatment of Wilms' tumor: Results of the Third National Wilms' Tumor Study. Cancer 64:349–360, 1989.

Favorable Histology

The treatment of favorable histology (FH) Wilms' tumor reflects the excellent prognosis of this tumor. The 4-year survival for patients treated on the third National Wilms' Tumor Study (NWTS III) was 96% for patients with stage I FH, 92% for patients with stage II FH, 87% for patients with stage III FH, and 73% for stage IV FH. The goal is to deliver therapy with as few short-term and long-term sequelae as possible while maintaining the excellent prognosis. Not only is this philosophy reflected in the treatment regimens, doses of radiation, and dose intensity chemotherapy, but it also should dictate the clinical and therapeutic decisions during the course of therapy. The standard treatment of stage I FH tumors is a combination of vincristine and dactinomycin given for 6 months. Radiation therapy is not required for stage I tumors. The standard treatment of stage II FH tumors is a combination of vincristine and dactinomycin given for 15 months. Radiation therapy is also not required for stage II tumors. The standard treatment of stage III FH tumors is a combination of vincristine, dactinomycin, and doxorubicin given for 15 months. Radiation therapy at a dose of 1080 cGy in six fractions to the tumor bed is required for stage III tumors. The standard treatment of stage IV FH tumors is a combination of vincristine, dactinomycin, and doxorubicin. Radiation therapy is delivered to the lungs for those with pulmonary disease and to the flank depending on the extent of the primary tumor. The fourth National Wilms' Tumor Study (NWTS IV) is investigating for all stages whether the chemotherapy given in 1 day each course (pulse intensive therapy) is as efficacious as the traditional fractionated schedule. For stages II, III, and IV, the NWTS IV is also evaluating whether 6 months of therapy is as efficacious as 15 months.

Anaplastic Histology

The treatment of anaplastic histology Wilms' tumor is also related to stage. Treatment of focally anaplastic tumors follows the guidelines for favorable histology tumors. Patients with stage I anaplastic tumors fare very well with 6 months of therapy with vincristine and dactinomycin. Radiation therapy is not required for stage I anaplastic tumors. The standard treatment for patients with stages II through IV diffuse anaplastic tumors is 15 months of therapy with vincristine, dactinomycin, doxorubicin, and cyclophosphamide. The radiation therapy that is given is related to stage and age, but at more aggressive doses than for favorable histology tumors. Children with diffuse anaplastic tumors fare considerably more poorly than comparably staged patients with favorable histology, except for those with stage I tumors. The outcome for patients with stage IV anaplastic tumors is very poor. As a result, new aggressive regimens, similar to those being evaluated for metastatic and high-risk sarcomas, are being considered for this group of patients.

Clear Cell Sarcoma

The treatment of clear cell sarcoma of the kidney has improved significantly in the last 10 years. The current standard therapy for all stages is a chemotherapy regimen of vincristine, dactinomycin, and doxorubicin for 15 months following surgical excision of the tumor. Radiation therapy is delivered to all stages. The current recommendation for stages I and II is to deliver a limited dose (1080 cGy) to the flank, although the need for radiation in these low-stage, completely resected tumors has not been established in a clinical trial. Supplemental doses may be required to areas of bulk disease. The new combination of ifosfamide and etoposide is particularly active against clear cell sarcoma of the kidney. Cures of children with recurrent metastatic disease to bone have been reported using this regimen.

Rhabdoid Tumors

The optimal treatment of rhabdoid tumors within or outside the kidney has not been established. Except for very young children with stage I rhabdoid tumors that are confined to the kidney and completely resected, the outcome for rhabdoid tumors remains poor. Standard Wilms' tumor therapy with vincristine, dactinomycin, doxorubicin, and moderate radiation doses has been almost uniformly unsuccessful. Newer, more aggressive chemotherapeutic approaches include the following drug combinations: ifosfamide and etoposide; ifosfamide or cyclophosphamide combined with etoposide and carboplatin; carboplatin and etoposide; and cisplatin and etoposide. For stage I rhabdoid tumors, it may be appropriate to incorporate some of the standard Wilms' tumor agents with these newer combinations into a moderately aggressive treatment regimen.

Bilateral Wilms' Tumor

Bilateral Wilms' tumor (Stage V) is a unique and challenging clinical problem. Just as for unilateral Wilms' tumor, the stage of the primary tumors, presence or absence of metastases, and histology are the important prognostic factors. The guidelines for treatment of stage V Wilms' tumor are generally the same as the guidelines for unilateral tumors except that every attempt must be made to maintain adequate renal function. To accomplish this, the multidisciplinary team of pediatric oncologists, surgeons, radiologists, radiotherapists, and nephrologists must work very closely together. Innovative surgical approaches, including bench surgery and heminephrectomy, and innovative radiation therapeutic approaches, including intraoperative and interstitial radiation, are being explored. Careful imaging, multiple surgical explorations, and repeated biopsies are often required to determine the optimal timing and extent of the resections. In spite of these challenges, the prognosis for patients with bilateral favorable histology Wilms' tumor is very good. Bilateral Wilm's tumor occasionally requires total renal ablation, although this should be the last resort. Dialysis and subsequent transplantation are then indicated because of the good prognosis.

Recurrent Wilms' Tumor

The treatment of recurrent Wilms' tumor is complicated and based on a number of prognostic factors, the most important of which are the site of relapse (limited lung disease is most favorable), infradiaphragmatic local recurrence without prior radiation (favorable), timing of the relapse (a relapse more than 12 months after completion of therapy is better than an on-therapy relapse), histology (favorable histology is better than unfavorable histology), and the number of prior relapses (first relapse is better than subsequent relapses). For those patients who have not been treated previously with doxorubicin, this agent should almost always be included in the regimen. The combination of ifosfamide and etoposide has an excellent response rate (65% to 70%) in recurrent Wilms' tumor, with a cure rate as high as 25% to 35% even for high-risk relapses. Thus, this is an important treatment regimen to consider. The combinations of cyclophosphamide and etoposide and of carboplatin and etoposide also have demonstrated efficacy. The use of high-dose alkylating agent therapy followed by autologous bone marrow or peripheral stem cell rescue for patients with high-risk relapses should be strongly considered once a second remission is achieved. Preliminary data suggest that this approach may be efficacious.

OTHER MALIGNANT TUMORS OF THE KIDNEY

The treatment of other malignant tumors of the kidney is determined by the specific histology and stage of the disease. Because of its excellent prognosis, mesoblastic nephroma is almost always treated with surgery alone. Localized renal cell carcinomas usually are treated with surgery alone because of the lack of clear evidence that adjuvant therapy is of benefit. Immunologic approaches to treating this tumor show some promise. Treatment of neuroblastomas that arise within the kidney is determined by the same factors that determine therapy for this disease arising elsewhere: N-*myc* oncogene amplification, histology, age, and stage of disease. Treatment of rhabdomyosarcomas arising in the kidney, as for those tumors arising outside the kidney, is determined by histology and stage. Primitive sarcomas and primitive neuroectodermal tumors arising in the kidney must be treated aggressively. Chemotherapy combinations commonly used are vincristine, doxorubicin, and cyclophosphamide; and ifosfamide and etoposide.

13

Bones and Joints

CRANIOFACIAL MALFORMATIONS

CHARLES H. THORNE, M.D.
LEONARD B. KABAN, D.M.D., M.D.
MICHAEL T. LONGAKER, M.D.

Jaw surgery (orthognathic surgery) and neurosurgery evolved independently until the 1960s, when Paul Tessier, a French plastic surgeon, developed techniques that bridged the gap by allowing simultaneous exposure and surgical manipulation of the cranium and the facial bones. The specialty of craniofacial surgery was born. In the 1970s, multidisciplinary craniofacial teams were established in the United States. In the 1980s, craniofacial techniques, originally developed for adult patients, were adapted to infants in an effort to improve growth potential, minimize secondary distortion, and aid in self-image development. Principles of craniofacial surgery also have been applied in the last two decades to the treatment of acute craniofacial trauma, acquired posttraumatic deformities, and reconstruction after tumor resection. Advances in imaging techniques, particularly computed tomography (CT scanning), with three-dimensional reconstruction have resulted in improved diagnostic accuracy and more precise treatment planning.

The decade of the 1990s challenges investigators to improve our understanding of the developmental biology of normal and abnormal facial morphology, to futher elucidate the genetics of craniofacial anomalies, and to develop new therapeutic methods that will enhance growth of the abnormal craniofacial region. With advances in molecular biology and genetics, it may be possible to prevent certain craniofacial anomalies. Recent developments in fetal surgery provide the possibility that selected anomalies may be treated in utero. More likely, the study of fetal wound healing will result in knowledge and techniques that can be employed after birth to manipulate the wound healing response.

The most common types of congenital craniofacial anomalies are the following.

1. Craniosynostosis (isolated and syndromal)
2. Hemifacial microsomia (first and second branchial arch syndrome)
3. Treacher Collins syndrome
4. Facial clefting syndromes (e.g., hypertelorism)
5. Anomalies secondary to cleft lip and palate

CRANIOSYNOSTOSIS

The estimated incidence of craniosynostosis is 1 in 1000 live births. Cranial sutures are not primary sites of bone growth. Rather, they are passive structures that allow the cranium to expand in response to rapid brain growth during the first few years of life. Consequently, premature fusion of a cranial suture prevents the normal symmetric expansion of the skull, and the resultant skull deformity depends on which suture is involved. Most commonly, craniosynostosis involves a single suture. For example, with premature fusion of the sagittal suture, a long, narrow skull develops (scaphocephaly) because of restriction to growth in the transverse dimension. Trigonocephaly describes the narrow, pointed forehead that results from synostosis of the metopic (midforehead) suture. Synostosis of a single coronal suture results in plagiocephaly, in which the ipsilateral forehead is recessed and the contralateral forehead is often excessively prominent. Unilateral lambdoid synostosis results in skull asymmetry that is most pronounced posteriorly but that may result in some compensatory asymmetry in the frontal region as well.

If more than one suture fuses prematurely, increased intracranial pressure develops, and treatment is essential not only to correct the skull deformity but also to expand the cranial volume and prevent deleterious effects of increased intracranial pressure. The intracranial pressure situation is not as clear when a single suture is involved. Marchac and Renier have shown that intracranial pressure is elevated in a certain percentage of single-suture craniosynostosis cases. These patients, however, are generally asymptomatic, and the significance of the measured increase in pressure is unknown.

Craniosynostosis may present as an isolated problem or as part of a syndrome in association with other anomalies. The syndromal cases involve multiple suture synostosis and, therefore, result in increased intracranial pressure. In addition to cranial deformities, the development of the facial bones is affected, resulting in midface hypoplasia and retrusion. The orbits are shallow, and patients tend to manifest prominent ocular globes (exorbitism).

Two of the most common craniosynostosis syndromes are the Apert and Crouzon syndromes. The major distinguishing characteristic between them is the complex syndactyly of the fingers and toes that occurs in Apert syndrome. Although exorbitism may occur in all syndromal synostosis, it tends to be most severe in Crouzon syndrome and may result in exposure keratitis and corneal injury. Unlike the isolated craniosynostoses that occur sporadically, Apert, Crouzon, and Pfeiffer syndromes are all inherited in an autosomal dominant fashion. Genetic counseling, therefore, is an essential component of management.

Treatment of isolated, single-suture craniosynostosis is generally recommended to be done in a child between 6 months and 1 year of age. The surgical procedure requires reshaping the cranial vault and the frontoorbital region depending on the suture involved and the location of the deformity. The procedure, which requires a craniotomy, is generally performed by a plastic surgeon in conjunction with a neurosurgeon. Treatment of the single-suture cases is extremely reliable, and the complication rate in experienced hands is low. Patients generally require no further surgery, with the exception of occasional, minor touchup type procedures to smooth irregularities or, occasionally, to remove a protruding wire or plate. The 6- to 12-month period is chosen for the primary procedure because the bone is pliable and easy to work with. In addition, any small defects resulting from surgery tend to ossify spontaneously if the procedure is performed before 1 year of age. Because intracranial pressure does not appear to be a significant issue, the procedure can probably be delayed without risk to the patient.

Treatment of the multisuture synostoses is an entirely different situation. These patients tend to have increased intracranial pressure, as well as more severe deformities of the cranial vault. The treatment protocol for these patients remains in evolution but, in general, consists of the following.

1. Cranial vault reshaping to increase intracranial volume at 6 months of age or earlier if increased intracranial pressure dictates.
2. Secondary cranial vault remodeling at 2 to 3 years of age, particularly in the Apert and Pfeiffer patients, who tend to have abnormal cranial development regardless of the initial procedure.
3. Midface advancement by the Le Fort III osteotomy or monobloc frontofacial advancement at 5 to 7 years of age.
4. Definitive jaw surgery when the patient is skeletally mature. This may involve a secondary Le Fort III osteotomy or monobloc osteotomy.

This protocol is flexible and must be individualized for each of these complex cases. The syndromal patients also may have airway obstruction requiring tracheostomy immediately after birth, hydrocephalus requiring shunting, as well as problems specifically related to each syndrome, such as syndactyly in the Apert patients.

HEMIFACIAL MICROSOMIA

Hemifacial microsomia has been called craniofacial microsomia, first and second branchial arch syndrome, and lateral facial dysplasia. The deformity involves hypoplasia of one or both sides of the face. It is always asymmetric. The hallmark of the deformity is the hypoplasia of the mandibular condyle, although the spectrum of the deformity is large and may involve ear anomalies, partial or complete facial nerve paralysis, hypoplasia of the soft tissue of the face, and asymmetric deformities of both the maxilla and mandible.

Hemifacial microsomia is not usually an inherited disorder.

Because of the variability in presentation it is difficult to outline a protocol of treatment that is applicable to all patients with hemifacial microsomia. Patients with an isolated ear deformity, therefore, would not require soft tissue augmentation of the cheek. In general, the approach is as follows.

1. Removal of preauricular skin tags and correction of macrostomia, if present, in the first year of life.
2. In cases of severe mandibular asymmetry, elongation of the hypoplastic mandible, either by the newer bone lengthening technique described by McCarthy et al.[2] or by the more traditional bone grafting technique at age 2 to 4 years. This unilateral elongation of the mandibular ramus results in an open bite on the side of the deformity. An orthodontic appliance is then inserted that allows downward growth of the maxilla on the affected side, leveling the occlusal plane.
3. Reconstruction of the ear deformities beginning at age 6 years. In cases of severe asymmetry, the ear deformity may be of secondary importance when compared with the hypoplasia of the cheek. In these cases, the ear reconstruction is best postponed until later in life.
4. Soft tissue augmentation by microvascular transfer of adipose tissue at age 8 to 12 years.
5. Definitive orthognathic (jaw) surgery when the patient is skeletally mature.

Patients with hemifacial microsomia must be divided by the craniofacial team into mild and severe types. In the milder cases, orthognathic surgery is best delayed until adolescence, when a single, definitive procedure can be performed. In the severe cases, it is best to initiate treatment early (age 2 to 4 years) so as to make the child more presentable during the school years and, hopefully, to reduce the deformity that is eventually treated in adolescence.

TREACHER COLLINS SYNDROME

The Treacher Collins syndrome is inherited as an autosomal dominant trait. Like hemifacial microsomia, the deformity involves hypoplasia of the facial tissues, but it is symmetric. Characteristic features include ear deformities involving both the external ear and the middle ear, zygomatic (cheek bone) hypoplasia, deficiency of the lower eyelids, and deformities of the maxilla and mandible. The jaw deformities involve a short posterior facial height, a steeply inclined mandible, and a recessed chin. The combination of features, although variable, make Treacher Collins an easily recognized pattern of deformity.

In general, the treatment protocol is as follows.

1. Attention to the airway, which may be inadequate and require tracheostomy shortly after birth. Although infant tracheostomies are prone to obstruction and time consuming for families to care for, the risk of *not* performing the procedure frequently far outweighs any disadvantages.
2. Bone conduction hearing aids as soon as possible (within the first few months of life). Hearing is essential for speech development and can be evaluated by brainstem auditory evoked response testing (BAER) before the mother and child are discharged from the hospital after birth.
3. Reconstruction of the cheek bones at age 5 to 7 years or at skeletal maturity, depending on the severity. This can be either with traditional bone grafting procedures or with vascularized bone transfers. Conventional bone grafts tend to resorb dramatically if followed long enough, and, therefore, the vascularized bone transfers are generally preferred.[3]
4. Reconstruction of the external ear deformities beginning at approximately age 6 years. CT scans of the temporal bones are performed to see if the patient is a candidate for reconstruction of the ear canal and middle ear, but the middle ear deformities tend to be severe and unreconstructable in this syndrome.
5. Definitive jaw surgery when the patient is skeletally mature.

FACIAL CLEFTING SYNDROMES

Numerous craniofacial deformities exist that are difficult to categorize but that fit into the general category of craniofacial clefting syndromes. Some of these cases demonstrate an obvious linear soft and hard tissue deficiency that resembles a cleft. In other cases, there may be *excess* hard and soft tissue occurring in a linear fashion (e.g., hypertelorism). Tessier has developed the most useful classification of facial clefts that numbers the clefts from 0 to 14 depending on the location relative to the orbit.

One of the most common facial clefts, which involves widening of the midline and lateral displacement of the orbits, is called hypertelorism. In some cases, there is a midline cleft of the upper lip and bifidity of the nose in association with the widened intraorbital distance. The hypertelorism may be associated with craniosynostosis (craniofrontonasal dysplasia syndrome).

Surgical correction of hypertelorism involves combined intracranial and extracranial exposure of the orbits, which are mobilized by osteotomies and moved toward the midline. This surgery is best performed in children 5 to 7 years of age, when growth of the orbital region nears completion. A full description of the treatment of craniofacial clefting syndromes is beyond the scope of this section.

ANOMALIES SECONDARY TO CLEFT LIP AND PALATE

Jaw deformities secondary to cleft lip and palate are strictly facial and do not really belong in a discussion of craniofacial malformations. Cleft lip and palate, however, are the most common of all congenital deformities involving the face and are mentioned here because of that frequency.

Cleft lip and palate, if left untreated, result in normal or nearly normal facial growth. It is the surgical correction of the cleft palate, however, that results in retardation of midface growth, presumably related to scar contracture. Approximately 15% to 25% of patients will have growth restriction sufficient to warrant Le Fort I advancement in adolescence.

FETAL INTERVENTION FOR CRANIOFACIAL MALFORMATIONS

The diagnosis and treatment of fetal anomalies have improved dramatically in the past 15 years. Advances in imaging, specifically fetal ultrasound, combined with the observation that fetal skin wounds heal without scarring (early in gestation) has led surgeons to consider the possibility of in utero correction of craniofacial malformations.

One anomaly where in utero correction may be possible is cleft lip and palate. Fetal ultrasound is a reliable technique to diagnose this anomaly as early as 15 weeks' gestation. Such a repair may result in scarfree healing and possibly prevent the restriction of midface growth that accompanies standard treatment. Fetal surgery is still in the experimental stage, and before it is applied in humans with craniofacial malformations, the benefits of the procedures and the safety for the fetus and mother must be demonstrated.[1]

An animal model has been developed to study fetal cleft lip surgery in rabbits. Following maternal hysterotomy and exposure of the fetal head, the cleft lips were created surgically and immediately repaired at 24 days' gestation (term gestation is 31 days). The fetuses were allowed to progress to term. The lip wounds healed without gross scarring and with a symmetric lip and nose. Histologic analysis revealed a lack of fibrosis and demonstrated muscle regeneration across the repair site. To evaluate midface growth, some animals were not killed at birth and were allowed to grow for 6 months, when rabbits normally complete facial growth. Clinical examination and radiologic measurements revealed no evidence of maxillary growth retardation. The findings are encouraging but not definitive because they refer to cleft lip repair, whereas it is cleft palate repair that generally is believed to cause growth retardation.

A similar model has been developed in the fetal lamb to create and repair defects in the lip. The lamb model offers advantages over the rabbit model. The large size of the fetal lamb makes fetal manipulation easier, and the long gestation (140 days) allows for comparison of lip repair at different gestational ages. The latest gestational age at which the fetal lip can be repaired and heal without scar formation can be defined. This model will also be used to determine the effect of lip repair on subsequent facial growth.

These preliminary results support the hypothesis that in utero repair of cleft lip and palate may result in scarless healing and may avoid the adverse effects on midface growth produced by postnatal repair. If successful, the techniques may be extended to more complex congenital anomalies. More likely, this research will lead to a better understanding of the biochemical and cellular events that make fetal healing unique, and that knowledge, in turn, will be employed to manipulate postnatal healing.

REFERENCES

1. Longaker MT, Golbus MS, Filly RA, et al: Maternal outcome after open fetal surgery. A review of the first 17 human cases. JAMA 265:737–741, 1991.
2. McCarthy JG, et al: Lengthening of the human mandible by gradual distraction. Plast Reconstr Surg 89:1, 1992.
3. Posnick JC, Goldstein JA, Waitzman AA: Surgical correction of the Treacher Collins malar deficiency: Quantitative CT scan analysis of long-term results. Plast Reconstr Surg 92:12, 1993.

DISORDERS OF THE SPINE AND SHOULDER GIRDLE

MICHAEL DAVID SUSSMAN, M.D.

Disorders of shoulder girdle and spine can be classified as those problems that are congenital, infectious or inflammatory, traumatic, and acquired or developmental. In the pediatric age group, one does not see degenerative changes. However, some of these disorders may predispose to degenerative problems in later life. Disorders of the spine may affect neurologic function by applying pathologic mechanical stresses on the spinal cord, and this may have a greater impact on function than has the primary deformity.

SHOULDER GIRDLE

Congenital Problems

Congenital Pseudarthrosis of the Clavicle. In this entity, there is a discontinuity, which is present at birth, in the midportion of the clavicle. Congenital pseudarthrosis can be easily distinguished from a birth fracture, in that it is painless. The abnormality is usually found on the right side and is probably related to impairment of the development of the clavicle as a result of the juxtaposition of the subclavian artery to the underside of the midportion of the developing clavicle. Congenital pseudarthrosis of the clavicle also may occur in a bilateral form in association with cleidocranial dysostosis.

No treatment is required in infancy, and elective surgical repair of the pseudoarthrosis to correct the cosmetic deformity is almost always successful (in contrast to congenital pseudarthrosis of the tibia, which is quite resistant to treatment). Repair can be accomplished when the child is old enough that the structures are large enough for the fixation devices used at the time of surgery. A recent report suggests that early repair without rigid internal fixation is successful if it is performed within the first few years of life. No specific treatment or handling of the child is required before repair.

Sprengel's Deformity. The scapula lies adjacent to the cervical region during early fetal development and subsequently descends to its normal position on the posterior thorax. Failure of complete descent of the scapula results in Sprengel's deformity. In this deformity, the scapula is in an elevated position and is small, malformed, and rotated so that the glenoid faces downward. It also has a superomedial portion that hooks over the upper portion of the thorax. This results in a cosmetic deformity, as well as limitation of the mobility of the shoulder because of the fixation and downward inclination of the glenoid. The deformity may be unilateral or bilateral. There is a female preponderance in most series, but this may be due to an ascertainment bias because of the cosmetic nature of this problem. Twenty percent to thirty percent of patients may have a supernumerary bone, known as the *omovertebral bone,* which connects the elevated, malformed scapula to the axial skeleton. All patients with Sprengel's deformity should be carefully assessed for anomalies of the spine by radiography and for anomalies of the kidney by ultrasonography.

One third of these patients have a mild grade I deformity in which the shoulder joints are almost level, and the deformity cannot be seen with the patient dressed. Those patients with mild deformities should be followed up throughout growth, as there may be progression in the severity of the deformity. One third of the patients have a grade II deformity, in which the asymmetry is mild to moderate but can be appreciated with the patient dressed owing to the asymmetry at the base of the neck. Another third of patients have more severe, grade III deformities, which are easily visible and can cause functional impairment.

Patients with grade II or III deformities may undergo surgery before age 5 or 6 years to correct the cosmetic appearance. In moderate cases, excision of the superomedial portion of the scapula in an extraperiosteal fashion, leaving the levator scapulae detached, and excision of the omovertebral bone, if present, may suffice. For more severe deformities, the Woodward procedure is recommended. With this technique, the origin of the trapezius is detached and moved caudally, in addition to excision of the superomedial angle of the scapula and omovertebral bone. If one waits to perform surgery until the child is older than 7 years, the risk of brachial plexus palsy from compression of the plexus between the scapula and the first rib is increased, so that surgery at a younger age is preferred.

The major goal of surgery is to reduce the cosmetic deformity. However, increased range of motion can also be expected. Scoliosis is common in such patients and may be due to congenital anomalies, or it may develop during the adolescent growth spurt in a pattern similar to that of idiopathic scoliosis. Other associated findings include Klippel-Feil syndrome, rib anomalies, and urogenital system abnormalities.

Snapping Scapula. In this syndrome, there is a palpable, audible, and sometimes painful click with elevation and declination of the scapula. This can be due to one or more osteochrondromas on the costal surface of the scapula or may be a forme fruste of Sprengel's deformity with a prominent and curved superomedial portion of the scapula. These lesions can be excised surgically when identified.

Acquired Problems

Birth-Related Brachial Plexus Palsy. The most common type of brachial plexus palsy affects the upper, or C5-C6, nerve distribution. This is usually found in large infants and is due to traction on the brachial plexus during delivery. These infants have limited active abduction, external rotation, and elbow flexion. Therefore, the arm is held in an adducted, internally rotated, and extended posture.

In the acute phase, no treatment is indicated, but the arm should be handled with care to avoid further traction on the injured nerves. At 2 to 3 weeks of age, gentle range of motion can be begun, with concentration on external rotation and abduction. Range of motion should not be forced, and long-term passive splintage should not be used. If elbow flexion is absent when sitting age is reached, an elbow splint should be used to maintain the elbow at 90 degrees to allow for development of active hand use. If the lower plexus is involved, a hand and wrist splint may also be used. Because there are areas that are insensate, close observation should be made to avoid injury to these insensate areas. Improvement is often seen until the age of 2 years. Subsequent to this, however, further improvement is unlikely. The percentage of children who achieve full recovery varies from 10% to 75%, depending on the series. If deficits persist, muscle releases or transfers or both may be done to improve range of motion.

In some cases, a rotational osteotomy of the upper humerus may be performed to improve function. Patients with severe defects persisting past 6 months of age may benefit from surgical exploration of the plexus and grafting to replace destroyed nerves.

Shoulder Dislocation. Congenital dislocation of the shoulder has been reported but is exceedingly rare. Traumatic shoulder dislocations, likewise, are rare in the pediatric age group but may occur in older teenagers. More frequently, proximal humeral fractures occur with traumatic episodes.

Voluntary dislocation of the shoulder, however, may be seen in children, and the dislocation may be multidirectional (i.e., posterior as well as anterior). In general, surgery should be avoided in these patients, and physical therapy should be used to strengthen muscles that maintain shoulder alignment. In addition, patients should be counseled not to dislocate their shoulders voluntarily.

Fractures

Fractured Clavicle. This is the most common fracture seen in the pediatric age group. Neonatal clavicular fractures occur with birth trauma, and usually no treatment is required other than gentle handling of the affected extremity. These fractures heal exceedingly rapidly, and infants are usually asymptomatic within a week to 10 days.

In children other than neonates, clavicle fractures can be treated with a figure-of-eight dressing to reduce the symptoms. Healing is almost universal, and generally no reduction is necessary because bone remodeling is usually complete. A large amount of fracture callus may occur at the healing site, which may be cosmetically apparent, since the clavicle is directly subcutaneous. However, patients can be counseled that this will resolve in 6 to 12 months.

Fractured Scapula. Fractures of the scapula are very rare in pediatric patients and are usually associated with major trauma. In most cases, scapular fractures can be treated by immobilization of the extremity in a sling until healing occurs.

Fractures of the Upper Humerus. Fractures of the upper humerus usually occur in the proximal metaphysis, 1 to 2 cm distal to the growth plate and not through the growth plate. Although these fractures may be completely displaced, no reduction of the fracture fragments is necessary, and manipulation is indicated only if the skin is in jeopardy. Treatment with a collar and a cuff and swathe for 3 to 4 weeks is sufficient. Even in severely displaced fractures, healing and subsequent remodeling can be anticipated, and full recovery of function is likely.

SPINE

Congenital Anomalies

Congenital anomalies can occur anywhere in the spine. They may include only a single level or multiple levels or may affect the entire spine. These deformities may affect the growth plate and, therefore, result in progressively increasing deformity.

Most spine anomalies can be classified as failure of segmentation of vertebrae, failure of formation of portions of vertebrae, or combinations of both. Failures of segmentation result in fusion of all or part of one vertebral body to an adjacent vertebral body. If this fusion is partial, the growth plate is absent in the area of fusion but may be present in the unfused area, leading to the development of a progressive deformity. Similarly, if a partially formed vertebra extends over only a portion of adjacent vertebral bodies, the deformity may increase with growth. This asymmetric growth will cause increasing deformity, resulting in progressive scoliosis, kyphosis, or both. Lordosis may occur in those rare cases in which there are multiple congenital fusions of the posterior elements with intact bodies anteriorly.

As with other congenital anomalies, when congenital scoliosis is discovered, the patient should be examined carefully to detect the presence of other anomalies. These may include hypothyroidism or hearing impairment with upper spinal anomalies and cardiovascular, gastrointestinal, or urogenital anomalies associated with anomalies lower in the spine. Spinal anomalies may also be associated with diastematomyelia or tight filum terminale, which may tether the spinal cord and result in progressive spinal cord dysfunction with growth. For patients with vertebral anomalies who show evidence of neurologic dysfunction or back pain, magnetic resonance imaging (MRI) should be used to demonstrate spinal cord anomalies, if present.

In most cases of congenital spine deformity, serial (usually yearly) radiographic follow-up is indicated until growth is finished. If significant progression occurs, posterior spinal fusion, usually without instrumentation, should be performed to prevent further progression of the deformity. Bracing may be indicated to control flexible curves adjacent to anomalous areas, but it is not efficacious in most cases of congenital scoliosis. If posterior fusion alone is insufficient to prevent progression of the deformity, anterior fusion may also be required.

Congenital anomalies in the cervical and upper thoracic spine tend to be less aggressive in terms of producing deformity than those in the lower thoracic and lumbar spine.

Klippel-Feil Syndrome. Any congenital fusion in the cervical spine is known as the Klippel-Feil syndrome. In most cases, this is a total failure of segmentation and, therefore, does not produce scoliosis or kyphosis but limits the linear growth of the cervical vertebrae, resulting in a short neck, low hairline, and limitation of motion of the cervical spine. A high percentage of such patients have hearing problems.

No treatment is necessary for most cases. In exceedingly severe cases in which the cosmetic appearance is unacceptable, resection of the upper two or three ribs, with skin grafting to alter the contours in the shoulder area, may improve the cosmetic appearance.

Occipitocervical Instability. This form of instability, which may present with headache or pain with neck motion, is exceedingly rare and may be seen in combination with fusions in the cervical spine. When detected and documented radiologically, the instability should be treated by fusion of the occiput to the upper cervical spine.

Atlantoaxial Hypermobility. Excessive motion between C1 and C2 may occur in otherwise normal children with an os odontoideum (a hypoplastic odontoid with an ossicle superior to it), in children with skeletal dysplasia due to a hypoplastic odontoid (particularly Morquio syndrome and spondyloepiphyseal dysplasia congenita), or in children with Down syndrome (owing to alteration and laxity of the restraining ligaments). Diagnosis is made by interpretation of *voluntary* flexion-extension radiographs of the cervical spine with measurement of the distance between the posterior border of the anterior arch of C1 and the anterior border of the odontoid (atlanto-dens interval). It is important not to obtain these radiographs by passively forcing flexion of the neck, since this maneuver could result in injury or even death of patients with hypermobility. An absolute distance of greater than 4 mm of the atlanto-dens interval is abnormal. In the absence of neurologic findings, patients with instability of less than 6 to 7 mm should be observed closely, and those with instability of greater amounts should undergo atlantoaxial fusion to prevent progressive myelopathy or acute spinal cord damage. If long tract signs, such as clonus, hyperreflexia, Babinski reflex, weakness, or incontinence, are present, MRI scan with flexion should be done to demonstrate cord compression, and C1-C2 fusion may be indicated.

Atlantoaxial instability is prevalent in patients with Down syndrome. Even if pathologic laxity is not documented in these patients, they should avoid activities that may place undue stress on the neck, such as tumbling and trampoline exercises. Patients may participate in most recreational sports, with the pediatrician recognizing that their risk of cervical injury is slightly increased. Patients with Down syndrome should undergo radiography initially at age 3 or 4. If the findings are within normal limits, radiography should be repeated every 2 to 4 years, or sooner if evidence of spinal cord compression is detected.

Pseudosubluxation of C2 to C4 in Children. After experiencing spinal trauma, many children exhibit what appears to be a subluxation of C2 on C3 or C3 on C4 (or both) on the lateral flexion radiograph of the cervical spine. If this reduces fully in extension, is not greater than 5 mm, and is not associated with other evidence of fracture, such as an increase in the prevertebral soft tissue space, this can be considered normal. Patients should not be overtreated when they exhibit this normal pseudosubluxation.

Developmental Disorders

Idiopathic Scoliosis. Idiopathic scoliosis may present in infancy, although this occurs rarely in the United States and infrequently in the juvenile years. The most frequent onset of idiopathic scoliosis is during the pubertal growth spurt. Small spinal curvatures may occur in 5% to 10% of the preadolescent population, but only 1 in 20 of these requires treatment.

Curves of small magnitude in immature individuals have the potential to progress to severe deformities, so that patients with clinical evidence of spinal asymmetry should be evaluated and treated if progression occurs. Serial radiographs of all patients with spinal asymmetry document the degree of deformity and identify progressive curves, but this approach is costly and results in unnecessary radiation to adolescent children. Therefore, radiography should be reserved for those patients with significant deformities, whereas those with milder deformities can be observed clinically.

The degree of deformity may be assessed by measurement of the rib hump or lumbar hump in the forward bend position by using the scoliometer, as described by Bunnell. This device, adapted from a nautical pitch gauge, is placed in the posterior midline at the point of maximum deformity with the patient in the forward bend position. The angle with which the trunk deviates from the horizontal is then read directly on the scoliometer. This angle of deformity is referred to as the "angle of trunk rotation" (ATR).

Patients with curves of greater than 20 degrees had an ATR of greater than 5 degrees in 99% of the cases examined by Bunnell, giving a very low false negative rate. There is, however, a significant false positive rate. Thus, some patients with mild curves have an ATR of 5 degrees or more. Therefore, patients with 5 degrees or less ATR do not require radiography. However, if these patients have growth remaining, they should be observed at 6- to 12-month intervals with clinical examination using the scoliometer to detect progression. If significant progression is detected (greater than 2 degrees ATR) or if the initial ATR is greater than 5 degrees, a single standing anteroposterior radiograph in boys or a posteroanterior radiograph in girls should be taken using high-speed screens. Girls are seven times more likely to experience progression than boys, and the more immature the patient at the time of initial curve detection, the more likely the curvature is to progress. In addition, there is a strong familial predisposition to scoliosis, and patients with a positive family history should be followed closely.

For patients with curvatures that measure less than 25 to 30 degrees on radiographs by the Cobb technique, no treatment is necessary. However, follow-up until relative skeletal maturity, which occurs 2 years after menarche in girls and voice change in boys, is indicated to ensure lack of progression. Curves that progress to the range of 25 to 45 degrees in skeletally immature individuals should be treated with an orthosis, usually of the underarm type, until skeletal maturity is achieved. The goal of bracing is to prevent progression of the curvature. In general, most physicians treating scoliosis prescribe 23 hours a day of brace wear, although there is some evidence that part-time brace wearing (16 hours per day) may be as effective as the 23-hour-a-day program that has been traditional.

Electrical stimulation has been advocated by several groups to prevent progression of scoliosis. This is done at night only by use of transcutaneous electrodes attached to a stimulating device. However, several studies have found this approach ineffective, and at present this approach is not recommended.

The Charleston Bending Brace is a scoliosis body brace that overcorrects the curves and is used only 8 hours at nighttime. Preliminary studies of this orthosis indicate it may be quite effective.

Curvatures greater than 45 degrees in most cases continue to progress following adolescence and require surgical treatment. Surgery consists of insertion of stainless steel rods onto the posterior (or, in some cases, other devices onto the anterior) spine, which partially correct the deformity and hold the curvature in the corrected position while the spine that has been prepared for fusion by removal of facet joints, decortication, and addition of bone graft heals solidly. The Cotrel-Dubousset system and similar systems that allow multiple sites for hook placement, as well as provide correction of sagittal contours, have replaced the Harrington rod in treatment of idiopathic scoliosis. These systems allow patients to be mobilized rapidly following surgery without the need for a brace. The patients are able to be discharged from the hospital within a week of surgery and are back in school within 2 weeks.

Neuromuscular Scoliosis. Scoliosis is found in a high incidence in quadriparetic cerebral palsy patients, as well as in patients with degenerative neuromuscular diseases, such as Duchenne muscular dystrophy and spinal muscular atrophy. Bracing may be indicated in younger patients with cerebral palsy and spinal muscular atrophy and may retard curve progression, but many of such children ultimately require surgery with sublaminar wiring by the Luque technique, which produces excellent curve correction and exceedingly stable fixation, allowing rapid mobilization following surgery.

Bracing is not effective in scoliosis associated with Duchenne muscular dystrophy and may only delay surgery in these boys, thereby subjecting them to surgery at a time when their pulmonary function has deteriorated. Therefore, spinal bracing is contraindicated in boys with Duchenne muscular dystrophy, and these patients should undergo early surgical stabilization as soon as it is apparent that a curvature is developing.

Postural Roundback. Postural roundback is an increase in the normal thoracic kyphosis found in children and adolescents. As long as the kyphosis is flexible, no orthotic treatment is necessary. These patients may respond to physical therapy in the form of thoracic hyperextension and pelvic tilt exercises. Occasionally, if the deformity is severe and progressive, an orthosis may be indicated. Patients should be followed radiologically for progression or development of structural changes.

Scheuermann's Disease. Scheuermann's disease is characterized by an increased thoracic or thoracolumbar kyphosis associated with changes in the vertebral body consisting of anterior wedging of greater than 5 degrees of at least three vertebra, end plate irregularity, and Schmorl's nodes. This usually presents in mid to late adolescence and may be associated with back pain and hamstring tightness. Boys are affected more frequently than girls. If the thoracic kyphosis is greater than 45 degrees and there is significant growth remaining, the patient should be treated with an orthosis and physical therapy. Unlike the goal of prevention of progression in patients with scoliosis, actual correction can be achieved and maintained in patients with Scheuermann's disease. Surgical correction may be indicated for patients with severe kyphosis.

Spondylolisthesis. Spondylolisthesis is forward slippage of a vertebral body relative to the adjacent distal vertebral body. This usually occurs when L5 slips forward on S1, and in children, this is usually due to a defect in the pars interarticularis, which appears in a predisposed individual during the first decade. Spondylolisthesis may also occur because of congenital deformity and elongation of the pars.

Patients with spondylolisthesis may present with back pain, posterior thigh pain, and evidence of tight hamstrings, or they may be asymptomatic but show evidence of deformity. Clinical examination demonstrates flattening of the buttocks, decreased range of flexion of the spine, and hamstring tightness. Oblique radiographs document the presence of the pars defect, and the severity of the forward slippage should be measured on a standing lateral film.

In order to measure the slippage, the upper border of the sacrum is divided into four quadrants. Grading ranges from grade I for slippage less than 25% to grade V for complete slippage of L5 on S1 (spondyloptosis). Patients with grade I and II spondylolisthesis without significant symptoms should be observed throughout growth for possible progression of the slippage by lateral standing radiographs of the lumbosacral spine on a yearly basis or more frequently if symptoms indicate. Recent studies, however, have indicated that progression is unusual following initial presentation. If there is no evidence of increased slippage, no treatment other than avoidance of high-risk activities, such as football and gymnastics, is required. If the patient is symptomatic, immobilization in a lumbosacral orthosis or cast may decrease symptoms, and the patients may be weaned from the orthosis when asymptomatic.

For patients with persistent symptoms or progressive slips of grade III or greater, spinal posterolateral fusion using a massive amount of autogenous graft, usually between L4, L5, and the sacrum, is performed. Only in very severe cases is decompression of the anterior sacrum, anterior fusion, or reduction indicated. Removal of the L5 lamina (Gill procedure) is not indicated and may actually aggravate the instability. When solid fusion is achieved, the symptoms, including the hamstring spasm, will resolve.

Traumatic Injury

Traumatic injuries to the spine may occur at any time during childhood and may be associated with injury to the underlying spinal cord. Injuries that occur at birth may be confused with anterior horn cell disease, since both of these conditions give signs of lower motor neuron damage. However, the spinal cord injury is nonprogressive. In infancy and childhood, spinal cord injury may occur following major trauma without radiographic evidence of bony injury.

The most common cause of vertebral and spinal cord trauma in children is motor vehicle accidents, and appropriate seat restraints are effective in prevention of these disastrous injuries. In the case of complete loss of spinal cord function, no recovery can be expected; with incomplete injuries, recovery may occur. Immediate postinjury treatment of patients with high doses of systemic steroids may reduce the magnitude of neurologic deficit. In either case, the bony injury and instability, if present, should be treated, and a rehabilitation program at a center accomplished in treatment of these patients should be instituted. Surgical decompression of the spinal cord is not of any benefit to patients with complete injuries, but in selected patients with incomplete injuries, surgery may enhance the resolution of the neurologic deficit by removal of pressure on the spinal cord. Surgery may be necessary to stabilize the associated bony injury. In preadolescents with spinal cord injuries of the upper thoracic and cervical spine, the incidence of scoliosis is exceedingly high, and treatment of progressive spinal deformity below the level of injury with an orthosis should be done prophylactically. If progressive scoliosis exceeds 40 degrees, spinal fusion with segmental instrumentation should be done.

Fractures of the Ring Apophysis. With hyperflexion or hyperextension injury of the spine, fragments of the ring apophysis may be separated from the main body of the vertebra and may impinge on the spinal cord, cauda equina, or nerve roots. These fragments can be seen on computed tomography (CT) or MRI studies. When this occurs, the fragments must be surgically removed.

Causes of Back Pain in Children

A variety of entities may cause back pain in children, and it is important to distinguish these from one another by careful history, physical examination, and follow-up of the clinical course. The major causes of back pain are described next.

Spondylolisthesis. Patients with spondylolisthesis usually present with pain that may begin with the back and radiate into the posterior thighs, rarely before the age of 10 years.

Spinal Cord Tumor. The most common presentation of spinal cord tumor is back pain. However, careful physical examination may demonstrate the presence of neurologic dysfunction, and anteroposterior spinal radiographs may show evidence of increased interpedicular distance. Diagnosis is made by MRI or myelography. Treatment consists of neurosurgical excision of the tumor.

Disc Disease. Disc disease may occur in young adolescents and is frequently due to a bulging annulus rather than a herniation of the nucleus. A trial of conservative therapy is indicated in most cases, but a high percentage of patients ultimately require surgical decompression. Because the bulging disc may be central rather than peripheral, patients may present with diffuse, nonradicular pain. Diagnosis can be made by MRI or myelography.

Osteoid Osteoma. Osteoid osteoma is an unusual condition that is thought to be neoplastic. Although the lesions of osteoid osteoma generally appear in the second or third decade, they can occur in young children. They present with nonradiating back pain, which is frequently more apparent at night and classically is relieved by salicylates. Diagnosis can be made by plain radiography, tomography, and technetium-99 scan and confirmed and precisely localized by CT. Treatment of these lesions is by surgical resection, which may be facilitated by injection of the patient with radionuclide and intraoperative use of a radiation-sensitive probe.

Discitis. Discitis may present as back pain with or without leg pain or as pseudoparalysis of the lower extremities. Radiographs may demonstrate a decreased disc space height and end plate irregularity. Although bacterial cultures of the disc are usually negative, many, if not all, of these cases may be secondary to focal osteomyelitis of the vertebral end plate. The usual organism is *Staphylococcus,* but occasionally other organisms, including gram-negative bacteria, may be responsible. In the past, many children with discitis were treated successfully with cast immobilization alone. However, 3 to 6 weeks of antibiotic coverage along with cast or brace immobilization of the spine is probably indicated in most cases. An effort should be made to obtain a bacteriologic diagnosis by serial blood cultures and, on occasion, needle biopsy of the vertebral body before institution of antibiotic therapy.

Cord Tether. Tethered cord may present with back pain, although it frequently presents with painless neurologic dysfunction in the lower extremities or secondary incontinence. Patients with a tethered cord secondary to a tight filum terminale also frequently have skin abnormalities, such as café au lait spot, hairy patch, or a dimple at the base of the spine. This entity may be diagnosed by MRI and is treated by surgical release of the tether.

Low Back Strain. Low back strain may be seen in teenagers with acute onset of low back pain without neurologic symptoms or radiographic evidence of bony abnormalities. This is not associated with radicular pain or neurologic changes. The usual treatment is with salicylates or nonsteroidal anti-inflammatory drugs, plus an active stretching program.

REFERENCES

1. Bunnell WP: Spinal deformity. Pediatr Clin North Am 33:1475, 1986.
2. Bunnell WP: An objective criterion for scoliosis screening. J Bone Joint Surg 66A:1381, 1984.

ORTHOPEDIC PROBLEMS OF THE EXTREMITIES

MICHAEL G. EHRLICH, M.D.
EDWARD AKELMAN, M.D.

UPPER EXTREMITY

Sprengel's Deformity

Congenital elevation of the scapula is often mistaken for scoliosis, with which it is often confused, because of the shoulder elevation. The patients usually have some limitation of shoulder abduction and a cosmetically unappealing prominence above the clavicle. Physiotherapy may aid abduction slightly, but the scapula is usually bound down by an omovertebral band and does not improve much unless there is surgical transfer of the scapula. This is a very successful procedure, improving cosmesis and shoulder function. This should be done before age 7, as later transfer may jeopardize the brachial plexus. It is important to look for associated problems, especially Klippel-Feil syndrome or fusion of the cervical vertebrae, and renal and cardiac anomalies.

Congenital Pseudarthrosis of the Clavicle

This is generally a right-sided lesion, which presents as a painless bump. It is distinguished from a fractured clavicle, since the fracture is usually painful or leads to pseudoparalysis of the arm in an infant. Further, clavicular fractures always heal regardless of the degree of displacement. The pseudarthrosis has been reported occasionally to cause some aching in the shoulder, and we have observed late cases of thoracic outlet syndrome in some patients. If the patient really has an unsightly cosmetic deformity or in cases where there is some discomfort or other problems, such as outlet syndromes, resection of the pseudarthrosis, interposition of an iliac graft, and plating give excellent results. This condition may be associated with neurofibromatosis, and if it occurs on the left side, it is usually associated with a cervical rib, which may give an outlet syndrome picture with paresthesia in the hand. Bilateral pseudarthrosis is associated with cleidocranial dysostosis.

Benign and Malignant Neoplasia

The proximal humeral physis is one of the fastest growing bones in the upper extremity and, therefore, is a frequent site of neoplasia. Chondroblastomas tend to occur in the epiphysis (i.e., the end of the bone), and unicameral bone cysts frequently occur in the metaphysis. One may also see aneurysmal bone cysts here. Osteosarcomas are not uncommon in the proximal humerus as well. One has to look carefully for the lesions when there is pain around the shoulder. Most benign lesions require open biopsy, curettage, and grafting, but unicameral cysts may be eradicated successfully in about half the cases by steroid injections into the cyst.

Congenital Dislocation of the Shoulder

Congenital dislocation of the shoulder is a rare upper extremity problem, and it is associated with underdevelopment of the upper extremity. The shoulders may be small in appearance, with total instability of the humerus. Most patients do not have symptoms of pain. Treatment in this condition is conservative, as no satisfactory surgical treatment has been shown to give functional improvement.

Recurrent Dislocation of the Shoulder

Traumatic shoulder dislocation tends to occur during the teen years and has a high rate of recurrence. Although good controlled studies are not available, we still treat the patient with a traumatic dislocation with the arm immobilized to the side for about 4 weeks for the first episode. If there are a number of subsequent involuntary dislocations when the arm is abducted and externally rotated, there should be surgical intervention.

A number of children can voluntarily subluxate or dislocate their shoulder on command. That particular group does not do well with surgery and should be treated with physiotherapy and, occasionally, psychotherapy to get them to break the habit of voluntary dislocation.

Panner's Disease

Osteochondritis dissecans of the capitellum usually presents between ages 4 and 8. It is the commonest cause of nontraumatic stiffness in the elbow in children. Later, in the preteen or adolescent years, one sees a similar picture as the result of repetitive trauma, for example, pitching in Little League elbow. In the young child, there is not much that one can do other than splinting, active range-of-motion exercises, and no passive stretching. In traumatic cases in teenagers, one may have to remove loose fragments or drill the joint surface. Better treatment is to prevent these late complications by avoiding overuse of the elbow. Although children are restricted in the numbers of innings they may pitch, they tend to log excessive extra hours by practicing.

Congenital Dislocation and Subluxation of Radial Head

This may occur spontaneously or as part of one of several dysplasias. Congenital dislocation has to be distinguished from traumatic dislocations. This sometimes proves difficult because the child may be several years old, and congenital dislocation is only first diagnosed at the time of an unrelated traumatic episode. The congenitally dislocated radial head can be distinguished because it has a bullet-shaped appearance, whereas the normal or traumatically dislocated one is shaped like a saucer. The range of motion is remarkably good with congenital dislocation, with very good pronation and supination and just slight restriction of flexion. We generally do not try to reduce these dislocations. In the rare case where there is pain or marked cosmetic deformity around adolescence, the radial head can be excised. This is never done in children who still have a great deal of growing because the wrist may subluxate as well.

Congenital subluxation of the radial head is somewhat different from traumatic subluxation in that the radial head is partially in the joint, and this is painful early, with loss of supination and pronation. The radial head is excised around adolescence.

Upper Limb Deficiency

The pediatric amputee population has a higher percentage of children with limb loss due to congenital limb deficiencies than to acquired amputation. Most child amputee clinics report 60% congenital and 40% acquired amputations. Congenital limb deficiencies occur with equal frequencies in males and females, with the upper limb being involved twice as often as the lower limb.

Madelung's Deformity

This condition is not a true congenital deformity because it is not present at birth. It is characterized by radiographic changes that appear at age 2, with the ulnar and volar half of the distal radial epiphysis growing more slowly than the radial half. The radius becomes shorter on the ulnar half than the radial half, with a slope toward the ulnar side. The distal ulna becomes prominent. These deformities are usually asymptomatic and require no surgical treatment.

LOWER EXTREMITY

Rotational Deformities in Children

There is a fair amount of conflict over whether these deformities should be treated. Probably most of the torsional deformities are related to intrauterine positioning, and they are exacerbated by patients sleeping prone with their feet turned inward. In Europe, where children traditionally were nursed on their sides, there are almost no torsional deformities. It is not uncommon, therefore, for children to have supple metatarsus adducts shortly after birth and then present between ages 1 and 2 with internal tibial torsion, and between ages 3 and 5 with turning in from the hips, with femoral anteversion. The diagnosis of anteversion is made by looking at the rotation of the hips with the thighs and legs in the extended positions. Normally, the hips and the knees should turn out more than they turn in. Patients with excessive anteversion rotate their hips in more than they turn out. Internal tibial torsion can be diagnosed by flexing the knee and supporting the foot in a neutral position. The foot should normally be facing forward, but in internal tibial torsion, it will rotate in. Metatarsus adductus is similarly diagnosed by pressing on the sole of the foot. The heel should align with the second metatarsal. If it faces in and can be easily reduced by gentle pressure on the first metatarsal, it is considered supple.

Many orthopedists maintain that internal tibial torsion disappears when children start to walk, and the natural history of femoral anteversion is to spontaneously improve with age. However, not all of the patients correct spontaneously, and many of the anteversion patients, although looking better, have artificial correction because they develop compensatory external tibial torsion. These may present with knee problems in adolescence because the hip faces in and the foot faces out. If one does not believe the torsional problems need treatment, at least it would be prudent to try to get the children to sleep on their backs so that gravity rotates the feet out. This can be assisted by sewing some bulk to the front of the pajamas to make the child uncomfortable if sleeping prone. Since the treatment is not particularly difficult, one could treat the supple metatarsus adductus with exercises or outflare shoes at night. The internal tibial torsion can be treated by an 8- to 12-inch night bar, with the feet facing out about 45 degrees, and the anteversion can be treated by adding knee immobilizers to the bar, so that the sleeping child does not flex the knees up underneath

and rotate the hip inward. Sometimes, a child will have severe persistent internal tibial torsion or persistent anteversion. If so, a tibial or femoral osteotomy is done. This usually occurs after about age 7 or 8. Since half of adult growth is completed by about age 2, there is an advantage to try to treat these conservatively early. After about age 5, there is little to recommend bracing, since growth is relatively slow, but it is worth allowing the children several years of backsleeping to see if they recover.

External rotational deformities are less of a problem. Most children rotate outward from their hips due to what is called the "external rotation contracture of infancy." This is not treated and usually corrects during the first full year of walking because the knees cannot be flexed efficiently if they are facing outward. External tibial torsion is rarely treated because the normal progression of the foot is about 10 degrees outward. If there is a great deal of external tibial torsion about age 2 years, use of a night bar may be considered. Surgery is rarely performed on the older child with external tibial torsion unless it is bilateral and interfering with activities, such as riding a bike or squatting.

Bowlegs (Genu Varum) and Knock-Knees (Genu Valgum)

Bowlegs are physiologic until about 18 months or 2 years of age. Children then go into a knock-knee phase, which peaks at about 3 years of age. Obviously, one does not treat mild deformities that are age appropriate. However, the physician should be equally careful not to ignore a significant deformity even if it occurs at an age-appropriate time. It is always necessary to be on the alert for renal rickets or phosphate diabetes when the bowing or knock-knees looks significant. There is a particularly virulent form of bowing known as Blount's disease, which is a combination of bowing and internal tibial torsion. It is often progressive, and even surgical intervention may not be adequate to prevent the progression. However, although many orthopedists consider Blount's disease to be a primary growth disturbance, the facts that it shows a predilection for heavy children, who are early walkers and tends particularly to be prevalent among children with less access to health care suggest that it may represent a particularly severe form of physiologic bowing, with early walking, increased weight, and delayed treatment playing a part. The pediatrician can treat early bowing if concerned that it may be a little more severe, along with the torsion, by using an extra long (about 14 inches [35 cm]) night bar. After age 3 years, a formal Blount's disease or bowing brace may be necessary.

Genu valgum is a little more difficult to treat and may require a formal night knock-knee brace. Because it is often associated with ligamentous laxity and pronated feet, some believe that wearing polypropylene inserts with a scaphoid pad tends to shift the weightbearing line slightly and help the valgus. Older children with knock-knees or bowlegs may have a hemiepiphyseodesis performed if they have enough growth left. This is usually done with stapling of the physis, a relatively atraumatic procedure. If growth is already finished or if the deformity is too severe early, one may have to do an osteotomy.

Osgood-Schlatter Disease

This disease is referred to as an osteochondritis or an apophysitis because there is fragmentation of the bone. Actually, Osgood-Schlatter disease probably represents a chronic low-grade fracture through the physis of the tibial tubercle. Children who are particularly active develop a prominence of the tubercle. It probably represents a chronic avulsion pull by the patella tendon, which is attached to the largest muscle in the body, the quadriceps. Traditionally, this has been treated with benign neglect because it has always been stated that the tubercle would bind down once growth was finished. Although that is true, a certain percentage of young children, usually in the teen years, will go through a period of persistent pain or discomfort that may last for a few years. A small percentage actually avulse small fragments that form a pseudojoint in front of the tubercle and continue to hurt even when growth stops. These may have to be surgically removed. If the children are uncomfortable with their Osgood-Schlatter disease, it is not enough to advise them to "take-it-easy." Most of these children interpret this to mean that they cut down their basketball from 3 hours to 2 hours a day. I often place them in a walking cast or a rigorously enforced knee immobilizer for 6 weeks.

Chondromalacia of Patella or Patellofemoral Compression Syndrome

This condition is almost ubiquitous in teenagers and some preteen groups. Although its symptoms resemble those of the chondromalacia seen in adults, at arthroscopy one does not usually see gross changes. Most of the children have audible crepitation and pain with flexion and extension or on patella compression. They also complain when they sit for a time with the knees severely bent, as in an automobile.

There are many different treatments for this. The British do not treat it, as fairly often it seems to disappear around early adult life. Many U.S. orthopedists treat it with isometric exercises, the presumption being that these exercises will strengthen the vastus medialis oblique muscle and realign the patella. Although the initiating cause may be partial malalignment of the patella, sometimes due to residual anteversion at the hip or to external tibial torsion, to some extent this is really another overuse syndrome. I have successfully managed great numbers of patients who did not respond to exercises by giving them 2 months of anti-inflammatories and stopping their sports during that time. This gives relief in about 90% of children. They are then allowed to return to sports, but some forbearance is urged. It probably is not wise for our children to play and train for a major team sport each season. They should have a down day or two during the week and maybe a down or off season each year.

Those who fail to respond to conservative measures will sometimes benefit from lateral release of the patella following diagnostic arthroscopy. It is not clear whether this functions by reducing the pressure on the patella, altering its alignment, or partially denervating it.

Recurrent Subluxation or Dislocation of Patella

The patella may slip partially or completely out to the lateral side. This is more common in girls. Although the initial episode usually is accompanied by swelling and medial pain (torn ligament attachments), subsequent episodes may present as a sudden giving way of the knee. This is sometimes difficult to distinguish from the buckling seen in chondromalacia. Usually, the child will be able to describe the patella moving out to the side. Episodes accompanied by swelling probably should lead to immobilization of the knee for 6 weeks to permit ligament healing. That can be done with a cast or a knee immobilizer. For recurrent problems, the first line of defense is again isometric exercises to strengthen the quadriceps, which may stabilize the patella. This is best done with straight leg raising, since moving through a full range of motion, especially with weights, aggravates arthritis under the patella and is very uncomfortable for the child.

When conservative treatment fails, milder cases of subluxation may be treated with a lateral release. For real dislocation, one usually has to add realignment of the patella tendon and the quadriceps tendon. Waiting for too long a time before repair may lead to irreparable damage to the patella and many years of pain.

Osteochondritis of Femoral Condyle

Children do not usually tear menisci until they are in their advanced teens, older than 15 or 16 years. Therefore, locking of the knee is more likely the result of a loose fragment from osteochondritis. This separation, involving both bone and cartilage, most often involves the lateral aspect of the medial femoral condyle. Some think that it represents avascular necrosis, with the cartilage outgrowing its blood supply, since it tends to occur in some overfed farm animals. Others, however, think that it represents trauma, since it affects race horses more than other types of horses. This is important in its implications for treatment. When this separation appears in children below the age of 10 years, we usually think that it is irregular ossification and may not treat it. After age 10, we are more concerned and initially treat it with a cast or knee immobilizer. The downside of knee immobilizers is that as soon as young patients are asymptomatic, they tend to remove

the knee immobilizer or take off any removable splint and, therefore, delay healing. It is important to try to make the diagnosis as early as possible. Radiographic changes may not be readily apparent on AP and lateral views, and one should obtain a tunnel or notch view.

When osteochondritis dissecans does not respond to conservative therapy, drilling of the lesion, possibly bone grafting, or screw fixation of the defect may be required. If the fragment has separated, sometimes only a salvage operation can be done, which has a poor prognosis.

Congenital Discoid Meniscus

This actually represents a very rare lesion but can be a cause of buckling or locking in the knee in children sometimes below the age of 10 and sometimes older. It tends to occur on the lateral aspect of the knee, and one may see a cyst there or feel popping in the knee. The diagnosis is best made with an MRI. Actual traumatic tears of the medial meniscus, so common in young adults and late teens, are rarely seen during the growing years. We try to save at least part of the meniscus, since we now appreciate it as a weightbearing structure.

Congenital Hyperextension of Knee

This is usually a benign, if grotesque appearing, lesion in which the knee is bent back on itself. It can usually be reduced manually and held with a cast. Reduction should be done soon after birth, that is, in a day or two.

Posterior Bowing of Tibia

This is a deformity whose main importance is to distinguish it from anterolateral bowing of the tibia, which usually implies a precursor to congenital pseudarthrosis of the tibia. In posteromedial bowing, the foot usually assumes a calcaneal position; that is, it appears somewhat pressed against the front of the tibia. This is considered a fairly benign condition, although in recent years, it has been associated with mild degrees of limb shortening. It may be treated with a cast or brace to bring the foot into more plantar flexion or to put pressure over the apex on the front of the tibia. Many just watch it, and there is usually slow, gradual improvement. Surgery is rarely necessary.

Congenital Pseudarthrosis of Tibia

This condition is often associated with von Recklinghausen's neurofibromatosis. Although there usually are no neurofibromas at the site of the lesion, the bone tends to be dysplastic in the area of involvement. Therefore, in the first 2 years of life, there may be anterolateral bowing of the tibia or the fibula or both. The foot tends to be in equinus. This should alert the pediatrician to radiograph the leg. There may be cystic changes, sclerosis, or narrowing of the medullary canal in the lower third of the tibia. Prevention of an ultimate fracture there sometimes can be done by prophylactic bracing, and some surgeons are using bypass allografts before the bone breaks to give extra support.

Once the tibia has fractured and conservative treatment with casting has failed, the options are intramedullary rods extending through to the ankle for extra stability, nonvascularized allografts to span the avascular site, vascularized fibula transfer, autografts with plates, and with all of these, either electrical coils, external electrical fields, or autografting. All of these techniques have some measure of success, none has a perfect record, and amputation still frequently results. Because many of these children have so many surgeries and still often must undergo amputation, some surgeons believe that it is kinder to do a below-knee amputation when the first treatment fails.

Congenital Absence of Tibia or Fibula

Obviously, there are many variants of this condition, as part or all of a bone may be lost. There is also a very extensive international nomenclature, and one may speak of incomplete terminal tibial meromelia, meaning loss of the end of the tibia, or intercalary fibula hemimelia, referring to loss of part of the fibula between the two ends. Obviously, the treatment will be different for partial absence.

With complete fibula loss (frequently associated with proximal focal femoral deficiency), the foot goes into extreme valgus, and attempts at reconstructing the ankle joint have been dismal failures. With complete absence of the tibia, there have been attempts to centralize the fibula under the femur. These also have been largely unsuccessful in terms of restoring anything approaching a normal knee joint. These children will benefit from early amputation and have a much more normal life. Partial losses of either bone may be better salvaged.

FOOT DEFORMITIES

Flatfoot

Flatfoot can be described as loss of the normal longitudinal arch or pronation of the foot, that is, weightbearing on the medial border of the foot with the heel in valgus. Loss of the arch occurs in 97% of infants because of infant distribution of fat and obviously should not be treated. Pronated feet occur in children who are loose ligamented and can be confirmed by the normal appearance of the arch when nonweightbearing or when standing on the toes so the muscles support the arch. This naturally is usually bilateral and can be further confirmed by laxity elsewhere (one can usually flex the thumb up to the forearm). As many of these children get older, the ligaments tighten up, and the flatfoot disappears. Children are sometimes treated with scaphoid pads or longitudinal arch inserts, but their only function is to have the children slide off the schapoid pad and wear the shoes out differently. In severe cases, a polypropylene scaphoid pad can be used to support the arch, and a UCB heel can be used to keep the child from sliding off the arch. The parents must be told that the child may still have a flatfoot, since the arch support does not tighten the ligaments. However, a large study of military recruits showed that a loose-ligamented or supple flatfoot is not painful in adults. There are other types of flatfoot that do become painful in adults.

Coalition Syndrome. This presents as a painful flatfoot between ages 10 and 16 years. There is usually a coalition between either the calcaneus and navicular, best seen on lateral oblique views, or the talus and calcaneus, best seen on CT scans. There is lack of inversion, with eversion of the foot. Because of pain over the peroneal tendons with inversion, it was known previously as peroneal spastic flatfoot. In early cases without secondary adaptive changes, one may consider resection of the coalition to try to regain motion. In older children, I still believe an arthrodesis has the best chance of resolving pain.

Congenital Vertical Talus. This looks like a rockerbottom foot, and again there is no inversion or eversion. The talus is prominent in the sole of the foot, and the navicular is dislocated on the talar neck. This is very painful in adult life if it is not treated. Early casting is done to loosen the ligaments, but the treatment is surgical reconstruction of the foot.

Flatfoot with Congenital Tightness of Heel Cord. To get the foot out of equinus, or plantar flexion, the child everts the foot, trying to get dorsiflexion at the subtalar joint. That is because the subtalar joint is an oblique axis joint, and it goes into dorsiflexion at the same time that it everts. As a result, the talus is again prominent in the medial sole of the foot, and this becomes painful as an adult. In fairly young children, heel cord lengthening and wearing a UCB insert may do the job. In older children, one has to reconstruct the foot, although some authors prefer an extraarticular subtalar arthrodesis.

Flatfoot with Accessory Navicular Bone. Ten percent of children have an extra navicular bone making a prominence on the medial border of the foot, but in 90% of these, the bone is bound down and is not painful. Of those with an unattached bone, it may be painful, with discomfort radiating up along the posterior tibial tendon that supports the arch. If wearing a UCB insert does not ameliorate the symptoms, some surgeons remove the extra bone. We have achieved better results when resection of the accessory bone is accompanied by reattaching the posterior tibial tendon under the foot to support the arch.

Clubfoot and Rigid Metatarsus Adductus

There is a type of positional clubfoot, and a more rigid form of metatarsus adductus, that do not respond to exercises. These usually can be treated by several sessions of serial casting that will restore a normal foot fairly quickly. The more rigid type of clubfoot has traditionally been treated by casting for a number of months. There is a strong tendency now not to continue casting much beyond 3 months. Continued casting beyond 3 months more frequently leads to a rigid small foot, with a high rate of recurrence. Earlier surgical intervention is performed more frequently, with a posteromedial and lateral release giving a good, albeit not perfect, foot with minimal recurrence.

If a simple metatarsus adductus is not corrected by several years of age and is developing callosities, it might require surgical intervention.

Cavus Foot

The cavus, or high arch, foot is frequently associated with clawing of the toes. Severe callosities develop under the metatarsal heads, especially the first. This is always painful in an adult if left untreated, so it should be surgically treated in a child.

This type of foot deformity is almost pathognomonic of an underlying neurologic disorder, and all appropriate attempts should be made to rule out the neurologic problem. These include doing MRIs and EMGs to look for tethered spinal cords, epidural lipomas, hereditary sensorimotor neuropathies (Charcot-Marie Tooth disease), polio, and cerebral palsy. It is a mistake to perform muscle transfers without knowing whether the transferred muscles will become involved later. In younger children, one can do muscle transfers. Older children usually need bone work as well.

Habitual Toe Walking

Children usually walk up on their toes in the first 6 months after starting to walk. If they continue to do so for 1 or 2 years, it is certainly worth ruling out spasticity or dystrophy. Traditionally, most physicians do not treat toe walking because they expect that the foot will come down flat ultimately. However, many children develop heel cord contractures and the type of painful flatfoot described earlier to compensate for the tight heel cord. Therefore, persistent toe walking by about age 3 is treated. We use a dorsiflexion assist brace to tire the foot and break the habit. Physiotherapy is used if there is any heel cord contracture. Other approaches involve casting of the foot for periods of several months or heel cord lengthening.

Toe Varus or Congenital Curling of Toes

This is thought to be an inherited tendency, with weakness of the small intrinsic muscles of the toes. It manifests itself by curling of the third, fourth, and fifth toes toward the center of the foot and usually overlapping of the second toe over the third. Sometimes, it presents as congenital overlapping of the fifth toe. If the curling is mild, no treatment is necessary other than one size wider shoes so as not to aggravate the curling. With severe conditions, the toes sometimes will underlap to the extent that they are compressed, and the children develop paresthesias. If the condition is severe, excellent results are obtained by transfer of the long toe flexor to substitute for the intrinsic muscles.

Bunion Deformities

Sometimes, the first metatarsal faces in, giving the child a wider foot. This would be fine if teenage girls, in whom it most frequently occurs, would wear broad shoes with a wide square toe. Since they do not wear such shoes, a number develop bunion deformities in their teen years. If it is painful, and it often is, and cosmetically disturbing to them, a surgical option is worth considering. It is not enough to remove the bunion, since the deformity will recur. An osteotomy of the first metatarsal is necessary to narrow the foot and to prevent recurrence.

Pump Bumps

Children have a tendency to respond to any irritation over a boney prominence with the generation of more bone. One area where this occurs frequently is the prominence over the back of the calcaneus. The painful bumps seen here are referred to as pump bumps because they were often seen in women wearing pumps, which are shoes that stay on by virtue of their tightness. In children, the condition is usually seen with very tight and firm shoes, such as ice skates, or soccer cleats. The pain can be relieved by stretching the shoes so they do not press over the bumps. If treatment is unsuccessful, the bumps may be surgically removed.

Sneaker Bursitis

This is an entity that is being seen more frequently in recent years. Children have pain, swelling, and local tenderness, but no erythema, just in front of the distal end of the Achilles tendon. This is caused by running while wearing high top sneakers. The sneakers sometimes strike the fat pad in front of the tendon and produce a chronic state of irritation. Treatment is wearing sandals or sneakers with a very large groove cut in the back of the heel to stop the trauma. Sneaker bursitis is fairly resistant to therapy and may take months of reduction of activity plus shoe changes to have an effect.

Osteochondritis of Tarsal Navicular (Kohler's Disease) and of Second Metatarsal Head (Freiberg's Infraction)

Kohler's disease occurs between ages 4 and 8 years and may present with limping, pain, or posterior tibial spasm. The treatment is purely symptomatic: casting, arch support, or anti-inflammatories. Ultimately, the symptoms will go away.

Freiberg's disease is often found in adolescent girls. It usually presents with pain in the second metatarsal head, and x-rays show fragmentation. Relief can sometimes be obtained by using a metatarsal pad to remove the weight from the metatarsal head. Surgery is necessary occasionally to deal with a loose fragment that is giving pain.

Leg Length Discrepancies

Many children are born with or develop leg length discrepancies. Actually 30% of all the people in the world are estimated to have ½ inch (1.25 cm) or less of difference. For anything under ½ inch, we do not even use lifts. The children compensate by bending the longer leg slightly when standing with double leg support, which actually occurs only during a small part of walking. For a ½- to 1-inch (2.5 cm) difference, we use lifts in growing children. One can put probably no more than a ¼-inch (0.65 cm) lift inside the heel. Otherwise, the heel will ride out of normal shoes. For greater differences, the lift has to be outside of the shoe.

Differences of 1 inch or greater can be corrected easily by stopping the growth of the longer leg. This can be done by stapling or by epiphyseodesis, which can sometimes be done percutaneously. Larger differences can be made up by this method or by leg lengthening. One should determine what the ultimate height of the patient is going to be before advising on this condition.

CONGENITAL HAND AND UPPER LIMB DEFORMITIES

PETER M. WATERS, M.D.
BARRY P. SIMMONS, M.D.

Congenital hand and upper limb differences occur in approximately 6% to 7% of live births, with about 1% being multiple anomalies. One in 626 live births have been estimated to have upper extremity anomalies, but only 10% of these differences have significant cosmetic or functional deficits. Of these congenital differences, 1% to 2% are caused by chromosomal abnormalities. A minor portion are secondary to defined genetic causes. The cause of the congenital malformations is unknown in the majority of cases.

There is a long-standing classification of upper limb malformations based on embryologic failures that divides the congenital differences into seven general categories:

1. Failure of formation of parts
2. Failure of differentiation of parts
3. Duplication
4. Overgrowth
5. Undergrowth
6. Constriction band syndrome
7. Generalized skeletal abnormalities

To best appreciate this classification system and the malformations it describes, it is important to understand the embryologic development of the upper limb. The arm bud appears 26 days after fertilization, 24 hours before the appearance of the leg bud. Growth is in a proximal to distal fashion, and development is guided by the apical ectodermal ridge inducing the mesoderm to condense and differentiate. The upper limb anlage initially is continuous and extends to a hand paddle by day 31. The digital rays develop by day 36 by fissuring of the hand paddle, initially with the central rays, followed by the border digits. Mesenchymal differentiation also begins in a proximal to distal fashion, with chondrification, enchondral ossification, joint formation, and muscle and vascular development. Joint formation and digital separation require programmed cell death. The entire process is complete by 8 weeks postfertilization. Obviously, major organ system development is occurring at the same embryonic time and accounts for the associated cardiac, craniofacial, musculoskeletal, and renal anomalies with upper limb malformations.

Management of the malformation is dependent on the individual condition, and specific discussion is reserved for each malformation. However, the present options for treatment include observation, occupational hand therapy including splinting, prosthetic care, and surgery. The caring surgeon should have a full armamentarium of these resources to offer each child to best suit the needs and unique situation.

In general, surgical intervention should maximize functional hand development. This is particularly true for thumb development of prehension. Opposition fine motor skills begin by 9 to 10 months of age and continue to mature through the second year of life. As surgical techniques and instruments have improved and pediatric anesthesia has become routine for infants, surgery for major congenital malformations has been performed routinely in the first 6 to 18 months of life. This allows the postoperative rehabilitation to be complete as the toddler enters the important age of exploration and independence with the reconstructed hand.

FAILURE OF FORMATION

Transverse Arrest

Congenital amputations occur at any level and include amelia (absence of a limb), hemimelia (absence of the forearm and hand), acheiria (absence of the hand), adactylia (absence of digits), and aphalangia (absence of phalanges). The most common upper limb congenital amputation is a forearm level amputation. These anomalies are quite rare, with forearm amputations being 1 in 20,000 live births and upper arm amputations being 1 in 270,000 live births. These amputations are sporadic events and are predominantly the only malformation present in these infants. Amputations related to constriction band syndrome are now classified as a deformation related to intrauterine amnionic bands.

The treatment options for these children include observation (i.e., leave the child alone), prosthetic use, and surgery. By and large, these children have minimal functional deficits. The cosmetic issues vary widely between children and need to be addressed on an individual basis. Frequently, treatment for forearm level amputees includes early prosthetic fitting when they are able to sit independently (sit to fit).

This enables the child to develop spatial orientation of two equal limb lengths for activities. The initial prosthesis is passive, with the introduction of an active opening or closing hand at approximately 2 to 3 years of age. Myoelectric prostheses are becoming more affordable and repairable but are still reserved for the adolescent or very functional prosthetic-using child. Unfortunately, the majority of amputees do not use their prostheses on a regular basis. The prostheses are insensate and require visual input to the central nervous system for functional use. The prostheses are still not cosmetically the equivalent of a normal limb. In addition, they can be cumbersome, fragile, and expensive. However, the option and trial of prosthetic use should be offered to all congenital amputees.

Longitudinal Deficiencies

Phocomelia

This is a rarely seen intercalary segment deficiency. Its renown was in the late 1950s and early 1960s when thalidomide was used to control nausea in pregnant women between the 38th and 54th post-fertilization days. Sixty percent of those women had phocomelic infants. At present, phocomelia is most often associated with craniofacial syndromes (Robert's syndrome). There are three types of phocomelia:

1. The hand attaches directly to the trunk.
2. The forearm and hand attach directly to the trunk.
3. The hand attaches directly to the humerus.

These children become facile from birth with using their feet as hands. Unfortunately, this is not often socially acceptable. Treatment options include a prosthesis or limb lengthening acutely (i.e., vascularized fibulae transfer) or chronically (i.e., distraction osteoclasis). The purpose of surgery is to improve upper extremity function.

Radial Club Hand

Radial dysplasia encompasses a broad spectrum of preaxial malformations that may involve the elbow, forearm, wrist, and thumb. The defects may be in isolation or may be associated with cardiac (Holt-Oram syndrome), hematologic (Fanconi anemia), musculoskeletal (VACTERL), or craniofacial (Nager) syndromes. It is usually a sporadic event, although it may be associated with chromosomal abnormalities (trisomy 18/21). The incidence ranges from 1 in 30,000 to 1 in 100,000 live births, and it is bilateral in half the cases. The degree of radial dysplasia ranges from complete absence of the radius and thumb to a foreshortened radius. Classification is

1. Short distal radius with delayed distal physeal growth
2. Hypoplastic radius with delayed proximal and distal physeal growth
3. Partial absence of the radius
4. Complete absence of the radius

Complete absence of the radius is the most common form (Fig. 1). It is always associated with preaxial deficiencies of muscles, tendons, nerves, and blood vessels, in addition to the obvious bone and joint defects evident on radiographs.

Treatment begins in the neonatal period with passive stretching exercises and corrective splinting. The goal is to correct the radial-side contracture and allow passive placement of the hand on the distal aspect of the ulna. In those infants in whom therapy, splinting, or casting is unsuccessful, distraction external fixators are being used to gradually correct the soft tissue contracture over 6 to 12 weeks. When the soft tissues are flexible, operative radialization or centralization can be performed. Generally, this occurs between 6 and 12 months of life. Operative correction improves forearm length, appearance, and hand grip function. It is imperative that these children have near normal elbow range of motion preoperatively. Otherwise, with forearm correction, they will lose the ability to feed and groom themselves with that extremity. Postoperative splinting and therapy may be necessary intermittently throughout growth to prevent recurrence of the

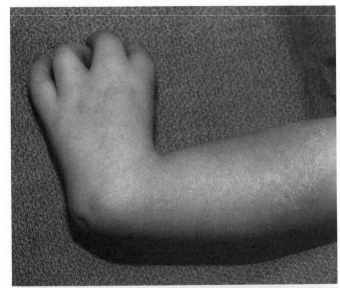

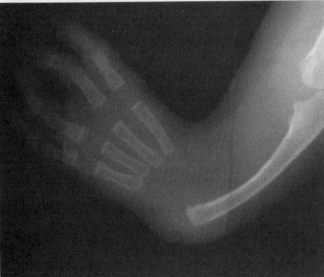

FIGURE 1. *A,* Infant with radial club hand with 90 degrees of radial deviation deformity. Treatment should consist of early stretching, splinting-casting, followed by operative centralization-radialization. Note the thumb aplasia. *B,* Radiograph of this child indicates a complete absence of the radius (type 4) and thumb.

deformity. It is extremely important that surgery not ablate the distal ulna physis, or the forearm will be markedly foreshortened in adulthood. In those situations, distraction osteoclasis to lengthen the forearm has been used.

The majority of these children have hypoplasia or aplasia of the thumbs. Reconstruction of the hypoplastic thumb includes skin Z-plasties, opponensplasty tendon transfers, and metacarpal-phalangeal joint ligamentous reconstruction or arthrodesis. Aplasia of the thumb is best treated with pollicization of the index finger (Fig. 2). In congenital absence of the thumb, this is better than microvascular toe transfer (Fig. 3). Thumb reconstruction or pollicization is generally performed between 6 and 18 months of age. The quality of the pollicized digit is definitively dependent on the quality of the original index finger in terms of tendon function and joint motion.

Ulnar Club Hand

Ulnar dysplasia is much less common than radial dysplasia. Often, it is sporadic. It may be associated with other musculoskeletal defects

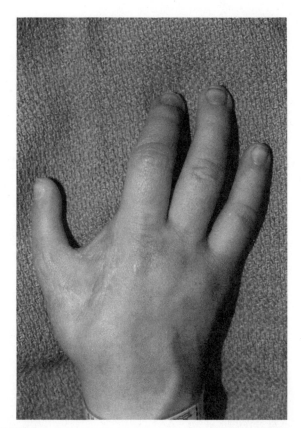

FIGURE 2. Postoperative photograph of patient 1 year after pollicization for thumb aplasia.

(ulnar-fibular syndrome) or syndromes (Cornelia de Lange). Since the ulna stabilizes the elbow and the radius stabilizes the wrist, these patients predominantly have elbow instability and dysfunction, whereas patients with radial dysplasia have wrist instability and dysfunction. Classification is based on the degree of ulnar dysplasia:

1. Hypoplasia of both proximal and distal ulna physis
2. Partial absence of ulna with radial bowing most common
3. Total absence of ulna
4. Total absence of ulna with radiohumeral synostosis

Treatment is based on improving hand or arm function and is dependent on the degree of elbow motion, forearm stability and position, wrist ulnar deviation posture, and thumb/digital function. Clearly, correcting progressive deformity, as in resecting the ulna anlage in types 2 and 4 deformities, is indicated. Similarly, improving thumb function by rotational osteotomy and web space-deepening procedures is worthwhile. However, some of these children are very functional without surgical intervention, and, therefore, all planned operations should have a specific functional goal. Preoperative videos of these children in activities of daily living is often useful in determining the value and potential success of surgery.

Cleft Hand and Symbrachydactyly

Central defects of the hand have been described in the past as typical or atypical. Since 1992, the International Federation of Societies of Surgery of the Hand has classified typical cleft hands as cleft hands and atypical cleft hands as symbrachydactyly.

Cleft hands generally have autosomal dominant inheritance. There are often associated anomalies, such as cleft lip and palate, congenital heart disease, and imperforate anus. There frequently are cleft feet. The hand is often V-shaped, and the middle ray is absent. The condition is generally bilateral.

Symbrachydactyly is a sporadic event without genetic inheritance. There are no associated anomalies. The feet are normal, and it is a unilateral process. The hand is U-shaped and often has many absent rays.

Flatt has called cleft hand a functional triumph and a social disaster. Treatment is dependent on improving both the cosmesis and functional condition of the involved hand. This includes cleft closure and deepening the first web space to improve thumb opposition. Often, this entails transposition of the index ray to the area of the absent middle ray. Associated first and fourth web space syndactylies need to be released. Axial malalignments and flexion contractures of the digits must be corrected.

Symbrachydactyly reconstruction is more complex and individualized. With multiple absent digits, nonvascularized or microvascular toe transfers are successful alternatives to provide pinch function. Digital lengthening techniques frequently are used also.

Aplasia of Thumb

The absence of the thumb is a significant cosmetic and functional deficit. As already mentioned, it is most commonly associated with radial club hand. It is similarly associated with the same syndromes that occur with radial club hand (Holt-Oram syndrome, Fanconi anemia). The goal of treatment is to provide prehension skills at an early age (less than 18 months). This is best achieved by pollicization of the index finger. The results are pleasing cosmetically and functionally, especially in the presence of a normal forearm. Pollicization is truly a masterful use of the index finger to create a thumb and is uniquely rewarding for surgeon, patient, and family.

FAILURE OF DIFFERENTIATION

Syndactyly

Syndactyly is the most common congenital hand malformation. It may occur in isolation or be associated with other congenital hand anomalies (polydactyly, brachydactyly) or systemic malformations (Poland, Apert). Syndactyly occurs in 1:2000 live births. It may be inherited in an autosomal dominant fashion. It is much more common in whites than in blacks. It is classified as simple, involving skin only (Fig. 4A), or complex, involving skin, bones, and joints. Syndactyly may be incomplete, involving only part of the web space, or complete,

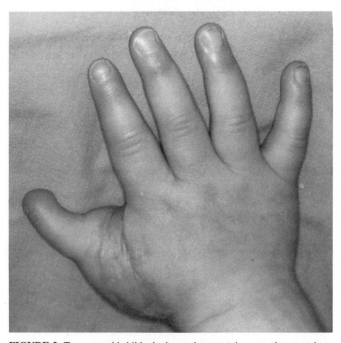

FIGURE 3. Two-year-old child who has undergone microvascular second toe transfer for traumatic amputation of thumb. This is to illustrate the appearance of a microvascular toe transfer. Its use in congenital differences is limited.

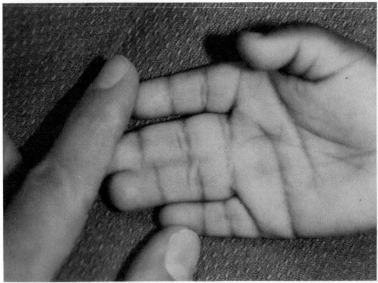

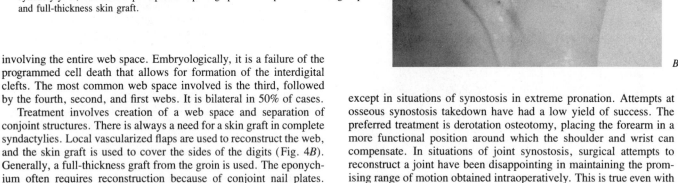

FIGURE 4. *A,* Simple, complete syndactyly of third web, the most common type of syndactyly. *B,* Immediate postoperative photograph of this patient outlining Z-plasties and full-thickness skin graft.

involving the entire web space. Embryologically, it is a failure of the programmed cell death that allows for formation of the interdigital clefts. The most common web space involved is the third, followed by the fourth, second, and first webs. It is bilateral in 50% of cases.

Treatment involves creation of a web space and separation of conjoint structures. There is always a need for a skin graft in complete syndactylies. Local vascularized flaps are used to reconstruct the web, and the skin graft is used to cover the sides of the digits (Fig. 4*B*). Generally, a full-thickness graft from the groin is used. The eponychium often requires reconstruction because of conjoint nail plates. Composite skin grafts from the toe can be used, in addition to local rotation flaps to improve the contour and appearance of the nail area.

The timing of surgery depends on the web space involved and the complexity of the deformity. Border digit syndactylies (first and fourth) are between digits of unequal length, and the syndactyly can cause growth deformity in the longer digit. Release should be early (3 to 6 months of age) in these situations. Simple, complete syndactylies are released and grafted between 6 and 18 months of age. Complex syndactylies are treated at 6 to 12 months of age. Incomplete syndactylies can be treated at any age before the child starts school. In all cases, the earlier the release, the higher the risk of recurrence of a mild syndactyly in the web space (web creep). Attempts at neonatal release have the highest risk of recurrence. In situations of multiple syndactylies (acrosyndactyly), each side of the involved digit should be released at a separate operation for fear of vascular compromise to the digit. The success of surgery is dependent on the degree of original deformity. Complex syndactylies may have residual limited range of motion or malalignment requiring further surgery. Simple syndactyly releases lead to normal function and pleasing cosmetic results, although skin graft is never the same as native skin in appearance. Attempts at tissue expansion have had too high a rate of complications to warrant its use.

Synostosis

Synostosis occurs with the failure of separation of embryologic conjoint structures. This can lead to failure of formation of a joint (humeral-ulnar synostosis, symphalangism) or of normal bones (radial-ulnar synostosis, complex phalangeal syndactyly). The most common upper extremity synostosis is proximal radial-ulnar synostosis. Treatment of this entity depends on functional impairment. The loss of forearm rotation can be compensated by shoulder and wrist motion,

except in situations of synostosis in extreme pronation. Attempts at osseous synostosis takedown have had a low yield of success. The preferred treatment is derotation osteotomy, placing the forearm in a more functional position around which the shoulder and wrist can compensate. In situations of joint synostosis, surgical attempts to reconstruct a joint have been disappointing in maintaining the promising range of motion obtained intraoperatively. This is true even with the advent of the distraction devices, such as the Ilizarov device.

DUPLICATION

Preaxial Polydactyly

Thumb duplication may be a misnomer, since it implies there are two normal thumbs. In reality, both are hypoplastic, and, therefore, split thumb may be a more accurate name for preaxial polydactyly. In isolation, split thumb deformity is usually a sporadic occurrence. It may be associated with genetic syndromes (acrocephalopolysyndactyly). The incidence of preaxial polydactyly is 0.08 in 100,000 live births. Classification is dependent on the number of bifid or duplicated phalanges or metacarpals. A duplicated proximal and distal phalanx is the most common type (Fig. 5). Reconstruction involves excision of the most hypoplastic thumb, generally the radial one, and reconstruction of the remaining thumb with the tendons, ligaments, and muscles that were shared or attached to the excised digit. This leads to a functional and cosmetic thumb. However, the need for further surgery with growth may be as high as 40%, with a Z-deformity of the proximal and distal phalanges being the most common problem. Surgical recombination of the distal phalanx and nail beds (Bilhaut-Clouquet procedure) has been disappointing and should be reserved for rare circumstances. Unlike postaxial polydactyly, thumb skin nubbin polydactylies should never be ablated in the nursery or office with suture ligature (Fig. 6). Almost always, the thenar musculature attaches to the radial polydactyly, even in the presence of a nubbin. Simple ablation can lead to deformity and opposition weakness.

Postaxial Polydactyly

Small finger polydactyly is very common. In the black population, its incidence is 1 in 300, and in whites, it is 1 in 3000. It has an autosomal dominant inheritance, and it may be associated with other systemic anomalies (Ellis-van Creveld, Laurence-Moon, and Bardet-Biedl syndromes). In a white infant with a negative family history, the presence of a postaxial polydactyly should warrant a screening for other anomalies. There are three types:

1. Soft tissue nubbin
2. Partial duplication, including bone
3. Complete duplication, including the metacarpal and phalanges

Most often, the skin nubbins are treated with suture ligature amputation in the nursery by the primary care physician. However, this frequently leads to a residual mass at the base of the digit that many adults complain about. Thus, it may be better to excise the entire remnant, including its broad base, under local anesthesia. Duplications that include bone should be reconstructed in the operating room after 6 months of age, when anesthesia administration is safer.

OVERGROWTH

Fortunately for both the surgeon and the patient, macrodactyly is very uncommon. It is a very difficult problem to reconstruct surgically with success, and its presence is disturbing cosmetically and socially to the patient. It is usually unilateral and predominantly on the radial side of the hand. It most commonly affects the index finger, and it more often involves multiple adjacent digits than an isolated finger. It is often associated with neurofibromatosis of the median nerve. Macrodactyly needs to be distinguished from overgrowth related to vascular or lymphatic malformations or hemihypertrophy.

Surgery is aimed at reducing the bulk of the digit. Soft tissue resection is always a major component of treatment, but recurrent deformity and gigantism are common. Epiphysodesis and phalangeal reduction in length or width or both are commonly employed. Amputation by ray resection may yield the best cosmetic and functional result in extreme cases. However, the patient and family should be forewarned that amputation may lead to accelerated growth in the

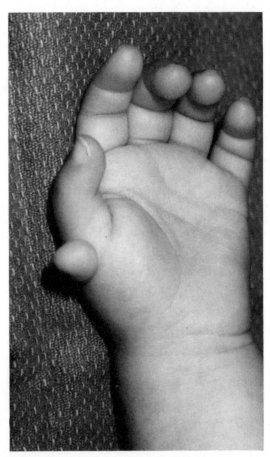

FIGURE 6. Unlike treatment for postaxial polydactyly, never excise a skin nubbin duplication of the thumb. The thenar musculature probably attaches to this duplication, and excision alone will lead to deformity and weakness.

adjacent digit. Most congenital hand surgeons view this as their most difficult problem. The best results may come with very aggressive surgical intervention at an early age.

UNDERGROWTH

Brachydactyly is a common malformation. In isolation, it has an autosomal dominant inheritance with variable penetrance. It is frequently associated with other syndromes (Turner, Larsen) or diseases (cretinism, sickle cell), especially with brachymetacarpia. It most often involves the middle phalanx, especially in the small finger. It may be in conjunction with symphalangism, camptodactyly, or clinodactyly. The presence of brachydactyly, especially brachymetacarpia, warrants systemic examination for associated malformations. Treatment options include digital lengthening, bone grafting, microvascular transfer, or osteotomies for malalignment.

Thumb hypoplasia may represent a significant deficit in prehension and grasp. It may involve hypoplasia of the metacarpal (Cornelia de Lange syndrome, diastrophic dwarfism) or phalanges (Rubinstein-Taybi syndrome, Apert syndrome). It is most commonly associated with other radial ray deficiencies (Holt-Oram syndrome, Fanconi syndrome). Thumb hypoplasia has varying components of thenar musculature atrophy, metacarpal-phalangeal joint instability with ulnar collateral ligament deficiency, decreased first web space, and interphalangeal joint instability or stiffness. These elements need to be reconstructed surgically by first web space four-part Z-plasty, opponensplasty, MCP joint collateral ligament reconstruction, or chondrodesis. In the extreme case of a ponce flottant, pollicization of the index finger rather than reconstruction of the thumb is best.

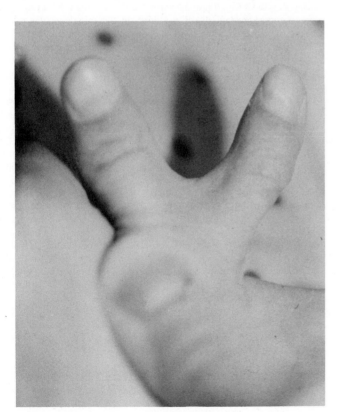

FIGURE 5. Thumb duplication, or preaxial polydactyly, preoperatively. This requires reconstruction of tendons, joints, and skin.

CONSTRICTION BAND SYNDROME

Constriction band syndrome is associated with acrosyndactyly and acral amputations (Fig. 7). It is most likely a mechanical deformation related to an abnormal intrauterine environment from early amnionic rupture and resultant oligohydramnios and amnionic bands. There is no inheritance pattern. It occurs in 1 of 9000 live births. It is associated with other deformations in 50% of cases, the most common being clubfoot. There may be devastating cleft lip and facial deformations as a result of constricting amnionic bands. In terms of hand involvement, the ring finger is affected most frequently with constriction bands. The constriction ring often will lead to distal edema and limited function. In acrosyndactyly associated with constriction band syndrome, there often are skin clefts that pass dorsal to volar, indicating the embryonic formation of a web space before the amnionic rupture and subsequent deformation. Treatment involves release of the constriction by Z-plasty, which frequently reduces the distal edema. In the presence of acrosyndactyly, separation of digits with Z-plasties and skin graft is performed.

GENERALIZED MUSCULOSKELETAL DISORDERS

Arthrogryposis

Arthrogryposis multiplex congenita is not a specific syndrome but rather a symptom complex of congenital joint contracture associated with neuropathic or myopathic problems. It may be best viewed as one of three types: classic musculoskeletal arthrogryposis, peripheral arthrogryposis involving hands and feet, or arthrogryposis associated with systemic malformations. The upper limb is classically postured in shoulder adduction and internal rotation, elbow extension, forearm hyperpronation, wrist palmar flexion and ulnar deviation, digital flexion, and thumb-in-palm deformity.

Physical and occupational therapy is the cornerstone of all treatment for these children. In the upper extremity, the goal is to improve passive range of motion of the elbow, wrist, and hand. If passive elbow flexion of 90 degrees is not achieved by 2 years of age, an operative triceps lengthening and posterior elbow capsulotomy should be performed. If active elbow flexion is not attained by 5 years of

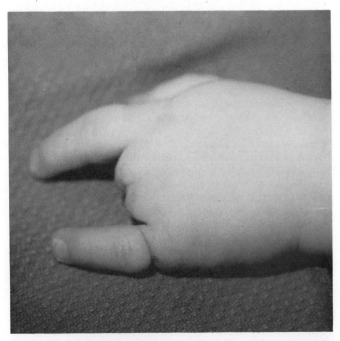

FIGURE 7. Constriction band syndrome with acral amputations and constriction rings. This is an intrauterine malformation. Surgical treatment requires Z-plasties of the constriction ring.

age, an elbow transfer of either the triceps, latissimus dorsi, or pectoralis major should be performed. The triceps may be the most functional but has the disadvantage of limiting pushoff and weight-bearing in patients with significant lower extremity involvement. The pectoralis major transfer probably should be limited to boys because of asymmetric breast development in girls. The wrist deformity that persists despite therapy and splinting should be treated with a radial or carpal closing wedge osteotomy and wrist extensor tendon transfer. The incomplete syndactylies of all four web spaces should be released with Z-plasties early. The goal of surgery is to provide these children, and subsequent adults, with independent function of hygiene, feeding, and self-care. Surgery is clearly warranted in these intelligent but physically challenged children.

OTHER CONGENITAL HAND DIFFERENCES

Camptodactyly

Camptodactyly translates from Greek to mean "bent finger." It involves a flexion deformity of the proximal interphalangeal joint, most commonly in the small finger. It may present in infancy or in adolescence. It may be associated with multiple systemic malformations. There is an anatomic imbalance between the flexor and extensor mechanisms. There may be abnormal insertions of the lumbrical, flexor digitorum superficialis, or retinacular ligaments. Treatment should attempt to restore normal flexor-extensor balance. In the infantile form, this may be best achieved by progressive extension splinting. The adolescent form is the most difficult to treat with either splinting or surgery. There frequently are bony changes present that preclude restoration of normal motion or alignment. Camptodactyly associated with systemic malformations may have the most successful surgical reconstructions by correction of aberrant anatomy.

Clinodactyly

Clinodactyly similarly translates from Greek to mean "bent finger" but represents abnormal radial deviation in the middle phalanx or distal interphalangeal joint. It most often involves the small finger and is usually bilateral. It commonly occurs in normal children. It has an autosomal dominant inheritance. It is frequently associated with other syndromes (Down) and may alert the primary neonatal examiner to look for associated malformations or problems. Treatment is based on the degree of deformity. Most are mild and nonprogressive and, therefore, do not warrant intervention. Progressive clinodactyly associated with a middle phalanx delta phalanx may require an osteotomy or physeal bar resection to improve alignment and function.

Trigger Thumbs

Trigger thumb represents an abnormality of the flexor pollicus longus and its tendon sheath at the A1 pulley. In this condition, the tendon either triggers on the pulley, creating a painful snap, or it becomes locked in flexion at the interphalangeal joint. There is a palpable mass (Notta's nodule) at the volar, proximal thumb crease over the metacarpal-phalangeal joint region. This nodule represents a size discrepancy between the larger tendon and the smaller pulley through which it must pass. In the past, trigger thumbs have been defined as congenital. However, the vast majority are probably acquired in the first 2 years of life, as evidenced by a recent prospective screening of neonates that failed to yield any trigger digits. Thirty percent of the cases are bilateral. In infants less than 9 months of age, 30% may have spontaneous resolution. In infants older than 1 year of age, less than 10% spontaneously resolve. Surgical release of the A1 pulley and flexor tendon sheath will resolve the flexion contracture and prevent permanent deformity. There have been no reported recurrences of trigger thumbs in infants or toddlers after surgical release.

REFERENCES

1. Bora FW: The Pediatric Upper Extremity. Philadelphia, WB Saunders Co, 1986.
2. Carter PR: Reconstruction of the Child's Hand. Philadelphia, Lea & Febiger, 1991:113–233.
3. Dobyns JH, Wood VE, Bayne LG: Congenital hand deformities. *In* Green DP (ed): Operative Hand Surgery. New York, Churchill Livingstone, 1988: 225–537.
4. Flatt AE: The Care of Congenital Hand Anomalies. St. Louis, Quality Medical Publishers, 1994.

THE HIP

PAUL G. DYMENT, M.D.

SEPTIC HIP

Septic arthritis of the hip joint is one of the true emergencies in pediatrics, as prompt surgical drainage of the joint space may prevent destruction of the femoral head and permanent loss of function. It is associated with an adjacent osteomyelitis, hematogenous seeding, or direct inoculation of bacteria into the joint from trauma. In neonates the most common organisms are *Staphylococcus aureus, Haemophilus influenzae,* group B streptococci, and gram-negative coliform bacteria. In infants and children from 4 weeks to 4 years of age, they are *S. aureus, Streptococcus pneumoniae, H. influenzae,* group B streptococci (especially if the child is under 1 year of age), and group A streptococci, and in children over 4 years of age, it is usually *S. aureus.*

Diagnosis

Diagnosis may be difficult in the neonate because the usual symptoms and signs are absent. Instead, the baby has symptoms like those of septicemia, with lethargy or irritability, refusal to feed, failure to thrive, cyanosis during the feeding, and no fever. The typical infant or child with a septic hip usually can be diagnosed readily, as pain and loss of motion are the presenting symptoms. These children look ill, and the older ones usually have fever, if not chills. The hip joint is kept in flexion, abduction, and slight external rotation, and any sort of passive motion of the infected hip is resisted because it causes pain. The child does not actively move the involved hip, and the proximal thigh may be swollen. A distant site of infection, such as paronychia, skin infection, or pneumonia, is frequently present. Palpation of the anterior hip joint will reveal tenderness.

The leukocyte count is of only limited value in helping with the diagnosis, as most patients will not have leukocytosis, and over one third will have a normal differential count. The erythrocyte sedimentation rate is a more useful test, being elevated in over 90% of cases, especially after the first 24 to 48 hours of symptoms. However, it is unreliable in the neonate. Ultrasonography may show signs of fluid in the joint space, and radiography may show signs of an adjacent osteomyelitis, although this is a late sign.

The suspicion of a septic hip should lead directly and immediately to an emergent consultation with an orthopedic surgeon to perform an aspiration of the joint. At the time of aspiration, it is critical to confirm that the joint has been entered in the event of a negative (dry) tap. For this reason, the procedure should be performed under fluoroscopic control, or radiopaque dye should be instilled into the joint after aspiration, and a radiograph should be obtained. The joint fluid will reveal a high cell count, mainly neutrophilic leukocytes, and decreased glucose. A gram stain may reveal microorganisms.

Treatment

Antibiotics should be commenced as soon as the diagnosis is made, the initial choice depending on the child's age, the most likely causative organisms, and the results of the Gram stain (Table 1). The

TABLE 1. Drug Doses

DRUG	ROUTE AND DOSE	DURATION OF TREATMENT
Septic Hip		
Neonates		
Methicillin *or*	IV or IM dose depends on age and prematurity	≥21 d
cefotaxime	IV or IM dose depends on age and prematurity	≥21 d
Infants and Young Children		
Cefuroxime	IV or IM 100–150 mg/kg/24h divided q8h	≥21 d
Children >4 Years		
Nafcillin *or*	IV 150–200 mg/kg/24h q6h (Max: 2000 mg q6h)	≥21 d
oxacillin	IV 150–200 mg/kg/24h q6h (Max: 2000 mg q6h)	≥21 d
Toxic Synovitis		
Ibuprofen	PO 40–50 mg/kg/24h t.i.d. or q.i.d. (Max: 2400 mg/d)	

initial antibiotic should be changed to a more specific one when the synovial fluid culture and sensitivity results are available.

Immediate arthrotomy, within 6 hours after the synovial fluid analysis confirms the diagnosis, should be performed to decompress the joint space to try to prevent destruction of the cartilage (which is permanent and leads to degenerative arthritis), and avascular necrosis, a consequence of arterial compression of the proximal femur.

TRANSIENT SYNOVITIS

Transient synovitis, or toxic synovitis, is a self-limited syndrome of acute hip pain of unknown etiology. An infectious cause has been postulated because of its frequent association with an upper respiratory infection. It has also been thought to be secondary to occult hip trauma, a sort of contusion of the hip. Its incidence is about 3 in 100, and boys are twice as likely to have it as girls. Most cases occur between ages 3 and 8 years.

Diagnosis

The cardinal presenting symptom is the acute onset of unilateral hip pain without any history of trauma. There is a limp, and the involved limb is kept preferentially in flexion and external rotation. The patient does not look sick, and there is usually no fever, although there may be an upper respiratory infection. The leukocyte count and sedimentation rate are either normal or only minimally elevated. Radiographs of the hips are obtained mainly to help exclude a more serious diagnosis. Ultrasound examinations can demonstrate the presence of a mild joint effusion, but this test is generally not necessary, nor is a bone scan indicated, since both increased and decreased regional activity can be seen. About 70% of patients undergo spontaneous resolution of their symptoms within a week, and almost 90% have done so by 4 weeks. There is a 10% chance of recurrence, generally within the first 6 months after the initial episode.

Treatment

Simple bedrest and insistence on no weightbearing of the involved joint are generally all that is necessary. This should be continued until there is no further pain and there is a full range of motion. At one time, many of these youngsters received skin traction of the joint as part of their initial treatment, but this is now believed not to be helpful. If symptoms do persist, such traction can be instituted, but it should be done with the hip flexed to 30 to 45 degrees, the position at which hip joint pressure measurements are at a minimum.

It is not known whether the use of a nonsteroidal anti-inflammatory drug will hasten resolution, but on theoretical grounds, it would be reasonable to prescribe one for its anti-inflammatory effect as well as for its analgesic action (ibuprofen 40 to 50 mg/kg/d, t.i.d. or q.i.d., max: 2400 mg/d) (Table 1).

DEVELOPMENTAL DYSPLASIA OF THE HIP

Developmental dysplasia of the hip (DDH), formerly called "congenital hip dislocation" or "congenital hip dysplasia," refers to a condition beginning in infancy in which there is hip instability and dysplasia. The clinical abnormalities range from simple instability, in which the femoral head can be dislocated and reduced out of and into the acetabulum, to a complete dislocation, in which there is loss of contact between the femoral head and acetabulum. The acetabular cavity frequently is both shallower and more vertical than normal, and the ossification of the proximal femoral epiphysis often is delayed, so the condition is not just a simple dislocated hip. There is a dysplastic component.

The incidence is about 1 in 1000 infants. It is more common in baby girls (1 in 300 compared with 1 in 2000 for boys), and this is consistent with one of the postulated etiologies based on experimental data. Neonatal ligamentous laxity may be induced by estrogen followed by progesterone in female guinea pigs but not in male guinea pigs exposed to the same hormones. This laxity, combined with neonatal positioning, appears to be the principal contributing cause, although there is another group of infants whose diagnosis is not apparent during the newborn screening examination who have frank acetabular dysplasia. Studies of twins have revealed a genetic component, with 34% of identical twins but only 3% of fraternal twins affected. The incidence is increased in certain high-risk groups: frank breech position (25% have DDH), coexisting torticollis (15%), positive family history (6%), and coexisting metatarsus adductus (1%). It is reasonable to screen high-risk newborn infants with ultrasonography. A single anteroposterior (AP) radiograph taken at 3 to 6 months of age (when the presence of ossification centers makes interpretation more reliable) can confirm the diagnosis.

Diagnosis

Although it is important for a hip examination to be performed on all newborn babies as at least 50% of DDH cases will manifest physical abnormalities of the hip during the newborn period, the other cases will be detected only several months later with only the finding of limited hip abduction. Hence, routine screening by physical examination of the hip should continue throughout the first year of life, with negative findings being recorded during each well-child visit.

Newborn

The Barlow modification of the Ortolani test is the standard examination procedure and should be performed as follows. Many examiners prefer the infant to be lying on the mother's lap. The physician stabilizes the pelvis by holding it between the thumb and fingers of one hand. The other hand grips the leg being examined, with the thumb over the femoral triangle, the web between the thumb and index finger over the knee, and the middle fingertip over the greater trochanter. The knee and thigh should be flexed to 90 degrees, and the hip is then abducted to the midabduction position. At that point, the examiner presses the middle finger forward over the greater trochanter, and if there is forward movement of the femoral head, the hip has been dislocated. The examiner then applies an up-and-down force with the thumb several times with the hip in both the midabduction and adduction positions. Hip instability can be detected by a "clunk" as the femoral head slides over the posterior rim of the hip socket. So-called clicks can be found in up to 10% of normal infants.

Infancy

This same examination should be performed throughout the first year of life. After the first few weeks of life, the signs of hip instability tend to disappear, and limited abduction and limb shortening become the most prominent clinical findings. Asymmetric gluteal folds are a good clue to the presence of limb shortening in such infants.

Radiography

By age 3 to 6 months, either a single AP radiograph of the pelvis or ultrasonography is the most definitive diagnostic test. Radiography should be performed on all infants with an abnormal Ortolani-Barlow test and on all infants at high risk, as listed previously, even if the hip examination is normal. The abnormal radiograph will show the acetabular slope to be more oblique than normal or the ossific nucleus to be either smaller than the normal side or absent or the metaphysis to be displaced laterally.

Treatment

Treatment should be prescribed and monitored frequently by an orthopedic surgeon. There is no justification for a primary care physician's advising triple diapers in an attempt to force continuous abduction, as was the practice for many years. This only wastes time when the infant can be treated successfully by conservative means using the Pavlik harness, a simple, effective, inexpensive, and comfortable treatment that has been successful in treating more than 90% of young infants with DDH. The earlier the treatment is started, the more likely that it will be successful and the less likely that the infant will develop avascular necrosis of the femoral head, a complication of splinting. The Pavlik harness works by keeping the hip flexed and abducted and by limiting extension.

If treatment is not begun until infants are over 6 months of age, they will probably require traction, reduction under anesthesia, and prolonged immobilization using a cast. Children newly diagnosed after age 2 years will probably require open reduction.

LEGG-CALVÉ-PERTHES DISEASE

Legg-Calvé-Perthes disease (LCPD) is an avascular necrosis of the femoral capital epiphysis of unknown etiology. Its incidence is 1 in 20,000, and it appears between the ages of 4 and 8 years. Boys are affected about four times as often as are girls. About 14% of cases are bilateral, and there is a familial predisposition with an incidence of 1 in 35 in family members. There are several associations with this condition: low birth weight, retarded bone age, and white race.

The natural history is for death of all or part of the epiphysis, followed by removal of the dead bone and replacement with new bone, a healing process that takes 2 or 3 years. The femoral head can regrow deformed, especially if there has been unrestricted weight-bearing or if the lateral part of the head is not contained within the acetabulum (with an indentation of the new bone resulting from pressure from the hard lateral border of the acetabulum). An abnormally shaped femoral head can lead to persistent limitation of motion and premature degenerative arthritis of the hip joint. Modern forms of treatment are designed to allow the femoral head to regrow in a round configuration and thereby prevent later arthritis.

Diagnosis

The insidious appearance of a limp is the most common presenting symptom. There is usually a history of pain in the hip, but sometimes the condition can present with the referred pain in the knee only. This pain is worse with activity and is relieved by rest. Physical examination will reveal an antalgic gait, one in which the patient takes a quick step to shorten the time of weightbearing on the affected side. The passive range of motion of the hip will reveal limited abduction and internal rotation. There may be atrophy of the thigh or calf muscles and, eventually, a shortened leg length as the femoral head flattens.

There are four radiographic stages:

1. In the *initial stage,* the femoral ossific nucleus is smaller than the contralateral one, and there is an apparent joint widening as seen in synovitis, probably actually caused by epiphyseal cartilage hypertrophy. The metaphyseal bone appears less mineralized than the epiphysis, and a subchondral radiolucent zone believed to be a stress fracture demarcates the extent of the necrotic fragment. At this stage, a radioisotopic bone scan may show decreased uptake on the affected side.

2. In the *fragmentation phase*, the epiphysis has areas of radiolucency and radiodensity, the latter presumably representing healing by new bone formation.
3. In the *reossification stage*, there is increasing homogeneity of the epiphysis and alteration in the shape of the femoral head and neck during the healing stages. A bone scan can show enhanced uptake.
4. In the *healed stage*, residual deformities are all that can be seen.

Treatment

Although half of patients with LCPD do not need any treatment, the decision whether or not to treat and the close follow-up of all of these patients whether treated or not require an orthopedic surgeon with experience in managing this condition. Earlier treatment programs were based on the belief that prevention of weightbearing would prevent the deformities of the head and, therefore, later degenerative arthritis. This required prolonged hospitalization, traction, strict bedrest, and a spica cast. However, not only has this resulted in much emotional trauma and financial cost, but also prolonged immobilization has not appeared to influence the radiographic course of the disease.

The basic premise of modern day treatment is *containment*, based on the concept that deformity of the affected epiphysis can best be prevented by containing the femoral head within the depths of the acetabulum, thus allowing the acetabulum to mold the new head. This can be accomplished by either a broomstick abduction long leg cast (Petrie cast) or an abduction brace (such as the Scottish Rite orthosis), both of which allow weightbearing and maintenance of hip range of motion. Such an orthosis allows free motion of the knee and ankle, and the child can walk. Such devices generally must be worn full time for 6 to 18 months until the radiographic stage of reossification is reached and there is no risk of additional deformity. Patients who do not even require bracing are those whose area of avascular necrosis is restricted to only a small portion of the femoral head, such as the anteromedial portion. If the necrosis involves either the lateral portion of the femoral head or the entire head, either a bracing program or surgical intervention is indicated.

Although a bracing program appears to be the treatment of choice, it does require a good deal of compliance on the part of the patient and family. Surgical containment procedures, such as a varus osteotomy of the proximal femur (to place the avascular area within the acetabulum), offer the hope of shorter treatment periods, but there are risks from these procedures, and there is no evidence that earlier surgery to contain the hip is preferable to prolonged bracing. The need for secondary procedures to remove surgical hardware also may make these techniques less desirable.

SLIPPED CAPITAL FEMORAL EPIPHYSIS

Slipped capital femoral epiphysis (SCFE), or adolescent coxa vara, is the condition in which the epiphysis of the proximal femur separates from the metaphysis, causing the femoral metaphysis to move anteriorly and proximally and the epiphysis to slip posteriorly and medially. Although SCFE can result acutely from severe trauma, generally it is a more gradual slip resulting from chronic abnormal shear forces. It can occur only before the epiphyseal plate closes during late puberty.

The incidence of SCFE is about 2 in 100,000, and it occurs twice as often in boys as in girls and in blacks more than in whites. About 50% of cases are bilateral, but only 25% are bilateral at the time of initial diagnosis. It is seen between the ages of 9 and 15, usually during early puberty, thus at a later age in boys than in girls. Almost 90% of affected patients are obese. There is a slight familial tendency, with 5% of patients with SCFE having a parent who also had the condition. If left untreated, a limp and limited hip motion will persist, and premature degenerative arthritis can develop by early adulthood.

Diagnosis

If there has been an acute slip, there is a history of trauma and the patient cannot walk. The affected femur is held in external rotation,

and passive movements of the hip are painful. In the chronic form, the pain is more varied and frequently is located in the anterior thigh or knee. The latter is a well-known clinical trap and is a reason all children and adolescents with knee pain should have their hips examined. Physical examination will show a limping child with the affected hip kept in external rotation. Internal rotation, abduction, and flexion of the hip are limited.

When the clinical picture is that of SCFE, anteroposterior, lateral, and frog lateral radiographs should be obtained. A mild slip is more obvious on the lateral view, where posterior displacement of the epiphysis is more apparent. Diffuse osteopenia of the metaphysis and widening of the physis are also radiographic characteristics.

Treatment

Once a diagnosis is confirmed radiographically, the patient should be hospitalized immediately, and further slipping should be prevented by surgical fixation of the epiphysis using threaded pins across the physis or another fixation technique. Manipulation may be attempted to reduce the amount of slippage, but this is associated with a considerable risk of avascular necrosis. For persisting deformity after physical closure, an osteotomy of the proximal femur to reposition the femoral head is the procedure of choice.

CONGENITAL DEFORMITIES OF THE ANTERIOR CHEST WALL

ROBERT C. SHAMBERGER, M.D.

STERNAL DEFECTS

Midline sternal defects can be divided into three categories. First, and most severe, is *thoracic ectopia cordis,* produced by defects of the sternum and overlying soft tissues of the chest, which results in the heart being entirely exposed and protruding from the thoracic cavity. Affected infants usually have intracardiac defects as well and, despite extensive surgical efforts, rarely survive.

Second, and less severe, is *thoracoabdominal ectopia cordis,* in which the inferior portion of the sternum is cleft, but the heart resides within the thoracic cavity and is covered by either a thin layer of skin or omphalocele. Such infants often have a constellation of anomalies termed the *pentalogy of Cantrell,* which consists of defects in the abdominal wall, diaphragm, pericardium, heart, and inferior sternum. Efforts should be made initially to achieve a dermal closure of the defect to prevent sepsis. The cardiac anomaly should then be repaired before soft tissue coverage of the defect with muscle flaps to minimize the risks of cardiac trauma. Many of these infants can be saved with recent advances in pediatric cardiac surgery. The prognosis is related primarily to the intrinsic cardiac anomaly.

Third, and least severe, is the *bifid or cleft sternum,* in which a V-shaped defect of the upper sternum or complete separation of two sternal halves is present but covered with normal skin and subcutaneous tissues. Echocardiography should be performed to exclude the rare associated cardiac anomaly. Closure of the defect is best achieved in infancy when the chest wall is pliable and can be closed primarily without compression of the heart. Closure provides protection from trauma to the underlying heart.

PECTUS EXCAVATUM AND CARINATUM

Pectus excavatum, posterior depression of the sternum and costal cartilages, is identified at birth or within the first year of life in 86% of infants who will have the defect. It is present more frequently in males than females by a 4:1 ratio, and a family history of chest wall deformities is often present (37%). Its etiology is unknown. Patients should be evaluated for scoliosis, which is seen in 15%. Although the severity of the depression may change with growth, it rarely resolves entirely. Individuals with particularly severe defects or young males with associated scoliosis should be evaluated for Marfan syndrome. Several series have evaluated cardiopulmonary function in these patients, particularly by means of exercise stress tests. They have demonstrated some impairment from this defect, but the role of conditioning is difficult to assess in these studies. A readily performed and reproducible test to evaluate the impact of the pectus excavatum deformity on cardiopulmonary function has not been defined. Decisions regarding repair must be based on patient and family desires and the severity of the defect. Long-term studies have demonstrated that persistent pulmonary abnormalities exist following repair of the deformity, presumably because of the narrow anterior/posterior dimensions of the chest in these children.

Pectus carinatum, anterior protrusion of the costal cartilages and sternum, is identified at birth in only a third of infants who will ultimately have the defect. In fact, in almost half the children, the defect is not identified until after the 11th birthday, when it appears with the pubertal growth spurt. It also has a male predominence (78%), and a family history of chest wall defects often is present (26%). The etiology is unknown. Indication for repair is primarily the severity of the local protrusion, which generally progresses until full stature is achieved.

POLAND SYNDROME

Poland syndrome is a constellation of anomalies that frequently occur in association. Each component of the syndrome can occur with varying severity. Absence of the sternal portion of the pectoralis major muscle, the pectoralis minor muscle, and subcutaneous tissue is found in most patients. Associated thoracic defects may include hypoplasia of the ipsilateral chest wall and, less frequently, depression of the chest wall or aplasia of the ribs. The last may require rib grafts for reconstruction. Brachysyndactyly of the ipsilateral middle fingers is seen with variable severity in two thirds of patients with this syndrome. Hypoplasia or absence of the ipsilateral breast (amastia) will necessitate reconstruction in females at puberty with a latissimus dorsi muscle flap and breast augmentation.

ASPHYXIATING THORACIC DYSTROPHY

Infants with asphyxiating thoracic dystrophy (Jeune's disease) are born with a hypoplastic, rigid, bell-shaped chest. Little respiratory motion is present due to the horizontal direction of the ribs. Infants frequently succumb in the perinatal period from pulmonary hypoplasia, but a spectrum of severity is seen in this anomaly. Surgical efforts have been made to enlarge the chest by dividing the sternum and interposing bone grafts or prosthetic material, but no clear improvement in the underlying pulmonary hypoplasia has been demonstrated. Because asphyxiating thoracic dystrophy is inherited in an autosomal recessive pattern, genetic counseling is critical.

REFERENCES

1. Shamberger RC, Welch KJ: Cardiopulmonary function in pectus excavatum. Surg Gynecol Obstet 166:383, 1988.
2. Shamberger RC, Welch KJ: Surgical repair of pectus excavatum. J Pediatr Surg 23:615, 1988.
3. Shamberger RC, Welch KJ: Sternal defects. Pediatr Surg Int 5:156, 1990.

BONE AND JOINT INFECTIONS

JOHN D. NELSON, M.D.

ACUTE BACTERIAL INFECTIONS

It is desirable that management of patients with bone and joint infections be a combined effort of the pediatrician or family physician, the orthopedic surgeon, and, when necessary, the physiatrist.

Surgical Management of Arthritis

Surgical evacuation of pus is done initially by needle aspiration. The pus is sent for bacterial culture. At the time of aspiration, it is desirable to flush the joint thoroughly with sterile normal saline to remove as much loculated pus, fibrin, and debris as possible. (It is not advisable to irrigate with antibiotic solutions, since they are usually irritating to synovium.) In most cases, two or three daily aspirations suffice. If substantial amounts of pus persist after a few days, open surgical drainage is performed.

There are situations in which needle aspiration of joint fluid is not satisfactory. With rare exceptions, open surgical drainage of hip joint pus should be performed immediately. The joint is especially vulnerable to permanent damage from pus itself and from vascular compromise due to pressure. There are recent reports of needle aspiration with copious irrigation of the hip joint instead of open surgery, but experience is limited. If the history suggests the possibility of a foreign body in the joint, open surgical drainage and exploration are advisable. The use of drains and the types of drains employed are a matter of the surgeon's personal preference and have not been subjected to the scrutiny of controlled trials.

Joints should be immobilized in a functional position of extension by sandbags, splints, or casts until pain is alleviated and range of motion exercises can be carried out.

Surgical Management of Osteomyelitis

The optimal surgical management of acute osteomyelitis is controversial. Our practice for many years is described, but it is possible that a less aggressive surgical approach would be as beneficial. If frank pus is encountered in a diagnostic aspiration, the patient undergoes surgical decompression through a cortical bone window. There are exceptions to this. In very young infants whose physis has not formed, metaphyseal pus often decompresses spontaneously into the contiguous joint, whence it can usually be removed by repeated needle aspirations. If the infected area abuts the growth plate, surgical intervention could conceivably cause damage. If the diagnostic aspiration yields only bloody material rather than pus, antibiotic therapy alone generally suffices.

The need for casts and immobilization must be determined in individual cases. If there is extensive involvement of a bone in the legs, weightbearing is prohibited to avoid the possibility of pathologic fracture.

Medical Management

Fluid and electrolyte therapy and medication for relief of pain are given as necessary. Initial antibiotic therapy in about half the cases can be guided by the results of gram-stained specimens of joint fluid or pus interpreted by an experienced microbiologist. Otherwise, initial therapy is empirical and based on likely pathogens at various ages (Table 1).

In the newborn infant, group B streptococci and staphylococci are the major pathogens, but coliform bacilli must be considered. Initial therapy with methicillin and either an aminoglycoside or an expanded-spectrum cephalosporin, such as cefotaxime, can be used. I prefer a cephalosporin because it is easier to use and safer than aminoglycosides. Furthermore, aminoglycosides have somewhat reduced activity in acid pH and decreased oxygen tension, both conditions that exist

TABLE 1. Etiologic Bacteria in Acute Suppurative Bone and Joint Infections

AGE	ARTHRITIS	OSTEOMYELITIS
Neonates	Group B streptococci*	*Staphylococcus aureus**
	*Staphylococcus aureus**	Group B streptococci*
	Coliform bacilli	Coliform bacilli
	Gonococcus	
Infants	*Haemophilus influenzae* b*†	*Staphylococcus aureus**
	Pneumococcus	Group A streptococci
	Group A streptococci	*Haemophilus influenzae* b
	Salmonella	
	Staphylococcus aureus	
Children	*Staphylococcus aureus**	*Staphylococcus aureus**
	Group A streptococci	Group A streptococci
	Pneumococcus	
	Gonococcus	

*Most common causes.

†In populations immunized with *Haemophilus* conjugate vaccines, this infection has become uncommon.

in pus. If cultures confirm group B streptococcal infection, treatment is changed to penicillin or ampicillin. For gonococcal infection, ceftriaxone is preferred until it is known whether the isolate is susceptible to penicillin.

In the past, arthritis in infancy was caused by *Haemophilus influenzae* type b in more than half the cases, but disease caused by that organism has become rare since the institution of immunization of infants with *Haemophilus* conjugate vaccines. A variety of organisms can be encountered. Cefuroxime is active against the usual organisms. Osteomyelitis in infancy is usually caused by staphylococci and streptococci, with occasional cases caused by *H. influenzae,* so cefuroxime is appropriate.

Beyond infancy, almost all cases of arthritis and osteomyelitis are caused by gram-positive cocci, and an antistaphylococcal beta-lactam drug or clindamycin is used. Clindamycin or vancomycin is used for patients with a history of allergy to beta-lactam drugs. Vancomycin is used for cases of methicillin-resistant staphylococcal infections. Gonococcal tenosynovitis in sexually active youngsters is treated with ceftriaxone. There are special situations discussed later in which alternative drugs are given as initial empiric therapy.

Antibiotic therapy is tailored to the culture and susceptibility test results. Suggested dosages are given in Table 2. Customarily, antibiotics are given parenterally for the entire course of treatment. However, several studies have shown that large-dosage oral antibiotic regimens can be employed successfully under rigidly monitored conditions. After several days when the clinical condition has stabilized and any necessary surgical procedures have been performed, an appropriate oral antibiotic is selected and given in doses two to three times greater than those recommended for less serious infections (Table 2). Approximately 1 hour after a dose of oral suspension or 2 hours after a dose of a tablet or capsule, a serum specimen is obtained either for measurement of antibiotic content or for serum bactericidal titer. The peak concentration of beta-lactam drugs or chloramphenicol should be at least 20 μg/ml and that of clindamycin at least 10 μg/ml. If the serum bactericidal titer test is done, it should be at least 1:8 against *Staphylococcus aureus* and *H. influenzae* and 1:32 or greater against streptococci. Five percent to ten percent of patients have poor gastrointestinal absorption of antibiotics and cannot be treated successfully by the oral route. The large doses of drugs are well tolerated and do not cause gastrointestinal side effects.

Response to therapy is judged by resolution of fever and local signs and by normalization of the erythrocyte sedimentation rate (ESR) and the C-reactive protein (CRP). In successfully treated patients, the CRP value normalizes in several days, whereas the ESR declines more slowly. Persistent elevation of these tests, even though clinical signs have improved, should prompt investigation for undrained pus or sequestrum.

The duration of antibiotic therapy is individualized. Pneumococcal, group A streptococcal, or *Haemophilus* arthritis usually responds to therapy promptly, and a 10- to 14-day course of antibiotics may suffice. A 3-day regimen has been reported to be successful for gonococcal tenosynovitis, but the Center for Disease Control Sexually Transmitted Diseases Treatment Guidelines recommends 7 days of antibiotic therapy for disseminated gonococcal infection. *Pseudomonas* osteochondritis of the foot can be treated with 7 to 10 days of antibiotics, providing that infected material has been thoroughly removed by curettage.

In most cases of osteomyelitis, antibiotic treatment is given for 3 weeks *providing that* the patient has shown good response of symptoms and physical findings and that the ESR and CRP have become normal. If this has not occurred, treatment is extended.

Chronic Osteomyelitis

Chronic osteomyelitis is usually a staphylococcal disease. Sequestrum is often present and has to be removed surgically. Medical therapy consists of an oral antistaphylococcal antibiotic given in a dose sufficient to attain peak serum concentrations of at least 20 μg/ml for beta-lactams and 10 μg/ml for clindamycin. Relapses are common after short courses of therapy. Most infections can be cured by appropriate surgical therapy and antibiotics given for 6 to 12 months depending on the clinical and radiologic responses.

SPECIAL SITUATIONS

In children with *sickle cell disease,* aseptic bone infarction can mimic osteomyelitis, and vice versa. Bone infarctions tend to be multiple, there is little fever and no bandemia, and the ESR is normal.

TABLE 2. Suggested Dosages of Antibiotics to Treat Bone and Joint Infections

ANTIBIOTIC	PARENTERAL DOSAGE	ORAL DOSAGE*
Beta-lactam Antibiotics		
Amoxicillin	—	100–150 mg/kg/d q6h
Ampicillin	150 mg/kg/d q6h	—
Cefaclor	—	100–150 mg/kg/d q6h
Cefazolin	75–100 mg/kg/d q8h	—
Cefotaxime	100 mg/kg/d q6–8h	—
Ceftriaxone	50–75 mg/kg/d q12–24h	—
Cefuroxime	100–150 mg/kg/d q8h	75–100 mg/kg/d q6h
Cephalexin or cephradine	—	100 mg/kg/d q6h
Cloxacillin	—	100 mg/kg/d q6h
Dicloxacillin	—	75 mg/kg/d q6h
Methicillin	200 mg/kg/d q6h	—
Oxacillin or nafcillin	150 mg/kg/d q6h	—
Penicillin	150,000 U/kg/d q4–6h	100 mg/kg/d q6h
Ticarcillin or mezlocillin	200–300 mg/kg/d q4–6h	—
Aminoglycosides		
Amikacin or kanamycin	15 mg/kg/d q8h	—
Gentamicin or tobramycin	6 (children)–7.5 (infants) mg/kg/d q8h	—
Miscellaneous		
Chloramphenicol	75 mg/kg/d q6h	50–75 mg/kg/d q6h
Clindamycin	30 mg/kg/d q8h	30 mg/kg/d q6h
Vancomycin	40 mg/kg/d q6h	

*Some dosages are greater than those recommended by the manufacturers for less serious infections.

Osteomyelitis usually affects one bone, fever is higher, bandemia may be present, and the ESR becomes elevated. When in doubt, a diagnostic aspiration can be done. Osteomyelitis is often caused by *Salmonella* or other coliform bacilli. Arthritis is often caused by the pneumococcus, which is an uncommon cause in normal hosts.

Hemophiliacs have an increased incidence of suppurative arthritis compared with the general population, and the pneumococcus is the most common cause.

Sacroiliitis is indolent on presentation and occurs in older children. It is almost always staphylococcal.

Discitis, a syndrome of unknown etiology, affects infants and young children and resolves spontaneously within a few weeks. It must be differentiated from vertebral osteomyelitis, which occurs in older children and is associated with more severe symptomatology. It is most often caused by staphylococci.

Brodie abscess, a subacute or chronic staphylococcal infection, can occur in the metaphysis or diaphysis. It can be difficult to differentiate from bone tumor without surgical curettage. If surgical removal is not performed, I treat Brodie abscess with antistaphylococcal antibiotics for several weeks or months until there is roentgenographic resolution of the lesion.

Granulomatous diseases due to mycobacteria, fungi, or *Brucella* tend to be indolent processes that cross the epiphyseal plate and cause disabling sequelae. Patients are treated with long-term antimicrobial drugs.

Infections secondary to *penetrating trauma* are usually polymicrobial. Cultures of sinus tracts are contaminated with skin bacteria that are not present at the site of infection. Specimens for culture need to be acquired by needle aspiration or surgical exploration through uninfected skin and soft tissue. Because *Pseudomonas* commonly is present in the spongy material in the soles of sneakers, penetrating trauma through them often inoculates bone or cartilage with that organism as well as skin bacteria.

Epiphysitis almost always affects the epiphyses in the knee joint and usually presents as a sterile knee joint effusion. It is generally a subacute process. *Staphylococcus aureus* is the most common cause.

FOLLOW-UP

Because the child's skeleton is growing, it may take many months before abnormalities of bone growth or joint function become apparent. Children with bone and joint infections should be examined periodically for at least 1 year by orthopedic surgeons because of their special expertise in evaluating the skeletal system.

MALIGNANT TUMORS OF BONE AND LIMB SALVAGE

JULIE A. KATZ, M.D.

Primary bone tumors are rare in childhood, representing the sixth most common group of neoplasms in children less than 15 years of age and accounting for approximately 5% of all childhood malignancies. When adolescents and young adults are considered, however, bone tumors represent the third largest group of malignancies, following leukemias and lymphomas. The age-adjusted annual incidence rates per million population for all childhood bone cancers are 5.5 for whites and 4.3 for blacks. This represents 1 chance in 12,000 of developing a bone malignancy before 15 years of age. When considered in aggregate, bone malignancies occur with equal frequency in both sexes and with peak occurrence in early adolescence, coinciding with the pubertal growth spurt. Osteosarcoma and Ewing sarcoma account for the vast majority of bone tumors (89%), with osteosarcoma occurring in over 60% of cases. Fibrosarcoma of bone, chondrosarcoma, and malignant fibrous histiocytoma occur infrequently.

Over the past two decades, major advances in therapy for children with bone sarcomas have resulted from the development of effective adjuvant therapy and advances in diagnostic imaging and surgical techniques. The development of computed axial tomography (CT) and magnetic resonance imaging (MRI) permits extremely accurate evaluation of local anatomy and has enhanced the possibility of safe resection. With improved surgical knowledge and experience, local control of the primary tumor can be achieved with less radical surgery, specifically limb salvage procedures.

OSTEOSARCOMA

Osteosarcoma is a primary malignant tumor of bone in which the malignant proliferating spindle-cell stroma directly produces osteoid or immature bone. Osteosarcoma represents half of bone cancers seen in children 14 years of age and younger, with an annual incidence of 3.4 cases per million in blacks and 2.5 cases per million in whites. A number of distinct variants of osteosarcoma have been defined on the basis of clinical, radiographic, and histologic features. The largest group, comprising 75% of cases, are the high-grade *conventional osteosarcomas,* which are the lesions usually seen in children and adolescents.

The etiology of osteosarcoma is unknown. The only environmental agent known to produce bone sarcomas in human beings is ionizing radiation, implicated in approximately 3% of osteosarcomas. Osteosarcoma is known to occur at sites of preexisting skeletal lesions and has been reported in patients with Paget's disease, solitary or multiple osteochondroma, solitary enchondroma or enchondromatosis (Ollier's disease), hereditary exostoses, fibrous dysplasia, chronic osteomyelitis, and regions of previous bone infarction. The peak incidence of osteosarcoma occurs in the second decade of life during the adolescent growth spurt, suggesting a relationship between rapid bone growth and development of this malignancy. Exciting data relevant to the etiology of osteosarcoma have emerged from studies of children with hereditary (bilateral) retinoblastoma. Secondary nonocular tumors, the majority of which are sarcomas (50% of these are osteosarcomas), have been described in many case reports and series of patients who survive retinoblastoma. The gene associated with retinoblastoma *(RB)* has been implicated in the generation of osteosarcoma as well, even in patients with no history of retinoblastoma.

Clinical Features and Staging

The evaluation of a suspected bone tumor begins with history, physical examination, and plain radiographs. The majority of patients with osteosarcoma complain of pain, with or without an associated soft tissue mass over the affected bone. Frequently, a history of trauma is present. Systemic symptoms are rare in the absence of widespread metastatic disease. Osteosarcoma characteristically involves the metaphyseal portions of the long tubular bones, with half of tumors arising adjacent to the knee joint. The distal femur, proximal tibia, and proximal humerus are, respectively, the most frequently involved sites. Physical examination is typically remarkable only for the soft tissue mass that is usually evident at the primary site. Regional and distal lymph node metastases are rarely observed.

The key to the diagnostic evaluation of the patient with a suspected bone tumor is radiologic evaluation of the lesion. Plain radiographs of osteosarcoma show permeative destruction of the normal trabecular pattern with indistinct margins. The lesions typically originate in the medullary cavity and are most often sclerotic due to neoplastic bone production, although patchy lytic areas may be identified (Fig. 1A and B).

If plain radiographs suggest an osteosarcoma, staging studies, including bone scintigraphy, CT, and MRI, should be performed *before* biopsy, as surgical manipulation of the lesion will influence results. Staging studies are required to delineate local tumor extent, vascular displacement, and compartmental localization and to plan for definitive surgery. Bone scintigraphy helps to determine polyostotic involvement, intraosseous tumor extension, and metastatic disease. CT

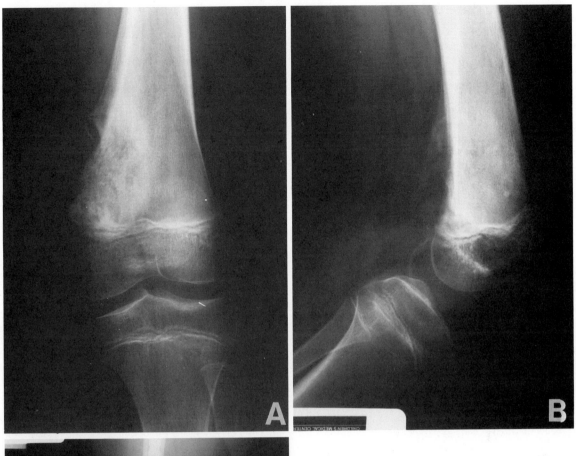

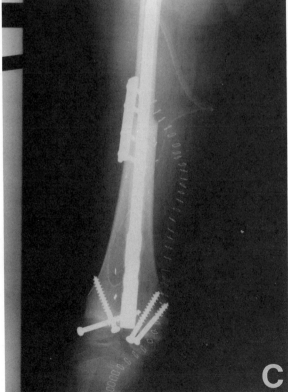

FIGURE 1. *A*, Posteroanterior, and *B*, lateral, radiographs of osteosarcoma of the distal femur. The tumor shows a mixed lytic and sclerotic appearance, along with periosteal reaction, formation of Codman's triangle, and an adjacent soft tissue mass. *C*, Posteroanterior radiograph depicting distal femur following en bloc resection of osteosarcoma of the distal femur and limb salvage procedure using an allograft affixed by orthopedic hardware.

provides excellent evaluation of both intraosseous and extraosseous extent of the tumor and demonstrates the relationship of the tumor to adjacent structures, such as vessels and nerves. MRI is superior to CT for showing the extent of the extraosseous component of the tumor into adjacent soft tissues and the tumor relationships to neurovascular bundles. Extension into the marrow cavity is exquisitely demonstrated by MRI.

The presence of metastases is an important prognostic variable with a major impact on management. Approximately 10% to 20% of patients present with macrometastatic disease. The majority of metastatic lesions are found in the lungs. Routine posteroanterior and lateral radiographs of the chest allow detection of metastases in most cases, but CT is more sensitive, especially for detection of pleura-based lesions. A small fraction of patients present with bone metastases, which should be delineated by bone scintigraphy.

Treatment

Although the radiographic findings in a patient with a suspected malignant bone tumor may be highly suggestive, biopsy is necessary for histologic confirmation. The biopsy should be performed by an orthopedic surgeon familiar with management of malignant bone tumors and preferably by the surgeon who will ultimately perform the definitive surgical procedure. Most patients require open biopsy to obtain an adequate and representative sample. A longitudinal incision is preferred, as the biopsy tract must be excised en bloc with the tumor during the definitive surgical procedure.

Because osteosarcoma is generally unresponsive to conventional dose radiotherapy, treatment includes *surgical management* of the primary tumor and *chemotherapy* to control micrometastatic disease. The goals of surgery are to eliminate all gross and microscopic tumor locally and to preserve or restore maximum function. Traditional surgery for local control of primary osteosarcoma of the extremity is amputation. With advances in diagnostic imaging techniques and improvements in survival of patients with osteosarcoma, surgeons have attempted to reduce the functional and psychologic morbidity associated with amputation by using limb salvage resection. Both approaches incorporate the principle of en bloc excision of the tumor and biopsy site through normal tissue planes with a margin of normal, uninvolved tissue.

The selection of surgical procedure involves consideration of several interrelated factors, including tumor location, size, extramedullary extent, presence or absence of metastatic disease, and patient factors, such as age, skeletal maturity, and lifestyle preference. The surgical approach to salvage the limb must not compromise the goal of removing all gross and microscopic tumor.

Tumors occurring in expendable bones, such as the ulna, patella, fibula, scapula, or ribs, although rare, provide a relatively straightforward opportunity for limb salvage. The majority of limb salvage procedures for osteosarcoma, however, require *three surgical phases:*

1. En bloc resection of the primary tumor, leaving clean surgical margins
2. Reconstruction of the surgical defect to restore the structural integrity of the involved extremity
3. Soft tissue and muscle transfers to cover and close the resection site and restore motor power (Fig. 2)

Restoration of the structural integrity of the involved extremity has centered around use of biologic materials and metallic endoprosthetic devices. Biologic approaches using autologous grafts or cadaver allografts should offer an enduring repair by providing a structural lattice for ingrowth of the patient's own bone (Fig. 1C). However, the large skeletal defects created by surgery have limited the use of autologous bone grafts, and longer segments of allografted bone may fracture or undergo dissolution. Endoprosthetic devices fabricated of metal and synthetic materials can be used both to provide a functional joint and to give immediate structural integrity to the limb. An expandable prosthesis incorporates a telescoping unit that expands with a gear device, permitting implantation of the endoprosthesis into skeletally immature children. Problems with loosening, fatigue fracture, and infection may limit the use of endoprosthetic devices.

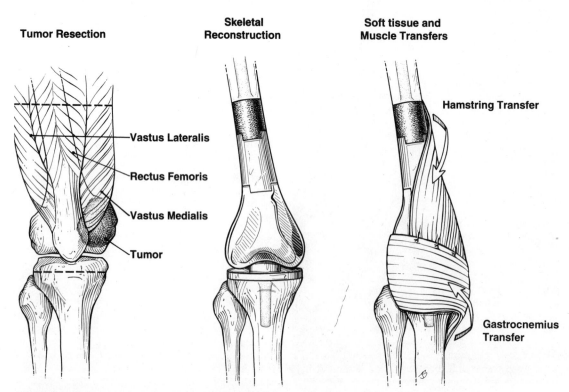

Tumor Resection

Vastus Lateralis
Rectus Femoris
Vastus Medialis
Tumor

Skeletal Reconstruction

Soft tissue and Muscle Transfers

Hamstring Transfer

Gastrocnemius Transfer

FIGURE 2. Three phases of a limb-sparing procedure for osteosarcoma of the distal femur. (From Aboulafia AJ, Malawer MM: Limb-sparing surgery for osteosarcoma. Contemp Oncol 2(3):24, 1992. Copyright © Medical Economics Publishing, Inc.)

Recent advances in surgical techniques for limb salvage have increased surgical options available for patients with osteosarcoma. Amputations are reserved principally for patients whose primary tumor is unresectable. Several studies have demonstrated that the risk of local recurrence in patients who have undergone limb salvage surgery by skilled orthopedic surgeons is the same as for those treated by amputation (<5%). Similarly, reported continuous disease-free survival rates are the same as for patients undergoing amputation alone. However, long-term functional results achieved by limb salvage surgery are yet to be assessed, and merit careful evaluation.

Although control of the primary tumor is reliably accomplished by surgery, historical studies suggest that the majority of patients with osteosarcoma have microscopic, subclinical metastatic disease at diagnosis, which can be eradicated by chemotherapy if it is initiated when the burden of metastatic tumor is low. The development of adjuvant chemotherapy regimens has been largely empirical, as osteosarcoma is a notoriously drug-resistant neoplasm. A number of uncontrolled trials of adjuvant chemotherapy conducted in the 1970s and early 1980s showed apparent improvement in outcome compared with dismal results with surgery alone. Two randomized, controlled trials conducted in the mid-1980s confirmed the favorable impact of adjuvant chemotherapy in the treatment of osteosarcoma. Most current regimens incorporate doxorubicin, cisplatin, ifosfamide, and high-dose methotrexate with leucovorin rescue.

The administration of chemotherapy before definitive surgery of the primary tumor (in addition to postoperative adjuvant chemotherapy) has evolved from consideration of limb salvage. Preoperative (neoadjuvant) chemotherapy provides an opportunity for reduction in size of the primary tumor, which increases the feasibility of limb salvage surgery and allows time for fabrication of a customized endoprosthetic device if needed for limb reconstruction. With current treatment regimens, approximately 60% to 65% of patients with nonmetastatic osteosarcoma of the extremity will survive without evidence of recurrence.

An aggressive therapeutic approach with curative intent is also indicated for patients who present with metastases to the lung. Removal of all overt metastatic disease, leaving microscopically clean margins, is a prerequisite for long-term survival. Patients with extrathoracic lesions (usually to bone) are rarely curable unless the lesions are surgically accessible.

PAROSTEAL OSTEOSARCOMA

Parosteal osteosarcoma is a low-grade malignancy that accounts for 1% to 2% of all bone tumors. The lesion typically arises on the cortical surface of long tubular bones, most commonly along the posterior aspect of the distal femur. Patients with parosteal osteosarcoma are usually young adults who have an indolent clinical course and a low propensity to develop metastatic disease. Most of these lesions are relatively well differentiated, and long-term survival exceeds 90% for patients undergoing wide surgical resection alone.

EWING SARCOMA

Ewing sarcoma is the second most common primary malignant tumor of bone in children, with an annual incidence of 2.4 cases per million white children. The median age at diagnosis of Ewing sarcoma is 11 years, and 80% of patients are younger than 20 years. The tumor is rare in both black and Asian children.

Ewing sarcoma was originally described in 1921 by James Ewing, who characterized it as a tumor of the shaft of long bones that, in contrast to osteosarcoma, was radiosensitive. He speculated that the tumor was of endothelial origin, but more recent evidence supports a neural origin. Ewing sarcoma is now recognized as the most undifferentiated tumor of a spectrum of histologic forms, which includes typical and atypical Ewing sarcoma, extraosseous (soft tissue) Ewing sarcoma, and peripheral primitive neuroectodermal tumors (PPNET). Both Ewing sarcoma of bone and soft tissue and PPNET express a consistent cytogenetic abnormality, a translocation between the long arms of chromosomes 11 and 22, specifically t(11;22) (q24;q12), which serves as a diagnostic marker. Molecular genetic studies have additionally shown that these tumors exhibit high levels of c-*myc* RNA with or without amplification.

Clinical Features and Staging

Pain, swelling, or both at the site of the primary tumor are the most common presenting symptoms at diagnosis. Extensive tumor necrosis may result in increased local temperature and swelling, mimicking infection.

Ewing sarcoma frequently arises in the weightbearing bones of the lower extremity or in the pelvis. In the long bones, it most often arises in the medullary cavity of the diaphysis. In this location, plain radiographs typically show ill-defined, permeative bone destruction, with laminated periosteal reaction that tends to create an onionskin effect. The surrounding soft tissue mass is often disproportionally large compared with the bony component. CT scanning of the primary site helps to define the extent of bony disease and soft tissue involvement, and MRI offers the best assessment of disease in the medullary cavity. Radionuclide bone scanning will screen for metastases to distant bone. A chest x-ray and thoracic CT will delineate pulmonary metastases. Approximately 25% of patients with Ewing sarcoma have metastatic disease to lung, bone, or bone marrow at diagnosis. Bone marrow aspiration and biopsy are necessary to detect metastatic disease in the marrow.

Treatment

The definitive diagnosis of the Ewing sarcoma family of tumors is made by histologic examination of a biopsy specimen. Successful treatment requires eradication of tumor at the primary site as well as at sites of gross metastatic or micrometastatic disease. Therefore, treatment has been conceptually compartmentalized into measures to affect both local and systemic control.

Local control of the primary tumor is generally accomplished by *radiotherapy* or *surgery* or both. No randomized studies are available to directly compare these two modalities. Effective local control by radiotherapy requires moderately high doses of radiation, approximately 45 to 50 Gy to the entire bone, with a boost of 10 to 15 Gy to the primary tumor. The application of *hyperfractionated radiation* (i.e., smaller radiation fractions delivered more frequently, generally twice daily) permits larger total radiation doses to be delivered over a shorter treatment course. Hyperfractionation exploits the superior radiation repair capacity of normal compared with malignant tissue, theoretically offering less long-term normal tissue damage and better tumor control.

The role of surgery for local control of Ewing sarcoma is evolving. The rationale for surgical intervention includes reducing the risk for local recurrence, eliminating tissue damage secondary to radiation, and reducing the risk of second malignant neoplasm. Conservative surgery is often used in conjunction with radiotherapy, and more radical surgery with wide excision or amputation may serve as an alternative to radiation therapy. Surgery is advantageous for lesions that arise in expendable bones, such as the clavicle, iliac wing, rib, or digital rays of the hands or feet. However, the application of limb salvage procedures for treatment of Ewing sarcoma is often limited by the extensive extraosseous soft tissue spread or intraosseous medullary cavity spread or both.

Before the routine use of adjuvant *chemotherapy* for treatment of the Ewing sarcoma family of tumors, only 10% of patients survived 5 years. In the 1960s, combinations of vincristine, cyclophosphamide, and dactinomycin were found in several small studies to improve survival rates as compared with historical controls. Most studies of chemotherapy in Ewing sarcoma since 1970 have used a combination of these three drugs, with or without doxorubicin, in varied schedules and doses. Five-year failure-free survival rates for patients with localized disease participating in multimodality studies range between 55% and 75%. Treatment results for patients with clinically overt metastatic disease at diagnosis are dismal. A novel approach to patients with metastatic disease using total body irradiation or high-dose chemotherapy or both with *autologous bone marrow rescue* has shown promise in a limited number of patients.

FIBROSARCOMA OF BONE

Fibrosarcoma of bone is a malignant fibroblastic tumor that may arise as a de novo lesion or may be associated with preexistent skeletal conditions, such as fibrous dysplasia, Paget's disease, bone infarct, and osteomyelitis. Fibrosarcomas arising in bone are quite rare in children and adolescents and may occur in either intramedullary or periosteal locations. Surgery is the primary treatment of choice, either radical en bloc resection or amputation. Patients with high-grade fibrosarcomas may benefit from preoperative and adjuvant chemotherapy. Those with medullary lesions have a uniformly worse prognosis, with 10-year survival rates of 20% versus 50% for those with periosteal lesions.

CHONDROSARCOMA

Chondrosarcomas appear most frequently in middle-aged or older adults. Their occurrence in patients under 21 years of age is rare. These slow-growing tumors may develop in any bone preformed in cartilage but are most frequent in the appendicular skeleton and pelvis. Surgery is the primary treatment, as chondrosarcomas in general are not radiosensitive, and chemotherapy yields less than satisfactory results. Cure is directly related to the ability for successful local control, but local recurrences are the rule if surgical excision is inadequate. Distant metastases to lung are rare but may appear years after diagnosis. Histologic grading, tumor location, and tumor size provide a reliable guide for predicting clinical outcome.

MALIGNANT FIBROUS HISTIOCYTOMA

Malignant fibrous histiocytoma is a predominantly pleomorphic sarcoma that generally occurs in patients between 40 and 60 years of age. Only 4% to 5% of cases occur in children. These tumors most frequently present as a painless mass deeply situated in the lower extremity. Local excision with histologically clean margins is the treatment of choice. Postoperative radiation therapy is recommended for site(s) of residual tumor. Reported 5-year survival rates in large series are poor, ranging between 27% and 53%. Several recent studies suggest that adjuvant chemotherapy may improve survival.

ORTHOPEDIC TRAUMA

TAHSIN M. ERGIN, M.D.

Children and adolescents, in the course of exploring their environment, testing their burgeoning skills, and feeding their competitive natures, will get hurt, and although safety considerations in supervision and equipment design are critical, it is not reasonable to expect the elimination of all injuries. Because of the peculiarities of the developing skeleton, they suffer from many injuries that are not found in adults. As a consequence, special attention must be given to the injured child to ensure that an injury that would be trivial to an adult does not develop into a major problem once the child's growth has been completed.

Children's bones are more porous, having a much greater number of haversian canals per unit area of cortical bone. Where an adult bone fails only in tension in the diaphysis and metaphysis, children's bones may fail in tension (greenstick fracture), compression (torus or buckle fracture), or a combination of the two (plastic deformation or bending fracture).

Biomechanical tests of the elements in the growing skeleton reveal that the strongest link is the thick periosteal sleeve, which most com-

monly remains intact despite large degrees of displacement. This helps to account for the rarity of open fractures from bone puncture of the skin and the ease with which reduction may be obtained by traction and simple manipulation, using the periosteal sleeve as a hinge. The joint capsule and ligaments around the joint are extensions of the periosteal sleeve and, as a result, are equally tough. They serve to transfer stress around a weak link, the epiphysis, which is also protected by joint congruity and a compressible shock absorber, the articular cartilage. The weakest link in the chain is the growth plate (physis), which is especially true during the adolescent growth period as the perichondrial ring at the periphery of the physis narrows. In general, children do not sprain ligaments or dislocate joints but rather fracture through the physis or metaphysis or both, making roentgenographic study of the injured extremity a necessary rather than a precautionary measure. Complete radiologic evaluation of the site of injury includes two views of the fracture at right angles to each other, as well as the joints proximal and distal to the fracture, with additional oblique or special views taken as needed. Comparison views (x-rays of the uninjured side) may be very helpful in defining the injury and should be used liberally. Supplemental information from CT scans, bone scans, MRI, arteriogram, or arthrogram may still be required. The diagnosis of musculoskeletal injury requires a clinical assimilation of the information from the history and physical examination (local swelling, deformity if present, and point tenderness over the fracture site on the bone), along with that culled from these ancillary studies. Reliance on the radiographic studies is simply not a substitute for a good examination of the child.

Salter and Harris presented a clinically useful system of five categories in which to classify injuries about the growth plate. A sixth category was later added by Rang (Fig. 1). In general, they are numbered in descending order of frequency and ascending order of risk of physeal closure. Type I and II fractures carry a low risk of growth arrest and are fairly easily reduced when recognized and treated acutely. Type III and IV fractures involve the joint surface, in addition to the growth plate, and very frequently require open reduction and fixation to accurately realign both the joint surface and the growth cartilage. These carry a higher risk of growth arrest, especially when brought to treatment at a later stage. Failure to achieve accurate reduction also portends poorly for health of the joint cartilage in the future. Type V and VI injuries are quite sinister in nature. Pure type V injuries do not involve disruption of the epiphysis or metaphysis and are, therefore, nearly impossible to diagnose at the time of injury. They are usually recognized at the time that growth arrest becomes clinically apparent, and, therefore, all injuries that potentially involve the growth plate and possible growth arrest need to be followed carefully with radiographic study to monitor for plate closure, bridge formation, or progressive deformity. Physeal arrest needs to be addressed promptly.

Growing bones have tremendous potential to remodel following injury due to longitudinal growth from the physis and periosteal bone formation to fill in angular deformities. Large degrees of angulation can be accommodated as the bone and cartilage respond to the application of stress. In general, remodeling can best be expected in fractures near the ends of long bones, with displacement of the fracture in the direction of the plane of movement of the joint, and in children with 2 years or more of skeletal growth remaining. Rotational malalignment, however, will not remodel and cannot be accepted in the reduction of a fracture.

Sometimes, the history of the fracture does not jibe with the radiographic evidence in terms of mechanism of injury or in the degree of trauma necessary. Fractures that occur with mechanisms of injury that do not generally produce a fracture are suspicious and need to be thoroughly investigated. Pathologic lesions within the bone, such as unicameral bone cyst, nonossifying fibroma, and enchondroma frequently are found in children's skeletons and can result in fracture even with minimal trauma. In most instances, these are best approached by treating the fracture, then the underlying lesion as needed. Other conditions noted to predispose to skeletal injury include fibrous

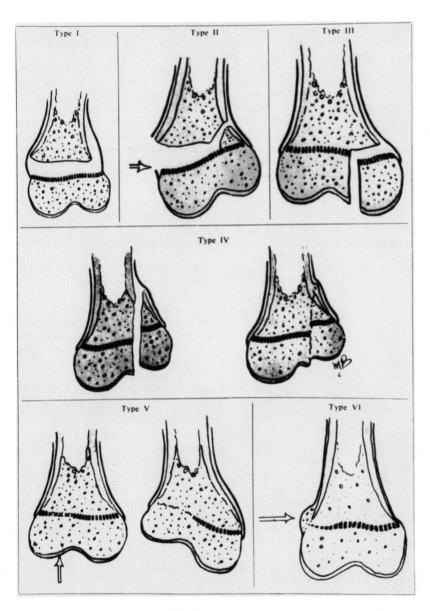

FIGURE 1. The Salter-Harris classification of physeal fractures, as modified by Rang with the addition of a type VI. See text for a complete discussion of the fracture types. (From Rang M: The Growth Plate and Its Disorders. Baltimore, Williams & Wilkins, 1969.)

dysplasia, osteogenesis imperfecta, Ehlers-Danlos syndrome, rickets, renal disease, cerebral palsy, and muscular dystrophy.

CHILD ABUSE

The careful physician must have a high index of suspicion regarding injuries to children under the age of 2 years. A regular percentage of fractures in this age group will be associated with abuse. Suspicion should be raised when any part of the history of the child's injury is questionable or does not mesh with the physical examination, including the behavior of the child. Dispassionate parents, delay in seeking treatment, insufficient trauma to have caused the injury seen, and multiple sites of injury or serial injuries are causes for concern. All such children should be admitted to the hospital for observation and thorough testing, including a skeletal radiographic survey, and the social work network should be contacted immediately. Fractures characteristic of child abuse are posterior rib fractures (crush injury), fractures of the humerus or femur (twisting injury) in a child under 2 years of age, corner epiphyseal fractures (pulling injuries), and the presence of subperiosteal new bone (minimal injury but evidence of trauma to bone). Other manifestations may be found, including skull and spine fractures, bruises, bites, and burns of the cigarette tip or

hot water variety. The risk to the child for missing a case of child abuse is a 10% chance of death from battering within 1 year.

MULTIPLE TRAUMA

More and more frequently, children are the victims of major or multiple trauma. They may be hurt when hit by a car as a pedestrian or cyclist, while riding in a car, and in recreational activities in falls from heights, all-terrain vehicles, and dirt bikes. Care for these patients begins in the field and continues on arrival at the hospital. An adequate airway, effective ventilation, and circulating blood volume must be established, monitored, and maintained. The cervical spine is stabilized, and the patient is transported with the use of a backboard. Long bone fractures are immobilized temporarily with splints, and the wounds are dressed. Evaluation in the hospital continues with assessment of head, thoracic, abdominal, and pelvic injuries, in addition to the spine and extremities. Orthopedic evaluation includes complete documentation of neurologic function, palpation and assessment of all portions of the spine, pelvis, chest, and appendicular skeleton, examination of open wounds, and formulation of a plan of management of all injuries in conjunction with the other members of the trauma team. Portions of the evaluation may best be accomplished after induction of anesthesia to avoid unnecessary pain to the child. Regional trauma centers are more prevalent in the management of severely injured patients and are best equipped to handle the myriad of problems in these children.

Open fractures (a break in skin continuity over a fracture site) require prompt and effective management. Measures to be undertaken in the emergency ward should include administration of tetanus toxoid (if more than 5 years have passed since the last booster) or hyperimmune globulin and intravenous antibiotics, and application of a dressing. Opinions vary whether a culture of the wound is necessary. The child should be moved to the operating room within 6 hours of the time of injury, where the wound is debrided of devitalized tissue along with crushed or necrotic skin margins and copiously irrigated with pulsatile lavage. Volume is key. Antibiotic solutions may be used at the surgeon's discretion. The wound is thoroughly explored, and the bone ends are exposed and mechanically cleaned. The type of closure depends on the degree of soft tissue injury and the amount of contamination present. The wound may need to be left open, with delayed primary closure or redebridement or both performed in 1 to 5 days as needed and resolution of soft tissue coverage problems, possibly requiring skin grafts or flaps. Stabilization of the fractures may take many forms depending on the type and location of injury and the presence and severity of other injuries, such as head or abdominal injuries. Simple cast or splint immobilization may be sufficient for some injuries, whereas others may require skeletal traction or smooth pin, external, intramedullary, or plate fixation. Decision making in fracture care in these situations is often complex and must be individualized.

SOFT TISSUE INJURIES

Soft tissue injuries to the extremities can be classified as contusions, sprains, and strains. Contusions involve direct impact, with crush injury of tissue and associated bleeding. Because of their abundant blood supply, muscles are most susceptible to severe contusion, with hematoma formation and inflammatory response. Sprains occur when a ligament or joint capsule becomes stretched or torn. These tissues are viscoelastic, undergoing both stretch in continuity and disruption, with the amount of damage done dependent not only on the amount of force applied but also on the rate of application of that force. Sprains may be graded based on the remaining integrity of the structure. Grade I sprains involve some tearing of the fibers, although the ligament integrity is essentially intact, with no change in the range of motion and no increase in joint laxity. Grade II sprains involve damage to a substantial portion of the ligament, with a concomitant increase in joint laxity and loss of motion, but some ligament integrity remains when the joint is stressed. Grade III sprains are complete tears and show clear-cut joint instability to stress. Strains are injuries to a muscle-tendon contractile unit. These injuries occur in the muscle belly, the tendon, or at the junction of the two. They may be graded like sprains based on the amount of muscle and tendon injured, with complete rupture of a muscle considered a grade III strain.

Rest, ice, compression, and elevation (RICE) should be the mainstay of management in these soft tissue injuries. Rest allows for pain relief in addition to preventing further tissue damage and, when accomplished by immobilization, encourages reduction in use of the injured part. This should be adhered to over the initial 2 to 3 days following the injury. Ice (cryotherapy) causes vasoconstriction, with a decrease in bleeding and inflammation, edema reduction, and relief of pain. Heat causes vasodilatation and hyperemia, increasing swelling and inflammation and frequently pain and should be avoided in the acute phase of management. Ice chips or ice/water mixtures are effective and economical and should be applied immediately after the injury when possible and for 20 minutes two to four times daily for 2 to 3 days thereafter. Compression aids in the control of edema both by limiting the volume of the injured compartment and by increasing the interstitial pressure reducing fluid transudation from the capillary bed. Compression (with, for example, an elastic bandage) should be

firm and even and should not result in reduction of arterial supply to or venous return from the affected part. This is particularly true when used about the elbow and the knee, as the bandage can bunch if it is applied carelessly. Elevation also plays a role in control of edema by improving venous and lymphatic return from the site of injury. This is best accomplished by raising the body part above the level of the heart. Any elevation, however, is better than none at all.

As the soft tissue injury begins to respond to treatment in the acute phase, there is a gradual transition to the rehabilitative phase. Use of RICE is continued while restoration of function is developed in stages. Recovery of range of motion is foremost, followed by functional return of strength, endurance, and agility. The time frame may range from several days to 2 to 3 months.

A special class of soft tissue injury involves the muscle contusion resulting in heterotopic bone formation, or myositis ossificans. With a severe muscle injury, a contained hematoma may be present as a discrete mass. Clinical findings include swelling, pain exacerbated by contraction or passive motion of the muscle, and warmth, often remarkable. The ranges of motion of the joints proximal and distal to the contusion are reduced. Initial treatment consists again of RICE. Passive range of motion exercises and massage, which may increase the trauma and bleeding, should be avoided. Active range of motion exercises are begun once active muscle control is obtained. Gradually, muscle strengthening through progressive resistance exercises is introduced, and work continues on active range of motion. Anti-inflammatory medication, such as indomethacin, may have a role in decreasing the likelihood of bone formation. If bone that remains in the muscle is symptomatic, it may be excised, but only after the mass has matured completely, generally within 12 to 18 months.

COMPARTMENT SYNDROME

Fractures and crush injuries may result in large amounts of muscle damage and bleeding. Muscles in the extremities are enveloped by a fairly inelastic fascia, and with rapidly increasing bleeding and muscle edema, the pressure in the fascial compartment in turn increases. Blood flow to the muscles and nerves in the compartment is gradually compromised and is cut off when pressure in the compartment exceeds the capillary perfusion pressure. Suspicion of a compartment syndrome should be raised initially by pain out of proportion to the type of injury, with later findings including pain with passive stretch, lack of active muscle control, and paresthesias or reduction of two-point discrimination in sensory distributions. Absence of a palpable pulse is a very late finding. Suspicion should result in the physician immediately splitting encircling dressings, and compartment pressures should be measured if the symptoms are unresolved. Various recommendations have been made for the threshold pressure at which fasciotomy is indicated, with many authors recommending that compartment pressures over 30 mm Hg be carefully monitored and fasciotomy performed at pressures over 40 mm Hg. Some have recommended fasciotomy at compartment pressures that rise to within 40 mm Hg of mean arterial pressure. The key is rapid action, as irreversible changes in muscle and nerve occur after 6 hours of ischemia and may occur in far less time. The most common sites of compartment syndrome are in the volar forearm and the compartments of the lower leg, although the syndrome may also be found in the hand, foot, thigh, and upper arm.

SPECIAL WOUNDS

Occasionally, a laceration of the skin with or without bony involvement requires special attention. The most notable example of this is the human bite wound, which most often occurs when hand meets tooth in an altercation. Skin puncture usually is found on the dorsum of the fourth or fifth metacarpophalangeal joint and may penetrate skin, extensor tendon, joint capsule, and even bone. Any puncture wounds on the hands should be considered possible human bite wounds unless the history is clearly contradictory. Management consists of irrigation for large lacerations, splinting, intravenous antibiotics to include coverage of both gram-positive aerobic (cefazolin) and anaerobic (penicillin G) organisms. Surgical treatment is necessary when presenting late with abscess formation and joint or tendon involvement.

Puncture wounds to the foot, from stepping on a nail, for instance, can cause problems due to development of deep bone or joint infection with *Pseudomonas aeruginosa*. The presence of deep infection requires debridement, irrigation, and treatment with intravenous antibiotics for 2 to 6 weeks, with bone involvement dictating the latter course. A puncture wound to the foot mandates close vigilance and initial antibiotic coverage.

SPLINTING

There are a wide variety of splinting techniques available for temporary immobilization and sometimes treatment of extremity injuries. Initial care of an injury often involves immobilization for pain relief, protection from further damage, and reduction of swelling—not simply to "let the bone heal." A simple splint may be fashioned with several layers of cast padding, 10 to 12 layers of plaster bandage, and a stretch gauze roll or elastic bandage, although care should be taken not to apply the latter too tightly. Various prepared splint materials are readily available in both Fiberglas and plaster and are simple to apply. Children's skin is sensitive and burns easily. Plaster and Fiberglas splints set in an exothermic (heat-producing) reaction, so cold water should be used, with care taken to avoid contact with the skin. When applying a splint, the position of the splint and extremity must be maintained until the material has set completely.

In the upper extremity, useful emergency splints include the volar forearm splint for wrist and hand injuries, radial and ulnar gutter splints for injuries on the thumb or small finger sides of the hand, coaptation splints, and forearm and upper arm sugar-tong splints for humeral and forearm fractures. The arm can be positioned, in most cases, with the elbow flexed 90 degrees, the forearm in neutral rotation, the wrist in slight dorsiflexion, and the hand positioned with the thumb slightly opposed and the metacarpophalangeal and interphalangeal joints slightly flexed, as if the child were holding a can of soda. If the position of immobilization compromises neurovascular status, it must be immediately changed. At the time of definitive treatment, the position of the extremity may be changed depending on the type of injury.

In the lower extremity, useful emergency splints include the long posterior or long U-splint placed medial and lateral on the leg for femoral and tibial fractures, medial and lateral coaptation or Jones splints for injuries about the knee, and the short leg posterior and short U-splint for ankle and foot injuries. The leg may be positioned with the knee extended and the ankle in neutral dorsiflexion.

STRESS FRACTURES AND OVERUSE INJURIES

Children, like high-performance athletes, will perform activities repetitively and occasionally to the exclusion of all other activities and, as a result, are sometimes the victims of stress or overuse injuries. In general, these will respond to rest, ice, and possibly mild anti-inflammatory medication to reduce the initial pain, with alteration or elimination of the activity that precipitated the injury. To prevent recurrences, rehabilitation should involve stretching and strengthening the surrounding muscles, followed by a gradually advancing program to allow return to participation. Common sites of stress fracture, in addition to those overuse injuries to be addressed, are the metatarsals, distal fibula, calcaneus, and proximal medial tibial metaphysis in runners and, in the spine, the pars interarticularis in the vertebral bodies of gymnasts, divers, and football linemen.

Osgood-Schlatter Disease

Not truly a disease, this overuse injury is seen in 10% of adolescent athletes and occurs at the infrapatellar tendon insertion into the tibial tubercle apophysis. Repetitive high-stress activity results in microfractures of the apophysis at the tendon insertion. The highest stresses

in this area happen when landing from a jump and decelerating while running. Osgood-Schlatter, therefore, is found commonly in the left leg of right-handed basketball players and right-footed soccer players. The patient experiences pain with direct pressure over the tibial tubercle and when running, jumping, or going up or down stairs. Radiographs are necessary in unilateral disease to rule out other pathology and may reveal fragmentation and enlargement of the tibial tuberosity or heterotopic bone within the substance of the infrapatellar tendon. Treatment consists of restriction of painful activity and ice to the tender area when the knee is painful. A Neoprene knee support for activities may help, primarily to protect the knee from incident trauma and to identify the injury for the coach. Stretching for tight hamstrings and quadriceps muscles and straight leg resistance exercises (isometric quadriceps contraction) progressing to 10% of the patient's weight for resistance help to maintain function and reduce stress on the apophysis. The patient should be allowed to participate in sports if not limping. Any limp, however, indicates a need for further rest. There is absolutely no indication for steroid injection or a cast. A cast results in more disability and loss of function than the disease itself. The problem ultimately will resolve completely at the time of physeal closure. If the patient's symptoms continue, radiographs often reveal an ossicle within the tendon, and symptoms resolve following excision.

Sinding-Larsen-Johanson Syndrome

The counterpart to Osgood-Schlatter disease, this is an overstress injury of the infrapatellar tendon insertion to the inferior pole of the patella. Small avulsion ossicles occasionally may be seen at the inferior pole. Treatment of the problem is similar to that for Osgood-Schlatter disease, although pain more often may persist beyond growth plate closure.

Sever's Calcaneal Apophysitis

The Achilles tendon is attached to the vertically oriented calcaneal apophysis through numerous Sharpey's fibers, and the apophysis is subject to high shear stress when children run and jump. As with Osgood-Schlatter disease, the repetitive trauma causes microfractures around the tendon insertion. Symptoms (pain in the heel with running and jumping) are seen in 1% of adolescent athletes, and tenderness with local pressure is found over the insertion of the Achilles tendon. Tight heel cords are commonly found, with ankle dorsiflexion limited to neutral or less with the knee extended, not the normal 15 degrees. Rest when painful, use of viscoelastic heel inserts, and heel cord and plantar stretching exercises help to resolve the problem. Occasionally, a nighttime dorsiflexion splint is needed in young athletes. Fragmentation and sclerosis of the calcaneal apophysis on radiographs are normal, but the films are taken to rule out other pathology.

Little League Elbow

There are many different forms of Little League elbow, the most widely recognized of which involve overstress of the medial elbow stabilizing structures or repetitive compression injury of the lateral radiocapitellar articulation. On the medial side, physeal overstress or even complete separation of the medial epicondylar apophysis can occur. Point tenderness at the medial epicondyle with loss of complete extension may be found. Radiographs reveal widening of the physis and, occasionally, fragmentation. On the lateral side, irregular fragmentation of the ossific nucleus of the capitellum or even osteochondral fracture of the capitellum may occur. Pain is primarily on the lateral side, and there is often loss of motion. Loose bodies from fragmentation of the capitellum may cause locking of the joint.

The milder forms of Little League elbow are treated with rest. Once the injury heals, which may take 3 to 6 weeks, progressive rehabilitation is followed by a graduated throwing program. Surgical treatment is needed if the medial epicondyle is displaced or the elbow is unstable to valgus stress. Removal of loose fragments within the joint may be required. An ounce of prevention is worth a pound of cure, however, and the amount of hard throwing young pitchers do should be monitored carefully. Pitchers should pitch no more than six innings per week, with 3 days rest between outings. Managers should closely observe the throwing mechanics of their pitchers and watch for signs of fatigue.

Little League Shoulder

A fatigue fracture of the proximal humeral physis has been referred to as Little League shoulder. Previously, many of these injuries went undiagnosed. The symptoms are nonspecific. Pain with throwing or aching in the shoulder after throwing is usual. The proximal humeral physis may be widened radiographically or may show subperiosteal new bone formation, although a bone scan may be needed for diagnosis. Rest is followed by a progressive rehabilitation and then a throwing program, and again managers need to ensure that their players throw using proper mechanics.

Swimmer's Shoulder

High levels of training are necessary in competitive swimming, even in young age groups, and as a result, shoulder pain in childhood and teen swimmers is very common. After the rotator cuff and muscles of the shoulder girdle fatigue, the athlete's ability to control shoulder motion and position is diminished. As swimming continues, shoulder mechanics deteriorate and result in friction injury of the rotator cuff and subacromial bursa in the subacromial space. This is exacerbated by the fact that swimmers, due to their demands, already have increased laxity in the shoulder ligaments and capsule. Tenderness is found over the supraspinatus tendon and subacromial bursa and, occasionally, over the biceps tendon. Pain is produced by forward flexion of the shoulder, with adduction and internal rotation. Radiographs of the shoulder are normal. Treatment consists of rest and anti-inflammatory measures, along with a strength program for the rotator cuff, with gradual return to swimming when the pain subsides. Practice should end for the swimmer when muscle fatigue causes the athlete to lose proper stroke mechanics.

Femoral Neck Stress Fracture

Although far less frequent than other overstress injuries, especially in children, femoral neck stress fractures have great clinical importance. A femoral neck stress fracture that becomes a complete fracture is a serious complication. The clinical presentation may be nonspecific, with a generalized ache in the groin in the early stages and a limp later. Examination may show loss of hip motion, and radiographs may show the stress fracture. If x-rays are negative, a bone scan is diagnostic. The stress fracture may occur on the inferior part of the neck (compression side) or superior part of the neck (tension side). Treatment for inferior neck stress fractures present on bone scan only is with partial weightbearing crutch ambulation for 4 to 6 weeks. The patient may perform nonimpact aerobic exercise if it is not painful. Tension side fractures and all fractures radiographically present should be internally fixed in situ to prevent completion of the fracture.

UPPER EXTREMITY TRAUMA

The upper extremity is very susceptible to injury in children, as there are thousands of ways in which children of all ages can fall onto their outstretched arms. Indeed, when the patient presents to the emergency ward, the history taken frequently reads, "Fell from the monkey bars landing on . . . ."

Clavicle

Injuries to the medial end of the clavicle are rare and are also difficult to visualize on routine radiographs. Occasionally, they are seen with cephalic tilt views of the clavicle, although a CT scan may be required. Because the medial clavicular epiphysis remains open until age 22, these injuries are commonly epiphyseal fractures, not dislocations. They, therefore, heal and remodel well, and intervention should be considered only for posterior irreducible displacement with compromise of the great vessels. Management consists of a sling for comfort, with gradual return to activities after 3 to 6 weeks.

Clavicle shaft fractures in childhood may be difficult to see on radiographs, but they can be found easily by looking for the clinical signs of fracture (swelling, local tenderness, and deformity) in the physical examination. A sling for comfort is frequently sufficient, although a figure-of-eight clavicle brace is used to maintain the length of the clavicle in displaced fractures with overlap. Protection is maintained for 3 to 5 weeks, and remodeling depending on the age of the patient and complete recovery are the rule.

Birth fractures of the clavicle occur more frequently in large infants and in breech presentation. These are usually noted incidentally or because of a lack of arm movement by the infant. They are treated for comfort and heal fully but must be differentiated from proximal humeral epiphyseal separation, osteomyelitis of the shoulder, and brachial plexus traction injuries.

Acromioclavicular Joint

Injuries to the acromioclavicular (AC) joint in the skeletally immature are most commonly epiphyseal fractures rather than ligament disruptions. Because of the presence of an intact periosteal tube and intact coracoclavicular ligaments, these injuries heal and remodel readily despite wide displacement. Treatment is by clavicle brace or sling for comfort. True ligament injuries of the AC joint (shoulder separations) are very rare, if they occur at all, but may be seen in late adolescence. They are treated as in adult AC separations, with operative reduction and repair considered only in the case of complete or wide displacement of the clavicle. Generally, return to activities may be pursued in 4 to 6 weeks.

Scapula

Scapula fractures are rare, although the scapula may appear radiographically to be fractured due to the appearance of secondary centers of ossification from ages 10 to 22. For that reason, careful assessment of radiographs, with comparison views if necessary, is essential. Fractures are treated conservatively with rest and gradual mobilization when comfortable, unless displacement of a large intra-articular glenoid fragment is noted. In these cases, operative intervention should be considered to avoid problems of late arthritis or shoulder instability.

Shoulder Dislocation

True traumatic dislocation of the shoulder is rare in children and is more common in adolescents. In the younger age group, physeal injuries to the proximal humerus are much more common. The history of the dislocation is vital, as atraumatic involuntary dislocation may occur in patients with congenital joint laxity or structural problems, whereas atraumatic voluntary dislocations occur in those with psychiatric or emotional problems. Atraumatic involuntary dislocation is best treated with rehabilitation, with emphasis on strengthening all shoulder girdle muscles, especially the internal rotators. Surgery is considered if a diligent exercise regimen fails to solve the problem. Voluntary dislocation requires attention to the underlying emotional disorder, although rehabilitation may also be beneficial.

Traumatic anterior dislocation disrupts the capsulolabral attachments to the glenoid, injuring the middle and inferior glenohumeral ligaments. Treatment is by reduction and immobilization for 3 weeks in adduction and internal rotation. Rehabilitation to correct muscle atrophy is necessary before resumption of competitive sports, especially for the muscles of the rotator cuff. Despite treatment as outlined, recurrence of the dislocation takes place over 50% of the time. Adolescent athletes show an 82% redislocation rate, and dislocations in children recur 100% of the time. Late reconstruction of the shoulder is often required. Numerous repair techniques have been described and used effectively. The gold standard is anatomic reconstruction via the Bankart procedure.

Posterior dislocation is rare, with traumatic posterior dislocations being rarer still. They are often missed at first, and careful physical and radiographic assessment is crucial to prompt diagnosis. Initial management of traumatic posterior dislocation is conservative, with reduction and immobilization.

Humerus

Proximal humeral fractures are Salter-Harris type II fractures, with type I injuries occurring in children less than 5 years old. As 80% of the longitudinal growth of the humerus results from this physis, these fractures remodel readily. Manipulative reduction is required only with complete displacement of the humeral shaft in older patients. The arm is immobilized at the side or in a spica cast if necessary. Healing is in 3 to 6 weeks depending on the age of the patient and the degree of displacement, with a gradual progression of activities to follow.

With all extremity trauma, a complete neurologic assessment of the extremity is mandatory. This is especially true for humeral shaft fractures, where for much of the humeral diaphysis, the radial nerve lies in close proximity and is most vulnerable at the junction of the middle and distal thirds of the humerus. Humeral shaft fractures are managed closed, with reduction rarely required. Immobilization in coaptation splints and sling, or occasionally a hanging cast, is usually sufficient. Open treatment is rarely required. Remodeling is most reliable if the fracture is close to the proximal physis or in younger patients. The neurologic status should be assessed both before and after reduction, with particular attention to the function of the radial nerve. Loss of radial nerve function is often due to neuropraxia in continuity. An intact nerve usually recovers, with signs of recovery evident in 8 to 12 weeks. The nerve should be explored if recovery does not ensue.

Elbow

This remains a frequent site of childhood injuries and also one of the more difficult to manage. Distal humerus fractures are difficult to evaluate radiographically for several reasons. True AP and lateral views are difficult to obtain in a child in pain. In addition, the distal humerus has four separate ossification centers: the medial epicondyle, lateral epicondyle, capitellum and lateral trochlear ridge, and medial trochlea. The appearance and development of these centers may give the normal distal humeral epiphysis a fragmented or even fractured appearance, making nondisplaced and minimally displaced fractures difficult to characterize. Comparison views of the opposite elbow are nearly always helpful, and an arthrogram, CT, or MRI of the injured elbow may be required.

Several radiographic keys can help in the diagnosis. On the AP view, the width of the proximal and distal fragments at the fracture should be equal. The fragment is rotated if they are not. On the lateral view, a line along the anterior humeral cortex should pass through the middle of the lateral condylar epiphysis, which in turn should form an angle of about 30 degrees with the humeral shaft. Extension at the fracture site is present if these are not aligned properly. Finally, a posterior olecranon fossa fat pad visible with the elbow flexed is, with few exceptions, indicative of the presence of a joint effusion.

With displaced fractures, the brachial artery and radial, median, and ulnar nerves may become damaged by traction, laceration, or entrapment within the fracture site or joint. The function of these structures should be determined both before and after reduction or fixation or both. Arteriography may be necessary for a complete evaluation.

Supracondylar humeral fractures are usually due to a fall on an outstretched arm, most often with the elbow extended. These occur most often in those 5 to 8 years of age, and there is a gradual decrease in incidence until about age 15. The extension fracture is far more common than the flexion type and may be nondisplaced, greenstick with an intact posterior cortex, or completely displaced. Treatment for the first two types consists of simple cast or splint immobilization, with a minimal reduction occasionally necessary by flexing the elbow, with a careful watch on the neurovascular status of the arm. Children with displaced supracondylar fractures should be admitted to the hospital to monitor their neurovascular status for the development of compartment syndrome and should be seen immediately by an orthopedist who regularly takes care of this injury. These injuries are best treated with closed reduction and immobilization or percutaneous Kirschner wire (K-wire) smooth pin fixation, using either two parallel lateral pins or one medial and one lateral pin to hold unstable fractures or those in which reduction may be maintained only in marked flexion. Open reduction may be needed for irreducible fractures, open fractures, and neurovascular compromise uncorrected by reduction. The pins are removed at 3 to 4 weeks, and the cast is replaced for an additional week. The advantages of pin fixation are improved stability of the reduction, and, thus, the elbow may be extended slightly to lessen the risk of neurovascular compromise. Disadvantages include difficulty in accurate pin placement, pin-related problems, and potential ulnar nerve injury with a medial pin. Lateral or overhead skeletal traction may be used in grossly swollen elbows, with hospitalization to monitor reduction. Late complications are not infrequent and may include cubitus varus (gunstock deformity), stiffness, and nerve embarrassment. Most neuropraxias recover with observation, and corrective osteotomy may be used to treat malunion.

Fractures of the lateral condyle and epicondyle are fairly common and are usually Salter-Harris type IV fractures. Displaced fractures require accurate open reduction and internal fixation with K-wires to realign the growth plate and articular surface, whereas nondisplaced fractures may be immobilized but must be checked early for loss of position. These fractures carry a higher risk of late arthritis and growth arrest. True lateral epicondyle fractures are rare, although elbow radiographs will often have this appearance. Careful clinical examination is crucial, and comparison views may be necessary.

Distal humeral physeal separations (Salter-Harris type I or II) occur in children less than 7 years old and look clinically like an elbow dislocation. The child should be admitted to closely monitor the neurovascular status. The treatment of choice is closed reduction with casting in extension for 3 weeks. Open reduction can lead to cubitus varus and loss of function, although percutaneous K-wire fixation is sometimes required to maintain reduction.

Medial epicondyle avulsion fractures occur under valgus stress or in association with elbow dislocations. The avulsed epicondyle may be displaced from the distal humerus and can become lodged within the joint, as can the median nerve. A thorough neurologic assessment is, therefore, essential. Comparison views, arthrography, or MRI may be needed to fully describe the injury. Undisplaced fractures are treated in a long arm cast, with open treatment and internal fixation if the epicondyle is displaced, the elbow remains unstable, or the epicondyle or nerve is trapped within the joint. For closed treatment, the elbow is flexed, and the forearm is pronated to relax tension on the epicondyle from the common flexor origin.

Medial condyle fractures can present difficulties in diagnosis, as the ossific nucleus of the trochlea does not appear until age 9 to 11 years. The principles of management are identical to those for lateral condyle fractures. Elbow stiffness and, occasionally, growth disturbance may result regardless of treatment.

Elbow dislocations do happen to children, although most often they occur in association with a fracture. Following reduction, the joint is carefully examined for congruency, elbow stability, and fluidity of motion. Soft tissue or bone may be interposed in the joint, or unstable fractures may be present. If so, operative reduction is required. An MRI or arthrogram may best delineate the injury. After a true dislocation, the elbow should be immobilized for 1 week in a sturdy splint, followed by the return of elbow motion gradually within the stable range.

Fractures of the proximal radius are common, but unlike adult injuries, damage to the articular surface of the radial head is rare. A fall on the outstretched arm is the usual cause, with the radiocapitellar articulation accepting the force. The fracture is most commonly Salter-Harris type I or II. True AP and lateral views of the proximal radius are needed, as treatment is based on the relative position of the radial head. Less than 30 degrees angulation can be accepted and treated with a cast for 3 weeks, with full motion after remodeling expected.

For more than 30 degrees, the radial head should be reduced (closed or open) and the elbow casted. Complications, such as synostosis of the proximal radius and ulna or avascular necrosis of the radial head, may follow even with closed treatment.

Olecranon fractures may be treated with cast immobilization, though displaced fractures may require tension band wire fixation. It is essential to perform a thorough examination to ensure that this is the only injury.

Pulled elbow (nursemaid's elbow) may be the most common elbow injury in children. Parents and caretakers often use a forceful pull on the arm to direct a recalcitrant child and should be advised of the cause of the problem. Distraction of the joint allows the annular ligament to slip over the top of the radial head, and the child will not use the arm. The interposed ligament may be reduced as the radiology technician supinates the forearm to obtain the AP radiograph. The elbow is reduced by gentle traction in extension, supination, and then flexion, and a click is sometimes palpable as reduction occurs. The joint is fully reduced if full flexion is reestablished, and the child resumes using the arm a short time later. If the problem recurs repeatedly, casting the elbow in flexion and supination with the elbow reduced will allow the stretched annular ligament to shorten.

Forearm

Fractures of the ulnar shaft associated with a dislocation of the radial head are *Monteggia fractures*. Equivalent injuries in children include plastic bending of the ulna with radial head dislocation and ulna fracture with separation of the proximal radial epiphysis. The ulna fracture is readily noted at presentation, and care must be taken to look for the radial head dislocation. The radiographs, therefore, need to include both the joint above (elbow) and joint below (wrist) the fracture, a valuable practice in the evaluation of all fractures. Treatment in children involves closed manipulation to realign the ulna and reduce the radial head. Traction is applied to the arm in extension, followed by supination, followed by flexion to 90 degrees and cast immobilization, with close follow-up to ensure maintenance of the dual reduction. Occasionally, the ulna must be fixed to maintain the radial head reduction. If the radial head dislocation is posterior, reduction may best be held in extension.

Greenstick fractures of the forearm may be treated by closed reduction. The fracture should be completed by cracking the intact cortex to reduce risk of recurrence of deformity in the cast and late refracture. Healing occurs in 4 to 6 weeks, and less than 10 degrees angulation must be maintained to avoid loss of forearm rotation. *Displaced fractures of the forearm* bones should be reduced closed, with attention to correct rotation and angulation, and the intact periosteal sleeve can be used as a hinge to aid reduction. Cortex-to-cortex apposition is adequate provided the alignment and rotation are correct. The arm is immobilized, with the long arm cast or sugar-tong splint carefully formed to provide three-point fixation. Open reduction and internal fixation may be needed if an acceptable reduction cannot be obtained or in adolescents.

Buckle fractures of the distal radius or ulna or both occur with compression failure of the young bone. The buckle is usually found just proximal to the distal radial physis, and radiographs may show only a subtle ripple along one cortex or soft tissue swelling. Treatment is with a short arm cast for 3 weeks.

Fractures of the distal radius and ulna are usually Salter-Harris type I or II and are found primarily from ages 6 to 12. Type I injuries occur in younger children and are frequently nondisplaced. Radiographs are either normal or show subtle widening of the physis. The clinical examination is, therefore, the key. Reduction is performed for large amounts of displacement, as remodeling is the rule, and the child is protected for 3 weeks in a cast. Type II injuries are more common in older children and adolescents and usually are treated closed with reduction if necessary and cast immobilization. Growth disturbance is rare but can result, and the patient should be checked with radiographs for 6 to 12 months to monitor the result.

Hand

Several principles are important in the care of hand fractures in children. Fractures of the shafts of the metacarpals and phalanges must be aligned properly, with special attention to the rotation of the digits. A reliable check of rotation is to flex the finger metacarpophalangeal (MP) joints 90 degrees and check the fingernails, which should be aligned evenly. Enough immobilization should be provided to ensure that even the most active patient cannot dislodge the fracture. The period of immobilization should be for 3 weeks for almost all injuries. In hands of children, this will be sufficient for clinical but not radiographic union of the fracture.

Fractures of the base of the thumb metacarpal occur with hyperextension or abduction of the thumb. These may be metaphyseal fractures or physeal fractures of the basal thumb physis. Angulation of less than 30 degrees is acceptable due to the mobility of the basal thumb joint and requires only thumb spica cast immobilization. Salter-Harris type II fractures may require open reduction if widely displaced, and type III injuries (an adult Bennett fracture equivalent) require reduction and K-wire fixation.

A frequent skiing injury is the so-called *gamekeeper's thumb*. Valgus stress is applied to the thumb across the MP joint and results in tearing of the ulnar collateral ligament of the joint in adults and a type III physeal injury in children. A displaced fracture or a stress view demonstrating over 45 degrees of angulation at the joint is best treated with repair.

Metacarpophalangeal joint dislocation may occur with hyperextension of the joint and may be simple (reducible) or complex (irreducible). Complex dislocations require an operative reduction, with removal of the interposed volar plate from the joint and extraction of the metacarpal head from a Chinese finger trap of palmar fascia and flexor tendons. Radiographically, the metacarpal usually is found to be parallel to the proximal phalanx on the lateral view in the complex dislocation.

Injuries to the tip of the finger and nailbed are very common in children of all ages. Crush injuries to the distal phalanx require thorough irrigation, with repair directed at preservation of length, the nailbed, and the proximal nailfold. Mallet finger deformity in young children is usually a type I physeal separation and also often open. Thorough irrigation of the wound, antibiotic prophylaxis, and reduction of the nail back underneath the proximal nailfold is required, in addition to reduction of the fracture. In older children, a type III injury of the distal phalanx epiphysis, through avulsion by the pull of the extensor tendon, is common. Repair with K-wire fixation is required if the fragment is displaced.

LOWER EXTREMITY TRAUMA

Hip

Dislocation of the hip occurs more often than fracture in children, requires less force than in adults, and is found primarily in the 12 to 15 year age group. Posterior dislocation is far more common than anterior dislocation. Dislocations are usually reduced closed, and the patient is treated in Buck's skin traction for 1 to 2 weeks. The patient walks with crutches, avoiding the positions of flexion and adduction for approximately 3 weeks. It is crucial to ensure that a concentric reduction of the hip is obtained, as bone or cartilage fragments may become trapped in the joint. A careful search for fractures of the femoral head and acetabulum must be performed, and CT scans frequently are needed for complete assessment. Open reduction is performed if a concentric closed reduction cannot be established, through an anterior approach for anterior dislocations and posterior approach for posterior dislocations. Dislocation can recur in patients with excessive ligament laxity in conditions such as the Ehlers-Danlos syndrome. The risk of avascular necrosis following this injury is approximately 8% to 10%, less than that for adults, although still significant.

Femoral neck fractures require significant trauma in children and are fairly infrequent, fortunately, as the risk of complications is high. Major complications include avascular necrosis (AVN), which occurs in 30% to 50% and is highest in patients over 8 years of age; coxa vara due to malunion, which is found in 20% to 30% of patients and may require corrective osteotomy later; and premature physeal closure, which depends on the type of injury and can occur in up to 60%. Traumatic slipped capital femoral epiphysis (SCFE) may be reduced gently at the time of positioning the hip for fixation and pinned in place with cannulated screws under image-intensifier control. The pins should not penetrate the subchondral bone, as chondrolysis of the articular cartilage will result, and vigorous reduction can result in further damage to the epiphyseal vascular supply and increased risk of AVN. If the epiphysis is dislocated, AVN is certain. Transcervical femoral neck fractures are treated with closed reduction and cannulated screw fixation, and a spica cast is used for protection for 4 to 6 weeks. There is a 50% risk of AVN with displaced fractures. Basicervical fractures, with better blood supply to the femoral neck and head, may be treated with a hip spica cast if nondisplaced and closed reduction, internal fixation, and a spica cast if displaced.

Femur

With *fractures of the femoral shaft,* it is important to check for the presence of other injuries, particularly to the ipsilateral hip and knee in trauma victims and to other bones in the possible victim of child abuse. The hip and knee should be included routinely on the radiographic studies. Careful neurovascular assessment is also required, although it is frequently negative. Femoral shaft fractures heal without difficulty as long as the proximal and distal ends of the fracture remain in the same thigh. Overlap or bayonet apposition of the fragments in most cases is sufficient, as overgrowth of the femur can make up for up to 2 cm of shortening. Small deformities are well hidden by the bulk of the thigh muscle.

Treatment is age dependent. In children less than 3 years of age, an immediate spica cast may be applied, usually with the hip flexed 90 degrees and abducted 45 degrees, and maintained for 4 to 6 weeks. On cast removal, the fracture callus will be easily palpable in the thigh. Skeletal traction using a distal femoral traction pin can be used in those patients 3 to 10 years old. Radiographic studies guide positioning and weight application, and the setup is maintained for 2 to 3 weeks until the fracture becomes sticky, when a spica cast is applied. Recent efforts to provide earlier mobilization and reduced hospitalization of the patient have led to trials of immediate spica cast application in these patients. Ischial weightbearing cast braces and external fixation have been used by some, with good results. Adolescent patients, if close to the end of growth, may be treated as adults with intramedullary rod fixation and early mobilization. Internal or external fixation is used in the head injury patient, as these patients are unable to cooperate with care.

Supracondylar fractures and fractures of the distal femur may be very difficult to align in traction. The pull of the gastrocnemius muscle flexes the distal fragment. Internal fixation may be required if adequate reduction cannot be established.

Knee

Distal femoral epiphyseal separation may be seen in the adolescent football player subjected to a clip while playing. Where an adult would tear the medial collateral ligament, the player with open growth plates sustains a type I or II epiphyseal separation. Valgus stress radiographs may aid in the diagnosis. The popliteal artery is closely applied posteriorly and may be damaged at the time of injury. The vascular supply of the limb should be carefully checked, and an arteriogram may be required. Treatment is through closed reduction and a cast, although open reduction may be required if the injury is irreducible due to interposed soft tissue. Internal fixation may be beneficial if arterial exploration is required. The patient should be admitted for observation

for compartment syndrome or vascular embarrassment. The knee may become stiff, and the incidence of growth arrest is 50%.

Patella fractures are rare in children. These may be treated with a cast in extension if the fracture is nondisplaced and if the extensor mechanism is intact. Displaced fractures or the inability to actively extend the knee indicates a need for operative care. A tension band wire technique is used for fixation. A patella fracture variant is the sleeve fracture, in which the infrapatellar tendon avulses a fragment of bone from the inferior pole of the patella along with articular cartilage. Internal fixation is necessary if the fracture is displaced.

Lateral patellar dislocation is a common problem in childhood and adolescence and most often is related to malalignment of the lower limb. Increased knee valgus, persistent femoral neck anteversion, external rotation of the tibial tubercle, excess tightness of the lateral retinaculum of the knee, congenital ligament laxity, hypoplasia of the trochlea, or a combination of these factors may be found. A hemarthrosis is routinely present. Initially, the knee is aspirated, radiographed, and immobilized, and subsequently it is rehabilitated. Articular damage can result as the patella dislocates and then relocates, and osteochondral fractures may require removal if they are small or internal fixation if they are large. A large tear in the medial retinaculum may require operative repair early, and realignment procedures are indicated for recurrent dislocation.

Intercondylar eminence fractures of the tibia are the child's equivalent of the torn anterior cruciate ligament. They occur with hyperextension, hyperflexion occasionally, or valgus rotational stress on the knee and result in an impressive hemarthrosis. Tibial eminence fractures may be nondisplaced, hinged, or displaced. The knee is aspirated for comfort, and the leg is casted with the knee in full extension for nondisplaced or reducible hinged fractures. Displaced and irreducible fractures require reduction, which may be done open or arthroscopically, and internal fixation. Despite this treatment, increased laxity of the ACL may be seen following healing, although tightening can be expected as the child grows.

Fractures of the proximal tibial epiphysis, similar to distal femoral injuries, may be associated with vascular compromise. The popliteal artery is tethered to the epiphysis by the geniculate vessels and is easily injured. Careful assessment is required. The presence of pulses does not preclude the presence of arterial injury with an intimal tear. Displaced fractures dictate admission to the hospital and arteriography, with observation for compartment syndrome. Types I and II are most common and can be treated with reduction and a cast. If a vascular repair or reconstruction is needed or if the fracture is type III or IV (intraarticular or across the physis), open reduction and internal fixation are necessary.

Avulsion of the tibial tubercle at the infrapatellar tendon attachment is found primarily in patients 14 to 16 years of age. These require open reduction and internal fixation if displaced or occurring at the level of the tibial physis. Nondisplaced or minimally displaced fractures may be treated with a cast in extension.

Meniscal tears do occur in children and can be treated with arthroscopic resection or repair as appropriate. MRI of the meniscus is very helpful, although the greater vascularity of the meniscus in children can present difficulty in reading the study. Vertical tears through the meniscosynovial junction or in the most peripheral 33% to 50% of the meniscus are repairable. The rest of the meniscus may not be sufficiently vascular to heal following repair. Discoid lateral meniscus may cause a snapping knee and can be a cause of knee pain and locking when torn. Loose fragments that cause symptoms should be removed, with meniscoplasty to form a more normal appearing meniscal rim performed along the remaining meniscal substance.

Tibia and Fibula

Fractures of the tibial shaft can be treated with long leg cast immobilization and heal readily in young patients in 6 to 8 weeks. Care is taken to avoid varus or valgus angulation of more than 5 to 10 degrees, and the foot should be rotated to match the foot/thigh angle of the uninjured limb. Wedging the cast can correct alignment problems. Operative treatment is rarely required, although to maintain length and alignment, intramedullary fixation may be chosen in those nearing skeletal maturity, and pins may be incorporated into the cast (pins and plaster) or external fixation may be necessary. If the fibula bows but remains intact with tibial shaft fracture, the cast must be carefully molded to avoid the fracture migrating into the varus or valgus.

A limping child less than 2 years of age may have a *toddler fracture*, a spiral, nondisplaced fracture of the tibia. These heal readily and without displacement but should be treated with a cast for 3 weeks for protection. Problem fractures include displaced proximal metaphyseal fractures, as damage to the vascular trifurcation can occur, and greenstick fractures of the proximal tibial metaphysis. These latter fractures, unless reduced well and carefully casted in extension, can result in overgrowth medially, with progressive deformity of the tibia.

Ankle

Type I epiphyseal separation of the distal fibula is the pediatric equivalent of the ankle sprain. Cast immobilization for 3 weeks is sufficient, and displacement is rare.

The *Tillaux fracture* is a type III epiphyseal injury to the lateral aspect of the distal tibial physis, occurring most likely as an avulsion injury at the site of attachment of the anterior tibiofibular ligaments under external rotation stress. Closed reduction and cast immobilization can be performed, although open treatment is required if displacement is 2 mm or more. This is an intraarticular fracture, and congruity of the articular surface of the ankle must be reestablished.

The *triplane fracture* of the ankle combines a type II injury with a type III injury (Tillaux). Radiographs can be difficult to interpret, and a CT scan can be invaluable to evaluate the fracture and subsequent reduction. If there is any question whether the closed reduction is adequate, open reduction and internal fixation should be pursued. Epiphyseal arrest and joint incongruity are potential complications, and the fracture must be treated aggressively.

A *type II separation* of the distal tibial physis can occur with greenstick fracture of the fibula. This fracture can be treated closed, and despite angulation of up to 20 degrees, results are good due to remodeling. Growth disturbance is a rare complication.

Medial malleolar fractures are type III or IV physeal injuries and should be treated with accurate reduction to align the physis and articular surface and internal fixation to maintain it. There is a high incidence of bridge formation (partial physeal closure) with these fractures, especially those treated nonoperatively.

Foot

Several fractures in the foot should be mentioned. Most fractures not mentioned will respond to cast immobilization for 3 to 6 weeks until healed. Phalangeal fractures require little more than buddy taping, perhaps with reduction, as all will heal readily. Fractures of the bones of the great toe may require more aggressive care if displaced or intraarticular or to prevent early degenerative change.

Stress fracture of the fifth metatarsal base can occur with residual clubfoot deformity due to transfer of weightbearing to the lateral border of the foot. The base of the fifth metatarsal may also suffer an avulsion injury with inversion injury due to the pull of the peroneus brevis, although displacement is rare. These may be treated with weightbearing casts. However, in the residual clubfoot situation, the deformity ultimately may need to be addressed.

Fractures of the talus are rare and result from high-energy trauma and may be divided into neck and body fractures. Talar neck fractures are usually nondisplaced and heal with a cast. Reduction and internal fixation may be needed in displaced fractures. Body fractures are frequently displaced and require open reduction and internal fixation and are associated with an increased incidence of AVN.

Calcaneus fractures are rare in children and most often can be managed closed with nonweightbearing cast immobilization. Admission to the hospital may be necessary, since marked swelling can be anticipated.

Osteochondral fractures of the dome of the talus occur following 1% of ankle injuries. They are frequently picked up late as symptoms continue, and acute stage and even delayed radiographs may not be diagnostic. The common sites of occurrence are the anterolateral and posteromedial dome of the talus. Persistent ankle pain or a joint effusion following injury should signal the possibility, and a CT scan, bone scan, or MRI usually is diagnostic. The lesions may be staged, with compression injury (bone bruise) without delineation of an osteochondral fragment amenable to conservative cast treatment. Partial or complete delineation of an osteochondral fragment, with or without separation, requires arthroscopic treatment, including drilling of the defect and perhaps debridement of cartilage and bone fragments. A scar fibrocartilage will form in the defect.

14

Muscles

TORTICOLLIS

RICHARD J. MIER, M.D.

Torticollis means *twisted neck* and describes a situation in which the head is persistently laterally flexed and rotated on the neck.

CONGENITAL TORTICOLLIS

The most common cause of congenital torticollis is fibrous shortening of the sternocleidomastoid (SCM) muscle (congenital muscular torticollis). The reason for the shortening is unknown, but postulated mechanisms include abnormal intrauterine positioning, hemorrhage, birth trauma, and a compartment syndrome. Muscular foreshortening draws the head into lateral flexion and produces rotation to the contralateral side, with the chin pointing away from the lesion. Other positional deformities may be present, including hip dysplasia (in 20%) and facial asymmetry if the restriction is persistent. An olive-shaped fibrous mass often appears during the early postnatal period and usually regresses by the end of the first year even if the torticollis persists.

Occipitocervical malformations, including vertebral fusion (the Klippel-Feil syndrome), odontoid aplasia, hemiatlas, and basilar impression, may cause torticollis presenting at birth. Affected children may have low hairlines, short necks, and neck webbing. Failure to make the correct diagnosis may result in a neurologic catastrophe if physical therapy is attempted. One case of quadriplegia resulting from spinal manipulation in an infant with a spinal cord astrocytoma has been described. Computed tomography (CT) or magnetic resonance imaging (MRI) may be necessary to exclude these anomalies, since the immature spine may not demonstrate the abnormality radiographically. Such spinal malformations are predisposed to injury. Therefore, in children presenting with torticollis at birth, a fracture or dislocation must be considered a possible etiology even if the delivery is not traumatic in the usual sense of the word.

Gastroesophageal reflux may be associated with abnormal torticollis-like head and neck positioning as the baby reacts to the discomfort of reflux esophagitis (Sandifer syndrome). This may be present early enough to represent a congenital lesion.

ACQUIRED TORTICOLLIS

Acquired torticollis can result from serious cervical trauma but is more frequently due to such benign causes as minor soft tissue trauma or viral myositis. An inflammatory condition affecting any of the tissues of the neck may cause torticollis, including adenitis, pharyngitis, retropharyngeal abscess, cellulitis, or sinusitis.

It is sometimes difficult to distinguish these from true rotatory atlantoaxial subluxation, which is not rare in children and may itself be related to an upper respiratory tract infection, minor trauma, or chronic inflammation of the atlantoaxial joint as occurs with juvenile rheumatic arthritis.

Other less common causes of acquired torticollis include medications (particularly the phenothiazines), cervical disc disease, myositis ossificans progressiva, ocular strabismus, syringomyelia, and tumors of the posterior fossa, brainstem, or cervical spine (including osteoid osteoma and osteoblastoma). One case due to pseudotumor cerebri has been reported.

Spasmodic torticollis may be the manifestation of a segmental or focal dystonia. These dystonic reactions can occur after head trauma, but most often their cause is unknown. A small number of children have been described with paroxysmal torticollis, sometimes associated with headache, vomiting, or ataxia. They sometimes manifest more typical symptoms of migraine subsequently. There frequently is a family history of either paroxysmal torticollis or classic migraine.

DIAGNOSIS AND TREATMENT

Radiographs should be performed on all infants with torticollis before therapy is attempted. CT scanning should be performed on all infants with radiographic occipitocervical abnormalities, physical stigmata of cervical spinal abnormalities (such as webbing, short neck, low hairline), a rigid deformity, or neurologic abnormality, or if there is *no* olive or shortening of the SCM muscle.

CT (for suspected bony lesions) or MRI (for soft tissue or cord lesions) is useful in the older child with acquired torticollis if symptoms are severe or persistent or if the cause is not apparent.

Congenital muscular torticollis generally (90% of the time) responds well to physical therapy, assuming that vertebral anomalies have been excluded. Therapy can be performed at home by gentle but persistent lateral flexion of the head to stretch the contralaterally tightened SCM muscle. Rotation of the head toward the side with the tightness can be done simultaneously. Ten to twenty repetitions, holding momentarily at maximal range, usually will suffice if performed three or four times daily. A referral to a physical therapist is a good idea in order to monitor progress and compliance.

Children who fail conservative measures or who present after 1 year of age (particularly if they exhibit significant facial asymmetry) will most often require surgery (usually SCM release) followed by postoperative physical therapy and splinting. Tong traction and facial reconstruction may be necessary in long-standing cases.

Painful acquired torticollis can be associated with osteoid osteotomy or osteoblastoma best diagnosed by technetium bone scan and localized by CT. Rotatory atlantoaxial subluxation will often respond to traction, although open reduction and fusion are sometimes necessary in children with long-standing refractory symptoms. Botulinum toxin and rhizotomy have been used for patients with intractable spasmodic torticollis.

REFERENCES

1. Canale ST, Griffin DW, Hubbard CN: Congenital muscular torticollis: A long-term follow-up. J Bone Joint Surg 64:810, 1982.
2. Shafris Y, Kaufman BA: Quadriplegia after chiropractic manipulation in an infant with congenital torticollis caused by a spinal cord astrocytoma. J Pediatr 120:266, 1992.

CONGENITAL MUSCULAR DEFECTS

RICHARD J. MIER, M.D.

Congenital muscular defects comprise a large number of disparate conditions. These disorders may be subgrouped as representing either embryologic absence of a specific muscle or group of muscles (e.g., Poland's anomaly) or intrinsic abnormalities of muscle itself (e.g., central core myopathy).

PRIMARY DEFECTS

Disability due to these abnormalities varies widely depending on the site and degree of the defect and may be of trivial importance, of cosmetic importance only, or of serious functional significance. Therapy, when available, is primarily surgical and is oriented to reparative or tendon transfer procedures.

An archetypical example of isolated congenital lack of muscle development is Poland's anomaly, consisting of unilateral absence of the costal and sternal portions of the pectoralis major muscle, often with synbrachydactyly of the ipsilateral hand and other mesodermal defects of the upper ipsilateral chest (skin hypoplasia, nipple absence, or hypoplasia). Thought to be a local defect of mesodermal development, Poland's anomaly is generally not hereditary, and there is no specific therapy.

Similar congenital hypoplasia syndromes have been described for the depressor anguli oris muscle, resulting in the asymmetric crying facies syndrome, important because of its association with congenital heart disease and genitourinary and other anomalies. Electrophysiologic studies may be required to distinguish muscular absence from true facial nerve palsy.

Duane's syndrome represents replacement of the ocular abducens muscle by a fibrous band and causes failure of abduction of the affected side, with retraction of the globe when adduction is attempted. Congenital absence of the trapezius, quadratus femoris, and serratus major muscles has been described.

SECONDARY MUSCULAR DISRUPTION SYNDROMES

Secondary muscular disruption syndromes are not uncommon at birth and manifest themselves as a result of other more primary processes. This occurs, for example, in congenital limb deficiency syndromes (such as radial hypoplasia) or as a result of massive fetal urinary tract dilatation, which inhibits development of the muscles of the anterior abdominal wall (the prune-belly syndrome of Eagle and Barrett).

INTRINSIC MUSCLE DISEASE

Intrinsic muscle disease may manifest itself at birth as well. Included here are such "benign" causes of early proximal hypotonicity as nemaline myopathy, central core disease, and myotubular myopathy. Elevations of muscle enzymes often are modest, if present at all, and electrophysiologic studies often are normal. Structural and ultrastructural changes on microscopy permit categorization and prognostication, which is often, but not invariably, good.

Several of the muscular dystrophies may be present at birth, including, most prominently, congenital muscular dystrophy, inherited as an autosomal recessive with a slow, somewhat unpredictably progressive course. One variant is associated with mental retardation (Fukuyama), and one is associated with striking congenital joint contractures (Ullrich disease). Diagnosis is dependent on muscle biopsy.

Additionally, several of the dystrophic myotonic disorders may present at birth, including Thomsen's disease (myotonia congenita) and the congenital form of myotonic dystrophy. Usually hypotonic at birth, these babies have a weak cry and suck, often exhibit arthrogryposis, and frequently are mentally retarded. Therapy is supportive, and orthopedic procedures may be necessary to improve function.

BENIGN CONGENITAL HYPOTONIA

DAVID K. URION, M.D.

The floppy infant presents the clinician in neurologic practice with a classic problem in localization. Decreased tone can occur from dysfunction at any level of the neuraxis. Hence, the problem of determining the cause of reduced tone in an infant is one of correct localization. This often can be achieved by a process akin to triangulation in navigation. One can establish the likeliest level of the affliction of the nervous system by examining what other features are seen in association with the hypotonia.

Oppenheim (1900), one of the great neuropsychiatrists of the late nineteenth and early twentieth centuries, attempted to distinguish a

TABLE 1. Causes of Reduced Tone in Infants

LEVEL	CAUSES	ASSOCIATED FEATURES
Cortex	Cerebral dysgeneses	
	Agenesis of the corpus callosum	May be associated with seizures, retinal anomalies
	Midline dysgenetic syndromes	May be associated with neuroendocrine defects
	Aminoacidopathies	May be associated with seizures
	Organic acidemias	Systemically quite ill; unexplained metabolic acidosis
	Urea cycle defects	May be associated with seizures
	Hypothyroidism	Check cord blood thyroid
Subcortical white matter	(Evolving) periventricular leukomalacia	Symmetric; more common among premature infants; evolves toward spastic diplegia
	Periventricular hemorrhagic infarct	Usually asymmetric
	Dysmyelinating syndromes	Progressive
	Hypomyelinating syndromes	
Brainstem	Structural defects (e.g., Moebius)	Associated cranial neuropathies
Spinal cord	Traumatic injury	Diagnosable level
Anterior horn cell	Infantile spinal muscular atrophy	Fasciculations; fibrillations; areflexia; mild elevation of serum CPK; aldolase
	Infectious poliomyelitis	Asymmetric; CSF pleocytosis
Dorsal root	Landry-Guillain-Barré-Strohl syndrome	Elevated CSF protein without CSF pleocytosis

TABLE 1. Causes of Reduced Tone in Infants *Continued*

LEVEL	CAUSES	ASSOCIATED FEATURES
Nerve	Congenital neuropathies	Areflexia; may be insensitive to pain
Neuromuscular junction	(Transient) neonatal myasthenia	Mother with myasthenia gravis
	Congenital myasthenia	Abnormal muscle on electron microscopy
Muscle	Muscular dystrophies X-linked (Duchenne/Becker)	Males only; CPK highest in newborn period
	Myotonic dystrophy	Mother usually symptomatic
	"Congenital" myopathies, e.g., nemaline, central core	Typical findings on biopsy
	Mitochondropathies	Often present with seizures; serum pyruvate/lactate elevated
	Peroxisomal disorders	Elevated long-chain fatty acid concentrations in blood; facies characteristic

group of infants with benign forms of congenital hypotonia from those with more serious, progressive diseases, such as infantile spinal muscular atrophy (Werdnig-Hoffmann disease). After more than 50 years of fractious debate regarding the legitimacy of this diagnostic entity, Walton proposed the term *benign congenital hypotonia* to describe a group of infants with decreased muscle tone in the newborn period who have a relatively good developmental outcome.

Most pediatric neurologists now accept the existence of such a group of infants, who present with reduced muscle tone at or shortly after birth and who do not succumb to their condition. Some authors, such as Dubowitz,[1] prefer the concept of *central hypotonia*, emphasizing that the condition probably comes from dysfunction at the level of the cortex or subcortical gray matter, is not necessarily benign for the child or parent, and is often associated with mild to moderate cognitive dysfunction. All authors in this field concur that the diagnosis of benign congenital hypotonia or central hypotonia is one of exclusion and that other causes of decreased tone must be excluded.

Table 1 lists causes of reduced tone in the infant, organized by level of usual presentation in the nervous system. Common associated findings that help in generating a localizing hypothesis are also included. These principles may be used as the basis for a diagnostic paradigm that can help the clinician in approaching the infant with reduced tone (Fig. 1). If one follows this decision tree and ends in a point without a specific diagnosis supported by laboratory data, a

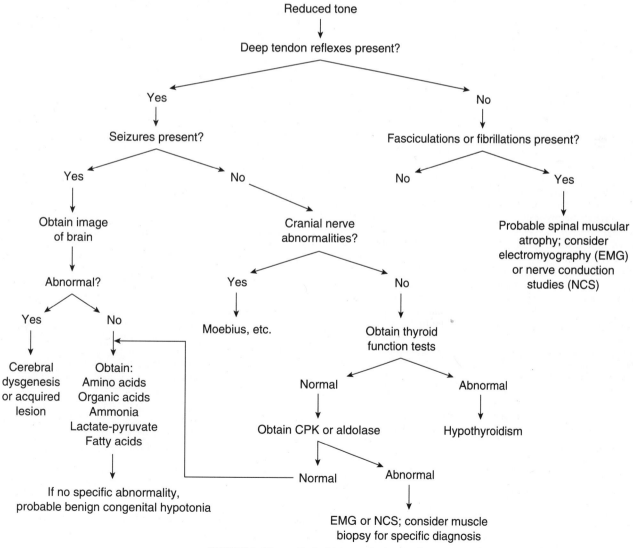

FIGURE 1. Diagnostic decision tree for hypotonia.

diagnosis of benign congenital hypotonia may be tendered. This approach may also improve the cost-effective nature of an evaluation, leading the clinician away from diagnostic maneuvers unlikely to shed light on the underlying process.

Several points are worth bearing in mind. A diagnosis of benign congenital hypotonia must always be considered provisional. The child should be followed at regular intervals to make certain that some more definitive sign has not presented itself, leading the clinician to reinstitute an evaluation for a specific cause of reduced tone.

TREATMENT

Infants with reduced tone appear to benefit from physical and occupational therapy services. Families may learn to do these therapies at home under the guidance of a trained physical or occupational therapist, or such services may be provided directly by appropriate personnel.

Finally, as such children appear to be at risk for other sorts of developmental problems, such as delayed speech and language acquisition, the practitioner should keep close watch over other aspects of development. Delay in other domains should be investigated sooner, rather than later, and may lead the clinician to reconsider the issue of ultimate causation.

REFERENCE

1. Dubowitz V: The floppy infant: A practical approach to classification. Dev Med Child Neurol 10:706, 1968.

MUSCULAR DYSTROPHY AND RELATED MYOPATHIES

PETER T. HEYDEMANN, M.D.

Conditions of muscular weakness in children include the congenital myopathies, metabolic myopathies, inflammatory myopathies, and muscular dystrophies. Some diseases have specific treatments, and all have a common need to deal symptomatically with weakness.

Polymyositis is treated with prednisone and other anti-inflammatory medications plus intravenous immune globulin in certain circumstances. Metabolic myopathies, such as ragged red myopathies, may be treated with coenzyme Q plus carnitine and vitamins that are involved in mitochondrial respiration. Myotonia can be treated with phenytoin, acetazolamide, or quinine. Hyperthyroid or hypothyroid myopathy is treated successfully by addressing the underlying disease.

Duchenne muscular dystrophy (DMD) is the most common of the childhood muscular diseases. It occurs in 1 in 3500 male infants, who typically present in the late toddler years with mild proximal weakness, Gower's sign, large rubbery tough calves, and a 100- to 300-fold creatine phosphokinase (CPK) elevation. Becker muscular dystrophy is a milder allelic condition that occurs at the same Xp21 site of the X chromosome. Proper diagnosis is made by the cited clinical features and a blood test that shows a deletion or duplication anomaly of the gene (70% of affected children) or dystrophic features on muscle biopsy plus altered or absent dystrophin (100% of affected children). Common differential diagnoses are Kugelberg-Welander disease (childhood spinal muscular atrophy), acid maltase deficiency, Emery-Dreifuss dystrophy, and polymyositis.

The following discussion concentrates on DMD except where specifically noted, and the reader may make extrapolations in regard to similar care for other forms of muscular weakness.

INITIAL FAMILY DISCUSSION

After establishing a specific diagnosis of DMD, the initial approach should include an open discussion with the parents. As with any situation in which medical personnel deliver difficult news to families, information should be shared simply and directly with both parents together by a physician with enough time, sympathy, tolerance, and expertise to deal confidently with the parents' emotional response and limitations of understanding. The discussion should include the natural history of the disease: relative early normalcy, progressive difficulty walking in the early school years, loss of independent ambulation in mid to late grammar school years, more visible arm weakness in the teen years, cardiac and respiratory muscle weakness, and death due to respiratory or cardiac causes in the late teens to 20s. Parents are told that the disease is treatable though not curable at this time. It is emphasized that genetic tests can help to prevent future cases of DMD in the family. Family members at risk for having affected children should be notified by the parents of the availability of testing to assess their carrier state before further family pregnancies ensue. The child should receive a simple explanation that his slow running or stair climbing is due to sick muscles, not laziness, of which many such boys have been accused. The message is that he is a good kid with an illness of the muscles.

It is important to counsel the parents to deal with their sense of loss in an effort to treat their son relatively normally in the early years of diagnosis, which is the time when he will be able to participate happily in many normal peer activities.

GENERAL CARE

Interdisciplinary care is helpful and may include neuropediatricians, orthopedic specialists, geneticists, occupational and physical therapists, physiatrists, psychologists, social workers, and dietitians, as well as additional subspecialists in cardiac, pulmonary, and scoliosis care.

ORTHOPEDIC INTERVENTION

Aggressive orthopedic and orthotic intervention at the right times in the DMD natural history can prolong ambulation and probably minimize the incidence and severity of scoliosis. It is remarkable how some children can maintain a center of gravity and an upright posture with minimal pelvic girdle and paraspinal strength by locking their skeletal joints (especially knees and spinal facets) in a balanced posture and thereby continue to ambulate in the home. Contractures are a common aspect of chronic muscular weakness. Passive stretching exercises of Achilles and hip flexor tendons may prevent or delay the need for surgical procedures.

Surgical release of lower extremity contractures should be considered when a child is beginning to fall frequently. This excludes the 5- to 6-year-old child who is falling because he still has the mindset of an active mobile preschooler and has not yet adapted to his limitations. Percutaneous release of contractures at the Achilles tendon, hip flexors, and tensor fascia latae is helpful when properly timed.

Orthotic bracing is needed as part of follow-up care. Ankle foot orthoses (AFOs) are used to keep the feet plantigrade. Knee ankle foot orthoses (KAFOs) are used to help keep the knees locked when upright. These braces allow a boy to stand and walk slowly for short distances, so they should seldom be used in the child who can walk independently in the community. Although the procedures are operatively simple, it takes a surgeon experienced with muscular dystrophy to know when a contracture is compensatory (actually beneficial) and when it should be released. Rapid ambulation after any surgical procedure is essential because bedrest results in progressive disuse weakness, which can be catastrophic for children who are tenuously compensated. Knee sleeves may be helpful in the child whose knees buckle occasionally. Some contractures clearly aid in function and should not be released. For example, the biceps contracture (elbow flexion) aids the DMD child in feeding and grooming activities that require him to reach toward the head.

The younger a DMD child is when he becomes wheelchair bound, the more likely he is to develop scoliosis. In other neuromuscular diseases, scoliosis may develop during the ambulatory phase of illness (e.g., fascioscapulohumeral dystrophy). Scoliosis results in added respiratory impairment, back discomfort, poor sitting posture, and cosmetic impairment and makes it harder to use the hands functionally. The candidate for a spinal stabilization procedure is the child with a progressive curve over 35 to 40 degrees and adequate pulmonary function. Molded thoracic shells or molded seating systems may be used to help limit the progression of scoliosis less invasively (and less successfully).

Scapular fixation to the ribcage is a surgical procedure that can allow arm elevation in the fascioscapulohumeral dystrophy patient who has lost that ability.

Secondary orthopedic problems are common in DMD. Fractures occur due to a combination of disuse osteopenia, low muscle mass, and weak protective responses. Early mobilization is an important part of fracture management. Occasional arthritic changes at chronically deformed joints may be treated with seating adjustments, nonsteroidal anti-inflammatory agents, and contracture release procedures.

MEDICATIONS

Treatment with prednisone 0.75 mg/kg/d may prolong independent ambulation up to 2 years in DMD. The rate of muscle weakening is decreased. The benefits of such therapy are balanced against predictable steroid side effects. Prednisone therapy should be considered for selected early school age boys who demonstrate an ability for weight control.

WHEELCHAIRS

Wheelchairs improve mobility and independence. Families often dread the time when the wheelchair will be necessary, and occasional resistance is encountered. This is highlighted in the teenager whose high concern with body image outweighs the realistic benefit of increased mobility. Power chairs must be used when older children do not have adequate arm strength for pushing on carpets, for moderate distances, or up mild inclines. Tray tables, mobile arm supports, and molded seating systems can be helpful power chair adaptations.

HOME ADAPTATION

Single-level homes or elevator apartments are preferable. When stairs are unavoidable, it is often necessary to install a ramp or lift for wheelchair access. Doctors may recommend in-home devices, such as hydraulic lifts for transferring heavy immobile children, commode chairs, electric beds, devices for reaching, and lever-style door knobs that are easier to manipulate. A home visit by an experienced occupational therapist can be helpful in making these recommendations.

RESPIRATORY CARE

Severe proximal muscular weakness is commonly accompanied by decreased lung capacity due primarily to chest muscle weakness and to scoliosis to a lesser extent. Daytime tiredness, night sweats, nightmares, and nocturnal shortness of breath indicate hypoventilation. Pulmonary function tests and polysomnograms may be helpful in diagnosis. Therapy may include oxygen, rocking beds, nocturnal continuous positive airway pressure (CPAP) by mask (especially Bipap) or tracheostomy and a ventilator.

Pneumonia prevention is important beginning early in the course of weakness. To this end, we recommend polyvalent pneumococcal vaccination, yearly influenza vaccinations, home chest physiotherapy, and incentive spirometry.

CARDIAC CARE

All boys with DMD have cardiac muscle involvement. A minority have symptomatic cardiomyopathy, rarely before age 9 years. The low level of physical activity in the teenage dystrophic child is cardioprotective. Cardiac therapy with digoxin, diuretics, afterload reduction, and dietary measures can be helpful but seldom for more than 1 to 2 years. A teenager with a resting pulse rate over 100 needs more detailed cardiac assessment with ECG, chest x-ray, and echocardiogram and possible referral to a cardiologist.

DIET

Prevention of obesity is critical. The muscles of ambulation cannot carry an overweight person as easily as a light one, and parents may be injured trying to lift or transfer a heavy, nonambulatory child. Wheelchair-bound children often drink low volumes because of difficulty getting to the toilet. Nonconstipating, high-fiber foods are helpful because the chairbound lifestyle promotes constipation.

GENETICS

Modern genetic testing for Duchenne dystrophy using multiplex polymerase chain reaction (PCR) and Southern blot analysis can give definitive carrier and prenatal information for most affected families. With the use of blood lymphocytes or other tissues, such testing is based on identification of a deletion or duplication in the dystrophin gene on the X chromosome. When a specific gene abnormality cannot be detected, linkage analysis techniques can be used. In some cases, carriers may be identified by dystrophin analysis of a muscle biopsy specimen. Many other muscle diseases are inherited. Specific gene defects have been identified in DMD, myotonic dystrophy, and mitochondrial myopathies, and the list is lengthening. Occasionally, none of the modern techniques are informative, and genetic counseling is based on blood CPK, clinical features, and mendelian probabilities.

EDUCATION

Special educational services often are needed to help the child with muscular weakness get from class to class and to perform fine motor manipulations and to give support for learning disabilities, which are common in DMD. Although the large majority of these boys have normal intellect, the average scores on intellectual testing are reduced from the norm even accounting for motor disability. The school should provide psychoeducational testing, occupational and physical therapy evaluations, and other assessments on a periodic basis in order to offer services appropriate for the child's weakness and level of cognitive function.

DEFINITIVE THERAPY

No definitive therapy is available for treatment of any muscular dystrophy. Techniques of gene transfer (e.g., by adenoviral vectors or myoblast transfer) are rapidly developing in muscular dystrophy. Some success has been shown in animal systems in which dystrophin becomes expressed and muscle degeneration is prevented by transfer of a healthy dystrophin gene into the organism. Gene transfer therapy within the next decade seems within reach.

MYASTHENIA GRAVIS

DAVID M. DAWSON, M.D.
DAVID LACOMIS, M.D.

Myasthenia gravis (MG) begins before a child is 17 years of age in about 11% of all cases. The illness may be *acquired* (autoimmune) or *genetic* in origin.

ACQUIRED MYASTHENIA GRAVIS

Acquired MG includes *transient neonatal* MG and *juvenile* MG. Antibodies to acetylcholine receptors (AChR) in muscle are believed to be present in both types. However, they are not always measurable. Antibodies to AChR cause a postsynaptic impairment in neuromuscular transmission, resulting in fatigue and weakness.

Transient Neonatal Myasthenia Gravis

In transient neonatal MG, the antibodies originate in the affected mother and cross the placenta. Symptoms last days to weeks and occur in only 10% to 15% of the infants of myasthenic mothers. The severity of the illness in the mother may not be correlated with the child's symptoms. Therefore, mothers with only mild or moderate MG may have a severely affected child.

Treatment

Supportive Care. In transient neonatal and all other types of MG, supportive care is crucial. Airway protection and oxygenation must be maintained, and nutritional status must be optimized. Intubation, mechanical ventilation, and enteral feeding may be required. Good general nursing care, aimed especially toward preventing infection, is equally important.

Anticholinesterase Drugs (ACEDs). These agents are the mainstay of therapy, and they may be required for days to weeks. ACEDs should be started if bulbar or respiratory symptoms occur, as happens in about 80% of cases. Neostigmine was introduced first and has been used successfully for diagnosis and treatment of MG in neonates. However, most clinicians now prefer pyridostigmine (Mestinon) for all forms of MG, mainly because it has fewer muscarinic side effects. Intubated neonates can be given pyridostigmine either intramuscularly or slowly intravenously (Table 1). When symptoms are severe but oral feeding is possible, intramuscular pyridostigmine can be given 30 minutes prior to feedings. If oral medication can be tolerated, the syrup form of pyridostigmine is most convenient. It is best to start with lower doses and to increase the dose or frequency of dosing gradually while monitoring for muscarinic and nicotinic types of cholinergic toxicity. Muscarinic toxicity manifests itself by diarrhea, salivation, vomiting, lacrimation, and bradycardia. Atropine generally reverses these effects. Nicotinic side effects may occur later. They include weakness, fasciculations, and cramps.

Because of the transient nature of the disorder and the exogenous source of antibodies, steroids and immunosuppressive agents are not indicated. However, exchange transfusions have been shown to be effective in several cases.

Juvenile Myasthenia Gravis

Juvenile MG generally begins after 1 year of age, with a mean age of onset of 8 years. The clinical characteristics are similar to those of the adult form.

Treatment

Anticholinesterase Drugs. ACEDs, usually oral pyridostigmine, are the first line of treatment (Table 1). They often result in good, although not total, control of symptoms. Generally, this is the only form of treatment for purely ocular weakness. The dose is titrated upward to control symptoms without causing significant toxicity. Few patients require more than 500 mg/d, and many manage well on 180 mg/d. If there is bulbar weakness, a dose should be given just before meals. Dose effects generally last 3 to 4 hours. The timed-release preparation is often useful when given at bedtime. If patients cannot take oral medications (e.g., perioperatively) or if only swallowing function is impaired, parenteral pyridostigmine can be administered (slowly if given intravenously).

Edrophonium (Tensilon) is short-acting and is used primarily for the diagnosis of MG (Table 1). One fifth of the total dose is administered intravenously while heart rate and blood pressure are monitored. If there is no significant bradycardia or increase in respiratory secretions, the rest of the dose is given either incrementally (in young children) or in one or two doses (in older children). Clinical signs and symptoms such as vital capacity and muscle strength and fatigability should be checked before and after edrophonium is given. The increase in strength occurs within 2 to 5 minutes and lasts about 30 minutes.

Steroid Therapy. If symptoms are disabling, despite optimal pyridostigmine dosing, prednisone is usually begun. Several empiric regimens are in common use. If the illness is mild, a slow increase in dose starting at 15 mg every other day and increasing over several weeks is employed. Efficacy usually is evident near a dose of 1 mg/kg every other day. With more severe weakness, the patient should be hospitalized and begun on 1 to 2 mg/kg as a single morning dose. An alternate-day regimen can be instituted in 3 to 4 weeks. Potassium supplements, antacids or H_2-blocking agents, and vitamin D plus calcium supplements often are required with long-term steroid use. Maintenance steroids are needed in about half the patients, often at a dose of 0.5 mg/kg every other day.

Thymectomy. The indications for thymectomy are somewhat controversial. Clearly, the procedure is indicated for all patients with a thymoma, but this is a very rare problem in childhood. Older studies recommended thymectomy only for severe MG that did not respond to optimal medical management. The current trend is toward earlier thymectomy,[1] either after treatment with ACEDs alone or after stabilization with other treatment modalities. Prospective, randomized trials have not been done, but retrospective data indicate that 60% to 70% of adult myasthenics improve after thymectomy.

Thymectomy is best performed in centers that have demonstrated low morbidity from the procedure. In this setting, the morbidity from a successful, potentially curative thymectomy is lower than the morbidity from long-term steroid use. Optimally, all thymus and mediastinal fat are removed. Either a transsternal or a transcervical approach may be used. To control symptoms throughout the perioperative period, *plasmapheresis* is usually performed before surgery.

TABLE 1. Anticholinesterase Drugs Used for Diagnosis and Treatment of Myasthenia Gravis

DRUG	ROUTE	AVAILABILITY	DOSE IN INFANTS	DOSE IN CHILDREN	COMMENT
Pyridostigmine (Mestinon)	IV, IM	5 mg/ml in 2-ml ampules	0.05–0.15 mg/kg up to q3–4h	1–1.5 mg per dose q3–4h	IV/IM dose is equivalent to 1/30 of PO dose
Pyridostigmine (Mestinon)	PO	12 mg/ml syrup; 60-mg tablet 180 mg sustained-release tablet	4–10 mg up to q3–4h	30–60 mg q3–8h	Each dose is typically effective for 3–4h Sustained-release tablets may be most useful at bedtime in adolescent patients
Neostigmine bromide (Prostigmin)	PO	15-mg tablet	1–2 mg up to q2–4h	7.5–15 mg up to q2–4h	IV/IM dose is 1/30 of PO dose
Edrophonium (Tensilon)	IV	10 mg/ml in 1-mg ampules	0.15–0.2 mg/kg total	0.2 mg/kg total; maximum: 10 mg	For diagnosis only. Give 1/5 total dose as test dose; if tolerated, give remainder incrementally; monitor BP and heart rate; atropine (0.01 mg/kg up to 0.4 mg) can block or reverse muscarinic effects

Myasthenic Crisis. This refers to severe weakness with bulbar and respiratory compromise occurring during the course of the disease. Myasthenic crisis is often difficult to separate from *cholinergic crisis* resulting from ACED toxicity. The presence of muscarinic side effects usually indicates toxicity, and an edrophonium test (Table 1) can be helpful. The test dose (0.04 mg/kg) is given while monitoring muscarinic effects, strength in multiple muscle groups, and respiratory function. If there is improvement in all measures, the patient may be in myasthenic crisis and should benefit from higher doses of ACEDs. If there is worsening in any measure, overdose nicotinic effects may be present at some receptors (cholinergic crisis). However, in crisis situations, there is often a combination of myasthenic and cholinergic-induced weakness. Thus, the best solution is to discontinue ACEDs, institute supportive care, and begin plasmapheresis. Three to five exchanges are performed during the course of a week. Improvement occurs within a few days in most patients. Once the patient improves, other forms of medical treatment (including ACEDs and steroids) can be restarted, and thymectomy can be considered.

Immunosuppressive agents, such as azathioprine, have not been well studied in children and are not recommended, although they are effective in long-term care of adults. Improvements in MG have been reported in uncontrolled trials with high-dose intravenous IgG (0.4 g/kg × 5 doses). This form of treatment is as expensive as plasma exchange but requires less specialized equipment. Further study of this program is warranted.

Problems Associated with Treatment. *Pitfalls in the treatment of all forms of MG include administration of drugs that can exacerbate weakness. These include aminoglycosides, procainamide, quinidine, curare, succinylcholine, and possibly calcium channel blockers and beta-blockers.* Sedatives and narcotics may be dangerous if respiratory or bulbar symptoms are present. Infections should be managed aggressively. Other associated autoimmune disorders, such as hyperthyroidism and diabetes mellitus, should be sought and treated appropriately.

GENETIC MYASTHENIA GRAVIS

Genetic forms of MG are very rare and generally present at birth or during infancy as the clinical entity of *congenital myasthenic syndrome.* An affected relative may be identified. Antibodies to AChR are absent, and the diagnosis is made by neurophysiologic or sophisticated ultrastructural techniques.[2] Numerous defects involving presynaptic and postsynaptic transmission of AChR have been observed. Some presynaptic defects involve abnormal AChR resynthesis or transport or abnormal uptake of choline by the nerve terminal. These disorders are usually responsive to modest doses of ACEDs. Congenital end-plate acetylcholinesterase deficiency, however, is a postsynaptic defect that is refractory to ACEDs. Similarly, there is no known effective treatment for another postsynaptic disorder, the so-called slow channel syndrome. Corticosteroids or other immunomodulators are not helpful in treating genetic forms of MG.

REFERENCES

1. Adams C, Theodorescu D, Murphy EG, Shandling B: Thymectomy in juvenile myasthenia gravis. J Child Neurol 5:215–218, 1990.
2. Engel AG: Congenital myasthenic syndromes. J Child Neurol 3:233–246, 1988.

PERIODIC PARALYSIS

Michael A. Nigro, D.O.

Management of the periodic paralyses is determined by an accurate diagnosis of an elusive condition. This group of autosomal dominant disorders is better understood than in the past but is still underrecognized. An abnormal level of or unusual sensitivity to potassium in the presence of episodic muscle weakness is the basis for diagnosing periodic paralysis. The condition is suspected when the child exhibits intermittent muscle weakness lasting minutes to hours, often ascending or asymmetric, occurring after a rest following exercise. Restoration of strength is usually complete, although in older patients, permanent weakness and atrophy may develop. Sustained muscle contraction after voluntary effort (myotonia) may also occur with episodic weakness. Serum potassium values during an event should substantiate hyperkalemic or hypokalemic paralysis, although in rare instances serum potassium values may be normal.

Both absolute values and marked sensitivity to relatively abrupt potassium fluctuations are the basis for provocative diagnostic tests. These tests must be done with caution in view of potential cardiac arrhythmias. In unusual cases, periodic paralysis is accompanied by chronic ventricular arrhythmia and warrants cardiac evaluation and comanagement when indicated. Hyperthyroid periodic paralysis must be identified, since treatment of thyroid dysmetabolism is usually sufficient to reduce or abolish the symptoms. In the past several years, potassium-sensitive periodic paralysis has been linked to variable alleic deletions on the long arm of chromosome 17. This locus on 17q is the site of the skeletal muscle sodium channel. Direct or indirect effects of potassium on the sodium channel are the presumed pathogenic basis for hyperkalemic and normokalemic paralysis and for paramyotonia congenita. The gene locus for the hypokalemic form is undefined. Molecular genetic testing ultimately should be the specific diagnostic study. Treatment of the periodic paralyses is aimed at preventing attacks, restoring strength, and preventing complications during severe attacks.

Hyperkalemic periodic paralysis is prevented in most patients by the use of acetazolamide (Diamox), a carbonic anhydrase inhibitor. The mechanism of action of acetazolamide is not completely understood but is probably due either to its plasma potassium-lowering effect (through kaluresis) or to its stabilizing effect on intracellular potassium. Dosage is titrated according to symptoms and ranges between 10 and 15 mg/kg/d divided into two or three doses. Side effects (including paresthesias, polyuria, sedation, gastrointestinal irritation, and uric acid calculi) may prevent long-term use. In this event, chlorothiazide (Diuril) can be substituted at 10 to 20 mg/kg/d divided into two doses. With chronic use, thiazides can also have a number of undesirable side effects (e.g., blood dyscrasias, pancreatitis, hyperbilirubinemia), and children receiving thiazides should be monitored as clinically warranted. Thiazide-induced hypokalemia is a side effect capable of inducing muscle weakness, and as a result, the thiazide dose should be maintained at the lowest amount sufficient to keep the patient normokalemic and free of weakness. Dichlorphenamide, another carbonic anhydrase inhibitor, has been used in adults.

A diet high in carbohydrates and relatively low in potassium may help avert attacks. If the diet contains 60 mEq or less of potassium, caloric, vitamin, and mineral supplementation usually is necessary. Fasting and sudden exposure to cold should be avoided. Children with coexisting ventricular arrhythmias should be evaluated and comanaged by a cardiologist. Exercise is limited more by cardiac disease than by intermittent weakness. In other children, gradual incremental exercise is recommended, and warmup exercises before exertion may help prevent bouts of weakness and myotonia.

In an acute attack of hyperkalemic periodic paralysis, oral ingestion of a potassium-free glucose-rich solution (2 g/kg) may be adequate to alleviate symptoms. One to two puffs of albuterol (Proventil) inhalant, a beta-adrenergic, can abort an impending attack. The dose may be repeated after 4 to 6 hours. However, caution should be used in view of the potential for this drug to induce a cardiac arrhythmia. If weakness is too severe to permit adequate intake, intravenous solutions containing glucose (0.5 g/kg with 0.3 U insulin per gram of glucose) should be given over 2 hours. Sodium bicarbonate 1 to 3 mEq/kg is administered once over 5 minutes. Intravenous calcium gluconate (10%) 0.2 to 0.5 ml/kg given over 15 minutes can also abort an attack. Cardiorespiratory monitoring is mandatory until the patient is improved and stable.

Paramyotonia congenita is associated with a mutation on the long arm of chromosome 17. Cold-induced stiffness (myotonia) and weakness are attributed to greater temperature sensitivity of the mutant sodium channels. Hyperkalemia may accompany periodic attacks of paramyotonia. Acetazolamide may increase the frequency and severity of attacks and should be avoided. Mexiletene, an antiarrhythmic structurally similar to lidocaine (but orally active), can reduce the myotonia and cold-induced weakness. Mexiletene probably acts by inhibiting inward sodium current. Side effects of mexiletene (gastrointestinal and CNS) are dose related. Chlorothiazide is needed to prevent weakness associated with hyperkalemia. Another orally effective agent, tocainide (an amine analog of lidocaine), is also reported to be effective in paramyotonia.

Hypokalemic periodic paralysis is effectively prevented in most patients by daily administration of acetazolamide 4 to 20 mg/kg/d in two or three divided doses. In this condition, the benefit of acetazolamide may be related to induction of a mild metabolic acidosis. Patient sensitivity to the drug is quite variable and can be defined only by a therapeutic trial. In rare instances, the use of acetazolamide can exacerbate the weakness. In this case, spironolactone (Aldactone), an aldosterone antagonist that spares potassium and induces a mild metabolic acidosis, can be used (1 to 3 mg/kg/d in two to four divided doses). Diet can be important, and the patient should avoid high carbohydrate intake (60 to 80 g/d) and restrict sodium intake to 10 mEq/d. Triamterene has been used when acetazolamide and spironolactone are ineffective or not tolerated. Supplemental potassium has not been proven effective as a preventive measure.

In the event of acute moderate to severe paralysis, the patient should be carefully monitored in the emergency room or intensive care unit. If the patient can adequately and safely swallow, a chilled unsweetened oral solution of potassium chloride 0.2 to 0.35 mEq/kg can be given initially and repeated as often as needed to produce normokalemia and improve strength. Because of poor absorption, tablets of potassium should not be used. If unable to swallow, the patient should be given intravenous potassium chloride 0.25 mEq/kg in a glucose-free solution (0.3N saline or 5% mannitol) over 30 to 60 minutes. This can be repeated after 1 hour if necessary.

Normokalemic periodic paralysis is treated in the same manner as hyperkalemic paralysis.

Acquired secondary systemic hyperkalemia and hypokalemia must be identified and treated appropriately.

Not all patients require chronic prophylactic medication, but when it is used, the physician should be aware of potential side effects and anticipated benefits. Doses required for chronic and acute use need to be defined by patient tolerance and response. Carefully monitored aggressive therapy may help prevent chronic myopathy associated with repeated paralytic attacks.

INFLAMMATORY MYOPATHIES

OWEN B. EVANS, M.D.

Juvenile dermatomyositis is the most common inflammatory myopathy and the most frequent cause of acquired muscle disease of childhood. Eighty percent of children with juvenile dermatomyositis respond to therapy. The other major inflammatory myopathies, adult dermatomyositis, polymyositis, and inclusion body myositis, are rare in childhood and have a less predictable response to treatment. There is no effective therapy for inclusion body myositis.

It is generally agreed that steroids are effective in ameliorating the signs and symptoms of dermatomyositis. The starting dose is 2 mg/kg/d of prednisone in two divided doses. Within days, the fever usually remits, and within a week, the serum enzyme concentrations are reduced. After about 2 weeks, there is improved strength. At this point, the steroid dose can be changed to alternate-day therapy, with tapering of the alternate daily dose over 1 week to reduce the probability of adrenal suppression. Some recommend continued daily therapy to achieve maximal effectiveness. The total daily dose can be reduced by 10 mg/wk until 50 mg/d and then reduced by 5 mg/wk until a maintenance dose of about 5 to 10 mg/d is achieved.

During the initial period, the child should be followed frequently to evaluate strength and serum enzyme concentrations and to monitor for side effects of therapy. If there is clinical deterioration, the dose of prednisone should be increased to 2 mg/kg/d and tapered more slowly. The typical treatment period is 2 years for those who respond to steroids. If the drug is discontinued too soon, there may be relapses, and the long-term prognosis may be worse.

Complications of steroid therapy are potentially serious but are usually well tolerated. Cushingoid appearance and temporary growth delay are common. Hypertension, hyperglycemia, cataracts, and increased susceptibility to infections are uncommon in my experience. However, varicella exposure should be avoided. Osteoporosis is encountered occasionally, and vertebral compression fractures can occur. One pitfall of high-dose steroid therapy is a superimposed steroid myopathy that may obscure the clinical signs of the underlying disease.

If the child has not responded within 3 months to prednisone doses of greater than 1.0 mg/kg/d, requires more than 0.25 mg/kg/d of prednisone to control the disease, or develops intolerable side effects, alternative therapy must be considered. The use of cytotoxic drugs has been found to be beneficial in some patients as an adjunct to steroids. Methotrexate 1 to 2 mg/kg/wk either PO or IM (maximum of 25 mg/wk) can be given, with regular monitoring of liver function studies and complete blood counts. The prednisone can be tapered by 5 mg/wk until a maintenance dose is achieved with minimal side effects. Azathioprine or cyclophosphamide 2.5 mg/kg/d can be used in a similar fashion. Patients who clearly are deteriorating despite maximal doses of steroids and cytotoxic therapy pose special problems. Our experience with immunoglobulins has been good in refractory cases. The recommended dose is 1 g IV over 12 hours every 4 weeks. Cyclosporine is reported to be useful in selected cases at 2.5 to 7.5 mg/kg/d in two divided doses. Serum cyclosporine levels and renal function studies must be carefully monitored in these children. Plasmapheresis and total body radiation have been reported to be useful, but clinical trials of the former and complications of the latter argue against these therapies.

The typical rash does not improve as rapidly as the muscle weakness. It does not normally require specific therapy, and steroid application is of no benefit. Patients should use sunscreens generously, since the rash is photosensitive. Hydroxychloroquine 2 to 5 mg/kg/d is reported to be useful as adjunctive therapy, especially in children with severe dermatologic manifestations. Calcinosis is a severe complication and can practically encrust the patient when extensive. Systemic steroids may reduce the subcutaneous deposits but have not been effective in my experience, nor has chelation therapy. A serious complication is secondary bacterial infections of the ulcerative vasculitic lesions or areas where calcium deposits have protruded through the skin. Vigorous antibiotic therapy and wound care may be necessary to prevent local or systemic spread of the infection.

Physical therapy must be instituted early in the course of the illness to help prevent contractures and to maintain mobility. Patients who have a chronic, unremitting course are in need of rehabilitation services to provide occupational therapy and orthopedic appliances to maintain mobility and independent function.

15

Skin

ALLERGIC CONTACT DERMATITIS

SUSAN BAYLISS MALLORY, M.D

Allergic contact dermatitis (ACD) is a form of eczematous dermatitis in which a chemical agent, such as a plant, medicine, cosmetic, fabric, or metal, is the local inciting factor. The configuration of skin lesions and the site involved often give clues to the causal agent. Patch testing confirms the diagnosis but is usually not necessary in the more common causes of ACD, such as poison ivy.

TREATMENT

Treatment can be divided into two major categories: prevention and management.

Prevention

Avoidance of the provocative allergen is necessary in curing contact dermatitis. Cross-reacting allergens should also be avoided. A detailed history may be needed to find the offending agent. Patients should understand that they may become allergic to a substance or chemical at any time after initial exposure and that it actually takes time to become sensitized to a certain agent.

Oral hyposensitization to poison ivy is not practical or recommended. Side effects, such as vesicular or urticarial eruptions and pruritus ani, occur in the majority of patients, and complete desensitization is rarely accomplished.

Barrier creams, such as polyamine salts of a linoleic acid dimer, can be used as topical prophylaxis if applied before exposure. This type of agent is available as Stokogard-Gard Outdoor Cream* and should be washed off within 8 hours.

Management

The pruritus and oozing of acute ACD may be treated with compresses for debridement and a cooling effect. Simple baths or wet wraps with tap water are satisfactory. Burow's Solution (aluminum sulfate and calcium acetate, Domeboro) can be added for a drying effect. Towels or bandages should be moist but not dripping. They should be left in place for 15 minutes to 1 hour but not allowed to dry. This procedure can be repeated as many times as needed. Plain calamine lotion also has a drying effect.

When the acute weeping eruption subsides or if the dermatitis is mild, potent topical steroid creams, lotions, or ointments can help reduce inflammation. Weaker topical steroids, in classes 6 and 7, such as hydrocortisone 1% have little effect on significant ACD. Potent topical steroids are more effective (e.g., Diprolene, Lidex, Temovate) and are recommended except on the face, groin, and axillae. In these areas, hydrocortisone 1% is adequate. Adult-sized patients should be cautioned if using more than 45 g/wk of a potent steroid because of potential suppression of the pituitary-adrenal axis.

Systemic administration of corticosteroids may be indicated for severe or very extensive dermatitis (oral prednisone beginning at 1 mg/kg/d and tapering slowly over 2 to 3 weeks). Intramuscular triamcinolone has a prolonged effect, is erratically absorbed, and therefore is not recommended. Oral dose packs of steroids (e.g., Medrol Dosepak) usually last 6 days. However, in ACD, lesions can continue to form up to 2 to 3 weeks after a single exposure. Therefore, oral steroids should be given for a 2- to 3-week period.

Administration of an oral antihistamine, such as hydroxyzine or diphenhydramine, may decrease pruritus mainly because of its soporific effect and may, therefore, be most useful at bedtime. Topical anti-itching preparations that contain benzocaine or diphenhydramine (Benadryl) are of only temporary benefit and may be potential sensitizers. Therefore, these preparations are not recommended.

The most common contact allergens in childhood differ from country to country. In the United States, poison ivy, neomycin, nickel, rubber chemicals, formaldehyde, balsam of Peru, and benzocaine are the most common contact allergens. Neomycin is found in otic preparations, topical antibiotic creams, and some prescription topical medications. Nickel can be found in earrings, jewelry, and snaps on clothing, including infant clothing. With pierced ears becoming more popular in boys, nickel dermatitis of the ear lobes is likely to increase. Rubber chemicals are found most often in shoes. Clothing, particularly that made with permanent press materials, can contain formaldehyde and may need to be washed several times before they are worn to decrease the amount of formaldehyde in the clothing. Cosmetics and hand lotions can contain formaldehyde releasers, balsam of Peru, or other fragrances. Benzocaine is found in topical anti-itching creams, particularly those for sunburn or poison ivy.

Educating a sensitive patient to avoid appropriate substances can greatly reduce the number of episodes of ACD. Recognizing local plants that cause contact dermatitis is also beneficial. Occasionally, an extensive history may be needed to find the source of ACD. For instance, a dog may run in the woods and pick up and carry poison ivy oleoresin (plant sap) to its owner by means of its fur. Only by diligently searching for these sources of ACD will a physician find them.

If a child has recurrent or persistent ACD, patch testing for specific allergen identification may be useful. Patch testing involves placing the suspected substance in a standard percentage on the skin under a patch for 48 hours, removing the patch, and reading it at 72 hours, looking for the typical eczematous dermatitis. Because false positive and false negative results are common, patch tests should be performed by a physician skilled at reading them, such as a dermatologist. When a contact allergen is confirmed by this method, avoidance of the substance is necessary for the dermatitis to clear. Lists of products that contain these chemicals are usually available in a dermatologist's office where patch testing is routine.

---

*Manufactured by Stockhausen and available through Dermatologic Lab and Supply, Inc., 201 Ridge, Council Bluffs, IA 51503, or 1-800-831-6273.

ATOPIC DERMATITIS

CYNTHIA GUZZO, M.D.

Atopic dermatitis is a chronic inflammatory skin disorder most prevalent during childhood. Ninety-five percent of pediatric cases are apparent by age 5. It is a common disorder, and current estimates of the cumulative incidence range from 10% to 15% in children up to age 14. Atopic dermatitis frequently is associated with elevated IgE levels and a personal or family history of atopy, including atopic dermatitis, allergic rhinitis, and asthma. The clinical lesion of eczema is nonspecific, and diagnosis is based on a combination of personal and family history and multiple morphologic findings.

TRIGGER FACTORS

Patients with atopic dermatitis generally experience exacerbations followed by periods of less severe disease. Trigger factors associated with disease flares have long been recognized. Wool (lanolin) and harsh detergents are irritating to the skin. The role of house dust mites has been investigated in recent years. Patients have a high frequency of IgE antibodies and T cells, which detect house dust mite antigens. There is a positive correlation between the magnitude of exposure to dust mites and the frequency of disease. Microbes are important also. In atopic individuals, the carriage rate of *Staphylococcus aureus* is high, and infection with *S. aureus* is associated with flaring of the disease. Patients are more prone to viral infections, and localized herpes simplex can produce generalized exacerbation of dermatitis. Food allergens in a selected group of patients have produced a cutaneous flare. Psychic stress has been implicated, and recently recognized imbalances in neuropeptides may mediate this state.

CLINICAL FEATURES

The skin symptoms of atopic dermatitis present as an erythematous, papulovesicular eruption that progresses to a scaly, lichenified dermatitis secondary to persistent scratching. The distribution varies with age, beginning with facial and extensor involvement in infants and progressing to flexural disease with time. The diagnosis can be made in adults and children if the patient has all of the following major features.

1. Typical morphology and distribution
   a. Flexural lichenification or linearity in adults
   b. Facial and extensor involvement in infants
2. Chronic or chronically relapsing course
3. Personal or family history of atopy
4. Pruritus

If only three major features are present, the patients must have three or more minor features, including xerosis, pityriasis alba, palmar hyperlinearity, keratosis pilaris, high serum IgE, recurrent conjunctivitis, Dennie-Morgan infraorbital fold, and other atopic stigmata.

In infancy, the criteria for diagnosis are modified. Two major features or one major and one minor feature are required. The major features are as follows.

1. Family history of atopic disease
2. Evidence of pruritic dermatitis
3. Typical facial or extensor eczematous or lichenified dermatitis

Minor features for infants include xerosis-icthyosis-hyperlinear palms, perifollicular accentuation, chronic scalp scaling, and periauricular fissures.

THERAPY

Nonspecific Measures

It is important to reduce pruritus and scratching, prevent irritation, and hydrate the skin. Fingernails should be trimmed short. Patients should bathe in tepid water, avoid soap, and pat dry with soft absorbent towels. Bathing should be followed by application of a lubricating ointment or cream. Lotions should be avoided, since they contain alcohol and water. Lubrication should be repeated frequently. Sweating generally leads to pruritus and should be avoided. Lightweight, nonocclusive clothing, such as that made of cotton, is preferred.

Corticosteroids

Topical corticosteroids are the cornerstone of therapy. In general, for acute disease, midstrength corticosteroids, such as 0.1% triamcinolone ointment, are optimal. Occasionally, higher potency steroids are necessary. However, only low-potency steroids (1% hydrocortisone cream or ointment) should be used on the face and intertriginous regions. As the disease improves, reduction of the steroid strength and frequency is recommended to prevent side effects, such as cutaneous atrophy, telangiectasias, striae, and systemic absorption. This is particularly true in infants and young children.

Systemic steroids should be avoided if possible. Many patients experience a rebound flare after a short course. If steroid use seems necessary, it should be combined with intensive topical therapy as the steroids are tapered.

Antipruritics

Antihistamines are widely used in atopic dermatitis, but their level of efficacy is not clear. Sedating antihistamines and tricyclic antidepressants are generally thought to be more effective than nonsedating antihistamines, but recent studies have produced conflicting results. Hydroxyzine 2 mg/kg/d divided every 6 hours and diphenhydramine 5 mg/kg/d divided every 6 hours are used frequently in infants and children. Sedation is the limiting side effect, and often only a nighttime dose is possible.

Control of Skin Infection

Treatment of bacterial skin infection is an important mainstay for control of a flare. Ninety-five percent of atopic patients are colonized with *S. aureus*. Initiation of treatment with erythromycin 30 to 50 mg/kg/d divided every 6 hours (maximum 1 g), followed by dicloxacillin 12.5 mg/kg/d divided every 6 hours (maximum 1 g) if there is a poor response, is appropriate in the absence of culture and sensitivity information.

Herpes simplex infection can present as shallow ulcerations. A Tzanck smear or culture will confirm the diagnosis. Patients should be treated with oral acyclovir 1200 mg/m²/d divided every 4 hours for limited skin lesions. Patients are at risk of ocular involvement and widespread dissemination, called *eczema herpeticum*. Eczema herpeticum is a serious complication requiring hospitalization and IV acyclovir 750 mg/m²/d divided every 8 hours.

Diet

Double-blind placebo-controlled food challenges in atopic dermatitis patients have demonstrated that food allergens can trigger pruritic, erythematous rashes in some patients. Eggs, milk, peanuts, soy, and wheat are the most commonly offending foods. In patients in whom specific food allergies have been documented by careful testing, an appropriate avoidance diet can result in substantial improvement. More generalized food avoidance diets do not have a good response/risk ratio.

Other Measures

Both ultraviolet B (UVB) and psoralen with ultraviolet A (PUVA) phototherapies are effective for atopic dermatitis. Inflammatory components of the disease should be controlled before initiation of therapy. UVB is preferable in the pediatric population and should be limited to prevent actinic damage.

Hospitalization for severe disease unresponsive to outpatient management is appropriate. Removal from the environment, intensive topical therapy, antibiotics, and at times a coal tar and UVB combination are highly effective. Experimental agents include cyclosporine, interferon gamma, thymopentin, and Chinese herb therapy.

PROGNOSIS

It is often stated that most children "outgrow" atopic dermatitis. However, 50% of patients can have persistent disease as adults. Risk factors favoring this outcome include early disease in childhood, a family history of atopic dermatitis, associated asthma or allergic rhinitis, female sex, and onset before 1 year of age. Finally, breast feeding, with allergen avoidance diets in the mother and subsequently in the child, may reduce the incidence of atopic dermatitis in children at high risk.

REFERENCES

1. Cooper KD: Atopic dermatitis: Recent trends in pathogenesis and therapy. Prog Dermatol 27:1–15, 1993.
2. Sampson HA: Atopic dermatitis. Ann Allergy 69:469–79, 1992.

URTICARIA

ELLIOT F. ELLIS, M.D.

Urticaria, or hives, is a common skin disorder characterized by well-circumscribed, sometimes coalescent, localized, or generalized erythematous skin lesions (papules) of various sizes. Although lesions are generally pruritic, the degree of itching can vary from intense to little, if any. Resolution of the individual hives generally occurs within 48 hours, but new or multiple lesions may continue to appear. Individual lesions persisting longer than 48 hours suggest a diagnosis of urticarial vasculitis, a much more serious condition than classic common urticaria. If urticaria persists for longer than 6 weeks, it is considered to be chronic. In angioedema, the deeper layers of skin or submucosa or subcutaneous or other tissues are involved. The gastrointestinal and upper respiratory tracts are common target organs. The distinction between urticaria and angioedema is unclear, and the lesions appear to differ only in the depth of tissue involvement and lack of pruritus in angioedema. Urticaria and angioedema occur secondary to the release of a diverse array of vasoactive mediators that arise from activation of cells or enzymatic pathways. Although a hive is the typical dermal manifestation of IgE-mediated allergy, an allergic etiologic diagnosis is established in a minority of cases of acute urticaria and only rarely in cases of chronic urticaria.

TREATMENT

Nonspecific Treatment

Identification of the cause of the urticaria and its elimination is the best treatment. However, as noted, the etiology is not often established. There are certain factors that need to be considered that aggravate cases of urticaria causing cutaneous vasodilatation. These include alcohol, aspirin, becoming overheated, exertion, and, in some cases, emotional stress. By definition, acute urticaria is a self-limited disease that generally resolves in a few weeks. During the symptomatic period, suppression of the urticarial lesions is the goal of therapy. If the child is receiving drug therapy, usually an antibiotic, it should be discontinued, and an alternative should be sought. If a food is involved, the parents may have made the diagnosis before coming to see the physician and have eliminated the food from the diet.

Acute Urticaria

Since histamine is the best established mediator of urticaria, antihistamines given orally are the drugs of choice. Diphenhydramine (Benadryl), hydroxyzine (Atarax, Vistaril), and cyproheptadine (Periactin) are widely prescribed agents. Diphenhydramine may be given

in a dose of 5 mg/kg/d in two divided doses, hydroxyzine may be given as 2 mg/kg/d in two divided doses, and cyproheptadine may be given in a dose of 0.2 mg/kg/d in three or four divided doses, all for the first few days of therapy. Both hydroxyzine and diphenhydramine have long half-lives, and, therefore, treatment may be continued thereafter on a once a day dosing regimen. Cyproheptadine often can be decreased to a twice a day dosing interval. Children generally do not complain of adverse central nervous system (CNS) symptoms, such as sedation, and if they do, this problem generally resolves over the course of a week to 10 days while the drug is continued. However, if sedation persists or other evidence of CNS impairment becomes evident, a switch to one of the newer so-called nonsedating agents may be considered. Drugs currently marketed in the United States are terfenadine (Seldane), astemizole (Hismanal), and loratadine (Claritin). None of these agents is labeled for use in children under 12 years of age, although they are certainly being used in this age group. Largely on the basis of safety considerations, loratadine is the drug of choice among the nonsedating drugs.

It is generally recommended, particularly in the more severe outbreaks of acute urticaria, that antihistamine therapy be continued a week to 10 days after the lesions have resolved and then gradually withdrawn. It is hoped that this may prevent the development of chronic urticaria, although there are no firm data on this point. If the patient is particularly distressed by the acute urticaria and does not have sufficient relief from the antihistamine therapy, injection of epinephrine 1:1000, 0.01 ml/kg to a maximum of 0.3 ml per dose, usually affords rapid, although temporary, relief of acute urticaria. Epinephrine not only has a favorable effect on the skin vasculature but also may inhibit mediator (histamine) release from tissue mast cells. If epinephrine therapy needs to be continued, SusPhrine (epinephrine 1:200) may be given in a dose of 0.005 ml/kg SC, administered no more often than every 6 hours. In some cases of acute urticaria secondary to drug allergy, systemic corticosteroid therapy is required. The suggested dose of prednisone or prednisolone is 1 to 2 mg/kg/d generally in divided doses initially, then given once daily early in the morning usually in decreasing dose until the urticaria subsides and for a few days thereafter.

Chronic Urticaria

When urticaria persists longer than 6 weeks, it is considered to be chronic in nature. At the outset, it is important to appreciate that in less than 10% of cases is an etiologic diagnosis established in individuals suffering from this enigmatic disorder. However, chronic urticaria is much less common in children than in adults. There appears to be a consensus among many dermatologists and allergists that hydroxyzine is the drug of choice for initial treatment of chronic urticaria, although diphenhydramine and cyproheptadine are acceptable alternatives. As with acute urticaria, if CNS adverse effects occur, one of the nonsedating antihistamines may be tried. If antihistamine therapy is unsuccessful, doxepin (Sinequan), a tricyclic antidepressant with H_1- and H_2-blocking effect, is worth trying. It is important to note that the drug is not labeled for use in urticaria or for children under 12 years of age. The usual adult dose is 10 to 25 mg three times a day. Several reports in adults indicate that since the human skin vasculature possesses both H_2 and H_1 receptors, a combination of an H_1 and H_2 antihistamine is more effective than an H_1 antihistamine alone in controlling chronic urticaria. The adult dose of cimetidine (Tagamet) is 300 mg four times a day, and that of ranitidine (Zantac) is 150 mg twice a day. Neither ranitidine nor cimetidine is labeled for use in urticaria. Additionally, ranitidine is not labeled for any indication in children. Cimetidine is not recommended for use in children under 16 years of age, but on the basis of limited studies, a dose of 20 to 40 mg/kg/d has been prescribed.

As in acute urticaria, corticosteroid therapy is sometimes indicated in severe cases of chronic urticaria to provide temporary relief. It is often a problem to withdraw the steroids. Pharmacologic doses of 1 to 2 mg/kg/d are given initially, and if the patient responds, an alternate-day regimen, adjusted to as low a dose as possible, is used.

Dietary manipulation rarely is of benefit in chronic urticaria. Psychologic support of the patient with chronic urticaria is important in this distressing disorder. The prognosis is generally good.

Hereditary Angioedema

Hereditary angioedema (HAE) is an autosomal dominant disorder caused by a deficiency of the inhibitor of the first component of complement, C1 esterase inhibitor. HAE is a life-threatening disorder because of the frequency of occurrence of upper airway obstruction due to glottic edema. Hives do not occur. Treatment is not very satisfactory, and although subcutaneous epinephrine is often administered intermittently, its efficacy is open to question. Fresh frozen plasma and partly purified C1 esterase inhibitor have been used, but their role in acute therapy has not been established. Tracheostomy is indicated if laryngeal edema occurs. The prophylaxis of attacks of angioedema has been much more successful than treatment of acute episodes. Administration of impeded androgens, such as danazol or stanozolol, has been successful in preventing attacks of angioedema and in inducing synthesis of normal C1 esterase inhibitor and returning the serum level of C4 (useful as a screening test for the disorder) to normal. Unfortunately, the impeded androgens are not labeled for use in children.

Other Forms of Childhood Urticaria

Papular urticaria presents as pruritic erythematous papules with or without an erythematous urticarial flare. The clusters of lesions usually are found over the shoulders, upper arms, buttocks, and particularly on the anterior aspects of the legs. The disorder occurs predominantly between the ages of 18 months and 7 years. The lesions represent cell-mediated reactions to a variety of biting insects. Dog and cat fleas are most commonly involved. Treatment of papular urticaria involves avoidance of the insect. Oral antihistamines are worth trying. Topical application of low-potency corticosteroid creams also appears to be useful in providing symptomatic relief. Contact urticaria due to skin contact with urticariogenic agents, for example, stinging nettles, is seen occasionally. Treatment of this self-limited form of urticaria involves avoidance and antihistamines.

Other Conditions Associated with Urticaria

Urticaria also occurs in a number of other so-called physical allergies, which are discussed in Chapter 19.

DRUG REACTIONS AND THE SKIN

PAUL J. HONIG, M.D.

Drug reactions occur at a rate of 3 per 1000 courses of therapy in the general population. Hospitalized patients are more likely to experience a reaction to a drug than are outpatients because of their frequency of exposure. The rate of adverse events depends on the particular medication used (e.g., 50 adverse events per 1000 drug courses of trimethoprim-sulfamethoxazole compared with 0.2 reactions per 1000 courses of chloral hydrate). Children are less likely to experience undesirable side effects than adults as a result of their decreased exposure to drugs and a reluctance of physicians to use systemic therapy in the pediatric population.

Drug reactions occur on an immune or nonimmune basis. Many of the four types of immunologic mechanisms (immunoglobulin E-mediated, immune complex, cytotoxic, or cell-mediated) can be involved. Adverse reactions also occur on the basis of overdoses, specific toxicity, common side effects of a particular drug, or unusual drug interactions. Many times, the exact pathophysiology is not identified.

The appearance of drug reactions is nonspecific and may mimic almost any known dermatosis. Therefore, one cannot make a diagnosis of a drug reaction on the basis of the appearance of the rash alone. However, certain patterns should make one suspicious of the presence of an adverse reaction.

1. Urticaria constitutes the most common expression of drug sensitivity. Association of urticaria with arthritis or arthralgias indicates the presence of a serum sickness-like syndrome. A number of medications may be at fault (e.g., amoxicillin, cephalexin, trimethoprim-sulfamethoxazole), especially cefaclor in children less than 5 years old who have received the medication for the second or third time.
2. Maculopapular eruptions similar to a viral exanthem are the second most common skin change seen. This pattern poses a difficult problem because children are frequently infected by viruses.
3. Erythema multiforme often occurs secondary to drugs. However, recent observations suggest that the majority of cases of erythema multiforme minor may be due to herpes simplex virus or other infectious agents.
4. Vasculitis may occur.
5. Erythema nodosum may occur.
6. Photosensitive cutaneous eruptions may occur.
7. Toxic epidermal necrolysis may occur.
8. Fixed drug eruptions (i.e., recurrent, circumscribed, erythematous to brown plaques that recur at the same site with each exposure to the offending medication) may occur.

THERAPY

Essential to the management of any drug reaction are the identification and elimination of the offending medication. Historical information frequently overlooked includes the following.

1. Drugs ingested by the mother during pregnancy (newborn with skin changes)
2. Medications given to nursing mothers (the amount of drug excreted in mother's milk varies from drug to drug)
3. Topically applied preparations (enhanced absorption through children's skin due to greater surface area/body weight ratio, e.g., steroids or salicylic acid)
4. Medications for other family members ingested accidentally
5. Over-the-counter preparations not considered to be "medications" by patients

Treatment must be individualized. Minor reactions frequently disappear once the offending agent is discontinued. Persistent pruritus can be controlled with oral antihistamines. More severe, persistent reactions may respond to oral antihistamines (e.g., diphenhydramine, hydroxyzine) or oral steroids or both. If blistering occurs, attention to fluid and electrolyte balance and secondary infection is important. With mucous membrane involvement, an ophthalmologist must be consulted to rule out the presence of corneal changes. Hospitalization should be considered in toxic patients with severe skin involvement that may include extensive exfoliation.

Acyclovir may have a role in the treatment of erythema multiforme minor, especially if herpes simplex is the cause, although there have been no studies indicating efficacy of this medication for this purpose.

Stevens-Johnson syndrome and drug-induced toxic epidermal necrolysis (conditions at the most severe end of the drug reaction spectrum) demand special consideration. The literature suggests that steroid therapy of these conditions is of no value, will prolong hospital stays, and may be harmful. However, many clinicians think that steroid preparations are helpful. Steroid therapy (an equivalent of prednisone 1 to 2 mg/kg/d) should be reserved for the toxic patient whose condition is rapidly worsening. Steroids must be started within the first 2 to 3 days of the eruption to be effective. Thereafter, existing damage probably cannot be reversed. If the patient continues to progress after 5 days of steroid therapy, the medication should be discontinued. Patients receiving steroids must be monitored carefully for infection (complete blood cell count, periodic wound and blood cultures if fever occurs).

When skin denudation involves greater than 20% of the child's body surface area, steroid therapy should not be used at all. Open lesions respond to wet dressings of Burow's Solution or application of topical silver sulfadiazine. Broad-spectrum antibiotic coverage is started if patients have unusual temperature fluctuations or changes in the level of consciousness. Urethral involvement may produce urinary retention and secondary infections. Therefore, urinary output must be monitored. If denudation progresses to greater than 25% of body surface area, the patient should be transferred to a burn unit. Plasmapheresis has been used when all else has failed.

REFERENCES

1. Arndt KA, Jick H: Rates of cutaneous reactions to drugs: A report from the Boston Collaborative Drug Surveillance Program. JAMA 235:918–923, 1976.
2. Hebert AA, Sigman ES, Levy ML: Serum sickness-like reactions from Cefaclor in children. J Am Acad Dermatol 25:805–808, 1991.
3. Orton PW, Huff JC, Tonnesen JG, et al: Detection of a herpes simplex viral antigen in skin lesions of erythema multiforme. Ann Intern Med 101:48–50, 1984.
4. Weston WL, Brice SL, Jester JD, et al: Herpes simplex virus in childhood erythema multiforme. Pediatrics 89:32–34, 1992.

ERYTHEMA NODOSUM

PAUL J. HONIG, M.D.

Nodose lesions are described as raised, hot, erythematous, poorly marginated subcutaneous nodules that are tender. Erythema nodosum (EN) lesions are found most commonly on the shins and other extensor surfaces. They are usually bilateral and vary in size from 2 to 10 cm in diameter. Crops appear over a 3- to 6-week period, with individual lesions taking 2 to 3 weeks to clear. Their color fades from red to yellow-purple, looking very much like a bruise. The condition is uncommon in children less than 6 years old but has been reported to occur in the first year of life. There is a slight female:male predominance in children unlike the 10:1 ratio in adults.

The cause of EN is found in less than 50% of patients. Many of the associations are shown in Table 1. The workup of a patient with EN depends on which etiology is most likely, as determined by a history, physical examination, age of the patient, location in the United States, and country of immigration. Table 2 contains a list of routine screening tests that should be performed, as well as other tests as determined by history, age of the patient, state of residence, and so on. A chest film is helpful in states where fungal infections are common. Chest films are also indicated when considering tuberculosis or sarcoidosis. An extensive gastrointestinal workup is not warranted for every patient. However, if signs and symptoms referable to the gastrointestinal tract are present or the child is not growing well (a frequent presenting feature in children with inflammatory bowel disease), a gastrointestinal workup should be considered.

Therapy is usually not necessary for EN because it is a self-limited condition, resolving in 2 to 3 weeks. However, if a condition asso-

TABLE 1. Conditions Associated With Erythema Nodosum

Streptococcal infection	Behçet's disease
Drugs (e.g., sulfonamides, contraceptives)	Blastomycosis
Inflammatory bowel disease	Cat-scratch disease
Ulcerative colitis, 4% of patients	Leprosy
Crohn's disease, 6.8% of patients	Leukemia
Coccidioidomycosis	Lymphoma
Histoplasmosis (5% of patients)	Sarcoidosis
Tuberculosis	Systemic lupus erythematosus
Acute and chronic Epstein-Barr virus infections	Vasculitis
	Yersinia infection

TABLE 2. Workup of Child With Erythema Nodosum

ROUTINE SCREEN	OTHER STUDIES
Throat culture	Chest radiograph
Streptozyme	Extensive gastrointestinal workup
Tuberculin skin test	
Review of growth chart	
Sedimentation rate	

ciated with EN is identified, therapy can be specific, hastening resolution of the EN. Nonspecific treatment of EN includes salicylates, nonsteroidal anti-inflammatories (e.g., indomethacin, ibuprofen, naproxen), and intralesional or oral steroids as a last resort. Iodides, dapsone, and colchicine have been used to treat EN but are not recommended in children. Decreased activity, leg elevation, and elastic wraps are helpful for the pain secondary to tissue distention.

ERYTHEMA MULTIFORME

BRETT P. GIROIR, M.D.
CHARLES M. GINSBURG, M.D.

Erythema multiforme is a descriptive term for a syndrome of diverse etiologies that is characterized by an acute onset of fixed erythematous *target* or *iris* lesions of the skin. Although the term "erythema multiforme" has been used to describe a spectrum of pathologic conditions, the syndrome can generally be subdivided into three clinical entities: *EM minor,* in which systemic symptoms are minimal or absent, mucosal lesions are not present or are mild, and recurrences are common, *EM major* (erythema exudativum, Stevens-Johnson syndrome), a syndrome characterized by fever and varying degrees of systemic toxicity, mucous membrane involvement of two or more mucosal surfaces, and widespread cutaneous lesions that often evolve into blisters and bullae, and *toxic epidermal necrolysis (TEN),* a severe form of EM major, commonly induced by drugs, that is characterized by large bullae and diffuse partial to full-layer skin involvement invariably accompanied by extensive and widespread mucous membrane involvement.

EM minor is a benign illness with no important complications. By contrast, EM major and TEN are potentially life-threatening conditions whose mortality rates generally correlate with the degree and depth of epidermal and dermal involvement. Frequent complications that may lead to increased morbidity and mortality include

1. Volume depletion from poor intake and increased insensible losses
2. Hypoproteinemia from transdermal plasma losses, protein catabolism, and insufficient dietary protein intake
3. Infectious complications, including sepsis and urinary tract infection
4. Gastrointestinal hemorrhage
5. Ophthalmic complications, including symblepharon, keratitis sicca, and corneal ulceration, leading to permanent visual impairment.

Less frequent complications, such as hepatitis, pneumonitis, phlebitis, hypothermia, and pulmonary thrombosis, also have been reported.

The majority of patients with EM minor have, by definition, an acute self-limited disease that usually requires no intervention. For the small number of patients who are prone to relapsing EM minor secondary to recurrent herpes simplex infection, there is evidence from studies conducted on adolescents and young adults that early therapy with oral acyclovir may abort the cutaneous syndrome or at least reduce the morbidity and the duration of illness of EM minor. Treatment of the more severe forms of erythema multiforme depends on the extent of mucocutaneous involvement and the degree of systemic toxicity. Although there is a notable lack of prospective, blinded, randomized trials of therapy for these syndromes, retrospective studies have demonstrated that meticulous and aggressive supportive care and avoidance of iatrogenic complications yield outcomes equivalent to or superior to any proposed specific therapy.

Potential putative stimuli, such as antimicrobial or anticonvulsant agents, should be immediately discontinued and permanently avoided. If an anticonvulsant is suspected to be the provocative factor and there is a requirement for continued anticonvulsant therapy, an alternate agent with a different chemical structure should be instituted. Additionally, if possible, all other medications should be stopped.

Meticulous care of the skin is the cornerstone of therapy for patients with the severe forms of erythema multiforme. Patients with severe disease should be nursed on a specialized hospital bed that assures equal distribution of pressure to avoid ulceration and further skin breakdown. The skin should be cleansed daily to reduce bacterial colonization and inspected at least twice daily for evidence of cellulitis or infected lesions. Blisters and bullae should be left intact, and moist compresses with aluminum acetate solution (Burow's Solution) should be applied to any lesions that are oozing. All necrotic skin should be debrided, and deep open wounds should be covered with silver nitrate cream or other reasonable dressings, such as petrolatum gauze or 2nd Skin. These dressings may, if necessary, be covered with additional dressings and secured with a conforming bandage. Patients with widespread skin involvement, particularly those with partial or full-thickness lesions, should be admitted to a burn unit where the affected areas can be covered by biologic dressings, such as autologous cultured keratinocytes or porcine xenografts. Because fever is an invariable concomitant of EM major and TEN, it is important to obtain baseline blood and urine cultures and to repeat these on a daily basis if fever persists or recurs. In one study of infants and children with Stevens-Johnson syndrome who had indwelling urinary catheters, 10% of patients developed an acute urinary tract infection.

Ophthalmic consultation should be requested routinely for all patients with any evidence of eye involvement. The eyes should be irrigated as needed with physiologic solutions. Although many clinicians choose to instill topical antibacterial agents on the surface of the eye to prevent secondary infection or to use corticosteroid-containing eyedrops, the efficacy of either of these treatment modalities has not been rigorously evaluated.

Patients with EM have increased fluid requirements because of increased insensible losses that are the result of fever and the loss of the epidermal barrier. Patients may also experience increased plasma losses through large areas of denuded skin. Therefore, the patient's intravascular volume status should be assessed frequently by clinical examination of heart rate, pulses, capillary refill, and urine output. Fluids should be aggressively replaced either enterally or parenterally. Although the resting energy expenditure of these patients has not been quantified, it is believed to be greatly increased over that of normal individuals and comparable to that of patients with thermal burns. Unfortunately, because of painful oral and esophageal ulcerations, patients rarely consume sufficient protein and calories to meet increased needs. Oral feedings should be attempted. However, if the number of calories consumed is below the amount required for maintenance, a soft small-bore nasogastric tube should be placed to provide sufficient nutrients. Parenteral nutrition should be considered if enteral feeding fails. Packed red blood cells, plasma, and albumin should be administered as needed.

Because of the painful oral mucosal ulcerations, patients with severe EM may have difficulty clearing oral and nasal secretions. Therefore, suction should be available at the bedside, and secretions should be suctioned as needed. Mouthwashes with hydrogen peroxide both provide cleansing of the oral and gingival mucosa and also help to relieve the pain of the oral lesions. Since urinary tract infection and urosepsis are frequent complications, indwelling bladder catheters should be avoided unless urinary retention cannot be relieved by other noninvasive methods (such as sitting the child in a tub of warm water and encouraging voiding into the tub).

Secondary infection leading to sepsis, shock, multiorgan failure, and death is the major life-threatening complication of EM. Accordingly, some clinicians advocate the use of prophylactic antibiotics for patients with moderate to severe erythema multiforme, although there is no evidence to support or discredit this practice. The use of prophylactic antibiotics may increase the potential for selecting infections with resistant organisms.

Because of the high risk for infection in these patients, it is imperative that cultures of blood, urine, and, if appropriate, wounds be obtained when there is any evidence of infection. Broad-spectrum gram-positive and gram-negative coverage (e.g., nafcillin plus tobramycin) may be instituted before culture results are obtained if there is clinical suspicion of infection. When culture results are available, the selection of an antimicrobial agent should be based on the antibiotic sensitivity pattern of the organism.

The role of corticosteroids in the treatment of EM remains controversial. Arguments in favor of steroid use in EM major or TEN are based on small numbers of subjective, uncontrolled clinical experiences. The preponderance of available medical evidence, including six retrospective studies on hundreds of pediatric and adult patients, demonstrates that corticosteroids do not improve outcome and may actually worsen it. In one prospective, nonblinded study of 30 patients with TEN admitted to a burn center, administration of corticosteroids resulted in a doubling of mortality. Although all but one small study on corticosteroids and EM were uncontrolled, the best evidence available indicates that steroids are ineffective and possibly harmful for patients with these conditions.

DISCOID LUPUS ERYTHEMATOSUS

BERNARD A. COHEN, M.D.

Discoid lupus erythematosus (DLE) defines a pattern of clinical disease characterized by disc-shaped or coin-shaped cutaneous lesions found most commonly on sun-exposed sites. Although findings in DLE are usually confined to the skin, nearly 15% of individuals with systemic lupus erythematosus (SLE) will develop discoid lesions, and many patients with DLE experience at least mild systemic symptoms.

CLINICAL FINDINGS

DLE is a chronic persistent disease that may last for years. The eruption develops most commonly on the face, followed by the scalp and ears. Occasionally, lesions spread to the extremities and trunk. Localized lesions are only rarely associated with SLE. However, widespread involvement both above and below the neck may impart a higher risk for systemic disease.

The cutaneous eruption begins with slightly infiltrated, erythematous, violaceous papules and plaques with adherent scale and prominent follicular hyperkeratosis. When the scale is peeled away, the undersurface reveals a characteristic carpet tack appearance from the retained follicular keratin plugs. Expanding plaques develop peripheral hyperpigmentation and central atrophy and hypopigmentation. Lesions may become confluent on the face and scalp, producing extensive, disfiguring scarring and pigmentary changes. Thick, warty scale (hypertrophic DLE) may develop in old burned-out plaques, particularly at their periphery. Malar plaques on the face may demonstrate a butterfly pattern. Follicular destruction on the scalp leads to widespread, permanent, cicatricial alopecia. Involution of the eruption without scarring may also occur. The lips and mucous membranes, particularly the buccal mucosa and gingiva, may develop silvery white scaling and ulceration. Patients with chronic scarring in these sites require close observation because of the risk of development of squamous cell carcinoma.

LABORATORY FINDINGS

Diagnostic changes of DLE on cutaneous biopsy of involved sites include hyperkeratosis with follicular plugging, thinning and flattening of the outer layers of the epidermis, lymphocytic perivascular and periappendageal infiltration of the dermis, edema, vasodilatation, and mild hemorrhage in the upper dermis. However, histologic findings may be subtle and may vary with the evolution of clinical lesions.

Some individuals with DLE demonstrate a biologic false positive result for syphilis, positive rheumatoid factor, low-titer antinuclear antibody, slight increase in gamma globulin, minimal decrease in complement, and mild hematologic abnormalities. However, progressive laboratory changes should suggest the possibility of SLE.

TREATMENT

Although fewer than 5% of patients with DLE will develop SLE, all patients with active cutaneous lesions should be evaluated at least twice yearly with a thorough interval history, physical examination, and selective laboratory studies (complete blood count, erythrocyte sedimentation rate, platelet count, antinuclear antibody, urinalysis, and complement).

Individuals who give a history of exacerbation of disease after sun exposure should be counseled regarding sun avoidance and the use of sunscreens and sunblocks. Protective clothing with tightly woven materials, hats, long sleeves, and long pants are particularly useful during the summer months. Beach vacations and midday exposure should be discouraged. Sunscreens with a sun protective factor of 15 or higher should be applied to all exposed surfaces at least 15 minutes before going outdoors from April until October. Opaque makeup provides an excellent sun shield, and many enhancement cosmetics contain sunscreens. Patients living in the Sun Belt states may require year-round sunscreen protection. Extra precautions should be taken at high elevations, in arid climates, in windy conditions, and while skiing because of increased exposure to ultraviolet light.

In all patients, medical coverup cosmetics may be a useful adjunct to therapy. Excellent cosmesis is achieved with products such as Covermark (Lydia O'Leary) and Dermablend (Florey Roberts). These agents are hypoallergenic, relatively water-resistant, and blend well with normal pigment. They are, however, occlusive and consequently comedogenic.

Limited discoid plaques may respond within several weeks to medium-potency topical steroids (e.g., Aristocort 0.1%, Valisone 0.1%). Thicker plaques may require high-potency topical agents (e.g., Diprolene, Psorcon, Temovate), which also may be used for several weeks with close clinical monitoring. Overzealous application of topical agents may result in atrophy and hypopigmentation. Resistant localized plaques may be treated with small quantities (0.1 to 0.2 ml per papule) of intralesional steroids (e.g., Kenalog 10 mg/ml diluted with 2% lidocaine to 2.5 to 5 mg/ml) before proceeding to systemic therapy.

In patients with widespread or resistant cutaneous disease, antimalarials, chloroquine (250 mg/d) or hydroxychloroquine (200 to 400 mg/d), are the most effective treatment. Ophthalmologic examinations should be obtained before starting therapy and every 6 months during treatment because of the risk of antimalarial retinopathy. If possible, therapy should be discontinued during winter remissions. Lesions resistant to individual agents may respond to a combination of chloroquine, hydroxychloroquine, and quinacrine.

Individuals with rapidly progressive, disfiguring DLE, particularly on the face, improve quickly with oral prednisone 0.5 to 1 mg/kg/d in two divided doses in combination with a single dose of an antimalarial. The systemic corticosteroid can usually be tapered over 4 to 6 weeks while the antimalarial begins to take effect.

When active lesions settle down, old scars and postinflammatory hyperpigmentation may soften and lighten with the daily application of retinoic acid cream (Retin-A 0.025% cream) over 4 to 6 months.

PAPULOSQUAMOUS DISORDERS

JO-DAVID FINE, M.D., M.P.H.
PAMELA J. GUEST, M.D.

All papulosquamous disorders are characterized by the presence of scale. It should be realized, however, that some nonpapulosquamous disorders may have focal scale formation as a reflection of a secondary response to treatment or healing. Careful inspection of the color and pattern of scale may be highly informative. For example, the scale of psoriasis is usually silvery white and rather confluent overlying well-demarcated, red plaques and can be easily induced on the surface of nonscaling plaques by gentle scratching. Because of the resemblance of psoriatic scale to the mineral mica, such scale is often referred to as micaceous. In contrast, rather confluent yellowish (or greasy-appearing) scale is characteristically observed in seborrheic dermatitis. Other more unusual scale patterns are discussed with their respective diseases.

SEBORRHEIC DERMATITIS

Seborrheic dermatitis is probably the most common papulosquamous disorder seen in infants and children. It may run the spectrum from very localized and self-limited disease to generalized exfoliative dermatitis. The most common presentations in a pediatric population are cradle cap and diaper dermatitis. The former is characterized by the presence of rather adherent yellowish scale to the mid and posterior aspects of the scalp. Such scale should be softened with mineral oil for 20 to 30 minutes and gently debrided using a soft toothbrush and tap water or a mild shampoo. This can be repeated two to three times weekly as needed. For most infants, a mild baby shampoo will be sufficient. Only rare children will need to be treated with one of the medicated (i.e., containing salicylic acid, selenium sulfide, zinc pyrithione, or tar) shampoos. Infrequently, some children will continue to have recurrent red patches and scaling of the scalp, eyebrow areas, or postauricular skin folds. Application of 1% hydrocortisone solution or cream to the involved areas should be performed daily for about 3 to 5 days or until all scaling and redness have resolved. Infrequently, some children, usually as they approach young adulthood, may require intermittent (i.e., 3 to 7 days) application of a medium-potency corticosteroid solution to less responsive scalp areas. Recurrent scaling of the eyelashes can be safely corrected with warm water compresses and careful manual debridement.

The diaper eruption of seborrheic dermatitis can be distinguished from an irritant (i.e., secondary to urine or stool) or allergic contact dermatitis by the usual sparing of skin folds by the former. Similarly, the lack of exudate or peripheral (satellite) pustules usually easily distinguishes seborrheic dermatitis from a candidal diaper dermatitis. As in virtually all skin areas involved by seborrheic dermatitis, the inguinal and perianal areas usually can be easily treated or controlled by the intermittent application of 1% hydrocortisone cream. In those few cases not responding to the latter, a trial of 2.5% hydrocortisone is indicated. As a general rule, a fluorinated corticosteroid is never required for the treatment of a child with localized seborrheic dermatitis. Localized cases not responding to such treatment should be biopsied to exclude the possibility of histiocytosis X, which clinically may mimic seborrheic dermatitis in children.

Another common site for seborrheic dermatitis is within the axillary vault. This should respond readily to the intermittent use of 1% to 2.5% hydrocortisone cream.

PSORIASIS

It has been estimated that some 3% of the American population will experience some form of psoriasis during their lifetimes. Although psoriasis is associated with significant morbidity in all age groups, it is often most devastating when it occurs in infancy and childhood, since many of the more effective therapeutic modalities are difficult or impossible to employ in childhood.

Several forms of psoriasis have been described. The most common form, psoriasis vulgaris, is characterized by the symmetric development of thick, red, well-demarcated plaques over extensor aspects of the body or scalp or both. Nails are commonly involved and are often thickened and disfigured. A second type, seen most often in children and young adults, is referred to as "guttate psoriasis." Usually a sequela of streptococcal pharyngitis, guttate psoriasis is characterized by the rapid onset of numerous small circular or oval red plaques, especially over the trunk, in a paint-splattered distribution. Other less common forms of psoriasis include pustular psoriasis (either localized or generalized) and psoriatic exfoliative erythroderma. Any of these psoriasis variants may be associated with an often debilitating if not mutilating distal symmetric arthropathy (pustular arthritis).

Most forms of psoriasis respond, albeit slowly, to the application of medium-potency (Synalar, Lidex, Valisone) or high-potency (Halog, Diprolene, Temovate) halogenated corticosteroids, especially when sparingly applied two to four times daily to affected skin sites. Penetration of the active corticosteroid is enhanced if occlusion is applied, either in the form of an ointment base or with the use of wet towel wraps or plastic food wrap occlusion following application of the corticosteroid-containing cream to affected body sites. Because of the potential for development of cutaneous atrophy secondary to the application of potent corticosteroids to the face, breasts (both areolar and inframammary), genital regions, and other selected body folds (to include the axillary vaults), such areas are best treated instead with 1% or 2.5% hydrocortisone cream or ointment. Chronic widespread application of medium- to high-potency halogenated corticosteroids to the skin of infants and small children is to be avoided because of the significant risk of adrenal gland suppression.

Scalp psoriasis is usually treated with the daily use of tar-containing shampoos (such as Neutrogena T/Gel, Sebutone, Ionil T, DHS-Tar, Pentrax), followed by application of several drops of a medium-potency corticosteroid solution (such as Synalar or Lidex) or gel (Lidex) to affected scalp sites (daily for 5 to 7 days or until clear of psoriasis). A keratolytic gel (such as Keralyt) applied under shower cap occlusion to the moistened scalp for 1 or more hours nightly for several days may be highly effective in stripping the scalp of psoriatic scale, thereby facilitating penetration of the chosen corticosteroid preparation into the underlying psoriatic plaques. An alternative to Keralyt gel is Baker's P & S solution, which can be applied to the premoistened scalp at bedtime, occluded overnight under a shower cap, and rinsed out the following morning with a conventional shampoo. Like Keralyt, Baker's P & S solution should be used nightly for 3 to 7 days until all scale has been debrided and then used as needed thereafter. Intralesional corticosteroid injection with 3 to 5 mg/ml of triamcinolone may be highly effective if used to treat very localized or recalcitrant psoriatic plaques. Unfortunately, it is difficult to administer to children.

Application of tar to selected affected skin areas may act synergistically with other topical measures. For example, we commonly have our psoriasis and eczema patients soak in bath water containing small volumes of a tar-containing solution (such as Balnetar) once or twice daily before local application of a topical corticosteroid. A variety of tar-containing topical medications are commercially available as shampoos, ointments, creams, gels, emulsions, and solutions. Unfortunately, tar-containing ointments are messy to apply, stain clothing, and are malodorous. In addition, localized occlusion folliculitis may occur in some hair-bearing sites after repeated applications of tar ointments. Although many commercial preparations of tar are available to the practitioner, one can also use crude coal tar [in, for example, the form of liquor carbonis detergens (LCD)] compounded at a final concentration of 2% to 5% in some bland ointment base, such as Aquaphor. In addition, small amounts of tar can be added easily to most of the commercially prepared medium-potency corticosteroid ointments if simultaneous therapy is desired. For aesthetic reasons, tar preparations are most often applied overnight and then removed the following morning.

Another topical alternative or addition to corticosteroids is anthralin. Anthralin is a primary irritant and may cause staining of clothes and skin, especially when applied for longer periods of time. Because of these potential problems, anthralin treatment should be employed only under strict supervision. When applied for only brief periods of time (short-contact therapy, usually about 20 minutes) directly to lesions, the concentration of anthralin-containing creams (Lasan, Drithocreme) or ointment (Anthra-Derm) can be increased slowly (initial concentration 0.1%, maximum concentration 1%) until either improvement or irritation is experienced. The frequency of anthralin application can be subsequently reduced from daily to once or twice weekly as maintenance therapy once all lesions have been cleared.

Systemic antistreptococcal antibiotics are often used empirically for 10 to 14 days in patients with new onset of guttate psoriasis, especially in the presence of a history of recent pharyngitis and, ideally, after confirmation by throat culture or serology.

Frequent (four to six times daily) application of wet-to-damp compresses with normal saline to pustule-containing psoriatic plaques may be remarkably beneficial in debridement of crusts and pustules and may help in reducing the fever associated with generalized pustular psoriasis.

Children with severe generalized psoriasis may benefit from outpatient or inpatient treatment with ultraviolet light (either UVB or UVA with systemic psoralens, PUVA therapy). Unfortunately, phototherapy is particularly difficult to perform on children and may be associated with the risk of potentially severe second degree burns in uncooperative patients. Either type of phototherapy should be administered only by a dermatologist experienced in these techniques and only to those patients who are old enough and sufficiently mature to reliably cooperate with such intensive therapy.

Severe generalized psoriasis (including pustular, erythrodermic, and arthritis-associated forms) often responds well to systemic methotrexate, administered in low doses on one of two weekly schedules. Administered only by dermatologists with extensive experience with the use of this drug in psoriasis, methotrexate therapy is particularly risky in small children and, therefore, is used only rarely. Systemic etretinate (Tegison), when administered daily at usually 1 to 1.5 mg/kg/d, may be beneficial, especially in cases of pustular psoriasis. Unfortunately, several potential side effects, most noticeably premature closure of the epiphyses, teratogenicity, injury to liver and bone marrow, and elevation of serum lipids, limit its use to only brief windows of time in children. Use of either methotrexate or etretinate requires careful serial laboratory evaluations to monitor for evidence of early drug toxicity.

LICHEN PLANUS

Lichen planus, a usually markedly pruritic eruption, may be either localized or generalized in distribution. Lesions are characteristically described as individual polygonal, purplish, flat-topped papules, which in some cases may merge into larger plaques. Careful examination of the surface of such a lesion with a hand lens usually reveals the presence of several small white lines (referred to as Wickham striae), which may be observed also within asymptomatic patches along the buccal surfaces of the oral cavity. A lichen planus-like eruption also may result from a variety of systemic medications. Therefore, the evaluation of any lichenoid eruption should include a careful review of all medications taken within 1 to 2 weeks prior to the onset of the rash. Treatment involves the use of systemic antihistamines (such as diphenhydramine or hydroxyzine) for control of pruritus and frequent (two to four times daily) application of a medium-potency corticosteroid ointment. Systemic prednisone usually at a dose of up to 1 mg/kg/d administered once daily may be required in those rare patients with intractable pruritus who do not respond to more conventional therapy. Unfortunately, most patients treated with systemic prednisone flare unless very slow tapers are attempted.

PITYRIASIS ROSEA

Pityriasis rosea may be seen at virtually any age, although it is distinctly uncommon in small children and infants. The classic eruption is first characterized by the appearance of a large (up to several centimeters in diameter) circular or oval, pruritic plaque, which is usually located on the trunk and is pink or slightly tan in color. Such a lesion, referred to as the herald patch, is often mistaken for localized eczema (lichen simplex chronicus). Classically, however, up to hundreds of smaller (usually ≤2 cm diameter), scaly, oval patches or papules will later erupt primarily over the trunk and follow normal skin tension lines (Langer's lines) in symmetric, bilateral array, simulating the appearance of branches of a fir tree. Although not always observed, the hallmark finding is the presence of a peripheral collarette of scale on individual lesions. It should be remembered that the use of some medications may result in a pityriasis rosea-like rash and that the cutaneous eruption of secondary syphilis may closely mimic that seen in pityriasis rosea. Therefore, we recommend careful history taking, examination of mucous membranes for evidence of syphilitic involvement, palpation for regional adenopathy, and the performance of a VDRL in all sexually active adolescents who present to the pediatrician with a pityriasis rosea-like eruption.

Treatment of pityriasis rosea is usually confined to symptomatic control of pruritus with oral antihistamines (diphenhydramine, hydroxyzine) and simple emollients containing low concentrations of menthol with or without phenol (such as Sarna lotion), since the course of this disorder is usually unaffected by topical or systemic intervention. In rare individuals with uncontrollable, widespread pityriasis rosea, however, one or two treatments with suberythemagenic doses of artificial UVB, which is available in most dermatologists' offices, may be highly effective in relieving pruritus and hastening resolution of the eruption itself.

SCABIES

The typical presentation of scabies is not papulosquamous. However, scabies may masquerade as a rather nondescript, generalized papulosquamous disorder, referred to as Norwegian scabies, usually in immunocompromised or institutionalized individuals. Such a diagnosis is most often made by examination of a KOH preparation of the scale, since it may be mistaken for a dermatophyte infection. The treatment of Norwegian scabies is identical to that of more routine scabies, as discussed elsewhere in this book, although recurrences are common because of the widespread involvement of the skin in Norwegian scabies.

LUPUS ERYTHEMATOSUS

Lupus erythematosus (LE) may have many different cutaneous presentations. Two papulosquamous presentations common in adulthood, discoid and subacute cutaneous LE, are observed only rarely in children. Localized discoid LE may be treated by several modalities, including intralesional corticosteroids (i.e., Kenalog 3 to 5 mg/ml, total volume per lesion usually <0.4 ml) or topical application of medium-potency corticosteroid ointment or Cordran tape. More extensive cases of discoid LE and subacute LE may require the use of systemic antimalarials (Plaquenil or Atabrine) or systemic corticosteroids (0.5 to 1 mg/kg/d) or both. Dapsone may be of some benefit in rare cases of generalized subacute LE. In adults the usual dose of dapsone is 100 to 150 mg/d. The dose in children should be reduced accordingly. The use of dapsone is best confined to those specialists having extensive experience with this drug. In patients with G-6-PD deficiency, dapsone therapy may lead to severe or even life-threatening hemolytic anemia. In addition, dapsone may cause generalized malaise and headaches and rarely may produce significant increases in hepatic enzyme levels, a mononucleosis-like syndrome, or even agranulocytosis.

Other cutaneous papulosquamous cutaneous manifestations of LE include neonatal LE and systemic LE. Both usually respond readily to systemic prednisone.

All patients with cutaneous and systemic LE should chronically wear sunlight-protective clothing and use sunscreens with broad-spectrum coverage and SPF ratings of at least 15.

DERMATOPHYTOSIS

Dermatophyte infections (also referred to as tinea infections) usually present as papulosquamous disorders. Frequently, the lesions exhibit annularity and central clearing, explaining the origin of the name "ringworm." Confirmation can be made easily if a KOH preparation is made of the scale. Localized cutaneous involvement is easily treated with twice-daily application of any of the broad-spectrum imidazoles formulated in cream base (Micatin, Lotrimin, Loprox, and Spectazole). Therapy should be continued for at least 2 weeks after apparent total clearing of the rash. Widespread involvement or scalp infection is best treated with 4 to 6 weeks of PO griseofulvin 125 to 250 mg/d of ultramicrosized drug for adults, 5 mg/kg/d for children weighing ≤50 lb. The tablet should be crushed and then given with a fatty meal (such as ice cream). Long-term use of griseofulvin, especially needed when fingernail infections are being treated, dictates careful serial monitoring of hematologic and hepatic functions, since either may be injured by this agent. Patients should be advised about potentially experiencing photosensitivity while on griseofulvin.

TINEA VERSICOLOR

Tinea versicolor, a usually widespread papulosquamous eruption of the trunk and more proximal portions of the extremities, is caused by superficial infection with the fungus, *Malassezia furfur*. Although a variety of cutaneous presentations may occur, tinea versicolor is most often characterized by the presence of small (about 1 cm diameter) and usually discrete patches that are slightly tan or fawn-colored. A very fine, tannish scale (sometimes referred to as "furfuraceous") is present overlying each patch. This scale is easily disrupted by gentle scraping of a lesion. The diagnosis can be confirmed readily by observation of tangles of small hyphae and clusters of spores on KOH examination of the scale. Postinflammatory hyperpigmentation or hypopigmentation is commonly observed. Although there are several effective methods of treatment, we normally have the patient apply 2.5% selenium sulfide suspension (Exsel) to all affected areas (and usually to the entire trunk and upper halves of the extremities) nightly for 10 consecutive days, with removal of the medication each evening after only 20 minutes of skin contact. This approach is as effective as but less expensive than the use of any of the imidazole antifungal agents. In many individuals prone to have recurrences, the latter may be decreased or prevented by the once or twice monthly use of a sulfur-containing (Fostex) or zinc pyrithione–containing (ZNP bar) soap in the shower.

EXFOLIATIVE DERMATITIS (EXFOLIATIVE ERYTHRODERMA)

As implied by its name, exfoliative dermatitis is characterized by marked shedding of scales from erythrodermic skin. It may be caused by numerous otherwise unrelated diseases or exposures, including psoriasis, lichen planus, atopic dermatitis, seborrheic dermatitis, contact dermatitis, drug eruptions, pityriasis rubra pilaris, mycosis fungoides, and some internal malignancies (Hodgkin's disease). Initial therapy involves the frequent use of oilated baths to rehydrate the skin, followed by the liberal application of emollients or lubricants. A low-potency or medium-potency topical steroid may be used, followed by the application of wet (tap water) dressings. Whenever possible, the underlying cause, if identified, should be treated. Rare patients with exfoliative erythroderma require treatment with low-dose systemic methotrexate given weekly in a manner identical to that employed in psoriasis.

PITYRIASIS LICHENOIDES CHRONICA (PLC) AND PITYRIASIS LICHENOIDES ET VARIOLIFORMIS ACUTA (PLEVA)

PLC and PLEVA are two rare papulosquamous disorders that probably represent opposite poles of a spectrum of conditions that may either present de nova or evolve from pityriasis rosea. Both conditions have been reported in children, and each usually resolves spontaneously within months to years. Treatment of both disorders usually involves the judicious use of medium-potency topical corticosteroid ointments and systemic antihistamines. In addition, patients with PLEVA are usually also treated empirically with high-dose oral erythromycin, since the latter has been shown to be beneficial in many chronic cases. UVB and PUVA have been reported to be effective in selected patients.

ERYTHEMA ANNULARE CENTIFUGUM (EAC)

EAC is an uncommon papulosquamous disorder characterized by the presence of one or usually only a few slowly expanding, asymptomatic annular or circular red areas that typically have a fine rim of scale along the receding edge of each lesion. A careful search for cutaneous fungal infection elsewhere on the body is warranted, since EAC is usually a hypersensitivity reaction to such an infection. Furthermore, the evaluation is best done by a dermatologist, since the lesions of EAC may be inadvertently confused by dermatophyte infection, granuloma annulare, or the skin findings of Lyme disease by physicians lacking experience with each of these different entities. Treatment of the underlying cause reportedly causes spontaneous involution of the lesions of EAC. Unfortunately, in the majority of cases, the etiology of EAC is not found. Topical measures are usually of no benefit for EAC, although occasional lesions do appear to fade more quickly if treated judiciously once or twice daily with triamcinolone or another medium-potency corticosteroid cream or ointment.

OTHER TYPES OF UNCOMMON OR RARE PAPULOSQUAMOUS DISORDERS

Secondary syphilis typically presents with cutaneous findings that are morphologically similar to those of pityriasis rosea, although usually the papulosquamous lesions of syphilis are unaccompanied by either pruritus or a herald patch, appear more copper-colored, and may be associated with other cutaneous manifestations of secondary syphilis. These skin lesions rapidly respond to conventional systemic therapy of the underlying treponemal infection.

Each of the major forms of *ichthyosis* is characterized by a papulosquamous component. In some, as best typified by ichthyosis vulgaris, shedding of scales is of minor importance, whereas in others, such as lamellar ichthyosis, widespread desquamation may be visible. Considering the lifelong nature of the ichthyoses, most patients are best treated with frequent hydrating baths (in lukewarm oatmeal tub baths for 20 minutes daily), followed by the liberal application of a bland emollient or lubricant (Eucerin cream, Aquaphor ointment, Lubriderm lotion, or even solid Crisco shortening). Such preparations can be reapplied once or twice more each day after brief rehydration of the skin with a damp washcloth. If desired by the patient, an attempt can be made to intermittently chemically debride the skin of scale in a limited area by daily use (for 3 to 5 days, as needed) of a keratolytic-containing preparation (Lac-Hydrin lotion) or 40% propylene glycol solution. The latter can be applied for 1 or more hours per day under plastic food wrap occlusion to enhance its absorption and efficacy. Unfortunately, any of the keratolytic agents may prove to be irritants if they are used too frequently. Rare patients with severe generalized forms of ichthyosis may benefit from intermittent therapy with systemic etretinate, a synthetic retinoid derivative. Etretinate should be employed only by a skin specialist, since it has many potentially severe side effects, including teratogenicity, and if used chronically, it may stimulate premature closure of the epiphyses.

Drug eruptions are infrequently papulosquamous. When they present in this manner, they most often resemble lichen planus. Psoriasiform eruptions have been primarily attributed to beta-blockers. The pruritus associated with drug eruptions is rather easily controlled with oral antihistamines. Occasionally, the use of just a topical medication containing menthol (such as Sarna lotion) may be sufficient. No other topical therapy is necessary other than possibly the application of an emollient or lubricant following an oilated sponge or tub bath if the skin is beginning to desquamate. In particular, the use of topical corticosteroids does not appear to have any influence on the natural course of most evolving drug eruptions.

Erythema multiforme may rarely present as a papulosquamous eruption. The rash itself is best managed as is described for drug eruptions. The use of systemic prednisone remains controversial. Most clinicians who employ this drug in erythema multiforme reserve it for patients with severe, generalized disease, particularly those with evolving Stevens-Johnson syndrome or early toxic epidermal necrolysis.

Pityriasis rubra pilaris (PRP) is a rare, generalized, papulosquamous disorder that often has rather abrupt onset. Rarely seen in children, PRP is distinguished from psoriasis vulgaris by the presence of orangish thickening of the palms and soles and the presence of islands of sparing appearing within large pinkish-red plaques. Topical corticosteroids and ultraviolet light therapy are rarely effective. Most patients require systemic methotrexate, etretinate, or vitamin A, the last at nearly toxic doses.

Pemphigus foliaceus, a superficial, autoimmune, vesiculobullous disease, may rarely present as a papulosquamous disorder resembling seborrheic dermatitis. Although rarely controlled with oral antibiotics (such as erythromycin) and topical corticosteroids, most cases require treatment with systemic prednisone, usually at a dose of about 1 mg/kg/d.

Mycosis fungoides (MF), also known as cutaneous T cell lymphoma, is a cutaneous manifestation of a malignant lymphoma that is presumably of systemic origin at the time of its initial presentation, even in the absence of definable sites of internal involvement at that time. MF rarely has been described in children, although it is most commonly observed in adults. In the earliest (or premycotic) stage, MF may mimic other often chronic generalized dermatoses, including nummular eczema, PRP, contact dermatitis, and psoriasis. An erythrodermic variety, usually associated with generalized exfoliation, may occur occasionally. Diagnosis may be particularly difficult in the earlier stages of MF and may require the performance of numerous skin biopsies before confirmation. Therapy is usually complicated, and the response is often unpredictable or short-lived. Treatment of MF should be reserved to those specialists with particular experience with this disease. Unfortunately, data suggest that the therapies currently employed in MF have no influence on the overall course or duration of this usually progressive disease.

CHRONIC NONHEREDITARY VESICULOBULLOUS DISORDERS

KARYN L. GROSSMAN, M.D.
KENNETH A. ARNDT, M.D.

Blistering diseases in children can present a confusing diagnostic dilemma as well as a therapeutic challenge. The differential diagnosis of a child with a blistering disorder is extensive. One must consider both congenital and acute blistering diseases before entertaining a diagnosis of one of the more rare chronic vesiculobullous disorders. Hereditary diseases include incontinentia pigmenti, epidermolytic hyperkeratosis, acrodermatitis enteropathica, and the epidermolysis bullosa groups. Acute lesions can be seen in various infections, such as congenital syphilis, bullous impetigo, herpes virus infections, staphylococcal scalded skin syndrome, and toxic epidermal necrolysis. Bullous lesions may also be seen in erythema multiforme and bullous urticaria pigmentosa.

CHRONIC BULLOUS DISEASE OF CHILDHOOD

This is the only bullous disease that is found exclusively in children. There is controversy surrounding this disorder, and some people believe that it is a form of dermatitis herpetiformis or childhood cicatricial pemphigoid. However, others argue that it is a distinct entity. The lesions consist of moderately pruritic vesicles and bullae located predominantly over the pelvic and perioral areas. Eye involvement may lead to conjunctival scarring, with subsequent blindness. Lesions have been described as a "cluster of jewels," with new bullae forming around older lesions. On immunofluorescent examination of a biopsy, a linear deposit of IgA is seen in the basement membrane zone, which localizes to the roof of the bullae on salt split skin. Many patients are HLA-B8 positive, but no associated celiac disease is reported. The mean age of onset is 4 to 5 years, and the disease spontaneously remits, leaving hyperpigmentation but no scarring.

If the decision to treat the lesions is made, the primary recommendation is to start dapsone. Dapsone is generally well tolerated and is not thought to have an effect on subsequent growth and development of the child. The usual dose is 2 mg/kg/d to a maximum of 400 mg/d. Most patients require 20 to 125 mg/d for effective control. The primary side effects are hemolysis, toxic hepatitis, the development of a peripheral neuropathy, crystalluria, headache, and lethargy. Before commencement of treatment, a G-6-PD level, CBC, liver function tests, BUN, creatinine, and urinalysis should be performed. Caution should be taken in those individuals with low G-6-PD levels, methemoglobulin reductase deficiencies, and diabetes mellitus. A CBC should be checked weekly for the first month, then monthly during the following 6 months. After this time, the frequency can be reduced. Liver function tests should be checked periodically. During follow-up examinations, special attention should be paid to signs and symptoms of developing neuropathies. There have been reports in adults of the benefit of taking vitamin E with dapsone to prevent hemolytic anemia.

Sulfapyridine, one of the original sulfonamides, may be used as a primary treatment, although it is not readily available. Sulfapyridine is given in an initial dose of 100 to 200 mg/kg/d in four divided doses to a maximum of 4 g/d. Sulfapyridine may cause the same hematologic and hepatic side effects as dapsone, as well as bone marrow suppression, and laboratory tests should be monitored in a similar fashion. If the lesions are not responsive to these medications, oral corticosteroids may be added.

DERMATITIS HERPETIFORMIS

Dermatitis herpetiformis (DH) is a chronic, recurrent pruritic eruption consisting of pleomorphic erythematous papules, vesicles, and bullae symmetrically distributed primarily over extensor surfaces. Shoulders, elbows, knees, and buttocks are typical locations. The disease most commonly presents in the second and third decades but has been known to occur in younger children. It persists for life and is characterized by chronic remissions and exacerbations. Many patients also have a gluten-sensitive enteropathy. Unlike patients with celiac disease, patients with DH do not have diarrhea or malabsorption. Many patients with the enteropathy have been noted to be HLA-B8 or HLA-DRw3 positive. On biopsy, a subepidermal blister with a mixed cellular infiltrate, including eosinophils, is seen. On direct immunofluorescence, a deposition of IgA is seen at or near the basement membrane zone. The most common picture is a granular pattern in the superficial dermal papillae. If a linear pattern is noted, it may be referred to as linear IgA disease, although this may or may not be a separate entity.

Treatment should be dietary restriction with or without the addition of pharmacologic agents. It is estimated that 75% of patients can be controlled by the complete elimination of all gluten-containing products from their diet. This requires referral to an experienced dietitian and strict compliance and cooperation from patients, as they will not experience abdominal pain or diarrhea with nonadherence as do patients with celiac disease.

For limited disease, application of topical corticosteroids may diminish lesions. With more extensive involvement, systemic medications will be needed. Dapsone and sulfapyridine are the two most effective agents. Patients respond rapidly with improvement and clearing within 4 to 48 hours. Subsequently, the amounts of medications may be tapered to keep the disease under control. As little as 25 to 50 mg/d of dapsone may be all that is required to keep the disease quiescent. In cases where the diagnosis is unclear, the rapid response to dapsone has been used to help confirm the diagnosis.

HERPES GESTATIONIS

Herpes gestationis is a rare autoimmune disorder that occurs during pregnancy. Although it is the mother who is primarily affected, the infant may be born with a similar eruption. It is postulated that this is due to the passive transfer of a C3 binding serum factor (HG factor) across the placenta. The lesions in the mother may develop any time during pregnancy but are most common during the second trimester. They are described as polycyclic pruritic vesicles and bullae that frequently start at the umbilicus. On biopsy, a subepidermal blister is seen, and on direct immunofluorescence, a linear deposition of C3 is noted at the basement membrane zone. There is an increased incidence of HLA-DR4, HLA-DR3, and HLA-B8 in these patients. Lesions usually resolve spontaneously several days postpartum but may recur in subsequent pregnancies, with the use of oral contraceptives, or during menses.

In the mother, treatment should be with systemic corticosteroids. If possible, medication should be withheld during the first trimester and tapered close to the time of delivery to avoid adrenal axis suppression in the fetus. There are some reports of successful treatment with hormone manipulation and with plasma exchange. The infant requires no treatment, for the disease is self-limited and resolves spontaneously.

BULLOUS PEMPHIGOID

Bullous pemphigoid (BP) is an acquired immunobullous disease that usually affects the elderly, although slightly over 30 cases have been reported in children. Childhood BP mirrors that of adults, with lesions that begin as urticarial, irregularly bordered erythematous plaques that develop tense variable sized bullae. Bullae may also arise on nonerythematous skin. The lesions frequently are pruritic, and the pruritus may even develop before the skin lesions. Areas frequently affected include the mucous membranes, palms, soles, inner thighs, flexural aspect of the arm, axillae, and groin. BP usually follows a benign course, with spontaneous remissions and an average disease duration of 1 year. On biopsy, a subepidermal bulla is seen, and on direct immunofluorescent examination, a linear deposit of IgG or C3 or both is seen at the basement membrane zone in the lamina lucida. Titers of the BP antigen obtained by indirect immunofluorescent techniques may not reflect disease activity.

The treatment of this disease is complex. Prednisone is the treatment of choice, with the initial dose being 1 to 2 mg/kg/d. It is thought that the effects of prednisone are mediated through its antiinflammatory abilities, as well as through the inhibition of lysosomal enzyme release, decrease in leukocyte chemotaxis, and decreased B lymphocyte function with subsequent lowered Ig production. Once the disease is controlled, the dose should be tapered to decrease the long-term side effects of chronic steroid use. For limited disease, application of class I topical steroids under occlusion has been used successfully. An area 5 cm around the lesion must be treated also to help clear the bullae as well as to prevent new ones. Treatment should continue for 1 week beyond clearing, and one should watch for the development of steroid-induced cutaneous atrophy. Dapsone and sulfapyridine have not been shown to be very effective as single therapeutic agents but are useful as adjunctive therapy, particularly for patients with lesions containing numerous neutrophils. Azathioprine has been used as a steroid-sparing agent in adults, but its efficacy has recently been disputed. It is probably not a reasonable medication to use in children because of its potential long-term complications.

Recently, programs that avoid the use of systemic corticosteroids have been tried in adults, although their efficacy and use in children have not been determined. Erythromycin, tetracycline, niacinamide, and plasma exchange programs may be promising alternatives to drugs with severe potential side effects.

PEMPHIGUS VULGARIS

Pemphigus is rare in children and classically has been considered a more severe disease because of its persistent nature and its rate. The lesions consist of flaccid bullae with a positive Nikolsky's sign. The lesions may also present as erosions. Oral involvement may be severe, causing problems with feeding. On biopsy, an intraepidermal bulla is seen with acantholytic cells, and direct immunofluorescence reveals epidermal intracellular deposition of IgG and C3. The mainstay of treatment is systemic corticosteroids. High doses are often required to control the disease. Once control has been obtained, the dose should be tapered. Immunosuppressive drugs, such as azathioprine, methotrexate, and cyclophosphamide, have been used as steroid-sparing agents, although the long-term effects of chronic administration of these medications have not been determined.

FUNGAL INFECTIONS OF THE SKIN

RICHARD E. FITZPATRICK, M.D.

DERMATOPHYTE INFECTIONS

Dermatophytes are fungi with an enzymatic system that allows invasion and colonization of keratinized tissue. This factor limits infection to the skin, hair, and nails. Clinical infections are classified according to body location. Some dermatophyte species are so highly specialized that they exclusively infect humans and tend to cause very chronic infection *(Trichophyton rubrum)*, whereas other species are predominantly animal parasites and, when involved in human infection, may produce an intense acute inflammatory reaction *(Microsporum canis)*.

Dermatophyte infections are extremely common worldwide, to the extent that 90% of adult men are infected at least transiently at some time during their life, and 20% of the population has an ongoing chronic infection. Though tinea infections are considered rare or unusual in infants and young children, an appropriate index of suspicion is necessary to make the diagnosis, as these infections are often overlooked or misdiagnosed. Tinea capitis, tinea faciale, and tinea corporis are common in children aged 5 to 12 years, whereas tinea cruris and tinea pedis are common in adolescents (Table 1).

Most of the dermatophyte infections, but especially tinea capitis, behave as a familial disease. The presence of a dermatophyte in one

family member acts as a source of infection for others. The spread of infection is either through direct contact with infected lesions or through contact with flakes of skin, nail fragments, or hair infected with dermatophytes. Such contact is often indirect, through sharing of contaminated combs, brushes, clothing, shoes, socks, towels, blankets, sheets, and headgear or even through house dust and flooring surfaces. Repeated contact over a prolonged period is generally necessary to spread the infection from one person to another, but this may occur in as many as 75% of family members.

Moisture, skin hydration, and heat are critical factors in the establishment of clinical infection. The incidence of infection, the severity of symptoms, and the extent of lesions are all directly proportional to environmental heat and humidity. When these two conditions are not present, infections may be subclinical and asymptomatic, and infectivity and spread are low.

A secondary skin eruption representing an allergic reaction to the dermatophyte, termed an "id" reaction, occurs in some patients. In children, this occurs most commonly with tinea capitis and is predominantly truncal and may be scarlatiniform, seborrhea-like, eczematous, or similar to pityriasis rosea or erythema multiforme. In adolescents, it occurs with inflammatory tinea pedis and presents as papular and vesicular lesions on the sides of the fingers, palms, and wrists.

Diagnostic Procedures

Because the clinical presentations so closely simulate a variety of other dermatologic diseases, confirmation of the presence of dermatophyte hyphae by microscopic examination or culture is essential. The active margin of the lesion should be scraped with a No. 15 Bard-Parker blade to obtain relatively large pieces of keratinous material. Suppurative or macerated areas should be avoided. Scrapings for culture can be placed in a dermatophyte test medium or on a glass slide with 20% potassium hydroxide (KOH) preparation and a coverslip in place for direct examination. These laboratory procedures have an 80% to 90% accuracy rate if performed correctly.

Hyphae are visible as highly refractile, long-branching threads that course through cells. Chains of spores are often visible as well (Fig. 1). The major artifact to be differentiated is the very visible interlacing periphery of keratinized epidermal cells. This artifact diminishes if the scraping is given adequate time (10 to 15 minutes) to soak in the KOH preparation.

Tinea Capitis

Tinea capitis is primarily a disease of black children younger than 11 years of age. It occurs most commonly in urban, overcrowded areas. The racial prevalence is poorly understood. The essential feature is invasion of hair by the dermatophyte, resulting in broken-off hairs. Two types are seen (Table 2).

In the United States, "black-dot" tinea capitis, caused by *Trichophyton tonsurans,* is the most common clinical presentation. A chronic noninflammatory course follows. Black dots appear from hair breaking at the skin surface, resulting in patches of baldness studded with black dots. Lesions are small (often only two to three hairs per lesion) and result in polygonal indistinct lesions with normal hairs intermixed. If extensive, a diffuse alopecia results. Scaling of the scalp mimics seborrheic dermatitis. Infected family members, often asymptomatic, represent the main source of infection. Because adult scalps can be

TABLE 1. Relative Incidence of Dermatophytoses

YEARS	TINEA CAPITIS	TINEA CORPORIS	TINEA FACIALE	TINEA PEDIS	TINEA CRURIS	TINEA UNGUIUM
0–4	+	+	+	−	−	−
5–12	+ + + +	+ + +	+ + +	±	±	−
13–18	+	+ +	+	+ +	+	±

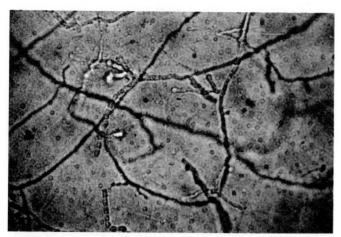

FIGURE 1. Potassium hydroxide preparation of epidermal scraping. Highly refractile, branching hyphae can be seen coursing through these epidermal cells.

infected, the mother may act as a continuing source of infection for other children.

"Gray-patch" ringworm is the more classic disease pattern, caused primarily by *Microsporum canis* and *Microsporum audouini*. This pattern involves hairs breaking off a few millimeters above the scalp, usually affecting about 95% of the hairs in an area, and a dense scale on the scalp surface. This results in a clinical picture of several distinctive annular patches of hair loss and scale. It is uncommon for more than 50% of the scalp to be involved.

The differential diagnosis of these conditions includes seborrheic dermatitis, psoriasis, alopecia areata, trichotillomania, traction alopecia, impetigo, pyoderma, secondary syphilis, and cicatricial alopecia.

Tinea Corporis

Tinea corporis refers to lesions on the glabrous skin of the trunk or limbs. In children, these lesions most commonly occur from contact with lesions of an infected animal (usually a kitten or puppy) or as secondary spread from lesions of tinea capitis. In adolescents, lesions result from the spread from other primary sites of infection: tinea pedis, tinea cruris, or tinea unguium.

Characteristically, the lesion is a red, scaly, annular patch with central clearing and an active advancing margin—classic "ringworm." Some lesions may persist for years, but the majority will resolve spontaneously after a few months. The more inflammatory the lesion, the shorter the duration.

The differential diagnosis includes psoriasis, nummular eczema, contact dermatitis, granuloma annulare, impetigo, and pityriasis rosea. One source of confusion in diagnosis is alteration of the appearance of lesions by the application of topical steroid creams after misdiagnosis. Bizarre clinical pictures may result, including hypopigmented lesions, acneiform papules, folliculitis, inflammatory papules, striae, and atrophy.

Tinea Faciale

This is simply tinea corporis located on the face. Some lesions may be light-sensitive and may simulate systemic lupus erythematosus or polymorphous light eruption. It occurs most commonly from contact with infected pets.

Tinea Cruris

Tinea cruris refers to lesions of the groin, perineum, and perianal region. It is rare in infants and children but more common in adolescents.

The upper, inner aspect of the thighs is usually involved in a bilaterally symmetric fashion. Lesions are normally absent from the scrotum but may extend to the intergluteal fold and even out onto the buttocks. The lesion is characterized by a sharply marginated, scaling border at the periphery and may be quite inflammatory.

The differential diagnosis includes flexural psoriasis, seborrheic dermatitis, intertrigo, erythrasma, neurodermatitis, and atopic dermatitis. In the infant, *Candida albicans* may produce similar lesions.

Tinea Pedis

Tinea pedis, or "athlete's foot," is by far the most common dermatophyte infection in humans. It is primarily an infection of the interdigital spaces and plantar surface of the feet related to the heat and maceration that result from wearing shoes. Prior to 7 years of age, the incidence is negligible and thereafter rises; 1% are infected at age 7 to 8, 6% to 9% by age 12, and 20% by age 20.

Peeling, maceration, and fissuring of the skin between the toes are typical. The lesions are very persistent but may be subclinical except during periods of high temperature and humidity. With successive exacerbations, the eruption spreads to the plantar surface, sides, and dorsum of the foot. *Trichophyton rubrum* tends to cause chronic infection with dry, scaling, hyperkeratotic patches of the soles. Nails are often involved as well. *Trichophyton mentagrophytes* tends to cause vesicular lesions, single or grouped, often on the instep. These lesions are very pruritic and rupture, leaving a jagged collarette scale.

The differential diagnosis includes erythrasma, intertrigo, psoriasis, ichthyosis, eczema, and contact dermatitis.

Tinea Unguium

Tinea unguium (or infection of the nails) usually occurs in association with tinea pedis. Infection begins in the lateral nail folds and extends under the lateral nail to the nailbed. The nailbed epithelium becomes irritated and produces soft keratin. This accumulation of subungual hyperkeratosis is the most characteristic feature of tinea unguium. Involvement is usually asymmetric and often includes only one or two nails. Early infection is characterized by subungual hyperkeratosis, brownish discoloration of the nail, and separation of the nail from the nailbed along the lateral borders, causing a yellow-white discoloration. Later in the course, the nail becomes thicker, and the distal edge crumbles and becomes irregular.

The differential diagnosis for dystrophic nails includes psoriasis, eczema, lichen planus, warts, contact dermatitis, and pyogenic granuloma.

TABLE 2. Tinea Capitis

CAUSATIVE DERMATOPHYTE	FLUORESCENCE WITH WOOD'S LIGHT	POTASSIUM HYDROXIDE EXAMINATION	CLINICAL PATTERN	INFLAMMATORY RESPONSE	SPONTANEOUS RESOLUTION	INFECTION OF ADULTS
Microsporum canis *Microsporum audouini*	Brilliant green	Hyphae inside hair Spores outside hair	Circular patches of hair loss	+ + Kerion formation "id" reaction	Months to years	No
Trichophyton tonsurans	None	Hyphae inside hair Spores inside hair (endothrix)	Irregular, ill-defined polygonal patterns of hair loss	± Asymptomatic carrier state described	Decades to lifetime	Yes

Treatment of Dermatophyte Infections

Topical Therapy

With the exception of tinea capitis, tinea unguium, and chronic tinea pedis, most lesions caused by dermatophyte infections respond to treatment with topical antifungal creams. Occasionally, these lesions require systemic therapy.

Treatment with topical agents should generally be continued for at least 1 week beyond clinical resolution because these medications are fungistatic and require elimination of fungal elements through turnover of the epidermis. For this reason, treatment generally should be continued for a minimum of 4 weeks.

Modern agents include the imidazoles: clotrimazole (Lotrimin, Mycelex), miconazole (Micatin), and econazole (Spectazole). Miconazole has been released as an over-the-counter agent, as has the non-imidazole haloprogin (Halotex). All of these agents are safe and effective broad-spectrum topical antifungal agents.

Cicloprox (Loprox) is another non-imidazole antifungal agent that has proven to be equally efficacious. Naftifine (Naftin), an allylamine, is at least as effective as the imidazoles and has been shown to have an earlier onset of action. In addition, it has fungicidal-type activity and because of its ability to concentrate in the epidermis, allows once-daily dosing without compromising effectiveness.

Recently, terbinafine (Lamisil), a synthetic allylamine derivative that is fungicidal rather than fungistatic, has become available in a 1% cream that may be effective with daily applications for as short a time as 1 week. There are no available data on the use of this agent in a pediatric population, however.

Systemic Therapy

The drug of choice for treatment of tinea capitis and tinea unguium is griseofulvin. Like the topical agents, griseofulvin is fungistatic, and, therefore, reliance is placed on noninfected griseofulvin-impregnated tissue replacing infected tissue through normal growth processes.

Griseofulvin is generally well tolerated, but side effects include headache, gastrointestinal disturbances, urticaria, pruritus, photosensitivity, and transient leukopenia. Laboratory monitoring with periodic complete blood count and SMA 20 panels is recommended.

The ultramicroscopic form (Gris-PEG, Fulvicin P/G) is absorbed better and is recommended. Doses are listed in Table 3. For tinea capitis, one single oral dose of 3 g has been shown to be effective and is useful when treating an unreliable patient. In addition, the use of selenium sulfide shampoo (2½% twice a week) is helpful in removing spores and fungal elements in the treatment of tinea capitis.

Ketoconazole is a newer broad-spectrum antifungal agent that has proven effective against dermatophytes. However, because of hepatotoxicity that occurs in a symptomatic form in 1 in 10,000 patients and has resulted in hepatic necrosis and death in 2 patients, it is generally considered a drug to be used in patients who are intolerant of griseofulvin or whose infection has been unresponsive to griseofulvin. Monitoring of hepatic function with periodic blood tests is essential.

Two new oral agents recently available may provide effective treatment for chronic dermatophytoses, although data relative to pediatric use are lacking. These two drugs are fluconazole (Diflucan) and itraconazole (Sporanox). Both drugs have an excellent safety profile (lack of liver toxicity) and proven efficacy in tinea unguium, as well as resistant tinea pedis and candidiasis, but both are very expensive. Both are absorbed better if ingested with a carbonated beverage.

CANDIDIASIS

Candidiasis or moniliasis is an acute or chronic fungal infection involving the skin or mucous membranes. *Candida albicans* exists most commonly as a nonpathogenic colonist on preexisting cutaneous lesions or in the gastrointestinal tract or vagina. Infection occurs by transmission from one individual to another. It is harbored in the vagina in up to 35% of normal women, and this is often the source of infection in newborns.

Clinical disorders caused by *Candida* can be classified as (1) infection of mucous membranes, (2) infection of the skin, and (3) chronic mucocutaneous candidiasis.

Diagnostic Procedures

Because *Candida* can be found in large numbers as a saprophyte, it is sometimes difficult to interpret the nature of its presence. The demonstration of true segmented mycelia (budding cells and filaments) in a KOH preparation (see discussion under dermatophyte infections) suggests a pathologic state, as these are formed only after invasion of tissue. The demonstration of *C. albicans* by culture on Sabouraud's media is of no significance by itself. The direct examination via KOH preparation is of much more significance because of the ability to document budding spores and mycelia. These laboratory data must be considered in relationship to the anatomic location of the lesion and the clinical presentation in order to arrive at a correct diagnosis.

Infection of Mucous Membranes

Thrush. Oral candidiasis is the most common manifestation of thrush. The tongue or other oral surfaces are covered with discrete patches of a creamy white pseudomembrane, which are almost pure colonies of the fungus. The lesions may extend to the corners of the mouth, forming cracks and fissures covered with the creamy material, a condition known as perleche.

Oral thrush in the newborn is usually a complication of vulvovaginal candidiasis present at the time of delivery. This can be prevented by administering a suspension of 100,000 units of nystatin in 1 ml of water into the infant's mouth on the second, third, and fifth days of life.

The presence of oral thrush in an infant other than a newborn requires investigation into the general health status of the patient, as it occurs much more readily in the presence of diabetes and other endocrine disturbances, immune disorders, vitamin deficiencies, malnutrition, or neoplasia.

Vaginitis. Newborn infants acquire candidal vaginitis in the same manner that they acquire thrush: from maternal infection during birth. A white or yellow curdy discharge is the most characteristic sign. Labial swelling and erythema with thrushlike patches may be present as well. As with thrush when it appears in an older infant or child, underlying systemic disorders need to be excluded.

Infection of the Skin

Candidal Intertrigo. The most characteristic lesion of candidal intertrigo is a well-defined weeping erosion with scalloped edges and an intense red base. Satellite flaccid vesiculopustular lesions outside the main plaque are common and make the clinical picture more diagnostic. The areas of involvement are the groin, axilla, prepuce and glans penis, intergluteal cleft, and interdigital spaces. Intertrigo,

TABLE 3. Griseofulvin Dose and Therapy

DOSE (7.3 mg/kg/24 h)		THERAPY	
WEIGHT (lb)	DAILY DOSE RANGE (mg)	SITE	DURATION OF THERAPY
35–60* (15.5–27 kg)	125–187.5	Scalp	4–8 wk
60–100 (27–45 kg)	187–375	Skin	3–4 wk
100–125 (45–56 kg)	317–453	Palms and soles	8–12 wk
		Fingernails	4–9 mo
		Toenails†	6–18 mo

*Dose has not been established for children 2 years of age or younger.
†Requires an increase in dose by a factor of 50% to 100%.

seborrheic dermatitis, psoriasis, contact dermatitis, tinea, and impetigo are in the differential diagnosis, but they may also be preexisting conditions that predispose to infection. Diabetes, obesity, and the use of systemic antibiotics also are predisposing factors.

Candidal Paronychia. Edema and erythema of the paronychial tissue and occasional purulent drainage from the nail fold are characteristic of candidal paronychia. Paronychial involvement always precedes nail changes in candidiasis. The absence of subungual hyperkeratosis and of thickening or crumbling of the nailplate differentiates this nail dystrophy from tinea. Candidal paronychia generally occurs in conjunction with mucous membrane involvement or as a secondary manifestation of the systemic disorders previously mentioned.

Diaper Dermatitis. This occurs most commonly during the second to fourth months of life. When *C. albicans* is a causative agent, the intertriginous areas usually are affected, and the lesions are typical of those described as candidal intertrigo. The eruption generally starts in the perianal area and spreads to involve the perineum and upper thighs. Predisposing factors include dampness and maceration, irritation from urine and feces, and contact or irritant dermatitis from rubber or plastic pants or laundry detergents and fabric softeners. Diaper dermatitis may also be a secondary infection in infants with oral or vaginal candidiasis.

In addition to treatment with appropriate antifungal creams, treatment includes keeping the area as dry as possible by changing diapers frequently, discontinuing the use of occlusive plastic or rubber pants, and using powder frequently.

Chronic Mucocutaneous Candidiasis

Chronic mucocutaneous candidiasis is a progressive infection associated with underlying lymphocytic disorders, especially congenital thymic disorders. Symptoms generally begin during infancy with thrush or intertrigo, which are very resistant to therapy and spread to the scalp and glabrous skin. Large polycyclic plaques, resembling ringworm or psoriasis but with thick hyperkeratotic crusts, are typical. *C. albicans* proliferates in the crusts.

Defective cell-mediated immunity is a constant feature of this syndrome, but systemic candidiasis rarely occurs. When cell-mediated immunity is restored to normal, the cutaneous lesions resolve.

Treatment of Candidiasis

The first principle in treatment of candidiasis is to look for an underlying condition and to correct it. Once this has been accomplished, treatment of candidiasis will be successful using the following measures.

The treatment of all cutaneous infections requires avoidance of excessive moisture and maceration. Application of antifungal creams will then effectively eliminate *C. albicans*.

In thrush, nystatin (100,000 units four times per day for 10 days) is administered by oral suspension and may be placed directly on lesions. Nystatin may be administered as a vaginal tablet containing 100,000 units and should be inserted twice daily for 7 to 14 days for vulvovaginal candidiasis.

The newer antifungal creams, the imidazoles, have a broad spectrum and are effective against *C. albicans*. This group includes miconazole (Micatin, Monistat) and econazole (Spectazole). In addition, the newer non-imidazoles are equally effective and include cicloprox (Loprox) and naftifine (Naftin). These creams and lotions should be used on areas of infection involving the skin for a period of 7 to 14 days.

TINEA VERSICOLOR

Tinea versicolor is a noninflammatory, asymptomatic, superficial fungal infection of the stratum corneum. It causes whitish to brown macular patches of superficial scale, often becoming confluent and covering large areas of the torso and proximal extremities. Direct examination of the scale reveals the causative fungus, *Malassezia*

furfur. Its characteristic appearance on KOH examination is that of "spaghetti and meatballs": short filaments and grapelike clusters of budding cells. This fungus has beeen shown to be identical to the fungus *Pityrosporum orbiculare*, a normal inhabitant of the skin. This suggests that the condition is actually an overgrowth during conditions of heat and moisture of an organism that is part of the normal skin flora. In some typical areas, as many as 50% of the population may be affected.

Tinea versicolor is common in adults and adolescents but has been considered rare in children by most authors. However, a recent survey of a mycology clinic in Italy found the condition not infrequent in patients aged 5 months to 13 years. One significant difference in pediatric patients was facial involvement, which was found to be present in 50% of the pediatric cases but unusual among adults.

Treatment

All of the topical broad-spectrum antifungal creams are effective against tinea versicolor, including the imidazoles: miconazole (Micatin, Monistat), clotrimazole (Lotrimin, Mycelex), econazole (Spectazole), ketoconazole (Nizoral), and oxiconazole (Oxistat) and the non-imidazoles: cicloprox (Loprox) and naftifine (Naftin). These should be applied once or twice daily for 2 to 3 weeks until the infection has cleared. Selenium sulfide suspension is effective as well. Recurrences are common, as the source of infection appears to be from the normal skin flora.

REFERENCES

1. Fitzpatrick RE, Newcomer VD: Dermatophytosis and candidiasis. *In* Feigin RD, Cherry JD (eds): Textbook of Pediatric Infectious Diseases, 2nd ed. Philadelphia, WB Saunders Co, 1984:818–855.
2. Roberts DT: Itraconazole in dermatology. J Dermatol Treat 2:155–158, 1992.
3. Stiller MJ, Sanquerza OP, Shupack JL: Systemic drugs in the treatment of dermatophytoses. Int J Dermatol 32:16, 1993.

WARTS AND MOLLUSCUM CONTAGIOSUM

JOSEPH W. LANDAU, M.D.

WARTS

Warts are skin tumors produced by the human papillomavirus (HPV). More than 60 different types of HPV have been identified on the basis of their DNA sequences. These types have been associated with a variety of different clinical entities, including common, flat, plantar, and anogenital warts. The vast majority of these warts are benign. Certain HPV types, such as 16, 18, and 31 found in some anogenital warts, have been associated with genital dysplasias and carcinomas. Malignant transformation is more likely to occur in warts in patients with the rare genetic disorder epidermodysplasia verruciformis and with various other types of immunosuppression.

Treatment

Common, flat, and plantar warts, particularly in children, will usually resolve spontaneously in several years. Treatment is often desired, however, to remove painful or cosmetically disfiguring warts and to prevent spread. No currently available treatment is specific, completely safe, and totally effective. The selection of any treatment must consider the age and pain tolerance of the child and the location of the wart. Treatment should produce negligible scarring and minimal disability. Warts in immunosuppressed patients occur more frequently, are widespread, and are difficult to treat.

Common and Plantar Warts

Initial treatment of common and plantar warts with salicylic acid or lactic acid or both in liquid vehicles, in plaster dressings, or in a karaya gum patch is relatively safe for home use. As part of this treatment, paring of the warts and application of 25% trichloroacetic acid every few weeks in the physician's office is helpful. Common warts on the extremities can be treated with liquid nitrogen applications. This treatment is very effective if the patient can tolerate the pain. Several applications at 2- to 3-week intervals may be required. The application of cantharidin in collodion is another office method that is sometimes effective. Electrodesiccation is an excellent method of removing one or two common warts. Local anesthesia is necessary with this method, and scarring may occur.

Aggressive therapy is not recommended for plantar warts because any scarring on the sole may be very painful. Caution is always advised in patients with compromised peripheral circulation.

Flat Warts

Flat warts can be treated with mild peeling agents containing benzoyl peroxide, salicylic acid and lactic acid preparations, and tretinoin. Slight peeling and erythema are desirable. Several months of treatment are often required. Liquid nitrogen and electrodesiccation must be used with extreme caution on the face.

Recalcitrant Warts

Additional methods of treating recalcitrant warts are being studied. These methods include CO_2 laser vaporization, topical 5-fluorouracil, intralesional bleomycin, sensitization to dinitrochlorobenzene or squaric acid dibutyl ester, interferons, and systemic retinoids. The superiority of these methods over conventional modalities and their safety in children have not been established.

Anogenital Warts

Management of anogenital warts is more complex. The usual transmission is sexual, and additional studies are indicated to exclude other possibly coexistent sexually transmitted diseases. Women should have a pelvic examination and a Papanicolaou smear. Most cervical HPV infections and some lesions in men may be entirely invisible without the application of 3% to 5% acetic acid and magnification. In children, the presence of anogenital warts may indicate the possibility of sexual abuse. Perianal warts in the absence of other genital warts are suggestive of anal intercourse and, in men, of homosexuality.

Office treatment of external anogenital warts includes local application of cryotherapy, 50% trichloroacetic acid, podophyllin, and electrosurgery. Other methods include 5-fluorouracil, interferon, and laser ablation. A topical solution of podifilox, a purified derivative of the active ingredient in podophyllin, has been approved for self-treatment of genital warts by patients older than children. Patients with cervical, vaginal, intraurethral, and rectal warts should be managed by appropriate specialists.

MOLLUSCUM CONTAGIOSUM

Molluscum contagiosum is a common skin disease produced by a member of the poxvirus group. It is characterized by single or multiple, asymptomatic, translucent, pearly papules from 2 to 15 mm in diameter with central umbilication. Some papules may become inflamed before they disappear. The usual sites of involvement are the trunk, face, and extremities in children and the anogenital region in sexually active adolescents. In young children, the presence of the papules predominantly in the anogenital region may denote sexual abuse. The disease is benign and generally clears spontaneously within several years.

Treatment

Treatment is not absolutely essential but may be desired to prevent spread and improve appearance. Neither systemic nor specific antiviral therapy is available. Daily topical application for 4 to 6 weeks of weak peeling agents, such as benzoyl peroxide gels, salicylic acid and lactic acid preparations, and tretinoin, is sometimes successful. Some mild degree of irritation is expected and is desirable. Daily application of adhesive or similar tape for several weeks may remove

TABLE 1. Selected Drugs for Treatment of Warts and Molluscum Contagiosum

Benzoyl Peroxide	**Podofilox**
Benzac	Condylox
Benzagel	
Desquam	**Salicylic Acid**
PanOxyl	Duofilm
Persa-Gel	Duoplant
Xerac BP	Occlusal HP
	SalAc Plasters
	Trans-Plantar
Cantharidin	Trans-Ver Sal
Cantharone (currently unavailable in the United States)	
	Tretinoin
	Retin-A
Lidocaine and Prilocaine	
EMLA Cream	

some lesions. The office application of cantharidin in collodion at 2- to 3-week intervals is effective and reasonably well tolerated. Other procedures include the removal of each papule with a sharp curet and the superficial incision of each papule followed by expression of the contents with a comedo extractor. These minor surgical procedures can be performed rapidly, often without local anesthesia, although the prior application of a topical anesthetic cream containing lidocaine 2.5% and prilocaine 2.5% under occlusion may help reduce discomfort. Table 1 lists selected drugs used in the treatment of warts and molluscum contagiosum. Light electrodesiccation and application of liquid nitrogen are other methods of destroying the lesions. Treatment often must be repeated several times at monthly intervals as new lesions appear. Patients with AIDS may have multiple lesions located characteristically on the face that persist even with treatment.

SCABIES AND LICE

BERNARD A. COHEN, M.D.

SCABIES

Scabies is an infestation by the mite *Sarcoptes scabei*. Definitive diagnosis requires identification of the viable mite, usually a female, from scrapings obtained from burrows that are typically present on the web spaces of the hands, wrists, genitals, breasts, and feet. In any child with new onset pruritus, particularly at night, the diagnosis should be considered. After several weeks to several months of infestation, many patients will develop a widespread eczematous rash that may camouflage the primary lesions. Infants are a good barometer of disease activity in the family because they are ineffective scratchers, and burrows are often widespread, with involvement of the palms, soles, trunk, scalp, and extremities.

Most cases of scabies will respond to a single overnight application of 5% permethrin cream (Elimite, 2-oz tube), followed by a thorough rinsing bath in the morning. This synthetic pyrethrin has an excellent safety profile and has been approved for use in infants as young as 2 months old. Scabies is spread by intimate physical contact, resulting in the need to treat all family members, bunkmates, and close physical contacts in institutional settings. Pruritus, which results from a hypersensitivity reaction to the mite, eggs, and fecal material, will wane over 2 to 4 weeks. Antihistamines (diphenhydramine 5 mg/kg/d, hydroxyzine 2 to 5 mg/kg/d) may be useful, particularly at bedtime. Mild irritation is a common complication of treatment and should be treated with the liberal use of lubricants (Vaseline, Keri lotion, Lubriderm lotion, Cetaphil lotion). Secondary infection should be treated with antistaphylococcal antibiotics (cephalexin 30 to 50 mg/kg/d in three divided doses, cefadroxil 30 mg/kg/d in one or two divided doses, dicloxacillin 25 to 50 mg/kg/d in four divided doses, amoxicillin-clavulanic acid 20 to 40 mg/kg/d in three divided doses, erythromycin 30 mg/kg/d in three divided doses).

Lindane or 1% gamma benzene hexachloride (Kwell, Scabene) lotion is an effective alternative treatment for scabies. However, lindane should be used with caution in infants and small children because of increased percutaneous absorption of this potentially neurotoxic substance. Five percent precipitated sulfur in petrolatum is another effective option (and many consider this the treatment of choice in pregnancy for medical-legal reasons) but requires unpleasant, nightly applications for 3 to 5 days. The use of 10% crotamiton (Eurax lotion) has been associated with treatment failure rates exceeding 30%.

Persistent pruritic postscabicic nodules that occur commonly on the diaper area, genitals, and axillae do not require therapy. However, symptoms may respond temporarily to the application of high-potency topical steroids (fluocinonide 0.05%, betamethasone diproprionate 0.05 to 0.1% cream or ointment). Occasionally, adolescents will require intralesional steroids (triamcinolone acetonide 10 mg/ml, 0.1 ml per nodule). These lesions represent a local hypersensitivity reaction to the mite and may take 6 to 12 months to resolve.

Although fomites are not a major source of reinfestation in most cases, mites can remain viable for 48 to 72 hours off the host. Clothing and bedsheets should be laundered with hot water, and blankets and comforters can be put aside in plastic bags for 7 to 10 days.

Crusted Scabies

In compromised individuals (HIV infection, patients on chemotherapy, institutionalized individuals), the scabies mite may produce an explosive infestation in which thousands of organisms cover the skin surface, resulting in diffuse scaling and crusting. Crusted scabies, also known as Norwegian scabies, is extremely contagious and can spread by even casual exposure. Patients may have little or no pruritus because of immunosuppression. The key to preventing an epidemic is early recognition of the condition and identification of all contacts for treatment. Patients should be isolated until scrapings fail to reveal viable mites. Several treatments with permethrin or lindane should be administered at weekly intervals. Secondary infection is invariably present.

PEDICULOSIS

Head Lice

In the United States, pediculosis capitis is the most common form of louse infestation. Epidemics occur in schools, day care centers, and other settings where hair to hair contact is frequent. Young children are most often affected. Girls are slightly more likely to acquire lice than boys. No socioeconomic group or geographic area is spared. However, blacks are affected only rarely in North America. In South America and Africa, pediculosis capitis is endemic regardless of age and race.

For over 30 years, 1% gamma benzene hexachloride or lindane (Kwell) shampoo has been used affectively and safely as a 4-minute rinse. One to one and one-half ounces should be massaged into the hair and then lathered with a small amount of water before rinsing thoroughly. All members of the household and close contacts should be treated simultaneously. Anywhere from a third to a half of the nits may survive, necessitating a second treatment 1 to 2 weeks later. When used appropriately, the risk of neurotoxicity is remote. Most reports of toxicity have been associated with ingestion or repeated use. Rare cases of lindane resistance have been reported.

Alternative pediculocides include the naturally occurring pyrethrins (RID liquid, Lice-Enz shampoo, A-200 shampoo and gel, R & C shampoo) and synthetic pyrethroid (Nix 1% permethrin cream rinse). These over-the-counter agents are comparable in overall efficacy to lindane. However, they kill the lice more quickly than lindane and have better ovicidal activity. Unlike lindane and the natural pyrethroids, Nix has good residual activity for 7 to 10 days. Despite these advantages, some nits may survive even with the synthetic

pyrethroid, and a second treatment may be required 1 to 2 weeks later.

Although the presence of nits does not necessarily signify active infestation, many schools have a "no nit policy" for readmission. A 10- to 15-minute soaking with dilute acetic acid (vinegar) will help to loosen the cement that binds the eggs to the hairshaft before vigorous brushing with a fine tooth comb. Formic acid 0.5% solution (Step 2) is an expensive alternative.

Associated pruritus responds well to oral antihistamines, and secondary bacterial infection, usually streptococcal and staphylococcal, should be treated as for scabies.

Pubic Lice

Although crab lice most commonly infest the genital hair in sexually active adolescents and adults, nonsexual transmission from viable lice and eggs in clothing and bedsheets and nonsexual close physical contact may be sources of transmission. However, the diagnosis of pediculosis pubis in children should prompt an investigation for possible abuse. Occasionally, the mustache, beard, axillae, scalp, and eyelashes are involved. Identification of the 1- to 2-mm crab louse *Phthirus pubis* or the tiny nits, which are less than 1 mm long, in the pubic area is diagnostic. Viable lice, nits, and fecal material also can be found in other hair-bearing areas of the body.

Treatment options include a single 10-minute application of a pyrethrin liquid (RID) or a 4-minute application of lindane 1% shampoo. A second treatment 1 week later occasionally is necessary. When the eyelashes are infested, the safest treatment consists of the application of petrolatum (Vaseline) three to five times a day for 7 to 10 days. In recalcitrant cases, physostigmine 0.25% (Eserine) has been applied to the lashes three to five times a day for 3 days. However, this agent should be used with extreme caution, particularly in infants and young children, because of the risk of ocular effects and systemic absorption.

Body Lice

Although pediculosis corporis is not a common pediatric problem, the surge in families with children joining the ranks of the homeless will undoubtedly result in an increasing number of cases. Asymptomatic 2- to 3-mm urticarial red papules on the trunk at the site of bites may be the only sign of infestation. However, chronic pediculosis usually leads to intense pruritus and itching, with a high risk of secondary infection.

Diagnosis can be made by searching for the louse or eggs in the seams of clothing and bedding. Clothing can be disinfected by exposure to uniform heat (65°C) in a standard washer and dryer. Patients should be treated with a single overnight application of 5% permethrin cream (Elimite) or 1% lindane lotion (Kwell, Scabene). Regular bathing will reduce the risk of reinfestation.

DISORDERS OF PIGMENTATION

LAWRENCE F. EICHENFIELD, M.D.

Disorders of pigmentation are due to changes in pigment amount or manner of dispersion in the skin. Skin color is due to effects of light absorption and scattering by cutaneous chromophores, compounds in the skin that absorb specific wavelengths of light. Hemoglobin (red) and melanin (brown, blue-gray, or black) are examples of intrinsic chromophores, and carotene (yellow) is an example of an external agent that may affect skin color. This section is limited to melanin pigment disorders.

Pigmentary disorders may be very common and range from those of primarily cosmetic effect to those signaling serious systemic disease. Treatment is based on understanding the pathogenesis of the pigmentary change and awareness of the potential adverse effects on a child's psychosocial development and self-image.

HYPERPIGMENTATION

Freckles

Freckles (ephelides) are small (generally 2 to 4 mm), light tan to brown macules that appear on sun-exposed skin. Freckles are generally seen on individuals who burn easily and tan poorly and are seen more commonly in children with fair skin and red hair. Freckles are not present at birth and develop during later infancy or early childhood. They vary seasonally with sun exposure and may fade during winter months. Although the lesions are primarily of cosmetic significance, some studies have reported freckles to be a risk factor for melanoma. Freckling during early infancy may be a sign of xeroderma pigmentosum or other photosensitivity diseases.

Histologic evaluation of freckles reveals increased epidermal melanin without an increase in melanocyte number. Prevention of new lesions is advised. Sun avoidance and regular application of sunscreens or opaque sunblocks with a sun protection factor of 15 or above should be advised for all children who freckle easily. This may minimize the risks of ultraviolet light skin damage, both acute (sunburn) and chronic (photoaging and skin cancer). Treatment of existing lesions with light freezing with liquid nitrogen or hydroquinone bleaching agents may be effective but is not commonly done in children because of discomfort, irritation, and sensitization.

Lentigines

Lentigines are medium to dark brown macules, similar in size to freckles, that may be congenital or acquired. Lesions differ from freckles in having distinct borders and not darkening on sun exposure. Mucosal and lip lesions are not uncommon. Histologic examination shows increased melanocytes along the basal layer of the epidermis and elongated epidermal rete ridges. Most lentigines are sporadic and of no health significance, although they may be seen in several syndromes, including Peutz-Jeghers syndrome, LEOPARD (Lentigines, ECG conduction defects, Ocular hypertelorism, Pulmonary stenosis, Abnormalities of genitalia, Retardation of growth, and Deafness) syndrome, LAMB (Lentigines, Atrial myxomas, Mucocutaneous myxomas, and Blue nevi) syndrome, and Moynahan syndrome.

Treatment of lentigines is not necessary, although therapy if desired may be effective with cryotherapy with liquid nitrogen, hydroquinone bleaching agents, shave excision, or laser photocoagulation (Q-switched Nd:YAG, pulsed-dye laser at 504 nm, or CO_2 laser at low powers).

Café au Lait Spots

Café au lait spots are even-colored, tan to brown macules seen in 10% to 20% of normal children. Lesions range in size from a few millimeters to over 20 cm and may be present anywhere on the body. Although most children with café au lait spots are healthy, multiple lesions may be seen with neurofibromatosis type 1 (NF-1) and other syndromes. Six or more café au lait spots greater than 0.5 mm in diameter in prepubertal children or greater than 1.5 cm in diameter in adolescents or adults are presumptive evidence of NF-1. Multiple, small, 1- to 4-mm café au lait spots in the axillary area (Crowe's sign) and inguinal area, termed "freckling," is another cutaneous sign of neurofibromatosis in children. Large café au lait spots, often in a segmental distribution, are suggestive of polyostotic fibrous dysplasia (McCune-Albright syndrome), which may include precocious puberty and endocrine dysfunction. Other disorders with increased numbers of café au lait spots include tuberous sclerosis, Russell-Silver syndrome, Watson's syndrome, and Turner's syndrome. A single large macule that develops on the shoulder just before puberty is characteristic of a Becker nevus. For lesions of cosmetic importance, pigmented lesion laser therapy may be effective (useful lasers include Q-switched ruby laser at 694 nm and pulsed-dye laser at 510 nm).

Postinflammatory Hyperpigmentation

Postinflammatory hyperpigmentation is probably the most common cause of hyperpigmentation in children. It occurs from an increase in melanin formation following skin inflammation from a variety of causes, including trauma, eczematous eruptions, irritants, insect bites, psoriasis, pityriasis rosea, drug eruptions, pyoderma, and various exanthems. It is more prominent in children with dark skin and who tan easily. Postinflammatory hyperpigmentation lasts for weeks to months, although it may persist for longer periods, especially in heavily melanized individuals. Pigment may reside in dermal macrophages or drop below its normal epidermal placement into the dermis (melanin incontinence), correlating with slower improvement. Wood's light examination will enhance melanin in the epidermis, whereas dermal melanin will display less contrast.

Antiinflammatory therapy with topical corticosteroids may be helpful, especially if there is active or recurrent inflammation. Topical hydroquinone bleaching agents in 2% to 4% topical creams or lotions may be effective used twice daily over several months. However, continuous use of these agents may result in a paradoxic ochronosis-like hyperpigmentation or hypopigmentation. Tretinoin (Retin-A) cream may be effective alone or compounded (0.1%) with hydroquinone (2% to 5%) and hydrocortisone (1%). Cosmetic coverups (Dermablend, Covermark) may be useful for severe hyperpigmentation.

Melasma (Chloasma)

Melasma is a patchy, dark brown hyperpigmentation located on the faces of women who are pregnant or take estrogens. The condition becomes more obvious after sun exposure. Treatment is generally unsatisfactory. Potentially responsible medications should be discontinued. Sunscreens, cosmetic coverups, and agents described for postinflammatory hyperpigmentation may be helpful.

Incontinentia Pigmenti (Bloch-Sulzberger Syndrome)

Incontinentia pigmenti is an X-linked dominant disorder that is almost exclusively seen in females, as it is prenatally lethal to males. It is characterized by four phases of cutaneous findings: linear inflammatory vesicles, acral verrucous papules, whorled macular hyperpigmented lines and swirls, and hypopigmented patches. The hyperpigmented phase is highly characteristic, with slate-brown to blue-gray macular pigmentation with a marble-cake pattern. The disease name is derived from the histology of this phase, with melanin "incontinence," appearing to have dropped from the epidermis to the dermis. Pigmented streaks generally fade over years, and no treatment is required. Appropriate evaluation of other systemic manifestations (central nervous system, ocular, dental, musculoskeletal) and genetic counseling are indicated.

Dermal Melanocytosis: Mongolian Spots and Nevus of Oto and Ito

Dermal melanocytosis is the term used for lesions that are composed of melanocytes in the dermis. Because of the Tyndall effect on light scattering, these lesions have a characteristic bluish to gray color. *Mongolian spots* are macular lesions present at birth, usually located in the lumbosacral area, buttocks, and occasionally limbs or trunk of normal infants. Occasionally, they are mistaken for bruises associated with child abuse. Lesions generally fade by late childhood, and no treatment is necessary. *Nevus of Ota* is a large, blue-gray discoloration surrounding the eye in the distribution of the first and second branch of the trigeminal nerve, often with ipsilateral coloration of the sclera. These lesions are permanent and generally benign, although rare cases of malignant transformation have been reported. *Nevus of Ito* has the same clinical features located on the shoulder and neck region. The nevus of Ota and the nevus of Ito may be diminished or fully cleared with laser surgery (Q-switched Nd:YAG or Q-switched ruby lasers).

HYPOPIGMENTATION

Hypopigmentation disorders may be divided into those with congenital hypopigmentation and those with depigmentation or loss of pigment in areas with previously normal amounts of melanin. Acquired hypopigmentation includes postinflammatory hypopigmentation, pityriasis alba, tinea versicolor, and vitiligo. Congenital hypopigmentation may be seen with albinism, piebaldism, tuberous sclerosis, hypomelanosis of Ito, and a variety of syndromes with generalized pigmentary dilution (e.g., Chediak-Higashi syndrome, Griscelli syndrome).

Vitiligo

Vitiligo is a common, acquired condition characterized by patterned depigmentation with melanocytes in involved areas. Lesions are macular, oval, or irregular ivory-white patches, often symmetric, with sharp demarcation from uninvolved areas. Although the etiology is unknown, it is generally categorized as an autoimmune disease, and the incidence of vitiligo is higher in patients with other autoimmune disorders. The course of vitiligo is variable, although spontaneous resolution is unusual. Lesions of shorter duration and facial and truncal lesions may be more responsive to therapy than lesions on the fingers, hands, and feet. Topical corticosteroid treatment may be useful in inducing repigmentation, using midpotency to high-potency agents over several months. Less potent corticosteroids should be used for facial, eyelid, or intertriginous areas. Ultraviolet light (UVA) with systemic or topical psoralen compounds (PUVA) may be used in older children. Treatment may take months and requires motivated, compliant children because of problems with photosensitivity, visual damage (cataracts, retinal damage), and cumulative phototoxicity. Phenylalanine and natural light exposure have been advocated by some authors, but studies are limited. Vitiliginous skin is devoid of the natural protection from sunlight of melanin and is vulnerable to sunburn. Routine sun protection is mandatory and will minimize differences in pigmentation between affected and nonaffected areas. Dye formulations (Dy-O-Derm, Vitadye) and cosmetic coverups (Dermablend, Covermark) may be used to camouflage lesions. Surgical treatment of areas with punch grafts and melanocyte cultures with autotransplantation has been attempted, but these new techniques are of limited use in pediatric patients.

Piebaldism

Piebaldism, also known as partial albinism, is a dominantly inherited disorder manifested by patterned depigmentation due to congenital absence of pigment. Presence at birth, consistent pattern, and proportionate growth with the child may differentiate this from vitiligo. Treatment is limited to sun avoidance and sunscreen preparations and cosmetic coverups and aniline dyes to minimize the abnormal appearance.

Waardenburg's Syndrome

This congenital depigmentation resembles piebaldism except that it is associated with sensorineural deafness, laterally displaced medial canthi, and heterochromic irides. A white forelock is present. Protection from sunburn should be stressed.

Tuberous Sclerosis

Hypopigmented macules with a characteristic oval, ash leaf shape may be seen with the neurocutaneous syndrome, tuberous sclerosis. Tuberous sclerosis is an autosomal dominant disease, with other cutaneous findings including angiofibromas, connective tissue nevi (Shagreen patch), and periungual fibromas. Other system problems may include central nervous system disease (seizures, retardation, intracranial calcification), cardiac rhabdomyomas, and renal cysts and tumors. Hypopigmented ash leaf spots and larger hypopigmented patches may be accentuated by a Wood's light. There is no need for treatment of these hypomelanotic lesions.

Hypomelanosis of Ito (Incontinentia Pigmenti Achromians)

Hypomelanosis of Ito is the phenotypic expression characterized by whorled, marble-cake macular hypopigmentation, usually present at birth or early infancy. Hypomelanosis of Ito may be associated with multiple system problems, including the central nervous system, ocular system, and skeletal system. A variety of chromosomal abnormalities has been documented in patients with this condition. No treatment of the hypopigmented areas is necessary.

Disorders of Generalized Pigment Dilution

Abnormalities of melanin synthesis or transport to keratinocytes results in generalized pigment dilution.

Albinism is a heterogeneous group of genetic disorders, characterized by hypopigmentation of the eyes, skin, hair, and meninges. Photophobia, translucent irides, hypopigmented fundi, decreased visual acuity, nystagmus, and strabismus are common findings. Albinism is classified by clinical findings, fundoscopic examination, and assay of hair bulb tyrosinase activity. *Chediak-Higashi syndrome* is a rare autosomal recessive disorder characterized by partial oculocutaneous albinism, recurrent bacterial infections, neutropenia, giant lysosomes in all granular cell types, and a lymphoma-type accelerated phase. Hypopigmented skin and silvery hair are due to abnormalities of melanosome packaging and problems with transport of giant melanosomes to keratinocytes. Other disorders with congenital generalized hypomelanosis include *Menkes' kinky hair syndrome,* an X-linked disorder characterized by growth retardation, seizures, hair abnormalities, and cerebellar degeneration, *phenylketonuria, histidinemia, homocystinuria, Elejalde disease,* and *Griscelli syndrome.* There is no satisfactory treatment for pigment dilution in these disorders. Skin protection from chronic ultraviolet radiation is essential in patients with depigmentation and hypopigmentation. Sun avoidance, proper clothing, and sunscreens should be used.

Pityriasis Alba

Pityriasis alba is a common condition in children, manifesting as hypopigmented, slightly scaly patches most commonly seen on the cheeks. Lesions are often evident with sun exposure as nontanning annular areas. Pityriasis alba is more common in children with atopic dermatitis. The ashy appearance is most distressing to parents of darkly pigmented individuals. Lesions should be differentiated from the hypopigmented plaques of tinea versicolor. Treatment of pityriasis alba includes mild topical corticosteroids (1% hydrocortisone) and moisturizers.

Postinflammatory Hypopigmentation

Postinflammatory hypopigmentation may be observed after a variety of conditions, including eczematous conditions (atopic dermatitis, contact dermatitis, irritant dermatitis), psoriasis, burns, and bug bites. Ongoing inflammatory conditions may be treated with appropriate strength topical corticosteroids. Postinflammatory hyperpigmentation generally is self-limited.

Tinea Versicolor

Tinea versicolor is a superficial fungal infection caused by *Pityrosporum orbiculare (Malassezia furfur)* and presents as hypopigmented areas on the neck, shoulders, back, and occasionally the face. Lesions may be hypopigmented or hyperpigmented, thus versatile in color (versicolor). It is a common disorder in adolescents and young adults, although it may be seen at any age. A potassium hydroxide preparation of scrapings from lesions shows hyphae and spores in clusters (spaghetti and meatball pattern). Treatment with topical antifungal solutions, such as selenium sulfide 2.5%, or topical antifungal creams may adequately treat patients, but persistent colonization is common. Oral ketoconazole is highly and rapidly effective, though generally not advised because of concerns with drug hepatotoxicity.

PHOTODERMATOSES

JEFFREY S. DOVER, M.D., F.R.C.P.C.

Light exposure causes a wide variety of photosensitive disorders. Some are photoaggravated dermatoses (light aggravates but does not cause the disorder, e.g., herpes simplex and lupus erythematosus), whereas others are primary photosensitivity disorders that do not develop without sun exposure (polymorphic light eruption is the most common of these).

Visible light (wavelengths 400 to 700 nm) is rarely implicated in photosensitivity. The shorter wavelength and higher energy of ultraviolet A (UVA) (wavelengths 320 to 400 nm) and ultraviolet B (UVB) (wavelengths 290 to 320 nm) induce most photosensitivity reactions.

Effective management of the photosensitive patient includes a detailed history because the role played by sunlight in photosensitivity reactions is not always immediately obvious to the physician or, occasionally, to the patient. The history should supply such information as the age at which the photosensitive reaction first occurred, the temporal relationship between sun exposure and the eruption, the duration of the eruption, the nature of associated symptoms, the relationship to potential photosensitizers, including recent medications, and a family history. An important clue on physical examination is that regions of the body that receive relatively more ambient light are typically more involved in a photodermatosis. These classically involve the forehead, malar region, nose, rims of the ears, sides and back of the neck, V of the chest, and extensor surfaces of the distal extremities. Absence of the eruption in areas of partial sparing (the area below the alae nasae, the recessed area of the eyelids, the nasolabial line, the web spaces of the fingers, and skin that is covered by fixed jewelry, such as a watch band) is also important diagnostically.

Evaluation and treatment of the photosensitive patient may be aided by phototesting. The patient is exposed to various doses of visible, UVA, and UVB bands at different sites on the skin with or without systemic administration of a drug or topical application of a photosensitizer if drug- or chemical-induced photosensitivity is suspected. Test sites are evaluated within 1 hour and 1 to 2 days later. The range of wavelengths (action spectrum) and dose of light that produce the biologic response (erythema, edema, papules, or vesicles) can, therefore, be determined.

Sunburn, which is primarily due to UVB, is more easily prevented than treated. Recommendations include wearing protective clothing, avoiding outdoor activities between 10:00 AM and 2:00 PM, and using sunscreens with a sun protection factor (SPF) (defined as the minimal dose of light required to produce erythema in protected skin divided by the minimal erythema dose in unprotected skin) of at least 15, liberally applied repeatedly throughout the day. The pain of a severe sunburn can be blunted with nonsteroidal anti-inflammatory drugs, such as aspirin and indomethacin. Nonblistering sunburn reactions can be treated topically with bland emollients, such as hydrated petrolatum, or potent topical corticosteroids that induce vasoconstriction and sometimes reduce patient discomfort. Blistering sunburn reactions should be treated as second-degree thermal burns with topical antibiotic ointments.

Polymorphous light eruption (PMLE) is a pruritic eruption consisting of papules, macular erythema, plaques, vesicles, or eczematous plaques that are usually confined to sun-exposed body areas and that develop 1 to 72 hours following sun exposure and last days to weeks. PMLE, which may be caused by light in the visible, UVA, or UVB wavelength ranges, affects 10% of the population and is especially common in individuals under 30 years of age. Protective clothing in combination with broad-spectrum sunscreens and avoidance of solar radiation is the treatment of choice for PMLE. Once symptoms develop, potent topical corticosteroids may be helpful. Systemic corticosteroids and antimalarials can be useful in preventing and treating PMLE, but potential toxicities limit their long-term and frequent use. The treatment of choice, which depends on the known ability of many PMLE patients to become less photosensitive over the summer from increasing exposure to ultraviolet light, is a course of increasing doses of UVB or PUVA (psoralen plus UVA) beginning 4 to 8 weeks before spring.

Drug- or chemical-induced photosensitivity results from a combination of light and a topically or systemically administered drug, causing tissue damage. A wide variety of compounds produce photosensitivity eruptions, including *para*-aminobenzoic acid (in sunscreens), musk ambrette (in perfumed agents), coal tar derivatives, furocoumarins, such as psoralens (in limes, fragrances, and moldy celery), and drugs, such as quinidine, tetracyclines, phenothiazines, sulfonamides, thiazides, and amiodarone. The best therapy for drug-induced phototoxicity is discontinuation of the offending compound. If, however, a drug necessary for the patient's well-being is implicated and if the photosensitivity is mild, avoidance of sun exposure and the use of opaque sunscreens effective against UVA and visible light, such as Clinique Continuous Coverage, may be adequate.

Solar urticaria, an immunoglobulin E-related reaction, develops within seconds to minutes following sun exposure and subsequently resolves over minutes to hours. Protective clothing, sunscreens, corticosteroids, nonsteroidal anti-inflammatory drugs, antimalarials, and beta-carotene are of little use in treating solar urticaria. Patients with solar urticaria are often so light sensitive that sun avoidance is ineffective. Antihistamines appear to delay the onset and limit the severity of the urticarial reaction in a subset of individuals. Desensitization, using incremental doses of the implicated wavelengths, is an effective, albeit time consuming treatment.

The *porphyrias* are a group of diseases in which porphyrin-heme biosynthesis is altered in such a way that porphyrins, some of which are photosensitive compounds, accumulate in erythropoietic tissues or in the liver and skin. Patients with porphyria cutanea tarda (PCT) are often unaware that sunlight plays a role in producing their lesions, since there is no acute photosensitivity reaction. In contrast, acute photosensitivity with pain and swelling is seen in erythropoietic protoporphyria (EPP). The best treatment for PCT is strict avoidance of exacerbating agents, including sunlight and alcohol. Second-line therapies are phlebotomy, low-dose chloroquine, or both. Sun avoidance, sunscreens, and beta-carotene are the basis of treatment for EPP.

Xeroderma pigmentosa (XP), a group of autosomal recessive disorders with a major defect in the ability to correctly repair UVB-induced defects in DNA, is associated with excessive sunburn reactions to minimal light, with early onset of freckling and with severe actinic damage. The cornerstone of managing XP involves early diagnosis (now possible in utero) and protection from UV irradiation. Potent sunscreens (SPF 30 or greater), combined with restricted sun exposure and protective garb, can reduce actinic damage to the skin. The eyes of XP patients should be protected constantly with wrap-around UV-absorbing glasses. Cutaneous neoplasms should be detected and treated as early as possible.

A large number of rare or incompletely described processes are also associated with photosensitivity in children. *Hydroa vacciniforme* is an extremely rare photodermatosis that first presents in late infancy or early childhood. The action spectrum is in the UVA range. Natural or artificial UVA exposure results in vesicles that heal with chickenpox-like scarring. Patients with *Bloom syndrome*, an autosomally recessive disease associated with a high frequency of chromosomal rearrangements and breaks, are prone to a host of internal malignancies. *Rothmund-Thomson syndrome* is a hereditary oculocutaneous photosensitivity disorder with an increased risk of cancer and cutaneous poikiloderma. Sun avoidance is the mainstay of treatment of all these conditions. *Pellagra* is a photodermatitis caused by niacin deficiency. Intake of isoniazid, a niacin analog, can cause a similar photodermatitis.

NEVI AND NEVOID TUMORS

BERNETT L. JOHNSON, JR., M.D.

A nevus is defined as a new growth of skin of congenital origin, a tumor that may be formed from any tissue, cell, or substance of the skin. The definition includes those developmental elements that are acquired. Nevus is also used by some to mean a hamartoma, a tumor of elements of tissue. This term was further defined by Albrecht as tumorlike malformation showing a faulty mixture of the normal components of the organ in which they occur. In the usual meaning, nevus refers to those tumors with melanocytes or the hamartomatous varieties defined by prefix, for example, vascular nevus, neural nevus.

MELANOCYTIC CONGENITAL NEVI

Melanocytic nevi may be congenital or acquired. Congenital melanocytic nevi give the most cause for concern because of the potential to develop melanoma. Congenital melanocytic nevi are divided into two major groups, small congenital nevi (less than 3 cm in diameter) occurring approximately 1 in every 18,000 to 20,000 births, and large congenital nevi (greater than 3 cm in diameter) occurring in 1 in every 500,000 births. Congenital nevi occur in 1% of all newborns and consist of tumors of melanocytic cells. These cells are found in all layers of the skin from the epidermis to the subcutis. Congenital nevi occur in all people. The incidence in the pigmented races is approximately 2 to 1 over that of nonpigmented people. Small, large, and giant congenital nevi, should be evaluated systematically and repeatedly. The incidence of melanoma arising in each of these nevi is controversial. Some studies quote 3% to 15% for small congenital nevi. One study estimates that the incidence of congenital nevi associated with melanoma is 2.8%. Small congenital nevi, depending on the site, can be removed entirely by surgery, which is the treatment of choice. When the site of the tumor precludes total removal, follow-up, including serial photography, is essential. Suggested management guidelines for congenital nevi follow.

1. Repeated observations (e.g., every 6 months) with photographic documentation
2. Surgical management
   a. Small congenital nevi
      (1) Excise in toto when the site permits; surgery should be performed at an age when the risk to the patient is least
      (2) When total excision is not possible, excise those areas in the nevus that are clinically changed
   b. Giant (large) congenital nevi
      (1) Biopsy or partially excise any area in which there is
         (a) Color change
            i. Hyperpigmentation
            ii. Loss of pigment
            iii. Pigment diffusion into the surrounding normal skin
         (b) Inflammation
         (c) Atrophy
         (d) Associated adenopathy
         (e) Ulceration

In the management of congenital nevi, histologic examination is the only way to differentiate benign from malignant change. Neither clinical inspection, palpation, nor oiling of the skin with macro-magnification will ensure the detection of malignant change. The presence or absence of hair has no bearing on the malignant potential of a pigmented lesion and should never be used as a gauge of this attribute. Therapeutic alternatives that should never be used in the treatment or evaluation of congenital nevi include electrocautery, cryotherapy, dermabrasion, chemical destruction, and laser ablation. These methods preclude the availability of tissue for histologic evaluation and place the patient and the physician at risk.

MELANOCYTIC ACQUIRED NEVI

Acquired nevi are those not present at birth that develop later in life, usually appearing around the age of 4 to 7 months. Acquired nevi occur in almost 90% of people, with the incidence being less in the pigmented races. Acquired nevi are classified as junctional (melanocytic cells only in the epidermis), dermal (melanocytic cells only in the dermis), and compound (melanocytic cells in the epidermis and dermis). These types of acquired nevi do not usually require any therapy unless there is cosmetic concern or clinical change. The majority of these are removed for cosmetic reasons.

Spindle and Epithelioid Cell Nevus (Spitz)

Spitz was the first person to describe this nevus, using the term "juvenile melanoma" and later the term "benign juvenile melanoma." More recently, this melanocytic tumor has been termed spindle and epithelioid cell nevus by Kernen et al. This is an uncommon lesion in children, less common in adults, and is rarely seen after the fourth decade of life. Spindle and epithelioid cell nevi occur in either sex and are less common in the pigmented races. Clinically, these nevi do not resemble more common acquired nevi in that they are seldom pigmented. Most often, they are red to pink in color with well-defined even borders. They occur frequently on the head and neck, as well as the extremities. These nevi are not usually recognized clinically as nevi but are thought to be verrucae or vascular tumors. The clinical differential diagnosis for these tumors includes pyogenic granuloma, hemangioma, xanthogranuloma, mastocytoma, and sarcoidosis. Although the vast majority of these lesions are nonpigmented, there is a small percentage that are pigmented and verrucous and may be confused with verruca, epidermal nevi, dermatofibroma, and other keratosis. Sudden growth is frequently the reason for removal of these tumors. The histology of these nevi may be atypical and can be confused with melanoma, hence the prior name, benign juvenile melanoma. The treatment is excision, since they are rarely larger than 10 cm in diameter.

A diagnosis of melanoma from a lesion in a child who does not have a congenital nevus should alert the physician to the possibility of this being a spindle and epithelioid cell nevus, and review of the histology would be prudent. Spindle and epithelioid cell nevi that are incompletely excised should be reexcised with a modest margin (5 mm). Recurrent spindle and epithelioid cell nevi often have more atypical histology than the original specimen and may be a cause for erroneous interpretation.

Halo Nevi

Halos (areas of depigmentation) can occur around any type of nevus whether single or multiple. Halo nevi are more common in children than in adults. Halo nevi may be associated with vitiligo, pernicious anemia, and the Vogt-Koyangi-Harada syndrome, although they occur most commonly without any associated conditions. Clinically, there is an oval zone of depigmentation surrounding a central pink to red-brown papule. This papule represents the nevus. As the lesion progresses, the central papule disappears, leaving only the depigmented halo. These areas of depigmentation are more sensitive to ultraviolet light and should be protected from sun exposure. Histologically, halo nevi may have atypical melanocytes within the dense lymphocytic infiltrate. There has been discussion as to whether these lesions all should be excised and reexcised if the initial excision was inadequate. I believe that this is not necessary, since the usual course of these nevi is benign.

DYSPLASTIC (ATYPICAL) NEVUS

Dysplastic or atypical nevi are a variant of acquired nevi. They were first described in families in which at least two members had developed melanoma. Clinically, these are rather large nevi, being on average greater than 0.5 mm in diameter. They have a variegated light brown to dark brown color. The borders are irregular and not well defined. These nevi may have a papular component but are most often flat and plateau-like, with the center being the highest point, and fading to an imperceptible nonpapular border. Dysplastic nevi usually occur after puberty and are rare in prepubertal children. They can occur on sun-exposed as well as unexposed sites.

The significance of dysplastic nevi is that they are indicators of a risk for the development of melanoma. Those at greatest risk are families with a history of melanoma and dysplastic nevi and those individuals without a family history of melanoma who do develop melanoma and also have increased numbers of dysplastic nevi. There are those individuals who have neither melanoma nor a family history of melanoma who develop random dysplastic nevi. The risk of melanoma in this latter group is uncertain.

Histologically, dysplastic nevi show a disordered array of melanocytes, some of which may be cytologically atypical. These cells are usually found within the epidermis, although dysplastic atypical melanocytic cells also have been described in the dermis. The management of patients with dysplastic nevi, with or without associated melanoma history requires the following steps.

1. Cyclic clinical follow-up with photographs
2. Excision of nevi that are clinically suspicious
3. Excision of nevi that have changed since the last evaluation
4. Examination of the scalp and genitalia for unsuspected nevi
5. Diligent sun protection
   a. Avoidance of excessive exposure
   b. Use of sunscreens

DERMAL MELANOCYTOSES

Dermal melanocytoses are those conditions in which there are pigmented, spindle-shaped melanocytes in the dermis. The dermal melanocytoses are the mongolian spot, the nevus of Ito, the nevus of Ota, and blue nevi.

Mongolian spots are congenital and occur with greater frequency in people of African and Asian descent. They are found in the sacral and gluteal areas and are blue-black in color and flat. Melanocytes within the mongolian spots are in the superficial dermis. These lesions usually fade after puberty. They do not require treatment.

The *nevus of Oto* (nevus fuscoceruleus ophthalmomaxillaris), sometimes congenital in origin, is found in the distribution of the first and second divisions of the trigeminal nerve and may involve the opposite sclera, lips, nasal mucosa, and oral mucosa. Its color is a deeper blue-black than that of the mongolian spot, and this is because the melanocytes found within this tumor are in the deeper dermis. The nevus of Oto occurs most commonly in people of African or Asian descent and favors females over males. The significant clinical association with the nevus of Oto is the possibility of melanoma of the leptomeninges or ocular melanoma. One should be aware of these associations and follow patients accordingly. The other major concern of these patients is that of the cosmetic appearance of the lesion. Appropriate cosmetic coverage, such as Dermablend or Covermark, may be used.

The *nevus of Ito* is similar in color to the nevus of Oto, is located usually over the shoulder or scapula, is unilateral, and may be congenital. The clinical significance is mainly cosmetic, and it requires no treatment.

BLUE NEVI

Blue nevi are dermal melanocytic tumors in which there are spindle melanocytes in the dermis associated with dermal fibroplasia. Clinically, these tumors are blue-black, dome-shaped papules or nodules. A variety of the blue nevus is the cellular blue nevus. This tumor rarely contains pigment, its cells are found deeply within the dermis and subcutis, and it is larger. Cellular blue nevi occur commonly on the buttocks and have been associated with the development of melanoma. Cellular blue nevi may be congenital. The usual blue nevus is rarely associated with malignant potential, and its treatment is observation. Blue nevi can be confused with vascular tumors, tattoos,

dermatofibroma, and metastatic melanoma. When the diagnosis is in doubt or there is a clinical change in the lesion, a biopsy is essential. Cellular blue nevi should be followed on a regular basis. Any change in the clinical presentation requires a biopsy. In these nevi, the biopsy must be deep, down to fascia, so that the subcutaneous fat is included, since the cells of the cellular blue nevi are found in this location.

ORGANOID NEVI: NEVUS SEBACEOUS

Nevus sebaceous is an organoid hamartoma of epidermis, papillary dermis, sebaceous glands, and apocrine sweat glands. They may be congenital or appear shortly after birth as a hairless, red-yellow plaque on the scalp or face. There is no racial or sexual predominance. Sebaceous development and epidermal verrucous hyperplasia occur after puberty. Biopsies of these tumors before puberty will not show all of the characteristic features. Basal cell carcinoma and nevus syringocystadenoma develop in nevus sebaceous at a frequency of about 10% to 20%. The treatment of choice when necessary is complete excision or multistage excision when primary excision cannot be done because of the site or size of the tumor.

EPITHELIAL NEVI

Epithelial nevi represent congenital hyperplasia of the epidermis and papillary dermis. As these nevi develop, there is increased epidermal hyperplasia, which reaches its zenith after puberty. Clinically, these nevi appear as linear, raised verrucous plaques, devoid of hair and slightly darker than the patient's normal skin. They are rough to the touch. Epithelial nevi may be many centimeters in length, along the length of an extremity or in small localized plateau-like areas. Epithelial nevi occur at birth or develop shortly after birth and may be associated with bony or nervous system defects. These defects are well documented in the literature. The epithelial nevus has less propensity than nevus sebaceous to develop cutaneous malignancies, although basal cell carcinoma and squamous cell carcinoma have been described. When these changes occur, excision is the treatment of choice. Treatment is removal of the entire nevus. This has been frustrating, since epithelial nevi often recur after incomplete excision, especially if the underlying papillary dermis is not removed.

Treatment is usually directed at the verrucous hyperkeratosis, its appearance, and odor. Vinegar and water soaks and topical antibiotics (Bactroban, Polysporin) reduce bacterial growth and odor. The keratolytics (urea products, salicylic acid products, and ammonium lactate products) smooth the nevi and reduce the stratum corneum, thereby decreasing the media in which organisms grow.

VASCULAR NEVI

Vascular nevoid proliferations comprise the most common new growth in children. The incidence of vascular nevi is approximately 35% to 40% of infants; both sexes and all races are affected. Vascular nevi may be ectatic (dilatations) or proliferations (tumors). All are composed of vascular channels, lined with normal endothelium, that, during growth, show marked endothelial proliferation. Vascular malformations may be associated with underlying structural abnormalities. The most common structural abnormalities are bone growth changes due to the increased blood supply of the affected bone.

Hemangiomas

Capillary (strawberry) hemangioma is the most common proliferative vascular tumor of children. They occur at or shortly after birth, beginning as a red macule. At some point, usually several weeks after the initial appearance, the lesion begins to grow and may become several centimeters in size. The tumor is red-purple in color and studded with small red capillary protrusions, giving the tumor the appearance of a strawberry. These tumors are usually single (80%), although about 20% of the children have more than one tumor. Capillary hemangiomas grow rapidly during the first 6 months of life, becoming stable, and do not grow further after the age of about 1 year. During the growth phase of these tumors, only a small percent triple or quadruple in size. The majority grow to at least double their size. The most common sites of these strawberry hemangiomas are the head, neck, and trunk. Involution of capillary and cavernous hemangiomas occurs spontaneously after the first year of life. The early sign of involution is a dull red color. The tumors become somewhat blue-red and then develop areas of gray and white foci. Fifty percent of the tumors resolve within the first 5 years, approximately 70% resolve by the seventh year, and by age 9, 90% have resolved. After resolution, there may be residual erythema, hypopigmentation, or redundant skin. Tumors may ulcerate during regression. Treatment for an ulceration includes the use of drying agents (compresses with vinegar and water 3% solution) and avoiding infection. The use of systemic broad-spectrum antibiotics or topical antibiotics (Bactroban) should be initiated. Large lesions that involve the orbit should be treated by both pediatrician and ophthalmologist.

OTHER VASCULAR SYNDROMES

Blue-Rubber Bleb Nevus Syndrome

Blue-rubber bleb nevus syndrome is a syndrome composed of blue, raised, wrinkled, soft, compressible cutaneous vascular tumors that are tender or painful on pressure. They feel rubbery and spongy to the touch. The cutaneous tumors are associated with angiomas of the gastrointestinal tract, mainly the small intestine or colon. The complications of this syndrome are bleeding from the gut and anemia. Treatment is directed at the complications of bleeding and may require resections of portions of the affected intestine. Early recognition of this condition and aggressive treatment of gastrointestinal lesions may prove lifesaving.

Kasabach-Merritt Syndrome

Kasabach-Merritt syndrome is a syndrome in which there is platelet sequestration in giant hemangiomas, resulting in anemia and thrombocytopenia. The hemangiomas may enlarge suddenly and compress underlying vital structures, or there may be sudden massive hemorrhage. These can be life-threatening complications. Cutaneous lesions may not be a major component of this syndrome. Treatment is directed at blood replacement when needed for anemia or thrombocytopenia. Systemic prednisone 2 mg/kg/d in one dose for a period of 2 to 3 weeks and intralesional corticosteroids (triamcinolone 40 mg/ml) injected into various sites under local or general anesthesia have been used for suppression of hemangioma growth. Intralesional therapy can be given monthly depending on the response and side effects. The response rate is from 20% to 70%. As with all steroid therapy, careful consideration of risks versus benefits should be weighed, since these drugs have significant side effects that are well documented in the literature. This treatment should not be undertaken by the inexperienced.

Interferon alfa-2a has been used in hemangioma therapy in patients who have not responded to corticosteroids or as an initial trial in other patients. The doses have ranged from 2 to 3 million U/m^2. The results have not been striking, but some patients have responded with 45% to 50% tumor regression. Therapy has been given for as short as 1 month or as long as 12 months. Radiation has been and is still being used for hemangioma shrinkage. This should be performed by a pediatric radiotherapist.

Diffuse Neonatal Hemangiomatosis

Hemangiomas are usually present at birth and involve the liver, gastrointestinal tract, lungs, and central nervous system (CNS). The cutaneous component of this syndrome is minimal, with the presence of small red-purple cutaneous papular nodular angiomas. Treatment is not usually effective, and children often die secondary to vascular and circulatory complications that include hemorrhage, arteriovenous shunts, cardiac failure, hepatic failure, and CNS hemorrhage. Corticosteroids used as in the Kasabach-Merritt syndrome have been used to suppress vascular growth in this condition.

Maffucci Syndrome

Maffucci syndrome is more common in males than in females. Vascular osseous malformations consist of dyschondroplasia, hemangiomas, phlebectasias, and lymphangiomas. Patients develop nodules of the fingers and toes, with or without fractures. The incidence of malignancy in the tumors is increased, and patients may develop chondrosarcoma or angiosarcoma. Treatment is directed at management of the cutaneous nodules and malignancies.

Cobb Syndrome

This syndrome consists of CNS and vascular malformations. The vascular changes consist of cutaneous cavernous hemangiomas, angiokeratomas, angiolipomas, and nevus flammeus. The nevus flammeus or angiokeratomas may be in a dermatomal distribution on the trunk or extremity and associated with angiomas of the spinal cord. This condition occurs more commonly in males. The neurologic changes are paralysis, hyperesthesias, and numbness. There may also be bony erosion of the spinal column. Treatment is directed at controlling the spinal angioma, with embolization (ethylene vinyl alcohol) or surgery. With surgical treatment, it is not always possible to effect a complete cure.

Gorham Syndrome

The Gorham syndrome is an osteovascular syndrome in which osteolysis is associated with cutaneous angiomas. Bones may be replaced with fibrous tissue. The cause of the bone loss and of the association with the angiomas is unknown. There is no known effective treatment.

Klippel-Trenaunay-Parks-Weber Syndrome

This syndrome consists of vascular malformations associated with hypertrophy of bone and soft tissue of an extremity. The vascular malformations are capillary hemangiomas or cavernous hemangiomas, arteriovenous shunts, or phlebectasias. Males are more commonly affected than females. Skeletal deformity is a complication of this syndrome. There is no satisfactory treatment.

VASCULAR ECTASIAS

The salmon patch is the most common vascular malformation, occurring in approximately 45% of all newborns. Such patches are found most commonly at the nape of the neck (40%), the glabella, and the eyelid. Salmon patches are macules, pink to red in color, with and without telangiectasia. These lesions redden on crying, do not grow (proliferate), and resolve within the first year of life, except for the nuchal lesions, which often persist into adulthood. No treatment is necessary.

Nevus Flammeus

Nevus flammeus (nevus telangectaticus) or port-wine stain is a vascular malformation present at birth and most commonly located on the face. Nevus flammeus is composed of increased numbers of dilated superficial vascular channels with normal endothelium. These vascular lesions do not proliferate as do capillary hemangiomas, nor do they fade as the child ages. Nevus flammeus becomes darker with age (more purple in color), and the surface becomes verrucous. They are most commonly unilateral in location. Since these vascular malformations do not involute, there have been many types of therapies, almost all unsuccessful. Laser therapy holds the most promise. The argon laser seems to be best suited to correct this malformation, although other dye lasers are being developed. Laser therapy requires multiple treatments and is painful. Children must be prepared for the treatment. The use of EMLA (topical lidocaine 2.5% and prilocaine 2.5%) with occlusion ½ hour before treatment will provide topical anesthesia that will make laser therapy less painful and easier for the patient, parent, and therapist.

Associated Nevus Flammeus Syndrome

Sturge-Weber (encephalofacial or encephalotrigeminal angiomatosis) *syndrome* is characterized by a nevus flammeus in the distribution of the first branch of the trigeminal nerve, as well as associated ipsilateral vascular malformations of the meninges or cerebral cortex. There can be associated focal motor seizures and hemiparesis contralateral to the facial lesions. If the nevus flammeus does not involve the upper eyelids or forehead, an association with CNS involvement is less likely. Patients with CNS involvement have seizures (80%), retardation (60%), hemiplegia (30%), and glaucoma (45%). The cutaneous vascular malformations can be treated with the laser as desired.

MALIGNANT MELANOMA IN CHILDREN

Malignant melanoma, when compared with other cutaneous malignancies, is an uncommon tumor. There appears to be some increase in the incidence of this tumor type owing to today's behavior of continued and persistent sun exposure. In children, the greatest source for the development of malignant melanoma is the congenital nevus. The predicted incidence for the development of melanoma in those with congenital nevi is almost two and a half times that for those who do not have similar lesions. Melanomas in children also arise from acral sites, including the nailbed, palms, and soles. There is a reported increased incidence of melanoma in patients with dysplastic nevus syndrome. True dysplastic nevus syndrome is relatively uncommon, although there are many reports of sporadic dysplastic nevi. Whether the presence of sporadic dysplastic nevi indicates an increased risk for melanoma is debatable.

Treatment

The treatment of malignant melanoma in children is the same as for adults. The critical issue in the treatment of melanoma is its early recognition and diagnosis. In large congenital nevi, early recognition of small areas of malignant change is often difficult, if not impossible, because of the milieu in which the melanoma has developed. Those areas in congenital nevi that become nodular, grow suddenly, or change their characteristics (including becoming inflamed and pruritic) should be attended to with haste. A biopsy of the lesion should be performed. Because congenital nevi of the large garment type often occupy large body areas, excisional surgery for the entire nevus containing the melanomas is not feasible. Melanomas that arise in dysplastic nevi or on acral surfaces should be removed in toto. The histologic assessment provides an aid for further therapy. Malignant melanomas that are in the radial growth phase and occupy only the superficial layer of the papillary dermis (level II thin melanoma) are considered zero-risk melanomas, and complete excision is the treatment of choice. Malignant melanomas that are considerably thicker (>1 mm) should also be totally excised, and the patient should be followed. Whether one should perform a node dissection at the time of primary surgery or later is still open to question. There are some clinicians who believe that if nodes are palpable at the time of the primary excision, a node dissection should be done along with the excision of the melanoma.

New therapies are on the horizon for melanoma, including interferons, interleukins, vaccines, and cancer therapeutic drugs. The use of oral tamoxifen has been introduced for melanoma therapy, and studies are early but promising. Combined therapy with cisplatin, dacarbazine (DTIC), and the nitrosoureas (carmustine) also is being used to treat melanoma and disseminated melanoma. There are specific protocols used by hematology-oncology and cooperative melanoma groups for the various combinations of these agents, including tamoxifen, in treating melanoma and disseminated melanoma. The National Cancer Institute continues to lead in the development of new and innovative therapies in melanoma, including autologous melanoma cell vaccines.

The therapy of melanoma should not be viewed with pessimism, especially when lesions are diagnosed early and the histologic as-

sessment is that of a thin melanoma. Perhaps the most disconcerting patients to treat are those children who have large congenital nevi whose potential risk for the development of melanoma is always in the fore. The best means of treating melanoma is for a physician to engage in judicious, prudent, and prompt follow-up and to watch for change and detail.

OTHER SKIN TUMORS

CYNTHIA GUZZO, M.D.

Cutaneous tumors are common in children, particularly the pigmented lesions already discussed. Fortunately, the majority of tumors in childhood are benign, although each lesion must be carefully evaluated. The cosmetic effect is often of prime concern. Association with underlying syndromes must be excluded with select lesions, and the potential for malignancy, although rare, must be considered.

Cutaneous tumors can be divided into those differentiated from the epidermis, epidermal appendages, dermis, and fat and muscle. The more common lesions are reviewed.

EPIDERMAL TUMORS

The *epidermal nevus* is a benign congenital disorder apparent at birth or in early childhood. Its location is often on the trunk or limb. The lesion is velvety or papillomatous, grayish to yellow brown in color, and round, oval, or linear. Nevus unius lateris refers to extensive and systematized lesions that may appear as whorled patterns over large areas of the body. Epidermal nevus syndrome is a congenital syndrome that includes deformities of the skin (epidermal nevi, hypopigmentation, café au lait spots), skeletal system, central nervous system (CNS), and cardiovascular system.

Malignant degeneration of epidermal nevi is rare. Treatment is difficult and cosmetic in nature. Excision of localized lesions is sometimes possible. Cryosurgery, dermabrasion, or electrodesiccation results in improvement, but subsequent recurrence is frequent.

Basal cell carcinoma is the most common cancer in adults but, with increasing sun exposure, is appearing in adolescents. It is slow-growing, locally invasive, and usually nonmetastasizing. Often located on the face and upper trunk, it appears as a pearly erythematous papule with telangiectasias that can develop central necrosis with growth. Variants, including pigmented forms, exist. Its occurrence in childhood is seen with xeroderma pigmentosum, nevus sebaceus of Jadassohn, and basal cell nevus syndrome. Basal cell nevus syndrome is an autosomal dominant disorder often presenting with multiple basal cell carcinomas appearing in puberty. Associated abnormalities include temporal bossing, dental cysts, bifid ribs, intracranial calcification, ovarian fibromas, and, rarely, medulloblastomas. Basal cell carcinomas should be removed completely, or local recurrence occurs. Lesions can be surgically excised or removed by curettage and electrodesiccation.

Squamous cell carcinoma is a malignant tumor rarely seen in children except in those affected by xeroderma pigmentosum. Lesions arise as solitary nodules with central ulceration and an indurated base in sun-exposed skin. Metastatic potential is greater than that for basal cell cancers. Treatment is by surgical excision or curettage and electrodesiccation.

TUMORS OF EPIDERMAL APPENDAGES

Nevus sebaceus usually presents at birth or early childhood as a yellow to orange, oval or linear plaque on the scalp or face. It often becomes verrucous at puberty. Also during adolescence or adulthood, 10% to 15% of lesions develop secondary neoplastic changes, most commonly basal cell carcinoma. Local prophylactic excision is recommended.

A *trichofolliculoma* is a benign, solitary, flesh-colored papule with a central pore and protruding hair on the face. It is derived from the hair follicle. It is rarely seen in children. Excision is for cosmetic reasons.

Trichoepithelioma may present as a solitary nonhereditary tumor in early adult life or as a dominantly inherited disorder with multiple lesions appearing in early childhood or at puberty. A firm 2- to 5-mm flesh-colored papule on the face characterizes the solitary form. Hereditary, multiple trichoepitheliomas are located on the central face. Surgical excision is the treatment of choice for solitary lesions. Therapy of multiple lesions is difficult, and electrodesiccation, cryotherapy, or dermabrasion is followed by recurrence. Differentiation from basal cell carcinoma is necessary.

Syringomas, tumors of eccrine ducts, frequently present during puberty as 1- to 3-mm skin-colored papules on the lower eyelids. Generalized lesions can occur on the neck, upper thorax, abdomen, extremities, and genitalia. Lesions are frequent in Down syndrome, affecting up to one third of individuals. Treatment is cosmetic by electrodesiccation, cryotherapy, or excision.

The *pilomatrixoma,* an uncommon benign tumor of hair structures, usually develops during childhood or adolescence. It appears as a reddish blue 0.5- to 2-cm, hard nodule on the head, neck, or upper extremities. Treatment is by excision for cosmetic purposes.

The *eccrine poroma* is a benign tumor arising from the sweat duct. Usually appearing in adulthood, it can occur in adolescence, presenting as a firm, reddish nodule usually less than 1 cm on the foot or occasionally the palm. Surgical excision is the treatment of choice.

DERMAL TUMORS

Angiofibromas occur rarely as solitary lesions not associated with systemic disease or more commonly as multiple lesions and, therefore, a cutaneous sign of tuberous sclerosis. Pink or flesh-colored papules (1 to 4 mm) appear on the central face, generally in early childhood but occasionally not until puberty. They are hamartomas of fibrous and vascular tissue. Treatment for cosmetic improvement is best accomplished with cryosurgery, electrodesiccation and curettage, or dermabrasion. Recurrence is common.

Connective tissue nevi may be single or multiple, skin-colored papules or nodules, 0.5 to 2 cm in size, occurring anywhere on the body and appearing at birth or in early childhood. They are localized malformations of dermal collagen or elastic fibers. The solitary lesion is usually not associated with underlying disease. In the Buschke-Ollendorff syndrome, multiple widespread connective tissue nevi are associated with osteopoikilosis. The shagreen patch is a large connective tissue nevus seen in tuberous sclerosis. After diagnosis by biopsy, treatment is unnecessary.

Juvenile xanthogranulomas are yellow to red-brown papules and nodules on the head, neck, proximal extremities, and trunk, occurring at birth or within the first year of life. Numbers may vary from 1 to several hundred. Lesions are composed of histiocytes. The majority of cases resolve within several years and are limited to the skin. Systemic involvement may occur, most often in the eye and less frequently in the lung, pericardium, meninges, liver, spleen, and testes. Ocular tumors can result in glaucoma, hemorrhage, or blindness. Children with the disease should be examined by an ophthalmologist.

Mastocytosis is a group of clinical disorders characterized by the accumulation of mast cells within the skin. The most common variants in children are localized lesions, mastocytomas, and multiple diffuse lesions, urticaria pigmentosa. A mastocytoma is a 1- to 5-cm, light brown to yellow nodule often localized on the arms, neck, or trunk. Lesions of urticaria pigmentosa are red-brown, 3- to 5-mm papules scattered symmetrically, often on the trunk. Solitary and multiple lesions display Darier's sign, urtication after stroking. Common cutaneous symptoms include pruritus and blistering. Systemic disease with infiltration of mast cells in the bone marrow, gastrointestinal track, bone, and liver occurs and can be associated with flushing,

hypotension, and diarrhea. Resolution occurs in some children as they grow older. Antihistamines are helpful, but therapy of cutaneous lesions is difficult.

Neurofibromas are tumors of connective tissue and nerve fiber that often first appear in childhood as solitary lesions not associated with systemic disease or as multiple lesions seen in neurofibromatosis. Solitary neurofibromas are soft, polypoid, flesh-colored papules that invaginate with pressure. Lesions associated with neurofibromatosis usually increase in number and may grow to large sizes. Therapy is by surgical excision for cosmetic or comfort purposes.

Dermatofibromas are benign growths of connective tissue appearing as red-brown, 1- to 3-mm nodules fixed to the skin and movable over the subcutaneous fat. They usually occur on extremities more commonly in adults than in children. Treatment is by excision for cosmetic purposes only.

Recurring digital fibromas of childhood, tumors of fibroblasts and collagen, appear as smooth, shiny, erythematous nodules on the distal phalanges of infants and young children. Management is controversial. Spontaneous resolution has been reported, and observation is suggested by some. If surgery is necessary, recurrence is frequent, and dissection down to the periosteum is necessary.

Epidermal cysts are skin-colored, 0.5- to 5-cm nodules, often with central pores, appearing after puberty on the head or upper torso. They result from proliferation of surface epidermal cells situated within the dermis, with subsequent production of keratin. Excision is the treatment of choice.

A *keloid* is an exaggerated connective tissue response to skin injury that is composed of dense bundles of collagen. It appears following injury to the skin and may occur at any age, although it is more frequent between puberty and age 30. It is more common in darkly pigmented races. Lesions are firm and smooth and extend irregularly beyond the original scar. Intralesional corticosteroids are the therapy of choice. Excision followed by corticosteroid injections can be attempted, but recurrence is frequent.

TUMORS OF FAT AND MUSCLE

A *lipoma* is a benign tumor composed of mature fat cells seen at any age but usually first occurring at puberty. Located on the upper body, the lipoma is a soft nodule of variable size. Treatment is usually not required but, if necessary, is by excision.

A *leiomyoma* is a benign tumor composed of smooth muscle that is uncommon in children. Lesions may be solitary or multiple. They are pink or dusky brown, firm nodules associated with intermittent episodes of pain. Multiple lesions are located on the face, back, or extremities, whereas solitary lesions are often on the genitalia, breasts, and lower extremities. Treatment is by wide surgical excision, but recurrence is frequent.

REFERENCE

1. Hurwitz S: Clinical Pediatric Dermatology: A Textbook of Skin Disorders of Childhood and Adolescence, 2nd ed. Philadelphia, W.B. Saunders Co, 1993:198–241.

GENODERMATOSIS

JAMES E. RASMUSSEN, M.D.

The genetic diseases that primarily affect the skin number in the hundreds, and there are thousands of syndromes that feature some cutaneous manifestations. Our genetic makeup also determines how we handle environmental factors, diseases, and responses to drugs. Although the number of identified genes and chromosomes responsible for skin diseases is approximately two dozen (Table 1), the list will undoubtedly become much longer. For most of these diseases, there

TABLE 1. Skin Disease and the Human Genome

1p	Dysplastic nevus syndrome		11q	Albinism
	Ehlers-Danlos VI			Tyrosinase-negative
2q	Ehlers-Danlos			Tyrosinase-positive
	XP-B		11q22-23	Ataxia telangiectasia
	Waardenburg's syndrome		12q	EBS (K5), EHK
3p	Dystrophic epidermolysis		13q	XP-G
	bullosa		15q	Albinism, Tyrosinase-positive
	Dominant			tive
	Recessive		16p	Tuberous sclerosis
4q	Piebaldism		17p	Squamous cell carcinoma,
6p	Bullous pemphigoid Ag1			BCC
9p	Melanoma		17q	EBS (K14), EHK (K10),
9q	BCC, keratoacanthoma			Neurofibromatosis type I
	Tuberous sclerosis		19q	XP-D
	XP-A		Xp	Lamellar ichthyosis (x-linked recessive)
	Nail-patella syndrome			(steroid sulfatase)
			Xq	Ectodermal dysplasia

BCC = basal cell carcinoma, EBS = epidermolysis bullosa simplex, EHK = epidermolytic hyperkeratosis, XP = xeroderma pigmentosum.

is little therapy other than palliation. Knowledge of specific genes and their protein products at least offers hope for early diagnosis and holds tremendous future promise for more rational development of drugs and, eventually, genetic manipulation.

Every component of the skin can be affected by genetic diseases, but only a small number, with a few examples in each category, are considered in this brief review of therapy.

EPIDERMIS

Mild Ichthyosis

The two milder types of ichthyosis are dominant ichthyosis vulgaris and X-linked ichthyosis. The scaling in these conditions can be treated with lubricants, such as petrolatum (Vaseline), hydrophilic petrolatum (Aquaphor), and creams (Eucerin, Nivea, and many others). It is important to realize that water is the best lubricating agent and is the quickest way to soften scaly skin. However, unless something is put on to prevent the evaporation of water, its effects are short lived. Consequently, prolonged bathing followed by lubricants is an excellent way to keep the skin hydrated. Climates with high humidity and heat, such as the southeastern United States, produce less severe manifestations of ichthyosis than do the colder, dryer portions of the midwest during the winter.

Another excellent group of lubricating agents is the alpha-hydroxic acids. Examples include lactic acid (Lac-Hydrin and Lacticare), glycolic acid (Aquaglycolic lotion and others), and salicylic acid (Keralyt and others). Urea at concentrations of 10% to 20% (Carmol, Aquacare) is also an excellent lubricant. However, alpha-hydroxic acids and urea can be irritating when applied to the skin.

It is also possible to treat these types of ichthyosis with topical preparations of transretinoic acid (Retin-A). In practice, however, this class of drug is so irritating that very few patients will continue with long-term therapy.

Severe Ichthyosis: Lamellar Ichthyosis (Recessive) and Epidermolytic Hyperkeratosis (Dominant)

These are the two most severe forms of ichthyosis, producing significant cosmetic and functional impairment. Consequently, therapy tends to be used somewhat more aggressively. In addition to the lubricants described, alpha-hydroxic acids and keratolytics, such systemic retinoids as 13-cis-retinoic acid (Accutane) and etretinate (Tegison) may be appropriate. Both these drugs are potent teratogens and have significant long-term skeletal effects. Earlier concern about premature closure of eiphyses has been reported on only a few occasions,

and apparently these do not, in general, interfere with normal growth and development.

Darier's Disease

This dominant condition does not usually manifest itself until later childhood or midadolescence, when a tremendous number of dirty-brown papules appear on the face and midline areas of the trunk. They are objectionable in appearance and are commonly accompanied by an unpleasant odor. In addition to treatment with lubricants and keratolytics, topical and systemic antibiotics and degerming agents are often successful in reducing the odor. Iodine-containing soaps (Betadine and others), chlorhexidine (Hibiclens), and baking soda are useful topically. Occasionally, patients with severe Darier's disease will benefit from treatment with systemic retinoids, such as 13-cis-retinoic acid and etretinate. These have significant long-term and short-term side effects and should be used with great care in the pediatric population.

Epidermal Blistering Diseases

Epidermolysis bullosa simplex (dominant) has been shown to be due to genetically abnormal keratins 5 and 14, which provide internal structure and support for the keratinocytes. These defects produce epidermal blisters at sites of trauma. Soft shoes, a cool environment, and local wound care are of some benefit. Some cases improve at puberty.

MELANOCYTES: ALBINISM

Both dominant and recessive forms of albinism have been described, and although there is no specific treatment, it is important to emphasize sun protection. People with albinism are exquisitely sensitive to the acute and chronic effects of sunburn, skin aging and carcinogenesis. Affected children should be encouraged to avoid sun exposure and to use protective clothing and sunscreens throughout life. A hat, long-sleeved clothing, and development of lifestyles that avoid sun exposure are the mainstays of preventive therapy. Sunscreens are available in a wide choice of vehicles (creams, lotions, gels, sprays, and ointments) and are appropriate for children at any age. In addition to increasing the potency of sunscreens (an SPF of at least 15 should be a minimum), several new sunscreens cover both the UVA and UVB spectra (Shade UVA, Photoplex).

Patients with albinism usually have severe visual problems that should be evaluated at a very early age. A very small percentage also will have other systemic abnormalities, such as deafness and coagulation disorders. Patients with albinism should be screened on a regular basis for the premature development of actinic keratoses, basal cell carcinomas, squamous cell carcinomas, and melanomas.

HAIR DISORDERS

There is a wide variety of hereditary hair disorders that feature fragile shafts (monilethrix and others), sparse hair (hereditary hypotrichosis, anhydrotic ectodermal dysplasia), absent scalp hair (congenital atrichia), and acquired hair loss (androgenetic alopecia). In addition, genetics play a significant role in patients with alopecia areata and tumors of the hair germ (trichoepitheliomas). There is no specific therapy for any of these disorders, except for androgenetic alopecia. Topical minoxidil (Rogaine) is the first and only scientifically proven drug to help regrow hair and decrease the rate of loss. This condition can be present during later teenage life, and the availability of somewhat effective therapy is important. Minoxidil is applied twice daily, with about 10% of patients achieving a satisfactory result. Another 40% to 50% will notice a significant reduction in hair loss, and the other 50% will notice no significant improvement. Minoxidil is not known to be associated with any significant side effects. Undoubtedly, more effective compounds will be marketed.

SWEAT GLANDS

Decreased to absent glands and diminished function occur in anhydrotic ectodermal dysplasia, an X-linked syndrome featuring sparse to absent scalp hair, protuberant ears, flattened nasal root, prominent lips, periorbital hyperpigmentation, and short stature. The most significant manifestation is anhydrosis, which produces increased sensitivity to febrile illnesses and changes in ambient temperature. Patients should be encouraged to avoid stressful physical activity, and vigorous therapy with antipyretics should be used, especially during childhood. Special suits similar to those used by astronauts are available for close environmental monitoring in very hot climates.

DERMIS

The primary function of the dermis is to provide support and containment for the skin, blood vessels, nerves, and appendages. Disturbances of collagen metabolism can manifest as lack of formation (Goltz syndrome), dermal blistering (epidermolysis bullosa dystrophica), and disorders of elasticity (Ehlers-Danlos syndrome).

Goltz Syndrome

Goltz syndrome (focal dermal hypoplasia) is inherited as an X-linked recessive disorder. Affected females show a tremendous variety of cutaneous, skeletal, and ophthalmologic problems. The main treatment is surgical correction.

Epidermolysis Bullosa Dystrophica

This is inherited as either a recessive or (less commonly) a dominant disease. It features deeply placed bullae that heal with minor or severe degrees of scarring because of abnormalities of type 7 collagen (anchoring fibrils). No effective therapy is known except for providing optimum conditions for wound healing. Parents and patients should be made aware of the local chapter of DEBRA (Dystrophic Epidermolysis Bullosa Research Association), which can be a valuable source for commonsense information on wound management, dental hygiene, and nutrition. Surgical correction may be necessary for scarring syndactyly. Any chronic scarring disease can develop the late complication of squamous cell carcinoma. Although initial uncontrolled reports indicated that phenytoin was effective in reducing the blistering by an inhibitory effect on collagenase, a recent blinded and controlled study showed no effect.

Ehlers-Danlos Syndrome

Ehlers-Danlos syndrome has a variety of genotypes and phenotypes. Affected individuals may show severe disorders of elasticity in the skin, arterial vessels, or ligaments. These may be manifest as hyperelastic skin, double jointedness, or poor wound healing and by the late development of arterial aneurysms and ruptures. No specific therapy is available, although some types may be responsive to high doses of vitamin C.

BLOOD VESSELS

Osler-Weber-Rendu syndrome features the autosomal dominant inheritance of a tendency to form superficial ectasias of arterial capillaries. These manifest as small, red telangiectasia on the face, mucous membranes, trunk, extremities, palms, and subungual areas. The disease has its onset in childhood or adolescence with excessive nosebleeds that may progress to severe blood loss. These superficial telangiectasias can be treated with any type of surgical modality, although the CO_2 laser is commonly used on mucous membranes. The tunable dye laser is also useful for both cosmetic and functional improvement.

NERVES

Neurofibromatosis, inherited in an autosomal dominant fashion, is one of the most common genetic diseases, although 30% to 50% of patients have no family history of the disease. Type I features the development of cutaneous café au lait spots and neurofibromas, with relatively milder expression in other organs. Type II features acoustic neuromas. Each is inherited independently. Some of the newer types of lasers (pigmented lesion laser, copper vapor laser) may be used for eradicating café au lait spots. Neurofibromas may be surgically removed if located in cosmetically important sites or if they result in functional impairment, as they may with plexiform neurofibromas. Symptomatic neurofibromas located in deeply seated organs should be surgically removed. Patients with neurofibromatosis can have other systemic manifestations that are not directly related to the development of neurofibromas, such as hyperthyroidism and pheochromocytomas resulting in hypertension. Low intelligence, short stature, and generalized pruritus have been noted in a small percentage of patients.

IMMUNE SYSTEM

Although not commonly thought of as genetic disorders, atopic dermatitis and psoriasis are probably primary disorders of the immune system that have a tendency to affect the skin.

Atopic Dermatitis

Of patients with atopic dermatitis, 60% to 80% have a family history of asthma, hayfever, or atopic dermatitis. Primary therapy is involved with lubricating the skin (Aquaphor and others) and suppressing inflammation (topical corticosteroids, such as 1% hydrocortisone, 0.1% triamcinolone, and 0.025% triamcinolone). In addition, patients with atopic dermatitis may have a component of allergic reactions to foods, cutaneous microorganisms *(Pityrosporum ovale),* and environmental allergens (house dust mite). Avoidance, immunotherapy, or in the case of *Pityrosporum,* treatment with antifungal agents (Nizoral) may be appropriate. Other therapies for patients with more severe atopic dermatitis include systemic corticosteroids, ultraviolet light, and in the case of life-threatening disease, interferon gamma or cyclosporine.

Psoriasis

Psoriasis has its onset in childhood or the teenage years in approximately 30% to 40% of patients. About 40% to 60% of patients have an affected first-degree relative. The disease can be treated topically with corticosteroids, such as 0.1% triamcinolone (Kenalog, Aristocort, and generics), desoximetasone (Topicort), and clobetasol (Temovate). Potent corticosteroids are not appropriate in intertriginous sites or the diaper area or for prolonged use in any patient. They are not usually given to very young patients. Psoriasis also responds to ultraviolet light from the sun or artificial light cabinets. Coal tar preparations are historically of interest, although they probably contribute relatively little to improvement of the disease. They are available in the forms of ointments (crude coal tar 2% to 5% in petrolatum), creams (10% L.C.D.), gels (Estar gel, Psorygel), and bath additives (Balnetar and others). Finally, anthralin 0.1% to 1% (Anthra-Derm and others) is definitely a useful agent in the treatment of psoriasis. Because of its tendency to produce irritation and discoloration of the skin, it is usually used in a fashion that bears the acronym SCAT (short-contact anthralin therapy), 15 to 30 minute applications followed by vigorous removal.

Systemic agents available for the treatment of psoriasis include methotrexate, sulfasalazine, and psoralen and ultraviolet light A (PUVA) and for those severe life-threatening cases, cyclosporine and retinoids. Because of the long-term consequences of PUVA, methotrexate, cyclosporine, and retinoids, these agents are usually not given to children except in the case of erythroderma or pustular psoriasis.

DISORDERS OF PHOTOSENSITIVITY

The classic recessive genetic disease in this category is xeroderma pigmentosum. Patients are usually noted in early childhood to have severe photosensitivity, followed within a few years by the onset of bizarre hyperpigmented freckles. In later childhood or early adolescence, patients will develop a variety of premalignant and malignant tumors, such as basal cell epithelioma, squamous cell carcinoma, and melanoma. Patients also are susceptible to more deeply seated tumors of fibrous and vascular tissue, such as sarcomas.

Many different clinical varieties of disorders of photosensitivity exist, but most feature an inability to repair ultraviolet-induced DNA damage, which is the basis of the laboratory diagnosis.

Treatment consists of prevention and removal of premalignant and malignant growths. Prevention should begin as early as possible in childhood as the diagnosis can be made because it involves a radical change in the patient's and parents' lifestyle. Outdoor daytime activities should be strictly forbidden. Standard preventive measures include a broad-brimmed hat, full body clothing, and a sunscreen with as high an SPF and as broad a coverage as is possible. Older children and adolescents should be encouraged to wear heavy titanium-containing sunscreens and makeup, such as Dermablend and Covermark. No one in the home should smoke. Premalignant lesions, such as actinic keratoses, are usually treated with liquid nitrogen cryosurgery, although topical use of 5-fluorouracil (Efudex, Floraplex) also may be helpful. Lesions suspected of malignancy should be biopsied and treated.

Although systemic retinoids, such as 13-*cis*-retinoic acid and etretinate, have been shown to be of value in reducing the development of malignant and premalignant lesions, a rebound effect occurs when these drugs are discontinued. In addition, since the dose necessary to achieve a significant reduction in the number of lesions is higher than normal, it will be associated with a significant number of side effects. Decisions whether to use this modality must be made on a case-by-case basis and not be taken lightly. Dermabrasion and skin peels show promise in preventing malignancies and are certainly of cosmetic appeal. Whether they are truly of value will be determined by longer-range studies.

GENETIC COUNSELING

Patients and their parents will benefit from long-term genetic counseling. At present, it is not possible to use a gene cream or a gene gun to correct the genetic defect. Rational family planning, however, cannot be made without a full knowledge of the scope and inheritance pattern of the disease. With the ability to identify affected carriers of recessive disorders, it may be possible to use in vivo fertilization techniques. In addition, prenatal diagnosis is practical for some of these disorders and theoretically possible for many others.

PATIENT-ORIENTED GROUPS

I think that individuals and their parents may benefit tremendously from contact with patient-oriented associations. These are often a source of commonsense tips for management of the disease and social get-togethers. In addition, they are proving to be potent lobbying agents for research funding of their particular diseases. The following is a list of a few of these organizations.

National Alopecia Areata Foundation
P.O. Box 150760
San Rafael, CA 94915
(415) 456-4644

National Foundation for Ectodermal Dysplasias
219 East Main Street, Box 114
Mascoutah, IL 62258
(618) 566-2020

Eczema Association for Science & Education
1221 S.W. Yamhill, Suite 303
Portland, OR 97205
(503) 228-4430

National Eczema Society
4 Tavistock Place
London WC1H 8Ra
England
071-388-4097

Ehlers Danlos National Foundation
P.O. Box 1212
Southgate, MI 48195
(313) 282-0180

DEBRA (Dystrophic Epidermolysis Bullosa Research Association of America, Inc.)
141 Fifth Avenue
New York, NY 10010
(212) 995-2220

National Epidermolysis Bullosa Registry Data Collecting & Coordinating Center
Rockefeller University
1230 York Avenue, W214
New York, NY 10021-6399
(212) 327-8280

Alliance of Genetics Support Groups
Suite 440
35 Wisconsin Circle
Chevy Chase, MD 20815
(301) 652-5553

FIRST (Foundation for Ichthyosis & Related Skin Types, Inc.)
P.O. Box 20921
Raleigh, NC 27619-0921
(800) 545-3286

National Neurofibromatosis Foundation
141 Fifth Avenue, Suite 7-S
New York, NY 10010
(800) 323-7938
(212) 460-8980

National Psoriasis Foundation
6443 S.W. Beaverton Highway, Suite 210
P.O. Box 9009
Portland, OR 97221
(503) 297-1545

NORD (National Organization for Rare Disorders)
Box 8923
New Fairfield, CT 06812-1783
(203) 746-6518

National Tuberous Sclerosis Association
8000 Corporate Drive, Suite 120
Landover, MD 20785
(800) CAL-NTSA (225-6872)
(301) 459-9888

National Vitiligo Foundation
P.O. Box 6337
Tyler, TX 75711
(903) 534-2925

Xeroderma Pigmentosum Registry
Department of Pathology
UMDNJ-New Jersey Medical School
185 South Orange Avenue
Newark, NJ 07103
(201) 456-4405

REFERENCE

1. Alper JC (ed): Genetic Disorders of the Skin. St. Louis, Mosby-Year Book, 1991.

DISORDERS OF THE HAIR AND SCALP

STEPHEN E. GELLIS, M.D.

Disorders of the hair and scalp can be categorized into congenital or acquired. Only the most common of these are discussed.

CONGENITAL ABNORMALITIES OF THE SCALP

Nevus Sebaceous

Nevus sebaceous, a birthmark of unknown etiology, appears as a well-circumscribed patch with an orange-yellow color and a sticky uneven surface. In some instances, it may be linear in shape and have a raised cobblestone surface. Apart from a rare association with central nervous system (CNS) abnormalities (linear nevus sebaceous syndrome), it is significant for a high degree of malignant degeneration later in life. Management includes either prophylactic excision or close surveillance for changes.

Aplasia Cutis Congenita

Aplasia cutis is a birthmark that usually appears as a single erosion or crusted lesion near the vertex of the scalp. As it gradually heals, it is replaced by a hairless, atrophic, shiny area of scalp that is often indented. On palpation, there is a lack of subcutaneous tissue, and the bony structures of the skull may be easily appreciated. The cause of this congenital defect is usually unknown, although there occasionally is a history of a twin pregnancy and the fetal demise of one twin earlier in the pregnancy. In rare instances, there may be associated CNS abnormalities. Treatment is not required unless the defect is cosmetically undesirable, in which case surgical excision can be undertaken.

Meningocele, Encephalocele, and Dermoid Cysts

These lesions may present as subcutaneous masses often in the midline of the scalp. There may be overlying abnormalities in the scalp, including defects in the surrounding hair pattern. Radiologic imaging or ultrasonography to rule out intercommunication with the CNS is essential before surgical intervention.

CONGENITAL ALOPECIA

There are many causes of alopecia. Among these are a group of congenital syndromes displaying distinct abnormalities of the hair shaft. These can be appreciated on microscopic examination (trichorrhexis nodosa, monilethrix, trichorrhexis invaginate). Some have a metabolic abnormality (trichothiodystrophy, Menkes' syndrome). There is no therapy for most of these conditions.

ACQUIRED ALOPECIA

Alopecia Areata

Alopecia areata is a common cause of hair loss in children. It usually presents with the sudden appearance of a bald spot. It may resolve spontaneously over several months or progress to involve large areas of scalp. Tapered short hairs less than 1 cm long resembling exclamation points may be seen early in the disease and are diagnostic. There may be a positive family history of alopecia or a history of other autoimmune diseases. In severe cases, complete loss of scalp hair, as well as eyebrows, eyelashes, and body hair, may occur. The natural history is unpredictable.

Although many therapies have been tried, none are proven effective in every case, and in many instances, nothing works. There is no evidence to suggest that therapy will alter the natural history of the disease in a particular patient. A potent topical steroid solution can be applied once or twice a day to the involved scalp for 2 to 3 months. If no response is seen, a topical sensitizer may be tried next. Anthralin has been used with some success, as have dinitrochlorobenzene and squaric acid. These therapies should be prescribed by a clinician familiar with their use. Phototherapy with either oral or topical psoralen in combination with ultraviolet light has had some success. Systemic corticosteroids usually produce a regrowth of hair that cannot be maintained without continuation of this medication. Because of the development of long-term side effects, corticosteroids should be avoided. Intralesional injection of corticosteroids is often effective but painful and not appropriate for small children.

Trichotillomania

Trichotillomania may occur in children of all ages. The hair loss is caused by the child who surreptitiously or unconsciously pulls out or breaks off hair by twisting or rubbing. The areas of hair loss are well defined and often of a bizarre pattern. Hairs of varying lengths may be a clue to the diagnosis. In some cases, the child will admit to manipulating the hair. Children who display this tendency often may be emotionally disturbed and need psychologic evaluation. Treatment may include psychopharmacologic intervention.

INFLAMMATORY CONDITIONS

Tinea Capitis

Tinea capitis is a common problem in children living in urban settings. There are two clinical presentations in children. Some children present with diffuse hair loss and a fine scaling of the scalp. In other children, there is a sudden appearance of pustules and crusting and the occasional development of a large boggy mass (kerion).

Treatment should not be initiated without a definitive diagnosis. This can be accomplished either by microscopic examination of hairs for fungal spores or by culture. The appropriate specimen of hair consists of a "black dot," a tiny stubble less than 1 mm long. Normal length hairs will usually not show infection. Wood's light fluorescence is often misinterpreted and is only diagnostic in the minority of cases (*Microsporum canis*). After establishing the diagnosis, systemic therapy (oral griseofulvin) is required. Topical antifungals will not eradicate tinea capitis. There are two forms of griseofulvin: micronized and ultramicronized. The ultramicronized form has a greater bioavailability and is equivalent to twice the micronized dose. The recommended dose is 15 mg/kg/d for the micronized form and 7.5 mg/kg/d for the ultramicronized preparation. The liquid suspension is micronized and available as 125 mg/5 ml. The daily dose can be divided into two or three doses and is best absorbed with fatty meals. The usual course of treatment is 6 weeks. Success of treatment can be assessed by the absence of scaling and broken-off hairs and regrowth of hair.

Complications of treatment include the rare possibility of pancytopenia and elevation of liver function tests. Monitoring laboratory tests (complete blood count with differential and liver function tests) may be recommended when the course of treatment is prolonged beyond 6 weeks. The appearance of a generalized, fine, papular rash at the onset of treatment is an occasional problem and usually represents a hypersensitivity reaction to the release of fungal antigens. Differentiating this rash from a drug-induced eruption may be difficult and may require the discontinuance of the drug and careful reinstitution. Treatment failures may occur because of poor absorption of the medication or interference from another medication that affects the cytochrome P450 system (anticonvulsants). Relapses are also a problem and are usually due to failure to diagnose and treat other family members. Treatment of inflammatory lesions (kerions) is controversial. A combination of antibiotics, systemic corticosteroids, and griseofulvin has been used in this condition. However, this combination has not been proven to be more effective than griseofulvin administered alone.

Psoriasis

Psoriasis of the scalp usually appears in association with a generalized eruption. On occasion, it may be isolated to the scalp. Its appearance is characterized by either patches of fine white scale or thick clumps of adherent gray scale. There may be associated pruritus. The treatment can be messy and difficult. It first consists of removing the thick scale, which can be accomplished by applying keratolytic gels or lotions (Keralyt, Epilyt). These products are most effective if applied to dampened hair and left on overnight under the occlusion of a shower cap. In the morning, the hair is washed with a tar-containing shampoo. After several days of treatment when the scale has been removed, the keratolytic is discontinued, and a potent topical steroid lotion (Diprolene, Temovate) can be applied to the scalp after shampooing. In stubborn cases, overnight treatment with a combination of a topical steroid in an oil base (Dermasmoothe-FS) may be helpful. As the condition improves, the strength of the topical steroid should be reduced. There is some evidence implicating *Pityrosporum* colonization as a cause of psoriasis. Therefore, ketoconazole-containing shampoo can be tried and can be used several times per week for 1 to 2 months.

DISORDERS OF THE SEBACEOUS GLANDS AND SWEAT GLANDS

STEPHEN E. GELLIS, M.D.

DISORDERS OF THE SEBACEOUS GLANDS

Acne, a common skin problem that is seen to some extent in almost all patients, may begin in children as young as 8 years of age. Whereas some teenagers may be overly concerned about what appears to be mild acne, others may deny the presence of a severe problem. Often, it is the parent who expresses the most concern and whose involvement may be viewed negatively by the adolescent.

It is important to obtain a history that includes the date of onset of the problem, family history, presence of other medical problems, including endocrine disorders, current medications, prior therapies, and external factors, such as activities that may exacerbate acne (e.g., athletic endeavors requiring helmets or shoulder padding or involvement in food preparation with exposure to grease-filled kitchens).

Next, an assessment of the type and degree of skin involvement is made. *Mild acne* is characterized by open and closed comedones (plugged sebaceous follicles) with little erythema. *Moderate acne* cases show pustules, papules, and erythema, with early scar formation. *Severe acne* cases involve multiple inflamed nodules with significant scarring.

The treatment should be individualized. A patient who has a tendency to produce postinflammatory hyperpigmentation following minor comedonal acne may require aggressive systemic treatment.

Mild Acne

Mild acne can be successfully managed with topical preparations. These include benzoyl peroxide, retinoic acid, and topical antibiotics. It is important to explain to the patient that topical preparations are applied not only to the lesions but also to the areas in which the lesions tend to form.

Benzoyl Peroxide

The easiest and least expensive treatment for mild acne is benzoyl peroxide, which reduces bacteria, produces desquamation, and lowers sebum production. It is available over the counter and by prescription in soaps, washes, creams, gels, and scrubs. The concentration ranges from 2.5% to 10%. Benzoyl peroxide is usually applied to the skin twice a day. The main side effect is excessive drying, which can be avoided by selecting the lower-strength products or those that are compounded with emollient bases and by decreasing the frequency of application.

Retinoic Acid (Retin-A)

For extensive numbers of comedones not responding to benzoyl peroxide, retinoic acid can be added. Retinoic acid produces desquamation and reduces comedones. It is available in various strengths. The cream forms are less irritating than the gels and the liquid preparation. The available forms are, in increasing strength and irritancy: 0.025% cream, 0.05% cream, 0.1% cream, 0.01% gel, 0.025% gel, and 0.05% liquid. The medication is usually applied at night, confining the application of benzoyl peroxide to another time of day. Simultaneous application of both agents may produce inactivation. Retinoic acid should be applied to dry skin to minimize irritation. Some redness and peeling are desired. If irritation occurs, the frequency of application should be reduced. Patients should be told to expect some possible worsening of the condition in the first 1 to 2 months of use. Use in fair-skinned individuals during the summer may have to be curtailed because of increased sensitivity to the sun.

Topical Antibiotics

If a small number of inflammatory lesions are present, a topical antibiotic can be used along with benzoyl peroxide and retinoic acid. The most commonly prescribed topical antibiotics include erythromycin and clindamycin. They are available in gels, creams, and solutions and are applied twice a day.

Moderate Acne

Moderate acne characterized by extensive inflammatory lesions often necessitates initial treatment with systemic antibiotics to avoid the development of scarring. This is undertaken in combination with the previously discussed topical preparations.

Oral Antibiotics

The most commonly used oral antibiotics include tetracycline, erythromycin, minocycline, and doxycycline. The initial choice may be determined by cost and convenience.

Tetracycline is best absorbed on an empty stomach. Because an empty stomach is an unusual occurrence in most male teenagers, erythromycin may be a better choice in this patient population. The starting dose for both tetracycline and erythromycin is usually 1 g/d divided into two, three, or four doses. School schedules and other activities make twice-a-day administration the most practical. The dose can be increased to 1.5 g.

Tetracycline may cause an increased tendency for vaginal yeast infections to develop. It can also cause a photosensitivity in some patients. Another potential complication of both tetracycline and erythromycin is interference with the effectiveness of birth control medication. This may be due to alterations in the metabolism of the oral contraceptive. Patients should be warned to take additional contraceptive precautions if breakthrough bleeding occurs. Once improvement occurs, the antibiotic dose may be lowered.

For minocycline and doxycycline, an initial dose of 50 to 100 mg is prescribed. This can be increased up to a total of 200 mg/d. Minocycline can produce dizziness and hyperpigmentation, which is first noticeable along the hard palate or over the anterior tibias. If such side effects occur, the drug should be discontinued.

Severe Acne

13-cis-Retinoic Acid

For severe acne consisting of inflammatory nodules and scarring that fails to respond to conventional treatments, 13-*cis*-retinoic acid (Accutane) may be considered. It should be prescribed only by those familiar with the potential complications. Accutane must not be used in patients who are pregnant or who may become pregnant while undergoing treatment.

Major fetal abnormalities related to Accutane have been reported. Women of childbearing age should be counseled on the risk to a fetus if the drug is taken while pregnant. A negative pregnancy test should be obtained 2 weeks before initiating treatment. Treatment can begin on day 2 or 3 of the next menstrual cycle. An effective form of contraception should be used beginning 1 month before treatment and continuing until 1 month after its cessation. The usual course of treatment is 20 weeks.

Other side effects include dry skin causing epistaxis, cheilitis and conjunctivitis, pseudotumor cerebri (particularly when Accutane is given with tetracycline), depression, fatigue, muscle ache, and skeletal hyperostosis. Abnormal laboratory findings seen in some patients include hypertriglyceride and elevated sedimentation rates. The usual dose is 1 mg/kg.

Steroids

Intralesional steroid injections offer another useful therapy for inflammatory nodules. Triamcinolone acetonide at a concentration of 2.5 to 5.0 mg/ml can be injected intralesionally into a nodule. Resolution usually results within 24 hours.

Before commencing any form of acne treatment, it is important to be sure that the patient and parent have a clear understanding of the pathophysiology of acne. The most commonly held misconceptions relate to the role of greasy food and poor hygiene.

DISORDERS OF THE SWEAT GLANDS

Foot

Hyperhidrosis of the feet is usually exacerbated by occlusive sneakers, boots, or shoes. From a repetitive cycle of wetting and drying, fissuring may develop. In the acute stage, treatment consists of application of emollients or, in some instances, topical steroids. Prevention of hyperhidrosis can be accomplished with the use of absorbent powders (Zeasorb), avoidance of occlusive footwear, frequent changes of shoes and socks, and application of emollients to prevent drying.

Axilla and Palm

Hyperhidrosis of the axillae and palms can be a socially upsetting condition. Aluminum hexahydrate (Drysol), applied nightly for up to 1 week, will reduce sweating, which can then be maintained by less frequent application. When no response is seen, Drysol can be applied and occluded by plastic wrap overnight for several consecutive nights until the sweating is reduced. In unresponsive patients, an alternative is iontophoresis, which produces physical blockage of sweat ducts. Iontophoresis can be accomplished with a battery-powered home unit (Drionic).

SUN PROTECTION

CYNTHIA GUZZO, M.D.

Skin cancer is increasing at a dramatic rate. In the United States, 500,000 new cases of skin cancer are reported each year, most of which are basal cell or squamous cell carcinomas. However, the rise in malignant melanoma is of a great concern because this cutaneous cancer carries a serious prognosis. The lifetime risk for developing melanoma has risen from 1 in 1500 for a person born in 1930 to 1 in 100 for one born in 1990.

The increase in skin cancers is likely related to multiple factors. Ultraviolet radiation, delivered in sunlight, is clearly incriminated as a contributing factor to skin cancer. Increase in the ultraviolet exposure of today's society is the result of several occurrences, including the popularity of suntans, an outdoor-oriented lifestyle, the shift of the United States population southward, and the depletion of the ozone layer.

PHOTOBIOLOGY

Acute effects of sun exposure include sunburn and drug-induced phototoxic reactions. Chronic effects include photoaging and skin cancer. The solar radiation that reaches the earth is divided into three segments based on wavelength: ultraviolet (290 to 400 nm), visible (400 to 760 nm), and infrared (760 to 1800 nm). It is the ultraviolet spectrum that is responsible for the majority of skin problems we see. Ultraviolet C (UVC, 200 to 290 nm) is adsorbed by the upper atmosphere and does not reach the earth. There is concern that depletion of the ozone layer may change this in the future. Ultraviolet B radiation (UVB, 290 to 320 nm) causes sunburn, skin cancer, and photoaging. Ultraviolet A radiation (UVA, 320 to 400 nm) contributes to photoaging and photosensitivity diseases, enhances UVB erythema, and increases the risk of UVB carcinogenesis.

SUN EXPOSURE

It is estimated that two thirds of an individual's lifetime ultraviolet radiation dose is received by 18 years of age. Because of extensive summer sun exposure, the average child receives three times the annual UVB dose of the adult. Young children may be harmed more by equivalent UVB doses than adults. Painful or blistering sunburns in childhood or adolescence more than double the risk of developing malignant melanoma. Intrinsic factors that increase a child's susceptibility to sun exposure include skin that burns easily and does not tan, light eyes and hair color, multiple nevi, and a tendency to freckle. Finally, the acute effects of sunburn can be more serious in childhood, especially in the infant, because a small child's skin represents a greater percentage of total body mass than an adult's.

SKIN CANCER PREVENTION

Sunscreens

Topical sunscreens are chemical or physical blockers of UV radiation. Chemical sunscreens prevent sunburn by absorbing the UV radiation. They include PABA esters, cinnamates, benzophenones, and others. There are more effective UVB absorbers than UVA absorbers. Most sunscreens contain combinations of two or more chemicals. Physical sunscreens are opaque and reflect ultraviolet and visible radiation. Examples include titanium dioxide and zinc oxide. In general, they are cosmetically unacceptable. However, recently micronized titanium dioxide in a cream base is available.

Sunscreens are evaluated for sun protection factor (SPF) and substantivity. The SPF is the ratio between the dose of ultraviolet radiation required to produce minimal erythema (MED) on sunscreen-protected skin and the dose required to produce it on unprotected skin. This evaluates protection against UVB. There is no standard test for UVA protection. Substantivity grades the sunscreens resistance to removal by water. *Water-resistant* implies that a sunscreen continues to function after 40 minutes in water. *Waterproof* sunscreens withstand 80 minutes in the water. Children 6 months of age or older should use waterproof sunscreens of SPF15 or greater when outdoors. They should be reapplied every 2 hours. Chemical sunscreens can be irritating to the eyes. Therefore, sunscreens with micronized titanium dioxide are often better on the faces of young children. Infants should be kept out of sunlight entirely.

Outdoor Exposure Time

Sunscreens do not supply absolute protection and are not an excuse for excessive outdoor exposure. Outdoor activities should be limited between 10 AM and 2 PM, when the sun is most intense. Clearly, this requires significant rethinking of summer camp and recreational activities. Reflected light off sand, water, and concrete can reach children in the shade. Therefore, the beach under the umbrella is still a dangerous place for the skin.

Protective Clothing

Cotton clothing offers increased protection to sun exposure and is lightweight. Long sleeves and pants should be worn when tolerated. Caps and visors protect facial skin and eyes.

Tanning Salons

Many salons advertise the safety of UVA for tanning and lure teens into treatment. UVA is not safe, particularly in the large doses used, and contributes to photoaging and carcinogenesis. It is the duty of pediatricians and dermatologists alike to educate parents and children about skin protection and change attitudes about tanning if we are to limit the increase of skin cancer.

16

The Eye

THE EYE

David S. Walton, M.D

Careful assessment of a child's eyes should be a component of each well child examination and also is indicated when a complaint or symptom suggests an ocular causation. Often, this appraisal can be brief and done in the pediatrician's office, but sometimes, referral to an ophthalmologist will be necessary for a more complete examination and determination of treatment. Occasionally, the ophthalmologist will have to repeat an examination under general anesthesia to obtain sufficient diagnostic information about a child's eye problem.

OPHTHALMIC HISTORY

As in general pediatrics, the direction of history taking depends on the age of the child and the astuteness of the parents. A parent may recognize bilateral decreased vision by noting the inability of the infant or child to fixate on an object. The eyes may appear to wander in wide swings suggesting searching movements. Such pendular nystagmus suggests an early onset of abnormal vision. Parents may also recognize the failure of the infant or child to pick up or recognize small objects or the child's desire to hold objects very close to the face.

Loss of vision in one eye may be less apparent. A clue to the time of onset of decreased vision in one eye may be gained by determining when an eye first turned either in (esotropia) or out (exotropia) or when nystagmus was first observed in the abnormal eye. When an eye deviates early in life, suppression and decreased visual acuity of the deviated eye may result secondarily. When an eye deviates later in childhood, after 6 years of age, diplopia may become symptomatic because the child cannot suppress the second image.

When a younger child has an irritative ocular condition, parents will report such symptoms as rubbing of the eyes, blinking, squeezing of the eyes (blepharospasm), tearing, injection of the conjunctiva, and photophobia. An uncomplicated conjunctivitis usually causes only a gritty sensation, redness, and sticking together of the eyelids caused by a mucopurulent discharge. Involvement of the cornea and inflammation of the iris or ciliary body usually induce the triad of pain, photophobia, and lacrimation. Tearing may result either from an increased output of the tear gland (lacrimation) or from a decreased outflow through the lacrimal duct system (epiphora). If a parent asserts that a difference in pupil size has become evident, ask for old photographs with which to compare the condition. Anisocoria may be normal and occurs in approximately 7% of the population.

Headache and "failure to do well at school" often suggest to parents a possibility of an eye problem. Certainly, such children should have an eye examination. However, headaches caused by refractive errors or extraocular muscle imbalance (heterophorias) account for only a small percentage of all headaches.

Ocular abnormalities may be caused by systemic diseases (e.g., juvenile rheumatoid arthritis, diabetes mellitus) or by nonocular treatment programs (e.g., steroid preparations, radiation). Perinatal considerations also are important (e.g., prematurity, evidence of prenatal anoxia). Careful review for familial hereditary ocular and nonocular abnormalities is essential.

The chance of the ophthalmologist's finding an ocular abnormality in a child said to have dyslexia is approximately the same as in a normal population of a similar age group. Dyslexia, in almost every instance, is not caused by a disorder of the eyes and cannot be treated effectively by the ophthalmologist or optometrist.

OCULAR EXAMINATION

Well Child Eye Examinations

Evaluation of visual function and the integrity of the ocular structures should be an integral portion of the pediatrician's routine examination.

Newborn Period. Rule out an obvious eye abnormality by careful inspection of each eye and surrounding structures. Are the pupils equal in size, and do they respond to light? Are the corneas of normal size and clarity? Are eye movements full in response to passive head turning? Examine the red reflex with the ophthalmoscope to screen for opacities in the media, such as cataract, as well as for fundus lesions. Is there evidence of a worsening conjunctivitis? Remember that the chemical conjunctivitis caused by 1% silver nitrate prophylaxis improves rapidly after the first 48 hours of life, so this does not adequately explain persistent or progressive signs of conjunctivitis.

Infancy. Look for the development of vision. By testing each eye, determine if there is good fixation and willingness to follow the movement of toys. Are the pupils reactive to light on each side? Does the child show an interest in toys and reach for them? Such visual behavior is expected by 4 months of age but may be seen even earlier. This examination of the infant's vision is best done by an experienced examiner and alert patient. Are the eye movements full? Does the light reflex reflect from a symmetric position on each cornea, suggesting straight eyes? This test for an eye deviation is especially helpful during the first year of life. Check for the presence of clear corneas of equal size. Corneas of unequal size are always abnormal. Confirm that a red reflex from the ocular fundus of each eye is present.

Childhood. The ocular examination techniques suggested for infancy are continued until the child is approximately 3 years of age. By this age, most children can have a subjective visual acuity test. Picture targets work best, for example, Allen cards (Ophthalmex, LaGrange, Indiana). Test each eye separately. By 4 years of age, children will be able to identify the orientation of Es in various positions when instructed to point toward the direction that the E points. Visual acuity should be at least 20/30 in each eye by this test. By third grade, letters or numbers are familiar enough to young patients to be useful for visual acuity testing. The visual acuity of each eye should be checked in this way annually. Normally, a visual acuity of 20/25 is present in each eye. These subjective measurements may be done carefully by a trained assistant. The rest of the routine eye examination should follow the visual acuity testing. The eyelids, conjunctiva, and anterior segments should be inspected. Pupillary function should be estimated. Ocular motility should be assessed, and the presence of an eye deviation should be ruled out. The fundi should be examined, and specific structures, especially the discs and macular regions, should be inspected.

Careful documentation of pertinent findings (e.g., visual acuity) and normal findings (e.g., red reflex) during well child examinations represents important record keeping in respect to the adequacy of eye care.

Referral to an Ophthalmologist

Pediatricians should consult ophthalmologists liberally and early when a puzzling or difficult ocular abnormality is suspected. In infancy, this may be manifest by delayed development of visual activity, recognition of an ocular congenital anomaly, or history of prematurity.

At any age, referral is indicated for any abnormality of ocular motility, such as an ocular deviation, or for a suspected intraocular abnormality. Family history of eye disease or of systemic conditions complicated by eye disease may suggest the need for a thorough ocular evaluation. A complicating neonatal experience may dictate that an eye examination be done.

External inflammatory disease of the lids or conjunctiva may be treated by the pediatrician. Failure to respond to treatment should suggest the need for ophthalmic consultation in respect to etiologic diagnosis, extent of disease, and the best treatment.

Parents may feel the need for ophthalmic consultation more strongly than their pediatrician for certain problems. Their needs should be respected. Parents are especially desirous of ophthalmic consultation when faced with a recurrent or persistent childhood eye problem. Pediatricians should be sensitive to their concerns and facilitate such consultation. After facial trauma associated with possible eye injury, eye consultation also should be recommended.

OCULAR DISORDERS

Significant eye disorders in children rarely go away spontaneously, and most get progressively worse and complicated (e.g., amblyopia complicating an untreated esotropia). Treatment often can be more successful and less difficult if initiated promptly when signs or symptoms are first seen. It is appropriate for the pediatrician also to be especially sensitive to the significant parental anxiety caused by a suspected childhood ocular abnormality. Careful ocular examination can be expected to establish the integrity of the visual system or identify the type of problem if one is present and facilitate development of an appropriate care plan.

The "Red Eye"

The evaluation of the young patient with a "red eye" centers initially on determining the primary focus of inflammation. Is one faced with an orbit abnormality, lid problem, conjunctivitis, corneal inflammation (keratitis), or an intraocular inflammatory disease? Each of these possibilities must be considered, and a clinical decision must be made before treatment is begun.

Diseases of the Eyelids

Blepharitis is an inflammatory condition of the skin of the eyelids. The most common type is *seborrheic blepharitis*. Rarer causes also must be considered.

Seborrheic-Staphylococcal Blepharitis. Some individuals have a seborrheic condition of the eyelashes that produces a chronic redness and scaling along the eyelashes. The severity of scaling and the amount of discomfort associated with the condition usually wax and wane but may never completely disappear. Superimposed staphylococcal infection of the eyelids may aggravate the condition. The seborrheic condition can be kept under control (but not cured) by lash scrubs, followed by routine instillation of an antibiotic, such as erythromycin or sulfacetamide ointment. Lash scrubs are performed with a clean cotton-tipped applicator dipped into equal parts of a tearless baby shampoo and water. The cotton-tipped applicator is passed horizontally along the lid margins in a back-and-forth maneuver to dislodge crusts and scales. When the condition is severe, lash scrubs and antibiotic ointment may be applied three times a day. Once the condition is improved, an application each night at bedtime might suffice.

Increased lid margin redness and associated keratitis and conjunctivitis suggest significant *staphylococcal blepharitis*. Chalazia also occur with these abnormalities. Long-term topical antibiotic medication, usually best in ointment form, frequently is helpful. Short-term oral antimicrobials also can help this condition. For example, lid cleansing daily combined with a topical ointment mixture of bacitracin and polymyxin for 6 weeks is often helpful. If uncontrolled lid rubbing occurs, a short-term topical steroid preparation (e.g., dexamethasone phosphate 0.05% ointment) may be indicated.

Herpetic Blepharitis. This is characterized by the appearance of multiple eyelid and facial vesicles that become crusted or ulcerated and are surrounded by a zone of erythema. Conjunctivitis and keratitis also may occur. New lesions appear for approximately 5 days and are usually predominantly on one side. Moderate lid swelling can occur. This illness usually represents a primary herpes simplex infection, and fever is present early in the clinical course. Blepharospasm and photophobia signal the presence of associated keratitis, dictating prompt referral to an ophthalmologist for consideration for specific topical antiviral medication. Adenine arabinoside (Vira-A) ointment is used until the corneal lesions are healed, usually within 7 to 14 days. With significant lid margin involvement, this preparation is indicated three times per day for prophylaxis against spread to the cornea. When the patient is seen early, especially in the presence of eczema, the use of acyclovir (Zovirax) is indicated by mouth or optimally by vein to lessen spread and hasten recovery. Young family members should be protected from contact, and older family members with history of recurrent active herpes simplex lesions (e.g., fever blisters) should know the risks of such lesions for young children.

Other Virus–Induced Lesions. *Molluscum contagiosum* and *verruca viruses* produce small tumorlike growths on the lid margins and secondarily induce chronic keratoconjunctivitis. Excision of the lesions is the treatment of choice.

Periorbital Cellulitis Versus Orbital Cellulitis. In the evaluation of lid inflammation, the possibility of cellulitis confined to the eyelids (periorbital cellulitis) or eyelid cellulitis in continuity with orbital inflammation (orbital cellulitis) must always be carefully considered.

Periorbital cellulitis represents an acute bacterial tissue infection of the eyelids. Staphylococcal, streptococcal, or *Haemophilus* infection is most likely. Rapid swelling of the eyelids, erythema, and tenderness occur with fever. The eye itself, however, retains full range of movement and is not proptotic or otherwise affected.

Orbital cellulitis denotes the infection of tissues posterior to the orbital septum, with involvement of the retrobulbar structures, producing proptosis, chemosis, limitation of eye movement, and possibly reduction of vision. The orbit usually is infected from a contiguous structure, and often sinusitis is the cause. In a young child, *Haemophilus* infection must be considered. Blood cultures and consultation with an otolaryngologist are indicated. This is a life-threatening condition, since infection may spread posteriorly to the cavernous sinus and require emergency treatment. Drainage of the orbit itself usually is not indicated immediately but may be necessary later in the course if an abscess forms. Frequently, orbital abnormalities occur secondary to a subperiosteal abscess adjacent to the periorbita. When this does not clear with medical treatment or when prompt orbital decompression is indicated, subperiosteal drainage is indicated. Evaluation of such lesions is assisted by computed tomography (CT). The possibility of an intraorbital foreign body should always be considered. History and CT usually can rule out this possibility.

For both periorbital cellulitis and orbital cellulitis, hospitalization is indicated for intravenous antibiotics against staphylococcal and *Haemophilus* agents.

Sty, Hordeolum, and Chalazion. A sty or an infection (usually staphylococcal) at the base of the eyelashes is also called an external hordeolum. It can be treated with warm compresses and a topical antibiotic preparation, such as erythromycin or bacitracin (ophthalmic) ointment four times a day. Warm compresses can be applied using a clean washcloth soaked with hot tap water. Wet heat should be maintained on the eyelid for 10 to 15 minutes with each application. The water should be warm but not so hot that the skin is scalded.

Each of the tarsal plates in the eyelids contains a large number of vertically oriented sebaceous glands called meibomian glands. These glands secrete material at the lid margin, just behind the eyelashes. If the duct of one of these glands is plugged, the normal product of the gland accumulates within the eyelid. A chronic inflammatory lipogranuloma develops as a foreign body response to this accumulated material and may produce a painless swelling in the tarsal portion of the eyelid (chalazion). The mass periodically may become inflamed and tender. Warm compresses are indicated during the acute inflammation. Some physicians like to prescribe a topical antibiotic preparation as well. If a chronic, noninflamed, palpable mass has persisted on the lid for months, it is reasonable for an ophthalmologist to incise and curette the granuloma. Young children require a brief outpatient general anesthesia for this procedure, but cooperative children over 12 or 13 years of age need only injected local anesthesia.

Conjunctival Disorders

Subconjunctival Hemorrhages. Subconjunctival hemorrhages are in themselves of no consequence. Over a period of many weeks, they gradually dissipate to a yellow discoloration and then vanish altogether. One should, however, ascertain that the hemorrhage was indeed spontaneous. A child or even a family may suppress a history of trauma in a situation in which subconjunctival hemorrhage is the only obvious external sign of ocular damage. Elevated systemic blood pressure, bleeding dyscrasia, increased cranial venous pressure (for example, from bouts of coughing), and viral or bacterial conjunctivitis may also be associated with subconjunctival hemorrhages.

Conjunctivitis. Conjunctivitis is common in childhood and must be differentiated from more serious intraocular inflammation or keratitis. Conjunctivitis is known by the laity as pinkeye and may be bacterial, viral, allergic, chemical, or secondary to foreign material. Redness of the conjunctiva associated with discharge but with little or no light sensitivity is typical of these disorders. Pain and tenderness are minimal.

ACUTE INFECTIOUS CONJUNCTIVITIS. This is the most common type of conjunctivitis and may be viral but is usually of bacterial etiology. Routine cultures and smears are not usually done but can be informative in respect to inflammatory cell type (neutrophils with bacteria) and bacterial etiology. If there is something clinically unusual about the conjunctivitis or if it is severe, a culture may be helpful. Bacterial conjunctivitis is caused by *Staphylococcus aureus,* but other frequent bacterial causes include *Streptococcus pneumoniae, Haemophilus influenzae,* and *Moraxella catarrhalis.* An associated tender preauricular node suggests a viral or chlamydial etiology. Bacterial or viral conjunctivitis may be associated with pharyngitis or otitis media. Appropriate treatment of infectious conjunctivitis is to prescribe a mixture of bacitracin and polymyxin (Polysporin) three times a day for 7 days. It is helpful to have the family telephone if the conjunctivitis is not significantly improved in 2 days or if it is not completely resolved in 5 days. Systemic antibiotics are generally unnecessary. Occasionally, the conjunctival and lid inflammation is intense, as occurs with some streptococcal infections. Copious discharge is present, with lid swelling and erythema accompanied by tenderness. Systemic and topical treatment is indicated accompanied by careful follow-up ophthalmic care.

ALLERGIC CONJUNCTIVITIS. Itching is a prominent symptom of allergic conjunctivitis and is common in youngsters with allergic disorders, such as hay fever and asthma. Rubbing the eyes in an effort to relieve the itching just makes matters worse. Cold compresses sometimes give relief. Mild vasoconstricting agents (Naphcon-A) can be given topically and may whiten the eye and provide brief symptomatic relief but should not be used continuously. Nonsteroidal anti-inflammatory preparations can be helpful (Acular). Preparations that stabilize mast cells, such as lodoxamide tromethamine (Alomide), can be used and lessen the need for topical steroids. In spite of the role of such agents, some patients will require topical steroid preparations. When they are administered, an ophthalmologist should be consulted to monitor the eye pressure and response to treatment.

Vernal conjunctivitis is a chronic, bilateral allergic conjunctivitis that causes itching, a stringy discharge, and hypertrophic papules on the palpebral conjunctiva of the upper lid. Corticosteroid therapy is very helpful. A mast cell-stabilizing agent (Alomide) may also be effective. Long-term treatment often is necessary. The corneal condition must be monitored carefully. Ophthalmic consultation is necessary for treatment of vernal conjunctivitis.

A 1- to 2-mm mass straddling the limbus, a red eye, and extreme photophobia suggest *phlyctenular keratoconjunctivitis.* Phlyctenula can occur anywhere on the bulbar conjunctiva or cornea and usually represent a hypersensitivity reaction in the limbal conjunctiva and cornea to bacterial components. A higher incidence of phlyctenula occurs in impoverished populations, and phlyctenula have been associated with tuberculosis. They usually respond dramatically to topical corticosteroids and antimicrobial agents.

CONJUNCTIVITIS IN THE NEONATE. The four most common types of conjunctivitis in the neonate are chemical, gonococcal, staphylococcal, and inclusion. The time of onset may provide a good clue to diagnosis.

Chemical Conjunctivitis. Chemical conjunctivitis usually begins on the first day of life, soon after silver nitrate is instilled. Gonococcal conjunctivitis usually begins on day 3 or 4, inclusion conjunctivitis usually begins on days 7 to 10, and staphylococcal conjunctivitis may begin at any time.

A mild conjunctivitis secondary to silver nitrate prophylaxis is common. Treatment of this chemical conjunctivitis, which is brief in duration, is unnecessary. A worsening conjunctivitis during the first week of life must be differentiated promptly from this condition.

Gonorrhea. It is wisest to consider all purulent conjunctivitis in the first few days of life as gonococcal until proved otherwise. The rapidity with which the gonococcus can penetrate the cornea has been well documented, and gonococcal conjunctivitis presents a truly urgent situation. The diagnosis is made by Gram stain of a conjunctival scraping, bacterial (Thayer-Martin medium) cultures, and tests for *Chlamydia* infection. Treatment should not be delayed if confirmation tests are unavailable, and the infant should be hospitalized for isolation, observation, and treatment.

Initial treatment of gonococcal conjunctivitis should be with a third-generation cephalosporin (cefotaxime for 7 days or single-dose ceftriaxone) to cover penicillin-resistant organisms. Topical erythromycin with saline irrigation every 4 hours should accompany systemic therapy.

The occurrence of neonatal conjunctivitis and resultant ocular complications and loss of vision have been decreased dramatically by topical use of prophylactic agents immediately after vaginal delivery. Routine use of silver nitrate 1% (Credé's maneuver) is highly effective. Erythromycin and tetracycline ointments also are used but may be ineffective against resistant organisms. Pretreatment of infected mothers is helpful when it is possible. Infants born to mothers with active untreated gonorrhea should be treated prophylactically with intravenous or intramuscular penicillin or a single dose of ceftriaxone (50 mg/kg), with the addition of topical erythromycin ointment four times per day for 7 days.

Chlamydial Infection (Inclusion Blenorrhea). Although chlamydial infection of the neonate is not the ocular emergency that gonococcal disease is, the differential diagnosis initially can be difficult. Credé's prophylaxis is not effective against the chlamydial agent. Chlamydial conjunctivitis usually commences 5 to 12 days after birth. The diagnosis is made by seeing cytoplasmic inclusions on a Giemsa stain of conjunctival scrapings. There is a mixed cellular response in these scrapings, both mononuclear cells and polymorphonuclear cells being present. Culture techniques are difficult and are not generally available, but monoclonal antibody or enzyme-linked immunoassay can be helpful.

Long-term follow-up has indicated that poorly treated individuals may develop a trachomalike corneal vascularization. The infected infant should receive topical erythromycin or tetracycline ophthalmic ointment four times a day for 3 weeks. Since chlamydial agents are present in the upper respiratory tract as well, systemic erythromycin (e.g., four times per day for 3 weeks) is also indicated for these children, who are also at risk for chlamydial pneumonitis. Both parents should be treated once the diagnosis is made in the neonate.

Chronic Bacterial Keratoconjunctivitis. Though staphylococci are an infrequent cause of acute conjunctivitis, this organism is the most common cause of chronic nonallergic conjunctivitis. Characteristically, the lid margins are red, the conjunctiva is injected, and corneal abnormalities may be present, causing a symptomatic foreign body sensation and opacities on examination. Lashes may be lost from rubbing. Irritation and other symptoms are worse in the morning. Evaluation consists of lid margin cultures for determining bacterial etiology and sensitivities. Aerobic, gram-negative bacilli may also cause acute or chronic conjunctivitis. Treatment consists of long-term antibiotic administration.

Inflammation of the Eyeball

Episcleritis and scleritis. Episcleritis and scleritis are rare in childhood and appear as localized areas of inflammation on the white of the eye, possibly accompanied by pain. Episcleritis is more common than scleritis and may be seen in association with regional enteritis. It usually responds well to topical steroid medication.

Keratitis. The acute onset of inflammation of the cornea (keratitis) causes extreme pain and light sensitivity. A variety of etiologic agents may be the cause.

VIRAL KERATITIS. Acute conjunctivitis with considerable discomfort and a preauricular node may be caused by adenovirus infection, called epidemic keratoconjunctivitis (EKC). The cornea may become involved and interfere with vision 10 to 14 days later. Conjunctivitis of this type is highly contagious, and it is quite important to instruct the patient and family in good hygiene and to take measures to prevent the examining office from becoming a vector of communicability. Handwashing and thorough cleansing of contaminated equipment are advisable.

Herpes simplex may present initially only on the eyelids, it may affect the lid margins and eyelashes (herpetic marginal blepharitis), or it may affect both the conjunctiva and the cornea (herpetic keratoconjunctivitis). The major reason it is such a serious cause of blindness in the United States is its tendency to leave scars in the cornea. Topical steroids significantly worsen the course of the corneal epithelial infection with herpes simplex and must be avoided at this stage. If an active corneal herpetic ulcer is suspected after fluorescein staining, an ophthalmologist should be consulted. Treatment of herpetic keratitis consists of topical trifluridine drops (Viroptic) or vidarabine ointment (Vira-A). If a child is known or suspected to have had ocular herpes simplex in the past, it is best to let an ophthalmologist evaluate and treat a new episode of red eye.

BACTERIAL OR FUNGAL KERATITIS. Bacterial infections of the cornea most commonly complicate a severe bacterial conjunctivitis or follow corneal injury. Fungal corneal infection is especially frequent after an injury to the cornea by plant life or prolonged topical steroid and antibiotic administration to the cornea for conjunctival or corneal disease. Rapid ulceration of the corneal stroma occurs, which may permanently destroy the optical clarity of the cornea. Whenever a

pediatrician sees a painful red eye in combination with a corneal infiltrate, an ophthalmologist should be consulted immediately. Most bacterial and fungal ulcers are treated with subconjunctival injections and multiple topical instillations of antibiotics or antifungal agents, in combination with cycloplegics.

Iritis, Iridocyclitis, and Posterior Uveitis. A red eye with little or no discharge may be the result of *acute iritis* rather than conjunctivitis. A characteristic circumlimbal or ciliary injection is present in both iritis and keratitis from conjunctivitis. Similarly, photophobia is quite characteristic of both keratitis and iritis and should alert the physician that a red eye is not caused by conjunctivitis. The pupil may be somewhat smaller and irregular in the eye with iritis.

Iritis and *iridocyclitis* in the adult are almost always accompanied by pain, lacrimation, and photophobia, but they may smolder asymptomatically in children. This is often the case in chronic iridocyclitis accompanying pauciarticular juvenile rheumatoid arthritis. Periodic examinations by an ophthalmologist are often necessary to monitor these children. Definitive diagnosis and management depend on slit-lamp examination. Acute iritis or anterior uveitis is usually of undetermined cause and is most often treated with nonspecific therapy consisting of cycloplegic agents (e.g., cyclopentolate or atropine) and topical steroid medications.

Posterior uveitis commonly causes decreased vision in the affected eye or eyes, and it can be an acute or chronic disease. Specific etiologic agents are more commonly recognized with posterior uveitis and include infection with *Toxoplasma* protozoa, herpes simplex or cytomegalic viruses, or *Toxocara canis* larvae. With chronic cyclitis, a causative agent is rarely determined. For *Toxoplasma* chorioretinitis, specific therapy consisting of pyrimethamide (Daraprim) and sulfadiazine is indicated when vision is threatened by a posterior pole lesion.

Ocular Trauma

Blunt Ocular Trauma

Black Eye. Despite the slight, even jocular, attention often given to a "shiner," a black eye may be the prominent initial sign of serious ocular injury. Blowout fracture of the orbital floor, retinal detachment, hyphema, dislocated lens, traumatic iritis, and other ocular injuries may be overlooked because the lids are so swollen that insufficient attention is paid to the globe itself. Some experts contend that all black eyes should be evaluated by an ophthalmologist. Certainly, if there is any other sign of ocular abnormality, such as conjunctival injection or diminished visual acuity, ophthalmic examination with detailed fundus examination is definitely indicated.

Ocular Abrasion. Even minor trauma from a fingernail, a comb, or the edge of a sheet of paper may produce a defect in the corneal epithelium (corneal abrasion). Abrasions require prompt attention because they are very painful and if unattended may become secondarily infected. Some corneal abrasions are caused by foreign bodies under the upper lid. This should be suspected particularly with a superior corneal defect that stains with fluorescein. Routine eversion of the upper lid usually will demonstrate the foreign body. A recent corneal abrasion can be treated with bacitracin-polymyxin ointment and a tight patch during awake hours. Systemic analgesics may be helpful during the first 24 hours. If the abrasion was extensive or if the child is not completely comfortable when the patch is removed in 24 hours, reevaluation is advisable. A corneal abrasion that has been neglected or that persists, especially if any corneal opacity is present, should be seen promptly by an ophthalmologist. The possibility of a herpes simplex keratitis must always be considered.

Contact Lens Abrasion. The corneal epithelium does not have a direct vascular supply but receives its oxygen from the air when the eyes are open and from the back of the eyelids when the lids are closed. When hard contact lenses are not permeable to oxygen, the corneal epithelium depends for its oxygen supply on the exchange of oxygenated tears under the contact lens. This exchange, in turn, depends on eye blink-induced movement of the contact lens and is more effective in some individuals than in others. When the patient falls asleep, the contact lens rests in one position on the cornea, exchange of tears is minimal or stops, and a corneal abrasion may occur. This abrasion is treated in the same manner as a traumatic abrasion.

Corneal Foreign Body. Corneal foreign bodies should be removed promptly. They are painful, and significant delays increase the chance of secondary infection. After a drop of local anesthetic (0.5% proparacaine) is placed in the eye, many superficial corneal foreign bodies can be brushed away with a cotton-tipped applicator or a blunt spatula. A cotton-tipped applicator may carry away more corneal epithelium and, therefore, leave a larger corneal abrasion that must heal, but since a cotton-tipped applicator is blunt, many physicians feel comfortable using it around the eye. A sharp needle is needed to remove embedded material. Any sharp object brought close to the eye should be kept tangential, not perpendicular to the cornea. Such care is best done by an ophthalmologist and only for a cooperative child. Without cooperation, general anesthesia is required for this care.

Metallic foreign bodies that have been on the cornea for a period of time often will leave a rust ring after the major foreign body has been removed. A large rust ring may retard satisfactory healing and should be removed. Foreign bodies leaving large rust rings, deeply embedded corneal foreign bodies, glass foreign bodies, and foreign bodies in the central cornea involving the visual axis should also be referred promptly to an ophthalmologist for removal. Once the foreign body is removed, the remaining defect is treated like a corneal abrasion, with antibiotic ointment and an eyepatch.

Traumatic Hyphema. Traumatic hyphema is bleeding into the anterior chamber of the eye secondary to injury. Although it may complicate a penetrating injury, it is more frequently a consideration in a nonpenetrating blunt contusion of the globe, for example, a fist or ball injury. The possibility of a hyphema is always a consideration with a history of significant trauma to the eye. Careful ophthalmic examination with slitlamp is indicated, and the finding of blood in the anterior chamber confirms that the injury is serious. The amount of blood may be minimal, evident only on slitlamp examination, or gross, with a significant part of the anterior chamber filled with blood.

Treatment of a traumatic hyphema by the pediatrician and ophthalmologist is to prevent further injury by the patient and to take all reasonable steps to prevent a secondary hemorrhage, which most often follows during the first 5 days after the primary injury. Bedrest with head elevated, cycloplegic agents, topical steroids, and an eyepad plus protective aluminum shield are often ordered. Sedation may be necessary, and the use of aspirin is strongly contraindicated. Hospitalization is appropriate if these measures and careful ophthalmic observation cannot be accomplished with the patient living at home. If a secondary hemorrhage occurs, it is often more severe and painful than the initial hemorrhage and may cause acute glaucoma followed by cataract formation, iris atrophy, and optic atrophy. This circumstance is a serious ophthalmic emergency.

Chemical Burns

Strong acids and, especially, strong alkali burns may be devastating to ocular tissues. Profuse irrigation of the eye with tap water should be instituted as soon as possible. If a family calls about such an injury, they should be instructed to irrigate the eye immediately at the site of the injury and then come to the office. Do not delay irrigation waiting for the patient to reach medical attention. The eye should be irrigated with water for several minutes continuously. It is important to retract both of the lids so that the chemical agent is not retained in the recesses of the conjunctival fornices. Particulate caustic material must not be overlooked in the fornices.

The irrigation can be repeated when the patient reaches medical attention. In the office, irrigation can be performed using an elevated bottle of saline with an intravenous tubing set. No needle is required, but the infusion tubing allows a controlled and copious flow of irrigation fluid with minimal inconvenience and special equipment. The

technique of doubly everting the upper lid is important to examine the recesses of the superior conjunctival fornix. Litmus paper touched to the conjunctival surface should register in the neutral range if the irrigation has been satisfactory. The extent of the injury then must be assessed by careful examination, including visual acuity assessment, examination with magnification and focused white light, and then fluorescein staining. Complete blanching of the conjunctival vessels at the limbus is an ominous sign. Corneal defects after serious chemical burns may not heal readily. Ophthalmologic attention is clearly indicated in these serious chemical burns.

The optimal approach to chemical burns is that of prophylaxis. Household caustic agents should be well out of the reach of inquisitive youngsters. The value of safety glasses in hazardous circumstances, such as chemistry laboratories or when learning how to jump start a car, should be taught from the earliest possible age.

Penetrating Ocular Trauma

History taking from traumatized children is notoriously unreliable. Not infrequently, the child feels guilty about the circumstances of the injury and gives an inaccurate or incomplete acccount of the accident. One must not be misled by an innocuous-sounding history but should be guided by physical findings and entertain a high degree of suspicion that the injury involves more than the presenting signs. For example, a lid laceration must be assumed to involve an intraocular injury until specifically proved otherwise. A full-thickness lid laceration should be fully evaluated and repaired by an ophthalmologist. The likelihood of an accompanying penetrating injury to the globe is great, and, if there is any doubt, it is best to treat the eye as if it has been penetrated.

Once the diagnosis of a penetrated globe is made or suspected, it is best to avoid direct pressure or excessive manipulation of the globe, since the intraocular contents may be extruded. The ophthalmologist may have definite preferences about management of the patient. In general, it is best to avoid ocular ointments in this situation, for it is undesirable for ointment to reach the intraocular structures. Topical antibiotic drops can be instilled, and a loose patch and a metal shield (Fox shield) should be placed over the eye to avoid accidental trauma until the ophthalmologist sees the patient.

The history of an ocular injury from a flying foreign body generated by metal striking metal must be taken very seriously. A sliver of metal may make a surprisingly subtle entry into the eye and leave only a small area of conjunctival injection as evidence of its entry site. Occasionally, it may pass through clear cornea in a self-sealing manner. The vision may still be 20/20 immediately after an intraocular foreign body enters the eye, but intraocular foreign bodies can cause extensive and irreparable intraocular damage. They need to be evaluated by an ophthalmologist on an urgent basis.

Ocular injuries with glass and other transparent foreign bodies pose special optical problems in identification of all the particles. They are best evaluated and treated by an ophthalmologist with the aid of a slitlamp biomicroscope.

Newly Diagnosed Ocular Deviation

The sudden onset of an ocular deviation usually occurs in children with healthy eyes but may be the initial presentation of the potentially life-threatening intraocular tumor, retinoblastoma, or a manifestation of severe neurologic disease. In general, ocular deviation due to neurologic disease will be of the paretic type, with the amount of deviation changing according to direction of gaze, and there often will be limitation of full movement of at least one eye. In comitant strabismus, there is full movement of each eye, and the amount of deviation is roughly the same in all fields of gaze. Comitant strabismus is the most common type of eye deviation. It may be caused by or the cause of poor vision in one eye, however, so that one must test the visual acuity in each eye and specifically examine the maculae and optic nerves to rule out retinoblastoma or other serious ocular disease that needs immediate attention. If the nonophthalmic physician is certain that the strabismus is comitant and that the visual acuity and fundus are normal in the deviating eye, referral to an ophthalmologist should be immediate but on a nonurgent basis. There are no advantages and numerous disadvantages in delaying the referral for many months for children with eye deviations. If the deviation is neurologic in origin, referral to a pediatric neurologist is suggested.

Tear System Disorders
Lacrimal Duct Obstruction, Dacryocystitis, Congenital Dacryocele

Congenital lacrimal duct obstruction may remit spontaneously— 80% of cases will remit spontaneously during the first 6 months of life. During the first 6 months, it is best to prescribe antibiotic ointment (e.g., erythromycin ointment t.i.d.). Treatment is directed toward avoiding infection and minimizing stagnation. If tearing persists after 6 months of age, probing of the nasolacrimal duct should be considered. Probing can be done while restraining a youngster, or brief general anesthesia can be used.

Dacryocystitis, characterized by swelling, tenderness, and erythema below the medial canthus, should be treated with systemic antibiotics to cover the occurrence of gram-positive organisms and *Haemophilus influenzae.*

Once the infection has cleared, the obstruction and cause of the problem can be relieved by probing the nasolacrimal duct. Congenital dacryocele can be relieved by probing during the newborn period. At this age, probing without general anesthesia usually can be done.

Dacryoadenitis

Acute suppurative dacryoadenitis may look like orbital cellulitis, except that the greatest swelling is seen in the upper outer quadrant of the anterior orbit under the lid. Treatment of the two conditions is similar. (See earlier section in this chapter on orbital cellulitis.) Subacute dacryoadenitis may be seen secondary to mumps, sarcoid, and lymphomas.

Dry Eye Syndrome

Such entities as erythema multiforme, toxic epidermal necrolysis, familial dysautonomia, exposure keratitis, and neuroparalytic keratitis may result in a dry eye syndrome caused by diminished tear production, diminished production of mucin from diseased conjunctival goblet cells, inadequate blinking, or inadequate protection of the cornea by the lids. Drying of the cornea ensues. Once a cornea becomes dry, its epithelial layer degenerates, and corneal scarring, with or without infection, soon occurs. Tear replacement in the form of artificial tears may help to alleviate the conditions. Tarsorrhaphy and punctal plugs are also helpful.

Cloudiness of the Cornea

The cornea normally is beautifully transparent, and alteration of this characteristic should be considered an abnormality. The possible causes of corneal cloudiness or opacification are many and include acute glaucoma, corneal injury, storage diseases, inherited corneal dystrophy, band keratopathy, corneal infection, and vitamin A deficiency. In a pediatric examination, the transparency of the parents' corneas can be used for comparison to help decide whether or not a corneal transparency defect is present. Whenever this abnormality is suspected, an ophthalmologist should be consulted.

Infantile Glaucoma (Congenital Glaucoma)

Public awareness of glaucoma has increased so that most people know that it affects a significant portion of the adult population over 40 years of age (variably estimated as 2% to 5%). Regrettably, there is not the same awareness that glaucoma exists in childhood. It is crucial to make this diagnosis early in life before vision is irreparably lost. To make the diagnosis, it is important to maintain a constant vigil and to consider glaucoma routinely in the differential diagnosis of ocular problems in childhood.

The classic signs of infantile glaucoma are tearing, photophobia, cloudy cornea, or corneal enlargement in one or both eyes. The signs may be present in the newborn period, or they may develop in the first few months of life. Only one sign may be present initially, and

it is important not to wait for the full constellation before making a complete evaluation for glaucoma. It is worthy of note that after 2 years of age, the corneas generally do not enlarge even if the intraocular pressure is elevated. After age 2 years, the configuration of the optic nerve cupping and, in particular, the asymmetry between the cupping in the two eyes become important diagnostic signs of glaucoma. The diagnosis of glaucoma is confirmed by pressure measurements.

Glaucoma may be primary and often caused by an inherited or inheritable defect of the aqueous humor filtration mechanism, or it may be secondary and caused by other ocular disease, such as an intraocular tumor, inflammation, or an ocular injury.

Although glaucoma is unusual in childhood, the pediatrician must be sensitive to the signs of glaucoma in early life and consider it when a young patient has an eye condition or family history of childhood-onset glaucoma that places the child in jeopardy for its occurrence.

The treatment of primary glaucoma in early childhood is often surgical, whereas medical therapy is used more frequently for secondary glaucoma. A topical beta-adrenergic blocker (Timoptic) and acetazolamide are frequently used.

Proptosis

Anterior protrusion of an eye in childhood is an important abnormality and may be caused by infection, neoplasm, idiopathic inflammation, trauma, and hyperthyroidism.

Rhabdomyosarcoma

Rhabdomyosarcoma is a rare tumor, but it is the most common primary malignancy of the orbit in childhood. Rapidly developing proptosis from rhabdomyosarcoma may mimic an inflammatory condition. On occasion, early diagnosis and treatment have been delayed by therapy mistakenly directed toward a presumed orbital cellulitis. Radiotherapy combined with chemotherapy has replaced radical exenteration as the principal form of therapy, but there continues to be a significant mortality from this aggressive tumor.

Hemangioma of Orbit and Eyelid

Hemangiomas of the orbit or eyelid or both appear during the first 6 months of life. They are upsetting to parents and may become complicated by refractive or occlusion amblyopia. Displacement of the eye and proptosis are common.

Like strawberry hemangiomas elsewhere on the body, those that involve the lids have a tendency to grow during the first year of life and then tend to regress spontaneously. In terms of minimizing scarring and side effects of therapy, one should delay intervention as long as possible, but if the eye is completely occluded by a hemangioma, one must intervene, however young the infant. Infants with these lesions should always be referred to an ophthalmologist. If treatment becomes necessary, injected or systemic steroids and, rarely, even radiation for very rapidly growing lesions should be considered. Surgery rarely is initially advisable during the first few years of life for these abnormalities.

The White Pupil (Leukokoria)

The pupil normally appears black, but with the development of a lens opacity (cataract) or with the occurrence of an opacity in the anterior vitreous behind the lens, the pupil will appear gray or white. Parents frequently report this abnormality as "seeing something in the eye." This so-called cat's eye reflex pupillary sign is a complaint or sign that should be followed by prompt referral of this patient to an ophthalmologist. The most serious cause of the white pupil is a retinoblastoma tumor.

Retinoblastoma

The earliest sign of this ocular malignancy may be a faint whitish discoloration in the pupil (leukokoria). The parent may comment on this, or it may be noted during a well baby examination. Retinoblastoma is the most frequent ocular malignancy in children. If untreated, the tumor is fatal, and the success of therapy in preserving life and vision depends on early diagnosis. Retinoblastoma must be considered in the early differential diagnosis of an acquired strabismus, even without a white pupil, since early involvement of the macula may interfere with central fixation and disrupt fusion. Since retinoblastoma is inherited in a dominant fashion, children born in a family known to have retinoblastoma should be seen by an ophthalmologist shortly after birth and be reexamined periodically thereafter.

Cataracts in Childhood

Cataracts are an important cause of visual loss in childhood. A cataract may cause leukokoria or disturb the red reflex. There is no medical treatment for most congenital cataracts. Cataracts secondary to galactosemia, if diagnosed early, may regress following dietary control. The ophthalmologist must decide whether a cataract in infants and young children is severe enough to cause a permanent amblyopia. If this is the circumstance, surgery will be considered regardless of the child's age. Treatment of cataracts in older children may be indicated if a significant limitation of visual function is present or if visual preference is occurring secondary to an asymmetry in the severity of the cataracts. The visual potential of the eye being considered for surgery must always be considered. For instance, some infants with unilateral congenital cataracts in microphthalmic eyes may develop useful vision even if cataract surgery is performed early in life, followed by optical correction. Surgery of traumatic cataracts also dictates careful consideration by the surgeon of possible associated eye injuries. In some instances, cataract surgery is indicated for cosmetic purposes to remove the white pupil.

Retinal Disease

The possibility of a retinal abnormality must be considered frequently in the evaluation of eye disease and always as a component of a normal eye examination. The health of the optic nerve head also is of primary importance in the examination of the ocular fundus. Retinal detachment after ocular injury, a retinoblastoma in an infant with a newly recognized eye deviation or leukokoria, a retinal degeneration in a patient with familial night blindness, decreased vision with color blindness, and the risk of retinopathy of prematurity in premature infants are relationships that must not be disregarded.

Retinopathy of Prematurity

The risk of retinopathy of prematurity is greatest in premature children with a birth weight of less than 1200 g. Prolonged episodes of hyperoxemia increase the incidence still further. All such premature infants should be examined for retinopathy of prematurity by 6 weeks of age. Treatment of the active stage of this disease represents an important frontier of pediatric eye care. At present, prevention of premature delivery and careful control of oxygen administration to premature infants represent the most important measures in the control of this disease. Active retinal disease may be halted by cryotherapy or laser treatments.

17

The Ear

HEARING LOSS

ROBERT J. RUBEN, M.D.

Hearing loss is one of the most prevalent conditions seen in infancy and childhood. Such loss can range from mild to total hearing loss. Hearing losses can affect one ear more than the other or only affect one ear. Unilateral losses, as well as bilateral losses, carry substantial morbidity. The amount of loss and the susceptibility of the patient to its effects are factors in the magnitude of the end result of the hearing loss on the child. Infants and young children with developmental delay or with either acquired or intrinsic language delays or with other sensory system disorders are vulnerable to the effects of the smallest of hearing losses. The difference in susceptibility in children to the effects of hearing loss precludes the assignment of conventional categories, such as mild and moderate, for what may be mild for one child may be disabling for a child with an expressive language deficiency or who is retarded. Thus *therapy for hearing loss must consider the child's susceptibility to the effects of the hearing loss*. The susceptibility will determine the form and the extent of the therapeutic intervention.

The major symptom of hearing loss in the infant or toddler is language or speech delay. For all infants, any indication or suspicion of language delay, particularly observations by the baby's caretaker that the child is not progressing adequately, must be taken as a serious indication of hearing loss that must be explored. The human central nervous system (CNS) is so constructed that there is a critical period for the acquisition of language and the establishment of critical auditory discriminations underlying the development of oral language. This critical period is in the first 2 years of life, with some extension into the third and fourth years. If the opportunity for normal hearing is missed during this time period, there will be a permanent loss in language function and auditory discrimination. These linguistic and long-term discrimination morbidities are preventable by the timely recognition and treatment of hearing loss.

A number of developmental scales have been constructed that can be used by the practitioner to screen for language or speech abnormalities in children. The Early Language Milestone Scale[1] (ELM), an easy test to administer, has been developed and validated to screen for the language and speech development of infants and children from birth to 36 months of age. It is recommended that the ELM or a similar screen be used periodically at well baby visits for every child from birth to 36 months. If at any visit there is any suspicion of abnormality in hearing, speech, or language, the screen should be applied immediately. If the child fails the language screen, it is imperative to obtain a definitive assessment of the child's hearing, speech, and language functions.

No child is too young or too impaired to have an accurate and detailed evaluation of hearing in each ear (Table 1).[2] Infants from birth to 6 months of age can be assessed by means of auditory evoked potentials (AEP), which can be carried out for different frequencies, at different intensities, using both air and bone conduction for each ear. Infants and toddlers who are developmentally 6 months or older may be tested behaviorally at each frequency, in each ear, by bone and air conduction using the technique of Visual Reinforced Audiometry (VRA). The results of VRA are similar to those of audiograms in older children. Patients older than 3 years usually can be tested by routine audiologic procedures.

There are two other assessments used for the evaluation of ear function in children. The most common is tympanometry, of which the most common form is the tympanogram. Tympanometry does not measure hearing. It measures various parameters of the physical characteristics of the tympanic membrane and middle and external ears. The tympanogram is useful in diagnosing and documenting the probability of fluid in the middle ear. Tympanograms that are type B (i.e., flat) are most often associated with otitis media with effusion (OME). A second test is the recording of spontaneous or evoked cochlear emissions. This new form of assessment measures the function of the outer hair cells. It does not measure hearing.

Hearing losses can come about from disease processes that affect the outer, middle, or inner ear (Table 2). Some diseases affect the auditory nerve, and others affect the CNS. The location of the pathologic process determines the type of hearing loss and the appropriate therapy. Those losses that come about because of dysfunction of the external or middle ear are called conductive losses, the term "conductive" referring to the ability of the patient to hear well through direct sound stimulation of the bone but not through stimulation of the cochlea by airborne sound. The second type of loss, sensorineural hearing loss (SNHL), is the result of a defect in the inner ear or the auditory nerve. A third type, CNS hearing loss, is caused by abnormalities in that system. A fourth type is a mixed loss, with components

TABLE 1. Assessments of Hearing

ASSESSMENT	AGE	FUNCTION
ELM	0–36 mo	Language and speech
ABR	All ages	Hearing and central nervous system integrity
VRA	6–36 mo	Hearing
Audiometry	>36 mo	Hearing
Tympanometry	All ages	Physical characteristics of the middle ear, e.g., probable presence or absence of OME; *this is not a test of hearing*
Cochlear emission, spontaneous or evoked	All ages	Outer hair cell function; *this is not a test of hearing*

ABR, auditory brainstem evoked potential; ELM, early language milestone scale; OME, otitis media with effusion; VRA, visual reinforced audiometry.

TABLE 2. Types of Hearing Loss

TYPE	LOCATION OF DEFECT	TEST TO DEFINE	TEST FINDING	COMMON CAUSES
Conductive	External or middle ear	ABR	Increased latency of response	OME Cholesteatoma Malformation Trauma
		VRA	Bone conduction greater than air conduction	OME Cholesteatoma Malformation Trauma
		Audiogram	Bone conduction greater than air conduction	OME Cholesteatoma Malformation Trauma
		Tympanogram	Type B	OME Cholesteatoma Malformation Trauma
SNHL	Inner ear	ABR	Decreased threshold	Genetic, meningitis, autoimmune disease, PLF, sound trauma, ototoxicity
		VRA	Decreased threshold	Genetic, meningitis, autoimmune disease, PLF, sound trauma, ototoxicity
		Audiogram	Decreased threshold	Genetic, meningitis, autoimmune desease, PLF, sound trauma, ototoxicity
		Cochlear emissions	Absence	Genetic, meningitis, autoimmune disease, PLF, sound trauma, ototoxicity
Mixed	External, middle, and inner ear	ABR	Bone conduction decreased but better than air conduction	SNHL with OME
		VRA	Bone conduction decreased but better than air conduction	SNHL with OME
		Audiogram	Bone conduction decreased but better than air conduction	SNHL with OME

ABR, auditory brainstem evoked potential; OME, otitis media with effusion; PLF, perilymphatic fistula; SNHL, sensorineural hearing loss; VRA, visual reinforced audiometry.

of both conductive loss and SNHL. Accurate, noninvasive techniques are widely available to determine which hearing losses are sensory from the loss of hair cells, which are neural from defects in the auditory nerve, and which are central because of defects in the CNS. Effective therapies are available for all of these hearing losses.

THERAPY OF OTITIS MEDIA WITH EFFUSION

The most common form of hearing loss is associated with middle ear infections and is caused most often by fluid remaining in the middle ear, resulting in a conductive hearing loss—otitis media with effusion (OME). Hearing losses associated with OME are variable, ranging from none to a loss of greater than 40 dB pure tone average (PTA) of 500, 1000, and 2000 Hz. The loss level varies from day to day. In determining therapy for OME, there are two critical considerations. Who should be treated? What should the treatment be? In addition to the hearing loss, other important indications for treating OME include recurrent acute otitis media, otalgia, otorrhea, severe tympanic membrane retraction, and incus necrosis. The therapies discussed are indicated solely on the basis of the hearing loss that is a consequence of OME. These interventions should be undertaken to restore normal hearing in all patients in whom the hearing loss is definitely or probably interfering with aural or oral communication. Because of the critical period for language development, the timeliness of the restoration of hearing must be emphasized for those less than 36 months of age and especially for those less than 24 months of age. An infant or toddler who has an absolute or relative delay in expressive or receptive language, as measured by a scale such as the ELM, or whose caregiver believes that the child may be having language or speech problems and who has an associated OME must be considered for therapy directed at restoring normal hearing. Because of the fluctuations inherent in the disease, hearing evaluations of these children at any particular time may or may not show hearing loss. The presence

of OME, either by history or examination or both, and a language problem make the child a candidate for intervention to maintain normal hearing. In some cases, the patient may be followed with hearing and language assessments to monitor the disease and its effects. Infants, toddlers, or children who have a persistent loss of greater than 15 dB PTA should have hearing restored. The object of the therapy (Table 3) is to restore or enable normal hearing as quickly as possible.

Meta-analysis[3] of 10 randomized studies of OME, with the outcome of either tympanometry or otoscopy or both (but not hearing), showed only a 10% to 35% advantage of an antibiotic over a placebo. The antibiotic resolution of OME occurs over weeks, and may be effective in 10% to 33% of patients. These data indicate that antibiotics do *not* restore normal hearing in a timely fashion in most patients with OME. Substantial sequelae from the use of antibiotics include the creation of antibiotic resistance and the development of antibiotic allergy in 5% to 10% of patients so treated.

Restoration of hearing can be brought about in a timely fashion either by the removal of the fluid and insertion of a tympanostomy tube or by the use of hearing aids. Most often, operative intervention should be used. This should be combined with an adenoidectomy when indicated so as to decrease the rate of recurrence of OME after extrusion of the tympanostomy tubes. Adenoidectomy should not be performed in patients with cleft palate or in those with submucosal clefts of the palate, the latter often evidenced by a bifid uvula. In such patients, removal of adenoidal tissue may result in the development of velopharyngeal insufficiency. For most patients, removal of the middle ear fluid with the insertion of the tympanostomy tube and subsequent aeration of the middle ear by the tympanostomy tube will result in a return to normal hearing. Sequelae associated with the operative procedure, which include the problems of general anesthesia and postoperative bleeding from the adenoidectomy, occur in about 2% of the patients, and otorrhea following tympanostomy tube insertion will occur in 10% to 15% of the patients. In addition, the

TABLE 3. Therapies for Hearing Loss from OME

THERAPY	EFFECTIVENESS	SEQUELAE
Antibiotics	10%–35% effective as measured by otoscopy or tympanometry; hearing may be restored in weeks	Allergy (5%–10%) and the creation of antibiotic-resistant organisms
Tympanostomy tubes with or without adenoidectomy	Effective for restoration of hearing within a day	Operative morbidity (1%–2%), otorrhea (10%–15%), precautions against water entering the ear, otorrhea, long-term changes in the tympanic membrane
Hearing aids	Immediate restoration of hearing	Expense, lack of acceptance, and loss by young patients

operated ear(s) must be protected against water entering, which will necessitate the use of earplugs while swimming or bathing. Long-term sequelae include otorrhea, changes in the tympanic membrane, and tympanic membrane perforations. The incidence of the long-term sequelae varies with different populations. Patients with a tympanostomy tube(s) in place must be cared for until the tympanostomy tube(s) has been extruded or has been removed.

Tympanostomy tubes cannot be used in patients with constant otorrhea or in those with immune deficiency, for example, patients with cilia dyskinesis (Kartagener's syndrome). To avoid the chronic hearing loss these patients would have as a result of their middle ear fluid, they should be fitted with low gain hearing aids. These have functioned well in the restoration of normal hearing and development and maintenance of normal language. Problems connected with hearing aids are expense, maintenance, loss, otitis externa, and poor acceptance by teenagers. Whether a tympanostomy tube or hearing aid is used to enable adequate hearing, the efficacy of the intervention can be gauged by the child's hearing and, most importantly, by the child's language and speech development. For children less than 36 months of age, the ELM or similar screen can be used at periodic follow-up visits to monitor language and speech development.

Acquired conductive hearing losses can result from infection, cholesteatoma, a benign tumor, or trauma. Hearing loss from these causes is corrected by surgical intervention or the use of hearing aids or both. Congenital conductive hearing losses resulting from malformation, some of which can be progressive, are cared for in the same manner, with greater dependence on the hearing aid than on surgical intervention, especially in complex malformations.

THERAPY OF UNILATERAL HEARING LOSS

In the past, the educational and linguistic significance of unilateral hearing loss was not recognized. It is now established that children with a unilateral sensorineural hearing loss (SNHL) or any significant unilateral loss will be at an educational disadvantage. This is demonstrated, for example, by the finding that a child with a unilateral hearing loss has a 20 times greater probability of repeating one of the first few years of school than have normal hearing children. These children with unilateral hearing loss are found to have linguistic deficits and a decreased ability to perceive speech in noise. The most effective therapy for unilaterally hearing-impaired children includes early identification of the problem, language therapy, and the use of an FM or similar system in the class room. With the FM system, the teacher uses a microphone that transmits her or his speech via FM to the good ear of the unilaterally hearing impaired child wearing an appropriate receiver. This arrangement enhances the signal—the teacher's voice — which compensates for the child's unilateral handicap of signal in noise detection.

THERAPY OF SENSORINEURAL HEARING LOSS

There are effective therapies for all forms of SNHL. Successful therapy for either congenital or acquired SNHL at all levels of loss is dependent on early detection and prompt institution of the appropriate therapy. Most often, therapy will be the use of hearing aids

and intensive language habilitation. There are three areas in which effective medical or surgical therapies are now available (Table 4).

Progressive SNHL in children occurs as a result of *autoimmune diseases*. The hearing loss may be the sole manifestation of the condition, or there may be other signs, among which the most common are conjunctivitis and arthritis. The diagnosis depends on the detection of autoimmune antibodies against inner ear tissue. These cases, which are rare, are treated with immunosuppressive therapies. Corticosteroids are used primarily in children. Such therapy has resulted in the restoration of some hearing and the probable arrest of further loss. These patients must be monitored closely for changes in hearing acuity and the sequelae associated with immunosuppression. They should be cared for in a manner similar to patients undergoing tissue transplantation.

Another cause of progressive SNHL in infants and children is *perilymphatic fistula* (PLF). The hearing loss results from a loss of perilymph into the middle ear. Perilymph is the fluid that surrounds the inner ear and is derived from and is in contact with the cerebrospinal fluid through the perilymphatic aqueduct. The loss of fluid will most often be through the oval window or the round window or both. These PLFs occur because of congenital, acquired, or genetic abnormalities. PLFs are found in families, identical twins, and brother and sister, as well as sporadically. They may occur as a result of head trauma, sometimes modest, in an infant or toddler. They have been seen in infants who have fallen from a bassinet or been hit in the head by a car seat, without an associated hematotympanum or temporal bone fracture. PLF is found in children with temporal bone fractures. Cases of PLF will present as progressive or fluctuating hearing loss. Usually, speech discrimination is poorer than would be expected from the audiogram. Fistula testing is specific (few false positives) but not sensitive (many false negatives). The treatment is surgical repair of the fistula. The surgical results can be remarkable[4] (Fig. 1) but commonly may only stop the progression of the loss. Early detection of a PLF allows for better hearing to be salvaged and probably increases the opportunity for restoration of hearing.

Acquired profound SNHL resulting from meningitis, ototoxicity, trauma, progressive nonsyndromic hereditary hearing loss, or other causes in children who have developed language (i.e., >24 months

TABLE 4. Medical and Surgical Therapies for Acquired SNHL

TYPE OF SNHL	THERAPY	COMMENT
Autoimmune SNHL	Immunosuppressive agents	Need for definitive diagnosis by means of inner ear antibody test
Perilymphatic fistula	Surgical repair	Etiology can be genetic or traumatic; fistula test is specific but not sensitive
Postlingual profound deafness	Cochlear implant	May be used in children >24 mo of age; has benefit in speech production and reception; patient requires extensive habilitation

SNHL, sensorineural hearing loss.

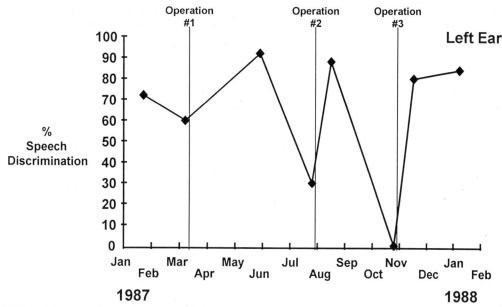

FIGURE 1. A 10-year-old boy who underwent three exploratory tympanotomies for fluctuating hearing loss. Discrimination scores (%) are plotted against time. After each surgical intervention (vertical lines), the patient's discrimination improved. (From Ruben RJ, Yankelowitz SM: Spontaneous perilymphatic fistula in children. Am J Otol 10:198–207, 1989.)

of age) can be cared for with a cochlear implant (CI). CIs have their best results in the area of speech production and to a lesser extent in speech reception in postlinguistically deafened children. CIs have not had a substantial effect on the children's language development. Children with acquired profound SNHL with a CI require the same extensive habilitative education as other profoundly deaf children who use hearing aids or other means of communication. However, the children with CIs can benefit from the limited increased abilities in speech production and reception.

Recently, molecular biologic manipulations have been developed that result in regeneration of the heretofore considered end-stage transducer cells of the inner ear, the hair cells. Because this and other advances hold promise for biologic repair of the inner ear, children should not have both ears implanted with a CI because that would probably permanently destroy or greatly impair the chances for subsequent repair of the inner ear.

REFERENCES

1. Copland J: Early Language Milestone Scale: Examiner's Manual, 2nd ed. Austin, Texas, Pro-ed, 1993:1–95.
2. Gravel JR: Assessing auditory system integrity in high-risk infants and young children. *In* Gravel JR (ed): Seminars in Hearing. New York, Thieme Medical Publishers Inc., 1989;10:213–292.
3. Rosenfeld RM, Post JC: Meta-analysis of antibiotics for the treatment of otitis media with effusion. Otolaryngol Head Neck Surg 106:378–386, 1992.
4. Ruben RJ, Yankelowitz SM: Spontaneous perilymphatic fistula in children. Am J Otol 10:198–207, 1989.

OTITIS MEDIA

JACK L. PARADISE, M.D.

Next to the common cold, otitis media is the most prevalent childhood illness in developed countries. In the United States in 1990, otitis media was the principal diagnosis at over 19 million nonhospital office visits by children under age 15. The peak incidence and prevalence occur during the first 2 years of life. Factors identified as increasing the risk of otitis media include young age, male sex, low socioeconomic status, strong history of the disease in a parent or sibling, non-breast-milk feeding, day-care attendance, and cold weather. Other possible risk factors include white (as compared with black) race, respiratory allergy, and household smoking. Important characteristics of otitis media are its propensity to become chronic and to recur. In general, the earlier in life the first episode of otitis media develops, the greater the degree of subsequent difficulty with the disease.

Accurate diagnosis of otitis media in young children is often problematic. Symptoms may be absent or inapparent, especially during early infancy and in chronic stages of the disease. Cerumen often obscures the eardrum, and removing it may be difficult and require forcible restraint of the child. Once the eardrum is visualized, abnormalities may be subtle and difficult to interpret accurately.

Adverse effects of otitis media include the illness, discomfort, and potential suppurative complications and sequelae associated with acute and chronic middle ear infection and the transient reduction in hearing acuity that accompanies middle ear effusion. Long-term developmental consequences of otitis media remain uncertain, controversial, and the subject of continuing investigation.

ACUTE (SUPPURATIVE) OTITIS MEDIA VERSUS SECRETORY (NONSUPPURATIVE) OTITIS MEDIA (OTITIS MEDIA WITH EFFUSION)

For working purposes, the otitis media disease spectrum traditionally has been divided into two components:

1. Infection, termed *suppurative* or *acute* otitis media (AOM)
2. Usually noninfective inflammation accompanied by effusion, termed *nonsuppurative* or *secretory* otitis media, or *otitis media with effusion* (OME).

These two main types of otitis media are interrelated. Infection usually is succeeded by residual noninfective inflammation and effusion, which, in turn, predispose to renewed infection. Any schema for distinguishing between AOM and OME is somewhat arbitrary, as each may evolve into the other without any surely differentiating physical findings. Both types are accompanied by physical signs of effusion.

Bulging and redness of the tympanic membrane are likely to be prominent in AOM but absent or slight in OME. Ear pain usually is indicative of infection.

ACUTE OTITIS MEDIA

Advisability of Antimicrobial Treatment

Children with AOM should routinely receive antimicrobial treatment for three reasons: (1) a large majority of cases are caused by pathogenic bacteria, particularly *Streptococcus pneumoniae*, nontypeable *Haemophilus influenzae*, and *Moraxella catarrhalis*, (2) symptomatic improvement and resolution of infection occur more promptly and more consistently with antimicrobial treatment than without (even though most untreated cases eventually also resolve), and (3) the secular decline in suppurative complications, particularly mastoiditis, must be attributed mainly to the widespread routine use of antimicrobials for AOM. The policy advanced in some quarters of withholding antimicrobial treatment unless symptoms persist or worsen neither adequately takes these considerations into account nor is adequately supported by the studies cited by proponents.

Choice of Antimicrobial Drugs

Factors governing the choice among available antimicrobial drugs include, most prominently, safety and efficacy, and also cost, palatability, and required frequency of administration. Obviously, no child should receive a drug to which he or she has experienced a serious untoward reaction. Amoxicillin remains the drug of first choice under most circumstances, despite increasing resistance by some strains of bacteria in some regions, because of its excellent record of safety, its relative efficacy, and its low cost. In vitro studies to the contrary notwithstanding, none of the alternative drugs listed in Table 1 has been shown in well-controlled clinical trials to be significantly more effective as first-line treatment for AOM than amoxicillin. Nonetheless, of general concern regarding efficacy are the production of beta-lactamase by many strains of *H. influenzae* and most strains of *M. catarrhalis* and resistance on the part of certain strains of pneumococci to sulfonamides and, increasingly, to amoxicillin and other drugs, resulting from alterations in penicillin-binding proteins rather than from production of beta-lactamase.

Each of the drugs listed in Table 1 has advantages and disadvantages. Amoxicillin-clavulanic acid enjoys the safety of amoxicillin while at the same time being resistant to beta-lactamase, but it often causes troublesome diarrhea and is quite expensive. The various orally administered cephalosporins, all also quite expensive, differ in a number of characteristics. Cefaclor is palatable but may not be effective against beta-lactamase-producing organisms or resistant pneumococci and may occasionally cause serum sickness. Cefixime requires only once-daily administration but may be less effective against pneumococci than other available drugs. More recently available semi-synthetic orally administered cephalosporins—cefpodoxime, cefprozil, cefuroxime, and loracarbef—may prove useful in individual instances. Of these, cefpodoxime and cefuroxime seem most promising. Unfortunately, none of the cephalosporins is likely to be more effective against penicillin-resistant pneumococci than amoxicillin. Trimethoprim-sulfamethoxazole (TMP-SMX) is relatively inexpensive and requires only twice-daily administration, but it lacks efficacy against beta-hemolytic streptococci and many strains of pneumococci and, rarely, may cause severe reactions, such as bone marrow suppression or Stevens-Johnson syndrome. Erythromycin-sulfisoxazole also may cause such reactions, but it is more effective than TMP-SMX against gram-positive cocci. Clarithromycin, a newer macrolide, is effective against beta-lactamase-producing organisms as well as some resistant pneumococci. It also requires only twice-daily administration and appears less likely to cause diarrhea than some of the other antibiotics, but it is quite expensive. The efficacy of a single dose of intramuscular ceftriaxone remains to be evaluated definitively. With patterns of bacterial resistance changing, the relative efficacy of each of these drugs will require periodic reappraisal.

TABLE 1. Antimicrobials for Treating Otitis Media

DRUG	DAILY DOSAGE
Amoxicillin	40 mg/kg in 3 doses
Amoxicillin-clavu-lanic acid	40 mg/kg amoxicillin with 10 mg/kg clavulanic acid in 3 doses
Cefaclor	40 mg/kg in 2 or 3 doses
Cefixime	8 mg/kg in 1 or 2 doses
Cefpodoxime	10 mg/kg in 2 doses
Cefprozil	30 mg/kg in 2 doses
Cefuroxime axetil	250 mg in 2 doses (<2 y); 500 mg in 2 doses (≥2 y)
Clarithromycin	15 mg/kg in 2 doses
Erythromycin-sul-fisoxazole	50 mg/kg erythromycin with 150 mg/kg sulfisoxazole in 4 doses
Loracarbef	30 mg/kg in 2 doses
Trimethoprim-sul-famethoxazole	8 mg/kg trimethoprim with 40 mg/kg sulfamethoxazole in 2 doses

It must be noted that just as many cases of AOM resolve without any treatment, many cases also resolve after treatment with a drug or drugs that show less than optimal in vitro efficacy against the particular causative organism.

Bullous Myringitis

Bullous myringitis is a physical manifestation of AOM and not an etiologically discrete entity. Treatment is appropriately that of the underlying AOM.

Duration of Antimicrobial Treatment

The duration of treatment of AOM has often been set at 10 days in an apparent extrapolation from the optimal duration of treatment of streptococcal pharyngitis with penicillin. However, 10 days may be longer than necessary for some children and not long enough for others, depending on the severity of the infection and the child's degree of proneness to otitis. Study results in support of treatment periods of less than 10 days have not been convincing. For most episodes in most children, treatment for 10 days would seem advisable, and longer periods would be appropriate for children whose previous experience with AOM had been problematic.

Unsatisfactory Response to Initial Treatment and Deciding on "Second-line" Drugs

Complicating treatment are the facts that AOM is essentially a closed-space infection and that its resolution depends not only on eradication of the offending organism but also on restoration and maintenance of the ventilatory function of the eustachian tube. Unsatisfactory response to initial first-line treatment is thus usually attributable to factors other than inadequate antimicrobial efficacy. These factors include poor compliance, concurrent or intercurrent viral infection, persistent middle ear underaeration despite bacterial killing, reinfection from other sites or from outside sources, and immature or impaired host defenses. Nonetheless, switching to an alternative, or second-line, drug would seem reasonable when there has been inadequate improvement in symptoms or in middle ear status, as reflected in the appearance of the eardrum, or when the persistence of purulent nasal discharge suggests less than optimal efficacy of the antimicrobial drug being used. Second-line drugs also may be reasonably used when AOM develops in a child already receiving antimicrobial prophylaxis or in an immunocompromised child or in a child with severe symptoms whose previous experience with otitis has been problematic.

Myringotomy and Tympanocentesis

Myringotomy is a time-honored treatment for AOM but is usually not necessary in the antimicrobial era. Myringotomy is unquestionably effective in providing prompt relief of pain, but in a clinical trial limited to children with severe AOM, those who received amoxicillin plus myringotomy fared no better overall than those who received amoxicillin only. However, the study population was not large enough to have excluded the possibility that myringotomy had been marginally beneficial. Reasonable indications for myringotomy would include severe, refractory pain, hyperpyrexia, inadequate clinical response to vigorous antimicrobial treatment, complications of AOM, such as facial paralysis, mastoiditis, labyrinthitis, or CNS infection, and immunologic compromise from any source.

In very young infants with AOM who show systemic signs of illness, such as fever, vomiting, or lethargy, one cannot properly presume that AOM is the sole cause of the illness. In such infants, a sepsis workup is mandatory, and this should include tympanocentesis and culture of the middle ear aspirate. Tympanocentesis or myringotomy should be performed in those older infants and children in whom AOM has been refractory to empirically selected antimicrobial treatment.

Follow-Up

The appropriate interval for follow-up of an individual episode of AOM depends on the overall clinical circumstances and on the patient's symptomatic response. In the patient with only a sporadic episode and prompt symptomatic improvement, follow-up 1 month after initial examination is early enough. On the other hand, follow-up within days would be advisable in the young infant with a severe episode or in a child of any age with continuing pain or within 1 or 2 weeks in a child who is immunocompromised or has had frequent recurrences that have been resistant to treatment. In all cases, follow-up should be maintained at reasonable intervals until normal middle ear status has been achieved.

Early Recurrence after Treatment

Recurrence of AOM after treatment may be due either to incomplete eradication of infection in the middle ear or upper respiratory tract or to reinfection by the same or a different bacterium or bacterial strain. For recurrence within 60 days, treatment may be best guided by the response to treatment of the antecedent episode. If it had seemed to respond to a first-line antimicrobial, that drug would again be appropriate. If it had failed to respond to a first-line drug but seemed to respond to a second-line drug, use of a second-line drug from the outset might be advisable. Recurrence developing 2 or more months after a treated episode of AOM is usually caused by a different organism. Accordingly, use of a first-line antimicrobial irrespective of previous responses to treatment is appropriate.

SECRETORY OTITIS MEDIA

OME may occur either as the aftermath of an episode of AOM or apparently de novo as a presumed consequence of impaired middle ear ventilation. In most cases of OME, the effusion is sterile, but in a minority, the effusion contains pathogenic bacteria. Rational treatment of OME depends on knowledge of its natural history, its possible complications and sequelae, and the efficacy of available treatment modalities. Unfortunately, information in each of these areas is limited.

Natural History

Most cases of OME resolve with or without treatment within 3 months or less. Virtually no data are available concerning the subsequent long-term course of children in whom resolution does not occur within that time frame and who do not receive surgical intervention.

Possible Complications and Sequelae

Except in the minority of children who are discomfited by the variable conductive hearing loss, the main reason to consider treatment for OME is to prevent possible complications and sequelae: heightened risk of developing AOM, pathologic middle ear changes (e.g., tympanic membrane retraction pockets, adhesive otitis, ossicular discon-

tinuity, and cholesteatoma), cochlear damage with resulting SNHL, and long-term adverse effects on speech, language, cognitive, and psychosocial development. The extent to which these constitute real or merely hypothetical risks and the circumstances that might influence whether and to what degree they develop are not known.

Variables Influencing Treatment Decisions

In deciding whether and how vigorously to treat individual cases of OME, it may be useful to take into account both patient-related and disease-related variables that may affect the degree of morbidity and the prognosis. The patient-related variables include age, the frequency and severity of previous episodes of AOM and the interval since the last episode, the nature of prior treatment and of the child's response, and the presence or absence of a history of adverse drug reactions, concurrent medical problems or risk factors, and environmental risk factors, such as day care attendance or other exposure to infectious disease. The disease-related variables include whether the episode is newly developed or the aftermath of an attack of AOM, whether the effusion is unilateral or bilateral, the apparent quantity of effusion, the duration if known, the degree of hearing impairment, the presence or absence of other possibly related symptoms, such as vertigo or disturbance of balance, and the presence or absence of mucopurulent or purulent rhinorrhea, which would be indicative of concurrent nasopharyngeal or paranasal sinus infection that might be contributing to continuing compromise of middle ear ventilation.

Medical Treatment Options

Antimicrobials have definite but limited efficacy in resolving OME, presumably because they help eradicate nasopharyngeal or inapparent middle ear infection or both. The reported degree of efficacy of antimicrobials has varied, probably because of differences between studies in design, in the drug used, and in the constellations of patient-related variables. Because the efficacy of antimicrobials for OME is at best limited, because most cases resolve without treatment within a reasonably short period, and because of growing concern about the contribution of antimicrobial usage to the survival and spread of resistant bacteria, particulary *S. pneumoniae*, routine antimicrobial treatment of OME, as previously recommended by some authorities, no longer seems reasonable. Instead, treatment should be limited to cases in which there appears to be associated bacterial upper respiratory tract infection or in which chronicity or troubling hearing loss prompts consideration of tympanostomy tube placement. Should antimicrobial treatment be decided on, the choice of drugs is appropriately governed by the considerations reviewed previously in relation to AOM. Two weeks would usually constitute an appropriate duration of treatment. When the response to a first-line drug seems unsatisfactory, a trial of treatment with a second-line drug would be reasonable, although evidence to support greater efficacy of second-line drugs is lacking.

The efficacy of *corticosteroids* in the treatment of OME remains to be determined. Some studies have found substantial efficacy, whereas others have found none. One must keep in mind that the administration of steroids to children who have not yet had chickenpox but who have been recently exposed may have disastrous consequences.

Antihistamine-decongestant combinations are not effective in treating children in general with OME, but their efficacy has not been tested adequately in specifically allergic children. Antihistamines alone, decongestants alone, and mucolytic agents are unlikely to be effective. Allergic management might prove helpful in children with problematic OME who also have clear-cut manifestations of upper respiratory allergy, but supporting data are lacking. In children without clinical evidence of allergy, allergy testing is not indicated.

Myringotomy and Tympanostomy Tube Placement

Benefits and Risks. When OME persists despite both adequate antimicrobial treatment and an ample period of watchful waiting, the question arises about surgical intervention. Myringotomy alone, without tympanostomy tube placement, permits evacuation of middle ear effusion but often is followed, because the incision heals before eustachian tube ventilatory function has been restored, by reaccumulation of effusion. Adding tube placement, on the other hand, offers the likelihood that middle ear ventilation will be sustained for at least as long as the tube remains in place and functional, usually about 6 to 12 months. However, tube placement is not consistently innocuous. Common complications include obstruction of the tube lumen, premature extrusion, and secondary infection with otorrhea through the tube. Sequelae following tubal extrusion include residual perforation of the eardrum, tympanosclerosis, localized or diffuse atrophic scarring of the eardrum that may predispose to the development of retraction pockets or atelectasis or both, residual conductive hearing loss, and cholesteatoma. Currently, it appears that the more serious of these sequelae are the exception rather than the rule. Recurrence of middle ear effusion following the extrusion of tubes has not been studied systematically but develops frequently.

When To Consider. Given the uncertainties concerning possible otologic and developmental consequences of long-standing OME and given the costs and risks of surgical intervention, the point at which surgical intervention should be considered remains conjectural. Examples of reasonable approaches, subject to modification based on the specifics of the patient-related and disease-related variables discussed previously, particularly on the degree of hearing loss, would be to consider myringotomy with or without tube placement after 3 months of continuous bilateral OME or, alternatively, myringotomy with tube placement after 6 months of continuous bilateral OME.

SPECIAL POPULATIONS

Persistent OME, often punctuated by episodes of AOM, is virtually universal among infants and young children with cleft palate, although morbidity may be reduced to an extent by breast milk feeding. Antimicrobial treatment of OME in infants with cleft palate rarely results in clearance of effusion, and most such infants require tube placement on one or more occasions to maintain middle ear ventilation and normal or near-normal hearing. Children with Down syndrome also are at greater risk of developing both recurrent AOM and persistent OME than are children in general and also more often become appropriate candidates for tube placement.

PREVENTION OF OTITIS MEDIA

General measures to prevent otitis media consist of breast milk feeding, avoidance, insofar as possible, of exposure to individuals with respiratory infection, maintenance of general hygiene, and, probably, avoidance of environmental tobacco smoke. In children who have developed frequent episodes of AOM, *antimicrobial prophylaxis* with subtherapeutic doses of one or another antimicrobial—usually an aminopenicillin or a sulfonamide—has been shown in a number of studies to provide considerable protection against recurrences. Therefore, until recently, prophylaxis using amoxicillin or sulfisoxazole (use of TMP-SMX for this purpose is cautioned against in *Physicians' Desk Reference*) has seemed an appropriate routine intervention for such children. However, again because of the probable contribution of antimicrobial usage to bacterial, particularly pneumococcal, resistance, subjecting such children routinely to sustained antimicrobial prophylaxis now seems somewhat dubious, its risks potentially outweighing its likely benefits. This seems to be so, particularly for children in day care, who in any case are at increased risk of colonization with multiply resistant *S. pneumoniae*. How best to manage the individual child who is severely affected must remain a matter of individual judgment, with the alternatives to prophylaxis being either continued reliance on episodic treatment, which seems preferable where feasible, or referral for tympanostomy tube placement, with its own, previously noted risks. In such severely affected children, the parents properly should participate in decision making after being apprised of the relative risks. Also in such children, both

polyvalent pneumococcal vaccine and influenza vaccine may provide limited protection.

Finally, in children who have undergone tube placement and in whom, after extrusion of tubes, otitis media continues to be a problem, adenoidectomy is efficacious to a limited extent in reducing the risk of subsequent recurrences.

REFERENCES

1. Friedland IR, McCracken GH Jr: Management of infections caused by antibiotic-resistant *Streptococcus pneumoniae*. N Engl J Med 331:377–382, 1994.
2. Kaleida PH, Casselbrant ML, Rockette HE, Paradise JL, Bluestone CD, Blatter MM, Reisinger KS, Wald ER, Supance JS: Amoxicillin or myringotomy or both for acute otitis media: Results of a randomized clinical trial. Pediatrics 87:466–474, 1991.
3. Lieberman JM: Bacterial resistance in the '90s. Contemp Pediatr 11:72–99, 1994.
4. Mandel EM, Rockette HE, Bluestone CD, Paradise JL, Nozza RJ: Efficacy of amoxicillin with and without decongestant-antihistamine for otitis media with effusion in children: Results of a randomized, double-blind trial. N Engl J Med 316:432–437, 1987.
5. Mandel EM, Rockette HE, Bluestone CD, Paradise JL, Nozza RJ: Efficacy of myringotomy with and without tympanostomy tubes for chronic otitis media with effusion. Pediatr Infect Dis J 11:270–277, 1992.
6. Murray BE: Can antibiotic resistance be controlled? (Editorial). N Engl J Med 330:1229–1230, 1994.
7. Paradise JL: Otitis media in infants and children. Pediatrics 65:917–943, 1980.
8. Paradise JL: Does early-life otitis media result in lasting developmental impairment? Why the question persists, and a proposed plan for addressing it. Adv Pediatr 39:157–165, 1992.
9. Paradise JL, Bluestone CD, Rogers KD, Taylor FH, Colborn DK, Bachman RZ, Bernard BS, Schwarzbach RH: Efficacy of adenoidectomy for recurrent otitis media in children previously treated with tympanostomy tube placement: Results of parallel randomized and nonrandomized trials. JAMA 263:2066–2073, 1990.

FOREIGN BODIES IN EXTERNAL AUDITORY CANAL

ELLEN M. FRIEDMAN, M.D.

Young children frequently put foreign objects in their external auditory canal. Commonly retrieved foreign objects are beads, earrings, pieces of food, wads of paper, and toy parts. These foreign bodies may not cause any symptoms or, depending on the position, may inflict pain, vertigo, or hearing loss.

Anatomically, the size, shape, and curvature of the external auditory canal are highly variable. The external auditory canal is innervated by cranial nerves V, VII, and X and has a substantial vascular supply covered by rather thin skin. These anatomic factors, as well as the degree of patient cooperation, can make the removal of a foreign body from the external auditory canal a challenge. One's first attempt is the most likely to be successful, as subsequent attempts may be compounded by pain, bleeding, external canal swelling, poor visibility, and even poorer patient cooperation. Therefore, the initial attempt at foreign body removal is enhanced by proper illumination, patient restraints, appropriate-sized instruments, and possibly sedation. General anesthesia is rarely necessary when adequate sedation is achieved during the early stages of management. Multiple attempts with additional trauma, however, may necessitate that the procedure be performed in the operating room. If the patient is not immobilized with either medication or adequate restraints, the result may be a laceration of the external auditory canal skin, perforation of the tympanic membrane, or ossicular dislocation.

Chloral hydrate is a suggested sedative that has been used with great success. The papoose may be used to further limit patient mobility. The office microscope is useful for this procedure, although an otoscope with an operating head may also yield adequate illumination. Microinstruments, such as the alligator, the Tobey forceps, and the angled ear pick, will be necessary. Alternatively, irrigation may successfully flush out a foreign body. However, this technique should be avoided when the object is hydrophilic and may swell with irrigation. Live insects, which are common foreign bodies in the external auditory canal, may be removed by placing several drops of mineral oil in the external auditory canal and then flushing out the now dead insect. Forceful removal of live insects should be avoided because a portion of their barbs may remain embedded in the skin of the external auditory canal.

LABYRINTHITIS

MARGARET A. KENNA, M.D.

The term "labyrinthitis" refers to inflammation of the labyrinth, or bony and membranous inner ear structures, which include the cochlea and three semicircular canals. It does not specify whether the perilymph, endolymph, or bony labyrinth is the site of involvement. However, symptoms will not occur unless the membranous labyrinth is involved in the inflammatory process. The initial location of the etiology of the labyrinthitis may also determine the presenting symptoms.

Most labyrinthitis in children is due to acute or chronic bacterial or viral infections. Such types of labyrinthitis can be divided into several categories: suppurative, serous, viral, syphilitic, fistula related, and autoimmune.

SUPPURATIVE (PURULENT) LABYRINTHITIS

Suppurative labyrinthitis occurs when bacteria invade the inner ear from the middle ear, mastoid, other areas of the temporal bone, meninges, or cerebrospinal fluid (CSF) or by hematogenous spread. Symptoms include severe vertigo, often accompanied by nausea and vomiting, and sensorineural hearing loss (SNHL). The most common causes of acute bacterial suppurative labyrinthitis are acute otitis media (AOM) and meningitis. Other less common etiologies include lateral semicircular canal fistula (secondary to cholesteatoma or trauma) and surgery that injures the lateral canal or oval or round windows. Treatment of suppurative labyrinthitis requires identification of the bacterial organism involved. If AOM is the cause, tympanocentesis or wide myringotomy (sometimes with the placement of a ventilating tube) to drain the middle ear and obtain material for culture should be performed, and appropriate systemic antimicrobials should be given. If the patient does not improve using these measures, mastoidectomy may be indicated (especially if other complications of AOM are impending, such as meningitis). If bacterial meningitis is the cause of suppurative labyrinthitis, the acute labyrinthitis usually resolves when the meningitis is treated with the appropriate systemic antimicrobial agent. In some studies, systemic steroids have been shown to be of benefit in hearing preservation. However, there are conflicting reports, and final recommendations are inconclusive. If the meningitis is thought to result from a suppurative otitis media, the middle ear also may need to be cultured and drained. If a lateral canal fistula associated with chronic suppurative otitis media (with or without cholesteatoma) is identified, mastoidectomy, culture of mastoid contents, and systemic antimicrobials are recommended. No matter what the underlying cause, the vertigo may be slow to resolve, and if incapacitating vertigo persists despite appropriate treatment, labyrinthectomy may need to be considered.

Suppurative labyrinthitis is nearly always associated with some degree of SNHL, frequently severe. This loss may or may not improve with treatment, but the hearing rarely returns to normal. All children need to undergo complete audiometric evaluation when the acute disease process has stabilized. Evaluation of hearing in each ear sep-arately is necessary, as there may be profound loss in one ear but usable hearing in the other. If the child cannot cooperate for behavioral testing, auditory brainstem evoked response testing (ABR) should be performed. If the child is comatose or poorly cooperative, ABR or otoacoustic emission testing may be useful. If hearing loss is identified, the child needs immediate counseling for habilitative/rehabilitative purposes. If a profound, bilateral hearing loss is detected and the child is over age 2 years, he or she may be a good candidate for a cochlear implant. If a conductive hearing loss associated with persistent middle ear fluid is identified, insertion of ventilating tubes may be indicated. If the child has persistent dysequilibrium, vestibular evaluation should be undertaken. Such youngsters may benefit from physical therapy. Since the hearing loss that occurs secondary to meningitis may improve or progress, audiometric follow-up for several years after the infection has resolved is mandatory.

If the suppurative labyrinthitis resulted from acute or chronic middle ear and mastoid disease, the child may need further middle ear or mastoid surgery, such as tympanoplasty or ossicular reconstruction, after the acute labyrinthitis has been treated.

SEROUS LABYRINTHITIS

Serous labyrinthitis is a sterile inflammatory process that usually occurs secondary to a contiguous infection, such as otitis media or mastoiditis (acute or chronic). It is currently thought that bacterial toxins or inflammatory mediators cross the round or oval window membranes or may enter through a congenital or acquired defect, but that actual bacterial or viral or fungal invasion does not occur. The symptoms of serous labyrinthitis may include dysequilibrium and SNHL, although not usually as severe as in suppurative labyrinthitis. The management of serous labyrinthitis consists of treating the underlying disorder, which includes systemic antimicrobials and, in the case of otitis media, wide myringotomy. Hearing should be evaluated as soon as the child is well enough, as although it is uncommon to develop total deafness from a serous labyrinthitis, permanent SNHL can occur. The use of systemic steroids in the treatment of serous labyrinthitis has been helpful.

VIRAL LABYRINTHITIS

Viral labyrinthitis occurs as a result of invasion of the inner ear by a virus, with loss of cochlear hair cells. The viruses best known to cause labyrinthitis include mumps, measles, influenza, varicella-zoster, parainfluenza, adenoviruses, cytomegalovirus (CMV), and herpes viruses.

If a child is noted to have measles, mumps, chickenpox, or other definable viral illness associated temporally with the onset of the hearing loss, an audiometric and otoscopic evaluation should be conducted as soon as possible, since prompt initiation of treatment may improve or save the hearing. If the patient is seen soon (within 10 to 14 days) after the onset of the hearing loss, systemic steroids should be considered, as they have been used with some success in enhancing the chances of hearing recovery and preservation.

The patient may experience the acute onset of vestibular symptoms without hearing loss. This is termed "vestibular neuronitis." If the child has acute symptoms of dysequilibrium, bedrest, fluids, and such medications as meclizine, dimenhydramine, diazepam, or droperidol may be effective. If there is not prompt resolution of symptoms, other causes of inner ear dysfunction should be considered, with the evaluation to include CT, MRI, and vestibular function studies.

Congenital rubella and CMV also are associated with sensorineural hearing impairment. It is suspected that other viruses, especially in utero, may be responsible for some of the hearing losses noted at or shortly after birth. It has been difficult to identify these viruses as the causative agents because the in utero event occurs remotely from the time of diagnosis of the hearing loss. As with all other children with hearing loss, audiometric evaluation should be performed as early as possible so that amplification and educational intervention can be initiated.

SYPHILITIC LABYRINTHITIS

This is a very specific type of labyrinthitis that often can be identified and treated, with improvement in the hearing and vertigo. The histopathology is twofold. First, syphilis may cause a meningoneurolabyrinthitis in early congenital syphilis and in the acute meningitides of secondary and tertiary syphilis. Second, osteitis of the temporal bone may be the predominant form, with secondary involvement of the membranous labyrinth.

Diagnosis is made by serum FTA-ABS and positive CSF serology. The symptoms include sudden, fluctuating or progressive hearing loss, with or without vestibular symptoms. Treatment includes high-dose penicillin and high-dose, long-term steroids. Symptoms of hearing loss and vertigo may stabilize or improve on this regimen but may relapse (especially the hearing loss) if steroids are discontinued.

PERILYMPHATIC FISTULA

A perilymphatic fistula (PLF) is a connection between the middle and inner ears, and it can act as a conduit to the inner ear for viruses, bacteria, or toxins, resulting in labyrinthitis or meningitis or both. PLFs can be congenital or acquired (usually traumatic) in nature and may be silent. Symptoms include fluctuating or progressive SNHL and vertigo. A fistula may not be suspected until multiple bouts of meningitis have occurred and even then can be very difficult to identify. Treatment consists of middle ear exploration and closure of the fistula, as well as management of any associated infectious complications.

AUTOIMMUNE LABYRINTHITIS

Autoimmune labyrinthitis may occur in association with a known systemic autoimmune disorder, such as polyarteritis nodosa, rheumatoid arthritis, Wegener's granulomatosis, or Cogan's syndrome. Inner ear disease may be the principal manifestation of autoimmunity without other systemic symptoms. The diagnosis of autoimmune inner ear diseases is often made, especially if other manifestations of autoimmune disease are absent, only when there is a positive clinical response to systemic steroids and immunosuppressive therapy.

Other diseases that are associated with inner ear disease and may be autoimmune in nature include Meniere's disease, otosclerosis, and multiple sclerosis.

REFERENCES

1. Gulya AJ: Infections of the labyrinth. In Bailey BJ, (ed): Head and Neck Surgery—Otolaryngology, Philadelphia, JB Lippincott, 1993:1769–1781.
2. Schuknecht HF: Disorders of the immune system. In Pathology of the Ear. Philadelphia, Lea and Febiger, 1993:345–364.

MIDDLE EAR TRAUMA

SCOTT A. ESTREM, M.D.
DAVID S. PARSONS, M.D.

Injuries to the middle ear can have devastating lifelong effects. The majority of injuries to the ear in children involve the external pinna and ear canal, and these usually do not produce problems beyond cosmetic deformity. Middle ear injuries can potentially damage the facial nerve, resulting in facial paralysis; dislodge the ossicular chain, causing conductive hearing loss; tear the round or oval window membrane, leading to vertigo, tinnitus, or sensorineural hearing loss; or injure the base of the skull, producing all of the preceding problems with a cerebrospinal fluid leak. This section focuses on injuries to the middle ear, which also necessitates discussion of injuries to the tympanic membrane and inner ear.

ANATOMY

The middle ear is a simple cavity with vital structures around its periphery. The main structures of the middle ear are the ossicles: the malleus, incus, and stapes. The facial nerve courses along the medial wall of the middle ear cavity and into the mastoid, usually covered by bone. The lateral border of the middle ear is the tympanic membrane. The medial wall is composed of the bony surface of the cochlea, with its membranous entrances to the middle ear, the round and oval windows. The brain is just superior to the middle ear, and the eustachian tube exits the ear anteriorly (Fig. 1). The carotid artery and the jugular vein reside inferiorly. The middle ear connects to the mastoid, its posterior border.

ETIOLOGY

The middle ear may be injured by blunt trauma, penetrating injuries through the ear canal, or even by sudden, marked pressure change. The possibility of child abuse must always be considered when evaluating such injuries.

Trauma has become more and more a part of our life, with ever increasing violence. Advancing technology may also facilitate otologic trauma. The most common cause of injuries to children remains automobile accidents. Three- and four-wheeled, motorized pleasure vehicles are commonly driven by preteen and teenage children, and the incidence of severe ear injuries has dramatically increased, including base of skull and temporal bone fractures. Such fractures are common with serious closed head injury and can involve damage to the tympanic membrane, ossicular chain, round or oval window membrane, inner ear, and facial nerve and cerebrospinal fluid leakage with associated complications.

A slap to the side of the head may induce a sudden pressure change in the external ear canal, with resultant transmission of this energy to the tympanic membrane, ossicles, round and oval windows, and inner ear. Each of these anatomic parts thus may be disrupted, with associated conductive or sensorineural hearing loss. A slap may be from such events as physical abuse or a fall while water skiing, in which the side of the head hits the flat surface of the water.

Penetrating injuries most commonly result from attempts at cleaning or itching the ear, either by the child or by a parent. Q-Tips remain the worst offender despite public education to refrain from placing "anything smaller than the elbow" in the ear. Usually, the scenario involves a child or parent cleaning the ear when a sneeze, an opened door, or a slip results in injury to the tympanic membrane or ossicles. Iatrogenic injury to these same structures occurs with mechanical cleaning using a curette or even with water irrigation methods. Interestingly, branches of trees and bushes are a source of injury to the external canal and tympanic membrane. The child may be walking when a branch suddenly whips back and strikes the external auditory canal. Bullet wounds also can occur, resulting in a variety of middle and inner ear injuries, as well as other injury.

Rapid changes in pressure transmitted to the ear canal can result in middle and inner ear disruption. Barotrauma may occur during airplane travel, with the onset noted during descent when the eustachian tube is unable to equalize the pressure in the middle ear to that of ambient cabin pressure. This occurs despite the fact that the airlines have pressurized cabins. Any preexisting eustachian tube difficulty, including recent upper respiratory infection, predisposes to this problem. Even significant straining, as in weightlifting, can result in rupture of the round or oval window membranes, leading to a sensorineural hearing loss or dizziness or both. Blast injury to the ear from explosions can result in disruption of the tympanic membrane, ossicles, round and oval window membranes, and the inner ear. Patients struck by lightning often show injury to the ear, with the pattern similar to that of a blast injury.

DIAGNOSIS

Hemotympanum implies blood behind an intact tympanic membrane, resulting from trauma to the underlying middle ear mucosa

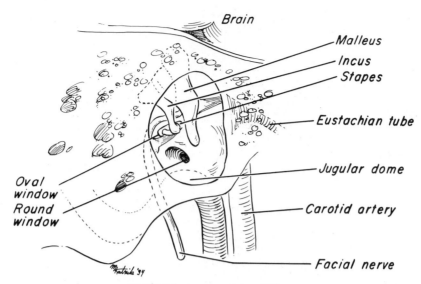

FIGURE 1. Anatomy of the middle ear.

with rupture of the vessels and extravasation of blood. This may result from barotrauma or blunt trauma. Examination of the ear reveals a purple discoloration behind the tympanic membrane with decreased mobility, as one would expect with any middle ear effusion. The blood may fill the middle ear or may be noted only in the dependent portion of the middle ear. Tuning forks will indicate a conductive hearing loss, if this is the only abnormality, with bone conduction greater than air conduction (Rinne test) and Weber testing showing a lateralization to the affected ear. Tympanometry will indicate a flat tracing, suggesting reduced compliance. An audiogram should be obtained to confirm the conductive hearing loss and to determine the possibility of a concomitant sensorineural hearing loss.

If a sensorineural hearing loss is also noted on initial evaluation, one must be concerned about the possibility of a rupture of the oval or round window membranes or a concussive injury to the cochlea. Either condition may be associated with dizziness or tinnitus. A rupture of either membrane could result in a fistula between the inner ear perilymphatic compartment and the middle ear. This can sometimes be detected by using pneumatic otoscopy, obtaining a very good seal, and slowly presenting significant positive and then negative pressure to the ear canal. Subjectively, the patient will describe dizziness with positive or negative pressure, and examination of the eyes might reveal a conjugate deviation of the eyes away from the affected ear with positive pressure but toward the affected ear with negative pressure. A brief period of nystagmus may occur after release of the pressure.

The presence of hemotympanum may imply a fracture of the skull base. This temporal bone fracture may be associated with an injury to the facial nerve because of disruption to the bony canal in which it travels in the middle ear or mastoid. Injury to the facial nerve may not be apparent initially, as the delayed onset may result secondary to edema of the nerve with compromise of its blood supply. One would then suspect the nerve to be intact. In many cases of severe head trauma, the patient is comatose the first day or two, or the patient is sedated for care. This makes it difficult to assess the function of the facial nerve. An immediate facial paralysis presents a greater concern, as it may imply actual physical disruption of the nerve.

Tympanic membrane perforation may occur with blunt or penetrating trauma or with rapid pressure change. It is important to determine if there is an associated perilymphatic fistula from rupture of the round or oval window membranes. The leakage from such a fistula is microscopic and not usually discernible on routine otoscopy. One must maintain a high index of suspicion for this often missed entity by being vigilant for a sensorineural hearing loss or the presence of dizziness. It is important to obtain an audiogram. Tympanometry would indicate a flat tracing, as in the case of hemotympanum or middle ear effusion with chronic serous otitis media, but would show a large volume, representative of the volume of the middle ear and mastoid in addition to the volume of the ear canal. This testing should not be performed if a temporal bone fracture is suspected.

With temporal bone fracture, one may note cerebrospinal fluid leaking through the torn eardrum into the external auditory canal. This clear fluid with a watery consistency may be mixed with blood from the middle ear and external ear canal, making the diagnosis more difficult. Such drainage often has a halo sign, a clear zone surrounding the bloody spot on the bedsheets or filter paper. Laboratory testing for beta$_2$ transferrin is confirmatory, with fluid collected on a cotton pledget or in a tube.

The carotid artery and the jugular vein course along the inferior aspect of the middle ear but are usually bone covered. It is unusual to see injury to these structures.

MANAGEMENT

With any condition involving the possibility of middle ear injury, one should inquire about hearing loss, tinnitus, dizziness, and otorrhea. All patients should have full audiometric testing, with pure tone testing of air and bone conduction, as well as testing of word discrimination. Tympanometry may be helpful in defining the underlying pathology. Tympanometry might demonstrate discontinuity of the ossicular chain with a tracing showing greater than normal peak amplitude (A$_d$ curve), indicating increased compliance. This is not always present, as some children with ossicular disruption may have a normal tympanogram.

Blunt trauma to the head may result in hemorrhage within the middle ear and resultant conductive hearing loss. Isolated hemotympanum will resolve without any treatment, and the patient's ear will return to its normal preinjury condition. Follow-up audiometric testing is important at a 2-month interval to determine the presence of associated ossicular chain disruption following clearance of blood from the middle ear. It is important to note that resolution of the conductive hearing loss may follow resolution of the hemotympanum clinically by 1 month. Therefore, one should not be too hasty in the determination of ossicular disruption until at least 1 month following clinical resolution of the hemotympanum.

Repair of the ossicular disruption is an elective procedure. The most common type of ossicular interruption is disruption of the incus from the stapes. Other injuries include disruption of the incus from the malleus and fracture of the stapes. These can be repaired by a surgical procedure under local or general anesthesia on an outpatient basis. The procedure consists of an incision deep within the ear canal and elevation of the eardrum to allow complete visualization of the ossicles of the middle ear. Repair of the ossicles usually requires removal of the disrupted ossicle and replacement with a synthetic prosthesis. Although prostheses are made from a variety of materials, the current material of choice is hydroxyapatite, the mineral matrix of our living bone. This is extremely biocompatible, allowing stability over long periods of time.

One must not forget the possibility that the conductive loss might have been preexistent. Fixation rather than disruption of the ossicles by processes, including childhood otosclerosis and other diseases, may have been present before the injury. The trauma may have called attention to the ear, with an audiogram obtained for the first time identifying the coincidental underlying disease process.

If the hemotympanum is related to barotrauma, one does not need to consider ossicular disruption but must be concerned about associated perilymph fistula from damage to the round or oval window membranes. If the hemotympanum occurs in the face of blunt or pentrating trauma, one must consider both possibilities in addition to the possibility of facial paralysis, which occurs commonly with temporal bone fracture.

If an assymetric sensorineural hearing loss is noted on initial audiometric testing or if symptoms of increased tinnitus or dizziness are reported, there may be an underlying perilymph fistula. This can mimic a concussive phenomenon to the inner ear. The ability to differentiate these two clinical entities is dependent on further fluctuation of the sensorineural hearing loss. Progression of the hearing loss would support a diagnosis of perilymph fistula, prompting more aggressive management. Bedrest with elevation of the head of the bed to at least 30 degrees may allow the fistula to heal spontaneously. Surgical management would be indicated with further progression of the hearing loss or persistence of dizziness. This involves an operation through the ear canal similar to that used for ossicular repair, performed under general anesthesia or even local anesthesia for older children. The tympanic membrane is reflected forward to identify the round and oval windows. Careful observation of these two areas under microscopic view, following a Valsalva maneuver or other similar method to increase intracranial pressure, may reveal a microfistula. Patching of these two sites with fascia or similar collagen tissue is performed, even without positive identification, since a fistula might be intermittent and difficult to identify with certainty.

A postraumatic perforation in the tympanic membrane should make one alert to the possibility of other otologic injuries, including perilymph fistula and ossicular injury. If purulent otorrhea is noted, antibiotic eardrops should be used to prevent secondary external otitis and to allow direct bathing of the middle ear through the perforation. Concerns about ototoxicity from otic eardrops are prompted by animal studies but rarely supported by clinical experience when there is infection. This may be because of a thickening of the round window membrane, which deters transfer of the ototoxic antibiotic to the inner ear.

One must be aware of the possibility of cerebrospinal fluid leakage, which courses through a tear in the dura, through the fracture site, with exit through either the tympanic membrane perforation or the eustachian tube. In such cases, instrumentation in the ear canal must be avoided to obviate contamination and possible meningitis. Eardrops should not be used in this situation. The use of systemic prophylactic antibiotics is controversial, with the primary issue being concern about selection of resistant organisms. Cerebrospinal fluid leakage usually stops spontaneously with bedrest and elevation of the head of the bed to at least 30 degrees. Placement of a lumbar subarachnoid drain or surgical closure seldom is required.

Examination of the perforation under the microscope may reveal the edges of the perforation to be folded toward the middle ear, decreasing the possibility of self-healing and increasing the chance of the eardrum skin growing into the middle ear itself, resulting in cholesteatoma formation. If this occurs, elevation of the edges of the perforation with placement of absorbable Gelfoam packing in the middle ear to support the edges or placement of a paper patch over the perforation may facilitate spontaneous healing of the perforation. Enough time for self-closure must be allowed, as most perforations do heal spontaneously. If no progress is noted after 2 months, surgical closure may be indicated. The edges of the perforation are freshened, and temporalis fascia is harvested from behind the ear to be placed under or over the perforation, serving as a bridge for the skin to grow across.

Facial paralysis may occur with temporal bone fracture either on presentation or during the next several days. Electrical stimulation testing is used to determine the integrity of the nerve and the survival of its axons. This testing may be quite uncomfortable, making it more difficult to follow young children. General anesthesia may be required to obtain maximal electrical stimulation of the facial nerve and allow EMG electrodes to be placed to monitor for the presence of viable motor units. This is referred to as electroneuronography (ENoG), and it allows objective assessment of the function of the facial nerve. Multiple tests are often required to follow the condition of the nerve. If there is greater than 90% degeneration by this form of testing, the patient should be considered for surgical decompression and possible repair of a severed nerve. The surgical method indicated would be dependent on the presence or absence of hearing. The use of steroids in the patient with facial paralysis is controversial. This medication may help reduce edema of the nerve, thereby maximizing the vascular supply that runs through the nerve within its epineural sheath.

Any hearing loss, dizziness, or tinnitus following trauma deserves workup. A thorough history is essential to elicit symptoms suggesting these problems. Neurologic, ophthalmologic, and otoscopic examinations with pneumotoscopy and tuning forks should be performed. If any findings suggest pathology, an audiogram with tympanogram must be obtained. Plain radiographs offer little assistance in determining the site of injury, and CT is the radiographic imaging of choice. If a pathologic state is identified, referral to an otologic surgeon is appropriate.

REFERENCE

1. Parisier SC: Injuries of the ear and temporal bone. *In* Bluestone CD, Stool SE (eds): Pediatric Otolaryngology, 2nd ed. Philadelphia, W.B. Saunders Co., 1990:578–595.

18

Infectious Diseases

NEONATAL SEPSIS AND MENINGITIS

Kenneth M. Boyer, M.D.

Neonates, particularly those born prematurely, are compromised hosts. During the first months of life, they are subject to infections by a unique list of pathogens, including group B streptococci, coagulase-positive and coagulase-negative staphylococci, coliform organisms, *Listeria*, and *Candida*. Impaired localization of infections by these neonatal pathogens commonly leads to septicemia. Untreated, these infections are usually fatal. Even with current therapy, death occurs in 5% to 10% of infected infants. Presenting symptoms may be vague or nonspecific, a feature that leads to septic workups and empiric antimicrobial therapy of the majority of infants admitted to neonatal high-risk nurseries. A discussion of therapy of neonatal sepsis, then, must address not only the management of babies with proven bacteremic disease but also a rational empiric approach to sick babies with a provisional or unsubstantiated diagnosis of sepsis.

The blood culture is the key microbiologic test in diagnosing neonatal sepsis. When the culture is positive for a recognized neonatal pathogen, particularly after a relatively short incubation (24 hours or less) in both bottles of a set, there is little etiologic doubt. Problems arise in interpretation of late positives (cultures that turn positive after 48 hours), isolates of uncertain pathogenicity (e.g., alpha-streptococci or coagulase-negative staphylococci), or discordant results (only one of several culture bottles positive). Such results often imply technical errors in collection or inoculation of blood specimens but occasionally may be the only tip to an occult infection, such as an infected central venous catheter, osteomyelitis, or abscess. Thus, a broader focus than just the blood culture is desirable in diagnosing and managing neonatal sepsis.

The results of complete blood counts, particularly studies done serially, can be a helpful guide to the presence of bacterial infection and therapeutic response. Elevated neutrophil counts or, more impressively, an initial low count followed by a dramatic response after initiation of therapy favors bacterial etiology. An immature/total neutrophil ratio of ≥ 0.2, an absolute band count of $\geq 1500/mm^3$, and thrombocytopenia of $\leq 100,000/mm^3$ are helpful hematologic indicators. Detection of group B streptococcal or *Escherichia coli* K1 polysaccharide antigens in urine by latex agglutination may be a useful confirmatory adjunct to blood culture. A positive blood culture with a negative concomitant urine antigen test suggests transient bacteremia. On the other hand, positive urine antigen tests with negative blood cultures may imply occult infection (e.g., group B streptococcal osteomyelitis) or partial treatment by intrapartum therapy.

Evaluation of the baby's mother is another useful diagnostic adjunct, particularly when early-onset neonatal infection is suspected. Pediatricians need to encourage their obstetric colleagues to obtain blood cultures from febrile parturients, in addition to other cultures (e.g., vagina, urine, lochia, amniotic fluid at cesarean section, placental surfaces), to define maternal infections that imply intrapartum exposure of the neonate. This is particularly important if maternal antimicrobial therapy is initiated. In turn, obstetricians must communicate situations to the pediatrician in which a suspicion of intrapartum infection exists.

Most important, evaluation of the neonate for infection should include an effort to identify the extent of spread and the portal of entry. Because meningitis is a common concomitant of neonatal bacteremic infection, lumbar puncture should be a part of the septic workup. However, because cerebrospinal fluid (CSF) cultures are seldom positive in the absence of bacteremia, there are a few circumstances in which a lumbar puncture can be deferred. Lumbar puncture may be deferred, for example, in an intubated, asphyxiated, premature newborn whose cardiorespiratory condition is unstable or in an asymptomatic full-term baby in whom a blood culture is being done solely because of maternal prolonged membrane rupture. If blood cultures are positive in such situations, however, subsequent reevaluation should always include lumbar puncture. Even if therapy has rendered cultures negative, results of cell counts, chemistries, and antigen detection are likely to identify the baby who has meningitis. In contrast, the neonate with meningomyelocele and (shunted or unshunted) hydrocephalus may well have meningitis without a positive blood culture and requires examination of the CSF whenever infection is suspected.

The urinary tract is rarely the portal of entry for bacteremia in a neonate less than 72 hours of age. In the older baby, identification of a urinary source for gram-negative sepsis is important because it may permit early correction of a structural anomaly. Clean-catch, catheterized, or suprapubic tap urine specimens are vastly superior to bagged urine specimens for culture. In contrast to CSF obtained after treatment, however, urine specimens need to be obtained before therapy to provide useful information.

Other potentially helpful bacteriologic information regarding portal of entry is often overlooked. A predominant organism in a gram-stained gastric aspirate indicates significant growth of organisms in the amniotic fluid and an infectious challenge to the neonate's lungs during labor and delivery. Gram stains and cultures of tracheal aspirates obtained shortly after intubation also have a high correlation with etiology in neonatal pneumonia. Intravascular catheter tips should always be cultured at the time of removal using the semiquantitative roll-plate technique. More than 15 colonies on the plate imply a catheter source for bacteremia. Stool cultures, if processed to identify predominant aerobic species, may be useful in guiding broad-spectrum therapy in babies with necrotizing enterocolitis. Cultures of skin lesions, including pustules, intravenous catheter exit sites, surgical wounds, or weepy umbilical stumps, may identify the source of bloodstream invasion or focus attention on sites that require removal of hardware, local treatment, or surgical intervention.

EMPIRIC THERAPY

Empiric therapy with combinations of antibiotics is the usual starting point in managing neonatal sepsis. As a general rule, *a decision for workup is a decision for intensive parenteral treatment,* despite the fact that only 5% to 10% of blood cultures from sick infants will prove to be positive. Broad coverage of likely infecting organisms, CSF penetration, safety, and selective pressures for development of drug resistance are the key considerations in choosing regimens. Because actual doses are tiny, drug costs are not a consideration. Factors that determine likely infecting organisms include the patient's age, birthweight, environment (home or hospital), prior courses of treatment, perinatal or nosocomial exposures to specific pathogens, the presence of hardware (e.g., catheters, drains, or endotracheal tubes), and the identification of specific sites of infection (e.g., pneumonia, meningitis, thrombophlebitis, or necrotizing enterocolitis).

Empiric therapy for early-onset sepsis (onset before 7 days of age) is predicated on the origin of virtually all infecting organisms in the maternal enteric or genital flora. The usual pathogens include group B streptococci, *E. coli,* enterococci, alpha-hemolytic streptococci, *Haemophilus influenzae,* and *Listeria monocytogenes.* Anaerobes are not uncommon, but positive blood cultures generally clear with or without treatment. Staphylococci, hospital "water bugs," and fungi are rare. The standard regimen for early-onset disease is ampicillin and an aminoglycoside, generally gentamicin or tobramycin. This combination not only provides broad coverage but is synergistic against streptococci and *Listeria.* Cephalosporins, regardless of their generation, are not active against *Listeria* or enterococci and should not be used without concomitant ampicillin. Used with ampicillin, moreover, they do not offer the advantage of synergism.

Late-onset disease (onset after the age of 7 days) is more heterogeneous in its epidemiology and clinical presentation than early-onset disease and may reflect maternal, family, community, or, most commonly, nosocomial sources for infecting organisms. Consequently, the pathogens involved cover a broad taxonomic spectrum. Bacterial infections in normal infants who have been discharged home may include late-onset group B streptococcal, *E. coli,* or *Listeria* septicemia, local or disseminated *Staphylococcus aureus* infections, urosepsis caused by coliforms, or community-acquired *H. influenzae* type b disease. The combination of ampicillin and a third-generation cephalosporin (cefotaxime or ceftriaxone) is recommended for empiric therapy of occult infection in these older neonates.

The older premature infant often has had his maternally derived flora eradicated by at least one course of therapy with ampicillin and an aminoglycoside and is particularly prone to nosocomial pneumonia related to prolonged intubation, necrotizing enterocolitis when feedings are introduced, and intravenous sepsis related to central or peripheral intravascular catheters. Major pathogens include coagulase-negative and coagulase-positive staphylococci, relatively resistant coliforms, including *Klebsiella* and *Enterobacter,* highly resistant opportunists, such as *Pseudomonas* and *Serratia,* and *Candida.* Selection of empiric regimens for such babies is difficult and should be individualized according to the drugs used previously to treat the infant, clinical presentation (e.g., occult infection, suspect necrotizing enterocolitis, pneumonia, or inflamed Broviac tunnel), gram stains, surveillance cultures (e.g., throat, skin, ostomy stomas, catheter exits, or endotracheal aspirates), and annual reviews of bacterial isolates from the nursery and their sensitivities. The combination of ampicillin, gentamicin, and clindamycin is recommended for suspected necrotizing enterocolitis. Vancomycin and ceftazidime are recommended for patients with occult infection, suspected catheter sepsis, and exacerbations of respiratory disease. An aminoglycoside should be added for overwhelming disease or slow response. Fungal infection should seldom be treated empirically. Amphotericin B and flucytosine are best reserved for well-documented invasive fungal infection.

Empiric antibiotics are a therapeutic first approximation and should be stopped or modified depending on the baby's clinical course and diagnostic workup. As a general rule, empiric antibiotics should be stopped after 72 hours if cultures, clinical course, and ancillary tests do not support the diagnosis of infection. Even if the blood cultures are sterile, however, treatment should be continued in focal infections and in situations in which bacterial infection continues to offer a plausible explanation for a baby's clinical status. Clinical judgment determines the fine line between the use and abuse of antibiotics in the nursery.

SPECIFIC THERAPY

Specific therapy in the septic neonate is determined by whether or not the infection can be identified as to site and specific infecting organism(s). From the welter of currently available antibiotic alternatives, the list of drugs that can be comfortably recommended for use in the neonatal period is relatively short (Table 1). A number of once-popular agents have been superseded because of limitations in spectrum, distribution, or toxicity. Included among these are carbenicillin, kanamycin, chloramphenicol, moxalactam, and virtually all first- and second-generation cephalosporins. Other recently licensed drugs have not been well studied in newborn infants and should be avoided unless sensitivity data provide no alternatives. Such drugs include the quinolones, azlocillin, piperacillin, imipenem, aztreonam, ticarcillin-clavulanate, and piperacillin-tazobactam. The third-generation cephalosporins cefotaxime, ceftriaxone, and ceftazidime, however, have been well studied in neonates and have achieved a major role in therapy. (Note that ceftazidime is the only third-generation cephalosporin with reliable activity against *Pseudomonas aeruginosa.*)

A number of infecting organisms are best treated with combination therapy. The addition of gentamicin to ampicillin for treatment of listeriosis or enterococcal infection provides synergistic activity and more rapid killing of a large initial inoculum. The same synergism has been documented for group B streptococci, but most centers stop the aminoglycoside and change to meningitic doses of penicillin G after initial improvement. The addition of gentamicin to a semisynthetic penicillin dramatically improves bactericidal activity against tolerant strains of *S. aureus.* Combination therapy for infections by *P. aeruginosa* is important because of the emergence of resistance with single-drug treatment. The addition of flucytosine to amphotericin B for treatment of disseminated candidiasis permits smaller doses of amphotericin (0.5 to 0.75 mg/kg/d) to be employed.

The duration and route of therapy are often issues, particularly in our current climate of cost efficiency and parent-infant bonding. However, in my opinion, isolation of a pathogen from the blood of a sick newborn mandates a minimum 10-day course of parenteral therapy. Longer courses of treatment are necessary for meningitis (14 to 21 days or longer depending on organism and clinical response), osteomyelitis (4 to 6 weeks or more), and disseminated candidiasis (6 weeks, or a total dose of 20 to 30 mg/kg of amphotericin B). Clinical judgment determines the duration of treatment in patients with asymptomatic bacteremia, culture-negative sepsis, antigenuria, or focal infections without bacteremia. Oral treatment is not appropriate for a newborn recovering from a serious infection because of the uncertainty of absorption of oral medication. Daily intramuscular ceftriaxone and home intravenous therapy with ceftriaxone or other drugs are possible alternatives to prolonged hospitalization that can be used in selected cases if vascular access is secure, nursing supervision is adequate, and the family is reliable.

SUPPORTIVE THERAPY

Major therapeutic considerations in neonatal sepsis other than antibiotics include cardiorespiratory, nutritional, and immunologic status. Blood pressure measurements are mandatory in the septic newborn. The presence of shock should prompt aggressive volume expansion with saline, albumin, or fresh frozen plasma and often will require the use of pressors. Disseminated intravascular coagulation is a common concomitant of septic shock and should be treated with platelet infusions in addition to fresh frozen plasma. Persistent fetal circulation, manifested by profound hypoxemia, is a common feature

TABLE 1. Dose Recommendations for Antimicrobial Agents Commonly Used in Treatment of Neonatal Sepsis and Meningitis

		DOSES (mg/kg/d) AND INTERVALS OF ADMINISTRATION			
		BODY WEIGHT <2000 g		BODY WEIGHT >2000 g	
DRUG	ROUTES OF ADMINISTRATION	AGE 0–7 DAYS	>7 DAYS	Age 0–7 DAYS	>7 DAYS
Amikacin*	IV, IM	15 div q12h	22.5 div q8h	20 div q12h	30 div q8h
Amphotericin B*	IV				
Endocarditis†		1 q24h	1 q24h	1 q24h	1 q24h
Endophthalmitis†		1 q24h	1 q24h	1 q24h	1 q24h
Other diseases		0.5–1 q24h	0.5–1 q24h	0.5–1 q24h	0.5–1 q24h
Ampicillin	IV, IM				
Meningitis‡		200–300 div q12h	300–400 div q8h	200–300 div q8h	300–400 div q6h
Other diseases		50 div q12h	75 div q8h	75 div q8h	100 div q6h
Aztreonam	IV	60 div q12h	90 div q8h	90 div q8h	120 div q6h
Cefotaxime	IV, IM	100 div q12h	150 div q8h	100 div q12h	150–225 div q8h
Ceftazidime	IV, IM	100 div q12h	150 div q8h	100 div q12h	150 div q8h
Ceftriaxone	IV, IM	50 q24h	50 q24h	50 q24h	80 q24h
Clindamycin	IV, IM	10 div q12h	15 div q8h	15 div q8h	20 div q6h
Flucytosine*	PO	100 div q6h	100 div q6h	100 div q6h	100 div q6h
Gentamicin*	IV, IM	5 div q12h	7.5 div q8h	5 div q12h	7.5 div q8h
Methicillin	IV, IM				
Meningitis		100 div q12h	150 div q8h	150 div q8h	200 div q6h
Other diseases		50 div q12h	75 div q8h	75 div q8h	100 div q6h
Metronidazole	IV	15 div q12h	15 div q12h	15 div q12h	30 div q12h
Mezlocillin	IV, IM	150 div q12h	225 div q8h	150 div q12h	225 div q8h
Oxacillin	IV, IM	50 div q12h	100 div q8h	75 div q8h	150 div q6h
Nafcillin	IV	50 div q12h	100 div q8h	50 div q8h	150 div q6h
Netilmicin*	IV, IM	5 div q12h	7.5 div q8h	5 div q12h	7.5 div q12h
Penicillin G	IV				
Meningitis‡		200,000–400,000 U div q12h	300,000–500,000 U div q8h	200,000–400,000 U div q8h	300,000–500,000 U div q6h
Other diseases		50,000 U div q12h	75,000 div U q8h	50,000 div U q8h	100,000 U div q6h
Ticarcillin	IV, IM	150 div q12h	225 div q8h	225 div q8h	300 div q6h
Tobramycin*	IV, IM	4 div q12h	6 div q8h	4 div q12h	6 div q8h
Vancomycin*	IV	20 q12h	30 q8h	20 q12h	30 q8h

Abbreviations: IV, intravenous; IM intramuscular; div, divided; q12h, every 12 hours.

*Serum concentration or toxicity monitoring desirable, particularly with birth weights less than 1200 g. See Prober et al: Pediatr Infect Dis J 9:111, 1990.

†Gradual dose buildup recommended. Give 0.25 mg/kg first day; 0.50 mg/kg second day; 0.75 mg/kg third day; then 1 mg/kg/d. Dose may be maintained at 0.5 to 0.75 mg/kg/d if flucytosine used concomitantly.

‡Consider the higher recommended dose for positive cerebrospinal fluid gram stain or if lumbar puncture deferred because of critical illness or clinical instability.

of early-onset group B streptococcal infection and generally requires high concentrations of inspired oxygen, mechanical ventilation, and possibly extracorporeal membrane oxygenation. Respiratory failure may be a consequence of the combination of birth asphyxia, neonatal pneumonia, hyaline membrane disease, and shock lung. Babies with this combination of problems, if they survive, often become the long-term residents of neonatal nurseries because of their development of bronchopulmonary dysplasia. Aggressive early management is an important preventive measure.

Nutritional status, particularly in the infected premature infant with limited metabolic reserves, is a major consideration during a prolonged course of antimicrobial therapy. Such babies have increased nutritional demands created by thermoregulatory disturbances, cardiopulmonary stress, frequent blood drawing, and surgical procedures. Depending on the site of infection, enteral feedings are generally not introduced or are interrupted during treatment. Delays in starting parenteral nutrition and the often marginal caloric intake provided by peripherally administered intravenous fluids generally lead to weight loss and a negative nitrogen balance at a time when reparative needs are greatest. Despite perceived infection risks, early central hyperalimentation is warranted for most of these babies.

Augmentation of the neonate's marginal supplies of white cells, antibodies, and nonspecific opsonins (e.g., complement, fibronectin) is a logical but as yet unproven adjunct to antimicrobial therapy. Fresh frozen plasma is the volume expander of choice for the septic newborn because of its content of IgG and IgM immunoglobulins and nonspe-

cific opsonins. White cell transfusions pose difficult logistic problems for the blood bank, with only minimal benefit in terms of therapeutic outcome. Colony-stimulating factors (G-CSF and GM-CSF) are an as yet experimental alternative. The prophylactic and therapeutic use of intravenous gamma globulin theoretically permits correction of deficiencies in transplacental specific immunoglobulins, thereby enhancing localization of infection and preventing depletion of marrow neutrophil reserves. Controlled trials have been disappointing, however. Current interest lies in the use of specific immunoglobulins directed against group B streptococcal polysaccharides and gram-negative endotoxins. Elucidation of the network of proinflammatory cytokines in the septic cascade has led to further studies of blockade of IL-1 and TNF, which may have application to the treatment of neonatal sepsis in the future.

MONITORING THERAPY

Babies with clinical signs suggestive of bacterial infection deserve hospitalization in an observation unit, intensive care nursery, or pediatric ward, not in a normal nursery or at home. In addition to monitoring therapeutic response, monitoring such infants involves recognition of complications and drug toxicity.

Adequate treatment of a septic neonate generally results in a dramatic response within 24 to 48 hours, as manifested by improved activity, respiratory effort, temperature regulation, and peripheral perfusion. White blood cell counts and proportions of segmented neu-

TABLE 2. Suggested Target Levels of Selected Antibiotics to Optimize Efficacy and Minimize Toxicity

DRUG	PEAK (μg/ml)	TROUGH (μg/ml)
Gentamicin	4–8	<2
Tobramycin	4–8	<2
Netilmicin	4–8	<2
Amikacin	15–25	<6
Vancomycin	15–30	?
Flucytosine	50–100	?

trophils often rise with treatment, a short-term response that generally is a favorable sign. Babies who do not respond to treatment may have a resistant organism, an occult focus of infection, or a viral or non-infectious problem. The blood culture should be repeated at the first report of a positive result to document sterilization. Measurement of serum bactericidal activity provides a more reliable indication of treatment efficacy than the usual in vitro susceptibility tests (which are based on bacteriostatic activity). Occult bacterial infections associated with slow response or persistence of bacteremia include meningitis, osteomyelitis, abscesses (intraabdominal, renal, brain, subperiosteal), and intravascular infection (suppurative thrombophlebitis, endocarditis). Computed tomography (CT), ultrasonography, echocardiography, and gallium scans may be helpful in identifying such problems. Disseminated neonatal herpes and enteroviral infections, in the absence of skin lesions or CNS abnormalities, can resemble bacterial sepsis. Striking elevations of serum transaminase values are a useful clue to these entities. It should always be kept in mind that the patient who does not respond to antibiotics or whose condition deteriorates during therapy may, in fact, have a noninfectious condition (e.g., hypoplastic left heart syndrome, pneumothorax, intraventricular hemorrhage, or intestinal obstruction).

Monitoring serum concentrations of aminoglycosides has become a standard of care in many nurseries, although the occurrence of ototoxicity and nephrotoxicity from these drugs has been difficult to study because of confounding by other conditions, such as shock, asphyxia, acidosis, or hyperbilirubinemia. Peak (at conclusion of intravenous infusion or 30 minutes following intramuscular injection) and trough (immediately before the next dose) concentrations should be measured in all infants with uncertain renal function or birthweights less than 1500 g. Waiting to measure concentrations until after the third dose of drug is reasonable to ensure equilibration. Target peak and trough antibiotic concentrations in serum are summarized in Table 2. Other drugs requiring measurement of serum concentrations during therapy are vancomycin and flucytosine. Vancomycin has been well studied in newborns, whereas experience with flucytosine is anecdotal. Amphotericin B concentrations are difficult to measure and not well correlated with toxicity. Safe use of amphotericin is best monitored by serial measurements of serum potassium, urea nitrogen, creatinine, and hematologic values and by careful documentation of urine output.

PREVENTION

The key elements in the prevention of early-onset neonatal sepsis are prevention of prematurity and proactive obstetric management of labor and delivery. Selective intrapartum chemoprophylaxis provides an effective approach to preventing early-onset group B streptococcal sepsis (see section on group B streptococcal infection). Prevention of late-onset disease can be best accomplished by giving close attention to handwashing, adhering to guidelines for isolation of communicable conditions in mothers, infants, and personnel, and minimizing antibiotic abuse and overuse in the nursery setting.

BACTERIAL MENINGITIS AND SEPTICEMIA BEYOND THE NEONATAL PERIOD

RALPH D. FEIGIN, M.D.
TERI LEE TURNER, M.D.

BACTERIAL MENINGITIS

Bacterial meningitis continues to be a significant problem in the pediatric population despite the decreased incidence of disease brought about by the advent of routine immunization against *Haemophilus influenzae* type b. *Streptococcus pneumoniae, Neisseria meningitidis,* and *H. influenzae* are the pathogens encountered most frequently in the normal child over 1 month of age.

Children with bacterial meningitis may present with fever, headache, photophobia, nausea, vomiting, lethargy, and excessive irritability. Signs and symptoms are variable, and often findings are very subtle in infants. Therefore, diagnosis depends on the physician, who must maintain a high index of suspicion for the possibility of bacterial meningitis. The diagnosis of bacterial meningitis is dependent on lumbar puncture, with careful examination of cerebrospinal fluid (CSF) using gram stain, culture, cell count with differential, glucose (with simultaneous serum glucose for comparison), and protein. In children between 1 and 12 years of age, the normal CSF contains less than 6 WBC/mm³, and in 95% of the normal population, no polymorphonuclear leukocytes are present. Rapid diagnostic tests, such as countercurrent immunoelectrophoresis or latex particle agglutination, may be used, but the results should not be used to change the initial choice of antibiotics until identification and sensitivities of the infecting organism are known.

If the lumbar puncture is traumatic, the ratio of leukocytes to red blood cells should be considered. If the peripheral red blood cell count and leukocyte count are normal, 1 leukocyte per 700 red blood cells may be subtracted from the total CSF white blood cell count. However, management decisions should not be based solely on the CSF leukocyte count when the lumbar puncture is traumatic.

Initial Therapy

Antibiotic treatment should be initiated empirically before the results of CSF cultures are obtained. Currently, most centers use either cefotaxime at 200 mg/kg/24 h IV divided in four doses or ceftriaxone at 100 to 150 mg/kg/24 h IV divided in two doses for children older than 3 months of age (Table 1). Previously, therapy with ampicillin 300 mg/kg/24 h divided in six doses and chloramphenicol 100 mg/kg/24 h divided in four doses was the treatment of choice. Long-term results with this treatment are well documented and are at least equivalent to the results achieved with the use of third-generation cephalosporins.

Chloramphenicol should be avoided in patients with persistent hypotension or shock. Once an organism and its sensitivity have been identified, antibiotic coverage can be adjusted accordingly. The duration of antibiotic therapy is based on the causative agent and the clinical response to therapy. Intravenous antibiotics should be continued until the patient is afebrile for 5 days but for at least 7 to 10 days total in all cases. The duration of therapy may be prolonged if the child is not improving or has complications that may result in delayed sterilization of the CSF.

In recent years, some physicians have been prompted to complete a course of antibiotic therapy for bacterial meningitis at home in a patient who appears well and who has been afebrile for 48 to 72 hours. Home therapy may be provided with ceftriaxone given IV or IM in a dose of 80 mg/kg/24 h once daily. Alternatively, chloramphenicol has been given PO in a dose of 75 mg/kg/24 h in four divided doses. When chloramphenicol is used, serum concentrations should be measured and maintained in a range of 10 to 20 μg/ml. There are no

TABLE 1. Drugs and Doses Recommended for Bacterial Meningitis and Septicemia beyond the Neonatal Period

Cefotaxime	200 mg/kg/d IV in 4 divided doses
Ceftriaxone	100–150 mg/kg/d IV or IM in 2 divided doses
Ampicillin	300 mg/kg/d IV in 4–6 divided doses (meningitic dose is q4h)
Chloramphenicol	100 mg/kg/d IV in 4 divided doses
	75 mg/kg/d PO in 4 divided doses
Aqueous penicillin	500,000 units/kg/d IV in 6 divided doses
Vancomycin	40–60 mg/kg/d IV in 4 divided doses
Nafcillin	150–200 mg/kg/d IV in 4–6 divided doses
Cefuroxime	150–200 mg/kg/d IV in 3 divided doses
Ticarcillin	200 mg/kg/d IV in 6 divided doses
Piperacillin	200–300 mg/kg/d IV in 6 divided doses
Clindamycin	30 mg/kg/d IV in 4 divided doses
Gentamicin	5–7.5 mg/kg/d IV in 3 divided doses
Amoxicillin	100 mg/kg/d PO in 3 divided doses
Amoxicillin-clavulinic acid	50–75 mg/kg/d PO in 3 divided doses
Trimethoprim-sulfamethoxazole	8 mg/kg/d PO of the trimethoprim component in 2 divided doses
Rifampin	10 mg/kg q12h for 4 doses for *N. meningitidis* prophylaxis
	(<1 mo of age, dose is decreased to 5 mg/kg q12h)
	20 mg/kg once daily for 4 days for *H. influenzae* prophylaxis
	(<1 month of age, dose is decreased to 10 mg/kg/24 h)
Dexamethasone	0.15 mg/kg per dose IV q6h for 16 doses (meningitis)
Phenytoin	5–20 mg/kg IV divided in 2 doses
Diazepam	0.2–0.5 mg/kg per dose IV (max: 5 mg in children <5 and 10 mg in children >5 y of age)
Lorazepam	0.03–0.05 mg/kg per dose IV (max: 4 mg per dose)

long-term prospective studies to document the equivalent efficacy of this form of therapy to a complete 7- to 10-day course of antibiotics provided intravenously.

When meningitis is caused by *S. pneumoniae*, Kirby-Bauer disc testing followed, if necessary, by tube dilution sensitivity tests must be performed. Fifteen to twenty percent of *S. pneumoniae* isolates in the United States are no longer completely susceptible to penicillin. Some pneumococci have intermediate resistance to penicillin (sensitivity only in concentrations of 0.1 to 1 μg/ml). Other pneumococcal isolates show even greater resistance to penicillin (sensitive only at 1 to 10 μg/ml or greater concentrations). Pneumococci with intermediate sensitivity to penicillin may be treated with aqueous penicillin G in a dose of 500,000 U/kg/24 h in six divided doses. If the organism is resistant to penicillin but sensitive to chloramphenicol or a third-generation cephalosporin, these options may be used in the following doses: chloramphenicol 100 mg/kg/24 h in four divided doses IV, cefotaxime 200 mg/kg/24 h in four divided doses IV, or ceftriaxone 100 mg/kg/24 h in two divided doses IV. In the last 7 years, strains of pneumococci resistant to third-generation cephalosporins have been reported in the United States. Some of these strains have retained their sensitivity to chloramphenicol, whereas others are resistant to multiple antibiotics. Multiply resistant pneumococci have retained their sensitivity to vancomycin, which should be provided IV in a dose of 60 mg/kg/24 h in four divided doses. A repeat lumbar puncture is not mandatory unless the clinical course is complicated or shows a lack of improvement after 24 to 48 hours of therapy.

Corticosteroid use has been suggested as an adjunct to antibiotic therapy because some studies have noted that its use is associated with a decreased frequency of neurologic handicaps and hearing loss. Other studies, including a recent multicenter study carried out in the United States, could not document therapeutic efficacy definitively.

The current recommendation includes the use of dexamethasone 0.15 mg/kg IV every 6 hours for a total of 16 doses initiated immediately before or at the same time as antibiotic therapy. Steroids should be withheld if CSF studies suggest a viral or other nonbacterial cause of infection. If steroids are administered, the patient should be monitored for bleeding from the gastrointestinal tract. If melena or gross blood is observed, steroids should be discontinued.

Supportive Care

The first 3 or 4 days of treatment of bacterial meningitis are the most critical. Initially, vital signs should be monitored every 15 minutes until the patient is stable and then hourly for the next 24 to 48 hours. On admission, a complete neurologic examination should be performed, and neurologic vital signs should be assessed at least every 4 hours for the first several days. Head circumference measurements, along with complete neurologic examinations, should be performed daily.

Prospective studies have documented that almost 60% of children with bacterial meningitis develop the syndrome of inappropriate secretion of antidiuretic hormone (SIADH). In an attempt to determine the presence and severity of SIADH, serum electrolytes and serum and urine osmolalities should be measured at the time of admission. Daily weights, along with careful measurement of fluids, are strictly monitored. Initially, the rate of fluid administration is restricted to 800 to 1000 ml/m²/d unless the patient is hypotensive or dehydrated. The patient should be given nothing by mouth for at least the first 24 hours, since vomiting may ensue, and aspiration is best avoided. Electrolyte, urine specific gravity, and urine and serum osmolality determinations should be repeated several times during the first 24 to 36 hours and then daily thereafter. These measures are continued until the possibility of inappropriate secretion of ADH can be excluded or, if it is present, until its effect is no longer detectable.

Complications

Seizures occur before hospitalization or during the first several days of treatment in approximately 30% of afflicted children. Seizures that are focal, difficult to control, or persist beyond the fourth hospital day are of greater significance. These children are more likely to have a permanent seizure disorder or other neurologic sequelae of their disease. If seizures are noted, a patent airway should be secured, and diazepam at 0.2 to 0.5 mg/kg per dose (max: for patients less than 5 years of age is 5 mg, and for those greater than 5 years of age 10 mg) or lorazepam at 0.03 to 0.05 mg/kg per dose (max: 4 mg total dose) may be used to control the seizure activity. This regimen is followed by IV phenytoin at 5 to 20 mg/kg provided in two divided doses. Phenytoin generally does not depress the respiratory center to the same extent as phenobarbital, and it may also benefit the patient by inhibiting the secretion of ADH. If seizure activity is no longer apparent after the second hospital day and there are no focal neurologic signs at the time of discharge from the hospital, anticonvulsants may be discontinued. A CT scan or MRI should be obtained in children with focal neurologic signs, prolonged mental status changes, increasing head circumference, or persistence of the disease process. Subdural effusion may be detected by these techniques but can be assessed by the physician at much less cost using transillumination. Subdural paracentesis should be performed only if it is thought that the effusion is responsible for abnormalities in the neurologic status of the child or if a subdural empyema is suspected. If a subdural tap is performed and the symptoms remain unchanged, repeated subdural paracentesis is not indicated. Subdural effusions generally resolve within 1 week to 3 months following identification of the effusion.

Shock or disseminated intravascular coagulation (DIC) or both may further complicate the clinical course of meningitis and should be treated as needed with vasopressors and circulatory support. Fifteen to twenty percent of children with bacterial meningitis develop some form of auditory nerve dysfunction, with the highest prevalence (30%) occurring with *S. pneumoniae* meningitis. Therefore, audiologic studies should be performed on all children with bacterial meningitis at the time of or soon after discharge. Brainstem evoked response audiometry can be used to assess auditory nerve dysfunction in the infant and young child, and pure tone audiometry may be used in older children and adolescents.

Prevention

Rifampin prophylaxis at a dose of 10 mg/kg every 12 hours for four doses is indicated as soon as possible for all nonpregnant contacts, including day care and hospital personnel who have had intimate contact with a child diagnosed with *N. meningitidis* meningitis. Also, nonpregnant contacts of children with invasive *H. influenzae* infection are considered candidates for rifampin prophylaxis if there is a child less than 4 years of age living in the patient's household and for day care attendees when 2 or more cases of invasive *H. influenzae* disease have occurred within 60 days. Rifampin should be given in a dose of 20 mg/kg once daily for 4 days to avoid reintroduction of the organism. The patient also should receive prophylaxis before discharge because of the frequency of carriage of the organism in the nasopharynx even after a course of intravenous antibiotics. The dose of rifampin is decreased to 10 mg/kg/24 h for infants less than 1 month of age for both diseases, following the same dose schedule.

Active prevention with vaccination is available for *S. pneumoniae*, *N. meningitidis* (A, C, Y, W135) and *H. influenzae* type b. Immunoprophylaxis is not available for group B meningococcus. The efficacy of these vaccines in children <2 years of age limits their use except for the group A meningococcus and *H. influenzae* type b conjugate vaccines. The use of conjugate *H. influenzae* vaccines beginning at 2 months of age in the United States has been followed by a marked decrease in the frequency of meningitis and septicemia caused by this organism. Future research will hopefully produce additional vaccines that are effective for other organisms in this high-risk group of children.

SEPTICEMIA

Septicemia beyond the neonatal period may be caused by any organism but most frequently has been caused by *S. pneumoniae* or *H. influenzae* type b. In general, a careful history and physical examination will provide clues to a bacteriologic diagnosis. Septicemia is a severe form of bacteremia and may progress to septic shock. Clinically, patients in septic shock present with hyperventilation, tachycardia, cutaneous lesions, temperature instability, and changes in mental status. Secondary manifestations can include inadequate tissue perfusion and DIC, especially in gram-negative septicemia.

Whenever septicemia is suspected, two or three sets of blood cultures should be obtained over a period of several hours. A careful search for possible sites of infection should be performed, along with cultures of suspicious foci. If no obvious source of infection is found, a chest radiograph and cultures of urine and CSF (if indicated) should be obtained. Ancillary tests, such as a complete white blood cell count with differential, platelet determination, prothrombin time, partial thromboplastin time, and fibrin-fibrinogen degradation products (such as D-dimer), should be performed if DIC is suspected.

Initial Therapy

Antibiotic treatment should be initiated empirically whenever septicemia is suspected. Treatment should be based on the most likely causative organisms and the patient's underlying host defense status. In those children older than 2 to 3 months of age with suspected sepsis due to community-acquired organisms, broad-spectrum coverage with a combination of nafcillin 150 to 200 mg/kg/d or another semisynthetic antistaphylcoccal penicillin plus cefotaxime 150 to 200 mg/kg/d or ceftriaxone 75 to 150 mg/kg/d should be initiated until a bacteriologic diagnosis is established. If meningitis is *excluded*, one may substitute cefuroxime 150 to 200 mg/kg/d for the third-generation cephalosporin. This regimen covers a broad range of organisms, such as *Staphylococcus aureus*, *H. influenzae* type b, *Streptococcus pyo-*

genes, and *S. pneumoniae*. Cefotaxime, ceftriaxone, or cefuroxime may be used alone in children older than 2 to 3 months of age only if septicemia due to *Pseudomonas aeruginosa* or *S. aureus* or both is not suspected. These antibiotics do confer some gram-positive coverage (second-generation greater than third-generation cephalosporins). However, if *S. aureus* is suspected, an antistaphylococcal drug should be added.

In children with indwelling central venous catheters or for infections thought to be due to methicillin-resistant *S. aureus*, vancomycin 40 to 60 mg/kg/d should be added or used in place of the semisynthetic antistaphylococcal penicillin.

It is also important to consider the host's defense status when choosing antibiotic coverage. Infection with *S. pneumoniae*, *H. influenzae*, or other encapsulated pathogens is more likely in patients who have been splenectomized. Infection with *S. pneumoniae* or *Salmonella* is more frequent in children with sickle cell disease or other hemoglobinopathies. Immunosuppressed children require antibiotic coverage for gram-negative enterics, *P. aeruginosa* and *S. aureus*. Suggested combinations include an antistaphylococcal semisynthetic penicillin or vancomycin plus an aminoglycoside. An antipseudomonal beta-lactam, such as ticarcillin 200 mg/kg/d or piperacillin 200 to 300 mg/kg/d, may be used to act synergistically against *Pseudomonas* species. Another combination includes an aminoglycoside plus an antipseudomonal beta-lactam or a third-generation cephalosporin or both. Third-generation cephalosporins can be substituted for aminoglycosides for empiric therapy, but they are not uniformly effective against *P. aeruginosa*. Vancomycin plus ceftazidime is another regimen that adequately covers the most likely pathogens that would produce disease in the immunocompromised host.

When an anaerobic organism is suspected, clindamycin 30 mg/kg/d should be added to the initial regimen. For example, in suspected intraabdominal or gastrointestinal pathology, one would use ampicillin 200 to 300 mg/kg/d, gentamicin 5 to 7.5 mg/kg/d, plus clindamycin. The most important consideration is to use broad-spectrum antibiotic coverage. Once an organism has been identified, antibiotic coverage can be tailored accordingly.

Shock and bleeding are common in septicemia, particularly when gram-negative organisms are implicated. In those patients with inadequate tissue perfusion, aminoglycoside dosing should be based on renal function. The routine first dose should be given at the beginning of therapy, and blood levels should be monitored within the first 24 hours to optimize the dose. The length of therapy is dependent on the focus of infection and response to antibiotic treatment. Generally, at least a 7- to 10-day course of antibiotics is completed for documented septicemia.

Bacteremia Without a Focus

Children Older Than 2 to 3 Months of Age

A syndrome commonly known as *occult bacteremia* has been described in children between the ages of 6 and 24 months of age who appear clinically well, with no obvious focus of infection. Approximately 5% of these children are bacteremic, usually with *S. pneumoniae*. These children typically have temperatures greater than 103°F to 104°F, with a white blood cell count of 15,000/mm³ or greater. We recommend a blood culture in children who meet these criteria to identify those who are bacteremic. Urine culture also should be obtained in all females less than 2 years of age and in all males less than 6 months of age.

Current debate is focused on the initial outpatient treatment of febrile children between 3 months and 3 years of age who do not appear septic. The decision to treat these children should be made on a case-by-case basis, including an assessment of the likelihood of adequate follow-up. When recall of patients is less than optimal or when a patient has a temperature greater than 39°C and a white blood cell count greater than 15,000/mm³, we advocate the initiation of antibiotic therapy after appropriate cultures have been obtained. Regimens suggested previously include amoxicillin 100 mg/kg/d, amoxicillin-clavulinic acid at 50 to 75 mg/kg/d, or trimethoprim-sulfamethoxazole (8 mg/kg/d trimethoprim) for those patients allergic to penicillin. Many physicians use ceftriaxone in a single IM dose of 50 to 75 mg/kg. Regardless of the decision to initiate treatment, careful follow-up at 24 to 48 hours and repeat physical examination should be performed. If the blood culture is reported to be positive and the child has persistent fever on follow-up examination, the patient should be admitted for evaluation for septicemia and meningitis, and parenteral antibiotics should be administered pending additional cultures. If the patient is afebrile and well, outpatient antibiotics can be continued.

Children Less Than 2 to 3 Months of Age

This group of infants represents one of the most challenging problems that a physician faces. They are challenging because of the nonspecificity of clinical symptoms or lack of symptoms other than fever. Despite their well appearance, such children have been admitted routinely to the hospital after a careful history and physical evaluation, along with cultures of blood, CSF, and urine. Various investigators have attempted to identify those infants who would be at low risk for serious bacterial illness, with the hope that criteria could be established that might permit outpatient management of some of these children.

There are no laboratory tests that will definitively resolve this issue. At this time, we recommend routine hospitalization of those infants up to 6 weeks of age. Blood, urine, stool, and CSF cultures are obtained, and parenteral antibiotic therapy is initiated. Ampicillin 200 to 300 mg/kg/d and cefotaxime 200 mg/kg/d may be prescribed IV every 6 hours.

Children older than 6 weeks but less than 3 months of age may be hospitalized as indicated clinically. They are evaluated carefully by history, physical examination, and laboratory data. Additional data, such as radiographs of the chest and investigative studies for other sources of infection, are based on clinical symptoms. If these children were previously healthy, are nontoxic in appearance, have no focal infection other than otitis media on physical examination, have a normal lumbar puncture examination, a normal white blood cell count, normal urinalysis, and when diarrhea is present, have less than 5 WBC/hpf, ceftriaxone 50 mg/kg IM up to 1 g may be administered, and the patient may be followed on an outpatient basis. These patients should be reevaluated in 24 hours. A small percentage of these low-risk infants will subsequently have bacteremia or other serious manifestations of their initial disease process. Thus, the most important consideration in the treatment of such children is careful and frequent evaluation for the primary source of infection until the disease process or symptoms or both have resolved.

REFERENCES

1. Feigin RD: Bacterial meningitis beyond the newborn period. *In* Oski FA, et al (eds): Principles and Practice of Pediatrics. Philadelphia, JB Lippincott, 1990:1028–1035.
2. Feigin RD, McCracken GH Jr, Klein JO: Diagnosis and management of meningitis. J Pediatr Infect Dis 11:785–814, 1992.
3. Kaplan SL: Bacteremia and endotoxin shock. *In* Feigin RD, Cherry JD (eds): Textbook of Pediatric Infectious Diseases, 3rd ed. Philadelphia, WB Saunders, 1992:863–875.

CELLULITIS

MICHAEL L. FORBES, M.D.
EUGENE MOWAD, M.D.
KENNETH SCHUIT, M.D.

Cellulitis, an infection of the skin and, on occasion, its underlying structures ranges in severity from a self-limited infection to severe disease progressing to bacteremia. Although cellulitis is caused most often by gram-positive cocci, gram-negative bacilli, anaerobes, and even fungi can sometimes act as skin pathogens. In this section, cellulitis occurring in the newborn is treated separately, not because of great differences in etiology but because of potentially different presentations and the greater likelihood of dissemination or even death.

A number of diseases presenting with erythroderma can mimic cellulitis but are actually the cutaneous manifestation of illness caused by exotoxin-producing gram-positive cocci, such as scarlet fever and toxic shock syndrome.

NEONATAL CELLULITIS

Cellulitis in the newborn frequently is a complication of otherwise trivial trauma, but because of the neonate's immunonaivete, such trauma can represent the focus for bacteremia and even sepsis. In this section, we discuss (1) mastitis, (2) cellulitis caused by obstetric misadventures, and (3) omphalitis.

Mastitis neonatorum is easily recognized by inflammatory changes in the breast. This infection usually is caused by *Staphylococcus aureus,* although gram-negative bacilli, such as *Escherichia coli,* have been implicated. After cultures have been obtained, broad-spectrum coverage (e.g., with a beta-lactamase-resistant penicillin and an aminoglycoside) should be initiated until definitive culture results allow narrowing of the regimen. Incision and drainage also may be needed. The duration of therapy can be predicated on the rate of response.

Scalp abscesses are a complication of fetal monitoring. The etiology can include any of the inhabitants of the birth canal. Although some authorities recommend only drainage, one should have a low threshold for using broad-spectrum antibiotics until culture and sensitivity results are available. The risk of underlying osteomyelitis argues against the use of topical preparations alone. The same can be said for the treatment of *facial lacerations,* which can occur as a complication of forceps-associated delivery. If a cellulitis develops, broad-spectrum parenteral therapy is indicated to prevent spread to deeper structures.

Omphalitis is a serious infection that begins in the umbilical stump and spreads to the umbilical vein and then to the liver. The pathogens that cause omphalitis include groups A and B streptococci, staphylococci, and enteric gram-negative bacilli. The complications of hepatic abscess, peritonitis, and necrotizing fasciitis justify the aggressive use of broad-spectrum parenteral antibiotics with gram-positive, gram-negative, and anaerobic activity. The clinician's high index of suspicion for diagnosing and treating the neonate with even mild signs of umbilical infection may be lifesaving.

CELLULITIS IN INFANTS AND CHILDREN

Skin infections in children most often occur via direct inoculation. Infections of the skin are best classified with respect to the depth of the inflammation. The most superficial epidermal infection is impetigo. In the past, the appearance of the impetiginous lesion had etiologic significance. For example, a flat, erythematous lesion covered by a honey-colored crust typified streptococcal impetigo. Inflamed bullae with yellow turbid fluid suggested a staphylococcal infection. Because of the changing bacteriology of impetigo, all clinical presentations are now more likely to be due to staphylococci and should be treated with an oral antistaphylococcal antibiotic or with a topical preparation.

Erysipelas, an infection of the superficial lymphatics of the skin, presents as a rapidly expanding, brightly erythematous plaque with a palpable, sharply demarcated margin. Erysipelas often presents with systemic complaints and high fever. The etiology is most often group A *Streptococcus* and should be treated accordingly. Once common, erysipelas now is an unusual occurrence. It remains to be seen whether the increased virulence of group A streptococci will influence the incidence of erysipelas.

Infections that extend into the dermis are properly termed "cellulitis." The clinical presentation is marked by the classic *tumor, dolor, calor,* and *rubor,* that is, a tender, warm, erythematous induration of the skin. The commonest causes are again the gram-positive cocci, streptococci, and staphylococci. There is often direct inoculation via a wound, but the initial injury may not be recalled or found at the time of presentation. In severe cases of cellulitis, the recommended treatment is a parenteral antistaphylococcal drug.

Skin structures can also be the seat of an infection. These, however, tend to form isolated abscesses (furuncles) or, as in the case of a carbuncle, an interconnected, insinuating tract of infection involving several skin structures. These are often caused by staphylococci, with the exception of perirectal abscesses, which may be due to gram-negative bacilli. Any long-standing abscess may involve anaerobic bacteria. Therapy for these special cases should be individualized and often involves surgical intervention.

UNCOMMON FORMS OF CELLULITIS

A number of unique skin infections should be mentioned because treatment is different from that for the more common cellulitides. For example, infections acquired in fresh water can be caused by gram-negative bacilli, such as *Aeromonas hydrophilia.* Thus, an aminoglycoside should be added to the usual regimen until culture results are available.

Necrotizing fasciitis refers to a rapidly progressing cellulitis that also involves underlying fascial planes and, on occasion, muscle. This condition can develop from a surgical wound infection or omphalitis and usually has a polymicrobial etiology. Treatment consists of broad-spectrum coverage for gram-positive cocci, for aerobic gram-negative organisms, and also for anaerobes, including *Bacteroides* sp. Surgical intervention frequently is necessary early in the course of this emergency situation.

PNEUMONIAS

JEROME O. KLEIN, M.D.

Therapy should be initiated promptly once bacterial pneumonia is diagnosed or strongly suspected. Initial therapy may be guided by the examination of the gram-stained smear of sputum or tracheal aspirate. If these materials are unsatisfactory or unavailable, other criteria must be used. The relative frequency of respiratory pathogens in the various age groups may provide guidelines for initial therapy for the child with pneumonia who has no significant underlying pulmonary systemic illness or defect in immune function.

INITIAL CHOICE OF ANTIMICROBIAL AGENTS IN VARIOUS AGE GROUPS

Neonatal Pneumonia

The treatment of neonatal pneumonia is similar to that of other forms of severe neonatal infection, including sepsis and meningitis. Initial therapy must include coverage for gram-positive cocci, particularly group B *Streptococcus,* and gram-negative bacilli.

A penicillin is the drug of choice for the gram-positive organisms. If there is reason to suspect staphylococcal infection, a penicillinase-

resistant penicillin is chosen. If there is no significant risk of such infection, ampicillin is used. The latter drug also has activity against some enterococci and some gram-negative bacilli, particularly *Escherichia coli* and *Proteus mirabilis,* when used alone or in combination with an aminoglycoside.

The choice of therapy for suspected gram-negative bacillary infection depends on the antibiotic susceptibility pattern for recent isolates obtained from newborn infants. The patterns vary in different hospitals or communities and from time to time within the same institution. At present, an aminoglycoside, gentamicin, tobramycin, or amikacin, is the preferred drug. Based on antibiotic susceptibility patterns of recent isolates of gram-negative enteric bacilli at Boston City Hospital, we use gentamicin to initiate therapy for severe neonatal infections. Because of the rapid changes in renal function during the first few weeks of life, different dose schedules for selected antibiotics should be used for infants 6 days of age or younger and for infants 1 to 4 weeks of age (Table 1).

The initial therapy should be re-evaluated when the results of cultures are available. The duration of therapy depends on the causative agent. Pneumonia due to gram-negative enteric bacilli or group B *Streptococcus* is treated for 10 days. Disease caused by *Staphylococcus aureus* requires 3 to 6 weeks of antimicrobial therapy according to the severity of the pneumonia.

Pneumonia in Children 1 Month to 5 Years of Age

The vast majority of bronchopneumonias at this age are caused by respiratory viruses. If the initial clinical findings are consistent with viral infection and the child can be observed closely, antibacterial therapy may be withheld pending the results of bacterial cultures. *Streptococcus pneumoniae* and *Haemophilus influenzae,* both type b and nontypable strains, are the major bacterial agents responsible for pneumonia in this age group. Strains of *H. influenzae* resistant to amoxicillin have been isolated throughout the United States, but at present, amoxicillin is still appropriate initial therapy for the young child with mild disease. If the child is moderately or seriously ill, drugs with uniform efficacy against *S. pneumoniae* and *H. influenzae* should be administered by parenteral routes. These include cephalosporins (cefuroxime, ceftriaxone, cefotaxime, or ceftazidime) or chloramphenicol. Therapy must be reevaluated when results of cultures and antibiotic susceptibility tests are available.

S. aureus has been an uncommon cause of acute pneumonia in the past 15 years. However, if clinical signs compatible with staphylococcal disease are present (such as empyema, abscess formation, or pneumatoceles), initial therapy should include a parenteral penicillinase-resistant penicillin (methicillin, nafcillin, or oxacillin).

TABLE 1. Daily Dose Schedules for Parenteral Antibiotics of Value in Treating Bacterial Pneumonia in Newborn Infants*

	DAILY DOSE SCHEDULE	
ANTIBIOTIC	≤6 DAYS OF AGE	1–4 WEEKS OF AGE
Penicillin G	25,000–50,000 U/kg q12h	25,000/kg q6–8h
Ampicillin		
Methicillin		
Nafcillin	25 mg/kg q8–12h	25 mg/kg q6–8h
Oxacillin		
Cefotaxime	50 mg/kg q12h	50 mg/kg q8h
Gentamicin	2.5 mg/kg q12h	2.5 mg/kg q8h
Tobramycin	2 mg/kg q12h	2 mg/kg q8h
Amikacin	7.5 mg/kg q12h	7.5–10 mg/kg q8h
Chloramphenicol†		
Premature	25 mg/kg in 1 dose	25 mg/kg in 1 dose
Full-term	25 mg/kg in 1 dose	25 mg/kg q12h
Vancomycin	10 mg/kg q12h	10 mg/kg q8h

*IM or IV routes are satisfactory except where specifically noted.
†IV route only, inadequate absorption from IM sites.

Chlamydia trachomatis is a common cause of pneumonia in the first 6 months of life. Erythromycin or a sulfonamide appears to be effective in ameliorating signs of illness for infants who have pneumonia caused by this organism.

Pneumonia in Children 5 Years of Age and Older

S. pneumoniae is the major bacterial cause of pneumonia in this age group. *H. influenzae* is less common than in the preschool-age child but should be considered in initial therapy.

Infection by *Mycoplasma pneumoniae* is frequent in the schoolage child, adolescent, and young adult. Erythromycin and the tetracyclines (for use in the child 8 years of age or older) are effective in reducing the duration of illness, and once the diagnosis is made or strongly suspected, treatment with one of these agents is appropriate. The new macrolides, clarithromycin and azithromycin, are effective in vitro against *S. pneumoniae* and *M. pneumoniae* but are not approved for treatment of children with pneumonia (March 1995).

CHEMOTHERAPY FOR SPECIFIC PATHOGENS

Pneumococcal Pneumonia

Penicillin G is the drug of choice for children with pneumococcal pneumonia, except those considered to be allergic to that antibiotic. For most children with mild to moderately severe disease, an oral penicillin is suitable. Phenoxymethyl penicillin (penicillin V) provides significant serum antibacterial activity (the peak is approximately 50% of an equivalent dose of intramuscular aqueous penicillin G).

Children who appear toxic or who have underlying disease or complications, such as abscesses or empyema, require the higher serum and tissue antibacterial activity provided by a parenteral form of penicillin. Intramuscular aqueous sodium or potassium penicillin G is rapidly absorbed, high peak levels occurring within 30 minutes. The levels thus attained make this route optimal for treatment of severe pneumococcal disease. However, since the intramuscular preparation is painful, the intravenous route should be used if therapy of any duration is anticipated.

Intramuscular procaine penicillin G attains lower peak levels (approximately 10% to 30% of those achieved with the sodium or potassium salt), but activity is sustained for 6 or more hours. Since the level of antibacterial activity in the serum may be exceeded manifold by oral penicillins, the use of parenteral procaine penicillin G is restricted to patients who cannot tolerate the oral form (those who vomit or are comatose). A single dose of benzathine penicillin G provides a low level of serum antibacterial activity for a period in excess of 14 days. Although this salt often has been effective in pneumococcal pneumonia, failures are frequent, and it is not recommended.

The dose schedule listed in Table 2 may be used to initiate therapy. The duration of therapy depends on the clinical response, but the drug should be continued for at least 3 days after defervescence and significant resolution of the radiologic and clinical signs.

Strains of *S. pneumoniae* with diminished susceptibility to penicillins and cephalosporins are now occurring throughout the United States and Europe. In contrast to susceptible strains with minimal

TABLE 2. Daily Dose Schedules for Antibiotics of Value in Bacterial Pneumonias of Infants* and Children

ANTIBIOTIC	ROUTE	RECOMMENDED DOSE PER DAY	SCHEDULE
Penicillin G	PO	100,000 U/kg	4 doses†
	IM or IV	100,000–200,000 U/kg	4–6 doses
Penicillin V	PO	100 mg/kg	4 doses
Methicillin	IM or IV	200 mg/kg	4–6 doses
Oxacillin	PO	100 mg/kg	4 doses†
Nafcillin‡	IM or IV	200 mg/kg	4–6 doses
Cloxacillin	PO	50–100 mg/kg	4 doses†
Dicloxacillin	PO	25–50 mg/kg	4 doses
Amoxicillin	PO	40 mg/kg	3 doses
Ampicillin	IM or IV	200 mg/kg	4 doses
Amoxicillin-clavulanate	PO	40 mg/kg	3 doses
Ticarcillin	IV or IM	50–300 mg/kg	4–6 doses
Cephalothin	IM or IV	200 mg/kg	4–6 doses
Cephalexin	PO	50 mg/kg	4 doses†
Cefazolin	IM or IV	50–100 mg/kg	4 doses
Cefamandole	IM or IV	50–150 mg/kg	4 doses
Cefaclor	PO	40–60 mg/kg‖	2–3 doses
Cefuroxime	IV or IM	75–200 mg/kg	3 doses
Cefuroxime axetil	PO	40 mg/kg	3 doses
Cefotaxime	IV or IM	100–200 mg/kg	3–4 doses
Ceftriaxone	IV or IV	50–75 mg/kg	1 dose
Ceftazidime	IV or IM	75–150 mg/kg	3 doses
Gentamicin	IM or IV¶	5 mg/kg	3 doses
Tobramycin	IM or IV¶	3–7.5 mg/kg	3 doses
Amikacin	IM or IV¶	15 mg/kg	2–3 doses
Chloramphenicol	PO	50–75 mg/kg	4 doses
	IV	50–100 mg/kg	4 doses
Clindamycin	PO	20–30 mg/kg	4 doses
	IM or IV	15–40 mg/kg	4 doses
Erythromycin	PO	20–50 mg/kg	3–4 doses
	IV	20–50 mg/kg	4 doses
Vancomycin	IV	40–60 mg/kg	4 doses

*1 month of age and older.
†Schedule at least 1 hour before meals or 2 hours after meals.
‡Manufacturer's precaution: There is no clinical experience available on the IV use of nafcillin in neonates and infants.
§This dose may exceed that recommended by the manufacturer.
‖The manufacturer's schedule for serious infection is 40 mg/kg/24h, with a maximum daily dosage of 1 g.
¶IV administration over 30 to 60 minutes.

inhibitory concentrations (MICs) of less than 0.1 μg/ml, intermediate strains have MICs of 0.1 to 1 μg/ml and resistant strains have MICs of ≥2 μg/ml. In some areas of the United States, up to 25% of pneumococcal strains have been intermediate or resistant. For patients with mild to moderate illness, no change is necessary now for initial therapy, but the pneumococcus isolate should be screened for penicillin resistance, and therapy should be changed if the patient does not respond appropriately. For patients with severe illness, vancomycin should be incorporated into the initial regimen. At present, there are no penicillin-resistant strains to vancomycin, and this drug provides assured efficacy.

Staphylococcal Pneumonia

The high incidence of penicillin G-resistant staphylococci in the hospital and the community requires the use of a penicillinase-resistant penicillin whenever staphylococcal pneumonia is diagnosed or suspected. Later, if the culture and sensitivity data indicate that the organism is sensitive to penicillin G, it should be used because of its efficacy and lesser expense.

Since 1961, laboratories in western Europe have reported varying proportions of strains of staphylococci resistant to methicillin and cross-resistant to the other penicillinase-resistant penicillins and some of the cephalosporins. The incidence of these resistant strains is low (approximately 1% or less) in the United States, but outbreaks have occurred in hospitals, including intensive care units. If a child with staphylococcal disease is given appropriate doses of one of these penicillins and does not respond as expected, resistance to the antibiotic must be suspected, and the sensitivity of the causative organism must be reevaluated. Vancomycin is an effective antistaphylococcal agent and may be used for the patient with pneumonia due to methicillin-resistant *S. aureus*.

The rapid evolution of staphylococcal pneumonia and the frequent association of empyema, pneumatoceles, and abscesses demand close observation and meticulous nursing care. The duration of antibiotic therapy depends on the initial response, the presence of pulmonary and extrapulmonary complications, and the rapidity of resolution of the pneumonic process. A large parenteral dose schedule should be used for 2 to 3 weeks, followed by an oral preparation for 1 to 3 weeks.

Haemophilus Influenzae

Amoxicillin should be considered the drug of choice in young children with mild-to-moderate pulmonary disease. It provides coverage for both *S. pneumoniae* and *H. influenzae* when there is uncertainty as to the bacteriologic diagnosis, and the high dose schedule needed for severe forms of disease can be given without concern for dose-related toxicity (Table 2).

Because of concern for ampicillin-resistant strains of *H. influenzae*, a cephalosporin with stability to beta-lactamase (cefuroxime, cefotaxime, ceftriaxone, or ceftazidime) or intravenous chloramphenicol should be used as initial therapy for patients with severe disease when *H. influenzae* is known or suspected to be the pathogen. The appropriate regimen is chosen when results of cultures and antibacterial susceptibility tests are available.

The child with mild-to-moderate pulmonary disease is treated until a period without fever of at least 3 days and a minimum of 10 days ensues. The child with severe disease is treated for at least 2 to 3 weeks.

Pneumonia due to Gram-Negative Bacilli

Initial therapy must be guided by the following factors: the source of infection, the underlying disease process (burn, cystic fibrosis), host susceptibility (deficient immune mechanisms), and the antimicrobial susceptibility pattern for gram-negative organisms in the community and hospital. The basis for the choice of antibiotic is similar to that outlined for suspected gram-negative bacillary pneumonia in the neonate. The regimen is modified if indicated by the results of

the cultures and the susceptibility of the causative organism. The duration of therapy must be tailored to the clinical course and the response to therapy. Pneumonias with minimal pulmonary lesions and symptoms should be treated for at least 3 days after defervescence. Severe pneumonias should be treated for a period of 2 to 3 weeks.

THERAPY FOR THE PENICILLIN-SENSITIVE CHILD

Any patient with a significant history of allergic reaction to any of the penicillins must be considered sensitive to all of them. Thus, alternative antimicrobial agents should be considered. Cephalothin and cefazolin have been used with success in the treatment of staphylococcal and pneumococcal pneumonias, and cefuroxime, ceftriaxone, cefotaxime, and ceftazidime are effective for pneumococcal and *Haemophilus* pneumonias.

Erythromycin and clindamycin are active in vitro against gram-positive cocci and are effective in the treatment of pneumococcal and staphylococcal pneumonias. Since some staphylococci may be resistant to these antibiotics, it is important to test the organism for susceptibility. Vancomycin may be considered for use in the patient who is allergic to penicillin and who has severe staphylococcal disease.

Tetracycline should not be used in children under the age of 8 years because of the frequency of tooth staining. For those over the age of 8 years, it may be of value in infection due to *Mycoplasma pneumoniae*. The small proportion of pneumococci and the significant number (approximately 30%) of streptococci resistant to tetracyclines limit their use in infections by these agents.

ADJUNCTS TO CHEMOTHERAPY

Antibiotics are only part of the management of the pediatric patient with pneumonia. Supportive measures, including the following, are also of the utmost importance.

1. Maintenance of fluid and electrolyte balance.
2. Humidification provided by cool mist.
3. Oxygen for severe dyspnea or cyanosis.
4. Maintenance of mouth hygiene.
5. Antipyretics should be used sparingly, since the temperature course may provide a guideline for the therapeutic response.
6. Bronchoscopy is limited to instances in which a foreign body, tumor, or congenital anomaly is considered.
7. Tracheal intubation or tracheostomy may be considered when there is laryngeal obstruction or when the patient is having difficulty clearing tracheal secretions and more efficient suctioning is warranted.
8. Drainage of pleural effusions may be necessary when the accumulation of fluid embarrasses respiration. Single or multiple thoracocenteses may be adequate when the volumes of fluid are small. If larger amounts are present, a closed drainage system with a chest tube should be removed as soon as its drainage function is completed, since delay may result in local tissue injury, secondary infection, and sinus formation.
9. Intrapleural instillation of antibiotic should be considered in early cases of empyema, particularly if the fluid is loculated and the presence of fibrous adhesions is a possibility. If a chest tube is in place, antibiotics are instilled following irrigation through the tube. In susceptible infections, aqueous crystalline penicillin G 10,000 to 50,000 units, ampicillin 10 to 50 mg, or a penicillinase-resistant penicillin or a cephalosporin 10 to 50 mg may be inoculated in 10 ml of diluent (sterile water or normal saline) after the tube is clamped. The clamp is maintained for 1 hour and then released for drainage. The instillations should be repeated three or four times each day that the tube remains in place. If thoracocenteses are performed, antibiotic is introduced after pleural fluid is aspirated.

VULVITIS, VAGINITIS, AND URETHRITIS

PAMELA J. MURRAY, M.D., M.H.P.

Vulvovaginitis is the most common gynecologic problem in children of all ages. The anatomy, physiology, and microbiology of the vulva and vagina vary with age. The approach to diagnosis and treatment of vulvitis, vaginitis, and urethritis differs according to the physiologic maturity of the patient and behavioral issues, particularly sexual activity. Although the diseases causing these problems differ by age, all require a careful history and physical examination and are not amenable to telephone diagnosis or treatment.

In the prepubertal child, the normally low estrogen level results in little stratification of the outer squamous layer of the vaginal epithelium. Therefore, it is relatively thin. The vagina maintains a neutral pH. Prepubertal labia are small. They neither cover nor protect the central structures from trauma or irritation. Even normal hygienic practices permit contamination by both stool and respiratory pathogens. In contrast, the prepubertal chemistry and anatomy limit the growth or spread of some pathogens. *Candida* rarely infects the prepubertal vagina, and *Chlamydia* and gonococci do not ascend into the upper genital tract to produce serious pelvic infections.

In adolescents, the external genital tissue and the internal reproductive organs are under the influence of estrogen and other sex hormones. The pH of the vagina becomes more acidic and supports a different constellation of normal flora. The mature vulva provides physical protection from trauma and minimizes contamination from enteric flora. Increasing glandular activity produces secretions that provide lubrication and naturally cleanse the genital tract. The presence of this normal discharge, physiologic leukorrhea, is a hallmark of increasing estrogen levels.

Physiologic leukorrhea begins during puberty. The discharge is clear to milky and mucoid. It may be profuse and bothersome in the perimenarchal young girl. It may leave a yellow stain on underwear as it dries. Microscopy reveals squamous epithelial cells without excessive inflammatory cells.

In adolescents, dysuria and vulvovaginal complaints of itching, discharge, odor, and pain are very common. A correct clinical diagnosis rarely can be made from history alone. Almost all conditions are more common in, but not necessarily exclusive to, sexually active teens. Multiple infections often coexist. In patients who have one sexually transmitted disease (STD), there is a high likelihood that a second sexually transmitted pathogen will be found. The presentation of any sexually related problems provides an opportunity to discuss the broader scope of reproductive health concerns, including STD prevention and contraception.

VULVITIS

Prepubertal Vulvitis

Vulvar inflammation per se in the prepubertal child is most commonly a manifestation of a generalized vulvovaginitis. However, because the majority of presenting symptoms reflect vulvar irritation and discomfort, a discussion of nonspecific vulvovaginitis is included. *Nonspecific vulvovaginitis* in the prepubertal child is most often the result of irritation or inflammation rather than a true infection. Perineal itching, burning, and discomfort are observed by the parent or described by the child. Rubbing or scratching in response to the discomfort may further irritate or damage the normally thin vaginal mucosa and may even result in bleeding. Small amounts of a stain or discharge may be found on underwear and toilet paper, but usually no discharge is visible.

The initiating causes must be identified and addressed. Nonspecific vulvovaginitis may be caused by mechanical or chemical irritation. Friction from tight clothing, masturbation, or sand, inadequate hygiene, or the use of perfumed and colored toilet paper, detergents, bubble baths, soaps, or shampoos can initiate the local inflammatory process. Secondary infection with normal enteric pathogens may occur. Less often, a primary infectious process occurs. When a discharge is present, infection must be considered. Specific infectious agents are discussed in detail under prepubertal vaginitis. Topical agents used for symptomatic relief or inappropriately prescribed therapies may further irritate inflamed tissue. A detailed history of prior efforts to treat the problem may reveal additional etiologies for the current problem.

Treatment should include a discussion of hygiene, including avoidance of irritants and offending agents, proper wiping techniques after toileting, and careful drying of the area to allow for healing. Sitz baths provide temporary symptomatic relief, as well as control of pain and pruritus. Antipruritics (pheniramine maleate or hydroxyzine) or analgesics (acetaminophen or ibuprofen) decrease discomfort reported at night or after prolonged sitting. If other measures have failed, an estrogen cream sparingly applied twice daily to the vulva for 7 days accelerates healing. Occasionally, breast buds appear with the use of estrogen cream, and discontinuation precipitates vaginal bleeding secondary to estrogen withdrawal. If a secondary bacterial infection is suspected, treatment with an antimicrobial, such as trimethoprim-sulfamethoxazole, for 7 to 10 days is advised.

Labial adhesions are most often found in 2 to 6 year olds with independent toileting. Local irritation or inflammation is thought to remove the protective external layers of the epidermis. As the skin reepithelizes, apposing tissues literally stick together or agglutinate. A central line of fusion connects otherwise normal looking genitalia. Adhesions are prominent posteriorly, and obstruction of the anterior urethral opening is very rare. True adhesions are benign and resolve spontaneously with puberty. Many resolve within 6 to 18 months of recognition. Specific therapy is not necessary unless parents cannot be easily reassured. Susceptible individuals have a tendency to have their labia readhere. If desired, treatment may be undertaken with estrogen cream (e.g., 0.01% estradiol vaginal cream or 0.625 mg/g conjugated estrogens) applied sparingly to the midline twice daily for 2 weeks. Temporary vulvar pigmentation, breast tenderness or enlargement, and estrogen withdrawal vaginal bleeding may occur. Gentle traction on the labia facilitates separation. Permanent removal of irritants discourages readhesion. Zinc oxide or petroleum jelly applied at bedtime to the recently separated labia for several months provides a barrier to reagglutination.

Pinworms (Enterobius vermicularis) located in the rectum or vagina may be recognized by sight or by characteristic nighttime perianal and perineal itching. Anal infection with this nematode is very common among preschool and school-aged children. Vaginal infestation is less common but occasionally produces a discharge in addition to pruritus. Scratching induces a secondary vulvitis. Perianal Scotch tape tests are helpful when they are positive. When the clinical presentation strongly suggests pinworm infestation, a single course of relatively benign and inexpensive therapy is advised. Single-dose treatment with either PO pyrantel pamoate 1 mg/kg (max: 1 g) or 100 mg mebendazole is effective for rectal infestations. Douching may be required if vaginal infestation is heavy. The appropriate dose should be taken by each family member over 2 years of age and repeated 2 weeks later. Reinfection is common, and retreatment is recommended with the same regimen used initially.

Urethral prolapse occurs when the urethral mucosa prolapses through the urethral meatus. It occurs most frequently among obese prepubertal school-age females. Increased intraabdominal pressure caused by coughing, straining, or crying often accompanies the onset of the problem. The prolapsed tissue becomes swollen and hemorrhagic. Bleeding and pain are common symptoms. On examination, the urethral opening is encircled by a red, swollen doughnut of mucosal tissue. The urethral mucosa is estrogen responsive, and twice-daily application of estrogen cream, as for labial adhesions, usually stimulates resolution of the problem. Sitz baths provide symptomatic relief. Elimination of the precipitating factors—obesity, cough, constipation, and crying—minimizes the chance of recurrence.

Lichen sclerosis presents insidiously as a chronic perineal itch that is eventually accompanied by skin breakdown, with bleeding or ulcers. The perineal and perianal areas are the primary sites of this skin disorder of unknown etiology. Dysuria and pain occur with more destructive lesions. A skillful history taking may avoid confusion with chronic sexual abuse. Diagnosis is made by a skin biopsy of the lesion, which should be optimally timed to avoid the effects of local or systemic anti-inflammatory agents. Moderate- to high-potency steroids and sex hormone-containing creams are recommended for treatment, with variable results. The side effects of the hormonal preparations must be considered in the context of the age of the patient. Some individuals respond well to therapy, and generally the condition improves with puberty. No potential malignant risks have been identified. Because of the chronicity of the condition and its potential confusion with other obscure dermatologic diseases that can present similarly, both biopsy and dermatologic consultation are advised.

Vulvitis in Prepubertal and Postpubertal Children

Trauma, either accidental or secondary to abuse, can result in injuries that present as inflammation. Abuse deserves consideration in the evaluation of almost all gynecologic complaints and in all cases of trauma. A low threshold for suspicion should encourage questioning of the patient and other family members individually. Whenever abuse is suspected, an attempt to have the patient interviewed and examined by child abuse specialists, if they are available, is recommended. Meticulous documentation of both the history and physical examination is critical. With adolescents, the individual's previous sexual history or behavior should not bias evaluation of the current problem. Half of all rapes involve adolescent females, and exploitative relationships are common among female teens. Accidental injuries deserve similar documentation of the mechanism of injury and the physical findings.

The perineal area is very vascular. Minor injuries bleed profusely and usually heal rapidly. Whenever internal injuries are suspected because of the history or physical examination, surgical exploration under anesthesia is necessary.

Trauma caused by consensual sexual activity, at first intercourse or otherwise, may cause vulvar irritation. The circumstances of the traumatic event should be elicited by sensitive and nonjudgmental questioning. Strategies to prevent further pain or irritation include ensuring adequate lubrication or using supplemental lubrication and limiting the duration of intercourse. An examination to check for any damage is indicated. Teens need to be adequately reassured of the normality of their own anatomy and sexual functioning.

Irritation occurs with chronic friction from sports (e.g., running), obesity, poor aeration and maceration (e.g., enuresis, wet bathing suits), and masturbation. Drying, healing, and protection from reinjury are curative.

Dermatologic conditions with a more general distribution may also cause vulvitis. Eczema, psoriasis, seborrhea, and acneiform conditions can involve the vulva and surrounding skin areas. Skin damaged by any of these disorders is more vulnerable to superinfection with yeast, human papillomavirus (HPV), and skin pathogens. Once the integrity of the cutaneous surface is restored, secondary infections respond better to treatment. Dermatologic consultation may be indicated.

Systemic immunodeficiencies, including those caused by HIV infection, chemotherapy, and high-dose steroids, may alter the presentation and treatment response of the other gynecologic conditions described. A thorough medical and medication history should reveal most sources of immunosuppression. The possibility of HIV testing should be addressed if concerns are raised.

Viral infections present as a systemic illness or as a localized rash or ulcer. Some of the more common viruses that cause vulvar infection include herpes simplex virus (HSV), molluscum contagiosum, HPV, and varicella-zoster virus. Less frequently, adenovirus, echovirus,

measles virus, and Epstein-Barr virus (EBV) cause vulvar symptoms. Viral cultures are recommended when HSV is suspected. Once HSV is clinically suspected, treatment with acyclovir 200 mg PO five times daily for 7 to 10 days is initiated immediately. Episodes of recurrent genital herpes may be treated with a 5-day course of acyclovir 200 mg five times a day or 400 mg three times a day. This regimen initiated during the prodromal phase, or the first 48 hours of disease, may attenuate the episode in some individuals. Acyclovir PO 20 mg/kg per dose four times a day for 5 days (max. single dose: 800 mg) is recommended for varicella infection when the patient is over 12 years of age or has a chronic skin or pulmonary disorder. Maximum effectiveness is obtained when treatment is initiated within 24 hours of the onset of infection. Acyclovir treatment will cause a decrease in severity and duration of both HSV and varicella-zoster infections. Salicylates are contraindicated with varicella infection.

Molluscum contagiosum is diagnosed clinically by the presence of waxy papules with an umbilicated center containing a small amount of white, firm to cheesy material in the core of the lesion. Lesions may resolve spontaneously. Treatment eliminates inoculation of other sites and contacts. Mechanical destruction of the central core with a needle or chemical destruction with trichloroacetic acid, cantharidin, liquid nitrogen, or wart removal preparations of salicylic or lactic acid usually is effective.

Scabies infestation occurs in all age groups. Among adolescents and adults, it may be sexually acquired. Intense itching that increases at night may be localized at the site where the mite is burrowed or generalized in response to sensitization to the proteins of the parasite. Excoriation often obliterates the mite's burrows. Characteristic red-brown nodules, less than 5 mm in size, are reactive granulomas to dead mite products. A definitive diagnosis is made by visualizing the mite or its eggs or feces by scraping an intact burrow with a scalpel after oil or water has been applied to the lesion. Recommended treatments include 5% permethrin, lindane, and crotamiton. Permethrin is both safe and effective in all age groups and in pregnancy. It is applied to the whole body and removed by bathing 8 to 14 hours later. Treatment of household members and environmental cleansing recommendations are discussed in Chapter 15. Both the nodules and the pruritus may persist after adequate treatment. Follow-up is recommended if symptoms do not abate.

Human papillomavirus (HPV) can infect the entire genital tract. It is acquired at birth, through sexual activity, and least frequently, by nonsexual contact. In the prepubertal child, the vulva is the most common site for genital infection. Warts appear as flat, papillary or verrucous growths. Warts identified in the first year of life are less likely to be caused by sexual abuse than those first appearing later in childhood. However, at any age, all possible sources of contact deserve consideration. Before any warts appear, the vulva may itch and give the impression of a nonspecific, noninfectious vulvovaginitis. Small painful fissures are sometimes noted in the perineal or perianal areas. In adolescents, clinically evident or subclinical HPV infection can extend throughout the entire lower genital tract. Pap smears may support the suspicion of HPV infection. The etiology of atypical presentations and of HPV infection in prepubertal patients is confirmed by biopsy of the tissue. Cultures are not generally available for clinical use.

Trichloroacetic acid 40% to 85% applied directly to lesions causes several minutes of moderately painful discomfort and burning but produces little subsequent pain. Pretreatment with 20% benzocaine (Hurricane) anesthetic spray significantly lessens the immediate discomfort. Weekly retreatment for up to 6 weeks may be needed to eradicate extragenital warts. Other treatment options include the use of 10% to 25% podophyllin or podofilox 0.5% solution (Condylox). Careful application is needed to avoid damage to healthy tissue. Podophyllin compounds do not cause pain at the time of application but are likely to cause pain and burning in subsequent days. Because of risks associated with systemic absorption, trichloroacetic acid is preferred by many clinicians.

Dermatologic techniques of electrical or thermal destruction also may be effective. Laser treatment is preferred for extensive lesions, and anesthesia may be required during such treatment for physical and psychologic reasons. Treatments most likely to be effective in a single session may be preferred for some younger children. None of the treatment modalities completely eradicates the virus, and recurrences are common. HPV infections of the lower genital tract, including the cervix, vagina, and vulva, are associated with dysplasia and an increased risk of neoplasm. Careful follow-up and referral are essential to the care of patients with HPV infection.

Ulcers and mucosal inflammation are known to appear as the initial manifestations of a chronic systemic illness or autoimmune process, such as Crohn's disease, systemic lupus erythematosus, Behçet's disease, and Stevens-Johnson syndrome. A comprehensive history and physical examination are required. In the absence of other features of these illnesses, laboratory testing and biopsies are necessary to secure a proper diagnosis before treatment can be initiated. STDs causing ulcers are discussed in the next section.

Neoplasms of the vulva are extremely rare but are more common in individuals with a history of HPV infection. The incidence of vulvar intraepithelial neoplasm (VIN) is increasing. Atypical and suspicious lesions, especially when accompanied by pigmentation changes, rapid growth, bleeding, or necrosis, deserve a specialist's attention, biopsy, and a definitive diagnosis.

Postpubertal Vulvitis

Nonspecific vulvitis in the adolescent may be caused by irritants, including menstrual pads, tampons, spermicides, deodorants, douches, and other feminine hygiene products. Elimination of the irritant and the symptomatic treatments described previously are curative.

Folliculitis and hidradenitis afflict some teens in the pubic area and may extend to the vulva. Warm soaks facilitate healing and drainage from infected lesions. When surrounding tissues become secondarily infected, antibiotic treatment directed at skin pathogens is indicated. When chronic discomfort and infection occur, suppressive therapy with antibiotics decreases the severity of the problem. A subset of patients with elevated androgens are likely to benefit by treatment with oral contraceptive pills that suppress excess ovarian androgen production.

Bartholin's and Skene's gland abscesses present as inflamed masses adjacent to the vulva and are usually caused by sexually transmitted organisms, most commonly *Neisseria gonorrhoeae*. Other sites should be cultured for STDs. Bartholinitis is treated as a complicated gonococcal or chlamydial infection. Surgical drainage relieves pain and facilitates response to treatment.

Bartholin's duct cysts can present as large labial swellings with a notable absence of inflammation. Symptomatic treatment, such as analgesics and local heat, are effective. These masses usually resolve spontaneously.

Genital ulcer disease in the adolescent may be caused by some of the less prevalent sexually transmitted infections, in addition to the systematic illnesses previously discussed. Individuals with any genital ulcer are at greater risk of infection with and transmission of HIV. HIV antibody determination should be strongly encouraged in these patients.

The chancre of primary *syphilis* appears as a firm, painless ulcer. A presumptive diagnosis is made by an elevated nontreponemal specific titer (VDRL or RPR) and further supported by a positive specific treponemal antibody test (FTA-ABS or MHA-TP). The diagnosis of early syphilis is confirmed by a positive darkfield examination for *Treponema pallidum* or a positive direct fluorescent antibody test of exudate or tissue from a suspect lesion. Consultation is recommended before specimen collection to maximize diagnostic accuracy. Treatment for primary and secondary syphilis is a single dose of benzathine penicillin G 2.4 million U IM.

Chancroid, in contrast to syphilis, presents as one or more painful genital ulcers. A third of patients also have tender inguinal adenopathy. A definitive diagnosis is made by the growth of *Haemophilus ducreyi*, but almost all diagnoses are made on the clinical presentation

and the absence of evidence for syphilis and herpes. Single-dose treatments include 1 g of azithromycin PO or 250 mg of ceftriaxone IM. Erythromycin base 500 mg four times a day for 7 days is also recommended. Other causes of genital ulcers, such as lymphogranuloma venereum, are much less common in the United States.

Pediculosis pubis (pubic lice or crabs) is the most common infestation in this age group. The louse lays its eggs on the shafts of human hair, preferring thick terminal hairs as its habitat. Most commonly transmitted by sexual intimacy, the lice can be transferred also by fomites, such as towels. Itching is the major symptom. All hairy areas, including facial hairs, underarms, eyebrows, and eyelashes, and the scalp should be checked for infestation. Egg cases can be visualized with the naked eye on hair shafts. Lice can be removed with gloved hands or an instrument. They may hold tenaciously to the skin and look like simple brown macules. Treatment consists of a pediculicide, as for head lice. Permethrin 1% cream is the least toxic and easiest to use, and both nits and eggs are killed. A 10-minute application to all infested hair is recommended for children older than 2 years of age and where there is no risk of pregnancy and no lactation. One percent lindane shampoo is applied for 4 minutes and then thoroughly washed off. Hand removal of nits and lice is recommended only for eyelashes, where pediculicide application is contraindicated. Retreatment in 8 to 10 days is recommended. Clothes and linens should be washed in hot water. Sexual contacts need treatment.

VAGINITIS

Prepubertal Vaginitis

Nonspecific vaginitis frequently accompanies nonspecific vulvitis, as previously discussed.

Infections more prevalent in the prepubertal child may be caused by respiratory pathogens, bowel pathogens, normal bowel flora, and skin microbes. A discharge is commonly present in infectious vaginitis. Sexually transmitted pathogens that cause cervicitis in mature females produce a vulvovaginitis in prepubertal girls. Proper specimen collection is critical. If at all possible, cultures should be taken when the discharge is visible. The hymen is very sensitive, and direct contact should be avoided. Small swabs moistened with nonbacteriostatic saline or soft catheters attached to a syringe minimize discomfort. Frogleg positioning with labial traction and the knee-chest prone position expose the hymenal opening and provide easier visualization and access.

Sexually transmitted pathogens, specifically gonorrhea and *Chlamydia,* can cause a vulvovaginitis clinically identical to that caused by nonsexually transmitted infections. Laboratory specimens for these pathogens should be submitted with special attention to proper collection technique and transport. *Chlamydia* cultures, rather than the antigen detection systems, are strongly recommended for the detection of *Chlamydia* infections in prepubertal females.

Respiratory and skin microbes infect the vaginal and vulval tissues. The most common pathogens in this category are *Streptococcus pneumoniae, Streptococcus pyogenes, Staphylococcus aureus,* and *Haemophilus influenzae.* They cause a superficial vulvovaginitis with purulent discharge. Streptococcal infections cause a more invasive local infection with clinical features of erysipelas or cellulitis. The pharynx may also be colonized with *S. pyogenes*. Routine cultures of the vaginal discharge will define the pathogen, and sensitivities may guide treatment.

Enteric pathogens and microbes normally found in stool cause vulvovaginal infections. Many of the organisms capable of causing urinary tract infections, such as *Escherichia coli,* also may cause a vaginitis. Toileting and other hygienic practices need to be modified to decrease the risk of reinfection. Cultures and sensitivities provide treatment guidance.

Shigella is the most frequent cause of acute and chronic infectious vulvovaginitis accompanied by a bloody discharge. Specific bacteriologic methods must be used to culture for this organism. There may be no history of diarrhea in some patients. In others, diarrhea may precede or accompany the onset of *Shigella* vulvovaginitis. However, stool cultures taken at the time of evaluation for vulvovaginitis are usually negative. These *Shigella* species have high rates of resistance to ampicillin and trimethoprim-sulfamethoxazole. Sensitivities are critical to the choice of appropriate antibiotics, and third-generation cephalosporins may be needed to eradicate the infection. A high rate of coinfection with pinworms has been reported.

Postpubertal Vaginitis

In the adolescent, 97% of all vaginitis can be attributed to one of three entities—candidiasis, bacterial vaginosis, and trichomoniasis. All three are more common in the sexually active teen, as are both urinary tract infections and cervicitis. Vulvar or vaginal pruritus and increased vaginal discharge or a change in its color or odor are the presenting complaints. In addition to the sexual and menstrual history, the practitioner should inquire about recent medication use, especially antibiotics and oral contraceptive pills, diabetes, steroid use, hygiene practices, pregnancy, immune compromise, and a history of previous infections, including urinary tract infections, vulvovaginitis, pelvic inflammatory disease (PID), and other STDs. In the sexually active adolescent, a full examination, including inspection of the external genitalia, and a speculum and bimanual examination are indicated. Cervical cultures and a vaginal specimen are essential. In the virginal adolescent, a sample of discharge for both microscopic and microbiologic evaluation can be obtained by carefully inserting a cotton-tipped swab through the hymenal ring. Application of a small amount of lidocaine to the hymenal ring may ease discomfort.

Bacterial vaginosis (BV) is a noninflammatory condition that occurs when the vaginal anaerobic bacteria, *Gardnerella vaginalis* and *Mycoplasma hominis,* replace the normal *Lactobacillus* population. The overall concentration of bacteria increases 100-fold. Vaginal odor and an abnormal discharge are reported in 75% to 90% of women with BV. Pruritus, dysuria, and pelvic and abdominal pain are not features of this condition. If they are present, consideration must be given to other vaginal and cervical infections.

The diagnosis is made by meeting three of the following four criteria: homogeneous white discharge, a positive whiff test (a fishy amine odor after addition of 10% KOH to a sample of vaginal fluid), clue cells (epithelial cells stippled with bacteria) representing more than 20% of the epithelial cells on a saline wet preparation, and vaginal secretions with a pH>4.5. Vaginal cultures are not helpful in diagnosis. Both *Haemophilus* and *Gardnerella* species, implicated historically in this disorder, are found among normal vaginal flora. Standard treatment for nonpregnant individuals has been oral metronidazole 500 mg twice daily for 7 days. Significantly lower cure rates (73%) are obtained with a 2 g single PO dose. Metronidazole 0.75% gel (5 g) may be applied intravaginally twice daily for 5 days. Alternatively, clindamycin 300 mg PO twice daily for 7 days or intravaginal clindamycin 5 g of 2% cream at night for 7 days is effective. The intravaginal preparation contains mineral oil, which can weaken latex condoms. Clindamycin in any form should not be used in individuals with a history of colitis. Partner treatment does not decrease reinfection and is not recommended. Recurrence rates are high, and retreatment with a different antibiotic or preparation is recommended. Multiple recent studies have confirmed an association between bacterial vaginosis and pregnancy complications, such as preterm labor.

Candidiasis, or yeast vaginitis, is an inflammatory reaction caused by overgrowth of yeast that often colonize the vagina. Ninety percent of such infections are caused by *Candida albicans.* Other *Candida* species and *Torulopsis glabrata* also cause a similar clinical picture. Symptoms include vulvar burning, a thick or milky adherent discharge, and pruritus that is most often reported in the perimenstrual period. Dysuria and dyspareunia may also be present. On examination, the vulva and vagina may be erythematous. A thick adherent discharge may be seen on the vaginal walls or cervix. The vaginal pH is low, between 3.5 and 5. Hyphae or spores are seen in 50% to 80% of patients with candidiasis on either the saline or the KOH preparation.

Torulopsis does not form characteristic hyphae. Routine bacterial cultures may yield fungal species. Yeast found on Pap smears in asymptomatic individuals does not need to be treated.

Intravaginal clotrimazole tablets 100 mg or 5 g of 1% cream, available without prescription, are 90% effective in the treatment of vaginal candidiasis using a 7-day course. Similar efficacy is attained with terconazole, miconazole, and butoconazole. Terconazole is available in a 3-day course of an 80 mg intravaginal suppository and 3-day or 7-day courses of intravaginal cream (0.8% or 0.4%). Terconazole in the 3-day suppository formulation and all miconazole preparations, tioconazole, and butoconazole contain oil-based vehicles and may weaken latex diaphragms and condoms. A 5-g, single-dose preparation of tioconazole in a 6.5% ointment has become available. The other single-dose alternatives, recommended for uncomplicated mild to moderate candidiasis, include 500 mg clotrimazole intravaginal tablets. Single-dose preparations improve compliance but do not produce a more rapid clinical response. Oral treatments for yeast vaginitis include ketoconazole and fluconazole. A longer course of oral therapy may be needed for recalcitrant and complicated vaginal yeast infections. Nystatin is least effective in eradicating vaginal fungal infections. Treatment of partners does not improve cure rates or decrease recurrence rates. Individuals with more than three or four proven episodes in a year have recurrent candidiasis and should be treated initially with a nonclotrimazole fungicide. If this fails to prevent recurrences, a longer course of curative therapy is followed by a monthly preventive or suppressive dose. For example, ketoconazole 400 mg daily for 2 weeks is followed by the same daily dosing for 5 days each month at the onset of menses. Alternatively, a 500-mg clotrimazole suppository is prescribed daily for 2 weeks, followed by one suppository monthly at the end of menses. Birth control pills or pregnancy increase the frequency of candidiasis in some women. A pill formulation with a lower estrogen content may prevent the recurrence of vaginitis.

Trichomoniasis is caused by a flagellated protozoon that thrives in the vaginal environment and can live on moist surfaces outside the host for 1 to 3 hours. There is a very high rate of asymptomatic colonization of the male genital tract with small numbers of trichomonads. Ten to twenty-five percent of infected women are asymptomatic. The majority of cases are sexually transmitted, but other modes of spread occur. Trichomonads have been found in postpubertal teens who have not been sexually active. The incubation period is 4 to 8 days. Pruritus is the most common presenting symptom (75%), and half of infected women have a greenish yellow vaginal discharge with a foul odor. Dysuria is a complaint in 20% of women, and about 5% will have abdominal pain. On pelvic examination, a frothy discharge at the vaginal opening commonly is found. Vulvar inflammation extending onto the perineal skin occurs. The discharge may be copious and require removal with a large cotton swab to visualize a red vagina and strawberry cervix with punctate hemorrhages. A saline wet preparation of the discharge will show motile trichomonads in 50% of infections. A sample of urine sediment viewed under the microscope has a slightly higher yield in females and males. Reports of trichomonads on Pap smears have a high rate of both false positives and false negatives and should not be used as a sole indication for treatment. Latex and DNA-probe office-based tests are now available. *Trichomonas* cultures, considered the gold standard of diagnosis, are not in common use in most clinical settings.

The preferred treatment consists of metronidazole 2 g PO in a single dose for the patient and her partner. A 7-day course of 500 mg twice daily is also effective. Metronidazole in the vaginal gel form has not been approved for treatment because there is not sufficient absorption to destroy trichomonads, which frequently coexist in the urethra and Skene's glands. Some individuals with resistant infections require a prolonged oral regimen of 2 g daily for 3 to 5 days, with supplemental intravaginal applications. Infections that persist require consultation with a specialist and culture and sensitivity testing of the organism.

Pregnant patients cannot be treated in the first trimester. Clotrimazole (Gyne-Lotrimin) cures a smaller percentage of trichomonal infections. There may be some correlation between *Trichomonas* infection in pregnancy and low birthweight. Patients should be warned of the disulfiram-like effect when alcohol consumption coincides with metronidazole therapy.

Allergic vaginitis in the adolescent is most often caused by a reaction to spermicides. Commercial or homemade douches, intravaginal medications, and latex also can precipitate an allergic reaction. Itching, dyspareunia, and dysuria are the most common symptoms. The vaginal walls may be erythematous, edematous, and tender. An inflammatory exudate may be present. A saline wet preparation may show white blood cells in the absence of organisms or positive cultures. Symptomatic treatment with a short course of oral antihistamines and topical hydrocortisone applied to the vulval and distal vaginal tissues is recommended. Care to avoid reexposure to suspected allergens is critical. A suspicion of allergy to spermicide can be confirmed with the application of a small amount of spermicide to the inner aspect of the arm. A local contact dermatitis will be produced in sensitized individuals.

URETHRITIS

Females

Dysuria, or pain on urination, may be due to acute bacterial cystitis, urethritis, or vulvitis and is the most common symptom of urethritis. Between 10% and 20% of adolescent females have at least one episode of dysuria per year. Internal dysuria describes pain on initiation of and during voiding felt primarily internally. External dysuria refers to pain continuing after the cessation of voiding and felt when the urine touches the skin. Self-report of internal or external dysuria has not been shown to distinguish reliably between urinary tract and gynecologic infections in adolescents. Frequently, multiple sites of infection and multiple etiologies coexist. Because this symptom is often ascribable to infections that are sexually transmitted, the approach to evaluation must include a sexual history and a pelvic examination. Several different studies confirm that among adolescents, vulvovaginitis is a more common etiology than bacterial urinary tract infections (UTIs) for dysuria. Vulvovaginitis is discussed in detail in the preceding section.

Acute bacterial cystitis (ABC) is characterized by the rapid onset of severe dysuria, frequency, and urgency. The most common pathogens are bacterial and include *E. coli, Staphylococcus saprophyticus,* and *Proteus, Klebsiella,* and *Enterobacter* species. Pyuria is the best indicator of bacterial infection. Microscopic hematuria is present in approximately 50% of patients. Suprapubic tenderness, when present, strongly suggests ABC. Nitrites produced by the usual uropathogenic gram-negative rods are highly specific for bacterial UTI. Nitrites, as well as pyuria and hematuria, can be positively identified on a urine dipstick.

Initial urine cultures may not be cost effective in females with frequency and dysuria who demonstrate both pyuria and bacteriuria. To treat without culturing the urine, both the history and physical findings should clearly support the diagnosis. Both the patient and the clinician should agree on a plan for follow-up purposes. When there is any doubt or complicating circumstances, a culture is recommended. Bacterial colony counts of a single organism as low as 100/mm³ in a symptomatic woman are associated with ABC. Tests of cure are not routinely indicated.

The ideal duration of therapy is controversial. Five days of antibiotic treatment is usually sufficient for lower tract UTIs. Excellent cure rates are produced by trimethoprim alone and in combination with sulfamethoxazole, nitrofurantoin, amoxicillin-clavulanic acid, and the new quinolones and cephalosporins (Vantin, Suprax). In some communities, there may be significant resistance to trimethoprim-sulfamethoxazole. Treatment of longer duration (7 to 10 days) is recommended if the ABC is associated with a fever, costovertebral angle tenderness, or symptoms preceding treatment for more than a week. The possibility of pregnancy must be considered before anti-

microbial selection. The timing of the last menses and sexual intercourse, the use of contraception, and the results of a urine pregnancy test will determine the risk of pregnancy and influence antibiotic choices.

The *acute urethral syndrome,* or dysuria-sterile pyuria syndrome, is clinically less acute than ABC. It has a gradual and often prolonged onset and is most often associated with STDs that can infect the female urethra (*Chlamydia,* gonorrhea, HSV). Patients who have had intercourse with a new partner or who report STD symptoms in their partner are more at risk. Since the causative organisms are often sexually transmitted, a pelvic examination with appropriate specimen collection must be performed in female patients. Specimen collection should include a clean-catch midstream urine for urinalysis (microscopy or dipstick or both) and culture, culture from the endocervix for *N. gonorrhoeae,* an endocervical specimen for detection of *Chlamydia,* and a wet mount from cervical-vaginal secretions for saline and KOH preparations. Samples for viral culture and Pap smears, if indicated, should be obtained. The increasing availability of polymerase chain reaction (PCR) determination for *Chlamydia* is changing diagnostic options. Currently, urine specimens are acceptable for Chlamydiazyme and *Chlamydia* PCR tests for males only. Treatment of gonorrhea and *Chlamydia* infection is discussed later.

Males

Urethritis is the most common manifestation of STDs in males. The presenting complaints are those of urethral discharge (drip), dysuria (burning), and pruritus of the meatus. Urethritis is classified as gonococcal urethritis when that organism is implicated and nongonococcal urethritis (NGU) when *N. gonorrhoeae* cannot be identified. *Chlamydia trachomatis, Ureaplasma urealyticum,* and *Mycoplasma hominis* are the most frequent pathogens identified in NGU. HSV and *Trichomonas* both cause dysuria, but much less frequently. With more widespread testing for *Chlamydia,* nonspecific urethritis (NSU) usually refers to nongonococcal, nonchlamydial urethritis. Although gonococcal urethritis typically produces a more profuse and purulent discharge with a shorter incubation than other nongonococcal infections, it is not possible to distinguish between the entities on clinical grounds alone.

Urethral discharge can be green, yellow, brown, or white. It may be visible at the urethral meatus or only when expressed by milking the distal urethra. If a discharge is present, a culture for gonorrhea and a gram stain are performed. If a discharge is not seen, an endourethral swab is obtained to streak on selective *N. gonorrhoeae* culture media or placed in specific transport media. An endourethral swab is obtained and sent for detection of chlamydial infection (PCR or enzyme immunoassay or culture). If white blood cells and intracellular gram-negative diplococci are noted on gram stain, the patient is treated for gonorrhea as well as chlamydial infection because of the high coincidence of infections. If more than 5 white blood cells per high power field are identified without finding gram-negative intracellular diplococci, a diagnosis of NGU is made, and appropriate treatment is initiated.

In males with dysuria but with minimal or no discharge, the sediment of the first 10 to 15 ml of a urine specimen can be examined for white blood cells. The presence of 15 or more white blood cells per high power field is abnormal and suggestive of the diagnosis of urethritis. On the basis of this finding, specimens for diagnosing gonorrhea and chlamydial infection from an endourethral swab are obtained. Presumptive treatment adequate for infection due to both of these organisms is begun. Sexual partners are evaluated and treated. In some settings, asymptomatic males are screened for urethritis with a dipstick test of the first 10 to 15 ml of urine. When the leukocyte esterase determination is positive, STD testing and treatment are recommended. The Centers for Disease Control issued new treatment guidelines for STDs in 1993.[1] The new monograph has been expanded to include HIV infection and discussion of clinical entities. Access to an up-to-date edition is strongly advised.

Gonococcal urethritis, compared with other etiologies, has a shorter incubation of 2 to 6 days and a more purulent and painful discharge. Assessment of the discharge is discussed in the preceding paragraphs. Treatment should begin presumptively whenever there is suspicion of sexually transmitted urethritis. Single-dose treatment options for uncomplicated gonococcal urethritis include cefixime (Suprax) 400 mg PO, cefpodoxime proxetil (Vantin) 200 mg PO, ceftriaxone (Rocephin) 125 mg IM, ciprofloxacin (Cipro) 500 mg PO, or ofloxacin (Floxin) 400 mg PO. None of these regimens eradicates coexisting *Chlamydia* infection. Ceftriaxone and ciprofloxacin are more effective than the alternatives in the treatment of suspected pharyngeal infection caused by *N. gonorrhoeae*. Ceftriaxone is most likely to treat incubating syphilis. One of the cephalosporins is recommended for infections acquired in Asia or other areas where higher levels of quinolone resistance have been reported. The quinolones are contraindicated for pregnant or nursing women and are not recommended for individuals under 18 years of age.

Spectinomycin 2 g IM is the single-dose alternative for individuals in whom the aforementioned regimens are contraindicated. Single-dose treatments are not adequate for the treatment of complicated infections or for infection in the immunocompromised host. A test of cure is not recommended for individuals who are asymptomatic and where the risk of reinfection has been eliminated by partner treatment and appropriate prevention. Abstinence is advised until partners have completed therapy and are without symptoms. Partners who need to be evaluated and treated include all contacts within the 30 days before the onset of a symptomatic infection or the most recent sexual partner if it has been longer than 60 days since last intercourse.

Chlamydial infection is the most prevalent treatable STD. The highest rates of chlamydial infection are among adolescents and young adults. *Chlamydia* accompanies the gonococcus in about 30% of infections. Because of the frequency and seriousness of complicated infections and the long-term sequelae, presumptive treatment is recommended if gonococcal or chlamydial infection is suspected. Recommended regimens include doxycycline 100 mg PO twice daily for 7 days or azithromycin 1 g PO in a single dose. When pregnancy is suspected, erythromycin base 500 mg PO four times daily for 7 days is suggested. This regimen often is not well tolerated because of gastrointestinal side effects. Alternatives include erythromycin 250 mg four times daily for 14 days or amoxicillin 500 mg three times daily for 10 days. When doxycycline, erythromycin, or amoxicillin is prescribed, a test of cure is recommended because of lower efficacy and poorer compliance with these courses of treatment. Alternatives with less efficacy and clinical experience include ofloxacin, sulfisoxazole, and other erythromycin preparations. Consult reference books for the limitations of nonstandard choices.

Nonspecific urethritis (NSU) may be caused by *U. urealyticum* or *Mycoplasma* infections, most of which are eradicated by the regimens recommended for *Chlamydia* infections. Currently, neither cultures nor other diagnostic tests for these organisms are performed routinely in clinical practice. *Trichomonas* infection should be considered when symptoms do not respond to conventional therapy. The diagnosis is made by microscopy, culture, or confirmation of a partner's infection. Treatment, as for trichomonal vaginitis in the female, is 2 g of metronidazole PO in a single dose. When a female exhibits a *Trichomonas* infection, the male partner is often the source, harboring a low-grade infestation of trichomonads, which when transmitted to the female, inoculate the vagina, cervix, vulva, or urethra.

Complications of urethritis are less common in males than in females. Epididymitis and disseminated gonococcal infection require more prolonged antibiotic therapy. Rarely, an infected individual develops an immunoreactive arthritis. Urethritis may accompany a more generalized immune-mediated process, such as Stevens-Johnson or Reiter's syndrome.

HSV urethritis is usually accompanied by genital ulcers, a profuse and serosanguineous or mucoid discharge, marked local pain, and systemic symptoms of fever, malaise, and lymphadenopathy. Both diagnostic techniques and treatment protocols are the same as for vulvovaginitis in the female.

REFERENCES

1. Centers for Disease Control and Prevention: 1993 Sexually Transmitted Diseases Treatment Guidelines. MMWR 42 (No. RR-14), 1993.
2. Peter G (ed): American Academy of Pediatrics: 1994 Red Book: Report of the Committee on Infectious Diseases, 23rd ed. Elk Grove Village, IL, American Academy of Pediatrics, 1994.

SHIGELLOSIS

LARRY K. PICKERING, M.D.
GUILLERMO M. RUIZ-PALACIOS, M.D.

Shigellosis is an acute infection of the intestinal tract mainly involving the terminal ileum, colon, and rectum. The spectrum of illness is broad, extending from asymptomatic shedding to mild, watery diarrhea to dysentery manifested by high fever, chills, toxemia, tenesmus, and the passage of multiple, scanty stools containing blood and mucus. Four species of *Shigella* are recognized: *Shigella sonnei* (the most frequent type isolated in industrialized countries), *Shigella flexneri* (which accounts for the majority of the rest of the episodes), *Shigella boydii*, and *Shigella dysenteriae*. One serotype, *S. dysenteriae* 1, the so-called Shiga bacillus, causes particularly severe disease in less developed countries and has been associated with hemolytic-uremic syndrome.

TREATMENT

Therapy for shigellosis can be divided into four phases: (1) emergency treatment of life-endangering complications, (2) specific antimicrobial drugs, (3) supportive measures, and (4) health education.

Potentially Life-Endangering Emergencies

The early stage of clinical illness due to *Shigella* is often characterized by watery diarrhea that can lead to dehydration in infants, particularly when it is accompanied by fever. Severe dehydration must be treated vigorously with IV infusions of 30 to 40 ml/kg of Ringer's lactate solution, isotonic saline, or similar solutions to restore the intravascular volume and to correct shock and acidosis. This should be followed by continued oral rehydration with a glucose-electrolyte solution.

Sequelae include convulsions, lethal toxic encephalopathy (ekiri syndrome), colonic perforation, hypoglycemia, bacteremia, and hemolytic uremic syndrome (with *S. dysenteriae* 1 only). During convulsions, airway obstruction due to aspiration of stomach contents may occur consequent to loss of consciousness. The high fever that may cause convulsions in young children may be lowered with oral acetaminophen and by sponging the child in a tepid water bath.

Specific Antimicrobial Therapy

Results of multiple placebo-controlled clinical trials have shown that certain antimicrobial agents significantly decrease the duration of fever, diarrheal illness, and excretion of *Shigella* in infections due to susceptible strains. This cumulative experience, bolstered by the fact that humans are the natural reservoir and host of this infection, constitutes a compelling rationale for treating all persons suffering from *Shigella* dysentery with antimicrobial agents. However, this must be tempered by the realization that only a few antimicrobial agents have proven clinical efficacy, even though many more show considerable anti-*Shigella* activity in vitro. In addition, increasing use of these effective antibiotics eventually results in the emergence of resistant *Shigella* strains. The increasing prevalence of resistance has been a recurring theme in the treatment of shigellosis. For example, sulfonamides, the drug of choice in the 1940s, were of little practical value by the mid-1950s. Oral ampicillin became the treatment of choice for pediatric shigellosis in the 1960s, but ampicillin resistance is now common. Oral trimethoprim-sulfamethoxazole (10 mg/kg/d of trimethoprim and 50 mg/kg/d of sulfamethoxazole in two divided doses for 5 days) currently is the first-line therapy. For strains that are resistant to trimethoprim-sulfamethoxazole, cefixime, ceftriaxone, cefotaxime, ciprofloxacin, and ofloxacin may be used.

The usual clinical indication for treatment with antibiotics is the child who presents with fever and overt dysentery (blood and mucus in stools). Trimethoprim-sulfamethoxazole is considered the antimicrobial agent of choice in the treatment of *Shigella* dysentery. If an epidemic strain or local endemic strains are known to be susceptible to ampicillin, that drug also may be used. In the situation in which a child has illness due to a *Shigella* strain that proves to be resistant to the first-line antimicrobial agents, cefixime may be used. Experience suggests that parenteral ceftriaxone 50 mg/kg given once daily IM or IV for 5 days constitutes effective therapy. The fluoroquinolone antibiotics, such as ciprofloxacin and ofloxacin, are useful in treating shigellosis in adults but are not approved for individuals less than 18 years of age. It is possible that in the future, short courses (2 to 3 days) of therapy with these antibiotics will be shown to be safe and effective in treating *Shigella* dysentery in children.

Supportive Measures

Agents that suppress intestinal motility, such as diphenoxylate, loperamide, and tincture of opium, should not be given to children with dysentery, since clinical data suggest that these agents may exacerbate the infection. There is no convincing evidence that common antidiarrheal preparations, such as attapulgite formulations, lactobacilli, or bismuth salicylate, have a significantly beneficial effect on the clinical or bacteriologic course of shigellosis, nor is there evidence that these agents are deleterious or contraindicated.

Health Education

Shigella infections are transmitted readily from person to person by direct contact with minute numbers of bacteria (as few as 10 *Shigella* organisms can initiate clinical infection). Consequently, it is imperative to impress on patients and their family contacts the importance of handwashing with soap after defecation or diaper changing.

UNUSUAL COMPLICATIONS

In addition to the sequelae mentioned, several other complications are recognized to be associated with shigellosis. However, they are rare. The hemolytic-uremic syndrome, leukemoid reactions, and hypoproteinemia are well recognized as complications of infection with *S. dysenteriae* 1, which occurs in many less developed countries. Reiter's syndrome, which consists of reactive arthritis, conjunctivitis, and urethritis, rarely occurs in patients with *S. flexneri* or *S. dysenteriae* infections who have histocompatibility antigen HLA-B27. Rectal prolapse can occur in infants with severe dysentery. It must be emphasized that these severe complications are uncommon, and their treatment is not considered in this section.

REFERENCES

1. Ashkenazi S, Amir J, Waisman Y, et al: A randomized double-blind study comparing cefixime and trimethoprim-sulfamethoxazole in the treatment of childhood shigellosis. J Pediatr 123:187–221, 1993.
2. Pickering LK: Therapy for acute infectious diarrhea in children. J Pediatr 118:S118–128, 1991.
3. Varsano I, Eidlitz-Marcus T, Nussinovitch M, Elian I: Comparative efficacy of ceftriaxone and ampicillin for treatment of severe shigellosis in children. J Pediatr 118:627–632, 1991.

CHOLERA

INA STEPHENS BURROWS, M.D.
MYRON M. LEVINE, M.D., D.T.P.H.

Cholera is a diarrheal disease that in its severe form, cholera gravis, is characterized by voluminous watery diarrhea that rapidly leads to dehydration, acidosis, hypovolemic shock, and death if prompt and appropriate therapy is not initiated.

EPIDEMIOLOGY

Cholera often occurs in explosive outbreaks and is one of the few bacterial infections that is capable of true pandemic spread. Until recently, it was believed that only *Vibrio cholerae* of serogroup 01 was capable of causing cholera. There are two biotypes of *V. cholerae* 01, classic and el'tor, and two serotypes, Ogawa and Inaba. Since the early 1960s, El Tor cholera has progressively spread throughout the less-developed world, resulting in the seventh pandemic. In 1991, El Tor cholera finally invaded Latin America, causing an epidemic of enormous magnitude. Since January 1991, more than 750,000 cases of cholera have been reported in Latin America. Several score travel-associated cases of cholera have been reported in relation to travel to South America since 1991. Secondary transmission of cholera is rare in well-sanitated industrialized countries, such as the United States.

Beginning in late 1992, large-scale epidemics of typical clinical cholera were reported in the Indian subcontinent. However, these epidemics were found to be caused by a new serogroup, 0139. This constitutes the first example of epidemic cholera resulting from infection with *V. cholerae* of a serogroup other than 01. This 0139 cholera has already disseminated to many other countries in Asia.

V. cholerae infection is transmitted by ingestion of contaminated food or water, particularly where sanitation and monitored water supplies are lacking. For each case of cholera gravis that presents to health care facilities during an outbreak, there are present in the community many other individuals harboring mild clinical and subclinical cholera infections.

Within the United States, there exists an endemic focus of cholera in the states bordering the Gulf of Mexico consequent to an environmental reservoir of an unusual strain of *V. cholerae* 01 el'tor inaba that persists in the brackish waters of the Gulf. Gulf Coast cholera is typically transmitted when raw or improperly cooked seafood is ingested.

PATHOGENESIS

Recognition of a few fundamental aspects of the pathogenesis of cholera forms the basis for rational therapy. Although many virulence properties of *V. cholerae* contribute to the molecular pathogenesis of cholera, it is the induction of copious secretion by the intestinal mucosa due to the effect of cholera enterotoxin that is paramount. This enterotoxic effect results in voluminous watery diarrhea that can culminate in hypotensive shock and death within 8 hours of the first symptoms.

The incubation period is usually 18 to 40 hours but can be as short as 12 hours or as long as 72 hours, depending on the inoculum ingested and the susceptibility of the host. Cholera gravis occurs more frequently in individuals with reduced gastric acidity (a potent nonspecific defense against acid-sensitive *V. cholerae*) and in persons of blood group O (the molecular explanation for this latter susceptibility is not known).

V. cholerae 01 and 0139 colonize the intestinal mucosal surface without invading epithelial cells or causing structural damage. During cholera, secretion is maximal in the proximal small intestine. Cholera stool is rich in electrolytes, but the precise composition depends on the age of the patient and the purge rate. At peak purge, the isotonic,

TABLE 1. Electrolyte Content of Cholera Stools in Older Versus Younger Children

	TEENAGER OR OLDER CHILD	YOUNG CHILD
Na^+	135 mEq/L	100 mEq/L
Cl^-	100 mEq/L	90 mEq/L
K^+	15 mEq/L	30 mEq/L
HCO_3^-	40 mEq/L	30 mEq/L

rice water stools of older children and teenagers have a high Na^+ (about 135 mEq/L) and bicarbonate (about 45 mEq/L) concentration (Table 1). In young children the Na^+ concentration typically does not exceed 100 mEq/L at peak purge.

The acidosis of cholera is predominantly the consequence of hypovolemia and diminished renal perfusion but is exacerbated by the potassium and bicarbonate losses in the diarrheal stools. Metabolic acidosis is increased as extracellular H^+ ions are exchanged for intracellular K^+. The acidosis is further exacerbated by lactic acid accumulation secondary to tissue hypoperfusion and anaerobic glycolysis, with depression of blood pH and plasma HCO_3^- and increased serum anion gap.

CLINICAL FEATURES

The clinical features of pediatric cholera include the passage of voluminous watery stools in children beyond infancy accompanied by signs of moderate or severe dehydration. In severe cases, cholera stools quickly become clear, with flecks of mucus resembling rice water. Ordinarily, cholera stools do not contain inflammatory cells or erythrocytes. Cramping of peripheral skeletal muscles and of abdominal muscles consequent to acute potassium and calcium losses may cause severe discomfort. Vomiting is common early in the illness.

Severe isonatremic dehydration is the most common life-threatening clinical feature of cholera. The patient manifests an increased pulse rate with a decrease in pulse volume, hypotension, sunken eyes, increased respiratory rate, dry mucous membranes, decreased skin turgor, decreased urine output, and thirst. Severely dehydrated patients typically have altered mental status, lethargy, and stupor.

TREATMENT

The therapy of patients with cholera gravis comprises three broad components: (1) aggressive rehydration therapy, (2) administration of antibiotics, and (3) treatment of complications. Aggressive rehydration by oral and intravenous routes to repair fluid and electrolyte deficits and to replace the prodigious ongoing diarrheal losses is the cornerstone of therapy. Appropriate antimicrobials are an important adjunct to fluid therapy, as they diminish the volume and duration of abnormal fluid losses and rapidly curtail the excretion of vibrios, thereby diminishing the chance of secondary transmission. Finally, as rehydration therapy has become increasingly effective, patients surviving from hypovolemic shock and severe dehydration manifest certain complications, such as hypoglycemia, that must be recognized and promptly treated.

Fluid Therapy

Fluid therapy is divided into two phases: (1) *rapid* replacement of water and electrolyte deficits and (2) maintenance fluids to replace ongoing losses. Rehydration therapy to repair fluid and electrolyte deficits should be accomplished as rapidly as possible (within 2 to 4 hours of initiation). Such rapid rehydration of pediatric and adult cholera patients is safe and effective. Patients suffering from severe dehydration with or without overt shock should be rapidly rehydrated with intravenous fluids. It is common for pediatric patients with cholera gravis to require several liters of intravenous fluids to stabilize them to the point where oral rehydration can then begin. At this point,

they are carefully weaned from intravenous fluids. Cholera patients with mild or moderate dehydration usually can be managed with oral rehydration alone.

Intravenous Fluids

The ideal intravenous solutions for treating cholera have a polyelectrolyte composition similar to that of the cholera stool, and such solutions (e.g., Dhaka solution) are available in some endemic areas. However, in overall practice, the most extensively used intravenous rehydration fluid worldwide for treatment of cholera is Ringer's lactate, which is widely available commercially. Ringer's lactate contains Na^+ 130 mEq/L, K^+ 4 mEq/L, Ca^{2+} 3 mEq/L, Cl^- 111 mEq/L, and lactate (precursor of HCO_3) 29 mEq/L. Because the concentration of K^+ in Ringer's lactate is too low, supplemental K^+ must be administered either by adding a sterile KCl (or similar potassium salt) solution to the Ringer's solution to increase the concentration of K^+ to 15 to 20 mEq/L or, if sterile potassium supplements are not available, by initiating oral rehydration as soon as possible (with one of the solutions described subsequently that contains K^+ in a concentration of 20 mEq/L). It is particularly important to replace potassium adequately in treating overtly malnourished children whose total body stores of potassium are notoriously low. The serum K^+ concentration may fall during the early hours of rehydration as treatment of acidosis drives K^+ intracellularly. The inclusion of glucose in intravenous fluids is desirable to diminish the risk of hypoglycemia in patients with cholera.

Aggressive rehydration with adequate volumes of fluid and appropriate electrolytes leads to rapid clinical improvement in the patient (e.g., stronger pulse, elevation of blood pressure, increase in skin turgor, and improved state of consciousness), which is reflected in simple laboratory assays (e.g., fall in hematocrit and in plasma specific gravity). Ensuring that an adequate volume of rehydration fluid is administered is the more critical determinant of outcome in patients with cholera than the precise electrolyte content of that fluid. Once renal perfusion is reestablished in the severely dehydrated patient, normal homeostatic mechanisms begin to play an important role in combating acidosis and regulating serum electrolyte concentrations.

An estimate of the total fluid deficit of the pediatric cholera patient in liters is made by multiplying the admission weight of the child by the clinical degree of dehydration (severe = 10%, moderate = 7%, mild = 5%). Thus, a 30-kg child with severe (10%) dehydration would have an estimated total fluid deficit of approximately 3 L (i.e., 3 kg). Patients with severe dehydration are administered 30 ml/kg as a push over 20 to 30 minutes. An additional 40 ml/kg should be administered over the next hour, and the rest of the estimated deficit should be administered at a rate to ensure that the entire fluid replacement has been completed within 4 hours of initiation. Once hypovolemic shock and severe dehydration have been adequately treated with intravenous fluids, oral rehydration solution should be initiated as soon as the patient can tolerate it. Patients with very high purge rates (>10 ml/kg/h) or persistent vomiting (uncommon) may require additional intravenous fluid therapy for a few hours in addition to oral therapy.

The volume of all diarrheal losses and vomitus must be measured in the patient with cholera. Once the patient has had replacement of the deficit and is in the stage of maintenance therapy, fluid management is generally based on 4-hour periods. The total fluid losses during the previous 4-hour period constitute the volume of fluids that will be administered to the patient during the next 4 hours. As diarrheal losses begin to diminish, the 4-hour replacement requirements will decrease accordingly.

Oral Rehydration

Even in the course of heavy purging, the small intestine of patients with cholera maintains its ability to absorb actively certain simple sugars, such as glucose and amino acids (such as glycine), by active transport mechanisms. Oral rehydration therapy was developed in the 1960s based on the discovery that glucose-mediated cotransport of sodium and water across the mucosal surface of the small intestine epithelium remains intact during cholera infection despite the effect of cholera toxin. This observation forms the basis of oral rehydration therapy with glucose-electrolytes or cereal-electrolytes solutions. The active transport of glucose or certain other substrates in the rehydration fluid leads to a cotransport of Na^+. Absorption of Cl^- and HCO_3^- then follows for electrostatic reasons. Absorption of H_2O occurs for osmotic reasons. Thus, even during cholera diarrhea, considerable absorption of electrolytes and water can be accomplished using oral rehydration solutions.

The tactics of oral rehydration follow the same general approach as parenteral rehydration. In overtly dehydrated patients, the estimated fluid and electrolyte deficits are rapidly replaced. Thereafter, therapy is directed to replace ongoing losses to keep the patient in balance. Cholera patients with only mild or moderate dehydration usually can be treated with oral rehydration alone. However, large volumes of rehydration fluids must sometimes be consumed to keep up with ongoing losses.

Pediatric cholera patients with moderate dehydration should be administered 150 ml/kg during a period of 4 hours or less. The patient is then evaluated clinically, using simple laboratory tests if available, to monitor the progress of rehydration. If the patient has been completely rehydrated at this point, maintenance therapy is initiated to keep up with ongoing losses. If the deficit has been only partially replaced, rehydration continues with 75 to 100 ml/kg being administered over the next 4 hours, at which point the patient is reassessed. If there is no improvement in the state of hydration despite two such cycles of oral rehydration, supplementary intravenous rehydration should be instituted. The regimen for calculating the amount of oral rehydration solution to be administered to replace ongoing losses differs by age. In older children, the Na^+ concentration in cholera stools is about 135 mEq/L. Therefore, one and one-half volumes of oral rehydration solution containing 90 mEq/L must be replaced for every volume of rice water diarrheal stool passed to adequately replace Na^+ losses. In contrast, in young children in whom the Na^+ concentration of cholera stools is only approximately 90 mEq/L, ongoing losses can be replaced on the basis of a 1:1 ratio of oral rehydration solution/volume of diarrheal stool. In older children and teenagers, there is a practical limit to the volume of oral rehydration solution that can be consumed on an hourly basis. The upper limit is approximately 750 ml/h.

Occasionally, there may be difficulty in promptly introducing an intravenous line in a cholera patient with severe dehydration. In such patients, the patient's head and upper torso should be elevated and a nasogastric tube should be inserted to initiate rehydration with oral rehydration solution until venous access can be obtained.

Composition of Oral Rehydration Solutions. The oral rehydration solution popularized by the World Health Organization (WHO) is composed of Na^+ 90 mEq/L, Cl^- 80 mEq/L, K^+ 20 mEq/L, citrate or HCO_3^- 30 mEq/L, and glucose 111 mmol/L, providing an osmolality of 331 mOsm/L. Packets containing sufficient salts and glucose to prepare 1 L of rehydration solution are widely available in developing countries. Each packet contains 3.5 g NaCl, 2.9 g of sodium citrate (or 2.5 g of $NaHCO^3$), 1.5 g of KCl, and 20 g of glucose. Inclusion of citrate rather than bicarbonate allows a longer shelf-life for the packaged material.

In some areas of the world, cereal-based oral rehydration solutions have become popular for the treatment of cholera. Starches and cereal proteins, such as those in rice powder, are broken down in the gastrointestinal tract, releasing glucose, actively transported amino acids, and other organic solutes that enhance the absorption of sodium and water. The advantage of cereal-based oral rehydration solutions is that they provide multiple actively transported substrates. Several randomized double-blind clinical trials comparing glucose-electrolytes solution with rice powder-electrolytes rehydration solution in the treatment of pediatric and adult cholera have revealed that the rice powder solutions are somewhat superior, decreasing by 50% the duration and

volume of diarrhea during therapy. This advantage has not been found for diarrhea due to other etiologies, such as rotavirus.

Antimicrobial Therapy

Appropriate antibiotics significantly decrease the duration of diarrhea, the total diarrheal stool volume, and the duration of excretion of *V. cholerae* and, therefore, serve as an important adjunct to rehydration therapy. Except for East Africa and a few other areas where tetracycline-resistant vibrios are endemic, tetracycline remains the drug of choice for all ages. The recommended dose is 50 mg/kg/d in four divided doses for 5 days, whereas the regimen for teenagers and adults is 500 mg four times a day for 5 days. Doxycycline has the advantage of being administered once daily in a dose of 4 to 6 mg/kg for children or 300 mg for teenagers and adults for 3 to 5 days. The short course of tetracycline therapy precludes staining of teeth and other adverse reactions encountered with long courses of this antibiotic.

In areas where tetracycline-resistant *V. cholerae* are prevalent or where antibiotics other than tetracycline are deemed preferable for the treatment of cholera in pediatric patients, alternative antimicrobial regimens that are usually effective include (5-day courses of therapy) erythromycin (pediatric dose 40 mg/kg/d in four divided doses, adult dose 250 mg four times daily), trimethoprim-sulfamethoxazole (pediatric dose 8 mg/kg/d of trimethoprim and 40 mg/kg/d of sulfamethoxazole in two divided doses, adult dose 160 mg of trimethoprim and 800 mg sulfamethoxazole twice daily), furazolidone (pediatric dose 5 mg/kg/d in four divided doses, adult dose 100 mg every 6 hours), and ampicillin (pediatric dose 50 mg/kg/d in four divided doses, adult dose 500 mg every 6 hours).

In endemic areas or epidemic areas where secondary transmission within households is shown to be a frequent event, a short (3-day) course of tetracycline (or another antibiotic cited previously) administered to household contacts can greatly diminish transmission within households. *However, such use of antibiotics must be strictly controlled and supervised because indiscriminate use in the community can rapidly lead to antibiotic-resistant strains of V. cholerae.* This was the situation in Guayaquil, Ecuador, in 1991 following the introduction of cholera into that community. An attempt at mass chemoprophylaxis rapidly led to the appearance of *V. cholerae* 01 strains that had acquired resistance to tetracycline, as well as several other antibiotics.

Adjunct Therapy with Nonspecific Agents

Although some antidiarrheal drugs, such as chlorpromazine, have been shown to reduce stool output somewhat in clinical trials, none are sufficiently potent to warrant adding them to the current treatment regimens for cholera. For example, the sedative effect of chlorpromazine interferes with oral rehydration therapy. Antiperistaltic agents, such as loperamide and diphenoxylate hydrochloride, are specifically contraindicated in cholera, as they may lead to pooling of fluid in the intestine.

COMPLICATIONS

Glucose Derangements

Cholera patients of all ages exhibit a mild fall in serum glucose concentration in the course of rehydration. On the other hand, severe hypoglycemia is relatively rare, and when it occurs, it is almost always seen in pediatric patients who manifest acute convulsions. The hypoglycemia of pediatric cholera is associated with high case fatality. Coma, as well as seizures, can accompany severe hypoglycemia, especially if serum glucose concentrations fall below 1 mmol/L. The hypoglycemia of cholera is believed to result from inadequate gluconeogenesis and exhaustion of glycogen stores.

The risk of hypoglycemia associated with cholera can be minimized if the intravenous solutions administered to cholera patients with severe dehydration contain 2% to 5% glucose. Such glucose-containing rehydration solutions will not cause an osmotic diuresis even if they are administered rapidly. Early initiation of an oral rehydration solution to children with diarrhea also will help prevent the complications of hypoglycemia, as will early feeding.

Renal Insufficiency

In patients with severe dehydration, a marked decrease in renal perfusion and glomerular filtration with a resultant decrease in urine production, prerenal azotemia, acute tubular necrosis, and eventual anuria can occur. Acute renal failure is much less common now than it was previously because of the institution of rapid rehydration.

Pulmonary Edema

Very rarely, pulmonary edema can occur if large volumes of intravenous fluids without bicarbonate are rapidly infused in a patient with severe acidosis. The severe acidosis causes peripheral vasoconstriction, which allows a notable proportion of the administered fluid to remain in the large vessels, resulting in increased pulmonary blood flow. In fact, this is a very rare complication, and the opposite clinical situation is much more frequent, that is, a failure to administer intravenous fluids in volumes adequate to correct the extreme deficits encountered in the severe dehydration associated with cholera gravis.

VACCINES

The parenteral inactivated whole cell cholera vaccine that has been in use for many decades plays no role in control of cholera in endemic or epidemic situations or in immunization of travelers because it confers only a moderate level of short-term protection. Two new oral vaccines have become available in some countries in Europe for use in travelers. These include a recombinant attenuated *V. cholerae* 01 strain, CVD 103-HgR, used as a single-dose live oral vaccine (Orochol), and a nonliving vaccine consisting of a combination of inactivated *V. cholerae* organisms and the B subunit of cholera toxin (cholera vaccine, peroral). The latter vaccine is administered as two or three doses spaced 2 to 6 weeks apart. It is anticipated that these vaccine may become available in the future for use in U.S. travelers.

CLOSTRIDIUM DIFFICILE

NATHAN M. THIELMAN, M.D. M.P.H.
RICHARD L. GUERRANT, M.D.

Clostridium difficile, an obligate anaerobic gram-positive rod, was first identified as part of the normal intestinal flora of healthy neonates in 1935. It is now recognized as the predominant etiologic agent of pseudomembranous colitis and the most commonly identified cause of antibiotic-associated diarrhea in adults. Its role in pediatric diarrhea and enterocolitis is more ambiguous because of the variable but high rate of carriage in asymptomatic children. Nevertheless, in the setting of inflammatory, antibiotic-associated diarrhea, a positive cytotoxin assay for *C. difficile* argues in favor of the pathogenicity of this organism in a given pediatric patient.

C. difficile causes diarrhea and colitis almost exclusively in the setting of antibacterial therapy that alters the microecology of the gut, leading to the overgrowth of toxigenic strains of *C. difficile*. Although almost all antibiotics have been associated with *C. difficile* disease, reports of broad clinical experiences (primarily in adults) most commonly implicate the aminopenicillins, cephalosporins, and clindamycin (Table 1). Rarely or inconsistently, the administration of tetracyclines, chloramphenicol, sulfonamides, and trimethoprim-sulfamethoxazole leads to *C. difficile*-mediated disease. Toxigenic strains produce an enterotoxin (toxin A) that elicits an intense inflammatory response with associated mucosal damage and fluid accumulation in animal models and a potent cytotoxin (toxin B). Toxin B lacks significant enteropathic activity but has proven useful for detecting the presence of toxigenic *C. difficile*. Its exact role in disease is uncertain.

TABLE 1. Antimicrobial and Chemotherapeutic Agents Associated with *C. difficile* Diarrhea or Colitis

MORE FREQUENTLY ASSOCIATED AGENTS	LESS FREQUENTLY ASSOCIATED AGENTS
Cephalosporins	Chloramphenicol
Penicillins	Metronidazole
Especially broad-spectrum and beta-lactamase stable penicillins*	Amphotericin B
	Quinolones
Clindamycin	Rifampin
Tetracyclines	5-Fluorouracil
Erythromycin and other macrolides	Methotrexate
Trimethoprim-sulfamethoxazole	Doxorubicin
	Cyclophosphamide
	Aminoglycosides
	Sulfonamides

Data from Aronsson B, Molby R, Nord CE: Antimicrobial agents and *Clostridium difficile* in acute enteric disease: Epidemiological data from Sweden, 1980–1982. J Infect Dis 151:476–481, 1985; Bartlett JG: Antibiotic-associated diarrhea. Clin Infect Dis 15:574, 1992; Silva J, Fekety R, Werk C, et al: Inciting and etiologic agents of colitis. Rev Infect Dis 6(Suppl 1):S214–S221, 1984.
*Including ampicillin, amoxicillin, penicillin G, penicillin V, methicillin, nafcillin, carbenicillin, cloxacillin.

EPIDEMIOLOGIC CONSIDERATIONS

An understanding of the epidemiology of this organism is particularly relevant to the treatment and prevention of pediatric *C. difficile*-mediated disease. Whereas only 3% to 11% of healthy adults harbor *C. difficile*, between 15% and 70% of asymptomatic neonates carry the bacterium, sometimes with toxin as well. Thus, extreme care should be taken when interpreting positive laboratory tests for *C. difficile*. The striking age-related vulnerability to toxigenic *C. difficile* may be explained by the absence of intestinal brush border receptors for toxin A in neonates—a hypothesis supported by studies in tissues from humans and infant rabbits. It also has been suggested that infants may be protected by maternally acquired antibodies.

Although *C. difficile* is often found as a part of the normal gut flora, a growing body of literature emphasizes person to person and environmental acquisition of toxigenic strains. Biotyping techniques have demonstrated patient to patient transmission, and the organism has been cultured from nearly 60% of health care personnel caring for *C. difficile*-infected patients. In addition, outbreaks have been reported in day care centers and chronic care facilities.

CLINICAL MANIFESTATIONS

The intestinal manifestations of *C. difficile*-mediated disease may be quite varied. In many patients, diarrhea is brief and self-limited, others produce cholera-like volumes of stool, and, rarely, patients with *C. difficile* colitis present with an acute abdomen or toxic megacolon without diarrhea. The onset of symptoms is usually 5 to 10 days after the initiation of antibacterial therapy, but disease has occurred as late as 10 weeks after cessation of therapy. Findings suggestive of colitis include cramping abdominal pain, leukocytosis, fever, hypoalbuminemia, fecal leukocytes, and fecal blood. Other complications include extreme dehydration, intestinal perforation, peritonitis, and sepsis. Mortality rates of 10% to 20% are reported in fulminant *C. difficile* colitis left untreated. Occasional relapses of inflammatory bowel disease may be associated with *C. difficile* toxin in the stool and may respond to antimicrobial therapy.

DIAGNOSIS

Direct visualization of pseudomembranes on colonoscopy or flexible sigmoidoscopy is considered the definitive means of diagnosing pseudomembranous colitis, and more than 90% to 95% of such patients will harbor toxigenic *C. difficile*. Of the various noninvasive means for detecting *C. difficile*, the cytotoxin assay remains the most reliable. FDA-approved ELISA kits for the detection of toxins A or B or both are now in use, and the sensitivity and specificity approach that of the cytotoxin assay. Although toxin assays quite reliably indicate the presence of toxigenic *C. difficile,* in children less than 12 months of age who have high rates of asymptomatic carriage, interpretation of positive test results requires careful scrutiny; infection with *C. difficile* should be considered a diagnosis of exclusion. In this population, corroborative evidence for the pathogenicity of *C. difficile* should be sought by examination for fecal leukocytes and blood or by direct visualization of colonic mucosa using lower endoscopy. The inexpensive latex particle agglutination test does not detect a protein specific to toxigenic *C. difficile,* and it should not be used alone to make the diagnosis of *C. difficile*-associated disease.

TREATMENT

Several general measures may obviate the need for specific anticlostridial therapy in patients with mild *C. difficile*-associated disease (Table 2). If the clinical situation allows, the offending antibiotic should be discontinued altogether or in favor of one less frequently associated with *C. difficile*-mediated disease (Table 1). Fluid and electrolyte losses should be monitored closely and replaced accordingly, and antimotility agents should be avoided. With these simple measures, most patients will recover within a few days.

More severely ill patients may need specific anticlostridial therapy. Though most *C. difficile* isolates are susceptible in vitro to rifampin, bacitracin, vancomycin, and metronidazole, only vancomycin and metronidazole have had widespread clinical use. In randomized, comparative double-blinded clinical trials, a 10-day course of either of these agents produced favorable initial clinical responses in 95% to 100% of adult patients, but relapse rates were as high as 20%. Some prefer oral vancomycin for severe disease. The usual daily dose is 10 to 40 mg/kg in four divided doses for 10 days. The total daily dose should not exceed 2 g. Although vancomycin is poorly absorbed after oral administration, rarely, serum levels may be detectable in the anephric patient with inflammatory enterocolitis. Serial vancomycin

levels should be considered in such patients. Oral metronidazole offers an effective inexpensive option for treating *C. difficile* diarrhea and colitis. In addition, its use as an alternative to vancomycin mitigates the potential threat now arising of promoting vancomycin-resistant strains of *Enterococcus* species. Metronidazole lacks Food and Drug Administration approval for *C. difficile* disease in children but is considered safe and effective in treating amebiasis. The pediatric dose of metronidazole is 5 mg/kg four times daily for 10 to 14 days. If the patient is unable to take medicines by mouth, anticlostridial therapy should be given via nasogastric tube if at all possible. When enteral administration is hindered by intestinal obstruction, metronidazole alone or in combination with vancomycin may be given intravenously until an oral agent is tolerated. In such patients, either drug can sometimes be administered via long intestinal tube, enema, or direct instillation through enterostomy sites.

Once adequate anticlostridial therapy has been delivered, clinical improvement is generally prompt. Fevers typically abate within 24 hours, and diarrhea resolves over 4 to 5 days. However, because of both the persistence of hearty *C. difficile* spores in the colon or in the environment and the nosocomial acquisition of new strains, up to one quarter of patients treated successfully initially experience recurrent disease. In patients with mild relapsing disease, cholestyramine (½ tsp/kg three or four times daily), which binds *C. difficile* toxins, may be effective, especially when given following specific anticlostridial therapy. (However, because cholestyramine also binds vancomycin, it is not recommended for use with simultaneous low-dose vancomycin therapy.) Frequently, relapses require more aggressive anticlostridial therapy with prolonged oral vancomycin or metronidazole, followed by a slow taper or pulse therapy with vancomycin.

A variety of novel biotherapies introduce competing nonpathogenic organisms aimed at reconstituting the normal intestinal flora. Cures have been reported with the oral administration of *Lactobacillus* preparations or nontoxigenic *C. difficile* and with the use of fecal enemas from healthy donors. In an open trial, lyophilized *Saccharomyces boulardii* was studied recently in infants with persistent *C. difficile*-associated intestinal symptoms. With doses of 250 mg two to four

TABLE 2. Therapy for *Clostridium difficile* Enterocolitis

MEDICATION	ROUTE	INTERVAL	SINGLE DOSE	DURATION
Antibiotics[1]				
Vancomycin				
Initial/relapse	PO/PR/IV	q.i.d.	2.5–10 mg/kg	10 d
Maximum[2]			125–500 mg	
Metronidazole				
Initial/relapse	PO/IV	q.i.d.	5 mg/kg	10 d
Maximum			250–500 mg	
Toxin-binding agent				
Cholestyramine[3]				
Relapse	PO	t.i.d. or q.i.d.	750 mg = ½ tsp/kg	14 d or longer
Maximum			4 g = 1 tbs	
Recolonizing agents				
Lactobacillus[4]				
Relapse	PO	q.i.d.	10 mg/kg	21 d
Maximum			1 g	
Saccharomyces boulardii				
Refractory/relapse[5]	PO	b.i.d. or q.i.d.	250 mg	15 d
Adult[2]	PO	b.i.d.	500 mg	2 mo

[1]Approximate pediatric oral doses. Rectal or intravenous administration is only indicated when oral therapy cannot be given.
[2]Usual adult dose.
[3]Should not be administered simultaneously with vancomycin.
[4]Lactinex from Laboratories Biocodex, France.
[5]Dosing regimen successfully used in infants by Buts, JP, Corthier G, Delmee M: *Saccharomyces boulardii* for *Clostridium difficile*-associated enteropathies in infants. J. Ped. Gastro. Nutr., 16:419–425, 1993.

Modified from Vinton NE: *Clostridium difficile. In* Burg F, Ingelfinger J, Wald E (eds): Gellis and Kagan's Current Pediatric Therapy, 14th ed. Philadelphia, W.B. Saunders, 1993:641.

times daily, 18 of the 19 infants had decreased bowel movements and improved physical condition, and within 15 days, 16 no longer had detectable cytotoxin activity in stool specimens. Such measures are potentially promising but remain experimental at this time.

REFERENCES

1. Bartlett JG: *Clostridium difficile:* Clinical considerations. Rev Infect Dis 12(Suppl 2):S243–S251, 1990.
2. Fekety R, Shah AB: Diagnosis and treatment of *Clostridium difficile* colitis. JAMA 269:71–75, 1993.
3. Qualman SJ, Petric M, Karmali MA, et al: *Clostridium difficile* invasion and toxin circulation in fatal pediatric pseudomembranous colitis. Am J Clin Pathol 94:410–416, 1990.

HELICOBACTER PYLORI

BENJAMIN D. GOLD, M.D.

The health care costs and economic impact of peptic ulcer disease in adults and children have resulted in an increased awareness of the morbidity and mortality of this entity. *Helicobacter pylori,* a gram-negative, microaerobic rod, colonizes the gastric antral mucosa and is a cause of primary, chronic-active gastritis in children as well as adults. This organism is associated with a significant proportion (90% to 100%) of duodenal ulcers and, to a lesser extent, gastric ulcers in children. Furthermore, recent epidemiologic evidence has linked chronic *H. pylori* infection (likely beginning in childhood) with the development of gastric carcinomas, adding an increased patient morbidity and mortality, as well as a possibly preventable burden, to these rising health care costs.

EPIDEMIOLOGY

H. pylori has been isolated from the gastric antrum of children and adults with chronic-active gastritis worldwide. The prevalence of *H. pylori* varies with age, ethnic group (higher in African Americans and Hispanics), and socioeconomic status. There is an increased prevalence with increasing age and lower socioeconomic status (independent of ethnicity). There is a particularly high prevalence in developing countries, where greater than 50% of children are colonized by age 10. The age of *H. pylori* acquisition appears important in its role in the potential development of gastric cancer. In addition, *H. pylori* infection is seen in family clusters, which suggests either a common source of infection or that close personal contact is necessary for transmission of the organism (either oral-oral or fecal-oral).

CLINICAL MANIFESTATIONS, DIAGNOSIS, AND TREATMENT CRITERIA

Once a child is colonized by *H. pylori,* there is a significant likelihood of maintaining this infection over his or her lifetime. Because of poorly defined host and bacterial factors, *H. pylori* infection results in variable clinical expressions of gastroduodenal diseases. Chronic infection with *H. pylori* is commonplace, as spontaneous clearance seldom occurs.

H. pylori infection is strongly associated with duodenal ulcers and, to a lesser extent, gastric ulcers. Although a small proportion of individuals infected with *H. pylori* develop ulceration, nearly 100% of patients with primary duodenal ulcers are colonized with this organism. Additional evidence for a causal role of *H. pylori* is that there is a significant decrease in the recurrence rate of ulcers following its eradication. Finally, the role of *H. pylori* acting as a cofactor in the development of stomach metaplasias is becoming increasingly clear, with the attributable risk of *H. pylori* infection to gastric cancer estimated to be as high as 60%.

Commonly reported symptoms are persistent abdominal pain, nausea, occasional vomiting, and anorexia. In addition, weight loss, iron

deficiency anemia, and halitosis have been reported. Prospective studies of symptoms in children undergoing upper endoscopy are required to assess both the clinical significance of *H. pylori*-associated chronic-active gastritis and selection criteria for treatment.

A fundamental principle of specific antimicrobial therapy is accurate diagnosis. There are numerous invasive and noninvasive methods used to diagnose patients with *H. pylori* infection. The invasive tests, considered the gold standard for diagnosis, include endoscopy followed by gastric biopsy and histologic demonstration of the organisms, biopsy with direct detection of urease activity in the tissue specimen, and biopsy with culture of the *H. pylori* organism. Noninvasive tests have revealed excellent sensitivities and specificities, particularly in adults (in some assays >95% for both sensitivity and specificity), for the initial diagnosis of *H. pylori* infection. These assays include serologic tests for immunoglobulin G antibodies to *H. pylori* antigens and breath tests of urease activity using orally administered ^{14}C- or ^{13}C-labeled urea. However, a readily available and accurate noninvasive method by which eradication of *H. pylori* can be monitored is lacking at present.

The therapy of *H. pylori* infection poses several unique challenges. First, the organism resides under the mucus gel layer bound to gastric epithelial cells, where rapid removal of ingested antimicrobials may occur in the acidic milieu of the stomach. These factors may contribute to the variable correlation between in vitro and in vivo antimicrobial effectiveness. Second, most accepted treatment regimens require at least 2 weeks of therapy with multiple agents. Thus, cost and patient compliance pose difficulties. Third, resistance to antimicrobials, in particular to nitroimidazoles such as metronidazole (as high as 50% in developing countries), is an important problem and a cause of treatment failure. Alternative treatment and prevention strategies, therefore, deserve research and development.

It is recommended that a child with refractory abdominal symptoms and documented *H. pylori* infection with histopathologic findings (chronic-active gastritis) should be treated with antimicrobial agents. Patients who have failed empiric acid blockade therapy (H$_2$-receptor antagonists) should be evaluated by a pediatric gastroenterologist for *H. pylori* infection before initiation of antimicrobial therapy. Patients who are undergoing maintenance antisecretory therapy and are subsequently diagnosed with *H. pylori*-associated peptic ulcer disease also should be treated for this infection, regardless of whether they are suffering from the initial disease presentation or from a recurrence. Controlled prospective studies are needed to assess the benefits of treating nonulcer dyspeptic patients with *H. pylori* infection. Furthermore, no patient should be treated for *H. pylori* infection unless one of the sensitive and specific tests mentioned previously demonstrates infection.

TREATMENT

The optimal treatment combines a bismuth preparation with one or two antibiotics (amoxicillin and metronidazole). Triple-therapy regimens combining bismuth with two antibiotics have been studied extensively in adults and can yield eradication rates of approximately 90%. However, care must be taken when using triple therapy in children because of potential side effects. In addition, tetracycline, which is one of the antibiotics often used in triple-therapy regimens, is contraindicated in children less than 10 years of age.

Bismuth salts all have in vitro activity against *H. pylori.* Bismuth subsalicylate (Peptobismol), however, is the only bismuth product available in the United States. The recommended dose is 5 ml per dose in 3- to 6-year olds, 10 ml per dose for 6- to 9-year olds, and 15 ml per dose for 9- to 12-year olds. The recommended adolescent and adult dose is 30 ml per administration. Bismuth compounds should be given four times per day for the duration of therapy.

H. pylori is sensitive to amoxicillin, metronidazole, tetracycline, and erythromycin in vitro. Most of these antimicrobials maintain effective activity at a low pH. As first-line therapy, amoxicillin should be administered at a 25 to 50 mg/kg/d dose divided into three daily administrations. Ampicillin should be administered at 50 mg/kg/d (max.: 1 g/d) in four divided doses. Antibiotic monotherapy using amoxicillin alone is not successful in long-term eradication of *H. pylori* in children. Similarly, it has been shown that bismuth alone is ineffective in the long-term clearance of this organism. Metronidazole 15 mg/kg/d in three divided doses or erythromycin 50 mg/kg/d should be considered as second-line adjuvants to the double therapy outlined, particularly if symptoms persist or there is a documented recurrence of infection.

Omeprazole in combination with antimicrobial agents has been suggested as an alternative therapy for *H. pylori* infection. This medication is in the class of antisecretory compounds directed at the H^+-K^+-ATPase inhibitors (i.e., proton pump antagonists). Omeprazole, like the bismuth salts and antimicrobials mentioned previously, also has in vitro inhibitory activity against *H. pylori*. Omeprazole combined with amoxicillin or clarithromycin has produced eradication rates as high as 90%. Conversely, omeprazole therapy alone has been shown to be unsuccessful in the eradication of *H. pylori*. Dosing regimens of omeprazole are 20 mg/d in a single dose to children 5 to 10 years old, and 40 mg/d in a single dose or in divided doses (of 20 mg) twice daily to children 11 years of age and older. There are, however, a number of important questions that remain to be answered with respect to the long-term side effects, dosing, and efficacy of this medication, given the chronic nature of *H. pylori* infection.

The duration of therapy yielding successful *H. pylori* eradication is uncertain. Regimens have varied from high-dose, single administration of antimicrobials to 8 weeks of triple therapy. The most common duration of therapy appears to be 2 weeks, although a recent pediatric study evaluating duodenal ulcers associated with *H. pylori* demonstrated a very high eradication rate with double therapy (amoxicillin and bismuth subsalicylate) of 6 weeks duration. It is essential that further case-matched, controlled, therapeutic trials are instituted to determine the optimal dose and duration of therapy necessary to eradicate *H. pylori* infection.

In summary, infection with *H. pylori* is common worldwide and is associated with a variety of gastroduodenal diseases. Symptoms are nonspecific and variable in severity. It is recommended that double therapy for a minimum of 2 to 4 weeks be used for *H. pylori* eradication. Therefore, proper screening, subspecialty referral, and patient selection are necessary for treatment regimens to be instituted.

REFERENCES

1. Blaser MJ: *Helicobacter pylori:* Its role in disease. Clin Infect Dis 15:386–393, 1992.
2. Drumm B: *Helicobacter pylori* in the pediatric patient. Gastroenterol Clin North Am 22:169–182, 1993.
3. Israel DM, Hassall E: Treatment and long-term follow-up of *Helicobacter pylori*-associated duodenal ulcer disease in children. J Pediatr 123:53–58, 1993.

NONTYPHOIDAL SALMONELLOSIS

MARGARET B. RENNELS, M.D.

Salmonella is a large and clinically important genus that is differentiated biochemically into three species: (1) *Salmonella typhi,* (2) *Salmonella choleraesuis,* and (3) *Salmonella enteritidis.* *S. enteritidis* contains over 2000 serotypes that are identified on the basis of their cell wall (O) and flagellar (H) antigens. This section deals with the nontyphoidal *Salmonella* infections.

EPIDEMIOLOGY

Infections with nontyphoidal *Salmonella* are widespread and frequent. The highest reported incidence is in children less than 1 year of age. Transmission is most commonly by fecal contamination of foods, which are then improperly cooked or stored, allowing the organisms to grow to high numbers. Large outbreaks in the United States have occurred from contaminated eggs. Fewer organisms are necessary to induce infection and invasion in persons with compromised defenses. Direct fecal-oral transmission to these individuals can occur from infected people or animals.

CLINICAL SYNDROMES

There are a number of different *Salmonella* syndromes, determined by both host factors and the infecting bioserotype: (1) acute or chronic asymptomatic infection or carriage, (2) simple gastroenteritis, (3) dysentery, (4) bacteremia, (5) sepsis, (6) focal infection (e.g., meninges, bone, lungs, kidneys), and (7) enteric fever. Enteric fever is a prolonged bacteremic illness accompanied by fever, malaise, and, typically, constipation. It is caused by *S. typhi* and *S. paratyphi* A, B, and C. Infection with *S. choleraesuis* carries a high risk of bacteremia with metastatic seeding. *S. enteritidis* bioserotypes typically cause uncomplicated gastroenteritis, although some serotypes of *S. enteritidis* (e.g., *S. dublin, S. oranienburg*) are particularly virulent, often leading to bacteremic illness in young children. Host factors predisposing to invasive, systemic disease include gastrointestinal abnormalities (achlorhydria, ulcerative colitis) and immunocompromise from (1) infancy (≤3 months), (2) hemoglobinopathy, particularly sickle cell disease, (3) leukemia or lymphoma, (4) immunosuppressive therapy, (5) congenital immunodeficiency, and (6) HIV infection.

DIAGNOSIS AND MANAGEMENT

The diagnosis of suspected *Salmonella* infection is made by culture of the appropriate material (stool, blood, urine, CSF, pus, bone marrow). Proper management of *Salmonella* infections often is unclear because randomized prospective studies either have not been or cannot be performed. There is general agreement that uncomplicated gastroenteritis in healthy children over 3 months of age does not require antibiotic therapy and that antibiotics are indicated for (1) gastroenteritis in immunocompromised children, including infants less than 3 months of age, (2) sepsis or enteric fever, and (3) focal, suppurative infection.

The following is a suggested approach to a child with signs or symptoms compatible with *Salmonella* infection. This is offered as a guideline only. Clinical judgment is always required, and other courses of action may be appropriate.

I. Initial visit
   A. Obtain stool culture if the child is toxic or immunocompromised or has prolonged diarrhea, dysentery, or blood and leukocytes in the stool.
   B. Draw blood culture if the child is ≤3 months old, immunocompromised, toxic, or ill-appearing or has dysentery.
   C. The decision to admit and begin antibiotics is based on general clinical principles that apply in any situation.
   D. A child with dysentery should be treated for suspected *Shigella* infection with an oral antibiotic, such as trimethoprim-sulfamethoxazole.
II. Follow-up visit of child with positive cultures
   A. Stool culture positive
      1. Admit, work up (CBC, blood culture, assess for focal infection, including meningitis), and begin parenteral antibiotics if the child is systemically ill, immunocompromised, or ≤3 months of age.
      2. Do not give antibiotics for uncomplicated gastroenteritis in immunologically normal children over 3 months of age who are systemically well. Do not repeat the stool culture in this situation unless required for public health reasons.
      3. Continue treatment of children with dysentery with an oral antibiotic to which the isolate is sensitive.

TABLE 1. Treatment of *Salmonella* Infections

ANTIBIOTICS	DOSES AND ROUTES
Ampicillin	200–300 mg/kg/d IV divided q6h, max: 8 g/d
Amoxicillin	40 mg/kg/d PO divided q8h
Trimethoprim-sulfamethoxazole	TMP 10 mg/kg/d, SMX 50 mg/d PO or IV divided q12h, max: TMP 160 mg q12h, SMX 800 mg q12h
Chloramphenicol	75 mg/kg/d PO or 100 mg/kg/d IV divided q6h, max: 3 g/d
Cefotaxime	150 mg/kg/d IV divided q6h, max: 12 g/d
Ceftriaxone	100 mg/kg/d IV or IM q24h or divided q12h, max: 4 g/d

B. Blood culture positive
1. Admit, work up, and give parenteral antibiotics if the child is young (definition sometimes used is <12 months), febrile or ill or has focal infection.
2. Management of the older child who is well on reexamination is controversial. Unfortunately, the presence or absence of *Salmonella* bacteremia cannot be predicted by temperature or WBC counts. Judgment is required based on the age, underlying health, species and serotype, and reliability of the family. Management options include
   a. Admit, reculture, and treat with parenteral antibiotics.
   b. Reculture and, pending results, give IM ceftriaxone or PO trimethoprim-sulfamethoxazole (TMP-SMX) depending on sensitivities. If the repeat culture is positive, admit and treat parenterally.
   c. Reculture and send home with no therapy but follow-up daily pending 72 hours of negative cultures.

The antibiotics listed in Table 1 are effective at the indicated routes and doses if the *Salmonella* sp. is sensitive. A third-generation cephalosporin is preferred for meningitis therapy. Antibiotic resistance is increasingly a problem in many parts of the world. Outbreaks of serious *S. enteritidis* infection in the United States have been caused by resistant strains that were traced to cattle fed subtherapeutic doses of antibiotics for growth promotion. The length of therapy for the *Salmonella* syndromes has not been adequately studied but generally is based on the type of infection being treated, for example, 4 to 6 weeks for osteomyelitis, 3 to 4 weeks for meningitis, and 10 to 14 days for bacteremic illness. Because recurrent *Salmonella* sepsis is a problem in HIV-infected children, some advocate chronic oral amoxicillin prophylaxis once *Salmonella* infection has been documented.

CAMPYLOBACTER INFECTIONS

GUILLERMO M. RUIZ-PALACIOS, M.D.
LARRY K. PICKERING, M.D.

Five species of *Campylobacter* produce disease in humans: *Campylobacter fetus*, *Campylobacter jejuni*, *Campylobacter coli*, *Campylobacter laris*, and *Campylobacter upsaliensis*. *C. fetus* is an infrequent cause of systemic disease in debilitated hosts and newborns. *C. jejuni* and *C. coli* cause diarrhea worldwide and, in many geographic areas, are the most prevalent bacterial enteropathogens. The incidence of *C. jejuni/C. coli* infection in developed nations is highest during infancy, with a second peak in early adulthood. *C. laris* and *C. upsaliensis* are rare causes of diarrhea.

TRANSMISSION

The chief reservoir for *C. jejuni* and *C. coli* species is the animal kingdom, including cattle, sheep, pigs, and fowl. The main source of human infection is through ingestion of contaminated poultry. Additional sources of infection include ingestion of unpasteurized milk or contaminated water and exposure to household pets with diarrhea. Person-to-person transmission has been documented, particularly involving young children. Perinatal infections with *C. fetus* have been associated with maternal infections during pregnancy or at the time of delivery.

CLINICAL MANIFESTATIONS

Acute diarrhea is the most common clinical manifestation of *Campylobacter* infection, with more than 90% of the episodes due to *C. jejuni*. Clinically, the disease is difficult to distinguish from disease from other bacterial causes. After an incubation period of 1 to 7 days, a nonspecific prodrome of fever, headache, and myalgia occurs. Diarrhea typically is accompanied by crampy abdominal pain, nausea, and occasionally vomiting. Less than half of the patients have blood in their stools. Usually, the illness is benign and self-limited, although colitis, abdominal pain that mimics appendicitis and chronic diarrhea, may occur. A wide variety of extraintestinal complications, including reactive arthritis, Guillain-Barré syndrome, Reiter's syndrome, and erythema nodosum, have been reported to occur following gastrointestinal tract illnesses.

Bloodstream and extraintestinal infections can occur, including bacteremia, endocarditis, phlebitis, and meningitis, especially in immunocompromised hosts or those at the extremes of age. Both *C. jejuni* and *C. fetus* can cause severe neonatal disease, with *C. fetus* being more common. It is believed that transmission generally occurs at delivery, but there is evidence for intrauterine infection as well.

TREATMENT

Rehydration and correction of electrolyte abnormalities are the mainstay of treatment of patients with diarrhea. Prospective trials in both adults and children have demonstrated that erythromycin terminates gastrointestinal tract shedding of *Campylobacter* within 24 to 72 hours. However, bacteriologic cure is not accompanied consistently by relief of symptoms. This lack of observed efficacy may be due to delayed initiation of antibiotics. Treatment does not appear to lead to a prolonged carrier state. Treatment with antibiotics is advisable in day care or preschool settings to diminish shedding and prevent potential spread. A trial of antimicrobial therapy also is warranted for patients with severe or persistent symptoms and for individuals who are immunocompromised.

Erythromycin is the drug of choice in a dose of 30 to 50 mg/kg/d divided in four doses for 5 to 7 days. Macrolides, such as azithromycin and clarithromycin, may simplify management because of the potential shorter courses and fewer side effects. In adults, tetracycline, ciprofloxacin, and ofloxacin represent reasonable alternatives. Women in the third trimester of pregnancy who have suspected or proven *C. jejuni* diarrhea should be considered for erythromycin treatment.

Infections with *C. fetus* usually are systemic and require antibiotic therapy. Aminoglycosides are the first-line treatment for systemic illness. The dose of gentamicin is 7.5 mg/kg/d IV divided every 8 hours, preferably in combination with a third-generation cephalosporin, such as cefotaxime or ceftriaxone. Duration is dependent on the underlying immune status of the host, the response to antimicrobial therapy, and the site of infection. Generally, treatment is given for 2 to 4 weeks. Chloramphenicol or cefotaxime is the preferred agent for meningitis caused by susceptible strains.

Prevention is achieved through use of appropriate handwashing practices, milk pasteurization, water treatment, thorough cooking of meat, and proper disposal of soiled diapers in hospital and day care settings.

REFERENCES

Campylobacter

1. Calva JJ, Ruiz-Palacios GM, Lopez-Vidal Y, et al: Cohort study of intestinal infection with *Campylobacter* in Mexican children. Lancet 1:503, 1988.
2. Penner JL: The genus *Campylobacter:* A decade of progress. Clin Microbiol Rev 1:157, 1988.

YERSINIA ENTEROCOLITICA INFECTION

STEVE KOHL, M.D.
MARGARET B. RENNELS, M.D.
MELVIN I. MARKS, M.D.

Yersinia enterocolitica is an enteropathogen that both produces toxins and may invade the intestinal mucosa. It is then taken up by the mesenteric lymphatics and from there may reach the bloodstream. Yersinial infection is more common in Canada and northern European countries than in the United States. It is more common in cooler climates and winter months. The organism may be acquired by the fecal-oral route from infected humans or animals or from contaminated animal products, milk, food, or water. Recently, the preparation of chitterlings from pork intestine has been associated with infection in children. There are also reports of transmission through packed red blood cells transfusions. Presumably, the donors had transient, asymptomatic bacteremia, with growth of the organism in the cold during blood storage.

CLINICAL FEATURES

Clinical manifestations of infection depend on the age and immune status of the individual and the virulence of the infecting strain. The most common presentation in young children is enterocolitis, typically consisting of fever, malaise, anorexia, abdominal pain, vomiting, and diarrhea (which may contain blood and leukocytes). Enterocolitis is usually self-limited, with resolution of symptoms within 2 weeks of onset. Older children and young adults may present with fever and right lower-quadrant abdominal pain from involvement of the terminal ileum and mesenteric lymph nodes. This so-called pseudoappendicitis syndrome is difficult to distinguish from appendicitis and has resulted in "outbreaks" of appendectomies. Sepsis and metastatic seeding, including meningitis, osteomyelitis, pneumonia, pyomyositis, and focal abscesses, may occur in immunocompromised, iron-overloaded, or, rarely, normal individuals. Postinfectious manifestations are more common in adults and include polyarthritis, Reiter's syndrome, and erythema nodosum. The pathogenesis of these entities is unclear.

TREATMENT

In Vitro Sensitivities

Because *Y. enterocolitica* is capable of producing beta-lactamase, typically it is resistant to most penicillins and first-generation cephalosporins. Most isolates are sensitive to aminoglycosides, chloramphenicol, tetracycline, trimethoprim-sulfamethoxazole (TMP-SMX), quinolones, third-generation cephalosporins, aztreonam, ticarcillin-clavulanic acid, and imipenem. Sensitivity in vitro (Table 1) does not necessarily mean that the antibiotic will be effective in vivo. Yersiniosis is largely an intracellular infection. Thus, only antibiotics that penetrate cells in active forms may be suitable. Optimal antibiotic choice, dose, and length of therapy have not been determined through prospective clinical trials. One must rely on anecdotal experience and retrospective series for guidance.

Recommendations

There is general agreement that uncomplicated gastroenteritis and mesenteric adenitis in normal children do not necessitate antibiotic therapy. A blinded, placebo-controlled prospective trial using TMP-SMX, begun after a mean of 12 days of symptoms, showed no clinical or bacteriologic advantage of therapy in children with yersinial gastroenteritis. A similar study in adults with either uncomplicated gastroenteritis or reactive arthritis did not demonstrate clinical or bacteriologic efficacy of antimicrobial therapy. It is possible that earlier therapy would be beneficial. It is prudent to treat high-risk individuals, such as persons with hemoglobinopathy, iron overload, immunodeficiency, and young infants (Table 2). Antimicrobial agents that may be useful (Table 3) are TMP-SMX 10 mg/kg/d of TMP PO divided in two doses or, in children over 8 years of age, doxycycline 2 to 4 mg/kg/d PO divided into two doses. The quinolones may prove to be useful in adults but are not recommended for use in children because of the potential for damage to articular cartilage.

Bacteremic disease and extraintestinal infection require antibiotic therapy. These manifestations of yersinial infection have been treated successfully either with gentamicin 5 to 7.5 mg/kg/d IV in three divided doses, TMP-SMX 10 mg/kg/d TMP IV divided in three doses, or chloramphenicol 75 to 100 mg/kg/d PO or IV in four divided doses. It is recommended that at least one of these drugs be used to treat serious infection. Although most isolates are sensitive in vitro to third-generation cephalosporins and they have been used successfully in some reports, failures have been reported with these drugs. Until more experience is gathered, a third-generation cephalosporin should probably not be used alone for treatment of serious *Y. enterocolitica* infections. Length of therapy is extrapolated from experience with other gram-negative enteric infections. For example, meningitis should be treated for a minimum of 3 weeks after documentation of negative cerebrospinal fluid cultures, and sepsis is treated for 2 weeks.

Iron therapy or chelation therapy in patients receiving such for anemia or iron overload should be discontinued for the duration of treatment of serious *Yersinia* infections. Enteric isolation precautions are indicated for the duration of illness.

Postinfectious syndromes have not been shown to benefit from antimicrobial therapy, although the recent demonstration of yersinial antigens in synovial fluid cells suggests that a relatively prolonged trial of antibiotic therapy may be warranted.

TABLE 1. In Vitro Susceptibilities of *Yersinia enterocolitica*

USUALLY SUSCEPTIBLE TO	ALWAYS OR OFTEN RESISTANT TO
Trimethoprim-sulfamethoxazole	Ampicillin
Aminoglycosides (gentamicin, amikacin, and tobramycin)	Penicillin
Tetracyclines (doxycyline)	Cloxacillin, oxacillin
Chloramphenicol	Erythromycin
Third-generation cephalosporins (cefotaxime, ceftriaxone, ceftazidime)	Cephalothin, cefazolin
	Clindamycin
Quinolones (ciprofloxacin, norfloxacin, ofloxacin, pefloxacin)	Vancomycin
	Amoxicillin-clavulanic acid
Aztreonam	
Ticarcillin-clavulanic acid	
Imipenem	

TABLE 2. Indications for Antibiotic Therapy of *Yersinia enterocolitica* Gastroenteritis

Under 3 months of age
Leukemia or lymphoma
Acquired or congenital immunodeficiency disease
Moderate or severe malnutrition
Thalassemia or other chronic hemolytic anemias
Iron overload
Appendicitis
Ulcerative colitis or other inflammatory bowel disease
Associated symptomatic intestinal parasitosis

TABLE 3. Therapy for *Yersinia enterocolitica* Infections

	ROUTE OF THERAPY	
RECOMMENDED DRUG	GASTROENTERITIS*	SEPSIS OR FOCAL INFECTION
Trimethoprim-sulfa-methoxazole	PO	IV
Doxycycline†	PO	
Gentamicin		IV
Chloramphenicol		IV

*Not recommended for uncomplicated illness in the otherwise normal child.
†Not recommended for children 8 years of age or less.

REFERENCES

1. Cover TL, Aber RC: *Yersinia enterocolitica*. N Engl J Med 321:16–24, 1989.
2. Kihlstrom E, Foberg U, Bengtsson A, et al: Intestinal symptoms and serological response in patients with complicated and uncomplicated *Yersinia enterocolitica* infections. Scand J Infect Dis 24:57–63, 1992.
3. Kwaga J, Iversen JO: In vitro antimicrobial susceptibilities of *Yersinia enterocolitica* and related species isolated from slaughtered pigs and pork products. Antimicrobial Agents Chemother 34:2423–2425, 1990.
4. Pai CH, Gillis F, Tuomanen E, Marks MI: Placebo-controlled double-blind evaluation of trimethoprim-sulfamethoxazole treatment of *Yersinia enterocolitica* gastroenteritis. J Pediatr 104:308–311, 1984.

INFECTIONS DUE TO ANAEROBIC COCCI AND GRAM-NEGATIVE BACILLI

LISA M. DUNKLE, M.D.

INCIDENCE

Anaerobic infections occur less frequently in infants and children than in adults, probably because the compromise of tissue health and integrity due to trauma or disease (which predisposes to invasion by anaerobic organisms) is less common in children. When anaerobic infections do occur, they generally involve flora endogenous to the child's skin or gastrointestinal tract and frequently are polymicrobial. Aerobic organisms commonly coexist in such infections and may contribute to the pathogenicity of the anaerobes by further reducing the oxygen tension of devitalized tissues.

TREATMENT

Prompt and thorough surgical debridement, as well as adequate antimicrobial therapy, is required for these pathophysiologically com-plicated infections. Hyperbaric oxygen therapy has been advocated for some deep-seated infections. However, there is little experience with this modality in children and under no circumstances can it replace appropriate surgical and medical intervention. Although surgical debridement may be the only therapy required in some localized abscesses or decubitus ulcers without signs of systemic involvement, antibiotics are indicated whenever systemic manifestations of infection are present or when suppuration has either extended into or threatened to spread into surrounding tissue.

Selection of Antimicrobials

Selection of antimicrobial agents for anaerobic or mixed infections is simplified when culture results of reliable specimens are available. This is rarely the case, however, because of the difficulty encountered in obtaining appropriate specimens and the relatively slow growth of anaerobes in the laboratory. Therefore, most patients must be treated empirically on the basis of suspected, rather than established, pathogens. Fortunately, the types of organisms involved in many anaerobic infections and their antimicrobial susceptibility patterns tend to be predictable. Gram-stained smears of infected material, together with the observation of foul odor, may be invaluable in the rapid identification of anaerobic infection.

Other factors to be considered in the choice of antimicrobial agents include the pharmacologic characteristics of various drugs, their potential toxicities, their effect on normal flora, and their bactericidal activity. The antimicrobial agents chosen should provide for adequate coverage of most expected pathogens at the site of the infection. Some commonly used broad-spectrum agents possess these qualities, but for most anaerobic infections, agents should be chosen specifically for their activity in these circumstances.

Specific Antimicrobial Drugs

Table 1 lists the antimicrobial agents most useful for the infections that commonly involve anaerobic organisms and the appropriate doses and route(s) of administration. Choices of other agents should be relied on only when specific results of culture and susceptibility testing are available.

Penicillins

Penicillin G is the drug of choice for infecting strains that are susceptible to this drug. These organisms include most gram-positive and most gram-negative anaerobic strains other than *Bacteroides fragilis*. Some strains of *Bacteroides*, such as the *Bacteroides melaninogenicus* group and *Bacteroides oralis*, as well as strains of *Clostridium, Fusobacterium* species, and microaerophilic streptococci, occasionally demonstrate resistance to penicillin, usually resulting from beta-lactamase production. Some of these strains are inhibited by concentrations of 8 to 32 U/ml of penicillin G. In these instances,

TABLE 1. Antimicrobial Agents for Anaerobic and Mixed Infections

SITE	DRUG	DOSE	ROUTE OF ADMINISTRATION
Pulmonary	Clindamycin	20–40 mg/kg/d	IV, PO
Parapharyngeal	Penicillin G	10–12 million U/m²	IV
Abdominal	Clindamycin (with aminoglycoside)	20–40 mg/kg/d	IV, PO
Pelvic	Cefoxitin	100–150 mg/kg/d	IV
Skeletal	Clindamycin	20–40 mg/kg/d	IV, PO
Soft tissue	Cefoxitin	100–150 mg/kg/d	IV
Central nervous system	Chloramphenicol	50–100 mg/kg/d	IV, PO
	Metronidazole (with penicillin)	30 mg/kg/d	IV, PO
Minor soft tissue (bites)	Amoxicillin-clavulanate/(Augmentin)	20–40 mg/kg/d	PO
Others	Imipenem	No pediatric dose available	IV

administration of very high doses of penicillin G may eradicate the infection. Although ampicillin, amoxicillin, and penicillin generally are equally active, methicillin, nafcillin, and the isoxazolyl penicillins have unpredictable activity and frequently are inferior to penicillin G. Carbenicillin and ticarcillin are active against most strains of *B. fragilis* because of the high serum concentrations that can be achieved. However, penicillin G is also active against *B. fragilis* in these concentrations. Resistance to these agents is present in up to 30% of *B. fragilis* strains.

Clavulanic acid, sulbactam, and tazobactam are beta-lactamase inhibitors that resemble the nucleus of penicillin but differ in several ways. They irreversibly inhibit beta-lactamase enzymes produced by some Enterobacteriaceae, staphylococci, and beta-lactamase-producing *Bacteroides* species (*B. fragilis* group and some strains of *B. melaninogenicus* and *B. oralis*). When used in conjunction with a beta-lactam antibiotic, they render the antibiotic effective in treating infections caused by beta-lactamase-producing bacteria. Combination of amoxicillin or ticarcillin with clavulanate or sulbactam or of piperacillin with tazobactam results in agents to which over 98% of the *B. fragilis* group are susceptible. However, resistance to penicillins due to other mechanisms is present in a small number of aerobic and facultative bacteria. Nonetheless, the amoxicillin-clavulanic acid combination probably represents the most useful agent available in the treatment of simple animal and human bite wounds that commonly involve a multiplicity of organisms, including aerobic and anaerobic and gram-positive and gram-negative strains.

Chloramphenicol

Although it is a bacteriostatic drug, chloramphenicol is one of the antimicrobial agents most active against anaerobes. Resistance is rare. Failures to eradicate infection, including bacteremia, with chloramphenicol have been reported. However, this drug has been used for more than 25 years as first-line therapy for anaerobic infections. It is regarded as a good choice for treatment of serious anaerobic infections when the nature and susceptibility of the infecting organisms are unknown, especially infections involving the central nervous system (CNS). The potential toxicity of chloramphenicol must be borne in mind, including the low risk of aplastic anemia, dose-dependent leukopenia, and gray syndrome in newborns and patients with impaired hepatic glucuronidation.

Cephalosporins

First-Generation. The first-generation cephalosporins are less active than penicillin G, and most strains of *B. fragilis* and many of *B. melaninogenicus* are resistant on the basis of cephalosporinase production.

Second-Generation. Cefoxitin, a second-generation cephalosporin, is relatively resistant to cephalosporinase and is, therefore, effective against most *B. fragilis* strains. Cefoxitin is active in vitro against at least 95% of strains of *B. fragilis* at a level of 32 µg/ml but is relatively inactive against most species of *Clostridium* (including *Clostridium difficile*) other than *Clostridium perfringens*. Clinical experience with cefoxitin has shown it to be effective in eradication of most anaerobic infections. It is used successfully for surgical prophylaxis because of its complementary activity against aerobic enteric gram-negative rods. Cefoxitin does not cross the blood-brain barrier and should not be used for CNS infections.

Third-Generation. Cefotetan exhibits a spectrum of activity similar to that of cefoxitin but is less active against some members of the *B. fragilis* group, which may constitute as many as 30% to 50% of the *Bacteroides* isolates from patients. Other third-generation cephalosporins exhibit unpredictable activity against anaerobes and may be effective against as few as 50% of *B. fragilis*.

Clindamycin

Clindamycin exhibits a broad range of activity against both gram-positive and gram-negative anaerobic organisms and has proved its efficacy in clinical trials. Approximately 95% of the anaerobic bacteria isolated in clinical practice are susceptible to easily achievable levels below 3 µg/ml. There are reports of resistant strains associated with clinical infections, although these are uncommon. Because clindamycin cannot be demonstrated to cross the blood-brain barrier efficiently, it should not be administered in cases of CNS infections. It is frequently used in combination with aminoglycosides for infections of the abdominal cavity and pelvis and represents first-line therapy for these infections. It is particularly useful in deep-seated purulent infection, such as osteomyelitis, because of its ease of entry into leukocytes. Because of the increasing frequency of penicillin resistance among oral anaerobes, clindamycin represents an excellent choice for the treatment of necrotic pulmonary infection, such as lung abscess due to aspiration. Although the primary toxicity recognized with clindamycin is colitis, it should be kept in mind that colitis is associated with a number of other antimicrobial agents, such as ampicillin and all of the cephalosporins, and may occur in seriously ill patients in the absence of previous antimicrobial therapy. The occurrence of colitis in pediatric patients is very rare.

Metronidazole

Metronidazole shows excellent bactericidal activity against most obligate anaerobic bacteria, such as *B. fragilis,* other species of *Bacteroides, Fusobacterium,* and *Clostridium.* More than 90% of gram-negative obligate anaerobes are susceptible to less than 2 µg/ml of metronidazole. However, most strains of gram-positive anaerobes, including gram-positive cocci, nonsporulating bacilli, microaerophilic streptococci, *Propionibacterium acnes,* and *Actinomyces* species, are almost uniformly resistant. Aerobic and facultative anaerobes, such as coliforms, are usually highly resistant. Therefore, metronidazole should not be used alone as therapy for clinical anaerobic infections that are usually mixed.

Clinical experience in adults and limited experience in children indicate the efficacy of metronidazole in the treatment of infections caused by gram-negative anaerobes, including intraabdominal sepsis, infections of the female genital tract, and especially infections of the CNS. However, it is not effective in therapy of gram-positive anaerobic pulmonary infections. Thus, when gram-positive or mixed infection is suspected, additional agents effective against these organisms, such as penicillin G, should be administered. Metronidazole may be particularly advantageous in CNS infections because of its excellent penetration into the CNS. Penicillin must be administered concurrently in these cases.

Other Drugs

Carbapenems. Imipenem is active against a wide variety of aerobic and anaerobic gram-positive and gram-negative organisms. It possesses excellent activity against beta-lactamase-producing *Bacteroides* species and is effective as a single agent for the treatment of mixed aerobic-anaerobic infections. However, data in children are limited, and this drug is not yet approved for use in this age group. Meropenem, a carbapenem currently undergoing clinical trials, appears to be even more active than imipenem versus certain cefoxitin-resistant or clindamycin-resistant *Bacteroides* and *Clostridium* isolates.

Tetracyclines. Because of the development of resistance by virtually all types of anaerobes, tetracyclines no longer represent useful therapeutic alternatives for anaerobic infections. The new tetracycline analogs, doxycycline and minocycline, are more active than the parent compound, but the use of any of these agents is not recommended in children under 8 years of age because of adverse effects on teeth and bone.

Erythromycin. Like tetracycline, erythromycin should no longer be relied on for empiric therapy because resistance has developed in a large proportion of strains.

Vancomycin. Vancomycin is effective against all gram-positive anaerobes but is inactive against gram-negative species. Little clinical experience has been gained in the treatment of anaerobic bacteria using this agent.

Quinolones. The quinolones (ciprofloxacin, norfloxacin) are active against most gram-positive anaerobic species but generally are not active against gram-negative species. Even for adolescents for whom quinolones may be used appropriately, they generally do not represent a satisfactory choice for the treatment of mixed anaerobic infections.

INFANT BOTULISM

MARGARET C. FISHER, M.D.

Infant botulism is a toxicoinfection. Disease occurs following ingestion of spores of *Clostridium botulinum*, colonization of the gut, production of botulinum toxin, and absorption of toxin from the bowel. The toxin acts on cholinergic nerve endings and blocks the release of acetylcholine. A spectrum of disease occurs, from sudden infant death to a gradual onset of descending paralysis to mild constipation with no other signs. Symptoms often progress rapidly. It is essential to consider the diagnosis in any hypotonic, weak, or constipated infant. Infant botulism has been reported in all states but is overrepresented in Hawaii, California, Utah, and Pennsylvania.

TREATMENT

The mainstay of therapy is meticulous supportive care. Antitoxin has no neutralizing effect on bound toxin. Recovery of function requires growth of new receptors. The goal of the health care team is to support the infant until these new receptors are generated. This requires days to months. Most children will require hospitalization for monitoring and observation, and intensive care must be readily available.

RESPIRATORY CARE

Respiratory management begins with careful and repeated evaluations of the child's ability to maintain adequate ventilation and avoid aspiration. Elective intubation is performed in the child whose gag reflex is lost or who has apnea or respiratory failure. Atelectasis is common and often migratory and increases the risk for bacterial pneumonia. Positioning of the patient and suctioning are important. Monitoring of cardiac and respiratory function is continued throughout the hospitalization. Respiratory support is continued until the child has regained the gag reflex. Although ventilatory support is often required for several weeks, tracheostomy is rarely necessary.

NUTRITION

Feedings are given orally only if the child has a normal gag reflex and is able to suck and swallow. Enteral feedings via nasogastric or nasojejunal tube should be started in the child who is too weak to take foods orally. Early implementation of feedings is helpful in minimizing the need for intravenous catheters and in contributing to the recovery of normal peristalsis. Oral feedings are reinstituted only after the child has a normal gag and swallow.

NURSING CARE

Many children with botulism will be totally paralyzed, and frequent changes in position are needed to avoid the development of pressure sores. It is essential to ensure that the endotracheal tube is secured to avoid inadvertent extubation. Passive range of motion and physical therapy are useful. Most parents can be taught to pass a nasogastric tube and administer tube feedings. Families require a great deal of emotional support, and social services should be involved as soon as possible.

ANTITOXIN

Antitoxin is not recommended for several reasons. Antitoxin neutralizes circulating toxin but has no effect on bound toxin. In infant botulism, toxin is present in the gut or bound to neuroreceptors. Orally administered antitoxin has not been studied. The organism colonizes the colon and constipation is a major symptom. Thus, orally administered antitoxin would probably not get to the colon in a timely fashion. Enemas of antitoxin might be more successful. Saline or mineral oil enemas to eliminate toxin by purging have not proven useful and may be harmful. The use of enemas should be reserved for obtaining the initial stool sample needed to confirm the diagnosis.

ANTIBIOTICS

Antibiotic therapy has not proven useful and is often harmful. Aminoglycosides potentiate neuromuscular blockade, and their use has been associated with respiratory deterioration and apnea in infants with botulism. Oral antibiotics have not proven useful in eliminating the organism. Antibiotic therapy is potentially harmful as toxin might be liberated from dying cells. Broad-spectrum antibiotics alter flora and predispose the patient to colonization with resistant flora. The use of antibiotics should be limited to therapy of nosocomial infection.

NOSOCOMIAL INFECTION

The infant with botulism is at great risk for nosocomial infection. Catheter-related infections are common. The best way to avoid these is to avoid catheters. Intravenous catheters should be removed as soon as possible. The practice of having a catheter in place "just in case" must be abandoned. Autonomic dysfunction sometimes causes urinary retention, and intermittent catheterization is preferable to the use of an indwelling catheter. Nasogastric tubes occlude or partially occlude the eustachian tube and sinus ostia, thus increasing the risk for otitis media or sinusitis. There are no data regarding the optimal care of nasogastric tubes, for example: Should the tube be changed every few days, or is it better to leave the tube in place? Viruses that are circulating in the community are often transmitted to the patient by visitors or staff. Handwashing before all patient contact is essential to minimize the spread of agents from child to child or staff member to child. Isolation or special precautions for the child with botulism are not necessary. Although toxin continues to be present in the gut and is shed in the stool, there have been no reported cases of nosocomial infection. This may be related to the fact that most children with botulism are constipated. More likely, it reflects the fact that other children are not susceptible to colonization by the organism. Recent studies in adults suggest that the bowel flora can be altered by surgery, gastric achlorhydria, or antibiotic therapy so that *C. botulinum* replicates in the gut, leading to infant botulism. Handwashing, common sense, and routine handling of diapers should be sufficient to prevent transmission of the organism from one patient to another.

PREVENTION

Prevention of infant botulism is probably not possible. The organism is widespread in the environment. Spores are present in soil and in some foods, notably honey and corn syrup. It is recommended that children under a year of age not be fed honey.

REFERENCES

1. Long SS: Botulism in infancy. Pediatr Infect Dis 3:266–271, 1984.
2. Schreiner MS, Field E, Ruddy R: Infant botulism: A review of 12 years' experience at The Children's Hospital of Philadelphia. Pediatrics 87:159–165, 1991.

BRUCELLOSIS

MOSES GROSSMAN, M.D.

Brucellosis is a contagious disease of animals, principally ungulates, that is occasionally transmitted to humans. The infective organism (a gram-negative bacillus) is transmitted through handling of infected meat (in slaughterhouses) and infected placentas (farms, veterinarians) and by ingestion of nonpasteurized milk or milk products from infected animals. Human infection is rare in the United States (less than 200 cases in a year) and is particularly rare in children. Brucellosis is often featured in the differential diagnosis of prolonged fever despite its rare occurrence. Diagnosis depends on culturing the organism from blood, bone marrow, or a focal site of infection or on a fourfold increase in agglutination titer measured in paired specimens of sera.

TREATMENT

Specific antimicrobial treatment serves to shorten the course of the disease and to prevent complications and relapses. The drug of choice by virtue of the greatest clinical experience and the best antimicrobial activity is tetracycline. The World Health Organization has recommended the addition of rifampin to tetracycline because of its good intracellular levels and excellent activity against *Brucella*. Although there is no well-documented series of children treated with this regimen, the preferred therapy for children older than 9 years is a combination of tetracycline 30 to 40 mg/kg/24 h divided into three or four doses and rifampin 20 mg/kg/d PO divided into two doses, both administered for 4 to 6 weeks. Doxycycline 4 to 5 mg/kg/d divided into two doses may be preferable to tetracycline based on ease of administration and effectiveness.

Children under the age of 8 or 9 years should not receive tetracycline because of its effect on tooth enamel and growing bone. The best alternative for this age group is trimethoprim-sulfamethoxazole 10 mg/kg/d of trimethoprim and 50 mg/kg/d of sulfamethoxazole in two divided doses PO. Some authors have used this medication alone successfully. Others have used trimethoprim without sulfamethoxazole, alone or in combination with other drugs. The largest series used trimethoprim-sulfamethoxazole combined with gentamicin for 5 days.[1] The combination of trimethoprim-sulfamethoxazole with rifampin for the younger child has theoretical appeal.

Many other drugs have been tried, including the new cephalosporins and the quinolones, but none have been shown to be effective. Response to treatment is apt to be slow. Relapses with a recurrent positive blood culture may occur and require retreatment. Besides specific antimicrobial therapy, children require supportive therapy, attention to nutrition, and an individualized approach to bedrest and school attendance depending on the severity of the disease.

REFERENCE

1. Lubani MM, Dubin KI, Sharda DC, et al: A multicenter therapeutic study of 1100 children with brucellosis. Pediatr Infect Dis 8:75–78, 1989.

CAT-SCRATCH DISEASE

J. JEFFREY MALATACK, M.D.

Although cat-scratch disease (CSD) has been recognized since its description by Debre in 1950, it was not until Carithers published his experience with 1200 patients that a more expanded description of CSD was elucidated.

The majority of patients suffering from CSD present with chronic lymphadenitis. Most often, a single node, the axillary node, is involved, but occasionally two or more nodes are affected. The adenitis is caused by an infecting organism carried by domestic cats and introduced into the host either through breaks in the integument or directly across mucous membranes. Scratches from a cat carrying the organism inoculate and infect the victim. Scratches from other animals allow inoculation and infection if intimate cat contact occurs following the injury. The adenitis is an infected node from the region draining the inoculation site.

Three to five days after contact with a cat, a papule, the inoculation site, appears on the skin. A mild flu-like illness occurs in 75% of patients. The inoculation papule evolves through a vesicular and crust stage over 2 to 3 days. The regional adenopathy appears within 1 to 2 weeks of the inoculation. The affected node usually regresses over weeks to months, although occasionally it will suppurate and then regress.

The peak occurrence of CSD is in children between 3 and 12 years of age in the months of July through December. The domestic cat appears to be the only vector, and immature cats, less than 1 year of age, are more frequently the vector than are mature cats. The cat carrying the disease is not sick.

ATYPICAL PRESENTATIONS

At least 10% to 15% of CSD patients have atypical clinical manifestation, including the oculoglandular syndrome of Parinaud, fever, hepatic and splenic involvement, thrombocytopenia, erythema nodosum, and lytic bone lesions.

DIAGNOSIS

Cat-scratch disease can be diagnosed in most instances on clinical grounds. The Carithers rule of five, modified for the recent development of serologic testing is helpful. The patient receives a score of one for the presence of a single node or regional lymphadenopathy. Two points accrue if there is a history of intimate cat contact. Two additional points are given if an inoculation site is found. Finally, two points are scored for a positive cat-scratch skin test, which may now be modified to be either a positive skin test or positive serology. Five points strongly suggest that diagnosis, and seven points are definitive.

ETIOLOGIC AGENT

The discovery of the putative organism of CSD was first described by Wear et al. in 1983. Subsequent work at the Armed Forces Institute of Pathology (AFIP) by English et al. demonstrated that the Wear organism met Koch's postulates as an etiologic agent for clinical CSD. The organism was named *Afipia felis* in recognition of the AFIP's discovery. Controversy arose when recent work by Regnery et al. showed that a second organism, *Bartonella henselae* (formally *Rochalimaea henselae*) was the cause of CSD. Serologic evidence supports *B. henselae* as the most frequent cause of CSD. Ninety percent of CSD patients have serologic evidence of a *B. henselae* infection.

THERAPY

The majority of cases of CSD are mild and self-limited and require no therapy. Warm compresses for 10 to 15 minutes four to six times daily may speed involution. Trauma to the node should be avoided. Needle aspiration may be helpful in cases of significant pain or if the contents of the node liquefy. Aspiration is accomplished by moving the needle around the node, since the caseating material is often loculated. The aspirated sample may be sent for bacterial cultures to rule out pyogenic infection. Surgical incision or excision is not recommended unless there is concern that the mass may be malignant.

Treatment with antimicrobials is indicated for patients with (1) a severe systemic illness due to CSD, (2) an underlying immunodeficiency complicating CSD, or (3) an underlying medical illness complicated by CSD. The choice of antibiotics is based on past anecdotal responses to various antibiotics. Intravenous gentamicin sulfate, has trimethoprim-sulfamethoxazole, rifampin, and ciprofloxacin all have been used and appear efficacious. In vitro susceptibility data generally are unavailable.

REFERENCES

1. Carithers HA: Cat-scratch disease: An overview based on a study of 1,200 patients. Am J Dis Child 139:1124–1133. 1985.
2. English CK, Wear DJ, Margileth AM, Lissner CR, Walsh GP: Cat-scratch disease: Isolation and culture of the bacterial agent. JAMA 259:1347–1352, 1988.
3. Regnery RL, Olson JG, Perkins BA, Bebb W: Serological response to *Rochalimaea henselae* antigen is suspected cat-scratch disease. Lancet 339:1443–1445, 1992.

DIPHTHERIA

BENOOSH AFGHANI, M.D.
MELVIN I. MARKS, M.D.

Although diphtheria is rare in the United States, it poses a constant threat in developing countries, especially among subgroups with low vaccination levels. Patients with toxigenic diphtheria infections can deteriorate rapidly, and clinical attention should be directed toward signs of airway obstruction and systemic toxicity. Patients with pharyngeal diphtheria present with low-grade fever and pharyngitis initially. Within 1 or 2 days, a white or gray membrane may cover the pharyngeal wall and extend to the larynx, leading to progressive stidor and hoarseness. Cutaneous diphtheria is less common. Skin lesions appear ulcerative, with sharply defined borders and a membranous base.

TREATMENT

The recovery of a child with diphtheria depends on prompt administration of specific antitoxin, since only the circulating exotoxin that is not yet bound to tissues is neutralized. A single dose should be administered intravenously if this clinical diagnosis is likely, even before culture results are available. Since the antitoxin is a horse antiserum, each patient should be tested for sensitivity before its administration. Sensitivity testing is performed by using a 1:10 dilution of antitoxin in the conjunctiva or a 1:100 dilution intradermally. Persons with positive reactions should be desensitized by trained personnel and in a facility fully equipped to manage adverse reactions, especially anaphylaxis. Negative tests do not absolutely rule out sensitivity, and animal sera should always be administered with caution. The dose of antitoxin depends on the site of infection and severity of illness. Antitoxin administered within the first 2 days of illness is associated with a substantial reduction in case fatality rates compared with administration later in the course of illness (16.3% versus 1.3%). However, it is recommended that antitoxin be administered even if symptoms have persisted for several days.

The current American Academy of Pediatrics dose recommendations for antitoxin are 20,000 to 40,000 U for pharyngeal and laryngeal disease, 40,000 to 60,000 U for nasopharyngeal lesions, and 80,000 to 100,000 U for extensive disease, disease of more than 2 days duration, or brawny swelling of the neck. The use of antitoxin is debatable in patients with cutaneous diphtheria, but a dose of 20,000 to 40,000 U should be used if there are any signs of toxicity.

Although intravenous immunoglobulin often contains diphtheria antibody, no comparative data are available to establish its efficacy, and lot-to-lot variation in antibody titers precludes accurate dosing.

Antimicrobial therapy is recommended to eradicate the organism and decrease transmission. Penicillin G 100,000 to 150,000 U/kg/d IV in four divided doses or procaine penicillin 25,000 to 50,000 U/kg/d IM in two divided doses for 14 days is required. Erythromycin 40 to 50 mg/kg/d PO or parenterally also is effective. If three consecutive negative cultures cannot be documented after completion of therapy, a second 5-day course of oral penicillin or erythromycin is recommended.

Strict isolation is indicated in patients with respiratory diphtheria, but contact isolation is sufficient for those with cutaneous disease. Isolation can be discontinued after two negative cultures are documented.

Although steroids have been used in severe cases of diphtheria, no controlled trials have been performed to prove their effectiveness. Their use should be considered in patients with severe respiratory distress due to upper airway obstruction.

Nontoxigenic *Corynebacterium diphtheriae* also can cause disease, especially in patients with underlying risk factors, such as immunodeficiency, indwelling foreign body, or chronic disease. Clinical syndromes most commonly associated with nontoxigenic *C. diphtheriae* include osteomyelitis, septic arthritis, endocarditis, bacteremia, meningitis, and wound infection. Patients infected with nontoxigenic diphtheria rarely present with pharyngeal or laryngeal diphtheria or toxin-related phenomena, such as myocarditis or neuritis. The pathogenicity and optimal therapy for infections due to nontoxigenic *C. diphtheriae* are poorly understood. However, all *C. diphtheriae* infections should be presumptively managed with antimicrobials until nontoxigenicity can be confirmed. Antitoxin is indicated if there is any evidence of invasive disease or toxicity. Testing for toxigenicity is done in vitro by Elek test or in vivo by animal inoculation and requires 24 to 72 hours.

COMPLICATIONS

Close observation for complications is important. The most common complications are myocarditis and neuritis. Myocarditis occurs in about 50% of cases, usually in the first week of illness. Bedrest and cardiac monitoring are necessary if myocarditis is suspected. Peripheral neuritis occurs after the second week, is usually self-limited, and requires supportive care. A few cases of hemolytic-uremic syndrome have been reported as a complication of toxigenic diphtheria infection. Most of these have been severe and required dialysis.

CONTACTS

Transmission of toxigenic diphtheria infection is directly related to the duration and intensity of exposure to the infected patient. All cases of diphtheria should be reported to the local public health authorities, and contact investigation should be started as soon as possible.

Although the efficacy of chemoprophylaxis has not been firmly established, all close contacts of diphtheria patients, irrespective of their immunization status, should be treated with penicillin or erythromycin and observed closely for 7 days. The recommended treatment is a single dose of 600,000 to 1,200,000 U benzathine penicillin G given IM, especially if compliance or follow-up cannot be assured. Erythromycin 40 to 50 mg/kg/d for 7 days is an alternative. Cultures of the nose and throat are strongly recommended before therapy. Antimicrobial prophylaxis is not 100% efficacious, and persistent colonization is possible. Contacts with positive cultures initially should have a repeat culture 2 weeks after the completion of therapy. Those who continue to be carriers should receive an additional 10-day course of erythromycin. Contacts with inadequate immunization or no immunization within the last 5 years should also be given a dose of DTP, Td, or DT depending on age.

PREVENTION

Immunization is the most important control measure. Although immunization decreases the carriage rate of toxigenic *C. diphtheriae* significantly, fully immunized individuals may still be carriers or may develop mild disease. Primary immunization consists of DTP vaccine at 2, 4, and 6 months of age and booster doses 6 to 12 months after the third dose and again between 4 and 6 years of age.

Primary immunization of children more than 7 years of age may be carried out using Td (adult type tetanus and diphtheria toxoid). Two doses are given 1 month apart, and a third dose is given 1 year later. The Td preparation contains no more than 2 Lf units of diphtheria toxoid per dose compared with 7 to 25 Lf units in the DTP preparation and is less likely to produce reactions. The incidence of reactions, such as erythema and swelling at the injection site, is less than 15%. Booster immunization with Td is recommended every 10 years.

GONOCOCCAL INFECTIONS

BARRY DASHEFSKY, M.D.

Infection with *Neisseria gonorrhoeae* is the most common reportable infectious disease in the United States. An estimated one-half million reported and 1 to 2 million unreported cases occurred in 1992. Although the infection is most prevalent among young adults, more than 25% of reported cases involve pediatric-age patients, especially teenage girls between the ages of 15 and 19 years. Although, as with sexually transmitted diseases (STDs) in general, most cases of childhood gonococcal infection are attributable to voluntary (albeit frequently unacknowledged) sexual activity, practitioners must be highly alert and responsive to the less frequent cases associated with perinatal transmission and sexual abuse.

The most significant recent change in the management of gonococcal infections reflects a decade-long increase in the number of isolates that are resistant to traditionally used antimicrobial regimens. Thirty-two percent of gonococcal isolates assessed by the Gonococcal Isolate Surveillance Project (GISP) in 1991 were resistant to either penicillin or tetracycline. *As a consequence, as of 1989, ceftriaxone has supplanted penicillin (or ampicillin or amoxicillin) as the empiric antimicrobial of choice for treating most proven or presumed gonococcal infections.* Certainly, penicillin or other candidate agents remain appropriate therapeutic alternatives when specific susceptibility data so signify.

GENERAL MANAGEMENT CONSIDERATIONS

Because multiple STDs often coexist, the suspicion or diagnosis of gonococcal infection should generally result in testing for the presence of other STDs, including *Chlamydia trachomatis,* syphilis, and depending on local prevalence, human immunodeficiency virus (HIV). With a similar rationale, sexually active patients diagnosed as having an STD should be vaccinated against hepatitis B virus.

Because *C. trachomatis* frequently coinfects patients with gonococcal infection (in up to 25% of men and 45% of women with acute urogenital gonorrhea), in the absence of accurate test data that definitively exclude this possibility, patients who are treated for suspected or documented gonococcal infection should also be routinely treated concomitantly with a second agent effective against *C. trachomatis* according to one of the following regimens:

- *Nonpregnant patients 16 years of age or older* (some would say adolescents of any age): azithromycin 1 g PO in a single dose.
- *Nonpregnant patients 9 years of age or older:* doxycycline 100 mg PO twice daily or tetracycline 500 mg PO four times daily for 7 days.
- *Nonpregnant patients 18 years of age or older:* ofloxacin 300 mg PO twice daily for 7 days. Ofloxacin is the only quinolone with proven efficacy against *Chlamydia.*
- *Pregnant patients or patients younger than 9 years of age:* erythromycin 10 to 12.5 mg/kg (max: 500 mg) PO four times daily for 7 days (max: 500 mg). An alternative, albeit less effective choice, if erythromycin cannot be given would be either amoxicillin 15 mg/kg PO three times daily for 7 to 10 days or, in patients older than

1 month of age, sulfisoxazole 37.5 mg/kg (max: 2 g) PO four times daily for 10 days.

A serologic test for syphilis (STS) should be performed on all patients with documented or suspected gonococcal infection. Although all regimens recommended for treatment of *N. gonorrhoeae* using penicillins or cephalosporins are adequate to treat incubating syphilis, the same cannot be said for therapies using spectinomycin, tetracylines, erythromycin, or quinolones. Therefore, if such agents are used, an STS should be repeated 6 to 12 weeks after treatment.

Hospitalization and parenteral therapy generally are indicated for at least initial treatment of all forms of gonococcal infection in neonates, as well as for systemic infection in older patients. In addition, because of substantial risks of poor compliance with prescribed treatment and long-term morbidity among adolescent patients with complicated genital infection, such as pelvic inflammatory disease (PID), a low threshold for hospitalization of this population is advised. Admission is warranted whenever the diagnosis of PID is uncertain, abscess is suggested, compliance with or tolerance of oral medication is suspect, the patient is pregnant, or a previous attempt at outpatient management has failed. Any patient with PID who is managed as an outpatient should be reassessed within 2 to 3 days.

Newborns and prepubertal children who are hospitalized with gonococcal infection require contact isolation precautions until 24 hours of effective therapy has been completed.

Because involuntary sexual contact after the neonatal period is the most likely mode of acquisition of gonococcal infection in prepubertal children younger than 9 years of age and because it must also be suspected in adolescents who are not sexually active, documentation of gonococcal infection in these populations mandates a careful and thorough evaluation for sexual abuse. Genital, rectal, and pharyngeal specimens should be obtained for culture. Diagnosis of gonococcal infection in cases of suspected abuse should be established by positive cultures confirmed by at least two different biochemical, enzymatic, or serologic tests. Because sexually abused children are considered to have a low but uncertain risk of acquiring STDs, in the absence of demonstrated infection, they need not be treated presumptively unless the perpetrator is known to be infected, the parents prefer treatment, or follow-up cannot be ensured.

SPECIFIC TREATMENT REGIMENS

Both the clinical manifestations and the appropriate specific therapies for childhood gonococcal infections vary with age. For the most part, treatment regimens have not been evaluated in pediatric populations, and recommendations are based on controlled observations in adult patients. Adult dose routines are used for children weighing more than 45 kg. Selected recommendations deriving from a large number of options for management of specific clinical problems due to gonococcal infection follow. For more detailed guidance, the reader is referred to the most recent recommendations of the U.S. Centers for Disease Control and Prevention[1] or the Committee on Infectious Diseases of the American Academy of Pediatrics.[2]

Neonatal Infections

Gonococcal infections of neonates include ophthalmia, scalp abscesses, and disseminated disease, such as sepsis, meningitis, arthritis, and endocarditis. Gonococcal disease at any site should prompt a careful evaluation for systemic infection. With the presumption that infection was acquired from the mother, both the mother and her sexual contacts should be evaluated and treated for the implicated STDs.

Both *uncomplicated neonatal gonococcal ophthalmia and scalp abscess* should be treated with either a single daily dose of ceftriaxone 25 to 50 mg/kg IV or IM (max: 125 mg) or cefotaxime 25 to 50 mg/kg IV or IM twice daily for 7 days. Penicillin G 100,000 U/kg/d IV in two to four divided doses for 7 days is an acceptable alternative for treating infection associated with susceptible isolates. Gonococcal ophthalmia should be managed also with eye irrigation using buffered saline at least hourly until the discharge has resolved. Topical antibiotics are inadequate alone and unnecessary adjuncts to parenteral therapy. Disseminated gonococcal infection, including meningitis, should be treated with either ceftriaxone 25 to 50 mg/kg IV or IM in a single daily dose or cefotaxime 25 to 50 mg/kg IV or IM two or three times daily for 10 to 14 days. Penicillin G 100,000 to 150,000 U/kg/d IV in two to four divided doses for 10 to 14 days is an alternative for susceptible isolates. Some nonmeningitic infections can be treated adequately in 7 days.

Ceftriaxone must be used cautiously in neonates with hyperbilirubinemia. The pain associated with intramuscular injection of ceftriaxone may be ameliorated by the use of a lidocaine diluent.

Infections in Prepubertal Children and Adolescents

After the neonatal period, gonococcal infection most frequently affects the genital tract. In prepubertal girls, this is most commonly manifest as vaginitis and, in boys, as urethritis. Following puberty, endocervicitis, urethritis, and PID are the most common expressions in female adolescents, and urethritis and epididymitis are the most common expressions in adolescent males. Pharyngeal, rectal, and conjunctival infection, as well as systemic disease, including pyogenic arthritis and tenosynovitis, arthritis-dermatitis syndrome with sepsis (also referred to as disseminated gonococcal infection), and, less commonly, osteomyelitis, pneumonia, meningitis, and endocarditis, also occur in children and adults of all ages.

For uncomplicated urogenital, rectal, or pharyngeal gonococcal infection, outpatient management consisting of a single IM 125-mg dose of ceftriaxone is recommended. Oral cephalosporins have not been sufficiently evaluated in young children to justify their routine use in this age group. However, cefixime 400 mg PO in one dose represents a very attractive alternative for treatment of older adolescents and adults (except for pharyngeal infection, for which ceftriaxone alone affords reliable treatment). In exceptional circumstances, cefixime 8 mg/kg PO in a single dose (max: 400 mg) can be considered for treatment of uncomplicated gonococcal infection in younger children, provided follow-up and test of cure culturing are assured. Following are other effective regimens:

- *Older patients:*
  - cefuroxime axetil 1 g PO taken once with 1 g of probenecid.
  - cefpodoxime 200 mg PO taken once.
  - cefotaxime 1 g IM as a single dose.
  - ceftizoxime 500 mg IM as a single dose.
- *Patients who are allergic to penicillins and cephalosporins:*
  - spectinomycin 40 mg/kg IM (max: 2 g) as a single dose.
- *Nonpregnant patients 18 years of age and older:*
  - ciprofloxacin 500 mg PO taken once.
  - ofloxacin 400 mg PO taken once.
- *Penicillin-susceptible isolates:*
  - procaine penicillin G 100,000 U/kg IM (max: 4.8 million units) as a single dose.
  - amoxicillin 50 mg/kg PO taken once (max: 3 g) administered with probenecid 25 mg/kg (max: 1 g) (a well-established treatment option).

PID is usually caused by infection with *N. gonorrhoeae, C. trachomatis,* gram-negative enteric bacilli, or anaerobes, either alone or in combination. Because of the difficulty of determining the specific cause in a given case, empiric therapy should consist of a broad-spectrum antimicrobial regimen that is sufficient to treat most, if not all, candidate pathogens, such as cefoxitin or cefotetan, combined with doxycycline. (See discussion on pelvic inflammatory disease in Chapter 22.)

Similarly, *epididymitis* is usually attributable to *N. gonorrhoeae, C. trachomatis,* or gram-negative enteric bacilli. Following are recommended treatments:

- *Children 9 years of age or older:* ceftriaxone 250 mg IM as a single dose, followed by 7 days of either doxcycline 200 mg/d PO in two divided doses *or* tetracycline 2 g/d PO in four divided doses.

- *Patients 16 years or older:* azithromycin 1 g PO in one dose.
- *Children younger than 9 years:* 7 days of erythromycin at 50 mg/kg/d PO in four doses (max: 2 g/d).

Nonsepticemic gonococcal ophthalmia usually can be treated successfully with a single dose of ceftriaxone 50 mg/kg IM (max: 1 g) and saline irrigation. Patients with severe disease may require hospitalization and ceftriaxone at the same dose schedule for 5 to 7 days.

Systemic gonococcal infection other than meningitis and endocarditis should be treated with the following:

- ceftriaxone 50 mg/kg/d IV or IM once daily (max: 1 g) for 7 to 10 days.
- cefotaxime 50 mg/kg/d IV or IM in three doses (max: 3 g/d) for 7 to 10 days.
- ceftizoxime 50 mg/kg/d IV or IM in three doses (max: 3 g/d) for 7 to 10 days.
- *Penicillin-allergic and cephalosporin-allergic patients:* spectinomycin 40 mg/kg IM in two divided doses (max: 4 g/d) for 7 to 10 days. Penicillin G 150,000 U/kg/d (max: 10 million U/d) IV in four to six divided doses or equivalent penicillin agents may be substituted when the susceptibility of the isolate permits.

Following substantial symptomatic improvement with parenteral therapy and subject to age and pregnancy restrictions, the rest of therapy may be completed on an outpatient basis using one of the following:

- cefixime 400 mg PO twice daily.
- ciprofloxacin 500 mg PO two times daily.
- cefuroxime axetil 500 mg PO twice daily.
- doxycycline 100 mg PO twice daily, depending on susceptibility data.
- tetracycline 500 mg PO four times daily, depending on susceptibility data.

Management of gonococcal arthritis may require additional therapeutic modalities appropriate for any case of pyogenic arthritis. (See discussion on septic arthritis in Chapter 13.) However, antimicrobial treatment alone typically suffices to effect an excellent outcome.

Patients with disseminated gonococcal infection should be evaluated carefully for evidence of meningitis or endocarditis. *Meningitis* should be treated with one of the following:

- ceftriaxone 50 to 100 mg/kg IV or IM in one or two doses (max: 2 g/d) for 10 to 14 days.
- cefotaxime 200 mg/kg/d IV in three or four doses (max: 8 to 10 g/d) for 10 to 14 days.

Alternative agents for susceptible strains include the following:

- Penicillin G 250,000 U/kg/d IV in four to six doses (max: 10 to 20 million U/d) for 10 to 14 days.
- *Penicillin-allergic and cephalosporin-allergic patients:* chloramphenicol 100 mg/kd/d IV in four doses (max: 2 to 6 g/d) for 10 to 14 days, with careful monitoring of blood levels.

Treatment for *endocarditis,* using the same agents and dose schedules, should be extended to at least 4 weeks. The occurrence of gonococcal meningitis or endocarditis or recurrence of disseminated gonococcal infection should prompt an evaluation for possible complement deficiency.

CONTROL AND PREVENTIVE MEASURES

Early detection of gonococcal infection affords the best chance for a satisfactory therapeutic outcome. Accordingly, routine screening of sexually active adolescents, as well as all pregnant women (at the time of the first prenatal visit and again late in pregnancy), is recommended. Infected pregnant women may be treated with standard regimens, except that doxycycline and tetracycline should be avoided.

Universal ophthalmic prophylaxis is indicated to prevent gonococcal ophthalmia neonatorum. Either 1% aqueous silver nitrate solution, 1% tetracycline ointment, or 0.5% erythromycin ointment should be instilled once in the eyes as soon as possible but no later than 1 hour after birth; the eyes should not be subsequently irrigated. These regimens do not prevent chlamydial infection. Despite the high degree of efficacy of ophthalmic prophylaxis, newborns delivered to women with untreated gonorrhea should receive a single dose of ceftriaxone 25 to 50 mg/kg (max: 125 mg) IM or IV.

All cases of gonococcal infection should be reported to public health authorities to facilitate surveillance and contact tracing. Sex partners of infected patients should be identified, evaluated, and usually presumptively treated for the implicated STDs.

Although currently recommended regimens are reliably effective in curing gonococcal infection, to permit timely recognition of the emergence of resistant strains, at least a representative sample of gonococcal isolates should be subjected to antibiotic susceptibility testing, and data from ongoing national antibiotic susceptibility surveillance programs should be regularly reviewed. (Fluoroquinolone-resistant isolates of *N. gonorrhoeae* were detected by the GISP surveillance program in Ohio and Hawaii in 1992–1994.) Likewise, all isolates associated with treatment failure should be evaluated to guide retreatment.

Because therapeutic failure following treatment with the combination of ceftriaxone and doxycycline is very rare, test of cure cultures are not routinely required for gonococcal infections treated with this regimen. However, a second specimen should be obtained for culture approximately 4 to 7 days after completion of any other therapeutic regimen. In addition, the selective use of rescreening cultures obtained 1 to 2 months after treatment is recommended irrespective of treatment regimen in order to permit the early detection of reinfection.

Education regarding issues of sexuality and transmission of STDs is the most important and potentially most beneficial element of strategies for controlling and preventing infection. Infected patients need to be instructed to defer additional sexual activity until after successful completion of a course of treatment. Harder still is teaching adolescents the lesson that, barring sexual abstinence, the (proper) use of barrier contraceptives, such as condoms, affords the only available means of minimizing (not eliminating) the risk of acquiring STDs.

REFERENCES

1. Centers for Disease Control: 1993 Sexually transmitted diseases treatment guidelines. MMWR 42(No. RR-14):56–67, 1993.
2. Committee on Infectious Diseases. American Academy of Pediatrics: Gonococcal infections. *In* Report of the Committee on Infectious Diseases, 23rd ed. Elk Grove Village, IL, American Academy of Pediatrics, 1994:195–202.

INFECTIONS CAUSED BY *HAEMOPHILUS INFLUENZAE* TYPE B

LILLY CHENG IMMERGLUCK, M.D.
ROBERT S. DAUM, M.D.

The recent introduction of effective immunization has resulted in a dramatic decrease in the occurrence of invasive infection, including meningitis, caused by *Haemophilus influenzae* type b, in young, preschool children beyond the neonatal period. At present, it is still appropriate to consider therapy of *H. influenzae* type b infections in some detail, although their importance may decline as they become increasingly rare.

TREATMENT

For many years, ampicillin was the drug of choice for all invasive *H. influenzae* type b disease. However, in the late 1970s, isolates of *H. influenzae* type b that produced beta-lactamase were identified in increasing numbers. The most recent multicenter collaborative surveillance of *H. influenzae* type b isolates, completed in 1988, found that 29.5% of *H. influenzae* type b isolates in the United States produced beta-lactamase. Additionally, rare isolates have been identified that are ampicillin resistant but do not produce beta-lactamase. The mechanism of resistance in this instance is the production of a penicillin-binding protein with decreased affinity for beta-lactam compounds.

When ampicillin resistance was first recognized in 1974, chloramphenicol became the agent of choice for the therapy of invasive *H. influenzae* type b disease. Advantages of chloramphenicol include low cost and good penetration into cerebrospinal fluid (CSF). Moreover, the compound is effective against most isolates of *H. influenzae* type b irrespective of beta-lactamase production. Chloramphenicol is usually well absorbed from the gastrointestinal tract. Accordingly, adequate concentrations of this drug may be achieved in the serum and even the CSF after oral administration. Disadvantages of chloramphenicol include the necessity for monitoring and the often emotionally held views regarding the rare occurrence of idiosyncratic aplastic anemia.

Resistance to chloramphenicol is usually associated with the elaboration of chloramphenicol acetyl transferase (CAT), although a few resistant isolates do not produce this enzyme. Chloramphenicol-resistant *H. influenzae* type b isolates have remained rare in the United States and most other countries, although they have been found more commonly in a few areas, for example, Barcelona and Taiwan.

Treatment with chloramphenicol must be carefully monitored. Serum concentrations should be monitored in all patients except those receiving very short courses of therapy, for example, 1 to 2 days. Peak concentrations (obtained 30 minutes after completion of an intravenous dose or 90 minutes after an oral dose) should be about 15 to 25 μg/ml. High serum chloramphenicol concentrations are associated with predictable, dose-dependent suppression of the bone marrow. In addition, especially in very young infants, high serum concentrations of chloramphenicol (usually >50 μg/ml) may lead to cardiovascular collapse and the so-called gray baby syndrome. Idiosyncratic aplastic anemia rarely may also complicate therapy at a frequency similar to that associated with fatal anaphylaxis after penicillin administration. Concurrent administration of anticonvulsants, such as phenobarbital, phenytoin, carbamazepine, or rifampin, may alter the metabolism of chloramphenicol. Conversely, chloramphenicol can interfere with the metabolism of certain drugs, such as phenytoin, tolbutamide, and dicumarol.

Isolates resistant to both chloramphenicol and ampicillin have been identified occasionally. Worldwide, the most recent tabulation identified 39 cases of ampicillin- and chloramphenicol-resistant *H. influenzae* type b meningitis in 1987. In the United States, fewer than 1% of isolates were resistant to both compounds. Extended spectrum cephalosporins, such as cefotaxime or ceftriaxone, have proven highly efficacious against *H. influenzae* type b and have become increasingly popular in the United States. These compounds offer advantages over chloramphenicol in their ease of administration, infrequent toxicity, and, thus far, lack of resistance. To date, only a single report of delayed sterilization of the CSF has been documented even though the relevant isolate was susceptible. Because of its long half-life, ceftriaxone administered once or twice daily has been widely used to treat serious *H. influenzae* type b infections and has even been used for outpatient therapy of selected patients.

Specific Antimicrobial Regimens

Because there is usually a delay until the causative organism is identified and its antimicrobial susceptibility determined, parenteral antimicrobial therapy of suspected invasive *H. influenzae* type b infections often is initiated empirically. Several considerations are relevant. First, other bacteria (for example, *Streptococcus pneumoniae* and *Neisseria meningitidis* in the case of meningitis) may produce clinical illnesses in children similar to those caused by *H. influenzae* type b. Thus, these species should also be targeted by the empiric antimicrobial regimen. Second, because of rare reports of isolates from the blood and CSF differing in their antimicrobial susceptibility pattern, susceptibility testing should be performed on all isolates that are recovered from normally sterile sites. Third, the chosen empirical antimicrobial regimen must be active against ampicillin-susceptible and ampicillin-resistant *H. influenzae* type b isolates. Regimens in widest clinical use include a single parenteral agent, such as cefotaxime or ceftriaxone or ampicillin and chloramphenicol. Once the organism is isolated and its antimicrobial susceptibility is ascertained, therapy should be directed against the responsible isolate. To minimize the development of resistance and contain costs, therapy with extended-spectrum cephalosporins should be reserved for use against isolates that are resistant to ampicillin.

Near the completion of antimicrobial therapy for many *H. influenzae* type b clinical syndromes, except meningitis, drugs are sometimes administered orally. In this instance, depending on available susceptibility testing, suitable agents include amoxicillin, amoxicillin-clavulanate, cefixime, or cefaclor. Some practitioners may wish to use chloramphenicol because of its low cost. Chloramphenicol has been used in the treatment of meningitis (see below).

Duration and Mode of Treatment

The recommended duration of treatment for *H. influenzae* type b infection is often based on custom rather than on scientific data. Therefore, the recommendations given here should be viewed as guidelines and should be modified when the clinical illness is severe or the course is complicated by other factors.

Meningitis

H. influenzae type b meningitis is usually treated with antimicrobials for 10 to 14 days. More recently, adequate treatment has been demonstrated with 7 to 10 days of antimicrobial therapy. Treatment should be administered intravenously for the entire duration, presumably because the concentration of an antimicrobial in the CSF must be maintained. Furthermore, as the meninges heal and the patient's clinical condition improves, the antimicrobial concentration attained in the CSF may be decreased even more. An exception is chloramphenicol, which is well absorbed when administered orally, with high concentrations attained in the CSF (~50% of the concentration in serum) independent of meningeal inflammation. Consequently, some may choose to complete a course of therapy for meningitis with chloramphenicol administered orally. In general, however, this approach should be reserved for situations in which the patient is not vomiting, there is a compelling reason that antimicrobials cannot be administered parenterally, serum concentrations of chloramphenicol can be monitored, and compliance can be ensured.

A proportion of patients with meningitis manifest the syndrome of inappropriate antidiuretic hormone (SIADH) secretion. Therefore, the input and output of fluids and electrolytes should be carefully monitored initially. If SIADH is documented by decreased serum osmolality, hyponatremia (serum sodium concentration <130 mEq/L), and increased urine osmolality, patients should be restricted to one-half to two-thirds maintenance fluid intake (800 to 1000 ml/m^2/24 h) and receive nothing by mouth. Care should be taken to adjust fluid requirements when the patient is febrile. Additionally, fluids should not be excessively restricted to the extent that cerebrovascular perfusion pressure is compromised. Routine fluid restriction in the absence of clinically manifest SIADH is probably not warranted. In the rare instance of SIADH with a serum sodium concentration <120 mEq/L, hypertonic saline may be given slowly, with the goal being to raise the serum sodium concentration to about 125 mEq/L. Once SIADH resolves, fluid administration should be increased toward the normal maintenance (1500 ml/m^2/24 h) requirement. Oral intake can then be resumed, and parenteral fluid volumes can be adjusted as appropriate.

It is estimated that 6% of patients with *H. influenzae* type b meningitis will be left with some form of hearing impairment. The pathogenesis is believed to be related to early inflammatory involvement of the cochlea and labyrinth. The results of several studies indicate that dexamethasone 0.6 mg/kg/d divided every 6 hours for 4 days,

particularly when given shortly before or concurrent with the initiation of antimicrobial therapy, may decrease the incidence of bilateral hearing loss associated with *H. influenzae* type b meningitis. Dexamethasone may not prevent hearing loss from meningitis caused by other bacterial species, and, therefore, the likelihood that *H. influenzae* type b is the etiologic agent should be considered before dexamethasone administration.

Supraglottitis (Epiglottitis)

Because of the risk of sudden, unpredictable airway obstruction, *H. influenzae* type b supraglottitis is a medical emergency. Carefully conceived and easily implemented written protocols for transport, diagnostic investigation, and treatment of patients with supraglottitis will diminish the rate of occurrence of serious complications. Most deaths occur in transit to the hospital or within the first few hours after arrival. Once this diagnosis is suspected, the patient should be constantly attended by individuals skilled in resuscitation and airway/ventilatory support. All patients with epiglottitis should be managed initially by electively securing the inflamed airway via nasotracheal or orotracheal intubation or by tracheotomy when intubation is not possible. This procedure is best accomplished by a trained expert under controlled conditions in an operating room. Unnecessary stress, for example, blood tests, extensive history taking, and transport delay, should be eliminated before securing the airway.

In the days following intubation, direct observation is often used to monitor epiglottic inflammation. The endotracheal tube may be removed when the inflammation has subsided (usually within 2 to 3 days). Antimicrobial therapy should be directed against *H. influenzae* type b, since this bacterium is the major cause of epiglottitis, and should be administered intravenously only after the airway is secure. Oral therapy may be substituted when the patient can take fluids by mouth. The duration of therapy customarily has been 7 days.

Uvulitis

H. influenzae type b uvulitis may occur alone or may be a concomitant of pharyngitis or epiglottitis. Like supraglottitis, infection of the uvula most likely arises by direct invasion by *H. influenzae* type b. The child may present with a gagging sensation or spitting. Unlike epiglottitis, there is generally no associated respiratory distress. When uvulitis occurs with concomitant epiglottitis, symptoms and signs are more typical of the latter: high fever, dysphagia, and progressive respiratory distress. A lateral neck radiograph may help to exclude involvement of the supraglottic laryngeal structures, and after appropriate surface and blood cultures are obtained, the patient with uvulitis should be started on parenteral antimicrobials. These should be targeted against *H. influenzae* type b and *Streptococcus pyogenes*.

Arthritis and Osteomyelitis

H. influenzae type b more frequently causes septic arthritis than osteomyelitis. Although septic arthritis typically involves a single joint, most commonly the hip or knee, multiple joint involvement does occur in about 6% of cases. A diagnostic lumbar puncture should be considered, given the potential for bacteremia and resultant involvement of the meninges. Parenteral treatment with an appropriate antimicrobial is administered for at least 5 to 7 days. If the clinical response is good (as evidenced by the absence of fever and decreased signs of inflammation) and compliance can be ensured, the rest of the course of antimicrobial treatment may be provided orally (amoxicillin 100 mg/kg/d divided in three doses if the isolate is susceptible or cefixime 8 mg/kg/d given as a single dose or divided into two daily doses of 4 mg/kg). Alternatively, therapy may be provided as a single daily dose of ceftriaxone 50 mg/kg (max: 2 g/d). Some experts believe that the dose should be adjusted so that the serum bactericidal titer is ≥1:8.

A 3-week course of therapy is probably adequate for uncomplicated arthritis. Some experts believe that the erythrocyte sedimentation rate should be normal before cessation of therapy. Needle aspiration of the infected joint probably provides adequate drainage in uncomplicated cases except for involvement of the hip or shoulder joints (which should receive prompt, additional surgical drainage).

H. influenzae type b is an infrequent cause of osteomyelitis. Adjacent, concomitant arthritis may be present. Treatment guidelines are similar to those for arthritis except that a 4-week course is preferred. Surgical drainage and debridement of infected bones generally is not required.

Cellulitis

About 75% of paitents with *H. influenzae* type b cellulitis have involvement of the face, head, or neck. Buccal cellulitis is classically erythematous with a violaceous hue, although this sign may be absent. Children with *H. influenzae* type b cellulitis may be clinically ill and bacteremic. A diagnostic lumbar puncture should be considered at the time of diagnosis because of the high incidence of concurrent meningitis, particularly when the patient is very young (younger than 18 months of age) or febrile or both. Antimicrobials should be administered parenterally. Fever usually resolves promptly on initiation of treatment, but local inflammation may not begin to decrease until 24 to 48 hours later. After the child becomes afebrile and the signs of inflammation decrease, an orally administered antimicrobial may be substituted. A 7- to 10-day course has been customary. Prolonged fever may be a sign of distant, concomitant infection, such as meningitis or arthritis.

Orbital and Preseptal Infections

The differential diagnosis of the clinical syndrome of the red and swollen eye includes several infectious diseases. Those that involve the superficial tissue layers anterior to the orbital septum are best termed *preseptal cellulitis*. Infectious processes that involve the orbit and its contents include *orbital cellulitis, orbital abscess,* and *subperiosteal abscess*.

Preseptal cellulitis does not have risk for visual impairment or direct CNS extension, although this is not the case when infection involves the orbit. *H. influenzae* type b preseptal cellulitis is characterized by edema, tenderness, warmth of the lid, and, occasionally, purple discoloration. There also may be conjunctival drainage. Evidence of interruption of the integument is usually absent. When infection involves the orbit, an event that occurs rarely, there may variably be lid edema, proptosis, chemosis, impaired vision, limitation of the extraocular movements, decreased mobility of the globe, and pain on movement of the globe. On occasion, the distinction between preseptal and orbital cellulitis may be difficult to make. In this instance, the extent of the infection often can be delineated by computed tomography (CT) or ultrasound.

For preseptal and orbital infections, parenteral antimicrobial therapy is indicated initially. Since *Staphylococcus aureus, S. pneumoniae,* and group A beta-hemolytic streptococci also may cause such syndromes, an empiric regimen should include agents active against these pathogens. Children with uncomplicated preseptal cellulitis who are older than 5 years of age may not require therapy directed against *H. influenzae* type b. Patients with preseptal cellulitis without concurrent meningitis customarily receive parenteral therapy for about 5 days until fever and erythema have abated. A similar but more conservative approach is suggested for orbital cellulitis in that parenteral therapy is continued for the duration of treatment. For both syndromes, in uncomplicated cases, antimicrobial therapy should be instituted for a total duration of 10 days. Abscesses in the orbit usually require prompt surgical drainage and more prolonged antimicrobial therapy, although there are published anecdotes that attest that some patients improve without surgical intervention. If an abscess is not found initially, but a patient fails to improve on parenteral antimicrobial therapy, the necessity for surgical exploration to drain a subperiosteal or orbital abscess should be reconsidered.

Pneumonia

As with cellulitis and arthritis, initial treatment of *H. influenzae* type b pneumonia is generally with a parenterally administered an-

timicrobial. Children younger than 12 months of age particularly, should receive parenteral antimicrobial therapy initially because of their increased risk for bacteremia and its complications. However, children who are not severely ill and, therefore, are unlikely to be bacteremic are often managed with an orally administered antimicrobial. If the child responds well to parenteral therapy, as evidenced by prompt defervescence and decreased respiratory distress, an orally administered agent may be substituted to complete a 7- to 10-day course of combined parenteral-oral therapy.

Uncomplicated pleural effusion associated with *H. influenzae* type b infection generally requires no special intervention. However, children with *empyema* may require drainage, which usually is accomplished by insertion of a chest tube. A prolonged course of antimicrobial therapy should be considered in this instance.

Bacteremia Without Focality—So-Called Occult or Walk-In Bacteremia

Because blood for culture is often obtained from febrile outpatient infants with no apparent focus of infection, physicians sometimes will be informed that a child was bacteremic with *H. influenzae* type b 24 to 48 hours earlier. There has been controversy about how such children should be managed, since the outcome ranges from spontaneous recovery to the development of *H. influenzae* type b meningitis. It has been estimated that 26.6% of children with occult *H. influenzae* type b bacteremia will develop meningitis if left untreated. Therefore, all children found to have *H. influenzae* type b bacteremia in this clinical setting should be reevaluated, and a careful search for a focus of infection should be made.

Subsequent management should depend on the clinical picture at reevaluation. If no source of infection is found but the child remains febrile or appears ill, a follow-up blood culture, diagnostic lumbar puncture, and chest radiograph are recommended. Such a patient should be hospitalized and treated with a parenterally administered antimicrobial pending the results of susceptibility testing. If no focus is identified, oral antimicrobial therapy may be substituted after 2 to 5 days to complete a 7- to 10-day total course. If, at reevaluation, no focus is found but the child is afebrile and appears well, blood for culture should be obtained again. However, further diagnostic evaluation, such as a lumbar puncture, may not be necessary. Many experts believe that even in this instance, an oral antimicrobial agent may not be adequate due to the risk of developing a serious focal infection. Therefore, the afebrile, previously bacteremic patient may be managed with a single daily dose of ceftriaxone 50 mg/kg until the second blood culture is known to be sterile and it is apparent that the fever will not recur and no focus of infection has developed. This therapy is sometimes provided in an outpatient setting if availability and reliability of follow-up clinical assessment can be ensured. The necessity for more prolonged, subsequent oral treatment for such children is uncertain.

Other Infections

Children with *H. influenzae* type b *pericarditis* generally need to have a partial or complete pericardiectomy and prolonged antimicrobial treatment. *H. influenzae* type b endocarditis is usually treated with antimicrobials for 6 weeks, although shorter courses have not received clinical evaluation. *Purpura fulminans* associated with *H. influenzae* type b bacteremia requires intensive supportive therapy. *H. influenzae* type b also has been reported to cause epididymo-orchitis, primary peritonitis, urinary tract infection, and endophthalmitis; these infections require regimens lasting 10 to 14 days, 7 to 10 days, 14 days, and 14 days of parenteral antimicrobial therapy, respectively.

PREVENTION

Chemoprophylaxis

Before the introduction of *H. influenzae* type b conjugate vaccines, it was realized that close contacts, younger than 48 months of age, of patients with invasive *H. influenzae* type b infections were at increased risk of invasive infection when exposed to an index case. The degree of increased risk was inversely related to age (for children older than 3 months). About half of secondary disease among susceptible household contacts occurred in the first week after hospitalization of the index patient, although new cases of disease in susceptible household contacts occurred from 1 to 11 months after illness in the index patient. More than 25% of secondary cases were recognized after 30 days. These realizations prompted widespread use of chemoprophylaxis in exposed household contact groups. However, the excellent efficacy associated with conjugate vaccine administration in the United States has allowed important changes in the recommendations for chemoprophylaxis of household contacts. Many children are now protected against spread of *H. influenzae* type b by prior immunization with a licensed conjugate vaccine against *H. influenzae* type b. Moreover, with the widespread use of conjugate vaccines, the rate of colonization with *H. influenzae* type b has decreased among immunized children.

The goal of chemoprophylaxis presumably is to prevent a susceptible child from acquiring *H. influenzae* type b from contacts by eliminating colonization in all members of the relevant group of close contacts (usually household contacts). Rifampin is the prophylactic agent of choice and should be administered as soon as possible after hospitalization of the index patient. Prophylaxis initiated 7 days or more after hospitalization of the index patient may still be of benefit, since adults and older children in such groups may transmit *H. influenzae* type b to susceptible children even though they are at little risk for invasive infection themselves. Therefore, rifampin prophylaxis should be provided to all members of the household contact group if the household contains one or more children younger than 48 months who are not fully immunized. *Fully immunized* in this instance is defined as having received at least one dose of an *H. influenzae* type b conjugate vaccine at 15 months of age or older, two doses at 12 to 14 months of age, or two or more doses when younger than 12 months of age with a booster dose at 12 months of age or older. An exception is made when the household contact group includes a fully vaccinated immunocompromised child because the vaccination may have been ineffective. The household contact group is defined as individuals residing with the index patient or a nonresident who spent 4 or more hours with the index patient for at least 5 of the 7 days preceding the day of hospitalization of the index patient. When the household contact group requires prophylaxis under these guidelines, the index patient also should receive rifampin prophylaxis.

Although recommendations for chemoprophylaxis to prevent secondary *H. influenzae* type b infections in household contact groups have been widely accepted, there has been disagreement about the use of rifampin for children enrolled in day care centers. First, because the data on the risk of secondary *H. influenzae* type b infection among children who attend group day care are conflicting, some believe that the risk is too low to justify the effort associated with rifampin administration in the day care setting. Second, because of the many different caretakers and physicians involved, it is often difficult to institute a uniform policy. Third, in the day care setting, children who are treated may soon become recolonized with *H. influenzae* type b from untreated siblings. A few general guidelines for chemoprophylaxis might be useful in evaluating a day care setting for possible rifampin administration.

1. Contacts in day care homes resembling households, such as those with children younger than 2 years of age in which contact is at least 25 hours per week, may benefit from rifampin prophylaxis.
2. When two or more cases of invasive disease have occurred within 60 days among attendees, administering rifampin to all attendees and supervisory personnel is recommended regardless of the size of the center.
3. If all day care contacts are older than 2 years of age, prophylaxis need not be given.

The dose guidelines for rifampin are as follows:

- *0 to 1 month:* 10 mg/kg once a day for 4 days.
- *>1 month:* 20 mg/kg (max: 600 mg per dose) once a day for 4 days.

Rifampin is not recommended for pregnant women because its effects on the fetus are not established. Rifampin induces the production of enzymes that metabolize oral contraceptives and, thus, may reduce their level of effectiveness. Other methods of contraception should be used for the duration of rifampin administration. Also, rifampin turns urine, saliva, and tears a reddish orange color and may permanently stain soft contact lenses.

Immunoprophylaxis: Vaccines

There are four licensed *H. influenzae* type b conjugate vaccines that differ in the carrier protein used, the polysaccharide molecular size, and the spacer that conjugates the saccharide to the protein: PRP-D (ProHIBiT, Connaught Laboratories) employs diphtheria toxoid as the carrier protein; HbOC (HibTITER, Lederle-Praxis) has an oligosaccharide linked to a nontoxic mutant diphtheria toxin called CRM_{197}; PRP-OMP (PedvaxHIB, Merck, Sharp & Dohme) has an outer membrane protein complex of *Neisseria meningitidis* group B as the carrier, and PRP-T (ActHIB/OmniHib, Pasteur Merieux Vaccine, Smith-Kline Beecham) employs a tetanus toxoid carrier. Two combination vaccines containing *H. influenzae* type b conjugate vaccines have been licensed in the United States. In one, HbOC is combined with DTP (TETRAMUNE). In the other, PRP-T is reconstituted with Connaught DTP immediately before administration. These combination vaccines contain the same concentration of immunogens as the individual vaccines.

The recommended regimens for the primary series are as follows:

- *Children younger than 7 months of age:* a three-dose series of HbOC or PRP-T or a two-dose series of PRP-OMP is given at 2-month intervals starting at 2 months of age. PRP-D is not recommended for children younger than 12 months of age. A booster dose of vaccine at 12 to 15 months of age is recommended for those who have completed the primary series. The same conjugate vaccine should be used for all the doses in the primary series, but any conjugate vaccine may be used for the booster dose.
- *Children starting immunization at 7 to 11 months of age:* three doses of HbOC, PRP-T, or PRP-OMP are recommended for all three conjugate vaccines. Two doses are given at 2-month intervals, and a booster dose is given at 12 to 18 months of age, preferably at least 2 months after the second dose.
- *Children starting immunization at 12 to 14 months of age:* two doses are recommended at a 2-month interval.
- *Children starting immunization at 15 to 59 months of age:* a single dose of any licensed conjugate vaccine is given.
- *Unvaccinated children older than 59 months of age with underlying conditions that predispose them to H. influenzae type b disease,* for example, sickle cell disease or asplenia: a single dose of any licensed conjugate vaccine. Special circumstances may require additional doses of vaccine. For example, two doses of any conjugate vaccine, 1 to 2 months apart, are recommended for children older than 59 months of age who are immunocompromised by HIV, IgG2 deficiency, malignancy, or bone marrow transplant. In this last instance, a two-dose regimen administered at 12 and 24 months produces the highest anticapsular antibody concentration.

Children who have had invasive *H. influenzae* type b disease when younger than 24 months, regardless of vaccination status, should be revaccinated during the convalescent period, 1 month after the onset of disease, according to the age-appropriate schedule for an unvaccinated child. For those 24 months of age or older who experience invasive *H. influenzae* type b disease, no further immunization is necessary, since the disease most likely generates a protective immune response.

H. influenzae type b infection may occur in children who were immunized. In some of these children the onset of disease will occur within a week of conjugate vaccination, before the vaccination is able to elicit a response. In others, *H. influenzae* type b infection will occur 2 or more weeks after vaccination. In this instance, when vaccination was provided at 15 months of age or older, quantitative immunoglobulins should be measured to eliminate the possibility of an immunodeficiency syndrome. Whether such evaluation is required for children who experience invasive disease during or after the primary series should be individualized.

LEPTOSPIROSIS

MICHAEL GREEN, M.D., M.P.H.

Leptospirosis is an uncommon but important infectious syndrome characterized by biphasic timing and protean manifestations. The illness is caused by spirochetes belonging to the genus *Leptospira*, of which *Leptospira interrogans* is the major pathogenic species. Animals are the major reservoir of leptospirosis. Historically, the risk of contracting this disease is limited to individuals exposed to ill animals or to stagnant pools of water contaminated with urine from infected animals, most commonly rats. However, more recently, acquisition has occurred increasingly in urban settings in children or adults exposed to dogs with chronic leptospiruria. *Leptospira* enters the human bloodstream after exposure to contaminated water or infected animal tissue, with subsequent penetration through intact mucous membranes or abraded skin.

Leptospirosis typically presents abruptly with a nonspecific, influenza-like illness characterized by fever, headache, myalgia, and conjunctival suffusion. This initial stage spontaneously resolves 4 to 7 days later. After an afebrile interval of several days, a second, or immune, phase occurs. It has been characterized as either anicteric (associated with aseptic meningitis, uveitis, rash, and fever) or the more severe icteric, or Weil's syndrome (jaundice, hemorrhage, renal failure, and myocarditis). The immune phase lasts from 1 to 30 days and may appear to be continuous with the initial phase in patients manifesting icteric leptospirosis. Fatalities are uncommon and occur only in patients experiencing icteric leptospirosis.

The role of antimicrobial therapy in the treatment of leptospirosis remains controversial. The vast majority of infectious episodes appear to be self-limited. This, along with the inadequate nature of many of the published treatment trials in humans, explains the lack of conclusive data regarding antimicrobial therapy of leptospirosis. Data obtained from in vitro susceptibility testing, as well as from experimental models of infections in animals, suggest that penicillin or tetracycline (doxycycline) should be effective therapy in humans. Animal studies have demonstrated improved survival even with the delayed use of antimicrobials, thus challenging the long-standing perception that therapeutic benefit is limited to cases treated within the first 4 days of illness. Results of two small but well-designed controlled trials in humans provide the best available data. In the first of these studies, doxycycline therapy resulted in a decreased duration of illness compared with placebo controls in adults presenting early in the illness (average duration of symptoms of 45 hours). In the second study, penicillin was shown to shorten the period of illness (including fever, renal insufficiency, and hepatic tenderness) compared with placebo in patients presenting with late (average 9 days) symptoms, supporting the results of late treatment from the animal model.

Most authorities recommend antibiotic therapy if the diagnosis of leptospirosis is considered possible or probable in a patient who has been ill for less than 5 to 7 days. The recent study demonstrating benefit in patients with late disease suggests that treatment in this group should be considered as well. Tetracycline or doxycycline may be the drug of choice for older children and adults. The dose of tetracycline is 20 to 40 mg/kg/d in four divided doses given either PO or IV. The dose of doxycycline is 5 mg/kg/d in two divided doses given PO or IV (max: 200 mg/d). The dose of penicillin is 250,000 U/kg/d in four to six divided doses given either IV or IM (max: 12 million units per day). The duration of therapy is 7 days regardless of therapeutic regimen. Clinicians treating patients who have leptospirosis should be aware that a Jarisch-Herxheimer reaction has been observed in some patients receiving penicillin, but this appears to be uncommon and not severe enough to prevent the use of penicillin.

In addition to antimicrobial therapy, supportive care may be necessary for patients with icteric leptospirosis. Attention should be paid to the potential development of renal failure, hemorrhage, or myocarditis. These complications are much more likely to occur in severely jaundiced patients. Correction of abnormalities in fluid and electrolyte status and the implementation of dialysis in cases of severe or prolonged renal failure are necessary. Although electrocardiographic changes may occur frequently in patients during the leptospiremic phase, pathologic involvement of the heart is uncommon. However, congestive heart failure and cardiovascular collapse may occur. Early recognition and appropriate treatment for these complications should result in improved outcome in those patients with more severe disease.

REFERENCES

1. Edwards CN, Nicholson GD, Hassell TA, Everard COR, Callender J: Penicillin therapy in icteric leptospirosis. Am J Trop Med Hyg 39:388–390, 1988.
2. McClain BL, Ballou WR, Harrison SM, Steinweg DL: Doxycycline therapy for leptospirosis. Ann Intern Med 100:696–698, 1984.

LEPROSY (HANSEN'S DISEASE)

ROBERT H. GELBER, M.D.

Leprosy (Hansen's disease) is a chronic infectious disease caused by *Mycobacterium leprae*. It is only rarely fatal but, owing to the predilection of the causative agent for peripheral nerves, may cause insensitivity (particularly to temperature, pain, and fine touch), myopathy, and resultant deformity. The World Health Organization (WHO) estimates that there are 5 to 6 million cases worldwide.

The successful treatment of leprosy requires long-term compliance with an appropriate antimicrobial regimen, recognition of and considered intervention for a variety of immunologically determined reactional states, the patients' cooperation in protecting insensitive parts from further damage, and skilled reconstructive and cosmetic surgery for established disabilities and deformities. Compliance in any disease requiring prolonged therapy is often inadequate. This may be a special problem in leprosy because of the lack of troublesome symptoms both initially and particularly after some months or years of treatment and, also, because of reactional symptoms often perceived by the patient to be the result of therapy itself. Because of social stigma, patients and their parents are often fearful of institutionalization and rejection by other family members and friends, do not seek medical attention for a diagnosis that they suspect, or reject the diagnosis and therapy when offered by a professional.

Sociocultural fears and expectations decidedly affect patients' lives. Many patients believe their disease is a result of some wrongdoing. On diagnosis, patients frequently remove themselves from the life of their families. They may begin to use separate dishes and toilet facilities and to sleep alone. Because of the belief in certain cultures that the disease is in the blood and because in some countries it had been the practice to separate children at birth from affected parents, patients frequently believe that they should not parent children. Children with established deformities become stigmatized and often are ridiculed by their peers. Both functional and cosmetic repairs are integral to the success of medical therapy and allow patients to live normally in society. Education and counseling are necessary initially and on a continuing basis to help patients comply with therapy and not allow certain cultural and psychosocial aspects of the diagnosis to contribute to debilitation.

Leprosy is a disease with a distinct clinicopathologic spectrum. The great majority of pediatric patients, fortunately, have the generally milder tuberculoid (paucibacillary) form of the disease. Patients with tuberculoid leprosy have one or a few hypopigmented, anesthetic macules often with erythematous borders or evidence of asymmetric peripheral neuropathy, most commonly of the ulnar nerve. Tuberculoid patients have dermal granulomas, few if any acid-fast bacilli, and demonstrable cellular immunity to *M. leprae*. On the other pole of the spectrum, lepromatous (multibacillary) patients have nodular and infiltrated skin lesions, later but more symmetric peripheral neuropathy, and frequently *chronic nasal congestion*. On skin biopsy, lepromatous patients have numerous acid-fast bacilli in the dermis and highly vacuolated or foamy macrophages. There is an absence of protective cellular immune responses to the causative *Mycobacterium*. Patients in the middle of the spectrum, borderline leprosy, have features of both polar forms.

TREATMENT

Chemotherapy

The mean age of onset of leprosy is in the 20s, and in many patients, the first signs of the disease develop in the first decade or two of life. Pediatric disease is generally mild and without substantial peripheral neuropathy. Because initiation of therapy largely arrests subsequent neuropathy and deformity, early disease detection and initiation of treatment are critical to prevention of serious neuromuscular sequelae. Unfortunately, the very places where the disease is most prevalent are poor and lacking in medical infrastructure—hence, the unavailability of the long-term therapy and care required for a salutary outcome. As a consequence, fewer than half of the patients worldwide receive any therapy whatsoever.

Dapsone

Because of the enormous numbers of *M. leprae* and the lack of cell-mediated immunity to *M. leprae*, the lepromatous form of leprosy presents the greater therapeutic difficulty. Dapsone (4,4'-diaminodiphenylsulfone, or DDS) is still the agent of choice for treating all forms of leprosy (Table 1). It is the only agent approved for general use as treatment of leprosy in the United States and has the virtues of being relatively safe, effective, and inexpensive. Dapsone is available in 25-mg and 100-mg tablets. In lepromatous leprosy, administration of dapsone should be initiated and maintained as a single adult daily dose of 100 mg. Suggested pediatric doses are the following: for ages 2 to 5 years, 25 mg three times weekly, for ages 6 to 12 years, 25 mg daily, and for ages 13 to 18 years, 50 mg daily. Although previously leprologists had built up to the maintenance dose slowly and discontinued dapsone during reactions, particularly erythema nodosum leprosum (ENL), these measures no longer appear

reasonable. Dapsone is cross-allergenic with sulfonamides and should not be initiated in patients with a history of sulfa allergy. It may cause a hemolytic anemia, particularly in patients deficient in glucose-6-phosphate dehydrogenase (G-6-PD), and may result in dose-related methemoglobinemia and sulfhemoglobinemia in certain patients. Early in therapy, the sulfone syndrome (associated with an initially morbilliform rash, followed by an exfoliative dermatitis and at times a mononucleosis-type blood picture, fever, lymphadenopathy, hemolytic anemia, and hepatic dysfunction) uncommonly occurs, and corticosteroids in addition to discontinuation of dapsone may be necessary.

Dapsone monotherapy of lepromatous leprosy may result in the development of dapsone-resistant relapse. This becomes clinically apparent with the development of new lesions despite continued dapsone administration and occurs at a minimum of 5 years after the initiation of dapsone therapy. The risks for dapsone-resistant relapse vary between 10% and 40% in different series. Regular full-dose dapsone monotherapy results in the lower percentage of dapsone-resistant relapse, whereas lower-dose regimens and intermittent adherence to therapy predispose to the higher percentage of resistant relapse. Because of the potential of resistant relapse, borderline and lepromatous leprosy ideally should be treated with at least two effective agents. Furthermore, even after 10 or more years of dapsone therapy, lepromatous leprosy patients harbor viable, dapsone-sensitive *M. leprae* "persisters." *It remains unclear what risk these persisters pose for clinical relapse if therapy is discontinued, and hence the safety of ever discontinuing treatment for lepromatous leprosy is uncertain.*

In certain remote regions, where patients do not have access to medical facilities and cannot be expected to take medication regularly, the repository sulfone DADDS* (225 mg IM every 77 days in adults and proportionally less according to weight in children) might be substituted for dapsone in all forms of leprosy. However, resulting plasma levels of DDS are low, and the potential for developing dapsone resistance is of sufficient magnitude that treatment of the lepromatous form of the disease with this agent alone should be avoided if at all possible.

Rifampin

In both animal and human studies, rifampin has proved to be significantly more potent than dapsone against *M. leprae*. It is available in 150-mg and 300-mg capsules. A single daily adult dose of 600 mg is recommended, and proportionately less is used for children, generally 150 mg/d for ages 2 to 5 years, 300 mg/d for ages 6 to 12 years, and 600 mg/d for ages 13 to 18 years, depending on body weight (10 to 20 mg/kg, not to exceed 600 mg/d). Rifampin turns the urine orange-red. Because it may be hepatotoxic, rifampin should be avoided in all patients with established liver dysfunction. *Discontinuation of rifampin followed by reinstitution has been associated with severe and even fatal episodes of thrombocytopenia and renal failure.* There is no available information on what duration of rifampin together with dapsone will prevent drug-resistant relapse and whether such combination chemotherapy for any duration will allow discontinuation of therapy without subsequent relapse from persisters. Furthermore, the cost of daily rifampin, about $300 per adult patient-year, is prohibitively expensive in most developing nations where leprosy is a problem. Hence, the WHO recommends monthly rifampin for the therapy of leprosy.

Second-Line Drugs

Particularly because of allergy to sulfones and in the therapy of sulfone resistance, other second-line antimicrobial agents may be necessary to treat leprosy.

TABLE 1. Pediatric Doses of the Most Important Antimicrobials for Leprosy

| DRUG | DOSE | | |
	2–5 YEARS OF AGE	6–12 YEARS OF AGE	13–18 YEARS OF AGE
Dapsone	25 mg three times weekly	25 mg/d	50 mg/d
Rifampin*	150 mg/d	300 mg/d	600 mg/d

*Dose is 10–20 mg/kg, not to exceed 600 mg/d.

---

*DADDS (4-4'diacetyl-diaminodiphenylsulfone) is not available in the United States.

Clofazimine* (Lamprene) appears as potent as dapsone against *M. leprae*. In adults, 50 to 100 mg/d or two to three times weekly PO is an effective alternative to dapsone administration. Its administration, unfortunately, is associated with a red-black discoloration of the skin, which may be unnoticeable in blacks and other dark-skinned persons but is cosmetically unacceptable to many people with lighter complexions. Clofazimine-induced gastrointestinal side effects of a mild to moderate degree affect some patients.

Ethionamide† is even more active than dapsone against *M. leprae* and, when used, should be given in a once-daily adult dose of 250 to 375 mg and proportionally less in children. Unfortunately, gastrointestinal intolerance to ethionamide is common, as is liver dysfunction, particularly when it is used together with rifampin. Indeed, if such a combination is used, liver function tests should be carefully monitored.

Streptomycin 1 g three times weekly IM in adults and proportionally less in children is as potent as dapsone against *M. leprae*. However, because of its potential for nephrotoxicity and eighth nerve damage, no more than 1 year's therapy can be recommended. Hence, streptomycin should be used only with another agent that can be administered on a longer-term basis.

New Agents

Minocycline, some of the newer macrolide antibiotics, particularly clarithromycin, and a number of fluoroquinolones have been found to be bactericidal against *M. leprae* in mice. Minocycline, clarithromycin, and three of the fluoroquinolones, pefloxacin, ofloxacin, and sparfloxacin, have been more rapidly effective than either dapsone or clofazimine in clinical trials. Thus, there are prospects that new antimicrobials may emerge to further improve the therapy of leprosy.

Response to Therapy

On therapy, tuberculoid macules may resolve somewhat, disappear entirely, or remain unchanged. Their anesthetic or hypoesthetic properties may also respond variably to therapy. Lepromatous infiltration does not begin to improve noticeably for a few months. Effective antimicrobials, however, do prevent new lesions and the progressive neuropathy of untreated disease from appearing. It is important that both clinician and patient understand these expectations.

Regimens to Treat Leprosy

Because of growing concerns with the emergence of secondary and even primary dapsone resistance, the WHO in 1981 developed some novel treatment recommendations. Triple-drug therapy was suggested for adults with multibacillary leprosy: rifampin 600 mg once monthly supervised, dapsone 100 mg/d, clofazimine 300 mg once monthly supervised, plus 50 mg/d. The WHO recommends that this therapy be maintained for at least 2 years, preferably until skin smears are bacteriologically negative (negativity generally occurs in 5 years) and that all therapy then be discontinued. For adult patients with paucibacillary disease, dapsone 100 mg/d and rifampin 600 mg monthly, supervised, are recommended for a total of 6 months. My own experience suggests that primary dapsone resistance is most uncommon, the few resistant strains being only partially resistant and sensitive to levels achieved by generally recommended dapsone doses. Furthermore, patients harboring partially dapsone-resistant strains respond clinically to dapsone. In the United States, I recommend dapsone sensitivity studies in newly diagnosed patients. If high-level dapsone resistance is found, multibacillary patients should receive rifampin daily and clofazimine three times weekly, and paucibacillary patients should receive rifampin daily alone.

Monthly rifampin and the reduced duration of therapy recommended by the WHO for both tuberculoid and lepromatous leprosy are largely a result of important economic considerations in developing countries. Because such economic considerations are not particularly relevant in the United States and Western Europe and because there is limited clinical experience with these reduced durations, I have not adopted monthly rifampin or these reduced courses of therapy. For multibacillary leprosy, I and authorities at the G. W. Long Hansen's Disease Center advise rifampin daily for 3 years and dapsone daily lifelong. I treat paucibacillary leprosy with dapsone daily for 5 years. Authorities at the G. W. Long Hansen's Disease Center treat adult paucibacillary leprosy with dapsone 100 mg/d for 3 to 5 years and with rifampin 600 mg/d for the first 6 months.

Reactions and Their Management

In about 50% of patients with lepromatous leprosy, the syndrome of erythema nodosum leprosum (ENL, lepra type 2 reaction) may develop, generally within the first few years of antimicrobial therapy. This syndrome may consist of one or a number of the following manifestations: crops of erythematous, painful skin papules that remain a few days and may pustulate and ulcerate, being most commonly found on the extensor surface of the extremities, fever that may be as high as 105° F (40.5° C), painful neuritis that may result in further nerve damage, lymphadenitis, uveitis, orchitis, and occasionally large joint arthritis and glomerulonephritis. Histopathologically, this syndrome is secondary to a vasculitis and is probably the result of immune complexes. The clinical manifestations may be mild and evanescent or severe, recurrent, and occasionally fatal.

Patients with borderline leprosy may show signs of inflammation, usually within previous skin lesions, and painful neuritis, which may cause further nerve damage and occasionally fever (lepra type 1 reactions). If these occur before therapy, they are termed "downgrading reactions." If they occur during therapy, usually within a few weeks of months of the start of treatment, they are termed "reversal reactions." Therapy is required in the presence of neuritis, with skin inflammation of a sufficient extent that ulceration appears likely, or for cosmetic reasons, especially if lesions involve the face.

Because the majority of cases of childhood leprosy are tuberculoid and because the described reactional states occur in borderline and lepromatous leprosy, reactions are not really as much a problem in affected children as they are in adults.

Corticosteroids are effective in ENL, and generally even the most severe cases can be controlled with adult doses of prednisone (60 mg). In this respect, I have not found alternate-day steroids useful. Individual ENL papules resolve in a matter of days, and control can be best judged by assessment of the prevention of new manifestations. When episodes are controlled, steroid doses can be tapered and then discontinued, generally in 1 to 4 weeks. If ENL appears to be recurrent, thalidomide is the drug of choice for its control and prevention. The dose must be individualized, and the minimal amount necessary to control ENL manifestation is advised. In adults, generally 100 to 400 mg in a single evening dose is sufficient. In the United States and Canada, thalidomide is available to licensed physicians participating as coinvestigators on the investigational license sponsored by Dr. Robert Hastings, G. W. Long Hansen's Disease Center. In the United States, there are a number of National Ambulatory Hansen's Disease Clinics and private physicians licensed to prescribe thalidomide. (For information, call 800-642-2477.) An occasional patient, despite thalidomide therapy, may still require corticosteroids to prevent recurrent ENL.

Because of thalidomide's potential for causing severe birth defects, including phocomelia, it should not be administered to women in the childbearing years. Side effects include tranquilization (to which tolerance generally develops rapidly), leukopenia, and constipation.

Clofazimine, although slow in onset of action and only moderately effective in adult doses of 300 mg/d, may enable one to reduce the steroid requirement for therapy of ENL.

Thalidomide is of no value for lepra type 1 reactions. Corticoste-

---

*Clofazimine is available from the G. W. Long Hansen's Disease Center, Carville, LA 70721.
†This use of ethionamide is not listed by the manufacturer.

roids are usually effective in controlling these reactions in adult doses of prednisone 40 to 60 mg/d, but generally they must be maintained at a lowered dose for a few months to prevent recurrence. Clofazimine may be of some value in decreasing the steroid requirement in these reactions in the same dose as in the treatment of ENL, but it is not as effective in lepra type 1 reactions.

Rehabilitation

Follow-up visits should always include examination of the feet, and plantar ulcers must be vigorously treated with specific antibiotics, debridement, and either bedrest or a total-contact walking cast until healed. Judicious use of extradepth shoes with molded inserts or specially molded shoes is crucial to prevent recurrence. Tendon transfers to permit substitutions of innervated for denervated muscles may provide patients with more functional use of hands, correct footdrop, and enable them to close their eyes so that corneal trauma and its sequelae will not lead to blindness. If maximal results are to be expected, reconstructive surgery should not be initiated until patients have received at least 6 months of therapy directed against *M. leprae* and at least 6 months have passed since signs of reaction have abated. When possible, mechanical devices may help the severely deformed patients, and special job training may be necessary to prevent trauma and further disability.

Prophylaxis

The close, prolonged, intimate contact of household members of lepromatous patients poses some risk for the development of subsequent disease (about 10% in endemic countries and 1% in nonendemic locales). Although tuberculoid leprosy is not contagious, family members of tuberculoid patients may be incubating disease obtained from the same source. I recommend that household contacts of patients be examined annually for 5 to 7 years, preferably by a physician experienced in leprosy. Health workers and casual contacts appear to be at no significant risk. Therefore, when patients are hospitalized, no isolation requirements are necessary.

Trials of chemoprophylaxis with sulfones have at most been marginally effective. Thus, they are not generally recommended. Bacille Calmette-Guérin (BCG) vaccination has been moderately successful in some locales and unsuccessful in others. It is not generally recommended. Unfortunately, a recent vaccine trial using the combination of killed *M. leprae* with BCG has proved no more effective than BCG alone. On the other hand, vaccination of mice with *M. leprae* subunits, largely proteinaceous and devoid of certain immunosuppressive *M. leprae* carbohydrates and lipids, has proved to result in far improved vaccine immunity than killed *M. leprae* itself. Thus, there are prospects that a truly effective human vaccine against leprosy may yet be developed.

LISTERIA MONOCYTOGENES

STEPHEN BAUMGART, M.D.
BARBARA IANNI, D.O.

EPIDEMIOLOGY

Listeria monocytogenes is reemerging as a commonly recognized and virulent pathogen in neonatal infection. Four major epidemic outbreaks of listeriosis have been identified in relation to food product contamination since 1981. Sporadic occurrences also have been reported, which were perhaps related to food contamination, particularly of unpasteurized milk and milk products. Current estimates suggest that newborn infection with *Listeria* occurs in 5 to 12 per 100,000 births.

CLINICAL MANIFESTATIONS

Maternal Infection

Newborn infections are sometimes heralded by maternal symptoms of a flu-like illness occurring 3 to 30 days before birth in approximately 45% of cases. Amniotic fluid with a dark appearance of meconium or hemorrhagic staining is frequently reported. *L. monocytogenes* is often recovered from cultures of amniotic fluid in infected pregnancies. Gram stain of amniotic fluid or meconium has been suggested in endemic outbreaks of listeriosis to screen for intrapartum infection.

Early- and Late-Onset Neonatal Infections

Neonatal infection with *L. monocytogenes* is an often fatal disease. *Neonatal listeriosis* is similar to *sepsis neonatorum* caused by group B streptococci, and two forms are often described:

1. Early-onset septicemia with severe respiratory failure and shock, which is acquired perinatally and is manifest before 72 hours of age
2. Late-onset bacteremia with meningitis, which occurs after 5 days of life

The overall survival for infants with listeriosis treated conventionally varies from 50% to 97%, since early-onset and late-onset syndromes are often combined in one series. However, mortality is probably higher in newborn babies with early-onset disease due to *L. monocytogenes*, who manifest severe respiratory failure, pneumonia, pulmonary hypertension, and septic shock more often than do those with late-onset bacteremia.

Necropsy and Pathogenesis

At autopsy, early-onset neonatal sepsis includes a process of necrotizing pneumonitis and miliary lung abscess formation known as *granulomatosis infantisepticum*. In the pathogenesis of this disorder, the *L. monocytogenes* bacillus is first phagocytized by the lung and tissue macrophages, which activates and proliferates a systemic inflammatory response. In animals, the bacteria resist being killed and may actually become persistent intracellular parasites. Diffuse and generalized tissue microgranulomatosis results, particularly in the lung, with extensive suppurative parenchymal necrosis. Inflammation of the lungs, liver, spleen, adrenals, skin, and meninges occurs in up to 80% of those infants with systemic sepsis and severe respiratory failure exacerbated by pulmonary hypertension.

ANTIMICROBIAL THERAPY

Usually in severe *Listeria* infections, particularly in the immunocompromised host (e.g., the neonate), parenteral administration of ampicillin 100 to 200 mg/kg/d divided into two or three doses is recommended. Initially, this therapy is given in combination with an aminoglycoside (gentamicin 5 mg/kg/d divided similarly, with monitoring of serum levels at peak and trough intervals), since animal studies indicate synergy. Therapy is continued for at least 14 days. *Listeria* may be sensitive to chloramphenicol, tetracyclines, and sulfonamides, but potential neonatal toxicities have been demonstrated for these agents. Cephalosporins are not useful for treating *Listeria* infections.

RECENT ADVANCES IN SUPPORTIVE THERAPY: ECMO

Since 1987, extracorporeal membrane oxygenation (ECMO), an aggressive new therapy, has been employed to treat infants with overwhelming early-onset *Listeria* infection. ECMO is long-term cardiopulmonary bypass used predominantly in neonates experiencing severe respiratory failure, pulmonary hypertension, and shock refractory to conventional treatments. Three- to five-day courses of ECMO are often sufficient to rescue babies from a variety of life-threatening neonatal conditions. Longer durations of 10 to 20 days, however, may be required for pneumonia with *L. monocytogenes*.

Hirschl et al.[1] recently reported 9 infants with severe respiratory failure and sepsis caused by *L. monocytogenes*. The diagnosis of pneumonia was made in all patients based on radiographic appearance or secretions producing *L. monocytogenes* on culture. Antibiotic sensitivity demonstrated susceptibility to ampicillin and gentamicin, and all infants were treated accordingly with at least 2 weeks of antibiotic therapy. All 9 infants experienced progressive respiratory deterioration despite hyperventilatory management, and patients developed hemodynamic instability, including hypertension, poor capillary perfusion, and acidemia. Infants were placed on ECMO for 14 to 96 hours. All patients required venoarterial extracorporeal support to treat pneumonia and septic shock. The duration of ECMO therapy for infants with *L. monocytogenes* sepsis or pneumonia ranged from 6 to 19 days, which is longer than the duration of ECMO for other neonatal bacterial infections. Lung recovery ensued with survival in 6 infants, and death followed failure to improve in 2 patients and after massive intracranial hemorrhage in 1 infant. Surviving infants required an additional 2 to 24 days on mechanical respirators after discontinuation of ECMO support. Neonatal follow-up revealed normal development in 5 survivors, with 1 infant found intellectually normal but suspect for mild hypotonicity in the lower extremities delaying gross motor milestone achievement. This child is now ambulatory at 4 years, with normal motor and cognitive function.

Flexible bronchoscopy for persistent atelectasis may be performed during cardiopulmonary bypass without the need for simultaneous ventilation, since the lungs are at rest. Segmental lung lavage performed under direct visualization allows mobilization of copious inspissated secretions and necrotic debris, with subsequent lung reexpansion.

CONCLUSION

ECMO intervention in neonatal respiratory failure provides support while pulmonary hypertension associated with early-onset, acute lung disease in this population is reversed. With *Listeria* infection, however, pulmonary hypertension is compounded by an underlying granulating parenchymal process that may prolong resolution of the respiratory failure. Nevertheless, necrotizing pneumonitis with *Listeria* infection is potentially a reversible process, and lung healing is an eventual expectation with appropriate antimicrobial therapy. A prolonged but often successful course may be expected when supporting patients with *Listeria* on ECMO.

REFERENCES

1. Hirschl R, Butler S, Corcoran L, Baumgart S: *Listeria monocytogenes* and severe newborn respiratory failure supported with extracorporeal membrane oxygenation. Am J Dis Child 148:513–517, 1994.
2. Pinner RW, Schuchat A, Swaminathan B, Hayes PS, Deaver KA, Weaver RE, Plikaytis BD, Reeves M, Broome CV, Wenger JD, The Listeria Study Group: II. Microbiologic and epidemiologic investigation. JAMA 267:2046–2050, 1992.
3. Schuchat A, Deaver KA, Wenger JD, Plikaytis BD, Mascola L, Pinner RW, Reingold AL, Broome CV, The Listeria Study Group: I. Case control of dietary risk factors. JAMA 267:2041–2045, 1992.

LYME DISEASE

Eugene D. Shapiro, m.d.

Lyme disease, caused by the spirochete *Borrelia burgdorferi*, is transmitted by ticks of the genus *Ixodes* (*Ixodes dammini*, the deer tick, in the eastern and midwestern United States, and *Ixodes pacificus*, the western black-legged tick, on the West Coast). Infection with *B. burgdorferi* results in a wide spectrum of clinical manifestations, from asymptomatic infection to encephalomyelitis. Because the disease has been recognized only recently, there are limited data

about optimal treatment regimens and about long-term outcomes after treatment, especially in children. It is likely that as more information becomes available and as new antimicrobials are licensed, some of the following recommendations will change. In addition, in many instances there are no data from clinical trials of treatment of children, so the recommendations are extrapolated from studies conducted with adults.

DIAGNOSIS

Although this text is not intended to address the issue of diagnosis, because of extraordinary publicity about this disease in the lay press, an exception must be made for Lyme disease, since misdiagnosis is so common.[1] Indeed, the most common reason for failure of treatment of Lyme disease is misdiagnosis. Methods of confirming that the organism is present in a patient (e.g., culture, antigen detection, or histopathology) have poor sensitivity or specificity or both and may require invasive procedures (e.g., biopsy of the skin) to obtain an appropriate specimen to test. Consequently, much reliance has been placed on serologic tests, such as enzyme-linked immunosorbent assays (ELISA), that measure the concentration of a patient's antibodies directed against the organism. Unfortunately, most of these tests are performed with prepackaged commercial kits that have been found to be unreliable, with unacceptably high rates of false negative and especially of false positive results. In addition, because patients often do not produce measurable concentrations of specific antibodies until 4 to 6 weeks after the onset of the infection, most patients with early Lyme disease will not have antibodies to *B. burgdorferi* that are detectable by conventional means.

Clinical manifestations are the most important factor in making the diagnosis. Physicians must evaluate the results of antibody tests critically. Patients with atypical symptoms (e.g., chronic fatigue or chronic arthralgias alone) are unlikely to have Lyme disease even if their antibody test is positive. In questionable cases such as these, the antibody test should be repeated in a reference laboratory (which periodically prepare their own fresh materials for the tests and use strict quality controls) and confirmed with a western immunoblot test (again performed by a reference laboratory rather than with a prepackaged commercial kit) before treatment is initiated. Hopefully, within the next few years, serologic tests that are more specific and better standardized will become more widely available.

TREATMENT

Appropriate treatment depends on the stage of the disease and the patient's clinical manifestations.[2] The stages of disease are generally divided into early and late disease.

Early Disease

Erythema Migrans

The first clinical manifestation of Lyme disease is erythema migrans, a characteristic expanding, erythematous, annular rash that occurs (typically within 7 to 10 days of the tick bite but occasionally up to a month later) at the site of the bite. The lesion may or may not demonstrate clearing in the center. The center may also become vesicular or, rarely, necrotic. The single erythema migrans lesion may or may not be accompanied by systemic symptoms, such as fever and myalgias. Often, dissemination occurs, with the development of multiple erythema migrans lesions accompanied by systemic symptoms. Occasionally, early Lyme disease manifests as a flu-like illness without erythema migrans (because the rash either is absent or is unrecognized). Because specific antibodies usually are not detectable at this stage of the illness, the diagnosis rarely can be made without the rash.

The recommended treatment regimens for early Lyme disease are shown in Table 1. Doxycycline and amoxicillin are considered to be equivalent in their therapeutic efficacy. Amoxicillin and doxycycline, respectively, have largely replaced penicillin and tetracycline as standard agents for treatment because they are better absorbed, are equally

TABLE 1. Antimicrobial Treatment of Lyme Borreliosis

1. Early Lyme disease
   a. Erythema migrans and disseminated early disease without focal findings
      Doxycycline 100 mg b.i.d. for 21 days (do not use in children <9 years of age)

      or

      Amoxicillin 50 mg/kg/d divided t.i.d. (max: 500 mg per dose) for 21 days
      An alternative agent for those who cannot take either amoxicillin or doxycycline is erythromycin 30–50 mg/kg/d divided q.i.d. (max: 250 mg per dose) for 21 days
   b. Facial nerve palsy
      Treat as for erythema migrans but for 21–30 days; do not use corticosteroids
   c. Carditis
      Treat as for late neurologic disease
   d. Meningitis
      Treat as for late neurologic disease
2. Late Lyme disease
   a. Neurologic disease*
      Ceftriaxone 50–80 mg/kg/d in a single dose IV or IM (max: 2 g) for 14–21 days

      or

      Penicillin G 200,000–400,000 U/kg/d IV divided q4h (max: 20 million U/d) for 14–21 days
   b. Arthritis
      Initial treatment is the same as for erythema migrans except treat for 30 days; if symptoms fail to resolve after 2 months or there is a recurrence, treat as for late neurologic disease

*For isolated palsy of the facial nerve, see 1b.

potent or more potent in vitro against *B. burgdorferi*, and may be administered less frequently. Doxycycline should not be administered to children less than 9 years of age because it may discolor their teeth. A slightly larger proportion of clinical treatment failures have been reported when erythromycin was used to treat early Lyme disease. Consequently, erythromycin should be used only when there are contraindications to the use of both amoxicillin and doxycycline. Although 21 days of treatment usually is recommended for early Lyme disease, a shorter course of treatment (10 days) may be effective but should be reserved for children with a single erythema migrans lesion and no systemic symptoms.

Because both amoxicillin and doxycycline are so effective in the treatment of early Lyme disease, it is not likely that newer antimicrobial agents will offer significant therapeutic benefits (Table 2). For example, studies of azithromycin (a macrolide antimicrobial) and of cefuroxime, conducted with a limited number of patients, have suggested that these drugs are at best equivalent in efficacy to amoxicillin and doxycycline in the treatment of early Lyme disease.

Facial Nerve Palsy

Paralysis of the facial nerve, which also is a manifestation of early disseminated Lyme disease, may develop while erythema migrans is still present and before antibodies to *B. burgdorferi* are detectable. The outcome of seventh nerve palsy due to Lyme disease (with or without antimicrobial therapy) generally is excellent, although varying degrees of paralysis may persist in a very small proportion of patients.

TABLE 2. Drugs Used to Treat Lyme Disease

Azithromycin
Amoxicillin
Doxycycline
Erythromycin
Cefuroxime
Ceftriaxone
Penicillin G

Resolution of the palsy usually occurs within 4 to 6 weeks. The purpose of antimicrobial treatment of facial nerve palsy is to prevent late manifestations of Lyme disease. If palsy of the seventh nerve is the only neurologic manifestation of Lyme disease, the outcome with orally administered antimicrobials is as good as the outcome with parenteral treatment, which, consequently, is not necessary. The oral regimens should be administered for 21 to 30 days as per Table 1. Corticosteroids are unnecessary and may be contraindicated. Although pleocytosis sometimes may be present in the cerebrospinal fluid, there is no evidence, without other neurologic symptoms (such as meningitis or radiculitis), that parenteral therapy is necessary for such patients. Nevertheless, some physicians prefer to treat patients who have a pleocytosis with antimicrobials administered parenterally.

Carditis

Lyme carditis, which usually presents with abnormalities of the conduction system (especially partial to complete atrioventricular block), is rare in children. If it does occur, it is a manifestation of early disseminated disease and should be treated as noted in Table 1.

Meningitis

Aseptic meningitis is an uncommon manifestation of early disseminated Lyme disease. It may be accompanied by other focal neurologic signs and symptoms. Treatment with parenterally administered ceftriaxone or penicillin is indicated.

Late Lyme Disease

Arthritis

Monarticular or oligoarticular arthritis of large joints (typically of the knee) is the classic manifestation of late Lyme disease. A number of different treatment regimens have been used for Lyme arthritis, the superiority of any one of which has not been demonstrated convincingly. Persistence of symptoms after treatment (treatment failure) occurs in a relatively small proportion of patients with either orally administered or parenterally administered antimicrobials. Presumably, in most instances, persistent synovitis is due not to the failure to kill *B. burgdorferi* but rather to either an autoimmune process or reactive inflammation.

If there are no concomitant neurologic symptoms, Lyme arthritis initially should be treated with orally administered amoxicillin or doxycycline. If symptoms persist or recur 2 months after treatment, a single course of parenterally administered penicillin or ceftriaxone should be administered.

Neurologic Symptoms

Encephalitis, encephalopathy, and radiculoneuritis are rare manifestations of Lyme disease in children. To make the diagnosis, it is desirable in the appropriate clinical and epidemiologic setting to document pleocytosis in the cerebrospinal fluid and, in a reference laboratory, the presence of elevated concentrations of serum antibodies against *B. burgdorferi,* as well as the production of specific antibodies against *B. burgdorferi* within the CNS. The latter is documented by determining the CSF index, which is defined as

$$\text{CSF Index} = \frac{\substack{\text{Concentration of } B.\ burgdorferi\text{–specific} \\ \text{antibodies in CSF/Concentration} \\ \text{of total IgG in the CSF}}}{\substack{\text{Concentration of } B.\ burgdorferi\text{–specific} \\ \text{IgG antibodies in the serum/Concentration} \\ \text{of total IgG in the serum}}}$$

A ratio greater than 1 suggests that antibodies against *B. burgdorferi* are being produced in the CSF rather than passively diffusing from the serum via inflamed meninges. Chronic fatigue alone and other nonspecific symptoms, in the absence of other objective abnormalities that are demonstrable by physical examination, nerve conduction tests, or psychometric tests, have not been shown to be associated with Lyme disease. The previously mentioned neurologic syndromes should be treated with parenterally administered antimicrobials, either ceftriaxone or penicillin. As with arthritis, it may take some time after treatment for the symptoms to resolve.

Tick Bites

There have been no studies that demonstrate that prophylactic antimicrobials are indicated for people in endemic areas who are bitten by *Ixodid* ticks.[3] Data indicate that the risk of developing Lyme disease after a recognized bite is very low. Even if a tick is infected, usually it must feed for at least 48 hours before transmission of the organism is likely. Since most people who recognize that they have been bitten will remove the tick within 48 hours, prophylactic therapy with antimicrobials after deer tick bites generally is unnecessary.

REFERENCES

1. Gerber MA, Shapiro ED: Diagnosis of Lyme disease in children. J Pediatr 121:157–162, 1992.
2. Rahn DW, Malawista SE: Lyme disease: Recommendations for diagnosis and treatment. Ann Intern Med 114:472–481, 1991.
3. Shapiro ED, Gerber MA, Holabird N, et al: A controlled trial of antimicrobial prophylaxis for Lyme disease after deer-tick bites. N Engl J Med 327:1769–1773, 1992.

MENINGOCOCCAL INFECTIONS

MARY P. GLODE, M.D.

Meningococcal infection was first described in the early 1800s in a manuscript entitled "The Disease Which Raged in Geneva During the Spring of 1805." Meningococcal infections continue to occur both endemically and epidemically, and fulminant meningococcemia remains a very frightening disease to all practitioners. The spectrum of meningococcal infections ranges from occult bacteremia to frank meningococcemia presenting with shock and purpura. The organism (*Neisseria meningitidis*) may also cause purulent conjunctivitis, septic arthritis, pericarditis, pneumonia, or meningitis. Chronic meningococcemia has been described, with a duration of symptoms of several months before the diagnosis. This illness is characterized by intermittent fevers, rash, and arthralgia or arthritis.

At least 10 serogroups of meningococci are recognized. These serogroup distinctions are based on differences in the chemical structure of the polysaccharide capsules. In the United States, almost half of all invasive disease is due to serogroup B and the rest to serogroup C. Serogroups W135 and Y are also recognized to occur in the United States. Under both endemic and epidemic conditions, most cases of meningococcal disease occur in young children less than age 2. The major reservoir for the organisms appears to be asymptomatic nasopharyngeal carriage by young adults.

PATHOGENESIS OF INFECTION AND PATHOPHYSIOLOGY OF DISEASE

Invasive disease occurs in exposed, susceptible hosts who lack bactericidal antibody to the organism and who acquire the organism from prolonged intimate contact with a colonized adult. Individuals with specific complement protein deficiencies also have an increased susceptibility to meningococcal infection. Current evidence suggests that the clinical illness seen in individuals with complement deficiencies may be less severe than that seen in normal hosts. It has been proposed that organisms are lysed less effectively in the absence of an intact complement system, and less endotoxin is released. A number of recent studies have suggested that a concurrent viral or *Mycoplasma* respiratory infection may enhance meningococcal invasiveness. Patients with systemic meningococcal disease were significantly more likely than colonized controls to have a concurrent nasal infection with respiratory viruses or *Mycoplasma* species. Nasopha-

ryngeal colonization with pathogenic meningococci may be an immunizing experience or may result in severe invasive disease.

The exact pathophysiology of meningococcemia is not completely understood, but it is recognized that meningococcal endotoxin is a very potent endotoxin relative to other gram-negative organisms. The pathologic lesions seen in fulminant meningococcal disease are similar to the generalized Shwartzman reaction induced in rabbits by endotoxin. Therefore, it is believed that the pathogenesis of tissue injury seen in this disease is mediated primarily through the effects of endotoxin. Current experimental animal work and human studies suggest that liberation of endotoxin results in release of a number of cytokines, including tumor necrosis factor (TNF), interleukin 1 (IL-1), and interleukin 6 (IL-6). These cytokines then initiate the release of other inflammatory mediators, such as platelet-activating factor (PAF), and arachidonic acid products. In addition, activation of the coagulation system and the kinin system occurs, and disseminated intravascular coagulation (DIC) is a frequent feature of meningococcemia. A pathologic study of 200 fatal meningococcal infections revealed myocarditis in 78% of the cases, acute meningitis in 68%, adrenal hemorrhage and necrosis in 48%, and cutaneous hemorrhages in 69% (ranging from isolated petechiae to diffuse purpura).

ANTIBIOTIC THERAPY

The ultimate therapy for meningococcal infections is anticipated to be disease prevention by immunization with polyvalent protein polysaccharide conjugate vaccines. These vaccines are currently under development. In the interim, efforts should be directed toward educating health care providers to recognize potential meningococcal infections and to initiate antibiotic therapy as early as possible. Fever and purpura in a young child or adult should be presumed to be meningococcemia until proven otherwise, and blood cultures should be obtained quickly and intravenous antibiotic therapy should be given. Penicillin remains the drug of choice for meningococcal infections in the United States. Occasionally, young infants presenting as clinical meningococcemia, with fever and purpura, may have infections due to the pneumococcus or *Haemophilus influenzae* (particularly in a splenectomized host, where pneumococcal infection is more likely to present in fulminant fashion), and, therefore, consideration should be given to broadening antibiotic coverage to include a drug effective against beta-lactamase-positive *H. influenzae* type b. A third-generation cephalosporin is most commonly used in these circumstances. Cefotaxime at 150 mg/kg/d in three divided doses or ceftriaxone at a dose of 100 mg/kg/d in two divided doses is a reasonable initial antibiotic choice. Chloramphenicol at a dose of 75 mg/kg/d in four divided doses with close monitoring of serum levels is also acceptable therapy and should be effective against infections due to the meningococcus, *H. influenzae* type b, or the pneumococcus.

Strains of *N. meningitidis* resistant to penicillin have now been reported from several countries, including Spain, South Africa, the United Kingdom, and Canada. Two mechanisms of resistance have been defined. The strains from Spain had an alteration in the penicillin-binding protein, thus affecting permeability of the organism to penicillin. These strains were beta-lactamase negative. Other penicillin-resistant strains reported from South Africa, the United Kingdom, and Canada were penicillinase-producing strains. A number of these strains had acquired a gonococcal plasmid encoding for the production of beta-lactamase.

Although penicillin remains the drug of choice for meningococcal infections it is appropriate for the laboratory to confirm the susceptibility of the organism to penicillin. In addition, one recently published randomized trial compared once-daily ceftriaxone to penicillin G. Forty-two children were randomly assigned to receive either ceftriaxone or penicillin G. The mortality rate in the ceftriaxone-treated patients was 5% compared with 9% in the group treated with penicillin G. This difference was not statistically significant. However, the investigators noted that necrotic skin lesions occurred significantly more frequently in the penicillin G group (8 of 22) compared with the ceftriaxone group (0 of 20). Other complications were not significantly different for the two treatment groups, and no adverse effects of either antibiotic were noted.

ADDITIONAL THERAPIES FOR MENINGOCOCCAL INFECTION

A number of pharmacologic agents have been used to attempt to modify the course of meningococcal infection. Several agents are readily available and routinely used in some medical centers, but their efficacy remains controversial. Several new agents that attempt to block mediators of inflammation are under development and may soon be commercially available.

The agents most commonly considered for use in patients with either meningococcal meningitis or overwhelming meningococcemia with purpura fulminans are corticosteroids. A number of randomized trials looking at the role of steroids in septic shock have been done. In general, it has been difficult to demonstrate any substantial efficacy of steroids in this setting. However, many authorities still recommend the use of steroids, particularly in individuals with overwhelming meningococcemia. Part of the rationale for this therapy is based on the adrenal hemorrhage seen commonly in fatal cases, although it has been difficult to demonstrate adrenocorticosteroid insufficiency at the time of presentation with disease. At our center, we have generally used pharmacologic doses of steroids in patients with overwhelming meningococcemia. A second rationale for the use of steroids derives from the recent trials of dexamethasone (Decadron) in children with bacterial meningitis. A number of studies now support the use of a short course of steroids in children with bacterial meningitis to reduce the frequency of sensorineural hearing loss and to improve neurologic outcome. Although this therapy was primarily studied in children with *H. influenzae* type b meningitis, many experts believe that the pathogenesis of hearing loss may be similar in patients with meningococcal meningitis. The dose of dexamethasone used for prevention of hearing loss was 0.15 mg/kg per dose IV given four times a day for 4 days.

The second controversial, but commonly used, agent in meningococcemia is heparin. A major sequela of meningococcemia with purpura fulminans relates to the DIC and microvascular thrombi that develop, with subsequent ischemia, gangrene, and loss of visible tissue. There are a number of children who survive meningococcemia each year but lose either portions of their extremities or entire extremities as a result of DIC. It is difficult to demonstrate the efficacy of heparin in this setting, and no large prospective, randomized, placebo-controlled trials are available. There are clinical trials comparing outcome in heparin-treated patients with historical controls using prognostic scoring systems. Some of these studies indicate that heparin may be effective in reducing the mortality rate from fulminant meningococcemia. At our institution, children with a clinical diagnosis of meningococcemia are heparinized using a bolus dose of 50 U/kg, followed by a dose of 15 to 20 U/kg/h. Further monitoring and dose adjustment are done by maintaining a level of 0.2 to 0.5 heparin units per milliliter. Complications of heparinization reported in the literature include retinal hemorrhage and cerebral hemorrhage. Other therapeutic modalities that have been reported in patients with DIC and meningococcemia with regard to correction of the coagulopathy include the use of fresh frozen plasma to replace clotting factors that are being consumed in the intravascular thrombosis. In addition, this disease has been demonstrated to result in an acquired deficiency of protein S and protein C, and there are now anecdotal reports of the use of protein C concentrate in patients with purpura fulminans.

Development of immunotherapies for meningococcemia is an area of intense investigation. *N. meningitidis* releases a potent endotoxin that binds to macrophages and initiates the release of various cytokines, including TNF and a variety of interleukins. Activation of the coagulation system and the complement system then ensues, and the host inflammatory response is believed to contribute substantially to the pathology seen in this disease. Initial attempts to intervene and disrupt the host response have included therapeutic trials of hyper-immune globulin prepared from individuals immunized with a vaccine from *Escherichia coli*. This hyperimmune plasma contained high titers of antibody directed against the core glycolipid, which is conserved among gram-negative organisms. However, when clinical trials were conducted, including a trial in 73 children with severe infectious purpura, administration of this hyperimmune plasma did not affect the course of disease or the mortality. Similarly, a study using intravenous immunoglobulin (IVIg) in a rabbit model of meningococcal endotoxin-induced shock concluded that IVIg did not significantly alter the physiologic response to endotoxin challenge, although it did significantly reduce endotoxin and TNF concentrations. No increased survival was seen with IVIg in this animal model.

Further attempts to interfere with the host response to infection have included development of IgM monoclonal antibodies against endotoxin. Although initial results in adults with suspected gram-negative sepsis were encouraging, reevaluation of these studies has led to serious concerns, and no product is available for clinical use. Investigational studies of the use of antibodies to TNF and IL-1 and the use of IL-1 receptor antagonist have shown benefit in animal models of septic shock.

A number of other therapies have been used in patients with fulminant meningococcemia and reported anecdotally to be successful. These should be considered in the category of heroic, unproven therapeutic modalities. They include plasmapheresis, topical application of nitroglycerin to purpuric areas, systemic or local infusions of tissue plasminogen activator, sympathetic blockade with caudal block, use of nifedipine, and use of hyperbaric oxygen to maximize oxygen delivery to ischemic tissue.

The mortality and morbidity from severe meningococcal infection will remain high until new therapeutic modalities are developed or until universal immunization with effective vaccines becomes available. In the interim, education regarding the clinical manifestations of disease and early initiation of therapy in patients with fever and petechiae or fever and purpura remain the current recommendation.

CHEMOPROPHYLAXIS

Transmission of meningococcal organisms occurs by prolonged intimate contact with an individual who has nasopharyngeal colonization with the organism. Approximately 90% of adults have developed anticapsular antibody against the major pathogenic *Neisseria* and, therefore, are not susceptible to infection. This acquisition of humoral immunity is age related. Thus, a higher percentage of young children may be lacking protective antibody and could develop invasive disease once exposed to the organism. The secondary attack rate is estimated to be approximately 3 per 1000, and those at highest risk include young children who are household contacts of a case and nursery school contacts. In general, schoolage contacts are not believed to be at significant risk for secondary disease, and no chemoprophylaxis is routinely recommended. However, outbreaks of disease have occurred among schoolage children. The major antibiotic used for eradication of the organism from the nasopharynx is rifampin. Two rifampin regimens are used, and both are effective in eradicating the organism. The first regimen is a 2-day protocol with rifampin at a dose of 10 mg/kg per dose twice daily for 2 days. The adult dose is 600 mg twice daily for 2 days. A single oral dose of 20 mg/kg/d given once daily for 4 days, with the adult maximum at 600 mg once a day for 4 days, also is effective in eradicating *N. meningitidis*.

Consideration should be given to treating the index patient, since intravenous penicillin may treat systemic disease but may not eradicate the organism from the nasopharynx, and the index patient may serve as a source of transmission to others even after discharge from the hospital. Several other antibiotics have been studied for carriage eradication and appear to be effective. A single dose of 250 mg of ceftriaxone for adults or 125 mg for children under 15 years of age has been studied and was highly effective in eradicting carriage of the meningococcus. In a trial comparing the efficacy of ceftriaxone to the standard dose of rifampin, ceftriaxone had a 97% eradication rate compared with 75% for oral rifampin. A single 750 mg PO dose of ciprofloxacin was also effective in adults in eradicating *N. meningitidis*. All contacts should be advised to seek medical attention immediately if they develop a febrile illness regardless of whether or not they have received chemoprophylaxis.

PREVENTION THROUGH IMMUNIZATION

A quadrivalent meningococcal vaccine is commercially available and contains purified polysaccharides from meningococcus group A, C, W135, and Y. The vaccine appears to be immunogenic and protective in children over age 2. However, children less than age 2 generally have not had a good immunologic response to the purified capsular polysaccharide. In a trial in Brazil, the group C meningococcal polysaccharide vaccine was not effective in preventing disease in children less than age 2. Meningococcal A vaccine may be effective in younger children. In the United States, approximately 50% of invasive disease is produced by serogroup C and 50% by serogroup B. Although extensive efforts have been extended in the development of a group B meningococcal vaccine, none is commercially available. The group B capsular polysaccharide is not immunogenic in animals or humans, and, therefore, attempts to produce a conjugate vaccine or outer membrane protein vaccine are still underway.

Patients at high risk for meningococcal disease, such as military recruits, individuals with recognized complement deficiencies, and splenectomized hosts, should receive the quadrivalent meningococcal vaccine. The question of whether splenectomized hosts have increased susceptibility to meningococcal disease is somewhat controversial, but we recommend meningococcal vaccine in addition to pneumococcal vaccine and *H. influenzae* type b conjugate vaccine for our splenectomized patients. Many physicians also recommend daily antibiotic prophylaxis with penicillin for splenectomized patients. Immunization may be recommended also for individuals traveling outside the United States to parts of the world with epidemic meningococcal disease. Contact the CDC for specific recommendations by country.

REFERENCES

1. Cartwright K, Reilly S, White D, Stuart J: Early treatment with parenteral penicillin in meningococcal disease. Br Med J 305:141–147, 1992.
2. Jafari HS, McCracken GH: Sepsis and septic shock: A review for clinicians. Pediatr Infect Dis J 11:739–748, 1992.
3. Schaad UB, Lips U, Gnehm HE, et al: Dexamethasone therapy for bacterial meningitis in children. Lancet 342:457–461, 1993.

NONTUBERCULOUS (ATYPICAL) MYCOBACTERIAL DISEASE

ANDREW M. MARGILETH, M.D.

Recently, nontuberculous mycobacterial (NTM) infections have been diagnosed and reported in the United States as frequently as *Mycobacterium tuberculosis* (tuberculosis, or TB) infections. Physicians will become more aware of NTM disease, since NTM disseminated disease is being reported more frequently in patients with acquired immunodeficiency syndrome (AIDS). Of the 26 known species of NTM, three (*Mycobacterium avium-intracellulare, Mycobacterium scrofulaceum,* and *Mycobacterium marinum*) account for the majority of NTM disease in children. Although NTM disease is rarely observed in daily practice, it is essential to distinguish patients with NTM disease from those with TB infection to avoid unnecessary and prolonged courses of drugs, as well as the stigma attached to labeling a child as tuberculous. It is also unnecessary for healthy children with a positive NTM-PPD (purified protein derivative) reaction or a suspected NTM infection to undergo prophylactic isoniazid (INH) therapy.

INCIDENCE IN CHILDREN

Atypical mycobacteria are acid-fast bacilli found in the soil, dust, water, and occasionally food (e.g., eggs, milk, and vegetables). Of the 26 species of NTM, none are pathogenic for guinea pigs, as are the human strains, *M. tuberculosis* and *Mycobacterium bovis*. Disease or latent infection produced in humans is usually caused by *M. avium-intracellulare* (MAC), *Mycobacterium xenopi, Mycobacterium fortuitum, Mycobacterium chelonei, M. scrofulaceum, Mycobacterium kansasii,* and *M. marinum*. NTM isolates obtained from closed aspiration of lymph nodes or abscesses and from tissue fluids (cerebrospinal fluid, blood, pleural, peritoneal) or resected tissue that culture more than a few colonies should be diagnostic.

The most common NTM disease in children is cervical lymphadenitis. During 35 years, our study of 145 patients with TB and NTM lymphadenitis showed a definite age-related difference. Most children aged 1 through 12 years had NTM adenitis, whereas most patients over 12 years of age had TB adenitis. MAC accounted for 75% of infected nodes, and 17% were due to *M. scrofulaceum*. Skin, joint, and bone disease are uncommon, and pulmonary NTM disease is rare in children and adolescents. In contrast, NTM pulmonary disease caused by MAC and *M. kansasii* occurs almost exclusively in adults.

Human-to-human transmission of NTM infection has not been documented. Most NTM strains are resistant to antituberculous drugs. Therefore, it is essential to perform mycobacterial cultures and drug susceptibility studies to determine appropriate antituberculous therapy (Table 1).

DISTINGUISHING TUBERCULOSIS FROM NONTUBERCULOUS MYCOBACTERIAL INFECTIONS

When tuberculosis or NTM infection is suspected and a diagnosis is supported by the history, physical examination, tuberculin testing, roentgenographic evidence, or laboratory test results [acid-fast bacillus (AFB) smear or tissue biopsy with DNA probes], physicians must make some therapeutic decisions while awaiting AFB culture reports. Weeks or months may pass before the organism is finally isolated and identified and its drug susceptibility is known. The use of commercially available DNA probes to distinguish the NTM species is strongly recommended. Often, mycobacteria fail to grow, especially the slow-growing NTM species.

Proper application of PPD-T and Mono-Vacc skin tests and accurate measurement of induration by the ballpoint method at 72 hours is essential.[3] If the Mono-Vacc test is reactive and PPD-T reaction is more than 15 mm of induration, infection with TB is probable (Table 1). If the PPD-T induration is less than 10 mm, NTM infection is more likely, especially if the PPD-T is negative and a Mono-Vacc test is positive (2 mm or more). Other clinical factors to help differentiate NTM from TB infection are noted in Table 1.

TABLE 1. Differentiation of Nontuberculous Mycobacterial (NTM) Infections From *M. tuberculosis* Disease in 145 AFB Culture-Positive Patients: 1957 to July 1, 1993

CLINICAL FEATURES	*Mycobacterium tuberculosis*	NONTUBERCULOUS MYCOBACTERIA
History of contact*	Common	Rare
Lymphadenitis, cervical	Uncommon, bilateral	Common, unilateral
PPD-T skin test (5TU)	≥16 mm†	0–15 mm‡
Chest roentgenogram§	Abnormal	Normal, usually
TBC chemotherapy	Effective	Ineffective, usually

*Person with active *M. tuberculosis* infection.
†*M. tuberculosis* isolated in 33 patients; PPD-T reactions (initial or repeat) were ≥15 mm in 100% of patients (33/33).
‡NTM isolated in 112 patients; 111 had a more positive (≥4 mm) PPD-NTM; PPD-T test was 0–15 mm in 65%, ≥16 mm in 35%.
§Abnormal in 25% (11/44) with TB and in 4% (8/196) with NTM disease.

MANAGEMENT

Lymphadenitis

Treatment initially depends on the presumptive diagnosis. The recommended therapy for excellent results is early surgical excision of only the larger infected nodes. Incisional biopsy or drainage or excision of all infected nodes is *not* recommended. I prescribe antituberculous drugs, such as INH and rifampin, when (1) the family refuses surgical excision, (2) the TB contact or family history is positive, (3) the PPD-T skin test of the patient or family is positive (especially if the reaction is 15 mm or larger or if the reaction is equal to or larger than the patient's NTM-PPD reaction), (4) the incisional or spontaneous drainage persists, (5) the drainage or prominent adenopathy persists over several months following surgery, or (6) the AFB culture is positive for *M. tuberculosis,* or an NTM species susceptible to INH or rifampin is isolated.

If prescribed, INH and rifampin should be administered until culture results and antibiotic susceptibilities are known or until healing is complete, usually in 2 to 6 months. To avoid hepatotoxicity, the recommended daily dose of INH is 10 mg/kg, and when combined with rifampin, the daily dose of rifampin is 15 mg/kg. If cultures are positive for TB, treatment is continued for 9 to 12 months or longer until healing is complete.

Skin and Soft Tissue Disease

Cutaneous NTM granuloma and abscesses may occur after skin abrasion from barnacles, shrimp, fish, or shellfish or after repeated exposure to fresh or salt water. These benign lesions usually manifest as mildly inflamed nodules, sporotrichoid nodules, small, crusted, wartlike excrescences, abscesses, or deep ulcers. Most NTM skin granulomas are self-limited, with spontaneous healing in several months or more. If persistent, cutaneous infections caused by the rapidly growing mycobacteria *M. chelonei* and *M. fortuitum* may be treated by surgical excision.[1] However, therapy with minocycline 2 mg/kg/d or doxycycline 2 to 4 mg/kg PO for 1 to 3 months can be effective against *M. chelonei* and *M. marinum* in children over age 7 years. All cultures of aspirated or biopsied material from such patients should be incubated for AFB at 30°C to 33°C and at 37°C in a carbon dioxide atmosphere to enhance growth of *M. marinum* or *M. chelonei.* Although the rapid growers are generally resistant to antituberculous drugs, the combination of ethambutol 15 to 20 mg/kg/d and rifampin orally for 6 to 12 months has been effective for *M. marinum* infections.

Application of local heat may hasten healing because these mycobacteria grow best at 30°C to 33°C. Alternatively, excisional biopsy of the lesion can be effective. Infection produced by *M. kansasii* is usually susceptible to rifampin, ethambutol, ethionamide, and streptomycin in the usual therapeutic doses. For deep-seated infection, removal of infected foreign bodies or catheter is essential. Oral erythromycin, clarithromycin, doxycycline, or trimethoprim-sulfamethoxazole for 3 to 6 months may be effective. Since the rapid growers are susceptible to clarithromycin, this agent should be considered in certain patients, especially in immunocompromised hosts.[2]

Pulmonary, Joint, Bone, or Disseminated Disease

Pulmonary, joint, bone, or disseminated NTM disease, rare in children, is usually due to MAC or *M. scrofulaceum.* Combinations of three or four antituberculous drugs, such as rifampin, ethambutol, ethionamide, streptomycin, and clarithromycin, based on susceptibility studies to the NTM isolated may be effective. Unfortunately, in patients with HIV infection, traditional drug regimens may fail. Newer drugs (amikacin, clarithromycin, clofazimine, and ciprofloxacin) may be tried (Table 2). Ciprofloxacin is limited for prolonged use in children. Surgical excision of localized disease, such as endobronchial tuberculous disease, lymphadenopathy, or bone, joint, or bursal lesions, is usually curative. In patients with uncomplicated disease, preoperative or postoperative chemotherapy is unnecessary. Owing to difficulty in testing visual acuity and red-green color discrimination in children under age 3, ethambutol should be used with caution. The potential toxicity of antituberculous drugs should be explained to each patient or to the parent or guardian, and written instructions regarding possible untoward reactions should be provided. Patients should be followed closely (monthly or bimonthly) to ensure compliance with chemotherapy. Ideally, to prevent drug-resistant tuberculosis from developing, patients should be directly observed by a health care professional while taking their daily or twice weekly multidrug preparations. Periodic monitoring for hepatotoxicity is recommended during the first 6 months of therapy, especially if the patient is taking both rifampin and INH.

Since more than 10% of children with AIDS develop disseminated NTM infection before death, one must consider the use of multidrug antimycobacterial therapy to increase the life expectancy of these unfortunate patients. Even though eradication of the nontuberculous infection is unlikely, the quality of life of such patients will be enhanced by a decrease in fever, malaise, and diarrhea with a temporary reduction in weight loss.

Isolation of the patient is not necessary. If large amounts of caseous material are being discharged from lesions or if cavitary pulmonary

TABLE 2. Antibiotic Doses for Nontuberculous Infection of Lymph Nodes, Skin, or Pulmonary Disease*

DRUG	DOSE (mg/kg/d) ROUTE OF ADMINISTRATION	MAXIMAL DAILY DOSE	NUMBER OF DOSES PER DAY	DURATION OF THERAPY (mo)	TOXICITY (PRIMARY)
Amikacin	15–30 IM	1.5 g	3	2–4	Otic, vestibular, renal
Clarithromycin	15–20 PO	1 g	2	6–12	Gastric
Ethambutol†	15–20 PO	1 g	1	≥12	Neuritis, optic
Ethionamide	15–20 PO	1 g	2	6–12	Gastric, hepatic
Isoniazid	10–20 PO	300 mg	1 or 2	≥12	Hepatic, renal
Minocycline	4 PO	400 mg	2	2–3	Dental, vertigo
Rifampin‡	10–20 PO	600 mg	1 or 2	6–12	Gastric, hepatic
or					
Rifabutin					
Kanamycin§	10–15 IM	1 g	1 or 2	2–4	Otic, vestibular, renal
or					
Streptomycin§	20–40 IM	1 g	1 or 2	2–4	Otic, vestibular, renal
Trimethoprim-sulfamethoxazole	8–20 TMP PO	2 g	2	3	Gastric, dermal, vasculitis

*Drug treatment to be continued if culture is positive for *M. tuberculosis;* excisional biopsy only is recommended for NTM adenopathy.
†Ethambutol to be used with caution for children under 3 years.
‡When sputum culture is negative for AFB, ethambutol may be substituted.
§For streptomycin and kanamycin, a single IM dose is given daily and then 3 times weekly after clinical improvement.

disease is present, respiratory isolation precautions should be considered until the results of cultures are available or until triple antituberculous therapy has been given for several weeks.

It is essential to distinguish patients with NTM disease from those with TB infections to avoid unnecessary and prolonged courses of drugs. Prophylactic INH therapy is unnecessary for healthy children with positive NTM-PPD reactions. Until special NTM-PPD antigens are available, repeat PPD-T testing 1 to 3 months after the initial PPD test will usually reveal a larger induration ($\geq$5 mm difference) than the initial PPD-T reaction, with an induration greater than 15 mm if the patient has an *M. tuberculosis* infection. If an NTM infection is present, the repeat PPD-T induration will usually be less than 15 mm. Close follow-up for several years is recommended for these patients.

REFERENCES

1. Alvi A, Myssiorek D: *Mycobacterium chelonae* causing recurrent neck abscess. Pediatr Infect Dis J 12:617–619, 1993.
2. Green PA, Fordham von Reyn C, Smith RP Jr: *Mycobacterium avium* complex parotid lymphadenitis: Successful therapy with clarithromycin and ethambutol. Pediatr Infect Dis J 12:615–617, 1993.
3. Margileth AM: Nontuberculous (atypical) mycobacterial diseases. Semin Pediatr Infect Dis 4:307–315, 1993.

PERTUSSIS

Sarah S. Long, m.d.

Pertussis continues to occur endemically in the United States as well as in 3- to 5-year epidemics, especially in areas where there is underimmunization of young children and crowded living conditions. Pertussis is not limited, however, by any age, socioeconomic stratum, or immunization status. *Pertussis should be considered in any patient with persistent paroxysmal cough.* Additional clues in young infants are apnea or cyanosis with or without a coughing paroxysm. Whooping is a pathognomonic feature but occurs reliably only in older infants and young children who are completely unimmunized. *Posttussive vomiting is suggestive of pertussis at all ages and is frequently the only distinctive feature in the schoolage child, adolescent, or adult.* *Bordetella pertussis* is the cause of pertussis, and other purported agents, such as *Bordetella parapertussis* and adenoviruses, play minor roles. Life-threatening effects of infection are obstructive or primary apnea, hypoxia leading to cardiopulmonary arrest, hypoxic or toxic encephalopathy, brain hemorrhage, and seizures. Life-threatening complications include massive aspiration following posttussive vomiting and secondary bacterial pneumonia from impaired ciliary function. Fatal and potentially fatal effects and complications of pertussis (except for secondary pneumonia) occur almost exclusively in very young infants, usually those under 3 months of age. In recently reported cases in infants younger than 12 months in the United States, pneumonia, seizures, and encephalopathy occurred in 17%, 2.5%, and 0.9%, respectively. Current case fatality in those younger than 6 months is 0.5%.

TREATMENT

Assessment and Supportive Care

At home or in the hospital, goals of therapy are to limit the number of paroxysms, to provide assistance when necessary during or after a paroxysm, and to maximize nutrition and rest. Infants are admitted to the hospital at age less than 3 months almost without exception, between 3 and 6 months of age unless they demonstrate an ability to sustain tone and color through paroxysms and have preserved nutrition and a sense of well-being, and older than 6 months (or any age) if complications occur or the family is unable to provide supportive care. Young infants born prematurely, those who have underlying cardiac, pulmonary, or neurologic problems, or those who have sub-

normal muscle mass or function have a particularly high risk of severe disease. In making the decision between hospital and home care, a paroxysm must be witnessed because even the infant with potentially fatal pertussis may appear completely well between episodes.

The specific, limited goals of hospitalization are to assess the likelihood of life-threatening events at the peak of disease, to prevent or treat complications, and to educate parents in the natural history of the disease and in the care that will be given at home. For the majority of infants without complications, this can be accomplished in 48 to 72 hours. Specific data required to safely make these judgments in hospital include continuous monitoring, detailed recording of coughing episodes, and documentation of feeding, vomiting, and weight change. Some very young infants have bradycardia, apnea, or hypoxemia without obvious coughing. Heart and respiratory rate and pulse oximetry are continuously monitored with alarm settings so that every paroxysm will be witnessed by health care personnel. A cough record allows tallying of the number of episodes during sequential 24-hour periods and is the critical assessment of severity and progression of disease and predictor of adverse outcome. Specific data recorded for each paroxysm include duration in seconds (less than 45 seconds and sequentially diminishing duration are good signs), color change (red is usual and is of no concern), change in heart rate (bradycardia of 70 per minute for a period not to exceed the actual paroxysm that is sometimes seen in young infants is of limited concern in the absence of other clinical abnormalities), change in pulse oximetry (oxygen desaturation during a paroxysm is expected but should spontaneously resolve immediately at its conclusion), posture, tone, and vigor of breathing at the conclusion of a paroxysm (whooping is a positive sign of sustained strength and self-rescue, whereas limpness, inactivity, and lack of gasping require urgent intervention), the presence and character of expectorated mucus (thick cast of trachea is more of a risk for airway obstruction), posttussive vomiting, posttussive demeanor (exhaustion is usual, but poor tone or activity is of concern), the need for stimulation to interrupt apnea or bradycardia, and the need for oxygen to correct hypoxia. These last assessments require skilled and experienced personnel who will wait watchfully to document the infant's ability for self-rescue but who will intervene rapidly and expertly when necessary. For infants with a history of cyanosis or a witnessed event, humidified oxygen is initially provided by nasal cannula or by handheld catheter during paroxysms until experience with the infant and knowledge of the complete clinical picture warrant careful assessment without intervention.

Within 48 to 72 hours, the direction and severity of disease usually are obvious by analysis of the recorded information. Occasionally, within 48 hours of hospitalization and antibiotic treatment, the infant is much improved, with fewer and less severe paroxysms. In my experience, these are usually 3- to 6-month-old patients, treated early in the course of infection, who have been removed from an aggravating environment, such as one with cigarette smoke, excessive stimulation and noise, or a dry or polluted heat source. More frequently, hospitalization is not associated with significant improvement in a coughing illness that can be expected to continue for weeks. *Discharge is appropriate if over a 48-hour period, disease severity is unchanged or diminished, no intervention is required during paroxysms, nutrition is adequate, no complication has occurred, and parents are adequately prepared for care at home.* It has been my experience that apnea or seizures unassociated with paroxysms occur early, in the incremental phase of disease, or in those inpatients with severe complicated illnesses. It is not my practice to send parents home with monitors, portable oxygen, or electrical suction apparatus. Parents of all children should be knowledgeable in cardiopulmonary resuscitation.

The benefit of a quiet, lowly lighted, undisturbed, comforting environment cannot be overestimated or forfeited in the desire to observe, monitor, and intervene. Dry air is detrimental. Mist by tent, religiously banned by some, is useful in some infants with thick tenacious secretions and excessively irritable airways and can be used safely if all other sight, sound, and electronic signals are diligently observed. Suctioning of the nose, oropharynx, or trachea always precipitates a coughing paroxysm, occasionally causes bronchospasm or apnea, and should not be performed on a preventive schedule. During a paroxysm, especially in very young infants, a single, brief attempt at suctioning performed by skilled personnel sometimes clears an offending mucous plug. Infants whose paroxysms repeatedly lead to life-threatening events require intubation, paralysis, ventilation, and frequent artificial clearing of the airway.

Feeding children with pertussis is a challenge. The risk of precipitating a paroxysm by nipple feeding does not warrant the use of nasogastric, nasojejunal, or parenteral alimentation. *If the infant is alert and able following a coughing paroxysm, feeding is best taken and retained during this brief period.* Small feedings avoid the added risk of regurgitation from gastric distention. In my experience, there is no thickness, thinness, or composition of prepared formula that affects secretions, protect against coughing, or predicts retention.

Therapeutic Agents

Antimicrobial Agents

An antimicrobial agent is always given when pertussis is suspected or confirmed for potential clinical benefit and to limit the spread of infection to others. Clinical efficacy is most evident in young infants who come to clinical attention quickly and in older individuals who are treated in the catarrhal or early paroxysmal stage. However, even those who have coughed for weeks may be infectious. Thus, all should be treated. Erythromycin 40 to 50 mg/kg/d PO in four divided doses (max: 2 g/d) for 14 days is standard treatment. Some experts prefer the estolate preparation, but ethylsuccinate and stearate also are efficacious. Small studies of erythromycin ethylsuccinate given at a dose of 50 mg/kg/d divided into two doses, at a dose of 60 mg/kg/d divided into three doses, and erythromycin estolate given at a dose of 40 mg/kg/d divided into two doses showed elimination of organisms in 98% of children.

In vitro, *B. pertussis* is exquisitely susceptible to erythromycin, quinolones, some newer macrolides, and third-generation cephalosporins. Ampicillin, rifampin, and trimethoprim-sulfamethoxazole are modestly active, but first- and second-generation cephalosporins are not. *B parapertussis* is less susceptible in vitro to all agents except erythromycin. In clinical studies, erythromycin is superior to amoxicillin for eradication of *B. pertussis* and is the only agent with proven efficacy. Activity of the drug at the site of colonization rather than intrinsic resistance is the usual limiting factor for pathogen eradication, although an erythromycin-resistant isolate has been reported recently.

Albuterol

A few small clinical trials and letters to editors have reported that the beta-$_2$-adrenergic stimulant albuterol reduces the symptoms of whooping cough. Its use is based on the assumption that by preventing bronchial obstruction or spasm, coughing paroxysms are lessened. Additionally, there is some evidence that pertussis is associated with a brisk IgE antibody response. No rigorous clinical trial has demonstrated a beneficial effect, and one small study showed no effect. In my experience, neither orally administered or aerosolized albuterol has a noticeable effect on the number or severity of paroxysms. The fussing associated with aerosol treatment triggers paroxysms.

Corticosteroids

No randomized, blinded clinical trial of sufficient size has been performed to evaluate the usefulness of corticosteroids in the management of pertussis. Studies in animals have shown a salutory effect on disease manifestations that do not have a corollary in respiratory infection in humans. Their clinical use is not warranted.

Pertussis Immune Globulin

Hyperimmune serum, derived from adults convalescing from pertussis, was widely prescribed and regarded as beneficial in the 1930s and 1940s. Later studies and the only placebo-controlled trial demonstrated little or no value. By the use of large intramuscular doses of hyperimmune serum (raised by immunization of adults with acellular pertussis vaccines in Sweden and selected for high antitoxin titer), whooping was significantly reduced in infants treated in the first week of disease compared with patients given placebo. The use of immunoglobulin preparations of any sort is not warranted unless further study confirms a beneficial effect.

COMPLICATIONS AND OUTCOME

In addition to the direct effects of *B. pertussis* infection on the respiratory tract and the probable obstructive and toxin-mediated events leading to apnea, hypoxia, encephalopathy, and sometimes death, secondary bacterial infection is common in hospitalized infants. Bacterial pneumonia and acute otitis media are suspected with changes in physical examination, occurrence of fever, or neutrophilia in the peripheral blood count. Inappropriate secretion of antidiuretic hormone can cause hyponatremia and seizures. Subconjunctival hemorrhage, facial edema, and petechiae on the upper body commonly result from forced coughing. Rectal prolapse occurs only rarely, in patients with premorbid malnutrition. It has been mistakenly attributed to pertussis in patients with prolonged coughing, but it was actually due to cystic fibrosis.

In general, the younger the child under 1 year of age with pertussis, the longer the convalescent phase. Many infants have recurring paroxysmal cough with simple viral respiratory illnesses in the months of convalescence (*B. pertussis* is not recoverable), and most have sporadic paroxysms for 6 to 12 months. One longitudinal study of children under 2 years of age with pertussis demonstrated persistently abnormal pulmonary function 6 and 12 months after disease.

CONTROL MEASURES

Isolation

The patient is placed in respiratory isolation for at least 5 days after initiation of erythromycin therapy. It is our practice to continue to isolate infants who require longer hospitalization to avoid any possibility of spread, to reduce noxious stimuli, and to avoid the protective concern of other families.

Care of Household and Other Close Contacts

Erythromycin 40 to 50 mg/kg/d PO in four divided doses (max: 2 g/d) for 14 days should be given promptly to all household contacts and other close contacts, such as those in day care, regardless of age or history of immunization. Repeatedly, studies have shown the efficacy of chemoprophylaxis and have elucidated that the majority of contacts in household or residential facilities are or will become infected when a case of pertussis is recognized. Visitation and movement of coughing family members in the hospital must be assiduously controlled until erythromycin has been taken for 5 days. Immunization is evaluated for close contacts younger than 7 years. Those who are underimmunized are given DTP vaccine, with further doses to complete the recommended series. Children who received a third dose 6 months or more before exposure or a fourth dose 3 years or more before exposure should receive a booster dose of DTP. If infection with *B. pertussis* is documented at any age, the individual is exempted from routine pertussis immunization. Antimicrobial prophylaxis is not routinely recommended for exposed health care workers. Recommendation for the use of acellular pertussis vaccine beyond 7 years of age awaits further study.

PSYCHOSOCIAL ISSUES

Parents of children with pertussis are frequently angry. The diagnosis in the child and in themselves often had been overlooked. Additionally, they may feel angry or guilty depending on whether the child received routine DTP immunization. They are always exhausted, sleep-deprived, overwhelmed by helplessness to stop the attacks, and truly terrified that the child will die during each paroxysm. The first messages to give are empathy for what the child and family has experienced, transfer of the burden of responsibility for the child's life to the health care team, and delineation of what assessments and treatments will be given. After 24 hours of assessment (and renewal of the family's strength), the cough record is used to explain the infant's progress. The family is recruited as part of the team of care-givers, and education is begun on expectations of the duration of illness and home care. The patient requires as much comforting as medical intervention. Older children and adults describe the feelings of strangling suffocation during a paroxysm, bursting headache, and fear of anticipation of coughing attacks. Ongoing communication and support are required over the weeks or months of recovery.

PLAGUE

MARIA D. GOLDSTEIN, M.D.

ETIOLOGY

Plague is caused by *Yersinia pestis,* a small, pleomorphic, gram-negative bacillus. In the United States today, *Y. pestis* is endemic in the rodent populations of 15 western states. Plague in this country is predominantly rural and is transmitted to humans by the fleas of infected wild rodents.

People living in the rural areas of the American Southwest may acquire plague by one of the following mechanisms: (1) the bite of the flea of an infected wild rodent or, less commonly, an infected domestic animal, (2) the inhalation of infected droplets from a case of pneumonic plague, and (3) direct bloodstream infection via a break in the skin during the skinning and eviscerating of an infected animal. Most cases of plague in the United States occur between April and September. There is no gender difference in attack rate, 60% of the cases occur in people under the age of 20, and 35% of cases occur in Native Americans.

CLINICAL MANIFESTATIONS

The bubonic form of plague is by far the most common presentation, the infection being localized in the regional lymph nodes and resulting in a bubo, an extremely tender, often visible swelling of the lymph nodes. The septicemic form of plague may or may not be associated with buboes. The onset of the illness is usually abrupt, with fever, malaise, weakness, headache, and, occasionally, gastro-intestinal symptoms. Meningitis may sometimes occur late in the course of the illness in spite of antibiotic treatment.

Pneumonic plague is very rare, especially as a presenting symptom, but is usually fulminant and very infectious. Therefore, all plague patients should be isolated until pneumonia has been ruled out or the patient has been treated with antibiotics for 48 hours. Health care workers tending plague victims in whom pulmonary disease has not been ruled out should wear face masks that include eye protection.

TREATMENT

Successful treatment of plague rests in its prompt diagnosis. Classic bubonic plague presentation in an endemic area is easy to diagnose. The nonspecific presentation of septicemic plague makes its early diagnosis more difficult, and, therefore, a high degree of suspicion is necessary. In endemic areas or in patients with a history of recent travel to endemic areas, treatment of community-acquired sepsis should include an aminoglycoside because of the possibility of plague.

Antibiotic Therapy

The antibiotics with the greatest proven efficacy in the treatment of plague are streptomycin and tetracycline.

Streptomycin, Tetracycline, Chloramphenicol

Streptomycin is the drug of choice for severe plague, including septicemic and pneumonic plague. It is given in a dose of 20 to 30 mg/kg/d IM, initially in four divided doses, in an effort to avoid sudden release of massive doses of endotoxin, and later in two divided doses, for a total of 10 days or for 2 to 4 days after fever lysis.

Tetracycline 30 to 40 mg/kg/d in four divided doses may be used in uncomplicated cases of bubonic plague in adults and children over 8 years of age.

Plague meningitis is best treated with chloramphenicol 50 to 100 mg/kg/d IV in four to six divided doses. Chloramphenicol may also be used as an adjunct to the other antibiotics.

Aminoglycosides and Sulfonamides

Aminoglycosides, such as kanamycin 15 mg/kg/d in three divided doses, up to 1.5 g/d, and gentamicin 7.5 mg/kg/d in children and 3 to 5 mg/kg/d in adults are also probably effective against plague, but experience with them is limited.

Sulfonamides, including sulfadiazine and the trisulfapyridines at a loading dose of 25 mg/kg and then 75 mg/kg/d PO in four divided doses also may be effective. Trimethoprim-sulfamethoxazole has been used successfully in a few instances.

Penicillins and Cephalosporins

Penicillins, semisynthetic penicillins, and cephalosporins, although effective in vitro, are considered to be only partially effective in vivo.

Intravenous Fluids and Glucocorticoids

Besides the prompt institution of appropriate specific antibiotics for treating the infection, in cases of shock, the usual supportive therapy with intravenous fluids and glucocorticoids should be considered.

PREVENTION AND CONTROL

Hospitalized patients with plague must be isolated with respiratory precautions to prevent secondary spread due to pneumonic plague until the patient has been receiving appropriate antibiotics for 48 hours. Contacts should receive chemoprophylaxis with tetracycline 0.5 g four times a day for 7 days if older than 8 years or a sulfonamide 150 mg/kg/d in four divided doses if younger than 8 years. A plague vaccine is available and recommended for laboratory and field personnel who are exposed to *Y. pestis* on a regular basis.

In areas of high endemicity, surveillance for epizootics and periodic community education must be high priorities. Other measures should include extensive use of insecticides in fields and housing areas, domestic animal flea control, and avoidance of wild rodents.

REFERENCES

1 Hull HF, Montes J, Mann JM: Septicemic plague in New Mexico. J Infect Dis 155:113–118, 1987.
2. Kaufman AF, Boyce JM, Martone WJ: Trends in human plague in the United States. J Infect Dis 141:522–524, 1980.

RAT-BITE FEVER

BARRY DASHEFSKY, M.D.

Rat-bite fever is a term applied to two similar but distinct clinical syndromes currently occurring rarely in the United States. Both are characterized by the abrupt onset of high, often intermittent fever, rash, musculoskeletal complaints, and constitutional symptoms that are caused by microorganisms usually transmitted by biting rodents or, occasionally, following more casual contact with colonized animals. The more common entity in the United States—streptobacillary fever—is caused by *Streptobacillus moniliformis*. It typically presents within 3 (up to 5) days after a rat bite that heals promptly without producing significant regional lymphadenopathy and features a pink maculopapular or petechial rash on the extremities (in 75% of cases) and nonsuppurative migratory polyarthritis or arthralgia (in 50% of cases). Streptobacillary fever may also be acquired by ingestion of contaminated food, milk, or water (Haverhill fever) and may be manifested additionally by pharyngitis. Untreated, the illness usually subsides within 3 weeks, although it may be complicated by a chronic, relapsing course of arthritis, the development of subcutaneous abscesses or other focal disease, most significantly endocarditis, and a mortality rate of 10%.

Less common in the United States, classic rat-bite fever (or *sodoku*) is caused by *Spirillum minus*. Typically, after an incubation period of 14 to 18 days (range 7 to 21 days), it presents with ulceration of an initially healed rat bite in association with prominent regional lymphadenopathy and a rash consisting of large purple to reddish brown macules and occasional indurated plaques. Joint involvement is rare. Untreated infection with *S. minus* usually resolves within 3 to 8 weeks. However, multiple relapses of fever and rash may occur over months or years. Suppurative complications and death are very rare.

TREATMENT

Both varieties of rat-bite fever are treated similarly and respond promptly and readily to antimicrobials. Recommended treatment is procaine penicillin G 20,000 to 50,000 U/kg/d, up to 1.2 million U, IM in one to two doses or penicillin G 50,000 U/kg/d, up to 2.4 million U, IV in four to six doses, for 7 to 10 days. Oral penicillin V 1 to 2 g/d in four divided doses for the same duration is considered to be a satisfactory alternative for at least the second half of a course of treatment.

For penicillin-allergic patients, options include tetracycline 30 to 50 mg/kg/d (max: 2 g/d) PO or IV in four doses for patients 9 years of age or older, streptomycin 20 to 30 mg/kg/d (max: 4/g/d) PO or IV in four doses, or chloramphenicol 50 to 75 mg/kg/d (max: 4/g/d) PO or IV in four doses. For treating endocarditis, penicillin G 150,000 to 250,000 U/kg/d (max: 20 million U/d) IV in four to six divided doses for at least 4 weeks is recommended. Streptomycin, or presumably another aminoglycoside, may be a helpful adjunct.

Additional treatment issues include care of local bite wounds, drainage of abscesses as necessary, and implementation of standard guidelines for tetanus prophylaxis. Gloves should be used for touching any infective material until 24 hours of effective antimicrobial therapy has been completed. The major preventive measure is rodent control. Some authorities recommend administering penicillin prophylactically following a rat bite (noting a risk of transmission of up to 10%), although there are no data addressing the efficacy of this strategy.

REFERENCES

1. Byington CL, Bason RD: Rat-bite fever. *In* Feigin RD, Cherry JD (eds): Textbook of Pediatric Infectious Diseases, 3rd ed. Philadelphia, WB Saunders Co, 1992: 1236–1239.
2. Holroyd KJ, Reiner AP, Dick JD: *Streptobacillus moniliformis* polyarthritis mimicking rheumatoid arthritis: An urban case of rat-bite fever. Am J Med 85:711–714, 1988.
3. Roughgarden JW: Antimicrobial therapy of rat bite fever. Arch Intern Med 116:39–54, 1965.

STAPHYLOCOCCAL INFECTIONS

MICHAEL RADETSKY, M.D., C.M.

Both *Staphylococcus aureus* and *Staphylococcus epidermidis* are part of normal human flora. Both are universal commensals that rarely cause disease except under unusual circumstances. *S. aureus* requires inoculation into skin breaks, and *S. epidermidis* requires the presence of either foreign bodies (catheters, prosthetic devices) or abnormal phagocytic defenses. Occasionally, *S. aureus* strains will produce biologically active products that mediate noninvasive toxin diseases (scalded skin syndrome, toxic shock syndrome, food poisoning). Lasting immunity does not occur for invasive disease. Successful therapy requires well-placed suspicions, identification of the causative organism, a proper choice of antimicrobials, and removal of the physical underpinnings of infection (draining of abscesses, removal of foreign body).

ANTIMICROBIAL FACTORS

Since the majority of *S. aureus* strains are resistant to penicillin, all infections in which *S. aureus* is isolated or suspected should be treated with antimicrobials impervious to beta-lactamase. In general, the antistaphylococcal penicillins (nafcillin, oxacillin, methicillin, dicloxacillin) or the first-generation cephalosporins (cefazolin, cephalothin, cephalexin) are the drugs of first choice because of their proven efficacy, safety, and long history of successful use. No evidence exists demonstrating the therapeutic superiority of any one of these standard drugs over another. Although methicillin is a cause of reversible nephritis, other penicillins and cephalosporins are reported to have caused the same condition. Second-generation (cefuroxime, cefoxitin) and third-generation (cefotaxime, ceftriaxone, ceftizoxime) cephalosporins have reduced activity against *S. aureus* and, based on this factor alone, are not generally recommended as premier antimicrobials. Nevertheless, studies have consistently demonstrated the successful therapy of invasive staphylococcal disease when these drugs are given in the recommended doses (Table 1). The use of linked antimicrobials, in which a beta-lactam drug is combined with a beta-lactamase antagonist (e.g., amoxicillin-clavulanate, ampicillin-sulbactam, ticarcillin-clavulanate) is widespread and successful despite a paucity of published studies that document efficacy. Clindamycin is an underused drug with good oral bioavailability, and although rarely considered as a first-line drug, it can be used in patients with moderately severe staphylococcal infections who are allergic to beta-lactam medications.

S. aureus resistant to all beta-lactam antimicrobials (methicillin-resistant *Staphylococcus aureus*, or MRSA) are encountered infrequently in childhood infections. When they do cause disease, it is usually in the context of nosocomial infections occurring in intensive care units. On the other hand, *S. epidermidis* resistant to beta-lactam antimicrobials (MRSE) is common and should be presumed. In either case, the choice for such infections is vancomycin, whose toxicity makes it an inappropriate selection for any other purpose except for those severely ill patients allergic to beta-lactam drugs.

Central nervous system infections due to *S. aureus* may be primary but are more commonly associated with prior head trauma or an indwelling foreign body, such as ventriculoperitoneal shunt. Such infections may be refractory to antimicrobial therapy alone. The efficacy of cephalosporins in treating such infections is limited because of poor penetration. Of the available drugs, nafcillin is the choice for CNS infections, with vancomycin for the allergic patient or the resistant organism. Higher doses of antimicrobials than in other staphylococcal infections generally are necessary. *S. epidermidis* infections of the CNS are invariably associated with implanted prosthetic devices, and vancomycin is the drug of choice. However, such infections are usually refractory to antimicrobials alone and generally require removal of the foreign body.

TABLE 1. Antimicrobials for Staphylococcal Infections

	DAILY DOSE, FREQUENCY		
	NEWBORNS*	CHILDREN	ADULTS
Parenteral Route			
Nafcillin	100 mg/kg/d, q6h	150 mg/kg/d, q6h	6–12 g/d, q4h
Oxacillin	100 mg/kg/d, q6h	150–200 mg/kg/d, q6h	6–12 g/d, q4h
Methicillin	100 mg/kg/d, q6h	150–200 mg/kg/d, q6h	6–12 g/d, q4h
Cefazolin	60 mg/kg/d, q8h	50–100 mg/kg/d, q8h	1–6 g/d, q6–8h
Cephalothin	80 mg/kg/d, q6h	75–125 mg/kg/d, q4–6h	2–12 g/d, q4–6h
Cefuroxime	NR	100–150 mg/kg/d, q8h	2–4.5 g/d, q8h
Cefotaxime	150 mg/kg/d, q8h	100–200 mg/kg/d, q6–8h	3–12 g/d, q4–8h
Ceftriaxone	75 mg/kg/d, q24h	50–100 mg/kg/d, q12–24h	1–4 g/d, q12–24h
Vancomycin	45 mg/kg/d, q8h	40–60 mg/kg/d, q6h	
Ampicillin-sulbactam	NR	100–200 mg/kg/d, q6h†	6–12 g/d, q6h
Ticarcillin-clavulanate	NR	200–300 mg/kg/d, q4–6h†	12–18 g/d, q4–6h
Clindamycin	20 mg/kg/d, q6h	25–40 mg/kg/d, q6–8h	0.5–3 g/d, q8h
Oral Route			
Dicloxacillin	NR	12–25 mg/kg/d, q6h	2 g/d, q6h
Cephalexin	NR	25–50 mg/kg/d, q6h	2 g/d, q6h
Amoxicillin-clavulanate	NR	40 mg/kg/d, q8h	1.5 g/d, q8h
Erythromycin	NR	40 mg/kg/d, q6h	2 g/d, q6h
Clindamycin	NR	20–30 mg/kg/d, q6h	1–2 g/d, q6h
Rifampin	NR	20 mg/kg/d, q12–24h	600 mg/d, q12–24h

*May require modification of dose or frequency in premature infants and newborns younger than 7 days of age.
†Not approved for use in children.
Abbreviations NR, not recommended.

In serious, invasive disease (e.g., endocarditis, overwhelming septicemia), the use of an antistaphylococcal penicillin plus an aminoglycoside or rifampin or both is thought to be advantageous because of an additive or synergistic effect.

For superficial skin infections, such as impetigo or paronychia, any of the oral antistaphylococcal drugs may be used. For impetigo, topical therapy with mupirocin is also effective. Rifampin should never be used as a single agent because of the rapid emergence of resistance.

APPROACHES TO THERAPY

Staphylococcal infections are notoriously tenacious and have a tendency to persist or recur. Explanations for this phenomenon are incomplete. The presence of viable, cell wall free forms (L-forms) in hypertonic debris is one attractive but unproven hypothesis. Antimicrobial tolerance, in which there is a dissociation between the minimal inhibitory concentration and the minimal bactericidal concentration, is another. In any event, because of these difficulties, certain management principles should guide therapy.

- Whenever possible, all accessible pus should be drained. If there is an infection associated with a deep vascular line or other foreign body, strong consideration should be given to removing it if feasible.
- All infections that fail to respond favorably to standard antimicrobials within 48 to 72 hours may require surgical drainage or debridement. Imaging studies, such as CT scan, gallium citrate scan, or indium-labeled white cells scan, can be useful in identifying occult foci that may benefit from drainage procedures.
- Parenteral antimicrobials should be given initially in all but minor staphylococcal infections.
- Oral antistaphylococcal drugs should be used as primary therapy only for minor infections unlikely to be associated with bacteremia.
- In selected circumstances, sequential oral therapy may be substituted for a parenteral antimicrobial in more serious infections, but only if the following guidelines are met.
  - The patient has exhibited a trend of steady, demonstrable improvement on the parenteral antimicrobial and is "almost well."
  - There is knowledge of the antimicrobial susceptibilities of the causative organism.

- There is an appropriate oral antistaphylococcal agent available that the patient can tolerate.
- Compliance with the oral dosing of drug and medical follow-up is assured.
- The dose of oral antistaphylococcal antimicrobial is usually 2 to 3 times the normal amount, e.g., 75 to 100 mg/kg of dicloxacillin or cephalexin.
- Sequential oral therapy is primarily reserved for more serious skin, soft tissue, bone, or joint infections. Staphylococcal septicemia, endocarditis, or meningitis/ventriculitis should be treated entirely with parenteral antimicrobials.
- Total duration of treatment of staphylococcal infections has not been standardized. In general, superficial infections should be treated for 7 to 10 days. As a rule of thumb, more serious infections should be treated for 2 weeks beyond the resolution of all clinical and laboratory signs of infection (e.g, focal findings, fever, blood culture, sedimentation rate), with a minimum duration of 3 weeks.
- Relapsing disease not associated with an undrained focus of infection may be due to cell wall-deficient L-forms and may respond to a 5- to 7-day course of antimicrobials that act at the level of the ribosome, such as clindamycin or rifampin.

CLINICAL INFECTIONS

Skin Infections

Impetigo and Cellulitis

Impetigo is an infection of the superficial epidermis; 60% are caused by *S. aureus*. Cellulitis is an infection of the skin that involves the dermis and subcutaneous tissues and presents as a red, painful, edematous area with indistinct borders. Most cases are due to either group A streptococci or *S. aureus*. The diagnosis is usually made by inspection, but in cases of severe cellulitis, cellulitis not responding to conventional therapy, or cellulitis in immunocompromised hosts, aspiration to recover the etiologic agent should be attempted. Recovery of organisms by aspiration occurs in two thirds of cases.

CARDINAL FEATURES

- Red, painful, edematous skin and soft tissues
- Predisposing trauma, skin abrasions, or other skin lesions (e.g., varicella)
- Fever

Treatment consists of topical mupirocin for impetigo, an oral antimicrobial for either impetigo or minor cellulitis, and a parenteral antimicrobial for more extensive cellulitis or any soft tissue infection in a toxic child.

Scalded Skin Syndrome

The staphylococcal scalded skin syndrome comprises a spectrum of dermatologic conditions caused by the epidermolytic toxin of *S. aureus*, primarily phage group II. The toxin causes lysis of the intracellular attachment between cells in the granular layer of the epidermis. The pathogenic organism may be a focal colonizer only (e.g., of nose or umbilical stump), may be causing minor local infection (e.g., conjunctivitis, infected abrasions, infected circumcision), or may be a part of a serious infection (e.g., bacteremia, endocarditis, omphalitis, wound infection). The toxin is absorbed from the site of colonization or infection and disseminates to distant sites. The manifestations of disease are a function of age and the presence of circulating antitoxin antibody. In newborns with no passive maternal antitoxin, the disease is severe and is known as Ritter's disease. In older susceptible children, the disease is called staphylococcal scalded skin syndrome and consists of a painful erythroderma, purulent conjunctivitis, and separation of the superficial epidermis into bullae and desquamating sheets. Lateral traction on the involved skin with the thumb will remove the superficial epidermis and is termed Nikolsky's sign. The children are febrile and irritable and look moderately ill. The older susceptible child may present with a scarlatinaform rash and mild conjunctivitis (staphylococcal scarlet fever). Focal inoculation of a skin site with a toxin-producing staphylococcus produces a local bullous lesion, bullous impetigo.

CARDINAL FEATURES

- Diffuse painful erythroderma or focal flaccid bulla
- Nikolsky's sign
- Conjunctivitis, often purulent
- Gross desquamation
- Normal oral mucous membranes

In general, the disease is self-limiting. Fluid support and analgesia for the painful erythroderma are supplemented by the use of an antistaphylococcal antimicrobial. The use of corticosteroids may delay recovery.

Myositis

There are four types of bacterial myositis: tropical pyomyositis, acute bacterial myositis, clostridial gas gangrene, and nonclostridial crepitant myositis. Tropical pyomyositis is a condition characterized by single or multiple muscle abscesses. In over 95% of cases, *S. aureus* is the causative agent. Preceding trauma to the affected area is a common feature. The lumpy, tender lesions may be deep and elicit a minimal visual inflammatory response. Low-grade fever is common. Acute bacterial myositis is usually caused by the group A streptococcus, but cases due to *S. aureus* have been reported. Abscesses are not seen. Rather, the infection extends diffusely through one or more muscle groups, with pain and swelling. Systemic spread of the organism with multiple organ involvement and septic shock may occur. Gas gangrene and nonclostridial crepitant myositis are not due to *S. aureus*.

CARDINAL FEATURES

- Focal pain and swelling of muscle
- Fever
- Systemic toxicity
- Preceding traumatic muscle injury or wound

Bacterial myositis of all types require surgical exploration, drainage, and debridement. A gram stain is useful as a guide for choice of an antimicrobial agent. In tropical pyomyositis and acute bacterial myositis, an antistaphylococcal penicillin or first-generation cephalosporin should be chosen. The use of hyperbaric oxygen may be indicated if surgical debridement is likely to be incomplete or mutilating.

Respiratory Infections

Pneumonia

Acute, severe, or fulminant pneumonia occasionally is caused by *S. aureus* and may be primary or secondary. Primary pneumonia is most common in infants under 1 year of age. Pneumonia secondary to *S. aureus* bacteremia can also occur, usually in older children. A pleural effusion is present in over 80% of cases. Although lobar pneumonia is most common, bronchopneumonic and hemithoracic patterns are also seen. Without appropriate therapy, infection is rapidly progressive, with a fatality rate approaching 25%. Failure to use an antistaphylococcal antimicrobial is the major risk factor for severe disease. The causative agent is usually isolated through cultures of blood and pleural fluid.

CARDINAL FEATURES

- Respiratory distress, hyperpnea, or tachypnea
- Fever and systemic toxicity
- Extensive parenchymal disease
- Pleural effusion

Treatment of pneumonia consists of both supportive and specific therapies. Oxygen supplementation is the mainstay of supportive care. However, because the degree of pulmonary shunting may be large in extensive pneumonia, response to increasing levels of ambient oxygen may be blunted. In sick young infants or in severe pneumonia at any age, presumptive antimicrobials active against *S. aureus* should be started once appropriate specimens are obtained for culture. Chest tube drainage of pleural effusions is usually required. The advantages of chest physiotherapy are unproven.

Bone and Joint Infections

Acute Suppurative Arthritis

Outside of the newborn period, the most common cause of primary monoarticular septic arthritis is *S. aureus*. *Haemophilus influenzae* type b remains a potential pathogen of joints in unimmunized children. The constellation of fever, joint pain, and decreased range of motion of any joint should prompt appropriate investigative steps. Imaging studies add little to the physical examination, except in septic arthritis of the hip joint. However, even in the hip, normal radiographs cannot exclude the diagnosis of septic arthritis. Definitive diagnosis is made by arthrocentesis. The gram stain may reveal organisms that subsequently may not grow on culture because of the bacteriostatic effect of joint fluid. For this reason, up to 30% of septic joints may be sterile on culture. A blood culture will be positive in approximately 50% of patients.

CARDINAL FEATURES

- Fever
- Joint pain or limb disuse
- Restricted range of motion
- Swelling and redness (later finding)

Unless contradicted by the gram stain, presumptive monotherapy with an antistaphylococcal antimicrobial should be adequate at most ages in normal children. In newborns, an antistaphylococcal antimicrobial, ampicillin, and an aminoglycoside should be used in combination. Adjunctive surgical drainage of infected joints commonly is performed but has not been proven to be superior to repeat needle aspiration of the joint. However, whether by open drainage or closed aspiration, evacuation of the joint space must be accomplished. Since repeat aspiration of the hip joint is technically difficult, open drainage of that joint is advised.

Acute Osteomyelitis

Although any bone may be involved, hematogenous osteomyelitis tends to occur in the metaphysis of long tubular bones and the metaphyseal equivalent areas of flat bones (e.g., pelvis, vertebral bodies). S. aureus accounts for 80% of all cases of osteomyelitis. The appropriate clinical findings may be supported by conventional radiography. Loss of bone density or periosteal elevation and reaction may be seen. However, radiographs may be falsely negative or misleading in 40% of cases. In older children, bone scans with technetium-99m compounds have a sensitivity of over 90%. False negative bone scans are seen routinely in newborn osteomyelitis, for which sensitivity is only 30%. Bone scan-negative osteomyelitis may be localized by a gallium-67 scan. Definitive diagnosis requires isolation of bacteria from the site of infection by aspiration of the bone, the subperiosteal space, or the joint. Such cultures will be positive in 80% of cases. A bone biopsy is also definitive. Alternatively, focal bone disease with a positive blood culture confirms the diagnosis.

CARDINAL FEATURES

- Fever
- Specific bone pain
- Disuse or pseudoparalysis of the affected limb
- Refusal to stand or walk in pelvic or vertebral infection
- Soft tissue swelling as a late finding

Antimicrobial therapy alone is successful in the majority of cases. In newborns, ampicillin, an antistaphylococcal antimicrobial, and an aminoglycoside should be started. In normal older children, an antistaphylococcal antimicrobial alone is adequate. For traumatic osteomyelitis, antistaphylococcal coverage should be combined with an aminoglycoside. Traumatic osteomyelitis also demands surgical debridement, since cure is rarely possible with antimicrobials alone when infection resides in dead or devitalized bone.

Cardiac Infections

Infective Endocarditis

Native heart valves without demonstrable abnormalities may become infected by S. aureus. Any organism, including such weakly pathogenic organisms as S. epidermidis, may infect prosthetic devices. When the clinical findings are suggestive of infective endocarditis, the presence of reliably positive blood cultures confirm the diagnosis. In infective endocarditis, continuous bacteremia is present. Multiple blood cultures are essential to separate endocarditis with bacteremia from mere bacterial contamination, since S. epidermidis, a frequent contaminant, may cause true disease. The use of echocardiography to detect valvular vegetations has a sensitivity of only 60%, and false positive tests are not infrequent.

CARDINAL FEATURES

- Fever (98%)
- Murmur (90%)
- Splenomegaly (50%)
- Petechiae (33%)
- Emboli (28%)
- Hematuria (35%)
- Malaise/anorexia (66%)
- Heart failure (30%)
- Neurologic signs (18%)

If a child with presumed infective endocarditis is toxic, an antistaphylococcal penicillin should be used in addition to standard therapy with penicillin and an aminoglycoside. If a prosthetic valve is present, vancomycin and an aminoglycoside is the appropriate combination for the additional possibility of S. epidermidis. Therapy for specific organisms should be individualized based on culture results. Once the causative organism has been isolated, serum bactericidal titers should be obtained. Optimal therapy is achieved with a peak $\geq 1:64$ and a trough $\geq 1:32$. Repeated daily blood cultures should be drawn until sterile cultures are obtained. Fever that persists beyond 1 to 2 weeks despite appropriate antimicrobial therapy should prompt an investigation for more extensive disease, including valve ring and myocardial abscess. Surgery may be necessary in refractory heart failure or multiple serious embolic events, as well as in most cases of prosthetic valve endocarditis and local suppurative complications, such as a myocardial abscess.

Purulent Pericarditis

Bacterial infection of the pericardium may result in inflammation, effusion with or without tamponade, and fibrosis with or without constriction. Infection arises either by direct extension of involved lung or pleura or by hematogenous spread from a distant focus. A chest radiograph will reveal an enlarged heart. The absence of increased pulmonary vascular markings supports the diagnosis, as does the separation of the mediastinal and subepicardial fat stripes. Electrocardiograms provide little benefit compared with echocardiography, which not only reveals the presence of the pericardial fluid but also gives an indication of cardiac function. Aspiration of pericardial fluid by a subxyphoid approach provides the definitive diagnosis and samples of fluid for cell count, gram stain, and culture. Blood cultures will usually reveal the infecting organism.

CARDINAL FEATURES

- Cardiomegaly
- Shock or congestive heart failure
- Patient with septicemia or a focus of infection (e.g., pneumonia, meningitis)
- Chest pain and pericardial friction rub (not universal in children)

Antimicrobial therapy alone is insufficient for the successful treatment of purulent pericarditis. Pericardial drainage must be performed. Percutaneous pericardial catheters may be able to drain thin effusions, but if the pus is thick, surgical drainage will be necessary. Antimicrobial choice should be guided by a gram stain of the pericardial fluid. When there is doubt, both an antistaphylococcal antimicrobial and a third-generation cephalosporin should be started.

Systemic Infections

Septicemia

Disseminated staphylococcal septicemia is an unusual entity. It is seen most often in the previously healthy older child or adolescent. It is characterized by bacteremia associated with multiple foci of infection, including the lung, bone, joints, skin, CNS, kidney, and heart. These children can be critically ill, with depressed myocardial function and a fall in stroke volume. Maldistribution of available cardiac output results in regional ischemia and lactic acidosis. There is a loss in capillary integrity with a flux of plasma constituents into the interstitial space. Septic shock becomes evident. The high-grade bacteremia seen in this condition is quickly documented in blood cultures. Chest x-ray and a gallium-67 scan are useful for the identification of multiple foci.

CARDINAL FEATURES

- Fever (or hypothermia)
- Poor peripheral perfusion (mottled, cool extremities, delayed capillary refill)
- Tachycardia and tachypnea
- Multiple foci of infection

The therapy of septicemia requires both supportive care for shock and specific antimicrobials. Presumptive antimicrobials include an antistaphylococcal penicillin or cephalosporin plus an aminoglycoside. All foci may need to be drained before improvement is certain. There is no evidence that the use of corticosteroids alters the course of bacterial septicemia.

Toxic Shock Syndrome

Toxic shock syndrome (TSS) is a multisystem disease associated with *S. aureus,* usually phage group I. The precise pathogenesis of the syndrome is not fully known. Established facts include (1) focal infection with a phenotypic TSS strain of *S. aureus,* (2) high levels of microbial protease production facilitated by abscesslike conditions (e.g., found in sinusitis, soft tissue abscesses, septic arthritis, pneumonia, vaginitis during tampon use, wound infections), and (3) the presence of toxic shock syndrome toxin-1 (TSST-1), a marker exotoxin, in 100% of menstrual TSS and 50% of nonmenstrual cases. There is also evidence both for broad activation of plasma proteins with release of vasoactive cascades and for abnormalities in immunomodulation. TSS is a clinical diagnosis supported by the isolation of *S. aureus* from a focal or enclosed infection. Clinical and laboratory evidence of multiple organ involvement often appears only later in the course of TSS.

CARDINAL FEATURES

- Fever
- Nonpurulent conjunctivitis
- Inflammation of the lips and tongue
- Diffuse erythroderma (generalized, sunburnlike exanthem) with absence of Nikolsky's sign (desquamation with lateral skin traction)
- Focal infection with *S. aureus*

Untreated TSS may evolve to include shock, cardiomyopathy, pericarditis, hepatitis, adult respiratory distress syndrome (ARDS), renal failure, disseminated intravascular coagulation (DIC), and encephalopathy. Specific therapy for each of these complications may be necessary. The critical intervention that may avoid this multisystem disease is drainage of the focus of *S. aureus* infection. An antistaphylococcal antimicrobial should be started, and the adjunctive use of corticosteroids (1 mg/kg per dose methylprednisolone four times daily for 2 to 4 days) is recommended in severe cases. Intravenous immunoglobulin also has been used by some investigators.

Central Nervous System

Bacterial Meningitis

Bacterial meningitis due to *S. aureus* occurs only rarely and usually in the context either of a penetrating head wound or an intravascular infection, such as infective endocarditis or catheter-associated sepsis. Coexisting brain abscesses are not uncommon. The disease has a fatality rate as high as 50%. Recurrences following apparently successful therapy occur in as many as one quarter of patients, especially if a ventricular shunt is present.

CARDINAL FEATURES

- Fever
- Altered level of consciousness (age specific)
- Signs of increased intracranial pressure (bulging fontanelle, vomiting)
- Signs of inflammation (nuchal rigidity, seizures)
- Penetrating wound or intravascular infection

Nafcillin is the drug of choice for staphylococcal meningitis or brain abscess. Drug combinations have not been investigated extensively, but experience suggests that rifampin may be a useful addition to nafcillin. Vancomycin in a dose of 60 mg/kg in four divided doses should be used in patients allergic to penicillin or in infections caused by MRSA. The removal of infected ventricular shunts and the drainage of abscesses may be necessary for cure.

Ventricular Shunt Infections

Infections of ventricular drainage devices occur in approximately 10% of recipients. Seventy percent of such infections occur within 2 months of surgery and are usually caused by organisms that colonize the skin. *S. epidermidis* is recovered in 50% of these infections, and *S. aureus* is recovered in an additional 30%. Mixed infections occur one sixth of the time. No one shunt type is more prone to infection than another. The operative technique has a major impact on infection rates. Cerebrospinal fluid obtained from percutaneous aspiration of the shunt reservoir or tubing reveals the causative organism in 90% of cases. Cerebrospinal fluid may be culture positive in the absence of a pleocytosis.

CARDINAL FEATURES

- Fever
- Altered sensorium
- Irritability
- Shunt malfunction
- Abdominal pain or peritonitis (ventriculoperitoneal shunts)

The most successful management of shunt infections is the immediate removal of the device combined with appropriate antimicrobials. A temporary ventriculostomy for 3 to 5 days may be necessary before shunt replacement to sterilize the infected ventricle and allow the inflammation to subside. Once sterility has been achieved, a new shunt may be placed, preferably at a different site. Antimicrobial therapy with delayed removal of the shunt achieved a cure in 90% of cases. The use of antimicrobials alone is successful in less than half of cases, with relapses occurring weeks to months after discontinuation. For susceptible staphylococcal species, nafcillin is the drug of choice. However, because of nafcillin resistance in over half of the infecting *S. epidermidis,* vancomycin has emerged as the recommended initial therapy in shunt infections caused by gram-positive cocci. The addition of oral rifampin or the instillation of intraventricular vancomycin for recalcitrant *S. epidermidis* infections lacks proof of enhanced efficacy.

GROUP A STREPTOCOCCAL INFECTIONS

MICHAEL RADETSKY, M.D., C.M.

Group A beta-hemolytic streptococcus *(Streptococcus pyogenes)* is the most frequent cause of acute bacterial pharyngitis, the antecedent event to acute rheumatic fever (ARF). It also causes a spectrum of cutaneous infections, may spread to the lungs and other deep organs, and may lead to acute poststreptococcal glomerulonephritis. Severe invasive streptococcal syndrome, a systemic illness of high mortality, is the most recent manifestation of this highly pathogenic organism.

MICROBIOLOGIC PROPERTIES

Group A streptococci are gram-positive cocci that grow as pairs or short to moderate-length chains on 5% sheep blood agar plates. Organism recovery is enhanced when the medium contains trimethoprim-sulfamethoxazole to suppress the growth of normal oral flora. Colonies are 1 to 2 mm in diameter and are surrounded by comparatively large zones of complete (beta) hemolysis. Strains that produce abundant hyaluronic acid capsules appear mucoid. Organism virulence depends on the presence of the antiphagocytic M-protein cell wall antigen, which also forms the basis for classification into over 80 different serotypes.

Numerous extracellular products are produced by group A streptococci. Streptolysins O (oxygen labile) and S (oxygen stable) damage cell membranes and are hemolytic. Enzymes that degrade DNA (DNases A, B, C, D), hyaluronidase, streptokinase, and various proteases are spreading factors that facilitate the rapid propagation of organisms through tissue planes. Antibody to streptolysin O (ASO), DNase B (ADB), and multiple antigenic determinants (Streptozyme) are the serologic markers for recent (but not acute) streptococcal infection. Pyogenic exotoxins A, B, and C, formerly called "scarlet fever erythrogenic toxins," produce rashes and also are pyogenic, cytotoxic, mitogenic, and immunosuppressive. Pyogenic exotoxins have been implicated in the severe invasive streptococcal syndrome.

STREPTOCOCCAL PHARYNGITIS

Epidemiology

Streptococcal pharyngitis is a common infection of children and young adults. Serogroup A causes virtually all these episodes. Serogroup C, and perhaps G, may cause episodic pharyngitis in college-aged adolescents but only rarely, if ever, in younger children. M-protein strain-associated virulence defines the pattern of illness. M serotypes 1, 2, 4, and 12 cause uncomplicated pharyngitis, serotypes 1, 3, and 18 are associated with serious invasive infections, and M3 and M18 are linked with ARF. The infection is spread by direct contact via either saliva or droplets, but foodborne or waterborne outbreaks are well described. Acutely infected individuals readily transmit virulent M-protein-positive organisms. Even without therapy, the numbers of streptococci, the M-protein content, and the risk of person-to-person spread decline with time. An asymptomatic, noncontagious carrier state exists, which at times may represent 5% to 15% of schoolage children.

Clinical Manifestations

The prototype case of streptococcal pharyngitis begins 2 to 4 days after exposure with a sore throat, and abrupt fever, headache, and malaise. Vomiting and abdominal pain also occur. Physical findings include erythema and edema of the pharynx, exudative tonsillitis, characteristic (though infrequent) palatal petechiae, and tender, enlarged, symmetric anterior cervical lymphadenitis. In the absence of fever and pharyngitis, group A streptococci are rarely found. This classic presentation occurs only in the minority of cases, since the clinical spectrum of streptococcal pharyngitis is wide. Mildly symptomatic or asymptomatic infections occur and may induce subsequent seroconversion. If fact, one third to two thirds of ARF victims have no clear-cut memory of a preceding sore throat. The manifestations of streptococcal infection are more mild in infants and in individuals with prior tonsillectomies.

Scarlet fever occurs in a nonimmune individual infected with a pyogenic exotoxin–producing strain. The rash appears on the second day of illness as a diffuse, sunburnlike exanthem (diffuse erythroderma), with accentuation in the flexural folds (Pastia's lines) and relative sparing of the face, palms, and soles. Nikolsky's sign (denuding of the epidermis with traction) is negative. Sweat gland occlusion gives the rash a sandpaper texture. Mild conjunctivitis, circumoral pallor, and inflammation of the tongue (strawberry tongue) complete the disease profile. The rash fades over 5 to 7 days with desquamation that may be extensive and last for weeks.

Although ARF is unusual in young infants, mucosal streptococcal infection is not. Group A streptococci may be cultured in 10% of febrile children less than 3 years of age, of whom two thirds will develop a rise in antistreptococcal antibodies. Most of these infants present with colds, pharyngitis, or both. Excoriation and erythema of the nasal alae or philtrum are common.

Complications

Peritonsillar cellulitis, peritonsillar abscess, and retropharyngeal abscesses all may contain group A streptococci but usually contain mixed oral flora as well. Pharyngeal streptococci occasionally may participate in infections of adjacent structures, such as the sinuses, the preseptal orbital tissues, and the middle ear.

ARF and acute poststreptococcal glomerulonephritis (AGN) are the nonsuppurative complications of streptococcal pharyngitis. Appropriate antimicrobial therapy within 7 to 9 days of the onset of illness will reduce the subsequent risk of ARF by 90%. The risk of AGN, however, is not altered by the use of antimicrobials.

Diagnosis

A diagnostic strategy for streptococcal pharyngitis relies on certain established principles.

1. The basic purpose of diagnostic streptococcal testing is to prevent ARF.
2. The major risk factor for ARF is a personal or family history of prior ARF.
3. The general incidence of ARF in the United States is low, but rheumatogenic M-protein serotypes cause local epidemic disease.
4. Prompt treatment of streptococcal pharyngitis with antimicrobials is most likely to meaningfully accelerate patient recovery in severe clinical disease.
5. The contagious spread of streptococci is ablated with 24 hours of antimicrobial therapy.
6. The carrier rate of streptococci may be high, especially among schoolage children.
7. The clinical assessment of acute pharyngitis can predict the absence of group A streptococci with accuracy (negative predictive value of 97%) but cannot reliably predict its presence (positive predictive value of 36% at a prevalence of 15%).
8. The throat culture remains the gold standard for streptococcal detection. The ideal office medium is a 5% sheep blood agar plate containing trimethoprim-sulfamethoxazole, ideally incubated anaerobically.
9. Rapid streptococcal test kits are accurate when positive but may be falsely negative up to 40% to 60% of the time.

Therapy

Penicillin remains the drug of choice for confirmed streptococcal pharyngitis. Intramuscular benzathine penicillin G may be given in a single dose of 600,000 U for patients less than 60 lbs and 1,2000,000 U for patients greater than 60 lbs. Alternatively, penicillin V may be used in a PO dose of 250 mg three times daily for 10 days. Less frequent dosing intervals or a shorter duration of therapy has not been validated for the prevention of ARF. For penicillin-allergic patients, erythromycin estolate 20 to 40 mg/kg/d or erythromycin ethylsuccinate 40 mg/kg/d divided into three or four doses may be given for 10 days, with a maximum dose of 1 g/d. Alternatively, an oral cephalosporin may be substituted because of the low risk of cross-reactions in penicillin-allergic patients. Trimethoprim-sulfamethoxazole, sulfonamides, and tetracyclines will not cure streptococcal pharyngitis. Symptomatic, anti-inflammatory relief should be prescribed with acetaminophen 10 to 15 mg/kg per dose every 3 to 4 hours, salt-water gargles, hard candy, popsicles, and fluids.

Follow-Up

If the acute illness resolves, reculture of the throat is not recommended. Five to thirty percent of patients will have pharyngeal group A streptococci after proper therapy, but the risk of ARF in these patients and the protective efficacy of retreatment are not known and are thought to be small in normal individuals. Only if the patient has a history of ARF, if an outbreak of ARF is occurring, or if symptoms persist or recur should the throat be cultured again. Explanations for recurrent streptococcal pharyngitis include poor compliance, reacquisition from a family member, or occasionally inactivation of penicillin due to beta-lactamase-producing oral copathogens. If streptococci are found, a single retreatment course with an oral cephalosporin is a reasonable response, but no subsequent culture (proof of cure) should be obtained. In exposed families, the only members who require throat cultures are those who are symptomatic and those with a history of ARF. It is wise to avoid the reinforcement of a family's fears of streptococcal infection (strep phobia) through an excessive concern for either the disease or its documented eradication.

Prevention of Recurrent Acute Rheumatic Fever

Individuals who have already experienced one episode of ARF are at high risk for developing recurrent attacks. Recurrences may occur after asymptomatic infection. Prevention of further attacks depends on a policy of continuous antimicrobial prophylaxis (secondary prevention). The standard choice for this purpose is benzathine penicillin 1,200,000 U IM at 4-week intervals. However, because of declining serum drug levels toward the end of the dosing interval, experts now recommend that this schedule be shortened to every 3 weeks dosing in areas where the risk for ARF is high. Oral penicillin V 250 mg twice daily or sulfadiazine 0.5 g once daily for patients less than 27 kg (60 lbs) and 1 g once daily for patients greater than 27 kg are the recommended oral drugs for this purpose. For penicillin-sulfadiazine-allergic children, erythromycin estolate 250 mg twice daily is the drug of choice. For patients who have experienced rheumatic carditis, the risk of recurrent carditis is high, and such patients should receive prophylaxis well into adulthood and perhaps for life. For patients who have not had carditis, the risk of future cardiac involvement is lower, and prophylaxis may be discontinued when the patient reaches 20 years of age and 5 years have elapsed since the last rheumatic attack.

STREPTOCOCCAL PYODERMA

Inadvertent intradermal inoculation of colonizing group A streptococci and direct finger inoculation of sores, bites, or abrasions are the antecedents for streptococcal pyoderma. Depending on the depth of the skin involvement, the infection may produce clinical impetigo, ecthyma, erysipelas, cellulitis, fasciitis, or a mixture of clinical types. For unexplained reasons, ARF does not occur after streptococcal pyoderma. However, skin infections with nephritogenic strains do cause AGN regardless of antimicrobial therapy. *Staphylococcus aureus* may coinfect streptococcal pyoderma or be the primary infecting organism. In one recent culture survey, 60% of cases of acute impetigo were due solely to *S. aureus*.

Therapy

Antimicrobial therapy for culture-proven group A streptococcal pyoderma is penicillin. However, if a site culture is not definitive, antimicrobials suitable for both *S. aureus* and group A streptococcus must be chosen. Since cephalexin recently has become available as a generic drug, it has emerged as the oral antimicrobial of choice for the ambulatory therapy of pyoderma because of its pleasing taste, gastric tolerance, price, and suitable spectrum. For impetigo, erythromycin is an alternative choice, as is topical mupirocin. Deep tissue involvement requires parenteral antibiotics and possibly surgical debridement.

GROUP A STREPTOCOCCAL TOXIC SHOCK SYNDROME

This recently described syndrome has been seen both sporadically and in clusters throughout the United States. DNA restriction-enzyme analysis suggests that most cases are caused by a uniquely virulent clone. The pathophysiology of disease is not yet understood but involves the production of one of four types of pyrogenic exotoxins that cause nonspecific stimulation of T lymphocyte proliferation, enhance delayed hypersensitivity, suppress immunoglobulin synthesis, and release tumor necrosis factor-alpha and interleukin 6.

Clinical Features

An expert panel has recently proposed a consensus definition for group A streptococcal TSS.

1. Isolation of group A streptococcus from a normally sterile site (e.g., blood, CSF, pleural fluid, peritoneal fluid, tissue, surgical wound)
2. Hypotension
3. Two or more of the following clinical signs of severity:
   a. Renal impairment
   b. Coagulopathy
   c. Liver involvement
   d. Adult respiratory distress syndrome
   e. Generalized macular rash that may desquamate
   f. Soft tissue necrosis

Generally, the afflicted individual has no predisposing factor and develops either a focal, suppurative streptococcal infection of the soft tissues or lung (65%) or streptococcal bacteremia without a focus (35%). Infected varicella is one common setting for this sequence. The disease evolves rapidly. Bacteremia is documented 70% of the time. In 80% of cases, there is cutaneous evidence of pyogenic exotoxin in the form of erythema, bullae, or focal swelling. Reported mortality has been as high as 30%.

Therapy

Successful therapy consists of early recognition, antimicrobials, and full critical care support commensurate with the degree of illness. Surgical debridement of suppurative soft tissue foci is recommended when possible. The choice of antimicrobials is becoming controversial. Penicillin 300,000 U kg/d IV divided every 4 hours has been the mainstay of therapy. However, some experts have suggested that clindamycin may be useful because of its ability to impede toxin production and that ceftriaxone may have greater affinity for streptococcal penicillin-binding proteins. No comparative trials have been performed to validate these suggestions. There is also evidence that intravenous gammaglobulin may downregulate the aberrant cytokine response and decrease the pace and severity of disease expression.

GROUP B STREPTOCOCCAL INFECTIONS

KENNETH M. BOYER, M.D.

Streptococci of Lancefield group B (GBS) are the most frequent cause of life-threatening neonatal infection in the United States. GBS infections are classified according to the age of onset and clinical patterns. Both classification schemes reflect prevailing concepts of pathogenesis (Table 1). The major reservoir for neonatal infection is asymptomatic gastrointestinal and genital tract GBS colonization, present in approximately 20% and 15%, respectively, of pregnant women. Transmission to the neonate is vertical, most often from an amplified inoculum in contaminated amniotic fluid during labor. Amniotic fluid infection may lead to *early-onset* neonatal disease, manifested by pneumonia, bacteremia, sepsis, and, in about 20% of cases, meningitis. Amnionitis is also the usual intermediate step in pathogenesis of maternal GBS sepsis.

Surface colonization of the neonate's skin and mucous membranes, acquired at parturition by contact with maternal genital secretions, may lead to "middle" early-onset sepsis in the 2- to 7-day-old neonate, usually without pneumonia, as well as *late-onset* (after 7 days of age) disease. Meningitis is present in about 50% of these older affected babies. Late-onset disease may also manifest as the cellulitis-adenitis syndrome and as osteomyelitis or septic arthritis. Skeletal infections are believed most often to represent seeding of metaphyses or joints by transient bacteremia at birth. Neonatal surface colonization is believed to be the reservoir for nosocomial nursery transmission of GBS, a likely explanation for the fact that only about half of late-onset cases have a demonstrable maternal source.

TREATMENT

Empiric Therapy

Prompt and aggressive empiric antimicrobial therapy is mandatory in any newborn infant with sepsis or symptoms suggestive of sepsis. The first principle of therapy is *to kill the organisms at the site(s) of infection as rapidly as possible*. The empiric regimen chosen must, therefore, include bactericidal activity against GBS. The combination

TABLE 1. Classification, Mode of Acquisition, and Clinical Manifestations of Perinatal Group B Streptococcal Infection

CLASSIFICATION	ONSET IN RELATION TO BIRTH	USUAL MODE OF ACQUISITION	TYPICAL CLINICAL MANIFESTATIONS
Maternal sepsis*	Prior to delivery, up to 1 week postpartum	Ascending uterine infection, amnionitis	Chorioamnionitis, endometritis, bacteremia, sepsis, septic shock
Early-onset neonatal sepsis*	Prior to delivery, up to 2 days postpartum	Ascending uterine infection, aspiration of infected amniotic fluid	Pneumonia, bacteremia, sepsis, septic shock, meningitis
Early-onset neonatal sepsis "middle onset"*†	2–7 days postpartum	Surface colonization acquired during birth canal passage	Bacteremia, sepsis, septic shock, meningitis, scalp abscess
Late-onset neonatal sepsis	7–90 days postpartum	Surface colonization acquired during birth canal passage	Bacteremia, sepsis, septic shock, meningitis, cellulitis-adenitis syndrome
Late-onset neonatal sepsis	7–90 days postpartum	Transient neonatal bacteremia, birth trauma	Osteomyelitis/septic arthritis, endocarditis
Late-onset neonatal sepsis	7–90 days postpartum	Surface colonization acquired nosocomially	Bacteremia, sepsis, septic shock, meningitis, cellulitis/adenitis syndrome

*Amenable to intrapartum chemoprophylaxis (Boyer, Gotoff: N Engl J Med 314:1665, 1986).
†Amenable to postpartum chemoprophylaxis (Siegel, et al: Lancet 1:1426, 1982).

of ampicillin and gentamicin is used most often. Unless meningeal involvement has been excluded by lumbar puncture, doses of ampicillin should be meningitic, that is, 300 to 400 mg/kg/d. Such doses are justifiable based on the potential for permanent sequelae in neonatal meningitis, the relatively low penetration of penicillin drugs across even inflamed meninges, the decreased susceptibility of high inocula of GBS to penicillins, and the high therapeutic ratios of penicillins in neonates. Lower doses of ampicillin, in the 100 to 200 mg/kg/d range, are effective in infected infants with benign cerebrospinal fluid (CSF).

Gentamicin doses should range from 5 to 7.5 mg/kg/d (lower in infants with birthweights <1200 g). The dose should be adjusted based on level determinations (peak 4 to 8 μg/ml, trough <2 μg/ml) before and after the third dose. Although gentamicin alone is not active against GBS, it accelerates killing by ampicillin in vitro. Thus, in combination with ampicillin, it contributes synergy as well as a broader spectrum of antimicrobial activity. Other aminoglycosides have similar effects, but experience with them is less than with gentamycin.

Specific Therapy

GBS infection is confirmed by a positive blood or CSF culture. Equally valuable is a positive culture from another normally sterile site (e.g., tracheal aspirate, joint fluid, or bone). In any confirmed infection, at least a 10-day course of parenteral treatment is mandated. Penicillin G is generally viewed as the drug of choice, although GBS are also susceptible to ampicillin, the cephalosporins, particularly cefotaxime and ceftriaxone, and vancomycin. Optimal doses and durations of therapy are dictated by the severity of infection and the site(s) of involvement. Table 2 provides recommendations based on clinical experience. Comparative trials of the efficacy of various doses and regimens, however, do not exist.

The switch from empiric (combination) to specific (penicillin) therapy should take place in most instances when bacteriologic confirmation is certain (not based on gram stain results). In meningitis, the use of ampicillin-gentamicin empiric therapy should be continued until CSF sterility has been documented. For this purpose, a repeat culture of CSF should be performed 24 to 48 hours after initiation of therapy and incubated 48 hours before being considered negative. Ideally, all antimicrobial therapy should be administered intravenously through a secure central line (umbilical catheter, percutaneous central venous line, or Broviac are best). This prevents lapses in doses based on technical problems and decreases the risk of local morbidity from infiltrations and phlebitis.

Response to therapy requires close monitoring. At recommended doses, inadequate antimicrobial therapy is seldom the explanation for

TABLE 2. Antibiotic Therapy for Neonatal Group B Streptococcal Infections

TYPE OF INFECTION	ANTIBIOTIC (DOSE) FOR HOSPITAL MANAGEMENT	ANTIBIOTIC (DOSE) FOR HOME MANAGEMENT	DURATION
Suspected sepsis* (initial empiric therapy)	Ampicillin (100–200 mg/kg/d) *plus* Gentamicin (5–7.5 mg/kg/d)†	Inappropriate	Until documentation of bloodstream sterility or identification of organism
Suspected meningitis (initial empiric therapy)	Ampicillin (300–400 mg/kg/d)‡ *plus* Gentamicin (5–7.5 mg/kg/d)†	Inappropriate	Until documentation of cerebrospinal fluid sterility and identification of organism
Asymptomatic bacteremia*	Ampicillin (100 mg/kg/d) *or* Penicillin G (200,000 U/kg/d)	Ceftriaxone (50 mg/kg/d)	10 days
Septic shock or pneumonia*	Ampicillin (200 mg/kg/d) *or* Penicillin G (300,000 U/kg/d)	Inappropriate	14 days
Meningitis	Penicillin G (300,000–500,000 U/kg/d)‡	Inappropriate	14–21 days
Osteomyelitis or septic arthritis	Penicillin G (200,000–300,000 U/kg/d)	Ceftriaxone (80 mg/kg/d)	4–6 weeks
Endocarditis	Penicillin G (200,000–300,000 U/kg/d)	Inappropriate	6 weeks

*Assumes lumbar puncture has been performed and there are no cerebrospinal fluid abnormalities suggestive of meningitis.
†Monitor serum concentration to maintain a peak level of 6–10 μg/ml and a trough of less than 2 μg/ml.
‡Consider the higher recommended dose if cerebrospinal fluid gram stain is positive or if lumbar puncture has been deferred for critical illness or clinical instability.

failure to improve. Persistent positive cultures during therapy suggest undrained purulent collections (e.g., subdural empyema) or intravascular infection (e.g, endocarditis). Patients who do not improve immediately may be manifesting the pathogenic momentum of their original infections. The infant with GBS meningitis, for example, may not begin to show improvement until 3 to 5 days into therapy because the major clinical manifestations of meningitis are the result of host inflammatory responses rather than the presence of organisms per se.

A situation that is increasingly encountered is the *asymptomatic newborn infant* whose mother has received selective intrapartum chemoprophylaxis based on perinatal risk factors (such as premature labor, prolonged membrane rupture, or intrapartum fever) or the combination of a risk factor with maternal GBS colonization. The probability of neonatal GBS infection (had the mother remained untreated) ranges from less than 1% for the baby whose mother had premature labor only up to as high as 10% to 15% for the baby whose mother had the combination of GBS colonization with intrapartum fever. Blood cultures are likely to be rendered negative by maternal treatment, as are skin surface cultures. Thus, if maternal therapy has been given, the infant should be treated for 48 hours pending confirmation of intrapartum maternal GBS carriage and results of the baby's blood culture.

If the blood culture is negative, the most valuable indications for continuing therapy are a positive gastric aspirate gram stain at birth (indicative of a large intrauterine inoculum of organisms), an abnormal CBC (with an immature/total neutrophil ratio of ≥ 0.2 or an absolute band count of $\geq 1500/mm^3$), or a positive urine latex agglutination test for GBS antigen (relatively likely to represent a true positive because the chances of skin contamination are reduced by maternal therapy). Under any of these three circumstances, a 10-day course of treatment as for asymptomatic bacteremia is appropriate. If all three are negative, discontinuation of treatment is justified.

Supportive Therapy

Survival and therapeutic outcome in GBS disease are determined as much by supportive measures as by antibiotics. The principle on which supportive measures is based is *maintenance of normal oxygen delivery and nutrient delivery to the brain*. These issues are paramount from the moment a septic condition is first suspected. For this reason, initial management should take place in the environment of a neonatal or pediatric intensive care unit. The need for more aggressive supportive measures should be considered in the differential diagnosis of poor therapeutic response.

Respiratory failure in GBS disease may be a consequence of pneumonia, apnea, acquired respiratory distress syndrome (ARDS), or persistent pulmonary hypertension (PPH). Supplemental oxygen, mechanical ventilation, and positive end-expiratory pressure (PEEP) are the normal supportive measures. Arterial blood gases must be monitored. There have been some remarkable successes (but also failures) using extracorporeal membrane oxygenation (ECMO) for infants with ARDS or PPH associated with GBS pneumonia. Inhaled nitric oxide, a promising selective pulmonary vasodilator, is currently in therapeutic trials for these two conditions.

Circulatory failure in GBS disease is generally a consequence of birth asphyxia, septic shock, or a component of the syndrome of PPH. Resuscitation of circulating blood volume and pressure with colloid (albumin or plasma) or crystalloid, followed by the use of pressors, are the key therapeutic modalities. Normal blood pressure, peripheral pulses, capillary refill (<3 seconds), and urine output (>1 ml/kg/h) are the usual measures of effective circulation and must be monitored.

In GBS meningitis, correction of respiratory and circulatory failure or insufficiency takes precedence over all other supportive considerations. Other concerns in meningitis include cerebral edema, seizures, inappropriately high ADH secretion (SIADH), inappropriately low ADH secretion (diabetes insipidus), cerebrovascular accidents, and hydrocephalus. In GBS sepsis and septic shock, additional complications that usually require intervention include disseminated intravascular coagulopathy (DIC), metabolic acidosis, and multiorgan

system failure. A unique cause of persistent respiratory distress and pulmonary opacification in GBS pneumonia is right-sided diaphragmatic hernia. In this circumstance, surgical intervention is required.

Dexamethasone, white cell transfusions, and intravenous gammaglobulin to alter host immunity have been proposed as therapeutic adjuncts. None has been proven to be of benefit in the treatment of neonatal GBS disease.

Home Therapy

Home therapy is inappropriate for infants with suspected or confirmed sepsis, suspected or confirmed meningitis, pneumonia, septic shock, or endocarditis due to GBS. However, once clinical stability has been achieved, home therapy with ceftriaxone may be considered in babies with asymptomatic GBS bacteremia or skeletal infections. As in any decision regarding pediatric home therapy, the commitment and competence of the parents are key considerations.

PREVENTION

GBS early-onset sepsis can be prevented through the use of selective intrapartum chemoprophylaxis with ampicillin. This strategy is predicated on the observation that most early-onset sepsis has an intrapartum pathogenesis involving proliferation of organisms in contaminated amniotic fluid. A number of studies of this approach have been published, all demonstrating prophylactic efficacy. Based on these studies, selective chemoprophylaxis has been advocated and widely publicized by the American Academy of Pediatrics and the Centers for Disease Control and Prevention.

The strategy advocated by these organizations involves obtaining cultures for maternal GBS vaginal and rectal colonization at the 26- to 28-week prenatal visit. Ampicillin prophylaxis (2 g IV followed by 1 g every 4 hours until delivery) is advocated during labor for colonized women who also have the perinatal risk factors of premature labor (<37 weeks gestation) or prolonged membrane rupture (>12 hours). Ampicillin treatment is recommended for all women with intrapartum fever regardless of GBS colonization status. Intrapartum prophylaxis is also recommended regardless of colonization status or risk factors for any woman with a prior infant infected with GBS. Widespread implementation of these recommendations has the potential to substantially reduce the incidence of GBS early-onset disease, particularly in those premature infants at highest risk for fatal outcome.

Maternal vaccination with conjugate type-specific GBS polysaccharide vaccines holds promise for even further reducing the incidence of GBS neonatal disease. Tetanus toxoid and GBS "c protein" conjugates have been prepared, and preliminary studies indicate immunogenicity in unprimed adults. Vaccination has the potential for prevention of late-onset as well as early-onset disease. Efficacy studies of these vaccines are eagerly awaited.

SYPHILIS

PABLO J. SÁNCHEZ, M.D.

Since 1986, there has been a steady increase in the incidence of primary and secondary syphilis in the United States. This increase has been greatest among African Americans and Hispanics in such large urban areas as New York City, Miami, Los Angeles, and Detroit and is largely due to the exchange of drugs, particularly crack cocaine, for sex with multiple partners of unknown identities. Such practice makes partner notification, a traditional syphilis control measure, virtually impossible. In parallel with the rise in primary and secondary syphilis among women of childbearing age, there also occurred a resurgence of congenital syphilis. In 1993, over 3000 cases of congenital syphilis were reported to the Centers for Disease Control and Prevention (CDC). Recently, there has been a decrease in both early syphilis in adults and cases of congenital syphilis. This has been attributed to innovative, community-based methods that identify specific sex-for-drugs locations rather than only named sexual partners of persons with early syphilis. Such a strategy facilitates identification, serologic testing, and treatment of persons at high risk for syphilis because of behaviors associated with their crack use.

TREATMENT

Penicillin remains the drug of choice for treatment of both acquired and congenital syphilis. A serum concentration of 0.018 μg/ml is required to ensure adequate killing of *Treponema pallidum* and must be maintained for 7 days in early cases and up to 3 weeks in late disease. No penicillin-resistant isolate has been recovered.

All patients with reactive serologic tests for syphilis should be counseled concerning the risks of infection with the human immunodeficiency virus (HIV) and tested for HIV antibodies.

Persons Exposed to Syphilis

A person exposed sexually to a patient with early syphilis may be infected yet seronegative if the exposure occurred within the previous 90 days. In such a case, the person should be treated presumptively with benzathine penicillin G 50,000 U/kg IM (max: 2.4 million units). The efficacy of either doxycycline, tetracycline, or ceftriaxone is less. Combination therapy with ceftriaxone and doxycycline, which is recommended for treatment of gonorrhea, is probably effective against incubating syphilis.

Early Syphilis (Primary, Secondary, and Early Latent Syphilis of Less Than 1 Year's Duration)

The recommended treatment for early syphilis is a single IM injection of benzathine penicillin G 50,000 U/kg, not to exceed 2.4 million units. Alternative regimens for nonpregnant, penicillin-allergic adult patients include doxycycline 100 mg PO two times a day for 2 weeks and tetracycline 500 mg PO four times a day for 2 weeks. Both are equivalent therapies, although compliance is better with doxycycline, because fewer doses are required, it can be taken with meals, and it is associated with less gastrointestinal irritation. Tetracycline and doxycyline are not recommended for children younger than 9 years of age because of the dose-related risks of dental staining, enamelization defects in deciduous and permanent teeth, and depression of linear bone growth. The use of erythromycin has resulted in higher rates of failure as well as poor compliance secondary to gastrointestinal side effects. Ceftriaxone 250 mg IM once a day for 10 days also appears to be effective therapy, although clinical experience is limited. A single dose of ceftriaxone is not effective for the treatment of syphilis.

Nontreponemal antibody titers should decline fourfold by 3 months after treatment with primary or secondary syphilis or by 6 months with early latent infection. Persons whose serum nontreponemal titers fail to decrease appropriately should be retested for antibody to HIV. Unless reinfection is established as the cause, cerebrospinal fluid (CSF) examination and retreatment should be performed. Persons with persistent or recurrent signs and symptoms or who have a fourfold increase in their nontreponemal test titer either have failed treatment or are reinfected. They also should be retreated after evaluation for HIV infection. Unless reinfection is likely, a lumbar puncture should be performed as well.

Late Latent Syphilis of More Than 1 Year's Duration or Latent Syphilis of Unknown Duration

Benzathine penicillin G 50,000 U/kg IM (max: 2.4 million units) administered 1 week apart for 3 consecutive weeks is the treatment of choice. For nonpregnant penicillin-allergic patients, doxycycline 100 mg PO twice a day for 4 weeks or tetracycline 500 mg PO four times a day for 4 weeks may be given but only after CSF examination has excluded neurosyphilis. Other indications for performing a lumbar puncture in these patients include neurologic signs or symptoms, treat-

ment failure, serum nontreponemal antibody titer greater than 1:32, other evidence of active syphilis, such as aortitis, gumma, or iritis, and a positive HIV antibody test. If results of the CSF examination are consistent with neurosyphilis, a regimen appropriate for neurosyphilis is indicated. Tetracycline or doxycycline should not be given to children younger than 9 years for reasons outlined previously.

Quantitative nontreponemal serologic testing should be performed 6 and 12 months after treatment. If serologic titers increase fourfold or there is a recurrence or persistence of clinical signs, reevaluation for possible neurosyphilis and retreatment are recommended.

Tertiary Syphilis

Patients with gumma and cardiovascular syphilis who do not have evidence of neurosyphilis may receive benzathine penicillin G 2.4 million units IM administered 1 week apart for 3 consecutive weeks. Alternatively, patients with cardiovascular syphilis may be treated with a neurosyphilis regimen.

Neurosyphilis

The recommended treatment for neurosyphilis and syphilitic eye disease (uveitis, neuroretinitis, or optic neuritis) is IV aqueous crystalline penicillin G 200,000 to 300,000 U/kg/d or 50,000 U/kg every 4 to 6 hours for 10 to 14 days. The maximum adult dose is 12 to 24 million units per day (2 to 4 million units every 4 hours) administered IV for 10 to 14 days. If outpatient compliance can be ensured, an alternative regimen consists of daily aqueous procaine penicillin G 2.4 million units IM plus probenicid 500 mg PO four times a day, both for 10 to 14 days. Some authorities follow both of these treatment regimens with benzathine penicillin G 50,000 U/kg IM (max adult dose 2.4 million units). Patients with a history of penicillin allergy should be skin tested and desensitized if necessary. Amoxicillin 6 g combined with 2 g of probenicid daily, doxycycline 200 mg twice daily, and ceftriaxone 1 g daily for 14 days have been used as alternative regimens. However, insufficient clinical data and follow-up are available for any of these regimens to be recommended.

A follow-up CSF examination should be performed every 6 months until it is normal. CSF pleocytosis that has not improved significantly by 6 months or failure of the CSF examination to become normal by 2 years after therapy is an indication for retreatment.

Syphilis in HIV-Infected Patients

Patients coinfected with syphilis and HIV can be treated for syphilis with a regimen similar to that for patients who lack HIV antibody. Penicillin therapy, however, should be used whenever possible in these patients. Moreover, careful and frequent clinical and serologic follow-up at 1, 2, 3, 6, 9, and 12 months after treatment is indicated. If nontreponemal antibody titers have not declined fourfold by 3 months with primary or secondary syphilis or by 6 months in early latent syphilis or if the titer has increased fourfold at any time, a CSF examination should be performed, and the patient should be retreated with a neurosyphilis regimen unless reinfection can be established as the cause of the increased titer. Patients with late latent disease and HIV infection should undergo CSF examination before treatment. If the CSF is abnormal, a regimen for neurosyphilis is indicated.

Syphilis in Pregnancy

Pregnant women should be treated with the penicillin regimen appropriate for the stage of syphilis. Benzathine penicillin G remains the drug of choice for treatment of maternal infection and prevention of congenital syphilis. The efficacy in early syphilis is approximately 98%. Since transmission of *T. pallidum* to the fetus is highest following maternal secondary syphilis, a second dose of benzathine penicillin G 2.4 million units IM administered 1 week after the initial dose has been recommended by some experts. Tetracycline and doxycycline are contraindicated during pregnancy, since both can result in staining of decidual teeth. Tetracycline also has been associated with temporary impairment of long bone growth and with hepatic toxicity in pregnant patients who have impaired renal function. Erythromycin should not be used because of unpredictable maternal serum levels and transplacental transfer, leading to a high risk of failure to cure infection in the fetus. Pregnant women with a history of penicillin allergy should be skin tested and, if necessary, desensitized according to the protocol established by Wendel et al.[1]

Follow-up consists of monthly quantitative serologic testing until delivery. Criteria for retreatment are the same as for nonpregnant individuals.

Congenital Syphilis

The decision to treat an infant for congenital syphilis is based on the clinical presentation, previous serologic test results and treatment of the mother, and results of serologic testing of the infant and mother at the time of delivery. Evaluation of the infant for congenital syphilis and treatment at birth is required for the following situations.

1. The infant has abnormal physical examination and laboratory or radiographic studies that are consistent with a diagnosis of congenital syphilis.
2. The infant's nontreponemal antibody titer is fourfold or greater than the maternal titer.
3. Maternal treatment before delivery is nonexistent, cannot be documented, is inadequate for the stage of syphilis, or is within 4 weeks of delivery.
4. The mother was treated with an antibiotic other than penicillin.
5. The mother has been appropriately treated previously for syphilis, but there is evidence, either by physical examination or a fourfold increase in nontreponemal titer, of reinfection during the pregnancy.
6. The adequacy of maternal treatment for early syphilis during pregnancy cannot be fully evaluated, since insufficient time has elapsed for nontreponemal serologic titers to decrease fourfold.

Infants who are 4 weeks of age or less and who have proven or highly probable disease, that is, symptomatic infants or asymptomatic infants with an abnormal CSF examination, abnormal bone radiographs, abnormal laboratory evaluation, or a serum nontreponemal titer that is fourfold or greater than the mother's titer, should be treated for 10 days with either (1) aqueous crystalline penicillin G 50,000 U/kg IV every 12 hours for the first 7 days of life and every 8 hours beyond 1 week of age or (2) aqueous procaine penicillin G 50,000 U/kg IM once daily. If more than 1 day is missed, the entire course should be restarted. Although the CSF concentration of penicillin is higher among infants who receive intravenous aqueous penicillin G than among those treated with intramuscular procaine penicillin, the significance of this finding remains unclear, since both therapies have resulted in clinical and laboratory cure. Similar infants who have congenital syphilis or neurosyphilis and who are older than 4 weeks of age should receive aqueous penicillin G 50,000 U/kg IV every 6 hours for 10 days. Children diagnosed with syphilis should have their birth and maternal records reviewed to determine whether the child has congenital or acquired syphilis. Children with acquired syphilis should have a CSF examination performed to exclude neurosyphilis. They may be treated with a penicillin regimen appropriate for the stage of infection, as in adults.

The treatment of the asymptomatic infant with a normal physical examination, normal CSF examination, and normal laboratory and radiographic findings is dependent on maternal treatment history. If, at delivery, maternal treatment is nonexistent or unknown, a 10-day course of either aqueous penicillin G or procaine penicillin G is preferred by such authorities as the CDC. Alternatively, a single IM injection of benzathine penicillin G 50,000 U/kg can be administered, with follow-up serologic testing of the infant. Failure of a single injection of benzathine penicillin G administered to 3 asymptomatic infants has been reported. These infants were delivered of mothers with early syphilis and were not fully evaluated for evidence of congenital syphilis at delivery. These treatment failures have been attributed to the inability of penicillin to adequately penetrate and

achieve treponemicidal concentration in certain sites, such as the aqueous humor and CNS.

Asymptomatic infants whose physical examination, bone radiographs, and laboratory tests are normal can be treated with a single IM dose of benzathine penicillin G 50,000 U/kg under the following circumstances: (1) the mother was treated for syphilis during the pregnancy with erythromcyin, (2) the mother received adequate treatment for syphilis in the last 4 weeks of pregnancy, (3) the mother was treated with an appropriate penicillin regimen for the stage of infection during the pregnancy, but her nontreponemal titers have not yet decreased fourfold, (4) the mother has late latent infection with a low nontreponemal serologic titer ($\leq 1:2$), or (5) the infant's nontreponemal serologic test result is nonreactive, and maternal treatment is nonexistent or unknown. All of these situations involve infants who are at low risk for congenital infection. If the mother received adequate therapy more than 4 weeks before delivery, the infant does not require any treatment. Benzathine penicillin G is adequate therapy for these infants if the physical examination is normal and adequate follow-up cannot be ensured.

Infants born to mothers who are coinfected with syphilis and HIV may be at higher risk of infection with *T. pallidum* and HIV. Nonetheless, there are no data to support more aggressive or prolonged penicillin treatment beyond the regimen recommended for infants not exposed to maternal HIV infection. The necessity of serologic follow-up of these infants is paramount.

Infants with reactive serologic tests for syphilis require frequent clinical evaluation and serologic follow-up with RPR/VDRL (rapid plasma reagin/Venereal Disease Research Laboratory) titers and MHA-TP/FTA-ABS (microhemagglutination assay for *T. pallidum* antibody/fluorescent treponemal antibody-absorbed) tests. This can be incorporated into routine pediatric care at 2, 4, 6, 12, and 15 months of age. The nontreponemal serologic tests of most uninfected infants treated in the newborn period will become nonreactive within 6 months. Persistent stable titers beyond 1 year are an indication for reevaluation and retreatment with aqueous penicillin G 50,000 U/kg IV every 6 hours for 10 to 14 days. A reactive treponemal test beyond 15 months of age, seen in approximately 40% to 70% of symptomatic infants, is a retrospective method of confirming the diagnosis of congenital syphilis. For infants whose initial CSF findings are abnormal, a second lumbar puncture should be performed 6 months after therapy. A reactive CSF VDRL result, pleocytosis, or elevated protein content at this time is an indication for retreatment with aqueous penicillin G 50,000 U/kg every 6 hours for 10 to 14 days.

JARISCH-HERXHEIMER REACTION

The Jarisch-Herxheimer reaction is an acute systemic reaction that occurs in both adults and infants within several hours after the initial treatment of syphilis with antibiotics, especially penicillin. It is characterized by fever, myalgias, headache, vasodilatation with flushing, tachypnea, hypotension, tachycardia, accentuation of the cutaneous lesions, and death due to cardiovascular collapse. In pregnant women, uterine contractions, fetal tachycardia, and decelerations, as well as decreased fetal movements, may occur. Symptoms may last 24 to 36 hours and are usually associated with treatment of early syphilis. The exact etiology is unclear. However, the absence of lipopolysaccharides in *T. pallidum* and the recent recognition that its membrane lipoproteins possess inflammatory activities with induction of cytokines implicate the release of treponemal lipoproteins from dead or dying organisms as the likely inducers of this clinical phenomenon. There is no proven preventive treatment, although aspirin may ameliorate the symptoms.

REFERENCE

1. Wendel GD, Stark BJ, Jamison RB, et al: Penicillin allergy and desensitization in serious maternal/fetal infections. N Engl J Med 312:1229–1239, 1985.

TETANUS NEONATORUM

JEFFREY S. GERDES, M.D.

Neonatal tetanus, caused by infection with *Clostridium tetani*, is primarily a disease of developing countries, although rare cases are reported in the United States. The major risk factors for this condition are (1) birth outside of a medical facility with nonmedically trained attendants, (2) lack of maternal immunization, and (3) nonsterile umbilical cord care, including cutting of the cord with contaminated instruments or customary native poultices for cord care, such as cow dung or fermented milk.

Symptoms of neonatal tetanus are classic and unlikely to be confused with other diagnoses. Sepsis should always be ruled out, however, as it often accompanies tetanus in the newborn. The symptoms of neonatal tetanus include poor suck, abnormal cry, intermittent muscular spasms (tense abdomen, opisthotonos, trismus), and fever. The mortality rate can be as high as 75% but can be reduced to 10% through use of the following treatment regimen.

Supportive care with intensive bedside nursing and monitoring is of utmost importance. Since the major immediate causes of death from neonatal tetanus are aspiration and apnea or respiratory failure, attention must be paid to positioning and suctioning of oral secretions and to monitoring of oxygenation and ventilation. Mechanical ventilation should be instituted for frequent apneic or cyanotic episodes, hypercarbia, or marked inability to handle secretions or aspiration of feedings. Some centers report good results from early intubation, ventilation, and neuromuscular blockade for the first week until the disease begins to resolve. However, others report comparable outcomes with intense supportive care and heavy sedation. The infant should be nursed in a dark, quiet environment, with strict attention to minimizing external stimuli that can precipitate spasms.

Diazepam is the most effective sedative for control of tetanic spasms. An initial dose of 0.1 to 0.2 mg/kg IV is used to relieve an acute spasm, followed by a continuous IV infusion of 15 to 40 mg/kg/d, titrated to control the spasms. After 5 to 7 days, the dose can be tapered by 5 to 10 mg/d and given by the orogastric route.

Phenobarbital is used as an adjunctive therapy, with a loading dose of 20 mg/kg, and maintenance therapy of 5 mg/kg/d to achieve a serum phenobarbital level of 30 to 50 mg/dl. Significant apnea can be expected in up to 10% of neonates treated with this sedation regimen. Accordingly, the means to provide respiratory support should be immediately available.

Human tetanus immune globulin (TIG) should be administered as a single dose of 3000 to 6000 U IM to bind circulating tetanus toxin. If TIG is unavailable, equine tetanus antitoxin (TAT) could be considered. If therapy with TAT is undertaken, acute and delayed reactions to serotherapy should be anticipated. Intravenous immune globulin (IVIg) contains tetanus antibodies, but there is insufficient knowledge about dose and efficacy. The standard dose of IVIg for other indications is 400 to 500 mg/kg. Since tetanus infection does not elicit an antibody response in the host, infants with neonatal tetanus should be immunized with the *DPT* series, starting when recovery from active disease is complete.

Aqueous penicillin G 100,000 U/kg/d is given IV every 4 to 6 hours for 10 to 14 days. Penicillin therapy serves to eradicate the *C. tetani* that are infecting the umbilical stump. The umbilical stump should receive antiseptic cleansing, but surgical debridement is not usually indicated.

Although specific anticlostridial therapy with penicillin and TIG is essential, the key to survival for the neonate with tetanus is carefully managed intensive care.

REFERENCES

1. Einterz EM, Bates ME: Caring for neonatal tetanus patients in a rural primary care setting in Nigeria: A review of 237 cases. J Trop Pediatr 37:179–181, 1991.
2. Okuonghae HO, Airede AI: Neonatal tetanus: Incidence and improved outcome with diazepam. Dev Med Child Neurol 34:448–453, 1992.
3. Traverso HP, Kamil S, Rahim H, et al: A reassessment of risk factors for neonatal tetanus. Bull WHO 69:537–539, 1991.

TUBERCULOSIS

RICHARD F. JACOBS, M.D.

In 1992, reported cases of tuberculosis (TB) had increased to 26,673 in the United States, an increase of 1.5% from 1991. This case rate of 10.5 per 100,000 reflects an alarming increase in reported cases from 19 states. Although a decline of approximately 6% to 7% occurred from 1981 to 1984, in the period from 1985 to 1991, the number of reported cases increased by 18%. The largest increase in tuberculosis cases by age group occurred in the 25- to 44-year-old cohort (52% increase from 1985 to 1991), and cases increased 19% among 0 to 4 year olds and 40% among children 5 to 14 years of age. This recent increase in tuberculosis cases, the changing epidemiology of TB in children, human immunodeficiency virus (HIV) infection, and the emergence of drug-resistant and multidrug-resistant TB have necessitated several changes in the approach and treatment of tuberculosis in children.[3]

TREATMENT

The treatment of tuberculosis in children has undergone major changes during the past decade. As recently as the early 1980s, recommended treatment durations for pulmonary tuberculosis in children were 12 to 18 months. These long regimens were effective when properly followed, but failure rates were high because of poor adherence to therapy. Extensive new studies in children have shown that treatment durations as short as 6 months with multiple-drug regimens are successful for most forms of tuberculous disease. The key to this new approach is intensive initial therapy with several bactericidal drugs and better methods to assure adherence.

Laboratory observations of *Mycobacterium tuberculosis* and results of clinical therapy trials have led to a widely accepted hypothesis concerning the activity of the organism within the host and the mechanisms of action of various antimycobacterial drugs. Tubercle bacilli can survive in several host environments—open cavities, closed caseous lesions, and inside macrophages. The oxygen tension and pH are optimal for growth in open cavities, leading to a large bacterial population on the order of 10^9 organisms. Most children with primary pulmonary tuberculosis and all patients with extrapulmonary tuberculosis are infected with a smaller number of organisms because the cavitary population is not present.

The treatment of tuberculosis is affected by the presence of naturally occurring drug-resistant organisms (primary resistance) before chemotherapy. Although an entire population of bacilli may be considered susceptible to one or more drugs, a subpopulation of drug-resistant organisms is found at predictable frequencies. The estimated frequencies for drug-resistant mutations are: streptomycin 10^{-5}, isoniazid 10^{-6}, and rifampin 10^{-7}. A cavity containing 10^9 organisms has thousands of drug-resistant clones, whereas a closed caseous lesion with 10^6 bacilli will have few or none. These microbiologic characteristics explain why no single drug can cure cavitary tuberculosis. Fortunately, the current hypothesis concludes that the occurrence of resistance to one drug is unrelated to that for any other drug. The chance that an organism is naturally resistant to two drugs is 10^{-11} to 10^{-13}. Populations of this size rarely, if ever, occur in children, so organisms with primary resistance to two drugs are virtually nonexistent.

A major microbiologic determinant of the success of antituberculosis chemotherapy is the size of the bacillary population within the host. Children with extensive pulmonary infiltrates have large bacterial populations. Single drug-resistant bacilli will be present, and adequate treatment requires the use of at least two antituberculosis drugs. If a single effective drug is used, organisms naturally resistant to this drug will multiply and emerge as the dominant population, resulting in the creation of secondary drug-resistant tuberculosis.

This secondary resistance because of ineffective treatment or adherence to treatment is the major factor for increasing rates of isoniazid, rifampin, and multidrug resistance in the United States. Conversely, for children with tuberculous infection (positive tuberculosis skin test) but no radiographic or clinical evidence of disease, the bacterial population is small, drug-resistant organisms are rare or absent, and a single drug can be used as preventive therapy. Children with limited primary pulmonary tuberculosis or moderate extrapulmonary disease have medium-sized bacterial populations, significant numbers of drug-resistant bacilli may or may not be present, and, in general, these children are treated with at least two bactericidal drugs.

The various antituberculosis drugs differ in their primary site of activity and their mechanisms of action. The two major actions of antituberculosis drugs are bactericidal (killing organisms) and bacteriostatic (preventing the emergence of resistance to other drugs). Isoniazid and rifampin kill organisms in all three environments, and both are effective at preventing resistance to other drugs. Streptomycin kills rapidly multiplying organisms but is less effective at preventing resistance. Pyrazinamide contributes to killing organisms in an as-yet unidentified manner. It exerts its maximum effect during the initial 2 months of therapy rather than throughout the full duration of treatment. However, pyrazinamide is not effective in preventing the emergence of resistance to other organisms. Ethambutol is inhibitory to *M. tuberculosis* at a lower dose (15 mg/kg/d) but has some bactericidal activity at a higher dose (25 mg/kg/d).

The earliest treatment regimens for tuberculosis combined the action of a bactericidal drug, such as isoniazid, with a bacteriostatic drug that prevented the development of isoniazid resistance. A small number of drug-susceptible organisms survived, and a treatment period of 18 to 24 months was necessary to permit host defenses to eliminate persisting organisms. Despite this prolonged treatment period, relapse rates among patients were 5% to 10%. The use of rifampin with isoniazid led to cures in almost 100% of patients in a treatment period of only 9 months. When pyrazinamide was added to the isoniazid and rifampin regimen during the first 2 months of treatment of pulmonary tuberculosis, cure rates greater than 98% and relapse rates less than 3% were reported with 6 months of treatment. Over 1000 children have been successfully treated with this regimen for pulmonary tuberculosis. If pyrazinamide was excluded from the 6-month regimen in adult trials, the rate of bacteriologic failure rose to 7% to 10%. However, the addition of streptomycin added little to effectiveness. Regimens of less than 6 months duration were less effective even when four or five drugs were used initially.

During the past decade, several therapeutic trials for tuberculosis in children have been reported. In 1983, Abernathy et al. reported successful treatment of 50 children with tuberculosis using isoniazid 10 to 15 mg/kg and rifampin 10 to 20 mg/kg daily for 1 month, followed by isoniazid 20 to 40 mg/kg per dose and rifampin 10 to 20 mg/kg per dose twice weekly for 8 months (total duration of therapy 9 months). Some patients with only hilar adenopathy were successfully treated with these two drugs given for 6 months. However, the incidence of primary drug resistance is considerably lower in the patient population in Arkansas than in many other regions in the United States. A study from Brazil reported successful treatment of 117 children with pulmonary tuberculosis using isoniazid and rifampin daily for 6 months. Although these results are impressive, the two-drug, 6-month regimen has not been adopted for general use because of limited data and problems with potential drug resistance. The Brazilian study also highlighted the difficulties with adherence in taking long-term medications. Even with this fairly simple regimen, 17% of children did not complete treatment.

There have been several studies of a 6-month regimen of antituberculosis therapy using at least three drugs for drug-susceptible pulmonary tuberculosis in children. Although the combinations of drugs used in these various trials have differed slightly, the most common regimen consisted of a 6-month period of isoniazid and rifampin supplemented during the first 2 months with pyrazinamide. The success of these regimens was independent of the use of streptomycin. Most trials used daily therapy for the first 2 months, followed by daily or twice-weekly therapy for the last 4 months. Regimens that used twice-weekly therapy were as safe and effective as those using daily therapy. In all these trials, the overall success rate was greater than 95% for complete cure and 99% for significant improvement during a 2-year follow-up. The incidence of clinically significant adverse drug reactions, usually gastrointestinal upset or skin rash, was less than 2%.

On the basis of these trials, the American Academy of Pediatrics (AAP) has endorsed as standard therapy for intrathoracic tuberculosis in children a regimen of 6 months of isoniazid and rifampin, supplemented during the first 2 months by pyrazinamide.[1] It is desirable to have medications administered daily for the first 1 to 2 months. After this initial period, they can be administered either daily by the family or twice weekly under the direct observation of a health care provider (directly observed therapy, DOT). For patients in whom social issues or other constraints prevent reliable daily self-administration of drugs, even in the initial phase, DOT has been successfully used two or three times per week from the beginning of treatment. Direct observation means that a health care worker is physically present when the medications are administered to the patient. An alternative regimen uses only isoniazid and rifampin for 9 months. Possible disadvantages of the 9-month regimen include a greater likelihood that secondary resistance will develop during therapy, a slower bactericidal effect, and the need to continually monitor drug susceptibilities, with a greater likelihood of bacteriologic failure or relapse should the child become nonadherent later in therapy. Because adherence usually decreases as regimens become longer, the three-drug, 6-month regimen is currently preferred. Recommended drug regimens, treatment durations, and usual doses of antituberculosis medications are listed in Tables 1 and 2.

HIV Infection

The optimal treatment of tuberculosis in children with HIV infection has not been established. Adults with tuberculosis and HIV coinfection usually can be treated successfully with standard regimens (isoniazid, rifampin, and pyrazinamide) if the total duration of therapy is extended to 9 months or to 6 months after cultures of sputum smears become sterile, whichever is longer. Data for children are limited to isolated case reports. It may be difficult to determine whether a pulmonary infiltrate in an HIV-infected child who has a positive tuberculin skin test reaction or a history of exposure to an adult with infectious tuberculosis is due to *M. tuberculosis*. Treatment usually is presumptive and is based on epidemiologic and radiographic information, and it should be considered when tuberculosis cannot be excluded. Most experts believe that HIV-seropositive children with drug-susceptible tuberculous disease should receive isoniazid, rifampin, and pyrazinamide for 2 months, followed by isoniazid and rifampin to complete a total treatment duration of 9 to 12 months. Preventive therapy for HIV-seropositive children who have tuberculous infection should be 12 months of isoniazid. A difficult situation arises when an anergic HIV-seropositive child is exposed to an adult with tuberculosis. In this situation, tuberculous infection cannot be ruled out. The safest course of action usually is to treat the child for presumed tuberculous infection with isoniazid for 12 months.

Extrapulmonary Tuberculosis

Controlled clinical trials for treatment of various forms of extrapulmonary tuberculosis in children are virtually nonexistent. Several of the previous 6-month, three-drug regimen trials included cases of lymph node and disseminated tuberculosis, and all responded favorably. The basis for treatment of extrapulmonary tuberculosis comes from clinical trials in adults. Most nonlife-threatening forms have

TABLE 1. Recommended Treatment Regimens for Tuberculosis in Infants and Children

FORM OF TUBERCULOSIS	REGIMENS*	COMMENTS
Asymptomatic infection		1. At least 6 consecutive months of therapy with adherence is required
Isoniazid-susceptible	9I	2. If daily therapy is not possible, twice-weekly therapy may be used
Isoniazid-resistant	9R	for 9 months
Pulmonary (includes hilar adenopathy)	6-month regimen 2IRZ/4IR *or* 2IRZ/4I$_2$R$_2$	1. If drug resistance is possible, an additional drug (streptomycin or ethambutol) should be added to the initial therapy until drug susceptibility is determined 2. Drugs can be given two or three times per week under directly observed therapy
Extrapulmonary other than meningitis, disseminated (miliary), or bone/joint	6-month duration 2IRZ/4IR *or* 2IRZ/I$_2$R$_2$	Comments the same as those for pulmonary tuberculosis
Meningitis, disseminated (miliary), and bone/joint	2IRZS/10IR *or* 2IRZS/10I$_2$R$_2$	1. For patients who may have acquired tuberculosis in geographic locales where resistance to streptomycin is common, capreomycin 15–30 mg/kg/d or kanamycin 15–30 mg/kg/d may be used instead of streptomycin

*Treatment regimen codes show duration of initial daily phase of therapy, drugs used/duration of continuation phase, drugs used, and rhythm of administration. I, isoniazid; R, rifampin; Z, pyrazinamide; S, streptomycin. For example, 2IRZ/4I$_2$R$_2$ means 2 months of daily treatment with isoniazid, rifampin, and pyrazinamide, followed by 4 months of twice-weekly treatment with isoniazid and rifampin.
Adapted from American Academy of Pediatrics Committee on Infectious Diseases: Pediatrics 89:161–165, 1992. Reproduced by permission of Pediatrics, copyright 1992.

responded well to a 9-month course of isoniazid and rifampin or a 6-month regimen using three or four drugs in the initial phase of therapy. In general, the optimal treatment for most forms of extrapulmonary tuberculosis is the same as for pulmonary tuberculosis. Possible exceptions may be disseminated, meningeal, and bone and joint infections, which have been associated with higher failure rates when 6-month regimens have been used in anecdotal case reports. For these forms of extrapulmonary tuberculosis, many experts recommend 9 to 12 months of chemotherapy.

Cases of tuberculous meningitis usually have not been included in trials of extrapulmonary tuberculosis because of the serious nature and fairly low incidence of this disease. For drug-susceptible tuberculous meningitis, treatment with four-drug regimens that included isoniazid and rifampin for 12 months have been effective. A recent study from Thailand showed that the survival and morbidity rates are improved significantly if pyrazinamide, which crosses the blood-brain barrier very well, is included in the initial 2 months of treatment. Adding pyrazinamide may allow shortening the duration of successful therapy to 6 months. The recommendation of the AAP is 12 months of therapy including isoniazid, rifampin, pyrazinamide, and strepto-

mycin (Table 1). Many experts believe that a treatment duration of 6 to 9 months is adequate if pyrazinamide is included in the initial phase of treatment. Most experts add a fourth drug initially, usually streptomycin, ethambutol, or another aminoglycoside, to protect against unsuspected initial drug resistance.

Drug-Resistant Tuberculosis

The recent emergence of drug-resistant tuberculosis has become a serious problem for the effective treatment of tuberculosis. In New York City in 1991, 33% of tuberculosis cases were resistant to at least one drug, and 19% were resistant to both isoniazid and rifampin. Resistance to both isoniazid and rifampin substantially increases the cost and duration of treatment while decreasing the efficacy.

Based on surveys of all tuberculosis cases reported to the Centers for Disease Control (CDC) during the first quarter of 1991, cases of tuberculosis resistant to one or more drugs were reported from all 10 Health and Human Services/Public Health Service regions of the United States. Moreover, during the period 1982–1986, 0.5% of new tuberculosis cases were resistant to both isoniazid and rifampin. Preliminary analysis of data for the first quarter of 1991 suggests that

TABLE 2. Antituberculosis Drugs in Children

DRUGS	DOSE FORMS	DAILY DOSE (mg/kg/d)	TWICE-WEEKLY DOSE (mg/kg per dose)	MAXIMUM DOSE
Isoniazid*†	Scored tablets 100 mg 300 mg	10–15	20–40	Daily: 300 mg Twice weekly: 900 mg
Rifampin*	Capsules 150 mg 300 mg Syrup: formulated in syrup from capsules‡	10–20	10–20	600 mg
Pyrazinamide	Scored tablets: 500 mg	20–40	50–70	2 g
Streptomycin	Vials: 1 g, 4 g	20–40 (IM)	20–40 (IM)	1 g
Ethambutol	Scored tablets 100 mg 400 mg	15–25	50	2.5 g
Ethionamide	Tablets: 250 mg	10–20	–	1 g
Kanamycin	Vials: 1 g	15 (IM)	15–25 (IM)	1 g
Cycloserine	Capsules: 250 mg	10–20	–	1 g

*Rifamate is a capsule containing 150 mg of isoniazid and 300 mg of rifampin. Two capsules provide the usual adult (>50 kg) daily dose of each drug.
†Many experts recommend not using isoniazid syrup, as it is unstable and is associated with frequent gastrointestinal complaints, especially diarrhea.
‡Merrell Dow Pharmaceuticals (Cincinnati, Ohio) issues directions for preparation of this extemporaneous syrup.

this proportion was about 3%. From 1990 through 1992, the CDC investigated nine outbreaks of multidrug-resistant tuberculosis (MDR-TB) in hospitals and prison facilities in Florida and New York. A high mortality rate among patients with MDR-TB was documented (range 72% to 89%), with a short median interval between tuberculosis diagnosis and death (range 4 to 16 weeks).

Drug-resistant tubercle bacilli are transmitted in the same manner as drug-susceptible organisms. A four-drug regimen with isoniazid, rifampin, pyrazinamide, and streptomycin or ethambutol is preferred for the initial presumptive treatment of tuberculosis in these areas. When adherence with this regimen is assured, the four-drug regimen is highly effective even for isoniazid-resistant organisms. Based on the prevalence and characteristics of drug-resistant organisms, at least 95% of patients will receive an adequate regimen (at least two drugs to which their organisms are susceptible) if this four-drug regimen is used at the beginning of therapy. Even with susceptible organisms, sputum conversion is accomplished more rapidly from positive to negative with a four-drug regimen than with the standard three-drug regimen. DOT is more easily managed with the four-drug regimen, since it can be administered intermittently three times per week from the beginning of therapy. The four-drug regimen also can be administered two times per week following a 2-week induction phase of daily therapy.

Susceptibility Testing

M. tuberculosis cultures from all patients should be tested for drug-susceptibility. This is essential in all culture-positive patients on their first isolate. These results should be reported promptly to the health care provider and to the local health department. Drug-susceptibility testing should be performed on additional isolates from patients whose cultures fail to convert to negative within 3 months of beginning therapy, or if there is clinical evidence of failure to respond to therapy. In children, this may include cultures from sputum (when available in older children), early morning gastric aspirates, bronchoalveolar lavage fluid, pleural fluid, or cerebrospinal fluid. When cultures in children are not available, the information on these cultures should be actively sought from the adult contact case(s).

Initial Regimen

The initial treatment of suspect or proven drug-resistant tuberculosis should include four drugs. During the first 2 months, the drug regimen should include isoniazid, rifampin, pyrazinamide, and either streptomycin or ethambutol. When drug-susceptibility results are available, the regimen should be altered as appropriate. This regimen should be considered for all patients unless the local epidemiology, susceptibility patterns, and exposure make the likelihood of isoniazid and rifampin resistance low.

Analysis of local patterns of drug resistance provides the best basis for determining when the four-drug regimen might not be necessary. Local community rates of isoniazid resistance <4% can be taken as an indication that an initial regimen with less than four drugs may be acceptable. Institutions (e.g., health care and correctional facilities) or communities that are experiencing outbreaks of tuberculosis resistant to isoniazid and rifampin or that are restarting treatment in a patient from a resistant area with a prior history of antituberculosis therapy may need to begin five-drug or six-drug regimens as initial therapy. The treatment regimen of patients with drug-resistant organisms should be guided by consultation with physicians experienced in the treatment of drug-resistant tuberculosis. Where the prevalence of drug resistance is sufficiently high to justify starting all patients on the four-drug regimen (i.e., a prevalence of isoniazid resistance >4%), pyrazinamide should be discontinued at 8 weeks, but streptomycin or ethambutol should be continued with isoniazid and rifampin for a total of 6 months (for pulmonary disease).

Immunosuppressed Patients

HIV coinfection, primary or secondary immunodeficiencies, and immunosuppressive drugs are important considerations when clini-cians select the most effective regimen for the treatment of tuberculosis. These factors are particularly important with drug-resistant tuberculosis because of the potential for rapid disease progression and death when patients receive inadequate treatment. Most authoritative committees recommend that such patients be treated for a total of 9 months and for at least 6 months after sputum conversion (if available).

Directly Observed Therapy

A major cause of drug-resistant tuberculosis and treatment failure is patient nonadherence to prescribed treatment. Drug-resistant tuberculosis and treatment failures have a higher mortality, especially in immunosuppressed patients, and create other serious public health care risks because they can lead to prolonged infectiousness and increased transmission of tuberculosis in the community. DOT is an important method of ensuring adherence and preventing further development of secondary resistance. DOT requires that a clinician or other designated person observe while the patient ingests antituberculosis medications.

DOT should be considered for all patients because of the difficulty in predicting which patients will adhere to a prescribed treatment regimen. Decisions regarding the use of DOT should be based on the evaluation of local treatment completion rates. If the percentage of patients who complete therapy within 6 to 9 months is <90% or unknown, the use of DOT should be expanded. If >90% of patients beginning therapy complete a recommended course of therapy within 6 to 9 months, the expanded use of DOT may not be necessary. All patients with tuberculosis caused by organisms resistant to either isoniazid or rifampin and all patients receiving intermittent therapy should receive DOT.[2]

When tuberculosis is initially diagnosed, clinicians should explain the disease and treatment and the importance of completing the recommended course of therapy to the patient or parents or both. They should also confirm that the parents understand this information in their native language. When DOT is administered, the method must be specifically defined for each patient and must be based on a thorough assessment of each patient's needs, living conditions, and preferences. The parents and the clinician should agree on a method that ensures the best possible DOT routine and maintains confidentiality. Patients on daily therapy can be managed successfully with self-administered therapy. Public health officials responsible for tuberculosis treatment should be notified when patients not receiving DOT are suspected of not taking medication appropriately, miss appointments, or demonstrate other nonadherent behaviors. These patients should have all regimens administered two times per week or three times per week as DOT for the duration of therapy.

Effective use of DOT sometimes requires an outreach worker to go into the community to locate a patient or family and administer each dose of medication. However, most patients can receive the daily, two times per week, or three times per week treatment at a location agreed on by both the clinician and the family. DOT can be arranged and administered in various settings, including tuberculosis clinics, community health centers, migrant clinics, homeless shelters, prisons or jails, schools, drug treatment centers, hospitals, HIV/AIDS clinics or hostels, or occupational health clinics.

In some situations, another responsible person other than a health care worker may administer DOT. Persons administering DOT can include physicians, nurses, health care aids, correctional facility personnel, staff of community-based organizations, school nurses or teachers, reliable volunteers, drug treatment center employees, social and welfare case workers, and clergy or other community leaders. These arrangements require careful supervision by the clinician. The use of incentives or enablers (e.g., providing transportation or car/bus fare to the treatment site) may promote patient adherence to a DOT program.

Corticosteroids

Corticosteroids are beneficial in the management of tuberculosis in children when the host inflammatory reaction contributes significantly to tissue damage or impairment of function. Data exist to show that corticosteroids decrease mortality rates and long-term neurologic sequelae in patients with tuberculous meningitis by reducing vasculitis, inflammation, and intracranial pressure. Children with enlarged hilar lymph nodes that compress the tracheobronchial tree, causing respiratory distress, localized emphysema, or collapse-consolidation lesions, frequently benefit from corticosteroid therapy. Other forms of tuberculosis that may improve with corticosteroids include miliary disease with alveolar-capillary block, pleural effusion, and pericardial effusion. There is no convincing evidence that one corticosteroid is superior to another. Most commonly used is prednisone 1 to 2 mg/kg/d for 4 to 6 weeks, with a subsequent tapering dose over 1 to 2 weeks.

Preventive Therapy

The treatment of persons with asymptomatic tuberculous infection to prevent development of tuberculous disease later in life is an established practice. Placebo-controlled trials of 1 year of isoniazid preventive therapy involving more than 125,000 subjects have demonstrated a 90% reduction in the incidence of subsequent tuberculous disease among subjects with good adherence to treatment. In children, the effectiveness has approached 100%, and the effect has lasted for at least 30 years.

There is ongoing debate over the optimal duration of isoniazid preventive therapy. Trials among infected adults in Eastern Europe have shown that a 12-month duration of isoniazid preventive therapy is more effective than a 6-month duration, but the 6-month therapy is more cost effective because of fewer toxic reactions to the drug and less need for monitoring patients for toxic effects. There is little comparable data for children. The AAP recommends a 9-month period of isoniazid preventive therapy in children, although a high level of protection probably is achieved with a 6-month course. Rifampin given for 9 months is recommended for children with suspected isoniazid-resistant infection or intolerance to isoniazid therapy. Although controlled trials are lacking, either drug can be given twice weekly under DOT when adherence with daily self-administered therapy cannot be ensured.

Follow-Up During Antituberculosis Therapy

Nonadherence with drug therapy is a major problem in tuberculosis control because of the long-term nature of treatment. As treatment regimens become shorter in duration, adherence becomes even more important. Suspected cases of tuberculosis must be reported so that the local health department can compile accurate statistics, perform necessary contact investigations, and assist both families and clinicians in ensuring adherence to therapy. An assessment of potential nonadherence should be made at the initiation of therapy. Nonadherence and missed appointments should be brought quickly to the attention of the responsible public health officials, who may be able to use various incentives or behavior modification. In extreme cases, removal of the child from the home may be necessary to ensure adherence.

The clinician should take an active role in the care of children with tuberculosis. The three major reasons for following children carefully during their treatment are to (1) ensure adherence, (2) monitor for toxic effects or other side effects of the medications, and (3) be sure the tuberculosis is adequately treated. In general, patients should be seen at monthly intervals and should be given only enough medication to last until the next scheduled visit.

Anticipatory guidance in taking medications is crucial when treating children with tuberculosis. The clinician should anticipate difficulties for the family by the introduction of several new medications (often in inconvenient dosage forms for a young child). Children may receive inadequate medication in the first several weeks until the family develops a dosing scheme that works for them. A liquid suspension of isoniazid is available commercially, but its stability is variable and it can produce diarrhea. Rifampin can be made into a stable suspension by a pharmacist, which is helpful for treating small

children because the only commercially available forms are capsules. Isoniazid and pyrazinamide pills can be crushed and given with small amounts of food. Rifampin should be taken on an empty stomach.

The rates of adverse reactions to antituberculosis medications among children are low enough that routine biochemical monitoring usually is not necessary. Monitoring by signs and symptoms is preferable. If the patient or family reports anorexia, vomiting, abdominal pain, or jaundice, all medications should be discontinued until the child has had a complete physical examination and blood chemistry studies are performed. Serum liver enzyme elevations of two to four times normal occur rarely and do not necessitate discontinuation of treatment if all other findings are normal. All children taking ethambutol should have regular monitoring of visual acuity and color discrimination, if possible. Exceptions to clinical monitoring include children with severe disseminated disease, hepatic involvement, and postpubescent (especially postpartum) African-American and Hispanic females. Baseline serum liver enzymes and routine monitoring every 1 to 2 months should be considered in these groups.

Radiographic improvement of intrathoracic tuberculosis in children occurs very slowly, and frequent chest radiographs usually are not necessary. After chemotherapy is discontinued, hilar adenopathy frequently continues to resolve for 2 to 3 years. Most experts obtain a chest radiograph at diagnosis and 1 or 2 months into therapy to be sure that no unusual changes have occurred in the radiographic appearance. Another radiograph is not routinely necessary until the end of therapy, usually at 6 months. A normal-appearing chest radiograph is not a necessary criterion for stopping therapy. If significant improvement has occurred during treatment, medications can be discontinued, and the child can be seen at intervals of 3 to 6 months after the completion of therapy to follow improvement in the radiographic appearance.

REFERENCES

1. American Academy of Pediatrics Committee on Infectious Diseases. Pediatrics 89:161–165, 1992.
2. Centers for Disease Control and Prevention: MMWR 42:1–8, 1993.
3. Starke JR, Jacobs RF, Jereb J: Resurgence of tuberculosis in children. J Pediatr 120:839–855, 1992.

TULAREMIA

RICHARD F. JACOBS, M.D.

Francisella tularensis is a small, nonmotile, gram-negative coccobacillus and the etiologic agent of tularemia in humans. The organism is found primarily in wild animals, biting arthropods, and their environments. Although restricted regional distribution of *F. tularensis* biovar A (subspecies *tularensis*) and biovar B (subspecies *palaearctica*) was previously hypothesized, worldwide distribution of all strains recently has been proven. *F. tularensis* subspecies *tularensis* has traditionally been thought to be more virulent and potentially lethal, with subspecies *palaearctica* characterized by a link to waterborne disease of rodents, less virulence, and a protracted clinical course. Subspecies *tularensis* is the predominant strain identified in North America.

The transmission of tularemia is primarily by arthropods, with several tick species the most common transmitting vector. Other biting arthropods, animal tissues, and animal bites are also implicated in transmission, especially in high-risk groups (hunters, animal care handlers). The organism produces disease that may be difficult to diagnose, and the success of treatment may be affected by the capability of intracellular survival for extended periods of time.

The primary clinical presentations of tularemia involve infection of skin and regional lymph nodes. In children, cervical lymphadenitis is the most common site of infection, with inguinal lymphadenitis most common in adults. The clinical forms include ulceroglandular, glandular, oculoglandular, oropharyngeal, typhoidal, and pneumonic tularemia. A high index of clinical suspicion is required for early diagnosis and effective treatment, as there is a delay of 7 to 10 days in the seroconversion of standard tularemia serologic tests. Culture of *F. tularensis* has become more common with improved blood culture and basic microbiologic technology. A degree of risk remains for routine handling of cultures in the microbiology laboratory, and caution should continue to be emphasized for laboratory personnel.

Recent studies of tularemia in children from endemic areas have emphasized tularemia as a cause of pneumonia.[2] *F. tularensis* has to be added to the list of pneumonic pathogens that are unresponsive to beta-lactam antibiotics and should prompt a history of tick and animal exposure, season of disease, and local epidemiology.

TREATMENT

Streptomycin, gentamicin, tetracycline, and chloramphenicol have been used successfully in the treatment of tularemia (Table 1). The largest and most successful experience in the treatment of tularemia continues to emphasize streptomycin as the drug of choice. The dose of 20 to 40 mg/kg/d divided into two equal IM doses for the first 2 to 5 days until defervescence occurs, followed by 4 to 5 days of 20 mg/kg/d, completes a standard 7 to 10 day total course of therapy. The total daily dose should not exceed 2 g. The lower daily dose after 2 to 5 days has been used to reduce the most serious adverse effect, ototoxicity. Tinnitus will herald most cases of ototoxicity, which is primarily vestibular but includes hearing loss. Nephrotoxicity is a rare problem with standard dosing regimens.

Gentamicin is an effective alternative to streptomycin, although data are limited in children. The daily dose of 5 mg/kg is divided into two or three equal IV or IM injections. No comparative studies exist to evaluate gentamicin versus streptomycin therapy, but both agents are bactericidal for *F. tularensis,* with only rare cases of documented relapse or treatment failure. A 7- to 10-day course of therapy with 2 to 3 days of an afebrile clinical state is required for successful treatment. Vestibular and auditory ototoxicity and nephrotoxicity are adverse side effects found in a few patients. Other aminoglycosides have not been investigated adequately to evaluate their effectiveness in tularemia.

Tetracycline and chloramphenicol are also effective in the treatment of tularemia. However, these drugs are bacteriostatic, and relapses occasionally occur with treatment courses of less than 2 weeks. Relapses are more common than in patients treated with streptomycin. Tetracycline may be given PO in a dose of 30 to 40 mg/kg/d in four equally divided doses (max: 2 g/d), or doxycycline may be given as 2 to 4 mg/kg/d in two equally divided doses (max: 200 mg/d). The IV tetracycline preparation is given as doxycycline in a dose of 2 to 4 mg/kg/d in one or two daily doses as a 2-hour infusion (max: 200 mg/d). The debate continues among experts and practicing physicians

over administration of tetracycline preparations in infants and children less than 7 to 9 years of age because of the staining effect on developing teeth. Many infectious disease specialists would consider a single short course of tetracycline therapy appropriate in these children under specific circumstances. In general, repetitive use should be avoided. Chloramphenicol is given in a dose of 50 to 75 mg/kg/d PO or IV in four equally divided doses (max: 2 g/d). Aplastic anemia is a rare idiosyncratic complication, with cardiovascular collapse (gray baby syndrome) and reversible bone marrow hypoplasia being related to serum concentrations above therapeutic levels. The course of treatment in confirmed cases of tularemia with either tetracycline or chloramphenicol is usually 2 weeks. Serum chloramphenicol level monitoring is required, especially in more seriously ill children receiving higher doses of the drug.

New in vitro data have suggested that alternative agents might be effective in the treatment of tularemia. Antimicrobial susceptibility testing of *F. tularensis* has revealed quinolones and cephalosporins as potentially effective agents. In particular, ceftriaxone, cefotaxime, and ceftazidime were effective with MICs in the range of <0.12 to 16 µg/ml. Additionally, the MICs of 90% of the strains were inhibited with less than 8 µg/ml of ceftriaxone, 4 µg/ml of cefotaxime, and 0.5 µg/ml of ceftazidime. However, we have just described eight cases that represent documented failures of ceftriaxone in the treatment of tularemia in children.[1] Case reports of the successful use of norfloxacin and ciprofloxacin in adult patients with tularemia have been published.[3] No comparative data are available, and the use of quinolones as routine therapy in children is still restrained by concerns over potential side effects.

Although the potential spread in the microbiology laboratory of these virulent organisms is a serious concern, human-to-human transmission is considered a rare occurrence. No isolation is required for patients with tularemia pneumonia or other systemic forms of the disease. Contact isolation and body fluid precautions should be recommended for open lesions or lymph node drainage during therapy. Late suppuration of lymph nodes (over 2 weeks) occurs in up to 25% of children with tularemia cervical lymphadenitis, but positive cultures from drainage material have not been confirmed following successful antimicrobial therapy.

Clinical response and defervescence occurs within 48 to 72 hours in the majority of patients treated appropriately for tularemia. Relapses may occur in patients treated for less than 2 weeks or with a bacteriostatic drug or with a cephalosporin. Lifelong immunity should occur in nearly all patients following primary infection. The overall mortality rate in children with tularemia is less than 1%.

PREVENTION AND REPORTING

Documented cases of tularemia should be reported to local and state health departments so that high-risk areas can be identified for epidemiologic risk factor assessment and institution of control measures. A live, attenuated tularemia vaccine is available from the Centers for Disease Control and Prevention for use in special circumstances.

Proper handling of wild game (especially rabbits) and animal carcasses should include impervious gloves and proper carcass disposal. Meat should be consumed only after thorough cooking and preparation. *F. tularensis* survives freezing and low degree heat. Proper control and preventive measures for tick attachment and blood meal consumption should be employed to reduce or prevent transmission of tularemia. The use of prophylactic antibiotics for tick bites or contact with suspect animals is not warranted or proven to be effective.

REFERENCES

1. Cross JT Jr, Jacobs RF: Tularemia: Treatment failures with ceftriaxone. Clin Infect Dis (in press).
2. Jacobs RF, Condrey YM, Yamauchi T: Tularemia in adults and children. Pediatrics 76:818–822, 1985.
3. Scheel O, Reiersen R, Hoel T: Treatment of tularemia with ciprofloxacin. Eur Clin Microbiol Infect Dis 11:447–448, 1992.

TABLE 1. Drug Treatment for Tularemia

DRUG	DOSE AND ROUTE
Streptomycin	20–40 mg/kg/d IM divided b.i.d. for 2–5 d followed by 20 mg/kg/d to complete 7–10 d (max: 2 g/d)
Gentamicin	5 mg/kg/d IV or IM divided b.i.d. or t.i.d. for 7–10 d
Tetracycline*	30–40 mg/kg/d PO divided q.i.d. for 2 wk (max: 2 g/d)
Doxycycline*	2–4 mg/kg/d PO b.i.d. or over 2 h IV q.d. for 2 wk (max: 200 mg/d)
Chloramphenicol*†	50–75 mg/kg/d PO or IV divided q.i.d. for 2 wk (max: 2 g/d)

*Rate of relapse is higher than experienced with streptomycin.
†Serum concentrations should be monitored initially and weekly.

TYPHOID FEVER

IDALIA R. RIVERA, M.D.
THOMAS G. CLEARY, M.D.

Typhoid fever is a severe systemic disease caused by *Salmonella typhi*. Ingestion of contaminated water or food can cause human infection. Persons at risk to develop typhoid fever are those living in endemic areas, those with recent travel to endemic areas, and those in close contact with chronic carriers of *S. typhi*. Typhoid fever is relatively uncommon in the United States (0.2/100,000) compared with developing countries, which have rates as high as 540/100,000.

Usually, typhoid fever has an insidious onset of systemic complaints, including fever, malaise, fatigue, chills, headache, rose spots, coated tongue, abdominal pain, vomiting, hepatosplenomegaly, constipation, and rarely diarrhea. Relative bradycardia with toxic appearance, cough, and central nervous symptoms, such as delirium, lethargy, or abnormal mental status, also can be seen. Severe diarrhea or ulcerative colitis as an initial presentation can be seen in symptomatic HIV patients with typhoid fever. The diagnosis of typhoid is confirmed by positive blood or bone marrow cultures. In patients pretreated with antibiotics, bone marrow culture gives the highest yield. Late in the disease, the organism can be isolated from urine or stool. A positive Widal test can suggest clinical infection.

THERAPY

Patients with typhoid fever are usually hospitalized for enteric isolation, antibiotic treatment, and hydration. Antipyretic drugs should be avoided because of the risk of precipitous drops in temperature. There are many antimicrobials that are effective in typhoid. Initial therapy classically has been chloramphenicol 50 to 100 mg/kg/d IV or PO given in four divided doses or ampicillin 200 mg/kg/d IV given in four divided doses for 14 days. After adequate oral intake, therapy can be given by mouth. Amoxicillin 100 mg/kg/d PO in three divided doses may be substituted for ampicillin. Amoxicillin has been reported to be as effective as chloramphenicol, whereas oral ampicillin has a slower response and higher failure rate even in high doses. Alternatively, trimethoprim-sulfamethoxazole (TMP-SMX) trimethoprim 10 mg/kg/d plus sulfamethoxazole 50 mg/kg/d IV or PO in two divided doses for 14 days can be used.

The third-generation cephalosporins have been studied because of concern about multiresistant *S. typhi*. Cefotaxime 150 to 200 mg/kg/d IV (max: 12 g/d) given in four divided doses for 14 days or ceftriaxone 60 to 100 mg/kg/d IM or IV once daily or in two divided doses for 14 days is effective. Relapse after cefotaxime treatment has been described. A 3- to 7-day course of ceftriaxone has been reported to be as effective as a 14-day course of chloramphenicol, suggesting that shorter courses may become the norm. Cefoperazone 100 mg/kg/d IV or IM in two to four divided doses for 14 days is clinically and bacteriologically effective, with minimal side effects in children with typhoid fever. This drug is eliminated by biliary excretion and needs to be used carefully with hepatic impairment. First- and second-generation cephalosporins are not recommended for treatment of typhoid.

Other less commonly used agents available for drug-allergic patients include aztreonam, furazolidone, and quinolones. Aztreonam, a beta-lactam antibacterial agent, has been studied in children with antibiotic-resistant typhoid with clinical success, and 150 mg/kg/d is recommended IV in three divided doses for 14 days. Furazolidone can be used to treat typhoid fever, and it has low cost, reasonable oral absorption, good clinical response, minimal side effects, and a low rate of resistant organisms. Quinolones are considered very effective in the treatment of typhoid fever in adults. The use of quinolones in children has been controversial because of concern about damage to growing cartilage in juvenile animals. More data are necessary before the use of quinolones can be recommended in children.

Dexamethasone has been recommended for treatment of severe typhoid fever (characterized by delirium, stupor, coma, or shock). Such patients should receive an initial dose of 3 mg/kg per dose, followed by eight doses of 1 mg/kg per dose IV every 6 hours for 48 hours.

COMPLICATIONS

Relapse or recurrence after therapy is the most common complication. Retreatment is appropriate. Intestinal perforation and intestinal bleeding are among the severe complications of typhoid fever. When intestinal perforation occurs, surgical intervention with antibiotics and adequate hydration is indicated.

CHRONIC CARRIERS

Individuals with stool excretion of *S. typhi* for a period greater than 1 year after an episode of typhoid are considered to be chronic carriers. Patients with a normal gallbladder should be treated with ampicillin 100 mg/kg/d or amoxicillin 40 mg/kg/d PO in three divided doses and probenecid 25 mg/kg per dose (initial dose), followed by 40 mg/kg/d in four divided doses for 6 weeks. Patients with gallbladder dysfunction should be treated with intravenous ampicillin for 7 to 10 days, followed by cholecystectomy and an additional 30 days of amoxicillin or ampicillin.

VACCINATION

Vaccination is indicated only in the following groups: (1) travelers to areas where typhoid fever is endemic, (2) persons with close contact with known chronic carriers, and (3) laboratory workers with frequent exposure to the organism. The vaccines available for immunization in the United States are a heat-phenol *S. typhi* vaccine for parenteral administration and an oral live attenuated vaccine prepared from the Ty21a strain of *S. typhi*. The oral vaccine is preferred in the absence of specific contraindications because of its safety and efficacy.

The dose for heat-phenol parenteral vaccine in older children and adults is 0.5 ml SC on two occasions separated by a period of 4 weeks or more (children <10 years of age receive 0.25 ml per dose). Parenteral vaccine is contraindicated if severe local and systemic reactions have occurred with prior vaccination. Parenteral vaccine booster should be given every 3 years for patients at high risk.

Oral vaccines are not indicated for children less than 6 years old or for immunocompromised individuals, including HIV patients. One enteric-coated capsule on alternative days for four doses is recommended for children and adults, and a booster is recommended every 5 years.

REFERENCES

1. Edelman R, Levine M: Summary of an International Workshop of Typhoid Fever. Rev Infect Dis 8:329–349, 1991.
2. Keusch GT: Antimicrobial therapy for enteric infections and typhoid fever: State of the art. Rev Infect Dis 10:S199–S203, 1988.
3. Punjabi NH, Hoffman SL, Edman DC, et al: Treatment of severe typhoid fever in children with high dose dexamethasone. Pediatr Infect Dis J 7:598–600, 1988.

ROTAVIRUS

MARGARET B. RENNELS, M.D.

Rotavirus is a 70-nm virus that resembles the reoviruses. It is transmitted by the fecal-oral route, after which it infects enterocytes at the tips of microvilli throughout the small intestine. Infection leads to cell death and, thus, loss of brush border digestive enzymes. Approximately 48 hours after ingestion, susceptible children typically develop fever, vomiting, and watery diarrhea. The fever and vomiting subside in 1 to 2 days, but the diarrhea may persist for several days and be very profuse, leading to dehydration.

Rotavirus is the single most important cause of diarrhea in young children throughout the world. Virtually everyone has been infected by age 4 years, and most children develop infection during the first 2 years of life. Rotavirus is responsible for tremendous morbidity and mortality from dehydration. In the developing world, where safe rehydration practices are often not readily available, rotavirus is estimated to cause between 800,000 and 1,000,000 childhood deaths annually. In the United States, the yearly mortality figure is around 100. Morbidity estimates in the United States are staggering. There are between 70,000 and 100,000 hospitalizations due to rotavirus dehydration annually, and there is a 20% nosocomial transmission rate on infant wards during community outbreaks of disease. Efforts to develop a vaccine have been ongoing for over a decade. Candidate vaccines (consisting of animal-human rotavirus strain reassortments that are given orally), are in field trials, but their protective efficacy has been modest.

Infections occur throughout the year in tropical climates but are confined to late fall through late winter in temperate areas. A recently completed epidemiologic study by the Centers for Disease Control and Prevention revealed that infections in the United States begin in the southwest in November-December and then march from west to east, ending with infections occurring in the northeast in April-May.

DIAGNOSIS

Various methods can be used to detect rotavirus in the stool: (1) enzyme-linked immunosorbent assay (ELISA), (2) latex particle agglutination, (3) electron microscopy, and, (4) polymerase chain reaction. The most readily available of these is the ELISA. It should be kept in mind that asymptomatic infection and excretion of rotavirus are very common during outbreaks. Thus, detection of rotavirus in the stool is not absolute proof that rotavirus is the cause of the child's problems. In cases of mild, watery diarrhea in healthy children, it is usually not necessary or economically feasible to pursue the cause. Diagnosis of the etiology should be sought if the child is toxic, has bloody stools, is seriously dehydrated, has chronic diarrhea, or is immunocompromised.

TREATMENT

The most essential therapy for rotavirus diarrhea is restoration and maintenance of hydration. The combination of fever, vomiting, and watery diarrhea in young children puts them at significant risk of dehydration. The dehydration seen with rotavirus infection is usually isotonic. Children should be admitted for intravenous rehydration if they are severely dehydrated, cannot drink, or are vomiting so severely that they cannot absorb oral fluids. Once rehydration has been accomplished, the child can be maintained on oral fluids. The vast majority of children can be managed as outpatients with an oral rehydration solution, such as the WHO formulation or commercial fluid and electrolyte preparations designed for treatment of diarrhea. Details of fluid and electrolyte management are handled elsewhere in this text. Most authorities now agree that rapid reintroduction of feeding after rehydration is preferable to keeping a child on clear fluids for 24 to 48 hours. Nutrition is required to repair the damage to the intestinal mucosa.

Recent studies of bismuth subsalicylate and *Lactobacillus* preparations demonstrate that they may provide benefit in amelioration of diarrhea in young children. There has not been sufficient experience with either, however, to recommend their general use. There is no role for antimotility agents in the treatment of diarrhea in young children.

Rotavirus infection in severely immunocompromised children may lead to chronic infection and chronic, debilitating diarrhea. There has been limited experience suggesting that oral or duodenal feeding of immune globulin in some cases is associated with cessation of diarrhea or clearing of virus from stools. A dose used with success in one report was 150 mg/kg of immune serum globulin given as one dose.[1]

A therapeutic trial of enteral immunoglobulin for an immunocompromised child with chronic rotavirus diarrhea is reasonable.

REFERENCE

1. Guarino A, Guandalini S, Albano A, et al: Enteral immunoglobulins for treatment of protracted rotavirus diarrhea. Pediatr Infect Dis J 10:612–614, 1991.

ENCEPHALITIS

JULIA A. MCMILLAN, M.D.

Encephalitis is an inflammation of the brain, most frequently the result of extension of viral infection into the central nervous system (CNS). When there is simultaneous evidence of meningeal inflammation, the term "meningoencephalitis" is used. When the spinal cord is involved, myelitis or encephalomyelitis is the appropriate description. Fever, headache, seizure, alteration in state of awareness, agitation, and other signs of cerebral or cerebellar dysfunction are the clinical manifestations of encephalitis. They may be seen in association with evidence of acute infection (fever, respiratory symptoms, rash), or they may be part of a postinfectious or parainfectious immunologically mediated syndrome.

The clinical findings seen in patients with encephalitis may be seen also in a variety of other disorders affecting the CNS, and it is important that these other conditions be considered in the evaluation of such patients. Metabolic derangements, including hypoglycemia, uremia, hepatic encephalopathy, and inborn errors of metabolism, can be eliminated from the differential diagnosis with laboratory determination of serum electrolytes, hepatic enzymes, creatinine, and ammonia. Toxic ingestion and syndromes associated with toxic products, such as Reye syndrome and toxic shock syndrome (TSS), also should be considered. It is appropriate to include computed tomography (CT) or magnetic resonance imaging (MRI) or both in the evaluation of acute CNS disorders because of the possibility of tumor, abscess, or hemorrhage. An electroencephalogram (EEG) is indicated both to assess the possibility of status epilepticus, especially nonconvulsive status, and to evaluate the nature of CNS electrical dysfunction, if any.

A wide variety of infectious agents have been implicated as causes of encephalitis (Table 1). An encephalitic syndrome has been described following treatment with animal-derived antisera used in the treatment of infectious diseases, such as tetanus, diphtheria, and pneumococcal pneumonia and meningitis. Postimmunization encephalitis occurs infrequently following the administration of vaccines to prevent influenza, measles, and typhoid-paratyphoid. The CNS abnormalities observed in approximately 1 in 300,000 patients who receive whole-cell pertussis immunization have been described by some as encephalitis, but pathologic evidence in fatal cases is more consistent with encephalopathy (CNS derangement without accompanying inflammation).

Assignment of a specific etiology in patients with encephalitis depends most often on a constellation of clinical and epidemiologic findings. The viruses most frequently identified as causes of encephalitis because of direct infection of the brain include enteroviruses (echoviruses, coxsackie A and B, enterovirus 71, and poliovirus), arboviruses (in the United States these include Eastern equine, St. Louis, Western equine, Venezuelan equine, California, Powassan, and Colorado tick fever encephalitis viruses), and herpes simplex virus.

Laboratory evaluation should include examination of the cerebrospinal fluid (CSF), although the results are usually nonspecific. In patients with viral encephalitis, the CSF white blood cell count may range from zero to several thousand cells. There may be an initial predominance of polymorphonuclear cells, although usually mononuclear cells are in the majority. Localized CNS hemorrhage may

TABLE 1. Etiologic Agents in Acute Encephalitis and Acute Meningoencephalitis

ETIOLOGIC AGENTS	FREQUENCY*
Viruses	
Spread person to person only	
Adenoviruses	+ +
Herpes simplex types 1 and 2	+ + +
Varicella-zoster	+ +
Epstein-Barr	+
Cytomegalovirus	+ +
Variola	+
Enteroviruses	+ +
Reoviruses	+
Rubella	+ +
Influenza A and B	+ +
Respiratory syncytial	+
Parainfluenza 1–3	+
Mumps	+ + +
Measles	+ +
Hepatitis B	+
Human parvovirus	+
Spread to people by mosquitoes or ticks	
Arboviruses—those that occur in the United States are the following: St. Louis, Eastern equine, Western equine, Venezuelan equine, California, Powassan, Colorado tick fever	+ + +
Spread by warm-blooded mammals	
Rabies	+ + +
Herpesvirus simiae (herpes B)	+
Lymphocytic choriomeningitis	+ +
Encephalomyocarditis	+
Vesicular stomatitis	+
Bacteria	
Haemophilus influenzae, Neisseria meningitidis, Streptococcus pneumoniae, Mycobacterium tuberculosis, and other bacterial meningitides often have an encephalitic component.	+ + +
Spirochetal infections: syphilis, leptospirosis, Lyme disease, and other *Borrelia* sp. infections	+ + +
Brucella sp.	+
Actinomycosis and *Nocardia*	+
Cat-scratch disease	+
Other	
Chlamydia psittaci, Chlamydia pneumoniae	+
Rickettsial infections: Rocky Mountain spotted fever, ehrlichiosis, Q fever, and typhus	+ + +
Mycoplasma infections: *Mycoplasma pneumoniae* and *Mycoplasma hominis*	+ +
Fungal: *Coccidioides immitis, Cryptococcus neoformans,* and other fungal meningitides often have an encephalitic component.	+ +
Protozoal: *Plasmodium* sp., *Trypanosoma* sp., *Naegleria* sp., *Acanthamoeba,* and *Toxoplasma gondii*	+ + +
Helminths: trichinosis, schistosomiasis, *Strongyloides stercoralis*	+ +
Drugs: trimethoprim	+

*Frequency refers to the rate of occurrence of encephalitis or encephalitis component in the particular disease cited and not its relative overall occurrence; + + +, frequent; + +, infrequent; +, rare.
From Cherry JD, Shields WD: Encephalitis and meningoencephalitis. In Feigin RD, Cherry JD (eds): Textbook of Pediatric Infectious Diseases, 3rd ed. Philadelphia, WB Saunders Co, 1992:446.

occur during viral encephalitis, and there may, therefore, be red blood cells and hemoglobin present in the CSF. A mild elevation of CSF protein is often seen, but the CSF glucose is usually normal.

In patients with suspected viral encephalitis, specimens of CSF, stool, and throat swab should be sent to a laboratory capable of viral isolation. Isolation of arboviruses is performed in only a few labo-ratories, and contact with the Centers for Disease Control and Prevention should be made if arbovirus infection is likely. The CSF should be examined also for acid-fast organisms, fungi, or parasites, as well as bacteria. Serum should be collected acutely and at 14 to 21 days and tested for antibody against specific causative agents.

THERAPY

The care of patients with encephalitis includes treatment of secondary complications, such as seizures, increased intracranial pressure, and respiratory decompensation. Involvement of other organ systems depends on the cause of encephalitis. Close observation and monitoring of cardiac and respiratory function is indicated. An arterial blood gas determination should be obtained if there is any question about respiratory compromise. In patients with a decreased level of consciousness, parenteral fluids should be provided, with careful attention to the maintenance of appropriate fluid status, electrolytes, serum glucose, and serum osmolarity.

Seizures in patients with encephalitis may be difficult to control. An initial attempt should be made to treat seizures with diazepam 0.2 to 0.5 mg/kg IV (max: 10 mg) or lorazepam 0.1 mg/kg IV (max: 4 mg). Phenytoin 20 mg/kg IV given over 20 minutes (max: 1000 mg/24 h) should be administered if seizures persist or recur (Table 2). Seizures not controlled by intravenous phenytoin should be treated with phenobarbital 20 mg/kg IV given at a rate of 100 mg/min (max: 300 mg). Diazepam, lorazepam, and phenobarbital can cause hypoventilation and lethargy. The need for aggressive and prolonged use of antiseizure medication may thus necessitate ventilatory support. Phenytoin can cause hypotension and cardiac conduction defects.

Increased intracranial pressure may develop in patients with encephalitis. Treatment includes hyperventilation, as well as such maneuvers as raising the head of the bed and minimizing pain and other noxious stimuli. Mannitol 0.25 to 1 g/kg IV given over 20 minutes and repeated, if necessary, every 5 minutes and furosemide 1 mg/kg may be used to reduce intracranial fluid. The use of dexamethasone in patients with suspected viral encephalitis is not recommended because of the possibility that it may potentiate the infection.

Specific antimicrobial therapy depends on the likely causative agent. The only cause of viral encephalitis for which specific therapy of known efficacy is available is herpes simplex. Patients with acute encephalitic symptoms and fever should be treated presumptively with acyclovir 1500 mg/m²/d given in three divided doses. Antibiotics effective in treating the usual causes of bacterial meningitis should also be instituted until bacterial cultures of the blood and CSF are negative.

PROGNOSIS

The prognosis in patients with encephalitis depends entirely on the etiologic agent and the degree and duration of secondary CNS involvement. The mortality rate in individuals with herpes simplex encephalitis treated with acyclovir is 28%. The likelihood of severe

TABLE 2. Drugs and Doses

DRUG	DOSE
Lorazepam	0.1 mg/kg per dose IV (max: 4 mg), may repeat 0.05 mg/kg in 5 min if needed
Diazepam	0.2–0.5 mg/kg per dose IV (max: 10 mg), may repeat q15–20min if needed
Phenytoin	20 mg/kg IV (max: 1000 mg/24 h)
Phenobarbital	20 mg/kg per dose IV at rate of 100 mg/min (max: 300 mg)
Mannitol	0.25 g/kg IV, may repeat q5min and may increase to 1.0 g/kg per dose if necessary
Lasix	1 mg/kg IV
Acyclovir	1500 mg/m²/d IV, divided into q8h doses

permanent neurologic sequelae is about 25%. The prognosis in patients with arboviral encephalitis varies depending on the specific virus implicated, but both mortality and serious morbidity are high.

REFERENCES

1. Rantala H, Uhari M: Occurrence of childhood encephalitis: A population-based study. Pediatr Infect Dis J 8:426–430, 1989.
2. Whitley RJ: Viral encephalitis. N Engl J Med 323:242–250, 1990.

VIRAL HEPATITIS

KAREN L. KOTLOFF, M.D.

Five viruses designated as hepatitis A, B, C, D, and E are recognized as agents for which the liver is the primary site of replication. All are capable of inducing inflammation of the liver, manifesting as fever, malaise, anorexia, nausea, vomiting, diarrhea, abdominal discomfort, dysphoria, acholic stools, dark urine, and jaundice.

HEPATITIS A (ACUTE ENTERICALLY TRANSMITTED HEPATITIS)

Etiology

Hepatitis A virus (HAV) is a small (27 nm), nonenveloped, single-stranded RNA virus belonging to the family Picornaviridae, genus enterovirus (enterovirus 72).

Epidemiology

HAV is endemic worldwide, with the greatest prevalence in areas where there is crowding and inadequate sanitation. HAV causes approximately 50% of the cases of hepatitis reported in the United States each year. In populations where HAV is highly endemic, the peak age incidence is during early childhood, whereas in countries with low endemicity, such as the United States, most cases occur among young adults.

The primary mode of transmission of HAV is person to person by the fecal-oral route. The period of greatest communicability is during the last 2 weeks of the incubation period and the early prodrome. Spread occurs readily following intimate contact (household or sexual) and when hygiene is compromised, such as occurs in day care facilities attended by children in diapers. Common source outbreaks resulting from ingestion of fecally contaminated food and water and vertical transmission from mother to infant also can occur. Parenteral transmission is uncommon, presumably because of the limited duration of viremia.

Clinical Features

The incubation period of HAV is 15 to 50 days (average 28 days). Before 2 years of age, most infected children are asymptomatic or have nonspecific symptoms. In contrast, nearly all adults with HAV are clinically ill, sometimes severely, and approximately two thirds develop jaundice. Clinical signs and serum transaminase abnormalities may persist for several months but usually resolve in 2 to 4 weeks, and chronic hepatitis is not seen. Fulminant hepatic failure and death are rare (<1%).

Laboratory Diagnosis

The diagnosis of HAV is established by demonstrating specific anti-HAV IgM serum antibody. An IgM response is an excellent marker for acute infection because it is almost always present at the onset of illness and is typically short-lived (usually less than 4 months). IgG anti-HAV appears during convalescence and persists for long periods, indicating the presence of preexisting immunity.

Preexposure Immunoprophylaxis

Preexposure prophylaxis with pooled human immune serum globulin (ISG) is recommended for all susceptible travelers to developing countries. A single IM dose of 0.02 ml/kg of body weight is suggested if travel is for less than 3 months. For prolonged visits or residence in developing countries, a dose of 0.06 ml/kg should be repeated every 5 months.

Postexposure Immunoprophylaxis

ISG (a single IM dose of 0.02 ml/kg) given early in the incubation period (within 2 weeks of exposure) is highly efficacious (80% to 90%) in preventing clinical illness. Giving ISG more than 2 weeks after exposure is not recommended. Serologic confirmation of the infection in the index patient is suggested before providing prophylaxis for contacts.

Following exposure to HAV, ISG is recommended for household and sexual contacts of the index case. ISG should be administered to all staff and children enrolled in day care centers or homes that accept children in diapers if a case is detected in an enrolled child or staff member or if cases are identified in two or more household or center attendees. When an outbreak (three or more affected families) occurs, ISG should also be given to household contacts of enrolled children in diapers. In centers not enrolling children in diapers, ISG need only be given to classroom contacts of the index case.

Although the benefit is unproven, ISG should be considered for a newborn infant whose mother is HAV infected and jaundiced at the time of delivery. When an outbreak occurs in a school, institution for custodial care, or hospital, ISG given to close contacts may reduce spread of the disease but need not be administered routinely when isolated cases occur in these settings. If administration within 2 weeks is possible, ISG should be given after common-source exposure and in selected instances to contacts of infected food handlers.

Vaccination

Both killed and live vaccines are under development. Inactivated HAV vaccine was shown to be highly efficacious in preventing infection and disease in several recent trials, and licensure in the United States is expected in the near future.

HEPATITIS B (PARENTERALLY TRANSMITTED HEPATITIS)

Etiology

Hepatitis B virus (HBV) is a 42-nm, enveloped, double-stranded DNA virus belonging to the family Hepadnaviridae. The outer envelope expresses hepatitis B surface antigen (HBsAg), and the inner nucleocapsid contains both hepatitis B core antigen (HBcAg) and hepatitis B e antigen (HBeAg).

Epidemiology

HBV is transmitted via parenteral, percutaneous, or mucosal contact with infected blood or body fluids. The United States is a low prevalence country where nearly 300,000 acute HBV infections occur each year and approximately 0.2% to 0.9% of the population (nearly 1 million people) is chronically infected, with most infections (about 90%) occurring during adulthood. By contrast, in highly endemic areas of the world, most infections are acquired perinatally or during early childhood. Transmission in the United States occurs primarily among groups with risk factors for sexual and parenteral exposure, such as injecting drug users, persons with multiple sexual partners, hemodialysis patients, recipients of clotting factor preparations, residents of custodial institutions and prisons, and health care workers. However, more than one third of infected persons have no identifiable risk factor. In ethnic groups that have higher infection rates than the general U.S. population, such as immigrants from endemic areas, Alaskan natives, and Pacific Islanders, patterns of transmission resemble those found in countries with high endemicity.

HBsAg appears in serum 1 to 2 months after exposure and persists for variable periods. Any person who is HBsAg positive can transmit infection, although infectivity is threefold to fourfold higher when the donor is HBeAg positive. The efficiency of vertical transmission of HBV from an HBeAg-positive mother to her infant is 70% to 90%.

Clinical Features

The incubation period of HBV is 45 to 160 days (average 120 days). Although the clinical manifestations of HBV are similar to those of HAV, the illness has a more insidious onset, longer duration (1 to 8 months or longer), and increased severity. The case/fatality ratio for reported cases is approximately 1.4%. Extrahepatic manifestations, including arthritis, papular acrodermatitis (Gianotti-Crosti's syndrome), urticaria, and polyarteritis nodosa, may be seen. However, acute infection in children frequently is asymptomatic.

The risk of persistent HBV infection is inversely related to the age at infection. The risk of chronic infection declines from 70% to 90% during the perinatal period to 6% to 10% by age 6 years. Chronic carriers are at high risk of developing chronic active hepatitis, cirrhosis, and primary hepatocellular carcinoma later in life, which is a leading cause of death in adults worldwide.

Laboratory Diagnosis

HBsAg is present in acute and chronic infection. HBeAg indicates HBV replication and infectivity in serum, and the appearance of anti-HBe indicates lower infectivity. Detection of IgM anti-HBc, which is present during the acute and subacute phase of infection, can distinguish acute and chronic infection and can establish the diagnosis of acute infection during the window period when antigenemia has cleared but anti-HBs has not yet appeared. Patients with chronic hepatitis B remain HBsAg positive, often with raised serum transaminase levels, for more than 6 months. Anti-HBc is also detectable in this phase. Immunity after HBV infection or vaccine is characterized by the presence of anti-HBsAg antibodies. Anti-HBc antibody, which is present in patients with prior infection but not vaccination, can be used to distinguish natural immunity from vaccine-induced immunity.

Postexposure Prophylaxis

Hyperimmune hepatitis B immune globulin (HBIG) can be highly effective in preventing HBV infection after exposure in several situations. A dose of 0.5 ml IM should be administered within 12 hours of birth following perinatal exposure of an infant to a HBsAg-positive mother and following household exposure of an infant less than 12 months of age to a primary caregiver who has acute HBV. A single dose of HBIG (0.06 ml/kg IM) is recommended within 14 days of last sexual contact with an HBsAg-positive person or following blood exposure to an infected household contact. For accidental percutaneous or permucosal exposure to blood, the decision to administer HBIG depends on whether the source of blood is available, whether the source blood is HBsAg positive, and the vaccination and anti-HBsAg antibody status of the exposed person. Detailed recommendations have been published by the Advisory Committee of Immunization Practices (ACIP) and the American Academy of Pediatrics (AAP) Red Book. In each instance, concomitant HBV vaccination should be initiated.

Hepatitis B Vaccination and Other Control Measures

A comprehensive strategy for elimination of HBV has been adopted that includes (1) universal HBsAg screening of pregnant women, with immunoprophylaxis (HBIG plus vaccination) of infants born to potentially infectious mothers to prevent perinatal infections, and (2) incorporation of HBV vaccine into the routine childhood immunization schedule to prevent early childhood infections in high-risk populations and to provide immunity to adolescents and young adults before developing at risk behaviors for infection. In addition, vaccination of high risk persons is encouraged, as described by the ACIP and AAP.

The licensed HBV vaccines available in the United States contain purified HBsAg produced in yeast cells by recombinant technology. Neither HBIG nor HBV vaccines carry the risk of transmitting HIV. Three intramuscular injections into the deltoid region (any age) or anterolateral thigh (infants) given at 0, 1, and 6 months are required to induce a protective (anti-HBs ≥10 mIU/ml) response in at least 90% to 95% of children and adults. Infants born to HBsAg-positive mothers should receive their first dose at birth (within 12 hours). For routine immunization of children born to HBsAg-negative mothers, vaccine is initiated at birth to 2 months, a second dose is given 1 to 2 months later, and a third dose is given at 6 to 18 months of age. Vaccination of premature infants should be delayed until hospital discharge if discharge weight exceeds 2000 g or until routine immunizations are initiated at 2 months. The recommended dose of vaccine varies according to age, product, and route of infection.

Vaccine-induced protection against chronic infection and clinical illness persists for at least 10 years, even though antibody levels may wane. Serologic testing 1 to 6 months after the last dose is recommended for persons who may require additional doses of vaccine to achieve or maintain protective immunity or who may require HBIG following an exposure, for example, perinatally exposed infants, hemodialysis patients, and HIV-infected persons, and may be considered for health care workers at risk for percutaneous exposures. The presence of HBsAg on retesting indicates that infection has occurred.

Treatment

Interferon alpha has been used for treatment of adults and children with chronic HBV hepatitis. A 3- to 6-month course of 5 to 10 million U given to adults daily or three times a week can induce clinical, histologic, and virologic improvement in 25% to 45% of patients. Delayed long-term benefits, including loss of all evidence of infection and further histologic improvement, have been observed among subjects who became HBeAg negative as a result of treatment. However, reactivation may occur in 5% to 10% of responders, usually within 1 year of treatment.

Limited experience with children suggests that interferon alpha can interrupt viral replication, but the drug is not approved for this indication. Furthermore, it is not known whether treatment can prevent long-term liver complications. Patients with high initial serum transaminase levels are more likely to respond to treatment. Among those with low initial transaminase levels, pretreatment with corticosteroids may improve response. Liver transplantation has been performed in patients with cirrhosis caused by HBV. However, reinfection of the grafted liver may occur.

HEPATITIS C (PARENTERALLY TRANSMITTED NON-A, NON-B HEPATITIS)

Etiology

Hepatitis C virus (HCV) is a small (30 to 60 nm), single-stranded enveloped virus belonging to the family Flaviviridae.

Epidemiology

HCV is the major cause of non-A, non-B parenterally transmitted hepatitis in the United States, affecting an estimated 150,000 persons annually, mostly adults. Injecting drug use continues to be the major (and an increasing) mode of HCV transmission, accounting for about 45% of cases. Transmission by heterosexual contact, household and institutional contact, and occupational exposure among health care workers each accounts for less than 10% of cases. After institution of anti-HCV screening of blood donors in May 1990, the risk of transfusion-associated HCV declined from 3% to 4% to 0.6% of transfusion recipients. Perinatal transmission of HCV occurs rarely and may be more efficient in the presence of concomitant HIV infection. In about 35% of patients, no source of HCV infection can be found.

Clinical Features

Following an incubation period of 40 to 90 days, a relatively mild hepatitis illness begins insidiously. Jaundice is present in approximately 25% of patients. In some individuals, illness rapidly resolves, but in others, clinical symptoms and serum transaminases may wax and wane. Nonhepatic manifestations, such as serum sickness, membranoproliferative glomerulonephritis, and vasculitis with cryoglobulinemia, have been reported. Despite the mild acute presentation, approximately half of patients will go on to develop chronic hepatitis, 20% of whom will develop cirrhosis. As with HBV, chronic HCV infection, especially when acquired early in life, confers an increased risk for hepatocellular carcinoma.

Laboratory Diagnosis

The first serologic screening tests for detection of HCV antibody that became available in 1990 were limited by false positive and false negative results, highlighting the need for a sensitive screening system and a specific confirmatory test. Recently licensed second-generation screening assays contain additional recombinant HCV structural and nonstructural antigens and offer improved sensitivity by detecting a broader range of anti-HCV antibodies. Many of these use enzyme-linked immunosorbent assay (ELISA) or enzyme immunoassay (EIA) techniques, but those using particle agglutination and other methods are also available. Second-generation recombinant immunoblot assays (RIBA) appear to have a lower false positive rate than the screening tests and are frequently used to confirm HCV infection in an individual with a positive screening test, particularly in those at low risk for acquiring HCV infection. However, the role of confirmatory tests in routine diagnosis has not been clearly established. The reverse transcriptase polymerase chain reaction (PCR) to detect HCV RNA is probably the most sensitive method for detecting the replicative, or infectious, phase of HCV infection and can become positive early after infection before antibody appears. However, the lack of standardization limits the clinical usefulness of PCR at present.

Seropositivity does not distinguish acute, chronic, or resolved infection. Sequential serum transaminase determinations can provide additional information to discern acute (self-limited elevation) and chronic (elevation persisting >6 months) hepatitis. Repeatedly normal enzymes could mean resolved infection, false positive, or chronic HCV infection with no or minimal liver disease.

Prevention and Treatment

Available data suggest that immunoprophylaxis with ISG is not likely to be of benefit. Interferon alpha has been approved for therapy of adults with chronic HCV infection. Treatment has resulted in reduction of hepatic inflammation, normalization of serum transaminases, and loss of viral replication in about 40% of patients. However, relapse is seen frequently after therapy is discontinued. Preliminary results of trials with recombinant interferon alpha that have been initiated in children (3 million U/m² three times weekly for 24 weeks) suggest similar clinical efficacy, but further study is needed before definitive recommendations can be formulated. Interferon alpha should not be given to patients with advanced liver disease because it may precipitate fulminant hepatitis. Orthotopic liver transplantation has been performed in patients with HCV hepatitis, although infection may recur in the transplanted liver. A vaccine is not currently available.

HEPATITIS D (DELTA AGENT)

Etiology

Hepatitis D virus (HDV), also termed the delta agent, is a 35- to 37-nm particle consisting of single-stranded RNA and a delta inner core antigen encapsulated by HBsAg. HDV requires the helper function of a coinfecting HBV to support its replication and expression.

Epidemiology

Although found worldwide, HDV is most prevalent in the Mediterranean (northern Africa, southern Europe, and the Middle East), where most transmission is horizontal from intimate contact. In nonendemic areas, such as the United States, northern Europe, and the Far East, it is confined largely to injecting drug users and recipients of pooled blood products, although sporadic cases occur. Perinatal transmission occurs uncommonly. Overall, infections in children are rare. HDV complicates 20% to 30% of cases of chronic HBV, acute exacerbations of chronic HBV, and fulminant HBV.

Clinical Features

Two clinical scenarios are seen. When a person is simultaneously infected with both HBV and HDV, the incubation period is similar to that for HBV. Most illnesses are self-limited. However, the incidence of fulminant or severe hepatitis is higher than that for acute HBV alone, with mortality rates of 2% to 20%. However, coinfection usually resolves, and only about 5% of cases result in chronic hepatitis. The second presentation, acute HDV superinfection of a chronic HBV carrier, follows an estimated incubation of 2 to 8 weeks. Extensive HDV replication often occurs, may transform mild disease to severe illness, and commonly (75%) results in progression to chronic hepatitis. More than 60% of chronically infected patients will develop cirrhosis, and mortality approximates 1% to 3% per year.

Laboratory Diagnosis

HDV infection can be detected by measuring anti-HDV antibody using commercially available assays. IgM anti-HBc antibody can be used to determine whether HBV infection is recent, thereby distinguishing simultaneous acute HDV and HBV infection from HDV superinfection of a chronic HBsAg carrier.

Prevention and Treatment

It is hoped that universal HBV vaccination will prevent most HDV infections. Treatment is supportive.

HEPATITIS E (ENTERICALLY TRANSMITTED NON-A, NON-B HEPATITIS)

Etiology

Hepatitis E virus (HEV) is a single-stranded, 30- to 35-nm RNA virus that is structurally similar to the enteric agent, calicivirus.

Epidemiology

HEV causes large waterborne outbreaks in parts of Asia, North and West Africa, the Middle East, and Mexico. Recent reports suggest that HEV may also account for a substantial proportion of sporadic hepatitis resulting from person-to-person transmission by the fecal-oral route among adults and children living in these areas. Endemic transmission has not yet been reported in the United States, but cases in travelers are seen. Recent demonstration of a viremic phase suggests that parenteral transmission may also be possible.

Clinical Features

The incubation period is estimated to be 15 to 60 days (mean 40 days). The clinical illness is similar to that seen with HAV, but with an unusually high mortality (15% to 20%) among pregnant women. Chronic infection does not occur.

Laboratory Diagnosis

No serologic test is commercially available. HEV should be considered in any person with hepatitis who has traveled abroad but has no detectable serologic markers for hepatitis A, B, C, or D infection.

Prevention and Treatment

ISG prepared in the United States has not been shown to provide effective immunoprophylaxis. Therapy is supportive.

ASEPTIC MENINGITIS

LAURENCE B. GIVNER, M.D.

Aseptic meningitis generally describes a relatively benign form of meningitis most commonly caused by enteroviruses (coxsackieviruses and echoviruses). These viruses circulate primarily in the summer and early fall months, so most cases of aseptic meningitis will occur during this time. Even during these months, but especially at other times of the year, other etiologies must be considered in the differential diagnosis, including other infections, both viral (e.g., arboviruses, herpes simplex virus) and nonviral (e.g., *Listeria monocytogenes,* tuberculosis), as well as noninfectious causes (e.g., drug-induced).

In aseptic meningitis, the cerebrospinal fluid (CSF) usually contains less than 500 white blood cells (WBC) per cubic millimeter, the CSF glucose may be mildly decreased, and the protein may be mildly elevated. The gram stain should be negative for bacteria. WBC counts occasionally may reach 1000 to 2000/mm³. However, such counts are unusual in aseptic meningitis, and in these patients, other diagnoses must be considered. The majority of WBC in the CSF are usually mononuclear, although early in the infection, a neutrophil predominance may be noted. In the latter case, it may be helpful to perform a second lumbar puncture 12 to 18 hours after the first, by which time a mononuclear predominance should be evident. Close observation is required in the interval between lumbar taps, and antibiotics should be administered immediately if the patient deteriorates. This approach should not be considered for the toxic-appearing patient. Such patients should be treated immediately with parenteral antibiotics.

The lumbar puncture may alleviate the symptoms of increased intracranial pressure (headache, vomiting). This finding may be helpful in the differentiation of aseptic from more severe forms of meningitis, including bacterial etiologies. Older and less severely ill children may be treated as outpatients with antipyretics and analgesics as needed. In patients with more severe illness or those unable to tolerate oral fluids, hospitalization may be necessary. Fluid restriction may be helpful in these patients to decrease intracranial pressure and to avoid the inappropriate secretion of antidiuretic hormone. Fluid and electrolytes should be monitored closely, with special attention to serum sodium concentration.

In young infants, hospitalization should be considered routinely. In infants under a few months of age, meningitis due to *L. monocytogenes* may occur, which also may be associated with a mononuclear pleocytosis in the CSF. Thus, young infants should receive broad-spectrum antibiotics (such as ampicillin and cefotaxime) parenterally. If cultures for bacteria are subsequently negative, antibiotics may be discontinued. In the young infant, differentiation from herpes simplex viral infection (for which parenteral antiviral therapy is indicated) also may be difficult. As noted, these other causes of meningitis should be considered especially during the months when enteroviruses generally do not circulate.

Occasionally, enteroviral infection of the young infant may be life threatening. Enteroviral infection should be considered in the young infant with overwhelming sepsis when routine bacterial cultures are negative. Although the human IgG preparations for intravenous use contain antibodies against the common enteroviruses, their use in the treatment of overwhelming enteroviral sepsis in the young infant cannot be recommended at this time because of the lack of controlled studies. Patients with agammaglobulinemia and chronic enteroviral (usually echovirus) meningoencephalitis may benefit from periodic infusions of pooled human IgG intravenously. Intraventricular administration also may be necessary for some of these patients.

Following aseptic meningitis in the first year of life, some studies have demonstrated long-term neurologic sequelae, especially in language development. However, these findings have not been consistent in all studies. The outlook for the vast majority of children following aseptic meningitis is excellent.

REFERENCE

1. Cherry JD: Aseptic meningitis and viral meningitis. *In* Feigin RD, Cherry JD (eds): Textbook of Pediatric Infectious Diseases, 3rd ed. Philadelphia, WB Saunders, 1992:439–445.

VIRAL PNEUMONIA

MICHAEL GREEN, M.D., M.P.H.

Viruses are the most common cause of pneumonia in infants and children. The diagnosis of pneumonia is considered in patients with cough, tachypnea, fever, increased work of breathing, and the finding of crackles on auscultation. The diagnosis is confirmed by typical findings on chest radiograph. Viral pneumonia is most likely to occur in young children and in children with underlying pulmonary or immunologic abnormalities.

The most common pathogen associated with viral pneumonia in immunocompetent infants and children is respiratory syncytial virus (RSV), accounting for approximately 50% of all cases. Parainfluenza virus (types 1, 2, and 3) and influenza A and B viruses are responsible for the majority of remaining cases. Less common causes of viral pneumonia in children include adenovirus, enterovirus, cytomegalovirus (CMV), and measles virus. Immunocompromised patients have an increased likelihood of developing pneumonia caused by CMV and adenovirus or of experiencing more prolonged or severe disease due to the more common viral pathogens compared with immunocompetent children. Similarly, such patients may experience pneumonia in association with varicella or herpes simplex viral infection.

A precise etiologic diagnosis of viral pneumonia should be sought if specific antiviral therapy is contemplated. A nasopharyngeal wash or aspirate provides the best specimen from which to recover RSV, influenza, parainfluenza, and adenovirus. The diagnosis of RSV usually relies on antigen detection or direct fluorescent antibody methods, as the virus is fastidious in tissue culture. Tissue culture is the diagnostic method of choice for the other common respiratory viruses, although direct fluorescent antibody testing also may be used. To confidently diagnose CMV pneumonia, fluid obtained from bronchoalveolar lavage should be subjected to both histologic evaluation (for the presence of inclusions) and early antigen detection by shell vial. It is important to note that asymptomatic patients may shed CMV in the lower respiratory tract. The definitive diagnosis of CMV pneumonia requires both the presence of clinical symptoms and either a positive culture or positive histology in the absence of another potential pathogen.

TREATMENT

The management of the child with viral pneumonia includes both supportive measures and specific antiviral therapies. Supportive measures may include supplemental oxygen and administration of intravenous fluids to maintain adequate hydration. Consideration should be given to the use of bronchodilators in the patient with an apparent component of reversible bronchospasm or in the child with a personal or family history of bronchospastic disease. A child with severe disease may require observation in the intensive care unit or mechanical ventilation for respiratory failure.

Concern for the presence or development of secondary bacterial infections with *Staphylococcus aureus, Streptococcus pyogenes, Streptococcus pneumoniae,* or *Haemophilus influenzae* may lead to consideration of the use of antibacterial agents in highly febrile children with radiographic evidence suggestive of bacterial disease. Because differentiation between bacterial and viral disease is difficult and may require the use of invasive tests, empiric use of antibacterial agents may be warranted at the time of initial diagnosis. Antibiotics should also be considered in patients who are recovering from viral pneumonia and suddenly experience increasing fever and lower res-

TABLE 1. Dosing Recommendations for Antiviral Therapy for Viral Pneumonia

DRUG	INDICATION	DOSE	ROUTE	DURATION (days)
Ribavirin	RSV	20 mg/ml H_2O for 12–18 h/d	Aerosol	3–7
Amantadine	Influenza A	1–9 y: 5 mg/kg/d divided b.i.d. (max: 150 mg)	PO	2–7 (treatment)
Rimantadine		>9 y: 200 mg/d divided b.i.d.	PO	
Acyclovir	Herpes simplex	<1 mo: 30 mg/kg/d divided q8h	IV	10–21
		1 mo–12 y: 750 mg/m^2/d divided q8h		
		>12 y: 30 mg/kg/d divided q8h		
	Varicella	<1 y: 30 mg/kg/d divided q8h	IV	5–10
		1–12 y: 1500 mg/m^2/d divided q8h		
		>12 y: 30 mg/kg/d divided q8h		
Ganciclovir	Cytomegalovirus	>2 mo: 10 mg/kg/d divided q12h	IV	14–21

piratory tract symptoms, suggesting the presence of a secondary bacterial infection.

Ribavirin

Ribavirin is a nucleoside analog that demonstrates broad-spectrum antiviral activity in vitro. It has received FDA licensure for use as an aerosol in the treatment of lower respiratory tract infection due to RSV. Clinical studies have reported varying efficacies of this agent. In recently published investigations, it appears that the majority of infants and children with RSV pneumonia do not require ribavirin. The Committee on Infectious Diseases of the American Academy of Pediatrics has suggested using ribavirin in certain high-risk children, including young infants (<6 weeks of age), infants with congenital heart disease, children with bronchopulmonary dysplasia or other chronic lung diseases, certain premature infants, children with congenital or acquired immunodeficiency syndromes, and infants hospitalized with severe RSV lower respiratory tract disease. A recent study of aerosolized ribavirin compared with aerosolized water (as a placebo) in infants requiring mechanical ventilation due to RSV infection showed that ribavirin recipients required shorter periods of mechanical ventilation, less oxygen treatment, and shorter hospital stays. However, the study has been criticized for using aerosolized water as the placebo, since it can irritate the lower respiratory tract.

Ribavirin is delivered by a small-particle aerosol generator in an oxyhood, tent, or mask from a solution containing 20 mg of drug per milliliter of water. The aerosol is administered for 12 to 18 hours per day. The duration of therapy necessary for efficacy is unclear, but typically patients are treated for 3 to 7 days. In a small study of 9 children given high-dose, short-duration therapy (6 g/100 ml over 2 hours three times per day) for up to 5 days, ribavirin was well tolerated, decreased viral shedding, and permitted easier access for patient care. Further evaluation of this dosing regimen is necessary to establish it as an appropriate therapy.

Contamination of room air with ribavirin occurs when the drug is administered via a hood or tent. Accordingly, the use of an aerosol scavenger device to remove escaping ribavirin from the child's room has been recommended. Because ribavirin is teratogenic in laboratory animals, exposure of pregnant women should be avoided.

There is limited experience in the use of ribavirin for other respiratory viruses, including influenza and parainfluenza viruses. Although no data from formal clinical trials are available, the use of ribavirin may be considered for severely immunocompromised children experiencing pneumonia due to one of these agents. There are several published reports describing the use of aerosolized ribavirin in combination with intravenous immune globulin in the treatment of measles pneumonia in immunocompromised patients.

Amantadine and Rimantadine

Amantadine and rimantadine are closely related antiviral agents that have been shown to both prevent and modify infections due to influenza A virus. Neither of these agents has activity against influenza B virus. Amantadine has been approved for the treatment and pre-

vention of influenza A infections in the United States for over 20 years, and rimantadine was licensed by the FDA for the prevention of infection due to influenza A in 1993. Although rimantadine has not been licensed for the treatment of influenza A, it is believed that it will have similar beneficial effects to amantadine in the treatment of patients with infection.

The primary prophylaxis against influenza A infection remains immunization. However, amantadine or rimantadine should be used as prophylaxis in high-risk patients simultaneously with vaccine when vaccination has been delayed (6 weeks duration for primary vaccine or 2 weeks for booster doses), when the circulating influenza A virus is not in the vaccine, or in children who cannot receive vaccine.

Guidelines regarding the use of amantadine and rimantadine for treatment of influenza A infection are less clear. In patients with severe pneumonia or those at high risk for developing severe pneumonia caused by influenza A, amantadine and rimantadine are appropriate therapeutic considerations. This is recommended in the absence of controlled clinical trials or explicit evidence that these agents prevent complications or mortality. The potential for benefit in these high-risk patients and the relative lack of side effects support this recommendation. The clinician is encouraged to use amantadine or rimantadine when confronting patients with moderate or more severe illness during influenza A epidemics.

The dosing recommendations for amantadine and rimantadine are shown in Table 1. Rimantadine has similar activity to amantadine but appears to have fewer CNS side effects. Therapy is initiated on diagnosis of influenza A infection and is continued for 2 to 7 days.

Acyclovir

Acyclovir is a nucleoside analog with activity against herpesviruses. The drug is effective in the treatment of infections due to herpes simplex virus and varicella zoster virus. Dosing for infections due to herpes simplex virus and for varicella is shown in Table 1.

Ganciclovir

Ganciclovir is a nucleoside analog with in vitro activity against double-stranded DNA viruses, in particular herpesviruses. The drug has been licensed for use in patients with life- or sight-threatening disease due to CMV. Although few studies are available in children, experience among pediatric AIDS patients or transplant recipients confirms the activity of this agent in these children. Data in other patient populations are not available. Dosing recommendations are shown in Table 1. Ganciclovir is typically used for 14 to 21 days. Depending on the underlying disease of the patient, chronic maintenance therapy at a dose of 5 mg/kg/d given 5 days per week may be of benefit.

REFERENCES

1. Drugs for Non-HIV viral infections. Med Lett 36:27–32, 1994.
2. Henrickson KJ: Lower respiratory viral infections in immunocompetent children. Adv Pediatr Infect Dis 9:59–96, 1994.
3. Keating MR: Antiviral agents. Mayo Clin Proc 67:160–178, 1992.

CYTOMEGALOVIRUS INFECTIONS

CHARLES G. PROBER, M.D.

Infections caused by cytomegalovirus (CMV) are ubiquitous and generally self-limited in the normal host. The majority of these infections are either asymptomatic or cause a very mild, nonspecific illness. Some patients may develop a constellation of symptoms and signs virtually identical to those associated with infectious mononucleosis. These include pharyngitis, fever, adenopathy, splenomegaly, and fatigue. Even when associated with symptoms, there is no indication for the use of antiviral therapy of CMV infection in the normal host.

In stark contrast to infections in normal children, CMV infections in the compromised host can be associated with substantial morbidity and mortality. Therefore, prevention and treatment of these infections, when possible, is indicated. In broad terms, the two types of compromised hosts for whom CMV infections may be significant are the fetus and neonate and the child with impaired cellular immunity. These two types of hosts are considered separately.

INFECTION IN THE FETUS AND NEONATE

CMV is the most frequent cause of congenital viral infection. An estimated 1% of all neonates contract this infection. Fortunately, about 90% of these infections are asymptomatic in the neonatal period. The remaining 10% of infections cause some combination of microcephaly, intracranial calcifications, hepatitis with hepatomegaly, thrombocytopenia, leukopenia, and hyperbilirubinemia. The survivors of these symptomatic infections invariably have substantial long-term neurologic handicaps. In addition to these infected infants who are symptomatic in the neonatal period, 10% to 15% of infants with congenital CMV will develop mild to moderate late handicaps, which may include sensorineural hearing loss and neurobehavioral/developmental defects. These sequelae often do not manifest until the early school years. At the present time, it is not possible to prevent congenital CMV infections. Several antiviral agents, including fluorodeoxyuridine, iododeoxyuridine, cytosine arabinoside, adenine arabinoside, interferon, and acyclovir, have been used to treat small numbers of congenitally infected infants. Other than diminishing the quantity of virus shed in urine, none of these agents has been clinically effective. There are perhaps at least two reasons for this lack of demonstrable effectiveness. First, congenitally infected infants already are chronically infected and perhaps irreversibly damaged by the time of birth. Second, the in vitro activity of these various agents against CMV is quite limited and the toxic/therapeutic ratio is narrow. Theoretically, a more promising drug for the treatment of congenital infection is ganciclovir. It has considerable in vitro activity against CMV and has proved to be quite effective in the management of CMV infections in older compromised hosts. Therapeutic trials of ganciclovir in neonates are being conducted.

Cytomegalovirus also can be acquired by neonates as a result of perinatal transmission. The most common mode of perinatal transmission is vertical, either from contact with contaminated cervical secretions at delivery or from exposure to infected maternal breast milk. Perinatal transmission from blood derived from CMV-infected donors also can occur but is preventable by transfusing neonates only with blood derived from CMV-seronegative donors. Except for very premature infants, most perinatal CMV infections are asymptomatic or associated with only mild, nonspecific symptoms. Premature infants perinatally infected with CMV may develop life-threatening problems, including hematologic abnormalities, hepatosplenomegaly, pneumonitis, chorioretinitis, encephalitis, and a septic state manifest with a peculiar gray pallor with fever. Other than anecdotal reports of treatment with immunoglobulin, there are no data regarding the therapy of perinatally acquired CMV infections.

INFECTION IN THE COMPROMISED HOST

The greatest morbidity and mortality of CMV infections are observed in hosts with compromised cellular immunity, including those who have received transplanted organs and those with AIDS. The most frequent organs involved in severe CMV disease include the lungs, eyes, gastrointestinal tract, and liver. Manifestations of disease commonly include progressive life-threatening pneumonitis, sight-threatening chorioretinitis, esophagitis, gastritis, enteritis or colitis, hepatitis, and fever. In general, the greater the degree of immunosuppression, the more severe the infection. For example, in bone marrow transplant recipients, CMV is the single most important cause of death. About half of all such patients will develop CMV infection, and pneumonitis is the single most important manifestation of infection. Without treatment, 80% to 90% of bone marrow transplant recipients who contract CMV pneumonitis will die.

Clearly, there is a need for effective antiviral therapy of CMV infections in compromised hosts, but until recently, such therapy had been very disappointing. Trials of interferon, adenine arabinoside, acyclovir, and intravenous immunoglobulin all failed to demonstrate efficacy. However, two recently developed antiviral agents with superior in vitro activity against CMV have shown promise in the treatment of these infections. These agents are ganciclovir and foscarnet. Both agents are licensed for the treatment of CMV retinitis in patients with AIDS, but they also appear to be effective in the therapy of other forms of CMV infection. The majority of the anecdotal experience with these drugs and the data from controlled trials reflect experience with adult patients. However, it seems reasonable to assume that efficacy demonstrated in adults also would be applicable to children.

The most favorable experience with ganciclovir has been in the management of CMV retinitis and, to a lesser degree, gastrointestinal disease in patients with AIDS. The outcome of pneumonitis caused by CMV in bone marrow transplant recipients also seems to be improved with the use of ganciclovir *if* intravenous immunoglobulin is given with this antiviral agent. Foscarnet also has been shown to be effective in the therapy of CMV retinitis, including disease caused by ganciclovir-resistant isolates of CMV. Foscarnet actually offered a survival advantage in one recent study that compared the outcome in 234 patients with AIDS treated with either ganciclovir or foscarnet for CMV retinitis.[2]

The most frequent toxic effect of ganciclovir is granulocytopenia, and the toxicity of foscarnet is primarily renal impairment, as well as disturbances of mineral and electrolyte balance. In general, treatment with either drug needs to be prolonged for as long as the patient remains severely immunocompromised. This is lifelong for patients with AIDS and until marrow engraftment in recipients of bone marrow transplantation. The precise dose used depends on the site of the infection, the renal function status, and whether it is during the induction or maintenance phase of therapy.

PREVENTION

Some primary CMV infections in immunocompromised hosts may be prevented by using blood and blood products derived from CMV-seronegative donors and by avoiding transplanting an organ from a CMV-seropositive donor into a CMV-seronegative recipient. However, reactivated infections will continue to occur despite these precautions. The role of CMV vaccines in preventing primary and reactivated infections has not been established. Most efforts in trying to prevent CMV infections in compromised hosts have focused on antiviral agents or immunoglobulin or both, administered prophylactically.[1] The types of regimens that have been evaluated in controlled clinical trials and their effectiveness in reducing the incidence of CMV disease are summarized in Table 1. In general, reactivated infections have been easier to prevent than primary infections. Furthermore, it is important to recognize that the effectiveness of any of the preventive strategies outlined here is reduced if the immunosuppressive therapy

TABLE 1. Trials Evaluating Preventive Strategies for CMV Infections in Immunocompromised Hosts

TYPE OF PATIENTS	FORM OF CMV INFECTION	REGIMEN EVALUATED	EFFICACY
Renal transplant recipients	Primary	Oral acyclovir or intravenous immunoglobulin or both	Yes
Renal transplant recipients	Reactivated	Oral acyclovir or intravenous immunoglobulin or both	Yes
Heart or lung (or both) transplant recipients	Primary	Intravenous ganciclovir	No
Heart or lung (or both) transplant recipients	Reactivated	Intravenous ganciclovir	Yes
Liver transplant recipients	Primary	Intravenous immunoglobulin	No
Liver transplant recipients	Reactivated	Intravenous immunoglobulin	Yes
Bone marrow transplant recipients	Reactivated	Oral acyclovir	Yes
Bone marrow transplant recipients	*	Intravenous ganciclovir	Yes

*Therapy was given to asymptomatic patients who had CMV isolated from a bronchoalveolar lavage, routinely performed 35 days after transplantation, and efficacy was defined as a reduction in the incidence of pneumonitis.

is intensified. This is especially evident when antilymphocyte antibody therapy is incorporated into the antirejection regimen.

REFERENCES

1. Rubin RH, Tolkoff-Rubin NE: Antimicrobial strategies in the care of organ transplant recipients. Antimicrobial Agents Chemother 37:619–624, 1993.
2. Studies of ocular complications of AIDS research group, in collaboration with the AIDS clinical trials group: Mortality in patients with the acquired immunodeficiency syndrome treated with either foscarnet or ganciclovir for cytomegalovirus retinitis. N Engl J Med 326:213–220, 1992.

ENTEROVIRUSES

JAMES C. OVERALL, JR., M.D.

The enteroviruses (EVs) consist of 3 serotypes of poliovirus, 24 of coxsackie A, 6 of coxsackie B, 32 of echo, EV types 68 through 71, and hepatitis A (EV 72, see Viral Hepatitis). Infections are widely prevalent, occur mostly in infants and young children, peak during the summer and fall months in temperate climates, and are usually asymptomatic. Transmission is by fecal-oral spread or direct contact with infected respiratory or ocular secretions, but waterborne and foodborne outbreaks and nosocomial transmission have been reported.

DIAGNOSIS

Diagnosis is made by isolation in cell culture of an EV from a normally sterile body fluid (e.g., CSF in aseptic meningitis or serum in the neonatal sepsis syndrome) or from a throat swab (particularly with pharyngeal or respiratory symptoms). Although isolation rates from stool are higher than from other body sites, etiologic association with disease is made difficult by the frequent occurrence of asymptomatic or mild infections and shedding of virus for weeks. In addition, oral polio vaccine (OPV) virus also may be shed in the stool for weeks and result in a positive stool isolate. Isolation usually requires 5 to 7 days. EV typing is available only in reference laboratories. More rapid antigen detection methods are not available commercially, but work is in progress on polymerase chain reaction (PCR) amplification and DNA probe detection methods for CSF specimens. Documentation of infection by rises in antibody titer is generally not practical because a separate neutralizing titer must be performed against each suspected EV serotype.

CLINICAL SYNDROMES

The major clinical syndromes caused by the EVs include nonspecific febrile illness (especially in neonates and young infants), febrile exanthems, aseptic meningitis and, rarely, encephalitis, the hand-foot-mouth syndrome, herpangina, myocarditis, pericarditis, pleurodynia, acute hemorrhagic conjunctivitis, paralytic disease, and chronic infections in patients with antibody deficiency syndrome.

EV clinical syndromes follow the "one virus . . . many diseases; many viruses . . . one disease" pattern. One particular serotype (e.g., echo 9) may cause nonspecific febrile illness, a febrile exanthem, and aseptic meningitis among different individuals during a community outbreak or even within the same family. On the other hand, many different EVs can cause one disease, for example, the aseptic meningitis syndrome.

Nonspecific Febrile Illness

Fever, malaise, and myalgia without specific respiratory, gastrointestinal, mucocutaneous, or central nervous system (CNS) signs or symptoms (nonspecific febrile illness) is one of the most common syndromes caused by EV. When this syndrome occurs in neonates or young infants, it cannot be distinguished clinically from bacterial sepsis. Among 233 infants less than 3 months of age hospitalized for suspected sepsis, over 60% had viral infections, and over half of these (one third of the total) were due to EV. Defining an EV etiology in these infants can decrease the need for additional diagnostic tests, eliminate the requirement for antibacterial therapy, and shorten the duration of hospitalization.

When EV are acquired perinatally by the fetus or neonate and there is lack of type-specific antibody in the mother at the time of delivery, disseminated disease can occur. Manifestations include meningoencephalitis, pneumonitis, hepatitis, myocarditis, pericarditis, and disseminated intravascular coagulation (DIC).

The occurrence of pneumonitis with hepatitis in a seriously ill neonate (unusual in bacterial infections), particularly when bacterial and fungal cultures are negative, should strongly suggest viral disease. Since disseminated neonatal herpes simplex virus (HSV) infection can cause a similar picture and since HSV responds to therapy with acyclovir, it is important to establish an etiologic diagnosis.

Febrile Exanthems

The usual exanthem with EV infections is a discrete to grouped, erythematous, maculopapular rash beginning on the face and neck, with spread to the trunk and then to the extremities. Vesicular, petechial, and even urticarial rashes also have been reported. Exanthems may be caused by a number of EV serotypes, but those most commonly involved are coxsackieviruses A2, A4, and A9 (vesicles) and echoviruses 2, 9, and 16 (Boston exanthem). The most common erythematous, maculopapular rash can be considered characteristic of EV infections but may not be sufficiently distinctive to allow an accurate clinical diagnosis. The occurrence of other features suggestive of EV infections should provide assistance in the clinical diagnosis: summer-fall season, outbreak in the community, presence of aseptic meningitis.

Aseptic Meningitis and Encephalitis

The best known syndrome associated with EV infections is aseptic meningitis. EVs account for over 80% of the known causes of aseptic meningitis. The most common causative serotypes are coxsackie A7 and A9, coxsackie B5, and echoviruses 4, 6, 9, and 30. Most cases occur in infants and young children. Characteristic clinical features include fever, irritability, headache, nausea and vomiting, and signs of meningeal irritation. Typical CSF findings include a WBC count in the 100s, with a lymphocytic predominance, a normal glucose, a mildly elevated protein, and a negative gram stain and bacterial antigen detection test. However, up to 40% of cases may have neutrophil predominance on the initial CSF. In these instances, shift to a lymphocyte excess occurs in 24 to 48 hours in viral meningitis, but a neutrophil predominance continues in treated bacterial meningitis.

Encephalitis is part of the CNS syndrome spectrum with EV infections, but it occurs infrequently. The major EVs involved are echo 4, 6, 9, 11, and 30. Such features as semicoma to coma and seizures suggest brain involvement. Focal disease is rare. The differential diagnosis for EV encephalitis is lengthy, but it is important to rule out HSV, since treatment is available. With EV encephalitis, the course of illness is much less severe and the prognosis is much better than with HSV or arbovirus encephalitis.

Other than paralytic disease discussed below, additional neurologic syndromes that have been associated with EVs include Guillain-Barré syndrome, transverse myelitis, and cerebellar ataxia.

Hand-Foot-Mouth Syndrome

The clinical features of the hand-foot-mouth syndrome resemble its name: painful vesicular lesions of the ventral surfaces of the hands and feet and vesiculoulcerative lesions in the mouth. The oral lesions usually involve the anterior mouth: the buccal mucosa, tongue, and occasionally the gingiva. Approximately 30% of cases will have an erythematous, maculopapular rash on other parts of the body, particularly the buttocks. Fever and constitutional symptoms are mild to moderate in degree. Sometimes, lesions may be small and infrequent. A careful physical examination can enable a diagnosis in a case of fever of unknown origin. The usual causative EV is coxsackie A16, but A5, A10, and EV 71 also have been reported. The virus can be isolated from vesicle fluid, as well as pharyngeal secretions.

Herpangina

Herpangina is an ulcerative pharyngitis caused by the coxsackie A viruses. Typical features include fever, sore throat, variable dysphagia, anorexia, and constitutional symptoms. Lesions are on the tonsillar pillars and soft palate, beginning as maculopapules progressing to vesicles and then shallow, 2- to 3-mm, pink-based ulcers. This is in contrast to hand-foot-mouth syndrome and herpes gingivostomatitis, where lesions are in the anterior mouth.

Carditis

In most instances, the etiology of myocarditis and pericarditis is not defined. However, the coxsackie B viruses are the most common established agents and are known to cause myocarditis in experimental animals. Typical features include fever, radiating or nonradiating precordial pain, and signs and symptoms of congestive heart failure. Rarely, there may be acute fulminant disease leading to death. This is much more common in neonates. Chronic cardiomyopathy may also occur.

Pleurodynia

Pleurodynia, or Bornholm disease, is coxsackie B myositis of the intercostal muscles resulting in pleuritic chest pain. The course is self-limited, and prognosis is excellent.

Acute Hemorrhagic Conjunctivitis

Acute hemorrhagic conjunctivitis (AHC) is a highly contagious, rapidly spreading, eye disease caused by outbreaks and epidemics of EV 70 and, less frequently, coxsackie A24 and adenovirus type 11. The conjunctivitis is bilateral and painful but self-limited without long-term sequelae.

Paralytic Disease

An average of only 10 cases of paralytic poliomyelitis occur in the United States each year. Approximately 90% of these are due to

the vaccine virus, either in a close contact of a recently vaccinated infant or in the vaccine recipient, usually with the first dose. Immunocompromised contacts or recipients are at greater risk of paralytic disease. The risk of paralytic disease from OPV is extremely small: 1 per 7.8 million doses distributed in recipients and 1 per 5.5 million in contacts. Wild-type poliovirus disease in the United States occurs in cases imported from other countries.

Clinical features include a prodrome of upper respiratory, gastrointestinal, or influenza-like illness, followed by an aseptic meningitis syndrome with associated pain and muscle cramping and an ascending, asymmetric, flaccid paralysis. Bulbar polio may occur and may involve any combination of cranial nerves and the medullary respiratory center. Risk factors for paralytic disease include absence of antibodies for all three poliovirus serotypes, extremes of age, pregnancy, and recent tonsillectomy. Residual paralysis is significant or severe in approximately 80% of cases.

Paralytic disease can occur much less commonly with nonpolio EVs, particularly EV 71. Bulbar involvement is rare, and prognosis is excellent.

Chronic EV Infection in Antibody Deficiency Syndromes

Individuals with antibody deficiency syndromes can be chronically infected with several EV serotypes, but most commonly the echoviruses. Persistent features include enteritis, arthritis, encephalitis, and a dermatomyositis-like syndrome.

THERAPY

Although a few antiviral agents have shown promise against EV infections in experimental animals, none has reached the stage of clinical trials in humans. Treatment, therefore, is supportive.

Intravenous immune globulin (IVIg) has been considered for treatment of serious EV infections, since (1) antibody appears to be the major host defense mechanism in recovery from illness, (2) patients with antibody deficiency syndromes are susceptible to chronic EV infections, (3) commercial IVIg preparations contain appreciable neutralizing antibody titers against most EV serotypes, and (4) passive antibody immunotherapy has been shown to be protective in experimental EV infections of animals. IVIg therapy has resulted in improvement in clinical status and decrease in viral shedding in antibody deficiency syndrome patients with chronic EV disease. There are anecdotal reports of success with IVIg therapy or prophylaxis (or both) in serious neonatal EV disease, but controlled trial evidence of efficacy is not available.

PREVENTION

Paralytic poliomyelitis due to indigenous wild virus has been eliminated in the United States with the active polio vaccine program. Although there are rare cases of live OPV associated with paralytic disease, this remains the recommended primary vaccine. An enhanced-potency inactivated polio vaccine (IPV) is available for use where OPV is contraindicated (e.g., immunocompromised patients or households with these patients). Consult standard sources for the specifics of OPV and IPV use, for example, the report of the Committee on Infectious Diseases of the American Academy of Pediatrics and the Advisory Committee on Immunization Practices of the Centers for Disease Control.

Prevention of spread of all EV infections is best accomplished by use of appropriate infection control measures (particularly handwashing), personal and home hygiene, and public health attention to safe culinary and recreational water.

REFERENCES

1. Cherry JD: Enteroviruses: Polioviruses (poliomyelitis), coxsackieviruses, echoviruses, and enteroviruses. *In* Feigin RD, Cherry JD (eds): Textbook of Pediatric Infectious Diseases, 3rd ed. Philadelphia, WB Saunders, 1992: 1705–1753.

2. Dagan R, Hall CB, Powell KR, Menegus MA: Epidemiology and laboratory diagnosis of infection with viral and bacterial pathogens in infants hospitalized for suspected sepsis. J Pediatr 115:351–356, 1989.
3. Morens DM, Pallansch MA, Moore M: Polioviruses and other enteroviruses. *In* Belshe RB (ed): Textbook of Human Virology. St. Louis, Mosby-Year Book, 1991:427–497.

HERPES SIMPLEX VIRUS INFECTIONS

SUE J. JUE, M.D.
RICHARD J. WHITLEY, M.D.

Herpes simplex virus (HSV) infections in children can be primary or recurrent and are usually caused by HSV type 1. In contrast, most genital HSV infections in sexually abused children and adolescents and over three quarters of neonatal infections are caused by HSV type

Work performed and reported by the authors was supported by contracts NO1-AI-15113, NO1-AI-62554, and NO1-AI-12667 from the Antiviral Research Branch of the National Institute of Allergy and Infectious Diseases, a grant from the Division of Research Resources (RR-032) from the National Institutes of Health, and a grant from the state of Alabama.

2. In both normal and immunocompromised children, HSV results in a spectrum of clinical syndromes. Antiviral therapy is available for herpes simplex encephalitis (HSE), neonatal HSV infection, and HSV keratoconjunctivitis. Therapy is also available for adolescents with primary genital infection. Unfortunately, no clinical trials have addressed the value of therapy for primary HSV gingivostomatitis. Furthermore, therapy of recurrent HSV labialis is of little clinical benefit. Those infections for which therapy is of documented benefit are discussed. A summary of recommended drug doses by disease indication appears in Table 1.

TREATMENT

Herpes Simplex Encephalitis

Herpes simplex encephalitis is the most common cause of sporadic fatal encephalitis in the United States. Disease in the child beyond the newborn age and adult is localized at the outset, beginning as a unilateral hemorrhagic necrosis of the inferior-medial temporal lobe. Ultimately, disease progresses to involve the contralateral lobe in the absence of effective therapy. Children generally have altered mentation, behavioral disturbances, fever, focal neurologic findings, and cerebrospinal fluid (CSF) findings compatible with viral encephalitis. The electroencephalogram (EEG) will frequently demonstrate spike and slow wave activity emanating from one or both temporal lobes.

TABLE 1. Recommended Drug Doses for Herpetic Infections

INDICATION	ROUTE AND DOSE	COMMENTS
Encephalitis	Acyclovir 10 mg/kg IV q8h for 14 d	Alternative therapy: vidarabine 30 mg/kg/d IV over 12 h for 10 d
Neonatal herpes*	Acyclovir 10 mg/kg IV q8h for 14 d	Alternative therapy: vidarabine 30 mg/kg/d IV over 12 h for 10 d
Keratitis	Trifluorothymidine (TFT) 1% ophthalmic solution, 1 drop q2h (up to 9 drops/d), then 1 drop q4h (5 drops/d) for 7 d; use not to exceed 21 d	Considered the drug of choice and least irritating to the eye; topical steroids may worsen disease
	Vidarabine ½ inch (1 cm) ribbon of 3% ophthalmic ointment 5 times/d	If no improvement in 7 days, therapy should be switched to TFT
	Idoxuridine ½ inch (1 cm) ribbon of 0.1% ophthalmic ointment 5 times/d	If no improvement in 7 days, therapy should be switched to TFT
Gingivostomatitis* (severe)	Acyclovir 5 mg/kg IV q8h or 200 mg PO 5 times d for 7–10 d	Therapy not recommended for mild cases
Recurrent herpes labialis	Not recommended	Even with therapy, there is only modest clinical benefit if used early; therapy not recommended routinely for primary labialis in normal hosts
Genital herpes		
Initial episode	Acyclovir 200 mg PO 5 times/d for 10 d or 5 mg/kg IV q8h for 5–7 d	No effect on recurrence rates; IV therapy for patients requiring hospitalization or with neurologic or visceral complications
Recurrent	Acyclovir 200 mg PO 5 times/d for 5 d if severe disease (adults only)	No effect on recurrence rate; efficacy greater if used early in attack but only modest clinical benefit
Suppression	Acyclovir 200 mg PO 3–5 times/d or 400 mg PO b.i.d. for 6 mo up to 1 y (adults only)	Studies performed only in adults
Immunocompromised host		
Mild mucocutaneous HSV	Acyclovir topically, 5% ointment applied to lesions 6 times/d for 7 d or 200–400 mg PO 5 times/d for 10 d	Oral therapy is preferred
Severe mucocutaneous HSV	Acyclovir 5 mg/kg IV q8h for 7–10 d or 250 mg/m² q8h IV for children <12 y old	Dose for hospitalized children
CNS or disseminated HSV	Acyclovir 10 mg/kg IV q8h for minimum of 14 d	Duration of therapy dependent on clinical response and on healing state of lesions
HSV prophylaxis for seropositive patients undergoing transplantation	Acyclovir 200 mg PO 3–5 times/d or 5 mg/kg or 250 mg/m² IV q12h	Used successfully in modifying or suppressing HSV episodes in bone marrow transplant patients and those receiving induction chemotherapy for ALL; lesions recur when therapy is stopped
Eczema herpeticum*	Acyclovir 200 mg PO 5 times/d for 5–7 d or 5 mg/kg or 250 mg/m² IV q8h for 5–10 d	For severe or disseminated cases, use IV acyclovir
Herpetic whitlow*		
Primary	Acyclovir 200 mg PO 5 times/d for 10 d	Of some benefit in anecdotal reports
Recurrent	Acyclovir 200 mg PO 3–5 times/d for 7–10 d	

*Not an FDA-approved use for acyclovir.

Computed tomography (CT) scans can be normal or show edema and hemorrhage of the involved temporal lobe. The only unequivocal means of diagnosis is brain biopsy of the involved site and isolation of virus in appropriate tissue culture. However, the recent application of polymerase chain reaction (PCR) technology to CSF specimens should be of diagnostic use and likely will be the noninvasive diagnostic test of choice.

Vidarabine was the first drug proven useful for the treatment of HSE. Initially, through placebo-controlled studies, vidarabine significantly decreased the mortality of virologically confirmed encephalitis from 70% to 28% 1 month after disease onset. Subsequently, survival data for patients with biopsy-proven disease who were treated with vidarabine versus those for patients treated with acyclovir were compared. These data have shown that acyclovir is superior to vidarabine for the treatment of HSE, with the mortality for vidarabine recipients being 54% as compared with 28% in the acyclovir recipients. In addition to improved efficacy, most clinicians prefer acyclovir because of its ease of administration and lesser toxicity. The dose of acyclovir is 10 mg/kg IV every 8 hours for 14 days. Early institution of therapy before definitive diagnosis and before progression to semicoma or coma is recommended, as the level of the patient's consciousness at initiation of therapy will markedly influence the outcome.

In addition to antiviral therapy, meticulous intensive care monitoring is required to optimize the outcome. Fluid management to prevent overhydration is critical. Intracranial pressure monitoring and administration of diuretic agents may assist in management of cerebral edema. Anticonvulsant therapy is often necessary to control the all too common severe and prolonged seizures that these patients can develop. Obviously, ventilatory support in most patients is mandatory. The use of steroids remains controversial and is unstudied.

Neonatal Herpes Simplex Viral Infection

Neonatal HSV infection is usually acquired as a consequence of contact of the infant with infected maternal genital secretions at the time of delivery. Less commonly, infections result from nosocomial or postnatal HSV acquisition by contact of the baby with other infected individuals. Neonates with HSV infection are classified into three categories according to the extent of disease: (1) disease localized to the skin, eye, and mouth (SEM), (2) infection of the central nervous system (CNS) with or without SEM involvement, and (3) disseminated infection.

Neonates with vesicular lesions or suspected HSV infection should be treated immediately with antiviral therapy. A study comparing vidarabine with acyclovir demonstrated that acyclovir was no better than vidarabine for the management of neonatal HSV infection. With either therapy, mortality from disseminated disease is still in excess of 50%. Acyclovir is again preferred because of the lower fluid load required for administration. The dose of acyclovir used is 10 mg/kg IV every 8 hours infused over a 1-hour period, and vidarabine is given in a dose of 30 mg/kg/d in one dose infused over 12 hours. The recommended duration of therapy is 14 days. Five to ten percent of treated infants will develop a life-threatening recurrence of infection requiring retreatment in the first month of life, whereas approximately 50% will have recurrent skin lesions, a universally perplexing problem for pediatricians. These infants, as well as those who continue to have recurrent skin lesions during the first year of life, usually do not require therapy unless systemic disease occurs. In those infants with three or more skin recurrences in the first 6 months of life, oral acyclovir therapy may prove of some benefit to prevent the neurologic sequelae that some of these patients develop. A clinical trial using oral acyclovir for 6 months to prevent recurrences and possibly to improve outcome is ongoing.

Herpes Simplex Viral Infections of the Eye

HSV infection of the eye is recognized as one of the commonest infectious causes of blindness in the United States, causing blepharitis, conjunctivitis, keratitis, and retinitis. Keratoconjunctivitis of HSV etiology is characterized by tearing, photophobia, discharge, and char-

acteristic dendritic lesions on fluorescein staining of the cornea. In the absence of therapy, lesions progress to geographic ulcers.

Three licensed topical drugs have a beneficial effect on HSV keratitis. These include idoxuridine (Stoxil, Herplex, Allergan), vidarabine (Vira-A), and trifluorothymidine (Viroptic, trifluridine). Trifluorothymidine (1% ophthalmic solution) is the treatment of choice, being used as one drop per eye every 2 hours while awake (maximum 9 drops daily per eye) until reepithelization of corneal ulcers and then one drop per eye every 4 hours while awake (minimum 5 drops daily per eye) for 7 additional days. The maximum duration of therapy is 21 days. Side effects consist of local stinging, burning, and edema (3% to 5% of cases). The indications and side effects of vidarabine ophthalmic ointment are similar to those of trifluorothymidine, although the ointment preparation may make it more useful in children. The dose is one-half inch of ointment per eye every 3 hours five times a day. If there is no improvement after 7 days of therapy, trifluorothymidine is indicated. Idoxuridine (0.1% ophthalmic ointment or solution), although it was the first effective therapy for ocular HSV infections, appears less effective and more toxic than the other two alternatives. None of the topical therapies have been shown to prevent recurrences.

Special consideration should be taken with infants less than 1 month of age with HSV ocular involvement. These infants should receive intravenous acyclovir and topical ophthalmic therapy and should be evaluated for systemic HSV infection.

The concomitant use of corticosteroids with antiviral therapy should be undertaken only by physicians experienced in the management of herpetic eye infections. For practical purposes, the child presumed to have HSV infection of the eye should be followed most carefully by an ophthalmologist. Both topical interferon alfa and topical acyclovir are effective in the therapy of ocular HSV disease but are not licensed or available as ophthalmic preparations in the United States.

Mucocutaneous Herpes Simplex Viral Infections

Gingivostomatitis

Gingivostomatitis is the most common primary HSV infection of childhood. The illness, which typically lasts 7 to 10 days, is characterized by fever and painful oral and pharyngeal lesions that can lead to poor fluid intake. Symptomatic therapy includes antipyretics and oral hydration with bland liquids (apple, pear, or peach juice, ice slurries, popsicles). Occasionally, poor oral intake may require hospitalization of the child with more severe mucosal involvement for parenteral hydration therapy. The use of topical viscous lidocaine for pain relief is no longer recommended and has resulted in cases of self-injury as a result of children chewing on the anesthetized oral mucosa or lips. The majority of cases of gingivostomatitis are mild, and antiviral therapy is not recommended. However, in the severely ill child with extensive oral involvement or the child hospitalized for intravenous hydration, acyclovir 5 mg/kg IV every 8 hours for 7 to 10 days will probably shorten the duration of illness and viral shedding. Oral acyclovir suspension (200 mg/5 ml) is also available, but sizable controlled studies are lacking in children to define the optimal dose and duration of therapy. From studies performed in adults, it appears that oral acyclovir at 200 mg per dose four to five times a day, not to exceed 80 mg/kg/d, may prove of benefit in children to shorten the duration of illness. This is not an approved indication for acyclovir.

Herpes Simplex Viral Labialis

Recurrences of HSV are usually localized to the vermillion border of the lip (cold sores, fever blisters) and adjacent skin. Reactivation can be induced by fever, local trauma, stress, and exposure to ultraviolet light. Most patients with recurrent HSV labialis will have evidence of a prodrome, consisting of burning and tingling at the site of subsequent skin vesicles. Oral acyclovir at a dose of 200 mg five times daily for 5 days has modest clinical benefit in treating recurrent herpes labialis if it is initiated very early after recurrence, but it cannot be recommended for routine therapy of herpes labialis in normal hosts, especially in children.

Genital Herpes Simplex Viral Infection

Genital HSV infection, both primary and recurrent, is not a common problem encountered in the pediatric population. However, with increasing and earlier sexual activity among adolescents, genital HSV infections will become a more significant problem.

Symptomatic therapy should be directed toward reduction of local discomfort, promotion of healing, and prevention of superinfection. The most important local therapy is keeping the lesions clean and dry. Patients with genital HSV infection often complain of dysuria and refuse to void. Painful urination may be lessened by having patients urinate into a water-filled bathtub or sitz bath. Some experts advise Burow's solution sitz baths. Prolonged soaking will delay healing.

Primary Genital Herpes Simplex Viral Infection. All three forms of acyclovir, topical, oral, and intravenous preparations, have been shown to be effective in the treatment of primary genital herpes. In all studies, especially those using intravenous or oral routes of drug delivery, treatment accelerated clearance of virus, loss of pain, and time to total healing and decreased such complications as urinary retention syndrome and aseptic meningitis. Intravenous acyclovir 5 mg/kg every 8 hours for 5 days is the most effective treatment for primary genital herpes. It should be reserved for patients requiring hospitalization because of severe local disease or complications (e.g., meningitis, urinary retention, transverse myelitis). In routine cases, PO therapy 200 mg five times daily for 10 days is nearly as effective as intravenous acyclovir for primary HSV infection and has become the standard treatment. Unfortunately, neither intravenous nor oral acyclovir therapy of primary genital HSV infection alters the frequency of subsequent recurrences.

Topically applied acyclovir reduces the duration of viral shedding but has no significant clinical benefit as compared with systemic therapy.

Recurrent Genital Herpes. Recurrent genital herpes is less severe and resolves more rapidly than primary infection. However, if severe enough to warrant therapy, recurrent disease responds to PO acyclovir therapy one capsule (200 mg) five times a day for 5 days. Oral acyclovir treatment of recurrent genital infection decreases the duration of viral shedding but has little clinical benefit. In patients with frequent recurrences, suppression with the continuous use of acyclovir one capsule (200 mg) three to five times per day or 400 mg PO b.i.d. for 6 months up to a year has dramatically reduced the recurrence rate by as much as 80% to 90%. However, suppressive therapy is only used in adults. For patients in whom recurrences are associated with severe complications, such as erythema multiforme, recurrent aseptic meningitis, or eczema herpeticum, suppression is also of benefit. Daily suppressive regimens appear to be more effective than intermittent episodic regimens.

All of these recommendations are predicated on studies performed in adults. No data are available for the management of primary or recurrent genital HSV infections in the prepubertal child or adolescent. Although it is reasonable to assume that acyclovir would be similarly efficacious in these patient populations, caution is indicated. The toxicity and potential long-term adverse effects of acyclovir have not been documented in young children. Thus, acyclovir should not be employed routinely for genital HSV infections in children unless complications are apparent.

Immunocompromised Host

HSV infections in the immunocompromised host are significantly more debilitating than those encountered in the normal individual. The lesions tend to be more invasive and slower to heal and are associated with prolonged viral shedding. Intravenous, oral, and topical acyclovir therapy all have been shown to provide clinical benefit to immunocompromised patients with mucocutaneous oral-labial and genital infections.

Topical 5% acyclovir ointment applied to lesions six times a day for 7 days is effective in decreasing pain and viral shedding, as well as shortening the time to complete lesion healing in immunocompromised patients with mucocutaneous HSV infection that is not life threatening. We prefer to use oral acyclovir 200 to 400 mg five times a day for 10 days for the treatment of most mild to moderate localized mucocutaneous HSV infections in this patient population. If lesions are extensive or if patients are more severely ill, they should be hospitalized and treated with IV acyclovir 5 mg/kg every 8 hours for 7 to 10 days. A dose of 250 mg/m² of body surface area every 8 hours should be used for children less than 12 years of age.

Patients with CNS involvement or disseminated infection with visceral organ involvement (esophagitis, hepatitis, or pneumonia) should be treated with a higher dose of acyclovir (10 mg/kg IV every 8 hours for a minimum of 14 days). The duration of therapy is dependent on clinical response and on the healing state of the lesions.

Oral or intravenous acyclovir prophylaxis of HSV-seropositive immunocompromised patients, such as those undergoing induction chemotherapy for leukemia or organ transplant recipients, has been shown to effectively suppress or modify the course of recurrent HSV episodes. Chronically immunocompromised or immunosuppressed patients, such as those with AIDS or primary immunodeficiencies, who are at risk for frequent and severe HSV recurrences should also receive acyclovir prophylaxis 200 mg PO three to five times per day, not to exceed 80 mg/kg/d or 5 mg/kg IV every 12 hours. Many patients will develop new HSV recurrences shortly after prophylactic chemotherapy is discontinued. These patients often can be managed with daily suppressive acyclovir therapy. Although there are no data in children, acyclovir 200 mg PO given two or three times a day or 400 mg PO given twice daily to adult patients with genital herpes is effective in reducing the rate of recurrent episodes. Individuals maintained on long-term suppressive therapy should be cautioned, however, that recurrences will likely develop following discontinuation of therapy and that the first recurrence may be more severe than those experienced previously.

Acyclovir-resistant infections should be suspected when patients with mucocutaneous infections remain culture positive, clinically worsen, or fail to show clinical improvement within a week of initiating systemic therapy. Clinical isolates that are resistant to acyclovir are thymidine kinase negative or have an altered thymidine kinase or DNA polymerase substrate. Pending sensitivities, patients suspected of having acyclovir-resistant strains should be treated with foscarnet. The dose and use of foscarnet in children have not been adequately studied.

Other Herpes Simplex Virus Infections

Acyclovir appears to be effective therapy for other HSV infections. There are anecdotal reports of oral acyclovir suppression of frequent recurrent herpetic whitlow. Eczema herpeticum is a more serious herpetic complication of atopic children, particularly patients with Wiskott-Aldrich syndrome. Some patients with extensive involvement require intravenous fluids and, occasionally, blood transfusion to correct electrolyte losses and anemia (particularly in children with Wiskott-Aldrich syndrome). Antistaphylococcal systemic antibiotics are usually administered to prevent bacterial superinfection. If there is evidence of generalized herpetic skin involvement or encephalitic disease, intravenous acyclovir at the higher dose should be administered. For milder cases, acyclovir 200 mg PO five times per day for 5 to 7 days may be of some benefit.

Antiviral Drugs

The drug of choice for most herpetic infections is acyclovir because of its efficacy, relatively low toxicity, and ease of administration. Vidarabine can be used as alternative therapy but is significantly less efficacious in all cases except neonatal herpes. Acyclovir, 9-(2-hydroxyethoxymethyl) guanine, is a synthetic acyclic purine nucleoside

TABLE 2. Dose Adjustment for Intravenous Acyclovir in Patients with Impaired Renal Function

CREATININE CLEARANCE (ml/min/1.73 m²)	% OF STANDARD DOSE	DOSE INTERVAL (h)
>50	100	8
25–50	100	12
10–25	100	24
0–10*	50	24

* Administered after hemodialysis.

analog that is a selective inhibitor of HSV types 1 and 2 and varicella-zoster virus. It is converted by virus-encoded thymidine kinase to its monophosphate derivative, an event that does not occur to any significant extent in uninfected cells. Acyclovir is then further phosphorylated by cellular enzymes to its active triphosphate derivative. Acyclovir triphosphate interferes with HSV DNA polymerase and inhibits viral DNA replication. Because acyclovir is taken up selectively by virus-infected cells, it has very low toxicity for normal host cells. The major side effects of oral acyclovir are gastrointestinal (nausea, vomiting) and headache or rash.

The toxicity of topical acyclovir is limited to local irritation or transient burning when the preparation is applied to genital lesions. This may be caused by the polyethylene glycol base. The intravenous preparation appears to be tolerated quite well. Rarely, infusions have been associated with local phlebitis, rash, diaphoresis, nausea, vomiting, and hypotension. Intravenous acyclovir may cause transient renal dysfunction (rise in serum creatinine) in 5% to 25% of patients. This toxic reaction appears to be dose dependent and is more common when patients are not receiving adequate hydration. Patients with impaired renal function should have adjusted doses as outlined in Table 2. Less commonly, neurotoxicity, such as lethargy, coma, confusion, hallucinations, tremor, and seizures, may occur. These are associated with elevated drug levels and reverse on cessation of therapy.

Vidarabine (Adenine Arabinoside, Ara-A) is an analog of adenosine. Vidarabine is phosphorylated to the corresponding nucleotides within the cell and acts by inhibiting HSV DNA polymerase. As it is relatively insoluble, it requires large fluid volumes to administer, which is impractical in the neonate and in patients with CNS involvement. The major side effects involve the gastrointestinal tract and include anorexia, nausea, vomiting, diarrhea, and elevated liver transaminases. CNS disturbances reported at therapeutic doses include tremors, dizziness, hallucinations, confusion, psychosis, ataxia, headache, and encephalopathy. These adverse drug reactions have occurred mostly in patients with impaired hepatic or renal function. Hematologic reactions that may occur include anemia, thrombocytopenia, and neutropenia.

All three licensed topical antiviral agents for the treatment of HSV keratitis (idoxuridine, trifluorothymidine, vidarabine) may cause local irritation, photophobia, edema of the eyelids and cornea, and superficial punctate keratopathy. Idoxuridine is the least effective and the most toxic of the three. Available data favor trifluorothymidine as the treatment of choice for HSV infection of the eye. Although these agents are not of proven value in the treatment of stromal keratitis and uveitis, trifluorothymidine is more likely to penetrate the cornea. The indications and side effects of vidarabine ophthalmic ointment are similar to those of trifluorothymidine.

CONCLUSION

Over the past 15 years, successful antiviral therapy of HSV infection has emerged with safe therapeutics. In spite of the major impact of acyclovir on the severity of HSV infection, morbidity and mortality of herpes simplex encephalitis and neonatal herpes still exist. Improved therapeutics likely will emerge over the next decade.

REFERENCES

1. Whitley RJ, Alford CA Jr, Hirsch MS, et al: Vidarabine versus acyclovir therapy in herpes simplex encephalitis. N Engl J Med 314:144–149, 1986.
2. Whitley RJ, Arvin A, Prober C, et al: A controlled trial comparing vidarabine with acyclovir in neonatal herpes simplex virus infection. N Engl J Med 324:444–449, 1991.
3. Whitley RJ, Gnann JW: Acyclovir: A decade later. N Engl J Med 327:782–789, 1992.

HIV INFECTION

DELIA M. RIVERA-HERNANDEZ, M.D.
GWENDOLYN B. SCOTT, M.D.

Children infected with the human immunodeficiency virus (HIV) have a chronic multisystem disease that requires comprehensive multidisciplinary health care with coordination of medical, social, psychosocial, and community support services. There is no definitive cure for this disease. However, important advances in the diagnosis and treatment of HIV infection in children have resulted in improved quality and duration of life. This chapter describes current practices in the management of HIV infection for both inpatient and outpatient care of children.

MANAGEMENT OF INFANTS AT RISK

Early identification of infants and young children at risk for HIV infection is of utmost importance, so that monitoring of clinical and immune status and tests for diagnosis of HIV infection can begin at birth or shortly thereafter. Virtually all new cases of HIV infection in young children result from vertical transmission from mother to infant. Accordingly, identification of infected pregnant women is the first step in managing perinatally acquired HIV infection so that their offspring can be appropriately identified and monitored for clinical and immunologic status. HIV culture, polymerase chain reaction (PCR), and p24 antigen detection are commonly used for diagnosis of HIV infection in infants. Using these assays, HIV infection can be detected in the first week of life in about half of children with HIV infection, and 95% of infected infants can be identified by 3 months of age using either viral culture or PCR assays.

ANTIRETROVIRAL THERAPY

Infants and children with a definitive diagnosis of HIV infection should have clinical evaluation and immunologic testing to establish the need for specific therapies and prophylactic measures. The goal of therapy is to stop the immune destruction and neurologic dysfunction that are characteristic of HIV disease in children by arresting replication of the virus. The use of antiretroviral drugs has been associated with clinical improvement, delay in the rate of HIV disease progression, and longer survival. In addition to drugs approved for routine use in HIV-infected children, newer drugs and treatment regimens are being tested as part of clinical trials in both children and adults with HIV infection. (Information about the clinical trials available for children can be obtained by calling 1-800-TRIALS-A, the AIDS Clinical Trials Group, National Institutes of Health, or 301-402-0696, Pediatric Branch, National Cancer Institute.)

Treatment for HIV-infected children continues to evolve as new drugs and treatment regimens become available. In 1992, a consensus panel consisting of health care providers and parents was convened by the National Pediatric HIV Resource Center to develop treatment guidelines and to define optimal therapy for children with HIV infection.[3] Thus, the treatments described in this section are based both on these guidelines and on our own experience with treatment of children with HIV infection.

TABLE 1. CD4+ Lymphocyte Values for Initiation of Antiretroviral Therapy in Children with HIV Infection[2]

AGE (y)	CD4+ COUNT	%
<1	<1750/mm³	30
1–2	<1000/mm³	25
2–6	<750/mm³	20
>6	<500/mm³	20

Antiretroviral therapy is indicated for children who have an established diagnosis of HIV infection and who have evidence of significant immunodeficiency or HIV-associated symptoms. At this time, there is no information about the benefit of instituting antiretroviral therapy in children who are asymptomatic and who have a normal immune status. Children with lymphadenopathy, hepatomegaly, or hypergammaglobulinemia as their only finding are considered to be asymptomatic, since these symptoms do not imply a poor prognosis. Thus, such children are not candidates for antiretroviral therapy. Decisions regarding the institution of antiretroviral therapy and prophylactic measures in HIV-infected adults have been based on CD4+ lymphocyte counts because they correlate with the degree of immunodeficiency, risk of opportunistic infections, and survival. However, absolute CD4+ lymphocyte counts in children are age dependent, and since children have higher CD4+ lymphocyte counts during the first 5 years of life, the number of cells correlating with severe immunodeficiency in children differs from that in adults. As a general rule, if an infected child is on prophylaxis for *Pneumocystis carinii* pneumonia, he or she should also be on antiretroviral therapy. Absolute lymphocyte counts and percentages for initiation of antiretroviral therapy as well as *Pneumocystis* prophylaxis are presented in Table 1. There also are several clinical conditions that are indications for institution of antiretroviral therapy, independent of CD4+ lymphocyte count (Table 2).

The first successful compounds in arresting the replicative cycle of HIV were inhibitors of the virus-encoded reverse transcriptase.

TABLE 2. Clinical Criteria for Instituting Antiretroviral Therapy

1. AIDS-defining opportunistic infection
2. Recurrent septicemia or meningitis (two or more episodes)
3. Progressive encephalopathy attributable to HIV
4. HIV-associated malignancy
5. Wasting syndrome or failure to thrive (defined as crossing two percentiles over time or being below the fifth percentile for age and falling from the growth curve)
6. Thrombocytopenia (platelet count <75,000/mm³ on two or more occasions)
7. Hypogammaglobulinemia (total IgG less than 250 mg/dl)
8. The following clinical conditions may warrant initiation of antiretroviral therapy when observed as an isolated finding, with correlation with overall clinical profile
    a. Lymphoid interstitial pneumonitis or parotitis
    b. Symptomatic cardiomyopathy
    c. Nephrotic syndrome
    d. Significant elevation of transaminase levels (>5-fold increase over normal)
    e. Splenomegaly
    f. Hematologic abnormalities: neutropenia (<750/mm³) or age-corrected anemia on at least two occasions over a week
    g. Diarrhea that remains unexplained and is either persistent (3 or more loose stools per day for 2 wk or longer) or recurrent (2 or more episodes of diarrhea accompanied by dehydration over a 2-mo period)
    h. Oral candidiasis persisting >1 mo or that is recurrent in spite of appropriate therapy
    i. Chronic bacterial infections
    j. Two or more episodes of herpes simplex or varicella-zoster within 1 y

These agents are active against an early step in the viral replication pathway and decrease HIV replication. Two antiretroviral drugs have been approved by the Food and Drug Administration for use in children: zidovudine (3'-azido-2',3'-dideoxythymidine, azidothymidine, AZT, ZDV, Retrovir) and didanosine (2',3'-dideoxyinosine, ddI, Videx).

Zidovudine

Zidovudine was the first drug approved for treatment of HIV infection in children, has been the agent most commonly prescribed as initial monotherapy, and is frequently a component of combination chemotherapy regimens. Zidovudine syrup (10 mg/ml) is used in children. For infants 0 to 2 weeks old, the recommended dose is 2mg/kg per dose PO every 6 hours. For those 2 to 4 weeks old, 3 mg/kg per dose PO is given every 6 hours. For infants and children over 1 month of age, 180 mg/m² per dose is given every 6 hours. For adolescents, the currently recommended adult dose of 500 mg/d (100 mg PO five times daily) is appropriate. The 100 mg capsules may be used in older children and adolescents. If the patient is unable to ingest anything by mouth, the intravenous dose is 120 mg/m² per dose given every 6 hours.

Zidovudine is associated with improvement in the general well-being of the child, growth, neurologic function, and immunologic and virologic parameters. The therapeutic response should be determined using serial physical examinations that include anthropometric parameters and neurologic and psychometric evaluations, laboratory assessment with liver and kidney function tests, serum chemistries, complete blood cell counts, measurement of T cell subsets, and quantitation of immunoglobulin levels.

Zidovudine is generally well tolerated, although some patients experience toxicity, mostly in the form of bone marrow suppression, with clinically significant anemia and granulocytopenia. Therefore, clinical and laboratory monitoring for evidence of toxicity is recommended after the first month of treatment and, thereafter, every 4 to 6 weeks. The hematologic adverse effects are usually reversible with dose reduction to 120 mg/m² per dose every 6 hours. The therapy may be temporarily withheld, especially if there is significant neutropenia (granulocytes <750/mm³) or anemia (hemoglobin <8 g/dl) until the problem is controlled. If hematologic abnormalities persist despite these adjustments, one should consider alternative antiretroviral therapy or use of colony stimulating factor(s) or both. Other less common toxic effects of zidovudine include headache, nausea, insomnia, and a myopathy. The last effect is suggested by weakness, muscle tenderness, and elevation in creatinine phosphokinase. Confirmation of the diagnosis by muscle biopsy showing the characteristic histopathology is an indication for discontinuation of treatment with zidovudine.

Results of a recent clinical trial comparing zidovudine alone, didanosine alone, and the combination of didanosine and zidovudine as initial therapy showed that more patients on zidovudine had toxicities and disease progression over a median 24-month follow-up period. This does not mean that zidovudine is ineffective but indicates that its benefits may be limited by factors such as the development of drug resistance. Thus choosing the drug to use in initial therapy becomes more complex, and the child's clinical and immunologic status needs to be carefully considered in the decision-making process. This study is ongoing, and updated guidelines for initial therapy in children with HIV are not available at this time. In the interim, it is recommended that the practitioner consult their local HIV specialist for updated information and recommendations for therapy of newly diagnosed patients.

Zidovudine also was the first antiretroviral drug administered to HIV-infected pregnant women and their newborns in an attempt to prevent vertical transmission, with encouraging results. The Pediatric AIDS Clinical Trials Group, in conjunction with the European study sponsored by the French Institute of Health and Medical Research and the French National AIDS Research Agency, carried out a placebo-controlled trial that studied the efficacy, safety, and tolerance of zidovudine administered to pregnant women with CD4+ counts above 200/mm³, between 14 and 34 weeks of gestation and to their infants for 6 weeks after delivery. Preliminary results suggest that the rate of HIV transmission from mothers to infants decreased from 25.5% in pregnant women and their infants who received placebo to 8.3% in women and infants treated with zidovudine.

Official recommendations for use of zidovudine in pregnant women have been published recently.[2] Infants whose mothers have received zidovudine should receive zidovudine within the first 12 hours of life at 2 mg/kg per dose every 6 hours for 6 weeks. A complete blood count should be checked at 2 weeks, since anemia, granulocytopenia, and thrombocytopenia can occur. The drug should be discontinued if the hemoglobin <8g/dl, granulocytes <750/mm³, or platelets <50,000/mm.³ It is important to remember that we do not know the long-term effects of zidovudine therapy on the mother or the infant, particularly those without HIV infection, and it is uncertain that the same treatment effect will be seen in women with CD4+ cell counts <200/mm³. Also, as this therapy becomes more widespread, it is possible that zidovudine resistance may be more prevalent in women and may render this therapeutic regimen less effective.

Intolerance to zidovudine or failure of therapy, with progression of HIV disease in a patient who has been compliant with the therapeutic regimen for 4 to 6 months, is an indication for changing antiretroviral therapy. Development of viral strains resistant to the drug has been seen in both children and adults and is associated with progression of disease. These patients frequently have responded with improved growth and stabilization of their HIV-associated disease when alternative antiretroviral therapy is instituted. Table 3 shows the indications for changing antiretroviral therapy.

Didanosine

Didanosine is an alternative therapy for children with HIV infection and should be the first agent used in patients who are intolerant to zidovudine. As with zidovudine, many children have responded to this therapy with improved clinical status, neuropsychologic function, growth, and immunologic and virologic parameters. Didanosine is nonmyelosuppressive, and its long-term administration has been well tolerated in children. The usual recommended dose is 100 mg/m² per dose given twice per day (range of 90 to 135 mg/m² per dose administered twice per day). Didanosine is acid-labile and must be taken with an antacid to prevent degradation of the drug by stomach acid. There are several formulations of the drug, and the bioavailability of these formulations may differ. Didanosine comes as a powder for oral solution to be reconstituted with water and liquid antacid, as a buffered powder for oral solution in single-dose packages, and as chewable, dispersible, buffered tablets. The drug should be used cautiously in patients who are on sodium-restricted diets because each buffered tablet contains 264.5 mg of sodium and each single dose packet contains 1380 mg of sodium.

TABLE 3. Indications for Changing Antiretroviral Therapy

1. Persistent or severe adverse reactions attributed to antiretroviral agent in use
2. Therapeutic failure evidenced by
   a. Growth failure
   b. Progressive neurologic disease, with decline in brain growth, cognitive function, or clinical neurologic function
3. A change in antiretroviral therapy might be considered with development of
   a. Symptomatic cardiomyopathy
   b. Nephrotic syndrome
   c. Significant elevation of transaminase levels (>5 times above normal)
   d. AIDS-defining opportunistic infection
   e. Persistent or sharp decrease (40%–50% drop) in absolute CD4+ lymphocyte count confirmed by repeated laboratory evaluation*

*At this time, recommendations do not include changes in therapy based solely on worsening of laboratory markers.

Pancreatitis has occurred in a small proportion of children using didanosine. Therefore, careful monitoring with measurements of serum amylase and lipase every 1 to 3 months is indicated for patients taking didanosine, aside from the other clinical and laboratory evaluations for disease status described for patients taking zidovudine. Asymptomatic hyperamylasemia does not seem to be an indication to discontinue didanosine therapy because it is not a specific indicator of impending pancreatitis. However, therapy should be discontinued in patients who have elevations in amylase and lipase levels associated with signs and symptoms of pancreatitis, including nausea, vomiting, and abdominal pain. Didanosine should not be administered along with other medications that may induce pancreatitis, such as pentamidine. Other side effects of didanosine are peripheral retinal depigmentation, which has not been associated with visual impairment, and painful peripheral neuropathy. For these side effects, monitoring with retinal examinations with dilatation every 6 months and questioning about the presence of pain, numbness, or tingling of the hands and feet are indicated.

Other Antiretroviral Agents

There are ongoing clinical trials evaluating the use of combination therapies for patients who have been intolerant to zidovudine or who have had disease progression while taking it. One of the drugs being tested in children is the nucleoside analog zalcitabine (ddC). The drug is already licensed for use in combination with zidovudine in adults and adolescents. The suggested dose is 0.01 mg/kg per dose orally every 8 hours. When compared with zidovudine in adult clinical trials, zalcitabine has proven to be an inferior agent for monotherapy. The most common toxicity found in adults has been peripheral neuropathy. However, this has not been described in children. Rash and oral ulcerations also have been described. Concomitant or alternating use of zidovudine and didanosine or zalcitabine is under study, since these agents do not have overlapping toxicities.

Another nucleoside analog under study, stavudine (d4T, 2',3'-didehydro-3'-deoxythymidine), has in vitro antiretroviral activity similar to that of zidovudine. Dose-related peripheral neuropathy and hepatic dysfunction have been described with its use. Nonnucleoside antiretroviral drugs that inhibit the HIV reverse transcriptase, such as nevirapine, pyridinone, and atevirdine, have been developed. When used as single agents, these compounds are associated with rapid emergence of resistance. Therefore, they are being evaluated in combination with other drugs, such as zidovudine and ddI.

Other parts of the life cycle of HIV can be attacked. Some of the potential approaches to therapy for HIV infection include blockage of viral cellular receptors with the use of sulfated polysaccharide, interference with HIV replication using antisense oligonucleotides, Tat-inhibitors, or viral protease inhibitors, action against the release of virus from the surface of the target cell by use of interferons, and inhibition of intracellular factors and cytokines that enhance HIV replication using N-acetyl-L-cysteine.

Immunization with viral envelope proteins (glycoproteins 120 and 160) as postinfection therapy is being evaluated as part of multicenter trials sponsored by the AIDS Clinical Trials Group and the AIDS Vaccine Evaluation Units. These antigens stimulate humoral and cellular immune responses that may be important in suppressing or controlling HIV infection. Vaccine trials are ongoing in pregnant women to evaluate their effect in prevention of perinatal transmission and in infants born to HIV-seropositive women. Passive immunization using gamma globulin with a high titer of antibody to HIV (HIVIG) is presently being used in clinical trials in pregnant women in combination with zidovudine to determine if perinatal transmission of HIV can be further reduced.

SUPPORTIVE THERAPY

Intravenous Gamma Globulin

The use of intravenous gamma globulin (IVIg) should be reserved for children who meet the following criteria: hypogammaglobulinemia

(IgG <250 mg/dl), recurrent serious bacterial infections, two or more episodes of pneumonia, absence of antibody formation, chronic bronchiectasis, and lack of measles antibody while living in an endemic area. The dose is 400 mg/kg given as a slow intravenous infusion every 4 weeks. In a large, multicenter, double-blind, placebo-controlled study, it was shown that the use of IVIg can prolong the time to development of serious bacterial infection but does not affect overall survival. This benefit was found only in children with absolute CD4 + counts over 200/mm³. More recently, a large study conducted by the AIDS Clinical Trials Group showed that IVIg does not offer a significant benefit for patients on antiretroviral therapy who are also receiving trimethoprim-sulfamethoxazole therapy as prophylaxis for *P. carinii* pneumonia. Children with recurrent pneumonia or serious bacterial infections and lack of antibody formation who are on antiretroviral therapy, and who are not receiving PCP prophylaxis should also receive IVIg. Two additional groups of children that may benefit from IVIg therapy independent of CD4+ counts are those with chronic bronchiectasis and those with a lack of measles antibody who live in an endemic area.

Erythropoietin

Anemia is common in children with HIV infection. Although there are few published studies on the use of erythropoietin in this group of children, it has been shown to be useful for the treatment of anemia in adults with HIV infection with a low endogenous production of erythropoietin (erythropoietin level <500 IU/L). When children present with anemia, a complete workup should be done to determine its cause. If a child is receiving zidovudine and has a hemoglobin <8g/dl, the dose should be reduced by 30%. If the child is transfusion dependent, erythropoietin should be used if endogenous erythropoietine levels are low. This drug may be useful also as adjunctive therapy in children receiving other drugs that are associated with bone marrow suppression, such as ganciclovir. The dose is 50 to 150 U/kg SC administered three times a week.

Granulocyte Colony-Stimulating Factor

Children with HIV infection may develop low granulocyte counts as a result of drug toxicity or infection. Granulocyte colony-stimulating factor (G-CSF) is given to children with persistence of absolute granulocyte counts <500/mm³. It is given subcutaneously at a dose of 5 to 15 µg/kg/d, and white blood cell counts are checked twice weekly at the beginning of therapy. If the absolute granulocyte count rises above 1500/mm³, the drug is decreased or discontinued. G-CSF has been well tolerated and appears to be beneficial in the care of this group of children.

THERAPY FOR HIV-ASSOCIATED CONDITIONS

Developmental Delay and Neurologic Abnormalities

HIV exhibits tropism for the central nervous system (CNS), and some studies have suggested that this invasion of the CNS may occur during the earliest stages of the infection. Such invasion is responsible for the HIV-associated progressive encephalopathy of childhood that may occur in up to 10% of children with AIDS and that may be a presenting feature of HIV infection. This process resembles a neurodegenerative white matter disease. Because HIV infection in children occurs during the development of the CNS, the children should be monitored for mental and motor delays, loss of developmental milestones, and development of pyramidal tract signs and other neurologic abnormalities. Also, the associated brain atrophy may result in microcephaly, and imaging studies may disclose calcification of basal ganglia. A computed tomography (CT) scan of the brain with enhancement and a spinal tap are in order when hypotonia, hypertonia, microcephaly, or other neurologic abnormalities are present to rule out other infections. Children with severe encephalopathy should have a retinal examination for this same purpose. Therapy with zidovudine may stabilize or reverse the course of HIV encephalopathy. If neuroradiologic imaging studies demonstrate progression of disease,

change in antiretroviral therapy is indicated. An early stimulatory program with physical, occupational, and speech therapy should be instituted to maintain as much function as possible.

Lymphoid Interstitial Pneumonitis

Lymphoid interstitial pneumonitis (LIP) is the second most common AIDS-defining illness in children and generally occurs in those who survive infancy with a relatively high CD4+ count. The presence of a reticulonodular pattern with or without hilar adenopathy that persists on chest radiographs for 2 months or longer and that is unresponsive to antimicrobial therapy is considered presumptive evidence of LIP. Opportunistic infections that can give a similar radiographic image, such as miliary tuberculosis, *P. carinii* pneumonitis, and cytomegalovirus or other viral pneumonias should be ruled out. Generally the patient is asymptomatic or presents with the insidious onset of cough and shortness of breath as the lymphoproliferative disorder progresses. If the patient becomes symptomatic, with shortness of breath, chronic cough, and arterial oxygen desaturation, glucocorticoid therapy may be of benefit. For children with Pao₂ of less than 90 mm Hg, prednisone can be given at 2 mg/kg/d in divided doses for 2 weeks, tapering to 1 mg/kg/d. This therapy is continued for several weeks and its end point is determined by improvement of oxygen saturation, which is monitored with determination of arterial blood gases and the use of pulse oximetry to measure transcutaneous oxygen saturations. The child usually shows improvement after a few weeks of therapy, although in some instances, there is severe chronic lung disease that is refractory to steroid treatment, and the patient becomes oxygen dependent. Children with LIP tend to develop pneumonia, and when they present with fever and tachypnea, they should be aggressively evaluated, with arterial blood gas determinations and blood and sputum cultures. Broad-spectrum antibiotic therapy should be instituted pending culture results. The most common organisms isolated are *Haemophilus influenzae* type b and *Streptococcus pneumoniae*. *P. carinii* pneumonia is found only rarely in association with LIP.

Nephropathy

Some HIV-infected children develop a nephropathy that generally presents with proteinuria as an early finding, although not all children with proteinuria progress to frank nephrosis. Besides proteinuria, the clinical presentation includes edema and elevation of the blood urea nitrogen (BUN) and creatinine, usually without hypertension. When this occurs, symptomatic treatment with fluid restriction, a low-salt diet, and diuretics is in order. A renal biopsy is indicated in this condition, and the most common histopathologic finding is focal segmental glomerulosclerosis. Corticosteroid therapy does not seem to be of benefit. Patients should be assessed on an individual basis to determine the potential advantage of hemodialysis or of peritoneal dialysis.

Cardiomyopathy

Cardiac abnormalities are recognized increasingly in children with HIV infection. Dysrhythmias, hemodynamic abnormalities, and congestive heart failure are the most common presentations. The most common echocardiographic findings are ventricular dysfunction and pericardial effusion, which only rarely is complicated by tamponade. Overt signs of cardiac dysfunction usually occur later in the disease. Treatment is symptomatic, with fluid restriction, use of diuretics, and digitalization, and the use of captopril if there is congestive heart failure unresponsive to these other measures.

Thrombocytopenia

Thrombocytopenia occurs in about 10% to 15% of HIV-infected children. The principal causative mechanism appears to be immune-mediated platelet destruction. Zidovudine therapy seems to be the most promising treatment for HIV-associated thrombocytopenia, as platelet levels usually rise in patients who begin antiretroviral therapy while being thrombocytopenic. A response may be evident after 2 weeks of therapy, but it might not occur in patients with advanced disease. An initial course of therapy with high-dose IVIg may be needed in those children with extremely low platelet counts (<20,000/mm^3) until the treatment with zidovudine takes effect. In these cases, high-dose IVIg at 1 g/kg per dose for 3 to 5 days may be of transient benefit. If the thrombocytopenia remains unresponsive to antiretroviral and IVIg treatments, a course of steroids should be administered. Prednisone 1 to 2 mg/kg PO for 4 weeks, followed by tapering the dose over the next 2 to 4 weeks, has been used with some success.

Wasting Syndrome and Failure to Thrive

It is essential that infants and children with HIV infection maintain a good nutritional status, especially because malnutrition may enhance immunodeficiency. The toll that this chronic illness state takes on the growth and general nutritional status of these patients mandates close monitoring of anthropometric parameters, evaluation of dietary habits, detection of specific nutritional deficiencies, and timely intervention with dietary guidance and the use of high-calorie supplemental formulas. With disease progression, emergence of gastrointestinal complications, opportunistic infections, and intolerance of diet, the use of nasogastric feedings and parenteral hyperalimentation may be necessary.

Other Supportive Measures

As disease progression occurs, the child will require more frequent medical visits and hospitalization. It is important to keep the child's life as normal as possible and to maintain a good quality of life for as long as possible. As the child becomes terminal, it is important to ensure that the child and family have adequate support and that emphasis is placed on comfort and control of pain. Assessment of pain and plans for its management are best done with the help of the caretaker and the patient, so stepwise interventions are made. Mild analgesics, such as acetaminophen, can be prescribed, progressing in degree of potency as the need arises, with the use of acetaminophen with codeine up to oral methadone or intravenous infusions of morphine. Families should be aware of the therapeutic expectations and be informed when additional interventional efforts will be futile in prolonging or improving the quality of life of the child. Careful explanations about withdrawal or withholding of therapy, the implications of a do not resuscitate order, and supportive care with sustained nutrition, hydration, and pain management are essential. Referral to hospice care may provide needed support to the family.

TREATMENT OF OPPORTUNISTIC INFECTIONS

Pneumocystis carinii Pneumonitis

PCP is the most frequent opportunistic infection in children with HIV infection. In perinatally acquired infection, it frequently presents during the first year of life, usually after 1 month of age. The median age of onset of disease is 5 months, and this may be the presenting illness suggesting HIV infection in a child. PCP should be suspected in the child at risk for HIV infection with fever and tachypnea with or without pulmonary infiltrates. Bronchoscopy with lavage is the preferred method for obtaining a specimen for diagnosis. If a diagnostic procedure cannot be done on admission and PCP is suspected, therapy should be initiated. The drug of choice for treatment is trimethoprim-sulfamethoxazole (TMP-SMX) 20 mg/kg/d IV of trimethoprim divided every 6 hours for a period of 14 to 21 days. Alternative agents for therapy include pentamidine isethionate 4 mg/kg/d IV as a daily dose, atovaquone 40 mg/kg/d PO divided every 8 hours, or trimetrexate. Pentamidine-associated side effects include hypoglycemia, hypotension, and renal failure. In our experience, these side effects are more common in young infants. Such agents as didanosine should be discontinued during pentamidine therapy because of the potential for development of pancreatitis. The didanosine may be started 7 days after discontinuation of pentamidine therapy, with careful monitoring of the amylase and lipase levels. Atovaquone is well tolerated, but there is less experience with its use in children.

We reserve this drug for children who cannot tolerate or have failed therapy with TMP-SMX or pentamidine. Trimetrexate is a drug approved for treatment of PCP in adults. Although there is little experience with the use of this agent in children, it could be used as an alternative if the previously discussed drugs cannot be used. Children typically will remain stable or may show progression of disease over the first few days of treatment. A treatment failure is defined as a child who continues to have progression of disease after 5 to 7 days of appropriate therapy.

Although there are no published data on the use of steroids in children with PCP, their use in adults with early mild to moderate PCP infection has been shown to be beneficial. At our institution, steroids are used routinely in children with suspected PCP as we initiate PCP-specific medications. Usually, methylprednisolone (Solu-Medrol) or oral prednisone is begun for a 5- to 7-day course. Children are not placed in a room with other immunocompromised hosts during the first 24 hours of treatment of PCP. Children who have had an episode of PCP should be placed on PCP prophylaxis for the rest of their lives.

Recommendations for PCP prophylaxis for children with HIV infection have been published.[1] However, cases of PCP continue to occur, particularly in the first year of life, and new recommendations are being developed. In the interim, we recommend that all children under 1 year of age who are at risk for HIV infection or who are known to have HIV infection should begin prophylaxis at 4 to 6 weeks of age and continue until they are 1 year of age unless HIV infection can be ruled out. At 1 year of age, if a child is infected, prophylaxis should be continued if the absolute lymphocyte count was ≤1000/mm^3, the CD4% was ≤25% during the first year of life, or the child had a serious AIDS-associated condition. In children between the ages of 1 and 6 years with newly identified HIV infection, those who have not received prophylaxis, and those who had prophylaxis discontinued after they were 1 year of age, prophylaxis should be initiated if the absolute CD4+ lymphocyte count is ≤500/mm^3 or the CD4% <15%. For those 6 years of age or older, prophylaxis should be started if the absolute CD4+ lymphocyte count is ≤200/mm^3 or the CD4% ≤15%. Any child with a prior episode of PCP should receive lifelong prophylaxis.

TMP-SMX (TMP 150 mg/m^2/d with SMX 750 mg/m^2/d) PO in two divided doses on 3 consecutive days of the week is the recommended regimen in children over 1 month of age. However, other alternative schedules are acceptable (Table 4). Adverse reactions include rash, hypersensitivity, and bone marrow suppression. Leukocyte counts should be monitored, and the drug should be discontinued if

---

TABLE 4. Drug Regimens for *Pneumocystis carinii* Pneumonia[1]

Recommended Regimen (Children >1 Mo of Age)
1. Trimethoprim-sulfamethoxazole (TMP-SMX) 150 mg TMP/m^2/d with 750 mg SMX/m^2/d PO divided b.i.d. three times per week on consecutive days (e.g., Monday, Tuesday, Wednesday)
2. Acceptable alternative TMP-SMX Dose schedules
   a. 150 mg TMP/m^2/d with 750 mg SMX/m^2/d PO as single daily dose three times per week on consecutive days (e.g., Monday, Tuesday, Wednesday)
   b. 150 mg TMP/m^2/d with 750 mg SMX/m^2/d PO divided b.i.d. 7 d/wk
   c. 150 mg TMP/m^2/d with 750 mg SMX/m^2/d PO divided b.i.d. three times per week on alternate days (e.g., Monday, Wednesday, Friday)

Alternative Regimens if TMP-SMX Not Tolerated
1. Aerosolized pentamidine (child >5 y of age) 300 mg given via Respirgard II inhaler monthly
2. Dapsone (child >1 mo of age) 1 mg/kg (not to exceed 100 mg) PO q.d.
3. Dapsone may be combined with TMP 150 mg/m^2/d PO q.d.
4. If neither aerosolized pentamidine nor dapsone is tolerated, some clinicians use pentamidine 4 mg/kg IV every 2 or 4 wk

granulocytopenia occurs. Alternatively, colony-stimulating factors might be considered in this situation.

There are few published data on the use of alternative drugs for PCP prophylaxis in children (Table 4). The use of aerosolized pentamidine as prophylaxis in adults with HIV infection is well established. We have used this therapy in older children who can cooperate with the procedure. Aerosolized pentamidine can be given as 300 mg every 4 weeks using a Respirgard II jet nebulizer. Some patients on this treatment may develop bronchospasm, and such patients should be pretreated with a bronchodilator before their treatment and monitored carefully. Clinical trials of alternative therapies are being conducted in children through the multicenter AIDS Clinical Trials Group. Breakthrough cases of PCP have been described despite prophylaxis. Therefore, patients should be closely monitored for this infection.

Cytomegalovirus Infection

Cytomegalovirus may cause disseminated disease, for example, hepatitis, retinitis, encephalitis, and colitis, in children with HIV infection. Ganciclovir is the drug of choice for treatment, and most experience in therapy has been in the treatment of retinitis. Initially, 10 mg/kg/d IV is given in two divided doses for 2 or 3 weeks until remission occurs. The patient then is kept on maintenance therapy at 5 mg/kg/d IV as a single daily dose. Relapse may occur and is not uncommon. A major toxicity of ganciclovir is bone marrow suppression, and patients may require the use of colony-stimulating factors to maintain hemoglobin and neutrophil counts in the normal range. Zidovudine also suppresses the bone marrow, and hematologic values should be monitored frequently when it is administered in combination with ganciclovir.

Phosphonoformate (foscarnet) is an alternative therapy for CMV retinitis, but there is limited experience in children. Its use should be limited to those cases of retinitis unresponsive to ganciclovir. Adverse effects include bone marrow suppression and renal toxicity. A new drug, valacyclovir, is in clinical trials in adults and children.

Herpes Simplex and Varicella-Zoster Viruses

Children with HIV infection may have severe and recurrent episodes of infection with herpes simplex virus (HSV). Treatment with oral or intravenous acyclovir, depending on the extent of the oral lesions, is effective. Although there is little experience with the prophylactic use of acyclovir, we have used it as oral prophylaxis in children with recurrent herpes, with a resultant decrease in the number of episodes of disease. Varicella-zoster virus (VZV) infection in children with HIV infection can be severe, depending on the state of immunocompromise. Susceptible children should receive varicella-zoster immune globulin (VZIG) within 96 hours of exposure. The child with HIV infection who develops varicella should be given IV acyclovir at a dose of 1500 mg/m²/d in three divided doses for 7 days. Children with zoster may also benefit from a course of intravenous acyclovir. Some children will develop chronic and persistent varicella lesions or have recurrences of zoster. In our experience, these episodes will respond to intravenous acyclovir, and the child may benefit from suppressive therapy with oral acyclovir.

Mucosal Candidiasis

A significant number of children with HIV infection will develop oral candidiasis. This is treated with oral nystatin suspension 2 to 6 ml four times daily or clotrimazole troches five times daily. For young infants and children whose *Candida* infection does not respond well to oral nystatin suspension, a clotrimazole troche is crushed and dissolved in 2 to 4 ml of the nystatin suspension, and the mixture is administered to each cheek four times daily. It is important to caution the caretaker not to give the child a feeding for at least 30 minutes after administering the suspension. For more severe or refractory disease, ketoconazole 6 mg/kg as a daily dose or fluconazole 3 to 6 mg/kg as a daily dose is effective. These two drugs are also effective treatment for *Candida* esophagitis, a condition that requires at least

2 weeks of treatment. Invasive *Candida* infection should be treated with amphotericin B.

Mycobacterium tuberculosis Infection

A large number of *M. tuberculosis* infections are seen in conjunction with HIV infection in adults, and a few cases have been reported in children. In the treatment of tuberculosis, it is important to know the antibiotic susceptibility pattern and epidemiology of the organisms isolated in the specific region of the country. In some parts of the nation, organisms with multiple drug resistance have been identified. Since most children have acquired their infection from an adult, the susceptibility of the organism isolated from the index case should assist in guiding initial therapy whenever this information is available. In areas without drug-resistant tuberculosis, children with HIV infection and tuberculosis may be treated initially with three drugs: isoniazid 10 to 15 mg/kg/d as a single dose, rifampin 10 to 20 mg/kg/d as a single dose, and pyrazinamide 30 mg/kg/d as a single dose. Short-course therapeutic regimens are not recommended, and treatment should be continued for at least 1 year. In areas with multiple-drug resistant tuberculosis, four or five drug regimens should be begun initially pending culture and sensitivity test results of the organism. Potential drugs for therapy include isoniazid, rifampin, pyrazinamide, ethambutol, streptomycin, and ethionamide. It is important to isolate the organism so that the sensitivity can be determined. Adjunctive steroid therapy is indicated in cases of (1) pleural or pericardial effusions to hasten resorption of fluid, (2) endobronchial lesions to relieve obstruction, (3) meningitis, (4) tuberculomas, and (5) miliary disease with alveolar capillary block.

Mycobacterium avium Complex Infection

Mycobacterium avium complex (MAC) infection occurs most frequently in severely immunocompromised children (CD4+ lymphocyte counts <100/mm³). The most common presenting signs are fever, weight loss, and pancytopenia. Several drug combinations are available for therapy, although none is extremely effective. Potentially useful drugs include amikacin, ethambutol, rifampin or rifabutin, clofazimine, ciprofloxacin, cefoxitin, and the macrolides azithromycin and clarithromycin. Initial therapy should include at least two drugs, one of which should be a macrolide. It is important to isolate the organism and determine its sensitivity. Two large placebo-controlled, blinded studies showed that prophylaxis with rifabutin 300 mg/d decreased the incidence of MAC in adults with absolute CD4+ counts <200/mm³. We also offer prophylaxis to older children and adolescents with CD4+ counts <100/mm³, with some adjustment to dose based on weight.

Recurrent Bacterial Infections

Children with HIV infection who present with fever should have a thorough workup for infection. Bacteremia, meningitis, septic arthritis, osteomyelitis, pneumonia, and urinary tract infection have been described in children with HIV. Many of these infections are caused by common organisms, such as *H. influenzae* type b, *S. pneumoniae*, *Staphylococcus aureus*, and *Salmonella* species. Children with wasting syndrome, opportunistic infections, or signs of progressive disease frequently will have gram-negative enteric organisms, such as *Pseudomonas* species and *Enterobacter* species. Therapy is begun pending culture results, usually with broad-spectrum antibiotics.

Parasitic Infections

Children can develop gastrointestinal infection with a number of parasitic infections, such as *Giardia, Cryptosporidium, Isospora belli,* and *Microsporidium*. Frequently, these infections are not self-limited, are more difficult to treat than in an immunocompetent host, and may recur. In our experience, cryptosporidiosis has been the most difficult to treat. We use paromomycin as initial therapy. If the diarrhea does not respond to this treatment, other agents, such as spiramycin, azithromycin, or hyperimmune bovine colostrum, are used. Clinical trials with hyperimmune bovine colostrum are underway in children. There are a few published reports on the use of octreotide in adults with severe secretory diarrhea from *Cryptosporidium,* but there is no published experience in children. Octreotide may control the diarrhea but does not clear the infection. Giardiasis may be treated with metronidazole, quinacrine, or furazolidone. Furazolidone is the only drug available in liquid form and is more convenient for treatment of young infants and children. *I. belli* responds to treatment with oral TMP-SMX, and in cases of recurrence, prophylaxis with daily TMP-SMX is an alternative. There are no proven treatments for diarrhea caused by *Microsporidium.*

Toxoplasmosis

Toxoplasmosis is less common in children than in adults with HIV. However, if a mother is infected with *Toxoplasma,* particularly if she has active disease, the infant is at risk for infection. Although it is uncommon, children with HIV infection may present at birth with evidence of congenital toxoplasmosis, and some will present later with retinitis. Once toxoplasmosis is diagnosed, the child should be treated with pyrimethamine, sulfadiazine, and folinic acid. The child with congenital infection should be treated throughout the first year of life. The older child who presents with a cerebral abscess should be treated for at least 6 weeks. Prophylaxis with sulfadiazine and pyrimethamine should be used to prevent recurrence of disease. An alternative drug for prophylaxis is clindamycin.

REFERENCES

1. Centers for Disease Control: Guidelines for prophylaxis against *Pneumocystis carinii* pneumonia for children infected with human immunodeficiency virus. MMWR 40(RR-2):1–13, 1991.
2. Centers for Disease Control: Zidovudine for the prevention of HIV transmission from mother to infant. MMWR 43:285–287, 1994.
3. Working Group on Antiretroviral Therapy: National Pediatric HIV Resource Center: Antiretroviral therapy and medical management of the human immunodeficiency virus-infected child. Pediatr Infect Dis J 12:513–522, 1993.

INFLUENZA VIRUSES

DEBRA A. TRISTRAM, M.D.
ROBERT C. WELLIVER, M.D.

Influenza viruses have plagued mankind for centuries, often causing worldwide pandemics. Despite the use of control measures in recent years, more than 10,000 deaths due to acute influenzal infection or its complications have occurred during each epidemic in the United States, mostly in the very young or in the elderly. Besides mortality, influenzal disease causes significant morbidity, resulting in absenteeism from school and work. Although antiviral therapy for acute disease is available, identification and prophylaxis of individuals at risk are more effective control measures.

CLINICAL MANIFESTATIONS

Influenza viral infection is an acute febrile illness characterized by sudden onset, with prominent myalgias, headache, and variable upper and lower respiratory tract symptoms. The duration of acute symptoms is usually about 4 or 5 days, but respiratory symptoms or malaise may be much more persistent. Influenza infections cause similar symptoms and signs in all age groups. There is little difference in the clinical disease manifestations of infection with different influenza virus types, although influenza B or influenza C infection is often less severe and of shorter duration than influenza A infection.

COMPLICATIONS

In most cases, the clinical diagnosis of influenza viral infection is straightforward, and recovery is without incident. However, complications can occur, the most frequent one being pneumonia. Patients can experience primarily viral pneumonia or a combination of viral pneumonia with secondary bacterial infection. The most common superinfecting bacteria are *Streptococcus pneumoniae, Haemophilus influenzae,* and *Staphylococcus aureus.* Other less common complications include Reye syndrome (associated with aspirin use during acute influenza infection), otitis media, myocarditis, pericarditis, myositis, encephalitis, transverse myelitis, and Goodpasture syndrome. Susceptible hosts, such as the very young, the elderly, and patients of any age with underlying cardiac, respiratory, or immunodeficiency diseases, may experience severe, life-threatening infection.

DIAGNOSIS

A definitive diagnosis of influenza infection rests on the recovery of infectious virus from respiratory secretions by tissue culture methods or on a fourfold rise in influenza-specific antibody during convalescence. Rapid diagnostic tests are used in certain virus laboratories. Such tests employ patient respiratory secretions stained with fluorescein-conjugated influenza-specific antibody to identify influenza antigen in virus-infected epithelial cells from the respiratory tract. These tests can be performed in laboratories that have experience in immunofluorescence techniques and can help guide therapeutic decisions, including vaccination strategies.

NONSPECIFIC TREATMENT

Symptomatic therapy should consist of maintenance of adequate hydration and sufficient analgesia necessary to provide relief from myalgia and headache. Acetaminophen (Tylenol) is the preferred agent over aspirin for influenza infections because of the association of aspirin use with the development of Reye syndrome following the acute phase of influenza A infection. The acetaminophen dose for children is 10 to 15 mg/kg per dose orally or rectally every 4 to 6 hours as needed, up to 650 mg per dose. The use of nonprescription cold and cough medications is discouraged because they tend to dry respiratory secretions and may inhibit the clearance of secretions from the respiratory tract. Cough suppressants containing codeine should be reserved for those patients who are unable to sleep at night because of their cough and should never be used for children under the age of 3 years. Antibiotics are indicated only for those patients with evidence of bacterial complications, such as pneumonia or otitis media. Adequate rest is essential for recovery from influenza. Deaths may occur from physical stress during acute influenzal illness, as seen in military recruits.

ANTIVIRAL THERAPY

An effective antiviral agent, amantadine hydrochloride (Symmetrel), is available in the United States for the treatment of influenza A infections. Amantadine is most effective when instituted within the first 2 to 3 days of onset of infection and should be considered for high-risk individuals with strong clinical suspicion of influenza A infection even if a definitive diagnosis is not immediately available. The dose of amantadine is 200 mg/d PO in adults and 100 mg/d PO in teenagers. In children 1 to 9 years of age, the dose is 5 to 8 mg/kg/d PO (max: 150 mg/d) divided in two doses. There is no approved dose for children under 1 year of age. Amantadine should be used for at least 7 days. The recommended doses must be modified in patients with renal insufficiency or seizure disorders. Side effects of amantadine, particularly stimulation of the central nervous system, may limit the use of the drug, especially in elderly individuals.

Another antiviral agent, ribavirin, has shown some efficacy in trials

TABLE 1. Influenza Vaccine Dose by Age Group—United States, 1993–1994

AGE GROUP	PRODUCT	DOSE (ml)	NUMBER OF DOSES	ROUTE*
6–35 mo	Split virus only	0.25	1 or 2†	IM
3–8 y	Split virus only	0.5	1 or 2†	IM
9–12 y	Split virus only	0.5	1	IM
>12 y	Whole or split virus	0.5	1	IM

*The deltoid muscle is the recommended site for vaccine administration in adults; the anterolateral aspect of the thigh is the recommended site for children.
†Two doses administered at least 1 month apart are recommended for children less than 9 years of age who are receiving influenza vaccine for the first time.
From the 1993–1994 recommendations of the Immunization Practices Advisory Committee (ACIP).

of healthy individuals with influenza A and B infection when it is used in aerosol form. Although expense and mode of administration are limitations to its routine use for influenza infections, ribavirin aerosol may be considered for use as an adjunct to amantadine for seriously ill patients.

PREVENTION

In the United States, two measures are available to reduce the impact of influenza in the community: immunoprophylaxis and chemoprophylaxis with amantadine. Vaccination of high-risk individuals each year before the influenza season is the most effective preventive method available. When the vaccine and epidemic strains are closely matched, high rates of vaccination can reduce the risk of outbreaks by inducing immunity. There are two types of vaccines, split virus vaccine and whole virus vaccine. To minimize the risk of febrile reactions, only the split virus vaccine should be used in children, although both vaccines have been shown to be safe and effective in adults. The suggested schedule is shown in Table 1. Target groups who should receive influenza vaccination include persons >65 years of age, residents of nursing homes or other chronic care facilities, adults and children with chronic disorders of the pulmonary or cardiovascular system, including asthma, or with chronic metabolic diseases (such as diabetes mellitus), renal insufficiency, hemoglobinopathies, or immunosuppression (including that caused by medication). In addition, children and teenagers who are receiving long-term aspirin therapy for chronic conditions should be vaccinated to reduce the risk of Reye syndrome. Finally, vaccination of health care workers, employees of nursing homes, and those persons whose jobs or family responsibilities include care of high-risk individuals is recommended to reduce the spread of disease to susceptible persons. The major contraindication to vaccination is known anaphylactic hypersensitivity to eggs or to other components of the vaccine. At present, there is no recommended vaccine dose for infants under 6 months of age.

Chemoprophylaxis is available for the prevention or amelioration of influenza A infection. Amantadine hydrochloride is the antiviral agent previously approved for use in the United States for this purpose. Rimantadine (Flumadine), a related compound, has shown equal efficacy with less toxicity and was recently approved by the US Food and Drug Administration for prophylaxis. Neither of these drugs is effective against infection with influenza B virus. The dose for prevention is the same as noted previously for treatment with amantadine. Dosages for rimantidine are the same as for amantadine. Individuals among the target populations who are not able to be immunized should receive this medication for all or part of the influenza season (5 to 7 weeks) if there is no medical contraindication. Alternatively, a program of influenza immunization followed by amantadine or rimantidine for 2 weeks while antibody develops can be instituted within 24 to 48 hours of influenza exposure. Additionally, amantadine or rimantidine can be used in closed populations as an adjunct to vaccination when community outbreaks of influenza begin.

INFECTIOUS MONONUCLEOSIS

CHARLES GROSE, M.D.
BETTY J. EDMOND, M.D.

The disease infectious mononucleosis is well known. Its symptoms include malaise and low-grade fever, followed by the signs of lymphadenopathy and hepatosplenomegaly and the appearance of atypical lymphocytes in the peripheral blood. In this section, the discussion is restricted to the disease caused by the Epstein-Barr virus (EBV). In older children and adults, this diagnosis is usually made on the basis of a positive rapid heterophil test obtained 7 to 10 days after the onset of the illness. In infants and young children, the heterophil test frequently is negative. Thus, the EBV capsid antigen IgG and IgM antibody assays are the diagnostic tests of choice. Similarly, the classic symptoms associated with infectious mononucleosis are most commonly seen in adolescents, whereas young children with primary EBV infection typically are asymptomatic or have nonspecific symptoms, such as prolonged fever, mild malaise, and anorexia. Both children and adults occasionally manifest severe tonsillitis and pharyngitis, with subsequent life-threatening respiratory compromise.

For most children with infectious mononucleosis, the treatment need only be supportive. The degree of fatigue may be enormous; for example, it is not unusual for students to remain in bed for days because they are too tired even to walk about the room. Loss of appetite may be accentuated by the mild to moderate hepatitis that frequently accompanies the disease. Therefore, a diet with increased carbohydrates and reduced fat content can be encouraged to maintain adequate caloric intake. Patients with jaundice should supplement their diet with a daily multivitamin tablet with zinc. They also need to maintain their fluid balance and can take acetaminophen for suppression of fever. Patients with tonsillar involvement should be screened for group A streptococcal infection and, if positive, should be treated with a 10-day course of penicillin V 250 mg three times per day or an oral cephalosporin (Table 1). Ampicillin should be avoided in a patient with infectious mononucleosis because it can produce a rash. Of importance, this period of acute disease can last for several weeks.

The convalescence can be prolonged, especially in otherwise active teenagers. Usually, we recommend that adolescents not return to rigorous athletic programs for one semester (3 to 4 months) after acute infectious mononucleosis: if a person is acutely ill in November, we recommend not returning to competitive athletics until the following summer. Obviously, patients with splenomegaly should not participate in any contact sports. If complaints about fatigue remain, we recommend a further 3-month respite from vigorous exercise. Only when a year has passed since the acute disease should there be undue concern about persistent lethargy. Since the relatively recent diagnosis of chronic infectious mononucleosis (or chronic fatigue syndrome) has become widely used, we have observed that it has been applied inappropriately to teenagers who are in the late convalescent stage of their acute EBV disease.

The use of antiviral agents for treatment of infectious mononucleosis in otherwise healthy children has no justification. Acyclovir is now approved for the treatment of herpes simplex viral infections and varicella-zoster viral infections, but this drug has no practical benefit for the management of EBV infection in the immunocompetent child. On the other hand, corticosteroids have been prescribed for treatment of symptomatic infectious mononucleosis for over two de-

TABLE 1. Drug Doses for Infectious Mononucleosis

DRUG	DOSE
Penicillin V	250 mg t.i.d. for 10 d
Prednisone	2 mg/kg/d with tapering on a daily basis

cades, especially in university student health clinics, although this regimen remains a subject of considerable dispute and usually is not recommended. However, one specific indication for corticosteroid therapy is to prevent or alleviate respiratory distress brought about by paratracheal lymphadenopathy and greatly enlarged tonsils. In the case of the patient with moderate lymphadenopathy and difficulty swallowing, a short course of prednisone is advocated to prevent the more severe respiratory complications. One schedule starts with 2 mg/kg on day 1, with a daily tapering over the next 6 days. When symptoms of respiratory distress abruptly occur as a result of obstructing lymphadenopathy, corticosteroids are given intravenously at an equivalent dose of 2 mg/kg of prednisone per day for several days, with rapid tapering over the following 7 to 10 days. Because the latter situation is an extreme medical emergency, the therapy should be initiated within an intensive care setting, as intubation may be required.

MEASLES

Barry Dashefsky, M.D.

CLINICAL FEATURES

Measles is an acute, highly contagious infection produced by a single antigenic type of RNA virus belonging to the group morbillivirus in the family Paramyxoviridae. Following an incubation period of 8 to 12 days, measles produces the abrupt onset of progressively severe fever, malaise, cough, conjunctivitis, and, after an average interval of 14 days from the time of exposure, a characteristic exanthem. Ordinarily, individuals infected with measles are contagious from 1 to 2 days before the onset of symptoms (3 to 5 days before the rash) to 4 days after the onset of the rash.

Complications of measles include otitis media, pneumonia (both viral and bacterial superinfection), laryngotracheobronchitis, diarrhea, and encephalitis (the last occurring at a frequency of approximately 1 per 1000 cases, often associated with permanent neurologic morbidity). The mortality rate is approximately 1 to 3 per 1000 cases, with most deaths caused by respiratory or neurologic complications mostly occurring among infants and adults. Subacute sclerosing panencephalitis (SSPE), a degenerative condition of the central nervous system (CNS) that is belatedly produced by measles infection (with a mean incubation period of nearly 11 years), has occurred very rarely since the advent of effective measles immunization.

PREVENTION

Active immunization with live virus measles vaccine is the primary instrument of preventing measles and, with few exceptions, is recommended for all children as part of the practice of routine childhood immunization. It can also be effective in preventing measles infection in a susceptible individual if administered within 72 hours of a discrete exposure, and, therefore, it is the recommended intervention for controlling outbreaks in schools. Passive immunization with immune globulin (Ig) that contains antibody against measles virus is effective in preventing or modifying infection if administered within 6 days of exposure. This modality is often used to protect exposed susceptible household contacts.

Active Measles Immunization

Further-attenuated live virus measles vaccine (e.g., Schwarz, Moraten, or Attenuvax strains) is the only measles vaccine available in the United States. It is available in the monovalent formulation and in combination with rubella vaccine (MR) but is most often used in combination with mumps and rubella vaccines (MMR), the formulation of choice for most indications since 1971.

Both killed and live attenuated measles vaccines were first licensed in 1963 and initially were recommended for routine administration at

9 months of age. Because of concern that lingering transplacentally acquired maternal antibody would neutralize the vaccine antigens and prevent an immune response, the recommended age for routine immunization was susbsequently changed, first to 12 months (1965) and then to 15 months (1976). In 1989, because of both the occurrence of epidemic rates of measles (among preschool and college-aged individuals) and an appreciation of the role of vaccine failure in abetting the outbreaks, it was recommended that a second dose of measles vaccine (administered as MMR) be given routinely at either of two times (see below). Finally, in 1993, because data had shown that antibody levels achieved following measles vaccination were lower than those associated with natural measles infection and noting the absence of the periodic natural boosting of measles antibody levels because of the rarity of exposure to natural measles, authorities again sanctioned the routine administration of the first MMR at any time from 12 to 15 months of age.

Recommendations for Use of Active Measles Immunization

Table 1 summarizes the AAP's recommendations (slightly modified) for measles vaccination as expressed in the 1994 *Report of the Committee on Infectious Diseases* (Red Book). The full text should be consulted for details.[1]

Routine Immunization Schedule

The first dose of measles vaccine, administered as MMR, should be given routinely at 12 to 15 months of age. The second dose (again as MMR because of both convenience and the opportunity afforded to ensure immunity for mumps and rubella as well) may be given either at grade school entry (4 to 6 years of age), as recommended by the Public Health Service, or middle school entry (11 to 12 years of age), as recommended by the AAP, but no earlier than 1 month after the first dose. In general, in deciding at which age the second dose of MMR should be administered, practitioners should be guided by local health department policy and by their perceptions of which option would result in greatest and most timely compliance among their patients.

Immunization Schedules in Special Circumstances

Other measles-susceptible individuals, including older children, adolescents, and young adults, should be immunized with two doses of measles vaccine (i.e., MMR) with no less than a 1-month interval between doses. Susceptible individuals are considered to be people born in or after 1957 (a year before which "everyone" is assumed to have had infection with wild measles virus) who lack documentation of physician-verified measles, laboratory evidence [usually by hemagglutination-inhibition (HI) or enzyme immunoassay (EIA) tests] of immunity to measles, or of receipt of adequate immunization.

All children who live in communities considered to be at high risk for measles should receive the first dose of MMR at 12 months of age. High-risk areas are defined by the Centers for Disease Control and Prevention as

1. Counties with more than five measles cases among preschoolers during each of the 5 previous years
2. Counties with a recent measles outbreak among unvaccinated preschoolers
3. Large innercity populations

During an outbreak, vaccine (preferably monovalent measles vaccine) may be given to children as young as 6 months of age. Because of their low rates of seroconversion, children who are immunized before age 12 months should later receive the standard two doses of MMR beginning at or after 12 months of age.

The following recommendations apply to those who were immunized according to pre-1989 guidelines. Those immunized before 12 months of age should be revaccinated according to currently recommended schedules. Those who were immunized between 12 and 14 months of age should receive a second dose. Those who received inactivated measles vaccine at any age or who were immunized with

TABLE 1. Recommendations for Measles Vaccination

GROUP	REMARKS
Unvaccinated (12–15 mo), no history of measles	A two-dose schedule (with MMR) is recommended if born after 1956; the first dose is recommended at 12–15 mo; the second is recommended during school years, either at grade school entry (4–6 y) or middle school or junior high school entry (11–12 y); local policy recommendations should be followed
Children 12 mo in areas of recurrent measles transmission	Vaccinate; a second dose is indicated during the school years
Children 6–12 mo in epidemic	Vaccinate (preferably with monovalent measles vaccine); if vaccinated before the first birthday, re-vaccination with (MMR) at 12–15 mo of age is necessary, and another dose is indicated during the school years
Children 11–12 y who have received one dose of measles vaccine at ≥12 mo	Revaccinate
Students in college and other post-high school institutions who have received one dose of measles vaccine at ≥12 mo	Revaccinate
History of vaccination before the first birthday	Consider susceptible and vaccinate
Unknown vaccine, 1963–1967	Consider susceptible and vaccinate
Further attenuated or unknown vaccine given with Ig	Consider susceptible and vaccinate
Egg allergy, nonanaphylactic	Vaccinate; no reactions likely
Neomycin allergy, nonanaphylactic	Vaccinate; no reactions likely
Tuberculosis	Vaccinate; vaccine does not exacerbate infection
Measles exposure within 72 h	Vaccination may protect; alternatively, Ig should be given if household exposure
HIV seropositive	Vaccinate
Immunoglobulin or blood product	Vaccinate at appropriate interval (see Table 2)

Modified from American Academy of Pediatrics Committee on Infectious Diseases: Measles. *In* Report of the Committee on Infectious Diseases, 23rd ed. Elk Grove Village, IL, American Academy of Pediatrics, 1994:313.

live measles vaccine within 3 months of having received inactivated measles vaccine should receive two doses of vaccine according to current guidelines. Patients who received Ig or measles immune globulin at the same time that they received measles vaccine after 1965 (when further-attenuated vaccine became available) should be considered susceptible and should be reimmunized according to standard guidelines.

Noting the prominence of imported measles in recent outbreaks in this country, it is important to ensure the immunity of those travelling to foreign countries where measles is prevalent. Those travellers born after 1956 who do not have documented immunity should receive a second dose of measles vaccine. For children less than 6 months of age who travel abroad, the presence of protective maternal antibody is assumed, and typically they are not immunized. Children between 6 and 11 months of age who travel abroad should receive monovalent measles vaccine. Those between 12 and 14 months of age should receive their first MMR. If it can be accomplished before departure, a second MMR should be given no sooner than 1 month after the first in children whose first MMR is given at 15 months of age or older.

Susceptible personnel employed in medical facilities who have direct patient contact should be immunized. (See Medical Settings discussion.)

Dose

In both monovalent and combination forms, measles vaccine is given in a dose of 0.5 ml SC. It may be given (in a separate syringe, at a separate site) at the same time as any of the other routinely administered childhood vaccines.

Vaccine Storage

Improper storage and handling of measles vaccine may render it inactive. To avoid heat inactivation before reconstitution, measles vaccine should be stored at 2°C to 8°C (35.6°F to 46.4°F) or colder temperatures. Freezing will not affect the lyophilized vaccine. Especially after reconstitution, vaccine should be shielded from ultraviolet light. It should be shipped at 10°C (50°F) or colder and may be shipped on dry ice. The vaccine diluent (sterile water) should not be frozen, since this may cause breakage of the glass container. Vac-

cine should be refrigerated after reconstitution and discarded if not used within 8 hours.

Vaccine Failure

When administered at or after 15 months of age, a single dose of measles vaccine produces protective antibody in at least 95% of recipients. Most cases of vaccine failure are thought to represent primary vaccine failure, that is, a failure to seroconvert following immunization. Such failure may be attributable to improper handling or storage of vaccine, administration too early when maternal antibody persists, or immunization at the same time as or in close proximity to Ig administration. A smaller number of vaccine failures are secondary, that is, a reflection of waning of antibody below protective levels (a phenomenon that is perhaps abetted by the absence of periodic boosting consequent to casual exposures to natural measles virus).

Adverse Reactions

The live attenuated measles vaccine, especially the further-attenuated varieties used since 1975, are safe and well tolerated. Approximately 5% to 15% of susceptible vaccine recipients experience a few days of fever (≥39.4°C), and 5% experience transient rashes, beginning 5 to 12 days after vaccination. Encephalopathy following measles vaccination occurs in less than 1 per million doses and is probably not causally related to the vaccine. Transient thrombocytopenia also has been reported occasionally after receipt of MMR. It is anticipated that all reactions occur much less frequently following revaccination because of the preexisting immunity that most vaccinees enjoy.

Measle vaccine is prepared in chick embryo cell culture. Allergic reactions and anaphylaxis attributable to egg antigen or trace amounts of neomycin contained in the vaccine occur very rarely.

Seizures, mostly simple febrile seizures, occur 5 to 12 days following measles vaccination, usually without long-term sequelae. SSPE has become exceedingly rare since the advent of measles immunization. Although a few cases have occurred in measles vaccine recipients who purportedly had never had natural measles, this association is dubious and does not represent a legitimate basis for foregoing immunization.

Up to 1 million doses of killed measles vaccine were given in some parts of the United States from 1963 to 1967 (and in Canada until 1964) before this biologic agent was abandoned. Although people vaccinated with killed vaccine who subsequently receive live measles vaccine may suffer more severe reactions than are typically experienced by live vaccine recipients, they should nonetheless be revaccinated according to the standard two-dose recommendations.

Precautions, Contraindications, and Special Considerations
Pregnancy

Although there are no data indicating that fetal infection occurs following administration of measles vaccine to a pregnant woman, for theoretical reasons, when administered as a monovalent product, measles vaccine should not be given to a pregnant woman or to one who may become pregnant within 1 month. When administered as MR or MMR vaccine, it should not be given during pregnancy or within 3 months before conception (the longer interval is dictated by concern for the very unlikely possibility of congenital rubella syndrome).

Allergies

A history of an anaphylactic reaction following ingestion of eggs represents a strong relative contraindication to administering measles vaccine. Skin testing and, possibly, desensitization of those demonstrating hypersensitivity to egg antigen might still permit vaccination to be performed safely and successfully. People with histories of nonanaphylactic reactions to eggs or allergic reactions to chickens or feathers may be immunized as per the usual recommendations.

Patients with histories of anaphylaxis following exposure to topical or systemic neomycin should not receive measles vaccine. However, those with histories of contact dermatitis in response to topical neomycin are not precluded from immunization. They may experience local reactions at the vaccine site 2 to 4 days after vaccination.

Recent Immune Globulin Therapy

Ig is known to interfere with the immune response to measles vaccine. Although previously there was a standard recommendation that measles vaccination should not follow receipt of Ig by less than a 3-month interval, the current recommended intervals following administration of immunoglobulin after which measles vaccination can be effectively accomplished vary with the particular immunoglobulin preparation (Table 2). Failure to observe these guidelines requires administration of an additional dose of measles vaccine at a later time unless seroconversion is documented.

Tuberculosis

Measles vaccine may be given concomitantly with the placement of a purified protein derivative (PPD) skin test. Because the vaccine may induce transient anergy, the PPD should be delayed for 4 to 6 weeks after administration of the measles vaccine if it is not placed concurrently. Unlike natural measles infection, measles vaccine does not exacerbate infection with tuberculosis.

Immunocompromised Hosts

Live measles vaccine virus may propagate and produce significant illness in recipients with altered immunity. Therefore, with the exception of HIV-infected persons, patients with immunodeficiency diseases or immunosuppression (e.g., those with leukemia, lymphoma, or generalized malignancy or those receiving alkylating agents, antimetabolites, radiation, or high-dose systemically administered corticosteroids) should not be immunized with the live measles vaccine. However, live measles vaccine may be given to patients with leukemia in remission who have not received chemotherapy for 3 or more months. Low to moderate doses of corticosteroid therapy for less than 2 weeks and, when given on alternate days for longer periods, topically applied corticosteroids (e.g., skin, intranasal) and corticosteroids in-

TABLE 2. Suggested Intervals Between Immune Globulin Administration and Measles Vaccination (MMR, MR, or Monovalent Measles Vaccines)

INDICATION FOR IMMUNE GLOBULIN (Ig)	ROUTE	DOSE		INTERVAL
		U OR ml	mg IgG/kg	(mo)*
Tetanus (as TIg)	IM	250 U	~10	3
Hepatitis A prophylaxis (as Ig)				
Contact prophylaxis	IM	0.02 ml/kg	3.3	3
International travel	IM	0.06 ml/kg	10	3
Hepatitis B prophylaxis†	IM	0.06 ml/kg	10	3
Rabies prophylaxis (as RIG‡)	IM	20 IU/kg	22	4
Measles prophylaxis (as Ig)				
Standard	IM	0.25 ml/kg	40	5
Immunocompromised host	IM	0.5 ml/kg	80	6
Varicella prophylaxis (as VZIG§)	IM	125 U/10 kg (max: 625 U)	20–39	5
Blood transfusion				
Washed red blood cells (RBCs)	IV	10 ml/kg	Negligible	0
RBCs, adenine-saline added	IV	10 ml/kg	10	3
Packed RBCs	IV	10 ml/kg	20–60	5
Whole blood	IV	10 ml/kg	80–100	6
Plasma/platelet products	IV	10 ml/kg	160	7
Replacement (or therapy) of immune deficiencies (as IVIg)	IV		300–400	8
ITP¶ (as IVIg)	IV		400	8
ITP	IV		1000	10
ITP or Kawasaki disease	IV		1600	11
Kawasaki disease	IV		2000	11

*These intervals should provide sufficient time for decreases in passive antibodies in all children to allow for an adequate response to measles vaccine. Physicians should not assume that children are fully protected against measles during these intervals. Additional doses of Ig or measles vaccine may be indicated after exposure to measles.
†Hepatitis B immune globulin.
‡Rabies immune globulin.
§Varicella-zoster immune globulin.
¶ITP, immune (formerly termed "idiopathic") thrombocytopenic purpura.
Modified from American Academy of Pediatrics Committee on Infectious Diseases: Measles. *In* Report of the Committee on Infectious Diseases, 23rd ed. Elk Grove Village, IL, American Academy of Pediatrics, 1994:319.

jected into joints or tendons are not immunosuppressive and do not contraindicate receipt of live measles vaccine. Immunoincompetent patients who are not themselves immunized against measles are afforded some measure of protection by vaccination of their household contacts. The vaccine virus is not transmissible from vaccine recipients.

Both asymptomatic and symptomatic HIV-infected patients should receive measles vaccine (as MMR) according to standard schedules because of both the severity of measles infection in that population and the accrued experience indicating that vaccine is well tolerated by HIV-infected persons. However, because of the inconsistency of their responses to immunization, HIV-infected patients who are exposed to natural measles infection should also receive Ig prophylactically unless they have received IVIg within the previous 3 weeks.

Personal or Family History of Seizures

Despite the slight increase in the rate of seizures (mostly febrile) in this population following measles vaccination, administration of MMR is recommended. Recipients should be alerted to the possibility of belated febrile illness 7 to 12 days after immunization, at which time prophylactically administered acetaminophen may be helpful.

Concomitant Illness

Minor illnesses, including those with fever, should not interfere with the routine administration of immunizations, including MMR. Immunization should be deferred in response to more severe illness.

Recommendations for Use of Passive Immunization with Immune Globulin

Ig is effective in preventing or modifying measles infection if administered to a susceptible individual within 6 days after exposure. It is recommended especially for susceptible household, pregnant, immunoincompetent, and infant (6 to 12 months of age) contacts. Infant contacts 5 months of age or younger are presumed to enjoy protection from maternally derived antibody and ordinarily need not receive Ig unless the source of exposure is the mother.

The recommended dose of intramuscularly administered Ig for hosts with normal immune competence is 0.25 ml/kg (max: 15 ml). For immunoincompetent hosts, the recommended dose is 0.5 ml/kg (max: 15 ml). If not otherwise contraindicated, measles vaccine should be given to those who receive Ig as prophylaxis against measles 5 months (for those who received 0.25 ml/kg) or 6 months (for those who received 0.5 ml/kg) after the administration of Ig, provided the vaccine is at least 12 months of age. IVIg at a dose of 100 to 400 mg/kg would also afford protection against measles if given 3 weeks or less before exposure.

Patients with symptomatic HIV infection who are exposed to measles should receive Ig 0.5 ml/kg irrespective of prior measles vaccination unless IVIg had been given within the previous 3 weeks. Both asymptomatic and symptomatic HIV-infected susceptible household contacts of measles, especially those younger than 1 year of age, should be given Ig.

MANAGEMENT OF A MEASLES OUTBREAK

A single case of measles constitutes an outbreak. All suspected cases should be promptly evaluated and reported to public health authorities for further investigation and initiation of control measures. All susceptibles, or those who cannot document immunity, should be vaccinated or excluded from settings where they might acquire or transmit measles (e.g., schools) until they are vaccinated or until at least 2 weeks after the onset of rash in the last case of measles.

Schools and Child Care Centers

Revaccination with MMR is recommended during outbreaks in child care centers, schools, and institutions of higher learning. This intervention should also be considered for nearby, as yet unaffected institutions at risk for transmission. Revaccination should be given to all attendees and their siblings as well as to all personnel born after

1956 who cannot document receipt of two measles vaccinations administered at or after 12 months of age or evidence of immunity. Attendees and personnel may return to the institution immediately after revaccination or, in the case of those not previously vaccinated, after receipt of the first dose. Generally, it is not necessary to revaccinate the entire community, and only very rarely is it necessary to cancel institutional events or to quarantine.

Children Less Than 12 Months of Age

Because complications of measles may be very serious in children less than 1 year of age, infants between 6 and 12 months of age should be immunized against measles (monovalent vaccine is preferred, but MMR is acceptable) in the event of a high risk of exposure to measles. Such vaccinees should subsequently receive two doses of MMR following the first birthday as per routine schedules.

Medical Settings

If a measles outbreak occurs in a hospital or other health care facility, all employees with direct patient care who were born after 1956 and lack documentation of either receipt of two doses of measles vaccine given no earlier than 12 months of age or other evidence of immunity should be immunized. Because measles has been acquired even by medical personnel who were born before 1957, these older employees with occupational exposure to measles should be considered for revaccination. Susceptible personnel should not have direct patient contact from the fifth through the twenty-first day after exposure regardless of whether they received vaccine or immunoglobulin after exposure. Those who contract measles should avoid patient contact for 4 days after the onset of rash.

MANAGEMENT OF MEASLES INFECTION

Management of patients with measles is largely limited to supportive measures intended to afford symptomatic relief: analgesia/antipyresis, fluids, and bedrest. Patients hospitalized with measles should be placed in respiratory isolation for 4 days after the onset of the rash. Compromised hosts should remain in respiratory isolation for the duration of hospitalization because of the unpredictability of the duration of their contagiousness. In addition, vigilance for complications should lead to timely initiation of diagnostic and therapeutic measures appropriate for those specific developments (e.g., antimicrobial treatment for complicating otitis media or bronchopneumonia, respiratory therapies and support for laryngotracheobronchitis or pneumonia, extensive monitoring and supportive measures for encephalitis).

TABLE 3. Indications for Vitamin A Therapy in Patients with Measles

1. Patients 6 months to 2 years of age hospitalized with measles and its complications (e.g., croup, pneumonia, and diarrhea); limited data available regarding the safety and need for vitamin A supplementation for infants younger than 6 months of age
2. Patients older than 6 months of age with measles who have any of the following risk factors and who are not already receiving vitamin A
   a. Immunodeficiencies (e.g., AIDS, congenital immunodeficiencies, and immunosuppressive therapy)
   b. Ophthalmologic evidence of vitamin A deficiency, including night blindness, Bitot's spots (grayish white deposits on the bulbar conjunctiva adjacent to the cornea), and xerophthalmia
   c. Impaired intestinal absorption (e.g., biliary obstruction, short bowel syndrome, and cystic fibrosis)
   d. Moderate to severe malnutrition, including that associated with eating disorders
   e. Recent immigration from areas where high mortality rates from measles have been observed

From American Academy of Pediatrics Committee on Infectious Diseases: Vitamin A treatment of measles. Pediatrics 91:1015, 1993. Reproduced by permission of Pediatrics, copyright 1993.

There is no demonstrably effective antiviral treatment for measles. The virus is susceptible to ribavirin in vitro, and some anecdotal reports purport ribavirin to have been beneficial when administered either intravenously or by aerosol to severely ill, immunocompromised patients with measles. Although its selective use in such circumstances should be considered, ribavirin is not approved for treatment of measles by the U.S. Food and Drug Administration.

Studies in third world countries have demonstrated that administration of vitamin A to children with measles is associated with decreased morbidity and mortality. Accordingly, the World Health Organization and the United Nations International Children's Emergency Fund (UNICEF) have recommended that vitamin A be given to all children with measles in communities with vitamin A deficiency where the mortality from measles exceeds 1%. Although vitamin A deficiency is not a significant problem in the United States, studies have documented lowered concentrations in children in this country with severe measles infection. The AAP recommends consideration of its use in the circumstances listed in Table 3.

Vitamin A is available in the United States as an orally administered solution (50,000 IU/ml). When indicated, a single dose of 200,000 IU of vitamin A should be given orally to children 1 year of age or older, and 100,000 IU should be given to children 6 months to 1 year of age. The same dose should be repeated the next day and in 4 weeks for children who have ophthalmologic signs of vitamin A deficiency. Vomiting and headache have been reported side effects, especially following the higher dose of vitamin A.

REFERENCES

1. American Academy of Pediatrics Committee on Infectious Diseases: Measles. *In* Report of the Committee on Infectious Diseases, 23rd ed. Elk Grove Village, IL, American Academy of Pediatrics, 1994:308–323.
2. Centers for Disease Control: Measles Prevention: Recommendations of the Immunization Practices Advisory Committee (ACIP). MMWR 38:1–13, 1989.
3. Hussey GD, Klein M: A randomized, controlled trial of vitamin A in children with severe measles. N Engl J Med 323:160–164, 1990.

MUMPS

GREGORY F. HAYDEN, M.D.

No specific therapy is available for this self-limited illness. The selection of treatment, if any, depends solely on the presence and severity of particular signs and symptoms. The spectrum of clinical illness is broad. Many infections are subclinical and require no therapy. Many children with mild clinical cases also benefit from therapeutic restraint. Occasional antipyretic-analgesic therapy with acetaminophen or aspirin may be used for symptomatic fever and general discomfort. Those relatively few children with severe or complicated cases may require more intensive support measures, sometimes including hospitalization.

MANAGEMENT OF SPECIFIC FEATURES

Appropriate management varies according to the manifestations of mumps that are encountered.

Parotitis

A regular diet is often well tolerated, but if chewing is painful, a soft diet with generous fluids will be appreciated. If acidic, sour, or highly seasoned foods induce pain, a bland diet is advisable. Analgesic therapy with acetaminophen often relieves parotid discomfort. Aspirin can also be helpful but may make matters worse if it is allowed to dissolve in the mouth. Warm or cold compresses may provide local relief. Anecdotal reports suggest that a short course of corticosteroids may reduce intense parotid swelling and pain, but such therapy has not prevented the development of contralateral parotid involvement.

This mode of treatment remains experimental and cannot be recommended.

Meningitis and Encephalitis

The spectrum of central nervous system (CNS) involvement is broad, ranging from asymptomatic lymphocytic pleocytosis in the cerebrospinal fluid (CSF) (common) to severe encephalitis (rare). Acetaminophen or aspirin may relieve associated headache. Lumbar puncture sometimes relieves the headache associated with mumps but is indicated only for diagnostic purposes. Children with severe CNS involvement may require hospitalization for bedrest, analgesic-antipyretic therapy, and carefully monitored parenteral fluid therapy. Hospitalization is not required for mild, typical CNS involvement as long as the etiology has been established as mumps with reasonable certainty. Limited experience in the former Soviet Union suggests that interferon therapy can shorten the course of CNS involvement associated with mumps, but these preliminary findings need to be confirmed in a double-blind clinical trial.

Pancreatitis

Mild elevation of pancreatic enzymes in the absence of symptoms is frequent. Clinically apparent pancreatitis is unusual, but parenteral fluid therapy may be necessary for those children with abdominal pain and severe vomiting associated with pancreatitis. Acetaminophen therapy may sometimes relieve pain adequately. Narcotic agents can be used for severe pain but can potentially induce biliary spasm, with transient elevations of plasma amylase and lipase levels. Antiemetic therapy is not recommended.

Orchitis

About 20% to 30% of postpubertal male patients with mumps are affected by orchitis, usually unilateral. Analgesia with acetaminophen or aspirin may relieve the associated discomfort, but narcotic agents may be required. Bedrest, intermittent application of icepacks, and gentle support of the affected testis may also be helpful. Anesthetic block of the spermatic cord has been reported to relieve pain but should be reserved for severe cases refractory to less extreme measures. Treatment with systemic corticosteroids has been reported to decrease fever associated with orchitis but has not been documented to accelerate the resolution of orchitis or to reduce the incidence of subsequent atrophy. Diethylstilbestrol therapy and surgical incision of the tunica albuginea are likewise of largely unproven benefit and should be used infrequently, if at all.

There is no evidence that bedrest reduces the risk of orchitis. When given after the onset of illness, standard immunoglobulin (Ig) does not prevent orchitis or otherwise modify the clinical course. In previous years, a human hyperimmune globulin (mumps immune globulin, or MIg) was sometimes given to young men with early mumps in the hope of preventing the subsequent development of orchitis. The efficacy of such therapy was controversial, however, and this expensive preparation is no longer commercially available.

Patients and their parents may benefit from reassurance about normal reproductive function following mumps orchitis. Only about 25% of cases of orchitis are bilateral, and in only a fraction of young men with such cases does progressive testicular atrophy develop. Subnormal sperm counts have been observed occasionally among such patients, but this impairment of fertility is generally partial and may be temporary. Contrary to popular belief, mumps orchitis does not cause impotence and very rarely results in sterility.

Very limited experience in Germany suggests that interferon therapy may help to prevent the late complications of mumps orchitis. However, these preliminary observations need to be confirmed in larger, controlled studies.

Arthritis

Salicylate therapy is often ineffective in treating the arthritis occasionally associated with mumps. A short course of corticosteroids or nonsteroidal anti-inflammatory agents is more likely to be helpful.

Other Manifestations

Other rare manifestations of mumps may include myocarditis, thyroiditis, nephritis, hepatitis, mastitis, epididymitis, oophoritis, and thrombocytopenia. These manifestations may be treated with a combination of careful monitoring, general supportive care, and symptomatic therapy.

ISOLATION

Hospitalized patients should remain in respiratory isolation until the parotid swelling has subsided or other manifestations have cleared. Attempts to isolate patients at home and in the community are less useful because patients are often contagious before the onset of parotid swelling and because persons with inapparent infection can nevertheless be contagious.

TREATMENT OF CONTACTS

The comprehensive treatment of a child with mumps includes counseling family members and other close contacts about their risk for development of mumps and informing them what preventive measures are available. When one is planning a suitable course of action, the first step is to determine whether the exposed persons are likely to be susceptible to mumps. Laboratory testing is, unfortunately, of only limited value. The presence of mumps-neutralizing antibodies reliably indicates immunity, but this assay is time consuming, expensive, and not generally available. The mumps skin test and the commonly available serologic tests for mumps are not adequately sensitive to be clinically useful.

In most instances, estimation of susceptibility must, therefore, depend on simple historical information. A definite history of previous mumps illness or immunization strongly suggests immunity and provides grounds for reassurance. In contrast, a negative history of mumps illness is poorly predictive of mumps susceptibility. Approximately 90% of adults with such histories are immune on the basis of previous, unrecognized infection.

If susceptibility to mumps is nevertheless suspected, what can be done? Standard Ig is not effective in preventing mumps infection. The efficacy of even the higher potency MIg in this setting was questionable. It is uncertain whether the administration of live mumps vaccine after exposure can prevent or modify illness. In deciding whether to recommend vaccine, several considerations apply. On the positive side, adverse reactions to mumps vaccine are uncommon, and there is no increased risk of adverse reactions following the vaccination of an immune person. Vaccination after exposure is not known to increase the severity of incubating mumps. If the recognized exposure has not resulted in incubating infection, live mumps vaccination should provide protection against subsequent exposures. On the negative side, vaccination after exposure has never been demonstrated to be effective, and the vaccination (and vaccinator) may wrongly be blamed for the manifestations of mumps illness that develop after the vaccination. *Contraindications to live mumps vaccination include immunodeficiency, anaphylactic allergy to neomycin, severe febrile illness, pregnancy, and receipt of Ig or blood products within 3 months.* Persons with anaphylactic allergy to ingested egg should receive mumps vaccine only with caution according to published protocols for skin testing and rapid desensitization. If vaccination is considered, these limitations and uncertainties should be described in sufficient detail that the involved persons understand what benefits can reasonably be expected.

HUMAN PARVOVIRUS B19 INFECTIONS

JANE D. SIEGEL, M.D.
CHARLES M. GINSBURG, M.D.

Human parvovirus B19 was first identified in 1975 in about 30% of serum specimens from adults who were being tested for the presence of hepatitis B antigen. Since that time, seroepidemiologic studies have defined the clinical syndromes and diseases caused by this virus. In 1981, the first condition, aplastic crisis in patients with sickle cell disease, was attributed to B19 infection. The association of B19 with erythema infectiosum (fifth disease) and nonimmune hydrops fetalis was reported in 1983 and 1984, respectively. Subsequently, several clinical manifestations have been described in both immunocompetent and immunocompromised hosts (Table 1).

Seroprevalence studies have detected antibodies to B19 in 30% to 60% of adults. The prevalence of antibody in infants and children is variable and directly correlates with age. Investigations of community outbreaks have indicated that the highest infection rates among susceptible pregnant women were in schoolteachers, followed by day care workers and homemakers. Health care workers are at comparatively low risk. Contact with schoolage children at home or at work and age <30 years have been identified as independent risk factors for acquisition of new infection. Nosocomial transmission in the hospital setting is unusual, but in one report of two outbreaks in the same center, attack rates were 36% and 38% among susceptible caregivers who were exposed during the first few days of admission of two patients with aplastic crisis.

ERYTHEMA INFECTIOSUM

No specific treatment is recommended for erythema infectiosum or the arthropathy that is often associated with B19 infection. The rash and arthritis/arthralgia are believed to be immunologically mediated because their onset coincides with the appearance of circulating antibody and the cessation of viral shedding. If chronic arthritis develops after B19 infection, treatment with anti-inflammatory agents is advised. A role for B19 or other parvovirus agents in the development of rheumatoid arthritis has been questioned but is unproven.

TRANSIENT APLASTIC CRISIS

A recent infection with B19 is associated with 80% to 93% of transient aplastic crisis (TAC) episodes in patients with chronic hemolytic anemia (e.g., sickle cell disease, hereditary spherocytosis, thalassemia). These episodes usually consist of an acute, self-limited pure red cell aplasia with severe reticulocytopenia. Occasionally, transient thrombocytopenia and neutropenia also can occur. Management of the patient with TAC consists of support of the direct effects of a sudden decrease in hemoglobin: congestive heart failure, respiratory distress, and hypoxemia. Blood transfusion with packed red cells

TABLE 1. Clinical Manifestations of Human Parvovirus B19 Infections

HOST	CLINICAL DISEASE*
Normal	Asymptomatic, erythema infectiosum (fifth disease), arthritis/arthralgias (acute, chronic)
Chronic hemolytic anemia	Transient aplastic crisis (TAC)
Immunocompromised	Chronic, persistent anemia and reticulocytopenia
Fetus	Stillbirth, hydrops fetalis secondary to anemia or myocarditis, fetal death

*Other less frequent manifestations: myocarditis, pancytopenia, hemophagocytic syndrome, encephalitis, brachial plexus neuropathy, systemic vasculitis, fetal bowel obstruction with meconium peritonitis.

TABLE 2. Isolation Guidelines for Patients with Human Parvovirus B19 Infections

1. No isolation for patients with erythema infectiosum or arthritis/arthralgia
2. Contact isolation for duration of illness of patients with transient aplastic crisis or immunocompromised patients with chronic aplastic anemia
3. Gown, gloves, masks during close contact with patient materials likely to be soiled with respiratory secretions or blood
4. Handwashing after contact with patient or contaminated materials
5. Pregnant women are restricted from caring for these patients

is often required and may be lifesaving. Spontaneous recovery of the bone marrow occurs in 10 to 12 days and is indicated by a brisk reticulocytosis, leukocytosis, and thrombocytosis. Patients with TAC are able to mount an effective antibody response and will clear the virus. Thus, recurrent or chronic TAC does not occur. Contact isolation for hospitalized patients is indicated for the duration of illness (Table 2).

CHRONIC APLASTIC ANEMIA

In recent years, B19 has been demonstrated to be the cause of chronic aplastic anemia in immunocompromised hosts. A treatment regimen has been devised using commercially available preparations of intravenous immunoglobulins (IVIg) that contain neutralizing activity against the erythropoietic suppression induced by B19 infection. A B19 hyperimmunoglobulin is not yet available. A single infusion of standard IVIg produces a dramatic decrease in the quantity of circulating virus and a prompt reticulocytosis in patients with both acquired and congenital immunodeficiency states who have a B19-induced chronic anemia. It is likely that the frequent infusion of immunoglobulins administered to bone marrow transplant patients immediately after transplantation protects against chronic B19 aplastic anemia. Treatment courses of 400 mg/kg/d for 5 to 10 days are recommended to produce long-term remissions, but repeated administrations may be necessary to sustain the remission if the immunosuppression cannot be reversed. Some patients develop erythema infectiosum-like rash and arthritis/arthralgia following IVIg infusion. Contact isolation is indicated for the duration of this illness (Table 2).

INFECTION IN PREGNANCY

There is no adverse effect of B19 infection on the mother during pregnancy. The rate of maternal-fetal transmission of B19 infection is approximately 33%, and the risk of fetal death has been estimated to be as high as 4% to 9%. However, the risk of fetal death in a woman of unknown serologic status who has a household exposure to parvovirus B19 is estimated to be 1% to 2% or less. The association of B19 with nonimmune hydrops and fetal death, especially in the second trimester, is proven but is of very low incidence. There is no evidence to support an association between in utero B19 infection and an increased risk of birth defects among liveborn infants.

If a woman is exposed to parvovirus B19 during pregnancy, the first step is to establish her serologic status by performing IgM and IgG antibody tests. When a recent B19 infection is documented in the mother, the pregnancy should be monitored closely with serial sonograms and serial serum maternal alpha-fetoprotein determinations for signs of hydrops. Because of the very low risk of adverse outcome for the fetus, interruption of pregnancy is not recommended for women who have acquired a new B19 infection during pregnancy. Intrauterine transfusion and intrauterine digitalization were recommended as possible treatment options for hydrops fetalis before spontaneous resolution of fetal hydrops was recognized. Several recent reports of the spontaneous resolution of nonimmune hydrops associated with B19 infection 3 to 5 weeks after diagnosis have led to a more conservative approach. If the condition of the fetus with hydrops continues to worsen and it is too early in the pregnancy to deliver an infant likely

to survive, fetal hemoglobin is measured, and intrauterine transfusion of packed red blood cells is recommended for hemoglobin ≤5 g/dl. There is no experience with IVIg infusions during pregnancy.

PREVENTION

At present, there is no specific therapy that has been proven effective for postexposure prophylaxis or treatment of B19. Despite anecdotal claims, there are no data to support the use of immunoglobulin for passive protection following exposure to B19. A candidate recombinant vaccine for human parvovirus B19 is in the early stages of development.

Prevention of spread of infection within the community is difficult because exposure of at-risk susceptibles occurs before recognition of clinical infection. Most pregnant women will be exposed to B19 infection from schoolage children at home. Nevertheless, since infection rates are increased as much as 20-fold during a school outbreak, temporary transfer of pregnant employees away from direct child contact may be a consideration. Women who are pregnant or are contemplating pregnancy should be informed of the increased occupational risk associated with school and day care contact with children, but this information should be put into the perspective of the very low incidence of adverse outcome and the frequent exposure if there are schoolage children in the home. Routine serologic screening is not recommended at this time but may be performed in individual cases if this is judged beneficial by the physician. Sensitive and specific serologic (IgG and IgM) tests are commercially available. Standard hygienic practices, such as handwashing and proper disposal of facial tissues or other items soiled with respiratory secretions, will decrease transmission of infection. Household contacts of patients who are at risk for B19-associated red blood cell aplasia should also be advised of the importance of taking these precautions if they are contemplating pregnancy.

Isolation guidelines for hospitalized patients are summarized in Table 2. Viral particles are present in respiratory secretions and blood. The highest titer of virus is present in patients with acute red cell aplasia and HIV-infected patients with chronic anemia. Although many publications recommend *respiratory* isolation, it is, in fact, the *close contact* with respiratory secretions from which personnel must protect themselves. Similar to the prevention of transmission of respiratory syncytial virus, *contact* isolation is effective and emphasizes the importance of handwashing and gloves. Masks should be used when in *close contact*. Pregnant women should be restricted from caring for patients with parvovirus B19 infections.

Although no virus is detectable in the liveborn normal infants who have had in utero B19 infection, virus is present during the acute stage of in utero infection. Therefore, the products of conception at the time of spontaneous abortion should be handled with gloves and disposed of as infectious material.

REFERENCES

1. Adler SP, Manganello A-M A, Koch WC, et al: Risk of human parvovirus B19 infections among school and hospital employees during endemic periods. J Infect Dis 168:361–368, 1993.
2. Berry PJ, Gray ES, Porter HJ, Burton PA: Parvovirus infection of the human fetus and newborn. Semin Diagn Pathol 9:4–12, 1992.
3. Harris JW: Parvovirus B19 for the hematologist. Am J Hematol 39:119–130, 1992.

RABIES

MARK S. PASTERNACK, M.D.

Rabies is a viral zoonosis endemic among a variety of terrestrial mammals. It is transmitted to humans either through direct contact with infected wild animals or through infection of domestic animals and pets, with subsequent human infection. Disease in humans is manifest by progressive encephalitis that is virtually always fatal. Consequently, the management of rabies focuses on

1. The prevention of disease in exposed individuals through passive and active immunization (postexposure prophylaxis)
2. The preexposure immunization of individuals who are at increased risk of contracting rabies as a result of professional or recreational activities, including travel
3. The immunization of pets (to reduce the possibility of rabies in a household vector)

Although currently fewer than one human case is diagnosed each year in the United States, thousands of cases of animal rabies are reported to the Centers for Disease Control and Prevention (CDC) annually, and over 10,000 individuals are treated for possible exposure. Tens of thousands of cases of human rabies occur each year in underdeveloped countries.

HUMAN RABIES

As noted, within the United States, rabies in humans is extraordinarily rare. Because of the potentially long incubation period, past rabies exposures (e.g., attacks by animals abroad, exploration of caves) may not be recalled, and rabies may not be considered in the initial differential diagnosis. The incubation period of rabies is highly variable, depending on the inoculum and site of infection. Although the incubation period commonly ranges between 20 and 90 days, clinical rabies has been reported months or even years after presumed exposure.

Clinical Features

Illness begins with an initial febrile prodrome, with malaise, headache, and abdominal pain. In some cases, there may be paresthesias at the site of infection. The prodromal phase lasts from 2 to 10 days, when acute neurologic disease supervenes. Early encephalitic symptoms include intermittent agitation, hyperactivity, and disorientation and may include neck stiffness and seizures. Laryngospasm and spasms of the diaphragm and intercostal musculature after attempted ingestion of liquids are responsible for classic hydrophobia. In an acutely ill and febrile patient, the presence of prominent brainstem findings with relatively clear sensorium (without an alternative explanation) strongly supports the diagnosis of rabies. A variety of additional neurologic findings may be present, including hyperactive or absent deep tendon reflexes and flaccid symmetric or asymmetric paralysis (dumb rabies). A mild mononuclear pleocytosis is present in the cerebrospinal fluid (CSF) in the majority of patients, with variable CSF protein and fluid pressure. After several days, the encephalitic phase progresses to coma and subsequent death by respiratory arrest in untreated patients. Intensive care unit support has prolonged the lives of patients with rabies for weeks, usually until a fatal complication supervenes.

Diagnosis

The diagnosis of rabies is best confirmed by neck skin biopsy and immunofluorescence testing. The patient should be isolated, and staff should use barrier (gown and glove) and respiratory precautions. Caregivers who have wound or mucous membrane contamination by the patient's secretions or tissues or who are bitten must undergo postexposure prophylaxis.

Postexposure Management

Rabies virus is present in the saliva of rabid animals, and transmission usually occurs following bite wound injuries. However, virus may be present on animal claws and transmitted by scratch, by contamination of a preexistent wound or abrasion by animal saliva, or rarely by aerosol exposures in such areas as caves containing aerosolized virus from rabid bat secretions or in laboratories engaged in the study or production of rabies virus. Rabies transmission is typically initiated by an unprovoked attack by a rabid animal. All injuries inflicted by wild carnivorous animals should be evaluated for rabies prophylaxis. Bites sustained during the feeding or handling of an apparently healthy domestic animal are considered provoked. Documenting an unprovoked attack, especially with young children, may be problematic, and infected animals may shed rabies virus in saliva for several days before the onset of symptoms. Hence, in addition to the type of exposure, epidemiologic considerations are crucial in the management of possible rabies exposures.

Criteria for Prophylaxis

The decision to initiate postexposure prophylaxis is based on the animal species responsible for the initial attack, the prevalence of rabies in this species in the local area, the nature of the animal contact, the animal's rabies immunization status, and the availability of the attacking animal for monitoring or direct tissue examination. Generally, bites by carnivorous wild animals, particularly skunks, raccoons, bats, or foxes and other predators, require postexposure prophylaxis. Conversely, attacks by small rodents, such as squirrels, rats, and mice, do not require prophylaxis, although larger species, such as woodchucks, can harbor rabies. Rabbits, hares, and opposums have not been associated with rabies transmission to humans. Petting a rabid animal or contact with its excreta does not require prophylaxis. When rabies is present in wild animals in the local area, attacks by unimmunized dogs or cats also require prophylaxis unless the domesticated animal can be captured for 10-day quarantine (pets) or examination (strays). Fully vaccinated dogs or cats have only rarely been reported to develop rabies. Quarantined domestic animals should be monitored by a veterinarian or animal control officer and killed for examination if signs of disease develop. Captured wild animals should be killed, and the head should be submitted for rabies testing. In addition to performing brain immunofluorescence examinations to confirm animal rabies, local and state health authorities offer expert consultative advice regarding the prevalence of rabies in a given area among different animal species and the need for postexposure prophylaxis in individual cases.

Wound Care

Prompt and thorough local wound care is the foundation of postexposure management. Wounds must be copiously irrigated with soap and water, and puncture wounds should be irrigated by catheter. Tetanus immunization status should be reviewed and prophylaxis should be administered if indicated, and antibiotics should be administered as clinically indicated. Specific immunoprophylaxis should begin as promptly as possible, preferably within 24 hours of the attack. Passive immunization with human rabies immune globulin (HRIg) confers protection to the victim before rabies vaccine can elicit protective antibody. HRIg is administered at a dose of 20 IU/kg, with half of the dose infiltrated into the soft tissues around the wound and the rest administered IM in the gluteal area. If HRIg is not immediately available, it should be administered as soon as possible, although it probably offers little benefit if it is given beyond 7 or 8 days after active immunization with rabies vaccine is begun. HRIg is not required if complete preexposure prophylaxis or earlier postexposure prophylaxis has been administered.

Vaccines

In the United States, two inactivated, tissue culture-derived rabies vaccines are available for human use: a human diploid cell vaccine

(HDCV) and an aluminum phosphate-adsorbed vaccine (RVA) derived from fetal rhesus lung diploid cell culture. In both instances, 1 ml of vaccine is given intramuscularly initially and on days 3, 7, 14, and 28 days thereafter in the deltoid (or anterolateral aspect of the thigh in young children). The vaccine should not be given in the same limb as the HRIg. If the captured domestic animal is observed for 10 days and remains well or is killed and is negative for rabies by immunofluorescence testing, the immunization series initiated at the time of animal attack may be discontinued. Although both vaccines reliably evoke protective neutralizing antibodies in normal hosts, immunocompromised individuals receiving rabies immunizations should be tested for the development of neutralizing antibodies. Local side effects, such as pain, swelling, and induration, as well as mild to moderate systemic toxicity, including fever, headache, and myalgias, are common and should not interrupt the immunization series. Instead, symptomatic treatment with analgesics or anti-inflammatory, antipyretic agents, such as aspirin, as well as antihistamines, should be employed. A variety of postexposure immunization schedules are used outside the United States, including the use of equine antirabies antiserum, intradermally administered tissue culture-derived rabies vaccines, and vaccines derived from nerve tissue. If postexposure prophylaxis has been initiated abroad, additional therapy may be necessary when the patient returns to the United States, and state or local health departments should be consulted for specific advice.

Preexposure Prophylaxis

Individuals at increased risk of rabies exposure include veterinarians, animal handlers, laboratory workers engaged in rabies research and virus production, spelunkers, and travelers residing for extended intervals in areas where there is endemic canine rabies. Primary preexposure vaccination with HDCV or RVA can be administered in the deltoid with three 1-ml intramuscular doses on days 0, 7, and 21 or 28. Alternatively, HDCV can be given as three 0.1-ml intradermal doses in the skin over the deltoid area according to the same schedule. Immunocompromised recipients should undergo intramuscular vaccine immunization and be tested for the development of neutralizing antibodies. Individuals receiving chloroquine or mefloquine prophylaxis for malaria also require the intramuscular vaccine immunization regimen because chloroquine interferes with the antibody response to HDCV.

Individuals with the highest ongoing risk of rabies exposure should undergo serologic monitoring of their immune status at 6-month intervals and receive boosters as needed to maintain adequate neutralizing titers. Individuals at moderate risk should undergo serologic monitoring at 2-year intervals or simply receive booster immunizations at this interval. Serologic monitoring and booster doses are not required for those with low risks of exposure once the primary vaccination series is completed. If previously vaccinated persons are exposed to rabies, they should receive two additional doses of vaccine 1 ml IM in the deltoid on day 0 and 3 days thereafter. Such individuals do not require administration of HRIg and do not require the complete five-dose postexposure vaccine regimen. An immune complexlike reaction is seen in some individuals receiving booster doses of HDCV but is not common in primary immunization recipients. This reaction has been attributed to nonvirion constituents in HDCV, and if it occurs, subsequent boosters should be administered with an alternate inactivated diploid cell rabies vaccine. Rabies vaccine inactivated (diploid cell origin—dried; Connaught Laboratories, Stillwater, PA. Telephone 1-800-VACCINE). a purified human diploid cell vaccine, has not been associated with this reaction.

RUBELLA AND CONGENITAL RUBELLA SYNDROME

STANLEY A. PLOTKIN, M.D.

Rubella is a viral infection of the nasopharynx leading to viremia, lymphadenopathy, and a rash. If the infected person is a pregnant woman, the viremia may lead to transplacental transmission to the fetus, in which viral replication results in a distinct complex of abnormalities known as the congenital rubella syndrome (CRS). The association between rubella and CRS was discovered by Norman Gregg in 1941. Less than 30 years later, in 1969, vaccines were deployed against rubella. In the United States and other developed countries, application of a live attenuated vaccine has dramatically reduced the incidence of rubella, to the point where CRS is rarely seen, but pediatricians must remain alert to detect instances of a completely preventable disease.

RUBELLA

The typical course of rubella after exposure is 1 week of complete latency, 1 week of lymphadenopathy with low-grade fever, and several days of rash. The incubation period between infection and rash is 14 to 21 days. A frequent history is that the rash becomes more apparent after a warm shower. Arthralgia or arthritis is commonly seen in adult women after the rash has resolved.

Although the presence of postoccipital lymphadenopathy followed by the development of a pruritic maculopapular rash on the face, rapidly spreading to the extremities, is reasonably characteristic of the disease, clinical diagnosis is notoriously faulty and should never be relied on in a pregnant woman or her contacts. Many other viral infections mimic rubella, and the rash may be atypical, evanescent, or even absent.

Diagnosis should be attempted through antibody tests performed on acute and convalescent sera to detect titer rises and the presence of IgM antibodies to rubella. Virus will be present in the nasopharynx of the infected patient from a week before the rash to about 5 days after. Virus isolation can be attempted but requires many days to complete. In any case, it is important to remember that exposure of a pregnant woman may occur before the rash becomes apparent on her contact.

The two most frequent complications of rubella are thrombocytopenia and encephalitis. A mild to moderate decrease in platelets is seen frequently in rubella, and occasionally, the decrease is sufficient to cause concern. Fortunately, the outcome is almost always benign. Encephalitis has been reported in about 1 of 6000 cases but also is usually mild. However, rarely, infection of the brain leads to a late progressive rubella panencephalitis.

Acute rubella can be treated only with antipyretics, analgesics, and antihistaminics. Thrombocytopenia and encephalitis should be treated conservatively, awaiting spontaneous resolution. Persistent thrombocytopenia should be treated like idiopathic thrombocytopenic purpura.

There is no specific antiviral agent available for the rubella virus.

CONGENITAL RUBELLA SYNDROME

If the rubella virus infects a woman during the early stages of pregnancy, there is a risk that the virus will pass to the fetus, with resultant derangement due to replication of the virus. The virus may kill the fetal cells and, thus, lead to spontaneous abortion and to the local phenomenon of cochlear destruction. Chronic nonlytic replication in fetal cells is also frequent, leading to developmental and other abnormalities. The type of damage done is to some extent dependent on the time of gestation at which infection takes place. Infection during the first 2 months of gestation may damage as many as 40% to 90% of fetuses. (There are many published estimates for

TABLE 1. Typical Manifestations of Congenital Rubella Syndrome

> **Seen at Birth**
> Hepatosplenomegaly
> Thrombocytopenic purpura
> Osteitis and radiolucencies of bones
> Dermal erythropoiesis
>
> **Seen at Birth or Shortly Thereafter**
> Cataracts, glaucoma, chorioretinitis
> Patent ductus arteriosus
> Peripheral pulmonic artery stenosis
> Cochlear degeneration
> Central auditory imperception
> Encephalitis, mental retardation
>
> **Seen as Late Complications**
> Diabetes mellitus
> Thyroid disorders
> Progressive rubella encephalitis

the risk of abnormality after fetal rubella infection, but the figures cited are based on virologically confirmed maternal rubella.) The incidence of abnormality drops during the third month to about 25% to 33% and during the fourth month to about 10%, after which the risk is quite low.

The principal manifestations of CRS are listed in Table 1. The original syndromes described by Gregg were cataracts, congenital heart disease, and deafness, but the great epidemic of 1964–1965 led to the description of an expanded CRS, including manifestations of disseminated infection present at birth and late complications. It is important to understand that CRS may exist as a single abnormality or as various combinations of the abnormalities listed in Table 1.

At birth, the CRS infant may show involvement of the bone marrow and reticuloendothelial system, including hepatosplenomegaly, thrombocytopenic purpura, and dermal erythropoiesis (the blueberry muffin baby). These signs resolve spontaneously, although organomegaly may persist for many months. CRS infants excrete the virus at birth and gradually become virus negative over the course of the first year of life. Anatomic malformations may be present at birth or become evident later. Cataracts, congenital glaucoma, and chorioretinitis are the typical ocular problems, and the infant should be carefully followed for their development. Cataract surgery should be deferred until the second year of life for the best results, possibly because the virus persists in the lens for longer than anywhere else. The cardiac problem is typically patent ductus arteriosus or peripheral pulmonic artery stenosis, but other anomalies are seen. Surgery follows the same hemodynamic indications as in other syndromes. Deafness is the result of a combination of direct damage to the cochlear cells and central auditory imperception, an aspect of brain damage. The deafness is variable in severity and may be unilateral or bilateral. Early auditory testing and consultation are essential for the application of special training and amplifying devices to help the child overcome the handicap.

The 1964–1965 epidemic revealed the extent of CNS involvement in CRS. Rubella virus was often isolated from the cerebrospinal fluid, which showed signs of inflammation. CRS infants showed a variety of neurologic problems, ranging from opisthotonus to severe mental retardation. As might be expected, this left behind a variety of neurologic and behavioral problems, which could be treated only by the symptomatic application of various tranquilizers. Follow-up of children with CRS from that same epidemic also revealed several late complications, evidently stemming from replication of virus in epithelial cells of various endocrine organs. Insulin-dependent diabetes mellitus was found in about 20% of CRS children, and various thyroid inflammatory disorders have been common. These must be treated similarly to endocrine disorders arising from other causes.

The sole effective prevention of CRS is rubella vaccination of women and their contacts.

RUBELLA VACCINE

The live attenuated RA 27/3 strain of rubella virus is now used to prevent rubella in the United States and throughout most of the rest of the world, either as a monovalent vaccine or combined with measles and mumps vaccines. Routine vaccination is recommended at 15 months of age and again at 6 to 12 years of age. Although the need for a booster of rubella vaccine has not been demonstrated, the simplicity of offering the triple vaccine on the occasion of the needed measles booster has resulted in a routine two-dose regimen for rubella in the United States. A number of European countries have also gone to a two-dose schedule.

Application of the vaccine has resulted in a 99% decrease in reported rubella and the reduction of CRS to a rare disease. That vaccination is still necessary, however, was confirmed by recent significant outbreaks of rubella in immigrant communities, followed by the expected clusters of CRS.

The vaccine is well tolerated in childhood, but adult women commonly have transient arthralgia or arthritis. There is no evidence that the vaccine virus poses a problem to the fetus, and inadvertent vaccination during pregnancy is not an indication for abortion, although for theoretical reasons, women are advised against being vaccinated when pregnant.

The U.S. Public Health Service recommends rubella vaccination of seronegative women as part of routine medical care, premarital counseling, family planning counseling, postpartum care, admission to college, and other situations where young women may be exposed. Moreover, all hospital employees of both sexes in contact with patients should be vaccinated. Rubella and CRS could be eradicated by a conscientious application of these recommendations.

VARICELLA-ZOSTER VIRUS INFECTION

ALLAN M. ARBETER, M.D.
ANNE A. GERSHON, M.D.

Varicella-zoster virus (VZV) causes two diseases, varicella and zoster. Varicella is the primary infection, and zoster is the secondary infection, resulting from reactivation of latent VZV. Zoster develops in about 15% of individuals, but by far, most cases occur in the elderly rather than in the young. Zoster most often occurs in immunocompromised patients. Both diseases are characterized by a vesicular skin eruption, generalized in varicella but localized and unilateral in zoster.

Varicella is usually a mild, uncomplicated illness in healthy children that rarely is complicated by severe multiorgan system involvement. Recurrent varicella has been reported rarely in healthy children. Primary varicella can be severe, even fatal in the immunoincompetent patient.

A recent resurgence of secondary infection of varicella with virulent strains of group A beta-hemolytic streptococci has resulted in rapidly progressive severe fasciitis, systemic sepsis, and death. This complication must be appreciated expectantly by parents and physicians.

TREATMENT

For most varicella infections in children, no specific therapy is required. Itching can be alleviated with calamine lotion or appropriate doses of antihistamines. Aspirin should not be administered for fever to avoid the complication of Reye syndrome. Bathing is essential to prevent bacterial skin superinfection, and oatmeal baths may provide relief from itching. Superinfections of skin or lung (usually caused by staphylococci or streptococci) that follow varicella should be treated with an antistaphylococcal penicillin until the offending organism is identified.

Antiviral therapy for treatment of chickenpox is available in the form of the DNA inhibitor acyclovir, but whether to treat otherwise healthy children with oral acyclovir is problematic. Acyclovir shortens the clinical illness, but only by about 1 day. It has no effect on the incidence of complications nor does it hasten the return to school. Acyclovir may be more useful for treatment of adults, whose illness tends to be more severe, than of children, whose illness is most often mild and self-limited. It may be useful, however, to treat selected children, such as older adolescents, and secondary household cases. A recent report from Japan indicates the efficacy of postexposure prophylaxis with oral acyclovir for healthy children exposed to varicella. However, in the United States an effective dose schedule and duration of prophylaxis have not been established. The use of oral acyclovir for postexposure prophylaxis is contrary to an American Academy of Pediatrics recommendation (1992) and does not permit subclinical seroconversion in all of those receiving acyclovir. Until additional data are available, postexposure prophylaxis remains without official recommendation.

Acyclovir given orally must be administered within 24 hours after onset of the rash to have an effect. The dose is 80 mg/kg/d divided into four doses given for 5 days. Acyclovir is available as a suspension of 200 mg/5 ml and as 200-mg capsules. The adverse effects are minimal, consisting of maculopapular rash and abdominal discomfort. Long-term effects of acyclovir, although predicted to be inconsequential, are not fully known. Latent infection with VZV is not prevented or cured with any available antiviral drug. The cost of a course of oral acyclovir for a child is about $35.

Acyclovir is indicated mainly for treatment of immunocompromised patients who are at great risk for severe varicella infection. In this case, it should be given in a dose of 500 mg/m^2 IV three times a day (1500 mg/m^2/d) in patients with normal renal function. The dose of acyclovir for patients with abnormal renal function (creatinine clearance less than 50 ml/min/1.73 m^2) should be smaller (usually one half to one third) than that routinely employed to prevent toxic concentrations of the drug from developing.

Although recent reports described conflicting experiences, children who have acquired primary varicella infection perinatally and are HIV positive may be at high risk for serious multiorgan disease. Indications for complicated varicella include low CD4 T cell counts, clinically apparent AIDS, and initiation of acyclovir therapy after 72 hours from the onset of symptoms. Any child known to be HIV positive should be treated with acyclovir because the clinical course can not be predicted accurately. Immunocompromised patients with varicella who have not been passively immunized or received varicella vaccine previously should be admitted to the hospital and treated with acyclovir as soon as the diagnosis of varicella is made, even if there are only a few skin lesions. Successful antiviral therapy has been associated with administration of intravenous ACV within the first 3 days after onset of illness. Children at high risk for severe varicella include those with an underlying malignancy (especially leukemia and lymphoma) for which they are receiving therapy, children with congenital or acquired immunodeficiency, and those receiving large dosages of steroids for any reason (1 mg/kg/d or more of prednisone or its equivalent).

In children with an underlying malignancy, consideration would be given to temporary postponement of chemotherapy. Baseline chest radiographs plus evaluation of blood gases and serum transaminase levels should be performed. The dose of steroids should be decreased to physiologic levels if possible, but stress doses may be given to severely ill children. Steroids should not be stopped abruptly.

Intravenous acyclovir therapy is usually given for 3 to 10 days, although in some instances, a shorter or longer interval may be used. Discontinuing acyclovir in patients who cease experiencing new lesions for a period of several days, who have become afebrile, and who are clearly recovering is reasonable. It is not uncommon, however, for patients in the early stages of severe varicella to appear to be stable for 1 or 2 days and then to have new lesions, presumably secondary to another bout of viremia. Therefore, care should be taken not to stop acyclovir therapy too soon in immunocompromised patients.

Relatively common adverse effects of acyclovir include phlebitis due to the high pH of the intravenous solution (in about 15% of cases), reversible elevation of serum creatinine (in about 5% of cases), hive-like rash (in about 5% of cases), and nausea and vomiting (in about 1% of cases). Elevation of serum creatinine is a result of precipitation of the drug in the renal tubules when it is administered at a high concentration. This can be prevented by allowing at least 1 hour for infusion of each dose and maintaining good hydration. Rare toxicity includes encephalopathic manifestations, such as tremors, confusion, and agitation.

Because zoster is a secondary infection, the prognosis is generally better than for varicella, even in the immunocompromised. Otherwise healthy children in whom zoster develops rarely need specific antiviral therapy. Although it is usually not a lifesaving measure, it is prudent to treat immunocompromised children if zoster develops to hasten healing and prevent dissemination. Whether to treat with the oral or the intravenous formulation of acyclovir depends on the condition of the patient. Those with early and mild infections may be started on oral therapy and observed closely, but those with extensive rashes or toxicity (such as fever) should be given intravenous medication, at least to begin therapy. Doses of acyclovir for zoster are the same as those for varicella.

VZV is not as susceptible to acyclovir in vitro as is herpes simplex virus (HSV), and there is considerable variability of susceptibilities of different strains of VZV to the drug. A dose of 500 mg/m^2 IV results in blood concentrations that are significantly above levels inhibitory to VZV, but oral administration of acyclovir at the usual adult dose for HSV (200 mg five times a day) is usually not inhibitory to VZV. Therefore, the dose of oral acyclovir for a large adolescent (or adult) is 4 g/d in five divided doses (four capsules five times a day). Only about 20% of orally administered acyclovir is absorbed.

It is difficult to make recommendations concerning antiviral therapy for patients with central nervous system (CNS) involvement with VZV because the underlying pathogenesis of this complication is unknown, and no controlled studies of the efficacy of antiviral therapy have been performed. Some clinicians elect to treat only immunocompromised patients with CNS involvement. This rationale is based on the likelihood that at least part of the problem in immunocompromised patients is a result of viral multiplication. This would be unlikely in immunologically normal patients. Children with cerebellar ataxia as a complication of chickenpox invariably recover without specific treatment.

Vidarabine is now the second-line drug for treatment of VZV infections, mainly because it is more toxic than acyclovir. If for some reason acyclovir cannot be given, vidarabine can be used for high-risk patients. The dose is 10 mg/kg/d IV administered once a day over a period of 12 hours, usually for 5 days. There are no data concerning the simultaneous use of both drugs for VZV infections, and because of potential toxicity, simultaneous use is not recommended.

PREVENTION

Varicella-Zoster Immune Globulin (VZIg)

VZIg was licensed by the Food and Drug Administration (FDA) in 1981. It is distributed in Massachusetts by the Massachusetts Public Health Biological Laboratory and elsewhere by the American Red Cross through local blood centers. Although VZIg is effective when administered up to 3 to 5 days after exposure, it should be given as soon as possible. The dose is 125 U/10 kg, with a maximum dose of 625 U IM. The cost of one vial containing 125 U of VZIg is $75. VZIg should be readministered to high-risk children who are closely reexposed to VZV 3 weeks following a first exposure for which VZIg was given.

Since varicella is a self-limited illness, passive immunization should not be administered to otherwise healthy children. The amount

TABLE 1. Candidates for VZIg Provided Significant Exposure Has Occurred

1. Immunocompromised children without history of chickenpox*
2. Susceptible pregnant women
3. Newborn infant whose mother had onset of chickenpox within 5 d before delivery or within 48 h after delivery
4. Hospitalized premature infant (≥28 wk gestation) whose mother has no history of chickenpox
5. Hospitalized premature infants (<28 wk gestation or ≤1000 g) regardless of maternal history

*Immunocompromised adolescents and adults are likely to be immune, but if susceptible, they should also receive VZIg.

VZV antibody in VZIg is about 10 times higher than that in immune serum globulin (ISg). ISg, therefore, is of little use for prevention of varicella, since the amount that must be given is unacceptably high. The efficacy of intravenous immunoglobulin (IVIg) for passive immunization against varicella has not been determined.

VZIg is mainly used to prevent severe varicella in exposed susceptible children who are at high risk for development of severe or fatal varicella. This group includes immunocompromised children and newborn infants whose mothers have active varicella at the time of delivery and children who have received systemic corticosteroid just before or during the incubation period of the illness. Candidates for whom VZIg is recommended by the Centers for Disease Control and Prevention are listed in Table 1.

High-risk infants and children should receive VZIg if they have had a close exposure to varicella or zoster (Table 2). They should be considered to be susceptible to varicella if there is no prior history of chickenpox or there is uncertainty about the history. The decision to administer VZIg to an immunocompromised child should not be based on an antibody titer because of the possibility of a false positive antibody test. In contrast, however, VZIg is not indicated for healthy adults unless they are proven to be susceptible by laboratory testing because most adults are immune. It is, therefore, advised that the blood be tested for VZV antibodies in adults with no past history of varicella who are likely to be closely exposed to VZV. Then, should a close exposure occur, VZIg could be given.

Children with human immunodeficiency virus (HIV) infection are also at high risk for severe varicella infection. Management should be similar to that for immunocompromised children and adults. Even those children who have been receiving IVIg for treatment of AIDS should receive VZIg if there is no history of varicella and a close exposure has occurred.

Infants whose mothers have active varicella at delivery should receive VZIg. This includes infants whose mothers have the onset of

TABLE 2. Types of Exposure to Varicella or Zoster for Which VZIg Is Indicated*

1. Household: residing in the same household
2. Playmate: face-to-face† indoor play
3. Hospital
   a. Varicella
      (1) In same 2- to 4-bed room or adjacent beds in a large ward
      (2) Face-to-face† contact with an infectious staff member or patient
      (3) Visit by a person deemed contagious
   b. Zoster: intimate contact (e.g., touching or hugging) with person deemed contagious
4. Newborn infant: onset of varicella in the mother 5 d or less before delivery or within 48 h after delivery; VZIg is not indicated if the mother has zoster

*VZIg should be administered within 96 h (preferably sooner) after exposure.
†Experts differ in the duration of face-to-face contact that warrants the administration of VZIg. However, the contact should be nontransient. Some experts suggest a contact of 5 or more min as constituting significant exposure for this purpose; others define close contact as more than 1 h.

TABLE 3. Summary of Recommended Doses of Drugs for Varicella Infections

Acyclovir (ACV)
Oral: For healthy children with chickenpox (or zoster in selected patients): 80 mg/kg/d divided into four doses given for 5 d; maximum single dose 800 mg (four capsules); for large adolescent (or adult): 4 g/d divided into five doses (four capsules five times a day)
Intravenous: For immunocompromised patients with normal renal function: 1500 mg/m²/d divided into three doses (500 mg/m² per dose); for patients with abnormal renal function (creatinine clearance less than 50 ml/min/1.73 m²): dose should be smaller (usually one half to one third)

Vidarabine (Ara-A)
Intravenous: 10 mg/kg/d q.d. over a period of 12 h usually for 5 d

Varicella-Zoster Immune Globulin (VZIg)
Intramuscular: 125 U/10 kg body weight (max: 625 U; for infants, 125 U)

chickenpox 5 days or less before delivery or within 48 hours after delivery. The dose of VZIg for infants is 125 U IM (Table 3). Usually, varicella is mild after VZIg, although occasionally, severe varicella may develop in an infant. Passively immunized infants should be observed carefully, but usually this can be done on an outpatient basis. Should an infant develop an extensive skin rash (more than 100 vesicles) or evidence of pneumonia, intravenous acyclovir should be administered.

VZIg can be given electively to infants under 1 week of age if their siblings at home have active varicella, especially if the mother has no history of chickenpox. It might also be given to infants younger than 1 week of age whose mothers have varicella. Infants exposed to mothers with zoster are not expected to develop severe varicella because they have high antibody titers and, therefore, do not require prophylactic VZIg.

Nosocomial spread of varicella in neonatal nurseries is a rare phenomenon. Low-birthweight infants, however, may have undetectable titers of antibodies to VZV. Therefore, it is recommended that newborn infants exposed to VZV who weigh less than 1000 g or of less than 28 weeks' gestation be passively immunized (Table 1). Varicella has been observed in infants with preexisting maternal transplacental antibodies when exposed to VZV, but it is usually a modified illness. This may be one reason that varicella in infants between 1 and 6 months of age is characteristically mild.

Zoster occurs despite serum antibody to VZV, and patients with zoster manifest brisk increases in VZV antibody titer. VZIg, therefore, is of no use in treating or preventing zoster.

Varicella Vaccine

A live attenuated varicella vaccine was tested in Japan in 1970. The vaccine is licensed in some European countries and in Japan and Korea, but it is not licensed in the United States. The vaccine is highly protective in immunocompromised children and healthy adults, and there is great interest in vaccinating healthy children on a routine basis. Not all vaccinees are completely protected, however. Some experience a mild breakthrough illness following an exposure. However, varicella vaccine has been 100% effective in preventing severe varicella. It is rare to need to use antiviral therapy in vaccinated leukemic children with a breakthrough illness. Leukemic children can be given varicella vaccine if they have been in remission for at least 1 year. Two doses of vaccine 3 months apart are administered. Chemotherapy must be stopped 1 week before and after the first vaccination. In those who are immunized, there is a 50% chance of a vaccine-associated rash developing 1 month later. About half of the affected children require antiviral therapy, which may be given either orally or intravenously depending on the extent of the rash and other symptoms, such as fever. Leukemic vaccine recipients who have a rash may transmit the vaccine-type virus to about 15% of other varicella-susceptible individuals with whom they have close contact. Secondary cases from vaccine virus spread have been mild.

Virus reactivation as zoster is no more common in children with leukemia who received vaccine than in children with leukemia who had previous natural infection. Children who have a relapse of leukemia have a greater risk of virus reactivation (zoster) than children who remain in remission.

VARICELLA IN PREGNANCY

Varicella can be severe in pregnant women, and careful follow-up is indicated. Treatment with acyclovir should be used in severe cases, such as those complicated by pneumonia. An unusual fetal syndrome (low birthweight, skin scarring, hypoplastic limb, mental retardation) occurs in about 2% of infants born to women who had varicella in the first or second trimester of pregnancy. Ultrasonography may be used to assess the condition of the fetus. Usually, termination of pregnancy is not recommended, although each case must be individualized.

REFERENCES

1. American Academy of Pediatrics: Report by the Committee on Infectious Diseases, 1994.
2. Balfour HH, Kelly JM, Suarez CS, et al: Acyclovir treatment of varicella in otherwise healthy children. J Pediatr 116:633–639, 1990.
3. Dowell SF, Breese JS: Severe varicella associated with steroid use. Pediatrics 92:223–228, 1993.

ASPERGILLOSIS

Mark W. Kline, m.d.

Aspergillus is a ubiquitous saprophytic fungus that may contaminate the hospital environment. Infection in humans usually occurs after inhalation of airborne spores. Invasive aspergillosis occurs predominantly among immunocompromised hosts. Predisposing factors include conditions that produce prolonged and profound granulocytopenia (e.g., aplastic anemia, cytotoxic chemotherapy, or acute leukemia in relapse), immunosuppression accompanying solid organ or bone marrow transplantation, corticosteroid therapy, and certain phagocytic killing defects (e.g., chronic granulomatous disease). Invasive disease, as well as several localized forms of *Aspergillus* infection, occurs occasionally in normal hosts without underlying medical conditions.

Individuals with invasive aspergillosis almost invariably have pulmonary involvement. Hematogenous dissemination can result in disease at any other body site, including central nervous system (CNS), bones and skin, heart, and kidneys. Localized *Aspergillus* infection may involve the ear, nose and paranasal sinuses, or skin. Allergic bronchopulmonary aspergillosis and aspergilloma represent two forms of noninvasive pulmonary disease.

TREATMENT

Antifungal Chemotherapy

Amphotericin B is the mainstay of therapy for invasive aspergillosis. The drug is administered intravenously in electrolyte-free dextrose-in-water at a concentration of 0.1 mg/ml. An initial test dose of 0.1 mg/kg (max: 1 mg) infused over 1 to 2 hours often is recommended. The patient is monitored closely for acute adverse effects, including fever, rigors, respiratory distress, and convulsions. In children, we have observed such effects at initiation of therapy only in those patients who have had prior courses of amphotericin B. Therefore, particularly in amphotericin B therapy-naive children with rapidly progressive or disseminated aspergillosis, it may be reasonable to forego an initial amphotericin B test dose. In such children, we recommend an initial dose of 0.25 to 0.5 mg/kg, followed 12 hours later by another 0.5 mg/kg dose. These and all subsequent ampho-

TABLE 1. Drugs for Treatment of Aspergillosis

DRUG	DOSE
Amphotericin B	0.1 mg/kg (max: 1 mg) IV test dose, followed by successive escalating doses of 0.25 and 0.5 mg/kg IV at 12–24 h intervals, with full-dose therapy at 1 mg/kg IV daily
Flucytosine	75–150 mg/kg/d PO in four divided doses
Itraconazole	100–400 mg/d PO in one or two divided doses

tericin B doses are infused over 4 to 6 hours. Twenty-four hours later, the patient begins full-dose amphotericin B therapy at 1 mg/kg/d (Table 1).

Infusion-associated chills, fever, rigors, nausea, and vomiting sometimes occur among children receiving prolonged courses of amphotericin B therapy. These effects can be minimized by extending the infusion time or providing premedication with acetaminophen and diphenhydramine. Rarely, it may be necessary to add hydrocortisone 0.5 mg/kg to the amphotericin B infusion solution.

Other adverse effects of amphotericin B therapy include hypokalemia, renal insufficiency, and anemia. We generally recommend monitoring the serum electrolytes, serum creatinine, and complete blood count at least twice weekly during amphotericin B therapy. Oral or intravenous potassium supplementation often is required. The serum potassium concentration should be greater than 3 mg/dl before infusion of amphotericin B. The blood urea nitrogen concentration, which often rises during long-term therapy with the drug, generally is not clinically useful. We consider amphotericin B dose reduction or alternative therapy if the serum creatinine concentration exceeds 2 to 2.5 mg/dl during the course of amphotericin B therapy. Alternate-day therapy may be beneficial for patients who develop marked amphotericin B-associated renal insufficiency.

On the basis of in vitro and animal experimental data indicating synergistic anti-*Aspergillus* activity and improved outcome, some authorities recommend combination chemotherapy with amphotericin B and either flucytosine or rifampin for patients with invasive aspergillosis. For children who can tolerate oral medications, it is reasonable to include flucytosine 150 mg/kg/d in four divided doses in the therapeutic regimen for invasive aspergillosis. Adverse effects of the drug include hepatitis and bone marrow depression. Serum concentrations of the drug should be monitored in an effort to minimize toxic potential.

Amphotericin B lipid complex and liposome-encapsulated amphotericin B are investigational agents that appear to have better therapeutic indices than standard amphotericin B, permitting higher-dose and longer-term therapy in some cases. To date, only uncontrolled, anecdotal data support the use of these agents in invasive aspergillosis, but they should be considered in situations where appropriate medical therapy is limited by amphotericin B-associated intolerance or toxicity.

Of the azole antifungal agents, itraconazole appears to be more active in vitro versus *Aspergillus* than either ketoconazole or fluconazole. Successful therapy of invasive aspergillosis with itraconazole, in some cases after failure of amphotericin B therapy, has been reported. However, treatment failures also have been observed. Itraconazole should be considered for patients who have completed an initial course of amphotericin B therapy for invasive aspergillosis and in whom long-term suppressive therapy is desired, or in some cases of localized disease.

The duration of therapy for invasive aspergillosis is based on clinical response to treatment and resolution of any underlying immunocompromising condition, rather than an arbitrary total treatment duration or cumulative drug dose.

Granulocyte Transfusions

Granulocyte transfusions have been recommended by some authorities as adjunctive therapy for invasive aspergillosis in patients with persistent granulocytopenia or chronic granulomatous disease. Individual case reports have described both treatment success and failure, but controlled data are lacking. Unfortunately, concomitant administration of granulocyte transfusions and amphotericin B has been linked to severe (or even fatal) pulmonary reactions. At present, the precise association of these agents with, and the pathogenesis of, these reactions is unclear. Other risks of granulocyte transfusions include transmission of bloodborne pathogens and hemolytic reactions in patients with chronic granulomatous disease and the associated McLeod blood phenotype.

Surgery

Surgical excision or debridement may be helpful in the management of some forms of *Aspergillus* infection, including sinusitis, cerebral mycetoma, and endocarditis. Surgical excision of pulmonary aspergilloma may be indicated for patients with recurrent or severe hemoptysis. For most cases of invasive or disseminated aspergillosis, surgical debridement appears to offer little advantage over medical therapy alone.

Allergic Bronchopulmonary Aspergillosis

Allergic bronchopulmonary aspergillosis results from a hypersensitivity response to inhaled spores of *Aspergillus fumigatus*. In general, invasion of the bronchial wall and lung parenchyma does not occur, but chronic inflammation can lead to severe destructive changes of the lung. The treatment of allergic bronchopulmonary aspergillosis includes administration of corticosteroids, inhaled bronchodilators, and chest physiotherapy to enhance pulmonary clearance. In children, a daily prednisone dose of 30 to 45 mg is administered initially and until radiographic clearing of pulmonary infiltrates occurs. A prednisone dose of 0.5 mg/kg then is administered daily for 2 weeks, followed by alternate-day therapy for 3 months. Subsequently, corticosteroid therapy is tapered and discontinued over another 3-month period. Relapse of disease occurs commonly, and long-term (or even lifelong) corticosteroid therapy may be required in some cases. Systemic antifungal therapy generally plays no role in the treatment of allergic bronchopulmonary aspergillosis.

PROGNOSIS

In general, the prognosis of invasive aspergillosis is poor. Early diagnosis, prompt initiation of specific therapy, and resolution of any underlying immunocompromising condition (e.g., granulocytopenia) favorably effect outcome. Hematopoietic growth factors (e.g., recombinant granulocyte colony-stimulating factor) hold promise, but data in support of their use in the treatment of patients with invasive aspergillosis and granulocytopenia are preliminary. Patients who develop invasive aspergillosis while receiving immunosuppressive therapy (e.g., transplant recipients) should have such therapy withdrawn, if possible, but the prognosis of infection remains poor.

REFERENCES

1. Denning DW, Stevens DA: Antifungal and surgical treatment of invasive aspergillosis: Review of 2,121 published cases. Rev Infect Dis 12:1147–1201, 1990.
2. Walmsley S, Devi S, King S, et al: Invasive *Aspergillus* infections in a pediatric hospital: A ten-year review. Pediatr Infect Dis J 12:673–682, 1993.

BLASTOMYCOSIS

THOMAS G. MITCHELL, Ph.D.

Blastomycosis is a chronic disease characterized by granulomatous and suppurative lesions. The infection is initiated by inhalation of the thermally dimorphic fungus, *Blastomyces dermatitidis*. From the lung, dissemination may occur to any organ, but preferentially to the skin and bones. Blastomycosis is endemic to eastern parts of the United States, but little is known about its prevalence. *B. dermatitidis* cannot be readily isolated from nature, and a good skin test is not available for population surveys of exposure to *B. dermatitidis*. Unlike histoplasmosis and coccidioidomycosis, blastomycosis does not occur frequently in immunocompromised patients, such as those with AIDS. There are almost a dozen reports of outbreaks of blastomycosis that have been attributed to common exposure to *B. dermatitidis*, and many have been associated with river banks. Investigations of these outbreaks have yielded important information about the natural history of blastomycosis, and several pediatric cases have occurred during outbreaks of blastomycosis.

The primary pulmonary infection may be inapparent to severe. Even if it is inapparent, dissemination may ensue to the skin, bones, or other sites. If the pulmonary episode is severe, generalized systemic disease may develop and may involve multiple organs. Cases associated with outbreaks have indicated that the incubation period is 3 to 12 weeks and that spontaneous recovery can follow primary blastomycosis. Overall, most cases occur in adults and in males, but in pediatric blastomycosis, children of both sexes are equally susceptible.

Most pediatric cases are recognized as acute blastomycosis. Patients with symptomatic, primary pulmonary infection may present with symptoms of mild respiratory infection, including cough, chest pain, and high fever, as well as numerous other complaints. The primary pulmonary infection may persist locally, spread to other organ(s), or both. Alternatively, the pulmonary lesion may heal by fibrosis and absorption, leaving no residual evidence of infection. In patients whose pulmonary lesions have resolved, dissemination, generally to the skin, may already have occurred. If the pulmonary focus becomes more severe, an acute to chronic lung infection may develop. Patients with chronic pulmonary blastomycosis usually present with cough, low-grade fever, loss of weight, night sweats, and other problems. The most common forms of pulmonary involvement are infiltration, cavitation, pneumonia, and nodules.

A wide variety of symptoms, pathologic signs, and radiographic appearances may be observed in blastomycosis. After the lung, the most frequently involved organs are the skin, bones, and genitourinary tract, followed by the central nervous system (CNS), liver, or spleen. Less often, the lymph nodes, thyroid, heart, adrenal, omentum, gastrointestinal tract, muscles, and pancreas may become infected.

DIAGNOSIS

Blastomycosis is best diagnosed by positive culture of direct examination of sputum, skin lesion, or other specimen. *B. dermatitidis* grows on most routine culture media to produce a mold with variable macroscopic features and conidia. Its identification is confirmed by growth on a rich medium at 37°C and conversion to the characteristic yeast form. Alternatively, a *B. dermatitidis*-specific antigen (exoantigen A) may be extracted and identified by an immunodiffusion test using reference antisera and antigen. A DNA probe is now commercially available in kit form to identify cultures of *B. dermatitidis*, as well as other agents of systemic mycoses.

In culture at 37°C or in tissue, *B. dermatitidis* forms large (8 to 15 μm) single-budding yeast cells with highly refractory cell walls and a broad attachment between the bud and parent yeast cell. In histopathologic sections, the yeasts are better seen with periodic acid-Schiff or methenamine silver stains, and in sputa, skin scrapings, and other direct specimens, the yeasts can be seen with calcofluor white or KOH preparations. Since the tests for complement-fixing antibodies and delayed-type skin reactivity lack specificity and sensitivity, they are not helpful unless the patient is negative to heterologous fungal antigens. Even then, positive, monospecific serologic tests for *B. dermatitidis* may not indicate active infection. Serologic tests for antibodies to the specific antigen A, which can be detected by the immunodiffusion test or an enzyme immunoassay, are more suggestive of infection, but negative tests do not exclude blastomycosis.

TREATMENT

As confirmed by the outbreak cases, primary blastomycosis in immunocompetent individuals may not require therapy. However, the patient with proven, primary pulmonary infection that is mild and resolves spontaneously without treatment must be closely observed for at least 2 years after primary infection because of the possible occurrence of reactivation blastomycosis. Patients with protracted, severe, or progressive primary infection, chronic pulmonary blastomycosis, or disseminated blastomycosis require treatment. Depending on the manifestations of disease and the integrity of the underlying host defenses, chemotherapeutic success rates with amphotericin B, ketoconazole, and itraconazole currently vary between 70% and 95%.

Ketoconazole

Ketoconazole is recommended for immunocompetent patients with mild to moderately severe disease (e.g., blastomycosis that neither is life threatening nor involves the CNS). A dose of 400 mg/d PO for 6 months is effective in most adult patients, but patients must be closely followed because relapses have occurred on ketoconazole. Solubility and absorption are increased when ketoconazole is taken with an acid beverage, such as orange juice or carbonated soda. For difficult cases, treatment with higher doses (800 mg/d) for more than 6 months, if tolerated, may be effective. Successful treatment of blastomycosis has been achieved in 80% to 90% of adult patients. The adverse effects of ketoconazole include liver toxicity and reversible hormonal imbalances (e.g., gynecomastia), as well as nausea, pruritus, dizziness, and headache.

Itraconazole

Recent trials have confirmed the efficacy of itraconazole for the treatment of nonmeningeal, nonlife-threatening blastomycosis. When such adult patients were given oral doses of 200, 300, or 400 mg/d for at least 2 months, the rate of cure or improvement was 95%. Itraconazole should be taken with meals, and patients are treated for approximately 6 months, with follow-up for 1 year or longer. Toxicity from itraconazole occurs in less than one third of patients, is usually mild, and rarely necessitates cessation of therapy. The most common side effects are gastrointestinal symptoms, usually nausea, vomiting, or diarrhea. Minor reactions include weakness, dizziness, headache, chills, fever, tinnitus, skin rash, pruritus, paraesthesia, and rarely, transient, modest elevation of transaminase. Any relapse may be amenable to a second course of itraconazole.

In comparison with ketoconazole, itraconazole appears to be equally or more effective and better tolerated. For example, gastrointestinal symptoms were more than twice as frequent among patients receiving ketoconazole than those receiving itraconazole, although such symptoms occur more often in association with higher doses. Several treatment failures with ketoconazole have been managed successfully with itraconazole. Since studies on pediatric doses of ketoconazole and itraconazole have not been conducted, pediatric doses must be extrapolated from adult doses on a milligram per kilogram basis.

Amphotericin B

B. dermatitidis is quite susceptible to amphotericin B, which is the recommended treatment for patients with life-threatening or severe disease (e.g., involvement of multiple organs), those with meningitis, blastomycosis in immunocompromised patients, and patients who do not respond to ketoconazole or itraconazole. In adults, a total dose of at least 2 g is required to eradicate all the organisms. When a dose of 1.5 g or less is administered, the relapse rate is significant. The protocols for administration of amphotericin B and monitoring renal function are similar to those for its use for other mycoses. An initial test dose of 1 or 5 mg in adults is administered intravenously in a solution of 5% glucose, deoxycholate, and buffer. The dose is gradually increased by 5 to 10 mg/d to a maximal daily administration of 0.5 to 1.5 mg/kg body weight. Most patients experience adverse side effects, including renal dysfunction, fever, anorexia, phlebitis, hypokalemia, nausea, chills, headache, and anemia. Administration is interrupted when blood levels of urea nitrogen reach 40 to 50 mg/dl or 3 to 3.5 mg/dl of creatinine. Blastomycosis in patients with AIDS may require maintenance therapy following the initial course of treatment with amphotericin B, similar to the management of cryptococcosis and histoplasmosis in patients with AIDS. Adult respiratory distress syndrome due to overwhelming pulmonary blastomycosis requires aggressive treatment with amphotericin B.

For children, the test dose of 0.1 mg/kg (max: 1 mg) should be followed by 0.25 mg/kg at 4 hours later and 0.5 mg/kg after 24 hours. Beyond 48 hours, 1 mg/kg/d is administered. Pediatric patients must be closely monitored for adverse reactions, as must adult patients.

Blastomycosis has been reported in pregnant women, and the infection may or may not be transmitted to the infant. Pregnant patients have been treated with amphotericin B without congenital or toxic effects in the fetus. In an endemic area, blastomycosis should be considered in any neonate with a reticulonodular lesion on chest film or whose mother has evidence of blastomycosis.

Surgery

In cases of chronic pulmonary or cutaneous blastomycosis, surgery may be necessary as an adjunct to antibiotic treatment. Because of the occurrence of relapse or reactivation blastomycosis, patients should be observed for years after treatment and resolution of the disease.

CANDIDIASIS

KWANG SIK KIM, M.D.

Candida albicans is probably the most important *Candida* species pathogenic to humans. Other clinically significant *Candida* include *Candida tropicalis, Candida krusei, Candida lusitaniae, Candida pseudotropicalis, Candida stellatoidea, Candida parapsilosis, Candida guilliermondii,* and *Torulopsis glabrata. Candida* causes a wide spectrum of diseases. In general, *C. albicans, C. tropicalis,* and *C. krusei* are common in disseminated disease, and *T. glabrata* and *C. parapsilosis* less often invade organs, such as the lung.

CUTANEOUS AND OROPHARYNGEAL CANDIDIASIS

This form of *Candida* infection is common and, in immunocompetent patients, usually responds to topical antifungal agents. For diaper dermatitis, topical nystatin, clotrimazole, or miconazole applied four times a day is the recommended therapy. Thrush responds to 100,000 U/ml PO nystatin suppression. In infants, 1 ml should be applied to each side of the mouth four times a day until the lesions resolve. In older children, up to 4 ml four times a day can be given. Perleche and paronychia can be treated with one of the topical antifungal agents. When the nail is involved (onychia), oral antifungal therapy may be needed (e.g., ketoconazole).

Chronic Oral *Candida* Infection Associated with Chronic Mucocutaneous Candidiasis and Immunosuppression. In more persistent and extensive oral candidiasis in patients with underlying immunosuppression, particularly patients with severe neutropenia or severe mucositis, treatment usually includes fluconazole, ketoconazole, intravenous miconazole, or a short course of parenteral amphotericin B.

URINARY CANDIDIASIS

Candiduria may reflect bladder infection or renal parenchymal infection or may be a manifestation of disseminated disease. However, in most instances, the finding of yeast in urine indicates improper collection and processing of urine samples. For *Candida* infection confined to the bladder without indwelling catheter, oral flucytosine therapy may be adequate. For patients requiring indwelling bladder catheterization, continuous irrigation with amphotericin B in a concentration of 1 mg/dl (10 μg/ml) for 5 to 7 days is usually successful. If urine cultures continue to yield *Candida,* systemic antifungal therapy with flucytosine or amphotericin B plus flucytosine is indicated. Since fluconazole is excreted in high concentrations in the urine, it may be a suitable alternative. The combination of amphotericin B plus flucytosine is indicated for renal parenchymal infection and infections associated with fungus ball formation.

PERITONEAL CANDIDIASIS

There is no well-established therapy for peritoneal candidiasis. Intraperitoneal lavage with amphotericin B, along with removal of the catheter, has been used successfully for patients requiring peritoneal dialysis, but systemic amphotericin B should be employed, particularly when disseminated candidiasis cannot be excluded.

CATHETER-RELATED CANDIDEMIA

Removal of the catheter and initiation of parenteral amphotericin B therapy for a total dose of 5 to 10 mg/kg should be sufficient for most cases in which there is no evidence of deep-seated or disseminated candidiasis.

DEEP-SEATED OR DISSEMINATED CANDIDIASIS WITH OR WITHOUT CANDIDEMIA

This form of candidiasis continues to provide a major diagnostic and therapeutic challenge to clinicians and includes sepsis, pneumonia, arthritis, osteomyelitis, endocarditis, endophthalmitis, and hepatosplenic candidiasis. Disseminated candidiasis is most frequently encountered in immunocompromised hosts and premature infants with the following predisposing factors: broad-spectrum antibiotic therapy, malignant hematologic diseases, cytotoxic or steroid therapy, intravascular catheters, central parenteral alimentation, and gastrointestinal surgery or pathology. Amphotericin B for a total dose of 30 to 40 mg/kg with or without flucytosine is recommended. Hepatosplenic candidiasis or so-called chronic disseminated candidiasis is slow to respond to a combination of amphotericin B and flucytosine, but its response to fluconazole therapy appears promising.

ANTIFUNGAL AGENTS

Amphotericin B

Amphotericin B, despite its considerable toxicity, remains the principal antifungal agent for deep-seated or disseminated candidiasis. The basic mechanism of antifungal activity of amphotericin B has been ascribed to its binding to sterols in the fungus cell membrane, with a resultant increase in the membrane permeability. Most of the *Candida* species are inhibited by amphotericin B in vitro. The drug is fungistatic but can be fungicidal at high concentrations. Resistance to amphotericin B is rare, but there are several reports of amphotericin B-resistant yeasts, including *C. albicans, C. tropicalis, C. lusitaniae, C krusei, C. parapsilosis,* and *C. guilliermondii.*

Amphotericin B should be administered intravenously to patients for whom adequate medical supervision and nursing care are available. The drug is very irritating, and care must be taken that no perivascular or subcutaneous leakage occurs. The drug should be prepared in a concentration of 0.1 mg/ml or less in 5% dextrose in water (not in saline because the drug will precipitate). Infusion times can vary from 2 to 6 hours based on patient tolerance but must be no less than 1 to 2 hours per infusion. Light shielding of the infusion bottle is unnecessary during drug administration. Amphotericin B is usually started at a test dose of 0.1 mg/kg (max: 1 mg), which is advanced gradually in daily increments of 0.1 to 0.25 mg/kg/d or as rapidly as possible to a maximal dose of 1 mg/kg/d for severely ill patients. For a patient who requires aggressive therapy, if a test dose is well tolerated, the rest of an initial dose of amphotericin B (e.g., 0.25 mg/kg) can be completed on day 1 of therapy. The speed of incremental increase depends on the patient's tolerance of the drug and toxicity. The tolerance to amphotericin B varies substantially from patient to patient. The pharmacology of intravenously administered amphotericin B remains incompletely understood, but the drug has a long half-life. Thus, after the clinical response and tolerance to doses are established, it is possible to give the drug on an alternate-day schedule or two to three times per week for consolidation therapy.

Amphotericin B induces abnormalities of renal function and inhibits erythropoiesis. Hypokalemia, increases in BUN and creatinine, and anemia are common but are not indications for discontinuance. Dose adjustments are not necessary with preexisting renal impairment. Sodium supplementation may decrease the nephrotoxic potential of amphotericin B. The potential of pentoxifylline to obviate nephrotoxicity is promising, and we have used it successfully in some patients who develop nephrotoxicity while on amphotericin B therapy. If decreased renal function occurs, the daily dose can be decreased by 50%, or the dose can be given every other day. Interruption of amphotericin B therapy may be needed if rapid decline in renal function occurs. Careful monitoring of patients' renal and electrolyte status is required (at least biweekly determination). Concurrent use of other nephrotoxic agents, for example, aminoglycoside, cyclosporine, or diuretics should be avoided if possible. Concurrent administration of carbenicillin or ticarcillin may exacerbate the hypokalemia.

Fever, chills, headache, nausea, or vomiting may develop during the infusion of amphotericin B. Depending on the patient's tolerance, an antiemetic (e.g., diphenhydramine 1.25 mg/kg per dose PO or IV), antipyretics (e.g., acetaminophen 10 mg/kg PO), meperidine 1 to 2 mg/kg (for chills), or ibuprofen 10 mg/kg (for chills and fever, used with extreme caution in patients receiving methotrexate) may be required 30 minutes before the infusion. In some patients, hydrocortisone 25 mg may be added to the infusion to minimize severe reactions.

Flucytosine

Flucytosine (5-FC) is well absorbed orally, is excreted via the kidney, and has been used for urinary candidiasis as a single agent. 5-FC is, however, more commonly used in combination with amphotericin B in the treatment of disseminated candidiasis or prolonged candidemia. Many clinical isolates of *Candida* are susceptible to 5-FC concentrations of less than 5 μg/ml, but as many as 25% of isolates are reported to be resistant to 5-FC. Resistance to 5-FC frequently develops when the drug is used alone. Thus, determination of susceptibility of *Candida* to 5-FC should be done in all instances. If the organism is susceptible to 5-FC, this drug should be used to treat deep-seated or disseminated candidiasis, although no prospective data are available comparing the efficacy of combined amphotericin B plus 5-FC versus amphotericin B alone. 5-FC is usually given in a dose of 50 to 150 mg/kg in four divided doses. The major toxicity is bone marrow suppression (e.g., leukopenia), which seems to be related to serum concentrations >100 μg/ml. Thus, serum drug levels should be measured to be certain to keep the level below 100 μg/ml. For patients with renal impairment, the dose interval needs to be increased, for example, every 12 hours for a 50% decrease in renal function. When it is used with amphotericin B (a nephrotoxic drug), serum levels of 5-FC should be determined periodically.

IMIDAZOLES

Clotrimazole

A topical preparation is available for cutaneous and vaginal candidiasis.

Miconazole

A topical preparation is useful for cutaneous and vaginal candidiasis. An intravenous preparation 20 to 40 mg/kg/d in three divided doses has been used for selected cases of mucocutaneous candidiasis. However, it has had limited success and is associated with a rather high incidence of adverse reactions.

Ketoconazole

Ketoconazole is available only as an oral preparation. The drug has been used for chronic mucocutaneous candidiasis at 5 to 10 mg/kg/d PO in two or three divided doses for 5 to 6 weeks, but its efficacy for esophageal candidiasis is not established. The common side effects are gastrointestinal reactions, including hepatitis. If the latter develops, the drug should be discontinued.

Fluconazole

Fluconazole is well absorbed orally and can be given either parentally or orally. The dose is the same for both routes, 3 to 6 mg/kg/d. The drug has a long half-life and is given once daily. It is excreted into the urine in high concentrations. Thus, dose modification is required in patients with renal impairment. Fluconazole is approved for the treatment of oropharyngeal, esophageal, and urinary candidiasis, but its efficacy in children is not established. One important issue in the treatment of candidal infection with fluconazole is that certain species, such as *C. krusei,* exhibit a low level of susceptibility in vitro.

REFERENCES

1. Armstrong D: Treatment of opportunistic fungal infections. Clin Infect Dis 161:1–9, 1993.
2. Gallis HA, Drew RH, Pickard WW: Amphotericin B: 30 years of clinical experience. Rev Infect Dis 12:308–329, 1990.
3. Swerdloff JN, Filler SG, Edwards JE Jr: Severe candidal infections in neutropenic patients. Clin Infect Dis 17:S457–S467, 1993.

COCCIDIOIDOMYCOSIS

BERNHARD L. WIEDERMANN, M.D.

Coccidioidomycosis, or San Joaquin Valley fever, is a relatively common infection in the southwestern United States, with an estimated incidence of 50,000 to 100,000 newly infected individuals per year. However, most of these infections are undetected because they produce no symptoms or very mild, nonspecific symptoms. Treatment is reserved for the minority of infections where disease is disseminated or there is a significant risk of dissemination (Table 1). Amphotericin B is the drug of choice for all forms requiring therapy, but ketoconazole, itraconazole, and fluconazole all have anticoccidioidal activity and may be useful in some situations. Serial determinations of serum and cerebrospinal fluid (CSF), if appropriate, antibody to *Coccidioides immitis* by complement fixation is very helpful in gauging treatment response.

PULMONARY COCCIDIOIDOMYCOSIS

Treatment for primary pulmonary coccidioidomycosis is indicated for individuals at high risk for dissemination (significant immuno-

TABLE 1. Risk Factors for Dissemination of Coccidioidomycosis

High Risk
Major immunodeficiency disorders (HIV infection, immunosuppressive cancer chemotherapy, congenital T cell disorders)
Neonatal period

Moderate Risk
Ethnic origin (Filipino > Black > Native American > Hispanic > Asian)
Less severe immunodeficiency states (steroid therapy, diabetes mellitus, pregnancy)
High anticoccidioidal antibody titer
Persistent symptoms of primary infection > 6 weeks

deficiency states, neonates, and some non-Caucasian children) and for infection in those individuals in whom symptoms do not clear within a reasonable period of time (6 weeks). Most of these latter patients will have significant mediastinal adenopathy, with persistent fever, malaise, and progressive elevation of coccidioidal antibody titers.

Parenteral amphotericin B is the drug of choice for these patients and is given in doses similar to those used for treating other fungal infections. Typically, a test dose of 1 mg or 0.1 mg/kg is given IV over 1 hour. If there are no adverse effects, such as arrhythmia, anuria, hypotension, or hypersensitivity reaction, further drug is given the same day to total 0.25 mg/kg for the first day's treatment. An infusion time of 2 hours is probably sufficient. The following day, the dose is increased to 0.5 mg/kg, and further daily increases to 1 mg/kg can be performed over the subsequent 2 days. Maintenance therapy with 0.75 to 1 mg/kg/d infused over 2 to 4 hours is continued until a total dose of 10 to 15 mg/kg has been administered. Higher total doses may be indicated based on clinical response.

At the onset of amphotericin B therapy, renal function and serum potassium and magnesium concentrations should be monitored approximately every other day for evidence of renal insufficiency, hypokalemia, and hypomagnesemia. Later in the course, weekly monitoring is sufficient if the patient is stable. Hypokalemia is particularly common and may be managed with oral supplements in most cases. Sodium supplementation, by the parenteral route, the oral route, or both, may prevent or alleviate nephrotoxicity. At least 5 mEq/kg/d of sodium is recommended, with careful monitoring for signs of fluid or salt overload. Renal insufficiency ultimately may necessitate lowering the dose of amphotericin B administered, but excretion of amphotericin is not altered in oliguric states. Acute onset reactions, such as fever, chills, and nausea, usually are easily managed. Pretreatment with diphenhydramine hydrochloride 1.25 mg/kg or acetaminophen 10 to 15 mg/kg is helpful. Hydrocortisone 0.5 mg/kg may be given as an intravenous bolus. Ibuprofen also may be helpful but carries the theoretic risk of worsening nephrotoxicity and is not recommended. More severe reactions can be prevented with meperidine in a dose of 1 to 1.5 mg/kg given intravenously. Heparin 1 U/ml may be added to the infusate to minimize thrombophlebitis. If pretreatment for acute reactions is necessary, it should be noted that the reactions tend to diminish later in the course of therapy, and withdrawal of the pretreatment medications should be attempted after 1 or 2 weeks of treatment if further amphotericin therapy is indicated.

Some authorities have advocated the use of azole derivatives, such as ketoconazole, itraconazole, or fluconazole, for initial treatment of individuals with pulmonary coccidioidomycosis. However, published experience is minimal, and relapses and failures have been reported. Until further experience is available, parenteral amphotericin B is the preferred treatment for most patients requiring therapy. Rarely (and almost never in children), pulmonary coccidioidomycosis progresses to a more chronic form, with development of cavitary lesions. The roles of both medical and surgical therapies for these patients are very controversial. Overall, series in adults suggest that about one third of these patients have slow resolution of the lesions, and two thirds may develop bleeding, which occasionally requires emergent surgical excision.

DISSEMINATED COCCIDIOIDOMYCOSIS

Disseminated coccidioidomycosis requires parenteral amphotericin B therapy, usually aiming for a total dose of 30 to 40 mg/kg, with the same management issues as discussed previously. The total duration of therapy must be based on clinical response, and some normal hosts with limited dissemination may be adequately treated with a shorter course, perhaps followed by oral fluconazole administration at a dose of 3 to 6 mg/kg/d for several weeks thereafter. There is no clear role for combination chemotherapy in these patients.

COCCIDIOIDAL BONE AND JOINT DISEASE

Bone and joint infection due to *C. immitis* may be a feature of disseminated disease or a result of trauma with primary inoculation. Systemic medical therapy alone is probably insufficient to cure these individuals. Surgical debridement of sequestra and other debris or necrotic areas is important. Additionally, it is advisable to provide local application of amphotericin B. For osteomyelitis, an infusion/suction system to instill a 10% solution of amphotericin B in water may be tried, although there are often difficulties with the mechanics of bathing the bone. Intraarticular injections of amphotericin B starting at 5 mg in sterile water three times weekly initially, then less frequently for up to 6 months, and synovectomy may be necessary to eradicate coccidioidal arthritis.

COCCIDIOIDAL MENINGITIS

Coccidioidal meningitis is extremely difficult to cure and may require lifelong suppressive therapy. Initial treatment should always include parenteral amphotericin B, continued for a prolonged period, but adjuvant therapy is probably needed. The gold standard is to provide for instillation of amphotericin B directly into the CSF by either the lumbar, cisterna magna, or ventricular approach. All three routes of administration have drawbacks, although the intracisternal approach is thought to be desirable. It may be less likely to cause a chemical arachnoiditis, and it allows for drug delivery closest to the site of infection, the basilar meninges. However, this is a cumbersome procedure, and many patients are now treated via the intraventricular route with the use of an Ommaya reservoir, starting with a low dose of 0.025 mg in water and working up to 0.1 to 0.5 mg doses given three to four times weekly. Later, the frequency can be diminished to once every 3 or 4 weeks, and this can be continued for at least 1 year if tolerated. Miconazole has also been used for CSF instillation, but more appealing is the possibility of oral fluconazole to replace most or all instillation procedures. Fluconazole has excellent CSF penetration, but experience is lacking so far in coccidioidal meningitis. Early studies have shown good response, but relapses occur.

COCCIDIOIDOMYCOSIS IN IMMUNOCOMPROMISED HOSTS

Experience is accumulating in the treatment of disseminated coccidioidomycosis in immunocompromised hosts, primarily because of the AIDS epidemic. These patients require a full course of parenteral amphotericin B and probably require lifelong suppressive therapy with either itraconazole (dose not established in children) or fluconazole.

OTHER PROMISING TREATMENTS FOR COCCIDIOIDOMYCOSIS

Many newer antifungal agents are in various stages of clinical trials for treatment of coccidioidomycosis and other fungal infections. A planned comparative trial of itraconazole and fluconazole for primary treatment of nonmeningeal disease may answer whether amphotericin B can be eliminated as initial therapy of subacute disease. Newer and potentially less toxic formulations of amphotericin B, such as amphotericin B lipid complex, amphotericin B colloidal dispersion, and different forms of lamellar vesicles as carrier packages for the drug are under study. Newer triazoles and the nikkomycins may offer further advantages over existing agents. Combination therapy for disseminated disease, using both polyene and azole drugs, needs further evaluation.

SUMMARY

The majority of cases of coccidioidomycosis, including those with mild pulmonary infections, do not require any specific therapy. However, progressive pulmonary disease and disseminated infection require antifungal treatment. Evaluation of newer agents to replace amphotericin B as mainstay therapy is complicated by the tendency of coccidioidomycosis to persist and relapse years after treatment.

REFERENCES

1. Einstein HE, Johnson RH: Coccidioidomycosis: New aspects of epidemiology and therapy. Clin Infect Dis 16:349–356, 1993.
2. Fish DG, Ampel NM, Galgiani JN, et al: Coccidioidomycosis during human immunodeficiency virus infection: A review of 77 patients. Medicine 69:384–391, 1990.
3. Tucker RM, Galgiani JN, Denning DW, et al: Treatment of coccidioidal meningitis with fluconazole. Rev Infect Dis 12(suppl 3):S380–S389, 1990.

HISTOPLASMOSIS

Stephen C. Aronoff, M.D.
Fernando J. Rosas, M.D.

More than 90% of primary infections with *Histoplasma capsulatum* are asymptomatic and self-limited. Eighty percent of symptomatic infections present with mild respiratory symptoms or a flu-like illness following a typical history of exposure to birds or bat guano (e.g., spelunking, exposure to old buildings or demolition). These acute pulmonary infections are also self-limited. Extrapulmonary disease (disseminated infection), chronic pulmonary infections with cavitation, acute pulmonary infection with adult respiratory distress syndrome (ARDS), and mediastinal granuloma with obstruction represent forms of histoplasmosis that require therapy.

EXTRAPULMONARY HISTOPLASMOSIS (DISSEMINATED)

Approximately 80% of patients with extrapulmonary histoplasmosis are immunoincompetent. In pediatric practice, infants under 2 years of age, children receiving immunosuppressive therapy, and HIV-infected individuals comprise the largest risk groups. Amphotericin B 0.5 to 1 mg/kg/d to a total dose of 30 to 35 mg/kg is recommended for all children with disseminated infection except those with HIV. Although ketoconazole is highly effective against *H. capsulatum* in vitro, clinical efficacy is poor among immunocompromised patients and cannot be recommended as single-agent therapy. For infections in older patients, initial amphotericin therapy of 500 mg total dose may be followed by 400 mg/d for 6 months to 1 year. Experience with fluconazole and itraconazole is limited in children, although fluconazole was used successfully for the treatment of CNS histoplasmosis in an adolescent.

Extrapulmonary histoplasmosis in HIV-infected individuals is almost uniformly lethal. Although the administration of more than 500 mg total dose of amphotericin B reduces the mortality rate from 100% to 50% in this population, the relapse rate is almost 100% following the cessation of amphotericin B therapy. Currently, histoplasmosis in older HIV-infected individuals requires induction therapy with amphotericin B 15 mg/kg total dose and indefinite maintenance therapy with thrice weekly intravenous amphotericin at 0.5 to 1 mg/kg per dose, oral itraconazole 200 mg twice daily, or oral ketoconazole 400 mg/d. Preliminary studies suggest that fluconazole and ketoconazole are inferior to itraconazole in adults. Young infants should be maintained on intermittent intravenous amphotericin B.

CHRONIC PULMONARY HISTOPLASMOSIS WITH CAVITATION

This form of histoplasmosis is rare in children and typically occurs in children with underlying lung disease. Individuals with chronically progressive symptoms, such as cough, fever, weight loss, and dyspnea, as well as radiographic evidence of pulmonary cavities with more than a 2-mm thick capsule, are candidates for therapy. For these patients, administration of amphotericin B 0.5 to 1 mg/kg/d to a total dose of 35 mg/kg is associated with a 20% recurrence rate, compared with a 39% recurrence rate for lower total doses. Ketoconazole is inferior to amphotericin B for the treatment of chronic, cavitary pulmonary histoplasmosis. No data are available for the treatment with itraconazole or fluconazole of this entity in children.

ACUTE PULMONARY HISTOPLASMOSIS

Acute pulmonary histoplasmosis is the most common symptomatic form of *H. capsulatum* infection. Patients presenting with acute pulmonary symptoms accompanied by ARDS require immediate intervention. Ventilatory support for the hypoxemia, as well as aggressive monitoring within an intensive care setting, is required. In previously healthy individuals beyond 2 years of age, short-course amphotericin B therapy (total dose approximately 10 to 15 mg/kg, 500 mg in adults) coupled with high-dose intravenous corticosteroid therapy (800 mg of hydrocortisone per day in adults) is recommended.

MEDIASTINAL GRANULOMA

This rare, late complication of pulmonary histoplasmosis is the result of encasement of vital mediastinal structures within a reactive granulomatous mass. Since viable organisms are not recovered from these masses, antifungal therapy is of little value. Surgical intervention is required to alleviate symptoms of obstruction (e.g., superior vena cava syndrome, dysphagia, and respiratory distress) or to repair fistulas. Total resection of the mass is often difficult to impossible. Although no studies have examined the role of anti-inflammatory agents for the treatment of this entity, the observation that the granulomatous tissue is rich in CD3 lymphocytes suggest a use for these agents.

DRUG TOXICITIES

Amphotericin B has been used extensively in children. Hypokalemia due to kaluria and azotemia are well-recognized, dose-related toxicities of this agent. Using a daily dose of 0.5 to 0.6 mg/kg/d reduces the magnitude of renal toxicity. Alternate-day therapy with reduction of dose, as well as potassium supplementation, may be required. An idiosyncratic reaction of fever, chills, and rigors that accompanies drug infusion can be reduced by premedication with diphenhydramine 1 mg/kg per dose IM or IV or meperidine 1 mg/kg per dose IM or IV one half-hour before drug infusion.

Rapid intravenous administration of amphotericin can result in a shocklike syndrome, and minimal infusion times of 4 to 6 hours reduce the likelihood of untoward side effects. The administration of a test dose of 0.1 mg/kg to a maximum of 1 mg is recommended to screen for the rare individual who may develop anaphylaxis. Although investigational, liposomal encapsulation of amphotericin B permits higher daily doses of drug with less dose-dependent toxicity. This agent should prove useful for the treatment of histoplasmosis in children.

The azole antifungals (ketoconazole, fluconazole, and itraconazole) have similar toxicities that differ in magnitude among the three agents. Ketoconazole is the most toxic agent. Hepatotoxicity is the most familiar and most dramatic side effect of ketoconazole. Serial liver function testing and examinations for icterus are recommended, and discontinuation of therapy should be considered for individuals who developed hypertransaminasemia (three times the upper limit of normal). Gastrointestinal discomfort is greatest with ketoconazole, but many patients receiving orally administered triazoles may experience nausea and vomiting with increasing doses. Reduction of serum testosterone concentrations is well described with ketoconazole. Gynecomastia and temporary sterility in males, alopecia in both sexes, and dysmenorrhea in women are reversed with exogenous testosterone. Addison's syndrome has been described rarely in conjunction with ketoconazole therapy.

MUCORMYCOSIS (ZYGOMYCOSIS)

W. Thomas Corder, M.D.
Stephen C. Aronoff, M.D.

Mucormycosis, also known as zygomycosis, is an infection caused by fungi commonly found on bread, fruit, and soil. Mucormycosis is rare and is seen most often as an opportunistic infection in patients with diabetic ketoacidosis, debilitation, agranulocytopenia, or immunosuppression. Nearby construction activity may present an independent risk factor for susceptible individuals. In particular, the infection has reportedly been transmitted to a neonate by a contaminated parenteral feeding solution. Infections are usually acute and rapidly fatal.

The most common forms of mucormycosis are rhinocerebral, pulmonary, intestinal, and cutaneous.

CLASSIFICATION

Rhinocerebral Mucormycosis

The fungus is suspected to invade through the mucous membranes of the nasal passages or sinuses or through the soft palate. Symptoms can include unilateral headache, eye irritation, periorbital edema, epistaxis, nasal discharge, and pain over the affected sinus (maxillary or frontal). Areas of black necrosis can be seen in the nose, medial maxillary wall, and turbinates or on the palate. Ecchymoses and periorbital cellulitis can occur. A discharge of black pus is pathognomonic. Direct extension to the central nervous system (CNS) can occur, leading to lethargy and coma.

Pulmonary Mucormycosis

The course is similar to that of pulmonary aspergillosis and is characterized by fever and pulmonary infiltrates. Pulmonary vascular thrombosis and infarction are late sequelae. Extension to the CNS is not uncommon and is usually fatal.

Intestinal Mucormycosis

Intestinal disease follows ingestion of fungi by susceptible persons. Symptoms, which may vary according to site and extent, include abdominal pain, diarrhea, hematemesis, and hematochezia. Ulcers can be found throughout the intestinal tract and may result in thromboses and gangrene.

Cutaneous Mucormycosis

Cutaneous mucormycosis is a particular danger to burn patients. Skin infection also has been reported with the use of Elastoplast bandages over wounds and adhesive tape over an intravenous site.

DIAGNOSIS

Definitive diagnosis requires histologic examination of biopsy or affected material because blood cultures and direct cultures from affected tissue often are sterile. Negative cultures cannot exclude the diagnosis. Multiple biopsies may be needed to make the diagnosis. Histologically, broad, coenocytic hyphae are found invading tissue. The organisms are known to invade arterial walls to produce an arteritis and thrombosis that results in infarction of the distally perfused area.

TREATMENT

Therapy consists of correction of the underlying problems (such as diabetic ketoacidosis), surgical debridement, and drainage. Amphotericin B is the antifungal agent of choice. Hyperbaric oxygen has been used experimentally in the rhinocerebral form. Fluconazole has been used occasionally in adults, but there is no experience with this agent in treating children with mucormycosis.

Side effects from amphotericin B include bone marrow suppression, nephrotoxicity, hypokalemia, fever, chills, headache, nausea, anorexia, phlebitis, and hypomagnesemia. Hypercalciuria, renal tubular acidosis, and acute hepatic failure can also occur. Baseline renal function, liver function, hematologic values, and electrolytes should be obtained before administration, and these parameters should be followed throughout the course of therapy.

To minimize side effects, the patient can be premedicated with acetaminophen 10 to 15 mg/kg per dose and diphenhydramine 1.25 mg/kg per dose 30 minutes before and 4 hours after infusion. If toxic symptoms still occur, the patient may also be premedicated with hydrocortisone 1 mg/kg per dose up to 25 mg, or this can be added to the intravenous solution. Amphotericin B is mixed with 5% dextrose to a concentration of 0.1 mg/ml and pH >4.2. A test dose of 0.1 mg/kg (up to a maximum of 1 mg) is infused over 20 to 30 minutes. The patient's temperature and vital functions are followed for the next 4 hours. If the test dose is tolerated well, the rest of a 0.25 mg/kg dose may be given over the next 4 to 6 hours. The dose is increased in daily increments of 0.25 mg/kg until a daily dose of 0.4 to 0.6 mg/kg is reached. This dose is given daily until the patient's condition stabilizes or improves, and then it can be given every other day until the total dose is administered. In adults, the total dose is usually in the range of 2 to 4 g. The total dose for children is unknown. According to extrapolation of the adult range, the total dose for a child would be 15 to 30 mg/kg.

SUMMARY

Mucormycosis is a rapidly progressive fulminant disease that is usually associated with a fatal outcome. A high degree of clinical suspicion and a prompt histologic examination of material submitted for biopsy are needed to make an early diagnosis. Rapid diagnosis and early institution of therapy provide the best chance for improved outcome.

CHLAMYDIA

MARGARET R. HAMMERSCHLAG, M.D.

The genus *Chlamydia* comprises a group of obligate intracellular parasites with a unique developmental cycle and with morphologically distinct infectious and reproductive forms. All members of the genus have a gram-negative envelope without peptidoglycan, share a genus-specific lipopolysaccharide antigen, and use host ATP for the synthesis of chlamydial protein. The genus contains three species, *Chlamydia trachomatis*, *Chlamydia psittaci*, and the recently described *Chlamydia pneumoniae* (TWAR strain).

Diagnosis can be made by isolation of the organisms in tissue culture. Several nonculture methods are valuable for the diagnosis of *C. trachomatis* infection, including enzyme immunoassays (EIA), direct fluorescence antibody tests (DFA), and DNA probes. All three categories of tests are approved for detection of *C. trachomatis* in cervical and urethral specimens from adolescents and adults. The EIAs and DFAs have additional indications for use in conjunctival and nasopharyngeal specimens from infants with suspected chlamydial conjunctivitis and pneumonia. Antigen detection tests and DNA probes are not approved and should not be used on genital (vaginal or urethral) and rectal specimens from prepubertal children or for any forensic purposes. The tests are not accurate at these sites.

Since infection with *C. pneumoniae* has been described only recently, culture and serology are available at a limited number of research laboratories in the United States. The complement-fixation (CF) test can be of use for the serologic diagnosis of psittacosis and lymphogranuloma venereum (LGV).

INFECTIONS WITH C. TRACHOMATIS

Eye Infections

Neonatal inclusion conjunctivitis usually presents 5 to 14 days after birth. Clinical presentation is variable, ranging from minimal infection and discharge to severe infection with chemosis, pseudomembrane formation, and copious mucopurulent discharge. The conjunctivae may be quite friable and bleed when stroked with a swab. The treatment of choice is erythromycin suspension 50 mg/kg/d PO in four divided doses for 10 to 14 days. Topical therapy is not indicated and is generally ineffective.

Pneumonia

Infantile chlamydial pneumonia usually presents between 1 and 3 months of age. Infants are usually afebrile and tachypneic. Rales are usually heard on auscultation. Wheezing is rare. The chest radiograph shows hyperinflation with variable infiltrates. Peripheral eosinophilia (>400/mm³) is also present.

Infants with *C. trachomatis* pneumonia should be treated with erythromycin at the same dose schedule as for chlamydial conjunctivitis.

Uncomplicated Urethral, Cervical, and Rectal Infection

C. trachomatis is the major identifiable infectious etiology of nongonococcal urethritis, responsible for 30% to 50% of cases. In women, it can cause mucopurulent cervicitis and salpingitis. The latter may eventually lead to tubal obstruction, infertility, and an increased risk of ectopic pregnancy. However, the great majority of chlamydial genital infections are asymptomatic.

The treatment of choice in adolescents is doxycycline 100 mg twice daily for 7 days. Alternative therapies are erythromycin 500 mg four times daily for 7 days, ofloxacin 30 mg twice daily for 7 days, or azithromycin, 1 g PO as a single dose. Sexual partners should also be treated. In children, erythromycin suspension 50 mg/kg/d in four divided doses for 10 to 14 days is recommended.

Lymphogranuloma Venereum (LGV)

LGV is a sexually transmitted disease caused by the L_1, L_2, and L_3 serotypes of *C. trachomatis*. The infection is characterized by an initial transient genital papule or ulcer, followed by the development of inguinal adenopathy, which may break down and form fistulas. This presentation is more common in men. Because the lymphatic drainage of the vulva is to the retroperitoneal nodes, women are more likely to present in the tertiary stage of the disease with rectovaginal fistulas and strictures.

Tetracycline 500 mg four times daily or doxycycline 100 mg twice daily should be given for 3 to 6 weeks.

INFECTIONS WITH C. PNEUMONIAE (TWAR)

C. pneumoniae appears to be a primary human respiratory pathogen. It has been isolated from 10% to 20% of both children and adults with community-acquired pneumonia. Disease presentations include asymptomatic respiratory infection, a flu-like illness with pharyngitis, sinusitis and headache, bronchitis, and atypical pneumonia. The organism has been isolated from the pleural fluid of a patient with pneumonia. Spread appears to be person to person via aerosol droplets, and multiple members of households may be infected.

C. pneumoniae is resistant to sulfonamides, and its therapy is not well defined. In adolescents and adults, it appears that up to 21 days of either doxycycline 100 mg twice daily or erythromycin 500 mg four times daily may be necessary. Preliminary data in children suggest that erythromycin 50 mg/kg/d in four divided doses for 14 days or clarithromycin 15 mg/kg/d in two divided doses for 10 days is effective.

INFECTIONS WITH C. PSITTACI

C. psittaci is a ubiquitous pathogen infecting practically every known mammalian and avian species. Infection in humans is due to animal exposure, most commonly to birds. Individuals at highest risk are veterinarians, bird fanciers, and workers in the poultry industry. Infection is uncommon in children under 17 years of age. The onset is abrupt, with high fever, headache is frequent, rales are usually heard on auscultation, and the chest radiograph reveals variable infiltrates and, frequently, pleural effusions.

The recommended treatment is tetracycline 500 mg PO every 6 hours for 7 to 10 days. Erythromycin 500 mg every 6 hours for 7 to 10 days can also be used.

REFERENCES

1. CDC: Recommendations for the prevention and management of *Chlamydia trachomatis* infections, 1993. MMWR 42:No. RR-12, 1993.
2. Chirgwin K, Hammerschlag MR: *Chlamydia* pneumonia. *In* Feigin RD, Cherry JD (eds): Textbook of Pediatric Infectious Diseases, 3rd ed. Philadelphia, WB Saunders, 1992:265–270.
3. Grayston JT, Campbell LA, Kuo CC, et al: A new respiratory tract pathogen: *Chlamydia pneumoniae* strain TWAR. J Infect Dis 161:618–625, 1990.

MYCOPLASMA

JEROME O. KLEIN, M.D.

The mycoplasmas are a unique group of microorganisms that colonize mucosal surfaces, particularly those of the respiratory and genital tract. *Mycoplasma pneumoniae*, the agent of primary atypical pneumonia, is the only mycoplasma found in the respiratory tract that is unequivocally associated with human disease. The genital mycoplasmas, including *Ureaplasma urealyticum* and *Mycoplasma hominis*, are present in the genital tract of sexually active adults and have been associated with a variety of local and systemic infections. The genital mycoplasmas have been associated with lower respiratory tract infections and rare cases of meningitis in neonates. *M. hominis* may also cause abscesses in newborn infants, usually as a result of impregnation into the skin and soft tissues of surface organisms by fetal monitors or forceps at delivery.

M. pneumoniae and *U. urealyticum* are susceptible in vitro to erythromycin (and the new macrolides clarithromycin and azithromycin), tetracyclines, and chloramphenicol. *M. hominis* is resistant to erythromycin but susceptible to tetracyclines, chloramphenicol, and clindamycin. Because mycoplasmas lack cell walls, they are resistant to all penicillins and cephalosporins.

Tetracyclines, erythromycin, clarithromycin, and azithromycin are effective agents for respiratory infections due to *M. pneumoniae*. Erythromycin 50 mg/kg/d in four doses for 7 days shortens the clinical course of pneumonia due to *M. pneumoniae* and is the drug of choice for children younger than 9 years. Tetracyclines, including tetracycline, chlortetracycline, and oxytetracycline 25 to 50 mg/kg/d in four doses for 7 days, or methacycline or demeclocycline 10 mg/kg/d in two doses for 7 days, are effective and may be used for older children. Neither clarithromycin nor azithromycin is approved for treatment of pneumonia in children (March 1995). The adult dose for clarithromycin is 250 to 500 mg twice a day for 7 days, and the adult dose for azithromycin is 500 mg for the first day and 250 mg once a day for days 2 through 7. Antimicrobial therapy may suppress but not eliminate the organisms from the upper respiratory tract. The patient may relapse after conclusion of therapy and require a second course of the same drug.

The optimal therapy of infections due to *M. hominis* and *U. urealyticum* in neonates remains uncertain because of the paucity of cases. Serious infections due to *M. hominis* should be treated with chloramphenicol or clindamycin. Tetracycline is more effective than chloramphenicol in vitro and may be of value in the treatment of meningitis due to *M. hominis*. Chelation of the drug to bones and teeth limits the use of the tetracyclines to critically ill infants unresponsive to chloramphenicol or clindamycin. On diagnosis, mild *Ureaplasma* infection may be treated with erythromycin.

GENITAL MYCOPLASMAL INFECTIONS

GAIL H. CASSELL, Ph.D.
KEN B. WAITES, M.D.
JULIANE HENTSCHEL M.D.

Of the 14 species of mycoplasmas known to infect humans, *Ureaplasma urealyticum* and *Mycoplasma hominis* are the species most commonly found in the urogenital tract. Because of their ubiquity in asymptomatic individuals, the disease-producing potential of *U. urealyticum* and *M. hominis* has been surrounded by controversy. However, they have been conclusively shown to be an important cause of urogenital disease in selected populations and a rather common cause of extragenital infection in immunocompromised children and adults. In addition, they are an important cause of perinatal morbidity and mortality primarily because of the frequency with which they are transmitted in utero and their association with premature birth.

Experience with *U. urealyticum* and *M. hominis* in immunocompromised patients indicates that these organisms cause progressive and destructive disease often with a paucity of systemic signs of infection. They are often refractory to antibiotic therapy, requiring prolonged administration of a combination of intravenous antibiotics and intravenous immunoglobulin.

Little information is available concerning the efficacy of antimicrobial treatment of *U. urealyticum* and *M. hominis* in infants. This, coupled with limited options for treatment in pregnant females and infants, presents a major challenge. Likewise, identification of mothers and infants at risk for invasive infections with these organisms is a major need for future research.

Considerations pertinent to therapy of *U. urealyticum* and *M. hominis* pediatric infections are summarized subsequently. Although *Mycoplasma fermentans*, *Mycoplasma genitalium*, and *Mycoplasma penetrans* are also found in the urogenital tracts of humans and recent data suggest that they may be a cause of disease, there are no published data pertaining to their occurrence in infants and children. Therefore, these organisms are not discussed.

PERTINENT BIOLOGIC PROPERTIES

Individual mycoplasma cells range in size from 100 to 300 nm in diameter, approximately the size of the influenza or pox viruses. They are unique among procaryotes in that they lack a cell wall. Because of their small size and lack of a cell wall, mycoplasmas are not readily stainable by gram stain or easily visible by other staining methods using the regular light microscope. The extremely small size of the mycoplasmal genome also severely limits their biosynthetic capabilities, helps explain their complex nutritional requirements for cultivation, and necessitates a parasitic or saprophytic existence for most species. In mammals, mycoplasmas most commonly colonize mucosal surface, particularly those of the respiratory and genital tracts.

The biologic properties of mycoplasmas often lead to diagnostic difficulties in the routine laboratory. The limited availability of reference mycoplasmal diagnostic facilities and the impracticality of obtaining specimens for microbiologic study in some conditions makes it necessary for clinicians to be familiar with the syndromes for which mycoplasmas may be responsible and provide treatment likely to eliminate the organisms.

EPIDEMIOLOGIC CONSIDERATIONS

Following puberty, colonization of the male and female lower urogenital genital tract by *U. urealyticum,* and *M. hominis* usually occurs as a result of sexual activity. *U. urealyticum* can be found in the vagina of 40% to 80% of sexually mature, asymptomatic women, and *M. hominis* can be found in 21% to 53%. The incidence of each is somewhat lower in males. In females, colonization is linked to younger age, lower socioeconomic status, sexual activity with multiple partners, black ethnicity, and oral contraceptive use.

U. urealyticum and *M. hominis* can be transmitted from an infected female to a fetus either in utero or at the time of delivery by passage through an infected birth canal. Isolation of *U. urealyticum* in pure culture from the chorioamnion, amniotic fluid, and internal fetal organs in the presence of funisitis and pneumonia and a specific IgM response provides strong evidence that fetal infection can occur in utero. Acquisition of *U. urealyticum* and *M. hominis* can occur in utero either by an ascending route secondary to colonization of the mother's genital tract or transplacentally from the mother's blood. Both organisms have been isolated from maternal and umbilical cord blood at the time of delivery.

Colonization of healthy full-term infants is relatively transient, with a sharp drop in isolation rates after 3 months of age. In premature infants with invasive ureaplasma infection, persistence of the organism in the lower respiratory tract and cerebrospinal fluid (CSF) has been documented for weeks to months. Fewer than 10% of older children and sexually inexperienced adults are colonized. Colonization after puberty increases with sexual activity.

DISEASES OF THE UROGENITAL TRACT

Three conditions of the urinary tract definitively shown to be caused by mycoplasmas are urethritis in males due to *U. urealyticum,* urinary calculi due to *U. urealyticum,* and pyelonephritis caused by *M. hominis.* Although the exact proportion of cases of nongonococcal urethritis caused by *U. urealyticum* may still be debated, the ability of this organism to cause urethritis can no longer be disputed. Intraurethral inoculation of human volunteers and nonhuman primates produces urethritis. Only one entity of either the male or female reproductive tract has been shown to be caused by mycoplasmas. Although the exact proportion of cases is unknown, *M. hominis* is considered to be a cause of pelvic inflammatory disease (PID). The organism has been isolated in pure culture from the fallopian tubes and from the endometrium. In addition, a role for this organism in cases of PID not associated with either *Neisseria gonorrhoeae* or *Chlamydia trachomatis* is supported by significant increases in specific antibody. Although *U. urealyticum* can be isolated directly from affected fallopian tubes, it usually is found in the presence of other known pathogens.

EXTRAGENITAL INFECTIONS

Although *U. urealyticum* and *M. hominis* typically remain localized in the lower genital tract in a normal host, both organisms can cause extragenital infections. These infections have been reported in patients of both sexes, with a broad range of ages (14 to 76 years) and underlying diagnoses. The true incidence of extragenital infections due to either ureaplasmas or *M. hominis* is not known, since these organisms are not sought routinely. Disseminated infection has been reported in otherwise healthy hosts, but most infections follow genitourinary manipulation or trauma of the genitourinary tract or occur in individuals with underlying immunosuppression or hypogammaglobulinemia or both. Persistent and fatal mycoplasmemia due to *M. hominis* has been reported in patients with immunosuppression or other underlying disease. Infected surgical wound sites most often include sternotomies and pelvic and inguinal wounds. Heart-lung transplant recipients commonly develop sternal wound infections due

to *M. hominis* with associated mediastinitis and empyema. These infections are refractory to treatment and often require closure by muscle flaps after sternotomy. Peritonitis following renal transplantation and thrombophlebitis due to *M. hominis* also have been reported.

Approximately 8% of individuals with hypogammaglobulinemia develop septic joint inflammation. There is evidence to suggest that mycoplasmas may be responsible for the majority of these. *U. urealyticum* and *M. hominis* can be isolated repeatedly from the joints in the absence of any other microbial agent. Both *U. urealyticum* and *M. hominis* also cause arthritis in other types of immunosuppressed or otherwise compromised (i.e., those with prosthetic joints) patients. In most of the reported cases, the arthritis has been persistent, lasting from several months to over a year. Aggressive, erosive arthritis that progresses in the face of anti-inflammatory therapy and gamma globulin replacement can occur. In some of the cases involving *U. urealyticum,* the arthritis is associated with subcutaneous abscesses, persistent urethritis, and chronic urethrocystitis/cystitis. Most of these cases have required massive and prolonged antibiotic therapy, but some of the strains involved are or have become resistant to multiple antibiotics. Osteomyelitis has been reported in association with invasive infection with both *U. urealyticum* and *M. hominis,* with direct isolation of the organism from bone tissue. *M. hominis* has been identified in several cases of meningitis following trauma and in brain abscesses of immunocompromised patients. *U. urealyticum* is the predominant cause of sinopulmonary disease and progressive lung failure in hypogammaglobulinemic patients and in such cases has been isolated directly from the bronchus. *M. hominis* is a cause of pneumonia in immunosuppressed and other compromised patients and can be directly isolated from lung tissue at autopsy and from blood and pleural fluid premortem in cases in which no other infectious agent or cause of death can be identified.

INFECTION OF THE FETUS AND NEWBORN

Individual case reports provide compelling evidence that in at least some individuals, *U. urealyticum* alone plays a causal role in chorioamnionitis, spontaneous abortion, stillbirth, and premature birth. *U. urealyticum* can persist in the amniotic fluid as long as 2 months in the presence of intact membranes and an intense inflammatory response and in the absence of labor and other detectable microorganisms and can be demonstrated directly in the inflammatory infiltrates in the fetal membranes by immunofluorescence. A number of prospective studies based on direct culture of the affected site indicate that both *U. urealyticum* and *M. hominis* can cause invasive disease in infants and are a cause of perinatal morbidity and mortality, particularly in infants born prematurely.

Congenital and Neonatal Pneumonia

Although individual case reports suggest that *M. hominis* may be a cause of pneumonia in newborns, it has not been implicated as a common cause in prospective studies. In contrast, *U. urealyticum* is an important cause of pneumonia in the fetus and the newborn. Retrospective studies, as well as prospective studies, indicate an association of *U. urealyticum* with congenital pneumonia. *U. urealyticum* has been isolated from amniotic fluid repeatedly over a 7-week period (16 to 23 weeks' gestation) in the presence of intact membranes and the absence of other microorganisms. *U. urealyticum* has been isolated in pure culture from lung tissue at autopsy less than 24 hours after birth. Inflammatory changes compatible with a histologic diagnosis of congenital pneumonia were demonstrated in the lungs. Organisms have been identified by immunofluorescence and electron microscopy directly in the areas of pulmonary inflammation, and in the same infant, an increase in IgM antibody has been documented by metabolic inhibition, proving that *U. urealyticum* can cause congenital pneumonia.

U. urealyticum, in the absence of other microorganisms, can be isolated from endotracheal aspirates at birth from infants with evidence of respiratory disease. In these same infants, it can also be isolated from pleural fluid before death and from lung tissue at autopsy in the absence of other microorganisms but in the presence of histologically proven pneumonia. Isolation of *U. urealyticum* from endotracheal aspirates in the absence of other documented respiratory pathogens is significantly associated with radiographic evidence of pneumonia, increased numbers of circulating white blood cells, and increased numbers of neutrophils in the tracheal aspirate 2 days after birth. In some infants, ureaplasmas can be concomitantly isolated from blood and CSF.

Taken together, the available evidence provides a strong argument that *U. urealyticum* is a common cause of pneumonia in newborn infants, particularly those born before 34 weeks' gestation. The organism can be isolated from endotracheal aspirates of up to 34% of infants <2500 g, and radiographic evidence of pneumonia is twice as common in these infants as in *U. urealyticum*-negative infants. Many of these infections develop as a result of in utero infection. Cases of ureaplasma pneumonia have been clearly documented in term infants, but by comparison, it occurs much less frequently.

Chronic Lung Disease of Prematurity

Isolation of *U. urealyticum* from endotracheal aspirates of infants ≤1250 g within the first 24 hours of birth is associated with an increased risk for development of bronchopulmonary dysplasia, or chronic lung disease (CLD) of prematurity. Current knowledge of the pathophysiology of CLD of prematurity would suggest that *U. urealyticum* produces pneumonia that goes undetected and untreated and results in an increased requirement for oxygen and subsequent development of CLD as a result of oxygen toxicity. Several facts suggest that those infants who acquire *U. urealyticum* in utero may be the ones at greatest risk for development of CLD.

Although the available data provide very strong evidence that *U. urealyticum* can be a primary cause or a contributing cofactor in development of CLD in humans, the data are not definitive. Cohort studies allow follow-up of exposed individuals and thus reduce bias, but the designs of these studies cannot rule out the possibility that a third factor associated with *U. urealyticum* is the true cause of CLD. A randomized trial of exposure to infection in humans is not ethical or practical. Whereas a randomized trial of antibiotic treatment could provide critical information related to patient management, it would still not bring us closer to proving causality. Even if treatment is found to be efficacious, conclusions about causation will be limited by the fact that the third factor might also be susceptible to the antibiotic chosen. Nevertheless, a treatment trial is urgently needed to determine whether appropriate therapy can reduce the incidence of morbidity and mortality associated with CLD.

Infections of the Central Nervous System

U. urealyticum and *M. hominis* appear to be among the most common microorganisms isolated from the CSF of newborn infants. The incidence, ranging from 0 to 13%, depends on the cultural methods used and the patient population examined. *U. urealyticum* CSF infection, in particular, appears to be more common in premature infants. The clinical findings in infants with *U. urealyticum* and *M. hominis* infection of the CSF are variable. *U urealyticum* and *M. hominis* may produce CSF pleocytosis, with either polymorphonuclear or mononuclear cells predominating, or the inflammatory reaction in CSF may be minimal or absent. In some patients, the organisms are eradicated spontaneously from the CSF, whereas in others, the organisms have been shown to persist in the CSF for weeks and even months.

Lack of inflammation, when the presence of the organism has been verified in the CSF on multiple occasions, may logically lead to some skepticism about the significance of mycoplasmal CSF infection. However, it should be noted that early in the course of infection with a number of other proven bacterial pathogens that may infect the meninges, inflammatory reactions may be scant or absent. The severely ill infant with meningitis may in fact represent only a fraction of the total number of *Ureaplasma*- or *Mycoplasma*-infected infants, with the majority experiencing only a mild, often subclinical infection that may resolve spontaneously.

Prognosis and long-term neurodevelopmental outcomes of infants with mycoplasmal CSF infections has not been studied in depth. Knowledge is limited primarily to case reports and short-term observations from recent prospective studies. Infants have been described whose infections were subclinical or in whom there was only moderate illness followed by complete recovery. A decrease in hydrocephalus in preterm infants with CNS infection caused by either *M. hominis* or *U. urealyticum* has been documented after antibiotic treatment. The relative contribution of mycoplasmas to demise in some infected infants has not always been clear because of the concurrent presence of other conditions, such as extreme immaturity, intraventricular hemorrhage, respiratory disease, and concomitant bacterial infection. Permanent neurologic handicaps in survivors ranging from mild hemiparesis to profound spastic quadriplegia have been described. Studies of additional infants with detailed case-controlled neurodevelopmental follow-up are needed to establish the characteristics and risk of long-term effects of mycoplasmal CSF infections during the perinatal period.

Most of the case reports of mycoplasmal CSF infections have involved symptomatic infants with CSF pleocytosis for which no bacterial cause could be ascertained. A mycoplasmal infection was considered only as a last resort, often after suspicious colonies that did not gram stain were identified on routine bacteriologic media or the child failed to respond to conventional chemotherapy. The prevalence, risk factors, typical manifestations, and long-term effects of mycoplasmal CNS infections in the newborn remained an enigma until the recent publication of prospective studies that began to clarify these issues to some degree. Until there is widespread awareness of how common mycoplasmal infections of the CNS can be, knowledge of what group is at risk for infection, and development of improved diagnostic capabilities, it is likely that the majority of cases will not be identified.

Other Conditions in the Newborn Caused by Genital Mycoplasmas

Bacteremia, pericarditis, adenitis, osteomyelitis, and abscesses of the subcutaneous tissue in newborn infants can be caused by both *U. urealyticum* and *M. hominis*.

DIAGNOSTIC AND THERAPEUTIC IMPLICATIONS

Because of the frequency with which *U. urealyticum* and *M. hominis* can be isolated from the lower female urogenital tract, routine screening and treatment of infections of this site are not justified. However, isolation, determination of antibiotic susceptibilities, and treatment are recommended for ureaplasmal nongonococcal urethritis. It is clear that both organisms can produce invasive infections but only in a certain subpopulation of those colonized in the lower genital tract. If confirmation of the microbiologic etiology of PID is desired, it is necessary to culture the endometrium and fallopian tubes by methods that circumvent cervical contamination.

A positive culture for mycoplasmas, especially from a normally sterile site and particularly in the absence of other microorganisms, is sufficient justification for treatment of patients suffering from a condition known to be caused by or associated with mycoplasmas. However, the presence of mycoplasmas in clinical material obtained from patients without evidence of mycoplasma-associated disease does not warrant treatment.

Treatment of mycoplasmal infections in newborn infants deserves special consideration. Antibiotics are used at some point in most admissions to the neonatal intensive care unit and almost universally in the low-birthweight neonate because of the inability to clinically distinguish nonspecific aspects of respiratory distress of prematurity from systemic infection.

Although systemic ureaplasmal and mycoplasmal infections have been described that probably contributed to morbidity and even death in a relatively small number of neonates studied to date, there is very little experience on which to base treatment indications, choice of drug, expected outcomes, or potential complications. The single, most difficult issue to resolve is when antibiotics should be given to an infant from whom *U. urealyticum* or *M. hominis* is isolated.

Proven ability of mycoplasmas to induce inflammation in the lung and CSF and isolation from blood, CSF, pericardial fluid, and pleural fluid in pure culture are adequate justification for administering specific antimicrobial treatment in clinically ill neonates when the organisms are isolated from an affected site and when there are no other verifiable microbiologic etiologies of pneumonitis, meningitis, or nonspecific respiratory or other systemic problems typical of disseminated infection. Whether antibiotics should be administered to an infant with a positive CSF culture but in whom there is no evidence of inflammation (pleocytosis), progressive hydrocephalus, or other clinical illness is a contentious issue and probably should be handled on a case-by-case basis. However, the finding of any microorganism in a sterile body fluid, such as CSF, is by definition abnormal, and the natural history and potential long-term effects of such infections, if left untreated, have not been adequately studied. There is evidence that some neonates from whom *M. hominis* or *U. urealyticum* is isolated from the CSF in the absence of pleocytosis may spontaneously clear the organisms without antimicrobial intervention. Whether this clearance occurs commonly in the low-birthweight neonate has not been established. Since presumptive *M. hominis* or *U. urealyticum* infection often can be detected in the clinical laboratory within 24 to 48 hours after specimen collection, the neonatologist with mycoplasmal diagnostic facilities in-house may prefer to closely monitor the patient, repeat a lumbar puncture, reculture, and examine CSF for the presence of inflammation and organisms before committing to treatment with potentially toxic drugs in a neonate who is not clinically ill by the time initial culture results are known.

Clear-cut ureaplasmal pneumonia, with or without bloodstream infection, is adequate justification for therapeutic intervention, with appropriate microbiologic documentation whenever possible. Because of the problems in identifying pneumonia and assigning a microbiologic cause with certainty in the early neonatal period, some physicians are taking a less conservative approach and treating low-birthweight neonates from whom *U. urealyticum* is isolated from the lower respiratory tract and who have respiratory distress as evidenced by supplemental oxygen or ventilatory requirements. Such indiscriminate antibiotic use is without supportive data from large prospective studies to determine if there is a clear benefit in terms of either microbiologic efficacy in organism eradication or improved clinical outcome.

A few reports of clinical improvement have been described in critically ill infants infected with *U. urealyticum* who received antibiotics. However, a number of cases had fatal outcomes despite treatment, suggesting that the mortality of symptomatic neonates with systemic ureaplasmal infection may be high. The relative contribution of ureaplasmal infection to morbidity and mortality is difficult to interpret, since most cases have been either very low birthweight infants with multiple complications or infants with other clinical problems that would likely contribute to the poor outcome.

SELECTION OF ANTIMICROBIAL AGENTS

The susceptibility of *M. hominis* and *U. urealyticum* to some of the antimicrobial agents of choice for treating local or systemic infections can no longer be predicted with accuracy. Therefore, in vitro testing, which can be completed by reference laboratories in 3 to 5 days, can be valuable to guide therapy, particularly if potentially toxic drugs, such as a tetracycline or chloramphenicol, that may show variable susceptibility are considered. Other clinical settings in which susceptibility testing can be particularly important include patients in whom there is treatment failure or immunocompromise. Most of the time, a physician who has a patient with a suspected infection due to *M. hominis* or *U. urealyticum* will have to rely on empiric treatment pending results of microbiologic evaluations, if available.

There have been very few clinical trials evaluating antimicrobial treatment of genital mycoplasmal infections in pediatric patients or comparing drugs with one another. Therefore, treatment recommendations must be largely based on in vitro susceptibility data and limited case reports documenting microbiologic or clinical efficacy of individual drugs.

M. hominis and *U. urealyticum* are intrinsically resistant to many of the antimicrobial agents commonly used to treat pediatric infections, including sulfonamides, trimethoprim, rifampin, all beta-lactams, and other agents that impair synthesis of bacterial cell walls. Chloramphenicol often shows in vitro susceptibility and should be considered for CNS infections as an alternative to the tetracyclines. There are a small number of case reports of infants with meningitis due to either *M. hominis* or *U. urealyticum* successfully treated with chloramphenicol, but at least two reports of chloramphenicol treatment failures in infants with *M. hominis* meningitis have been described.

There have been no reports demonstrating clinical or microbiological efficacy of aminoglycosides despite occasional isolates showing susceptibility in vitro. Some neonates have remained culturally positive for *U. urealyticum* in the respiratory tract after treatment with aminoglycosides for other reasons. Therefore, these drugs are not recommended for use against mycoplasmas or ureaplasmas.

Tetracyclines have been the standard treatment for infections due to genital mycoplasmas in adults for many years, but within the past two decades, resistance has been described in 20% to 40% of *M. hominis* and 10% to 15% of *U. urealyticum* clinical isolates. Despite potential bone and tooth toxicity, doxycycline has been used successfully to treat neonatal CNS infections due to *M. hominis* and *U. urealyticum* when there was no other viable alternative. If an intravenous tetracycline is to be used, doxycycline is preferred because it is the best tolerated and achieves better concentrations in CSF than does tetracycline.

No naturally occurring strains of *M. hominis* have been reported as clindamycin resistant, but few studies testing large numbers of clinical isolates have been performed. Even though lincosamides are not drugs of choice for CNS infections, an infant with meningitis due to tetracycline-resistant *M. hominis* was successfully treated with clindamycin. Occasional clindamycin-susceptible strains of *U. urealyticum* occur, but the majority have minimal inhibitory concentrations (MICs) too high for this drug to be of clinical use.

Erythromycin remains the drug of choice for treatment of neonatal infections due to *U. urealyticum* that do not involve the CNS, and most isolates are at least intermediately susceptible, with MICs in the range of 0.125 to 2 μg/ml. Some cases of meningitis due to *U. urealyticum* have responded to intravenous erythromycin or a combination of erythromycin and chloramphenicol, even though macrolides do not usually achieve appreciable concentrations in CSF.

Optimal dose and intervals for administration of erythromycin in neonates have not been firmly established. Erythromycin lactobionate given in doses of 40 mg/kg/d in four doses divided at 6-hourly intervals to a small group of preterm neonates with respiratory infection due to *U. urealyticum* resulted in serum concentrations that exceeded the MICs and eradicated the organisms at least transiently in most instances. Concentrations in the lung may exceed those in serum.

Ototoxicity in adults, cardiac arrhythmias, and thrombophlebitis in neonates have been associated with the use of intravenous erythromycin. We observed no difference in the occurrence of abnormal hearing screens in preterm neonates who were given erythromycin when compared with matched neonates who had not received the drug. Cardiotoxicity and thrombophlebitis appear to be related to the rate of infusion of the drug. Administering each dose over 60 minutes should reduce the occurrence of these events. Neonates given erythromycin who are concurrently receiving theophylline should be monitored for the possibility of increased theophylline levels.

Clarithromycin and azithromycin have now been approved for pediatric use and are available in oral suspension but not intravenous formulations. Both of these drugs have in vitro activity equivalent or superior to erythromycin against *U. urealyticum* but have not been

TABLE 1. Treatment of Pediatric Infections Caused by *Mycoplasma hominis* and *Ureaplasma urealyticum*

DRUG	ROUTE	DOSE/kg/24 h	COMMENT
Standard Treatments			
Doxycycline	PO, IV	4 mg loading dose day 1, then 2–4 mg in 1–2 doses	Contraindicated in children <8 y of age unless no other alternative; if giving IV, infuse over 60 min to prevent thrombophlebitis
Erythromycin	PO	20–50 mg in 3–4 doses	Ineffective for *M. hominis*
	IV	25–40 mg in 4 doses	Infuse over 60 min to prevent thrombophlebitis and minimize risk of cardiac toxicity; may elevate serum theophylline concentrations
Clindamycin	PO	10–25 mg in 3–4 doses	Ineffective for *U. urealyticum*
	IV	10–40 mg in 3–4 doses	
		For neonates, do not exceed 15–20 mg in 3–4 doses	
Chloramphenicol	PO	Inappropriate	
	IV	50–100 mg in 4 doses	Frequent monitoring of hematologic parameters and blood levels of the antibiotic are necessary
		For neonates up to 2 weeks of age, use 25 mg in 1 dose, thereafter 50 mg in 1 dose	
Alternative Treatments			
Azithromycin	PO	1 g single dose	Ineffective for *M. hominis;* use for urogenital infections
	IV	Not available	
Ofloxacin	PO, IV	600–800 mg in 2 doses	Use for urogenital infections; not approved for use in persons under 18 y

evaluated in clinical trials for use in infections specifically due to this organism in children. Azithromycin has been approved for use in nongonococcal urethritis due to *chlamydia trachomatis.* Preliminary studies have shown it works as well clinically as doxycycline in adult women infected with *U. urealyticum. M. hominis* is resistant to both azithromycin and clarithromycin.

Some of the fluoroquinolones are active in vitro against *M. hominis* and to a lesser extent against *U. urealyticum.* They have the advantage of being active against tetracycline-resistant strains. Ofloxacin, in particular, has shown promise in the clinical setting when used in treatment of urethritis in males and uncomplicated PID in females. This class of antimicrobial agents is not approved for use in persons under 18 years of age because of the occurrence of arthropathies and osteochondrosis in experimental animals.

Once a decision to treat for a suspected or confirmed infection due to either *M. hominis* or *U. urealyticum* has been made, a drug can be selected from those listed in Table 1. In general, a course of therapy for a minimum of 10 to 14 days or longer is recommended, with the exceptions of azithromycin and ofloxacin for uncomplicated urogenital infections. Sexual partners of adolescents should be treated if the condition is sexually transmissible (i.e., urethritis).

Most neonates, particularly those born preterm, with clinically significant local or systemic infection due to genital mycoplasmas will require an intravenous formulation of antimicrobial because of the potential seriousness of the infection and frequent contraindications for administration of oral medications. Physiologic and metabolic processes of neonates, particularly those born preterm, undergo rapid changes during the first few weeks of life, resulting in differing clinical pharmacology of antimicrobial agents from those of older infants, children, and adults. Thus, doses and intervals must be adjusted accordingly when there are data to support and direct such changes (Table 1).

Septic arthritis, osteomyelitis, bacteremia, abscesses, wound infections, or other conditions in immunosuppressed children or adults warrant the use of parenteral drugs, at least initially. Persons with hypogammaglobulinemia who have septic arthritis due to either *M. hominis* or *U. urealyticum* are particularly prone to relapse and may require intravenous treatment followed by oral medication for weeks or months, despite apparent in vitro susceptibility. Because of the difficulty in eradicating mycoplasmas in compromised hosts and the potential development of resistance, simultaneous treatment with more than one antimicrobial may be warranted. Adjunctive treatment with antiserum prepared specifically against the mycoplasma in ques-

tion may be of benefit in recalcitrant cases. Irreversible joint and bone destruction may result if the infection is not treated aggressively. Follow-up cultures of the infected site should be obtained when possible to ensure the eradication of organisms, particularly if there is a poor response to treatment. Uncomplicated urogenital infections in otherwise healthy sexually active adolescents usually can be managed with oral antimicrobials.

REFERENCES

1. Cassell GH, Waites KB, Crouse DT: Mycoplasma infections. *In* Remington J, Klein J (eds): Infectious Diseases of the Fetus and Newborn Infant, 4th ed. Philadelphia, WB Saunders, 619–655, 1995.
2. Furr PM, Taylor-Robinson D, Webster ADB: Mycoplasmas and ureaplasmas in patients with hypogammaglobulinemia and their role in arthritis: Microbiologic observations over twenty years. Ann Rheum 53:183–187, 1994.
3. Waites KB, Sims PJ, Crouse DT, et al: Serum concentrations of erythromycin after intravenous infusion in preterm neonates treated for *Ureaplasma urealyticum* infection. Pediatr Infect Dis J 13:287–293, 1994.

RICKETTSIAL INFECTIONS

J. STEPHEN DUMLER, M.D.

Human rickettsial diseases of pediatric importance in the United States include Rocky Mountain spotted fever (RMSF), murine typhus, and ehrlichiosis. Documented cases of Q fever, other spotted fever group rickettsioses, and imported rickettsioses, such as Mediterranean spotted fever or scrub typhus, are rarely recognized in pediatric patients in the United States. The etiologic agents of these diseases are classified as rickettsiae because they are obligate intracellular bacteria and may inhabit an arthropod as part of their life cycle. Concepts of phylogenetic grouping are evolving for the rickettsiae. Generally, however, three genera contain important pathogens: the genus *Rickettsia,* with *Rickettsia rickettsii,* which causes RMSF, and *Rickettsia typhi,* which causes murine typhus, the genus *Ehrlichia,* with *Ehrlichia chaffeensis* as the agent of ehrlichiosis, and *Coxiella burnetii,* the only member of its genus and the agent of Q fever. Most of these bacteria are transmitted via an arthropod vector, ticks for RMSF and ehrlichiosis and fleas for murine typhus, except for Q fever, which is usually acquired by inhalation. Because of the low frequency of some rickettsial infections in the United States pediatric population, this discussion focuses on RMSF, ehrlichiosis, murine typhus, and Q fever.

ROCKY MOUNTAIN SPOTTED FEVER AND MURINE TYPHUS

Clinical Features

The presentation of the vasculotropic rickettsioses is often similar, and differentiating among RMSF, murine typhus, and other rickettsial infections may depend on history and specific serologic tests. Each presents as a nonspecific febrile illness, with abrupt onset of fever frequently associated with severe headache and myalgias. Gastrointestinal or respiratory features may be evident in up to 50% of patients, and evidence of central nervous system (CNS) infection may be found in a small percentage. Laboratory evidence of mild to moderate hepatitis, renal dysfunction, mild to profound leukopenia and thrombocytopenia, hyponatremia, and hypoalbuminemia may be present. A maculopapular rash often develops in pediatric patients with rickettsial infections and often precedes a petechial rash in RMSF. The rash may occur late or be absent. Thus, absolute dependence on rash as a diagnostic clue is dangerous. If untreated, the illness may persist for 3 weeks or longer, and fatalities may occur. Increasing morbidity and mortality are associated with delayed diagnosis and treatment. Therefore, antimicrobial therapy must be instituted based solely on clinical suspicion in most cases, since serologic confirmation may be made only in convalescence.

Treatment

Therapy for RMSF and murine typhus requires administration of either tetracycline, doxycycline, or chloramphenicol (Table 1). Because the use of tetracyclines in children is associated with a dose-dependent tooth discoloration and since RMSF may present with significant signs and symptoms of meningitis, chloramphenicol is often advocated for patients under 9 years of age. However, the infrequent development of severe or fatal chloramphenicol-associated aplastic anemia and the low therapeutic/toxic ratio make therapy with this agent less desirable. In fact, a recent survey has shown that the case-fatality rate in patients treated with chloramphenicol alone was significantly higher than in those treated with tetracycline alone and was similar to the case fatality rate of untreated patients. On balance, since RMSF and murine typhus may be severe or fatal and because of the suspect inefficacy of and increasing concern over side effects of chloramphenicol, tetracycline and doxycycline appear to be the most rational choices. The efficacy of fluoroquinolones for RMSF and murine typhus has not been evaluated by clinical trials, but ciprofloxacin has been used successfully in at least one patient with murine typhus. Combination trimethoprim-sulfamethoxazole therapy is contraindicated and may worsen the course of vasculotropic rickettsial disease. Specific therapeutic regimens are as follows: tetracycline 25 to 50

mg/kg/d PO divided into four doses or 15 to 25 mg/kg/d IV, chloramphenicol 50 to 75 mg/kg/d divided into four doses or 50 mg/kg/d IV. Doxycycline has been effective when administered to adults as 100 mg PO twice daily, although intravenous preparations are now available and may be useful for therapy of severe disease in children. Therapy should be continued for a minimum of 5 days total and until the patient is afebrile for at least 2 to 4 days, since relapse occurs in a small percentage of all cases, especially in those in whom therapy was initiated very early in the course of illness. With this regimen, febrile patients will often become afebrile within 48 hours, and the total length of therapy is usually 5 to 10 days.

In severely hypotensive patients or in those with severe end-organ dysfunction, intensive supportive care with attention to intravascular volume, including hemodynamic monitoring, may be necessary to avoid precipitating iatrogenic pulmonary edema. Severe CNS infection has been treated with corticosteroids to diminish cerebrovascular inflammation and edema, although no controlled studies evaluating this therapy have been performed. Too often, diagnosis and therapy are delayed such that the accumulated vascular damage leads to progressive clinical illness despite appropriate therapy.

EHRLICHIOSIS

Clinical Features

Recently recognized in the United States, ehrlichiosis is a tickborne infection that may affect both children and adults. Although similar in clinical presentation to the vasculotropic rickettsioses, ehrlichiosis is caused by a newly described rickettsial pathogen of mononuclear cells, *Ehrlichia chaffeensis,* or by an *Ehrlichia* closely related to *Ehrlichia equi,* which infects granulocytes. Ehrlichiosis closely mimics RMSF in history and physical examination, although rash is less frequent and rarely becomes petechial. Clinical clues for diagnosis include the laboratory findings of moderate leukopenia associated with thrombocytopenia and moderately elevated hepatic transaminases in a febrile, tick-exposed patient. As in RMSF, the diagnosis is clinical, and confirmation is mostly serologic. The observation of infected cells in peripheral blood is rare. Fatal and asymptomatic infections are known to occur in children. Severe infection may be linked to delayed diagnosis and therapy.

Treatment

As for RMSF, both tetracycline and chloramphenicol have been used, but many untreated patients recover spontaneously. Ill patients treated with either of these drugs have a more rapid clinical response than those treated with alternate therapeutic regimens. However, *E. chaffeensis* is not susceptible to chloramphenicol in vitro, a finding that supports several case reports in which clinical response with this antimicrobial was not achieved. Rifampin is effective in vitro, but no information about therapy in patients is available. Thus, tetracycline and doxycycline are the only antimicrobial agents that can be advocated for therapy of ehrlichiosis (Table 1). Intensive support may be required for severe infections with hypotension and organ failure. Vasculitis is not the underlying pathologic lesion, but increased vascular permeability is present and mandates careful titration of fluid balance. Dosing and length of therapy with tetracycline and doxycycline are the same as recommended for RMSF.

Q FEVER

Q fever is a febrile zoonosis transmitted by inhaling aerosols containing *Coxiella burnetii,* an obligate intracellular bacterial pathogen of mononuclear phagocytes. The strongest epidemiologic link associates parturient farm animals or pet cats with human infection. Although currently considered within the classification for rickettsiae, *C. burnetii* is in a distinct phylogenetic grouping. Likewise, the clinical features and therapeutic approach differ. Illness is uncommon in children, but infection may present in several different forms. Acute Q fever may occur as an undifferentiated febrile illness, pneumonitis,

TABLE 1. Therapy for Rocky Mountain Spotted Fever, Murine Typhus, and Ehrlichiosis*

DRUG	DOSE		
Rocky Mountain Spotted Fever and Murine Typhus			
Tetracycline	25–50 mg/kg/d	PO	4 doses
	15–25 mg/kg/d	IV	
Doxycycline (adults)	200 mg/d	PO	2 doses
Chloramphenicol	50–75 mg/kg/d	PO	4 doses
	50 mg/kg/d	IV	
Ehrlichiosis			
Tetracycline	25–50 mg/kg/d	PO	4 doses
	15–25 mg/kg	IV	
Doxycycline	4–5 mg/kg/d	PO	2 doses
	4 mg/kg	IV	

*Therapy should be continued for a minimum of 5 days total and until the patient is afebrile for at least 2–4 days; ensure compliance with PO regimens

or granulomatous hepatitis, and manifestations of chronic infection include endocarditis and meningoencephalitis. Acute infection is rarely recognized while it is active and often subsides without specific therapy. Chronic Q fever, especially endocarditis, may be indolent and progressive, associated with high mortality, and difficult or impossible to treat adequately. The clinical syndromes are not specific, but the inability to establish a microbiologic diagnosis may suggest consideration of Q fever, and specific serologic tests may confirm the impression.

Treatment

The goals of therapy and, thus, the choice of agents for acute and chronic Q fever differ. Bacteriostatic effects of doxycycline, tetracycline, rifampin, and fluoroquinolones arrest *C. burnetii* growth and shorten the course of illness in acute infection. The efficacy of other antimicrobials, such as chloramphenicol, erythromycin, combination trimethoprim-sulfamethoxazole, and cephalosporins, is controversial, and the use of these agents is not advocated. Therapy for acute infection is advocated for 3 weeks to completely eradicate the bacteria. Despite years of therapy with drugs effective in acute Q fever, chronic Q fever is characterized by relapses and persistence. In adults, doxycycline or tetracycline with or without a fluoroquinolone may suppress the infection, but therapy for an indefinite period may be needed. Recent trials of combined antimicrobials and agents, such as chloroquine, that alkalinize the phagolysosome in which *C. burnetii* resides have shown promise to improve the efficacy of doxycycline for chronic Q fever. Effective therapy for children or transplacental infection in neonates is uncertain. Therapy of chronic Q fever endocarditis may require more than 3 years. Removal of infected valves or prosthetic devices may improve hemodynamics, but it is unclear whether surgical intervention aids in cure.

PREVENTION OF VECTORBORNE RICKETTSIOSES AND EHRLICHIOSIS

Careful inspection for ticks is important, since transmission requires tick attachment for several hours. Clothing that covers exposed extremities and the use of tick repellents may aid in decreasing tick exposure. Embedded ticks should be removed promptly with forceps by firmly grasping the tick mouthparts and steadily retracting the intact tick from the skin. The surface should be cleansed with a topical antibacterial. Ticks removed in this manner may be infectious and should not be handled or squashed. Fleaborne murine typhus can be prevented only by methods that entail environmental control of fleas in the vertebrate hosts that harbor these arthropods. Household pesticide treatment and eradication of fleas on infested pets diminishes potential exposures. However, other flea-bearing animals that have adapted to suburban and urban life continue to pose control problems. Since Q fever is a risk for immunosuppressed or debilitated patients or patients with preexisting cardiac valvular damage, infection in at-risk individuals may best be prevented by avoiding exposure to farm animals. However, a subset of urban dwellers have acquired infection without known epidemiologic exposure. No effective vaccines are available for *R. rickettsii*, *R. typhi*, or *E. chaffeensis*. It must be emphasized that recovery from RMSF and murine typhus requires development of active immunity. Thus, the rickettsiostatic drugs, such as tetracycline and chloramphenicol, must not be used as prophylaxis after tick or flea bite.

ASCARIS LUMBRICOIDES

BASIL J. ZITELLI, M.D.

Ascaris lumbricoides is the largest roundworm infecting humans and grows to a length of 25 to 30 cm. It is estimated to cause the most prevalent helminth infection, affecting an estimated 1 billion people. Despite the availability of effective therapy, nearly 20,000 people worldwide die annually from ascariasis.

Ascaris infection is prevalent in tropical and temperate climates where poor sanitation leads to fecal contamination of water, fruits, and vegetables with *Ascaris* eggs. It is endemic in some parts of the southeastern United States, Puerto Rico, and especially underdeveloped countries where human feces is used as fertilizer. Although people of all ages are affected, young children who are exposed more often to contaminated soil and have greater hand-mouth activity are affected most frequently. *Ascaris* eggs can survive extreme cold and drying, may be resistant to chemical disinfectants, and are not readily destroyed by sewage treatment. Eggs can be destroyed by direct exposure to sunlight for 12 hours and are killed by exposure to temperatures over 40°C.

Ascaris infection usually is acquired by ingestion of embryonated eggs from contaminated water or food sources. Eggs hatch in the upper small intestine, yielding larvae that penetrate the intestinal mucosa and enter the capillary lymphatic and venous circulation. Larvae pass through the portal system, through the right heart, and into the lungs. They then penetrate the pulmonary capillary bed and enter alveoli, ascend the respiratory tree, and are swallowed when reaching the glottis and oropharynx. Maturation of larvae to adult worms occurs in the small intestine. Female worms produce a prodigious number of eggs—up to 200,000 eggs per worm per day—over their lifespan of 1 year. Eggs are passed into the feces in an unembryonated, noninfective state. Under conditions of warm, moist soil, eggs embryonate in 3 weeks and remain infective for several months. The entire cycle from ingestion to the mature worm takes approximately 2 months.

Infection with *Ascaris* usually is inapparent in most patients until the worm burden increases beyond 15 to 20 worms. The most common complaint is abdominal pain, which can progress to intestinal obstruction with a large number of worms. Pulmonary symptoms frequently are absent, although fever, cough, wheezing, and dyspnea associated with pulmonary infiltrates and marked peripheral blood eosinophilia can occur. Less commonly, aberrant migration provoked by such stimuli as fever, certain drugs, or general anesthetics can lead to biliary obstruction and pancreatitis. Children who are malnourished may be at greater risk for nutritional failure with *Ascaris* infection, since the worm secretes antitrypsin, competes for dietary protein, and induces fat and carbohydrate malabsorption.

Diagnosis of ascariasis is made by finding characteristic eggs in feces. This is not difficult because of the large number of eggs produced by the female and their distinctive appearance.

Treatment of *Ascaris* infection generally involves either pyrantel pamoate (Antiminth) or mebendazole (Vermox) (Table 1). Pyrantel pamoate is given as a single dose of 11 mg/kg of body weight (max 1 g for both children and adults). Its formulation as 50 mg/ml allows convenient dose calculation at 1 ml of pyrantel pamoate per 4.5 kg

TABLE 1. Drug Treatment for *Ascaris lumbricoides* Infection

DRUG	FORMULATION	DOSE
Pyrantel pamoate (Antiminth)	Solution: 50 mg/ml	11 mg/kg as single dose or 1 ml/10 lb (max: 1 g, 4 teaspoons)
Mebendazole (Vermox)	Tablets: 100 mg	100 mg b.i.d. for 3 days for both children and adults
Piperazine citrate	Solution: 500 mg/5 ml	75 mg/kg single daily dose for 2 days (max: 3.5 g/d)
	Tablets: 250 mg	

(10 lb) body weight up to a maximum of 4 teaspoons. Uncommon side effects of gastrointestinal disturbance, headache, rash, and fever may occur.

Mebendazole is administered as a 100-mg tablet given twice daily for 3 days for adults and children. This therapy may be preferred if a coinfection with *Trichuris trichiura* exists. Diarrhea and abdominal discomfort may accompany therapy. Mebendazole should be used with caution in children under 2 years of age and pregnant women.

Piperazine citrate is recommended when intestinal obstruction due to *Ascaris* occurs. When given in a single daily dose of 75 mg/kg (max: 3.5 g/d) for 2 days, the bolus of worms is paralyzed and relaxed and may be passed without surgical intervention.

CYSTICERCOSIS

LOUIS M. WEISS, M.D., M.P.H.
MURRAY WITTNER, M.D., Ph.D

The pork tapeworm, *Taenia solium,* is one of the most common tapeworms of humans. Infection with its larval form, *Cysticercus cellulosae,* is a common cause of CNS disease in endemic areas. When humans or hogs ingest mature eggs, the embryos hatch (stimulated by gastric juice, intestinal enzymes, and bile), enter the circulation, and are transported throughout the body. They then enter and encyst in striated muscle and other tissues, where in 10 to 11 weeks they become infected larvae, termed *Cysticercus cellulosae.* Cysticerci are bladderlike cysts in which an inverted scolex has developed. Symptomatic disease can result when these larvae become encysted in the CNS, eye, or heart. Often, symptoms occur when the cysts die and are believed to be due to the host inflammatory response and the loss of osmoregulatory ability of the cyst.

Human infection with cysticerci is found wherever adult *T. solium* infection is common. Thus, human cysticercosis is often encountered in Mexico, South and Central America, Africa, India, and parts of China. In Mexico, autopsy studies have demonstrated this parasite in 3.5% of the population. Although the usual onset of symptoms is within 7 years of acquiring the infection (median incubation period of 3.5 years), symptomatic disease with cysticerci has occurred in patients who have been out of endemic areas for 30 years. In some cases, disease has occurred within 6 months of exposure.

The clinical manifestations depend on the number and anatomic localization of the cysts and the inflammatory response of the host. Cysticerci have been found in almost every tissue and organ of the body. Except in eye lesions, the cyst often provokes the development of a fibrous capsule. Cerebral cysticercosis may remain asymptomatic for years, with symptoms becoming evident only on the death of the cyst due to the resultant inflammatory response. Such CNS lesions often result in seizures and, in endemic areas, may be the leading cause of seizure disorders. In some endemic areas, injury due to falling from cysticerci-related seizures is a major public health problem. If a cysticercus is located in the ventricles, noncommunicating hydrocephalus can occur, and, rarely, a ball valve mechanism causing sudden blockage and syncope can occur. In the basilar cisterns, cysts can cause communicating hydrocephalus and cranial nerve palsy. Racemose forms may occur in this location and have a poor prognosis. Heavy cyst burdens may be associated with dementia and personality changes. Ocular cysticerci can manifest as disturbances of vision, scotoma, free floating parasites in the vitreous, or retinal detachment. In some cases, the retinal lesion has been misdiagnosed as a retinoblastoma, and the eye has been enucleated. Rarely, myositis may also develop, although skeletal muscle involvement is usually asymptomatic.

In any person with CNS manifestations who is from an endemic area, the diagnosis of CNS cysticercosis should be entertained. CT scanning will demonstrate active cysts, with edema, old calcified cysts, or hydrocephalus in 70% to 80% of cases. Magnetic resonance imaging (MRI) may be more sensitive to active lesions with edema but is less sensitive to old calcified lesions. No comparative trials are available that determined the more useful imaging modality. Calcified cysticerci often can be seen by roentgenographic examination, and multiple, comma-shaped or arclike calcifications in the brain or soft tissues is suggestive of cysticercosis. Careful physical examination may reveal subcutaneous cysticerci that can be biopsied for diagnosis. In selected patients, for example, those with hydrocephalus or aseptic meningitis, myelography to demonstrate extraventricular cysts may be useful.

Lumbar puncture is useful in that serologic studies can be performed on the CSF and will aid in the diagnosis. In addition, the presence of an active meningitic profile in the CSF is an indication to treat the infection. CSF eosinophilia is present in some cases. Hypoglycorrhachia to levels as low as 2 mg/100 ml is seen.

Serologic studies are useful in the diagnosis of this infection. Specimens of both CSF and serum should be examined in suspected cases. Recently, a western blot technique replaced the IHA and ELISA tests as the diagnostic test of choice. The western blot technique has eliminated the previous problems of cross-reactivity with *Echinococcus.* The reported sensitivity and specificity of western blot are 98% and 99% or more, respectively. In the setting of an isolated cyst, the sensitivity of the test may be lower. These tests are available from the Centers for Disease Control and Prevention.

Even though the yield is low, patients with cysticercosis should have stool examinations for *T. solium.* In some cases, family members should also be screened. Heavy CNS infections may be due to autoinfection in children harboring adult *T. solium.*

With the advent of praziquantel, treatment of CNS cysticercosis changed dramatically. Praziquantel at 50 mg/kg/d in three divided doses for 14 days has been shown in controlled studies to be successful in reducing the number of cysts and in the reduction of CNS symptoms. However, severe reactions to this therapy from the death of the cysticerci and subsequent host inflammatory response have been reported. For this reason, treatment is indicated only in patients with symptomatic neurologic disease, active meningitis, or hydrocephalus. Ocular cysticercosis is a contraindication to therapy. Steroids should be administered to reduce inflammation (but have been reported to cause lower serum levels of praziquantel). Prednisone should be given 1 to 3 mg/kg/d, starting 2 to 3 days before therapy and continuing for the course of treatment. Praziquantel is of no benefit when all of the cysticerci are calcified. As the natural history of an isolated cyst is benign, there is debate about the use of praziquantel in this setting. However, many authorities now recommend treatment of such patients. Patients with seizures should continue on anticonvulsants during treatment, although prophylactic anticonvulsant therapy is not needed after instituting antiparasitic treatment.

Alternative drugs with reported success in CNS cysticercosis are albendazole 15 mg/kg for 10 to 30 days, metrifonate 7.5 mg/kg for 5 days, and flubendazole. Metrifonate has also been reported to be effective for ocular disease. In many parts of the world, albendazole has replaced praziquantel as the drug of choice for cysticercosis. Recent studies suggest that it is more effective than praziquantel, with fewer severe reactions and a greater resolution of cysts on follow-up. In a Brazilian study of 28 days of drug treatment for neurocysticercosis, albendazole use resulted in the disappearance of 85% of cysts, and praziquantel caused the disappearance of 60%. In addition, anecdotal data suggest that albendazole has efficacy in racemose disease. Steroids are used with albendazole in the same dose as those used with praziquantel but are reported to elevate serum levels of albendazole. Cimetidine also elevates serum albendazole levels. Albendazole is available as an investigative drug in the United States from Smith Kline Beecham (1[800]366-8900, ext. 5291). It may soon be available by prescription.

Patients with hydrocephalus often require shunts. If intraventricular cysts are present, shunt obstruction may occur. This can be treated by simple ventriculostomy, with removal of the cysts. Resection of parenchymal cysts should be reserved for intractable seizures unresponsive to medical therapy in order to remove an epileptic focus. Basilar cistern adhesions may require lysis if the optic chiasm is involved, with visual compromise.

Prevention of this infection is the same as for any fecal-oral-transmitted parasite.

AMEBIASIS

MICHAEL KATZ, M.D.

Amebiasis, the third leading cause of death due to parasite infections, is a potential multisystem infection, which is most often limited to the intestinal tract. The causative agent, *Entamoeba histolytica*, has a worldwide distribution and affects some 500 million individuals. Disease develops in only a small fraction of those infected. Symptomatic individuals may have nonspecific diarrhea, dysentery associated with ulcerations of the colon, or invasion of organs, such as liver, lungs, and brain.

The infectious form of the organism is the cyst, which allows the ameba to survive inclement environments for months to years. The invasive organism is the trophozoite. Humans become infected by ingestion of the cysts in food or drink. The ingested cyst, which contains four nuclei, is partially digested in the small intestine, and the liberated organism divides to produce eight trophozoites.

DIAGNOSIS

Amebiasis should be suspected in an individual whose diarrheal symptoms have been protracted, in all those who have bloody diarrhea, including patients with the putative diagnosis of idiopathic ulcerative colitis, and in those who have a liver abscess, unexplained pulmonary densities, or space-occupying lesions in the brain. Male homosexuals are at increased risk for amebiasis. Diagnosis depends on microscopic examination of the stools and on serologic tests. The test most frequently used is the indirect hemagglutination test. The most precise tests are countercurrent electrophoresis and enzyme-linked immunosorbent assay (ELISA). All are available in specialized regional laboratories and at the Centers for Disease Control and Prevention (CDC). An experimental ELISA test, based on the detection by monoclonal antibodies of an adherence protein antigen in the serum and stool, appears to be helpful in distinguishing amebic infections with a pathogenic strain from those that are not pathogenic.

CLASSIFICATION

If the diagnosis of amebiasis is made, the condition should be classified as follows: asymptomatic or mild disease (simple but protracted diarrhea), severe intestinal disease (dysentery, usually representing ulceration of the colon), or extraintestinal disease (hepatic abscess or invasion of other organs).

TREATMENT

Although in areas where amebiasis is endemic and the probability of a reinfection is high, asymptomatic infections tend to be left untreated, elsewhere any infection deserves therapy. Asymptomatic infection needs to be treated with a luminal amebicide, such as iodoquinol 40 mg/kg/d in three divided doses for 20 days. The adult dose of 1950 mg/d should never be exceeded because *iodoquinol, given in excess, can result in subacute myelooptic neuritis, an irreversible condition.* However, given as recommended, the drug causes no undesirable side effects. Mild intestinal disease is treated in the same manner.

All other cases of amebiasis, from the severe intestinal disease to the extraintestinal invasive disease, are treated with metronidazole 40 mg/kg/d in three divided doses for 7 days, not exceeding the max-

imum daily adult dose of 2250 mg/d. This drug has been shown to be carcinogenic when given in very high doses to experimental animals, and in concentrations approximating ordinary doses, it is mutagenic to bacteria. It is prudent, therefore, not to prescribe it to pregnant women, especially in the first trimester. The severity of the disease, however, may force its use in life-threatening conditions. Metronidazole has an effect similar to that of disulfiram, in that it interferes with the metabolism of alcohol. Patients taking this drug should be cautioned against ingesting alcohol in any form, including cough medications. Although metronidazole has not been officially approved for use in children, it has been used widely in pediatric patients throughout the world. Other related nitroimidazole drugs, such as ornidazole and tinidazole, have been used abroad.

After completion of treatment with metronidazole, the patient should be given a course of iodoquinol, as previously described, because metronidazole does not always eradicate amebae from the colonic lumen. Cases of severe extraintestinal amebiasis that have not responded to metronidazole should be treated with dehydroemetine, which is available only from the CDC, at a dose of 1.5 mg/kg/d in two divided doses IM for 5 days (max: 90 mg/d). This drug is cardiotoxic and can cause arrhythmias and even asystole.

PREVENTION

Prevention of the disease depends on being careful of what one ingests. Boiling of food or water kills the amebic cysts. Filtration removes them, but chemical disinfection does not.

REFERENCES

1. Abd Alla MD, Jackson TF, Gathiram V, et al: Differentiation of pathogenic *Entamoeba histolytica* infections from nonpathogenic infections by detection of galactose-inhibitable adherence protein antigen in sera and feces. J Clin Microbiol 31:2854–2850, 1993.
2. Guerrant FL: The global problem of amebiasis: Current status, research needs, and opportunities for progress. Rev Infect Dis 8:218–227, 1986.
3. Jain NK, Madan A, Sharma TN, Sharma DK, Madhana RG: Hepatopulmonary amoebiasis: Efficacy of various treatment regimens containing dehydroemetine and/or metronidazole. J Assoc Phys India 38:269–271, 1990.
4. Nazir Z, Moazam F: Amebic liver abscess in children. Pediatr Infect Dis J 12:929–932, 1993.

ENTEROBIASIS

MICHAEL KATZ, M.D.

Enterobius vermicularis, the human pinworm, is ubiquitous. Moreover, it is found equally in children of all socioeconomic classes. Its life cycle is simple. Adult worms live in the rectum. At night, when the body temperature drops, they emerge on the perianal skin, lay eggs, and die. The eggs, which tend to irritate and cause itching—rarely, it can be quite severe—are picked up by the scratching fingers and are thus later transmitted into the mouth. Swallowed eggs release larvae in the small intestine, and the larvae migrate into the colon, mature there into adult worms, and begin the cycle anew. The period from swallowing an egg to the maturation of the worm is approximately 2 weeks. Occasionally, a pinworm makes its way into the vagina, where it eventually dies. In the interim, it can cause vaginal itching. Because the eggs are very light, they readily float in the air and can be inhaled into the mouth and then swallowed. Thus, intrafamilial spread is likely.

It is important to note that only a minority of infected children experience severe itching. Most have minor symptoms or none at all. Although a variety of other symptoms have been attributed to this infection, for example, grinding of teeth and enuresis, only itching is its established manifestation. It is important to emphasize that the presence of pinworms is no reflection of poor hygiene of the household. The rate of reinfection is very high because of the high prevalence of the infection and frequent contacts among children.

The diagnosis is made by observation of threadlike worms on the perianal skin. It is confirmed by a low-power microscopic examination of a plastic transparent adhesive tape that has been applied to the perianal skin first thing in the morning and then stuck onto a glass slide. The presence of the characteristic eggs confirms the diagnosis.

Treatment consists of a single administration of pyrantel pamoate at 11 mg/kg or a single oral dose of 100 mg of mebendazole (irrespective of weight). Either treatment is effective. The drug should be administered for the second time 2 weeks after the initial treatment to kill those worms that may have hatched from eggs swallowed after that time because neither drug acts on the eggs. Itching in the vagina is self-limited and can be treated only symptomatically.

Prevention is unlikely because of the ease of transmission of this infection.

SCHISTOSOMIASIS

CHRISTOPHER L. KING, M.D., Ph.D.

Human infection with several species of schistosomes may result in significant morbidity in the gastrointestinal tract and liver. Furthermore, mortality due to the subsequent hemodynamic changes in the portal circulation and liver failure is considerable. Infection is usually acquired in endemic areas early in life as children experience contact with freshwater bodies that contain the infective cercariae. Peak prevalence and intensity are generally seen in young adults 15 to 20 years of age, whereas disease sequelae may be seen in association with a peak intensity of infection or later in life. Gastrointestinal and liver disease are caused by infection with either *Schistosoma mansoni* or *Schistosoma japonicum*. In the far east, the less prevalent *Schistosoma mekongi* resembles *S. japonicum* infection and disease. There is controversy whether liver disease may occur in *Schistosoma haematobium* infection. For individuals from nonendemic areas, such as the United States, exposure to infection usually occurs during visits overseas. Infection acquired overseas should be preventable if proper travel advice is given. There is, however, a segment of our population that may be unable to avoid infection, such as those involved in military operations overseas.

Infection with *S. mansoni* is endemic in the northern area of South America, in some Caribbean countries, and in rural areas of Puerto Rico. It is also prevalent in most African countries and all through the Middle East. *S. haematobium* is found throughout much of Africa and in the Middle East, often in the same areas as *S. mansoni*. Principal areas endemic only for *S. haematobium* are upper Egypt, northern and central Sudan, the coastal areas of Kenya and Tanzania, and western Angola. In contrast, *S. japonicum* is limited in its geographic distribution to China, the Philippines, and Indonesia. *S. mekongi* is found in sporadic foci in Southeast Asia.

EPIDEMIOLOGY

The epidemiology of schistosomiasis in nonendemic areas, such as North America and Europe, differs from its features in endemic communities. Individuals (usually adults) from nonendemic areas are exposed to infection because of lack of understanding of its mode of transmission. Contact with freshwater bodies in endemic areas, whether stationary, slow moving, or fast flowing, is the source of transmission. This mode of transmission results in infection of individual travelers or, rarely, a group traveling together, most of whom have had no previous exposure. Under such circumstances, the disease sequelae have a characteristic pattern. Invariably, these manifestations occur on return to the nonendemic area, thus providing a diagnostic and management challenge to an unfamiliar medical profession. Oc-

casionally, several individuals are exposed simultaneously, resulting in a miniepidemic presenting with the acute manifestations of disease.

CLINICAL FEATURES

Infection with *S. mansoni* or *S. japonicum* may result in gastrointestinal or hepatic disease or both. These manifestations are seen in association with the established chronic stages of infection. Since most infections are asymptomatic, disease manifestations are only appreciated in a small group of infected individuals, who usually are young people with heavy infection or with genetic susceptibility. In contrast, individuals from nonendemic areas often present early with signs and symptoms related to acute schistosomiasis. Physicians in North America, Europe, and other nonendemic areas may encounter disease due to established infection in immigrants and rarely in individuals who have had casual exposure.

The gastrointestinal tract is affected pathologically in most infected individuals. Eggs of *S. mansoni* are deposited mainly in the veins of the inferior mesenteric system, whereas those of *S. japonicum* are usually seen in the distribution of the superior mesenteric vein. Granuloma formation, subsequent scarring, and occasionally colonic polyposis are the main pathologic features. Clinically, infection may be associated with nonspecific symptoms, such as crampy abdominal pain, diarrhea, and passage of blood with stools. In most epidemiologic studies in endemic areas, it has been difficult to prove the specificity and causality of these symptoms. Colonic polyposis is a specific syndrome described in Egypt but not in other *S. mansoni* endemic areas. Similar lesions have been described in China in association with *S. japonicum* infection. Colonic polyposis may cause bleeding, but its association with colorectal carcinoma is not known. In individuals with chronic infection and portal hypertension due to liver fibrosis, portosystemic varices may develop at the lower end of the esophagus and rectum and around the umbilicus (caput medusa). Esophageal varices may cause considerable bleeding, which may be the first serious manifestation of hepatic schistosomiasis and its hemodynamic sequelae.

In cases of moderate or heavy exposure, an acute febrile reaction can occur lasting for several days to weeks (Katayama fever). This is most often seen with *S. japonicum* infection and less often with *S. mansoni*. Although rarely reported, similar acute episodes may occur with *S. haematobium* infection. The fever occurs at the time of egg deposition and results from immune complex formation between the antigens of the egg and adult worms with the rapidly rising antibody levels.

Liver disease in schistosomiasis mansoni or japonica represents the major pathologic effect. Schistosome eggs are carried by portal blood flow and are trapped at the presinusoidal level. They are encircled with granulomas, finally causing fibrosis and its hemodynamic sequelae. The first manifestation of liver disease is hepatomegaly, which may be seen in most individuals with heavy infection, as well as in others. Decompensation occurs late in the course of disease, or it may result from additional insults from viral infections or nutritional deficiencies that lead to hepatic encephalopathy. Portal hypertension is related to presinusoidal obstruction, which results in congestive splenomegaly, ascites (in late stages), and the development of portosystemic varices. Evaluations of these patients may demonstrate normal hepatic wedge pressure. In the late stages of liver disease, enlargement of the organ may not be detected because of extensive fibrosis. In most of these patients, extensive splenomegaly, esophageal varices, and ascites may be appreciated. Portal hypertension and even cirrhosis can be observed in children, especially in areas with high transmission where infection is acquired early in life.

DIAGNOSIS

Eggs in the stool *(S. mansoni, S. japonicum,* and *S. mekongi)* or in the urine *(S. haematobium)* are diagnostic. A direct stool smear of 1 to 2 mg of feces often misses lightly infected individuals. A Kato thick smear, which uses 20 to 50 mg of feces, is much more sensitive. In *S. haematobium* infestation, a spun sediment of at least 10 ml of urine should be examined for ova. The sensitivity of urine can be increased by obtaining the specimen at midday after light exercise. The absence of peripheral eosinophilia or of elevated serum IgE levels in a potentially infected individual from a nonendemic area makes the diagnosis of schistosomiasis unlikely.

MANAGEMENT

Individuals suspected of having schistosomal gastrointestinal or hepatic disease should be fully evaluated for geographic history, as well as duration and intensity of infection. A thorough physical examination and laboratory evaluation are mandatory. The chemotherapy of schistosomiasis has undergone tremendous development with the discovery of several effective oral compounds. Praziquantel is the drug of choice. For *S. mansoni* and *S. haematobium* infection, 40 mg/kg body weight as a single PO dose is recommended. For *S. japonicum* infection, the dose is increased to 60 mg/kg body weight given in divided doses. The side effects of praziquantel are minimal and do not usually interfere with the delivery of the drug to individual patients. Praziquantel administration will result in parasitologic cure in approximately 80% of cases and will induce an approximately 95% to 99% decrease in egg counts. When the drug is given to adolescents and young adults, it induces reversal of the pathologic lesions and regression of the hepatomegaly. In patients with chronic sequelae, specific chemotherapy does not reverse pathologic lesions. Patients with portal hypertension, esophageal varices, or liver failure are treated with the standard surgical and medical regimens. Care should be taken in prescribing immediate surgical intervention for the first bleeding episode from esophageal varices. These patients usually tolerate several episodes of bleeding without the development of hepatic encephalopathy. Since surgery is associated with major complications and does not reverse the pathologic sequences, it should be reserved for selected cases of recurrent bleeding. The recent introduction of a transhepatic intraportal percutaneous shunt (TIPS) may offer a less invasive approach in dealing with the consequences of portal hypertension.

Prevention and control of schistosomiasis are a complex medical, social, and economic problem. For the individual who is traveling to an endemic area, avoiding contact with freshwater bodies is sufficient. No other practical protective measure exists. For communities in endemic areas, determination of the goal of control is essential. When control programs were attempted to eradicate infection, very little success was achieved. A more realistic goal may be reduction in transmission and morbidity.

REFERENCES

1. Acute schistosomiasis: Clinical, diagnostic and therapeutic features. Rev Inst Med Trop Sao Paulo 35:399–404, 1993.
2. Adams L, Soulen MC: TIPS: A new alternative for the variceal bleeder. Am J Crit Care 2:196, 1993.
3. Anderson RM, May RM: Infectious Disease of Humans: Dynamics and Control. Oxford, Oxford University Press, 1991.
4. King CH, Mahmoud AAF: Drugs five years later: Praziquantel. Ann Intern Med 110:290, 1989.

TOXOCARA CANIS

PETER J. HOTEZ, M.D., Ph.D.

Human toxocariasis results from the accidental ingestion of eggs of the canine ascarid, *Toxocara canis*. The eggs are shed in the feces by dogs that harbor the adult worms. In the United States, young puppies have particularly high infection rates with the adult stage of *T. canis*. Consequently, human infection is usually associated with either intimate dog contact or with playing in sandboxes and play-grounds contaminated with dog feces. Both the habit of geophagia and having a litter of puppies in the home are risk factors for acquiring human toxocariasis.

The ingestion of *T. canis* eggs can result in either one of two distinct disease syndromes in children: visceral larva migrans (VLM) and ocular larva migrans (OLM).

VISCERAL LARVA MIGRANS

VLM is primarily a disease of toddlers and young children between 1 and 4 years of age. Each *T. canis* egg that is ingested by a young child releases a larva, which invades the intestinal mucosa and migrates through viscera before dying. Organ damage occurs initially as the invading larvae cause mechanical destruction. This phase is followed by a vigorous host eosinophilic inflammatory response to the dying larvae. The hallmark of VLM is, therefore, pneumonitis, hepatitis, and cerebritis that result from larval migrations through the lung, liver, and brain, respectively. These children present typically with fever, hepatomegaly, and pulmonary infiltrates accompanied by wheezing. Seizures and neuropsychiatric disturbances are common. In contrast, ocular involvement is not a common finding in patients with VLM. The major laboratory findings include a leukocytosis with eosinophilia and hypergammaglobulinemia. The diagnosis is usually made on the basis of clinical and laboratory findings in association with an enzyme-linked immunoassay, which measures serum antibody against antigens that are released from *T. canis* (available from the Centers for Disease Control and Prevention).

Since a large component of the symptomatology of VLM occurs because of the host inflammatory response to dead and dying larvae, there is controversy about the role of specific anthelmintic chemotherapy. Some cases are self-limited, and an anthelmintic could theoretically exacerbate the inflammatory response by killing large numbers of larvae. Others argue, however, that anthelmintic administration will limit further larval migrations and, therefore, prevent further damage.

In the past, the drugs of choice for the treatment of VLM have been either diethylcarbamazine (Hetrazan) 6 mg/kg/d in three divided doses for 7 to 10 days or thiabendazole 50 mg/kg/d (max: 3 gs/d) in two divided doses for 5 days. Both of these drugs are well absorbed and achieve therapeutic levels in the tissues, but they are associated with a number of toxicities. Thiabendazole commonly causes vertigo, nausea, and crystalluria and has been implicated as a cause of Stevens-Johnson syndrome. Diethylcarbamazine often causes hypersensitivity reactions in infected patients.

Some newer information suggests that agents of the benzimidazole class may offer promise in the therapy of VLM. Albendazole (Zentel) 10 mg/kg/d in two divided doses for 5 days was shown in a limited therapeutic trial of 34 patients with VLM and OLM to be as effective as thiabendazole in achieving clinical improvement (as judged by resolution of symptoms and eosinophilia) but caused somewhat fewer reactions.[3] Another benzimidazole, mebendazole, was used to successfully treat a case of adult toxocariasis.[1] High doses were administered (1 g three times daily for 21 days), presumably to overcome the poor absorption of this drug. The benzimidazoles are embryotoxic and teratogenic in experimental animals and have not been extensively tested in children less than 2 years of age in the United States. However, in at least one anecdotal report from Papua, New Guinea, many thousands of children were treated with mebendazole and albendazole, with no side effects[2] (Table 1). An entirely different class of anthelmintic agent, ivermectin (Mectizan) may also offer promise for the treatment of VLM.

Patients frequently develop allergic hypersensitivity symptoms either before or during anthelmintic therapy. For these patients, corticosteroids can be administered (e.g., methylprednisolone). If signs of severe respiratory distress develop, the child may also require treatment with epinephrine, nebulized beta-adrenergic agents, diphenhydramine, or theophylline. Thiabendazole can prolong the metabolism of theophylline preparations and cause theophylline toxicity.

TABLE 1. Specific Anthelmintic Chemotherapy for VLM/OLM*

DRUG	DOSE
Thiabendazole	50 mg/kg/d (max: 3 g/d) in 2 divided doses for 5 days
Diethylcarbamazine	6 mg/kg/d in 3 divided doses for 7–10 days
Albendazole†	10 mg/kg/d in 2 divided doses for 5 days
Mebendazole†	1 g t.i.d. for 21 days (adults)

*Specific anthelmintic chemotherapy frequently requires the coadministration of corticosteroids, sometimes in association with beta-adrenergic agents or theophylline (thiabendazole can raise theophylline to toxic levels).

†The benzimidazoles are associated with fewer toxicities but are teratogenic and embryotoxic in experimental animals and have not been extensively tested in young children.

No information is available about the newer benzimidazole agents with theophylline or other antihypersensitivity drugs.

OCULAR LARVA MIGRANS

In contrast to VLM, which is primarily a disease of very young children, OLM typically occurs in older children between the ages of 5 and 10 years. For unknown reasons, larval invasion in these children is restricted primarily to the subretinal space, where they elicit posterior pole and peripheral pole granulomas. Vitreous inflammation also can occur, resulting in a chronic endophthalmitis. There is little evidence for systemic involvement, and, consequently the child with OLM does not usually have an eosinophilia nor does he always have elevated antibody titers to *T. canis* antigens (the ELISA is often negative). Instead, children with OLM will often present initially with unilateral vision loss and a strabismus (frequently an exotropia). On fundoscopic examination, they have peripheral and posterior pole retinal lesions, sometimes accompanied by a diffuse endophthalmitis or a papillitis. The diagnosis is usually made by the ophthalmologist, who can identify the characteristic retinal granulomas or vermiform tracks.

Several medical and surgical treatment modalities have been proposed for the treatment of OLM. For patients with tractional macular detachment, improvements have been observed following vitrectomy. Improvement with steroids and thiabendazole has been observed in some patients but not in others. Systemically administered thiabendazole has been shown to enter the aqueous and vitreous of a minimally inflamed eye. This frequently is administered as adjunct chemotherapy in association with surgery. It is not known whether better results will be obtained with the newer benzimidazole agents. Decisions for optimal therapy in these patients should always be carried out in consultation with an ophthalmologist.

REFERENCES

1. Bekhti A: Mebendazole in toxocariasis. Ann Intern Med 28:24–28, 1984.
2. Biddulph J: Mebendazole and albendazole for infants. Pediatr Infect Dis J 9:373, 1990.
3. Sturchler D, Schubarth P, Fualzata M, Gottstein B, Ottli A: Thiabendazole vs. albendazole in treatment of toxocariasis: A clinical study. Ann Trop Med Parasitol 83:473–478, 1989.

TRICHINOSIS

JOSE IGNACIO SANTOS, M.D.
JOSE LUIS ROMERO, M.D.

Trichinosis is a systemic disease caused by the presence of the larvae of the tissue nematode, *Trichinella spiralis*, in skeletal muscle, heart, brain, and gastrointestinal tract of the susceptible host. Humans acquire trichinosis by the ingestion of undercooked meat, generally pork, containing viable, encysted *Trichinella* larvae. After ingestion, these larvae hatch in the intestine and mature into adults, which in turn produce and release larvae that invade the intestinal wall and enter the bloodstream, ultimately encysting in skeletal muscle cells.

Although trichinosis was common in the United States up until a few decades ago, autopsy studies reveal a marked decrease in parasitism from 16% to less than 1% in recent years. The same is true in Mexico, where trichinosis is reported only sporadically and is generally associated with outbreaks related to improperly cooked pork sausage.

The clinical manifestations of trichinosis correlate with the load of larvae in tissues and the degree of the host's allergic response to them, which may range from asymptomatic to fatal. The incubation period from the time of the ingestion of the infected meat also correlates with the number of viable larvae ingested. This may be as short as 2 days but generally ranges from 5 to 15 days.

STAGES OF DISEASE

There are three stages of disease:

- Intestinal
- Muscle
- Convalescent

The intestinal stage is associated with diarrhea, pain, nausea, and vomiting but may be asymptomatic.

Muscle invasion is the second stage, in which edema of the eyelids and face is the most consistent finding. Other features include fever, myalgias, weakness, and eosinophilia. Myocarditis is the most frequent and serious complication, and patients with 100 to 5000 larvae per gram of tissue may die from involvement of the heart between 4 and 8 weeks after infection. Abnormal electrocardiographic findings have been reported in up to 20% of cases of acute trichinosis.

The convalescent stage, which begins after the second month, is marked by continued myalgias and muscle weakness in untreated individuals.

DIAGNOSIS

From a laboratory standpoint, eosinophilia is the most common finding. Muscle enzymes, such as aldolase and creatine phosphokinase, commonly are elevated. Because antibody titer rises do not occur until 3 weeks into the illness, serologic studies with indirect immunofluorescence, enzyme-linked immunosorbent assay (ELISA), or the bentonite flocculation test may help to confirm the diagnosis but are not useful in the management of severely ill patients. Similarly, although there is a commercially available skin test antigen, the skin test becomes positive after the third week. Biopsy of a tender muscle often reveals *Trichinella* larvae under low-power microscopic magnification.

TABLE 1. Therapy for *Trichinella spiralis* Infection

DRUG	PEDIATRIC DOSE
Prednisone (for severe symptoms)	1–2 mg/kg/d
Thiabendazole	25 mg/kg b.i.d. for 5 d
Mebendazole	5 mg/kg/d for 5 d

TREATMENT (Table 1)

Although various drugs are active against the adult parasites in the intestinal tract, no drug has been shown to be effective in controlled clinical trials against circulating and encysting larvae. The drug of choice for treating the intestinal parasite and, thus, for helping to reduce the number of larvae reaching the circulation is thiabendazole (Mintezol). Thiabendazole also has some activity against the larvae in muscle, and its anti-inflammatory activity may produce symptomatic relief by reducing the fever and the inflammatory response. Thiabendazole doses have not been standardized for adults or children, and the dose regimen approved by the U.S. Food and Drug Administration makes no adjustment for weight or age. The dose commonly recommended for children is 25 mg/kg twice daily for 5 days.

Mebendazole (Vermox) also has activity against circulating and encysting larvae, making it a useful alternative. It may become the future drug of choice. The dose recommended by the World Health Organization for children is 5 mg/kg/d for 5 days. Simultaneous administration of prednisone (1 to 2 mg/kg/d) may prevent the paradoxical worsening of symptoms (Herxheimer reaction) associated with the initial phases of therapy in acute trichinosis.

Corticosteroids at pharmacologic doses may also be used in patients with severe central nervous system or myocardial involvement but should never be used alone because that may intensify the disease.

BABESIOSIS

Trenton K. Ruebush II, M.D.

Babesiosis is a tickborne disease of wild and domestic animals caused by intraerythrocytic protozoan parasites of the genus *Babesia*. Several species of *Babesia* can infect humans. The majority of human infections in the United States have been caused by *Babesia microti*, a parasite of mice, and have been acquired on islands off the coast of New England and the nearby mainland. Babesiosis can be transmitted by blood transfusion.

B. microti infections are usually asymptomatic or mild, with fever, chills, myalgia, and fatigue. More severe infections with hemolytic anemia, jaundice, and respiratory distress have been observed in patients with previous splenectomies, in older persons, and in immunocompromised patients. Symptomatic infections in children are uncommon, although several severe infections in infants have been reported. Parasitemia may persist for several months, and clinical manifestations are often more severe than might be expected by the level of parasitemia.

Since *B. microti* infections are generally self-limited, symptomatic therapy is recommended in most cases. Based on studies in animals and limited experience in human beings, the most effective treatment available for severe infections appears to be clindamycin 20 mg/kg/d PO, IV, or IM in four divided doses (max: 600 mg every 6 hours) and quinine sulfate 25 mg/kg/d PO in three divided doses (max: 650 mg every 8 hours) for 7 days (Table 1). Chloroquine, which is frequently used in the initial treatment of these cases because of the morphologic similarity of *B. microti* and *Plasmodium falciparum*, has no effect on the parasite. Exchange blood transfusion has been used with success in several asplenic patients with severe illnesses, but this technique should be considered only when more conservative therapy has failed.

TABLE 1. Drug Treatment for Babesiosis

DRUG	DOSE
Clindamycin *plus*	20 mg/kg/d PO, IM, or IV q.i.d.
Quinine sulfate	25 mg/kg/d PO t.i.d. for 7 d

GIARDIASIS

Michael Katz, M.D.

Giardia lamblia is a flagellate with worldwide distribution. Although it is a pathogen of humans, it is also capable of infecting other mammals, notably beavers, which act as a reservoir. Infection is acquired by ingestion of binucleate cysts, which are lysed in the small intestine, releasing two trophozoites. These line the villi and can lead to a malabsorption syndrome, characterized by villous atrophy and manifest clinically as protracted, severe diarrhea. The disease can be so overwhelming that the affected person spends most of the day defecating. Although the infection can be sporadic, affecting only a few individuals, it often appears in epidemic forms as a result of community exposure to water contaminated by *Giardia* cysts. Sporadic infection can also be acquired by ingestion of food contaminated with these cysts. There is evidence suggesting that deficiency of secretory IgA predisposes to infection and leads to a more protracted disease than that experienced by individuals with normal IgA levels. Children in day care centers, those in institutions for mentally retarded, and male homosexuals have an increased incidence of giardiasis. A majority of those infected with *Giardia* are free of symptoms, and there is no apparent need to treat them.

Diagnosis depends on identification of the organism. Direct microscopic examination of the stool will detect about half of those infected. Use of the so-called string test is more reliable in that it has few false negative results. This test entails swallowing a capsule containing a small sponge, which adsorbs the organism from the duodenal mucosa, attached to a string. By pulling the string, one removes the sponge, which is then applied to a microscope slide, and the slide is examined for the organism. An alternative to direct visualization of the organism is a capture ELISA test, which is commercially available, to detect *Giardia* antigen in the stools. A refinement of this test—still experimental—employing monoclonal antibodies against two different epitopes of the parasite apparently can distinguish between symptomatic and asymptomatic infections.

Treatment is not wholly satisfactory because there are failures with each of the available drugs. The most effective drug is quinacrine hydrochloride administered PO at 6 mg/kg/d in three divided doses for 5 days (max: 300 mg/d). The drug tends to irritate the stomach and is best taken after a meal. It can cause nausea and, in excessive doses, can intoxicate to the point of a transient psychosis, and it can cause transient yellow discoloration of skin. When used correctly, however, it is the drug of choice, affording cure rates approaching 90%. Metronidazole, one of the nitroimidazoles, is an alternative drug used at 15 mg/kg/d in three divided doses PO for 5 days. (See cautionary notes about this drug in the section on amebiasis.) Albendazole 400 mg/d for 3 to 5 days is an acceptable alternative to metronidazole. In one study, it had a 97% cure rate. A more palatable drug for children is furazolidone, administered PO at 6 mg/kg/d in three divided doses for 7 days. Its cure rate is much lower, and it has the disadvantage of being considerably more expensive than either of the other drugs, but its palatability makes it more attractive for children. Drug resistance has been reported recently, but failures of therapy can usually be overcome by treatment with an alternative drug.

The infection can be prevented by avoidance of drinking contaminated water or food. Chemical treatment of water does not eradicate cysts, but boiling or filtration does.

REFERENCES

1. Hall A, Nahar Q: Albendazole as a treatment for infections with *Giardia duodenalis* in children in Bangladesh. Trans R Soc Trop Med Hyg 87:84–86, 1993.
2. Ungar BL, Yolken RH, Nash TE, et al: Enzyme-linked immunosorbent assay for the detection of *Giardia lamblia* in fecal specimens. J Infect Dis 149:90–97, 1984.
3. Upcroft JA, Upcroft P, Boreham PF: Drug resistance in *Giardia intestinalis*. Int J Parasitol 20:489–496, 1990.

4. Vinayak VK, Dutt P, Mehta S: Uses and limitations of monoclonal antibodies to *Giardia lamblia*-specific 66-kDa copro-antigen in copro-immunodiagnosis of giardiasis. FEMS Immunol Med Microbiol 6:37–44, 1993.

MALARIA

COY D. FITCH, M.D.

Malaria is an ancient and well-understood disease for which there has been adequate treatment for several centuries. Cinchona bark, a source of quinine, was introduced by American Indians to the Jesuits, who then introduced it in Europe more than three centuries ago. Nevertheless, the disease continues to be a major threat to people who live in tropical and subtropical areas. *Each year, malaria infects over 250 million people, and over 1 million children die from the disease.* Efforts have been made to eradicate the disease by controlling mosquitoes, but those efforts have been unsuccessful.

MECHANISM OF INFECTION

Of the more than 100 species of malaria parasites, only four naturally infect human beings: *Plasmodium malariae, Plasmodium vivax, Plasmodium ovale,* and *Plasmodium falciparum.* These protozoan parasites have two hosts, human beings and female anophelene mosquitoes of several species. The parasites undergo sexual reproduction in the mosquito, and the progeny (sporozoites) are infectious for the human host when injected by the bite of the mosquito. In human beings, the parasite reproduces asexually, first in the liver and then in erythrocytes. As part of the erythrocytic stage, female and male gametocytes are produced and are available for ingestion by mosquitoes, thus allowing the life cycle to be repeated.

The periodic chills and fever of malaria coincide with the asexual, erythrocytic reproduction of parasites and probably result from the release of toxic substances when erythrocytes more or less synchronously rupture to release their broods of new parasites (merozoites). *P. vivax, P. ovale,* and *P. falciparum* produce a typical periodicity of chills and fever of 48 hours (tertian). For *P. malariae,* the typical interval is longer, 72 hours (quartan). *P. vivax, P. ovale,* and *P. malariae* usually cause self-limited disease if the patient remains untreated, although relapses or recrudescences may occur after long periods of time. In fact, patients infected with *P. malariae* may harbor parasites for decades and transmit them when they donate blood for transfusion. In the case of *P. vivax,* it is well established that the liver stage of the parasite persists asymptomatically and gives rise to multiple recrudescences many weeks or months after the initial attack. *P. falciparum* does not persist in the liver stage, but it is the parasite that causes severe disease, including death.

Early in the course of malaria, the characteristic periodicity of chills and fever may not be present, and the disease may easily be mistaken for influenza or another febrile illness. Indeed, *P. falciparum* infections often fail to produce tertian chills and fever before the parasitemia is so great that there is extensive morbidity with central nervous system (CNS) symptoms (cerebral malaria) or acute respiratory distress. Therefore, a travel history may be the key to early diagnosis of malaria in nonendemic areas. Once suspected, malaria usually can be diagnosed by examining Giemsa-stained thick and thin blood films. An experienced examiner can identify the species of malarial parasite from the blood film. Other diagnostic tests are available but are not in general clinical use.

Not only is *P. falciparum* the most virulent malaria parasite for human beings, but also it has a propensity to develop resistance to antimalarial drugs, including chloroquine, quinine, and pyrimethamine. Chloroquine resistance has been reported from most countries endemic for *P. falciparum.* In Southeast Asia and South America, the phenomenon is widespread. Fortunately, the parasites usually are not totally resistant, and parasitemia can be suppressed by chloroquine, quinine, mefloquine, or halofantrine. Recently, chloroquine-resistant *P. vivax* infections also have been reported, mostly from Papua, New Guinea. The other two species of malaria parasites show relatively little tendency to develop drug resistance.

TREATMENT

The best antimalarial drugs fall into three classes: (1) quinoline derivatives and related drugs (which include quinine, chloroquine, mefloquine, and halofantrine), (2) dihydrofolate reductase inhibitors, and (3) sulfonamides. The latter two classes show synergism against malaria when combined, as in Fansidar, which includes 25 mg of pyrimethamine and 500 mg of sulfadoxine in each tablet. Certain other antimicrobials, including tetracycline, erythromycin, lincomycin derivatives, and fluoroquinolines, have antimalarial activity, but they are relatively slow to act and otherwise are not superior to the other drugs in our armamentarium. Because of the threat of drug-resistant *P. falciparum,* several potential new antimalarials are under development, the most promising of which is the Chinese drug ginhaosu (artemisine).

Chloroquine is still the drug of choice for large areas of the world, including West Africa. It is given orally in four doses over a 3-day period to achieve a total dose of 20 to 25 mg of the base per kilogram of body weight. Approximately 300 mg of chloroquine base is contained in a 500-mg chloroquine phosphate tablet. For older children and adults, the maximum recommended dose of chloroquine base is 600 mg in the first dose, 300 mg 6 hours after the first dose, and 300 mg on each of the next 2 days. For young children, the dose should be kept on the low side because these patients are especially susceptible to chloroquine toxicity. Other drugs closely related to chloroquine (quinacrine, amodiaquine, hydroxychloroquine) may be used if chloroquine is not available.

When chloroquine-resistant *P. falciparum* is suspected, quinine sulfate, mefloquine hydrochloride (Lariam), or halofantrine hydrochloride (Halfan) may be used, despite the fact that the parasite may have a low level of cross-resistance to these drugs. The dose of quinine is 20 mg/kg of the salt daily for 10 to 14 days. This dose is divided into three parts and taken orally after meals. The maximum dose of quinine for older children and adults is 650 mg of the salt three times daily for 10 to 14 days.

The therapeutic dose of mefloquine is 15 to 25 mg/kg of the base as a single PO dose. The maximum recommended dose of mefloquine is 1250 mg. The therapeutic dose of halofantrine is 8 mg/kg of the base every hour for three doses. This dose is repeated after 7 days for nonimmune patients.

In addition to quinine, mefloquine, or halofantrine, Fansidar may be added to the treatment regimen. For adults, the dose of Fansidar is two to three tablets as a single dose; for children 9 to 14 years of age, two tablets; for children 4 to 8 years of age, one tablet; and for children under 4 years of age, one-half tablet. If Fansidar cannot be used because of hypersensitivity, one of the antimicrobials mentioned earlier may be added.

When the patient is gravely ill, as with cerebral malaria or acute respiratory distress syndrome from *P. falciparum,* and cannot take oral medication, quinine or quinidine intravenously is the drug of choice. Each drug is a stereoisomer of the other and is approximately equally potent as an antimalarial agent. Each carries significant risk when used intravenously, and its use by this route can be justified only in emergencies.

The IV dose of quinine is 20 mg of the base per kilogram per day. One third of this dose, not to exceed 600 mg of the base, is diluted in 200 ml or more of normal saline and infused slowly over a period of 4 hours. These infusions may be repeated at 8-hour intervals only for as long as the patient is unable to take oral medication. During the use of intravenous quinine or quinidine, the patient should be monitored for hypoglycemia, hypotension, cardiac arrhythmias, and neurologic toxicity.

If the patient has a prior history of intravascular hemolysis associated with the use of quinine, parenteral chloroquine may be used instead of quinine. An initial dose of 3.5 mg/kg of the base is administered IM. This dose may be repeated at 6- to 12-hour intervals, but the total daily dose of chloroquine base IM should not exceed 10 mg/kg. Alternatively, a continuous IV infusion of 0.83 mg of chloroquine base per kilogram per hour may be used for up to 30 hours. Overdosage with chloroquine may produce respiratory depression, cardiovascular collapse, shock, convulsions, and death, especially in infants and children. As soon as possible, therefore, oral treatment should be started, through a stomach tube, if necessary, and supplemental therapy with Fansidar or an alternative antimicrobial should be instituted.

Because the sporozoites of *P. vivax*, *P. ovale*, and possibly *P. malariae* may persist in the liver for long periods of time, it is necessary to eradicate them to achieve a complete cure (radical cure). For this purpose, the therapeutic armamentarium is limited to one drug, primaquine. Chloroquine, quinine, and the other drugs used to treat the erythrocytic stage are ineffective against the liver stage. To achieve a radical cure, in addition to the standard treatment with chloroquine, primaquine phosphate is given in a daily dose of 0.3 mg of the base (approximately 0.5 mg of the salt) per kilogram for 14 days. The maximum dose for older children and adults is 15 mg of the base (26.5 mg of the salt) daily for 14 days. It is not necessary to use primaquine to treat infections with *P. falciparum* because this parasite does not persist in the liver.

Side Effects from Antimalarials

In addition to the toxicities that have already been mentioned, each of the antimalarial drugs has side effects. For example, chloroquine may cause pruritus in blacks, and in very large amounts (prolonged use with a cumulative dose exceeding 100 g), it may cause retinal damage.

Quinine and quinidine may cause cinchonism (tinnitus, headache, visual disturbances, nausea) and sometimes severe gastrointestinal, neurologic, and cardiovascular symptoms. Primaquine may cause oxidative hemolysis of glucose-6-phosphate dehydrogenase (G-6-PD)-deficient erythrocytes. Pyrimethamine may cause megaloblastic anemia. Mefloquine may cause nausea and dizziness and, infrequently, psychoses and convulsions. Halofantrine prolongs the QT interval and may cause cardiac arrhythmias.

Finally, sulfonamides may cause the Stevens-Johnson syndrome or a serum sicknesslike syndrome. Severe toxicities are relatively unusual, however, except for the oxidative hemolysis provoked by primaquine in susceptible individuals.

PREVENTION OF MALARIA

International travelers to areas endemic for malaria should receive advice on how to avoid mosquito bites and on chemoprophylaxis of malaria. Because anopheline mosquitoes primarily feed at night, travelers are advised to wear clothing covering most of the body, stay indoors, or use mosquito nets at night. A mosquito repellent, such as *N,N*-dimethylmetatoluamide (DEET), may also be helpful.

Recommendations for chemoprophylaxis of malaria are difficult and change frequently because consideration must be given to the increasing geographic distribution of chloroquine-resistant *P. falciparum* and the toxicities of the available chemoprophylactic agents. Chloroquine is still the safest and most effective drug for malaria prophylaxis, although its use does not guarantee protection from chloroquine-resistant *P. falciparum*. When used prophylactically, chloroquine is taken in a single weekly dose of 5 mg/kg of the base, not to exceed 300 mg, beginning 1 week before travel and continuing for 4 weeks after leaving the malarious area. It is also prudent for the traveler to carry a single therapeutic dose of Fansidar to be taken if chills and fever occur and if medical help is not immediately available.

After travel to an area endemic for *P. vivax*, *P. ovale*, or *P. malariae*, it is prudent to recommend a course of treatment with

primaquine, as previously discussed, to eliminate the possibility of persistence of the parasites in the liver. The use of primaquine in this way should be limited to people who exhibit normal G-6-PD activity in the erythrocytes.

For travelers to areas where chloroquine-resistant *P. falciparum* is prevalent, mefloquine is the drug of choice. It is taken as a single weekly dose of 3 to 6 mg/kg, depending on weight, but should not exceed 250 mg, beginning 1 week before the travel and continuing for 4 weeks after leaving the malarious area. Mefloquine is not recommended for travelers with known hypersensitivity to the drug, for children under 30 pounds in weight, for pregnant women, for anyone involved in tasks requiring fine coordination and spatial discrimination, or for anyone with a history of epilepsy or psychiatric disorders.

Because the recommendations for malarial chemoprophylaxis change frequently, the physician giving advice to international travelers should keep abreast of the most current information. A country-by-country listing of the risk of malaria is published periodically in the *Weekly Epidemiological Record* by the World Health Organization, and recommendations from the CDC may be found in the *Morbidity and Mortality Weekly Report*. The CDC encourages consultation by maintaining a Hotline: phone number (404) 639-1610.

PNEUMOCYSTIS CARINII PNEUMONITIS

WALTER T. HUGHES, M.D.

Pneumonitis caused by *Pneumocystis carinii* is usually fatal if untreated. With specific antimicrobial therapy, about 75% of patients can be expected to recover if treatment is begun early. Because the infection usually occurs in immunocompromised patients and a definitive diagnosis requires an invasive procedure, such as bronchoalveolar lavage or open lung biopsy, management consists of close attention to complications from the underlying primary disease and the diagnostic procedures. Thus, associated or secondary viral, bacterial, or fungal infections may occur, and pneumothorax or pneumomediastinum may complicate the diagnostic procedure. Hypoxia with low arterial oxygen tension (Pao_2) is regularly present, whereas carbon dioxide retention is unusual and the arterial pH frequently is increased. Unlike other infections in the immunosuppressed host, *P. carinii* infection remains localized entirely to the lungs, with rare exception.

When *P. carinii* pneumonitis is recognized as the first illness of an infant or child, a careful search should be made for an underlying disease.

TREATMENT

Specific Therapy

Trimethoprim-sulfamethoxazole (TMP-SMZ)* and pentamidine isethionate are equally effective in the treatment of *P. carinii* pneumonitis, but TMP-SMZ is the drug of first choice because of its low toxicity.

TMP-SMZ may be given orally or intravenously. The PO dose is 20 mg trimethoprim and 100 mg sulfamethoxazole per kilogram per day divided into four parts at 6-hour intervals. It is advisable to give half of the calculated daily dose initially as a loading dose when the oral route is used. TMP-SMZ is available in tablet form (regular size with 80 mg trimethoprim, 400 mg sulfamethoxazole and as a double-strength tablet with twice these amounts). An oral suspension contains 40 mg trimethoprim and 200 mg sulfamethoxazole per 5 ml. The intravenous preparation is available in 5-ml ampules containing 80 mg trimethoprim and 400 mg sulfamethoxazole. Each 5-ml ampule

---

*Manufacturer's precaution: Not recommended for infants younger than 2 months of age.

must be added to 125 ml of 5% dextrose in water. The IV dose is 15 mg trimethoprim and 75 mg sulfamethoxazole per kilogram per day divided in three to four equal doses. Each dose is infused over a 60-minute period. From available data, peak serum levels of 3 to 5 µg/ml of trimethoprim and 100 to 150 µg/ml of sulfamethoxazole seem to be the optimal ranges.

The adverse and toxic side effects are essentially those of sulfonamides, and although they are uncommon, they include transient maculopapular rash, nausea, vomiting, diarrhea, neutropenia, agranulocytosis, aplastic anemia, megaloblastic anemia, hemolytic anemia, methemoglobinemia, Stevens-Johnson syndrome, allergic reactions, toxic nephrosis, and drug fever. Folic acid deficiency has occurred rarely. It is reversed by folinic acid 10 to 25 mg/d. Folinic acid does not interfere with the therapeutic effects of the drug. Patients with acquired immunodeficiency syndrome (AIDS) have a higher rate of adverse reactions than other patients.

Pentamidine is the drug of second choice because of its high frequency of adverse effects. Pentamidine is administered as a single daily IV dose of 4 mg/kg infused over a period of 1 hour for 10 to 14 days. If improvement is apparent after 5 days of treatment, this may be reduced to 3 mg/kg/d. The total dose should not exceed 56 mg/kg. The drug may also be given by intramuscular injection if use of the intravenous route is not possible. Intramuscular injections should be given deeply into the anterolateral aspect of the thigh because severe local reactions are common.

Adverse effects include induration, abscess formation, and necrosis at injection sites, nephrotoxicity, hypoglycemia or, rarely, hyperglycemia, hypotension, alteration in liver function, tachycardia, hypocalcemia, nausea and vomiting, skin rash, anemia, hyperkalemia, and thrombocytopenia.

Isolation

Animal studies indicate that *P. carinii* is transmitted by the airborne route. It is advisable to use respiratory isolation procedures to separate active cases of *P. carinii* pneumonitis from other compromised individuals at high risk for this infection.

Recently, a new hydroxynaphthoquinone compound, atovaquone, was approved by the FDA for the treatment of mild and moderate cases of *P. carinii* pneumonia in adults who cannot tolerate or who do not respond to TMP-SMZ. The dose for adults is 750 mg three times daily by mouth. The efficacy of this drug has not been studied in children. Limited pediatric studies suggest a dose of 40 mg/kg/d might provide adequate plasma concentrations for treatment. The only formulation currently available is a 250-mg tablet, but a suspension formulation is expected to be available in 1995.

Supportive Measures

Oxygen should be administered by mask as needed to maintain the PaO₂ above 70 mm Hg. The fraction of inspired oxygen (FIO₂) should be kept below 50 vol%, if possible, to avoid oxygen toxicity, since oxygen therapy usually is required for relatively long periods.

Assisted or controlled ventilation is indicated in patients with arterial oxygen tension less than 60 mm Hg at FIO₂ of 50% or greater. Those with acutely elevated PaCO₂, without pH changes and with or without hypoxemia should be considered candidates for ventilatory therapy.

Studies of adults with AIDS suggest that a corticosteroid, such as prednisone, given early in the course of patients with moderately severe *P. carinii* pneumonia (arterial-alveolar oxygen gradient of 35 mm Hg or greater) results in an improved survival rate. No detailed studies have been reported in children and non-AIDS patients. The dose recommended in patients older than 13 years of age with AIDS by an expert committee is prednisone 40 mg twice daily for 5 days and then 20 mg twice daily for 5 days, followed by 20 mg daily until the antimicrobial treatment is completed.

Fluid and electrolyte quantities are calculated by the patient's needs, but the solution should contain 5% or 10% glucose to help prevent hypoglycemia during pentamidine therapy. Metabolic acidosis must be corrected.

Bacterial pneumonia or sepsis may occur in association with *P. carinii* pneumonitis. In the seriously ill patient with marked neutropenia (absolute neutrophil count less than 500 mm³) or evidence of bacterial infection, antibiotics should be given.

Efforts should be made to improve the nutritional status of the patient by dietary means even during the acute stage of the disease. Multivitamins should be given empirically. The value of intravenous alimentation has not been determined.

A blood transfusion is given if the hemoglobin level is lower than normal. The hemoglobin content must be sufficient to result in an arterial oxygen content of 15 to 20 ml/dl of blood at an arterial oxygen tension of 100 mm Hg.

Pneumothorax may be a complication of the diagnostic procedures. If it is mild with no adverse effect on respiration, close observation is adequate. If it is more extensive, insertion of a thoracotomy tube with a water-seal drainage system is necessary.

Parameters to Monitor

1. Assess serum immunoglobulin. At the onset of the illness, administer immune serum globulin 0.66 ml/kg (165 mg/ml) if the immunoglobulin G level is below 300 mg/dl.
2. Perform roentgenograms of the chest daily until there is clinical evidence of improvement. If needle aspiration of the lung, lung biopsy, or endotracheal brush catheter technique has been used as a diagnostic procedure, chest roentgenograms should be obtained at 30 minutes, 4 hours, and 12 hours after the procedure to detect pneumothorax.
3. Determine hemoglobin, white blood cell count and differential, and platelets daily.
4. Measure body weight, intake, and output daily.
5. Measure arterial blood gases: pH, PaCO₂, PaO₂, and base excess or deficit initially and as often as necessary, according to the severity of the clinical course.
6. Measure serum electrolytes: sodium, chloride, potassium, and carbon dioxide content every 3 days or more frequently if indicated.
7. Monitor total serum proteins, albumin, and globulin every 3 days. Hypoalbuminemia may occur.
8. Monitor blood pressure, pulse, and respiratory rate every 4 hours or more often if the condition is critical.
9. For patients receiving pentamidine, check blood urea nitrogen (BUN), creatinine, and urine every 3 days. If the BUN exceeds 30 mg/dl or serum creatinine is greater than 1.5 mg/dl, withhold pentamidine for 1 or 2 days. Monitor blood glucose 4 to 6 hours after each injection of pentamidine. Administer glucose if the blood glucose value is less than 40 mg/dl. Monitor serum glutamic-oxaloacetic transaminase (SGOT) every 3 days, withhold pentamidine for 1 or 2 days if evidence of hepatic toxicity exists, and monitor the serum calcium and phosphorus every 3 days. If the serum inorganic phosphate level increases and the calcium level decreases from normal values on the basis of renal insufficiency, give calcium lactate 15 to 20 g/d or calcium carbonate 5 to 8 g/d PO. The diet should be low in phosphate, and 25,000 to 50,000 units of vitamin D are given PO. For patients with renal impairment who are receiving TMP-SMX, the dose should be regulated on the basis of serum drug levels. Measurement of serum levels of the sulfonamide is adequate. The level of free sulfonamide should be maintained with peak values between 100 and 150 µg/ml measured 2 hours after the oral dosage.

Experimental studies suggest that diaminodiphenylsulfone (dapsone), trimetrexate with leucovorin, sulfadoxine-pyrimethamine (Fansidar), primaquine-clindamycin, and atovaquone may be effective in *P. carinii* pneumonitis.

EXPECTED COURSE

Fever, tachypnea, and pulmonary infiltrates usually persist with little change for 4 to 6 days. If no improvement is apparent after a week of therapy, concomitant or secondary infection most likely exists. These infections have included bacterial pneumonia or sepsis, systemic candidiasis, aspergillosis, cryptococcosis, histoplasmosis, and cytomegalovirus inclusion disease, as well as other viral infections. *P. carinii* pneumonitis may recur several months after apparent recovery in 10% to 15% cases.

PREVENTION

P. carinii pneumonitis can be prevented by chemoprophylaxis with TMP-SMZ. The dose is one-fourth the therapeutic dose, 5 mg/kg of trimethoprim and 25 mg/kg of sulfamethoxazole per day in two divided doses. Protection is afforded only while the patient is receiving the drug. Aerosolized pentamidine has been found to be effective in preventing *P. carinii* pneumonitis in adults with AIDS. However, similar studies in children are lacking.

TMP-SMX prophylaxis is recommended for all who have had a prior episode of the pneumonitis, for HIV-seropositive patients 1 to 12 months of age regardless of CD4 lymphocyte counts, for those 1 to 5 years of age with counts less than 500/mm³, and for those 6 years of age and older with counts less than 200/mm³. HIV-indeterminate infants from 1 to 12 months of age should receive prophylactic therapy until they are proved to be uninfected. For patients 5 years of age or older who cannot tolerate TMP-SMZ, aerosolized pentamidine once or twice monthly is recommended. For those younger than 5 years of age, oral dapsone 0.5 mg/kg/d is prescribed.

TOXOPLASMOSIS

MARIAN G. MICHAELS, M.D., M.P.H.

Toxoplasma gondii is a ubiquitous parasite whose definitive host is the cat. Other animals and humans become infected when the organism is inadvertently consumed, inhaled, or transmitted with a blood transfusion or organ transplant. To understand prevention and treatment modalities, it is important to briefly review the natural life cycle of *T. gondii* and the diseases that occur with human infection.

LIFE CYCLE

The sexual phase of *T. gondii* occurs only in the intestinal tract of members of the cat family. An acute infection in a cat results in the shedding of millions of oocysts for several weeks. The oocysts, which can be stable in the environment for months to years, become infectious after sporulation, approximately 48 to 72 hours after being shed (at room temperature). Unintentional inhalation or consumption can occur when cleaning a kitty litter box or when playing or gardening in infected soil. The parasite can exist in humans or other animals in its extraintestinal forms: the tachyzoite and cyst forms. The tachyzoite form multiplies rapidly intracellularly and is carried by the blood and lymphatics to distant sites, where it develops into the latent cyst form. Whereas the tachyzoite can invade all mammalian cells, the dormant cyst form has a propensity for muscle, heart, and brain tissue. Other modes by which humans acquire infection include ingestion of undercooked meats containing the tissue cysts, organ transplantation, or blood transfusions. Congenital infection occurs when the organism crosses the placenta.

CLINICAL MANIFESTATIONS

In general, postnatally acquired infections are benign and without accompanying problems. Persons who develop associated symptoms usually have localized lymphadenopathy. Occasionally, disease is manifest by a mononucleosis syndrome of fatigue, fevers, sore throat, and lymphadenopathy. Immunocompetent hosts usually have a self-limited course, although rare instances of more severe manifestations, such as chorioretinitis, encephalitis, or hepatitis, have been documented. Serious disease occurs in two specific situations: infection of a developing fetus when a pregnant women undergoes primary

infection and reactivation or primary disease in an immunocompromised host.

Congenital Infection

Overall, approximately 50% of women who undergo a primary infection during pregnancy will transmit the parasite to the developing fetus. Timing of infection during the pregnancy is critical. Early in gestation, the risk of the parasite infecting the fetus is low, but it may lead to spontaneous abortion of the fetus or severe manifestations of infection (including the classic triad of hydrocephalus, chorioretinitis, and cranial calcifications). Late in gestation, as many as 90% of fetuses become infected, but disease at birth is minimal or absent. However, later manifestations, particularly development of chorioretinitis, prompt the consideration of treatment for even asymptomatic newborns.

Immunocompromised Hosts

Immunocompromised hosts can also have severe disease from either primary infection or reactivation of latent organisms. This has become a prevalent complication for patients with AIDS. Reactivated toxoplasmosis is the most common cause of neurologic disease in adult AIDS patients. Recently, transplacental infection with toxoplasmosis has been documented to occur after reactivation of infection in pregnant women with AIDS. The growing prevalence of HIV infection in women makes this an increasing concern.

Cardiac transplant recipients are at risk for severe toxoplasmosis because of the cyst's propensity for this organ. Unlike AIDS patients, these patients experience problems when they undergo a primary infection from the donor rather than reactivation disease. For this reason, pretransplant screening of donor and recipient blood for *Toxoplasma* antibodies is important. The seronegative recipient receiving a heart from a seropositive donor deserves prophylactic treatment and close observation.

TREATMENT

Pregnancy

Primary prevention of infection with *T. gondii* is essential. Seronegative pregnant women should be advised to avoid acquisition of *T. gondii* by not cleaning the kitty litter box, wearing gloves while gardening, and cooking meat thoroughly. Particular attention to good hygienic practices, such as washing fruits and vegetables before eating them and cleaning the chopping board after preparing meat dishes, also may help decrease transmission of *T. gondii*.

Congenital infection is almost always secondary to primary disease. Therefore, a healthy woman who is seropositive before becoming pregnant is not at risk for transmitting this parasite. Because primary infection can be asymptomatic, serial screening during pregnancy is the best way to determine whether an infection has occurred. The placenta, which is almost always infected, affords some protection for the fetus, allowing time for early institution of therapy in the mother. Spiramycin, a macrolide antibiotic, is the drug of choice for pregnant women with a primary infection, as it appears safe for both the woman and developing fetus (3 g/d PO). In the United States, spiramycin is only available by request from the Food and Drug Administration (FDA). It concentrates in tissue, so that the placental concentration is five times that of the blood. A large study by Desmonts and Couvreur demonstrated spiramycin to decrease transmission across the placenta. However, once infection has crossed the placenta, spiramycin is not as effective, since it does not reach high enough levels in the fetus. Likewise, it does not penetrate the central nervous system (CNS) well. For these reasons, it is critical to try to determine whether fetal infection is present. Ultrasonography may show evidence of hydrocephalus. Samples of amniotic fluid, chorionic villi, or fetal blood can be sent for more specific serologic testing or culture. If evidence of fetal infection is found, pyrimethamine 25 mg/d PO with a sulfonamide (sulfadiazine 1 to 2 g/d PO) is recommended. Both drugs are antifolates and act synergistically. Because mammals also use folic acid, untoward side effects, such as bone marrow suppression, commonly occur. Folinic acid (leucovorin calcium, *not* folic acid) administration can help avert this toxicity as the parasite cannot use preformed folinic acid, whereas humans can. The sulfonamide most commonly used is sulfadiazine. Although its use is approved by the FDA, its availability in the United States is limited. Currently, the Centers for Disease Control and Prevention has a European supply that can be obtained on request. Alternatively, trisulfapyrimidines can be used in conjunction with pyrimethamine.

Congenital Infection

Treatment is recommended for all infants with congenital toxoplasmosis, including those who are asymptomatic. This recommendation is based on long-term follow-up of untreated children that shows a significant risk for chorioretinitis or developmental delay or both. However, the efficacy of treatment for this latter group is not known, and the optimal duration of treatment has not been studied. Treatment consists of the combination of pyrimethamine 2 mg/kg/d for 2 days, then 1 mg/kg/d plus sulfadiazine or triple sulfonamides 100 mg/kg/d divided in 2 doses. Folinic acid 5 to 10 mg every other day should also be administered to offset the bone marrow-suppressive effects of the treatment drugs. Based on clinical experience and the relapse of disease in patients treated less than 3 months, therapy is usually continued for 12 months.

Immunocompromised Hosts

Treatment regimens similar to those for congenital infection have been used for adult AIDS patients with encephalitis and chorioretinitis due to *T. gondii*. Clindamycin 2.4 g/d PO has also been used with pyrimethamine 50 to 75 mg/d PO for encephalitis due to *T. gondii* if patients are unable to tolerate sulfonamides.

Prophylaxis for toxoplasmosis has been used in high-risk heart transplant recipients with apparent success. Pyrimethamine 1 mg/kg/d not to exceed 25 mg/d with folinic acid has been used in varying regimens for 6 weeks to 6 months. Prophylactic strategies to prevent toxoplasmosis in seropositive AIDS patients also are being evaluated. An Australian study showed that trimethoprim-sulfamethoxazole used for prophylaxis of *Pneumocystis carinii* also prevented the development of encephalitis due to *T. gondii* in seropositive HIV patients compared with those using aerosolized pentamidine. Other strategies for prevention include pyrimethamine with dapsone or clarithromycin.

Other Treatment

The drugs currently used to treat toxoplasmosis attack the trophozoite stage but not the encysted form of *T. gondii*. Therefore, they do not eradicate the organism. Active investigation of drugs that might eliminate the cyst are being conducted, motivated in part by the AIDS epidemic. Two of the new macrolides, azithromycin and roxithromycin, show promising results against the cyst form in vitro. Atovaquone, recently approved for treatment of *P. carinii* pneumonia, has activity against the *Toxoplasma* cyst, but early trials have not been successful in treating toxoplasmic encephalitis. Finally, trimetrexate, related to the chemotherapeutic agent methotrexate, is also being evaluated.

REFERENCES

1. Hohlfeld P, Daffos F, Thulliez P, et al: Fetal toxoplasmosis: Outcome of pregnancy and infant follow-up after in utero treatment. J Pediatr 115:765–769, 1989.
2. McCabe R, Chirurgi V: Issues in toxoplasmosis. Infect Dis Clin North Am 7:587–605, 1993.
3. Remington JS, Desmonts G: Toxoplasmosis. *In* Remington JS, Klein JO (eds): Infectious Diseases of the Fetus and Newborn Infant, 3rd ed. Philadelphia, WB Saunders Co, 1990.

SEPTIC SHOCK

KENNETH A. SCHENKMAN, M.D.
P. PEARL O'ROURKE, M.D.

Septic shock is a life-threatening host response to an overwhelming infectious illness. Shock commonly occurs in the setting of gram-negative sepsis but can also be associated with gram-positive, viral, or fungal infections. Bacteremia is often present but is not essential to the diagnosis, since localized sites of infection can lead to shock. Most cases are associated with an underlying illness or previous surgical intervention, although previously normal healthy children can develop septic shock. The common causative agents of septic shock are listed in Table 1.

Shock is generally defined as inadequate tissue perfusion. In septic shock, the early pathologic mechanism is primarily a vascular endothelial injury caused by toxins produced by the invading organism. With gram-negative infections, endotoxin is released from the bacterial cell walls during rapid cell growth and with cell wall lysis after death of the microbe. The immune response of the host to these antigens includes activation of neutrophils and release of various cytokines, interleukins, prostinoids, and leukotrienes, complement activation, and production of oxygen free radicals. This insult leads to vasodilatation and increased vascular endothelial permeability, or capillary leak. As shock progresses, the heart becomes a target organ, and myocardial failure develops.

Mortality from septic shock is highest in patients with immune system defects or when septic shock is superimposed on preexisting debilitating conditions. Extremes of age, malnutrition, chronic illness, immunodeficiency, and trauma are all risk factors. Surgery, invasive procedures, immunosuppression, and the use of broad-spectrum antibiotics are therapies that also predispose patients to sepsis. Early diagnosis and the prompt institution of appropriate therapy may significantly reduce mortality.

CLINICAL PRESENTATION

The clinical presentation of shock is often divided into two phases that represent stages on a continuous clinical spectrum. The early stage is characterized by vasodilatation with a hyperdynamic cardiovascular response. Patients in this stage have warm, flushed, dry skin and are tachycardic and tachypneic, often with bounding pulses. The mean arterial pressure is usually maintained in the normal range or may be decreased, with a widened pulse pressure. The patient may be irritable and restless. This stage is referred to as *warm shock*.

As the pathologic process proceeds, the vascular injury leads to

TABLE 1. Common Pathogens of Septic Shock in Children

GROUP	PATHOGENS
Neonates	Group B streptococci
	Enterobacteriaceae
	Listeria monocytogenes
	Herpes simplex
Infants and young children	*Haemophilus influenzae* type b
	Streptococcus pneumoniae
	Staphylococcus aureus
	Neisseria meningitidis
Older children	*Streptococcus pneumoniae*
	Staphylococcus aureus
	Neisseria meningitidis
	Group A streptococci
Immunocompromised children	Enterobacteriaceae
	Staphylococcus aureus
	Pseudomonas sp.
	Candida sp.

end-organ dysfunction. The heart, which has been working to compensate for the vasodilatation and decreased circulating volume, starts to fail. Hypotension develops, and peripheral vascular resistance rises in an attempt to restore adequate perfusion. *Cold shock* develops. Patients in this state are cool and clammy (with thready pulses) and become listless. Tachycardia increases, blood pressure falls, and the pulse pressure narrows. Oliguria, cyanosis, and metabolic acidosis develop.

Other end-organ damage becomes apparent as the shock state persists. Acute respiratory distress syndrome (ARDS) frequently develops. The decreasing level of consciousness may progress to obtundation or coma as the brain exhibits lack of adequate perfusion and oxygen delivery. Oliguria may progress to complete renal failure. Disseminated intravascular coagulopathy (DIC) develops, and petechiae or purpura may be seen. Although this is typically associated with meningococcemia, other bacterial and viral agents can also cause a full-blown picture of purpura fulminans. Sloughing of the gastrointestinal tract mucosa and both upper and lower gastrointestinal bleeding can occur.

TREATMENT

Once the diagnosis of septic shock is suspected, appropriate therapy must be initiated immediately. It should be emphasized that although rapid institution of therapy may allow for temporary stabilization of the patient, the disease process itself may progress, leading to rapid clinical deterioration. Early referral to a tertiary pediatric medical center, where invasive monitoring and medical and nursing personnel trained in pediatric intensive care are available, should be considered for any child in septic shock.

Management should follow the approach taken with any critically ill child, with attention first to airway and breathing, followed by hemodynamic stabilization. Attention then is directed to antibiotic therapy and management of other end-organ involvement. Constant reevaluation of the patient's condition and response to therapy should be performed.

Respiratory Stabilization

All children in shock should have supplemental oxygen administered as an immediate intervention. Obtunded children or children with hemodynamic instability may require intubation and mechanical ventilation to stabilize the airway and decrease the work of breathing. Once the airway is stabilized, an assessment of the adequacy of oxygenation and respiratory effort or ventilation must be made. Pulse oximetry can be helpful to determine the adequacy of oxygenation in children with reasonable peripheral perfusion. With poor perfusion, pulse oximetry may be unreliable, and arterial blood gas determination should be made promptly. Blood gas analysis is also necessary to determine the efficacy of ventilation. Profound hypoxemia and increasing hypercarbia are clear indications for intubation and mechanical ventilation. Blood gas analysis should be repeated frequently as part of the ongoing reassessment.

A chest x-ray should be obtained in patients requiring intubation to verify proper tube placement. Chest x-rays can also be helpful in evaluating the lungs in children with significant respiratory embarrassment and to rule out a pulmonary source for infection.

Hemodynamic Stabilization

Septic shock affects the circulating (intravascular) volume, the peripheral vascular resistance, and the myocardial function, as described previously. These are interdependent, as cardiac output is determined by the stroke volume and the heart rate. Stroke volume, in turn, is determined by intravascular volume (preload), systemic vascular resistance (afterload), and myocardial contractility.

Assessment of the intravascular volume status can be made by several methods, which should be used together for the most accurate estimate. Physical evidence of hypovolemia includes cool or mottled extremities, increased time for capillary refill, and decreased urine output. Placement of a Foley catheter allows for quantitation of urine output and gives fairly rapid feedback to the clinician on the efficacy of the therapy. The heart size on chest x-ray can be used as an estimate of intravascular volume status. An abnormally small heart shadow indicates hypovolemia. Arterial blood pH is the most useful laboratory variable that can be easily obtained. Metabolic acidosis indicates inadequate perfusion. Echocardiography can also be used to provide a good assessment of volume status, as well as information about myocardial performance.

Invasive monitoring gives the most accurate estimation of volume status, although correlation with the physical examination is essential. Placement of a central venous pressure (CVP) catheter allows determination of the preload or volume status of the right side of the heart. A single reading of the CVP may be difficult to interpret by itself, and no ideal CVP value exists for all children. In general, CVP readings below 5 cm H_2O indicate hypovolemia, whereas readings above 10 cm H_2O in the presence of poor perfusion suggest impaired cardiac function. Changes in CVP in response to administered therapy yield the most useful information. In most children, the CVP can reasonably be used also to estimate the filling pressure of the left side of the heart. In children with significantly compromised cardiac function or with poorly compliant lungs requiring positive pressure ventilation, a correlation between the left- and right-sided pressures can no longer be assumed, and placement of a pulmonary artery (Swan-Ganz) catheter to measure the wedge pressure may be necessary. An intraarterial catheter should be placed in any hemodynamically unstable child for continuous blood pressure monitoring. Radial artery catheterization is the preferred site, but ulnar, dorsalis pedis, and posterior tibial arteries often are used. More central placement of arterial lines in axillary or femoral arteries is associated with greater risk but should be considered if peripheral arterial cannulation is unsuccessful. Brachial arteries should be avoided if possible, as there is poor collateral circulation around these vessels.

In general, children in septic shock are quite hypovolemic and require vast quantities of fluid therapy. This necessitates the rapid establishment of adequate vascular access. Peripheral intravenous catheter placement may be difficult in children with poor peripheral perfusion. Emergent placement of an intraosseous needle should be considered in critically ill young children if venous access cannot be obtained within a few minutes. Resuscitation fluids and intravenous medications can be administered via this route. Central vein catheterization (femoral, internal jugular, or subclavian vein) and saphenous vein cutdown are other means of rapidly establishing access.

Initial fluid therapy should be directed at rapidly restoring an adequate circulating volume. Recent studies of fluid therapy in septic shock have demonstrated an increased survival in patients receiving 40 ml/kg of fluid or more in the first hour over those receiving less. Replacement fluid can be either crystalloid or colloid, but generally normal saline or Ringer's lactate solution is chosen initially. Frequent additional fluid boluses in 5- to 10-ml/kg aliquots should be administered liberally in response to decreasing urine output, cooling of extremities, decreasing CVP, or decreasing mean arterial pressure (MAP). After initial stabilization, correction of anemia, coagulopathy, and hypoalbuminemia can be achieved using the appropriate colloid or blood product. These fluids can also be helpful in maintaining the volume status of the patient.

Aggressive fluid therapy should be continued until clinical improvement in perfusion is noted. Careful attention to changes in the physical examination is warranted during this resuscitative phase of treatment to monitor for signs of decreasing cardiac function. A rise in CVP without improvement in perfusion suggests poor cardiac function. An enlarging liver size, jugular venous distention, or the development of rales also points to cardiac insufficiency. Respiratory decompensation may be seen during this resuscitative phase, and pulmonary edema or ARDS may develop. Of note, aggressive fluid therapy does not appear to increase the risk of either of these respiratory complications, and it does lead to increased survival.

Myocardial Function

Myocardial function is decreased in septic shock by several mechanisms. Initially, catecholamine stimulation increases cardiac output in an attempt to compensate for the vasodilatation and hypovolemia. With time, the increase in metabolic demand on the heart starts to take its toll, and with decreasing oxygen and nutrient delivery, ischemia develops. In addition, direct cardiotoxic effects of endotoxin and host immunologic factors lead to myocardial depression. Other myocardial cellular metabolic derangements have been reported in septic shock. Therapy directed at improving myocardial performance should address the maintenance of an appropriate heart rate, presence of sinus rhythm, and augmentation of contractility. In addition, efforts to restore normal systemic vascular resistance need to be undertaken.

Young children and infants attempt to compensate for inadequate cardiac output mainly by increasing heart rate, as stroke volume is relatively fixed. The increase in heart rate causes an increase in myocardial oxygen consumption, a relationship that should be kept in mind when administering drugs that have chronotropic effects. Arrhythmias are possible complications resulting from catecholamine stimulation or metabolic disturbances. Serum pH, electrolytes, calcium, magnesium, and glucose should be closely monitored and corrected when abnormal.

Hypoglycemia should be treated with 1 to 2 ml/kg of $D_{20}W$ IV. Repeat glucose determinations should be obtained, and levels should be followed closely until stable. Fluids used for volume resuscitation should not contain glucose, and a separate maintenance glucose containing intravenous solution should be administered. Calcium should be administered for documented hypocalcemia with either 100 mg/kg of calcium gluconate or 25 mg/kg of calcium chloride. Calcium infiltration into extravascular tissues can cause extensive tissue necrosis and even loss of affected extremities. For this reason, calcium should always be administered into a central vein. In an emergency, calcium gluconate can be administered peripherally into a freely flowing intravenous tube, but calcium chloride should never be given peripherally. Hypokalemia should be treated cautiously because these children are at risk for developing oliguric renal failure. Administration of sodium bicarbonate should be considered for metabolic acidosis that is unresponsive to fluid replacement therapy. $NaHCO_3$ 1 to 2 mEq/kg IV as a slow infusion is recommended when the pH is less than 7.2 or 7.25. Careful attention must be paid to the serum sodium when administering $NaHCO_3$, as hypernatremia may develop from the excess administered sodium.

After correcting the underlying metabolic abnormalities, it may become necessary to improve myocardial contractility further with pharmacologic therapy. Three aspects should be considered: adding inotropic agents, correcting systemic vascular resistance (SVR), and decreasing excessive afterload. The most useful positive inotropic agents for septic shock are the sympathomimetic amines and the methylxanthines. Dopamine, dobutamine, and epinephrine belong to the first class of agents. Their pharmacologic effects are mediated via the adrenergic receptors in the cardiovascular system. Alpha$_1$-receptors are found in the peripheral and coronary vasculature and in the lungs, and activation leads to vasoconstriction and bronchoconstriction, respectively. Beta$_1$-receptors are found in the heart, and stimulation causes increased contractility and heart rate. Beta$_2$-receptors mediate vasodilatation in the peripheral vasculature and bronchodilatation in the lungs. Dopaminergic (delta) receptors are found in the renal cortex and modulate renal blood flow.

Dopamine is beneficial in early septic shock and has several useful effects. At low doses (3 to 5 µg/kg/min), dopamine acts predominantly on the delta-receptors and leads to increases in renal blood flow. At moderate doses (5 to 15 µg/kg/min), the predominant effect is on beta$_1$-receptors, thus improving contractility. Higher doses (>15 µg/kg/min) result in more alpha$_1$-receptor effect, with improvement in peripheral vascular tone. The combination of inotropic and vasoconstrictor effects makes it a good first choice agent for septic shock.

Dobutamine has predominantly inotropic and chronotropic effects

(beta$_1$) but does have some vasodilatory effects (beta$_2$) as well. It is often helpful in conjunction with dopamine for improved inotropy. However, it may lead to excessive tachycardia, with increased myocardial oxygen consumption, thus negating its inotropic benefit.

Epinephrine is probably underused in septic shock and should be initiated early in critical septic shock. It has both alpha and beta effects, with more beta predominance at lower doses (0.1 µg/kg/min). Thus, it is a potent inotrope at lower doses, with increasing vasoconstriction seen at higher doses (0.5 µg/kg/min). The significant effect of increasing SVR is not only an increased MAP but also the increase in diastolic pressure that improves coronary artery perfusion.

Amrinone and milrinone are methylxanthines that inhibit phosphodiesterase. Amrinone has been shown to be an effective inotrope with vasodilatory properties. It is, thus, useful in the later stages of septic shock when increases in SVR have developed. An intravenous loading dose of 2 to 5 mg/kg should be given carefully, as profound hypotension may occur. A maintenance infusion of 5 to 10 µg/kg/min is then started. Amrinone is not recommended in hemodynamically unstable children, since it has a sustained action once administered. If hypotension develops, discontinuing the infusion will not rapidly reverse its effects. Thrombocytopenia is a common side effect, and platelet counts should be monitored every 12 hours while the drug is being administered.

In severe septic shock, the SVR may be dramatically elevated. This puts an extra stress, or increased afterload, on the failing heart. In this setting, pharmacologic attempts to decrease afterload may be considered. Vasodilating agents, such as sodium nitroprusside, can be beneficial, but their use is associated with substantial risk. Profound and sometimes untreatable hypotension may develop with afterload reduction. For this reason, complete hemodynamic data from a pulmonary artery catheter should be available to the clinician before this therapy is attempted.

Antibiotic Therapy

The choice of initial antimicrobial therapy depends on the age of the child and the presence of underlying defects in the immune system. Broad-spectrum antibiotics are usually administered while identification of the causative organism is sought. Various antibiotic combinations are available that provide appropriate empiric coverage for the different patient populations (Tables 2 and 3). Blood, urine, and cerebrospinal fluid (CSF) cultures should be obtained. Gram stains of urine, CSF, sputum, and other relevant body fluids should be prepared. Latex agglutination tests for bacterial antigens can be performed with samples of urine and CSF. A chest x-ray should be

TABLE 2. Empiric Antibiotic Therapy for Septic Shock in Children

PATIENT	ANTIBIOTIC	DOSAGE
Neonates 0–4 wk	Ampicillin	50 mg/kg per dose q8h <7 d q6h >7 d
	and	
	Gentamicin	2.5 mg/kg per dose q12h <7 d q8h >7 d
Infants 1–3 mo	Ampicillin	50 mg/kg per dose q6h
	and	
	Cefotaxime	50 mg/kg per dose q6h
Young children 3 mo–5 y	Cefotaxime	50 mg/kg per dose q6h
Older children >5 y	Cefotaxime	50 mg/kg per dose q6h
	and	
	Nafcillin	40 mg/kg per dose q6h
Immunocompromised children	Vancomycin	10 mg/kg per dose q6h
	and	
	Ceftazidime	50 mg/kg per dose q8h

TABLE 3. Doses of Medications Used in Treatment of Septic Shock

MEDICATION	DOSE
Ampicillin	50 mg/kg per dose IV q8h <7 d q6h >7 d
Amrinone	2–5 mg/kg IV loading dose 5–10 μg/kg/min IV infusion
Cefotaxime	50 mg/kg per dose IV q6h
Ceftazidime	50 mg/kg per dose IV q8h
Dobutamine	1–20 μg/kg/min IV infusion
Dopamine	1–20 μg/kg/min IV infusion
Epinephrine	0.1–1 μg/kg/min IV infusion
Gentamicin	2.5 mg/kg per dose IV q12h <7 d q8h >7 d
Nafcillin	40 mg/kg per dose IV q6h
Vancomycin	10 mg/kg per dose IV q8h

obtained for evidence of pneumonia. In the last few years, significant interest in the use of monoclonal antibodies as a treatment for septic shock has developed. The HA-1A antibody initially was thought to show clinical promise, but recent evidence suggests that this therapy has no overall benefit in septic shock, and its use is not recommended. Steroid use in septic shock has also experienced the mood swings of hope and rejection. Steroids are recommended currently only in sepsis associated with documented meningitis. In these children, there has been a demonstrated beneficial effect in reducing neurologic sequelae, notably hearing loss. Replacement steroids should be considered also if adrenal insufficiency is suspected, since adrenal hemorrhage is a known complication of meningococcemia. The routine use of pharmacologic doses of steroids in septic shock is not recommended.

Other Therapy

The hematopoietic system is often severely affected in septic shock, and evidence of a coagulopathy should be investigated. Oxygen delivery to the already impaired tissues should be maximized by maintaining a sufficiently high hematocrit. Transfusions of packed red blood cells should be performed to keep the hematocrit above 35% to 40%. Platelet counts are often quite depressed, and replacement therapy should be aimed at keeping the platelet count over 50,000/mm³ in the presence of any bleeding. Fresh frozen plasma (FFP) should be administered in 10 ml/kg aliquots to correct abnormalities in clotting factors. FFP can be used as volume therapy, but care should be taken during rapid administration, as severe hypocalcemia may develop.

Renal perfusion should be optimized by establishing adequate intravascular volume and, in appropriate situations, adding low-dose dopamine. Close attention should be paid to the urine output, which should be maintained at greater than 1 ml/kg/h if possible. Prophylaxis for gastrointestinal bleeding should be administered using either intravenous H₂ blockers or oral sucralfate. Frequent neurologic examinations should be performed to evaluate for evidence of intracranial pathology (meningitis, bleeding) or the development of seizures. Sedatives and antiepileptic medications should be administered cautiously if indicated. Narcotics, benzodiazepines, barbiturates, and phenytoin cause myocardial depression and may potentiate hypotension.

Good management of septic shock requires meticulous attention to detail. Septic shock is a systemic illness and necessitates evaluation and treatment of multiple organ systems. Assessment and therapy must be carried out simultaneously. Changes in therapy should be directed by continuous ongoing assessment of the patient's condition. The efficacy of the therapy should be determined by the clinical response.

IMMUNIZATION PRACTICE

Martin B. Kleiman, m.d.

Routine childhood immunizations have resulted in a spectacular reduction of the mortality and morbidity caused by a handful of common childhood illnesses. The development of future vaccines and further refinements of immunization strategies promise still more benefit. Routine immunization is, therefore, a dynamic topic that requires that health care practitioners periodically reevaluate and revise their practices rather than persist with established routines.

Although incorporation of new, safe, and effective vaccines into standard practice is an obvious and desirable goal, the most prompt and dramatic contribution to the health of children can be achieved by programs that deliver current vaccines to infants and children consistently and at appropriate times. This is especially true for the urban poor, some racial and ethnic minorities, and the working poor, for whom economic constraints often interfere with preventive care. Toward this end, practitioners in both the public and private sectors should periodically evaluate their immunization practices in accordance with the standards listed in Table 1. Most deferrals of vaccine administration result from mild, nonfever-associated respiratory illnesses at the times of physician visits. These illnesses are not contraindications to immunization. In my experience, the effectiveness of most immunization programs can be immediately and substantially improved if (1) deferral of immunization is based only on established contraindications, and (2) providers take advantage of opportunities to immunize children when they visit for reasons other than well child checkups.

The *Report of the Committee on Infectious Diseases* of the American Academy of Pediatrics (The Redbook) is a current and authoritative reference for most childhood immunization issues. Table 2 summarizes the committee's most recent recommendations for the routine immunization of infants and children. Although they differ from earlier recommendations, the principal changes are not the result of new vaccines directed against additional infections. Rather they are refinements of current vaccines or changes in the strategic approaches to vaccine use. Recent changes pertain to hepatitis B, the availability of acellular pertussis vaccine products, and the availability of vaccine products that consist of combined immunogens for infections currently vaccine preventable.

TABLE 1. Standards for Pediatric Immunization Practices

1. Immunization services are readily available.
2. Barriers or unnecessary prerequisites to immunization are eliminated.
3. Immunization services are available free or for a minimal fee.
4. All encounters are used to screen and immunize children.
5. Caretakers are educated in understandable terms.
6. Caretakers are informed about contraindications, risks, and benefits.
7. Only *true* contraindications are used to defer immunizations.
8. All vaccine doses for which a child is eligible are given at each visit.
9. Records are accurate and complete.
10. Immunizations are coscheduled with other health services.
11. Adverse events are reported promptly, accurately, and completely.
12. A tracking system is used.
13. Recommendations for vaccine storage and administration are followed.
14. Scheduled audits are conducted to assess effectiveness in specified patient groups.
15. Written immunization protocols are developed and updated at least annually.
16. Patient and community suggestions to improve approaches are solicited and seriously considered.
17. Vaccines are administered by properly trained individuals.
18. Providers receive ongoing education and training about current immunization recommendations.

From Centers for Disease Control and Prevention: MMWR 42(RR-5):1–13, 1993.

TABLE 2. Recommendations for Routine Childhood Immunizations*: United States, January 1995

VACCINE	BIRTH	MONTHS						YEARS		
		2	4	6	12†	15	18	4–6	11–12	14–16
Hepatitis B†	HB-1									
Diphtheria, tetanus, Pertussis‡		HB-2		HB-3						
		DTP	DTP	DTP	DTP or DTaP at ≥15 months			DTP or DTaP	Td	
H. influenzae§ type b		Hib	Hib	Hib	Hib					
Poliovirus		OPV	OPV	OPV				OPV		
Measles, mumps, rubella¶					MMR			MMR or MMR		

* Boxes indicate range of acceptable ages for vaccination.
† For newborns of HBsAg-positive mothers, HBIg and hepatitis B vaccine are given at birth. A second dose of hepatitis B vaccine is given at 1 mo and a third at 6 mo of age.
‡The fourth dose of DTP may be given as early as 12 mo if at least 6 mo have elapsed since the third dose of DPT was given. Combined DTP-Hib products may be used when these two vaccines are given simultaneously.
§Three Hib vaccines are available for use in infants: (1) oligosaccharide conjugate Hib vaccine (HbOC), (HibTITER). (2) polyribosylribitol phosphate-tetanus (PRP-T) toxoid conjugate, (ActHIB, OmniHIB), and (3) Haemophilus b conjugate vaccine (PRP-OMP), (Pedvax-HIB). Children who have received PRP-OMP at 2 and 4 mo do not need a dose at 6 mo. After the primary infant Hib conjugate vaccine series is completed, any licensed Hib conjugate vaccine may be used as a booster dose at age 12–15 mo.
¶The second dose of MMR should be given *either* at 4–6 y of age *or* at 11–12 y of age.
DtaP, diphtheria, tetanus, acellular pertussis; OMP, oligosaccharide meningococcal protein.
From Centers for Disease Control and Prevention: MMWR 43:959–960,1995. Data from Advisory Committee on Immunization Practices, American Academy of Pediatrics and American Academy of Family Physicians.

HEPATITIS B

The most important change from prior practice is a new strategy for using the hepatitis B vaccine. Hepatitis B vaccine is now universally recommended for administration to all infants. This approach should ultimately decrease the incidence of hepatitis B more effectively than targeting high-risk groups that are poorly compliant and difficult to identify. The two currently available vaccines are preparations of purified hepatitis B surface antigen (HBsAg) produced with recombinant techniques. Plasma-derived vaccines are no longer produced. Prenatal screening for HBsAg is still recommended, since it plays a critical role in identifying newborns at risk for vertical transmission. When hepatitis B is acquired in the newborn period, there is a very high risk of developing chronic hepatitis B and its complications. The two available vaccine products (Recombivax HB and Engerix-B) are given to children in schedules that vary with the HBsAg status of the mother. If the mother is HBsAg negative, the preferred regimen is an initial vaccine dose in the newborn nursery, the second dose 1 to 2 months later, and a third dose at 6 to 18 months of age. An alternative regimen for infants of HBsAg-negative mothers who do not receive the first dose at birth is a three-dose regimen in which the first is given at 1 to 2 months, the second is given at least 1 month later, and a third is given at least 2 months, optimally 4 months, following the second but before 18 months of age. Infants of HBsAg-positive mothers should be treated with hepatitis B immunoglobulin promptly following delivery. They should also receive the first hepatitis B vaccine dose shortly after birth, then at 1 month, and again at 6 months of age. Vaccine should be given intramuscularly in the anterolateral thigh or upper arm. Administration in the buttock should be avoided, since it has been shown to result in inadequate serologic response rates in adults. Hepatitis B vaccine may be administered simultaneously with other vaccines, such as DTP and *Haemophilus influenzae* type b vaccines but should be given at separate sites, one or more inches apart from other vaccines. Hepatitis B vaccine doses vary in older age groups and with some underlying medical conditions.

High-risk populations, such as recipients of certain blood products, intravenous drug abusers, those at high risk for sexually transmitted diseases, household or sexual contacts of HBsAg carriers, staff and residents of institutions for developmentally disabled citizens, chronic hemodialysis patients, and travelers to hepatitis B-endemic areas should continue to receive hepatitis B immunization regardless of age. A preadolescent visit is an excellent time to immunize susceptible children against hepatitis B.

COMBINED DTP AND *HAEMOPHILUS INFLUENZAE* TYPE b CONJUGATE VACCINE

Because of the increasing number of vaccines now recommended for infants, there is a high priority for the development of multivalent vaccines that combine antigens and thereby permit immunization to be accomplished with fewer injections. The FDA has recently approved a diphtheria and tetanus toxoid and whole-cell pertussis vaccine (DTP) combined with an *H. influenzae* type b conjugate vaccine. Tetramune combines two previously licensed products, Tri-Immunol and HibTiter. The combined vaccine has been licensed for use in children 2 months to 5 years of age when indications for immunization against all four infections coincide. Alternatively, one of the *H. influenzae* type b conjugate vaccines, PRP-T, may be reconstituted with DTP (made by Connaught Laboratories) to give the two vaccines in a single injection.

ACELLULAR PERTUSSIS VACCINE

Pertussis is a common, often undiagnosed, disease of children and adults. Substantial morbidity and mortality accompany infections, especially in young infants. Standard pertussis vaccines are whole-cell products of *Bordetella pertussis* cultures and contain many antigens. They effectively control pertussis. Whole-cell pertussis vaccines result in 80% vaccine efficacy rates after three doses. Mild to moderate adverse reactions following whole-cell pertussis vaccines are common, although serious reactions are rare, and brain damage does not occur. A complete series of five doses of pertussis vaccine is recommended to prevent pertussis. Concern about adverse reactions to the whole-cell products has prompted the development of a number of more purified acellular pertussis vaccine products that contain one or more immunogens derived from pertussis cultures. Two acellular pertussis vaccines, combined with diphtheria and tetanus toxoids (DTaP), have been approved for use but, at present, are only recommended as the fourth and fifth doses of the series. Acellular vaccine products are protective and are accompanied by lower rates of local reactions, fever, and systemic reactions than whole-cell products. Acellular pertussis products may not eliminate all serious pertussis reactions, and they should not be given to children who may have had serious adverse reactions to whole-cell vaccines. No pertussis vaccine product is currently recommended for adults or for children past their seventh birthday.

IMMUNIZATION OF IMMUNOCOMPROMISED CHILDREN

Children treated with immunosuppressive drugs or those with immunodeficiency disorders that affect the humoral or cell-mediated immune system should not receive vaccines that contain live microbial agents. Examples of the latter include bacille Calmette-Guérin (BCG), oral attenuated poliovirus (TOPV), measles, mumps, rubella (MMR), and yellow fever vaccines. Short-term courses of steroids (<2 weeks) in otherwise normal children and low to moderate doses of steroids over a longer term may be only relative contraindications and not preclude the use of these vaccines. The exact amount of systemic corticosteroids and the duration of their use that suppress the immune response of a healthy child are not established. However, the equivalent of 2 mg/kg/d of prednisone or daily doses exceeding 20 mg of prednisone are considered sufficiently immunosuppressive to warrant concern about the safety of live viral vaccines.[1]

Household contacts of immunocompromised children should receive MMR. Enhanced potency inactivated polio vaccine (eIPV) should be substituted for TOPV when immunizing household contacts of immunosuppressed patients, including those with HIV infection, against polio.

The efficacy of many nonlive viral vaccines in immunocompromised children is not established, and increased doses or boosters may be needed. Inactivated vaccines are not dangerous in immunocompromised persons and should be given.

Although live viral vaccines are not recommended for use in immunocompromised patients, an important exception is in protecting patients with HIV infection against measles. Live measles vaccine is recommended for HIV-infected children. This recommendation is based on the observation of severe morbidity and mortality from measles in these children and the absence of significant morbidity in those who have received the measles vaccine. Since measles vaccine efficacy may be reduced in HIV-infected children, it and other immunizing agents should be given early in the course of HIV infection while the immune response may still be relatively adequate. eIPV, not TOPV, should be used to protect HIV-infected patients against polio.

SIMULTANEOUS ADMINISTRATION OF VACCINES, LAPSED IMMUNIZATIONS

H. influenzae type b conjugate vaccines, DTP, eIPV, hepatitis B, and MMR may be given in any combination in different syringes at different sites on the same day with no apparent reduction in immune response to any of the vaccines. In addition, TOPV may be given by

TABLE 3. Available Vaccines Licensed in the United States but Not Recommended for Routine Use in All Children

BCG
Cholera
Hepatitis A
Influenza
Meningococcal polysaccharide
Plague
Pneumococcal polysaccharide
Rabies
Typhoid
Yellow fever
Varicella*

*Not licensed.

mouth simultaneously. In general, intervals longer than those recommended between doses do not substantially affect serologic responses, provided that all the recommended doses are given. Therefore, restarting a series after a prolonged delay is not necessary.

NONROUTINE IMMUNIZATION

Various immunizing agents are licensed in the United States but are not recommended for universal use (Table 3). Circumstances in which these agents may be considered include the control of disease outbreaks, anticipated travel to disease endemic areas, and in children at high risk for specific disorders, such as the administration of influenza and bacterial polysaccharide vaccines to children with asplenia or certain complement factor deficiencies.

FUTURE DEVELOPMENTS

Developments to be anticipated in the near future are (1) approval of a varicella vaccine, (2) new acellular pertussis vaccine products and new strategies for their use, (3) additional combined vaccines that further reduce the number of injections required for routine immunizations, and (4) recommendations for a combined schedule using TOPV with eIPV that would protect against polio, retain good mucosal protection, and eliminate vaccine-associated paralytic polio.

REFERENCES

1. Centers for Disease Control: Recommendations of the advisory committee on immunization practices (ACIP): Use of vaccines and immune globulins in persons with altered immunocompetence. MMWR 42(No.RR-4):1–18, 1993.
2. Centers for Disease Control: Standards for pediatric immunization practices. MMWR 42(No. RR-5):1-13, 1993.
3. American Academy of Pediatrics: Report of the Committee on Infectious Disease, 23rd ed. Elk Grove Village, Ill, American Academy of Pediatrics, 1994.

FEVER

LOUIS M. BELL, M.D.

Fever is one of the most common complaints prompting parents to seek medical care for their children. Fever is viewed by many parents as a potentially harmful sign, one that may cause brain damage, seizures, or even death. Fever is a concern to physicians as well (especially in the infant) because it may indicate the presence of a life-threatening infection. In this section, we examine the management of fever in infants and children (0 to 36 months of age) who have fever and no source of infection. Focal infections, such as preseptal cellulitis, buccal cellulitis, pneumonia, or meningitis, define the treatment plan. However, appropriate management of the febrile infant or child without a focus of infection remains somewhat controversial.

FEVER PHOBIAS AND REALITY

Fever phobias and misconceptions about the dangers of fever are very common in parents and physicians. In one recent study, 11% of parents feared that fevers could lead to death; 27% were concerned that fever in itself could produce brain damage or stroke, and 48% feared seizures and loss of consciousness in their febrile child. Parents need to be instructed that temperatures from 37.8°C (100°F) to 40°C (104°F) are not harmful and that fevers do not cause brain damage unless temperatures are >41.7°C (107°F) for prolonged periods (hours). Furthermore, untreated fevers from infection will not climb higher than 41.2°C (106°F). Programs designed to educate parents about fever in children have been shown to decrease the number of visits for fever by one third.

To begin, we need a definition of fever. The normal rectal temperature in adults ranges from 36.1°C to 37.8°C (97°F to 100°F). In normal children, temperature ranges from 36.1°C to 38°C (97°F to 100.4°F). Body temperature is higher in children and decreases to adult levels by age 13 to 14 years in girls and 17 to 18 years in boys. Body temperature fluctuates during the day (circadian rhythm), although this rhythm is not well established until 2 years of age. The maximum body temperature occurs between 17:00 and 19:00 hours (the minimum body temperature occurs from 01:00 to 06:00 hours). The temperature may normally be as high as 38.4°C (101°F) rectally in some patients. In general, children should be considered febrile if rectal temperatures are over 38°C (100.4°F).

THERAPY

The general approach to controlling the height of the fever is outlined in Table 1. Antipyretic treatment for low-grade fevers (38.2°C to 39°C [100.8°F to 102.2°F]) is not necessary. Fever in neonates less than 2 to 3 months of age requires evaluation by a physician. Parents should be warned not to overdress their children. At temperatures of greater than 39°C (102.2°F) to 39.4°C (103°F), approximately one quarter of children are uncomfortable and may feel better with pharmacologic therapy. Children who are playful or comfortable do not necessarily require antipyretic drugs. If antipyretics are given, acetaminophen is the drug of choice. Peak concentrations occur about 30 minutes to 1 hour after dosing. The efficacy of acetaminophen is dose dependent. Therefore, doses of 15 mg/kg every 4 hours are usually necessary. There are few adverse reactions.

Ibuprofen at a dose of 10 mg/kg every 6 hours provides a similar antipyretic effect to acetaminophen. Randomized, double-blind studies comparing the antipyretic efficacy of ibuprofen with that of acetaminophen have not, in general, used an adequate dose of acetaminophen (usually only 10 mg/kg per dose); accordingly, they are difficult to evaluate. No significant differences in adverse effects have been reported for acetaminophen versus ibuprofen. However, abdominal discomfort and renal dysfunction are reported with ibuprofen, and because experience with this drug in children is limited, it should be assigned a second-line position.

MANAGEMENT OF FEBRILE INFANTS LESS THAN 90 DAYS OF AGE

More than in any other group, fever in the infant causes anxiety in both the parents and the physician. A fever in this age group (<3 months) may indicate a serious infection or bacteremia in a signficant proportion of infants. Rates of serious infection in infants less than 3 months of age range between 6% and 31%. Rates of bacteremia range from 2% to 15%. Children in the first month of life have a higher rate of bacteremia (as high as 10%) than do children who are beyond the first month of life. In children older than 1 month, the rate of bacteremia falls to 3% to 4%, which continues through the second year of life. In a study at The Children's Hospital of Philadelphia in children between 1 and 2 months of age with temperatures over 38.1°C, serious bacterial infection was found in 8.7% of 747 infants studied. Bacteremia occurred in 2.5% of this group. (Baker MD et al: N Engl J Med 329:1437–1441, 1993).

Serious illness in most studies is defined as (1) bacterial pathogens found in blood, cerebrospinal fluid (CSF), urine, stool, joint fluid, or deep tissue, (2) pneumonia (chest x-ray with an infiltrate), or (3)

TABLE 2. Management of Febrile Infants 0 to 90 Days with Fever and No Focus of Infection

AGE	THERAPY

0–27 d	Admit to hospital
	Chest radiograph
	Blood culture
	Urine culture
	Lumbar puncture
	Parental antibiotics
	  Ampicillin: <1 wk, 100 mg/kg/d in 2 divided doses
	    ≥1 wk, 200 mg/kg/d in 4 divided doses
	  Cefotaxime: <1 wk, 100 mg/kg/d in 2 divided doses
	    1–4 wk, 150 mg/kg/d in 3 divided doses*

28–90 d	A group of low-risk infants is defined
	Step 1: Is child low risk by the following criteria?
	Clinical
	  Previously healthy
	  Nontoxic clinical appearance
	  No focus of infection
	Laboratory
	  WBC count 5000–15,000/mm³
	  Band/neutrophil ratio <0.2
	  Normal urine analysis
	  Normal chest radiograph
	  Normal lumbar puncture
	Step 2: If low risk, two options
	Option 1
	  No antibiotics
	  Return for reevaluation at 24 *and* 48 h
	Option 2
	  Ceftriaxone 50 mg/kg IM at initial evaluation
	  Return for reevaluation at 24 *and* 48 h
	  At 24-h revisit, a second IM injection of ceftriaxone may be given
	Step 3: If does not meet low risk *or* no phone *or* inadequate transportation, admit to hospital with presumptive antibiotics pending cultures. Antibiotics (cefotaxime at 180 mg/kg/d in 4 divided doses and ampicillin 200 mg/kg/d in 4 divided doses) may be withheld if the patient is admitted because of social reasons

*If the results of the lumbar punctures are normal, then ampicillin and gentamicin: <1 wk, 5 mg/kg/d in 2 divided doses; >1 wk, 5–7.5 mg/kg/d in 3 divided doses may be given.

aseptic meningitis. The management options for febrile infants have been changing rapidly. Recently, there has been an effort to select a subset of febrile infants who have a low risk for serious illness who could be managed without antibiotics while in the hospital or even managed as outpatients with or without antibiotics. These infants are selected using a combination of history, physical examination, and laboratory studies. In an effort to establish clinical and laboratory criteria that can be grouped to define this low-risk group of febrile infants, The Children's Hospital of Philadelphia's Emergency Department performed a study from July 1987 to June 1993. Patients were enrolled if they were age 29 to 56 days and had temperatures over 38.2°C rectally. In this study 747 febrile infants received a full sepsis workup, which included a complete blood count, urinalysis, urine culture, blood culture, lumbar puncture, and chest x-ray. Infants were judged to be low risk if they met the strict selection criteria listed in Table 2. If the infants were deemed to be low risk, they were managed either as outpatients without antibiotics or admitted to the hospital without antibiotics pending culture results. Using this method, we were able to select 291 (39%) of 747 febrile infants aged 28 to 60 days who could be managed safely as outpatients without antibiotics. Serious bacterial illness was found in 65 infants in the rest of the group, and 64 of the 65 were in the high-risk category. Only 1 of the infants was originally assigned to the low-risk group. This method of screening for low-risk infants had a negative predictive

TABLE 1. Antipyretic Therapy for Febrile Child Over 2 Months of Age

RECTAL TEMPERATURE*	THERAPY
38.2°C–39°C (100.4°F–102.2°F)	No treatment needed; child should not be overdressed
39.1°C–41.2°C (102.4°F–106°F)	Remove excessive clothing and blankets; maintain a cool environment Acetaminophen 15 mg/kg per dose q4h as first choice Ibuprofen 10 mg/kg per dose given q6h as second choice

*Depending on age and signs and symptoms, evaluation by a physician may be warranted for any degree of fever.

value of 99% (95% confidence interval: 98, 100). The cost savings for this group of low-risk patients who were treated as outpatients was substantial. Other studies from Children's Hospital in Boston (Baskin MN et al: J Pediatr 120:22–27, 1992) and Rochester University (Dagan R et al: J Pediatr 107:855–860, 1985) also have concluded that it is possible to safely and effectively manage febrile 1- to 2-month-old infants as outpatients. These protocols differ somewhat in the criteria used to define low risk and the use of presumptive antibiotics. Once the group of low-risk febrile infants is selected, the decision to use parenteral antibiotics presumptively while awaiting culture results must be made. Table 2 outlines the management options. Most clinicians agree that younger infants (0 to 28 days of age) require hospitalization following a laboratory investigation for sepsis. Most will receive presumptive intravenous antibiotics until cultures are proven to be negative for bacteria.

MANAGEMENT OF CHILDREN 3 TO 36 MONTHS OF AGE WITH FEVER WITHOUT A SOURCE

When children between 3 and 36 months are evaluated in the emergency department for fever greater than 39.4°C (103°F), there is a 3% risk of bacteremia if the history and physical examination do not reveal a source and the child otherwise appears well. Bacteremia occurs with the encapsulated organisms listed in Table 3. In most children the bacteremia clears without therapy. However, a percentage of those with occult bacteremia may progress to an invasive and serious infection. This observation prompts discussions of methods to identify children at risk and the consideration of presumptive therapy.

To identify the child at risk, we need to consider five different factors: the practice setting, age, height of fever, severity of illness, and immunocompetence. The issue of occult bacteremia was raised as a result of caring for children in busy, high-volume, urban emergency departments where follow-up is often difficult. If one's *practice setting* is an office or clinic where close communication with families can be easily maintained, the management plan for occult bacteremia may appropriately be changed to fit that practice setting.

Age is another factor that will influence our management plan. We must remember that children less than 24 months of age have a poor immunoglobulin G antibody response to encapsulated bacteria. Therefore, children are at highest risk for bacteremia in the 7- to 12-month age range.

Height of fever is an important consideration in developing a management plan for these children. It is known that the prevalence of occult bacteremia increases with increasing temperatures. On the other hand, the negative predictive value for temperatures less than 38.9°C (102°F) is about 99.3%; that is, the chance of having occult bacteremia with temperatures less than 38.9°C is 7 in 1000. Conversely, temperatures over 39.4°C (103°F) indicates a 3% risk for bacteremia in the 4- to 36-month age group. Investigations in the past have suggested that hyperpyrexia or core temperatures greater than 41.2°C (106°F) put the patient at increased risk for bacteremia (15%) and meningitis (10%). However, other reports do not substantiate an increased risk of bacteremia or meningitis with hyperpyrexia. Despite this conflicting data, the hyperpyrexic child may require a somewhat more careful evaluation for serious infection, including a full evaluation for sepsis.

Although some have conjectured that the response of fever to antipyretics discriminates between bacterial and viral disease, evidence does not support this hypothesis. Research has shown that a prompt response to acetaminophen does not eliminate the possibility that the child has occult bacteremia.

The *severity of illness* is an important component of developing a management plan for these patients with fever without a source. McCarthy, in a series of articles, has developed an acute illness observation scale that includes six different observations that, when scored together, have been used with some success in determining whether a patient appears well or ill and what his or her risk for serious illness or invasive bacterial illness might be (McCarthy PL et al: Pediatrics 70:802-809, 1982). The observations include quality of cry, reaction of crying to parent stimulation, state lability, color, hydration, and response to social overtones. This emphasizes that any patient, regardless of the height of the fever, who looks seriously ill needs aggressive care in the clinic or the emergency department, including assessment of airway, breathing, and circulation.

Finally, it is important to assess *immunocompetence* in children who present to the clinic or emergency department. Patients undergoing cancer chemotherapy, patients who have a history of nephrosis or splenectomy, or those children who might be at risk for HIV infection are at increased risk for invasive disease and will need more aggressive management when febrile.

Laboratory data have limited value in identifying which febrile child is at increased risk for bacteremia. A normal white blood cell count (5000 to 10,000/mm³) is helpful. In this situation, the chance that the child has bacteremia is 8 out of 1000 (i.e., negative predictive value equals 99.2%). If the white blood cell count is over 15,000/mm³, the risk of occult bacteremia is increased to approximately 10%. Jaffe and Fleisher showed that the best sensitivity and specificity for detecting children at risk for occult bacteremia is achieved when you consider both the temperature and the white count (Pediatrics 87:670–674, 1991). In their study, a temperature ≥39°C (102.2°F) and a white blood cell count of over 10,000/mm³ detected the highest number of cases of bacteremia while missing the fewest. This translated into a sensitivity of 92% and a specificity of 43%. It is important to note that the white blood cell differential, in particular the number of band forms, does not correlate to increasing risk for occult bacteremia.

Evaluation of the febrile child should include, in some circumstances, a urine culture. In a study by Roberts et al there was a 4.1% incidence of urinary tract infections in 195 febrile children less than 24 months of age (J Pediatr 103:864–867, 1983). In this study, 7.4% were girls and 0 were boys. In other studies, the urinary tract infection

TABLE 3. Common Bacterial Isolates Associated with Occult Bacteremia and Percentages of Invasive Infection

	BACTEREMIA (%)	INVASIVE INFECTION (%)
Streptococcus pneumoniae	60	4–5
Haemophilus influenzae type b*	20	20–50
Neisseria meningitidis	10	25
Salmonella sp.	10	25

*Percentages may be affected by recent success of the *H. influenzae* type b vaccines.

TABLE 4. Management of Febrile Children 3 to 36 Months of Age with Fever, Appearing Well, with No Focus of Infection*

RECTAL TEMPERATURE	MANAGEMENT
≤39.2°C (102.5°F)	No laboratory tests Ensure follow-up if worsens Antipyretic therapy†

≥39.4°C (103°F)	Ensure follow-up (phone or office) in 24–48 h
	Chest x-ray if respiratory rate >45/min or cough
	Urine culture
	  All females
	  Males if <6 mo of age
	Blood cultures if temperature ≥39.4°C‡
	Presumptive antibiotic therapy
	  Option 1: No antibiotics
	  Option 2: Ceftriaxone 50 mg/kg IM if temperature is ≥39.4°C *and* WBC ≥15,000/mm³

*Otitis media does not count as a focus of infection. Therefore the recommendations described in this table apply.

†See Table 1.

‡If the white blood cell count is normal (5000–10,000/mm³), no blood culture need be sent. However, obtaining a complete blood count in every case is not always possible.

TABLE 5. Management of Febrile Children with Proven Occult Bacteremia

	AFEBRILE AT FOLLOW-UP VISIT (<38°C or 100.4°F)	FEBRILE AT FOLLOW-UP VISIT (>38°C or 100.4°F)
Streptococcus pneumoniae	Repeat blood culture; treat with penicillin VK as outpatient	Hospital admission*
Haemophilus influenzae type b	Hospital admission*	Hospital admission*
Neisseria meningitidis	Hospital admission*	Hospital admission*
Salmonella sp.	Hospital admission*	Hospital admission*

*Admission following an evaluation for sepsis (which should include a lumbar puncture) and parenteral antibiotic until cultures are proven negative at 48 h.

in boys usually occurred in boys less than 3 months of age in equal frequency with girls. The etiology of the urinary tract infections in neonates is based on secondary spread from a bacteremia rather than ascending infection through the urethra, which is the etiology after 3 to 6 months.

Finally, in the evaluation and management of the febrile child, pneumonia should also be a consideration. As is often the case, the only sign of a pneumonia in febrile children in this age group is tachypnea and a history of cough. Very often, there will be no localizing auscultatory findings. For that reason, children who have a temperature ≥39.4°C (103°F) and a respiratory rate of over 45 breaths per minute with a history of cough should have a chest x-ray performed.

Once we have determined who may be at risk for occult bacteremia, the question of presumptive treatment needs to be addressed. There are several controlled studies that evaluate presumptive therapy in children at risk for occult bacteremia. The first two studies (Carroll et al: Pediatrics 72:608–612, 1981; and Jaffe et al: N Engl J Med 317:1175–1180, 1987) found no evidence to support presumptive therapy. There have been two multicenter studies (Fleisher et al: J Pediatr 124:504–512, 1994, and Bass et al: Pediatr Infect Dis J 12:466–473, 1993) that compared oral antibiotic therapy with ceftriaxone for presumptive therapy in children at risk for occult bacteremia. The data suggest that in some instances (high white blood cell count and temperature >39.4°C [103°F]), parenteral antibiotics are associated with fewer sequelae of occult bacteremia and reduction in the duration of fever.

THERAPY FOR OLDER CHILDREN AT RISK FOR OCCULT BACTEREMIA

For children 3 to 36 months of age with temperatures <39.3°C (102.8°F) who look clinically well, neither laboratory tests nor treatment with presumptive antibiotics is indicated. For children who have no focus of infection, who have temperatures of at least 39.4°C (103°F) rectally, and who look clinically well, ensuring adequate physician follow-up within 24 to 36 hours is the most important component of the management plan (Table 4). The next steps in therapy are controversial. Two articles related to treatment options for these children (Downes: J Pediatr 118:21–29, 1991, and Lieu: J Pediatr 118:11–20, 1991) both concluded that taking a blood culture and giving empirical antibiotics were the most clinically effective and cost-effective strategies for children at risk for occult bacteremia. However, these authors make certain assumptions about the efficacy of therapy that are not proven. The option of not using antibiotics is, therefore, recommended as long as adequate follow-up is ensured. Chest x-rays should be considered in patients with tachypnea (respiratory rate >45/min) and a history of cough. A urine culture should be sent for male infants less than 6 months of age or female infants of any age who have temperatures >39.4°C (103°F) without a source.

The management of those patients who have a positive blood or urine culture is described in Table 5.

REFERENCES

1. Baker MD, Bell LM, Avner JR: Outpatient management without antibiotics of fever in selected infants. N Engl J Med 329:1437–1441, 1993.
2. Baraff LF, Bass JW, Fleisher GR, et al: Practice guideline for the management of infants and children 0 to 36 months of age with fever without source. Pediatrics 92:1–12, 1993.
3. Drwal-Klein LA, Phelps SJ: Antipyretic therapy in the febrile child. Clin Pharmacol 11:1005–1021, 1992.

19

Allergy

SERUM SICKNESS

Frank J. Twarog, M.D., Ph.D.

The complex of symptoms referred to as "serum sickness" was first recognized at the turn of the century with the introduction of heterologous antiserum (especially horse) for the treatment of infectious diseases, such as diphtheria and scarlet fever. Originally, the condition was referred to as "antitoxin rash" or "serum exanthem." With von Pirquet and Schick's classic monograph, the term "serum disease" was adopted.

Clinically, patients present with malaise and fever, which may precede other symptoms by 1 or 2 days. Arthralgias with pain (generally in excess of the degree of objective findings), headaches, abdominal discomfort (occasionally associated with vomiting or diarrhea or both), lymphadenopathy, and a variety of cutaneous eruptions follow. Dermatologic findings may include erythema, urticaria, and a morbilliform eruption. Vasculitic, renal, and respiratory symptoms are infrequent.

The most recent clinical description of serum sickness in a group of patients being treated with horse antithymocyte globulin for bone marrow failure may have been modified by the underlying disease or the concurrent treatment with systemic steroids. However, this group of patients presented with fever and malaise (100%), cutaneous eruptions (93%), arthralgias (63%), gastrointestinal symptoms (67%), cephalgia (57%), myalgias (37%), blurred vision (37%), arthritis (30%), dyspnea and wheezing (20%), lymphadenopathy (13%), and hoarseness or anosmia (10%).[1] A characteristic serpiginous band of erythema and purpura was also seen along the sides of the fingers, toes, palms, and soles 12 to 48 hours before the onset of other serum sickness symptoms in 75% of these patients.

Symptoms generally develop approximately 6 to 10 days following exposure to the precipitating agent. An accelerated form may develop in 1 to 2 days if sensitization to the antigen was present previously. Symptoms usually remit in 1 to 2 weeks even without therapy, and fatalities are rare. Fatalities reported in earlier studies were primarily related to acute anaphylactic episodes.

The most frequent cause of serum sickness when originally described was heterologous antiserum. The volume of antiserum administered was directly related to the risk of developing serum sickness. Eleven percent of those receiving less than 10 ml of serum developed symptoms, whereas 85% of those receiving greater than 100 ml did so. Except for unusual circumstances, such as bone marrow failure, transplantation, and envenomations, however, there is now little need for this type of treatment. Currently, antibiotics are the principal cause of serum sickness. Occasionally serum sickness occurs after bee sting (Hymenoptera) reactions and during the prodrome of infections such as hepatitis B; it rarely occurs with allergy injection therapy. Recently it was reported following high-dose intravenous gamma globulin for Kawasaki's disease.

Cases of serum sickness are more common in children receiving cefaclor than in those receiving either amoxicillin or trimethoprim-sulfamethoxazole. Cefaclor appears to cause a serum sicknesslike syndrome that may not be immunologic in nature and is of longer duration than serum sickness from other causes. In particular, rather striking urticaria and dermatographism may persist for weeks following the acute episode. Most children developing serum sickness from antibiotics have previously received multiple courses of treatment. Frequently, the course of antibiotics presumed to precipitate the serum sickness episode has been preceded by prior antibiotic therapy within 3 weeks.

Following the onset of symptoms, the causative agent should be discontinued if it has been identified and is still being administered. This situation would be unusual, since symptoms are generally delayed for a week or more. Treatment of serum sickness has been relatively empirical. It is directed at relieving symptoms of pruritus, arthralgias, and malaise. Nonsteroidal anti-inflammatory agents or acetaminophen (in doses appropriate for age) are used for the relief of fever and arthralgias. At times, it has been reported that arthralgias respond poorly to this treatment. Antihistamine therapy should be initiated at the onset of symptoms and continued on a regular schedule until symptoms have entirely cleared. Response to antihistamine therapy is generally more efficacious with continued rather than intermittent administration. Ongoing therapy has the theoretical advantage of preventing further deposition of immune complexes (the primary etiology of serum sickness). The choice of a specific antihistamine is arbitrary. Diphenhydramine (5 mg/kg/d) is often used. However, hydroxyzine (2 mg/kg/d) may have some advantages. Nonsedating antihistamines, such as astemizole, loratidine, and terfenadine, can be considered for those older than 12 years of age. For children acutely distressed with urticaria, epinephrine 1:1000 0.01 ml/kg to a maximum dose of 0.3 ml can be administered. Response to this treatment is often prompt but transient. Antihistamine should always be administered concurrently with epinephrine.

As serum sickness is a self-limited, generally non-life-threatening condition, the degree of discomfort or disability should guide whether or not to employ more aggressive therapy. For more severely symptomatic cases, systemic steroid treatment may result in prompt remission of discomfort, particularly of urticaria and arthralgias. Generally, a dose of 1 to 2 mg/kg/d of prednisone or methylprednisolone in divided doses is administered until symptoms diminish. This should be tapered over the next 1 or 2 weeks depending on the severity and duration of full-dose therapy. If symptoms rapidly remit, steroids can be discontinued abruptly after a 4- to 5-day course. For extremely severe symptoms, particularly when heterologous serum appears to have been the precipitant, plasmapheresis to remove immune complexes has been suggested as an alternate treatment.

If heterologous serum is required in a setting likely to cause serum sickness, prophylactic therapy should be considered. The value of pretreatment with antihistamines or systemic steroids, however, is unclear. In fact, a large proportion of recipients of horse antithymocyte serum developed serum sickness in spite of concurrent steroid therapy in one series. The symptoms, however, may have been modified or decreased by the pretreatment program. Antihistamines and systemic steroids in doses as noted previously should be administered before and concurrent with administration of the antiserum if this is not specifically contraindicated by the pharmaceutical manufacturer.

In addition to the complication of serum sickness, the possibility of anaphylaxis in patients receiving heterologous antiserum must be considered. Skin testing for the species of origin of the antiserum is suggested. Appropriate precautions, especially the availability of epinephrine for treatment of anaphylaxis, should be taken.

REFERENCES

1. Bielory L, Gascon P, Lawley TJ, Young NS, Frank MM: Human serum sickness: A prospective analysis of 35 patients treated with equine anti-thymocyte globulin for bone marrow failure. Medicine 67:40–57, 1988.
2. Heckbert SR, Stryker WS, Coltin KL, Manson JE, Platt R: Serum sickness in children after antibiotic exposure: Estimates of occurrence and morbidity in a health maintenance organization population. Am J Epidemiol 132:336–342, 1990.
3. Lawley TJ, Bielory L, Gascon P, Yancey KB, Young NS, Frank MM: A prospective clinical and immunologic analysis of patients with serum sickness: N Engl J Med 331:1407–1413, 1984.

ALLERGIC GASTROINTESTINAL DISORDERS

JUDY BUCKMAN SPLAWSKI, M.D.

The human gastrointestinal tract is exposed to a large quantity and wide variety of food. Food is processed for uptake of nutrients, while pathogens and their toxins are excluded and normal bacterial flora are tolerated. A large portion of the immune system of the body is involved in the successful accomplishment of these tasks. It is not surprising, therefore, that occasionally there are adverse reactions to food, some of which are immunologically mediated. The diverse nature of the immune response and the large number of factors involving both gastrointestinal and nongastrointestinal sites that can modify the responses demonstrate the complexity of the system and the difficulties inherent in diagnosis and treatment. For the purpose of this discussion, allergy is defined as an inflammatory response to noninfectious agents. A brief background discussion will aid in understanding the approach to therapy.

TYPES OF REACTIONS

Adverse immunologic reactions to food can be divided into immediate and delayed-type (chronic) responses.

Immediate Responses

Immediate responses result from food protein binding to specific IgE on mast cells. Crosslinking IgE on mast cells results in the release of histamine and a number of other factors that increase vascular permeability and contraction of smooth muscle. Mast cell stimulation can result in a diverse set of symptoms, including rhinorrhea, urticaria, angioedema, vomiting, diarrhea, laryngospasm, wheezing, shock, and circulatory collapse (anaphylaxis). These responses by definition occur within 1 or 2 hours of exposure. Most patients or their parents will be able to identify the food or substance that causes such immediate and serious consequences.

Chronic Responses

These reactions are characterized by less immediate symptoms and are due to chronic antigen exposure, which results in the recruitment of other cell types, such as activated T cells and eosinophils, that can promote tissue destruction. The more insidious onset and delayed response make it difficult to identify the offending food and the im-

munologic mechanism responsible for the more complex symptoms. Enteropathy due to cow's milk or soy protein intolerance in infants is typical of this response but not unique. This type of enteropathy can result in malabsorption and failure to thrive. Biopsies of the small intestine demonstrate patchy villous atrophy. Colonic biopsies may demonstrate an inflammatory infiltrate characterized by eosinophils, and the affected patients may present with bloody stools. This gastroenteropathy responds to removal of the offending protein from the diet. The natural course is for a large number of children to outgrow this response when the protein is excluded from the diet for several months. A number of investigators have proposed that T cells are involved in the epithelial injury. It is not clear whether resolution of the problem results from maturation of the gastrointestinal tract with decreased macromolecular absorption, the development of IgA resulting in exclusion of antigens, or the development of suppressor T cells.

Food Hypersensitivity with Manifestations Outside the Gastrointestinal Tract

Food hypersensitivity may result in symptoms outside the gastrointestinal tract, especially in patients with an atopic disposition. A number of studies provide convincing evidence for the ability of food hypersensitivity to exacerbate atopic dermatitis and for the dermatitis to improve with withdrawal of the offending food. In addition, there are cases where asthma, glomerulonephritis, and otitis media have been demonstrated to be induced by food hypersensitivity. The mechanism whereby food antigens result in these widespread manifestations is not clear but must involve macromolecular absorption from the gastrointestinal tract, since circulating food proteins or immune complexes have been demonstrated in affected patients, which implies an increase in gastrointestinal permeability. Ongoing injury to the gastrointestinal tract by chronic ingestion of the offending protein probably permits absorption of a number of additional proteins that may contribute to problems outside the gastrointestinal tract. Removal of the offending protein has been shown to promote tolerance to other proteins, most likely due to healing of the gastrointestinal tract with decreased macromolecular absorption. It is unclear why some children have their major manifestations in the skin, some in the airways, and others in the gastrointestinal tract.

Eosinophilic Gastroenteritis

Eosinophilic gastroenteritis is a disorder characterized by infiltration of the gastrointestinal tract by eosinophils. Any area of the gastrointestinal tract may be involved, and the condition may involve the mucosa, submucosa, or serosa, thus resulting in diverse presentations, including vomiting and abdominal pain, gastrointestinal obstruction, or ascites. Elevated IgE levels and the eosinophil infiltration suggest that this entity may be an allergic enteropathy. However, a specific relationship to food hypersensitivity can be identified only in about 50% of the patients.

DIAGNOSIS

Diagnosis often goes hand in hand with therapy, since attempts at dietary elimination are involved.

History

A relatively small number of antigens result in the vast majority of allergic reactions to food. These include cow's milk, soy, egg, peanuts, nuts, fish, shellfish, corn, and wheat. Therefore, the history should pay special attention to these particular foods. Immediate reactions to food are usually fairly easy to sort out. However, the foods responsible for chronic reactions are much more difficult to derive from the history, since most of the offending foods are eaten on a routine basis. The nature of the adverse response should be delineated, and if possible, the relationship of the response to specific foods in the diet and the results of any trials of elimination of the suspected food should be ascertained. Allergic reactions should be distinguished from potential nonimmune pseudohypersensitivity reactions resulting from histamine release (alcohol, chocolate, fish, pineapple, pork, tomatoes, and strawberries), tyramine hypersensitivity (aged cheese, red wine, beer, beef, chicken liver, summer sausage, and brewers yeast), or vasoactive amines (chocolate, citrus fruits, cheese). Patients can also be sensitive to common food additives present in many different types of processed foods, resulting in a confusing picture. These include foods containing salicylates (most fruit and mint), dyes, especially tartrazine (yellow No. 5), monosodium glutamate, sulfites (vegetable freshener), and aspartame (artificial sweetener). Milk allergy must be distinguished from acquired or secondary lactase deficiency, which can be determined by a positive hydrogen breath test in response to lactose. Oral manifestations alone suggest that the patient has birch pollen hypersensitivity with cross-reactive sensitization to nuts, apples, and carrots.

Elimination Diets with Open Challenge

Many patients present with possible food-induced symptoms but an unclear idea of the offending protein. A strict elimination diet that results in a decrease in symptoms may suggest that the problem is indeed food allergy. Subsequent addition of a single food over a week's time may help to delineate potential foods to which the patient has been sensitized. These may then be further defined by a double-blind placebo-controlled trial. These are strict diets and should be short in duration (2 to 3 weeks) and should be undertaken in consultation with a nutritionist to ensure a complete diet with sufficient calcium intake in milk-free diets. The use of a hydrolysate or elemental diet is recommended. A careful food-symptom diary should be kept before starting the diet and during the diet so that a concrete assessment of the symptoms under study can be obtained. The patient or parents will have to be instructed on how to read labels to find the hidden antigens. Primary unprocessed foods should be used because they contain fewer additives (preservants and colorants) that may complicate the picture. It should be noted that intolerance to one food in the legume family, for example, peanuts, does not necessarily mean that other botanical family members (green beans, garden peas, kidney beans, carob, lentils, blackeye peas) need to be avoided. Open challenges are used mainly for common foods that the patient has already been ingesting without anaphylaxis. However, there is some evidence to suggest that strict avoidance of a food may increase the risk for anaphylaxis to small quantities of that food. Therefore, it may be advisable to have the patient supervised when a food is reintroduced into the diet. A few proteins, such as peanuts, give lifelong symptoms. However, the natural history of this problem is that many patients lose their sensitivity after avoidance. Therefore, periodic testing may allow expansion of the patient's diet.

Double-Blind Placebo-Controlled Food Challenge

If the results of the open dietary challenges are equivocal, a double-blind placebo-controlled food challenge (DBPCFC) should be done to either confirm or disprove that a particular food results in symptoms.[1] This test involves eliminating *all* suspected foods from the diet for a week before the test. The patient is fasted overnight and should be off antihistamines for at least 96 hours, beta-agonists for 12 hours, and theophylline and cromolyn for 12 hours. The food is administered in increasing increments in a double-blind placebo-controlled fashion, and any adverse occurrences are monitored. The test is limited by the number of foods that can be tested at one time. The foods tested should be common ones that will be important staples in the child's diet. The DBPCFC tests mainly for immediate to intermediate responses. If a patient does not have immediate adverse effects, the food is introduced into the diet and tolerance is evaluated over a longer period of time. Foods can induce fatal anaphylaxis. Therefore, *a food that has provoked a serious anaphylactic event in the past should not be tested in a DBPCFC.* These tests should be performed by someone who is ready and able to resuscitate the patient immediately should this be necessary.

Prick Skin Tests and RAST Testing

If a large number of foods are implicated, skin testing may be helpful as a screening maneuver to limit the number of food challenges to be done. A positive skin test only indicates that a person has IgE specific for the food antigen. It does not mean that the food will cause symptoms. However, negative skin tests strongly suggest that a particular food is not involved in an IgE-mediated allergic response and, therefore, will not be a likely candidate for causing a positive DBPCFC response. DBPCFC primarily tests for immediate or intermediate IgE-related immune responses to food. RAST tests are no better at predicting food hypersensitivity than skin tests, and they are considerably more expensive. Therefore, skin testing is the preferred method of investigating food-specific IgE.

TREATMENT

Avoidance

At present, the only accepted therapy for food hypersensitivity is strict avoidance of the offending food. If the food is a nutritionally important component of the diet (such as milk) or if multiple foods have to be eliminated, diets should be prepared with the help of a nutritionist so that the diet proposed will be nutritionally adequate.

Hypoallergenic Formulas

Although soy formulas were first marketed for milk protein intolerance, it has since been amply demonstrated that soy itself may result in allergic gastroenteropathy. Recent reports of anaphylaxis induced by hypoallergenic formulas have prompted more thorough evaluation of the antigenicity of these formulas. In infants who require both milk and soy avoidance, the availability of casein hydrolysates has been important.[3] Reports suggest that casein hydrolysates have very little residual allergenic activity. Even extensively hydrolyzed whey hydrolysates have more residual activity than the casein hydrolysates. It should be emphasized, however, that infants with immediate responses to cow's milk may still be at risk for anaphylaxis to the hydrolysates. Alimentum is a casein hydrolysate that is also corn free and, thus, may be of benefit in a child who still has symptoms on Nutramigen or Pregestimil. In some cases an elemental diet, such as Tolerex or Neocate, may prove helpful. However, most elemental formulas were not intended for use in infants. Thus, a nutritionist should be consulted on the provision of supplemental calcium and vitamins when these formulas are given to infants for extended periods. Reabilan is a whey and casein hydrolysate that is nutritionally complete and contains 1 kcal/ml, which may be appropriate for older children.

Immunotherapy

Immunotherapy has been tried in patients with allergy to peanuts, and induction of tolerance may result. However, this therapy is not without risk. Immunotherapy to birch pollen does not prevent food hypersensitivity to cross-reacting foods, such as apples and carrots.

Pharmacologic Treatment

Avoidance of multiple foods becomes a logistic problem for children attending schools and other institutions. It can put severe limitations on lifestyle and nutrition. Therefore, pharmacologic treatment of food hypersensitivity can be important.[2]

Epinephrine. Patients with serious food allergies should always be prepared for a severe food reaction. Strict avoidance is difficult even when the patient and family are adept at reading labels, as demonstrated by the unsuspected presence of milk in canned tuna. EpiPen and Ana-Kit provide epinephrine for self-administration, and parents should be taught how to use these preparations.

Antihistamines. Histamine release has been shown to occur with adverse food reactions. With the advent of newer nonsedating H_1 antagonists, there has been renewed interest in treatment of allergic manifestations of food allergy with a combination of an H_1 antagonist

TABLE 1. Formulary for Treatment of Food Hypersensitivity

DRUG	TYPE OF DRUG	DOSE	COMMENT
Terfenadine	Nonsedating H_1-antagonist	3–6 y: 15 mg PO b.i.d. 6–12 y: 30 mg PO b.i.d. >12 y: 60 mg PO b.i.d.	Arrhythmias in combination with ketoconazole, erythromycin, and cimetidine
Astemizole	Nonsedating H_1-antagonist	>12 y: 10 mg PO q.d.	Arrhythmias in combination with ketoconazole, erythromycin, and cimetidine
Loratadine	Nonsedating H_1-antagonist	>12 y: 10 mg PO q.d. 10 mg q.o.d. in place with liver disease	
Ranitidine	H_2-antagonist	2 mg/kg per dose q8–12h *Adults:* 150 mg PO b.i.d.	↓ Dose in renal impairment
Sodium cromoglycate	Mast cell inhibitor	<6 mo: 20 mg/kg/d divided q.i.d. (before feedings and at hs) 6 mo–2 y: 30 mg/kg/d >2 y: 40 mg/kg/d *Adults:* 800 mg/d	Takes months for full effect
Ketotifen	Mast cell inhibitor, H_1-antagonist, PAF inhibitor	<3 y: 0.5 mg PO b.i.d. ≥3 y: 1 mg PO b.i.d.	Takes months for full effect; not yet available in USA
Prednisone	Anti-inflammatory corticosteroid	1–2 mg/kg/d Alternate day, less side effects (requires tapering)	Suppression of pituitary adrenal axis, cataracts, hypokalemia, psychosis, poor wound healing, Cushing's syndrome, osteoporosis, growth retardation, glucose intolerance, hypertension

(e.g., terfenadine) and an H_2 antagonist (e.g., ranitidine), and early trials using this approach have met with some success (Table 1). Parents should be warned that arrhythmias may result from the combination of terfenadine and ketoconazole or erythromycin. Therefore, this combination of drugs is to be avoided. The newer nonsedating H_1 antagonist loratadine is not believed to cause this complication.

Sodium Cromoglycate (SCG, Gastrochrom). This agent blocks the release of mediators, such as histamine, from mast cells. An interesting study demonstrated that food hypersensitivity increased intestinal permeability and that this could be prevented by prophylactic administration of SCG. SCG does appear to offer some benefit in patients with food hypersensitivity. The drug is only marginally absorbed and fairly well tolerated, with minimal side effects. For infants younger than 6 months of age, the dose is 20 mg/kg/d dissolved in liquid in four divided doses 30 minutes before feedings and at bedtime. For infants 6 months to 2 years of age, the maximum dose is 30 mg/kg/d, and for those older than 2 years of age, the maximum dose is 40 mg/kg/d. Adolescents may require up to 800 mg/d. The full benefit of the drug may not be realized for several months.

Ketotifen (Zaditen). Ketotifen is an oral tricyclic benzocycloheptathiophene that blocks the release of chemical mediators, such as slow-reacting substance of anaphylaxis, neutrophil chemotactic factor, and histamine. In addition, it is an H_1-receptor antagonist and inhibits the actions of platelet-activating factor (PAF) and the flow of calcium. It has been shown to be a useful drug in the treatment of asthma and also in treatment of food allergy and eosinophilic gastroenteritis. The side effects of this medication include drowsiness (to which patients become tolerant) and weight gain. In addition, it has a long startup time before optimal benefits are seen (6 to 12 weeks). It does not appear that this drug will be available for use in the United States in the near future. The dose is 0.5 mg PO twice a day for children <3 years of age and 1 mg PO twice a day for children ≥3 years of age.

Corticosteroids. Corticosteroids are effective in ameliorating the symptoms of allergic gastroenteropathy and are very effective in the treatment of eosinophilic gastroenteritis. However, the side effects are substantial. Because of adverse effects on growth, corticosteroids should not be used when less toxic medications will do. Corticosteroids should be used for short periods of time at a dose of 1 to 2 mg/kg/d. Alternate-day therapy is associated with fewer side effects, and the dose must be weaned because steroids suppress the pituitary ad-

renal axis. Trials of newly developed nonabsorbable steroids for use in gastrointestinal allergy treatment hold hope for the future. Intravenous methylprednisolone is indicated in the treatment of anaphylaxis or severe acute allergic responses to food.

Potential Future Therapies

Food hypersensitivity results in a cascade of factors from activated mast cells, which in turn recruit additional inflammatory cell types, such as eosinophils, neutrophils, and activated T cells, that promote the delayed-type response. Delineation of the important mediators involved in hypersensitivity responses has allowed the development of specific antagonists with potentially fewer side effects than more nonspecific anti-inflammatory agents. Several of these new inhibitors or antagonists may play a role in the prevention or empiric therapy of hypersensitivity to food. Prostaglandin E_1 (PGE_1) has mucosal protective properties that have been promoted for the prevention of ulcers due to nonsteroidal anti-inflammatory drugs. In addition, PGE_1 has been shown to inhibit the release of mediators from rat mast cells. Mast cells and eosinophils release leukotrienes C_4, D_4, and E_4, which constitute the slow-reacting substance of anaphylaxis (SRA), which is a potent stimulant of vasoactivity, smooth muscle contraction, and mucous secretion. Competitive inhibitors of leukotrienes and SRA are, therefore, potentially useful agents for treatment of food hypersensitivity.

PAF has been shown to be an important immunoregulatory molecule in asthma and most likely plays a role in the pathology of food enteropathy. Therefore, antagonists of this molecule would appear to be of benefit in reducing inflammation in food allergy. Calcium plays an important role in the release of mediators from eosinophils and mast cells and in activation of T and B cells. Therefore, calcium channel blockers may be expected to have a therapeutic role in prevention of food hypersensitivity. The calcium channel blocker, nifedipine, has been shown to prevent fish-induced asthma. In addition, verapamil was shown to have a mucosal protective effect that was thought to be due to the reduction of leukotriene B_4 and increased PGE_2. Finally, conjugation of the human IgE alpha-receptor to a human IgG molecule has been shown to block passive cutaneous anaphylaxis in vivo. This molecule binds to the IgE receptor on mast cells and prevents crosslinking and release of mast cell mediators. This molecule, therefore, is a promising new agent that should cause little toxicity and specifically prevent IgE-mediated disease.

PREVENTION

It appears that the incidence of atopic disease is on the rise and, with it, the accompanying morbidity and financial burden. Therefore, prevention of the problem would be highly desirable. Sensitization rarely occurs in the fetus, and elimination of potential allergens from the mother's diet during pregnancy has not been shown to be effective in the prevention of allergic disease in the infant. Soy milk given from birth does not prevent the development of atopic disease. Breast feeding is associated with a moderately lower risk for allergy than is the administration of infant formula. Breast feeding may decrease allergic potential through prevention of infection and enhancement of neonatal gastrointestinal tract and immune system development. Sensitization can occur, however, from the passage of small quantities of intact food proteins in the breast milk. Studies have shown that avoidance of milk, egg, and soy in the maternal diet during lactation results in decreased gastrointestinal sensitization. The effect on respiratory symptoms, however, does not appear to be significant. Recent studies have shown that feeding a casein hydrolysate to infants at risk for the development of atopic disease significantly reduced the risk for atopic dermatitis even at 4 years of age, although there was no significant difference in the development of respiratory symptoms. Such results support the conclusion that decreased neonatal exposure to potential antigens either by providing casein hydrolysate or by removing sensitizing foods from the diet of a breast-feeding mother can provide significant protection to the infant for the prevention of dermatitis but not necessarily for the prevention of asthma. Dietary prevention appears to be worthwhile if there is a history of atopic disease in both parents. Consideration should be given also to the temporary use of hydrolysate formula for infants who have suffered gastrointestinal injury from either infection or protein intolerance to avoid increased uptake and sensitization to soy or milk proteins when the barrier function of the gastrointestinal tract has been altered.

REFERENCES

1. Bock S, Sampson H, Atkins F, Zieger R, Lehrer S, Sachs M, Bush R, Metcalfe D: Double-blind, placebo-controlled food challenge (DBPCFC) as an office procedure: A manual. J Allergy Clin Immunol 82:986–997, 1988.
2. Podleski WK: Pharmacotherapy of food allergy—A neglected option. Int J Immunopharmacol 11:311–326, 1989.
3. Wahn U, Wahl F, Rugo E: Comparison of the residual allergenic activity of six different hydrolyzed protein formulas. J Pediatr 121:S80–S84, 1992.

ADVERSE DRUG REACTIONS

KATHERINE TEETS GRIMM, M.D.

Most adverse drug reactions (ADR) are not allergic reactions. In fact, about 80% of ADRs are predictable and occur in normal patients who do not have a predisposition to ADRs.

ADRs can be divided into two categories: predictable and unpredictable. Predictable ADRs are usually dose dependent and are related to the pharmacologic properties of the drug. Examples of predictable ADRs include toxicity from overdose (e.g., vomiting with excessive theophylline intake), side effects (e.g., gastric distress with erythromycin), secondary effects (e.g., *Clostridium* overgrowth with toxin production in the presence of clindamycin use), and drug-drug interactions (e.g., erythromycin potentiating theophylline levels).

Unpredictable ADRs generally are not dose related and not related to the pharmacologic properties of the drug. Often, there is a genetic predisposition to the ADR. Examples of unpredictable ADRs include intolerance (e.g., tinnitus in the presence of a low dose of salicylate), idiosyncratic reactions (e.g., malignant hyperpyrexia with general anesthesia), pseudoallergic reactions (e.g., anaphylaxis to radiocon-

trast dye caused by direct mediator release and not an antibody-antigen reaction), and true allergic reactions (i.e., antibody-antigen interaction or T cell reaction to drug antigen).

The risk of an allergic reaction to a drug in adults is 1% to 3%. In children, allergic drug reactions are less common. Death from allergic drug reactions is rare, 1 in 10,000 or less. Although allergic ADRs are not very common, they are often overreported. For example, approximately 5% of parents will report that their children are allergic to penicillin. This diagnosis is based on a rash—often maculopapular—associated with penicillin or ampicillin administration. When the child is skin tested for penicillin allergy, the test is almost always negative and the child handles challenge with penicillin well.

True immunologic responses to a drug may occur by one of several mechanisms, as described by Coombs and Gell.

1. Anaphylactic or IgE mediated
2. Cytotoxic, in which complement is involved in the reaction
3. IgG immune complexes
4. Delayed hypersensitivity or T cell mediated

Some drugs, such as penicillin, are able to elicit all four different types of immunologic reactions.

The risk of an allergic reaction to a drug is associated with treatment factors and patient factors. Some drugs, such as penicillin, are known for their allergenic properties. Also, parenteral routes of administration (IV or IM) are known to be more likely to precipitate allergic reactions than is the enteric route of administration (PO). Patient factors include age and a history of prior drug reactions. It is not unusual for a patient to have multiple drug allergies. A family history of drug allergy can be valuable in identifying the at-risk patient (e.g., a child whose mother has had acute allergic reactions to two different classes of drugs may be genetically vulnerable).

The major challenge for a physician is to know how to diagnose ADR properly, categorize it properly, treat it, and prevent further occurrence. Diagnosis can be quite difficult, since a patient with a rash who is taking a drug may have a concurrent viral illness. Viral illnesses are often associated with rashes, including urticaria. Skin testing, if available, can be useful in distinguishing an IgE-mediated drug reaction from a viral illness, but unfortunately, testing is not available for most drugs and does not identify the non-IgE-mediated ADRs.

Treatment of a suspected ADR usually dictates withdrawal of the drug. If the symptoms are a classic anaphylactic reaction (urticaria, angioedema, respiratory distress, hypovolemic shock), the same medical treatment is used to stabilize the patient as with any other case of anaphylaxis, that is, epinephrine 0.01 mg/kg every 15 minutes, diphenhydramine 5 mg/kg/d, prednisone 1 to 2 mg/kg/d for 3 to 5 days, and volume expansion if there is hypotension. If the reaction is primarily urticaria and angioedema without other signs of a systemic reaction, antihistamines are usually sufficient to ameliorate the symptoms. The choice of which antihistamine to use is determined somewhat by trial and error and should be dictated by side effects in the particular patient, as well as efficacy. Often, one antihistamine will seem to work a little better than another, but the best one to use varies from patient to patient. Both patient and doctor, however, need to be prepared for a low-grade allergic reaction to continue for several days.

There are rare situations in which a patient must receive a medication to which he or she is allergic. In such a situation, premedication with antihistamines and steroids in an acute care environment, where the patient can be carefully monitored, is one approach that has been used (e.g., for such agents as radiographic contrast media). An approach used with medications that can be administered orally is oral desensitization, in which the patient is carefully monitored and challenged with very small but increasing doses every 15 minutes until a therapeutic dose is reached. Once desensitized, the patient must be maintained on the medication daily. Because of the complexities and risks in desensitization and premedication, an allergist should be involved, and there must be adequate monitoring.

REFERENCE

1. Deswarte RD: Drug allergy. *In* Patterson R, Grammer LC, Greenberger PA, Zeiss CR, (eds): Allergic Diseases—Diagnosis and Management. Philadelphia, JB Lippincott, 1993;395–552.

URTICARIA AND ANGIOEDEMA

ALLEN LAPEY, M.D.

Urticaria, or hives, involves the superficial layer of the dermis and is generally pruritic and evanescent in character, waxing and waning over a matter of hours. Angioedema is a deeper subcutaneous swelling, less pruritic and erythematous, and often involving the periorbital or perioral soft tissues. It, too, is evanescent and often coexists with urticaria.

It is necessary to differentiate acute from chronic (greater than 2 weeks in duration) forms of urticaria and angioedema. Whereas in acute instances, the inciting factor frequently is allergenic and generally obvious on simple history, over 95% of chronic urticaria is idiopathic. Chronic urticaria is best approached with a thorough history and physical examination and, if the patient is otherwise well, no exhaustive testing, since the yield will be nil. Patients with chronic urticaria need reassurance that the problem is more a nuisance than a disease, that it will "burn itself out," generally in a matter of months, and that groping for a cause is counterproductive. Recent evidence that histamine-releasing IgG autoantibodies against the high-affinity IgE receptor are present in the serum of patients with chronic urticaria has proven helpful in explaining disease mechanism to families.

In one's therapeutic approach to acute urticaria, recognition of the many inciting factors, allergic and nonallergic, is critical, so that avoidance can be practiced.

URTICARIA AND DIET

Although immediate IgE-mediated reactions are common to a variety of foods, additives are rarely implicated. In the first 24 months of life, reactions to milk, egg, soy, wheat, and peanut represent over 90% of food-induced incidents. Peanut, nut, shellfish, and fish assume greater significance in later years as diet is liberalized and also because these allergies are apt to persist. Fresh fruit often causes minor mediator release in the lips or tongue. Chocolate, on the other hand, is weakly antigenic and rarely causes urticaria.

Food additives, although anecdotally incriminated, almost never cause urticaria per se. Agents mentioned as involved include tartrazine, dyes, bisulfites, monosodium glutamate, nitrites, and natural salicylates.

INFECTIONS

Infectious mononucleosis and hepatitis B initially may present with urticaria in some cases. In children, viral respiratory infections commonly are accompanied by transient urticaria. On the other hand, chronic focal infections (sinus, teeth, genitourinary tract, fungal) almost never cause chronic hives.

INHALANTS AND CONTACTANTS

Inhalant allergy rarely triggers urticaria as an isolated finding. Exceptions are encountered at the height of pollen exposure in association with severe respiratory symptoms. In a susceptible individual, exercise when there are high pollen counts can precipitate urticaria and anaphylaxis. Contact urticaria frequently is brought on by the smearing of finger foods on and about the face by infants and toddlers. Periorbital reactions are particularly common and should not be misinterpreted as systemic reactions (anaphylaxis). Saliva of household pets also may cause local reaction. Outdoors, Portuguese men-of-war, tarantula hairs, and PABA in sunscreens are hazards that often cause urticaria on contact.

PHYSICAL URTICARIA

Environmental factors frequently are implicated in both acute and chronic urticarial reactions, specifically, mechanical pressure, light, cold, heat, exercise, and vibration. Indeed, these are much more likely to be causative in chronic urticaria than is allergy per se.

Pressure Urticaria

This condition is encountered occasionally at sites of constant pressure to the skin, for example, from tight garments or on the soles of the feet following prolonged exercise. The lesions are erythematous, deep, and at times painful, especially with sustained trauma. Treatment with antihistamines and corticosteroids is disappointing, and it is preferable to avoid the trigger.

Cold Urticaria

In this somewhat more common condition, patients experience an immediate urticarial rash at sites exposed to the cold, for example, the face and hands on a wintry day. The ice cube test is diagnostic. Within 5 to 10 minutes after application of an ice cube, a well-demarcated wheal appears at the site of application, with surrounding flair. Cold urticaria is often associated with angioedema. In instances of total body exposure (swimming), hypotension, shock, and drowning have been reported. Patients are instructed to protect exposed surfaces from the cold and to swim with caution, never alone. The antihistamine cyproheptadine traditionally has been recommended for this disorder and may be helpful if it is used before exposure. However, specific comparative efficacy studies using this agent are not convincing.

Cholinergic (Heat-Induced) Urticaria

In instances of a generalized increase in core temperature caused by such activities as bathing, hyperpyrexia, sustained exercise with perspiration, or emotional upset, this highly pruritic, morphologically distinct rash may occur. Lesions predominate in the axillae, groin, neck, and trunk where sweating is prominent. Wheals are minute and in clusters, surrounded by large areas of erythema. Care must be taken not to confuse this lesser syndrome with exercise-induced anaphylaxis, which results in generalized warmth, flushing, and urticaria and angioedema. The angioedema often occurs on the face, palms, and soles, leading to hypotension. Cholinergic urticaria usually responds well to hydroxyzine pretreatment.

Vibratory Angioedema

This condition is probably a variant of pressure urticaria, occurring most often on the palms while holding vibrating equipment (e.g., lawn mower, power tools). Treatment is avoidance, with consideration of hydroxyzine pretreatment.

Solar Urticaria

Sun or artificial light exposure may result in urticaria, with the onset at times within minutes. This entity should be differentiated from drug-induced photoallergic reactions, as are seen with sulfa agents, or photosensitivity reactions (enhanced sunburn), as may occur with tetracyclines or quinolones. Other than sunburn, sun exposure most commonly causes polymorphous light eruptions, most often in spring or early summer before acclimatization has taken place. Avoidance and sunscreens suffice to avoid this condition.

Acute urticarial syndromes can be reproduced experimentally at certain wavelengths of light. The ultraviolet spectrum from 280 to 320 nm (sunburn range) is filtered by ordinary glass and can be blocked by sunscreens with a sun protection factor of 15 or higher. Higher wavelength sensitivity is less common and more difficult to treat, requiring strict avoidance and the use of nonchemical blockers, such as titanium dioxide or zinc oxide.

EXERCISE-INDUCED ANAPHYLAXIS

Perhaps as a consequence of the renewed emphasis on fitness through regular physical exercise, exercise-induced anaphylaxis (EIA) is being seen with increasing regularity, most often among joggers. The typical subject is an athletic young adult who exercises regularly, often daily. In contrast to other forms of physical allergy, which are reproducible, EIA occurs inconsistently in otherwise identical circumstances. This raises the possibility that other, as yet unknown factors may play a role. Particular attention has been given to postprandial exercise, since many of the first patients described had eaten recently. The foods in question usually but not always were substances to which the patient showed immediate hypersensitivity on prick testing but to which the patient did not otherwise react. Alcohol, aspirin, and NSAIDS also have been implicated in EIA.

The evolution of symptoms is characteristic: diffuse warmth or pruritus followed by generalized erythema, urticaria, or angioedema, leading to vascular collapse and loss of consciousness. Stridor may occur but is never the sole feature.

Treatment of EIA involves the usual steps for anaphylaxis, including subcutaneous epinephrine, volume repletion, and oxygen administration. Equally important is prevention, which includes delaying exercise 4 to 6 hours after meals, avoiding alcohol and aspirin before exercise, and recognizing the earliest hints that a reaction is imminent (feeling flushed, itchy). If such signs occur, all activity must be stopped immediately.

EIA should not be confused with exercise-induced asthma or cholinergic urticaria. In the latter, also often triggered by exercise, minute urticarial lesions 1 to 2 mm in diameter appear in association with intense perspiration, generally in warmer body sites, such as the axillae or groin. Facial angioedema, vascular collapse, and stridor do not occur. The wheeze and cough of asthma, if present, are transient and are not a dominant clinical feature of EIA.

CHRONIC IDIOPATHIC URTICARIA

Urticarial reactions ongoing for more than 2 weeks are considered chronic and almost never have a specific external cause. Such reactions may have physical features; for example, they can be worsened by cold exposure or exercise. They may be adversely affected by aspirin or NSAIDS, perhaps related to aspirin's effect on prostaglandin metabolism, but those affected continue to have lesions even without taking aspirin. Affected individuals are usually not atopic, and IgEs are normal. Typically, these patients are as frustrated as their management is frustrating. However, management has been clarified by a recent observation on pathogenesis. The majority of patients with chronic idiopathic urticaria have a strongly positive immediate skin test response to autologous serum. This seems to be due to a histaminic releasing IgG antibody against the alpha-subunit of the high-affinity IgE receptor of mast cells, resulting in crosslinking of IgE receptors and mediator release.

Management of chronic urticaria generally involves maintenance therapy with long-acting second-generation antihistamines, for example, astemizole 10 mg daily, terfenadine 60 mg twice a day, or loratadine 10 mg daily. Maximal clinical benefit is achieved with conventional doses, and additional amounts of drug serve no purpose. Furthermore, astemizole and terfenadine may on rare occasions cause cardiac arrhythmias at high blood levels. Erythromycin and ketoconazole interfere with hepatic clearance of astemazole and terfenadine, constituting an additional risk factor for cardiac toxicity. Coadministration is contraindicated. Rapid-acting first-generation antihistamines, for example, hydroxyzine 10 to 25 mg or diphenhydramine 25 mg, are added every 4 to 6 hours for exacerbations. Brief 5- to 7-day pulses of systemic corticosteroids (prednisone 20 mg twice daily for 3 days, followed by 20 mg daily for 2 days) are added when symptoms are unbearable or so disfiguring (periorbital or perioral angioedema) as to result in time lost from school or work.

HEREDITARY ANGIOEDEMA

Hereditary angioedema (HAE) is an autosomal dominant inherited disease resulting in recurrent episodes of self-limited circumscribed subepithelial edema of the skin, respiratory tract, and gastrointestinal tract. Lesions typically occur at sites of cutaneous trauma or instrumentation of the upper respiratory tract (tooth extraction, tonsillectomy). Gastrointestinal tract involvement may be isolated, with symptoms of colic, nausea, and vomiting usually misdiagnosed in a previously unrecognized episode. Skin lesions are nonpruritic, a helpful differential point, often described as burning, and not particularly erythematous.

The lack of a family history of the disease does not rule out the diagnosis of HAE. Over 90% of affected children lack a serum protein, C1 esterase inhibitor, providing a basis for diagnosis. A rare subgroup (usually adult) of patients have normal but nonfunctional levels of C1 esterase inhibitor, so functional assays may be indicated. Therapy involves the prophylactic use of antifibrinolytic agents, such as epsilon-aminocaproic acid and tranexamic acid, or attenuated anabolic steroids, such as danazol. The latter is generally not advised in children because of its potential effect on growth.

REFERENCE

1. Hide M, Francis DM, Grattan CEH, Hakimi J, Kochan JP, Greaves MW. Autoantibodies against the high-affinity IgE receptor as a cause of histamine release in chronic urticaria. N Engl J Med 328:1599–1604, 1993.

ALLERGIC RHINITIS

GILBERT ANTHONY FRIDAY, JR., M.D.

Approximately 15% of the general population has allergic rhinitis caused by immediate hypersensitivity. Allergic rhinitis is most prevalent in children. Signs and symptoms consist of nasal mucous membrane edema, clear nasal discharge of a usually serous nature, frequent sneezing, nasal pruritus, itching of the eyes or throat or both, nasal obstruction with mouth breathing, and snoring. Occasionally, malaise, fatigue, and irritability are noticeable. Conjunctivitis may be seen along with edema and a darkening of the tissues under the eyes, called an "allergic shiner." Etiologic factors include inhalants, such as pollens from grasses and weeds, mold spores, housedust mites (*Dermatophygoides*), cat, dog, and other mammals (epidermal, saliva, and urine). Allergic individuals have cell-bound immunoglobulin E (IgE) that specifically interacts with antigens (allergens) to set off an inflammatory event. The conjugation of cell-bound IgE and allergen molecules results in the release of chemical mediators that are capable of causing vasodilatation, increased mucosal permeability, increased mucous production, influx of inflammatory cells, and increased sensitivity to subsequent allergen exposure (priming).

The pathophysiology includes both immediate phase and late phase reactions. Interaction of allergen with IgE on the surface of nasal mucosa mast cells causes the release of mediators of immediate hypersensitivity, which primarily include histamine but also include kinin, tryptase, prostaglandin D_2, and leukotriene D_4. The late phase reaction occurs in 50% of patients 3 to 11 hours later, when basophils are activated and histamine, kinins, and leukotrienes reappear. Plasma transudation brings in kinin vasoactive peptides. Chemotactic factors are released that include hydroxyeicosatetraenoic acids and the metabolite of platelet-activating factor lyso-PAF, which may be important in the recruitment of inflammatory cells. Cells include eosinophils, neutrophils, basophils, and mononuclear cells. The appearance of eosinophil-derived major basic protein and eosinophil-derived neurotoxin gives further evidence for eosinophil degranulation. The nonadrenergic, noncholinergic portion of the nervous system acts as a communication link between the immunologic and neuroelements via the production of neuropeptides. Neuropeptides regulate the release of mediators from mast cells. These include vasoactive intestinal peptide (VIP), tachykinin, substance P, calcitonin gene-related peptide, and somatostatin. Even days after significant exposure, the inflammatory changes may be noticeable in the nasal airway.

DIFFERENTIAL DIAGNOSIS

Other types of rhinitis may be seen in children, although much less frequently than allergic rhinitis. Infectious rhinitis secondary to viral upper respiratory infections may be seen rather frequently, especially in the early years of school.

Nonallergic rhinitis with eosinophilia syndrome resembles allergic rhinitis on examination. However, skin tests are negative. Nasal smears for eosinophils show greater than 25% eosinophils. The etiology is unknown. The problem is not recognized frequently in children.

Vasomotor rhinitis is a nonallergic rhinitis syndrome in which eosinophils are not present in nasal secretions. Skin tests are negative. It is probably due to autonomic dysfunction and frequently is a diagnosis of exclusion.

Nasal polyposis is another inflammatory problem of unknown etiology usually associated in childhood with a diagnosis of cystic fibrosis. It is rarely associated with allergic rhinitis.

Other structurally related rhinopathy can be due to trauma, deviated nasal septum, unilateral choanal atresia, tumors, foreign bodies, and adenoidal hypertrophy. More rare conditions in childhood include ciliary dyskinesia, rhinitis medicamentosa, CNS rhinorrhea, and distichiasis.

DIAGNOSIS

Allergic rhinitis is commonly caused by such inhaled allergens as housedust mites, pollens, fungal spores, insect emanations, and animal danders. Pollens produce symptoms during the spring, summer, and fall, whereas housedust mites and animal dander produce perennial symptoms. Food rarely causes nasal symptoms after age 3 years. Foods, such as milk, may be a cause of nasal congestion in early infancy. Mold spore allergy and animal protein allergy may be seen in infancy. Pollen sensitization may occur as the child grows older and passes through four or more pollen seasons.

Typically, symptoms of allergic rhinitis include sneezing, itching of the nose, eyes, palate, or pharynx, nasal stuffiness, and a clear nasal discharge that may be accompanied by postnasal drainage. Fatigue may be present, as may irritability. Physical findings are generally limited to the eyes, nose, and ears. Allergic shiners are dark circles under the eyes due to venous engorgement secondary to nasal congestion. Conjunctiva may be injected. A transverse nasal crease results from an allergic salute. The nasal mucous membranes may be erythematous, pale, or violaceous in color, with variable degrees of edema, nasal obstruction, and clear watery secretion. Mouth breathing may be present. Mild ear effusions may develop.

Diagnostic Techniques

Skin testing with potent allergens with positive and negative controls is the diagnostic procedure of choice. The prick test method is the fastest, least expensive, and least painful screening tool. Intradermal tests should be reserved for patients who have negative prick tests but in whom there is a high degree of suspicion for an allergic cause. Skin tests must correlate with the patient's history to be of value. Radioallergosorbent testing (RAST) can be used if the skin is extensively covered with rash. Total serum IgE concentration is elevated in one third of the patients, but this is of limited value in diagnosis because the concentration varies greatly and usually overlaps with normal values. Peripheral blood eosinophil counts may be mildly

increased, and a smear of the nasal secretions during active disease may show increased eosinophils but is not diagnostic.

TREATMENT

Avoidance

The allergens causing allergic rhinitis are housedust mites, mold spores, animal proteins, and pollens, and the most effective therapy is avoidance of the allergens. Table 1 gives dust mite avoidance guidelines. The gastrointestinal enzymes contained in the mite feces are the most important mite allergens. These enzymes not only act as antigens but also can cause destruction of tissue. Their control in individuals with skin sensitivity to them and perennial rhinitis is of the utmost importance.

Mold avoidance largely involves measures to decrease household humidity. Humidity between 30% and 50% is satisfactory for normal respiratory physiology. Bedroom humidifiers and vaporizers are to be avoided. Heating and cooling systems should be checked to eliminate mold reservoirs. Dehumidifiers are useful at times, especially in the basement.

Animal proteins are more likely to be a problem when pets have the run of the house. Dogs and cats are the most likely to cause problems, yet 60% of American homes have such pets. One must weigh the patient's or family's emotional attachment to a pet against the degree of allergy and possible relief through other modalities besides elimination of the pets from the environment. At the very least, any pet can be kept out of the allergic patient's bedroom. Frequent bathing of dogs and cats may be of some benefit in eliminating the animal antigen from the environment.

Pollens can be eliminated from the indoor environment and automobiles by air conditioning.

Environmental control measures are frequently ignored and must be stressed. Very significant changes in the individual's sensitivities can occur when these measures are conscientiously carried out. Instructions may be given by word of mouth, reading material, videotapes and in some instances, by home visits. Avoidance of irritants, such as tobacco smoke, perfumes, and any type of material providing strong odors, will help.

PHARMACOLOGIC INTERVENTION

Antihistamines

H_1-antagonist drugs are the most frequently used medication in the treatment of allergic rhinitis. In general, their onset of action is rapid, and they reduce sneezing, pruritus, and rhinorrhea but not congestion.

There are now two generations of antihistamines (Table 2). Both generations seem to be of equal potency, but the older antihistamines have more side effects in some persons. In general, the older antihistamines provide more sedation and central cholinergic blockade, manifest by irritability and possible adverse effects on coordination. Antihistamines have a quinidine effect on cardiac muscle that can prolong the QT interval. Occasionally, overdose can lead to a life-threatening ventricular arrhythmia (torsades de pointes). There have been a few reports, particularly with terfenadine and astemizole, of

TABLE 1. Dust Mite Avoidance Guidelines

- Encase mattress, boxsprings, and pillow in mite-proof cover.
- Remove carpeting from bedroom. If this is impractical, use an acaricide,* such as benzyl benzoate,† to kill mites or tannic acid to denature mite antigen.
- Wash bedsheets and blankets in 130°F water once a week.
- Decrease household humidity to <50%.
- Remove all upholstered furniture from bedroom.
- Minimize dust traps (e.g., stuffed animals, books).

*Acarosan, Fison Corporation, P.O. Box 1766, Rochester, NY 14603.
†Allergy Control Products, Inc., 96 Danbury Road, Ridgefield, CT 06877.

TABLE 2. Classification and Pharmacology of H₁-Receptor Histamine Antagonists

CHEMICAL CLASS	FIRST GENERATION (CLASSIC)	SUGGESTED DOSE FOR CHILDREN (mg/kg/24 h)*	SUGGESTED DOSE FOR ADULTS	ANTIHISTAMINE EFFECT	SEDATION EFFECT	ANTICHOLINERGIC EFFECT
Alkylamines	Chlorpheniramine	0.35	4 mg q.i.d.	+ + +	+	+ +
	Brompheniramine	0.5	4–8 mg q.i.d.	+ + +	+	+ +
	Triprolidine	0.6 ± 1.25 mg q.i.d.	2.5 mg q.i.d.	+ + +	+ +	+ +
Ethylenediamines	Tripelennamine	3	25–50 mg q.i.d.	+ + +	+ +	+
Ethanolamines	Diphenhydramine	5	25–50 mg q.i.d.	+ + +	+ + +	+
	Clemastine	0.5–1 mg b.i.d.	1–2 mg b.i.d.	+ + +	+ +	+
Piperazines	Hydroxyzine	2	10–20 mg q.i.d.	+ + +	+ / + +	+
Piperidines	Cyproheptadine	0.25	4–20 mg q.i.d.	+ + +	+	+ +
	Azatadine	?	1–2 mg b.i.d.	+ + +	+ +	+ +
Phenothiazines	Promethazine	0.5	12.5–25 mg q.i.d.	+ + +	+ + +	+ +
	SECOND GENERATION (NONSEDATING)†					
	Terfenadine	15–30 mg b.i.d.	60 mg b.i.d.	+ + +	0	0
	Astemizole	<6 y: 0.2 6–12 y: 5 mg/d	10 mg q.d.	+ + +	0	0
	Loratadine	not known	10 mg q.d.	+ + +	0/ +	0

*Unless otherwise listed.
†Not formally approved; doses from literature.
? = not known.

accumulation of the parent drug through overdose or blockage of the cytochrome P450 1114A isoenzyme that metabolizes these drugs. The concurrent use of erythromycin preparations and antifungal drugs, such as ketoconazole, that block the enzyme system may cause a buildup of the parent drug and consequent toxicity.

Decongestants

The oral decongestant sympathomimetic agents, such as pseudoephedrine and phenylpropanolamine, are useful in reducing nasal mucous membrane edema by their alpha-adrenergic vasoconstriction effect. They work well in conjunction with antihistamines. There are a large number of combination products. These drugs can be administered either topically or systemically. Topical administration produces a more rapid onset of action and is more effective than systemic administration and should be reserved for facilitating the introduction of topical steroids and for sleep during severe exacerbations of allergic rhinitis. Prolonged topical administration, however, leads to rhinitis medicamentosa.

These agents constrict vascular beds and can produce insomnia and irritability. They must be used with caution in children prone to seizures or who have heart disease or hypertension. The usual dose of pseudoephedrine hydrochloride given every 6 hours is 15 mg for children 2 to 5 years of age, 30 mg for those 6 to 12 years, and 60 mg for those above 12 years of age.

Mast Cell Stabilizing Drugs

Cromolyn sodium has been useful in the prophylaxis of allergic rhinitis and, at times, before episodic exposure. Its primary use has been during pollen seasons or before known exposures to other allergens, such as animal proteins. The side effects are minimal. It is delivered intranasally as a 4% spray through a metered dose inhaler four to six times per day. Some patients respond to cromolyn sodium as they do to antihistamines. Others do not respond at all. Nedocromil nasal preparations may soon be available.

Glucocorticoids

Intranasal corticosteroids are very effective in relieving nasal congestion, as well as nasal secretions, sneezing, and itching. The preparations available include beclomethasone, flunisolide, triamcinolone, and dexamethasone. Treatments with topical nasal corticosteroids will diminish both the immediate and late phase responses. These agents all act by regulating gene expression, which accounts for the delay between their administration and clinical activity. They appear to diminish histamine release and to alter the pathways that lead to the production of mediators from arachidonic acid. Dexamethasone is absorbed to a significant degree and should not be used routinely to treat allergic rhinitis. Intranasal beclomethasone is usually well tolerated either as an aerosol or in an aqueous preparation. The drug is very poorly absorbed from the mucosa, and any portion swallowed is absorbed and metabolized rapidly to an inactive form. Flunisolide is quite active, but the stinging side effects limit its use in children. Triamcinolone can be used as an aerosol once a day, whereas the others must be used two to four times per day. The onset of action is rather slow and may take 2 to 3 days to show a benefit. Once the symptoms are under control, the dose can be weaned to a once-a-day regimen. Young children generally do not tolerate topical nasal sprays very well, but schoolage and older children have little or no difficulty, and compliance is good, especially if the dose is limited to once or twice per day.

Systemic corticosteroid use should be reserved for very special cases when there is little or no response to antihistamines, decongestants, or topical corticosteroid preparations. A short course at the peak of the season may be worthwhile using 1 to 2 mg/kg/d of prednisone. Intramuscular steroid preparations or intranasal corticosteroids are contraindicated in children.

Immunotherapy

Immunotherapy should be considered for patients who do not respond to medications well, cannot tolerate medication side effects, or have severe multiseason allergic rhinitis. It depends on the accurate assessment of an individual child's allergen sensitivity.

Immunotherapy results in immunologic changes. There is an increase in the levels of allergen-specific IgG antibodies in the serum. Antigen-specific IgE antibodies rise initially and then fall with continued treatment. Immunotherapy induces generation of antigen-specific suppressor cells, decreases the production of lymphokines, and reduces the production of a mononuclear cell-derived histamine-releasing factor. It reduces the late phase response and influx of eosinophils.

The parents of patients selected for immunotherapy need to be informed about the regimen, duration of therapy, potential complications, and anticipated outcome. There are no absolute guidelines, but in general, injections are given weekly for 6 to 8 months until a maintenance concentration of the antigen mixture is achieved. Allergens can be combined, fortunately, so that children may need to receive only one injection. Once a maintenance level is reached, injections can be given at 2- to 4-week intervals. When a patient demonstrates that with injections at intervals of 4 weeks there are few or no symptoms during seasons of the year previously bothersome, immunotherapy may be discontinued. Improvement can occur within 3 to 6 months from the beginning of treatment, and the degree of improvement appears to increase over a period of 1 to 2 years. When injections are stopped, some patients remain asymptomatic for long term, and others have minimal symptoms that are easily managed pharmaceutically. Side effects with immunotherapy are relatively uncommon, although anaphylaxis may occur, so extreme caution must be taken when administering the injections (under the direct supervision of a physician). Current studies have proven the efficacy of immunotherapy with allergic rhinitis and, more recently, with pollen asthma.

REFERENCES

1. Druce HM: Allergic and nonallergic rhinitis. *In* Middleton E Jr, Reed CE, Ellis EF, Adkinson NF Jr, Yunginger JW, Busse WW (eds): Allergy: Principles and Practice. St Louis, CV Mosby Co., 1993:1433.
2. Naclerio RM: Allergic rhinitis. N Engl J Med 325:860–869, 1991.

ASTHMA

EDWARD J. O'CONNELL, M.D.
DANN K. HEILMAN, M.D.

The prevalence of asthma has increased for reasons that are not well known. Moreover, morbidity and mortality have increased in the last decade, particularly among certain patient groups, despite development of newer, more effective drugs for treatment. A greater emphasis on the inflammatory component of asthma and the wider selection of effective therapies have made the options for management more complex.

Asthma can be defined as a chronic disorder consisting of airway obstruction that is at least partially reversible, with bronchial hyperreactivity and varying degrees of bronchial inflammation. Environmental, infectious, and genetic factors have all been implicated in the pathogenesis of asthma, but the precise roles of each are poorly defined. Exacerbations of asthma can be provoked by allergens, respiratory infections, inhaled irritants, and exercise, with variation among individual asthmatics as to the relative importance of each factor. Asthma can also be classified as mild, moderate, or severe. This classification, outlined in detail by the National Heart, Lung, and Blood Institute, can be summarized as follows.

1. *Mild asthma* is symptomatic only once or twice a week, causes little interference with sleep or daily activities, and usually requires only intermittent bronchodilators or regular medications for only brief periods of time.
2. *Moderate asthma* is associated with at least low-grade symptoms on a daily or ongoing basis, is aggravated by even modest exercise, and usually requires continuous medication for prolonged periods of time and systemic corticosteroids for exacerbations.
3. In *severe asthma*, patients generally wheeze daily, require several emergency room visits or hospitalizations (or both) per year, have very poor exercise tolerance, and require multiple daily medications, which for some may include long-term use of oral corticosteroids.

TREATMENT

The treatment of asthma is directed at decreasing airway inflammation and reactivity by eliminating or minimizing triggering factors and by selecting appropriate medications in a stepwise manner. The number of steps in the process depends on the severity of the asthma and the assessment of the response to each preceding step. For mild asthma, the first step is usually a bronchodilator, most often a beta-agonist. For moderate or severe asthma, an anti-inflammatory agent in combination with at least one bronchodilator is used. Goals of therapy include (1) normal activities, (2) normal or nearly normal pulmonary function, (3) prevention of troublesome symptoms, (4) prevention of exacerbations, and (5) avoidance of medication side effects.

Environmental Control

For patients with an allergic component to their asthma, allergen avoidance by manipulation of the environment may be beneficial. Avoidance of any triggering factor when possible is by far the most effective therapy. Elimination of tobacco and wood smoke, chemical fumes, and other respiratory irritants can be of great benefit to most asthmatics.

Of all the indoor aeroallergens, the housedust mites, *Dermatophagoides pteronyssinus* and *Dermatophagoides farinae*, have received the most attention in the literature. Depending on the geography and climate, as many as 70% of asthmatics may be sensitive to these mites. Dust mites thrive best in humid climates, so controlling indoor humidity may reduce levels by decreasing growth rates. Efforts at decreasing housedust, particularly in the patient's bedroom, improve asthma symptoms and more objective measures of respiratory function. There is virtually no limit to the steps that can be taken to accomplish this, but in general, the more simple the measure, the better the compliance. Encasing the mattress, boxspring, and pillows in allergen-proof coverings is the most effective measure, together with regularly washing all bedding in hot water. Frequent vacuuming has only transient benefit, so elimination of carpeted flooring may be necessary. Various air filtration devices with a wide spectrum of efficiency are available. However, components of housedust settle out of the air quickly and may only be airborne when the room is being disturbed, thus limiting the usefulness of these devices. Acaricides are available that can kill mites and decrease allergen levels, but they must be applied repeatedly to be effective.

Cat and dog allergens can be found in housedust and may persist for months after the animal has been removed permanently from the house. Removal of the allergenic pet is ideal, but for families who will not get rid of their pet, banning it from the patient's bedroom is mandatory. Limited studies on regular washing of pets have suggested some decrease in allergen levels. The social benefits of owning pets must be weighed against the severity of the child's asthma and the likelihood of improvement in symptoms if the animal is removed.

Indoor mold can also be a problem for asthmatics, but because of the lack of quality of test extracts, the frequency of hypersensitivity is difficult to assess. Mold overgrowth may be a problem in any area of the home where water or moisture is allowed to stand, for example, in basements, bath and shower areas, and humidifiers. Thorough cleaning with a bleach and use of a dehumidifier in damp basements may help reduce the levels of this type of allergen.

As a rule, outdoor allergens, such as pollens and outdoor molds, have a smaller role in the exacerbation of asthma in comparison with the indoor environment. However, certain patients may have seasonal asthma. In fact, *Alternaria* has been linked to fatal and near-fatal attacks of asthma. These allergens are extremely difficult to avoid, and staying indoors with doors and windows closed may be the only recourse during the problem season.

Beta-Adrenergic Agents

Choice of Agents

Beta-adrenergic drugs act by stimulating $beta_2$-receptors that are abundant in bronchial smooth muscle. Ideally, they should cause only minimal stimulation of the $beta_1$-receptors in the myocardium. Historically, epinephrine, ephedrine, isoproterenol, isoetharine, and metaproterenol are beta-agonists that have been used extensively. Currently, they have limited clinical usefulness because of the extent of $beta_1$-receptor stimulation, routes of administration, or short duration of action.

Since the early 1970s, drugs with more beta$_2$-specific properties have been developed. Currently, terbutaline, albuterol, and pirbuterol cause generally less cardiac stimulation and more bronchodilatation than older nonselective agents, such as metaproterenol (Table 1). Also, they all appear to be longer acting. Most recently, salmeterol has become available. It is highly specific for beta$_2$-receptors and is a longer-acting drug that can be given at 12-hour intervals, making it an attractive option for daily management of chronic asthma.

The use of beta-adrenergic drugs is indicated (1) for the treatment of acute asthma symptoms, including status asthmaticus, (2) for prevention, as in exercise-induced bronchospasm, or anticipated exposure to a known asthma trigger, and (3) for chronic use in moderate to severe disease.

Routes of Administration

Oral. Of the newer beta$_2$-agonists, terbutaline and albuterol are available in oral preparations. The peak onset is approximately 2 hours, and the duration of action is 4 to 8 hours (Table 1). Albuterol also comes in sustained-release forms that can be given twice daily. Because of varying degrees of absorption and greater volume of distribution, large doses must be given, with greater potential for beta$_1$-receptor-mediated and extrapulmonary beta$_2$-receptor side effects when compared with other routes of administration. Advantages of oral therapy include convenience and better delivery to obstructed lung segments.

Aerosol. Aerosol delivery of beta-agonist bronchodilators allows maximum delivery of the drugs to the airways and less delivery to other tissues as compared with the oral route. All the beta$_2$-receptor-selective agents cited previously are available in aerosol form and can be given by either metered-dose inhalers or nebulizers (not pirbuterol or salmeterol). When used properly, inhalers allow even smaller doses than nebulizers, are portable, and are generally more convenient. A spacing device, such as an InspirEase or AeroChamber, makes metered-dose inhalers more effective and allows them to be used in young patients. Nebulizer treatments are used frequently in hospital settings but can be appropriate for home use with portable units that can go virtually anywhere. Nebulizers are useful if technique is a problem with metered-dose inhalers, particularly in very young patients.

Parenteral. Epinephrine and terbutaline are the two most common beta-adrenergic drugs given by the subcutaneous route. Although they have been replaced largely by aerosol medications, they still have a place in the emergency treatment of acute bronchospasm because of their rapid onset of action, especially in the treatment of acute allergic reactions.

Intravenous agents are rarely used, although continuous infusion of isoproterenol or albuterol has been used for resistant status asthmaticus when respiratory failure is imminent. The potential for serious cardiac toxicity makes this route risky, and it should be used only by experienced personnel and only with very careful monitoring in an intensive care setting.

Problems with Use

The most common side effect reported by patients is tremor that is due to stimulation of beta$_2$-receptors in skeletal muscle. With continued use, this side effect usually diminishes over time. A smaller number of patients report an increase in heart rate and palpitations that are due to reflex stimulation of the heart secondary to peripheral vasodilatation and direct stimulation of the few beta$_2$-receptors that are in the heart.

Overall, the short-term use of beta$_2$-adrenergic agents for symptomatic management of acute asthma is remarkably free of adverse effects, making these agents the most useful class of bronchodilators for this purpose. However, in recent years, controversy has arisen over the role of beta-adrenergic agents for the long-term management of asthma, and a relationship between their continuous daily use and the current increase in asthma morbidity and mortality has been suggested. Increases in airway responsiveness, cardiac arrhythmias,

tachyphylaxis, lack of anti-inflammatory effect, and a false sense of well-being have been cited as possible mechanisms for this observation. Currently, a prudent course would be to continue using beta-agonists for acute symptomatic therapy and, whenever possible, to avoid regular daily use except for situations where appropriate anti-inflammatory treatment is inadequate.

Theophylline

Theophylline is a methylxanthine derivative that has been used to treat asthma for the last 50 years. In the 1980s, concern arose about the potential for such side effects as nausea, anorexia, irritability, insomnia, and inattentiveness in school. This concern, together with greater emphasis on the anti-inflammatory aspects of asthma management and the advent of newer beta$_2$-receptor-selective drugs, has led to a decline in the use of theophylline, particularly as a first-line monotherapeutic agent. Although few authorities question the efficacy of this drug as a bronchodilator, its specific mechanism of action is not clearly understood. Also, the newer beta-agonists have a greater bronchodilator effect. However, methylxanthines may have other airway benefits, including reducing nonspecific airway hyperactivity, improving mucociliary clearance, and increasing ventilatory drive.[2] Theophylline is very effective for controlling nocturnal asthma, and several studies indicate improved control of symptoms in patients taking daily doses and a steroid-sparing effect in steroid-dependent asthmatics.

The problem with theophylline is its narrow therapeutic range. Although blood levels can and should be monitored, side effects are common even when drug levels are kept within the therapeutic range of 5 to 15 µg/ml (Table 1). In addition, more serious reactions, such as severe vomiting, seizures, and cardiac arrhythmias, can occur when levels exceed 20 µg/ml. Theophylline must be used cautiously, and blood levels must be monitored, especially in patients with liver disease or in those taking drugs known to affect theophylline metabolism; for example, erythromycin, cimetidine, and oral contraceptives can increase the level of theophylline in the blood.

Theophylline still has a place in the treatment of childhood asthma. The National Heart, Lung, and Blood Institute consensus report includes theophylline in its recommendations for when the combination of a beta-agonist and an anti-inflammatory agent has failed to control symptoms. Several studies have refuted claims about the adverse effect of theophylline on school performance.

Oral theophylline comes in both short-acting and long-acting forms. However, sustained-release tablets and capsules that can be opened and sprinkled on food have largely replaced the short-acting preparations. Initial doses should be calculated according to the age and weight of the patient, keeping in mind potential drug interactions and any disease states that might interfere with metabolism. Because maximum benefit with minimum risk occurs at a serum level of 5 to 15 µg/ml, a level in this range measured 4 hours after a morning dose and after 3 days of constant dosing at the same dose without missed or extra doses should provide a wide safety margin against serious adverse effects. Initiating therapy with lower doses may also help avoid side effects.

Theophylline is available also in parenteral form, both as theophylline and as the more widely used aminophylline, which is more water soluble but has only 80% of the activity of theophylline. Aminophylline traditionally has been used for the inpatient management of status asthmaticus. Recent studies, however, question the added benefit when treatment already consists of continuous or frequent inhaled beta-agonists and systemic steroids.

Theophylline rectal suppositories have notoriously erratic absorption, have been associated historically with serious and occasionally fatal toxicity, and have no place in the treatment of asthma.

Cromolyn and Nedocromil

Cromolyn and nedocromil are two nonsteroidal anti-inflammatory medications available in metered-dose inhaler forms for the treatment

TABLE 1. Medications Used for Treatment of Asthma

DRUG AND HOW SUPPLIED	ROUTE	DOSE
Beta-Agonist Drugs		
Epinephrine, 1:1000, aqueous	SC*	0.01 ml/kg (max: 0.3 ml), q20min × 3
Epinephrine, 1:200 (Sus-Phrine)	SC	0.005 ml/kg (max: 0.15 ml), may repeat in 6 h
Albuterol (Proventil, Ventolin)		
2 mg/5 ml syrup	PO	<6 y: 0.1 mg/kg per dose t.i.d. (max: 12 mg/24 h)
2- and 4-mg tablets		6–12 y: 2 mg t.i.d. (max: 24 mg/24 h)
		>12 y: 2–4 mg t.i.d. (max: 32 mg/24 h)
Sustained-release tablets (Proventil Repetabs, Volmax), 4 mg	PO	4–8 mg b.i.d.
MDI, 90 μg per puff	INH	1–2 puffs q4h p.r.n.
Rotacaps (Ventolin), 200 μg per capsule	INH	1 capsule q4h p.r.n.
Nebulizer solution		
Multidose 0.5% (5 mg/ml)	INH	Infants: 0.05–0.15 mg/kg per dose mixed with 2–3 ml NS q4h
		Child: 1.25–2.5 mg per dose mixed with 2–3 ml NS q4h
Unit dose 0.083% (2.5 mg/2.5 ml NS)		Child ≥5 y: 2.5 ml (1 vial) q4h p.r.n.
Metaproterenol (Alupent, Metaprel)		
10 mg/5 ml syrup	PO	0.3–0.5 mg/kg per dose q6h (max: 20 mg per dose)
10- and 20-mg tablets		
MDI, 650 μg per puff	INH	1–2 puffs q4h p.r.n.
Nebulizer solution	INH	0.1–0.3 ml of 5% solution
5% (dilute with NS)		*or* 2.5 ml of 0.4% or 0.6% solution
Single-dose solution, 0.4%, 0.6%		
Terbutaline (Brethine, Bricanyl)	PO	<12 y: 0.05–0.15 mg/kg per dose t.i.d. (max: 2.5 mg per dose)
2.5- and 5-mg tablets		>12 y: 2.5–5.0 mg/dose t.i.d. or q.i.d.
MDI (Brethaire), 200 μg per puff	INH	2 puffs q4h p.r.n.
Solution for injection (Brethine, Bricanyl), 1 mg/ml	SC	<12 y: 0.005–0.01 mg/kg per dose q20min × 3 (max: 0.4 mg per dose)
	or	>12 y: 0.25 mg per dose × 1 (max: 0.5 mg in 4-h period)
Nebulizer	INH	<2 y: 0.5 mg in 2.5 ml NS q4h
		2–9 y: 1 mg in 2.5 ml NS q4h
		>9 y: 1.5 mg in 2.5 ml NS q4h
Pirbuterol (Maxair Autohaler)	INH	1–2 puffs q4h p.r.n.
MDI, 200 μg per puff		
Salmeterol (Serevent)	INH	1–2 puffs q12 p.r.n.
MDI, 21 μg per puff		

of chronic asthma (Table 1). They are in the so-called prophylactic or preventive category. Cromolyn exists also in a nebulizer solution.

Cromolyn and nedocromil act by inhibition of mediator release from inflammatory cells. They also modify the early and late phase IgE (allergic) reactions. Both medications are effective in modifying allergic-induced asthma, such as occurs with cat exposure. However, their benefit is strictly preventive, and they are of no use for relief of acute symptoms.

Cromolyn or nedocromil is usually given in the dose of two puffs in a holding chamber (such as an InspirEase or AeroChamber) four times a day on a daily basis for at least 6 weeks and usually longer. The benefits of treatment often are not seen for about 10 days or more. When clinical improvement is achieved, the dose of cromolyn can be decreased to two puffs three times a day and that of nedocromil to two puffs twice daily. The dose of the nebulizer form of cromolyn is one vial containing 2 ml given four times a day. The nebulizer solution is compatible with most beta-agonists available in nebulizer form, including albuterol, metaproterenol, and terbutaline. Thus, when necessary, these agents can be given mixed together (Table 1). Side effects with these compounds are very uncommon.

Anticholinergic Agents

Anticholinergic agents are a group of bronchodilator medications given by inhalation, usually in conjunction with other bronchodilators. Beta-adrenergic agents are considered to be more potent bronchodilators, but when they are used in combination with anticholinergic agents, there is an additive effect. Ipratropium bromide (Atrovent) is available by metered-dose inhaler (two puffs every 6 hours as needed) and nebulizer (unit dose 500 μg every 6 hours as needed) and usually is given concomitantly with albuterol by metered-dose inhaler or neb-

ulizer (Table 1). Some patients in status asthmaticus also benefit from the added bronchodilator effect of ipratropium bromide. Ipratropium bromide appears to be more effective than atropine.

Steroids

One of the most basic pathophysiologic aspects of asthma is inflammation of the bronchial mucosa. For this reason, corticosteroids have become important in the management of moderate to severe chronic asthma and of asthma exacerbations. Preparations are available for various routes of administration, including oral, inhalation (metered-dose inhalers), intramuscular, and intravenous. Risks of the short-term and long-term side effects of corticosteroids must be considered. Side effects of oral or parenteral steroid treatment are many. Acute side effects include increased appetite and, occasionally, muscle pain, usually occurring toward the end of the 5-day course. Long-term side effects from continuous oral use include growth suppression, osteopenia, subcapsular cataracts, and excessive weight gain.

For acute exacerbations, prednisone, prednisolone, or methylprednisolone is the steroid of choice, with a dose of 1 to 2 mg/kg/d divided into two to four equal doses for 3 to 5 days. The drug is given until the patient shows significant clinical improvement. The steroid therapy then can be discontinued abruptly. However, if the degree of improvement is not sufficient, smaller doses can be given for a few more days.

The use of inhaled steroids should be considered for patients with chronic asthma that is not well controlled with beta-agonists. Inhaled steroids are available by metered-dose inhalers and are best used with spacers or holding chambers (for example, AeroChamber and InspirEase). For children 6 to 12 years old, the recommended dose of beclomethasone is 100 μg three or four times daily (max: 500 μg in children), of triamcinolone acetonide is 100 to 200 μg three

TABLE 1. Medications Used for Treatment of Asthma Continued

DRUG AND HOW SUPPLIED	ROUTE	DOSE
Anticholinergic Drugs		
Ipratropium bromide (Atrovent)		
MDI, 18 μg per puff	INH	2 puffs (36 μg) q6h p.r.n.
Nebulizer solution, unit dose 500 μg	INH	1 vial (500 μg) q6h p.r.n.
Methylxanthines		
Aminophylline (approx. 80% activity of theophylline)	IV	Loading dose—depends on admission theophylline level:
		If <3 μg/ml: 6 mg/kg
		If >3 μg/ml: 1 mg/kg for every 2 μg/ml of desired increase in level
		Maintenance—0.5–1 mg/kg/h by continuous infusion; use 0.5 mg/kg/ h for infants; monitor level 6 h after loading dose and q12–24 h as indicated by clinical course
Theophylline	PO	Starting dose (>1 y)—12–14 mg/kg/24 h up to 300 mg/24 h
Theo-Dur Extended-Release Tablets 100, 200, 300, 450 mg (q12h dosing)		Maintenance—increase in steps over 1 week to 20 mg/kg/24 h up to 600 mg/24 h; measure level after 3 d at this dose; if not 5–15 μg/ml, adjust accordingly, rechecking levels after 3 d at each successive dose
Theo-Dur Sprinkle 50, 75, 125, 200 mg (q8–12h dosing)		
Slo-Bid Gyrocaps 50, 75, 100, 125, 200, 300 mg (q12h dosing)		
T-Phyl (200 mg) and Uniphyl (400 mg) (q24h dosing)		
Nonsteroidal Anti-Inflammatory Drugs		
Cromolyn sodium (Intal)		
MDI, 800 μg per puff	INH	2 puffs q.i.d.; reduce to t.i.d. when asthma is stable
Nebulizer solution, unit dose, 20 mg/2 ml	INH	1 vial q.i.d.; reduce to t.i.d. when asthma is stable
Nedocromil (Tilade) MDI, 1.75 mg per puff	INH	2 puffs q.i.d.; when asthma is stable, reduce to b.i.d.
Corticosteroids		
Prednisone	PO	Acute flares—1–2 mg/kg/d up to 60 mg/d in 2–3 divided doses × 3–7 d
Prednisolone		
Methylprednisolone		Chronic—lowest effective dose given once in the morning q.o.d.
Methylprednisolone (status asthmaticus)	IV	1 mg/kg per dose q4–6h × 24 h, then decrease rapidly as patient improves
Hydrocortisone (status asthmaticus)	IV	4–6 mg/kg per dose q6h × 24 h; then decrease rapidly as patient improves
Beclomethasone (Vanceril, Beclovent) MDI, 42 μg per puff	INH	2 puffs q.i.d. (max: 500 μg/d)
Triamcinolone (Azmacort) MDI, 100 μg per puff	INH	2 puffs q.i.d. (max: 1200 μg/d)
Flunisolide (Aerobid) MDI, 250 μg per puff	INH	2 puffs b.i.d. (max: 2000 μg/d)

*INH, inhaled; IV, intravenously; MDI, metered-dose inhaler; NS, normal saline; PO, by mouth; SC, subcutaneously.

or four times daily (max: 1200 μg for children and 1600 μg for adults), and of flunisolide is 500 μg twice daily (max: 2000 μg for adults). It is necessary at times to give larger doses to achieve control (Table 1).

If control of asthma is not achieved with the combination of exposure control, beta-agonists, cromolyn or nedocromil, theophylline, and inhaled steroids, it is necessary to add oral prednisone, prednisolone, or methylprednisolone. As low a dose as possible should be given as a single morning dose every other day and only as long as it takes to achieve better control. Then, the drug should be tapered slowly to help assume more lasting relief. For the few patients who are steroid resistant or steroid dependent but who need even more aggressive treatment, additional options exist. These options include the use of oral methotrexate, troleandomycin in combination with methylprednisolone, intravenous gamma globulin, and others. Most of these additional options are performed at a medical referral center.

Asthma Exacerbations

Asthma is a condition characterized by frequent exacerbations. Many patients develop a pattern of flares that parents learn to recognize, and many exacerbations of asthma can be handled at home. The parents and patient are educated about the condition of asthma and its specific triggering factors for the patient. Excellent educational materials are available from the Asthma and Allergy Foundation of America (1125 15th Street NW, Suite 502, Washington, DC 20005 (800) 7-ASTHMA) and National Allergy and Asthma Network (3554 Chain Bridge Road, Suite 200, Fairfax, VA 22030-2709 (800) 878-4403). Parents are given a written *Asthma Action Plan* to follow during

flares of asthma. This includes an agreed-on method of monitoring, including the symptoms of sleep disturbance, exercise tolerance, and peak flow measurements if the patient is old enough and cooperative enough to use a peak flowmeter (Table 2). The medications to be used with a flare are discussed with the family and made available, and proper inhaler technique is reviewed.

When a peak flowmeter can be used to monitor asthma, three zones are identified. The first is the patient's personal best and is considered the top of the *Green zone*. A number calculated at 50% of this or lower is the *Red*, or danger, *zone*. The flow values between these numbers are designated as the *Yellow*, or caution, *zone*. The zones are identified to help obtain and objectify the patient's respiratory difficulty and response to the treatment. In very young children, the monitoring method is based on symptoms and respiratory rate.

Exacerbations are treated by adding doses of an inhaled beta-agonist given every 1 to 4 hours (metered-dose inhalers or nebulizers), by continuing the maintenance medications (if they are being used), and by adding, if necessary, prednisone or prednisolone in the dose of 1 to 2 mg/kg/d in two to four divided doses. The bronchodilator agent is continued on a regular basis only as long as necessary, and the steroid therapy is discontinued promptly in 3 to 5 days if significant improvement is noted (Table 1).

Status Asthmaticus

Status asthmaticus is defined as severe asthma not responding to emergency room treatment or to aggressive treatment by a physician. Usually, this means failure to respond in a short period of time to inhaled or injected beta-agonists. Because this is a potentially life-

TABLE 2. Estimation of Severity of Acute Exacerbations* of Asthma in Children

SIGNS AND SYMPTOMS	MILD	MODERATE	SEVERE
Peak expiratory flow rate†	70%–90% predicted of personal best *Green zone*	50%–70% predicted of personal best *Yellow zone*	<50% predicted of personal best *Red zone*
Respiratory rate, resting or sleeping	Normal to 30% increase above the mean	30%–50% increase above the mean	Increase over 50% above the mean
Alertness	Normal	Normal	May be decreased
Dyspnea‡	Absent or mild; speaks incomplete sentences	Moderate; speaks in phrases or partial sentences; infant's cry softer and shorter; infant has difficulty suckling and feeding	Severe; speaks only in single words or short phrases; infant's cry softer and shorter; infant stops suckling and feeding
Pulsus paradoxus§	<10 mm Hg	10–20 mm Hg	20–40 mm Hg
Accessory muscle use	No intercostal to mild retractions	Moderate intercostal retraction with tracheosternal retractions; use of sternocleidomastoid muscles; chest hyperinflation	Severe intercostal retractions, tracheosternal retractions with nasal flaring during inspiration; chest hyperinflation
Color	Good	Pale	Possibly cyanotic
Auscultation	End-expiratory wheeze only	Wheeze during entire expiration and inspiration	Breath sounds becoming inaudible
Oxygen saturation	>95%	90%–95%	<90%
Pco₂	<35	<40	>40

*Within each category, the presence of several parameters, but not necessarily all, indicates the general classification of the exacerbation.
†For children 5 years of age or older.
‡Parents' or physicians' impression of degree of child's breathlessness.
§Pulsus paradoxus does not correlate with phase of respiration in small children.
From National Asthma Education Program Expert Panel Report: Guidelines for the Diagnosis and Management of Asthma (NIH Publication No. 91-3042). Washington DC, U.S. Department of Health and Human Services, Public Health Service, 1991:105.

threatening condition, the patients need prompt treatment and monitoring. Monitoring should include determination of oxygen saturation or blood gases, chest auscultation findings, respiratory rate, and cerebral function. Oxygen should be administered to maintain Pao₂ between 65 and 100 mm Hg or O₂ saturation greater than 90%. It is vital to be able to identify developing respiratory failure (Table 3).

Treatment of status asthmaticus includes the administration of a beta-agonist by nebulizer on a regularly scheduled basis over 2 to 4 hours (albuterol 5 mg/ml 0.05 to 0.15 mg/kg/20 min for three doses, then 0.15 to 0.3 mg/kg up to 10 mg every 2 to 4 hours as needed) or continuous nebulization (albuterol 0.5 mg/kg/h). Intravenous steroids (hydrocortisone 4 mg/kg or methylprednisolone 1 mg/kg every 4 to 6 hours) are added (Table 1). Recent evidence suggests that adding intravenous theophylline has no significant benefit and only enhances the likelihood of side effects.

After each episode of status asthmaticus, the situation should be reviewed with the physician in an attempt to prevent subsequent hospitalization.

EXERCISE-INDUCED ASTHMA

Exercise can be a potent stimulus for bronchial smooth muscle constriction. For some patients, it may be the sole or major provocation factor for their asthma symptoms. Most asthmatics have exacerbations in response to exercise in addition to other triggering factors. The type of exercise may be influential; for example, swimming is the sport easiest for young asthmatics to tolerate. Exertion in cold dry air seems more likely to produce bronchoconstriction.

Bronchospasm that occurs with exercise is thought to be due to loss of heat or water (or both) from the airway. This leads to changes in osmolality in the bronchial mucosa and, thus, to an increase in neurally mediated airway reactivity. The diagnosis is usually obvious in most patients but may be subtle, in which case a formal or informal exercise challenge test may be confirmatory. After an accurate diagnosis is made, treatment is usually straightforward.

The majority of children and adolescents respond well to an inhaled beta₂-agonist, such as albuterol two puffs given 15 to 30 minutes before exercise, with protection that lasts for several hours. Inhaled cromolyn two puffs 30 minutes before exercise also works well, and for those patients who are more resistant, both cromolyn and a beta₂-agonist may be used. For chronic asthmatics, better overall control with appropriate maintenance medications may improve exercise tolerance. Some patients have a refractory period of improved airway function for up to 2 hours after an episode of exercise-induced asthma, so a warmup period before more vigorous exercise may also reduce the need for medication.

Immunotherapy

Many well-controlled studies have shown the benefit of immunotherapy for allergic asthma with allergens that have included grass pollen, dust mite, and cat allergen. After good attempts at allergen

TABLE 3. Respiratory Scoring System*

	0	1	2
Pao₂ (mm Hg)	70–100	<70 in room air	<70 in 40% O₂
Cyanosis	None	In room air	In 40% O₂
Paco₂	<40	40–65	>65
Pulsus paradoxus (mm Hg)	<10	10–40	>40
Use of accessory muscles of respiration	None	Moderate	Marked
Air exchange	Good	Fair	Poor
Mental status	Normal	Depressed or agitated	Coma

*Interpretation of respiratory scoring system: 0–4, no immediate danger; 5–6, impending respiratory failure; 7 or greater, respiratory failure. At the 5–6 range, all those caring for patients in respiratory failure should be notified that there is a patient who may require assisted ventilation.
From Ellis EF: Status asthmaticus during childhood. *In* Weiss EB (ed): Status Asthmaticus. Baltimore, University Park Press, 1978:310. By permission of the editor.

avoidance, it is appropriate to consider for immunotherapy any asthmatic in whom one suspects a clinical hypersensitivity confirmed by appropriate skin testing. It is more difficult to assess the efficacy of immunotherapy in asthma than in allergic rhinitis because of the multiple trigger factors that many asthmatics have. One must be aware that the risk of anaphylactic reaction to allergen immunotherapy injections is somewhat greater in asthmatics than in other allergic individuals. After immunotherapy is initiated, it may take 6 months or more to detect any significant improvement, but if no improvement is seen within 1 to 2 years, the therapy should be discontinued. If a good clinical response is seen, maintenance injections at intervals of up to 1 month should be continued for 3 to 5 years or until the patient is symptom free or much improved for 1 to 2 years.

SUMMARY

The increasing prevalence and mortality rates for asthma are very alarming. A newer understanding of asthma as an inflammatory disease has led to efforts to find better forms of treatment. With regard to treating asthma, a useful reference is *Guidelines for the Diagnosis and Management of Asthma,* the Expert Panel Report of the National Asthma Education Program.[4] With our expanded knowledge of the diagnosis, monitoring, and treatment of asthma, it is hoped that this very common condition can be brought under better control.

REFERENCES

1. Ellis EF: Asthma in infancy and childhood. *In* Middleton E Jr, Reed CE, Ellis EF, Adkinson NF Jr, Yuninger JW, Busse WW (eds): Allergy Principles and Practice, 4th ed. St. Louis, Mosby, 1993; 2:1225–1262.
2. Hendeles L, Weinberger M, Szefler S, Ellis E: Safety and efficacy of theophylline in children with asthma. J Pediatr 120:177, 1992.
3. Middleton E Jr, Reed CE, Ellis EF, Adkinson NF Jr, Yuninger JW, Busse WW (eds): Allergy Principles and Practice, 4th ed. St. Louis, Mosby, 1993.
4. National Asthma Education Program Expert Panel Report: Guidelines for the Diagnosis and Management of Asthma (NIH Publication No. 91-3042). Washington, DC, United States Department of Health and Human Services, 1991.

ANAPHYLAXIS

LYDIA CAVALES-OFTADEH, M.D.
DOUGLAS C. HEINER, M.D., Ph.D.

Anaphylaxis is a severe, unanticipated clinical syndrome that sometimes follows exposure to a foreign substance and results in the release of a variety of mast cell and basophil-derived mediators. It may be manifested by cutaneous (urticaria, angioedema), respiratory (bronchospasm, laryngeal edema), cardiovascular (hypotension, arrhythmia, myocardial infarction), or gastrointestinal (nausea, vomiting, pain, diarrhea) symptoms occurring singly or in combination. Death may occur secondary to airway obstruction or to irreversible vascular collapse.

Usually, anaphylaxis is mediated by specific IgE antibodies, but occasionally, it is mediated by other immunologic or nonimmunologic mechanisms. When it is nonimmunologically mediated, it is termed an *anaphylactoid reaction,* in which case it is not a true (Gell and Coombs type 1) reaction but one in which similar mediators are released with similar clinical manifestations indistinguishable from anaphylaxis. Treatment is the same for both types of reaction.

Non-IgE-mediated mast cell activation may involve activation of complement components C3a, C4a, and C5a as a result of the pharmacologic actions of substances, such as opiates, certain foods, radiographic contrast media, dextran, and medications.

APPROACH TO INCITING SUBSTANCES

The majority of substances that elicit systemic anaphylaxis are proteins, but polysaccharides occasionally are responsible. Haptens are low molecular weight substances that are not allergenic by themselves but may become allergenic when attached to a host protein.

Penicillin and aspirin are the two most common drugs to cause anaphylaxis. Penicillin is metabolized in the body into a major penicilloyl determinant and into several minor determinants, including benzylpenicilloate and benzylpen-illoate. Most instances of penicillin anaphylaxis are believed to be induced by minor determinants. About 5% to 10% of penicillin-allergic persons have a positive skin test reaction only to minor determinants. Skin testing for minor determinants may be accomplished using the products of penicillin alkaline hydrolysis and, somewhat less reliably, using aged aqueous penicillin from the pharmacy shelf. Cephalosporins have a beta-lactam ring and, consequently, may cross-react with penicillin. Unrelated drugs that also cause anaphylaxis, in decreasing order of frequency, include sulfonamides, tetracycline, macrolide antibiotics, and almost any other medication.

Foods may cause anaphylaxis in susceptible persons, particularly peanuts, tree nuts, fish, crustaceans, mollusks, soybean, cow's milk, and eggs. Food additives also have caused serious allergic reactions. These include the papain used in meat tenderizers and metabisulfite and related agents that often are used as preservatives in the preparation of beer, wine, shellfish, salads, fresh fruits, vegetables, potato, and avocado.

The sting of certain insects (bees, wasps, hornets, yellowjackets, fire ants) may cause anaphylaxis in sensitive subjects. Their importance varies geographically. Bees and yellow jackets are especially common in temperate climates, wasps and fire ants are found in warm coastal areas, and killer bees are in the southern United States and in Central and South America.

A major allergen in both bee and wasp venon is phospholipase A. There is some cross-reactivity between species. A history of a systemic reaction is associated with an approximately 60% risk of a similar or more severe reaction with a future sting by the same insect.

Heterologous animal-derived antisera used in the treatment of snake bites, botulism, gas gangrene, diphtheria, spider bites, certain hematologic disorders, or organ transplant rejection can cause anaphylaxis. Before such preparations are administered, skin tests may be applied to identify IgE antibodies. Negative skin tests indicate that the risk of anaphylaxis is very small. A positive prick skin test with the antiserum, in association with a prior adverse reaction to the antiserum, indicates the need for extreme caution and a planned hyposensitization program if antiserum therapy is deemed essential. This program can be carried out by preparing five vials containing sterile 10-fold dilutions of the antiserum, i.e., 1:10, 1:100, 1:1000, 1:10,000, and 1:100,000. The intravenous route is preferred: 0.5 ml of the 1:100,000 solution is added to the intravenous setup to be infused over 15 minutes. If this is well tolerated, 1 ml is infused over the next 15 minutes, followed by 2 ml over the ensuing 15 minutes. If each infusion is well-tolerated, the same sequence is carried out with the 1:10,000 dilution. Thus, a new dilution is used every 45 minutes, finishing with the undiluted antiserum. The entire process requires 4.5 hours, at which time the patient should tolerate the entire amount, infused as recommended by the manufacturer. If at any step in this desensitization procedure there is an adverse reaction, the same volume of a 10-fold lesser concentration should next be infused, and the process should be restarted from that point forward as described. In our experience with this protocol, an adverse reaction is seen rarely, and it is almost never necessary to abort the desensitization protocol.

General anesthesia is associated with anaphylaxis in about 1:10,000 operations, and deaths occur in 0.1% to 5% of these reactions. Muscle relaxants are an important cause of anesthesia-associated reactions. There have been recent reports of intraoperative anaphylaxis due to rubber (latex) sensitivity, particularly in patients with spina bifida or cogenital anomalies of the urinary tract in whom there has been frequent prior, or long-term, exposure to rubberized catheters.

Anaphylaxis during dialysis in some instances has been attributed to the ethylene oxide used to sterilize dialysis membranes. Such reactions have been presumed to be secondary to activation of complement anaphylatoxins.

Transfusion of blood and its derivatives, including human albumin and gamma globulin, cryoprecipitate, and factors VIII and IX, occasionally leads to anaphylaxis. Plasma expanders, protamine sulfate, and streptokinase also have been reported to cause serious IgE-mediated reactions.

Exercise-induced anaphylaxis is a unique syndrome, since it may be variable and need not occur after every exercise experience. The reaction begins during or after exercise and may occur when exercise is performed following ingestion of a particular food, such as celery, shrimp, chicken, or wheat. However, in many cases, no specific food can be incriminated.

Anaphylaxis after sexual intercourse has been reported in women who have IgE antibody directed against a glycoprotein in the partner's seminal fluid.

Life-threatening reactions after administration of radiographic contrast media occur in approximately 0.1% of procedures. These generally are immediate-type reactions but usually cannot be shown to be IgE mediated. Pretreatment with an antihistaminic and a corticosteroid before the procedure will reduce the risk in patients who have had a prior reaction. Systemic anaphylactic reactions and fatalities have occurred occasionally after allergy immunotherapy, with symptoms generally beginning within a half-hour of the injection. Thus, patients should remain in the office or clinic for one half-hour following immunotherapy injections. The percentage of subjects who experience systemic reactions from immunotherapy is extremely small but may increase if the immunotherapy schedule is accelerated.

There is a subset of patients who experience recurrent anaphylaxis of unknown etiology despite comprehensive evaluation. This is known as idiopathic anaphylaxis. The majority of such patients are atopic and have coexisting asthma.

TREATMENT

Treatment of anaphylaxis is of utmost importance and should be continued for a minimum of 48 hours. Basic principles of treatment follow.

Establish a clear airway and adequate gas exchange. Mouth-to-mouth respiration, intubation, oxygen administration, positive pressure ventilation, cricothyrotomy, and cardiac resuscitation occasionally may be needed.

Record vital signs and assess the level of consciousness frequently. Stop administration of any potential antigen, and establish a line of intravenous access. If the patient is hypotensive or unconscious, an arterial line for monitoring blood pressure is recommended.

Administer aqueous epinephrine 0.1 to 0.5 ml of 1:1000 (0.01 ml/kg or 0.1 ml/20 lb) to a maximum of 0.5 ml SC or IM. For IV use, the dose is 0.1 ml of a 1:1000 dilution of aqueous epinephrine diluted in 10 ml normal saline, given by drip at a rate sufficient to normalize the blood pressure. If intravenous access is not attainable, aqueous epinephrine may be given via an endotracheal or intraosseous route. The dose may be repeated twice at 5-minute intervals. Epinephrine given into the tracheobronchial tree elicits peak blood levels about one-tenth those obtained from the same doses given intravenously. Because of the shortage of data concerning endotracheal use, it is safer to give epinephrine intravenously. A recommended infusion volume is 1 ml of a *1:10,000* solution. Smaller volumes of 1:1000 dilutions of epinephrine are not recommended, since adequate amounts may fail to reach the vein. If there is cardiac standstill, epinephrine may be given directly into the heart, followed by external cardiac massage.

Epinephrine by continuous infusion may be helpful in correcting hypotension. It should be delivered via a well-secured peripheral vein or, preferably, via a central line at a beginning rate of 0.1 μg/kg/min. The infusion rate should be adjusted according to heart rate, blood pressure, other clinical signs, and symptoms. Epinephrine should not be added to a bicarbonate-containing solution, since catecholamines are inactivated by alkaline solutions. Sus-Phrine, a long-acting epinephrine formulation in a 1:200 dilution, may be given in a dose of 0.008 ml/kg or 0.08 ml/20 lb SC to provide sustained action.

If anaphylaxis is secondary to an insect bite or antigen injection, apply a tourniquet proximal to the site of entry if possible. Then inject 1:1000 aqueous epinephrine 0.01 ml/kg up to 0.2 ml into the site of entry or infiltrate proximal to and surrounding the entrance site.

If epinephrine leads to incomplete clearing of respiratory or cardiovascular symptoms, give aminophylline 7 mg/kg or 70 mg/20 lb IV slowly over 10 to 20 minutes (max: 500 mg) while monitoring vital signs. This may be repeated after 6 hours.

Diphenhydramine (Benadryl) 1 to 2 mg/kg (up to 50 mg), chlorpheniramine (Chlor-Trimeton) 0.25 mg/kg, or promethazine (Phenergan) 1 mg/kg should be given IV immediately after the initial doses of epinephrine or epinephrine plus aminophylline. Hydroxyzine 0.9 mg/kg may be used IM but not IV. An antihistamine should be repeated every 6 hours for 48 hours to minimize a late recurrence of symptoms. A satisfactory alternative, if the patient has stabilized and is able to take liquids orally, is to give a single dose of astemizole (Hismanal) 0.5 mg/kg (max: 20 mg), which will provide antihistamine coverage for the ensuing 48 hours. Ranitidine (Zantac), an H_2-antihistamine, may be given intramuscularly or intravenously in a dose of 1 mg/kg every 6 hours in cases of severe anaphylaxis. Care should be taken to administer it slowly (over 5 minutes) if it is given intravenously, since rapid administration may cause or aggravate bradycardia. In general, an H_2-antagonist is recommended only after an H_1-antihistamine has been administered and the patient has not responded well to this and the other listed measures over a period of 30 to 60 minutes.

An additional important measure in cases involving severe reactions is the use of methylprednisolone or hydrocortisone (Solu-Cortef) 1 mg/kg or dexamethasone sodium phosphate (Decadron) 0.2 mg/kg IV initially and every 6 hours for 2 days. Oral prednisone can replace intravenous administration after the patient is stable and can take oral medications. Corticosteroids help forestall recurrences. Steroid action becomes optimal only 1 to 2 hours after intravenous administration and 2 to 4 hours after oral administration. Thus, corticosteroids are not initial drugs of choice.

An intravenous drip of normal saline or half-normal saline in 5% dextran is maintained as long as there is hypotension or severe distress. Arterial cannulation may be needed to monitor blood pressure and oxygenation/ventilation. If the patient is hypotensive, 20 ml/kg of normal saline may be given rapidly over 10 to 20 minutes once intravenous access is obtained. A child in hypovolemic shock may require 40 to 60 ml/kg during the first hour of resuscitation, and occasionally up to 100 to 200 ml/kg may be needed in the first 2 to 3 hours. Ringer's lactate solution may be preferred, since it minimizes the risk of hyperchloremic acidosis that occasionally results from infusion of large amounts of sodium chloride solutions.

If hypotension persists, it is helpful to insert a line to determine central venous pressure (CVP). If CVP is low (<5 cm H_2O), further fluid may be necessary. If CVP exceeds 15 cm H_2O, inotropic agents may be indicated as follows.

- Isoproterenol or epinephrine: >0.1 to 1 μg/kg/min as required to maintain blood pressure (0.6 mg/kg in 100 ml IV fluid)
- Dopamine 2 to 20 μg/kg/min as required (6 mg/kg in 100 ml IV fluid)
- Dobutamine 5 to 20 μg/kg/min as required (6 mg/kg in 100 ml IV fluid)

One must be cautious when using isoproterenol in conjunction with epinephrine because of synergistic effects that may cause tachycardia, arrhythmia, or myocardial ischemia. Continuous cardiovascular monitoring is essential whenever the two drugs are used within an hour of each other or when either is given by continuous drip. Isoproterenol and epinephrine (Medihaler) also can be given by inhalation if respiratory distress is present or if an infusion is impractical.

The patient who is receiving concurrent therapy with beta-blocking agents may be refractory to epinephrine or isoproterenol. Persistent hypotension in such a patient may respond to glucagon 50 μg/kg as an IV bolus, which increases intracellular cyclic adenosine monophosphate (cAMP) by directly activating adenylate cyclase independent of beta-receptors. However, glucagon is a vasodilator and occasionally may cause hypotension, so it must be administered with caution.

PREVENTIVE MEASURES

The life-threatening nature of anaphylaxis makes prevention a cornerstone of patient management. A crucial step in prevention is obtaining an accurate history of previous allergic or anaphylactoid reactions and their causes, if known, as well as of recent exposures to drugs and other potential precipitating factors.

Patients experiencing anaphylaxis may be referred to an allergist for help in determining the etiologic agent, in performing desensitization or immunotherapy, and to assist in educating the patient or parent (or both) about prevention of future anaphylactic episodes. Skin testing is helpful in determining sensitivity to stinging insects, penicillin (occasionally other drugs), heterologous sera, foods, pollens, and certain hormones. Skin testing itself carries a risk and should be done by experienced personnel with resuscitation equipment at hand. Patient education concerning self-administration of epinephrine in preloaded syringes may be lifesaving. Patients with unpredictable anaphylaxis, including those patients whose symptoms follow stings or food ingestion and those with idiopathic anaphylaxis, should carry injectable epinephrine, an oral histamine, and a tourniquet (for bee stings) at all times in a purse or pocket. Commercial kits include Ana-Kit (a prefilled syringe that can deliver two doses of 0.3 ml 1:1000 aqueous epinephrine) and Epipen (regular or junior) (a prefilled automatic injection device delivering 0.3 ml or 0.15 ml of 1:1000 aqueous epinephrine).

The prevalence of systemic anaphylaxis secondary to food hypersensitivity is unknown. However, from a survey by Bock of emergency departments in Colorado, it was estimated that 1000 or more instances of severe food anaphylaxis may occur in the United States each year. Most of the involved children are asthmatic, have a previous history of reaction to the incriminated food, and unknowingly ingest the food allergen. Persons who have had a systemic reaction to a food should be cautioned to read labels on all food products to be certain that the offending food is not included. They should also be aware of the constant danger accompanying prepared foods in restaurants. They should carry epinephrine for self-injection whenever they eat away from home. Fortunately, the patient with anaphylaxis has a good prognosis if proper treatment is undertaken promptly. Adults are more likely than children to have a myocardial infarction or cardiac arrest in association with an anaphylactic reaction.

Anaphylaxis following ingestion of an allergenic food or drug may begin within minutes or may be manifest only after an hour or more has passed. A variable period of time may be required for absorption of intact food molecules or for their conversion to allergenic metabolic products in the gastrointestinal tract. The size of the molecule, its susceptibility to acid or proteolytic degradation, gastric emptying time, intestinal motility, the presence in the gastrointestinal tract of unrelated food, and emesis or diarrhea may alter the time that elapses before the onset of symptoms. Oropharyngeal absorption may account for a rapid systemic reaction in a highly sensitive subject. Symptoms of anaphylaxis also may vary widely owing to individual differences in chemical mediator release and varying reactivity of target organs in different subjects. Frequently, there is a tingling sensation, itching, or metallic taste in the mouth, followed by itching and tightness in the throat, hives, and angioedema of the face and extremities. This may be followed by a sensation of air hunger and wheezing, nausea, abdominal cramps, vomiting, a drop in blood pressure, and finally, loss of consciousness.

If an agent that previously has caused anaphylaxis, such as an antibiotic or antiserum, is needed for treatment of a particular disorder or if exposure is unavoidable, desensitization may be necessary. This should be carried out by experienced personnel with appropriate facilities. To prevent subsequent reactions to radiocontrast media, the

TABLE 1. Contents of Emergency Kit for Anaphylaxis

Epinephrine Hydrochloride Solution
1:1000, 1-ml ampules or 30-ml vials

Injectable H₁-Antihistamines — Two of the Following
Diphenhydramine (Benadryl), 50-mg ampules
Chlorpheniramine (Chlor-Trimeton), 10-mg vials
Promethazine hydrochloride (Phenergan), 25-mg ampules
Hydroxyzine (Vistaril), 10-mg vials (25 mg/ml)

Injectable H₂-Antihistamine
Ranitidine (Zantac), 25 mg in 1-ml vial

Normal Saline

Dextrose 5% in Normal Saline
Dextrose 5% in half-normal saline
Salt-poor serum albumin, 20-ml vials

Injectable Anticonvulsant Drugs
Amobarbital sodium (Amytal), 65-mg ampules
Diazepam (Valium), 10-mg and 50-mg ampules
Sodium bicarbonate, 50-ml ampules (45 mEq)

Equipment
Tourniquet
Equipment for intravenous infusions
Sterile syringes and needles
Several sizes of airway and endotracheal tubes
AmbuBag
Aspiration or suction bulb
Surgical instruments for venous cutdown

patient may be pretreated for 24 hours with corticosteroids, either alone or in combination with H₁- and H₂-antihistaminics. A few children with exquisite egg sensitivity may be at increased risk for anaphylaxis from MMR vaccine. However, most children with a clinical history of egg allergy can tolerate the immunization without reaction. According to Yuninger, most anaphylactic reactions to MMR occurring in children may be due to nonavian components of the vaccine.

Subjects with exercise-induced or cold-induced anaphylaxis or cold urticaria must be cautious when running or swimming (see discussion of urticaria and angioedema). The former should avoid any drinks, food, or medications that have been incriminated previously for 4 to 6 hours before physical exertion.

Patients with malignant idiopathic anaphylaxis may require ≥60 mg of prednisone every other day or ≥ 20 mg of prednisone every day to prevent the syndrome. Glucocorticoids may thus be of preventive as well as therapeutic value.

An emergency kit should be available in every physician's office for immediate use as needed for patients who require treatment of an anaphylactic reaction. Suggested contents of the kit are listed in Table 1.

THE IMMUNODEFICIENCY SYNDROMES

HANS D. OCHS, M.D.
JERRY A. WINKELSTEIN, M.D.

Primary immunodeficiency disorders are caused by intrinsic defects of the immune system and include defects of T and B lymphocytes, phagocytic cells, and the complement system. Most primary immunodeficiency disorders have a genetic basis. The immune system can also be affected secondarily by prematurity, malnutrition, metabolic diseases, viral infections, malignancies, and immunosuppressive drugs. As a result, recurrent bacterial, fungal, and viral infections, resulting in chronic disease of multiple organs, occur.

TREATMENT

Patients with immunodeficiency require special care to maintain general health and nutrition, to reduce exposure to infective agents, and to manage recurrent acute and chronic infections. The aim is to let affected children grow up with the least amount of restrictions and to allow adults to lead productive lives.

Genetic Counseling

Genetic counseling is an important component of the care of patients with a primary immunodeficiency disease and their families. Many of the primary immunodeficiency diseases are genetically determined. Of those that are, the majority are inherited as autosomal recessive traits, seven are inherited as X-linked recessive disorders, and in one, the mode of inheritance is autosomal dominant. Thus, it is critical that patients with a primary immunodeficiency disease and their families have an appreciation for the genetic implications of their disease. Precise molecular genetic diagnosis, carrier detection, and prenatal diagnosis are available for many of the primary immunodeficiency diseases and afford patients and their families the opportunity to examine their reproductive options from an informed perspective.

Use of Vaccines and Blood Products

Killed vaccines (diphtheria, tetanus, pertussis, *inactivated* polio, *Haemophilus influenzae*, hepatitis B vaccine) are often used for diagnostic purposes and may be given for protection if a patient has been shown to mount a detectable immune response. Live attenuated vaccines (oral polio, MMR, BCG, varicella) should be avoided in all patients with severe B cell (antibody) or T cell (cellular) deficiency [e.g., X-linked agammaglobulinemia (XLA), severe combined immunodeficiency disorder (SCID)] to prevent vaccine-induced disease. Parents, siblings, and other household members should not be given oral polio vaccine to avoid the spread of the virus to the patient. Patients with XLA are highly vulnerable to live attenuated polio vaccine, since they do not make antibodies and may develop paralytic polio. BCG vaccination may spread locally or systemically in patients with SCID or with neutrophil defects. Patients with phagocytic cell abnormalities [chronic granulomatous disease (CGD) and leukocyte adhesion deficiency (LAD)] or with complement component deficiency may be vaccinated with live vaccines (except BCG) if the injection site is carefully prepared to avoid the introduction of other infective agents.

Antimicrobials

Antibiotics, antifungals, and antiviral drugs are most important therapeutic interventions for patients with primary immunodeficiency disorders. Because the infectious course is often rapid and overwhelming, any symptom suggestive of infection requires prompt sampling of multiple sites for culture (bacterial, mycoplasma, protozoa, fungal, and viral) and therapy with broad-spectrum antibiotics at recommended doses. If symptoms suggest a systemic infection, the child should be admitted to hospital and treated by the intravenous route. Even if cultures are negative, a full course of antibiotic therapy must be completed if the symptoms suggest infection. If antibiotic therapy fails to achieve improvement, patients need to be recultured, and antimicrobials must be added to cover fungal, *Pneumocystis carinii*, or myocplasma infection. Consideration of the primary defect is useful in selecting the optimal antibiotic. Patients with mainly an antibody deficiency are often infected with gram-positive or gram-negative organisms present in the upper respiratory tract or with mycoplasma. Patients with chronic granulomatous disease are most susceptible to peroxidase-positive organisms, including *Staphylococcus*, *Klebsiella*, *Serratia*, and *Candida*. Patients with LAD are often infected with *Staphylococcus*, *Bacteroides*, and *Pseudomonas*. Individuals with complement component deficiencies should be covered for encapsulated organisms (e.g., *Neisseria meningitidis*, pneumococci, *H. influenzae*). If mycoplasma is suspected, the antibiotic therapy should include erythromycin or tetracycline.

Prophylactic antibiotic therapy may be of benefit for disorders known to cause overwhelming infections of rapid onset in young infants, such as in boys with CGD. Patients with chronic lung disease, sinusitis, or mastoiditis may require long-term antibiotic therapy. It is advisable to rotate three to five different antibiotics at regular intervals (e.g., every 2 weeks) to avoid the development of resistant organisms. If possible, a treatment-free interval of 2 weeks or more should be incorporated into this treatment scheme. Prophylaxis for *P. carinii* pneumonia is indicated in patients with X-linked hyper-IgM syndrome, SCID, and other severe T cell deficiencies. Most effective is oral administration of trimethoprim-sulfamethoxazole (TMP-SMX) given three times a week at a dose of 75 to 150 mg/m² of TMP and 375 to 750 mg/m² of SMX. In many instances, prophylactic antibiotic therapy can be reduced if the patients are treated prophylactically with immunoglobulin. Short courses of acyclovir in immunodeficient patients with recurrent herpes simplex infection or in patients with cellular immunodeficiency exposed to chickenpox are recommended.

Human Immune Globulin (gamma globulin)

Immunodeficiency syndromes affecting predominantly antibody production are treated most successfully with serum immunoglobulin (Ig) prepared by cold alcohol precipitation from pooled human serum. If provided at regular intervals with adequate doses of Ig before chronic lung disease has developed, antibody-deficient patients may remain asymptomatic and free of complications. The process of purifying serum immunoglobulin eliminates contamination with viruses. Commercially available preparations are safe and effective and well tolerated by most patients. These preparations consist mainly of IgG, with traces of IgM and IgA. The material is prepared from large lots of pooled human plasma and contains IgG antibody to common bacterial, viral, and fungal pathogens. Human serum immunoglobulin has been formulated for intramuscular injection or for intravenous infusion and has a half-life of 20 days or more.

Intramuscular Immune Globulin (IMIg)

IMIg is obtained from pooled human serum by alcohol fractionation and formulated as a 16.5% solution in glycine buffer and with thimerosal as preservative. IMIg can be given intramuscularly, or subcutaneously by slow infusion. The dose of immunoglobulin that can be given intramuscularly is limited by muscle size. The monthly dose should be at least 100 mg/kg and, if tolerated, may be increased to 200 mg/kg/mo. The material has to be injected carefully to avoid injuring a nerve or hitting a vein. The preferred site is the upper outer quadrant of the gluteal area or the lateral thigh. The amount per injection site should be limited to 10 ml for adults, and the injection should be given slowly after aspirating to avoid injecting the material intravenously. Inadvertent injection of IMIg into a vein may cause severe anaphylactic shock. Therefore, epinephrine should be available at the bedside. A loading dose of 1.2 ml/kg (200 mg IgG/kg) is followed by monthly doses of 0.6 to 1.2 ml/kg/mo. The bioavailability of IMIg may vary depending on absorption and local proteolytic destruction of the material.

Slow subcutaneous infusion of IMIg is an alternative to intramuscular injection. The material is infused overnight into the abdominal wall using a 23-gauge butterfly needle and an automatic pump. Frequent infusions of small amounts (up to 10 to 20 ml per infusion) are given overnight and are well tolerated. This technique allows infusion of 300 to 500 mg of IgG per kilogram per month. Possible complications include local inflammation or infection and lipid atrophy at the site of infusion. The fact that the IMIg preparations available in the United States contain mercury as preservative has to be considered.

Intravenous Immune Globulin (IVIg)

The infusion of immune serum globulin by the intravenous route is the preferred prophylactic therapy for most patients with antibody deficiency. This allows the administration of large doses of IgG, given directly into the bloodstream, thus avoiding delayed absorption and proteolytic destruction at the site of injection. The intravenous injection is less painful and not contraindicated in patients with a bleeding disorder. Furthermore, the serum levels that can be achieved are within the physiologic range. Up to 2 g/kg can be infused at one time without side effects. At least six preparations are licensed in the United States. All are well tolerated and effective. Some are lyophilized and need to be reconstituted, whereas other preparations are available in liquid form. At least two preparations are treated with detergent to reduce further the possibility of viral contamination. To eliminate reactions, immunoglobulin for intravenous use is prepared by eliminating high molecular weight complexes to reduce anticomplementary activity. The aim of using IVIg is to provide sufficient antibody to prevent recurrent infections and chronic tissue damage. This can be accomplished by adjusting the amount infused and the interval between infusions. The recommended dose is 400 mg/kg/mo. To avoid high peak and low trough values, the interval between infusions may be shortened, for example, 200 mg/kg every two weeks. Most patients do well if the IgG trough level measured just before an infusion is 300 to 400 mg/dl above the baseline (the IgG level measured before immunoglobulin therapy). There is considerable variation among patients in the relationship between dose and serum IgG levels achieved. Thus, the frequency and amount of immunoglobulin infused must be individualized and adjusted by following serum IgG levels before the infusion. The goal is to achieve stable physiologic serum IgG levels. If needed, the dose may be increased to 600 to 800 mg/kg/mo. The rate of infusion recommended is 100 to 200 mg/kg/h. To reduce costs, infusion at home by the patient (self-infusion) or by a family member or friend has been introduced in selected patients, with excellent results. More frequent infusions, for example, every 10 to 14 days, reduce the incidence of side effects. Newly diagnosed patients should be initially infused with IVIg in a hospital or emergency room setting, with careful monitoring of vital signs, since the first one or two infusions may be associated with adverse reactions due to the formation of immune complexes. If a patient is selected for home infusion, adequate training and instructions on how to handle side effects are required.

Leukocyte Transfusions

Patients with a phagocytic defect may benefit from white cell transfusions. This treatment is especially effective in patients with LAD (CD11/CD18 deficiency). Generally, one transfusion per day is sufficient, and depending on the severity of infections, 1 to 2 weeks of therapy is required. White cells are obtained by placing the donor on a pheresis device and allowing the collection of 1 to 10 × 10^{10} (average 3 × 10^{10}) leukocytes. The yield of leukocytes is increased by pretreating the donor with prednisone (20 mg at −17 hours, −12 hours, and −3 hours). Reactions during and after white cell transfusion can be controlled with diphenhydramine, aspirin, and corticosteroids. The development of antibodies to HLA antigens has been observed. The donors have to be carefully screened for viral infections, including HIV, hepatitis B and C, and cytomegalovirus (CMV). Radiation of the cells with 25 Gy is recommended and is required if the recipient has a T cell abnormality.

Enzyme/Growth Factor Replacement

Patients with adenosine deaminase (ADA) deficiency and SCID have been treated successfully with weekly intramuscular injections of bovine ADA conjugated with polyethylene glycol (PEG-ADA). The usual dose is 10 U/kg body weight, injected once weekly. On rare occasions, transient antibody to bovine ADA has been observed.

Recently, cytokines and other growth factors produced by recombinant techniques have become available. Patients with persistent neutropenia, including cyclic neutropenia, congenital neutropenia (Kostman), and neutropenia associated with the hyper-IgM syndrome, have responded favorably to treatment with G-CSF (Neupogen) 5 μg/kg/d or GM-CSF (Leukine) 250 μg/m²/d.

A large multicenter placebo-controlled trial in patients with CGD has shown clearly that interferon gamma given SC three times weekly at a dose of 50 μg/m² (if the body surface area is less than 0.5 m², the dose is 1.5 μg/kg) is effective and well tolerated and reduces the frequency of serious infection by approximately 50%.

Patients with IL-2 deficiency may respond to infusions of IL-2. The recommended dose established in such a patient is 30,000 U of recombinant IL-2/kg IV three times weekly.

Bone Marrow Transplantation

Bone marrow transplantation (BMT) as a source of stem cells is considered the only definitive therapy for patients with primary immunodeficiency disorders. Allogeneic BMT has been employed successfully in the treatment of SCID, the Wiskott-Aldrich syndrome, CGD, and LAD. The most frequent problems related to BMT in these disorders are failure of engraftment and graft-versus-host disease. To reduce the incidence of graft-versus-host disease, the donor has to be selected carefully and should be an MHC-matched sibling or unrelated donor. Slightly less successful are haploidentical transplants from a parent. Before BMT, patients with SCID are usually not conditioned with immunosuppressive drugs, but patients with remaining T cell immunity require cytoreduction with cytoxan-busulfan.

Gene Therapy

Gene therapy is still in the experimental stage. It has been attempted in patients with ADA deficiency, using virus-derived vectors to insert the ADA gene into peripheral blood T cells or, more recently, into stem cells.

HUMORAL IMMUNODEFICIENCIES

A predominant defect of B cell function results in depressed or absent antibody synthesis. The defect either may be intrinsic to B lymphocytes, as in XLA, or may be due to abnormal T cell help required for B cell proliferation and differentiation and the switch from IgM to IgG, as in most patients with common variable immunodeficiency and the hyper-IgM syndrome. Most of these patients have hypogammaglobulinemia and respond with depressed antibody titers to standard immunization. Replacement with immunoglobulin infusions is most effective in preventing recurrent bacterial infections.

X-Linked Agammaglobulinemia

The molecular defect of XLA has been identified as a defect involving a B cell-specific tyrosine kinase (btk). As a consequence, pre-B cells fail to develop into functioning B cells. Affected boys present with severe, recurrent bacterial infections during the first year of life after maternal antibodies have disappeared. Prompt replacement therapy with IVIg starting during the first year of life is important to prevent the development of chronic lung disease. Since IVIg therapy is required throughout the patient's life, many parents of patients prefer to infuse at home. If serious infections occur or if chronic disease is developing, the dose may be increased from 400 mg/kg/mo to 800 mg/kg/mo, and the intervals between infusions may be shortened. High-dose IVIg therapy is very effective in preventing chronic infection with enteroviruses, including echovirus–induced meningoencephalitis and dermatomyositis. If acute or chronic infection develops, broad-spectrum antibiotics must be provided for an appropriate length of time.

Common Variable Immunodeficiency

This is a heterogeneous group of patients. They have in common hypogammaglobulinemia and poor antibody responses, frequently caused by insufficient T cell help. In contrast to patients with XLA, many of these patients are able to produce some antibody, frequently limited to the IgM class. The preferred therapy is regular infusions of IVIg at doses between 200 and 400 mg/kg/mo, and the aim is to prevent chronic lung disease. Common variable immunodeficiency (CVI) patients have a higher rate of autoimmune disorders, gastrointestinal symptoms frequently caused by *Giardia*, and a higher incidence of malignancies. Recurrent infections may be due to gram-positive and gram-negative organisms, *Mycoplasma*, or *Chlamydia*, but rarely viruses. If long-term therapy with antimicrobial agents is required, a system of rotating different broad-spectrum antibiotics on a biweekly basis to prevent resistance is recommended.

Immunodeficiency with Hyper-IgM (HIgM)

The majority of patients with the HIgM syndrome are males. The molecular defect involves the gene encoding for CD40 ligand, a T cell activation molecule that is crucial for T-B cell interaction. HIgM patients fail to develop memory B cells and to switch from IgM to IgG. As a consequence, they present with recurrent bacterial infections during infancy. Prophylactic therapy with monthly infusions of IVIg at a dose of 400 mg/kg body weight and with TMP-SMX during infancy to prevent *P. carinii* pneumonia is recommended for all HIgM patients. Persistent neutropenia responds to daily injections with G-CSF (5 µg/kg/d).

Transient Hypogammaglobulinemia of Infancy

The immature immune system of the newborn undergoes maturation during the first 2 years of life. Transient hypogammaglobulinemia of infancy is caused by a delay in the onset of immunoglobulin synthesis and antibody production by the infant. As a rule, this syndrome corrects itself in the first few years of life. If symptoms are mild, no therapy is required. If the management of infections is difficult, a therapeutic trial with IVIg or IMIg for a limited time is indicated. A reevaluation of infants with this syndrome is important for management. IgG serum levels should be monitored every 6 months before the decision is made to continue therapy.

Selective Ig Deficiencies

Not all patients with selective IgG subclass deficiencies have symptoms. However, if selective deficiencies of IgG1, IgG2, and IgG3 (and complete absence of IgG4) are associated with clinical symptoms and if the patient does not respond appropriately to antibiotic therapy, treatment with IVIg 200 to 400 mg/kg/mo may be indicated. Selective IgG deficiencies, unless based on a genetic abnormality, are often transient. Treatment with IVIg has to be reevaluated at regular intervals, and its efficacy must be documented.

IgA deficiency is the most common B cell disorder, occurring in approximately 1 in 500 individuals. All other Ig isotypes except IgA are present, and antibody responses are normal. There is no specific treatment available. Ig therapy is contraindicated, since some patients with selective IgA deficiency will develop anti-IgA antibody and develop severe reactions if exposed to IgG preparations. A frequent complication of IgA deficiency is autoimmunity, and patients need to be monitored carefully.

Selective IgM deficiency is a rare condition. Most patients with selective IgM deficiency can make antibody of the IgG isotype and rarely require specific therapy.

CELLULAR IMMUNODEFICIENCIES

Patients with predominant T cell deficiency have more extensive infections than those with selective B cell deficiencies. Because T help is required for adequate antibody responses, these patients also have an antibody deficiency (combined T and B cell defects). Patients with cellular immunodeficiency are susceptible to bacterial, viral, and opportunistic infections starting in early infancy. The aim of therapy is to reduce the incidence and severity of infections and, if the defect is severe, correct the immune defect (e.g., bone marrow transplantation).

Severe Combined Immunodeficiency

The mode of inheritance may be X-linked, autosomal recessive, or sporadic. All patients with SCID have in common a severe defect of both T and B cell function. Affected infants present with failure to thrive, opportunistic infections, severe gastrointestinal symptoms, and skin rashes. Treatment with antimicrobial agents and IVIg is only partially successful. *P. carinii* pneumonia prophylaxis with TMP-

SMX should be initiated immediately. Because of the poor prognosis, BMT is the treatment of choice. The preferred donor is an HLA-matched sibling. Alternatively, a nonrelated matched donor may be selected. In recent years, one-haplotype-identical donors, usually a parent, have been used successfully as a source of stem cells. This requires the removal of mature T cells from the collected bone marrow to prevent graft-versus-host disease. If the marrow recipient does not receive cytoreduction, the grafted cells may be limited to T cells. As a result, many marrow-transplanted SCID patients remain B cell deficient and require IVIg substitution therapy for years after marrow transplantation. SCID patients often present with severe diarrhea, most likely due to viral infections of the gut. The use of IVIg by mouth has been effective in reducing diarrhea in a number of SCID patients. Attempts to reconstitute SCID patients with thymic explants, thymic epithelial cells, or fetal liver cells have been generally ineffective.

SCID patients are especially vulnerable to graft-versus-host disease and transmission of CMV and other viruses and to complications from live vaccines. Blood products need to be irradiated, blood donors have to be carefully selected, and live vaccines should be avoided. Appropriate antibiotics, antiviral agents, and antifungal agents are indicated if the source of infection has been identified.

Mucocutaneous Candidiasis

The precise immune defect responsible for mucocutaneous candidiasis is unknown. Symptoms are limited to infections with *Candida* and may be associated with endocrinopathies. The severity of the *Candida* infection may vary between mild and severe. Treatment with topical nystatin is adequate if the symptoms are mild. Nystatin pastilles or troches (Mycelex) are more effective for the treatment of oral lesions. In the severe form of mucocutaneous candidiasis, systemic treatment with antifungal agents (ketoconazole 200 mg once daily, fluconazole 100 mg once daily) may be necessary. If extensive esophageal lesions are present, these drugs may have to be given intravenously. These new antifungal agents have had a major impact on the course of mucocutaneous candidiasis. Nevertheless, affected patients need regular follow-up to detect endocrine disorders.

DiGeorge Syndrome

The DiGeorge syndrome is a congenital defect involving structures derived from the third and fourth pharyngeal pouches, affecting the parathyroid glands, the thymus, and the development of the large cardiac vessels. A close association between the DiGeorge syndrome and a deletion within chromosome 22q11 has been reported. The immune defect varies from mild to severe. Symptomatic therapy to correct hypocalcemia and surgical intervention to correct the cardiovascular defect are of prime urgency during the immediate postnatal period. Absolute numbers of lymphocytes, T cells, and T cell subsets are helpful in following the immune status. Most patients do not require specific therapy to correct their immune defect. The use of thymic transplants or thymus extracts has not been uniformly successful. BMT has resulted in improved immune responses in a few patients with severe immune defects.

Wiskott-Aldrich Syndrome

Wiskott-Aldrich syndrome (WAS) is an X-linked recessive disorder characterized by an increased susceptibility to infection, thrombocytopenia, and eczema. The gene responsible for WAS has recently been identified. The underlying immunologic defect involves both T and B lymphocytes and results in susceptibility to a wide variety of bacteria, viruses, and fungi. The thrombocytopenia may be severe, is characterized by small platelet size, and is usually associated with significant bleeding. WAS patients have an increased risk of malignancies and autoimmune disorders. BMT using HLA-identical marrow is the treatment of choice for the Wiskott-Aldrich syndrome. Successful transplantation results in correction of the immunologic defect, thrombocytopenia, and eczema. Results with haploidentical marrow have been less encouraging, but newer techniques offer promise for the future. In those patients in whom a BMT is not possible, splenectomy usually corrects the thrombocytopenia. It should be noted, however, that patients with the WAS have a highly significant risk for sepsis after splenectomy and, therefore, should receive continuing antibiotic prophylaxis. Treatment with IVIg may be indicated in those patients who have not been corrected with BMT, since patients with WAS have deficient antibody responses to both protein and polysaccharide antigens.

Ataxia Telangiectasia

Ataxia telangiectasia (AT) is an autosomal recessive disorder characterized by an increased susceptibility to infection, cerebellar ataxia, and telangiectasia of the skin and mucous membranes. Patients with AT have both T and B lymphocyte defects. Their neurologic defects include progressive ataxia, chorioathetosis, and muscle atrophy and weakness. The molecular defect, believed to interfere with DNA repair, is unknown. Treatment of AT is largely supportive. In some cases, hypogammaglobulinemia and antibody deficiency develop, and treatment with IVIg is indicated. Progressive pulmonary disease occurs in most patients, but it is unclear how much is due to the immunodeficiency and how much is due to impaired pulmonary mechanics that develop secondary to the neurologic defects. In any case, postural drainage and pulmonary hygiene are important elements in the care of AT patients. Attention also must be paid to rehabilitative care for the progressive neurologic impairment, so that their ability to participate in activities of daily living and activities outside the home can be optimized. AT patients have an increased incidence of malignancies, and therapy is hampered by their low threshold for antineoplastic drugs and ionizing irradiation.

Bare Lymphocyte Syndrome (MHC-II Deficiency)

Lymphocytes and macrophages of affected individuals fail to express MHC-II. Patients with this syndrome have normal numbers of circulating B cells but markedly depressed numbers of T cells. Because the lack of MHC-II affects both T and B lymphocyte function, the clinical presentation resembles that of patients with SCID. *P. carinii* pneumonia prophylaxis with TMP-SMX is recommended. Because antibody responses are depressed, IVIg therapy is indicated. The treatment of choice is BMT preceded by cytoreduction.

Cytokine Deficiency

Rare patients with a clinical presentation of SCID were found to be deficient in the synthesis of IL-2 or of multiple lymphokines, including IL-2, IL-4, IL-5, and interferon gamma. Treatment with intravenous infusions of IL-2 has improved the clinical symptoms, and BMT is the treatment of choice.

Adenosine Deaminase Deficiency

A subgroup of patients with SCID lack the enzyme adenosine deaminase (ADA), the result of a genetic defect within the gene encoding ADA. In the absence of ADA, toxic metabolites of the purine pathway (dATP) accumulate within cells, and as a result, T lymphocytes and, to a lesser extent, B lymphocytes become functionally defective. The treatment of choice is BMT. If a suitable donor is not available, treatment with weekly intramuscular injections of bovine ADA conjugated with polyethylene glycol (PEG-ADA) is effective. Several patients with ADA deficiency are enrolled in programs in experimental gene therapy.

Other Syndromes Affecting T and B Lymphocytes

Patients with the *hyper-IgE syndrome* present with recurrent staphylococcal abscesses, with little inflammation, lung abscesses and pneumatoceles, bony abnormalities, and high serum IgE levels. The inheritance may in some cases be autosomal dominant or due to a spontaneous mutation. The primary defect is unknown and may affect T-B cell interaction. Surgical intervention to drain abscesses is required. Symptomatic therapy with antibiotics covering staphylococcal disease and long-term treatment with ketoconazole are beneficial.

The immune deficiency associated with *transcobalamin II deficiency,* an autosomal recessive disorder, responds well to treatment with monthly injections of high doses of vitamin B$_{12}$.

COMPLEMENT DEFICIENCIES

Genetically determined deficiencies have been described for nearly all of the individual components of complement. In general, patients with complement deficiencies present with either an increased susceptibility to infection, rheumatic disorders, or angioedema. Which of these clinical presentations is expressed by the patient depends on which specific component is deficient and the role of that component in normal physiology. For example, the major activation product of C3 (C3b) is an important opsonin. Thus, patients who are deficient in C3 or who are deficient in one of the components of the classic or alternative pathways needed for the activation of C3 are unusually susceptible to encapsulated bacteria (e.g., pneumococci, streptococci, *H. influenzae*), for which C3b-dependent opsonization is a critical mechanism of host defense. Similarly, C5, C6, C7, C8, and C9 form the membrane attack complex and are responsible for bactericidal activity. Thus, patients with deficiencies of these components are susceptible to systemic *Neisseria* infections, such as the meningococcus, for which serum bactericidal activity is important. The early components of the classic pathway, C1, C4, and C2, as well as C3, are important in the clearance and processing of immune complexes. Therefore, patients deficient in these components have an increased prevalence of rheumatic disorders. Finally, C1 esterase inhibitor is one of the important control proteins of the complement system and the kinin system. Patients deficient in this component manifest angioedema.

Although there is no specific replacement therapy for most of the complement deficiency diseases, a variety of prophylactic and supportive therapies are available. If the deficiency predisposes the patient to infection, immunization against the polysaccharide capsules of pneumococci, meningococci, and *H. influenzae* is indicated. However, the very young patient (i.e., < 2 years) may not be able to respond adequately to polysaccharide vaccines that have not been conjugated to carrier proteins (i.e., pneumococcal and meningococcal vaccines). In addition, in the case of the pneumococcal vaccine, not all serotypes are included. Thus, in some instances, prophylactic antibiotics are indicated, especially in younger children. Treatment of rheumatic diseases, such as systemic lupus erythematosus and discoid lupus, in patients with complement deficiencies is largely supportive and is generally the same as it would be for patients with an intact complement system. The therapy of the angioedema seen in C1 esterase inhibitor deficiency (hereditary angioedema) can be divided into that for acute attacks and that for prophylaxis of attacks. Therapy for acute attacks is largely supportive. Although antihistamines or corticosteroids or both are not effective, epinephrine has been of benefit in some cases. Laryngeal involvement may occur during attacks and lead to respiratory obstruction, requiring tracheostomy in some patients. Chronic maintenance therapy may be indicated in those patients who have frequent life-threatening or disabling attacks. Antifibrinolytic agents, such as epsilon aminocaproic acid (EACA) or its cyclic analog tranexamic acid, have been used with some success. More recently, impeded androgens, such as danazol and stanozolol, have emerged as useful in the long-term prophylaxis of attacks. Even though their masculinizing effects are attenuated, they are not indicated in children who have not reached their growth potential or sexual maturity.

PHAGOCYTIC DISORDERS

Disorders of the phagocytic system can be divided conveniently into those disorders in which phagocytic cells are deficient in number (neutropenia) and those disorders in which phagocytic cells are deficient in function. This section deals with disorders of phagocytic function.

Chronic Granulomatous Disease

CGD is an intrinsic disorder of phagocytic cells in which the cells are unable to produce the reactive oxygen metabolites (e.g., hydrogen peroxide, superoxide, hydroxyl radicals, and hypochlorite) that are necessary for efficient intracellular killing of certain bacteria and fungi. As a result, patients with CGD have an increased susceptibility to a number of bacteria and fungi (e.g., staphylococci, *Salmonella*, *Candida*, and *Aspergillus*). The therapy of CGD begins with prevention of infection. Careful attention to personal hygiene and early treatment of superficial cuts and bruises are important first lines of defense against infection in this disorder. A number of studies have shown that long-term prophylaxis with TMP-SMX or dicloxacillin also reduces the number of infections in children with CGD. In a multiinstitutional study, children with CGD treated prophylactically with recombinant interferon gamma had fewer serious infections and fewer hospitalizations than CGD patients who had not received interferon gamma. Once there are signs of infection, every effort should be made to identify the etiologic agent and initiate appropriate antimicrobial therapy. In some instances, however, the causative organism is not identified, and broad-spectrum antibiotics (including coverage for staphylococci and gram negative bacteria) may need to be initiated. Infections with *Aspergillus* species or *Pseudomonas cepacia* are relatively common in these children. Therapy for a given infection often requires intravenous antimicrobials for prolonged periods. Abscesses require surgical drainage for diagnosis and therapy.

Leukocyte Adhesion Deficiency

Patients with this disorder have diminished or absent expression of certain cell membrane glycoproteins on their phagocytic cells. These proteins are designated CD11/CD18 and include the iC3b receptor (CR3), LFA-1, and p150,95. Each of these molecules contains an alpha (CD11) and beta (CD18) chain. They share a common beta-subunit, which is deficient in patients with LAD. As a consequence, those leukocyte functions that depend on this family of surface molecules, such as adherence and adherence-dependent locomotion, are deficient. Clinical severity of the disease varies and correlates with the degree of expression of the deficient proteins. Treatment for patients with LAD is largely supportive. Good oral hygiene to combat periodontal disease and meticulous care and treatment of superficial skin lesions are emphasized. Prophylaxis with TMP-SMX or dicloxacillin has been helpful in some cases. Leukocyte transfusions are of benefit during the course of deep-seated or severe infections. Finally, in those patients in whom the defect is severe, BMT is indicated and has proven successful. LAD patients are excellent candidates for future gene therapy.

SUMMARY OF TREATMENT

General

- Erythromycin or tetracycline for treatment of mycoplasma infection
- Trimethoprim-sulfamethoxazole (TMP-SMX) PO 3 times per week at a dose of 75–150 mg/m² of TMP and 375–750 mg/m² of SMX for *Pneumocystis carinii* prophylaxis
- Acyclovir 200 mg q4–6h PO (adult) for recurrent herpes simplex or chickenpox or 5 mg/kg q8h IV for severe disease

Intramuscular Immune Globulin (IMIg)

- Monthly dose of 100 mg/kg; if tolerated, may be increased to 200 mg/kg/mo
- Loading dose of 1.2 ml/kg (200 mg IgG/kg) followed by doses of 0.6–1.2 ml/kg/mo
- Epinephrine (Epipen) should be available at bedside

Subcutaneous Infusion of IMIg

- Infusion of 300–500 mg of IgG per kilogram per month given slowly (by pump) SC in q.d. or q.o.d. aliquots

Intravenous Immune Globulin (IVIg)

- Recommended dose is 400 mg/kg/mo in 1–4 aliquots
- Dose may be increased to 600–800 mg/kg/mo; recommended rate of infusion is 100–200 mg/kg/h

White Cell Transfusions

- Pretreatment of donor with prednisone 20 mg at 17 h, 12 h, and 3 h before leukopheresis
- Yield per run: 1–10 × 10¹⁰ leukocytes in 200–400 ml of plasma

Enzyme/Growth Factor

- Bovine ADA conjugated with polyethylene glycol (PEG-ADA) (ENZON, South Plainfield, New Jersey); usual dose is 10 U/kg injected once weekly in patients with ADA deficiency
- G-CSF (Neupogen) or GM-CSF (Leukine); recommended dose is 5 μg/kg/d (G-CSF) or 250 μg/m²/d (GM-CSF) for patients with neutropenia or cyclic neutropenia
- Interferon gamma three times weekly at 50 μg/m² (if body surface area is less than 0.5 m², dose is 1.5 μg/kg) to patients with CGD
- IL-2; recommended dose, established in a patient with IL-2 deficiency (whose in vitro lymphocyte responses improved following addition of IL-2 to cultures), is 30,000 U of recombinant IL-2/kg IV 3 times weekly

BMT

- Patients with remaining T cell immunity require cytoreduction with cytoxan-busulfan
- Cytoxan generally given at 50 mg/kg/d on 4 consecutive days; busulfan at 1 mg/kg q6h × 16 [dose is adjusted to reach a steady-state blood level of 200 ng/ml plasma (matched sibling donor) or 600 ng/ml (nonmatched donor)]

XLA

- IVIg at 400 mg/kg/mo in 1–4 doses (e.g., 200 mg/kg q2wk); if required, dose may be increased to 800 mg/kg/mo

CVI

- IVIg at doses between 200 and 400 mg/kg/mo in 1–4 doses
- Broad-spectrum antibiotics, including TMP-SMX, ampicillin, cephalexin, ciprofloxacin

HIgM

- IVIg at 400 mg/kg/mo; TMP-SMX prophylaxis for *Pneumocystis carinii* during infancy
- G-CSF (5 μg/kg/d) for patients developing neutropenia

Selective IgG Deficiency

- IVIg 200–400 mg/kg/mo if unmanageable with symptomatic treatment

SCID

- *Pneumocystis carinii* pneumonia prophylaxis with TMP-SMX 75–150 mg/m² TMP and 375–750 mg/m² SMX 3 times weekly
- Blood products need to be irradiated before infusion

Mucocutaneous Candidiasis

- Topical nystatin if symptoms are mild
- Nystatin pastilles or troches (Mycelex) are more effective for treatment of oral lesions
- In the severe form of mucocutaneous candidiasis, systemic treatment with antifungal agents (ketoconazole 200 mg once daily, fluconazole, 100 mg once daily) is indicated

DiGeorge Syndrome

- Calcium supplement PO

Wiskott-Aldrich Syndrome

- Antibiotics (broad spectrum) if indicated
- IVIg prophylaxis in patients with recurrent bacterial infections or autoimmune disease (in combination with steroids)

Bare Lymphocyte Syndrome

- *Pneumocystis carinii* prophylaxis with TMP-SMX is recommended

Hyper-IgE

- Ketoconazole 200 mg once daily for cutaneous fungal infections

Transcobalamin II Deficiency

- Monthly injections of high doses of vitamin B_{12}

Complement Deficiencies

- In patients with acute symptoms of angioneurotic edema: epinephrine 1:1000 0.1–0.3 ml SC, antifibrinolytic agents, such as epsilon aminocaproic acid (EACA) or its cyclic analog tranexamic acid; danazol 200 mg b.i.d. initially, then decrease dose and stanozolol 2 mg t.i.d.? then decrease to 2 mg/d

PHAGOCYTIC DISORDERS

CGD

- Long-term prophylaxis with TMP-SMX or dicloxacillin
- Interferon gamma SC 50 $\mu g/m^2$, or 1.5 $\mu g/kg$ in infants, 3 times weekly

LAD

- TMP-SMX or dicloxacillin
- Leukocyte transfusions

20

Accidents and Emergencies

PREVENTING CHILDHOOD INJURIES

Janice A. Lowe, M.D.
Paul H. Wise, M.D., M.P.H.

The prevention of childhood injuries is often undermined by the myth that injuries are a result of accidents. However, quite to the contrary, the epidemiology of injuries makes it clear that childhood injuries follow predictable patterns of risk associated with age, socioeconomic status, and geographic location, among other factors. To address the challenge of reducing injuries in childhood, injuries must be viewed as both *predictable* and, therefore, potentially *preventable*.

Injuries take a tremendous toll during childhood, in terms of both morbidity and mortality. Injuries are the leading cause of death in children ages 1 to 19 years, accounting for nearly half of all mortality in this age group. In 1989, unintentional injuries accounted for 18.7 deaths per 100,000 children 1 through 4 years of age, with almost half of these due to motor vehicle crashes. Among children aged 5 through 9 years, unintentional injuries accounted for 11.6 deaths per 100,000, nearly 60% due to motor vehicles. For adolescents, motor vehicle–related mortality and homicide far exceed other causes of death. In addition, a variety of studies have shown that for every injury-related death, there are approximately 50 hospital admissions and 1200 visits to emergency rooms. The number of visits to doctors' offices, days missed from school, and morbidity associated with injuries are enormous.

Injury is defined as *physical damage due to the transfer of energy or the deprivation of essentials, such as oxygen and heat.* The types of energy involved in injuries include kinetic, thermal, chemical, electrical, and radiation. Interventions to prevent injuries largely attempt to reduce the risk that an injury will occur by altering the *host* (the person involved in the injury), the *agent* (the energy that is transferred), or the *environment* (the context in which the injury occurs). Developing preventive initiatives should be based first on a careful definition of the type of injuries of greatest interest. Epidemiologic data can often provide important insights into the scale of morbidity or mortality associated with any particular form of injury. Second, a careful analysis of all possible means of preventing the identified injury should be analyzed. This requires a purposeful search for preventive opportunities associated with the host, agent, or environment, with special attention to local conditions and community characteristics.

Injury prevention strategies can take many forms and rely on a number of different methodologies. For clinicians, however, it is often useful to consider involvement in child injury prevention as falling into three general opportunities for influence: the office setting, the community, and legislation.

THE PRIMARY CARE OFFICE

Physicians and other primary care providers are in a unique position to provide safety counseling to parents and children. They see children at periodic intervals, they form relationships with parents and children, and because of their training, clinicians who see children are well acquainted with the nature of a child's developmental stage. Indeed, counseling regarding injury prevention is best approached developmentally, with the content of counseling directed at the current developmental stage and in anticipation of soon to be acquired cognitive and motor capabilities (Table 1).

Studies have shown that safety counseling by physicians during regular office visits for routine well child care increase patient compliance with safety practices. In addition, when safety devices (e.g., ipecac or smoke detectors) have been made available in the office, other safety-related practices also have been increased. Counseling at office visits should target types of injuries that are high risk considering the capabilities of the child, the dynamics of family life, and the child's environment. For example, the parent of a 2-year-old child in an inner-city neighborhood should be cautioned about window falls, fires, and pedestrian injuries, whereas the parent of a 4-year-old child in a rural area may need counseling regarding pond drowning or injuries involving farm machinery.

The Injury Prevention Program (TIPP) of the American Academy of Pediatrics includes a series of questionnaires and handouts for parents that can be distributed during office visits. Similar types of materials are available also from some state health departments. In general, these programs are designed for use in an office practice and include recommended schedules for safety counseling based on the specific risks associated with each age group.

THE COMMUNITY

Community-based efforts are an important means of addressing childhood injuries, as education and access to specific interventions (such as car seats or smoke detectors) are often best implemented with strong community support. Many police and fire departments have personnel assigned as safety officers, and many school systems have curricula that emphasize safety. In addition, physicians can find allies in injury prevention in community hospitals, local boards of health, building inspectors, and local governments.

A number of community efforts have been shown to be effective. Bicycle helmet use has been enhanced using public education efforts, school-based programs, and helmet distribution programs. Smoke detector and window guard installation and maintenance have been advanced through both education and links to public housing and real estate agencies. The use of motor vehicle child restraints has been enhanced through rental programs and hospital-based discharge programs for newborns. Successful community projects often rely on broad community coalitions that garner the support and active par-

TABLE 1. Childhood Safety Counseling Schedule

PREVENTIVE HEALTH VISIT AGE	MINIMAL SAFETY COUNSELING INTRODUCE	REINFORCE
Prenatal/newborn	Infant car seat	
	Smoke detector	
	Crib safety	
2–4 wk	Falls	Infant car seat
2 mo	Burns—hot liquids	Infant car seat
		Falls
4 mo	Choking	Infant car seat
		Falls
		Burns—hot liquids
6 mo	Poison	Falls
	Burns—hot surface	Burns—hot liquids
9 mo	Water safety	Poison
	Toddler car seat	Falls
		Burns
1 y		Poison
		Falls
		Burns
15 mo	Specific to need	Poison
		Falls
		Burns
18 mo		Poison
		Falls
		Burns
2 y	Falls—play equipment	Auto—restraints
	Tricycles	Poison
	Auto—pedestrian	Burns
3 y		Auto—restraints, pedestrian
		Falls
		Burns
4 y	Car seat, booster, or	Pedestrian
	seatbelt	Falls—play equipment
		Burns
5 y	Bicycle safety	Seatbelt use
	Pedestrian safety	Smoke detector
6 y	Fire safety	Bicycle safety
		Seatbelt use
		Pedestrian safety
8 y	Water safety	Bicycle safety
		Seatbelt use
10 y	Sport safety	Seatbelt use
		Bicycle safety
Adolescence	Violence prevention	Sport safety
	Motor vehicle safety	Seatbelt use
		Bicycle safety

Adapted from The Injury Prevention Program, American Academy of Pediatrics.

ticipation of an array of community agencies, organizations, and institutions.

LEGISLATION

In many respects, the most effective strategies to prevent childhood injuries operate at the legislative level. Some legislative measures that have been proven effective are the Poison Prevention Packaging Act, the Flammable Fabrics Act, state smoke detector legislation, and passenger safety laws. Physicians and other child health workers were important advocates for the adoption of these important measures and have led successful lobbying efforts for the passage of a host of local and statewide safety ordinances.

The National Committee for Injury Prevention and Control has delineated eight essential functions for collaborators in injury prevention at state and local levels.

1. Draw on the cooperation of a multidisciplinary group of community members.
2. Coordinate existing local and state resources for injury prevention.

3. Initiate the examination of injury data and support prevention and control strategies (including support for legislation).
4. Create a statewide plan to promote the development of injury control programs at the local level.
5. Provide initial state funding of programs based on local communities when possible and help identify other sources of funding.
6. Provide technical assistance and training to involved groups.
7. Stimulate injury prevention research and training.
8. Be aware of the incidence and distribution of injuries over time.

Physicians and other child health advocates have an important role to play in the collective effort to reduce childhood injuries. Since injuries are the leading cause of childhood death, injury prevention must represent a central component of comprehensive pediatric care and draw on efforts based in clinical practice, community action, and legislative initiative.

ACUTE POISONINGS

EDWARD P. KRENZELOK, PHARM.D., A.B.A.T.

INCIDENCE

Poisonings rank among the five most common causes of accidental death in the pediatric population, and 12.5 million poisoning emergencies were reported to American poison information centers over the last decade. Although the mortality associated with pediatric poisoning is unfortunate, the occurrence of fatalities due to accidental pediatric poisoning is low—only 237 fatalities (representing 5% of poisoning-related fatalities) involved children less than 6 years of age during the 10-year period.

Children less than 6 years of age account for approximately 60% of all incidents, making accidental poisoning a relatively common occurrence of early childhood. In contrast to early childhood, there is a precipitous decline in the number of incidents involving the 6 to 12 year (5.6%) and 13 to 17 year (4.5%) age groups. Put into perspective, approximately 70% of all reported poisonings occur in the pediatric age group. This magnitude of cases means that the pediatrician in general practice will encounter a substantial number of poisoning cases. Therefore, it is essential to have a thorough understanding of the therapeutic intervention associated with basic management of acute poisoning emergencies, as well as some of the most common and dangerous poisonings. Ultimately, the emphasis of poison treatment is to prevent death. Practically, the major goal is to intervene as early as possible to reduce the morbidity associated with acute poisoning emergencies.

INITIAL PATIENT MANAGEMENT

Well over 99% of all pediatric poisonings have a favorable outcome, and 89% of the patients have a nontoxic exposure or experience only minor effects from the poisoning exposure. Therefore, most accidental pediatric poisoning exposures can be treated with the proverbial "glass of milk or water for the child and a tincture of reassurance for the parent."

A limited number of exposures will require therapeutic intervention. Since there are only a finite number of specific antidotes for the common toxins encountered by children, the cornerstone of patient management is good supportive care. Aggressive medical care and attention to the ABCs of life support often will suffice as adequate therapy.

Airway/Intravenous Access

Although most pediatric poisoning exposures do not necessitate aggressive intervention, comatose patients and children with impending serious toxicity (e.g., because of tricyclic antidepressant or clonidine poisoning) require intravenous access at minimum and frequently need endotracheal intubation, as dictated by the level of consciousness and clinical condition. Establishing early intravenous access will permit administration of maintenance fluid and electrolytes, assure hemodynamic stability, and provide a safe route to administer other drugs and pharmacologic antagonists (antidotes) when necessary.

Coma Drugs/Antidotes

Coma is an uncommon presentation of accidental pediatric poisoning. However, if a toxin is suspected as the cause of a child's coma, the standard drugs used to treat coma, dextrose and naloxone, should be administered. Hypoglycemia that is secondary to the ingestion of oral hypoglycemic agents can be treated with IV administration of 25% dextrose in a dose of 2 ml/kg. The administration of thiamine before dextrose to avoid Wernicke's encephalopathy is unnecessary unless the patient is an older child or adolescent who is suspected of being a chronic alcoholic.

Naloxone (Narcan), the opioid antagonist, is also administered to the comatose patient for both diagnostic and therapeutic purposes. With the exception of precipitating narcotic withdrawal in the narcotic-dependent patient, there are no disadvantages to administering adult doses to children of all ages. Therefore, doses based on body weight can be abandoned in favor of an IV dose of 0.4 to 2 mg. This dose should be administered every 2 to 4 minutes until the desired response (increased level of consciousness, improved respirations, or both) is achieved or a maximum of 2 to 10 mg is administered. If intravenous access cannot be obtained, naloxone can be administered intramuscularly, via the endotracheal tube, or by an intraosseous infusion.

Contrary to popular belief, flumazenil (Romazicon) should not be administered routinely to the comatose patient unless ingestion of benzodiazepines (e.g., diazepam, flurazepam, chlordiazepoxide) is suspected because of the history and level of consciousness. Although specific pediatric doses of flumazenil have not been established, the adult dose protocol of 0.2 mg IV over 30 seconds can be used in children. If the desired effect (improved level of consciousness) is not achieved after 30 seconds, a second dose of 0.3 mg IV over 30 seconds can be administered. If the level of consciousness still does not improve, additional doses (0.5 mg IV administered over 30 seconds at 1-minute intervals) up to a maximum total dose of 3 to 5 mg can be administered. Flumazenil use is contraindicated if a concurrent cyclic antidepressant overdose is suspected, since it may unmask the convulsive effects of the cyclic antidepressants.

Most other antidotal agents do not influence the patient's level of consciousness and are addressed as part of the specific management of the drugs discussed. Central nervous system (CNS) stimulants, such as nikethamide, picrotoxin, and caffeine, have no role in the management of toxin-induced CNS depression.

Patient History

Whenever possible, it is important to obtain a history of the drug or toxin exposure. An accurate history and the presence or absence of signs of exposure may direct the need for further therapy. Since both children and anxious parents or caretakers are often poor historians, a number of clues can help determine the validity of the exposure.

If the toxin (e.g., a medication or household cleaning product) is sold in a container, that container should be examined to determine how many dosage units (tablets, capsules) or how much volume remains. The parents may be able to confirm how many doses of a medicine had been administered before the poisoning event. Therefore, by adding that amount to the quantity remaining and subtracting the sum from the total number of dosage units originally found in the container, the amount that was allegedly ingested can be determined. If prescription medications are ingested, perusal of the label and instructions, as well as a call to the pharmacy, may quickly resolve the problem.

Many toxins, such as fingernail polish remover, have distinctive odors. The lack of such an odor on the child's breath may be sufficient evidence to confirm that the child did not consume any of the product that he or she was found playing with. Young children do not have fully developed motor skills and have a tendency to spill large quantities of the toxin on the floor or on their clothing. These amounts should always be taken into consideration when assessing potential poisoning exposures. If a poison information center has referred the patient for treatment, the historical aspects of the exposure always should be discussed with the poison information specialist, since parents and caretakers have a tendency to minimize the exposure when speaking with the treating physician.

Poison Information Centers

The regional poison information center (RPIC) should be contacted for further information about the diagnosis, prognosis, and management of the poisoning exposure after supportive care has been initiated. (Certified Regional Poison Information Center locations and telephone numbers are listed in Table 1.) The RPIC provides 24-hour service by poison information specialists and clinical toxicologists to assist both the lay public and health professionals with specific product ingredients, toxicology information, and contemporary management of poisoning exposures. The RPIC should be contacted in all poisoning exposure cases.

Dermal Exposures

Removal of the contaminated clothing to avoid further exposure is the most critical aspect of dermal decontamination. The clothing should be removed cautiously to prevent both extended patient contamination and contamination of the person providing care. Contaminated clothing should be placed in containers (e.g., plastic bags) that are labeled with precautionary warnings (the RPIC can provide guidance). The contaminated skin and contiguous areas should be thoroughly irrigated with lukewarm tapwater and gently washed with soap and water to remove toxin residue. If the integrity of the skin is severely damaged (as in an exposure to a corrosive agent), washing of the skin with soap and water may not be feasible. Irrigation of the skin should continue until all evidence of the toxin is eliminated (a minimum of 15 to 30 minutes).

Ophthalmic Exposures

Ocular irrigation can be accomplished preferably by using sterile normal saline, but tepid tapwater also may be used in the home setting (this will eliminate delays in treatment). The eyelids should be fully retracted, and normal saline (easily instilled using intravenous tubing) should be used to irrigate the affected eye(s) for a minimum of 15 to 30 minutes. Ocular irrigation for caustic alkaline exposures may be necessary for several hours. An ophthalmology consultation should be sought for ocular exposures involving corrosive toxins. Neutralization of ocular exposures to corrosives with the corresponding acid (vinegar) or alkali (sodium bicarbonate) is absolutely contraindicated, since the neutralization process may produce blepharospasm and make further irrigation difficult. Furthermore, neutralization may be associated with an exothermic (heat-producing) reaction that may produce further ocular injury.

Inhalation Exposures

Inhalation exposures may include accidental exposure to toxic fumes, such as carbon monoxide, or intentional inhalation abuse of solvents by adolescents. The specific therapy for such exposures is to immediately terminate contact with the toxin, ensure an adequate airway, and administer oxygen. Systemic toxicity should be treated appropriately, and vigilance for specific respiratory injury should be enhanced.

Bites and Stings

Insect bites and stings are common occurrences that often have self-limited manifestations regardless of the therapeutic intervention.

TABLE 1. American Association of Poison Control Centers Certified Regional Poison Centers, February 1994

Alabama
Regional Poison Control Center
The Children's Hospital of Alabama
1600 7th Avenue South
Birmingham, AL 35233-1711
Emergency phone: (205) 939-9201, (800) 292-6678 (AL only), or (205) 933-4050

Arizona
Arizona Poison and Drug Information Center
Arizona Health Sciences Center, Room 3204-K
1501 N. Campbell Avenue
Tucson, AZ 85724
Emergency phone: (800) 362-0101 (AZ only), (602) 626-6016

Samaritan Regional Poison Center
Good Samaritan Regional Medical Center
1441 North 12th St.
Phoenix, AZ 85006
Emergency phone: (602) 253-3334

California
Fresno Regional Poison Control Center
Valley Children's Hospital
3151 N. Millbrook
Fresno, CA 93703
Emergency phone: (209) 445-1222

San Diego Regional Poison Center
UCSD Medical Center, 8925
225 Dickinson Street
San Diego, CA 92103-8925
Emergency phone: (619) 543-6000, (800) 876-4766 (in 619 area code only)

San Francisco Bay Area Regional Poison Control Center
San Francisco General Hospital
1001 Potrero Avenue, Building 80, Room 230
San Francisco, CA 94122
Emergency phone: (800) 523-2222

Santa Clara Valley Medical Center Regional Poison Center
750 South Bascom Avenue
San Jose, CA 95128
Emergency phone: (408) 299-5112, (800) 662-9886 (CA only)

University of California, Davis, Medical Center Regional Poison Control Center
2315 Stockton Boulevard
Sacramento, CA 95817
Emergency phone: (916) 734-3692, (800) 342-9293 (Northern California only)

Colorado
Rocky Mountain Poison and Drug Center
645 Bannock Street
Denver, CO 80204
Emergency phone: (303) 629-1123

District of Columbia
National Capital Poison Center
Georgetown University Hospital
3800 Reservoir Road, NW
Washington, DC 20007
Emergency phone: (202) 625-3333, (202) 784-4660 (TTY)

Florida
The Florida Poison Information Center at Tampa General Hospital
Post Office Box 1289
Tampa, FL 33601
Emergency phone: (813) 253-4444 (Tampa), (800) 282-3171 (Florida)

Georgia
Georgia Poison Center
Grady Memorial Hospital
80 Butler Street S.E.
P.O. Box 26066
Atlanta, GA 30335-3801
Emergency phone: (800) 282-5846 GA only, (404) 616-9000

Indiana
Indiana Poison Center
Methodist Hospital of Indiana
1701 N. Senate Boulevard
P.O. Box 1367
Indianapolis, IN 46206-1367
Emergency phone: (800) 382-9097 (IN only), (317) 929-2323

Maryland
Maryland Poison Center
20 N. Pine Street
Baltimore, MD 21201
Emergency phone: (410) 528-7701, (800) 492-2414 (MD only)

National Capital Poison Center (DC suburbs only)
Georgetown University Hospital
3800 Reservoir Road, NW
Washington, DC 20007
Emergency phone: (202) 625-3333, (202) 784-4660 (TTY)

Continued on following page

The Hymenoptera order of insects (which includes bees) accounts for the majority of exposures in this category. Anaphylactic reactions secondary to bee stings may require aggressive use of ventilatory support, epinephrine, antihistamines, and steroids. However, most stings produce only intense pain, which resolves within hours. If the stinging insect is a bee (rather than a hornet or wasp), the stinger frequently will be left at the site of the sting. Therefore, rapid removal of the stinging apparatus can limit further venom exposure. The stinger should be removed with a scraping motion by using the rigid edge of a credit card or dull butterknife. Never attempt to pull out the stinger using fingers or a tweezer, since this will result in the injection of more venom.

Snake bites from nonvenomous snakes should be thoroughly cleansed with soap and water, and antibiotic prophylaxis is unnecessary. Venomous snake bites, however, require more intensive scrutiny. Envenomation does not occur in up to 50% of bites from venomous snakes, and it is important to determine if it has occurred. Pain, swelling, and ecchymosis are the pathognomonic signs of envenomation. Tourniquets and excisional therapy with venom extraction (cut and suck) have no role in the management of venomous

snake bites. The development of local swelling and systemic toxicity manifest as coagulopathies, hemodynamic compromise, and neurologic involvement will dictate the necessity of using the antivenin. A regional poison information center should always be consulted about the administration of the antivenin. Furthermore, it is important to remember that the antivenin is a derivative of horse serum and has the inherent potential to produce serum sickness and allergic reactions.

GASTRIC DECONTAMINATION

Most pediatric poisoning exposures involve the oral route. Therefore, after the initiation of supportive care as described, some form of gastric decontamination should be implemented to prevent further absorption of the toxin(s). Before the last decade, choices for gastric decontamination in the pediatric patient were quite clear—alert children received syrup of ipecac to induce emesis, and those with a decreased level of consciousness were lavaged. Activated charcoal was used as an adjunct to therapy when convenient. However, recent research and clinical experience have changed the traditional dogmatic approach, and there are a number of controversies about the efficacy

TABLE 1. American Association of Poison Control Centers Certified Regional Poison Centers, February 1994 *Continued*

Massachusetts
Massachusetts Poison Control System
300 Longwood Avenue
Boston, MA 02115
Emergency phone: (617) 232-2120, (800) 682-9211

Michigan
Poison Control Center
Children's Hospital of Michigan
3901 Beaubien Boulevard
Detroit, MI 48201
Emergency phone: (313) 745-5711

Minnesota
Hennepin Regional Poison Center
Hennepin County Medical Center
701 Park Avenue
Minneapolis, MN 55415
Emergency phone: (612) 347-3141, TDD (612) 337-7474

Minnesota Regional Poison Center
St. Paul-Ramsey Medical Center
640 Jackson Street
St. Paul, MN 55101
Emergency phone: (612) 221-2113

Missouri
Cardinal Glennon Children's Hospital Regional Poison Center
1465 S. Grand Boulevard
St. Louis, MO 63104
Emergency phone: (314) 772-5200, (800) 366-8888

Montana
Rocky Mountain Poison and Drug Center
645 Bannock Street
Denver, CO 80204
Emergency phone: (303) 629-1123

Nebraska
The Poison Center
8301 Dodge Street
Omaha, NE 68114
Emergency phone: (402) 390-5555 (Omaha), (800) 955-9119 (NE)

New Jersey
New Jersey Poison Information and Education System
201 Lyons Avenue
Newark, NJ 07112
Emergency phone: (800) 962-1253

New Mexico
New Mexico Poison and Drug Information Center
University of New Mexico
Albuquerque, NM 87131-1076
Emergency phone: (505) 843-2551, (800) 432-6866 (NM only)

New York
Hudson Valley Poison Center
Nyack Hospital
160 N. Midland Avenue
Nyack, NY 10960
Emergency phone: (800) 336-6997, (914) 353-1000

Long Island Regional Poison Control Center
Winthrop University Hospital
259 First Street
Mineola, NY 11501
Emergency phone: (516) 542-2323, 2324, 2325, 3813

New York City Poison Control Center
N.Y.C. Department of Health
455 First Avenue, Room 123
New York, NY 10016
Emergency phone: (212) 340-4494, (212) P-O-I-S-O-N-S, TDD (212) 689-9014

Ohio
Central Ohio Poison Center
700 Children's Drive
Columbus, OH 43205-2696
Emergency phone: (614) 228-1323, (800) 682-7625, (614) 228-2272 (TTY), (614) 461-2012

Cincinnati Drug & Poison Information Center and Regional Poison Control System
231 Bethesda Avenue, M.L. 144
Cincinnati, OH 45267-0144
Emergency phone: (513) 558-5111, 800-872-5111 (OH only)

---

and application of syrup of ipecac, gastric lavage, activated charcoal, cathartics, and whole bowel irrigation. Understanding the indications for each of these modalities is critical to the successful management of pediatric poisoning emergencies.

Syrup of Ipecac-Induced Emesis

Syrup of ipecac is the only emetic that should be used. Previously used emetic agents, such as apomorphine and copper sulfate, are potentially toxic and have no role in the management of poisoning emergencies. Syrup of ipecac is an effective emetic but is also the focus of considerable controversy about its capacity to eliminate significant amounts of toxin or reduce morbidity and mortality. The recent use of syrup of ipecac in the nonpediatric population has dropped substantially, largely because of its failure to eliminate toxins that have passed into the small intestine. Activated charcoal is being used increasingly as the sole means of gastric decontamination. Research has demonstrated that in the adult patient, there is a hiatus of approximately 3 hours between toxin ingestion and treatment, thereby rendering the use of ipecac rather ineffective. This is not generally the case in the pediatric population, where ingestions are often witnessed and the time between poisoning exposure recognition and treatment is short, often only minutes. Therefore, the adult data are not directly extrapolatable to the pediatric patient population.

Syrup of ipecac is indicated in the management of accidental pediatric poisonings that can be treated in the home. In most circumstances, the time from recognition of the exposure to treatment will be less than 1 hour. These types of ingestions usually involve exposure to mild to moderately toxic substances in which the estimated amount has exceeded the toxic threshold only modestly (e.g., acetaminophen, multiple vitamins with iron, mushrooms and plants). The induction of emesis can prevent an unnecessary visit to the emergency department. The same indication can be used to treat children in the emergency department, since gastric lavage is inappropriate under these circumstances. Alternatively, activated charcoal can be used in the emergency department for most of the same indications as syrup of ipecac (notable exceptions are addressed in the activated charcoal discussion).

Syrup of ipecac is an effective emetic and will remove 25% to 50% of the stomach contents. The amount of toxin removed is dependent on the timing of administration of syrup of ipecac in relation to when the ingestion occurred—the shorter the temporal separation, the more effective the emesis.

SYRUP OF IPECAC DOSAGE

- <1 year of age: 15 ml
- >1 year of age: 30 ml

Syrup of ipecac should preferably be administered before water is given (rather than mixed with water) to ensure that the entire dose is administered. Children should be encouraged to drink a minimum of 4 to 8 ounces of water. Other clear fluids, such as carbonated beverages

TABLE 1. American Association of Poison Control Centers Certified Regional Poison Centers, February 1994 *Continued*

Oregon
Oregon Poison Center
Oregon Health Sciences University
3181 S.W. Sam Jackson Park Road
Portland, OR 97201
Emergency phone: (503) 494-8968, (800) 452-7165 (OR only)

Pennsylvania
Central Pennsylvania Poison Center
University Hospital
Milton S. Hershey Medical Center
Hershey, PA 17033
Emergency phone: (800) 521-6110

The Poison Control Center Serving the Greater Philadelphia Metropolitan Area
One Children's Center
Philadelphia, PA 19104-4303
Emergency phone: (215) 386-2100

Pittsburgh Poison Center
3705 Fifth Avenue at DeSoto Street
Pittsburgh, PA 15213
Emergency phone: (412) 681-6669

Rhode Island
Rhode Island Poison Center
593 Eddy Street
Providence, RI 02903
Emergency phone: (401) 277-5727

Texas
North Texas Poison Center
5201 Harry Hines Boulevard
P.O. Box 35926
Dallas, TX 75235
Emergency phone: (214) 590-5000, Texas Watts (800) 441-0040

Texas State Poison Center
The University of Texas Medical Branch
Galveston, TX 77550-2780
Emergency phone: (409) 765-1420 (Galveston), (713) 654-1701 (Houston)

Utah
Intermountain Regional Poison Control Center
50 North Medical Drive
Salt Lake City, UT 84132
Emergency phone: (801) 581-2151, (800) 456-7707 (UT only)

Virginia
Blue Ridge Poison Center
Box 67
Blue Ridge Hospital
Charlottesville, VA 22901
Emergency phone: (804) 924-5543, (800) 451-1428

National Capital Poison Center (Northern VA Only)
Georgetown University Hospital
3800 Reservoir Road, NW
Washington, DC 20007
Emergency phone: (202) 625-3333, (202) 784-4660 (TTY)

West Virginia
West Virginia Poison Center
3110 MacCorkle Avenue, S.E.
Charleston, WV 25304
Emergency phone: (800) 642-3625 (WV only), (304) 348-4211

Wyoming
The Poison Center
8301 Dodge Street
Omaha, NE 68114
Emergency phone: (402) 390-5555 (Omaha), (800) 955-9119 (NE)

---

and fruit juices, also are acceptable. Although the use of milk is not encouraged, since it interferes with the ability to observe the vomitus for evidence of the toxin(s), it will not inhibit the emetic effect of syrup of ipecac. Activated charcoal also does not interfere with the emetic effects of syrup of ipecac and can be administered concurrently. However, this combination produces a messy emesis. Customarily, activated charcoal administration is usually delayed until approximately 1 hour after emesis has ceased.

Emesis will occur within 15 to 20 minutes and subside in most children within 30 to 60 minutes of onset. Food and fluids should be withheld for 60 minutes following the cessation of emesis. Once the child is able to tolerate oral fluids (generally 60 to 90 minutes after completion of emesis), solid foods may be ingested. Over 99% of children will have successful emesis with the recommended doses of syrup of ipecac. If the first dose fails to produce emesis within 30 minutes, a second dose (the same as the first) may be administered accompanied by additional fluids.

Adverse Effects

The therapeutic use of syrup of ipecac is associated with little toxicity, and acute toxicity in children is virtually unrecognized. However, chronic toxicity from syrup of ipecac abuse is widely recognized as a problem in children with eating disorders, such as bulimia. Emetine, one of the active alkaloids in syrup of ipecac, accumulates with repeated use (60 to 90 ml [2 to 3 oz]/d for a prolonged period, e.g., weeks to months) and can produce cardiac or peripheral myopathies, as well as cardiac conduction defects.

Contraindications to Emesis

Syrup of ipecac is not recommended in children less than 6 months of age primarily because of age-related incompetence in protecting the airway. However, this is rarely an issue, since this age group represents less than 1% of pediatric poisoning exposures. The use of activated charcoal is a suitable alternative in these children.

Emesis is absolutely contraindicated in patients who have a decreased level of consciousness (e.g., those who are comatose or postictal), since syrup of ipecac exerts an emetic response irrespective of the level of consciousness and may place the patient at significant risk of aspiration. Furthermore, syrup of ipecac should not be used in patients who have been exposed to extremely toxic agents where impending coma or other complications, such as seizures, may occur (e.g., tricyclic antidepressants, clonidine, calcium channel blockers, strychnine).

The ingestion of corrosives, such as acids and alkali, is a contraindication to the induction of emesis. The emetic process may subject the esophagus and oral cavity to reexposure of the corrosive agent, and the mechanical aspects of vomiting may result in esophageal perforation. Furthermore, syrup of ipecac should not be used if hydrocarbons with little potential for absorption have been ingested. For example, gasoline and motor oil are largely composed of hydrocarbon fractions that are not readily absorbed and produce little or no local toxicity in the gastrointestinal tract. However, their physicochemical nature predisposes these agents to a high risk of being aspirated during emesis, and hydrocarbon aspiration may be life threatening in children.

Gastric Lavage

Gastric lavage is indicated in pediatric patients who have ingested substances that must be removed from the stomach and where emesis is not the preferred means of removing the toxin. Lavage is also indicated in patients who have ingested toxins associated with high morbidity and mortality (e.g., cyclic antidepressants, methanol). Gastric lavage has been of greatest value in the management of pediatric poisonings among adolescents because of the difficulty of inserting gastric tubes with a large enough diameter in younger children.

Under ideal circumstances, gastric lavage is superior to syrup of ipecac-induced emesis. Although earlier studies clearly demonstrated that emesis was superior to gastric lavage, these studies were flawed by the use of small nasogastric tubes (12 to 18 French) and inadequate fluid volumes. More recent research has focused on the use of large-bore orogastric hoses (34 to 40 French) and voluminous amounts of fluid. These data indicate that aggressive lavage can remove 45% to 90% of marker drugs in adult volunteers under simulated overdose conditions. Unfortunately, all the study models have examined the efficacy of lavage versus other gastric-emptying modalities in adults, not in children.

To maximize the effectiveness of gastric lavage in children, the largest tolerable lavage tube with an adequate number of orifices of sufficient size must be used. In younger children, a 24 to 28 French orogastric tube is advised. The orifices on the distal end of the tube should be large enough to allow the introduction of lavage fluid without resistance and to allow the retrieval of gastric debris. Most adolescents can tolerate adult size orogastric hoses, which have a diameter of 34 to 40 French (approximately the diameter of a dime). This is the most efficient size range and has the capability of introducing and withdrawing large volumes of lavage fluid and gastric contents with relative ease. Unfortunately, the physical size of the adult size tube is not compatible with pediatric anatomy, and this greatly impairs the effectiveness of gastric lavage in the younger pediatric patient. Even with the larger-bore tubes, gastric lavage is relatively ineffective in removing large pieces of gastric debris that may be associated with pediatric ingestion of mushrooms and plant fragments.

Use of the optimal size lavage tube cannot be overemphasized. Of equal importance, however, is the use of the appopriate type and volume of lavage fluid. In older adolescents, lukewarm tapwater is the lavage fluid of choice. However, younger children have a more delicate balance of fluids and electrolytes, and half-normal or normal saline (warmed to room temperature) must be used. Younger children should be lavaged with 10 to 15 ml/kg per lavage exchange to a maximum of 100 to 150 ml per exchange. Attention should be paid to both the volume of fluid that is introduced and the volume being removed to ensure that these volumes are relatively equivalent. The lavage process should be continued until the lavage returns are clear of gastric debris or until approximately 3 L of lavage fluid have been used. In adolescents, up to 300 ml of tapwater can be used per exchange to an end point of clear lavage returns and a total volume of 10 to 20 L. Activated charcoal (therapeutic dose) can be introduced during an early lavage exchange to adsorb any toxins remaining in the stomach. Activated charcoal also serves as an excellent marker to help determine the effectiveness of gastric lavage. When the gastric returns are clear of gross macroscopic evidence of activated charcoal, the lavage process can be terminated.

Additional factors that improve the effectiveness of gastric lavage include frequent repositioning of the lavage tube and early implementation of the procedure while the toxin still remains in the stomach.

The child should be placed in the Trendelenburg position on the left side. Comatose patients should always be intubated, preferably with a cuffed endotracheal tube, before the performance of gastric lavage. The process of gastric lavage is facilitated by the gravity flow lavage technique. Instead of using a large-volume syringe to introduce and retrieve lavage fluid, gravity is used to accomplish both tasks. A number of closed gravity flow lavage systems, which also limit exposure of the practitioner to the patient's bodily fluids, are available commercially. A receptacle containing the lavage fluid is elevated on an intravenous pole and is positioned over the patient, allowing the desired amount of fluid to flow via gravity into the child's stomach. When sufficient fluid has been introduced, the tube is clamped to prevent further fluid instillation, and the clamp on the tube leading to the receptacle on the floor is opened, allowing the gastric lavage fluid to flow out of the stomach. This procedure is repeated continuously until the lavage procedure is completed.

Contraindications

Gastric lavage is a safe procedure, and there are few contraindications to its use. Gastric lavage should not be used if the ingestion involved a strong corrosive agent, since introduction of the gastric lavage tube may result in esophageal perforation. The patient must be able to protect the airway, and if there is any potential for airway compromise, gastric lavage should not be performed until the child is intubated.

Activated Charcoal

Prior to the 1980s, activated charcoal was used only as an adjunct in the management of acute pediatric poisoning emergencies. Now, activated charcoal is indicated in the majority of poisoning exposures that are the result of toxin ingestion.

Activated charcoal is activated carbon that is capable of adsorbing organic and inorganic toxins with a molecular weight range of 100 to 1000 daltons. The activation of charcoal means that it has been processed with various acids and gases to remove adsorbed contaminants and that it contains a network of pores that increase the surface area. Commercially available activated charcoal has a surface area that ranges from 950 to 2000 m^2/g. Products with a greater surface area more effectively adsorb toxins. The primary debate regarding activated charcoal use focuses on whether or not it can be used as the sole means of gastrointestinal decontamination. Activated charcoal has a substantial advantage over emesis and gastric lavage if gastric emptying has occurred, since the activated charcoal is capable of catching up with the toxin and binding the toxin throughout the rest of the gastrointestinal tract. It is indicated as the sole decontamination intervention when the toxin is known to be adsorbed by activated charcoal, the toxin has mild to moderate toxic potential, or there has been a substantial delay between the time of ingestion and treatment that would render emesis or gastric lavage ineffective. As a routine, activated charcoal should not be used as the sole intervention in poisonings that involve agents associated with significant morbidity and mortality. If the patient is stable, an effort should be made to perform gastric lavage on these patients before administration of activated charcoal.

Although activated charcoal is capable of adsorbing most toxins that are commonly ingested by children, it is ineffective in binding a limited number of substances. These primarily include but are not limited to low molecular weight compounds and metals. Examples of agents that are not effectively adsorbed by activated charcoal include lead, iron, lithium, strong acids and alkali, alcohols, and petroleum distillates. Activated charcoal is not contraindicated when there is doubt about the identification of the specific toxin or when other toxins known to be bound by activated charcoal have been ingested.

The doses for activated charcoal have been assigned rather arbitrarily. Since activated charcoal is inert (not pharmacologically active) and not absorbed, there is little advantage or toxicologic rationale for being conservative with its use.

ACTIVATED CHARCOAL STANDARD DOSAGES

- <1 year of age 1-2 g/kg
- 1–6 years of age 25 g
- 6–12 years of age 25–50 g
- >12 years of age 50–100 g

In most poisonings, activated charcoal is administered in a single dose as indicated. It is advisable to administer an additional dose at

4 to 6 hours after the initial dose. The rationale for the second dose is that activated charcoal does not irreversibly bind the toxins and the second dose may adsorb any toxin that desorbed from the initial dose. It is also conceivable that unbound toxin present in the gastrointestinal tract may be adsorbed by the second dose.

Multiple-dose activated charcoal therapy (also known as gastrointestinal dialysis) is a popular and effective means of activated charcoal administration. However, it has very limited application. Some toxins (e.g., theophylline and phenobarbital) are secreted into the gastrointestinal tract as the body attempts to establish an equilibrium between the high toxin concentration in the blood and the much lower concentration in the gastrointestinal tract. If multiple doses of activated charcoal are administered, the toxin in the gastrointestinal tract is adsorbed, which inhibits its reabsorption and the subsequent establishment of an equilibrium between the blood and intestinal tract. In an attempt to establish the equilibrium, additional toxin is secreted into the intestinal tract and is continuously adsorbed by the activated charcoal, thereby enhancing its elimination. Drugs such as digitoxin, which undergo extensive enterohepatic circulation, are also effectively eliminated by the multiple-dose regimen. If vomiting is a problem, as may be the case in theophylline poisoning, smaller doses may be given more frequently. For example, rather than administering activated charcoal 50 g every 4 hours, a dose of approximately 12 to 13 g can be administered every hour. The doses for multiple-dose activated charcoal therapy are identical to those for single-dose therapy, but the activated charcoal is administered at 4- to 6-hour intervals until the appropriate end point is achieved, that is, clinical improvement and diminishing blood levels of toxin.

Activated charcoal is available as a powder, a commercially prepared aqueous slurry, or a slurry containing sorbitol. Aqueous slurries or prepared slurries using tapwater and activated charcoal powder are preferred over the products that contain sorbitol, especially in very young pediatric patients. Sorbitol, which is a potent cathartic, is present in a fixed amount and may produce profound fluid loss in young children if the sorbitol dose exceeds 1.5 to 3 g/kg. This is potentially a very serious problem if the sorbitol-containing product is used instead of the aqueous product in multiple-dose regimens. Aqueous slurries of activated charcoal settle with time, and the containers must be agitated vigorously for at least 60 seconds before patient administration to ensure that the entire dose is delivered to the patient. The container should be thoroughly flushed with water, and those contents should be administered to the patient as well.

Adverse Effects

Activated charcoal is pharmacologically inert and, therefore, is not associated with any systemic toxicity. Adverse effects, therefore, have been the direct consequence of its physical presence.

During the last decade, the American Association of Poison Control Centers has documented administration of activated charcoal to over 757,000 patients. Yet only 7 fatalities related to the aspiration of activated charcoal have been reported. Six of the cases were secondary to airway obstruction from the activated charcoal, and a single case of bronchiolitis obliterans has been attributed to activated charcoal aspiration. This problem, although rare, can be minimized by intubating high-risk patients before charcoal administration, vigorously shaking the container to eliminate clumps, and diluting the aqueous activated charcoal with more water.

Contrary to popular opinion, administration of aqueous activated charcoal is not associated with a high incidence of vomiting, although the incidence is higher when hyperosmolar cathartics, such as sorbitol, are added to the activated charcoal. Smaller, more frequent doses of activated charcoal may minimize this problem.

Activated charcoal is often implicated when constipation, obstruction, or paralytic ileus occurs in the toxicology patient. These problems, however, are most likely secondary effects from the toxic exposure itself. Activated charcoal is pharmacologically inert and incapable of producing such findings except in patients whose motility is already deranged. For example, agents with anticholinergic (cyclic

antidepressants) or opioid (heroin) effects decrease intestinal motility, which may then be complicated by administration of activated charcoal. Therefore, active bowel sounds are a prerequisite for charcoal administration.

Although reported as adverse effects of activated charcoal, diarrhea and dehydration are almost always associated with the use of the cathartics that are customarily administered in conjunction with the charcoal.

Contraindications

Contraindications to the use of activated charcoal are very limited. Patients without bowel sounds should not receive activated charcoal because of the dangers of obstruction. Comatose patients must be endotracheally intubated before charcoal administration. Known allergies to any excipients or preservatives in activated charcoal should preclude the use of the commercial product. In these rare instances, the activated charcoal slurry should be compounded with bulk powder and water. Activated charcoal is not advised for use in patients who have ingested corrosive agents, since the charcoal will not prevent the local tissue injury and may obscure endoscopic evaluation of lesions that are produced by the corrosive toxin. Activated charcoal may be used safely in patients with acetaminophen overdose. Charcoal has a high affinity for acetaminophen and does not effectively adsorb N-acetylcysteine, the oral antidote for acetaminophen poisoning.

Cathartics

Although activated charcoal adsorbs toxins and prevents their absorption, that binding process is reversible. Therefore, cathartics have been used in conjunction with charcoal to hasten the elimination of the toxin-activated charcoal complex through the bowel. Clinical research has demonstrated that the use of a cathartic with charcoal can reduce serum levels of marker drugs when compared with the use of activated charcoal alone. The clinical significance of this finding is controversial, however. Cathartics may be used in single doses after the administration of activated charcoal. They should be used very cautiously during multiple-dose activated charcoal therapy, since serious fluid and electrolyte derangement may occur.

A single dose of a cathartic may be administered following the administration of activated charcoal (concurrent administration is not contraindicated but is more frequently associated with vomiting). If a charcoal-laden stool is not evident within approximately 8 hours, the dose of cathartic may be repeated. Sorbitol is the most effective cathartic and is often a component of the activated charcoal product. However, this type of activated charcoal product should not be used in children, since the dose of sorbitol is fixed and may be toxic to younger children. Furthermore, it may complicate preexisting problems in multiple-dose therapy. Magnesium citrate is also an effective and acceptable cathartic. Other cathartics, such as magnesium and sodium sulfate, phosphate solutions, and emollients are not as effective.

CATHARTIC DOSES

- Sorbitol 1.5 g/kg
- Magnesium citrate 3–4 ml/kg

Adverse Effects

Fluid and electrolyte depletion may be a significant problem if excessive doses of cathartics are used. Sorbitol, in doses exceeding 10 g/kg, has been associated with severe fluid and electrolyte derangement and subsequent neurodevastation. Hypermagnesemia has been reported with the use of magnesium cathartics, especially in patients with compromised renal function.

Contraindications

Magnesium citrate should be avoided in patients with diminished renal function. The absence of bowel sounds presents a relative contraindication to the use of cathartics. Cathartics should be avoided in patients who have ingested corrosive agents.

Whole Bowel Irrigation

Whole bowel irrigation (WBI) involves the instillation of large volumes of isoosmotic polyethylene glycol solution (Golytely, Colyte) to flush the bowel of toxins. This procedure has little use in the basic management of most pediatric poisoning exposures. The use of syrup of ipecac, gastric lavage, or activated charcoal is preferred in most pediatric poisonings that require gastrointestinal decontamination. WBI has some use in accidental exposures that involve iron or sustained-release products, where the toxin resides in the intestinal tract for long periods of time. Furthermore, WBI may be of value in the adolescent who has swallowed a bag, vial, or condom containing illicit drugs to eliminate evidence and avoid criminal prosecution. Such containers must be eliminated rapidly to prevent toxicity.

The WBI solution is either consumed by the patient or administered via a nasogastric tube. The fluid is instilled at a constant rate over approximately 5 hours until the rectal effluent is clear and the toxins have been recovered (in the case of the swallowed contraband). An abdominal x-ray can be used to determine if the iron has been eliminated from the intestinal tract.

WHOLE BOWEL IRRIGATION DOSAGE

- <5 years of age: 20 ml/kg/h
- >5 years of age: 0.5–2 L/h

Adverse Effects

Since WBI solution is isoosmotic, it does not cause third-spacing of fluid into the gastrointestinal tract. Therefore, the fluid and electrolyte abnormalities associated with cathartic use do not accompany WBI. The large volume of fluid necessary to produce the bowel-flushing effect is responsible for the primary adverse effects, nausea, vomiting, cramping, bloating, and abdominal distention.

COMMON AND LETHAL PEDIATRIC POISONING EXPOSURES

Medications account for approximately 40% of all poisoning exposures in children less than 6 years of age. Toxicity and treatment information on some of the most common and lethal medications is presented in this section. All treatment recommendations assume that basic life support measures, as described previously, have been implemented. This information is not inclusive, and an RPIC should always be consulted for specific toxicity information and treatment recommendations (Table 1).

Analgesics

Analgesic preparations account for more pediatric poisonings than any other single category. Their ubiquitous nature and the relative complacency about their use are responsible for the large number of poisonings. Acetaminophen is the most commonly ingested analgesic and toxin by children less than 6 years of age. The association between Reye syndrome and the use of salicylates has significantly reduced the number of salicylate-related exposures and nearly eliminated it as cause of mortality in children. Ibuprofen is rapidly gaining acceptance for use in children, and a parallel rise in the number of ibuprofen ingestions is evident. With the wide variety of analgesics available, it is incumbent on the practitioner to determine what specific analgesic was ingested and the correct dose. For example, "aspirin-free" may be either acetaminophen or ibuprofen, and these analgesics have distinctly different toxidromes. Similarly, the term "extra strength" has different meanings for different manufacturers. Since the toxicity and treatment of acute poisoning by analgesics is based on milligram per kilogram amounts, it is essential to determine this basic information to treat the child properly.

Acetaminophen

Toxicity. Acetaminophen is partially metabolized to a toxic metabolite that depletes endogenous glutathione, resulting in hepatotoxicity in adults and adolescents. Younger children have a lower incidence of hepatotoxicity despite the ingestion of known toxic doses of greater than 150 mg/kg. It is postulated that acetaminophen is metabolized by alternative pathways in young children. However, the data are not conclusive, and all ingestions in excess of 150 mg/kg should be regarded as potentially toxic.

Manifestations. There are four stages to acetaminophen poisoning:

1. Over the first 24 hours, gastrointestinal symptoms of nausea and vomiting predominate and even lethargy may be present.
2. Between 24 and 48 hours, there may be subjective improvement, but liver function values will begin to rise if there is toxicity.
3. In this stage, the manifestations of severe liver injury (e.g., coagulopathies, jaundice) develop.
4. If the patient recovers, the liver function tests will begin to normalize by 5 to 7 days after the ingestion.

Renal failure also has been associated with acute acetaminophen toxicity.

Treatment. Gastric decontamination should be considered in recent ingestions. Syrup of ipecac is effective if administered within the first 60 minutes postingestion. Activated charcoal may be administered and will not interfere with the use of the oral antidote, *N*-acetylcysteine. A serum level should be obtained to determine if the acetaminophen level warrants the use of *N*-acetylcysteine (a glutathione precursor or surrogate that prevents hepatotoxicity). Contact a poison information center for interpretation of the serum level. If the acetaminophen serum level is in the toxic range, *N*-acetylcysteine must be administered orally for 3 days:

N-ACETYLCYSTEINE DOSAGE

- Loading dose: 140 mg/kg
- Maintenance dose: 70 mg/kg q4h for 17 doses

Ibuprofen

Toxicity. Like acetaminophen, ibuprofen has a very high therapeutic index and is relatively safe in children. An acute overdose of less than 100 mg/kg is considered nontoxic. Mild to moderate toxicity may occur with doses of 100 to 300 mg/kg, and serious toxicity is associated with doses in excess of 300 mg/kg.

Manifestations. Gastrointestinal irritation, drowsiness, and lethargy may be early manifestations. Apnea, seizures, and metabolic acidosis may occur with acute poisoning. The acid-base disturbance differs from that of salicylate poisoning in that respiratory alkalosis is not a component of ibuprofen poisoning.

Treatment. Gastric decontamination in the home is advised for children who ingest more than 100 mg/kg but less than 200 mg/kg of ibuprofen. Children who ingest more than 200 mg/kg should be treated and observed in an emergency department for at least 4 hours.

Salicylates

Toxicity. Although the incidence of salicylate poisoning has diminished, it is still associated with significant morbidity and mortality. The threshold for acute toxicity is 150 mg/kg. Ingestions in excess of 300 mg/kg are often associated with significant toxicity.

Manifestations. Since salicylates produce respiratory stimulation, children hyperventilate and often develop a respiratory alkalosis associated with the compensatory loss of bicarbonate, which is partially responsible for the development of a concurrent metabolic acidosis. The mixed respiratory alkalosis and metabolic acidosis are pathognomonic of salicylate poisoning. In addition to hyperventilation, children experience fever and vomiting, resulting in fluid and electrolyte disturbances. Tinnitus is a common manifestation of salicylism, but it is a difficult symptom to elicit from young children. Seizures may occur in the presence of high serum salicylate levels. Acute salicylism must be differentiated from chronic salicylism (the same symptoms may occur at significantly lower serum salicylate levels).

Treatment. Gastric decontamination is beneficial, even several hours after ingestion, since salicylates often have a long residence time in the stomach. Although one or two doses of activated charcoal should be administered, there is no compelling evidence that multiple-dose activated charcoal therapy will enhance the elimination of salicylates. Fluid and electrolyte replacement therapy is important. The Done nomogram is of little or no use in the assessment of salicylate poisoning. Alkaline diuresis is unnecessary in patients with mild to moderate toxicity and of no therapeutic value in cases of serious toxicity. Hemodialysis very effectively enhances salicylate elimination, but it should be reserved for use in children with serious salicylism.

Cough and Cold Preparations

Cough and cold preparations, which include but are not limited to decongestants, antihistamines, expectorants, and cough suppressants, are the second leading category of medication involved in pediatric poisoning exposures. In general, they are not associated with a high incidence of morbidity and mortality. Since many of the preparations are combination products, the amount of each ingredient must be determined, and this will dictate the necessity of treatment. One can never assume that cough syrup contains just a cough suppressant, such as dextromethorphan. The product may also contain diphenhydramine, phenylpropanolamine, acetaminophen, guaifenesin, and up to 25% ethanol! Phenylpropanolamine is one of the most common decongestants. Diphenhydramine has significant toxic potential, and dextromethorphan is abused by some adolescents.

Phenylpropanolamine

Toxicity. The minimum toxic dose of phenylpropanolamine in children is 8 to 10 mg/kg. Toxic manifestations are more common with doses exceeding 17.5 mg/kg.

Manifestations. Hypertension may occur. Tachycardia and even a reflex bradycardia (secondary to hypertension) may be present. Confusion, anxiety, headaches, and agitation are common when this drug has been used for its abuse potential. Seizures are uncommon in acute overdoses in young children.

Treatment. Gastric decontamination is recommended if greater than 10 mg/kg has been ingested. Since many of the cough and cold products are liquid preparations and rapidly absorbed, activated charcoal may be used as the sole therapy if there is a delay between ingestion and treatment. Significant hypertension may necessitate treatment with nitroprusside. If necessary, symptom-specific therapy should be used to treat additional problems.

Diphenhydramine

Toxicity. Children are exquisitely sensitive to the toxic effects of diphenhydramine. Adolescents have died following intentional ingestions of 1.5 to 7.5 g. Seizures have been reported with 50 to 150 mg (uncommon), and fatalities have occurred with as little as 500 mg in younger children. The topical use of diphenhydramine-containing lotions may produce overt toxicity.

Manifestations. Diphenhydramine poisoning may present with a typical anticholinergic toxidrome, which includes tachycardia, mydriasis, decreased intestinal motility, and delirium. Consistent with antihistamine toxicity, lethargy and drowsiness often accompany toxic doses. Seizures are uncommon following small accidental ingestions by children but are very prominent following large doses. Status epilepticus that is resistant to therapy may occur. Fatal cases often present with status epilepticus, and this is a poor prognostic sign.

Treatment. In asymptomatic children, gastric decontamination should be performed if the dose exceeds 15 mg/kg. Patients who are mildly symptomatic for several hours after ingestion may be treated with activated charcoal alone. Gastric lavage followed by activated charcoal should always be used in large overdoses. Acute seizure control may be accomplished with diazepam. If toxicity is secondary to topical diphenhydramine use, the contaminated skin should be

thoroughly washed with soap and water. Serious anticholinergic toxicity may be treated with the cautious use of physostigmine, although this is rarely necessary.

Dextromethorphan

Toxicity. Acute toxicity in young children is uncommon. Doses of 90 to 180 mg are generally well tolerated. Toxicity is more often a manifestation of other medications in combination cough and cold preparations. Adolescent abuse of dextromethorphan-containing cough syrups is well documented, and ingestions of 120 to 600 ml (4 to 20 oz) may be used to achieve the desired psychoactive effects.

Manifestations. Small overdoses in children may result in mild CNS depression and unsteadiness. Patients who intentionally abuse such substances may present with a spectrum of effects that range from inebriation to hyperkinetic behavior to seizures and coma.

Treatment. The appropriate form of gastric decontamination should be used in patients who have acutely ingested over 10 mg/kg. As always, this is dictated by the time of ingestion and the presence or absence of symptoms. Naloxone may be an effective antagonist in children with CNS depressant effects.

Vitamins and Iron

Multiple vitamin exposures occur with great frequency in the pediatric population. Children are attracted to the chewable products that are attractively packaged and enticingly flavored and colored. Accidental multiple vitamin exposures rarely result in toxic manifestations unless the product contains iron. Iron is currently the most common cause of pediatric fatalities associated with poisonings. Chronic abuse of fat-soluble vitamins, especially vitamin A, can be associated with significant toxicity. However, the treatment and diagnosis of chronic vitamin A poisoning is beyond the scope of this section.

Multiple Vitamins

Toxicity. Acute toxicity is rare following even large overdoses of multiple vitamins. The minimal toxic threshold in children for vitamin A ingestion is 300,000 IU or 25,000 IU/kg. Infants have tolerated 600,000 IU or 100,000 IU/kg of vitamin D without ill effects. Acutely toxic doses of water-soluble vitamins are difficult to achieve with the typical pediatric multivitamin preparations.

Manifestations. Multiple vitamin overdose may result in gastrointestinal symptoms, including nausea, vomiting, and diarrhea. Facial flushing may occur if significant niacin has been ingested. Acute vitamin A toxicity in infants may result in increased intracranial pressure manifest as vomiting, irritability or lethargy, and bulging fontanelles.

Treatment. Gastric decontamination is usually unnecessary. Emesis is indicated only if the toxic threshold for one of the vitamins is exceeded or if the product contains iron. An RPIC should be contacted for specific information.

Iron

Toxicity. The ingestion of less than 20 mg/kg of elemental iron is not associated with acute toxicity. Minor side effects may occur with ingestions ranging from 20 to 60 mg/kg. More overt toxicity may develop when the ingestion exceeds 60 mg/kg. The risk of developing serious toxicity increases with each increment beyond 60 mg/kg.

Manifestations. Iron poisoning symptoms can present in an insidious fashion over several hours or with amazing speed. Vomiting, diarrhea, and abdominal pain may develop early in the progression of symptoms, leading to hematemesis, bloody diarrhea, shock, acidosis, and coma. Severe hypotension also may occur.

Treatment. Aggressive gastric decontamination needs to be accomplished in all patients who have ingested over 60 mg/kg of elemental iron. Following syrup of ipecac-induced emesis or gastric lavage, an abdominal roentgenogram is necessary to determine if any iron remains in the gastrointestinal tract. X-ray studies are of no value if chewable multiple vitamins with iron have been ingested. Activated charcoal does not adsorb iron. If large amounts of iron have been ingested or if iron is visible on the abdominal x-ray film, whole bowel irrigation should be used to purge the bowel of remaining iron. Administration of phosphate or bicarbonate solutions to render gastric iron insoluble and nonabsorbable is ineffective and contraindicated. Patients with serum iron levels in excess of 500 μg/dl and those with elevated levels and symptoms may be candidates for deferoxamine therapy. Deferoxamine is administered intravenously at a rate not to exceed 15 mg/kg/h and a total dose of 6 g/d. Oral deferoxamine therapy is not advised.

Cardiovascular Medications

The number of exposures to cardiovascular medications is relatively low, but the morbidity and mortality associated with such ingestions are very high. There are many notable medications in this category, but two of the most common and potentially lethal drugs are clonidine and the calcium channel blockers.

Clonidine

Toxicity. Clonidine is very toxic, and all ingestions should be considered significant. A decreased level of consciousness may occur with the ingestion of as little as 0.1 mg, and there is extreme variability in the response to clonidine. Clonidine sustained-release dermal patches contain a large amount of active and bioavailable drug when they are discarded and present significant risk when accidentally ingested.

Manifestations. CNS depression is the hallmark clinical finding, manifest by coma and respiratory depression. Bradycardia and hypotension are prominent findings.

Treatment. Gastric decontamination is essential. Symptomatic patients should not have emesis induced. CNS depression may respond to naloxone administration. Bradycardia may be treated with atropine. Symptom-specific problems should be treated as appropriate.

Calcium Channel Blockers

Toxicity. Calcium channel blockers are extremely toxic, and all pediatric exposures should be regarded as significant. Sustained-release products may produce both delayed and prolonged toxicity.

Manifestations. Hypotension and cardiac conduction impairment (bradycardia, heart block) are the most serious manifestations of calcium channel blocker toxicity.

Treatment. Syrup of ipecac–induced emesis should be avoided, since rapid loss of consciousness may occur. Furthermore, emesis may evoke vagal stimulation, which can aggravate preexistent cardiac complications. Gastric lavage followed by activated charcoal use should be performed in any child with a substantial ingestion. Multiple-dose activated charcoal may be effective if sustained-release products are ingested. Calcium should be administered to symptomatic patients, but it is usually ineffective, since the calcium channels are blocked. The administration of atropine may not effectively resolve the bradycardia. Beta-agonists may be effective in the management of hypotension. The use of a pacemaker may be necessary.

Tricyclic Antidepressants

The tricyclic antidepressants are responsible for more fatalities in the adult population than is any other group of medications. This is largely a consequence of providing patients who are depressed with a medication that has a narrow therapeutic index (the therapeutic and toxic doses are similar). Young children account for 42% of the exposures but less than 2% of the fatalities, and adolescents account for over 7% of all antidepressant-related fatalities. The tricyclic antidepressants (e.g., amitriptyline, imipramine, doxepin) and the tetra-cyclic agent maprotiline produce catecholamine depletion and quinidine-like effects on the heart, which make them significantly more toxic than the newer antidepressants (e.g., fluoxetine, paroxetine), which inhibit the CNS neuronal uptake of serotonin. However, all antidepressant poisonings in children and adolescents should be considered emergencies until proven otherwise. An RPIC should always be consulted.

Toxicity. All exposures should be regarded as potential life-threatening emergencies. Serious toxicity has been reported with as little as 100 mg of desipramine and a fatality with only 250 mg of imipramine. Ingestions of greater than 10 mg/kg may result in moderate to serious toxicity.

Manifestations. Hypotension, cardiac conduction impairment, respiratory depression, profound coma, seizures, and death are all commonly associated with tricyclic antidepressant toxicity. Anticholinergic effects may be present.

Treatment. Aggressive supportive care is the cornerstone of management. Syrup of ipecac–induced emesis is contraindicated, since there may be a rapid progression to coma. Gastric lavage and activated charcoal are the primary means of gastric decontamination. Ventricular arrhythmias may respond to alkalinization, lidocaine, or phenytoin. Hypotension that is unresponsive to fluids may necessitate the aggressive use of pressors (norepinephrine is preferred). A single seizure does not mandate therapy, and multiple seizures should be treated with diazepam. Physostigmine has no role in the management of tricyclic antidepressant poisonings. Asymptomatic patients should be monitored for a minimum of 6 hours, after which it is unlikely that any manifestations of toxicity will occur. Symptomatic patients should be monitored until they are symptom free for 24 hours. Serum levels do not dictate therapy and are primarily of value in the establishment of a diagnosis.

BOTULINAL FOOD POISONING

BARRY H. RUMACK, M.D.

Botulism is most frequently due to improperly home-processed foods, such as vegetables, meats, fruits, pickles, and seafood. Commercial products rarely are involved, although there have been recent reports of contaminated fish and meat products and soups. Simple cooking for 6 to 10 minutes is capable of destroying the formed toxin.

TREATMENT

The stomach is emptied, with care taken to protect the airway, and activated charcoal and a cathartic are administered. The patient should be hospitalized if there are any symptoms (e.g., paralysis, ptosis, blurred vision, diplopia, sore throat). Laboratory testing for toxins must be done early in the course. Assays are positive in 40% to 44% of serum and stool specimens collected during the first 3 days and in 15% to 23% obtained thereafter. Antitoxin should be administered under the supervision of the Centers for Disease Control and Prevention or the state health department. Guanidine and penicillin therapies have dubious value. Treatment consists primarily of administration of antitoxin and respiratory support. Patients with mild neurologic findings, which do not progress, will not require therapy. Respiratory and other support is similar to that used in the treatment of any serious neurologic problem. With modern therapy, recovery is the rule.

LEAD TOXICITY

HERBERT L. NEEDLEMAN, M.D.

The diagnosis and management of lead exposure in children has undergone rapid and drastic changes over the past two decades. Lead affects many organ systems. The central nervous system (CNS) is the most critical target. Until the mid-1940s, it was believed that if a child did not die of acute intoxication, there were no CNS sequelae. Between 1943 and the late 1960s, it was believed that psychologic impairment only occurred in those cases with encephalopathy. At that time, a toxic blood lead level was considered to be >60 μg/dl. Because of studies showing intellectual decrements in children at lower blood lead levels, the current definition of lead toxicity has been set at 10 μg/dl by the Centers for Disease Control and Prevention. Furthermore, it is the recommendation of the CDC that all children be screened with a blood lead test at approximately 1 and 2 years of age.

Although blood lead levels in American children have declined since 1980 (primarily because of the removal of lead from gasoline), the prevalence of elevated blood levels, under the new definition, remains unacceptably high. The CDC Guidelines, summarized in Table 1, provide a useful classification to guide appropriate action.

TREATMENT OF SYMPTOMATIC LEAD POISONING

It is essential to begin treatment of lead toxicity by ending exposure. Pharmacologic therapy is an adjuvant and will have little efficacy if exposure continues. Many children receive chelating agents without proper attention to continuing exposure. When a child with a blood lead level >25 μg/dl is identified, a team effort should be started in concert with public health authorities to find the source and remove it or to permanently remove the child from the source.

Children with elevated blood lead levels (>25 μg/dl) who are symptomatic should be admitted to the hospital and treated on an urgent basis. The symptoms of lead toxicity are vague and may be expressions of early encephalopathy. They include headache, abdominal pain, clumsiness, and behavioral change, including irritability, sleep disturbances, and alterations of consciousness.

If the blood lead is greater than 70 μg/dl, even in the absence of symptoms, therapy should begin with calcium disodium edathamil (EDTA) by vein 1000 mg/m²/d. EDTA should be diluted to a concentration of 0.5% in a D_w solution and administered either as a continuous infusion or in two divided doses. Intramuscular administration of EDTA is painful, and if this route is necessary, the agent should be mixed with procaine or lidocaine. EDTA should never be given orally. If the child is symptomatic or if the blood lead level is greater than 80 μg/dl, BAL (British anti-lewisite) 500 mg/m²/d IM should be given in three divided doses. Treatment with both agents should continue for 5 days.

EDTA may produce a reversible lower nephron nephrosis, and daily urinalyses for blood and protein are indicated. Occasionally, a

TABLE 1. Centers for Disease Control and Prevention Blood Lead Level Guidelines

CLASS	BLOOD LEAD CONCENTRATION (μg/dl)	COMMENT
I	<10	Not poisoned
II	10–19	Mild poisoning
III	20–44	Require medical management
IV	45–69	Urgently require medical management
V	≥ 70	Medical emergency

febrile response or a rash is seen. BAL can produce a febrile reaction, transient granulocytopenia, and sterile abscesses. Iron therapy should be deferred until BAL administration has been completed because of the risk of toxic reactions. Since the carrier for BAL is oil, children with peanut allergies should not be given this drug.

When using EDTA or BAL, it is important that adequate hydration be maintained to ensure urinary output. In the presence of CNS signs, overhydration should be avoided. Children with signs of encephalopathy should be treated in an intensive care unit under the supervision of an experienced intensivist. After the course of chelation, patients should be given restorative doses of calcium, zinc, and copper.

TREATMENT OF ELEVATED BLOOD LEAD LEVELS WITH NO CLINICAL SYMPTOMS

In the past 3 years, a new agent, dimercaptosuccinic acid (succimer), has been licensed for use in children. This agent reduces blood lead levels, but it has not been established that reduction is associated with any clinical benefit. Similarly, it is also not known whether EDTA conveys benefits to children with asymptomatic levels of lead. Succimer is currently being evaluated in a placebo-controlled trial under the aegis of the National Institute for Environmental Health Sciences.

Children with blood lead levels between 35 μg/dl and 45 μg/dl should be considered for succimer therapy. Treatment should always begin in a hospital. Hospitalization accomplishes a number of objectives: it ends exposure and permits a thorough evaluation of the health status of the child, including liver and kidney function and developmental status. Furthermore, during hospitalization, the abatement of lead in the residence or the search for safe housing can begin. Children should not receive chelating agents unless it is certain that the exposure has ended and should not be discharged except to a lead-safe dwelling. During hospitalization, the mother or other caretaker should observe the administration of succimer and, under supervision, give it to the patient.

Succimer is administered in a dose of 30 mg/kg/d for 5 days, followed by 14 days of treatment at a reduced dose (20 mg/kg/d). The only dose form is 100-mg capsules that contain coated granules of the drug. The dose is calculated to the nearest 100 mg. For younger children, the contents of the capsule are emptied into a palatable food: peanut butter, applesauce, or ice cream. The preparation technique should be demonstrated to the mother and then performed by her under supervision. Side effects of succimer include alterations in liver function, rashes, neutropenia, nausea, and stomachaches. For these reasons, liver function studies should be obtained on admission and on the third and fifth day of hospitalization. White blood cell counts and differentials should also be obtained on days 3 and 5 of therapy. Most of these side effects are transitory, and drug therapy frequently can resume. It is noteworthy that no systematic data collection of the long-term sequelae of succimer therapy has been attempted.

The decision to use succimer in children whose blood lead levels range between 20 and 34 μg/dl depends on several clinical factors. Among those to be considered are the age of the child, the presence of any systemic findings (e.g., anorexia, malaise, iron deficiency), and whether exposure can be terminated. A younger child (below 18 months) with signs of mild illness would rate consideration for chelation, whereas an older, robust child would generally be observed, and the blood lead levels and clinical state would be followed.

DEVELOPMENTAL STATUS OF CHILDREN WITH LOW-LEVEL LEAD EXPOSURE

Because it is well established that lesser levels of lead affect children's intelligence, speech, attention, and behavior, a developmental assessment is indicated in children with blood lead levels above 20 μg/dl to decide whether special services are needed. The Denver Developmental Index can be useful. Because it appears that speech is a sensitive marker for delayed development in 2 year olds with lead exposure, a screening instrument, such as the Language Development

Survey (Rescorla, an inventory of words known and spoken by a 2 to 3 year old), provides a rapid and valid measure of language competence. Children who are suspect should be followed and referred to a developmental specialist if there is any question about their status.

PREVENTION

The lack of a satisfactory agent to reduce blood lead levels below 25 μg/dl and the compelling evidence that toxicity occurs below this concentration argue persuasively that the only sound response to this disease is primary prevention. Accomplishing this goal is not a utopian vision. Indeed, a plan to achieve it has been clearly spelled out in the Public Health Service's historic publication *Strategic Plan for the Elimination of Childhood Lead Poisoning.*[1] This document also presents a cost/benefit analysis that demonstrates that the abatement of lead in the houses built before 1950 would cost $32 billion. The net monetary benefit, derived from average health and special education costs and from increased wages as a product of increased IQ, would be $60 billion. The primary prevention of lead poisoning is, therefore, both practical and wise.

REFERENCE

1. Centers for Disease Control and Prevention: Strategic Plan for the Elimination of Childhood Lead Poisoning. Atlanta, Department of Health and Human Services, 1991.

INSECT STINGS

GILBERT ANTHONY FRIDAY, JR., M.D.

Allergic reactions to insect stings range in severity from local inflammation to systemic anaphylaxis. Stings of insects of the order Hymenoptera (honeybee, yellowjacket, hornet, polistes wasp, and fire ant) result in systemic manifestations in nearly 3% of children. Systemic manifestations commonly include pruritus, erythemia, or urticaria, although angioedema or life-threatening symptoms involving the respiratory tract and cardiovascular system (e.g., laryngeal edema, bronchospasm, and vascular collapse) can occur. Fortunately, fewer than 50 deaths from insect stings are recorded in the United States each year, only 1 or 2 of which are reported in children.

TREATMENT OF ANAPHYLAXIS[1] (Table 1)

Respirations and blood pressure should be carefully and rapidly assessed. The child should be placed in a recumbent position, and the lower extremities should be elevated. Epinephrine is injected subcutaneously (Table 2). This may be repeated in 20 minutes if necessary. Epinephrine is often sufficient to terminate a reaction, but one must be prepared to establish an airway if laryngeal edema is present. Supplemental oxygen may be necessary. Diphenhydramine or other antihistamines may be given to lessen urticaria or angioedema. Aminophylline is occasionally needed for treatment of bronchospasm.

Late phase reactions should be anticipated and prevented by the administration of corticosteroids. Severe reactions may require intravenous fluids and pressors to maintain the blood pressure.

TREATMENT OF LOCAL REACTIONS

For treatment of immediate immunoglobulin E (IgE)-mediated local reactions, ice and antihistamines should be used. To prevent (or, occasionally, to treat) the delayed hypersensitivity reactions (lymphocyte-mediated), a short course of prednisone 0.5 to 1 mg/kg/d can be given and continued for 72 hours (or longer) to relieve discomfort, especially in those who have experienced such reactions previously.

TABLE 1. Treatment of Anaphylaxis

1. Assess rapidly.
2. Place patient in recumbent position and elevate lower extremities.
3. Inject epinephrine 1:1000 0.01 ml/kg (max: 0.3–0.5 ml) SC or IM q10–20min up to three times.
4. Establish airway; may require racemic epinephrine or albuterol 0.5 ml of 0.5% solution in 2.5 ml of saline or isoetharine 0.5 ml of 1% solution in 2 ml of saline via nebulizer or endotracheal tube.
5. Provide supplemental oxygen if needed (40%–100%: $Po_2 \geq 60$ mm Hg).
6. Give diphenhydramine 1.25 mg/kg (max: 50 mg) IV over 3–5 min (blocks H_1-receptor).
7. Give cimetidine 5 mg/kg (max: 300 mg) or ranitidine 1 mg/kg (max: 50 mg) IV over 3–5 min q6h (blocks H_2-receptor).
8. Establish IV to maintain blood pressure with IV fluids (saline or volume expanders in the form of colloid solutions, albumin or hydroxyethyl starch), pressors (epinephrine 0.5–5 μg/min or norepinephrine bitartrate 0.05–0.1 μg/min).
9. Give aminophylline 5 mg/kg IV over 20 min, then 0.5–0.9 mg/kg/h for severe bronchospasm.
10. Provide hydrocortisone succinate 5 mg/kg (max: 250 mg) or methylprednisolone 1 mg/kg (max: 50 mg) IV q6h.
11. Glucagon 5–15 μg/min IV (refractory hypotension with patients taking beta-adrenergic blockers).

PREVENTION

Avoiding Stings

Hives and nests near the home should be eliminated. Children should wear shoes when running in the grass. Stinging insects are attracted to brightly colored or flowered clothing. Children with a history of a previous sting should be dressed in a manner that will not attract stinging insects. Perfumes, sweet drinks, and foods also attract stinging insects and should be considered when children are playing outdoors.

Identification

Children who have a known hypersensitivity to Hymenoptera should wear a bracelet or necklace indicating anaphylactic hypersensitivity.

Emergency Kits

Emergency epinephrine should be available for administration by the parent or responsible adult or, in the case of an older child, for self-administration. The emergency kits Ana-Kit and Ana-Guard contain a preloaded syringe that can deliver epinephrine doses of 0.3 ml or less. For those who fear needles, the EpiPen syringe offers a

TABLE 2. Summary of Treatment for Insect Stings

AGENTS	DOSES
Albuterol	0.5 ml of 0.5% solution in 2.5 ml of saline
Aminophylline	5 mg/kg IV over 20 min, then 0.5–0.9 mg/kg/h for severe bronchospasm
Cimetidine	5 mg/kg (max: 300 mg) IV over 3–5 min q6h
Diphenhydramine	1.25 mg/kg (maximum 50 mg) IV over 3–5 min
Epinephrine 1:1000	0.01 ml/kg (max: 0.3–0.5 ml) SC or IM q10–20min up to three times
	0.5–5 μg/min
Glucagon	5–15 μg/min IV
Hydrocortisone succinate	5 mg/kg (max: 250 mg) IV q6h
Isoetharine	0.5 ml of 1% solution in 2 ml of saline
Methylprednisolone	1 mg/kg (max: 50 mg) IV q6h
Norepinephrine bitartrate	0.05–0.1 μg/min
Racemic epinephrine	0.5 ml of 0.5% solution in 2.5 ml of saline
Ranitidine	1 mg/kg (max: 50 mg) IV over 3–5 min q6h

TABLE 3. Selection of Children for Venom Skin Testing and Immunotherapy

CLASSIFICATION OF STING REACTION BY HISTORY	VENOM SKIN TEST	VENOM IMMUNOTHERAPY
Local	±	No
Large local	±	No
Systemic (<16 y)		
Life-threatening	+	Yes
Cutaneous	±	No
Toxic	±	No
Delayed (24 h)	±	No

recessed needle and a pressure-sensitive spring-loaded injection device. EpiPen delivers 0.3 mg (0.3 ml) of epinephrine 1:1000, and EpiPen Jr. delivers 0.15 mg of epinephrine 1:2000 (0.3 ml) IM.

Planning

When a child is stung, he or she should be observed carefully for signs of a systemic reaction. The first sign is usually itching, redness, and hives distant from the sting site. Epinephrine should be administered immediately, and the child should be transported to the nearest emergency facility. A single injection of epinephrine may be totally ineffective in reversing severe anaphylaxis. However, the other measures noted in Table 1 are best given in an emergency facility. Parents should be aware of available emergency facilities when traveling or on vacation.

Venom Immunotherapy

The treatment of patients allergic to insect stings with insect venom injections has been shown to be 99% effective in reducing the risk of sting-induced anaphylaxis.[2] Fortunately, venom immunotherapy is unnecessary for most children who are allergic to insect stings (Table 3).[3] Large local reactions do not require immunotherapy, but the severity can be lessened by immunotherapy. Only approximately 10% of patients younger than 16 years of age with generalized cutaneous reactions have systemic reactions on repeat stings, and, in general, there is no progression to more severe reactions. However, children who exhibit life-threatening, immediate respiratory and cardiovascular symptoms should be referred to an allergist for skin testing to identify the culprit (honeybee, yellowjacket, yellow hornet, white-faced hornet, or paper wasp). Fire ant stings are not a diagnostic problem. Radioallergosorbent tests (RAST) may be useful in detecting venom hypersensitivity in instances of questionable Hymenoptera sting reactions, although it is 20% less sensitive than skin tests.

If a sting results in a life-threatening reaction and if venom testing results are positive, immunotherapy with the appropriate venom(s) should be started immediately. Increasing amounts of venom are given weekly for several weeks (15+) until a dose of 100 μg (equals two bee stings) is reached. Maintenance injections are given at 4-week intervals the first year and every 6 weeks thereafter for approximately 5 years. Immunotherapy increases the serum concentration of IgG blocking antibody and decreases the level of venom-specific IgE. The development of negative skin test or RAST results after immunotherapy suggest that therapy can be safely discontinued. If a child is stung during this time, epinephrine should be at hand but need not be given unless there are signs of anaphylaxis. Immunotherapy for fire ant hypersensitivity can be accomplished by whole-body extracts rather than the venom, which is not commercially available.

REFERENCES

1. Morris FC: Anaphylaxis. *In* Levin DL, Morns FC (eds): Essentials of Pediatric Intensive Care. St. Louis, Quality Medical Publishing, 1990:103.
2. Valentine MD, Lichtenstein LM: Anaphylaxis and sting insect hypersensitivity. JAMA 258:2881–2885, 1987.
3. Valentine MD, Schuberth KC, Kagey-Sobotka A, et al: The value of immunotherapy with venom in children with allergy to insect stings. N Engl J Med 323:1601–1603, 1990.

ARTHROPOD BITES AND STINGS

WILLIAM BANNER, JR., M.D., Ph.D.

In the phylum Arthropoda, the most clinically important classes are the arachnids (spiders and scorpions), the myriapods (centipedes and millipedes), and the insects. Members of this phylum contain species with venom delivery mechanisms in both the oral and tail areas and with varied venom components.

ARACHNIDS

Widow Spiders

All spiders have venom, but the vast majority of spiders do not possess sufficiently large fangs to deliver venom to human prey. The female widow spider of the genus *Latrodectus* is capable of delivering a potent venom. This spider varies in size but can have a leg span as large as 4 cm. The body, although generally black, may be red or cream colored. An hourglass shape on the dorsal surface is generally red but also may be brown or cream colored. These spiders favor weaving an irregular web in areas near water supplies that are relatively protected. Envenomation by this spider usually produces an immediate sharp pain, and occasionally two small puncture wounds with a circular target of erythema may be seen. It is not uncommon to fail to find the spider at the scene or see any fang marks in children. The spider venom acts to cause muscle spasm and severe pain that, in its worst form, can interfere with respiration. More generally, patients become sweaty, with a mildly altered level of consciousness and muscle rigidity that progresses from the extremity to the central body. One peculiar finding is periorbital swelling regardless of the site of the bite. Occasionally, abdominal pain becomes striking enough that it may be misinterpreted as an acute abdomen.

In the vast majority of cases, only simple oral analgesics and reassurance are needed. In more significant cases, parenteral narcotics and sedatives have been used to provide symptomatic relief. Methacarbamol (Robaxin), a muscle relaxant, has been used occasionally in the pediatric population, but benzodiazepines are more appropriate. In cases of severe distress not responsive to routine analgesics, some authors have recommended the use of calcium or the use of an antivenom preparation. Efficacy and clear indications for the use of these modalities remain controversial. Furthermore, the response to calcium varies widely. The antivenom (black widow spider antivenom) should be diluted and administered slowly to avoid toxic effects from the antivenom itself. It's use is clearly indicated in life-threatening bites, and it may be useful also in patients with extreme distress unresponsive to simple approaches. No prophylactic treatment is indicated.

Tarantulas

A variety of tarantula species live in the United States and are unique for the large amount of hair on their surface. These are in general very benign but may produce a painful bite if provoked. There is no specific treatment for tarantula bite. In addition to the bite, the hairs on the abdomen of the tarantula contain irritant materials that may be thrown into the face of predators and may produce mucous membrane irritation in humans.

Brown Spiders

Perhaps no spider has caused more confusion than the brown spider. In certain geographic areas of the United States, particularly the southeast, one species of the genus *Loxosceles, Loxosceles reclusa* or the brown recluse, has gained a reputation for being one of the most venomous of the brown spiders. This entire genus and many other spiders in different genera are capable of producing a necrotic skin area. Typically, the victim is unaware of having been bitten but notices a small vesicle that rapidly evolves to become a central necrotic area with a surrounding halo suggesting a target. The area of tissue necrosis may extend in an extremely variable fashion and (with or without intervention) typically regresses before forming an eschar. In severe cases, a flu-like illness may occur, and intravascular hemolysis has been described, most commonly with *L. reclusa*. There are case reports of death attributed to complications from this spider, but these are extremely rare and not well documented. Numerous medical conditions may mimic the necrotic lesion of the brown spider, and careful attention to other findings and drug therapies, such as warfarin (Coumadin), is important.

Treatment of brown spider envenomation is rife with mythology. To date, there have been no consistent animal or human trials that have documented the superiority of one treatment over others. Because of the potential cosmetic damage that can occur with this envenomation, patients typically have a desire for aggressive intervention even in the absence of data. Approaches recommended by varying authors include radical surgical excision, administration of dapsone, direct injection of phentolamine, or corticosteroids. The most conservative approach is to monitor the patient carefully for secondary infection, undertake good wound cleansing, and administer tetanus toxoid. For cosmetic repair of large areas of necrosis, referral should be made to a plastic surgeon. Apart from this, it is difficult to advocate any specific therapy.

Scorpions

There are numerous scorpion species in the United States. However, the only significant human danger has been described from a single species, *Centruroides exilicauda* (or *sculpturatus*). The natural range of this species is limited to the southwestern deserts of Arizona, Nevada, and Southern California, with much less frequent reports in New Mexico or Southern Utah. Occasional "hitchhikers," however, have shown up in all areas of the country. In endemic areas, envenomation is common, but the morbidity and mortality are extremely low. It is extremely difficult to identify the envenomation site in children. In older children with acute local pain, mild cold compresses (without subjecting the limb to hypothermia) and oral analgesics are indicated. In smaller children (<3 years), a unique presentation of extreme agitation and roving eye movements can occur after envenomation. Convulsions, tachycardia, hyperthermia, hypertension, and tachypnea may also be present. In these instances, supportive measures, including sedation using benzodiazepines in a well-monitored environment, are appropriate. Narcotics should be avoided. Severe tachycardia may be treated with beta blockers. An antivenom not approved by the Food and Drug Administration is manufactured in Arizona for local use. This product should be used only following consultation with someone experienced in the management of such envenomation.

MYRIAPODS

Centipedes

Centipedes are members of the arthropod family with multiple segments. Some of the larger members of this genus have fangs sufficiently large enough to penetrate human skin and can produce severe local pain and swelling. Muscle necrosis has been reported rarely. There is no specific treatment beyond good wound care.

Millipedes

Millipedes are a more primitive segmented arthropod with a secretory mechanism in their skin that can secrete a toxic material on contact. This may result in a dermatitis or a severe mucous membrane irritation if the liquid gets into the eyes or mouth. Flooding the area with fluid has been suggested. There is no specific therapy.

INSECTS

Insects of many types are capable of stinging human intruders. In general, the toxicity of these venoms is related to their antigenic potential and resultant anaphylaxis. Hypersensitivity reactions are discussed elsewhere in this text.

Ants

Members of the ant family are capable of delivering a sting or a bite. The secretory mechanisms of the mouth can elaborate a formic acid material that is extremely irritating. Furthermore, the tail ends of some species of ant contain a stinging mechanism that delivers an irritant material that may produce severe inflammatory reactions or anaphylaxis. There is no specific treatment for an ant sting apart from treatment of anaphylaxis. Some people have suggested a neutralizing bicarbonate paste for the formic acid component.

REFERENCES

1. Banner W: Bites and stings in the pediatric patient. Curr Probl Pediatr 18:1–69, 1988.
2. Banner W: Scorpion envenomation. *In* Auerbach PS, Geehr EC (eds): Wilderness and Environmental Emergencies. St. Louis, C.V. Mosby Co, 1989:603–616.
3. Clark RF, Wethern-Kestner S, Vance MV, Gerkin R: Clinical presentation and treatment of black widow spider envenomation: A review of 163 cases. Ann Emerg Med 21:782–787, 1992.
4. Smith RL: Venomous Animals of Arizona. Cooperative Extension Services College of Agriculture, University of Arizona, Bulletin 8245, 1982.

ANIMAL AND HUMAN BITES AND BITE-RELATED INFECTIONS

KEITH E. MANDEL, M.D.
CHARLES M. GINSBURG, M.D.

Virtually all humans (particularly young children) and the more than 100 million domestic dogs and cats in the United States have the potential to bite. Therefore, many clinicians consider bite injuries an occupational hazard of childhood. In fact, it has been estimated that bite injuries account for slightly over 1% of visits to hospital emergency rooms and free-standing emergency centers. The number of individuals who sustain a bite injury who seek medical attention in medical offices and free-standing primary care clinics is unknown but is thought to be comparable.

Between 1979 and 1988, there were 157 fatalities from dog bites reported in the United States; 70% of these occurred in children less than 10 years of age. The breed of dog involved in the attacks on children varied. German shepherds, pit bulls, and rotweillers accounted for nearly 50% of all bite-related injuries. During this same period, there was a trifold increase in the proportion of deaths from pit bull-related injuries.

Although children of any age and gender may be victims of attacks by dogs, the majority of dog-related attacks occur in children between the ages of 6 and 10 years, and boys are attacked more often than girls (1.5:1). Approximately two thirds of the attacks occur around the home, three quarters of the biting animals are known by the child, and almost one half of the attacks are said to be unprovoked. By contrast, the greater than 400,000 reported cat bites per year occur primarily in girls and are inflicted by known household animals. There is a paucity of data on the incidence and demographics of human bite injuries in pediatric age patients. However, preschool and early school-age children appear to be the age group at greatest risk to sustain an injury from a bite by a human.

Based on data from studies performed in hospital emergency rooms, the type of dog bite-related injuries can be divided into three categories of about equal frequency: abrasions, puncture wounds, and lacerations with or without an associated avulsion of tissue. The most common type of injury from a cat bite is a puncture wound. Human bite injuries are of two types, the typical occlusional injury incurred when the upper and lower teeth come together on a body part and, in older children and young adults, a clenched-fist injury that occurs when the fist, usually on the dominant hand, comes in contact with the tooth of another individual.

Management of the victim of a bite begins with a careful history and physical examination. Particular attention should be paid to the circumstances surrounding the bite (e.g., type and location of the animal, domestic or sylvatic, provoked or unprovoked), a history of drug allergies, and most important, the immunization status of the child. The physical examination should be thorough and complete, with careful attention paid to the type, size, and depth of the injury, the presence of foreign material in the wound, the status of underlying structures, and when the bite is on an extremity, the range of motion of the affected area. A diagram of the injury should be recorded in the patient's medical record. If there is a likelihood that a bone or joint could have been penetrated or fractured or if there is foreign material present, an x-ray of the affected part should be obtained. Additionally, the possibility of a fracture or penetrating injury of the skull should be considered in individuals, particularly infants, who have sustained dog bite injuries to the face and scalp.

The decision whether or not to obtain material for culture from a wound depends on several factors, including the species of the biting animal, the length of time that has transpired since the injury, the depth of the wound, the presence of foreign material contaminating the wound, and whether or not there is evidence of infection. Infection is the most common complication of bite injuries regardless of the species of biting animal. Although potentially pathogenic bacteria have been isolated from up to 80% of dog bite wounds that are brought to medical attention within 8 hours after the bite, studies indicate that the infection rate for wounds receiving medical attention in less than 8 hours is between 2.5% and 20%. Therefore, unless they are deep and extensive, dog bite wounds that are less than 8 hours old do not need to be cultured unless there is evidence of contamination or early signs of infection. By contrast, the infection rate in cat bite wounds that receive early medical attention is at least 50%, and it is prudent to culture all but the most trivial wounds. The rate of infection increases almost exponentially in animal bite wounds, regardless of species of the biting animal, that are not brought to medical attention within 8 hours. In contrast to animal bites, all human bite wounds, regardless of the mechanism of injury, should be regarded as high risk for infection and should be cultured. In the preantibiotic era, up to 20% of human bite victims required amputation of the affected part because of infection. Because of the large incidence of anaerobic infection following bite wounds, it is important to obtain material for anaerobic as well as aerobic cultures.

After the appropriate material has been obtained for culture, the wound should be cleansed and vigorously irrigated with copious amounts of normal saline. Irrigation with antibiotic-containing solutions provides no advantage over irrigation with saline alone and has the potential to cause local irritation of the tissues. Puncture wounds should be thoroughly cleansed and gently irrigated with a catheter or blunt-tipped needle, but high-pressure irrigation should not be used. Avulsed or devitalized tissue should be debrided, and any fluctuant areas should be incised and drained.

There is much controversy over whether or not bite wounds should undergo primary closure or delayed primary closure (3 to 5 days) or should be allowed to heal by secondary intention, and few data are available. Factors to be considered are the type, size, and depth of the wound, the anatomic location, the presence of infection, the duration of time since the injury, and the potential for cosmetic disfigurement. Although there is general agreement that infected wounds and those greater than 24 hours old should not be sutured, there is disagreement and clinical experience has varied about the efficacy and safety of closing wounds that are less than 8 hours old with no evidence of infection. All hand wounds are considered to be at high risk for infection, particularly if there has been disruption of the tendons or penetration of the bones. Therefore, delayed primary closure is recommended for all but the most trivial bite wounds of the hands. Surgical consultation should be obtained for all patients with deep or extensive wounds, those involving the bones and joints, and infected wounds that require open drainage. In contrast to hand wounds, facial lacerations are at less risk for secondary infection because of the more luxuriant blood supply to this region. Many plastic surgeons, therefore, advocate primary closure of facial bite wounds that have been brought to medical attention within 5 hours and have been thoroughly irrigated and debrided.

There are few studies that unequivocally demonstrate a clear-cut benefit to administering antimicrobial agents for prophylaxis of bite injuries. However, there is a general consensus that antibiotics should be administered to all victims of human bites and all but the most trivial of dog and cat bite injuries, regardless of whether there is evidence of infection. The bacteriology of bite wound infections is primarily a reflection of the oral flora of the biting animal and, to a lesser extent, a reflection of the skin flora of the victim. Since each of the multitude of aerobic and anaerobic bacterial species that colonize the oral cavity of the biting animal has the potential to invade local tissue, multiply, and cause tissue destruction, the majority of bite wound infections are polymicrobial. Despite the large degree of homology in the bacterial flora of the oral cavity between humans, dogs, and cats, important differences exist between the biting species, and this is reflected in the type of wound infections that occur. The predominant bacterial species isolated from infected dog bite wounds are *Staphylococcus aureus* (20% to 30%), *Pasteurella multocida* (20% to 30%), *Staphylococcus intermedius* (25%), and *Capnocytophagia canimorsus*. Furthermore, approximately one third of dog bite wound infections contain mixed anaerobes. Similar species are isolated from infected cat bite wounds, although *P. multocida* plays a larger role, being the predominant species in at least 50% of cat bite wound infections. In human bite wounds, nontypable strains of *Haemophilus influenzae, Eikenella corrodens,* alpha-hemolytic streptococci, and beta-lactamase-producing aerobes (50%) are the predominant species. Clenched-fist injuries are particularly prone to infection by *Eikenella* (25%) and anaerobic bacteria (50%).

The choice between an oral and a parenteral agent should be based on the severity of the wound, the presence and degree of overt infection, signs of systemic toxicity, and the immune status of the patient. Amoxicillin-clavulanate is an excellent choice for empiric oral therapy of human and animal bite wounds because of its activity against the majority of strains of bacteria that have been isolated from infected bite injuries. Similarly, ticarcillin-clavulanate is preferred for patients who require empiric parenteral therapy. First-generation cephalosporins have limited activity against *P. multocida* and *E. corrodens* and, therefore, should not be used for prophylaxis or empiric initial therapy of bite wound infections. The therapeutic alternatives for penicillin-allergic patients are limited because the traditional alternative agents are generally inactive against one or more of the multiple pathogens that cause bite wound infections. For example, erythromycin should not be used for human bite wounds because it is not effective against *E. corrodens.* Although erythromycin is commonly recommended as an alternative agent for penicillin-allergic patients who have suffered dog and cat bites, it has spotty activity against strains of *P. multocida.* Similarly, clindamycin and the combination of trimethoprim-sulfamethoxazole have limited activity against strains of *P. multocida* and anaerobic bacteria, respectively.

Although the occurrence of tetanus following human or animal bite injuries is extremely rare, it is important to obtain a careful immunization history and to provide tetanus toxoid to all patients who are incompletely immunized or in whom it has been longer than 10 years since the last immunization. The need for postexposure rabies vaccine in victims of dog and cat bites is dependent on whether or not the biting animal is known to have been vaccinated and, most important, on the local experience with rabid animals in the community. The local health department should be consulted for advice in all instances where the vaccination status of the biting animal is unknown and in instances where there is known endemic rabies in the community. Postexposure prophylaxis for hepatitis B should be considered in the rare instance where an individual has sustained a human bite from an individual who is at high risk for hepatitis B.

All but the most trivial bite wounds of the hand should be immobilized in a position of function for 3 to 5 days, and patients with bite wounds of an extremity should be instructed to keep the affected extremity elevated for 24 to 36 hours or until the edema has resolved. All bite wound victims should be reevaluated within 24 to 36 hours after the injury.

SNAKEBITES

KATHERINE M. KONZEN, M.D., M.P.H.

In the United States, snakebites can be divided into three categories: (1) nonpoisonous snakebites, (2) nonindigenous (exotic) poisonous snakebites, and (3) indigenous poisonous snakebites. The major focus of this section is on treatment of poisonous indigenous snakebites, but management of the first two categories is discussed.

There are five genera of venomous snakes in the United States. Three genera are in the family Crotalidae, the pit vipers. They include *Crotalus* (15 species of rattlesnakes), *Sistrurus* (pygmy rattlesnakes, massasauguas), and *Agkistrodon* (copperheads and cottonmouth moccasins). *Micruroides* and *Micrurus* belong to the family Elapidae, the coral snakes. At least one species of poisonous snakes can be found in every state but Maine, Hawaii, and Alaska.

Pit vipers are responsible for the great majority of the poisonous snakebites in the United States. The venom consists of a combination of metal ions, free amino acids, large and small proteins, enzymes, and various polypeptides. Most envenomations occur in older adolescents and young adults in the summer months, and 97% of snakebites are on the extremities. Envenomations can lead to the following clinical conditions.[1]

1. Damaged endothelial cells, leading to edema and increased permeability of tissues
2. Local tissue and muscle necrosis
3. Hemolysis
4. Coagulation defects and platelet sequestration
5. Hypovolemic shock
6. Pulmonary edema
7. Renal failure
8. Lactic acidosis
9. Neurologic abnormalities, including nausea, vomiting, excessive salivation, weakness, paresthesias, motor paralysis, ptosis, dyspnea, and respiratory depression (occurring from coral snakebites and those from the Mojave rattlesnake)

SNAKE IDENTIFICATION

Appropriate management of snakebites includes recognition of distinguishing features of pit vipers from nonvenomous snakes. These characteristics include the following.[3]

1. A pit or foramen located between each eye and nostril. It is a heat-sensitive organ that enables the snake to locate warm-blooded prey. Nonpoisonous snakes do not possess pits.
2. A triangular head caused by the venom glands located in the temporal region. Nonpoisonous snakes have more oval or egg-shaped heads.
3. Elliptical and vertically oriented pupils. Nonpoisonous snakes usually have round pupils.
4. Two long and curved fangs that are movable and retract posteriorly when the mouth is closed. Nonpoisonous snakes have a snout with teeth.
5. Scales on the ventral portion caudad to the anal plate continue in a single row, whereas nonpoisonous snakes have a double row. Rattlesnakes possess rattlers on their tails.

Coral snakes are responsible for relatively few snakebites each year. Coral snakes have black snouts, round pupils, and blunt heads and lack facial pits. They have a black snout, followed by a yellow then a black band. Red-yellow and black bands alternate down the entire body. Fangs are short and fixed. The venom, a potent neurotoxin, is injected by a series of chewing movements.

Venomous snakes are capable of regulating the amount of venom excreted from their fangs. The amount of venom injected is related to the size of the prey. A key point to remember is that almost one third of poisonous snakebites do not result in envenomation because (1) too little venom is injected, (2) the gland-fang mechanism fails, or (3) an indirect hit has occurred.[2]

PREHOSPITAL MANAGEMENT

1. It is important to remain calm and collected and reassure the patient.
2. Basic life support should be initiated if necessary.
3. The affected extremity should be immobilized and jewelry or clothing should be removed. The wound must be cleansed.
4. Bite victims should be rapidly transported to the nearest health facility. Death does not usually occur immediately, and of patients who die from snakebites, more than 60% die 6 to 48 hours after the bite. Persons who reach a health care facility within 2 hours have excellent chances for survival.[2]
5. An attempt should be made to kill the snake and bring it to the health facility. However, it is important not to waste time in this effort. It is important to never presume a snake is dead, since snakebites can occur from a severed head. The snake should not be directly handled but should be transported in a cloth bag or at the end of a long stick.
6. The patient's movement should be minimized, and the affected extremity should be kept below the level of the heart.
7. The patient should be given nothing by mouth, and the use of ice, aspirin, alcohol, or sedative drugs should be avoided.
8. Incision, suction devices, and tourniquets should not be used by laypeople. These measures are controversial and should be administered only by a physician or an individual who possesses specialized skills in snakebite management.

HOSPITAL MANAGEMENT

1. Rapidly assess the patient, keeping in mind airway, breathing, and circulation (ABCs). In children, blood pressure should not be used to assess early stages of shock. Peripheral perfusion and pulse rate should be assessed.
2. Secure intravenous access for fluid resuscitation with Ringer's lactate solution or normal saline. Two intravenous lines should be established, one to administer antivenin, if necessary. For patients with imminent signs of shock, central venous pressure monitoring should be considered.
3. Identify the snake to verify that it was poisonous.
   a. If poisonous, proceed to step 4.
   b. If nonpoisonous, the patient should be observed. Proper wound care should include tetanus prophylaxis, irrigation and debridement of the wound, and consideration of prophylactic antibiotics. If no signs or symptoms develop after 6 hours, the patient can be discharged with close follow-up.
4. Obtain a thorough history, and carefully examine the patient, with particular attention to the wound site. This should include a search for fang marks and determination if a poisonous envenomation has occurred (if no envenomation has occurred, treat as in 3b). Measure and record the circumference of the injured extremity at the most proximal area of edema and 10 cm proximal to this level. Assess the progression at 15- to 30-minute intervals. Bites on the head, neck, or thorax should be considered severe. Grading of the reaction may guide therapy.[2]

a. Grading for pit viper bites

Grade 0: No envenomation. Fang marks with minimal pain, edema of less than 1 inch. In about 25% of strikes, little or no venom has been released and only a fang mark will be present.

Grade I: Minimal envenomation. Fang marks and pain, 1 to 5 inches of erythema, and edema occurring in the first 12 hours. No systemic symptoms.

Grade II: Moderate envenomation. Fang marks, pain, 6 to 12 inches of edema, and erythema in the first 12 hours. Systemic symptoms may be present.

Grade III: Severe envenomation. Fang marks, pain, edema, and erythema of 12 to 24 inches in 24 hours, systemic symptoms present.

Grade IV: Severe envenomation. Rapid edema, erythema, ecchymosis, blebs, coagulation, and systemic symptoms.

b. Grading for coral snakes

Grade 0: No envenomation. Fang scratches, punctures with minimal local erythema or edema. No systemic symptoms within 24 hours.

Grade I: Moderate envenomation. Fang marks, minimal swelling, systemic symptoms but no complete respiratory paralysis within 36 hours.

Grade II: Severe envenomation. Same as for grade I, but respiratory paralysis develops within 36 hours. Note that coral snakebites do not cause local signs characteristic of pit viper bites. Systemic symptoms usually occur within hours and can consist of euphoria, nausea, vomiting, excessive salivation, weakness, paresthesia of the affected limb, abnormal reflexes, motor paralysis, ptosis, dyspnea, and respiratory depression.[2]

5. Laboratory investigation should include a complete blood count, platelet count, prothombin time, partial thromboplastin time, bleeding time, fibrinogen, fibrin degradation products, platelet count, electrolyte panel with serum creatinine and BUN, serum glucose, serum protein, creatinine phosphokinase levels, transaminases, bilirubin, blood crossmatching, and arterial blood gases. A baseline urinalysis should be obtained.

6. For patients with ≥grade I envenomations, antivenin should be considered. Antivenin is highly antigenic horse serum, and, therefore, skin testing is mandatory. The package insert must be read thoroughly before administration. The standard skin test involves an intradermal injection of 0.02 ml of 1:10 dilution. A saline control should be used in the opposite extremity. Resuscitation equipment, including airway equipment, oxygen, epinephrine, antihistamines, and steroids, must be immediately available. The following types of antivenin are available.

a. For pit viper snakebites, antivenin crotalidae polyvalent is effective. Dosing:

Grade 0 reaction: no antivenin
Grade I reaction: 10 ml (one vial)
Grade II reaction: 30–50 ml
Grade III reaction: 50–100 ml
Grade IV reaction: 100–150 ml

In children, this dose may need to be increased by 50%.

b. For coral snakebites, *Micrurus fulvius* antivenin is used. Dosing:

Grades I and II: 30–50 ml (usually only repeated once)

c. For exotic snakebites, many poison control centers subscribe to an index showing the availability of unusual antivenins.

For best results, antivenin should be given within 6 hours of a bite. In severe envenomations with coagulation defects, antiven can be given 24 hours after the bite. The initial dose of antivenin may be repeated every 2 hours until a clinical response is noted. There is no maximum dose of antivenin.

7. Skin testing is neither highly sensitive nor reliable. Consider the following approach.

a. Negative skin test. Reconstituted antivenin is diluted with normal saline in a 1:1 to 1:10 dilution depending on the total volume desired. Administer the intravenous antivenin slowly (15 drops per minute) during the initial 30 minutes, watching for signs of shock.

(1) If no reaction occurs, give at a rate of 10 to 50 ml/h. (Higher rates can be used for severe envenomations.) Record vital signs and measure the affected extremity every 15 minutes. The infusion should be completed in 2 hours.

(2) Repeat the initial intravenous dose every 2 hours until there is no further progression of swelling.

b. Positive skin test. Consult with a medical herpetologist.[3] If allergic signs begin with the infusion, stop the infusion and begin administration of treatment. For mild allergy, give 1 to 2 mg/kg IV diphenhydramine. If symptoms resolve, begin again, but at a slower rate. If the symptoms recur, the infusion should be stopped. Steroids and epinephrine infusion can be used during administration, but this should not occur without appropriate consultation.

8. Pain management should be considered. The use of acetaminophen or opiate analgesics is preferred. Aspirin should be avoided.

9. Continuous monitoring of the patient should be done in an intensive care unit until the patient is stable.

a. Monitor the victim's intravascular fluid status closely.

b. Monitor vital signs continuously.

c. Repeat laboratory evaluations, including complete blood counts and electrolytes, every 4 hours. Treat hemolysis and correct electrolyte abnormalities as necessary. Administer fresh frozen plasma and packed red blood cells (10 ml/kg) as needed. For more severe bleeding, platelets (0.2 U/kg) and cryoprecipitate (1 bag per 5 kg body weight) may be considered.

d. Watch closely for signs of respiratory distress and the need for mechanical ventilation.

e. Wound care should consist of cleaning the wound and application of a loose dressing. The affected extremity should be kept at a level below the heart and in a position of function.

10. Broad-spectrum antibiotic (ceftriaxone) should be administered. Snake mouths contain a variety of anaerobic and gram-negative organisms. The wound should be cultured, and further antimicrobial therapy should be tailored to the specific organisms.

11. Superficial debridement of the wound should be considered 3 to 5 days after the bite. Cleansing three times daily with dilute hydrogen peroxide and hydrooxytherapy are recommended.[1] Hydrooxytherapy consists of immersion of the limb three to four times daily in Burow's solution (aluminum acetate 1:20 dilution), with oxygen bubbled through an aquarium air stone at 6 L/min.

12. Fasciotomy should be considered only in cases of documented, abnormal intracompartmental pressures. It is rarely necessary and can lead to further complications and prolonged hospitalization.[1,3]

13. Tetanus toxoid or tetanus immune globulin or both should be administered, depending on the immunization status of the patient.

14. Physical therapy and rehabilitation should begin within 5 to 7 days after the bite.

15. Serum sickness can develop within 1 to 3 weeks and is associated with fever, malaise, edema, headache, arthralgias, arthritis, myalgias, and lymphadenopathy. Corticosteroid therapy is effective in such instances.

16. If the patient was bitten by a captive venomous snake, notify the police. Many states require a license for these animals.

REFERENCES

1. Blackman JR, Dillon S: Venomous snakebite: Past, present, and future treatment options. J Am Board Fam Pract 5:399–405, 1992.
2. Gold BS, Barish RA: Venomous snakebites. Current concepts in diagnosis, treatment, and management. Emerg Med Clin North Am 10:249–267, 1992.
3. Hodge E, Tecklenburg F: Bites and stings. *In* Fleischer, Ludwig (eds): Textbook of Pediatric Emergency Medicine, 3rd ed. Baltimore, Williams & Wilkins, 1993:838–857.

BURNS

ALIA ANTOON, M.D.

Epidemiologic studies show burns to be a leading cause of accidental death in children, second only to motor vehicle accidents. Although preventive measures, such as smoke detectors, have reduced the likelihood of death in house fires by 85%, a number of children continue to suffer fatal burns as a result of house fires. Hot water scalding has been reduced by legislation requiring new water heaters to be preset at 120°F, yet scald injury remains the leading cause of all burns in children. Clothing ignition has clearly declined since the Federal Flammable Fabric Act was passed requiring children's sleepwear to be flame retardant. Despite the most vigorous burn prevention program, some 2 million people in the United States require medical care for burn injuries each year, with 100,000 of these patients requiring hospitalization. Thirty to forty percent of these patients are under 15 years of age, with an average childhood age of 32 months. Scald burns account for 85% of total injuries and are most prevalent in children under 4 years of age. Flame burns account for 13%, and electrical and chemical burns account for the rest. Approximately 16% of burn injuries occur as a result of child abuse, making it important to assess patterns and site of injury and determine consistency with the history provided.

FIRST AID MEASURES

1. Flames should be immediately extinguished by falling and rolling or by covering the individual with a blanket or coat.
2. After the airway has been checked and found to be patent, smoldering clothing or clothing saturated with hot liquid should be removed. Hot tar may be removed with mineral oil. Jewelry, particularly rings or bracelets, should be removed or cut away to prevent constriction and vascular compromise during the edema phase in the first 24 to 72 hours postburn.
3. The burned area should be covered with clean, dry sheeting, and cold (not iced) wet compresses should be applied to small injuries. Significant large burn surface area injury (greater than 15% to 20% body surface areas, BSA) results in a decrease in body temperature control, which contraindicates the use of cold compress dressings.
4. The cardiovascular and pulmonary status should be rapidly reviewed, and preexisting medical conditions (e.g., asthma, congenital heart disease, renal or hepatic disease) should be documented.
5. Intravenous access is needed for patients with burns greater than 10% to 15% BSA, and a nasogastric tube should be placed. An indwelling urinary catheter should also be inserted to allow accurate measurement of urine volume, particularly if transport to a burn center is anticipated.

LIFE SUPPORT MEASURES

1. It is essential to maintain an adequate airway and provide sufficient oxygen, using either a mask or an endotracheal tube (particularly in patients with facial burns or if the burn was sustained in an enclosed space) before facial or laryngeal edema becomes evident.
2. Children with burns greater than 15% of BSA require intravenous fluid resuscitation to maintain adequate perfusion. All patients with inhalation injury, regardless of the extent of BSA involved, also require adequate venous access to control the fluid intake. Furthermore, all high-tension and electrical injuries require venous access to ensure forced alkaline diuresis in case of muscle injury.

   Lactated Ringer's solution 10 to 20 ml/kg/h (normal saline may be used if Ringer's lactate solution is not available) is infused until proper fluid replacement can be calculated. Consultation with a specialized burn unit should be made to coordinate fluid therapy—type of fluids, preferred formula for calculation, and preferences for the use of colloid (albumin or fresh frozen plasma)—during treatment, particularly if transfer is anticipated.

3. Evaluation for associated injuries should be quickly undertaken. Such injuries are quite common in patients with a history of high-tension electrical burns, especially if the victim has fallen from a height. Injuries to the spine, bones, and thoracic or intraabdominal organs may occur. There is a very high risk of cardiac abnormalities, including ventricular tachycardia and ventricular fibrillation, resulting from the conductivity of the high electric voltage. Cardiopulmonary resuscitation should be instituted promptly at the scene, and the patient should be placed on a cardiac monitor as soon as possible.
4. Patients with burns greater than 15% BSA should not receive oral fluids (initially) as such patient may develop an ileus. In the emergency room, it may be necessary to insert a nasogastric tube to prevent aspiration.
5. All wounds should be wrapped with sterile towels until a decision is made to treat on an outpatient basis or refer to an appropriate facility for definitive care.

Indications for referral to a hospital are outlined in Table 1.

ESTIMATION OF BODY SURFACE AREA OF BURN

It is critical to use appropriate burn charts for different age groups of children to estimate accurately the extent of BSA burned. The volume of fluid needed in resuscitation is calculated by estimating the extent and depth of the burn surface. The mortality and morbidity of burn outcome also depend on the extent and depth of the burn (Table 2). The varying growth of the head and extremities throughout childhood makes it necessary to use surface area tables (Table 3). The rule of nines used in adults may be used only in children over the age of 14 years or as a very rough estimate to institute therapy before transfer to a burn center. In small burns under 10%, the rule of palm may be used, especially in outpatient settings. (The area from the wrist crease to the finger crease in the palm of the child equal 1% of the child's BSA.)

Children with first- and second-degree burns under 10% of BSA may be treated as outpatients unless there is inadequate family support or there are issues of child neglect or abuse. Outpatients do not require a tetanus booster or prophylactic penicillin therapy. Children who are not up to date with their immunizations should have them updated. Blisters should be left intact and dressed with silver sulfadiazine cream (Silvadene). Dressings should be changed twice daily after the wound is washed with lukewarm water to remove any cream left from the previous application. Very small wounds, especially those on the face, may be treated with Neosporin ointment or bacitracin and left open. Debridement of the devitalized skin is indicated when the blisters rupture. Burns to the palm with large blisters usually heal beneath the blisters. The great majority of superficial burns heal in 10 to 20 days. Deep second-degree burns take longer to heal. Pain control should be accomplished by using acetaminophen with codeine an hour before dressing changes. Wounds that appear deeper than at initial assessment or that have not healed by 21 days may require a short hospital admission for grafting.

The depth of scald injuries is notoriously difficult to assess early, and conservative treatment is appropriate to allow determination of the real depth of the burn before surgical closure is attempted. This obviates the risk of anesthesia if the wound epithelializes or can heal by wound contraction. Skin grafting is necessary if larger open areas

TABLE 1. Indications for Hospitalization

Burns greater than 15% body surface area (BSA)
High-tension electrical burns
Inhalation injury regardless of the size of BSA burn
Inadequate home situation
Suspected child abuse or neglect

TABLE 2. Burn Depth Categories

PARAMETER	FIRST DEGREE	SECOND DEGREE PARTIAL THICKNESS	THIRD DEGREE FULL THICKNESS
Cause	Flash, flame, ultraviolet (sunlight)	Contact with hot liquids or solids Flame to clothing Direct flame chemical	Contact with hot liquids or solids; flame, chemical, electrical
Surface appearance	Dry, no blisters; no or minimal edema	Moist blebs, blisters	Dry with leathery eschar until debridement; charred blood vessels visible under eschar
Color	Erythematous	Mottled white to pink to cherry red	Mixed white, waxy pearly; dark khaki, mahogany; charred
Pain level	Painful	Very painful	Little or no pain; hair pulls out easily
Histologic depth	Epidermal layers only	Epidermis, papillary, and reticular layers of dermis; may include fat domes of subcutaneous layer	
Healing time	2–5 d with peeling, no scarring; may have discoloration	Superficial: 5–21 d with no grafting Deep partial: With no infection, 21–25 d; if infected, converts to full thickness	Wound heals only after grafting unless it is a small wound that heals by contracture

persist. The lack of painful sensation and capillary filling demonstrates the loss of nerve and capillary elements consistent with deeper injuries.

INITIAL MEDICAL MANAGEMENT

A protocol for immediate wound care in the emergency room or outpatient facility is necessary for efficient therapy of a thermal injury. An accurate history of the burn should include when and where the accident occurred and the burn agent (e.g., flame, hot liquid, electricity). The history should also elicit any possibility of smoke inhalation injury and if the injury occurred in an enclosed space. Evaluation for possible associated injuries also is important. The pertinent past medical history, including drug allergies, should be documented at this time.

Acute Treatment

Fluid Resuscitation

For most children, the Parkland formula is a good starting guideline for fluid resuscitation. This formula recommends infusing 4 ml of Ringer's lactate solution per kilogram of body weight per percent BSA burned. One half of the calculated fluid is given over the first 8 hours from the time of onset of the injury. The remaining half of the calculated fluid is given at an even rate over the next 16 hours postinjury. The rate of infusion is modified to the patient's response to therapy. Pulse and blood pressure are restored, and an adequate urine output (1 ml/kg/h) is achieved by varying the intravenous rate. Vital signs, acid-base balance, and mental status reflect the adequacy of the resuscitation. Because of interstitial edema and sequestration of fluid in muscle cells, patients may gain up to 20% over baseline preburn body weight. Patients with burns of 40% to 60% BSA require a large venous access (central venous line) to deliver the large volume of fluid required over the critical first hours. Patients with burns greater than 60% BSA may require two central venous lines, and such patients are best cared for in a specialized burn unit.

TABLE 3. Method for Estimating Percent of Body Burned

	NEWBORN	3 YEARS	6 YEARS	12+ YEARS
Head	18%	15%	12%	6%
Trunk	40%	40%	40%	38%
Arms	16%	16%	16%	18%
Legs	26%	29%	32%	38%

During the second 24 hours after the burn, patients will begin to reabsorb edema fluid, and a diuresis follows. One half of the first day's fluid requirement is infused as lactated Ringer's solution in 5% dextrose. Controversies exist over whether colloid should be provided in the early period of the burn resuscitation. In our own unit (Shriners Burn Institute, Boston), the preference is to use colloid replacement concurrently if the burn is greater than 86% total BSA. Colloid is usually instituted 8 to 24 hours after the burn injury. In children less than 12 months of age, tolerance to excess sodium is limited. Therefore, the volume and sodium concentration of the resuscitation solution should be diminished if urinary sodium concentration is rising. The adequacy of resuscitation should be reassessed constantly using vital signs, blood gases, hematocrit, and protein levels. Very few patients require arterial and central venous lines or pulmonary artery pressure monitoring provided that circulation and urine output can be sustained. Oral supplementation may start as early as 48 hours postinjury. Milk formula, artificial feedings, homogenized milk, or soy-based products can be given by bolus or constant infusion via a nasogastric or small bowel feeding tube. As oral fluids are tolerated, intravenous fluids are decreased proportionately in an endeavor to keep the total fluid intake constant, particularly if pulmonary dysfunction is present. Five percent albumin infusions may be used to maintain the serum albumin levels at a desired 2 g/dl concentration. The following rates have been shown to be effective for total BSA burns of 30% to 50%, 0.3 ml serum albumin per kilogram of body weight per percent BSA burn infused over a 24-hour period; 50% to 70%, 0.4 ml/kg of body weight per percent BSA burn infused over 24 hours; 70% to 100%, 0.5 ml/kg of body weight per percent BSA burn infused over a 24-hour period. Packed red cell infusion is recommended if the hematocrit falls below 24% (hemoglobin under 8 g/dl). At our unit, we recommend maintaining a hematocrit at 30% (hemoglobin 10 g/dl) in patients with systemic infections, hemoglobinopathies, cardiopulmonary disease, or anticipated (or ongoing) blood loss when early excision and grafting of full-thickness burns is likely. Fresh frozen plasma is indicated if clinical and laboratory assessments reveal a deficiency of clotting factors, a prothrombin level above 1.5 times control, or a partial thromboplastin time greater than 1.2 times control in patients who are actively bleeding or in those scheduled for an invasive procedure or a grafting procedure that could result in an estimated blood loss of over half the blood volume of that patient. Fresh frozen plasma is used for volume resuscitation within 72 hours of injury in patients under 2 years of age with burns over 20% BSA and associated moderate inhalation injury.

Sodium supplementation may be required for those patients with burns greater than 20% BSA, particularly if 0.5% silver nitrate so-

TABLE 4. Acute Burn Management and Transport Advice

1. It is critical that the airway be adequately controlled before transport. If there is *any* question of airway involvement, the patient should have a nasotracheal tube placed for prophylaxis before transport.
2. Patients with significant burns should be transported with a nasogastric tube, Foley catheter, and two well-secured venous lines in place.
3. Outlying facilities should be given advice regarding fluid administration. A reasonable starting point would include the following.

   Weight <10 kg: D_5/RL* at 4 ml/kg/h (maintenance rate of dextrose-containing fluid)

   plus

   RL at 3 ml/kg per percent burn over first 24 h; first half given in the first 8 h after burn

   Weight >10 kg: RL at 4 ml/kg per percent burn over first 24 h; first half given in the first 8 h after burn

   These are starting rates and should be modified based on urine output; goal is 1 ml/kg/h urine output
4. Patients must be kept warm during transport. Wounds should be covered with a clean, dry sheet.

*RL, Ringer's lactate solution.

---

lution is used as the topical antibacterial burn dressing. Sodium losses with silver nitrate therapy are regularly as high as 350 mmol/m^2 BSA. An oral sodium chloride supplement of 4 gm/m^2 burn area per 24 hours is usually well tolerated. The dose is divided into four to six equal doses to avoid osmotic diarrhea. The aim is to maintain serum sodium levels at greater than 130 mEq/L and a urinary sodium concentration over 30 mEq/L. Intravenous potassium supplementation is supplied to maintain a serum potassium level of over 3 mEq/dl. Potassium losses may be significantly increased if aminoglycoside, diuretic, or amphotericin therapy is required. Table 4 provides a summary of acute burn management and transport considerations.

Prevention of Infection

Controversy over the need to use penicillin therapy prophylactically for all acutely injured hospitalized burn patients continues. In our unit, we use a 5-day course of penicillin therapy for all acute burns. A standard dose of crystalline penicillin is given orally or intravenously in four divided doses. Erythromycin may be used as an alternative in penicillin-allergic patients.

Death following the burn injury is not related to the toxic biologic effect of thermally injured skin but to the metabolic and bacterial consequences of a large open wound, depletion of the patient's host resistance, and extensive malnutrition. These abnormalities set the stage for life-threatening bacterial infection originating from the burn wound. Prevention of wound infection and wound treatment promote early healing and improve the esthetic and functional outcomes. Topical treatment of burn wounds with 0.5% silver nitrate solution, silver sulfadiazine cream, or mafenite acetate (Sulfamyalon) cream aims at prevention of infection. The last two medications have the advantage of tissue-penetrating capacity (Table 5). Regardless of the choice of topical agent, it is essential that all third-degree burn tissue be fully excised (before bacterial colonization occurs). The area must be grafted as early as possible to prevent deep wound sepsis.

In our unit, patients with over 30% BSA burn are housed in a bacteria-controlled nursing unit to prevent cross-contamination and to keep the patient in a temperature- and humidity-controlled environment to minimize hypermetabolism. Deep second-degree burns greater than 10% BSA benefit from early tangential excision and grafting. Sequential excision and grafting of third-degree and deep second-degree burns are required in victims of large burns to improve the outcome. Prompt use of skin substitutes, such as allografts, artificial skin, xenografts, or epidermal cultured cells, may be important for wound coverage in patients with extensive injury in order to limit fluid, electrolyte, and protein losses. Skin substitutes also reduce pain and minimize heat loss. The safety of extensive excision requires an integrated experienced team, incorporating a skilled pediatric burn

surgeon, pediatric anesthesiologist, and intensive care burn nurses. Early excision can be carried out safely by an experienced burn team while burn fluid resuscitation continues. Important features for success include attention to (1) accurate preoperative and intraoperative determination of burn depth, (2) the determination of safe operative extent and appropriate timing, (3) control of intraoperative blood loss, (4) specific instrumentation, (5) choice and use of perioperative antibiotics, and (6) type of wound coverage chosen (Table 6).

Supporting the Patient's Increased Energy Requirements

The burn injury produces a hypermetabolic response characterized by both protein and fat catabolism. Children with a 40% total BSA burn experience resting energy expenditures approximately 50% above the predicted levels for age. Early excision and grafting can decrease such stress.

Pain, anxiety, and immobilization increase physiologic demands. Furthermore, cold stress provides additional demands, especially if humidity and temperature are not controlled. This is especially true in young infants, where the largest surface area/mass ratio allows for proportionately greater heat loss than in adolescents and adults. Calorie demands can be decreased by providing control of environmental temperatures at 28°C to 33°C, adequate covering during transport, and liberal use of analgesia and anxiolytics. Special units to control temperature and humidity may be necessary in patients with large BSA burns.

The objective of caloric supplementation programs is to maintain body weight by decreasing metabolic demands. This prevents the steady erosion of lean body mass resulting from negative nitrogen balance and lipolysis. Our own aim is to provide calories at one and a half to twice the basal metabolic rate along with 1.5 to 2 g of protein per kilogram of body weight. We assess the response, comparing intake with metabolic studies to more accurately tailor caloric demands than can be done using a simple formula calculation.

Additional calories are necessary to allow not only for stabilization but also for growth. Multivitamins, particularly the B vitamin group, vitamin C, vitmain A, and zinc, as well as caloric supplements, are necessary. Alimentation should be started as soon as practical, either orally or intravenously, after commencement of the resuscitative phase. Patients with a burn greater than 40% total BSA need a gastric or small bowel feeding tube to facilitate continuous delivery of calories and to allow stabilization without the risk of aspiration. Parenteral nutrition is discontinued as soon as possible (after delivery of calories is established) to decrease the risk of an infectious complication associated with parenteral nutrition.

PAIN MANAGEMENT GUIDELINE

The perception of pain is a unique, subjective experience for each patient, with both physiologic and psychologic components. Effective

TABLE 5. Guide to Topical Agents

AGENT	ADVANTAGES	DISADVANTAGES
Silver nitrate	Painless Wide spectrum No resistant strains No sensitivity	Poor penetration Electrolyte changes Potentially messy Immobility from dressings
Mafenide	Painless Active penetration Easy to use Allows mobilization	Systemic effects Some sensitivity
Silver sulfadiazine	Painless Sensitivity infrequent Wide spectrum Minimal inactivation	Intermediate penetration Supplemental medication required
Providone	Minimal pain Allows mobilization Wide spectrum	Possible inactivation by wound exudate

TABLE 6. Burn Size and Method of Prompt Excision and Immediate Wound Closure

	EXTENT OF INJURY (% BSA)	PROCEDURES REQUIRED FOR EXCISION	METHOD OF CLOSURE	AVAILABILITY OF DONOR SITES	USE OF ALLOGRAFT FOR PROMPT PHYSIOLOGIC WOUND CLOSURE AND DELAYED AUTOGRAFT CLOSURE
Small burns	0–19	One stage	Autograft sheet or mesh	Adequate	None
Moderate burns	20–49	Multiple stages, usually every other day	Autograft sheet or mesh for special areas	Adequate	None
Severe burns	50–79	Multiple stages, usually every other day	Autograft mesh supplemented with temporary allograft (sheet), replaced with autograft (mesh)	Special sites needed, usually scalp and feet	Allograft removed 2–3 d before rejection; replaced with autograft from reharvested donor site
Massive burns	80–95	Multiple stages, usually every other day	Autograft mesh supplemented with temporary allograft (sheet); replaced with autograft (mesh)	Special sites needed, usually scalp and feet	Allograft removed 2–3 d before rejection; replaced with autograft from reharvested donor site; cultured cells used when available

pain management strategies involve a combination of pharmacologic and psychologic interventions that are individualized to meet the patient's specific needs.

The focus of this guideline is on the pharmacologic aspect of the management of pain and anxiety. It is provided as a reference for those strategies that require a physician's order and aims at providing a collaborative consistent approach to pain management.

I. Pharmacologic management of the ventilated acute patient
  A. Pain
    1. Morphine sulfate intermittent IV bolus
    Dose: 0.05–0.1 mg/kg q2h; dose may need to be increased gradually for some patients, or consider continuous infusion
    2. Morphine sulfate continuous infusion
    Dose: starting at 0.05 mg/kg/h; often increased gradually as patient needs change
    3. Naloxone (Narcan) for reversal if needed for airway crisis
    Dose: 5–10 μg/kg per dose IM or IV
  B. Anxiety
    1. Midazolam (Versed) intermittent IV bolus for patients unable to achieve adequate comfort with analgesics
    2. Midazolam continuous infusion for patients with ongoing needs for anxiety management not alleviated by other interventions
    Note: Reversible neurologic abnormalities have been reported in critically ill children following long-term midazolam use.
    Dose: starting at 0.04 mg/kg/h
    3. Flumazenil (Mazicon) for reversal if needed for airway crisis
    Dose: 0.2–1 mg given at rate of 0.2 mg/min; may take 6–10 min for peak effect; wait >1 min between doses; too rapid administration may cause seizures
II. Pharmacologic management of the nonventilated acute patient
  A. Background pain
    1. Pain
      a. Morphine sulfate immediate release (MSIR) on consistent schedule
      Dose: 0.3–0.6 mg/kg enterally q4–8h
      b. Morphine sulfate intermittent IV bolus to supplement enteral morphine
      Dose: 0.05 mg/kg IV q2–4h
      c. Morphine sulfate continuous infusion when enteral administration is not effective or patient is NPO
      Dose: starting at 0.05–0.1 mg/kg/h
    2. Anxiety
      a. Enteral or IV lorazepam on consistent schedule for patients unable to achieve adequate level of comfort

from analgesics or other measures
      Dose: 0.04 mg/kg IV or PO q8h
  B. Painful procedure cover
    1. Pain
      a. MSIR 1 h before procedure
      Dose: 0.3 mg/kg enterally
      b. Morphine sulfate IV bolus ½ h before procedure
      Dose: 0.05 mg/kg IV
      Note: Use pulse oximetry monitoring for patients receiving multiple bolus doses; morphine effects may exceed the duration of the procedure.
    2. Anxiety
      a. Enteral or IV lorazepam ½ h before procedure for patients unable to achieve adequate level of comfort from analgesics or other measures
      Dose: 0.04 mg/kg IV or PO
  C. Transitional issue: Pharmacologic management during changeover from parenteral to enteral route; opiate weaning
    1. Pain: IV opiate is systematically reduced, and enteral analgesia is started until transition is complete
      a. Morphine sulfate infusions are weaned 10%–20% every 24–48 h
      Note: Be alert for signs and symptoms of opiate withdrawal.
      b. MSIR enterally may be added as morphine infusions are tapered
      Dose: 0.3–0.6 mg/kg q4–6h
      c. MSIR is gradually tapered at a rate of 10%–25% of dose every q24–72h
      d. Acetaminophen may be appropriate when tapering MSIR dose
    2. Anxiety: Lorazepam dose is tapered by 25%/d over 4–7 d, in consultation with psychiatry as needed
III. Pharmacologic management of the acute rehabilitation patient
  A. Pain
    1. MSIR on a consistent schedule
    Dose: 0.3–0.6 mg/kg q4h enterally
    2. Morphine sustained release (MS Contin) for patients able to swallow tablet
    Note: MS Contin available only in 15 and 30 mg tablets that must not be broken or chewed; dose and route make this appropriate for the larger or older child.
    Dose: Based on 24-dose requirements of MSIR, administer one-half daily dose as MS Contin every 12 h
  B. Anxiety
    1. Lorazepam on a consistent schedule
    Dose: 0.04 mg/kg q8h or consider different approach

2. Consider different or longer-acting medication, psychiatric consultation

IV. Pharmacologic management of the reconstructive or routine post-operative patient

A. Pain
1. MSIR on consistent schedule
   Dose: 0.3–0.6 mg/kg q4–6h enterally
2. Morphine sulfate IV bolus
   Dose: 0.05–0.1 mg/kg q2h
3. Patient controlled analgesia (PCA) considered for older children, same dose availability
4. Morphine sulfate (Roxanol) rectal suppositories
   Dose: 0.3–0.6 mg/kg q4h
   Note: Available as 5-mg or 10-mg suppository.

B. Anxiety
1. Lorazepam on consistent schedule
   Dose: 0.04 mg/kg per dose q8h

INHALATION INJURY

Inhalation injury is a serious cause of increased morbidity in the infant and child, particularly if preexisting pulmonary conditions are present. Mortality estimates vary depending on the criteria for diagnosis but are typically between 45% and 60% in adults. Mortality figures are not available for children. Airway evaluation aims at early identification of inhalation injuries.

Respiratory tract injury may occur from (1) direct heat (greater problems occur in steam burns), (2) acute asphyxia, (3) carbon monoxide poisoning, or (4) toxic fumes. Sulfur and nitrogen oxides and alkalies formed during combustion of synthetic fabrics produce corrosive chemicals that may erode mucosa and cause significant sloughing. Exposure to smoke may also cause degradation of surfactant and decrease its production, resulting in atelectasis. Inhalation injury and burn injury are synergistic in increasing morbidity and mortality.

The pulmonary complications of burns and inhalation can be divided into three distinct clinical syndromes with distinct clinical features and temporal patterns. (1) Carbon monoxide poisoning, airway obstruction, and pulmonary edema are the *early* major concerns. (2) The adult respiratory distress syndrome (ARDS) usually becomes clinically evident *between 24 and 48 hours,* although it can occur later. (3) *Late* complications (days to weeks) include pneumonia and pulmonary emboli.

The risk of inhalation injury should be assessed by historical evidence of obvious injury, (e.g. facial swelling or carbonaceous material in nasal passages) and laboratory determination of carboxyhemoglobin and arterial blood gases. Treatment should initially focus on establishing and maintaining a patent airway through prompt and early nasotracheal intubation and ensuring adequate ventilation and oxygenation. In patients with inhalation injury, as suggested by burns of the face and neck, upper airway obstruction can develop rapidly, and endotracheal intubation may be a lifesaving intervention. Aggressive pulmonary toilet and chest physiotherapy are necessary in prolonged nasotracheal intubation or tracheotomy. If tracheotomy has to be performed, it should be delayed until burns at and near the site have healed and then performed electively under anesthesia with optimal tracheal positioning and hemostasis. The availability of less irritating endotracheal tube materials and improved tube and cuff designs has allowed progressively longer periods of safe translaryngeal intubation. An endotracheal tube can be maintained even for months without the need for tracheostomy. Extubation should be delayed until patients meet the accepted criteria for maintaining their own airways.

REHABILITATION AND RETURN TO SCHOOL

The rehabilitation program starts on admission and includes the following.
1. Positioning and splinting
   a. Static splinting
   b. Dynamic splinting
2. Exercise and ambulation
3. Activities of daily living
4. Pressure therapy and skin care

Implementation of the rehabilitation program is instituted and carried on for each patient according to the patient's need. The program is modified as the patient's condition changes and on discharge. Most patients with severe burns will require outpatient rehabilitation programs.

REFERENCES

1. Boswick JA Jr. The Art and Science of Burn Care. Gaithersburg, Md., Aspen Publishers, Inc., 1987.
2. Herrin JT, Antoon AY: Burn injury and cold injury. In Behrman RE (ed): Nelson's Textbook of Pediatrics, 14th ed. Philadelphia, WB Saunders Co, 1992.
3. Martyn JAJ (ed): Acute Management of the Burned Patient, Philadelphia, WB Saunders Co, 1990.

NEAR DROWNING

JOHN T. SLADKY, M.D.

There are few modes of accidental injury in childhood that are associated with the severe degree of mortality and morbidity that accompany submersion injury. In some series, drowning was the third leading cause of death, accounting for approximately 2000 deaths per year in the United States among children under the age of 15.[2,3] Among those who are rescued but require admission to an intensive care unit, only approximately 50% recover with good neurologic function. Three fourths of the rest of the patients do not survive, and those who do have severe neurologic impairments. The populations at greatest risk for drowning and near drowning are toddlers and adolescent males.[2] Among children under 5 years of age, accidental submersion, usually in unsupervised residential swimming pools, is the commonest setting for drowning and near drowning. In temperate climates in such states as California, Florida, Texas, and Arizona, drowning is the most frequent cause of accidental death in children under 5 years of age. The tragedy of drowning deaths in young children is that the majority are wholly preventable. The primary goal of health care policy is not treatment but prevention of submersion injury. However, despite widespread awareness and public information campaigns in endemic regions, the incidence of accidental drowning among toddlers has not significantly declined.

The most important factors influencing the outcome of submersion-injured children are operational before the arrival of medical or paramedical personnel. The single greatest concern is duration of submersion. Rapid rescue and early resuscitation have a far more critical impact on outcome than has any subsequent medical intervention.

Initial resuscitative efforts should focus on establishing ventilation and perfusion. The patency of the airway needs to be guaranteed, especially if submersion occurred in water containing particulate matter. Ventilation should be undertaken with care to minimize mobilization of the cervical spine, since spinal cord trauma related to diving injury often plays a role in near drowning (particularly in adolescent boys). If heart sounds are not audible, femoral and carotid pulses are not palpable, or there is significant bradycardia, external chest compressions should be initiated and maintained during transport until adequate perfusion can be documented.

On arrival at the emergency department, the usual ABCs of resuscitation (airway, breathing, circulation) require immediate attention. A stable airway should be secured, and adequate ventilation, oxygenation, and perfusion should be confirmed. Placement of a nasogastric tube and evacuation of stomach contents is useful to prevent aspiration. Hypothermia is a frequent complication of cold water immersion and may cause asystole, arrhythmia, or myocardial hypofunction. Several techniques have been proposed for rewarming the hypothermic patient, including external warming, gastric and rectal lavage, warm intravenous fluids and inspired gases, warm peritoneal or pleural lavage, and cardiopulmonary bypass. Patients with severe hypothermia (core temperature <30°C) will have poor perfusion due to absent or ineffective myocardial contractility and peripheral vasoconstriction. In this circumstance, external warming will have only limited efficacy, and internal techniques will be required. Cardiopulmonary bypass has the advantage of providing direct cardiac support and will maintain perfusion in the asystolic, hypothermic patient until adequate rewarming has occurred. There is no prospective evidence, however, that these invasive maneuvers are translated into improved outcome.

The first phase of resuscitation is focused on the heart and lungs: correcting systemic acidemia and fluid and electrolyte imbalances and establishing oxygenation and perfusion. Once these goals have been achieved, a succinct neurologic evaluation is in order. The Glasgow Coma Scale is a simple instrument that requires no specialized tools, can be administered in less than a minute, and provides a relatively standardized assessment of the level of neurologic function in the brain-injured patient. Whereas an asphyxiated myocardium may remain persistently hypoactive, asphyxiated neurons commonly respond in the opposite fashion. Successful reestablishment of cerebral perfusion and oxygenation is often followed by seizures. If they occur, seizures should be treated aggressively with intravenous lorazepam. Under most circumstances, control of seizures with an intravenous benzodiazapine should be followed by administration of a loading dose of a longer-acting anticonvulsant. Phenytoin is usually the drug of choice in such circumstances because adequate anticonvulsant levels can be achieved with relatively limited central nervous system (CNS)-depressant side effects. In the face of hypoxic/ischemic cardiomyopathy, phenytoin may be contraindicated, and treatment with phenobarbital during the acute phase may be a safer option. Alternative anticonvulsant drug treatment can be instituted at a later date depending on the outcome.

After successful resuscitation, rewarming, and stabilization of vital signs in the emergency room, the patient should be transported to a pediatric intensive care unit. If the patient survives the first 24 hours, submersion injury is classified as a near drowning. These children will have sustained a hypoxic/ischemic insult to multiple organ systems, although the respiratory system and the CNS most often bear the brunt of the injury. Lung injury can be the consequence of several mechanisms. The first is aspiration of fresh or salt water. In experimental studies of drowning, osmotic factors are thought to play a role in transudation of fluid and osmolytes in both directions across the alveolar membrane, with concomitant hemodilution (with fresh water) and hemoconcentration (with salt water) after significant aspiration. The experience in humans has shown a much more modest effect on blood volumes and electrolyte shifts than in animal studies.[2,3] Despite different proposed mechanisms of pulmonary injury after aspiration of hypotonic and hypertonic fluids, the resulting physiologic abnormalities (pulmonary edema, diminished compliance, ventilation perfusion discrepancies, and difficulties in maintaining oxygenation) are quite similar in either case, with damage to surfactant and the alveolar basement membrane. Furthermore, although laryngospasm may prevent significant subglottic fluid aspiration during the actual drowning event, pulmonary hypoxia/ischemia alone can result in a clinical picture typical of adult respiratory distress syndrome (ARDS). This may evolve after a period of 24 to 48 hours during which the patient is demonstrating good neurologic recovery. Despite maximal mechanical ventilatory support, it may be difficult to maintain adequate oxygenation. In the patient who has demonstrated early neurologic improvement, extracorporeal membrane oxygenation may be warranted.

The principal therapeutic goal in the management of children after near drowning is to increase the incidence of neurologically intact survivors. As a corollary, it would be useful to have reliable prognostic indices that would permit identification of subpopulations of submersion-injured children in which aggressive resuscitative measures

either should or should not be initiated. Unfortunately, there is no single variable or constellation of variables that reliably predicts outcome early in the course of resuscitation. Those children who arrive in the emergency department with stable blood pressure, spontaneous respirations, and a Glasgow Coma Scale score of greater than 5 generally will do well. Those children who have sustained prolonged submersion, demonstrate severe acidemia, require prolonged cardiac resuscitation, and are comatose without brainstem reflexes usually will not survive.[1-3] Persistent cerebral hypometabolism has been documented in this latter group as opposed to those who survive with good neurologic recovery. Even this sophisticated measure, however, is an imprecise discriminator in the individual patient early in the course of the insult. There have been rare but dramatic exceptions to these general observations, particularly when the patient is profoundly hypothermic, but also in children with an admission core temperature >32°C.[1] These anecdotal reports are disquieting insofar as they underscore the limitations of our ability to predict outcome based on early indices. Conversely, the many reports of complete recovery after prolonged submersion and cardiopulmonary resuscitation in patients with profound hypothermia clearly indicate that there is a potential for therapeutic neuroprotective intervention with improved neurologic outcome.

Prior strategies for cerebral resuscitation have focused on preventing intracranial hypertension. These protocols have included intracranial pressure monitoring, volume restriction, neuromuscular blockade, hyperventilation, osmotic agents, hypothermia, and barbiturate coma. Unfortunately, these strategies individually and collectively have been ineffective. Furthermore, the inability of such measures to improve neurologic outcome should have been predictable for several reasons. First, the therapies are instituted and the drugs administered well after the drowning event has occurred. Ideal neuroprotective treatments should be administered before the hypoxic/ischemic injury or at least early in the course of resuscitation. Perhaps more important, the theoretical substrate for prophylactic treatment of intracranial hypertension is to prevent secondary ischemia due to impaired cerebral blood flow autoregulation and increased cerebrovascular resistance. This mechanism of secondary brain injury appears to play a role in trauma and other focal cerebral insults but plays little role in the outcome after global cerebral hypoxia/ischemia. Posthypoxic/ischemic cytotoxic cerebral edema is a manifestation of prior energy substrate deprivation and lethal failure of oxidative and glycolytic metabolism, with subsequent widespread neuronal necrosis and brain swelling. This type of cytotoxic cerebral edema is poorly responsive to therapeutic interventions. It comes as no surprise, therefore, that documented sustained intracranial hypertension is associated with a poor prognosis, as it reflects the severity of diffuse irreversible hypoxic/ischemic neuronal injury. Intracranial pressure monitoring, hyperventilation, and other strategies aimed at preventing intracranial hypertension have no demonstrated efficacy and a theoretical potential for harm and should not be incorporated routinely into the treatment plan for patients after near drowning. There is abundant evidence, however, that postischemic reperfusion injury plays a substantial role in determining the severity of hypoxic/ischemic neuronal damage and that this phase of ischemic cerebral insult is potentially amenable to various neuroprotective approaches.

There has been an enormous effort in recent years to characterize the ability of pharmacologic agents that alter calcium channel behavior, modulate free radical-mediated tissue injury, or prevent postischemic excitotoxic neuronal damage to minimize the extent of cerebral injury after hypoxic/ischemic insults in animal models and clinical settings. Unfortunately, there have been few successful efforts to apply insights from this research to the setting of near drowning, and none in submersion-injured children. As stated previously, the observation that hypothermia (core temperature <33°C) can be associated with good neurologic recovery despite prolonged immersion and absence of vital signs suggests that other neuroprotective tactics might be efficacious in near drowning victims. There are a number of agents that have demonstrated efficacy in experimental hypoxic/ischemic brain injury that could potentially be of use in near drowning victims. The most promising of these are drugs that modulate reperfusion excitotoxic injury by glutamaturgic pathways, including glutamate antagonists such as adenosine or agents that block NMDA and AMPA receptors, such as MK-801 and NBQX. In the future, resuscitation of the submersion-injured child will probably include a neuroprotective cocktail containing one of these or similar agents, along with free radical scavengers, possibly in combination with moderate brain cooling. At the present time, however, the most effective therapy is *prevention*. It is hoped that clinical research will proceed expeditiously to define new strategies to enhance survival and quality of life of victims of submersion injury.

REFERENCES

1. Lavelle JM, Shaw KN: Near drowning: Is emergency department cardiopulmonary resuscitation or intensive care unit cerebral resuscitation indicated? Crit Care Med 21:368–373, 1993.
2. Levin DL, Morriss FC, Toro LO, Brink L, Turner G: Drowning and near drowning. Pediatr Clin North Am 40:321–336, 1993.
3. Orolowski JP: Drowning, near-drowning and ice-water submersions. Pediatr Clin North Am 34:75–92, 1987.

PENETRATING, GUNSHOT, AND KNIFE WOUNDS IN CHILDREN

C. WILLIAM SCHWAB, M.D.
J. CHRISTOPHER DIGIACOMO, M.D.

Coincident with the epidemic rise in penetrating injury in this country, the incidence of gunshot and stab wounds in the pediatric population is increasing at an alarming rate.[1,3] Houston, Texas, had a 75% increase in 1991 alone.[1] Eighty-five percent of all firearm deaths occur in the home of the victim, a relative, or friend and are usually inflicted by handguns that are kept loaded in readily accessible locations. Strikingly, 99.5% of people killed in a home that had a firearm were residents of that home. Firearms are involved in 5% of infant homicides, 25% of young child homicides, and 60% of homicides in adolescents. Overall, firearms are involved in approximately 40% of child homicides, and knives are involved in 15%.[3] Firearms are the fourth leading cause of unintentional deaths in children under 14 years of age (roughly 1200 per year), and this exceeds deaths from poisonings.[3] Of the estimated 8000 nonfatal gunshot injuries in children per year, 25% to 50% will cause permanent physical or emotional injury.[3] It is, therefore, imperative that parents be aware that firearms will be present in over half of the homes their children visit, and one in four homes will contain a handgun. Parents should be encouraged to ask about the location of weapons, and gun owners should be admonished to keep their guns stored unloaded and locked and out of the reach of children.

Penetrating injury is a surgical disease that requires operative intervention until proven otherwise. In the pediatric population, penetrating trauma is complicated by the unique anatomy and physiology of children. Anatomic differences, as compared with adults, include a larger head/body ratio, a relatively ventral and short larynx, and poorly protected abdominal organs, including the liver, spleen, kidneys, and bladder. Because skin thickness is less than in the adult, BBs or pellets shot from airguns can penetrate into body cavities of children and injure internal organs. Children also have a smaller blood volume and decreased respiratory capacity and reserve, but their physiologic compensatory mechanisms remain generally unimpeded by disease or aging. Therefore, the child with active bleeding may appear relatively stable until abrupt decompensation occurs.

As with any major injury, the evaluation begins with the primary assessment of airway, breathing, and circulation, the ABCs of trauma.

The evaluation and resuscitation of a victim of penetrating trauma need to be efficient and aggressive, require an understanding of the trajectory of the penetration, and assume the presence of severe injury. There must be a high index of suspicion for hypovolemia. A surgeon should be called as soon as possible, since most patients require operation. The importance of the resuscitation effort cannot be overemphasized as 83.3% of inhospital pediatric deaths due to trauma occur during the resuscitation phase in the emergency department. To limit these deaths, a trauma team whose members are designated in advance should be summoned for any penetrating injury of the head, neck, torso, or proximal extremities. A physician experienced in the management of trauma, usually a senior surgeon, should be visibly in charge as the command physician and direct the resuscitation effort. This is important because personnel directly working on a patient tend to become focused on their specific task, and the external appearance of the injury may cause the caregivers to lose sight of the overall resuscitation.

EVALUATION AND INITIAL TREATMENT

The first priority in any trauma assessment is always the airway, regardless of the appearance of the patient's injuries. One hundred percent oxygen should be administered by face mask. Because of the narrow diameter of the larynx and trachea, mucosal edema or extraluminal swelling can rapidly obliterate the airway. Ventilation and even intubation may become impossible. Therefore, the patient who is suspected of requiring intubation should be intubated promptly by experienced personnel. A rapid sequence induction technique, consisting of (1) preoxygenation by mask of 100% oxygen, (2) continuous cricoid pressure, (3) pharmacologically induced paralysis and sedation, and (4) orotracheal intubation, allows rapid and safe control of the airway. It also minimizes Valsalva, elevated blood pressure, and elevated intracranial pressure, which are common with awake intubations. Endotracheal intubation should not be delayed in hope of avoiding intubation, since a lost airway can be fatal. In our experience, as well as that of others, nasotracheal intubation is rarely useful in the traumatized patient.

Breathing is assessed next. For penetrating injuries of the thorax and upper abdomen, pneumothorax must be ruled out. Tension pneumothorax can develop rapidly, especially with positive pressure ventilation or mask-assisted ventilation. In the hemodynamically unstable patient, needle catheter decompression of the chest should be performed for suspected tension pneumothorax and must be followed by insertion of a chest tube. The needle should be left in place until after the chest tube is in position. Gaping chest wall injuries should be covered with an occlusive petroleum gauze dressing, and a chest tube should be placed simultaneously through a separate site to prevent tension pneumothorax.

The next step of the resuscitation effort is directed toward assessing circulation. The primary response of the child to hypovolemia is tachycardia. Injured children are especially prone to hypovolemia because of their smaller blood volume, and a relatively small amount of blood loss may place children in shock. In addition to tachycardia, other signs of hypovolemic shock include hypotension, widened pulse pressure, weak and thready pulse, pallor, and cool extremities. Obvious external bleeding should be controlled with manual pressure. Hemostats should never be placed blindly into bleeding wounds, as they are rarely placed on the bleeding vessel and they damage adjacent tissue, including nerves and tendons. Impaled objects should not be removed because they may be providing tamponade to injured or transected vessels. Venous access needs to be obtained, ideally with two large catheters in separate extremities. Acceptable sites include the greater saphenous vein anterior to the medial malleolus, the median cephalic vein at the antecubital fossa, the main cephalic vein of the arm, the external jugular vein, and in children under 6 years of age, intraosseous access in the tibia. Lower extremity access is efficacious and entirely acceptable with abdominal and pelvic injuries. Central venous access, such as the internal jugular or subclavian vein, is difficult in children, especially during the resuscitation effort, and should be attempted only by experienced personnel. Blood for laboratory studies and crossmatching can be obtained from these catheters before intravenous fluids are begun.

The child in shock has lost approximately 25% of his blood volume, or approximately 20 ml/kg. An initial fluid bolus of 20 ml/kg of Ringer's lactate solution should be given and repeated if necessary. Crystalloid replacement of whole blood loss needs to be three times the shed blood volume to fully restore the circulating volume, assuming there is no further blood loss. Therefore, if the patient is still unstable or hypovolemic after the second fluid bolus, immediate transfusion should be given with type O Rh-negative blood until type-specific or fully crossmatched blood becomes available. Patients needing operative intervention require special consideration, since the induction of anesthesia causes a loss of sympathetic tone, leading to vasodilatation. This sudden increase in vascular capacity can result in profound hypotension, tissue hypoxia, and ischemia.

Emergency department resuscitative thoracotomy should be considered for all children who present in extremis from penetrating injury. Although the application needs to be selective, the decision whether to perform resuscitative thoracotomy must be immediate, since time is of the essence. Rare anecdotal reports of successful emergency resuscitative thoracotomies have fostered the false impression that children are more tolerant of ischemia than adults. Children have a higher oxygen demand per kilogram than adults and are not resistant to ischemic injury. Resuscitative thoracotomy in patients of any age without organized cardiac activity after penetrating trauma or in extremis after blunt trauma is futile. These patients have exsanguinated and sustained irreversible ischemic injury. Those patients who present with penetrating injuries below the diaphragm and organized cardiac activity or waning signs of life may benefit from resuscitative thoracotomy with crossclamping of the descending aorta if an operating room is not immediately available. Without rapid volume expansion and immediate operative control of bleeding, however, resuscitative thoracotomy is futile. Resuscitative thoracotomy for penetrating thoracic injury is most successful in the treatment of pericardial tamponade secondary to a stab wound to the heart. Cardiac gunshot wounds occasionally are amenable to this treatment, and given the smaller thoracic diameter of children, any penetrating injury of the chest has this potential.

Once the primary and secondary surveys have been completed, if the patient is stable, portable x-rays should be obtained of all body regions with suspected injury or containing a bullet. The patient should not be sent to the radiology department, where monitoring may be suboptimal. If blood for laboratory studies was not obtained when intravenous access was obtained, it should be obtained at this time. A nasogastric tube and Foley catheter will be needed if the patient is going to the operating room. Since these are noxious procedures, especially to an injured child, consideration should be given to placing these catheters after anesthesia has been induced in the operating room. The status of the child's tetanus immunization should be reviewed and supplemented as indicated. Antibiotic coverage should be considered in all patients, and a first- or second-generation cephalosporin should be given to all patients who require operative intervention. Judicious doses of intravenous analgesics should be given if the patient is not going to the operating room immediately.

SPECIFIC CARE

Penetrating injuries of the head that involve the brain are highly lethal and mandate immediate neurosurgical evaluation. The patient who is poorly responsive or in coma should be intubated and hyperventilated. Associated injuries must be identified and addressed promptly. Volume resuscitation should not be limited because of concerns for cerebral edema. The unavoidable elevation of intracranial pressure associated with direct brain injury requires an increased systemic blood pressure to maintain adequate cerebral perfusion and oxygen delivery during that time when the injured brain has increased oxygen demand and is exquisitely sensitive to hypoxemia.

Penetrating injuries to the face can compromise the airway by direct injury or through swelling that obliterates the airway. The patient should be intubated immediately before airway compromise occurs. Bleeding can be massive and difficult to control. If direct manual compression is ineffective in controlling bleeding, a Foley catheter can be carefully introduced through the wound to the level of the suspected bleeding site, and the balloon can be inflated. This will tamponade the bleeding until definitive therapy in the operating room. If a Foley catheter is used, a clamp must be placed across the catheter to prevent blood from draining retrograde through the lumen. Balloon catheter tamponade can also be used for nasopharyngeal bleeding either in combination with or in lieu of packing.

Penetrating injuries of the neck that violate the platysma muscle often require exploration in the operating room. The wound should never be explored in the emergency department because of the potential for renewed vigorous bleeding. In stable patients, direct laryngoscopy, bronchoscopy, esophagoscopy, angiography, and Gastrografin swallow will delineate most injuries and may obviate the need for exploration. The decision for nonoperative management should be made by the surgeon. All patients require careful inhospital observation.

Simple gunshot and stab wounds involving only the hemithorax and not the mediastinum usually can be managed with a chest tube. Suspected mediastinal injuries require a thorough workup that includes bronchoscopy, esophagoscopy and aortography. Thoracotomy is necessary in only 15% of thoracic injuries. It is reserved for unstable patients and those with defined injuries. Thoracotomy may be needed to control bleeding if the chest tube initially drains over 10 to 15 ml/kg of blood on initial placement or continues to drain blood at a rate in excess of 3 to 5 ml/kg/h.

Exploratory laparotomy is mandatory for all penetrating injuries of the abdomen. Injuries in the area of the mid and lower ribcage and upper abdomen have the potential for concomitant abdominal and thoracic injury. They present difficult management decisions but often may be managed with chest tube placement and exploratory laparotomy.

Gluteal gunshot wounds need to be assessed for passage of the bullet into the pelvis. The bullet trajectory may be ascertained by placing a radiopaque marker, such as a paperclip secured with tape, over the wound sites and obtaining an anteroposterior pelvic film. Often, a lateral or oblique pelvic film will clarify whether the pelvis has been violated. If the bullet is determined to have crossed the margin of the pelvis, the patient should undergo laparotomy. If the pelvic margin is not violated, the patient can be managed with local wound care and in-hospital observation. Penetrating injuries of the buttocks that involve only the gluteal musculature can lacerate gluteal vessels and may require surgery or angiography for hemostasis.

Bony fractures resulting from penetrating injuries may require open debridement and reconstruction. Initial management includes splinting, radiographic evaluation, and prompt orthopedic consultation. An intravenous first-generation cephalosporin is usually indicated.

The child's overall safety is paramount, and all pediatric patients who have been shot or stabbed should be admitted to the hospital. Personnel experienced in pediatric psychology, as well as individuals familiar with child abuse cases, should be consulted in all cases. The psychologic impact of the physical injuries can be severe and result in permanent psychologic disorders. If the injury was intentional, the child is unlikely to give an accurate account of the injury until some rapport has been developed with a member of the treatment team. Clearly, a child cannot be returned to an environment where he or she is at risk for repeat injury.

The management of penetrating pediatric trauma is best performed by a calm and organized team of responders to evaluate the patient's injuries and begin treatment. A surgeon needs to be part of the resuscitation team from the outset, since the vast majority of patients sustaining penetrating injury will require operative intervention. On a larger scale, trauma care requires the efforts of a multitude of specialties, and coordination of these specialists can be the most difficult aspect of the delivery of care. The pediatrician is in the ideal position to administrate the efforts of all the specialists and maintain the broad overview of the postinjury physical and psychologic rehabilitation needs of the injured child.

REFERENCES

1. Joy AM: Psychosocial complications. In Mattox KL (ed): Complications of Trauma. New York, Churchill Livingstone, 1993.
2. Pediatric Trauma. In American College of Surgeons Committee of Trauma: Advanced Trauma Life Support Course for Physicians Student Manual. Chicago, American College of Surgeons, 1988.
3. Wasserberger J, Ordog GJ, Schatz I, Owens D, Prakash A, Balasubramaniam S: Gunshot wounds in infants and young children. In Ordog GJ (ed): Management of Gunshot Wounds. New York, Elsevier, 1988.

21

Special Problems in the Fetus and Neonate

DISTURBANCES OF INTRAUTERINE GROWTH

DAVID W. BOYLE, M.D.
JAMES A. LEMONS, M.D.

Intrauterine growth is an important sign of fetal well-being. Abnormalities of intrauterine growth are associated with increased perinatal morbidity and mortality. Although advances in fetal ultrasonography have improved greatly over the past several years, the prenatal detection of abnormalities in fetal growth remains a challenge.

DEFINITIONS

Before beginning a discussion of intrauterine growth, several concepts should be defined. Low birth weight (LBW) infants are those with a birth weight less than 2500 g. Very low birth weight (VLBW) infants are those with a birth weight less than 1500 g. Extremely low birth weight (ELBW) infants are those with a birth weight less than 1000 g. These terms describe one important factor affecting neonatal outcome, birth weight, but do not take into account the effect of gestational age. A full-term infant is an infant born at greater than 37 completed weeks through 42 completed weeks of gestation. A preterm infant, then, is one born at less than 37 completed weeks, and a postterm infant is one born after 42 completed weeks of gestation. Again, these terms are inadequate for fully assessing neonatal risk. To incorporate both gestational age and birth weight, infants are classified as small for gestational age (SGA), large for gestational age (LGA), or appropriate for gestational age (AGA). SGA infants have birth weights that are two standard deviations (2 SD) below the mean for gestational age, whereas LGA infants have birth weights 2 SD above the mean for gestational age. Infants whose birth weight is within 2 SD of the mean for gestational age are AGA. Full-term AGA infants are at the lowest risk for perinatal morbidity and mortality.

Although intrauterine growth retardation (IUGR) is often used synonymously with SGA, IUGR should be reserved to describe the pathophysiologic process resulting in restriction of fetal growth. A SGA fetus is determined statistically based on a normal distribution of birth weights at a given gestational age without consideration of the pattern of fetal growth. SGA fetuses, thus, represent a heterogeneous group, including normally grown small fetuses and those whose growth potential has been impaired. An IUGR fetus, on the other hand, is one whose growth has slowed or stopped even if the fetus is not SGA. The implications for perinatal management, as well as for perinatal morbidity and mortality, postnatal growth, and neurologic outcome, vary widely between these two groups.

Finally, SGA infants may be described as symmetrically growth retarded if all parameters of growth (birth weight, length, and head circumference) are reduced proportionately or asymmetrically growth retarded if there is disproportionate reduction in the various growth parameters. In the latter pattern, weight is affected to a greater degree than length, with relative sparing of brain growth. The pathophysiologic processes that result in these two patterns of growth retardation may be very different and have considerable prognostic significance.

Symmetric growth retardation is considered to have its origins in early gestation and is related to a decrease in growth potential that may be either hereditary or acquired. Examples include constitutional small size, congenital viral infections, chromosomal abnormalities (especially trisomies), and various genetic syndromes. In contrast, assymetric growth retardation occurs later in gestation and implies a decrease in maternal nutrient supply to the placenta or a reduction in placental substrate or oxygen transfer (or both) to the fetus, commonly referred to as *uteroplacental insufficiency*. Examples of asymmetric growth retardation include maternal starvation, preeclampsia, chronic hypertension, and maternal diabetes associated with vascular disease. The specific causes of IUGR are discussed in more detail in subsequent paragraphs.

GROWTH CURVES AND LIMITATIONS

Intrauterine growth curves have been constructed for birth weight, length, and head circumference (occipital frontal circumference, OFC) from infants born at different gestational ages. Curves have been generated compiling cross-sectional data from a variety of populations. These curves represent static measurements in individual infants and do not reflect dynamic growth of a fetus over gestation.

Classification of infants as LGA, AGA, or SGA on the basis of where they fall on an intrauterine growth curve implies an accurate assessment of the gestational age of an infant. Gestational age may be assessed from historical data (i.e., first day of the last menstrual period) or from clinical observations (i.e., fundal height, appearance of fetal heart tones). Gestational age based on this information has a range of ± 2 weeks. More recently, the use of prenatal ultrasonography to assess gestational age based on fetal morphopometric data has improved gestational age determination to within ± 1 week. However, to be accurate, these measurements need to be performed before 12 to 16 weeks gestation, at a time before the presentation of many IUGR fetuses. Postnatal determination of gestational age is based on evaluation of physical characteristics and neuromuscular maturity. The timing after birth when this examination is performed will affect its accuracy, but when performed correctly, it may be accurate to within 1 to 2 weeks.

Another consideration affecting interpretation of intrauterine growth curves is the accuracy of the individual measurements of weight, crown-heel length, and OFC. The crown-heel length is the least precise measurement. However, accurate and precise measurement of the OFC in a vaginally delivered infant with significant molding also may be difficult.

Finally, measurements made postnatally may not be representative of true in utero growth. In fact, it is not normal to be born prematurely, so that morphopometric measurements of babies born prematurely may either overestimate or underestimate the growth of an ideal fetus. Keeping in mind the problems in interpretation of intrauterine growth curves, several features of fetal growth have been demonstrated, and these curves have been useful in identifying infants at risk for neonatal morbidity and mortality.

NORMAL INTRAUTERINE GROWTH

Normal intrauterine growth is dependent on the genetic potential of the fetus and is influenced by the environment in which the fetus develops. Examination of the currently available data demonstrates that intrauterine growth curves are sigmoidal in shape. Although the fetus gains approximately 20 g/d throughout the second half of gestation, the rate of weight gain is not constant. Fetal weight increases exponentially at a rate of approximately 15 g/kg/d (1.5%/d) from 20 to 34 weeks gestation. From 34 to 40 weeks, growth rate slows. The reasons for this slowing are not clear. In fact, this apparent slowing in the rate of fetal weight gain may be artifactual because of the manner in which the data are collected. Nonetheless, possible explanations for this apparent slowing of fetal growth include physical constraints imposed on the fetus by the uterus and a relative reduction in the ability of the placenta to provide the necessary oxygen and substrates to maintain the fetal growth rate.

The increase in fetal weight over the latter portion of gestation is accompanied by complex changes in body composition. Whereas the accumulation of all of the chemical components of the fetus (water, fat, protein, and minerals) parallels the increase in body weight, the proportion of fetal weight contributed by each of these components varies as a function of gestational age. Protein content increases from 8% at 20 weeks to 12% at 40 weeks. Most notable are the changes in total body water and fat. Total body water decreases from 90% of the body mass at 20 weeks to 72% at 40 weeks. In addition, there is a shift of water from the extracellular compartment to the intracellular compartment. The most dramatic change in body composition of the human fetus is the greater than 200-fold increase in fat from <1% at 20 weeks to 12% at 40 weeks. These changes in body composition over gestation are reflective of the physiologic maturation of the fetus as it prepares for adaptation to extrauterine life.

Accompanying the changes in body composition during gestation are alterations in the energy requirements for fetal growth. Total caloric requirements of the fetus has been estimated to be approximately 100 kcal/kg/d. Energy requirements include that necessary for maintenance of basal oxidative metabolism, as well as that needed for accretion of new tissue. The latter requirement can be further divided into the energy stored in new tissue and the energy cost of tissue accretion. Because of the much greater storage of fat, with its higher caloric density, the total rate of energy storage increases by approximately 2.5-fold after 34 weeks. Perhaps this increase in the energy storage requirement beyond 34 weeks is related to the slowing in fetal growth rate seen at this point of gestation; that is, growth becomes more efficient from an energy perspective. (Nutritional strategies for neonates are designed to mimic fetal growth patterns.)

Alterations in fetal fat accumulation appear to be responsible for the altered intrauterine growth patterns of LGA and SGA infants. Macrosomic infants of diabetic mothers have a higher fat content than AGA infants born to nondiabetic mothers without differences in the chemical composition of the fat-free body mass. In addition, the differences in body composition between SGA and AGA infants are more pronounced in terms of fat content than nonfat dry weight. This suggests that in the face of reduced nutrient availability, as might occur with maternal starvation or uteroplacental insufficiency, the

fetus may be able to conserve energy by limiting the deposition of fat. The mechanisms by which this alteration in body composition might occur, however, are not known.

ETIOLOGY OF ABNORMAL FETAL GROWTH

LGA

LGA infants represent a heterogeneous group composed of infants who are normally grown, large infants and those with growth disturbances. Infants of diabetic mothers are often LGA. These infants are macrosomic, with increased muscle mass and fat deposition due to disturbances in fetal glucose homeostasis and hyperinsulinism. Organomegaly occurs in insulin-sensitive tissues, such as the heart and liver. Brain growth is not affected so that these infants will have a normal head circumference at birth. Other disorders associated with hyperinsulinism, for example, Beckwith-Wiedemann syndrome and beta-cell nesidioblastosis-adenoma spectrum, also result in excessive fetal growth. Most of the morbidity of LGA infants is related to difficulties encountered at the time of delivery and is due to their increased size. LGA infants may be delivered prematurely because of an overestimation of gestational age. There is an increased rate of cesarean section delivery. In addition, there is an increased incidence of shoulder dystocia, asphyxia, and birth injuries. Infants of diabetic mothers are also at risk for hypoglycemia, hypocalcemia, polycythemia-hyperviscosity syndrome, respiratory distress syndrome, and congenital anomalies. Obstetric and pediatric management of these infants should be directed to anticipating these problems and intervening as indicated (see Infants of Diabetic Mothers later in this chapter). Although LGA infants are still at increased risk for perinatal and neonatal morbidity, term LGA infants do not have increased neonatal mortality.

SGA

The etiology of SGA or IUGR infants can be divided into three groups based on the nature of the growth-restricting process: maternal factors, placental factors, and fetal factors.

Maternal Factors

Maternal factors beyond genetic transfer of growth potential have been shown to influence fetal size. Many SGA infants are born to mothers who have previously delivered an SGA infant. In fact, many of these women were themselves SGA. Maternal prepregnancy weight and stature also have a direct effect on fetal growth. Big mothers tend to have big babies, and small mothers have smaller babies. Uterine capacity may be a limiting factor in these women.

Maternal nutrition can greatly affect fetal growth. Prepregnancy weight and pregnancy weight gain affect fetal growth independently. These factors become especially important during the second half of gestation, when fetal weight is increasing exponentially and the metabolic demands on the mother are greatest. Many studies in animal models, as well as in humans exposed to periods of famine due to natural disasters, have demonstrated the importance of maintaining maternal caloric intake to avoid IUGR.

Chronic maternal illnesses that adversely affect uterine perfusion or are associated with chronic hypoxia will result in IUGR. Diseases that cause uterine ischemia include chronic or essential hypertension, pregnancy-induced hypertension-preeclampsia, and advanced diabetes mellitus associated with end-organ disease. Maternal conditions that result in uterine hypoxia include cyanotic heart disease, sickle cell anemia, such chronic pulmonary diseases as asthma and cystic fibrosis, and delivery at high altitude. In addition, maternal smoking and maternal drug use can result in IUGR.

Placental Factors

Placental function is critical to normal fetal growth. The placenta acts as an organ of gas exchange and nutrient transfer between the mother and the fetus. Placental insufficiency may be due to decreased uterine or umbilical perfusion or to a maternal nutritional deficiency or may be a complication of maternal vascular disease. Other placental disorders that affect placental function include chorioangioma, villitis, abnormalities of the umbilical cord, multiple infarcts, chronic abruptio placentae, and abnormalities of implantation.

Fetal Factors

Genetic determinants of fetal size are inherited from both parents. The ultimate attainment of this growth potential is then modulated by various environmental factors. Fetal genetic factors account for approximately 20% of SGA infants. In general, these infants tend to be symmetrically growth retarded. In particular, trisomies of chromosomes 8, 13, 18, and 21 result in IUGR. In addition, aberration of the number of X and Y chromosomes are associated with IUGR. Single-gene defects and many syndromes are associated with poor fetal growth and may result in IUGR.

In addition to inherited fetal abnormalities, congenitally acquired viral infections may result in symmetric growth retardation if the infection occurs during early gestation. Most notable is the growth retardation associated with cytomegalovirus (CMV) and rubella virus. These agents affect fetal growth by impairing placental function through inflammation of the villi, by inhibiting cell division, and by causing cell death either by an obliterative angiopathy or by cytolysis.

Multiple Gestation

Multiple gestations may produce growth retardation of one or all of the fetuses through several mechanisms. One of the primary determinants of fetal size is the constraint exerted by uterine capacity. This effect is observed when the combined fetal weight approaches 3 kg. The number of fetuses is important in determining the onset of fetal crowding in these pregnancies. Maternal nutritional factors are important in maintaining an adequate substrate supply to multiple growing fetuses. This metabolic demand increases with the number of fetuses. In addition, placental factors, such as implantation site and vascular anastomoses, as may occur in diamniotic monochorionic twins, may be associated with IUGR. Arteriovenous anastomoses will lead to a twin-to-twin transfusion. The donor fetus may be anemic and growth retarded, whereas the recipient fetus is often plethoric and normally grown.

DIAGNOSIS AND MANAGEMENT OF IUGR

Management of IUGR should begin during the pregnancy. A history of poor nutrition, a preexisting condition associated with IUGR as outlined, previous delivery of an SGA infant, or diagnosis of a multiple gestation pregnancy should increase the level of suspicion of the potential for IUGR. Such women should be followed closely with frequent examinations and ultrasound evaluation of fetal size and amount of amniotic fluid. Nonetheless, even if this intensive evaluation is completed, as many as 40% of SGA/IUGR fetuses will go unrecognized.

When poor fetal growth is identified, nonstress testing should begin at 26 weeks, and contraction stress testing with evaluation of the biophysical profile (ultrasound evaluation of fetal movement, amount of amniotic fluid, and fetal breathing movements, together with fetal heart rate and posture and tone) should be performed as clinically indicated. Bedrest on the left side may be effective when it is thought that there may be impaired placental blood flow, as with hypertensive disorders. Diuretics should be avoided, since they tend to diminish placental blood flow. The use of low-dose aspirin and dipyridamole to prevent recurrent idiopathic fetal growth retardation is under investigation. A mother thought to be at risk of delivering an infant with severe growth retardation or chronic asphyxia should be referred to a high-risk center. Early delivery may be indicated to remove the infant from a less than optimal environment. During labor and delivery, problems with hypoxia may be minimized by careful fetal monitoring. At delivery, the clinician should be prepared to resuscitate the infant, as the incidence of birth depression in these infants is high. Meconium aspiration should be prevented by aspiration of the nasopharynx and trachea as indicated.

In the newborn nursery, the infant should be observed for signs and symptoms of chronic or acute hypoxia, such as seizures and other signs of hypoxic-ischemic encephalopathy, diminished urine output, respiratory failure, persistent fetal circulation, coagulation abnormalities, and congestive heart failure with mitral insufficiency.

Infants need to be screened early for hypoglycemia. Chronic malnutrition will result in decreased glycogen stores, and asphyxia will rapidly deplete whatever glycogen is present. Early feedings should be initiated by mouth or by gavage. If the infant has been seriously hypoxic or is also immature or otherwise impaired, however, intravenous administration of glucose may be indicated.

The infant is examined for birth defects and minor anomalies that led to the diagnosis of unsuspected major anomalies. Chromosome analysis should be done if the physical findings are suspicious for a chromosomal abnormality. Examination of the placenta is important and often helpful in ruling out intrauterine infection. TORCH screening of cord blood serum is not indicated. If intrauterine infection is strongly suspected, the maternal VDRL, hepatitis, HIV, and rubella status should be reviewed. Total serum IgM levels may be useful as a screen, and a urine culture for CMV should be obtained. Imaging of the brain for calcifications and examination of the spinal fluid for protein and cells also may be indicated.

Because the infant is small with relatively large metabolic demands, heat loss and heat production may be impaired, and temperature control may be defective. Careful attention should be paid to thermal environment, particularly when the infant is wet or exposed for examination or procedures. Other metabolic complications, such as hypocalcemia, should be watched for and treated.

Some infants with chronic in utero hypoxia have a high hematocrit level, and blood flow to various organs may be diminished because of increased blood viscosity. These infants are particularly susceptible to hypoglycemia. Plasma reduction exchange transfusion may be useful in infants with central venous hematocrits greater than 65%, especially if clinical manifestations suggest hyperviscosity syndrome (see Neonatal Polycythemia and Hyperviscosity later in this chapter).

Early postnatal weight gain and appropriate head growth may be indicators that an infant will do well. The ultimate prognosis for infants with extreme IUGR is guarded, however, particularly when the cause is unknown. In addition, perinatal events, such as asphyxia, will also contribute to the infant's neurologic development. The infant need not be kept in the hospital until a particular weight is achieved. When the infant is gaining weight well, feeding well, able to maintain heat balance, and free of other significant problems, he or she may be discharged home.

MANAGEMENT OF THE NEWBORN INFANT AT DELIVERY

Ian R. Holzman, M.D.

The uncomplicated birth of a newborn infant is an event occurring around the world innumerable times each day. The physiologic changes accompanying this process are exceedingly complex yet occur repeatedly without difficulty. Because of this, we often fail to appreciate them until we face a delivery gone awry. The need for prompt and skillful resuscitation demands a clear grasp of normal and abnormal physiology and the personnel and tools critical to the task.

CARDIOVASCULAR TRANSITION

Birth induces profound circulatory changes that can have an impact on resuscitation. Most obvious of these is the loss of the large, low-resistance placental circulation. This is accompanied by a decrease in pulmonary vascular resistance and an increase in pulmonary blood flow that occur in concert with an increase in systemic resistance.

These changes allow for a marked redistribution of blood flow that can be interrupted by asphyxia, acidosis, hypercarbia, and hypovolemia. The failure to decrease pulmonary vascular resistance will lead to right-to-left intraatrial and ductal shunting and systemic hypoxemia. There may also be significant tricuspid valve insufficiency contributing to the atrial level shunt.

PERINATAL ASPHYXIA

The use of the phrase "perinatal asphyxia" should denote a specific sequence of events in close proximity to the delivery of the infant. Asphyxia has a biochemical definition that includes an increase in blood lactic acid, an increase in carbon dioxide, and a decrease in arterial oxygen (usually measured as Po_2). It is the result of an inadequate supply of oxygen to the tissues regardless of the cause. The magnitude of the immediate perinatal insult, both in severity and duration, is usually reflected in the ease by which an infant can be resuscitated and in the totality of the organ damage. Infants who do not clearly fit into the known causes of perinatal asphyxia or who do not have a postnatal course consistent with a lack of oxygen to tissues or organs should not be labeled as asphyxiated.

DELIVERY ROOM

General Organization

The need for swift action requires that proper working equipment is immediately available. It is also essential that there be a clearly written procedure assigning responsibility for the care and maintenance of delivery room equipment.

There should be an area specifically designed for infant care in each delivery room. The location of that area will depend on what role the anesthesiologist is expected to play in resuscitation. A radiant warmer with temperature control probes that can be affixed to the right upper quadrant of the abdomen or rectum and adequate lighting are essential. A source of oxygen with a flowmeter normally set to 6 L/min and wall suction with a mechanism to prevent undue negative pressure (20 to 30 cm H_2O is normally adequate) must be easily reachable by the health care team. A visible clock is extremely helpful for counting heart rate and respiration, and an electronic Apgar timer is ideal.

Specific Equipment

The single, most crucial piece of equipment for resuscitation is a working neonatal bag-mask-valve assembly that can deliver 100% oxygen. An attached oxygen reservoir is usually required for this. The addition of a manometer into the system can greatly decrease the risk of pneumothoraces. A selection of face masks specifically designed for the premature and full-term infant is essential for effective ventilation.

Various devices for suctioning the nose, mouth, and endotracheal tube are available. Any suctioning device must allow for careful control of negative pressure (usually with a fingerhole) so as not to injure a fragile airway. Uncuffed endotracheal tubes of internal diameters ranging from 2.5 to 4 mm are normally sufficient (Table 1) and can be inserted orally or nasally (the former usually is preferred in an emergency). Stiff stylets should be avoided unless intubation proves to be extremely difficult, but it is possible to make a flexible stylet

TABLE 1. Suggested Endotracheal Tube Sizes

WEIGHT (g)	GESTATIONAL AGE (weeks)	ENDOTRACHEAL TUBE SIZE (ID in mm)
<800	<26	2.5
800–1500	26–31	2.5–3
1500–2000	31–34	3
2000–3000	34–38	3–3.5
>3000	>38	3.5–4

from the aluminum curets used to culture the deep nasopharynx for bacteria. Straight laryngoscope blades of sizes 0 and 1 can be used for all intubations.

A number of other items must be immediately available but are used less frequently. These include a simple tray equipped for rapid umbilical venous catheterization, a selection of large-bore Teflon over-the-needle catheters (16, 18, and 20 gauge) for drainage of air or fluid from the chest and abdomen, and tubes for gastric decompression (5 and 8 French). The need for medications in the delivery room has been overstated, since proper attention to airway management is always more critical to success. Nevertheless, there are occasions when medications can be critical. The choice of a volume expander is a matter of local preference. Any physiologic salt solution can restore circulating volume, including an isotonic bicarbonate solution prepared by diluting 1 part standard sodium bicarbonate solution (1 mEq/ml) with 5 parts water.

It is the unusual neonate who truly is asystolic in the delivery room unless death has occurred in utero before delivery. More often than not, the inability to hear or feel a heartbeat is a technical problem when examining a sick, wet neonate. Epinephrine, if required, should be available in a form specific for neonatal use (1:10,000 solution). If mothers have received a significant narcotic dose within 3 to 4 hours of delivery, neonatal respiratory and muscular depression can result, and a neonatal solution of naloxone hydrochloride (Narcan 0.4 mg/ml, 1 mg/ml) must be accessible.

APPROACH TO RESUSCITATION

Before the actual delivery of an infant, every attempt should be made to learn the obstetric history of the mother and the possible complications expected. Preparation does much to relieve anxiety, and checking that all necessary equipment is present and working is very reassuring.

Regardless of the condition of the infant, the priority (except in the presence of thick meconium) must be to dry the baby, with an emphasis on the head and trunk, to eliminate evaporative heat loss. With smaller infants, it is also useful to use a nonporous plastic wrap over the baby to further eliminate heat loss. Clear plastic bags commonly used for equipment storage serve this purpose, and often, tiny babies can be placed within the bag with only their face uncovered. Within 10 to 15 seconds, the baby's heart rate, respiratory effort, and color and perfusion should be evaluated, which will guide the subsequent care.

Assigning an Apgar score is a worldwide tradition as a way to quantitate the cardiopulmonary status and neurologic reactivity of an infant. Although the Apgar score was initially thought to be a reliable indicator of the degree of perinatal asphyxia, it has become clear that it is fraught with much uncertainty, especially in the low birth weight (LBW) infant. When points are assigned during resuscitation, it should be made clear whether the assigned points represent spontaneous responses or are the result of ongoing resuscitation. Furthermore, assigning the score should *never* take precedence over resuscitation.

Specific Steps (Fig. 1)

Once the infant is dried and under the radiant warmer, the head and neck should be placed in a neutral position to maximize airway opening. The nose and mouth should be gently suctioned (3 to 5 seconds), since the presence of significant quantities of fluid can lead to sudden obstructive apnea in an otherwise healthy infant. A brief period of stimulation, by gently rubbing the infant's back, may induce respirations, but if regular respirations have not begun, that attempt should be abandoned after a few seconds and replaced with bag and mask ventilation with oxygen. The proper use of the bag and mask can provide adequate ventilation in almost all infants if attention is paid to providing a good seal of the mask and preventing downward pressure on the mandible with subsequent airway obstruction. *Always draw the infant's face into the mask rather than pushing down on the mask.*

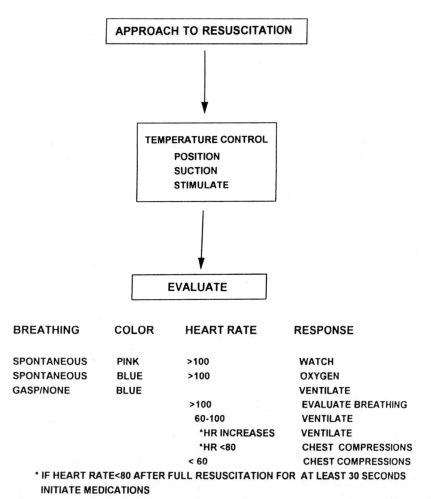

APPROACH TO RESUSCITATION

↓

**TEMPERATURE CONTROL
POSITION
SUCTION
STIMULATE**

↓

EVALUATE

BREATHING	COLOR	HEART RATE	RESPONSE
SPONTANEOUS	PINK	>100	WATCH
SPONTANEOUS	BLUE	>100	OXYGEN
GASP/NONE	BLUE		VENTILATE
		>100	EVALUATE BREATHING
		60-100	VENTILATE
		*HR INCREASES	VENTILATE
		*HR <80	CHEST COMPRESSIONS
		< 60	CHEST COMPRESSIONS

*** IF HEART RATE<80 AFTER FULL RESUSCITATION FOR AT LEAST 30 SECONDS
INITIATE MEDICATIONS**

FIGURE 21.2–1. A general outline of the steps to be taken in the assessment and resuscitation of a neonate in the delivery room.

A commonly employed algorithm for decision making in neonatal resuscitation is clearly delineated in the guidelines published jointly by the American Academy of Pediatrics and the American Heart Association.[1] Observations are made of respirations, heart rate, and color. If respirations are inadequate after the initial drying and suctioning, ventilation at a rate of 40 to 60 breaths per minute with 100% oxygen should be initiated for 15 to 30 seconds. Remember that initial breaths may require a pressure of 30 to 40 cm H_2O, but subsequent breaths can be less vigorous if there is chest expansion.

Heart rate is evaluated by auscultation or umbilical cord palpation, and three categories of response are assessed. If the heart rate is above 100 beats per minute, oxygen or continued ventilation or both are employed, depending on the infant's color. If the heart rate is between 60 and 100 beats per minute, ventilation is continued. Chest compressions are begun if the heart rate is between 60 and 80 beats per minute. It is recommended that compressions be interposed with ventilation in a 3:1 ratio so that there are 90 compressions each minute and 30 breaths. This rate of ventilation is lower than the 40 to 60 breaths per minute used if no chest compressions are required. When the heart rate is initially less than 60 beats per minute and no response has occurred to a trial of ventilation, chest compressions should begin immediately.

The use of medications in place of the proper attention to airway management interferes with resuscitation. Nevertheless, if an infant's heart rate remains below 80 beats per minute (not because of congenital heart block) despite adequate ventilation with 100% oxygen and chest compressions for at least 30 seconds, the use of epinephrine

is appropriate (Table 2). A dose of 0.1 to 0.3 mg/kg of 1:10,000 epinephrine is used intratracheally or intravenously, with the umbilical vein being the most rapid site of venous access. When given intratracheally, it is often necessary to dilute the epinephrine 1:1 with normal saline, and there is some evidence, as yet unconfirmed, that a somewhat higher dose may be necessary for intratracheal administration. Epinephrine may be given every 5 minutes during a resuscitation.

Failure to achieve the desired response with ventilation, chest compressions, and epinephrine should lead the physician to consider one of only a few possibilities. The need for volume expansion is often the reason for an inadequate response. In such a situation, the

TABLE 2. Management of Newborn Infant at Delivery

MEDICATION	CONCENTRATION	DOSE	ROUTE*
Epinephrine	1:10,000	0.1–0.3 ml/kg	IV/ET
Sodium bicarbonate	0.5 mEq/ml (4.2% solution)	2 mEq/kg	IV
Naloxone	0.4 mg/ml	0.1 mg/kg (0.25 ml/kg)	IV/ET IM†/SC
	1 mg/ml	0.1 mg/kg (0.1 ml/kg)	IV/ET IM†/SC

*ET, endotracheal.
†Acceptable but not preferred.

administration of a crystalloid solution through the umbilical vein in a dose of at least 10 ml/kg will often produce an immediate improvement. When an infant has had a response to volume expansion, it is important to search for the etiology of the volume loss (if such has occurred) and to monitor the changes in hematocrit that will occur hours later.

Mechanical causes for a lack of response to resuscitation should also be considered. The most likely problem is a pneumothorax, and the prompt evacuation of air with an 18 gauge Teflon over-the-needle catheter inserted in the second intercostal space in the midclavicular line can be lifesaving. A diaphragmatic hernia may produce a lack of breath sounds on one side of the chest (as can intubation of an individual bronchus) but will not respond to the removal of air. Other considerations include congenital lung defects, fluid in the chest or pericardium, or space-occupying lesions.

Once ventilation has been established, the possibility of a significant metabolic acidosis must be considered. The slow (over at least 2 minutes) intravenous administration of 1 to 2 mEq/kg of 0.5 mEq/ml sodium bicarbonate (not intratracheally) is recommended during prolonged resuscitation or in situations when there is ongoing production of lactic acid. On rare occasions, an infant has a depressed respiratory effort but little else to suggest a severe perinatal problem. If maternal administration of narcotics has occurred within 1 to 4 hours of birth, is is appropriate to give 0.1 mg/kg of naloxone either intravenously or endotracheally. The duration of action of the drug may be shorter than the action of the maternally derived narcotic, placing the infant at risk for recurrent respiratory depression hours after the initial dose. Close observation of these infants for at least 8 hours is mandatory. The management of deliveries accompanied by meconium is discussed in Meconium Aspiration Syndrome later in this chapter.

SUMMARY

Although the management of a sick neonate in the delivery room can be complex, planning, proper equipment, and trained personnel can ensure the best possible result. A rapidly stabilized warm infant with a secure airway should be the goal of every resuscitation. Once achieved, the next step is a careful consideration of all the diagnostic possibilities and close attention to cardiovascular and respiratory status. In most cases, it should be possible to predict the infant's subsequent course (e.g., hypotension, anemia, pulmonary hypertension, infection, seizures, renal failure) from a knowledge of the obstetric and perinatal events. Preparation again can be most reassuring.

REFERENCE

1. Chameides L (ed): Textbook of Neonatal Resuscitation. Chicago, American Heart Association, 1990.

PREPARATION FOR TRANSFER

MARY CATHERINE HARRIS, M.D.

The interhospital transfer of the critically ill neonate occurs at the most vulnerable period of his or her life. In the hours immediately after birth (or resuscitation and stabilization), plans must be made for the safe and effective transfer of the infant to a tertiary care facility. At the referring institution, preparation must begin the moment the need for transfer is realized. At the receiving institution, this preparation should begin the moment the transport call is received. From that point forward, the referring institution, the transport team, and the receiving hospital must coordinate accurate information regarding the status of the infant. With efficient communication between institutions, it may be possible to further stabilize and improve the infant's condition before transfer, making the transport a safer experience for

the neonate. Furthermore, effective communication may anticipate complications encountered on transport and promptly suggest additional management strategies.

In this section, we discuss some common neonatal problems necessitating interhospital transport of critically ill neonates. These include prematurity, respiratory and circulatory disturbances, congenital heart disease, and surgical anomalies. Using skilled personnel to provide ongoing consultation during transport and skilled members of the team to perform the transport, the vulnerable infant's prognosis can be enhanced.

GENERAL GUIDELINES

In all neonates being prepared for transfer, regardless of the underlying pathologic condition, several unifying concepts emerge. First, attention must be given to the ABCs of resuscitation and stabilization before transport. Second, it is important to anticipate problems likely to occur while the transport is in progress. For example, if the infant is at risk for apnea, persistent hypoxemia, or respiratory failure, it may well be best to perform an elective intubation and ventilate the infant during transport. Likewise, circulatory disturbances should be anticipated if the infant has received multiple infusions of crystalloid or colloid at the referring institution. The use of low-dose dopamine may provide additional circulatory stability during transport in certain circumstances. Furthermore, if either of these therapies (endotracheal intubation/ventilation, cardiovascular support) is found to be unnecessary, it can easily be discontinued at the receiving institution.

Third, one should consider the distance of the interhospital transport. The transport team should not plan to administer definitive or curative care at the referring institution. Rather, their job is to stabilize the infant and to ensure a safe transport to the receiving hospital, where definitive care is available. The decision to delay a transport while waiting for a reassuring laboratory value should be balanced against the danger of remaining in the field with an unstable infant. If the patient is being moved 20 minutes across town, it may not be appropriate to wait an additional 20 minutes for the blood gas results. Transcutaneous monitoring or pulse oximetry may be sufficient in the interim. On the other hand, if the transport is estimated to last 2½ hours, all aspects of respiratory and circulatory function should be stabilized and controlled before transfer. In certain circumstances, however, such as the referral of a critically ill neonate for extracorporeal membrane oxygenation (ECMO), it may be necessary to make the decision to transport a somewhat unstable patient, as definitive care is only available at the receiving institution. This may also be a situation when air transport becomes the preferred mode of transportation.

SPECIFIC GUIDELINES

The Premature Neonate

The premature infant has several common problems that can easily be anticipated. First, the premature infant has increased insensible water loss, necessitating attention to the maintenance of adequate hydration and electrolytes. In these infants, the establishment of venous access through either an umbilical vein or a peripheral venous line is mandatory before transfer. The infant's maintenance requirements for glucose (4 to 6 mg/kg/min), fluid (80 to 120 ml/kg/d), and electrolytes (see Fluid and Electrolyte Therapeutics later in this chapter) can then be delivered through this line. It is well known that premature infants have inadequate glycogen stores and, consequently, are at high risk for the development of hypoglycemia. Although an initial Dextrostix result should be confirmed with a serum glucose value, Dextrostix determinations may be useful during interhospital transport.

A second important need of the premature infant is temperature regulation. Maintenance of body temperature is critical to the survival of the infant in transport. Premature infants (and most term infants) are transported in heated isolettes for that reason. Skin temperatures are monitored during transport using axillary temperature readings or newly designed electronic skin probes.

Premature infants frequently are given the diagnosis of respiratory distress syndrome (RDS), and this often is the reason for transfer to a tertiary care facility. The course of this disease is characterized by gradual worsening of the infant's condition during the first few days of life. When RDS is present, the neonate should first be ensured a stable airway in preparation for transport. In addition, oxygenation and ventilation should be assessed using arterial blood gases and noninvasive monitoring. Today, many ambulances are equipped with ventilators for use in neonates, so that the infant can be stabilized on ventilator settings in the referring intensive care nursery, which are then duplicated in the ambulance during transport. In the neonate with severe RDS or pulmonary interstitial emphysema, the risk of a pneumothorax occurring during transport should be recognized, and appropriate equipment (e.g., needle, stopcock, and syringe) should be available for use if necessary. In premature neonates, respiratory illnesses are often accompanied by abnormalities of acid-base balance, including the development of metabolic acidosis. Ventilatory adjustments frequently can be made to control abnormalities of Pao_2 and $Paco_2$, but the presence of a metabolic acidosis often will require the administration of bicarbonate or tris-hydroxymethylaminomethane (THAM). If efficient communication has been established between institutions, many of these management strategies can be instituted while the team is en route. Likewise, if the infant's respiratory status has been stabilized before the team's arrival, this is likely to shorten the turnaround time for the team at the referring institution.

The Neonate with Congenital Heart Disease

The neonate with known or suspected congenital heart disease poses some special problems during transport. If the infant's heart disease has been diagnosed by fetal or neonatal echocardiography, management can be directed at the specific underlying pathology. For example, if the infant has a ductal dependent lesion that limits either pulmonary blood flow (pulmonary atresia with intact ventricular septum, tricuspid atresia) or systemic blood flow (hypoplastic left heart syndrome, coarctation of the aorta, or interrupted aortic arch), the infusion of prostaglandin E_1 to maintain ductal patency may be lifesaving. When prostaglandins are infused during transport, it is often safest to intubate the infant electively, because of the high risk of apnea with this medication. In situations where congenital heart disease is accompanied by shock, fluids and vasoactive drug infusions may be needed during transport.

In addition, the principles of management of oxygenation and ventilation in the infant with congenital heart disease are different from those in the infant with pulmonary disease. With some cardiac malformations, oxygen therapy may be contraindicated because it increases pulmonary blood flow, floods the lungs, and steals away from the systemic circulation. In addition, even though the infant may require ventilation for transport, $Paco_2$ values must be monitored closely, as a respiratory alkalosis may also increase pulmonary blood flow. In these infants, the best management is to maintain both Pao_2 and $Paco_2$ values around 40 mm Hg and to maintain the infant's pH in a neutral range with the use of sodium bicarbonate.

The infant with suspected congenital heart disease may be even more problematic for transport planning and management. One may arrive at the referring institution expecting to transport an infant with pulmonary disease, only to find that the diagnosis is more likely to be congenital heart disease. Furthermore, the chest radiograph may or may not be helpful in making that distinction. The diagnosis of cyanotic congenital heart disease may be confirmed by the hyperoxia test, in which the change in Po_2 in response to placement of the infant in 100% oxygen is assessed. Cyanosis from cardiac disease will not improve with the administration of 100% oxygen, although cyanosis from pulmonary disease should lessen. This distinction may be difficult in cases of pulmonary disease complicated by right-to-left shunting and pulmonary hypertension, as these infants may also fail the hyperoxia test. In these instances, a specific diagnosis may not be known during the transport process and may await definitive evaluation at the receiving institution.

The care for infants with suspected congenital heart disease on transport should be delivered in consultation with the most experienced neonatologists and cardiologists available. In this way, the best decisions can be made with regard to provision of oxygen, target parameters for ventilation, and administration of medications, such as prostaglandins and vasoactive agents. Moreover, excessive time should not be wasted at the referring institution attempting to obtain a specific diagnosis for the infant. Rather, care should be directed toward stabilization for the safest and fastest transport to the receiving institution where definitive care is available.

The Neonate with Surgical Disease

Many infants are transported for the evaluation of known or suspected surgical diseases. These include infants who are clinically stable but whose radiographs or clinical examination suggests a surgical lesion. On the other hand, many of the infants transferred for surgical evaluation require acute stabilization during the transport process and emergent surgical intervention on arrival at the receiving institution. Although the list of surgical anomalies prompting referral is extensive, some of the more common problems necessitating transport include congenital diaphragmatic hernia, abdominal wall defects, esophageal atresia and associated anomalies, intestinal obstruction, and necrotizing enterocolitis.

Congenital Diaphragmatic Hernia

The infant with a congenital diaphragmatic hernia (CDH) often presents as a true medical and surgical emergency. These infants usually exhibit signs of cyanosis and severe respiratory distress during the first several hours of life. This diagnosis may be suspected in the infant with diminished or absent breath sounds in the left chest, heart sounds auscultated in the right chest, and the presence of a scaphoid abdomen. If the referring physician is uncertain of the infant's diagnosis, the clinical examination can be confirmed with radiographs demonstrating air-filled bowel loops and the presence of the nasogastric tube in the chest. The abdomen is frequently gasless. As many newborn infants with CDH quickly progress to respiratory failure, their stabilization and transfer to a tertiary care facility become a matter of utmost urgency.

Although CDH is no longer considered an operative emergency, urgent stabilization is required to reverse the hypoxemia, hypercarbia, and metabolic acidosis associated with this condition. These management strategies must be initiated immediately on receipt of the transport call. Once the diagnosis is certain, the management of the infant should be directed toward reversal of the infant's hypoxemia and hypercarbia. Such management should include mechanical ventilation with 100% oxygen, alkalinization with hyperventilation and administration of sodium bicarbonate or THAM, and the use of sedation and paralysis as necessary to control oxygenation and ventilation. Fluid and vasopressor support may be necessary to correct hypotension. Decompression of the abdominal gas in the thorax should be accomplished using a nasogastric tube attached to suction.

It is extremely important to transfer these infants to a tertiary care facility where definitive therapies are available. Many of these infants are desperately ill and are not suitable candidates for immediate surgery. In these instances, ECMO may be used as a temporizing therapy until the pulmonary hypertension has abated and the infant's condition has stabilized.

Abdominal Wall Defects

The transport management of the infant with an abdominal wall defect also presents some special considerations. The most common abdominal wall defects are omphalocele and gastroschisis. If the diagnosis of gastroschisis or omphalocele has been made by antenatal ultrasound, the mother should be referred to a high-risk perinatal center for delivery. Similarly, infants born with gastroschisis or omphalocele should be transported to a tertiary care center as soon as possible after delivery for definitive care and repair of the abdominal wall defect.

The management of both lesions in the delivery room and nursery in preparation for transport is similar. The abdomen should be wrapped with saline-soaked gauze and covered by an outer dry layer of a thin plastic wrap for transport. The dressing should be kept moist. The outer plastic covering is applied to limit fluid and heat losses. Pressure should not be placed on the umbilicus in an attempt to reduce the defect, as this may diminish circulation to the affected bowel. A nasogastric tube should be placed to limit abdominal distention, and intravenous fluids should be administered to ensure adequate hydration of the infant. A blood culture should be obtained, and the infant should be started on broad-spectrum antibiotics. In infants with suspected omphalocele, attention should be directed to the possible presence of additional anomalies, including cardiac and chromosomal abnormalities.

Esophageal Atresia and Tracheoesophageal Fistula

Esophageal atresia may occur with or without an associated tracheoesophageal fistula. In the most common variety, there is atresia of the upper pouch of the esophagus with a distal tracheoesophageal communication. With esophageal atresia, there is often a history of polyhydramnios. Affected infants have excessive oral secretions that require frequent suctioning and that increase the risk of aspiration. The diagnosis of esophageal atresia is confirmed radiographically by visualizing the nasogastric tube coiled within a blind esophageal pouch. The presence of abdominal gas confirms the presence of a distal tracheoesophageal fistula. In infants with esophageal atresia without tracheoesophageal fistula, air is absent from abdominal radiographs and the abdomen is scaphoid in appearance. The management of infants with esophageal atresia involves the insertion of a sump suction catheter into the proximal pouch of the esophagus for the continuous evacuation of secretions. The infant should be placed NPO and maintained in an upright position to help avoid the aspiration of gastric secretions through the fistula and into the lungs. Maintenance intravenous fluids should be administered to ensure adequate hydration during transport. As associated anomalies may occur in as many as 40% of infants with esophageal atresia, a careful search must be made for any associated abnormalities. The most common associated malformations include cardiac and gastrointestinal anomalies.

Intestinal Obstruction

Intestinal obstruction in the newborn infant may occur secondary to a variety of causes. These include intrinsic lesions, such as atresias, stenoses, and meconium ileus, or extrinsic lesions, such as volvulus, peritoneal bands, annular pancreas, cysts, and tumors. Vomiting is a common sign and may occur soon after birth, particularly if the obstruction is high or complete. Abdominal distention frequently accompanies vomiting and is generally present by 24 to 48 hours. The failure to pass meconium indicates that the lesion is lower and more likely to be located in the colon.

In all these conditions, the infant should be promptly transferred to a unit where surgical expertise is readily available. During the period of acute stabilization, the infant should be resuscitated with intravenous fluids in preparation for transport. In addition, the infant should be made NPO, and a nasogastric tube should be inserted and kept attached to suction. It is not necessary, and may be harmful, to delay the infant's transport for the establishment of a definitive diagnosis. The specific etiology can be determined at the receiving hospital, where the surgical team is also prepared to take the infant to the operating room emergently.

Necrotizing Enterocolitis

Necrotizing enterocolitis (NEC) often presents as acute and fulminant sepsis and shock. These infants may quickly become acutely ill, and the planning and management of their transport may be an important determinant of survival. During the planning stages, the infant should receive fluid and blood products to maintain peripheral perfusion and blood pressure. It is a common mistake to administer inadequate amounts of intravenous fluids. Fluid losses are accentuated by third space capillary leak into the periphery and abdominal cavity. Blood pressure and perfusion may need support with inotropic agents, such as dopamine and dobutamine, which may also help to increase renal perfusion. Ventilatory needs must also be anticipated. These infants may develop apnea during the acute process, and in the ill-appearing infant with NEC, it is often best to perform an elective intubation before transport. Abdominal distention may limit thoracic expansion and interfere with mechanical ventilation. These infants frequently develop both respiratory and metabolic acidosis, which should be treated appropriately with ventilation and sodium bicarbonate. Before transfer, the infant should be placed NPO, the abdomen should be decompressed by insertion of a nasogastric tube, and broad-spectrum antibiotics should be administered after blood cultures have been obtained.

The Neonate with Shock

The emergency management and transport of the neonate in shock presents a special challenge. Regardless of the etiology, this diagnosis carries with it an extremely high morbidity and mortality, necessitating prompt recognition and early institution of aggressive support measures to avoid multiple organ system failure.

During the newborn period, shock is most frequently classified as hypovolemic, cardiogenic, or septic in origin. Although defining the etiology of shock in a particular infant may present some useful guidelines for management and treatment, many of the principles of management are the same regardless of the specific etiology. It is now recognized that the evolution of shock involves the interaction of a wide array of mediators, as well as physiologic derangements and adjustments in which the host immune system is an active participant.

When the transport call is first received, an assessment is made of the infant's hemodynamic stability. This assessment includes determination of blood pressure, heart rate, skin color and perfusion, capillary refill time, and urine output. It is important to remember that a neonate may maintain an adequate central blood pressure at the expense of intense vasoconstriction, making the blood pressure measurement less reliable than other clinical parameters for the diagnosis of shock. When one is communicating with the referring institution, it is important to try to assess these clinical parameters, as the prompt and early recognition of shock may result in improved morbidity and mortality and avoidance of multiple organ system failure.

One of the first steps in the management of shock is the establishment of adequate venous access for the administration of fluid. Although it may not be practical to place a central venous catheter at the referring institution, one, and optimally two, venous lines should be inserted for transport. The infant should be given a trial of fluid administration in the form of either crystalloid or blood products depending on the presumed etiology of the hemodynamic instability. The second venous line should be reserved for the administration of antibiotics and code medications should they become necessary. The infant should receive 20 to 40 ml/kg of fluid, following which a reassessment should be made. If there has been little or no clinical improvement or if the infant develops signs of congestive heart failure or pulmonary edema, it may be appropriate to initiate support with inotropic agents (dopamine or dobutamine). Similarly, if there are findings suggestive of a ductal dependent lesion, a prostaglandin E_1 infusion may be indicated (see section on Congenital Heart Disease). Antibiotics should be administered to all infants presenting with shock after a blood culture has been obtained, as bacterial infection has been known to present in the absence of identifiable risk factors.

The management of the neonate in shock also involves control of the infant's airway and ventilation. Even if the infant is not apneic or demonstrating signs of respiratory distress, it is usually safest to intubate the infant electively for transport. The infant in shock should receive aggressive ventilatory management and supplemental oxygen to ensure adequate tissue oxygenation. In situations where the etiology of shock is unknown, this management is best coordinated with the most experienced neonatologists and cardiologists at the receiving institution, who can help to make the best decisions for the infant's care.

The optimal management of the infant in shock should also include measurement of arterial blood gases to assess gas exchange and acid-base status. An ongoing respiratory acidosis should be treated with more effective ventilation strategies. The presence of a metabolic acidosis should be aggressively treated with ½-strength sodium bicarbonate (1 to 2 mEq/kg), and it may be necessary to administer additional doses of bicarbonate or use an infusion during the transport process.

It is important to understand that shock is an ongoing process, which is mediated through the release of vasoactive mediators into the circulation. This period of hemodynamic instability may continue long after the initiating problem has been corrected. Thus, therapies should be directed toward supporting the infant through this critical period of hemodynamic instability. It cannot be assumed that the infant is "out of the woods" if the blood pressure begins to stabilize. The team transporting this patient should have albumin, saline, and blood products available for administration. Additional inotropic medications and infusion pumps should be prepared.

PREPARATION OF THE PARENTS AND REFERRING PHYSICIAN FOR TRANSPORT

The transfer of the critically ill neonate occurs during one of the most vulnerable periods of his or her life. This may also be one of the most vulnerable periods of this infant's parents' lives. In this situation, honest and accurate communication with parents is crucial. They must be apprised of the infant's diagnosis and condition before departure of the transport team. The team should bring the infant in the transport isolette to visit the parents before leaving for the receiving hospital. This may be the last time the parents see their infant alive, and the few extra minutes taken for this event should never be omitted.

Finally, the transport team should prepare the referring physician by reviewing the infant's diagnosis, condition, and prognosis before departure. Optimally, there should be additional communication to confirm diagnosis and discuss ongoing management later during the same or the following day.

CONCLUSIONS

The preparation of the neonate for transfer involves optimal communication, attention to the specific disease process necessitating transfer, stabilization, and management of the infant. Using these modalities, the skilled members of the transport team can maximize this vulnerable infant's prognosis to prevent excessive morbidity and mortality.

REFERENCES

1. Day SE: Intratransport stabilization and management of the pediatric patient. Pediatr Clin North Am 40:263–274, 1993.
2. MacDonald MG, Miller MK (eds): Emergency Transport of the Perinatal Patient. Boston: Little, Brown & Company, 1989.
3. Sandman K: Emergency stabilization in transport of the critically ill neonate. Crit Care Nurse 8:14–15, 1988.

REWARMING AND HYPOTHERMIA

SHAUL SOFER, M.D.

Humans, since they belong to the homeothermic species, are able to maintain a constant body temperature in the presence of marked changes in environmental temperature. Breakdown of homeostasis, however, can occur from both environmental and pathologic causes, resulting in hypothermia or hyperthermia. Newborn infants are particularly prone to hypothermia because of a relative lack of movement and diminished shivering, increased heat loss because of impaired vasomotor reflexes, a large surface area/body mass ratio, and poorly developed subcutaneous fat. In developed countries, neonatal hypothermia is rare and is usually secondary to extremely cold winters or excessive air conditioning. In underdeveloped areas, even in subtropical climates, neonatal hypothermia is not uncommon and is closely related to poverty, home deliveries, and lack of medical assistance.

Premature and low birth weight (LBW) infants born during the cold season to young (inexperienced) mothers from lower socioeconomic strata are at particular risk for neonatal hypothermia. Other factors predisposing to hypothermia include perinatal stress, malnutrition, birth defects, immaturity of the immune system, leukopenia, and aspiration. These factors are also associated with neonatal infection, which is found in up to 60% of hypothermic infants. Infection can cause hypothermia by promoting tissue catabolism and disturbing normal hypothalamic temperature control mechanisms. Neonatal hypothermia is further associated with severe metabolic disturbances, bleeding tendency, and respiratory failure, which in turn may be related to severe infection. Therefore, neonatal hypothermia should not be termed "accidental hypothermia," since factors other than low environmental temperature are involved. This term should be reserved for adults and older children and does not apply to neonates and infants. In 1948, Nassau introduced the term "neonatal cold injury" to emphasize the uniqueness and severity of this syndrome. The morbidity and mortality of this condition correlate with the severity of the hypothermic episode. Mortality rates as high as 71% have been reported.

There is no agreement about the minimum body temperature required for a diagnosis of neonatal hypothermia. In our experience, the clinical signs of neonatal hypothermia are rarely observed in infants with body temperature above 34°C. However, the classic picture and severe complications are common in infants with rectal temperature of 34°C or below. Infants with a body temperature of 31°C to 34°C should be classified as mildly hypothermic, 28°C to 31°C as moderately hypotermic, and below 28°C severely hypothermic.

CLINICAL PICTURE

The clinical manifestations of this syndrome may be unrecognized for some time because the infant often does not appear critically ill. The early clinical signs usually are lethargy and decreased feeding. The infant is cold to touch, with edema of the extremities and a peculiar ruddy red appearance. The heart rate is usually slow, and respiration is slow and shallow. Periodic breathing and apneic episodes are not uncommon, although some infants may exhibit respiratory difficulty with tachypnea and cyanosis. In severe cases, the infant may be comatose or hypertonic and may exhibit focal or general seizures. Severe dehydration, oliguria, and shock may occur, and bleeding from injection sites and the gastrointestinal and respiratory tracts is not uncommon.

It should be emphasized that even when the infant's condition has become critical, the appearance of the infant can be deceiving, since the edema and redness of the face and extremities make the infant look healthy and pink. Most infants have a quiet and content appearance and do not draw the attention of caregivers. The most important alarming signs are coldness to touch and low body temperature.

DIAGNOSTIC MEASURES

Peripheral white blood cell counts frequently are abnormal, and thrombocytopenia is a common finding. A prolonged prothrombin time (PT) and partial thromboplastin time (PTT) are seen in about 50% of cases. Hyperglycemia or hypoglycemia may be present. Therefore, a blood glucose determination should be performed on arrival at the emergency department. Elevated blood urea nitrogen (BUN) and creatinine and electrolyte disturbances are common. A sepsis workup should be initiated promptly and should include blood, cerebrospinal fluid (CSF), urine, and stool culture. The lumbar puncture should be deferred in any infant who is clinically unstable. Arterial blood gases may demonstrate CO_2 retention, metabolic acidemia, or hypoxemia. Thyroid function must be assessed and should be repeated after recovery if triiodothyronine (T_3) or thyroxine (T_4) values are low. A chest radiograph is indicated in infants with respiratory disturbances and may show pulmonary overinflation and infiltrates. In the presence of pulmonary infiltrates, infections, atelectasis, and hemorrhage must all be considered diagnostic possibilities. The heart shadow is usually small, reflecting the state of dehydration. Electrocardiography usually demonstrates sinus bradycardia, and unlike adults, J waves and (ventricular) arrhythmias are uncommon. If respiratory syncytial virus is a diagnostic possibility, tests and appropriate cultures and rapid slide tests should be obtained. We have noted an association of neonatal hypothermia with respiratory syncytial viral infections. A cranial computed tomography (CT) scan and electroencephalogram (EEG) are indicated for infants in coma or for those with seizures.

TREATMENT

All infants with neonatal hypothermia should be admitted to a newborn or pediatric intensive care unit and closely monitored, even when vital signs are normal on arrival. Severe apneic episodes, bleeding, and shock with multiorgan system failure may develop later in the course of the disease, resulting in a fatal outcome.

Therapy should be focused initially on management of complications rather than correction of temperature. Securing a patent airway and establishing a normal breathing pattern and circulation are of utmost importance. Infants with respiratory failure should be intubated and mechanically ventilated immediately. Hypoxic infants with a normal ventilatory pattern (normal P_{CO_2} and normal pH) should be given supplemental oxygen. Infants with hypopnea or short apneic spells may be treated initially with methylxanthines (caffeine or theophylline). Infants with severe apneic episodes followed by cyanosis or bradycardia or those with frequently recurring apneic episodes unresponsive to methylxanthines should be mechanically ventilated. Patients with shock or severe dehydration should be mechanically ventilated and resuscitated with fluid. Inotropic therapy, such as dopamine or dobutamine, is indicated in infants with persistent shock that is refractory to fluid resuscitation.

Fresh frozen plasma, cryoprecipitate, and vitamin K can all be given when the PT and PTT are prolonged ($>$ 1.5 times the control value). In the absence of overt bleeding, platelets should be infused if counts are lower than $20,000/mm^3$. In the presence of bleeding, platelet counts should be kept $\geq 60,000/mm^3$. Serum electrolyte imbalance, especially hyponatremia or hypernatremia, should be corrected slowly, whereas hypoglycemia should be corrected immediately. Broad-spectrum antibiotics are given as soon as the diagnostic workup for sepsis has been completed. As in neonatal sepsis, ampicillin in combination with a third-generation cephalosporin or an aminoglycoside is usually used. In cases complicated by shock and renal failure, aminoglycosides should be avoided if possible. A nasogastric tube should be inserted in all infants, and no oral feeding should be introduced for at least 24 hours. An indwelling urine catheter should be used only in cases of shock and oliguria. Diazepam may be used for immediate seizure control, followed by conventional anticonvulsants.

REWARMING

The management of rewarming is controversial. Both active external rewarming and core rewarming have been advocated. Active external rewarming is easily available and can be delivered by (1) immersion in heated water, (2) electric blankets or a water bottle, or (3) a radiant heat source. An afterdrop of core temperature during external rewarming has been described in hypothermic adults under experimental conditions. Furthermore, the shunting of stagnant cool blood into the circulation due to peripheral vasodilatation may increase the risk of ventricular fibrillation. Owing to this potential danger, active core rewarming has been advocated by some investigators. Active core rewarming may be achieved by (1) irrigation of internal organs with warmed solutions (gastric, colonic, or mediastinal irrigation and peritoneal dialysis), (2) extracorporeal blood rewarming, or (3) inhalation of warm air. Experience with these techniques is limited in infants, and such techniques are not generally recommended. Furthermore, none of these techniques is free of complications, and all require special facilities and equipment. In addition, external rewarming has proven safe in infants, and afterdrop of core temperature and ventricular fibrillation have not been observed.

The optimal rewarming rate for hypothermic infants is also a subject of disagreement. In 1957, Mann and Elliot recommended slow rewarming to avoid the risks of hyperthermia and convulsions. This method is still advocated by some authorities. Slow rewarming is usually achieved in an incubator by maintaining the circulating air temperature 1°C above the infant's rectal temperature. The goal is to rewarm the baby at a rate of 0.5°C/h. Over the last two decades, however, rapid external rewarming using an incubator or radiant heat source has been performed repeatedly and successfully. When using a radiant heat source, the thermostat is taped to the infant's skin, and the servocontrol point is set at 37°C. In our experience, the mean increase of body temperature was 0.37 ± 0.2°C/h using the slow rewarming method and 2.26 ± 0.9°C/h using the rapid method.

Rapid rewarming has been associated with lower mortality and morbidity rates. Thus, rapid rewarming under a radiant heat source is safe, more effective, quicker, and easier to perform compared with the slow rewarming method. We have experienced no complications of rapid rewarming and, therefore, strongly recommend its use.

OUTCOME

The prognosis of the hypothermic infant is related to the primary pathologic condition, the severity of hypothermia, the severity of complications, and the availability of modern medical knowledge and technology. Of 120 hypothermic infants treated in our department during the last 10 years, 7 died (6%), 5 with severe hypothermia (body temperature ranging between 20°C and 28°C) and 2 with moderate hypothermia. Most fatalities were secondary to severe infections (sepsis and meningitis). Most survivors recovered completely. A minority (5%) demonstrated mild psychomotor delay or chronic renal failure (secondary to acute tubular necrosis).

PREVENTION

Young infants need constant warmth. Appropriate educational measures regarding warming of houses and dress of the newborn infant should be instituted in high-risk areas as early as possible, (preferably in the maternity unit). Parents of infants at risk, particularly premature and LBW babies born during the cold season to inexperienced mothers of low socioeconomic classes, should be aware of the possibility of hypothermia and should be advised about the signs and symptoms of that condition. Furthermore, they should be equippped with an appropriate thermometer with a scale reading below 35°C. Home visits by nurses and social worker may be appropriate in selected cases.

REFERENCES

1. Kaplan M, Eidelman AI: Improved prognosis in severely hypothermic newborn infants treated by rapid rewarming. J Pediatr 105:470–474, 1984.
2. Sofer S, Yagupsky P, Hershkowitz J, Bearman JE: Improved outcome of hypothermic infants. Pediatr Emerg Care 2:211–214, 1986.
3. Zabelle J, Dagan R, Neumann L, Sofer S: Risk factors for neonatal hypothermia in early neonatal life. Pediatr Emerg Care 6:96–98, 1990.

RESPIRATORY DISTRESS SYNDROME AND ATELECTASIS

ALAN R. SPITZER, M.D.
JAY S. GREENSPAN, M.D.

In spite of many significant recent advances in therapy, neonatal respiratory distress syndrome (RDS) remains the most commonly encountered problem in the newborn intensive care nursery. Furthermore, death from RDS is still the leading cause of mortality in the preterm infant, and the morbidity associated with this pulmonary disease is substantial. Chronic lung disease, or bronchopulmonary dysplasia (BPD), intraventricular hemorrhage with cyst formation or periventricular leukomalacia leading to cerebral palsy or developmental delay, retinopathy of prematurity (ROP), sepsis, necrotizing enterocolitis, and air leak syndromes are but a few of the complications commonly associated with RDS. The cost of care for such children is extraordinarily high.

The primary goals for the treatment of infants with RDS are, therefore, directed at minimizing complications while permitting adequate time for recovery and growth. Treatment begins with appropriate diagnosis, often made prenatally. Prenatal diagnosis, performed by extracting an amniotic fluid sample, allows the obstetrician and pediatrician/neonatologist to assess the likelihood of RDS in the first hours of life. A lecithin/sphyngomyelin ratio (L/S ratio) of less than 2:1, particularly in the absence of phosphatidylglycerol (PG) indicates a significant risk of RDS. A number of commercially available kits are used on many labor floors in place of the L/S ratio because of the enhanced speed of diagnosis.

If RDS is anticipated, the physician must be prepared to intervene quickly after birth. From many studies, it is evident that outcome is improved in infants with RDS when the lungs are kept inflated by the use of some form of ventilatory assistance, rather than allowing the characteristic atelectasis of RDS (from surfactant deficiency) to progress. Reinflation of atelectatic lungs is far more difficult. The physician in attendance should, therefore, be prepared to intubate, resuscitate, and ventilate in the delivery room complex. Consideration should be given to the administration of exogenous surfactant once the diagnosis of RDS is made. Surfactant currently must be given through an endotracheal tube placed with the tip above the carina. Two surfactants are approved by the FDA (Table 1). Exosurf, an artificial surfactant, is given in a dose of 5 ml/kg in two divided aliquots, positioning the infant with the right side down, then left side down. Survanta, a natural surfactant, is administered in a dose of 4 to 5 ml/kg, depending on the size of the infant. Survanta is given in four divided aliquots, in the head up and head down positions, in addition to the right and left side down positions. Surfactant should be infused into the airway slowly to avoid pulmonary decompensation in the infant. The doses of surfactant can be repeated every 12 hours for up to four more doses. Surfactant appears to work most effectively when given early (before 4 hours of life).

TABLE 1. Surfactants (FDA Approved)

DRUG	DOSE AND COMMENTS
Exosurf	5 ml/kg in two divided aliquots Patient should be turned right side down for half the dose, then the other half should be given left side down; dose may be repeated q12h for maximum of four doses
Survanta	4–5 ml/kg in four divided aliquots; one fourth of the dose with right side down, head up, then one fourth with head down; remaining aliquots are given similarly with left side down, head up, then head down

Surfactant allows better maintenance of lung volumes until the infant can generate adequate endogenous surfactant synthesis and release. Lung volume can also be maintained with continuous end-distending pressure, either with spontaneous breathing (continuous positive airway pressure, CPAP) or with positive pressure mechanical ventilatory assistance (positive end-expiratory pressure, PEEP). Oxygen is an essential part of care in these infants. Both oxygen and ventilatory assistance should be kept at the lowest levels that enable adequate gas exchange. The arterial oxygen tension (Pao_2) should be kept at 50 to 80 mm Hg, and the arterial carbon dioxide concentration ($Paco_2$) should be maintained between 40 and 50 mm Hg. The pH in these infants should be kept between 7.3 and 7.45. The use of excessive ventilatory pressures to improve oxygenation may result in air leak syndromes, such as a tension pneumothorax, pneumomediastinum, or pulmonary interstitial emphysema (PIE). Intentional underventilation, however, in which the $Paco_2$ is allowed to rise above 50 mm Hg, may create significant long-term complications with respect to neurodevelopmental outcome. Once ventilatory assistance is initiated, arterial blood gases should be monitored at least every 2 hours until stability is achieved. Blood gases can be determined less frequently as the child improves. Transcutaneous Pao_2 and $Paco_2$ monitoring and pulse oximetry are very helpful in reducing the number of blood gas samples drawn. These technologies have their limitations, however, and determination of arterial blood gases cannot be entirely eliminated. In particular, hypovolemia and hypothermia can result in erroneous values during transcutaneous measurements. Movement can affect the pulse oximeter when measuring oxygen saturation.

Ventilator weaning should be carried out as indicated in Figure 1. Changes should be made that have a minimal impact on the infant. It is preferable to use frequent small changes as opposed to infrequent larger changes to avoid flip-flop. Flip-flop refers to the circumstance in which one excessively decreases the degree of support that an infant requires, leading to poor gas exchange, following which the physician must then increase support back to an even higher level than was previously needed. This back-and-forth approach to therapy is characteristic of the inexperienced physician and can substantially prolong the duration of ventilatory support with its attendant complications. Paralysis of the infant for ventilatory support, in general, should be used only when a child cannot be ventilated adequately otherwise and all possible mechanical problems affecting either the ventilator or the infant have been considered and eliminated.

In cases of severe RDS, especially when complicated by pulmonary air leaks, other forms of ventilatory support may be beneficial. High-frequency jet ventilation (HFJV) or high-frequency oscillatory ventilation (HFOV) both use high frequencies (>150 breaths per minute) and low tidal volumes in an attempt to decrease pulmonary barotrauma. Both forms of treatment appear to offer advantages for the rescue treatment of most critically ill infants with RDS and air leak. Insertion of a chest tube (thoracentesis) may be needed in these circumstances to adequately evacuate intrapleural air.

Adjuncts to therapy for the infant with RDS include careful administration of intravenous fluids (often through umbilical arterial and venous catheters), screening for intraventricular hemorrhage, periventricular echogenicity (PVE), cyst formation, and periventricular leukomalacia (PVL) by ultrasound, cautious use of blood products to replace drawn specimens or to treat anemia, surveillance for infection, attention to nutritional needs of the infant, with administration of enteral calories as early as tolerated by the child, and sedation for pain relief from procedures and endotracheal tube suctioning. It is very important that the physician address the family's needs as well. Parents of critically ill, premature infants often carry substantial psychologic burdens from the guilt they feel by placing a child in such a distressing situation. Acknowledgment of these stresses and reassurance from the physician can be of the greatest importance in maintaining a strong parent-child relationship during this period. Ongoing involvement of the family during hospitalization appears to be a valuable, yet poorly investigated, determinant of neonatal outcome.

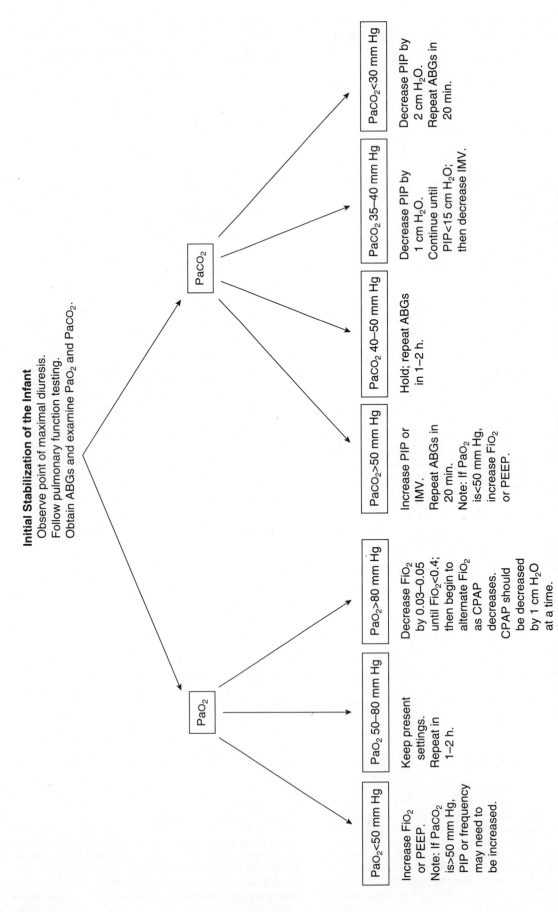

Initial Stabilization of the Infant
Observe point of maximal diuresis.
Follow pulmonary function testing.
Obtain ABGs and examine PaO_2 and $PaCO_2$.

PaO_2

$PaO_2 < 50$ mm Hg

Increase FiO_2 or PEEP.
Note: If $PaCO_2$ is>50 mm Hg, PIP or frequency may need to be increased.

PaO_2 50–80 mm Hg

Keep present settings. Repeat in 1–2 h.

$PaO_2 > 80$ mm Hg

Decrease FiO_2 by 0.03–0.05 until $FiO_2 < 0.4$; then begin to alternate FiO_2 as CPAP decreases. CPAP should be decreased by 1 cm H_2O at a time.

$PaCO_2$

$PaCO_2 > 50$ mm Hg

Increase PIP or IMV. Repeat ABGs in 20 min. Note: If PaO_2 is<50 mm Hg, increase FiO_2 or PEEP.

$PaCO_2$ 40–50 mm Hg

Hold; repeat ABGs in 1–2 h.

$PaCO_2$ 35–40 mm Hg

Decrease PIP by 1 cm H_2O. Continue until PIP<15 cm H_2O; then decrease IMV.

$PaCO_2 < 30$ mm Hg

Decrease PIP by 2 cm H_2O. Repeat ABGs in 20 min.

FIGURE 21.5–1. Management of ventilator weaning during respiratory therapy for RDS. ABGs = arterial blood gases; CPAP = continuous positive airway pressure; FiO_2 = fractional concentration of inspired oxygen; IMV = intermittent mandatory ventilation; PEEP = positive end-expiratory pressure; PIP = peak inspiratory pressure. (From Spitzer AR, Stefano J: Respiratory distress syndrome. *In* Workbook of Practical Neonatology. Philadelphia, WB Saunders, 1993:176.)

PNEUMOTHORAX AND OTHER AIR LEAKS

BRENDA R. HOOK, M.D.
RICHARD J. MARTIN, M.D.

Pulmonary air leak is a general term describing free air that has dissected beyond alveoli and presents as a pneumothorax, pneumomediastinum, pulmonary interstitial emphysema (PIE), pneumopericardium, pneumoperitoneum, or subcutaneous emphysema. The clinical presentation may range from an incidental radiographic finding in an asymptomatic infant to a life-threatening emergency requiring immediate intervention. Air leaks are more likely to require active intervention in infants with underlying lung disease, most notably respiratory distress syndrome (RDS), meconium aspiration syndrome, or other condition requiring positive pressure ventilation.

The diagnosis of a pneumothorax may be made on physical examination if there are decreased breath sounds on one side, shift of the cardiac impulse, abdominal distention, or asymmetric movement of the chest wall. Transillumination of the chest is a useful technique for rapid diagnosis of a tension pneumothorax requiring immediate therapy. However, accurate diagnosis typically requires radiographic confirmation using good radiographic techniques and experienced interpretation of the films to accurately localize accumulations of extrapulmonary air in the neonate.

Treatment of a pneumothorax depends on the infant's clinical condition. Infants who are asymptomatic or have mild respiratory distress with a transient oxygen requirement may be followed by repeated physical examinations and vital sign monitoring, including invasive or noninvasive assessment of blood gas status. Serial chest radiographs may be necessary to establish that the pneumothorax has resolved and the infant is ready for discharge. Any evidence of deteriorating clinical status, such as increasing respiratory distress, metabolic or respiratory acidosis, or inability to oxygenate, would require more aggressive intervention via placement of a chest tube, especially in the presence of underlying lung disease.

Evacuation of a pneumothorax should be done using sterile technique, local anesthesia, and a large-bore, multiholed chest tube. A small skin incision should be made at the anterior axillary line at the fourth or fifth intercostal space. Care should be taken to avoid the nipple area. Dissection over the top of the rib should be done using curved hemostats until the pleural space is entered. A trocar should not be used to guide the catheter into the pleural space, as this increases the likelihood of iatrogenic lung perforation. The chest tube should be anteriorly advanced into the pleural space and secured to the skin with a pursestring suture. The chest tube is connected to an underwater seal, initially at a suction pressure of 10 to 20 cm H_2O. If the air leak is large enough, additional chest tubes may need to be inserted to properly evacuate the pneumothorax. Chest tube suction should be maintained until fluctuations and bubbling of air have ceased. Before removal of the tube, it should be clamped for approximately 24 hours, and a radiograph should be done to exclude reaccumulation of the pneumothorax. If an air leak persists over many days, the diagnosis of a bronchopleural fistula should be considered, and surgical intervention may be needed. Failure of a pneumothorax to resolve after chest tube placement may also indicate the presence of underlying pulmonary hypoplasia.

Infants with a pneumomediastinum rarely require placement of a chest tube for decompression. Because they typically have underlying lung disease, most require close monitoring, and some need respiratory support. Pneumopericardium may also present as an incidental finding or an acute emergency due to cardiac tamponade. Diagnostic clues are muffled heart sounds, decreased pulse pressure, and low-voltage waveform on the cardiac monitor. Pneumopericardium causing cardiac tamponade should be decompressed immediately using an intravenous catheter inserted under the xiphoid process and advanced slowly while aiming for the left shoulder. Once air is recovered, the needle is removed, and the catheter is left in place. A persistent pneumopericardium is optimally treated with surgical placement of a pericardial tube. Neonatal pneumoperitoneum may present a real diagnostic dilemma. It may be very difficult to determine if the free air in the abdomen is from perforated bowel or represents dissection from the pleural cavity. Further diagnostic evaluation, such as paracentesis or contrast bowel studies, may be needed to avoid unnecessary surgical intervention.

PIE may be a localized or diffuse complication of neonatal assisted ventilation and may result in a vicious cycle of increasing ventilator pressures, thus aggravating the problem. PIE may spontaneously regress over time or be an early manifestation of bronchopulmonary dysplasia. During management of PIE, every effort must be made to reduce mean airway pressure by adjusting ventilatory parameters. Localized PIE may be treated successfully by positioning the infant with the emphysematous area of lung dependent, thus encouraging selective ventilation of the unaffected lobe(s). Although technically difficult, selective intubation of the mainstem bronchus on the uninvolved side may provide adequate ventilation and allow the diseased lung to heal. Surgical lobectomy may be needed if medical management of localized PIE fails and ventilatory status is severely compromised.

Fortunately, in both preterm and term infants with respiratory failure, newer therapeutic techniques have substantially improved respiratory therapy and reduced air leaks. Exogenous surfactant therapy for neonatal RDS has significantly decreased the incidence of pneumothorax and other air leaks. In neonates requiring assisted ventilation, high-frequency ventilation has had some success in decreasing air leaks (especially PIE), although optimal ventilator regimens for high-frequency ventilation are still being clarified.

REFERENCES

1. Gonzales F, Harris T, Black P, Richardson P: Decreased gas flow through pneumothoraces in neonates receiving high-frequency jet versus conventional ventilation. J Pediatr 110:464–466, 1987.
2. Jobe AH: Pulmonary surfactant therapy. N Engl J Med 328:861–868, 1993.
3. Miller MJ, Fanaroff AA, Martin RJ: Other pulmonary problems. *In* Fanaroff AA, Martin RJ (eds): Neonatal-Perinatal Medicine. St. Louis, Mosby-Yearbook, 1992:834–861.

MECONIUM ASPIRATION SYNDROME

THOMAS E. WISWELL, M.D.
WILLIAM W. FOX, M.D.

The pediatrician whose practice includes the delivery room setting frequently encounters infants with either meconium-stained amniotic fluid or suspicion of meconium aspiration. It has been estimated that 10% to 15% of all babies pass meconium-stained stool into the amniotic fluid before birth. Of this group, approximately 1 in 20 will develop the meconium aspiration syndrome (MAS), and approximately 10,000 infants a year in the United States with MAS will require mechanical ventilation.

PAST HISTORY AND PATHOPHYSIOLOGY

MAS has been a problem recorded throughout the ages. The passage of meconium has been known to be associated with fetal distress since the time of Artistotle. As many as 60% of babies born through meconium-stained amniotic fluid (MSAF) will require some form of resuscitation in the delivery room. Through the 1970s, the major mechanism of respiratory distress was thought to be obstruction of airways due to the viscosity of meconium. However, the frequent occurrence of pneumothorax among affected infants is likely due to a ball valve obstructive process initiated by the particulate material (thick meconium). Furthermore, inflammation due to meconium is thought to subsequently cause a chemical pneumonitis 24 hours or later following aspiration.

Meconium passage by the fetus was believed to be soley a reaction to some type of compromise. Fetal hypoxia or other adverse stimuli would cause increased intestinal peristalsis and relaxed anal sphincter tone, resulting in meconium passage. It was believed that infants only aspirated the substance with their first breaths shortly after delivery. The decline in the incidence of the MAS following near universal obstetric oropharyngeal suctioning, as well as intratracheal intubation and suctioning of the meconium-stained infant in the delivery room, was consistent with these suggested mechanisms. However, MAS still occurs. Approximately 5% of infants born through meconium-stained amniotic fluid will develop the disorder (contrasting with the 10% to 40% affected neonates before the reports of the efficacy of intratracheal suctioning). The fact that MAS still occurs is likely due to several factors: (1) As the fetus begins the transition to extrauterine life, the initial breaths may cause the meconium to be aspirated deep into the airways, where intratracheal suctioning cannot retrieve it. (2) Aspiration of meconium may have taken place in utero. (3) In utero hypoxemia may play a role in the development of respiratory distress. Antenatal insults can adversely affect the fetus' lungs and lead to respiratory distress associated with the presence of meconium but not primarily due to the substance itself. The respiratory distress may be in the form of clinical persistent pulmonary hypertension of the newborn (PPHN). Furthermore, in utero hypoxemia that is severe and prolonged enough may produce structural changes in the pulmonary vascular musculature, predisposing to a severe form of PPHN. Thus, the term MAS may be somewhat of a misnomer in a large proportion of infants, although it is generally used to describe respiratory distress in a neonate born through meconium-stained amniotic fluid whose symptoms cannot be directly attributed to another etiology. Recent in vitro studies have suggested that there is inactivation of surfactant by meconium, contributing to respiratory distress.

Other investigators have documented an intense pulmonary inflammatory response within a few hours of aspiration, suggesting that cytokines and other immunologic mediators may play a role in the pathophysiology of MAS. Whatever the mechanism for the clinical disorder, clinicians must be prepared for respiratory distress in all infants who are born through meconium-stained amniotic fluid.

SPECTRUM OF DISEASE

There is a continuum of disease among infants born through meconium-stained amniotic fluid and those who develop MAS. In the uncomplicated delivery, it is unusual for premature infants to pass meconium. After 37 weeks gestation, the passage of meconium becomes more frequent, and as gestation extends beyond 41 weeks into postmaturity, meconium passage becomes common.

It is known that meconium is made up of several components. The major components producing bulk are epithelial cell debris and mucopolysaccharides (these are typable by standard blood typing). In addition, there are bile acids and pancreatic secretions. Although bile acids are capable of causing airway edema, it is a combination of these substances that produces the pulmonary damage. Thick meconium fluid can cause physical obstruction of small or large airways. It is generally accepted that meconium passage commonly represents an intrauterine hypoxic or stress event, with relaxation of anal sphincter tone. For this reason, prepartum recognition of MSAF should alert the clinician to the possibility that the infant may need special attention (resuscitation) in the delivery room.

In many instances, the quantity of meconium passed will be small, especially when it is not associated with hypoxia. If the volume of amniotic fluid is normal, the result will be watery, thin-consistency MASF. The majority of infants born through thin MSAF will not develop respiratory illness. At the opposite end of the spectrum are infants who pass large quantities of meconium as a response to ongoing or severe compromise. Because of uteroplacental dysfunction, this

passage can be associated with oligohydramnios. The paucity of amniotic fluid may result in minimally diluted, thick amniotic fluid. Such neonates will be more likely to develop respiratory distress.

Whatever adverse stimulus led to the meconium passage may result in asphyxial damage to the lungs, structural vascular changes, or in utero aspiration. The most severely affected infants may be stillborn, die soon after birth, or have rapidly progressive respiratory failure. Their MAS may not be responsive to conventional therapy (mechanical ventilation at rates ≤60/min or hyperventilation to achieve alkalosis and hypocarbia). Many clinicians in the past were puzzled why some infants with mild aspiration on chest x-ray showed severe hypoxemia and others with extensive pulmonary infiltrates exhibited a milder or shorter clinical course. It is now clear that pulmonary hypertension is an important part of the syndrome, especially in the most critically ill infants. Unfortunately, there are no specific diagnostic tests to determine which infants have suffered postnatal aspiration versus those with in utero aspiration, asphyxial lung injury, or pulmonary vascular remodeling.

DELIVERY ROOM MANAGEMENT OF THE MECONIUM-STAINED INFANT

We are unsure whether there is a clear-cut group of meconium-stained babies for whom selective intubation is appropriate. Until well-designed, prospective investigations are performed to support selective intubation, we believe reasonable guidelines to follow are those established by a joint committee of the American Academy of Pediatrics (AAP) and the American Heart Association (AHA) in 1992 (Fig. 1). The committee recommends that all babies born through MSAF have adequate obstetric oropharyngeal suctioning before the shoulders and trunk of the child are delivered. In addition, intratracheal intubation and suctioning should be performed if (1) the meconium-stained fluid was thick or particulate in nature (including moderately thick MSAF), (2) there is prenatal evidence of fetal distress (abnormal heart rate tracing), (3) no obstetric oropharyngeal suctioning was performed, or (4) the neonate is depressed or requires positive pressure ventilation immediately after birth. The committee's recommendations include suctioning before any positive pressure ventilation. The remaining infants (those born through thin MSAF and apparently healthy in the delivery room) may not need intratracheal suctioning.

It has been suggested that several obstetric interventions may help to prevent MAS. Among these are the use of elective cesarean sections for women whose fetuses have MSAF and the use of intrapartum administration of narcotics to prevent fetal gasping. Neither of these

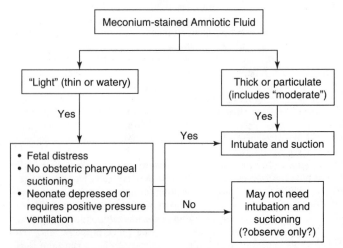

FIGURE 21.7–1. American Academy of Pediatrics–American Heart Association Guidelines for management of the neonate born through meconium-stained amniotic fluid. (From JAMA 268:2276–2281, 1992. Copyright 1992, American Medical Association.)

treatments has been proven to be effective. A third intervention, amnioinfusion, is more promising. With this therapy, warmed saline is infused into the uterus of mothers of fetuses with MSAF. It is believed that the additional fluid will either dilute the meconium or prevent umbilical cord compression. Although intriguing, the use of amnioinfusion remains controversial and needs to be evaluated in large clinical trials.

THE ROLES OF HIGH-FREQUENCY VENTILATION AND SURFACTANT THERAPY IN THE MANAGEMENT OF THE MECONIUM ASPIRATION SYNDROME

Several anecdotal reports have appeared concerning clinical improvement among babies with MAS following the use of either high-frequency ventilation (jet or oscillator) or exogenous surfactant therapy. To date, however, there have been no prospective, randomized trials that have validated the use of these adjunctive therapies. In fact, our animal data have shown no clear-cut clinical benefits with either of these modalities. We cannot recommend general use of these therapies in the management of MAS, but among those infants with respiratory failure due to the disorder who are not responding to conventional methods, the use of exogenous surfactant or high-frequency ventilation or both should be considered.

There are three relatively new or potential treatments for MAS that are confined to level III neonatal centers. For approximately 10 years, extracorporeal membrane oxygenation (ECMO) has been used in infants with MAS. This technique, which is essentially cardiopulmonary bypass (as used in open heart surgery), removes venous blood, oxygenates it through an artificial lung membrane, and returns it to the circulation. Because of the invasiveness of this therapy, ECMO has been reserved for the most critically ill infants and usually those with severe pulmonary hypertension and right-to-left shunting. The use of ECMO has resulted in a survival rate of 85% among infants whose predicted rate mortality was >80%.

Two additional approaches to severe MAS include nitric oxide therapy and liquid ventilation. It was discovered recently that nitric oxide is a biologic chemical with vasoregulatory properties. Endogenous nitric oxide provided by the vascular endothelium maintains vasodilatation and is the major mediator for vascular regulation. Current studies in animals and limited human studies suggest that nitric oxide may be given through a ventilator circuit in gas form (usually less than 80 parts per million concentration) to relieve pulmonary hypertension. The challenges that now exist include defining the most likely population of infants to respond, establishing the best method for delivery, and determining the optimum dose and side effects. Investigators have observed that the drug is more effective if administered earlier in the disease course.

Ventilating an animal or human with a liquid substance seems paradoxical when we have spent so many years trying to clear liquid from diseased lungs. Recent studies using perfluorochemical (PFC) compounds (similar to liquid Teflon) have demonstrated that these inert liquids can transport up to 20 times the amount of oxygen as blood, and because of low surface tension, alveolar pressures are lower during ventilation. Animal models of meconium aspiration have demonstrated excellent oxygen delivery and a cleansing effect of the PFC liquid during total liquid ventilation. In addition, antibiotics can be delivered with high efficiency to previously poorly ventilated areas. For total liquid ventilation, these liquids require special devices to ventilate humans, but prototypes are being developed. Another form of liquid ventilation (partial liquid ventilation) employs a combination of gas ventilation in a PFC liquid-filling lung. The method uses conventional ventilators and will be easier to apply but probably not as efficacious as total liquid ventilation for the critically ill term infant.

REFERENCES

1. Committee on Neonatal Ventilation/Meconium/Chest Compressions: Guidelines proposed at the 1992 National Conference on Cardiopulmonary Resuscitation and Emergency Cardiac Care, Dallas, 1992. JAMA 268:2276–2281, 1992.
2. Fox WW, Cox C, Farina C, Weis C, Wolfson MR, Shaffer TH: Liquid ventilation (LV) for pulmonary administration of gentamicin (G) in acute lung injury. Pediatr Res 35(4/Part 2):296A, 1994.
3. Katz VL, Bowes WA: Meconium aspiration syndrome. Reflections on a murky subject. Am J Obstet Gynecol 166:171–183, 1992.
4. Shaffer TH, Wolfson MR, Clark LC Jr: Liquid ventilation. Pediatr Pulmonol 14:102–109, 1992.
5. Wiswell TE, Bent RC: Meconium staining and the meconium aspiration syndrome: Unresolved issues. Pediatr Clin North Am 40:975–981, 1993.

PERSISTENT PULMONARY HYPERTENSION

JOHN P. KINSELLA, M.D.
STEVEN H. ABMAN, M.D.

Persistent pulmonary hypertension of the newborn (PPHN) is a clinical syndrome associated with various neonatal cardiopulmonary diseases, including meconium aspiration, group B streptococcal sepsis, and congenital diaphragmatic hernia. There is also an idiopathic variety. Despite the diversity of clinical settings of PPHN, marked pulmonary hypertension and altered pulmonary vasoreactivity are its central pathophysiologic features. High pulmonary vascular resistance (PVR) results in right-to-left shunting of blood across the patent ductus arteriosus and foramen ovale, often causing critical hypoxemia.

Descriptions of the management of PPHN have commonly focused on the subset of patients with idiopathic PPHN (often referred to as persistent fetal circulation or PFC). Patients with idiopathic PPHN have pulmonary hypertension of variable severity without concomitant lung disease.

However, PPHN frequently occurs with more common causes of neonatal respiratory distress, which are marked by moderate to severe lung disease (e.g., meconium aspiration and bacterial pneumonia). Moreover, sepsis neonatorum and perinatal asphyxia can severely compromise cardiac performance, leading to systemic hypotension in addition to severe pulmonary hypertension. The most difficult management cases of PPHN are complicated by both severe lung disease and hemodynamic lability with poor cardiac performance. Therefore, the therapeutic approach to PPHN requires meticulous attention to all aspects of the cardiopulmonary perturbations that characterize this syndrome (Table 1).

For the purpose of this section, it is assumed that the diagnosis of PPHN has already been established. The diagnosis of idiopathic PPHN should be considered when the severity of hypoxemia is disproportionate to the degree of parenchymal lung disease on chest radiograph. However, PPHN can also complicate diseases associated with severe lung disease (e.g., pneumonia, meconium aspiration syndrome). Patients with severe parenchymal lung disease without pulmonary hypertension can show marked lability in oxygenation. Therefore, this criterion is not sufficient to define PPHN. Measurements of preductal and postductal arterial oxygenation can provide clues to the presence of PPHN, but coarctation of the aorta may present with a markedly decreased postductal saturation without a reduced lower extremity blood pressure when the ductus arteriosus is widely patent.

The gold standard for determination of increased pulmonary vascular resistance involves direct assessments of pulmonary artery pressure and blood flow. However, instrumentation of the critically ill newborn with PPHN is imprudent because of the potential for vasospastic events causing acute deterioration. Moreover, the use of a Swan-Ganz catheter is impractical because of size limitations and the presence of ductal shunting (invalidating thermodilution measurements of cardiac output). In clinical practice, the gold standard defining PPHN rests on the echocardiographic (ECHO) findings of right-to-left shunting of blood at the foramen ovale or the ductus arteriosus or both and estimates of pulmonary artery pressure (applying the

TABLE 1. Clinical Categories of PPHN

PREDOMINANT PATHOLOGY	CLINICAL EXAMPLES	CLINICAL PRESENTATION
Decreased cross-sectional area of pulmonary vasculature Reactive pulmonary vasoconstriction in addition to fixed component	Congenital diaphragmatic hernia, pulmonary hypoplasia (oligohydramnios sequence)	Clear lung fields Marked postductal desaturation Increased risk of air leak (pneumothorax)
Reactive pulmonary hypertension without significant lung disease Reactive pulmonary hypertension with hemodynamic instability	Meconium aspiration syndrome Idiopathic PPHN Group B streptococcal sepsis	Changes on chest radiograph out of proportion to severity of hypoxemia Variable changes on chest radiograph: clear lung fields to marked pneumonia Severe hypotension
Reactive pulmonary hypertension with severe parenchymal lung disease: relative contribution of each to hypoxemia uncertain	Pneumonia Hyaline membrane disease Secondary surfactant deficiency	Diffuse parenchymal disease on chest radiograph: white out

modified Bernoulli equation to the peak velocity of the tricuspid insufficiency jet) (Table 2). Therefore, therapy for PPHN should be guided by the severity of illness, the presence of accompanying lung disease, hemodynamic variables, and the results of echocardiography. This section discusses pulmonary, pulmonary vascular, and cardiac problems pertinent to the management of PPHN.

MANAGEMENT

The goals of PPHN management are

1. To reduce pulmonary vascular resistance
2. To optimize lung inflation and treat any underlying pulmonary parenchymal disease
3. To sustain cardiac performance and systemic hemodynamic stability.

PPHN is a dynamic syndrome. Therefore, management should be based on serial assessments of PPHN and cardiac performance by ECHO and of lung disease by chest radiograph. Because of the diverse nature of diseases associated with PPHN, no single therapeutic approach will be effective in all patients.

Cardiac Management in PPHN

Systemic hypotension should be promptly treated initially with volume infusion of a colloid solution (5% albumin, Plasmanate, fresh frozen plasma) in 10 ml/kg increments. Although adequate systemic blood flow and substrate delivery should be determined by end-organ responses (e.g., urine flow rate, metabolic acidemia), these variables are time dependent, and rapid assessments of volume status are essential in the acute management of this disorder. Initial fluid resuscitation should be based on clinical observations of skin perfusion, heart rate, and blood pressure. Volume resuscitation should be used with extreme caution when systemic hypotension is related to poor cardiac performance, particularly when the heart is enlarged on chest radiograph. However, as a general rule of thumb, a mean arterial pressure less than 35 to 40 mm Hg in the term newborn should be considered hypotension.[3] In addition, a heart rate greater than 160 beats per minute (bpm) and capillary refill time that exceeds 2 seconds suggest intravascular volume depletion. Preferred solutions for vol-

ume replacement are 5% albumin or fresh frozen plasma (FFP is the solution of choice if there is evidence of a coagulopathy, e.g., prolonged prothrombin time, thrombocytopenia, clinical signs of bleeding diathesis).

If volume resuscitation alone is ineffective in maintaining normal blood pressure and systemic perfusion, cardiotonic agents (dobutamine or dopamine) should be administered (beginning at 5 μg/kg/min and increasing to 20 μg/kg/min) (Tables 3 and 4). If the heart rate is less than 140 to 150 bpm after initiating treatment with dopamine and dobutamine, the chronotropic effects of isoproterenol may be helpful in improving systemic blood flow, although this agent also reduces systemic afterload. If systemic vascular resistance is reduced more than pulmonary vascular resistance, right-to-left shunting across the ductus arteriosus could be exacerbated. Some clinicians use epinephrine infusions if systemic hypotension is refractory to dopamine and dobutamine therapy. We have found that the need for epinephrine portends refractory hemodynamic collapse, predicting the need for cardiac support with extracorporeal membrane oxygenation. However, in a subset of patients, epinephrine infusions are particularly useful. For example, in patients with systemic vasodilatation (e.g., sepsis) but with adequate cardiac performance, epinephrine causes systemic vasoconstriction and increased blood pressure without leading to cardiac failure.

Pulmonary Management in PPHN

The highest possible concentration of oxygen should be given initially in an oxygen hood (unless the infant is in clinically apparent respiratory failure) to allow measurement of the inspiratory oxygen concentration (F_{IO_2}). Usually, 85% to 95% oxygen is attainable in an oxygen hood if care is taken to loosely seal the hood at the neck with gauze. The infant's arterial oxygen saturation should be measured using pulse oximetry. Preductal (right arm) and postductal (lower extremity) oxygen saturation measurements will provide information about the presence of right-to-left shunting of blood across the ductus arteriosus. In many patients with PPHN, postductal oxygen saturation will be lower than preductal saturation (more than 3% to 4% difference should be considered significant). Simultaneous preductal and postductal blood gas measurements for determination of oxygen tensions provide equivalent information (a difference in Pa_{O_2} of 20 mm Hg

TABLE 2. Echocardiographic Findings in PPHN

MEASUREMENT	FINDINGS IN PPHN
Estimate of PA pressure using Doppler estimate of TR jet: 4 (V^2) + CVP	Elevated PA pressure reliably estimated (mm Hg), compare with simultaneous systemic pressure
Direction of PDA shunt (by pulsed and color Doppler)	Right-to-left or bidirectional PDA shunting
Direction of atrial shunt (by pulsed and color Doppler and bubble contrast)*	Right-to-left or bidirectional shunting through PFO

*Right-to-left shunt more likely determined with lower extremity contrast injection.

TABLE 3. Use of Catecholamine Drugs in PHN

CATECHOLAMINE DRUG*	DOSE (μg/kg/min)	INDICATIONS	COMPLICATIONS
Dobutamine	2–20	Hypotension Decreased cardiac performance	Tachycardia
Dopamine	2–20	Hypotension Decreased cardiac performance Selective renal effects at <5 μg/kg/min	Ectopy, tachycardia, severe hypertension with overdose Peripheral ischemia with IV infiltration
Isoproterenol	0.05–0.5	Decreased systemic perfusion with heart rate <140 bpm	Atrial and ventricular Arrhythmia Tachycardia
Epinephrine	0.05–0.5	Refractory hypotension despite dopamine and dobutamine therapy, with adequate cardiac performance	Intense peripheral vasoconstriction Increased SVR can offset improvement if cardiac performance is decreased Tachycardia Arrhythmia

*Note: Ensure adequate intravascular volume (preload) before initiating catecholamine drug therapy.

being significant). In general, a postductal arterial PaO_2 measurement greater than 150 mm Hg when inspired oxygen is near 100% makes the diagnosis of cyanotic congenital heart disease less likely. However, both severe PPHN and severe parenchymal lung disease may present with a low arterial PaO_2 while the infant is receiving a high inspired oxygen concentration. If respiratory failure occurs with increased work of breathing, a rising arterial $PaCO_2$, and decreasing arterial PaO_2 levels, mechanical ventilation should be instituted.

In idiopathic PPHN (i.e., without significant lung disease), the pulmonary management should be directed at minimizing overzealous mechanical ventilation and avoiding lung overinflation. Applying inappropriately high airway pressure to the normally compliant lung can lead to air leak (e.g., pneumothorax) and adverse cardiopulmonary interactions (decreased cardiac output from reduced venous return and cardiac filling). If adequate oxygenation (PaO_2 >80 mm Hg) cannot be obtained with moderate ventilator settings (peak inspiratory pressure <35 cm H_2O and inspiratory time <0.5 seconds), consideration should be given to a trial of respiratory alkalosis. Some patients will respond to alkalosis (pH 7.5 to 7.55) with marked improvement in oxygenation. However, if significant improvement is not promptly demonstrated, hyperventilation should be discontinued. Respiratory alkalosis can often be achieved with high-frequency ventilator devices, which may minimize peak distending pressures delivered to the lung.

In the setting of severe lung disease and PPHN, treatment of the underlying lung disease is essential (and sometimes sufficient) to cause resolution of the accompanying pulmonary hypertension. It is important to remember that airway pressure is poorly transmitted to the pleural space in the underinflated and poorly compliant lung. However, as lung inflation and compliance improve, ventilator support must be reduced accordingly to avoid injury.

Because of the diverse nature of diseases complicating PPHN, there is no single approach to mechanical ventilation in this syndrome. Ventilator adjustments must be made with attention to radiographic changes of the accompanying lung disease and hemodynamic status (including intravascular volume status, systemic perfusion, and cardiac performance).

Mechanical ventilation in PPHN should be initiated with conventional intermittent mandatory ventilation. However, there is increasing interest in the potential role of high-frequency ventilation in the management of PPHN. There are three high-frequency devices approved

by the United States Food and Drug Administration for use in the newborn. In our experience, the Infant Star High Frequency Ventilator lacks the power necessary to ventilate most newborns of greater than approximately 2 kg birthweight, and no studies have been published using this ventilator in the management of PPHN. The Bunnell Life Pulse Ventilator (high-frequency jet ventilator) is a very powerful device that can cause marked respiratory alkalosis while minimizing peak inspiratory pressure. However, we have found that this ventilator is often ineffective in recruitment of atelectatic lung and can lead to lung injury without vigilant attention to lung volume and air trapping. The Sensormedics 3100A high-frequency oscillator (HFOV) incorporates an active expiratory phase of exhalation, generating a sinusoidal (biphasic) pressure waveform superimposed on an adjustable mean airway pressure. This device is the only high-frequency ventilator shown to be effective in rescue therapy of term and near term newborns with severe respiratory failure in a randomized clinical trial.

In the patient with significant pulmonary parenchymal disease complicating PPHN, HFOV is an important adjunct in management. We have found that HFOV allows effective alveolar recruitment in diseases refractory to conventional ventilator therapy. However, the safe use of HFOV requires attention to lung volume and inflation on chest radiographs, and failure to reduce mean airway pressure in response to progressive improvement in lung inflation can lead to gross air leak and hemodynamic deterioration.

Pulmonary surfactant therapy may be beneficial in a subset of patients with PPHN and diffuse parenchymal lung disease. However, in idiopathic PPHN without accompanying lung disease, surfactant therapy has no role.

Much controversy surrounds the use of pharmacologic paralysis in the management of PPHN. We have employed a simple rule to guide the use of such agents as pancuronium and curare. We use pharmacologic paralysis if hyperventilation is instituted (because of the increased risk of air leak due to forceful expiration against mechanical inspiration) or if severe vasolability and arterial desaturation occur with routine interventions.

Pulmonary Vasodilators in PPHN

Current therapy to reduce pulmonary hypertension includes mechanical hyperventilation (as noted) to produce a respiratory alkalosis, the use of sodium bicarbonate or THAM (tris-hydroxymethylaminomethane) to induce a metabolic alkalosis, and vasodilator drug therapy. Pulmonary vasodilator drug therapy (e.g., tolazoline, sodium nitroprusside) is often unsuccessful because of concomitant systemic hypotension, adverse effects (e.g., gastrointestinal bleeding), or an inability to achieve or sustain pulmonary vasodilatation. Indeed, effective treatment of PPHN has suffered from the lack of an agent that causes selective and sustained pulmonary vasodilatation. However, recent breakthroughs in vascular biology have provided insights into

TABLE 4. Rapid Method for Calculating Catecholamine Drug Mixtures

(6 × body weight in kg × desired dose)/desired infusion rate = milligrams of agent to add to 100 ml of $D_{10}W$: then 1 ml/h = 10 μg/kg/min

Example: 3 kg infant: to deliver 10 μg/kg/min of dopamine using infusion rate of 1 ml/h: mix 180 mg dopamine in 100 ml $D_{10}W$

such an agent. Vascular endothelium elaborates a potent, short-acting substance (endothelium-derived relaxing factor, EDRF) that diffuses to the vascular smooth muscle, causing vasodilatation under basal conditions and in response to physiologic and pharmacologic stimuli. EDRF has been identified as nitric oxide (NO), which has subsequently been shown to play important roles in myriad physiologic systems and pathophysiologic states.

Recent reports suggest that inhaled NO improves oxygenation in newborns with severe PPHN, without causing systemic hypotension.[1,2] When administered by inhalation, NO diffuses to vascular smooth muscle, stimulating cyclic GMP production and causing vasodilatation. Its selectivity for the pulmonary circulation is due to the rapid and avid binding of NO by hemoglobin, decreasing its availability for causing systemic vasodilatation. Although marked right-to-left shunting is the major cause of hypoxemia in PPHN, some newborns also have altered ventilation-perfusion matching ($\dot{V}/\dot{Q}$) due to parenchymal lung disease (e.g., meconium aspiration). In addition to lowering PVR, inhaled NO further improves oxygenation by dilating pulmonary arteries associated with the best ventilated lung units, thereby enhancing $\dot{V}/\dot{Q}$ matching.

Inhalational NO therapy remains investigational. When it is approved for use in PPHN, however, this treatment will likely replace other vasodilator therapies because of its lack of systemic vascular effects. We have found benefits of inhaled NO to be possibly less successful without optimal pulmonary management. Conventional mechanical ventilation alone is often ineffective when PPHN occurs in association with severe parenchymal disease. In PPHN complicated by parenchymal lung disease (particularly homogeneous lung disease with underinflation), HFOV is an important adjunctive treatment, allowing adequate lung inflation while minimizing lung injury from tidal volume mechanical breaths.

Inhaled NO causes sustained improvement in oxygenation in severe PPHN when clinical management includes meticulous attention to the nature of the underlying lung disease. In patients with severe PPHN and parenchymal lung disease or pulmonary hypoplasia (e.g., congenital diaphragmatic hernia), optimal management may include HFOV to recruit and maintain lung volume, thus promoting effective delivery of the inhalational vasodilator NO. Moreover, loss of apparent NO responsiveness may occur due to deterioration in cardiac performance and progressive atelectasis (decreasing effective delivery of this inhalational agent to its site of action in terminal lung units). Finally, it is important to stress that not all neonates with hypoxemic respiratory failure have severe pulmonary hypertension. Pulmonary parenchymal disease can cause critical hypoxemia, and pulmonary vasodilator therapy would not be expected to be an effective therapy in this setting.

SUMMARY

PPHN occasionally presents as a relatively isolated pathophysiologic disturbance marked by severe pulmonary hypertension and altered pulmonary vasoreactivity without concomitant lung disease. However, PPHN is more commonly associated with variable degrees of pulmonary parenchymal disease (e.g. meconium aspiration, pneumonia, surfactant deficiency). Therefore, the therapeutic approach to PPHN requires attention to the cardiac and pulmonary vascular components of this syndrome, as well as the accompanying alveolar disease. Therapy must be tailored to the underlying diseases, with appropriate modifications in response to changes in the severity of illness.

REFERENCES

1. Kinsella JP, Neish SR, Shaffer E, Abman SH: Low-dose inhalational nitric oxide in persistent pulmonary hypertension of the newborn. Lancet 340:819–820, 1992.
2. Kinsella JP, Neish SR, Ivy DD, Shaffer E, Abman SH: Clinical responses to prolonged treatment of persistent pulmonary hypertension of the newborn with low-dose inhalational nitric oxide. J Pediatr 123:103–108, 1993.
3. Kitterman JA, Phibbs RH, Tooley WH: Aortic blood pressure in normal newborn infants during the first 12 hours of life. Pediatrics 44:959–968, 1969.

EXTRACORPOREAL MEMBRANE OXYGENATION

ROBERT E. SCHUMACHER, M.D.

Extracorporeal membrane oxygenation (ECMO) is the use of cardiopulmonary bypass techniques to provide a period of lung rest to a term or near-term infant with life-threatening respiratory failure. Such a period of rest allows time for lung recovery and survival of the infant. According to the Extracorporeal Life Support Organization's (ELSO) neonatal ECMO registry (Ann Arbor, Michigan), ECMO has been used in more than 9000 newborns, with an overall survival rate of 81%.

INDICATIONS

Inclusion Criteria

Because of regional variations in nurseries, every institution should have its own inclusion/exclusion criteria. However, certain criteria appear to be widely used. Gestational age should be greater than or equal to 34 weeks. Early experience with neonatal ECMO showed that premature infants had a higher incidence of intracranial hemorrhage and decreased survival when compared with term infants. Recent refinements in ECMO technique warrant consideration of ECMO for infants less than 34 weeks on a case by case basis. There should be no intracranial hemorrhage greater than grade I. Because ECMO alters cerebral blood flow patterns and requires systemic anticoagulation, the risk for intracranial hemorrhage (irrespective of gestational age) is increased. Infants with preexistent hemorrhage are at risk for extension of the hemorrhage. Some patients with preexistent hemorrhage have, however, been successfully managed on ECMO. There should be no significant bleeding or bleeding diathesis. With ECMO, systemic anticoagulation may render small, insignificant hemorrhages significant. Septic infants with preexistent coagulopathy and infants with prior surgery are at risk for severe bleeding episodes on ECMO.

Since ECMO provides a period for lung rest and recovery, infants considered for ECMO should have lung disease that is likely to be reversible within a short (2 weeks?) period of time. Some centers exclude infants who have been mechanically ventilated for more than 7 to 10 days, assuming that their lung disease is "irreversible."

Since ECMO will not cure congenital heart disease, major cardiac disease must be ruled out before institution of bypass for respiratory failure. ECMO has been used in patients with congenital heart disease as a temporizing agent or bridge to more definitive cardiac surgery.

Infants who are ECMO candidates should be at high risk of dying from respiratory failure. Quantitating the degree of respiratory failure is difficult. Since ECMO is now used at a rate of about 1 case per 3500 live births, most neonatal intensive care units will see only a small number of candidates in a given year. This makes generating high mortality rate criteria difficult. Because the risks and costs of ECMO are perceived by many as being high, most centers have arbitrarily selected an 80% mortality risk as being a prerequisite for ECMO. Criteria for ECMO or for transfer from a neonatal intensive care unit to an ECMO center should be made in an institution-specific manner, preferably in consultation with a local ECMO center. Following are the most commonly used neonatal ECMO criteria.

- An $AaDO_2$ ($PaO_2 - PaO_2$) ≥610 mm Hg, usually for several hours (which in many institutions has been equated with a predicted 80% mortality)
- An oxygenation index (OI = mean airway pressure × $FIO_2 ÷ PO_2$) ≥40 (range 25 to 60) over a period of several hours
- A PaO_2 chronically <35 to 59 mm Hg
- Significant barotrauma
- "Acute respiratory deterioration" accompanied by cyanosis

Since not all neonatal respiratory disease is alike, laboratory values that predict high mortality in some circumstances (meconium aspiration syndrome) may not be as predictive in another (respiratory distress syndrome). All criteria should be viewed as guidelines. Additionally, all ECMO centers invoke these criteria only after a fair trial of maximal medical management has been undertaken.

EQUIPMENT

With venoarterial (VA) ECMO, arterial outlet and venous inlet catheters are used. The venous catheter is surgically placed with its tip into the right atrium where blood is passively drained to the ECMO circuit. The arterial catheter returns blood from the circuit into the aortic arch via the carotid artery, which is ligated as part of the procedure. Typically, size 8 to 10 French catheters are used. In venovenous (VV) ECMO, a single double-lumen catheter is placed in the right atrium, where blood is both drained to and returned from the circuit. This is an isovolemic procedure in which some recirculation of blood is encountered. With VV ECMO, the heart is not bypassed, and an adequate native myocardial function is required. In both VA and VV ECMO, blood is drained from the right atrium to a venous silicone reservoir or bladder. This bladder acts as a bubble trap and provides a capacitance chamber that allows for continuous ECMO flow despite some variations in venous return. The bladder is used in conjunction with a sensor that serves to regulate the roller pump and prevent cavitation of the ECMO tubing under circumstances of low venous return. Two blood pumps are commonly used for neonatal ECMO, the roller occlusion pump (which is a positive displacement pump) and the centrifugal pump. Most ECMO centers prefer the former, as the centrifugal pump system can cause significant hemolysis in a neonate. The rotational speed of a roller head pump is used to calculate total system blood flow. The Scimed (Scimed Life Systems, Minneapolis, Minnesota) membrane lung is the only membrane lung currently approved for long-term cardiopulmonary bypass. The Scimed lung is a silicone rubber membrane envelope in which gas flows through the interior of the envelope and is separated from the blood phase by a silicone membrane. Countercurrent flow of blood and gas allows for maximum gas transfer. A blood warmer or heat exchanger is used before blood is returned to the patient.

PATIENT MANAGEMENT

The most common initial bypass problem is hypotension, which results from hypovolemia, hypocalcemia, or dilution of vasopressors. Moreover, catheters can be misplaced. Therefore, their position should be documented radiographically.

Once the infant is on bypass, ventilator settings can be weaned rapidly to "rest" settings. With VA bypass, high positive end-expiratory pressure has been shown to shorten bypass time. If the infant is on VV bypass, the wean must be made more cautiously as the infant may be dependent on myocardial function for oxygen delivery. Infants must be restrained while on bypass. The infant's head position is critical, and a head turned too far to the left will functionally occlude the left jugular vein (the right is ligated as part of the ECMO procedure). Sedation for the infant is usually required. Heparin is administered continuously into the circuit to prevent clotting. Infants are initially loaded with 100 U/kg of heparin before cannulation. A continuous drip of heparin (20 to 40 U/kg/h) is used to keep bleeding times one and one-half to two times normal. Bleeding times are usually measured with a bedside automated instrument that quantifies the activated clotting time (ACT). Results of the ACT are expressed in seconds (usual target 180 to 200 seconds).

The concept of parallel circulations (ECMO and native), each contributing a percentage of total cardiac output, is important in understanding VA ECMO. In VV ECMO, the two circulations are in series. Oxygen delivery is regulated by ECMO pump flow. In VA ECMO, oxygen delivery is evaluated with the aid of an indwelling O_2 saturation monitor placed in the venous return line. With VV ECMO, recirculation of blood precludes some of the usefulness of

venous saturation monitoring. Carbon dioxide removal is generally a function of ventilation or gas flow through the membrane lung. Carbon dioxide removal is often so efficient that carbon dioxide may need to be added to the system.

In most infants, a period of whiteout on chest x-ray, a decrease in functional residual capacity, oliguria, and increase in total body water, occurs shortly after placement on bypass. Fluid intake is restricted, and infants often are routinely given furosemide to facilitate diuresis. Hypokalemia is an unexplained but common finding. Parenteral nutrition, using high concentrations of dextrose, is delivered directly into the ECMO circuit and provides adequate calories without the need for large fluid volumes.

The entire circuit is inspected regularly for the presence of small clots. Coagulation studies and serum hemoglobin determinations are obtained routinely looking for evidence of consumptive coagulopathy and hemolysis. Platelets, plasma, cryoprecipitate, and red blood cell transfusions are administered judiciously. Cranial ultrasound studies are routine.

Weaning from ECMO

Patients are assessed for continued bypass need daily, using serial chest x-rays, blood gas values, and pulmonary function studies as measures of bypass need. A diuresis often occurs before clinical improvement in the patient. As blood gas values improve, the ECMO pump flow is typically weaned to 10% to 30% of estimated cardiac output. A trial off bypass is indicated at this point.

Complications

ECMO complications arise either from the interaction of blood with the large foreign body surface area or from ECMO changing patterns of blood flow throughout the body. Common complications include bleeding, hypertension, cholestatic jaundice, oliguria, hypertension, arrhythmias, brain infarction, seizures, and infection.

Procedures After Bypass

Once an infant is successfully removed from bypass, laboratory studies, including a complete blood count with platelet count and electrolytes, should be obtained until values are stable. Some centers routinely repair the carotid artery after ECMO. Although technically feasible, the risk of subsequent stenosis or embolization or both must be weighed against the theoretical benefit of reanastomosis. Because cranial sonograms can miss important lesions, infants should have a post-ECMO CT brain scan. The neck wound should be examined for signs of infection or bleeding. Postextubation vocal cord paresis has been reported. ECMO-treated infants are notoriously difficult feeders, but this is usually a temporary problem. Hearing screening and a thorough neurologic examination are indicated in every patient.

OUTCOME

Survival by the time of hospital discharge is 81%. Survival is diagnosis specific, with infants with meconium aspiration syndrome surviving at a 93% rate. Infants with sepsis and congenital diaphragmatic hernia do less well (76% and 58%, respectively). All infants require careful serial follow-up examinations. Medical problems commonly encountered during the first year of life include recurrent respiratory infections (usually wheezing associated respiratory illness), feeding difficulties and sensorineural hearing loss. Parents should be informed that infants with permanently ligated carotid arteries will have no palpable pulse in the right neck. Moderate to severe neurologic impairment is seen in 10% to 20% of infants, and cerebral palsy and seizure disorders are the most commonly reported problems. A similar percentage of infants are found to be developmentally or cognitively impaired, and several centers have noticed an increase in expressive language delay in these infants. Macrocephaly accompanied by ventriculomegaly and an increased size of the subarachnoid space have been noted in some infants. However, the developmental consequences of this finding are unknown. True external hydrocephalus with need for shunting is uncommon. Curiously, infants with diaphragmatic hernia seem to be particularly vulnerable to this finding. The accumulation of fluid over the cerebral convexities is noted occasionally in conjunction with thrombosis of the superior vena cava.

Follow-up post-ECMO is important. ELSO maintains a follow-up center directory and physicians requiring or wishing follow-up may contact an ECMO center for a local listing.

CONGENITAL DIAPHRAGMATIC HERNIA

CRAIG W. LILLEHEI, M.D.

Congenital diaphragmatic hernia remains one of the most common, yet lethal newborn surgical emergencies. The reported incidence varies from 1 in 2000 to 1 in 5000 live births. Most (85% to 90%) of the hernias are left-sided. Although the size of the defect varies, it is typically posterolateral, through the so-called foramen of Bochdalek. An anterior rim of diaphragm is usually present, but, posteriorly, the rim may be very narrow or absent. With left-sided hernias, the stomach, spleen, small intestine, colon, or left lobe of the liver may herniate into the chest. On the right, the hernia usually contains liver but may also involve small intestine or colon. A hernia sac is present in only about 20% of cases. The ipsilateral lung is hypoplastic and frequently does not immediately expand to fill the hemithorax. The number of airway generations, arterioles, and alveoli is substantially reduced. There is also increased muscularization around peripheral arterioles. These changes are often seen in the contralateral lung, although they are not as severe.

CLINICAL PRESENTATION AND DIAGNOSIS

Increasingly, diaphragmatic hernia is recognized in utero by prenatal ultrasonography, either done routinely or to evaluate polyhydramnios. Nonetheless, the most common presentation remains respiratory distress within the first few hours of life. Notable on physical examination is a scaphoid abdomen with an increased anteroposterior diameter of the chest. Breath sounds are absent on the side of the hernia, although bowel sounds can occasionally be heard. The cardiac apex is displaced away from the hernia. The chest radiograph is virtually diagnostic, demonstrating gas-filled intestinal loops within the chest and displacement of the cardiac silhouette.

TREATMENT

Preoperative Procedures

The extent of respiratory difficulty depends on the volume of herniated viscera and degree of pulmonary hypoplasia. Early insertion of a nasogastric tube is important to minimize gastrointestinal distention within the chest. It may also aid in radiographically confirming the intrathoracic position of the stomach. If the infant requires ventilatory assistance, prompt endotracheal intubation is essential to avoid further gaseous distention. Monitoring of arterial blood gases may be accomplished by an umbilical artery catheter to measure postductal gases or by a right radial arterial line to measure preductal gases. Supplemental oxygen is usually required. Rapid, gentle ventilation is used to optimize gas exchange yet avoid excessive barotrauma. *One needs to be constantly aware of the risk of an acute pneumothorax, particularly if high ventilatory pressures are needed.* Some physicians favor prophylactic placement of a chest tube in this setting.

Although, historically, prompt reduction of the hernia and repair of the diaphragmatic defect have been advocated, attention has recently been focused on preoperative stabilization. Extracorporeal membrane oxygenation (ECMO) has been used if necessary. Various predictors of survival have been studied, but precise prognostication remains elusive.

OPERATIVE PROCEDURES

Most pediatric surgeons favor a transabdominal rather than a transthoracic approach.

The entire abdomen and both chests are prepared and draped. A subcostal incision is preferred to allow optimal exposure of the diaphragmatic defect. When the peritoneal cavity is entered, the herniated viscera are reduced through the defect by gentle traction. A chest tube is inserted. The hypoplastic lung is inspected, but no attempt is made to hyperinflate this remnant. The posterior rim of the diaphragm is identified and unrolled. Barring excessive tension, primary closure of the diaphragmatic defect is achieved using interrupted, nonabsorbable sutures. Even if the hernia is quite large, it can often be closed medially, adjacent to the esophagus. The remaining defect is closed using a prosthetic patch or muscle flap. Although the intestinal fixation is often abnormal, a formal Ladd's procedure is not routinely performed. A gastrostomy may be inserted to facilitate postoperative gastrointestinal decompression and feeding. If closure of the abdominal fascia requires excessive tension or intraabdominal pressure, the skin alone is approximated. The resulting ventral hernia can be repaired at a later date, after the infant recovers.

Repair of a diaphragmatic hernia while the infant is on ECMO is feasible but necessitates meticulous hemostasis given the requisite anticoagulation.

Postoperative Procedures

Postoperative management of an infant with congenital diaphragmatic hernia can be exceedingly difficult. Initially, a "honeymoon" period may be seen during which oxygenation is satisfactory. However, the increased pulmonary vascular resistance resulting from a hypoplastic and reactive pulmonary bed typically produces pulmonary arterial hypertension. Right-to-left shunting may occur at the foramen ovale or ductus arteriosus or both, delivering desaturated blood to the systemic circulation. This hypoxemia and acidosis further aggravate pulmonary vasospasm, and a vicious cycle ensues.

The key elements in management are to optimize oxygenation and avoid acidosis. Hyperventilation may be useful, but excessive barotrauma should be avoided. Unfortunately, surgical repair of the diaphragmatic defect may acutely worsen pulmonary compliance, compromising effective ventilation. Intravenous bicarbonate or tromethamine (THAM) is used to correct acidosis. Vasodilators, such as tolazoline, may be used to reduce pulmonary hypertension, but they invariably cause systemic vasodilatation as well. Moderate fluid restriction is desirable to optimize oxygenation, yet systemic blood pressure must be maintained. High-frequency ventilation has been used with limited success. ECMO provides effective cardiopulmonary support. However, ultimate survival depends on successful weaning from the ECMO circuit with maintenance of satisfactory hemodynamics and gas exchange.

RESULTS

Despite dramatic advances in neonatal intensive care, the mortality rate of infants presenting with symptomatic diaphragmatic hernia within the first 6 hours of life remains nearly 50%. Those who present after 24 hours of age almost invariably survive. *Repair of the diaphragmatic defect has been successfully accomplished in utero, which offers promise for those most severely affected but without other life-threatening anomalies.*

BRONCHOPULMONARY DYSPLASIA

JEFFREY S. GERDES, M.D.
SORAYA ABBASI, M.D.
VINOD K. BHUTANI, M.D.

Bronchopulmonary dysplasia (BPD) is a chronic lung disorder, affecting both preterm (most commonly) and term newborn infants, that follows an acute pulmonary disease, such as respiratory distress syndrome (RDS). Although the definition of BPD is in transition, the infant classically considered to have BPD exhibits respiratory symptoms, has an abnormal chest radiograph, and requires supplemental oxygen at 28 days of age. The hallmark pathologic findings in this disorder are a chronic inflammatory and reparative cellular response to unresolved acute lung injury. Infants with BPD are characterized clinically by chronic respiratory distress, diminished blood oxygen concentration (hypoxemia), retention of carbon dioxide (hypercapnia), and an abnormal chest radiograph.

BPD is a unique phenomenon in pulmonary medicine in that it is a disease in which simultaneous lung injury and repair are superimposed on a system of ongoing organ growth and development. Although BPD is recognized in approximately 15% of preterm births, as many as 69% of babies of birth weight less than 1000 g may develop the condition. More significantly, 18% of those babies exhibit a severe form of the disease. These infants require a high level of care, and they often develop long-term pulmonary and neurodevelopmental complications. The etiology of BPD is multifactorial and includes inherent factors, such as lung underdevelopment (secondary to prematurity) as well as factors ensuing from therapies provided to the preterm neonate, such as oxygen administration and mechanical ventilation (Table 1).

The methods of treatment of BPD vary according to the severity of the disease. Therapeutic strategies are employed to specifically manage the pathophysiologic manifestations of chronic lung disease and to allow for lung growth and repair and eventual recovery of lung function.

PATHOPHYSIOLOGIC MECHANISMS AND THERAPEUTIC RATIONALE

Both the airways and pulmonary vasculature are abnormal in BPD, with mucosal metaplasia, lung inflammation, interstitial fibrosis, obliterative bronchiolitis, and smooth muscle hyperplasia. These changes lead to abnormalities of lung function (Table 2), the most important of which include bronchospastic and bronchomalactic airway disease, interstitial edema, increased work of breathing, and pulmonary hypertension.

TABLE 1. Factors Predisposing to Development of Bronchopulmonary Dysplasia

Anatomic lung immaturity
Biochemical lung immaturity (surfactant deficiency)
Genetic predisposition
Fluid overload
Patent ductus arteriosus
Pneumothorax
Pulmonary interstitial emphysema
Barotrauma from mechanical ventilation
Oxygen therapy and antioxidant insufficiency
Early development of increased airway resistance
Malnutrition
Lung inflammation and disordered fibrosis

TABLE 2. Pulmonary Pathophysiologic Changes in Infants with BPD

Decreased pulmonary compliance
Increased pulmonary resistance
Elevated driving pressure
Tracheobronchial airflow abnormalities
Expiratory airflow limitation: bronchospastic and bronchomalactic
Increased work of breathing
Air trapping and lung volume changes
Reactive airway disease
Pulmonary hypertension
Interstitial edema

Reactive Airway Disease

An exaggerated bronchoconstrictor response to various stimuli in infants with BPD has been attributed to airway hyperresponsiveness or hyperreactivity. The underlying assumption is that the change in bronchial smooth muscle tension leads to altered pulmonary functions. Other possibilities for the altered lung function are (1) mucosal edema, (2) engorged mucosal blood vessels, and (3) secretions. The physiologic consequences of the altered lung functions are decreased tidal volume, increased inspiratory time, and increased resistance to airflow. In addition, the critical opening pressure of the bronchioles is increased, thereby increasing the residual volume. The stiffening of the airway wall with the increased smooth muscle tone may actually prevent expiratory bronchiolar collapse. It is this reactive airway disease component that may be responsive to bronchodilator treatment.

Interstitial Edema

Interstitial water accumulation occurs in the lung of the infant with BPD for a variety of reasons, including capillary leak from the damaged epithelium, increased pulmonary capillary pressure, impaired lymphatic drainage due to the distorted architecture, and decreased plasma oncotic pressure from malnutrition or fluid overload. The majority of babies with BPD will benefit from the use of diuretics, even if there are no obvious signs of systemic fluid overload.

Increased Work of Breathing

In the infant with BPD, increased work of breathing is a major factor in the infant's ability to maintain gas exchange and to preserve adequate calories for growth and lung healing. Therapies that improve lung function will, therefore, also improve caloric balance. To compensate for the increased work of breathing, adequate caloric intake must be maintained, and in severe cases, mechanical ventilation must be provided to allow the infant adequate rest.

Pulmonary hypertension with subsequent cor pulmonale may result from smooth muscle hyperplasia and recurrent hypoxemia or hypercarbia. Infants with this complication of BPD require vigorous medical management, diuresis, and oxygen therapy to maintain relative nomoxemia.

THERAPEUTIC INTERVENTIONS

Oxygen Therapy

Owing to the propensity of hypoxemic episodes caused by reactive airway disease or other associated factors, such as feeding, straining, gastroesophageal reflux, crying, exercise, and colic, close monitoring by pulse oximetry is recommended for infants at risk. Oxygen supplementation is thought to correct delayed growth and improve weight gain. Bernbaum and Hoffman-Williamson[1] have defined the indications for oxygen supplement (Table 3). Oxygen saturation levels should be maintained at 92% to 96%.

In addition to fostering growth, the maintenance of adequate oxygenation may help forestall the development of pulmonary hypertension and right heart strain (cor pulmonale), the most feared irre-

TABLE 3. Commonly Used Indications for Supplemental Oxygen

Evidence of desaturation while breathing room air
Difficulty during oral feedings, associated desaturation
Apnea or bradycardia (reduced with O_2 supplement)
Poor growth rate
Poor exercise tolerance or chronic lethargy
Tachypnea or tachycardia (improved with O_2 therapy)

versible complications of BPD. Many infants with BPD exhibit sensitivity to oxygen administration and exhibit an acute decrease in pulmonary vascular resistance when the arterial Po_2 value is increased. Recurrent hypoxemia is likely to be harmful to the developing brain. Babies with chronic BPD and recurrent episodes of cyanosis are at significant risk for developmental delay.

Systemic Corticosteroid Therapy

Numerous studies have shown that administration of high-dose dexamethasone to ventilator-dependent infants with BPD facilitates weaning from respiratory support, with improvement in pulmonary function and attenuation of lung inflammation. These same studies indicate an acceptable level of side effects, ranging from no side effects in some studies to manageable degrees of hyperglycemia or hypertension in others. The theoretical risk of immune suppression and increased risk of infection has not been borne out in prospective studies. However, clinicians often withhold corticosteroid therapy from patients who are already infected. Preliminary data also indicate that corticosteroid treatment has no long-term adverse effects on neurologic outcome or pulmonary development. Although the use of corticosteroids clearly has short-term benefits, it is not yet clear whether the improvements in respiratory status of these babies translate into decreased mortality, morbidity, or hospital length of stay.

Initiation of dexamethasone therapy is usually considered between 2 and 4 weeks of age in the ventilator-dependent infant, although some recent studies are examining the possible benefits of commencing therapy in the first week of life. Most dexamethasone treatment protocols begin with a dose ranging from 0.25 to 0.5 mg/kg/d (for 3 days), followed by a reduction in dose every 3 days. Therapy is usually continued for 14 to 42 days. The literature is controversial as to the most beneficial dosage and course of treatment. Our usual approach is to start steroid therapy by 2 weeks of age in only the most severely ill infants. For all other ventilator-dependent babies, we begin dexamethasone by 1 month of age if they are not making progress despite optimal medical and respiratory management. However, if the baby is progressing and steadily weaning, we reserve treatment to allow the infant to heal on its own. The duration of treatment varies from 2 weeks in milder cases to several weeks for the most severely compromised neonates.

Symptomatic Pharmacologic Interventions

The overall goals of management and pharmacologic interventions are to (1) provide symptomatic control, (2) maintain normal activity levels, (3) ensure growth and neurodevelopmental maturation, (4) maintain pulmonary function as normal as feasible, (5) minimize acute exacerbations, (6) intervene early or prevent respiratory infections, (7) avoid adverse effects of medications, and (8) attempt to maintain home-based care.

The doses, routes of administration, and variety of drugs often used in BPD management during infancy are listed in Table 4. Reasonable unanimity has not been reached about the mode and basis for pharmacologic interventions. However, in a 1990 review, Davis et al. outlined broad guidelines.[2] A step-care approach, as used in the management of asthma, is often modified to increase the dose, frequency, and number of medications on a step-by-step, as-needed basis.

Bronchodilators

Theophylline, caffeine, albuterol, and terbutaline have all been shown to provide acute therapeutic relief for bronchospasm in these babies. Albuterol is the beta-agonist of choice because it has better beta-selectivity than terbutaline. Inhalation is the preferred route of administration of beta-agonists because the acute response is better than with oral dosing and side effects are minimized because of the

TABLE 4. Pharmacologic Agents in the Outpatient Management of BPD

DRUG	AVAILABLE FORM	DOSES
Inhaled Beta₂-Agonist		
Nebulized albuterol	Solution for inhalation: 0.5% (5 mg/ml)	0.1–0.15 ml/kg (max: 0.5 ml/kg/d)
Metered albuterol	Inhalation aerosol: 90 μg per puff	May repeat after 20–30 min (max: 2.5 mg/d)
Nebulized metaproterenol	5% (50 mg/ml)	0.1–0.3 ml (max: 15 mg/d)
Nebulized terbutaline (use injectable form)	0.1% (1 mg/ml) in 0.9% NaCl	0.25 ml (not FDA approved)
Systemic Beta₂-Agonist		
Albuterol	2 mg/5 ml	0.1–0.2 mg/kg/d in 3–4 divided doses
Terbutaline		
Oral	25 mg	1.25–2.5 mg in 3 doses q8h
Subcutaneous	1 mg/ml	0.01–0.5 mg/kg SC
Intravenous	1 mg/ml	Loading dose: 10 mg/kg Maintenance dose: 0.4 mg/kg/min; increase by 0.2 mg/kg/min to reach 3–6 mg/kg/min
Methylxanthines		
Theophylline	Aminophylline (80% of anhydrous theophylline)	Loading dose: 6 mg/kg (use 3 mg/kg with previous theophylline treatment) Maintenance dose: 1–2 mg/kg/d in 2–3 divided doses Desired drug level: range 12–15 mg/dl
Caffeine	Caffeine citrate 10 mg/ml	Loading dose: 20 mg/kg Maintenance dose: 2–7 mg/kg/d Desired drug level: 15–25 mg/dl
Diuretics		
Furosemide	IV PO	1 mg/kg q.d. or q.o.d. IV 1–5 mg/kg q.d. PO
Chlorothiazide	50 mg/ml	10–20 mg/kg/d in 2 divided doses PO
Spironolactone	10 mg/ml	1–3 mg/kg/d in 2 divided doses PO
Supplemental Medication		
Cromolyn sodium	Nebulized: 20 mg per ampule or capsule	20 mg per dose 3–4 times a day
Dexamethasone		0.25–0.5 mg/kg/d, then taper (see text)

selective effect on the bronchi. In infants with severe recurrent bronchospasm, theophylline is commonly used as well.

Reversibility of airflow limitations following administration of a bronchodilator helps to elucidate the pathology of airflow limitation. Improved airflow indicates increased bronchomotor tone as a contributing factor in airflow limitation. This test has been used for diagnostic evaluation and for defining the dose and frequency of a therapeutic agent. Worsening of airflow with the use of a bronchodilator may be due to several factors: undetected bronchomalacia, inadequate time for response to the drug, improper drug administration, or inappropriate testing. Several studies have indicated a paradoxical response to bronchodilator therapy in infants with bronchomalactic BPD. Thus, it would be appropriate to evaluate the response to short-term bronchodilator therapy before prescribing long-term outpatient bronchodilator treatment.

Diuretics

Furosemide has been the most frequently studied diuretic in BPD. The administration of furosemide results in a diuresis that minimizes total lung water and raises plasma oncotic pressure. However, furosemide also has important nonrenal effects on pulmonary function, which are evident soon after the dose has been given and well before the effect of diuresis has taken place. Furosemide causes venodilation, which increases venous capacitance and, therefore, decreases right ventricular end-diastolic volume and pulmonary capillary pressure. There are direct effects of furosemide on airway epithelium as well, which may result in decreased chloride and water transport across the epithelium and diminished airway reactivity. Studies of pulmonary mechanics have demonstrated improvement in both lung compliance and lung resistance. Most studies have used a dose of 1 mg/kg/d, but a recent investigation suggested that a dose of 1 mg/kg every other day can lead to a sustained improvement in pulmonary function with fewer side effects. The side effects of furosemide include fluid and electrolyte imbalance (chloride depletion and metabolic alkalosis, hyponatremia), hypercalciuria and nephrolithiasis, osteopenia, and ototoxicity.

Chlorothiazide in combination with spironolactone (Aldactone) results in a diuresis similar to that of furosemide, but the effects on pulmonary mechanics are less clear-cut. Whereas earlier studies showed improvement in lung compliance and airway resistance with this therapy, more recent studies have demonstrated an adequate diuresis but no improvement in pulmonary function or oxygenation. Chlorothiazide and spironolactone, however, may be advantageous because they produce fewer side effects than furosemide does.

Our current approach is to initiate therapy with furosemide in the early stages of BPD when weaning from the ventilator is a goal. When the infant is tolerating enteral feedings and is more stable, therapy is changed to chlorothiazide and spironolactone. Intermittent doses of furosemide are administered if respiratory deterioration or signs of fluid retention occur. Supplemental potassium chloride should be administered to prevent chloride and potassium depletion. Diuretics are generally continued until the infant no longer requires oxygen therapy.

PARENTAL COUNSELING

Parents of infants with BPD incur serious emotional trauma in dealing with prematurity, the intensive care nursery environment, repeated life-threatening illnesses, and separation from their baby. Discharge of an infant with BPD with the spectre of a possible chronic lung disorder adds to their grief and can contribute to a negative perception of the child. When these emotions are compounded by an inability to resume their normal lifestyle, parents and siblings may develop a resentment toward the infant. It is imperative to both educate and remind parents that most infants with BPD do recover and that the frequently cited sequelae are potentially not handicapping or life threatening.

REFERENCES

1. Bernbaum JC, Hoffman-Williamson M: Primary Care of the Preterm Infant. Philadelphia, Mosby–Year Book, 1991:97–98.
2. Davis JM, Sinkin RA, Aranda JV: Drug therapy for bronchopulmonary dysplasia. Pediatr Pulmonol 8:117–125, 1990.

DISORDERS OF THE UMBILICUS

FREDERICK J. RESCORLA, M.D.
RICHARD C. RINK, M.D.

Abnormalities of the umbilicus are uncommon but, when present, often manifest as a wet, edematous, enlarged umbilicus that will not slough. The differential diagnosis of umbilical disorders includes (1) urachal anomalies, (2) omphalomesenteric duct anomalies, (3) granulation of a healing umbilical stump, (4) umbilical hernia, (5) omphalitis, and (6) infected umbilical vessels. It is very rare to have both urinary and enteric drainage to the umbilicus simultaneously.

ETIOLOGY

Disorders in the umbilical region can be related to persistence of structures that normally obliterate before birth or failure of closure of the umbilical ring. The umbilicus in early gestation is made up of fusion of the body stalk containing the umbilical vessels and allantois with the extracoelomic yolk stalk containing the vitelline (omphalomesenteric) duct and vessels (Fig. 1). The vitelline duct normally obliterates between the seventh and eighth weeks of gestation. Failure of obliteration results in persistence of vitelline (omphalomesenteric) remnants that can lead to a wide variety of clinical disorders depending on the stage of arrest (Fig. 2). Failure of the allantois to form a cordlike urachus can result in urachal abnormalities (Fig. 3). The fetal midgut normally returns to the abdominal cavity between the tenth and twelfth weeks of gestation, and the abdominal wall proceeds to close. As mesoderm migrates to form the abdominal wall, the

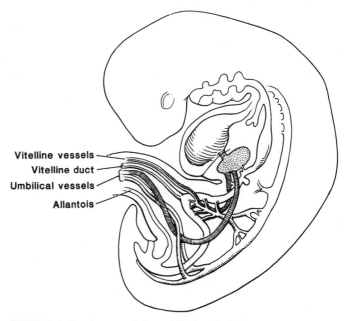

Vitelline vessels
Vitelline duct
Umbilical vessels
Allantois

FIGURE 1. Development of the umbilical cord. Structures present at approximately 35 days.

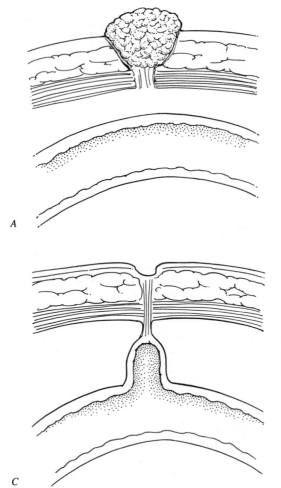

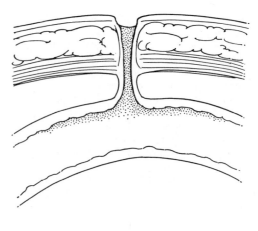

FIGURE 2. Omphalomesenteric (vitelline) duct remnants. *A,* Umbilical polyp. *B,* Umbilical fistula. *C,* Meckel's diverticulum with band of vestigial vitelline vessels to the umbilicus.

umbilicus closes to a small ring containing the insertion of the umbilical vessels and urachus. Failure of closure can lead to an omphalocele, hernia of the umbilical cord, or an umbilical hernia. The first two present at delivery as an abdominal wall defect and are not discussed in this section.

INITIAL EVALUATION

The initial evaluation is guided by the presenting signs and symptoms, as well as by careful inspection of the umbilicus. The character of the drainage (urine, intestinal contents) occasionally will confirm the diagnosis. If an opening is present, a radiographic contrast study can be obtained by placing a small catheter into the opening and gently injecting a water-soluble agent. As noted in Figures 2 and 3, contrast medium will enter into urachal or omphalomesenteric remnants that connect to the umbilicus. Ultrasound examination and a voiding cystourethrogram may be useful in evaluation of these urachal anomalies.

URACHAL ANOMALIES

Anomalies of the urachus are a result of failure of its normal involution. Initially, the allantois and cloaca are in communication. During formation of the bladder from the cloaca, there is descent of the bladder toward the pelvis. The apical connection of the bladder to the umbilicus is the urachus. The urachus resides between the peritoneum and transversalis fascia in the space of Retzius. Its investment in the umbilicovesical fascia usually limits extension of any urachal disorder. The urachus ultimately becomes a fibrous cord at 4 to 5 months gestation. Failure of all or a portion of the urachus to atrophy and obliterate results in four anatomic anomalies, three of which may present as an umbilical abnormality (Fig. 3).

The *patent urachus* (50% of cases) is a result of total lack of involution and presents in the neonatal period as urine draining from the umbilicus. The drainage may be intermittent or continuous. The umbilical cord is often quite enlarged and edematous (hydrops of the cord). Urachal anomalies have been noted to retract the umbilicus during voiding. Although bladder outlet obstruction is often suspected, it is present in only 14% of reported cases, although it has been seen in up to 50% of patients with prune-belly syndrome who also have a patent urachus. A *urachal cyst* (30% of cases) can form if there is incomplete involution of the urachus. Filling of the remaining lumen with desquamated epithelium results in this cyst formation. The urachal cyst per se does not present as an umbilical abnormality and is more often small and undetected. When noted, however, it is more common in older children or adults with an infraumbilical tender mass. If the cyst becomes infected, a *urachal abscess* may form. This abscess may tract to the umbilicus spontaneously, resulting in purulent umbilical drainage. Alternatively, it may drain into the bladder. Rupture into the peritoneum has resulted in an acute abdomen presentation, making correct diagnosis difficult. An external *urachal sinus* (15% of cases) may occur when the cranial aspect of the urachus does not involute or when a small infected urachal cyst dissects to the umbilicus. These generally present with intermittent periumbilical pain and tenderness. Intermittent drainage between the umbilicus and bladder is known as an *alternating sinus*. A *urachal diverticulum* (5% of cases) does not affect the umbilicus and, thus, is not discussed.

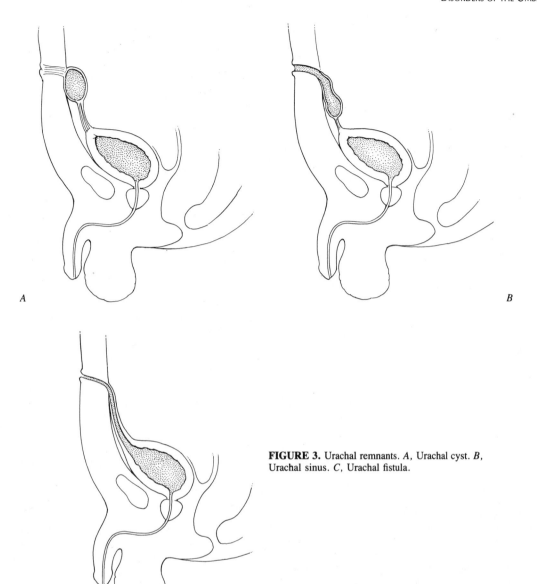

FIGURE 3. Urachal remnants. *A*, Urachal cyst. *B*, Urachal sinus. *C*, Urachal fistula.

Diagnosis

The diagnosis of patent urachus is generally confirmed by catheterization of the tract or fistulography. Intravesical injection of methylene blue is often helpful, as is analysis of the draining fluid for urea and creatinine. A lateral voiding cystourethrogram may reveal the patent urachus. The location of the urachus makes it ideal for evaluation by ultrasound or CT, the diagnostic procedures of choice for a suspected urachal cyst. A urachal sinus is defined by a lateral fistulogram or by probing the tract. Prenatal ultrasonographic diagnosis of a patent urachus has been reported. The normal urachal remnant has been noted in 62% of pediatric bladder ultrasound studies as a small, elliptical, hypoechoic structure above the bladder. This has no clinical significance.

Treatment

Treatment of urachal anomalies requires complete excision of the urachus along with a cuff of bladder. Cauterization or ligation of the tract has not been effective therapy. Any associated lower urinary tract obstruction should be dealt with first. Efforts at conservative management, such as drainage of urachal cysts, have resulted in a 30% recurrence rate. However, patients with an infected urachal cyst or urachal abscess may be better treated by initial incision and drainage or by percutaneous drainage of the abscess cavity. Following resolution of the inflammation, complete excision of the involved tissues is warranted. Broad-spectrum antibiotic therapy in this group of patients should begin before manipulation of the abscess. Although *Staphylococcus aureus* is the most common organism identified, other gram-positive and gram-negative organisms (including anaerobes) and fungi have been noted. Resection of the urachus and involved structures can be achieved through either a transverse midhypogastric incision or a vertical midline incision. The urachal attachment to the umbilicus should be removed at the dermis, preserving the umbilicus whenever possible. The umbilicus should be excised only if it is suppurative or severely involved in the process.

OMPHALOMESENTERIC DUCT ANOMALIES

The omphalomesenteric duct normally obliterates by the eighth week of gestation. Persistence of this structure most frequently leads to a Meckel's diverticulum. A Meckel's diverticulum usually has no connection to the umbilicus. However, occasionally, a vitelline vessel can extend from the Meckel's diverticulum to the umbilicus, which promotes volvulus of the intestine. In addition, the Meckel's diverticulum can remain attached to the umbilicus, presenting as an *umbilical fistula*. Other disorders include an *umbilical polyp, a sinus,* or an *enteric cyst* below the umbilicus. These may or may not have an attachment to the bowel (Fig. 2).

Diagnosis

The presence of intestinal contents draining from the umbilicus after cord separation confirms the diagnosis of an umbilical fistula. An umbilical polyp may appear initially similar to a granuloma, but the polyp does not respond to silver nitrate administration. Furthermore, the umbilical polyp can contain small bowel or gastric mucosa. Enteric cysts and sinuses are very uncommon anomalies. An enteric cyst may be asymptomatic or may present as an umbilical mass when the cyst fills with fluid.

Treatment

Excision of these structures can be accomplished with an intraumbilical incision. If a fistula is present, the ileum is delivered into the wound, the fistulous tract is excised, and the bowel is closed in a transverse fashion. If the intraumbilical incision is inadequate, an infraumbilical extension will allow delivery of the bowel into a larger opening to complete the excision. In cases of umbilical polyps, the excision is continued down to the center of the umbilicus. If the umbilical vessels and urachal remnant are encountered, they can be ligated. The base of the polyp will usually end outside the peritoneum. If it extends through the peritoneum, the peritoneum should be opened to determine if there is an enteric communication.

UMBILICAL HERNIA

Umbilical hernias are fairly common, occurring in approximately 1 in 6 children in some reported series. Complications of untreated umbilical hernias include incarceration and strangulation, although both are extremely rare. The natural history of untreated hernias in this area is unclear.

Most such hernias undergo spontaneous closure, usually by age 3 to 4 years, although some will close at an older age. Review of the literature reveals that hernias with an initial fascial defect of less than 0.5 cm are likely to close, whereas those with fascial defects greater than 1.5 cm are unlikely to close. The length of the observation period before surgical repair is, therefore, debated. Most umbilical hernias are repaired electively for failure of closure. Our current recommendation is to repair the hernia at age 4 to 5 years. However, defects greater than 1.5 cm in diameter and large proboscis-type hernias probably merit repair at a younger age (1 to 2 years), especially if no significant closure is noted after this period of observation.

Treatment

Repair is accomplished through an infraumbilical curvilinear incision. The fascia inferior to the hernia is identified, and the hernia sac is encircled at the level of the fascia. The hernia can then be handled in one of two ways. The sac can be transected and excised, with closure of the fascia, or the sac can be sharply dissected from the overlying skin and inverted, and the fascial defect can be closed without opening the peritoneal cavity. The undersurface of the skin at the center of the protruding skin is tacked to the fascia, and the skin is closed.

UMBILICAL GRANULOMA

A granuloma of the umbilicus is a common disorder that appears after cord separation as a mass of pink granulation tissue at the base of the umbilicus. It may be difficult to differentiate initially from an umbilical polyp. Treatment consists of topical application of silver nitrate. Several applications may be required. If the granuloma persists after several treatments, it should be treated with excision. If the lesion appears to extend through the base of the umbilicus, the center of the umbilicus should be excised, as it may actually represent an umbilical polyp.

MISCELLANEOUS DISORDERS

Infected umbilical vessels are rare. If they are present, excision of the vessel is the treatment of choice. Similarly, the incidence of *omphalitis* has been decreasing because of proper umbilical care. It is still noted in third world countries where antiseptic care is absent. Children with omphalitis should have cultures of the blood and cerebrospinal fluid and receive broad-spectrum antibiotics (ampicillin and an aminoglycoside) for 7 to 10 days.

ASCITES

SAMUEL A. KOCOSHIS, M.D.

PATHOGENESIS AND DIAGNOSIS

Ascites is "an abnormal accumulation of serous fluid within the peritoneal cavity."[1,2] Its development is the direct result of disequilibrium between osmotic and hydrostatic forces that govern fluid movement across the peritoneal capillary bed. Adequate mesenteric lymph flow and satisfactory portal venous blood flow play major roles in maintaining that equilibrium. Either mesenteric lymphatic obstruction or portal venous obstruction favors the development of ascites. Rupture of the biliary tree, the urinary tract, or gastrointestinal tract can flood the peritoneum with protein-rich fluid, defying adequate resorption. Primary inflammatory or infectious conditions of the peritoneum will increase capillary permeability and simultaneously retard resorption of peritoneal fluid. Finally, hypoalbuminemia can reduce plasma oncotic pressure sufficiently to produce both ascites and peripheral edema.

Successful treatment of neonatal ascites is predicated on correctly diagnosing the underlying conditions that produce abnormal fluid accumulation. Specific physical findings are characteristic of the disorders commonly associated with neonatal ascites. Jaundice and hepatosplenomegaly suggest underlying hepatic disease, portal hypertension, or bile duct perforation. Oliguria, hypospadias, or palpable kidneys suggest urinary tract pathology. Generalized edema is usually due to cardiogenic hydrops, hypoproteinemia, hemolytic disease, or oliguric renal failure.

Several radiographic tools may be helpful in differentiating generalized ascites from loculated fluid collections, such as abscesses or cysts. Abdominal ultrasonography is the easiest of these to perform and is free from ionizing radiation, although abdominal computed tomography (CT) and magnetic resonance imaging (MRI) may provide better-resolved images of pathologic solid organs. Urinary tract disease may be diagnosed by renal scintigraphy, intravenous pyelography (IVP), or voiding cystourethrography. Hepatobiliary scintigraphy will often identify a biliary leak.

Diagnostic paracentesis is extremely valuable in establishing the etiology of ascites. The procedure should be performed employing sterile technique at the midline just inferior to the umbilicus. A small-caliber angiocatheter is inserted by Z-tracking to minimize fluid leakage after removal of the catheter. Approximately 10 to 20 ml of fluid is withdrawn, and the catheter is removed. Complications are rare but include perforation of a hollow viscus or hemorrhage. Table 1 illustrates the characteristics of peritoneal fluid that point to a specific diagnosis. Table 2 lists laboratory tests that can be performed on peritoneal fluid to establish an etiology for the ascites.

A myriad of conditions (Table 3) is associated with the development of neonatal ascites. Management of the most common disorders is outlined.

URINARY ASCITES

Frank urinary tract perforation will be found in most but not all neonates with urinary ascites. The ascitic fluid may originate from

TABLE 1. Peritoneal Fluid Characteristics

APPEARANCE	DIAGNOSIS
Clear, yellow	Nonspecific
Dark green	Bile ascites
Milky	Chylous ascites (if patient has been fed)
Serosanguineous	Malignant ascites
Nonmilky, turbid	Inflammatory process

the retroperitoneum or from an intraperitoneal perforation. The site of perforation and level of obstruction dictate the management. Customarily, the serum creatinine and BUN are frighteningly high because of peritoneal reabsorption, but if the underlying condition has not produced renal dysplasia, kidney function may remain intact. Relief of obstruction may produce brisk diuresis and rapid correction of both creatinine and BUN. Percutaneous vesicostomy or nephrostomy is usually the initial therapeutic step unless posterior urethral valves (which can be primarily excised) are found. Timing of definitive urologic repair depends on the stability of the patient and the underlying disorder being treated.

MECONIUM PERITONITIS

Meconium peritonitis may be secondary to either in utero or postnatal small bowel perforation. If the perforation occurs during fetal life, the meconium is sterile and peritoneal irritation is not impressive, but abdominal distention will be present at birth. The ascites may produce fibroadhesive bands and a peel that seals off the fluid. A cystic cavity may be formed by adherent loops of bowel. Perinatal intestinal perforation usually produces generalized ascites. A rare neonate whose intestine has been perforated may appear healthy, but most develop vomiting and shock within hours of birth. Frank abdominal calcifications may be evident radiographically, or abdominal ultrasonography may reveal peritoneal fluid with a snowstorm appearance. Definitive therapy depends on the underlying etiology of the perforation, but initial medical therapy universally includes fluid resuscitation, nasogastric suction, and parenteral broad-spectrum antibiotics, such as ampicillin and gentamicin. Operative intervention may require bowel resection, but if the bowel is not frankly necrotic and bowel viability is in question, the surgeon may elect to forego resection, place appropriate enterostomies, and perform a second-look operation a short while after the initial decompressive procedure.

HEPATIC ASCITES

When liver dysfunction and portal hypertension cause neonatal ascites, an assiduous search for the etiology of the liver disease is imperative. The initial impulse to treat serious neonatal liver disease with immediate liver transplantation should be tempered by circumspection. Even though liver failure due to alpha$_1$-antitrypsin deficiency or neonatal hemochromatosis requires urgent transplantation, some metabolic liver diseases may clinically improve following initiation of appropriate dietary measures. For example, a lactose-free and galactose-free diet may be used for galactosemia, and a low-tyrosine, low-phenylalanine, low-methionine diet will improve the serum aminogram in tyrosinemia. These therapeutic measures should be instituted as soon as a diagnosis of galactosemia or tyrosinemia is established.

Whether the patient is a liver transplantation candidate or not, optimal pharmacotherapy of hepatic ascites is essential. Cornerstones of therapy are salt restriction and rational diuretic therapy. Sodium intake should be limited to 1 to 1.5 mEq/kg/d. Urinary electrolytes should be measured serially; the urinary sodium loss should approximate 2 to 2.5 mEq/kg/d to ensure weight loss. This can almost never be accomplished with salt restriction alone. Therefore, therapy with diuretics should be started early in the patient's course.

Spironolactone may be used alone at a dose of 3 mg/kg/d divided two or three times a day if ascites is not tense, but the onset of diuresis

may be delayed by several days or even weeks. The dose may be increased to 6 mg/kg/d or even 9 mg/kg/d if lower doses have not achieved maximal effect. Effectiveness can be judged by measuring the urinary sodium/potassium ratio, which will remain below 1 until the maximal spironolactone effect is attained.

Under more urgent clinical conditions, a combination of spironolactone 3 mg/kg/d and furosemide 1 mg/kg/d divided twice daily may be employed. The lack of a therapeutic response requires doubling or even tripling of the dose. Water balance, body weight, and serum electrolytes must be monitored daily during the first few days of therapy. Adult data suggest that 300 to 500 ml of ascitic fluid are likely to be mobilized per day if diuretics are used exclusively. In some infants, diuresis may be enhanced during the first few days of therapy by intravenously infusing 1 g of albumin per kilogram over 2 or 3 hours before intravenously administering each furosemide dose.

Two additional therapies of ascites deserve mention. Peritoneal-venous shunting of ascites was first popularized in the 1970s and 1980s. Unfortunately, adult-sized shunts are unwieldy for pediatric patients. In addition, a propensity for shunt occlusion and for shunt-induced coagulopathy has hampered their use in children. Most candidates for peritoneal-venous shunts are also candidates for liver transplantation and are better served by the latter procedure. Patients with stable liver function may benefit from transjugular portosystemic shunting, but few radiologists are skilled enough to perform such procedures in neonates.

BILE ASCITES

Most perforations of the extrahepatic biliary tree are at the junction of the cystic duct and common duct, and only occasionally is the perforation proximal to a distal obstruction. However, surgical exploration is essential. Unlike older individuals in whom bile peritonitis usually produces exquisite abdominal distress and rebound tenderness, most neonates with bile ascites experience an indolent course of gradual, nontender abdominal distention, failure to thrive, and mild jaundice. Bile leaks are initially confined to the porta hepatis as bilomas. Leakage into the peritoneum occurs gradually, and abdominal distention does not appear until several days or weeks after birth.

If biliary obstruction is identified surgically, a choledochoenterostomy may be necessary, but in the absence of obstruction, simple bile drainage usually is satisfactory therapy.

CHYLOUS ASCITES

The presence of milky, triglyceride-rich ascites in patients who have been fed is diagnostic of chylous ascites secondary to generalized

TABLE 2. Typical Laboratory Tests Performed on Ascitic Fluid and Their Significance

TEST	SIGNIFICANCE
Cell count	>250 cells = inflammation
	Lymphocytic predominance = tuberculosis
Serum albumin-ascitic fluid albumin gradient	Serum albumin–ascitic fluid albumin gradient >1.1 g/dl = cardiac, hepatic, myxedema
	Gradient <1.1 g/dl = bile ascites, peritoneal inflammation, bowel obstruction
Bilirubin level	>Serum level = bile ascites
Creatinine, urea nitrogen level	>Serum level = urinary ascites
Triglyceride level	>400 mg/dl = chylous ascites
Gram stain, fungal stain, acid-fast stain	Positive = infection
Bacterial, fungal, acid-fast bacillus culture	Positive = infection
L-Lactate level	>33 mg/dl = bacterial infection

TABLE 3. Causes of Neonatal Ascites

Urinary Ascites Urethral aplasia Extrinsic urethral obstruction Posterior urethral valves Neurogenic bladder Vescicoureteral reflux Ureteral obstruction Ureterocele Ureteropelvic junction obstruction Renal dysplasia Prune-belly syndrome	**Bile Ascites** Spontaneous bile duct rupture **Chylous Ascites** Localized mesenteric lymphangiectasis Generalized mesenteric lymphangiectasis Mesenteric lymphocele Malrotation of small bowel
Meconium Peritonitis Intestinal atresia Volvulus Intussusception Anal atresia Meckel's diverticulosis Meconium ileus Meconium plug	**Infectious Peritonitis** Toxoplasmosis Cytomegalovirus infection Herpes infection Syphilis Tuberculosis
Genital Tract Abnormalities Hydrometrocolpos Ruptured ovarian cyst	**Ascites Associated with Hydrops** Cardiac failure Hemolytic anemia Athyrosis Down syndrome Turner's syndrome Neural tube defects Achondroplasia Conradi's disease
Portal Hypertensive-Hepatic Ascites Galactosemia Nieman-Pick disease Tyrosinemia Neonatal hemochromatosis Neonatal hepatitis Gaucher disease Lysosomal storage disease Congenital hepatic fibrosis Polycystic liver disease Alpha$_1$-antitrypsin deficiency	

or localized mesenteric lymphatic obstruction. It must be emphasized that lymphatic obstruction may result in nonchylous ascites in patients who have not been fed.

If intestinal malrotation is identified as an associated finding, a Ladd procedure should be performed. Although relief of volvulus or lysis of mesenteric bands may facilitate lymphatic flow, lymph stasis may persist after surgery because of malformed mesenteric lymphatic channels.

A localized lymphocele can be excised surgically, with excellent results. However, diffuse mesenteric lymphangiectasis is not amenable to surgical therapy. In such cases, dietary therapy is the initial treatment. Fat intake is decreased to approximately 2 g/kg/d, and carbohydrate calories are increased. Some of the fat should be supplied in the form of medium chain triglycerides (MCT), whose transport is largely via the portal venous system rather than the lymphatics. Caution should be exercised to limit the quantity of MCT to 50% of dietary fat or less because excessive quantities may produce ketosis or essential fatty acid deficiency. Associated hypoproteinemia is common and may require intermittent infusions of albumin 1 to 3 g/kg/d.

If the volume of chylous ascites does not decrease after several weeks of a low-fat, high-MCT diet, or if the volume increases at any time, the use of total parenteral nutrition (TPN) and complete bowel rest should be considered. Many cases of chylous ascites resolve spontaneously if a low-fat diet or TPN is used, but refractory cases may require extracorporeal hemofiltration or peritoneovenous shunting. When shunting is contemplated for neonates, the shunt usually must be modified to permit venous insertion. Complications of shunting include shunt occlusion and disseminated intravascular coagulation.

THERAPEUTIC PARACENTESIS

Irrespective of the etiology of ascites, when tense fluid produces respiratory embarrassment, therapeutic paracentesis may become necessary. Controversy has raged for decades in the adult literature about the safety and efficacy of large volume paracentesis. The current consensus among hepatologists is that large volume (5 L) or even total paracentesis without plasma volume expansion is quite safe when performed on adult patients. In neonates, in whom intravascular fluid may be third-spaced quite rapidly, a more prudent approach is indicated. Fluid should be removed hourly, in smaller volumes by means of an indwelling catheter left in place for 12 to 18 hours. Simultaneous volume expansion with intravenous albumin will minimize the risk of developing shock. A caveat to this approach is that retention of the indwelling catheter for more than 12 to 24 hours heightens the risk of bacterial or fungal seeding of the peritoneal cavity.

REFERENCES

1. Fitzgerald JF: Ascites. *In* Wyllie R, Hyams JS (eds): Pediatric Gastrointestinal Disease. Pathophysiology, Diagnosis, Management. Philadelphia, WB Saunders, 1993:151–160.
2. Runyan BA: Care of patients with ascites. N Engl J Med 330:337–342, 1994.

FEEDING THE LOW BIRTH WEIGHT INFANT: ENTERAL AND PARENTERAL

SUDHA KASHYAP, M.D.
WILLIAM C. HEIRD, M.D.

Approximately 7% of infants born in the United States each year weigh <2.5 kg (low birth weight, LBW), and about 1% weigh <1.5 kg (very low birth weight, VLBW). Currently, the survival of infants weighing >1.5 kg at birth approaches 100%, and up to 75% of infants weighing <1.5 kg at birth survive. Providing adequate nutrition to satisfy the growth needs of these small infants is one of the pressing problems encountered by those responsible for their care. Of major concern is the possibility that failure to provide adequate nutrition to these infants when their organ systems (particularly the central nervous system, CNS) are undergoing rapid cellular proliferation may result in irreversible deficits and long-term sequelae.

The generally accepted goal for nutritional management of the LBW infant is to provide sufficient nutrients to support continuation of the intrauterine growth rate. The nutrient intakes recommended for these infants by the Committee on Nutrition of the American Academy of Pediatrics are based on this concept (Table 1).

The larger LBW infant frequently receives all nutritional intake exclusively by the enteral route. However, smaller infants, particularly those weighing <1.5 kg at birth, frequently are unable to tolerate enteral intakes because of gastrointestinal immaturity or respiratory distress or both. For these infants, parenteral nutrition usually is the

TABLE 1. Recommended Nutrient Intakes For Low Birth Weight Infants*

NUTRIENT	RECOMMENDED INTAKE†
	Amount/100 kcal
Protein (g)	2.7–3.1
Fat (g)	4.3–5.4
	(300 mg essential fatty acids)
Carbohydrate	—
Electrolytes and minerals	
Sodium (mEq)	2.3–2.7
Potassium (mEq)	1.8–1.9
Calcium (mg)	140–150
Magnesium (mg)	6.5–7.5
Phosphorus (mg)	95–108
Chloride (mEq)	2–2.4
Trace minerals	
Zinc (mg)	0.5
Copper (μg)	90
Manganese (μg)	5
Iodine (μg)	5
Vitamins	*Amount/d*
A (IU)	1400
D (IU)	500
E (IU)	5–25 (1 IU/g linoleic acid)
C (mg)	35
Thiamin (μg)	300
Riboflavin (μg)	400
Niacin (mg)	6
B₆ (μg)	300 (15 μg/g protein)
Folic acid (μg)	50
B₁₂ (μg)	0.3
Pantothenic acid (mg)	2
Biotin (μg)	35

*Committee on Nutrition, American Academy of Pediatrics: Pediatrics 75:976–986, 1985.
†Lower values are the recommended intakes for larger infants; higher values are the recommended intakes for smaller infants (BW <1250 g).

sole source of nutrition for the first several days to weeks after birth and is a supplement to tolerated enteral nutrition for some time thereafter.

ENTERAL NUTRITION

The types of feedings that are available for the LBW infants include human milk and bovine milk-derived formulas. Formulas designed specifically for LBW infants take into account both their nutrient requirements and their digestive limitations. For example, LBW infant formulas contain more protein (2.47 to 3 g/100 kcal), calcium (90 to 180 mg/100 kcal), and phosphorus (50 to 90 mg/100 kcal) than do term formulas. In addition, the protein content of all LBW formulas is modified bovine milk protein (whey/casein ratio of 60:40), which is less likely to result in metabolic acidosis and hyperaminoacidemia than unmodified bovine milk protein (whey/casein ratio of 18:82).

Fat provides approximately 50% of the nonprotein energy of both human milk and LBW infant formulas. Although poorer fat absorption by LBW infants has been reported and attributed to their relative deficiency of pancreatic lipase and bile salts, modern LBW formulas contain primarily unsaturated long chain triglycerides and medium chain triglycerides (MCT), both of which are reasonably well absorbed. The MCT content of current formulas varies from 10% to 50% of fat content.

Lactose is the major source of carbohydrate in human milk and in formulas for the term infant. The LBW infant may have difficulty in digesting lactose because of a developmental lag in intestinal mucosal lactase activity. Thus, LBW infant formulas contain a mixture of lactose and glucose polymers. Glycosidase enzymes involved in digesting glucose polymers are active in the LBW infant. In addition, glucose polymers have less of an osmotic load per unit weight than has lactose. The composition of the three commercially available formulas for LBW infants in this country is shown in Table 2.

Human milk has advantages over the commercially available formulas. Its immunologic properties, both cellular and humoral, are a distinct advantage. Recent studies show that the incidence of necrotizing enterocolitis and infections is lower in LBW infants fed human milk than in those fed formulas. An advantage in subsequent IQ at 7½ to 8 years of age also has been reported, but this finding needs to be confirmed. Evidence that human milk is nutritionally superior to commercially available formulas is lacking. In fact, growth rates of LBW infants fed their own mothers' milk (which has a 20% to 25% higher protein concentration than term milk for the first 3 to 4 weeks of lactation) are lower than the rates of infants fed LBW infant formulas. In addition, the calcium and phosphorus contents of human milk are insufficient to support adequate skeletal mineralization. Thus, the LBW infant fed human milk is at risk for development of rickets as well as fractures. Supplementation of human milk with commercially available human milk fortifiers that provide protein, calcium, phosphorus, and sodium appears to overcome these nutritional inadequacies.

In general, if a mother wishes to provide milk for her infant, she should be encouraged to express her milk for feeding the infant. This will provide the infant with the nonnutritional advantages of human milk and will provide potential psychologic benefits for the mother because of her involvement in the infant's care. This also will help ensure eventual success with breastfeeding. For infants weighing <1.5 kg, supplementation of human milk is strongly recommended. Infants weighing >1.5 kg at birth may not require supplementation but should be monitored closely for inadequate growth and development of rickets or fractures. Of infants whose mothers elect not to provide milk, those weighing <1.8 to 2 kg should be fed one of the LBW infant formulas. Larger infants can be fed term infant formulas. The LBW infant may be switched to unsupplemented human milk feeds or formulas designed for term infants when ready for discharge from the hospital.

Larger LBW infants without significant lung disease can be started on enteral feedings within the first 24 hours of life. For the smaller

TABLE 2. Composition (Amount/100 kcal) of Standard Formulas for Low Birth Weight Infants

COMPONENT	SIMILAC SPECIAL CARE*	ENFAMIL PREMATURE†	SMA PREMIE‡
Protein (g)	2.71	3	2.47
	(bovine milk)	(bovine milk, whey)	(bovine milk, whey)
Fat (g)	5.43	5.1	5.4
	(MCT, soy and coconut oils)	(MCT, soy and coconut oils)	(coconut, oleic and soy oils, oleo, MCT)
Carbohydrate (g)	10.6	11	10.5
	(lactose, glucose polymers)	(lactose, corn syrup)	(lactose, glucose polymers)
Calcium (mg)	180	117	90
Phosphorus (mg)	90	59	50
Magnesium (mg)	12	4.9	8.6
Iron (mg)	0.37	0.25	0.38
Zinc (mg)	1.5	1.5	1
Manganese (µg)	12	13	25
Copper (µg)	250	160	86
Iodine (µg)	20	7.9	10
Sodium (mg)	50	39	40
Potassium (mg)	140	111	90
Chloride (mg)	90	85	66
Vitamin A (IU)	680	1200	300
Vitamin D (IU)	150	330	60
Vitamin E (IU)	4	4.6	1.9
Vitamin K (µg)	12	13	8.6
Thiamine (B_1) (µg)	250	250	100
Riboflavin (B_2) (µg)	620	350	160
Vitamin B_6 (µg)	250	250	60
Vitamin B_{12} (µg)	0.55	0.3	0.3
Niacin (µg)	5000	4000	750
Folic acid (µg)	37	35	12.5
Pantothenic acid (µg)	1900	1200	450
Vitamin C (mg)	37	35	8.6

*Ross Laboratories
†Mead-Johnson Nutritional Division
‡Wyeth Laboratories

LBW infants who have significant respiratory distress requiring assisted ventilation, enteral feedings are often delayed because of the fear that necrotizing enterocolitis might develop. A number of randomized studies have shown that early minimal enteral feedings given along with parenteral nutrition may improve subsequent enteral feeding tolerance and shorten the time taken to achieve full enteral intake, thus reducing the time for parenteral nutrition. In no study was the incidence of necrotizing enterocolitis greater in infants who were randomized to receive early minimal feedings. Thus, for the smaller sick LBW infant (<1.5 g, ventilator dependent), early *minimal* feedings (which are not increased in volume) are recommended. However, there is no evidence that this approach is preferable to early enteral feeding with subsequent cautious slow increases in volume.

Large increases in feeding volume have been associated with development of necrotizing enterocolitis. For smaller LBW infants who are tolerating enteral feedings, rates of increase should not exceed 20 ml/kg/d. Feedings of larger LBW infants without any significant problems may be advanced more rapidly to achieve adequate enteral nutrition within 4 to 7 days.

Methods of Enteral Feeding

LBW infants born after 33 to 34 weeks gestation generally are able to nipple feed soon after birth. Smaller infants usually require gavage feedings, which may be given either intermittently or continuously. Infants weighing <1000 g at birth generally tolerate continuous feedings better than intermittent feedings. Intermittent gavage feedings may be administered by a nasogastric or an orogastric catheter, usually every 2 to 3 hours. As nasal tubes may affect pulmonary mechanics, oral tubes usually are preferred, especially if the tube is passed with every feeding. If the tube is to be left in place, a nasogastric tube is easier to secure. Continuous feedings may be infused directly into the stomach or into the duodenum (transpyloric feeding). In general, if intermittent feedings are not tolerated, a trial of continuous nasogastric feedings should be attempted. If this method of feeding is also unsuccessful because of regurgitation of residuals, a trial of transpyloric feedings should be considered. Before starting transpyloric feedings, the position of the catheter needs to be confirmed radiographically. This method of nutrient delivery may result in fat malabsorption probably because of bypassing the lipolytic effect of gastric lipase.

PARENTERAL NUTRITION

LBW infants comprise the largest single group of pediatric patients who receive parenteral nutrition. The nutrient regimen can be delivered by central venous infusion or by peripheral vein infusion. Regimens delivered by the central venous route can provide energy intakes exceeding 100 kcal/kg/d and, hence, support normal rates of growth and possibly even some catchup growth. Regimens delivered by peripheral vein usually provide only 50 to 80 kcal/kg/d. Such intakes maintain existing body composition and perhaps support some growth, but these intakes will not support rapid rates of growth. Generally, infants who seem likely to tolerate adequate enteral intakes within a period of 1 to 2 weeks should receive parenteral nutrition by the peripheral route. Infants who are expected not to tolerate feeds and thus require longer periods of time to achieve adequate enteral intakes should receive parenteral nutrition by the central venous route.

The nutritional infusate, whether for peripheral or central vein delivery, should include sources of nitrogen and energy, as well as sufficient electrolytes, minerals, and vitamins. Compositions of infusates suitable for both routes of delivery are shown in Table 3.

Several amino acid mixtures are available for use as the nitrogen source for parenteral nutrition. Some of these mixtures (TrophAmine, Aminosyn PF, and Neopham) were designed specifically for the pediatric patient. These pediatric mixtures result in plasma aminograms close to those of growing breastfed term infants and may be used more efficiently by the infant. An amino acid intake of 2.5 g/kg/d results in nitrogen retention comparable to that of the enterally fed term infant, but an intake of at least 3 g/kg/d is required to achieve intrauterine rates of nitrogen retention. When the LBW infant is initially started on intravenous alimentation, amino acid intakes less than 2.5 g/kg/d commonly are given and then gradually increased as the energy intake is increased. However, there is no convincing evidence that such a graded increase in amino acid intake is necessary.

Glucose is the predominant energy source of parenteral nutrition regimens. Most infants will not tolerate initial intakes greater than 12 to 15 g/kg/d. The ability of the very small LBW infant (<1000 g) to metabolize glucose is limited, and initial infusions of 10 g/kg/d frequently result in hyperglycemia. In these smaller infants, it is wise to begin with a lower glucose intake (5 to 8 g/kg/d) and then increase the intake as tolerated by the infant, usually by 2 to 5 g/kg/d.

LBW infants who receive fat-free parenteral nutrition develop essential fatty acid deficiency within a few days. To prevent this deficiency, parenteral lipid emulsions (0.5 to 1 g/kg/d) are indicated. Lipid emulsions of either soybean oil (Intralipid) or a mixture of safflower and soybean oils (Liposyn II) are available in both 10% and 20% concentrations. The ability to metabolize intravenous fat emulsions is related directly to the maturity of the infant. However, most LBW infants can tolerate the small doses required to prevent essential fatty acid deficiency. The 20% soybean oil emulsion (Intralipid) appears to be cleared more rapidly than the 10% emulsion. To use lipids as an energy source, the intake can be increased as tolerated (usually by about 0.5 g/kg/d) to a maximal intake of 2 to 3 g/kg/d.

Since electrolytes and mineral requirements vary considerably from infant to infant, the amounts suggested in Table 3 should not be interpreted as absolute requirements. Adjustments, made on the basis of close monitoring, are usually required. The calcium and phosphorus requirements for optimal skeletal mineralization are much higher and are not met with the amounts suggested. Furthermore, addition of higher amounts of these minerals to the parenteral nutrition is impossible because of the chemical incompatibility of calcium and phosphorus.

Zinc and copper should be added to the infusate of any infant who is likely to require parenteral nutrition for more than 1 to 2 weeks.

Other trace elements (e.g., selenium, chromium, manganese, molybdenum) should also be considered for patients who require parenteral nutrition for a longer time.

A pediatric multivitamin preparation is available that provides close to the recommended amounts of vitamins when added to the infusate at the dose suggested.

The parenteral nutrition infusate should be delivered at a constant rate using an infusion pump. Use of a 0.22-μm membrane filter between the catheter and the administration tubing is recommended. The lipid emulsion is piggybacked to the infusate beyond the filter.

The complications associated with parenteral nutrition are related to the technique per se (catheter related) or to the infusate. The major catheter-related complication is infection. Most often, improper care of the catheter or catheter site is the underlying cause. Rarely is contamination of the infusate a cause for the infection. With peripheral venous infusions, thrombophlebitis and skin and subcutaneous sloughs due to infiltration of the solution are the most common complications.

Metabolic complications may be related to the limited metabolic capacity of the infant or to the infusate itself. Some of the earlier reported complications (metabolic acidosis, hyperammonemia) related to the amino acid mixtures are no longer problems. Most metabolic complications related to the limited metabolic capacity of the infant (hyperglycemia, electrolyte or mineral abnormalities) can be avoided with close and frequent monitoring. The major concern is parenteral nutrition-associated hepatic disorders (cholestasis).

Adequate monitoring to detect metabolic and catheter-related complications is an absolute necessity. Some of the metabolic complications are unavoidable, but most can be controlled by careful monitoring and appropriate adjustments of the infusate. The monitoring required for safe and efficacious use of lipid emulsions is not clear. The usual practice of periodic visual or nephelometric inspection for lipemia does not reliably detect elevated plasma triglyceride and free fatty acid concentrations. However, serial monitoring of plasma triglyceride and free fatty acid concentrations may not be feasible. A reasonable compromise is to resrict the parenteral lipid intake to 2 g/kg/d (up to 3 g/kg/d for the larger stable infant) and to inspect the plasma visually or by nephelometry. This monitoring should be done more frequently when lipids are first started, when the intake is being increased, or when the infant develops a clinical condition that might interfere with triglyceride hydrolysis.

Weaning from parenteral nutrition should be considered once feedings are initiated. Enteral feedings should be introduced as soon as they are tolerated and advanced as tolerated by the infant. During the period of combined enteral and parenteral nutrition, care should be taken to ensure that the infant's tolerance for both fluids and nutrients is not exceeded. This requires careful attention to the total (enteral plus parenteral) intake and frequent adjustments downward of the parenteral intake as the enteral intake increases. Some LBW infants may require fluid restriction. In these infants, an enteral formula of high caloric density (81 kcal/dl) should be considered. When enteral intake of 2 to 2.5 g/kg/d of protein and 120 ml/kg/d of fluid (80 to 100 kcal/kg/d) is achieved, parenteral nutrition can be discontinued, and enteral feedings can continue to be advanced as tolerated by the infant.

TABLE 3. Composition of Parenteral Nutrition Infusates for Central Vein Infusion and Peripheral Vein Infusion

COMPONENT	CENTRAL VEIN (amount/kg/d)	PERIPHERAL VEIN (amount/kg/d)
Crystalline amino acids (g)	3–4	2.5–3
Glucose (g)	20–30	12–15
Lipid emulsion (g)	0.5–3	0.5–3
Sodium (mEq)	3–4	3–4
Potassium* (mEq)	2–4	2–4
Calcium (mg)	40–80	40–80
Magnesium (mEq)	0.25	0.25
Chloride (mEq)	3–4	3–4
Phosphorus* (mmol)	1–2	1–2
Zinc (μg)	300	300
Copper (μg)	20	20
Other trace minerals†		
Iron‡		
Vitamins (MVI-Pediatric)§ (ml)	1.5–2	1.5–2
Total volume (ml)	120–130	120–150

*Hyperphosphatemia frequently develops if phosphorus intake exceeds 2 mmol/kg/d, the amount given with a daily potassium intake of 3 mEq/kg as a mixture of KH_2PO_4 and K_2HPO_4. If a potassium intake of more than 2 mEq/kg/d is required, the additional potassium should be given as KCl.
†See text.
‡Iron dextran (Imferon, Fisons Corp., Bedford, MA) can be added to the infusate of patients requiring prolonged parenteral nutrition therapy. We arbitrarily limit the dose to 0.1 mg/kg/d. Alternatively, the indicated intramuscular dose can be used intermittently, either as the sole source of iron or as an additional dose.
§MVI-Pediatric (Armour Pharmaceutical Co., Chicago, IL) is a lypholized product. When reconstituted as directed, 5 ml added to the daily infusate provides 80 mg vitamin C, 700 μg vitamin A, 10 μg vitamin D, 1.3 mg thiamine, 1.4 mg riboflavin, 1 mg pyridoxine, 17 mg niacin, 5 mg pantothenic acid, 7 mg vitamin E, 20 μg biotin, 140 μg folic acid, 1 μg vitamin B_{12}, and 200 μg vitamin K_1.

NUTRITIONAL REQUIREMENTS OF LOW BIRTH WEIGHT INFANTS

GILBERTO R. PEREIRA, M.D.

In 1985, the Committee on Nutrition of the American Academy of Pediatrics recommended the optimal diet for premature infants as one that supports growth rates comparable to the third trimester of intrauterine life, without imposing stress on their immature metabolic and excretory functions. More recently, the concept of the optimal diet for infants has been expanded to include the need for favorable outcomes regarding long-term growth, health status, and neurologic development. This section provides guidelines for the nutritional care of low birth weight (LBW) babies during the immediate postnatal period and the rest of the first month of life, emphasizing differences in nutritional requirements according to birth weight and mode of alimentation, that is, enteral versus parenteral nutrition.

IMMEDIATE POSTNATAL PERIOD

Nutritional care of the LBW infant should start soon after birth. The goals for nutritional support during this period are the maintenance of fluid status, the control of glucose homeostasis, and the normalization of serum electrolyte and mineral concentrations. Guidelines for the initiation of intravenous fluids in neonates of different birth weights, when nursed at various environmental conditions, are presented in Table 1. Intravenous fluids containing 5% to 10% dextrose are provided for at least the first 24 hours of life until parenteral or enteral feedings can be established. Under conditions of inadequate dextrose intake, LBW infants are at risk to become hypoglycemic because of their limited glycogen stores. If, however, dextrose intake is initiated at rates exceeding the serum glucose disposal rates (4 to 6 mg/kg/min), these infants not infrequently develop hyperglycemia. The use of 5% rather than 10% dextrose solution is recommended for very low birth weight (VLBW) babies who have increased fluid requirements during the first 24 to 72 hours of life to prevent this complication. Sodium, potassium, and chloride are routinely administered after the first 24 to 72 hours of life, following documentation of adequate renal function. In practice, this is expressed by the following: (1) urine volume >1 ml/kg/h, (2) urine osmolality > serum osmolality, (3) fractional excretion of sodium <3%, and (4) urine specific gravity >1.012.

The LBW infant has decreased body stores of nutrients and, consequently, a limited capacity to tolerate prolonged starvation, especially if coupled with additional metabolic demands imposed by illness. For these reasons, nutritional support in the form of enteral or parenteral nutrition should be initiated by the second day of life, with the goals of preventing excessive weight loss and promoting earlier resumption of postnatal growth. Although a significant number of sick infants are maintained solely on parenteral nutrition during the first few days or weeks of postnatal life, an attempt should be made to institute enteral feedings as soon as the gastrointestinal tract is thought to be functional.

ENTERAL NUTRITION

Enteral nutrition is more suitable than parenteral nutrition, since it provides physiologic stimulation and preservation of the gastrointestinal mucosa, it is associated with a lower risk of medical complications, and it is more cost effective. Before the initiation of enteral

TABLE 1. Recommendations for Starting Parenteral Fluid Therapy in Low Birth Weight Infants

	WEIGHT	
	<1000 g	1000–1500 g
Radiant Warmer		
Water intake (ml/kg/d)*	100–140	90–120
Dextrose (%)	5–10	10
Incubator		
Water intake (ml/kg/d)*	80–120	60–80
Dextrose (%)	5–10	10

*Intake should be decreased 10%–20% with humidified incubator or artificial plastic shield placed over the infant. Intake should be increased 20%–30% with phototherapy.
Data from Baumgart, Costarino. Clin Pediatr 21:199, 1982, and Water and nutrition. *In* Nutritional Needs of the Preterm Infant. Baltimore, Williams & Wilkins, 1993: 1–14.

feedings, the LBW infant should be evaluated for signs suggesting readiness to tolerate enteral feedings, such as absence of abdominal distention, presence of active bowel sounds, and previous passage of meconium stools. After severe perinatal asphyxia, it is common practice to withhold enteral feedings for a minimal period of 3 to 5 days to decrease the risk of necrotizing enterocolitis.

Although the critically ill LBW infant is essentially dependent on parenteral nutrition for the first few days or weeks of life, the administration of minimal enteral feedings (trophic feedings) has gained wide acceptance for the nutritional management of these infants. These feedings are intended to prime the gastrointestinal tract before the initiation of more substantive enteral nutrition. The presence of intraluminal nutrients appears to stimulate the development of the gastrointestinal mucosa, the maturation of intestinal motor activity, and the secretion of regulatory peptides and hormones. Controlled studies in infants less than 1200 g have documented that the administration of trophic feedings at intakes varying from 2.5 to 20 kcal/kg/d results in a shorter time to attain full enteral nutrition and in a lower incidence of feeding intolerance. Additional benefits suggested by these studies include a shorter course of parenteral nutrition, a reduced length of hospitalization, and a lower incidence of cholestasis, jaundice, and metabolic bone disease. The risk of necrotizing enterocolitis associated with the use of minimal enteral feedings has not been adequately evaluated because of the small sample size of these studies.

Nutritional requirements during enteral feedings and the composition of feedings recommended for LBW babies are presented in Table 2. Preterm human milk is the preferred feeding for LBW infants because of its unique nutrient composition, increased bioavailability of nutrients, immunologic properties, and the presence of hormones, enzymes, and growth factors. Several studies have documented that preterm human milk has a higher concentration of calories, protein, sodium, and chloride and a lower concentration of lactose than mature human milk. These compositional differences, which persist during the first month of lactation, are regarded as nutritionally beneficial for premature infants. However, despite these differences, some studies suggest that preterm human milk does not consistently meet the needs of the growing premature infant for protein, calcium, phosphorus, sodium, iron, copper, zinc, and some vitamins. Therefore, supplementation of preterm human milk with a powder or a liquid fortifier is recommended after feedings have been established and the milk has matured. Supplementation of preterm human milk has been shown to improve growth, nitrogen retention, and bone mineralization in preterm infants. Table 2 describes nutrient requirements and the composition of preterm human milk with and without fortification.

In the absence of human milk, premature infant formulas are the most appropriate substitute. In comparison to formulas intended for full-term infants, premature infant formulas provide a higher concentration of whey-predominant protein, a reduced lactose load, a blend of fat containing 13% to 50% of medium chain triglycerides, and a higher concentration of minerals, vitamins, and trace elements. Multivitamin and folic acid supplementation may be necessary depending on the daily volume of formula ingested by the infant and individual nutritional status.

Gastric gavage feedings are indicated for LBW infants whose sucking and swallowing mechanisms are immature, as well as for those with severe respiratory distress or neuromuscular disease. These feedings are usually given intermittently, at 2- or 3-hour intervals, with the smaller infants being fed more frequently. Intermittent feedings are considered more physiologic than continuous feedings because they accommodate cyclic surges in gut hormones. In addition, intermittent feedings are easier to administer, require minimal equipment, and have a lower risk of nutrient precipitation in the delivery system. Continuous feedings are an alternative method for the extremely LBW infant (<1000 g) and for those with severe respiratory distress or intolerance to intermittent feedings. Transpyloric feedings are not indicated for routine use in LBW babies because they bypass the stomach, an important site for initiation of fat digestion. In addition, transpyloric feedings have been associated with decreased ab-

TABLE 2. Nutritional Requirements

	ENTERAL (kg/d)	COMPOSITION OF FEEDINGS (per 100 kcal)					
		PRETERM HUMAN MILK	HUMAN MILK +NAT. CARE	HUMAN MILK +ENF FORT.	ENFAMIL PREM.	SIMILAC SP. CARE	PREEMIE SMA
Water (ml)*	150–200	136	109	121	109	109	108
Energy (kcal)†	110–130	100	100	100	100	100	100
Protein (g)‡	3–3.8	2.4	2.6	2.9	3.0	2.71	2.34
Carbohydrates (g)	8–12	11	10.8	12.5	11.1	10.6	10.2
Fat (g)	3–4	5.3	5.4	4.4	5.1	5.4	5.6
Sodium (mEq)	2–4	1.9	1.8	1.9	1.6	1.8	1.7
Chloride (mEq)	2–4	2.2	2.1	2.4	2.1	2.1	1.6
Potassium (mEq)	2–3	2.1	2.9	2.3	2.9	3.6	2.5
Calcium (mg)	120–230	38	133	144	165	180	90
Phosphorus (mg)	60–140	22	68	74	83	90	50
Magnesium (mg)	8–15	5	8.9	5.4	6.8	12	8.6
Iron (mg)§	1–2	0.14	0.26	0.11	0.25/1.8	0.37/1.8	0.38
Vitamin A (IU)‖	700–1500	72	406	1250	1250	680	300
Vitamin D (IU)	150–400	12	88	270	270	150	60
Vitamin E (IU)¶	6–12	0.6	2.5	6.2	6.3	4	1.9
Vitamin K (µg)	7–9	3	8	8	8	12	8.6
Vitamin C (mg)	20–60	6.7	23	20	20	37	8.6
Vitamin B₁ (mg)	0.2–0.7	0.01	0.1	0.2	0.2	0.25	0.1
Vitamin B₂ (mg)	0.3–0.8	0.04	0.3	0.3	0.3	0.6	0.16
Vitamin B₆ (mg)	0.3–0.7	0.009	0.14	0.15	0.1	0.25	0.06
Vitamin B₁₂ (µg)	0.3–0.7	0.03	0.32	0.25	0.25	0.55	0.3
Niacin (mg)	5–12	0.3	2.8	4.0	4	5	0.75
Folate (µg)#	50	5	22.6	35	35	37	12.5
Biotin (µg)	6–20	0.8	20.7	4.1	4	37	2.2
Zinc (µg)	800–1000	560	1077	1350	1500	1500	1000
Copper (µg)	100–150	57	163	125	125	250	86
Selenium (µg)	1.3–3	—	0.9	—	1.8	1.8	—
Chromium (µg)	0.7–7.5	—	—	—	0.4	—	—
Manganese (µg)	10–20	0.54	6.8	6.3	6.3	12	25
Molybdenum (µg)	0.3	—	—	—	0.25	—	—
Iodine (µg)	30–60	27	15.5	22	25	20	12

*For immediate postnatal initiation of fluid therapy, use values presented in Table 1.
†Adjust according to weight gain.
‡Requirements increase with increasing degree of prematurity.
§Initiate between 2 weeks and 2 months of age. Some feedings are available with and without iron fortification.
‖Increased requirement (1500–2800 IU/d) in patients with bronchopulmonary dysplasia.
¶Supplementation (25–50 IU/d) might be necessary to maintain serum vitamin E levels between 1 and 2 mg/dl.
#Not present in oral multivitamin supplement.

sorption of fat and potassium, increased bacterial colonization of the upper intestinal tract, dumping syndrome, and intestinal perforation secondary to stiffening of the feeding tubes. For these reasons, the use of transpyloric feeding should be limited to infants who are intolerant of gastric feedings because of severe gastroesophageal reflux or other conditions resulting in delayed gastric emptying. Only Silastic feeding tubes should be used for transpyloric feedings so as to prevent complications related to stiffening of the feeding tubes.

PARENTERAL NUTRITION

Parenteral nutrition is indicated in all LBW infants when enteral feedings are either contraindicated or provided in insufficient amounts. Clinical conditions that commonly require the use of parenteral nutrition include extreme prematurity, congenital anomalies of the gastrointestinal tract, necrotizing enterocolitis, perinatal asphyxia, major surgical procedures, malabsorptive syndromes, and sepsis. Parenteral nutrition solutions should provide all nutrients necessary for growth and development, including amino acids, dextrose, fatty acids, vitamins, minerals, and trace elements. Nutritional requirements for LBW infants during parenteral nutrition and the composition of solutions used for these infants at the Children's Hospital of Philadelphia are presented in Table 3. The preparation of TPN solutions should be sufficiently flexible that nutrient composition can be altered according to the patient's metabolic tolerance and requirements. Pediatric amino

acid solutions are appropriate for LBW infants because they provide the conditionally essential amino acids, such as taurine, cysteine, and tyrosine, and reduced amounts of glycine, methionine, and phenylalanine. This composition is considered beneficial for LBW babies and has been demonstrated to enhance weight gain and nitrogen retention, as well as to normalize plasma amino acid levels.

The parenteral administration of amino acids early in the postnatal period is advantageous for premature babies because it enhances nitrogen retention by increasing the rate of protein synthesis and by decreasing the rate of protein degradation. A combination of dextrose and lipid is routinely used as the source of nonprotein energy during parenteral nutrition. Parenteral regimens that contain dextrose and lipids at isocaloric ratios are more energy efficient and promote greater nitrogen retention than regimens that contain only dextrose or lipid.

Dextrose solutions are started at concentrations of 10%, and if a central line is in place, daily increments of 5% are made until the desired caloric intake is achieved. The use of continuous insulin infusion (0.04 to 0.16 U/h) in conjunction with dextrose improves glucose tolerance and enhances weight gain in small premature babies who develop glucose intolerance during the course of parenteral nutrition.

Fat emulsions are manufactured in concentrations of either 10% or 20%. The use of 20% emulsions is preferred in LBW babies because the reduced concentration of phospholipid in these emulsions improves triglyceride clearance and lessens the accumulation of cholesterol and

TABLE 3. Parenteral Requirements and Composition of TPN Solutions for Low Birth Weight Babies

	PARENTERAL REQUIREMENTS (kg/day)	COMPOSITIONS OF TPN SOLUTIONS (per 100 ml)
Water (ml)	100–150	100
Energy (kcal)	90–110	51*–113†
Amino acids (g)‡	2.5–3.5	1.5/2/2.5/3
Dextrose (g)	10–15	10/15/20
Sodium (mEq)	2–3.5	4
Potassium (mEq)	2–3	2
Chloride (mEq)	2–3.5	4.6
Calcium (mEq)§	60–90	3–4.5
Phosphorus (mEq)§	40–70	1.4
Magnesium (mEq)	4–7	0.4
Zinc (μg)	400	500
Copper (μg)	20	60
Manganese (μg)	1	5
Selenium (μg)‖	1.5–2	3
Iodine (μg)	0–60	8
Iron (mg)	0.1–0.2	0.1
Vitamins, M.V.I. Pediatric (ml)	1.5 (<1 kg)	1.5
	3.3 (>1 kg)	3.3
Heparin (IU)¶	—	50
Fat emulsions (g/kg/d)#	1–3	1–3

*Using 1.5% amino acid, 10% dextrose, and 1 g/kg of fat emulsion.
†Using 3% amino acid, 20% dextrose, and 3 g/kg of fat emulsion.
‡Maintain serum amino acid pattern similar to that of breastfed infants. Higher requirements in more immature infants.
§Lower dose than that necessary to meet requirements is added to infusate to prevent precipitation.
‖Not present in standard trace element solution for neonates.
¶Reduced dose of heparin to prevent accumulation of serum free fatty acids following lipid infusions.
#20% fat emulsions contains a reduced amount of phospholipid and enhances blood lipid clearance compared with 10% fat emulsions. A minimum of 3% of daily caloric intake should be provided as linoleic acid to prevent essential fatty acid deficiency.

phospholipid in high density lipoproteins. Parenteral nutrition solutions are usually prepared with 1 U of heparin per milliliter to reduce the risk of clot formation in the catheter. Furthermore, the use of in-line heparin during parenteral nutrition has been shown to improve lipid clearance by releasing lipoprotein lipase from the endothelium of capillary vessels, which enhances the hydrolysis of the infused triglycerides to free fatty acids. A reduced concentration of heparin (0.5 U/ml) has been recommended for VLBW infants to prevent excessive accumulation of serum free fatty acids. There is general consensus that the adverse effects of lipid emulsions on pulmonary function, immune function, glucose metabolism, and bilirubin binding are minimized by the current practice of administering lipid emulsions at lower infusion rates for longer infusion periods (15 to 24 hours). None of the fat emulsions available for clinical use contain the omega-3 long chain polyunsaturated fatty acids that are deposited in the CNS of rapidly growing infants. The physiologic long-term consequences of this dietary deficiency are currently being investigated.

The concentrations of electrolytes and minerals in parenteral nutrition solutions need to be adjusted frequently in infants who are extremely premature, in those with renal dysfunction, excessive gastrointestinal losses, and fluid retention, and in those receiving diuretics. The amount of calcium and phophorus necessary to match intrauterine accretion rates is greater than that which can be safely delivered in parenteral nutrition solutions. Therefore, premature infants are at great risk for the development of osteopenia when the use of parenteral nutrition is prolonged. Newer formulations containing calcium glycerol-phosphate or monobasic phosphate may allow greater intake of these nutrients during parenteral nutrition. The requirements for vitamins in LBW infants are not clearly defined, but

recommended intakes during parenteral nutrition have been published recently. The pediatric multivitamin preparation available for parenteral use is administered to LBW infants in doses that vary according to the weight of the infant, 1.5 ml of the vial for infants weighing less than 1 kg and 3.3 ml of the vial for those weighing more than 1 kg. Trace elements should be routinely provided to patients requiring parenteral nutrition for more than 2 weeks. Selenium must be added to the infusate separately because it is not present in the standard neonatal trace element solution.

REFERENCES

1. Berseth CL: Effect of early feeding on maturation of the preterm infant's small intestine. J Pediatr 120:947–953, 1992.
2. Kashyap S, Schultz KF, Forsyth M, Dell RB, Ramakrishnan R, Heird WC: Growth, nutrient retention and metabolic response of low birth weight infants fed supplemented and unsupplemented human milk. Am J Clin Nutr 52:254–262, 1990.
3. Lucas A: Enteral nutrition. In Tsang RC, Lucas A, Uauy R, Zlotkin S (eds): Nutritional Needs of the Preterm Infant: Scientific Basis and Practical Guidelines. Pawling, NY, Caduceus Medical Publishers, Inc., 1993, pp. 209–223.
4. Van Lingen RA, Van Goudoever JB, Luijendijk HT, Wattimena JLD, Sauer PJJ: Effects of early amino acid administration during total parenteral nutrition on protein metobolism in pre-term infants. Clin Sci 82:199–203, 1992.
5. Wells DH, Ferlauto JJ, Forbes DJ, Graham TR, Newell RW, Wareham JA, Wilson CA: Lipid tolerance in the very low birth weight infant on intravenous and enteral feedings. J Parent Ent Nutr 13:623–627, 1989.

BREASTFEEDING

NANCY B. BRENT, M.D., I.B.C.L.C.
BEVERLY REDD, B.S., I.B.C.L.C.

Maternal and child health experts universally agree that breastfeeding is the optimal form of infant feeding. Often thought of as the first immunization, it offers the infant protection from a host of illnesses, ranging from infections to allergies to diabetes mellitus. The breastfed infant, even in industrialized society, suffers from fewer episodes of otitis media, gastroenteritis, and respiratory syncytial virus infection. If the infant is at risk for atopic disease, breastfeeding exclusively for the first 6 months of life, coupled with restriction of allergens in the maternal diet, offers protection. Many illnesses with etiologies as yet unclear are also decreased in the breastfed population, including pyloric stenosis, diabetes mellitus, and inflammatory bowel disease. Breastfeeding offers the mother a minimization of postpartum bleeding, a more rapid return to the prepregnancy state, and inhibition of ovulation and menses. The closeness between mother and baby that naturally occurs is uniquely enhanced and potentiated by the breastfeeding experience. Because of the many benefits of breastfeeding, all pregnant women should be given accurate and complete information about it so that they can make an informed choice on feeding methods.

INITIATION OF BREASTFEEDING

The initiation of breastfeeding education optimally occurs prenatally, with instruction of the expectant mother and evaluation for any potential problems. Flat or inverted nipples can be managed by wearing breast shells (plastic devices that encourage the nipples to protrude) for the last 4 to 6 weeks of pregnancy. Evaluation of postsurgical scars or abnormal early lactogenesis, as manifest by breast, areolar, and nipple changes, provides the opportunity to plan for potential breastfeeding difficulties.

Once the infant is born, breastfeeding management follows naturally from the physiology of lactogenesis and the maintenance of lactation. During pregnancy, the ductal system proliferates and differentiates under the influence of estrogen, and progesterone promotes an increase in size of lobes, lobules, and alveoli. Milk production begins with a complex sequence of events, triggered by the expulsion of the placenta at delivery. With the subsequent decrease of estrogen and progesterone, prolactin inhibitory factor (a dopamine-related substance) is also decreased, resulting in the release of prolactin from the anterior pituitary. With suckling, a neural reflux arc is initiated, resulting in surges of both oxytocin and prolactin. Oxytocin causes contraction of the myoepithelial cells surrounding the milk alveoli and allows delivery of milk into the ductal system and to the infant. This is referred to as the *milk ejection reflex*. Baseline prolactin is elevated throughout the entire period of lactation. In addition, prolactin surges with each nursing, thus ensuring continued milk production. This interplay of hormones and suckling activity translates easily into behavioral management of breastfeeding: the more the infant suckles, the more milk is made, and vice versa. It follows that to establish adequate milk production, the infant should nurse as soon and as frequently as possible after delivery. The physiology further dictates that no supplemental fluids be given, neither water nor breast milk substitutes. Supplementation decreases the amount of stimulation to the breast and, therefore, of milk production.

Questions have often arisen about duration of feedings in the first few days after birth. It was initially thought that decreasing the duration of the early feeds would decrease maternal nipple trauma. However, it has been found that nipple trauma occurs more from poor positioning at the breast than from prolonged time at the breast. Even 1 minute in the incorrect position can result in trauma, whereas 15 minutes in the proper position will not have a harmful effect. Of particular importance is maintaining the infant in the horizontal position, with face and abdomen facing the mother. The lips should be tickled to activate the rooting reflex, and then the infant can be latched on with as much of the areola in the mouth as possible. A large percentage of nipple trauma is caused by the infant's sucking only the tip of the nipple.

MANAGEMENT

Hospital Policy

Hospital routines and policy can have a significant impact on lactation success. The World Health Organization and UNICEF have developed guidelines to help maternity facilities promote, protect, and support breastfeeding. These guidelines, called the Ten Steps to Successful Breastfeeding, require that every facility providing maternity services and care for newborn infants should

1. Routinely communicate a written breastfeeding policy to all health care staff.
2. Train all health care staff in the skills necessary to implement this policy.
3. Inform all pregnant women about the benefits and management of breastfeeding.
4. Help mothers initiate breastfeeding within one half-hour of birth.
5. Show mothers how to breastfeed and how to maintain lactation even if separated from their infants.
6. Give newborn infants no food or drink other than breast milk, unless medically indicated.
7. Practice rooming-in, allowing mothers and infants to remain together 24 hours a day while hospitalized.
8. Encourage breastfeeding on demand.
9. Give no artificial teats or pacifiers (also called dummies or soothers) to breastfeeding infants.
10. Foster the establishment of breastfeeding support groups and refer mothers to them on discharge from the hospital or clinic.[3]

Home Management

Breastfeeding management after discharge from the hospital involves continuation of frequent, demand feeding and avoidance of bottle feeds for the first 4 weeks of life. By this time, breastfeeding is usually well established, and introduction of an occasional bottle feeding will not result in significant diminution of the mother's milk supply or in nipple confusion. Exclusively breastfed infants should be given fluoride and vitamin D. Fluoride is one of the few substances that is not transferred in mother's milk, and vitamin D levels in human milk vary with maternal intake and exposure to sunlight. Several documented reports of rickets in exclusively breastfed infants led to the recommendation from the Subcommittee on Nutrition During Lactation (The Institute of Medicine, National Academy of Sciences, 1991) of a daily vitamin D supplement of 5 to 7.5 μg for breastfed infants living in areas with decreased exposure to sunlight. Conversely, other fat-soluble vitamins are not influenced by maternal diet. These nutrients are supplied from stores in the maternal body tissue.

COMMON PROBLEMS

The three most prevalent reasons for discontinuing breastfeeding are nipple soreness, perceived or real milk insufficiency, and nipple confusion. It should be remembered that painful breastfeeding is not normal and is an indication for intervention.

To determine the problem, the mother and infant need to be evaluated together in the process of breastfeeding. Assessment of the mother's breasts and nipples, interpretation of the infant's cues, positioning, latch-on, areolar compression, signs of milk ejection reflex, audible swallowing, and adequate milk transfer are part of the breastfeeding evaluation.

Adequate intake is ensured if the infant is having six to eight wet diapers per day, a regular stooling pattern of yellow, seedy, unformed stools, and a weight gain of 15 to 30 g/d. Breastfed infants should regain their birth weight at 10 to 14 days and double their birth weight by 4 to 6 months of age.

Sore Nipples

Sore nipples are most commonly due to incorrect positioning and latch-on. Often, the infant fails to open the mouth wide during latch-on and sucks only the tip of the nipple. In addition, the infant may pull the nipple into the mouth gradually instead of taking it all at once, causing nipple trauma in the process. The mother should be taught that if it hurts, something is wrong, to break suction, to remove the baby from the breast, and to relatch. Most cases of nipple soreness can be corrected with proper technique.

For those cases in which severe nipple trauma has already occurred, several additional measures may be necessary. After learning proper positioning and latch-on technique, the mother should be instructed to air dry her nipples after feeds. She may then apply pure lanolin to the affected area. Wearing breast shells creates a layer of air between the damaged skin and her clothing, allowing more rapid healing. Occasionally, the mother is so sore that she cannot or will not put the baby to breast, yet does not want to wean. In this case, the baby can be taken off the breast while the mother expresses her milk for 24 to 72 hours to allow healing. During this time, attention should be paid to expressing the milk completely so that the milk supply does not falter. The infant can be fed the expressed milk or artificial formula or both without initiation of a bottle.

Real or Perceived Milk Insufficiency

Perceived or real insufficient milk production is another cause of cessation of breastfeeding even when weight gain is satisfactory. However, until breastfeeding becomes the cultural norm, it is easy for mothers to blame all the baby's fussiness on the nursing. These mothers need reassurance from their physician and breastfeeding support groups.

Real insufficient milk syndrome requires intervention. Interventions for increasing milk production include proper positioning, frequent feedings, pumping after feeding, supplementation at the breast with a nursing supplementer, and, on rare occasions, medication. The nursing supplementer consists of a bottle with feeding tubes instead of a nipple. The bottle hangs around the mother's neck and the tubes are attached to the breasts. The infant thus obtains milk from the supplementer and from the breast simultaneously. This ensures continued stimulation of the mother's milk supply and avoids nipple confusion.

Nipple Confusion

Nipple confusion is a commonly described entity, occurring when an infant refuses to breastfeed once a bottle has been offered. It is more prevalent in the first several weeks of life, and distressed mothers describe this breast refusal as a sudden change in feeding behavior often following one or more bottle feedings. Many infants adjust easily from breast to bottle with no apparent problems. Therefore, it is not possible to predict which infant will be affected.

The etiology of nipple confusion is unclear but may be related to the different mechanisms of suckling involved in bottle feeding and breastfeeding. As just reviewed, the infant must take the entire human nipple into the mouth, whereas bottle feeding is accomplished effectively by sucking only the tip of the nipple. With the introduction of subsequent bottles, the mother begins the downward spiral of decreased suckling and decreased milk production.

Nipple confusion can be managed in several ways. The use of a supplemental nurser allows immediate release of milk, encouraging the infant to suckle until the milk ejection reflex is initiated. Alternatively, a nipple shield, a soft flexible silicone device that covers the nipple, can be used. This device is closer to a bottle nipple and offers the infant a transition period to straight breastfeeding. Once the infant has successfully attached with the use of the shield and initiated feeding, the shield can be removed quickly, and the infant can be placed back onto the areola. Nipple shields limit milk transfer from mother to baby because of compromised areolar compression. With decreased transfer of milk, the mother's production declines, and the infant may fail to gain weight adequately. Supplementation may be necessary while using a nipple shield. It is wise to follow the use of a shield with bilateral pumping so that breast stimulation is maintained.

If neither of these interventions is successful, it may be necessary to take the infant off the breast and finger feed. A syringe with a feeding tube is attached to the mother's finger. As the infant suckles correctly, she depresses the plunger on the syringe. This trains the infant's sucking and avoids bottle sucking. Often the infant will return to the breast after 1 or 2 days of finger feeding. It is crucial that the mother maintain her supply during this period by expressing her milk.

BREASTFEEDING THE INFANT WITH A MEDICAL CONDITION

The incidence and duration of breastfeeding often are compromised when the infant has a medical condition. Overwhelmed by stress, grief, specialists, and appointments, mothers may not maintain milk production adequately or continue to breastfeed at all without help. Ironically, these babies benefit most from the immunologic properties human milk has to offer. Any method of feeding these infants may be difficult and time consuming. Mothers usually need to maintain their production through pumping and may need the help of breastfeeding devices, such as the supplemental nursing system or finger-feeding. Modifications of breastfeeding positions may also be helpful. Continued monitoring, contact, and support are imperative for breastfeeding success.

Breastfeeding the Low Birth Weight Infant

Breastfeeding the low birth weight (LBW) infant offers the breastfeeding dyad multiple advantages: nutritional, immunologic, and emotional. Even more than for the full-term infant, human milk is the best nutrition for the LBW infant. It also may help to ameliorate some of the complications of prematurity, such as necrotizing enterocolitis. It is critical that every mother of an LBW infant be given the opportunity to make an informed decision on infant feeding. She may not have considered the issue yet or may have erroneously assumed that an ill, hospitalized infant could not breastfeed.

Preterm human milk is higher in sodium, protein, and immunologic components than term milk. Despite this, deficiencies may still exist or may develop owing to the increased nutritional needs and decreased stores of the LBW infant. In particular, it has been found that preterm mothers' milk must be supplemented with protein to optimize growth. In addition, supplementation with calcium and phosphorus is necessary for optimal growth and prevention of rickets. These supplements may be provided by a powdered human milk fortifier or by a preterm formula. Breastfed LBW infants should be given multivitamin and trace mineral supplements. Iron (2 mg/kg/d) should be added at 2 to 8 weeks of age or at hospital discharge.

Lactation should be initiated as soon as possible after delivery. If the infant is too ill or small to tolerate oral feedings, mothers should be instructed on the use of the bilateral electric breast pump, as well as the proper sterile technique for collection, handling, and storage of human milk. Mother's milk should be expressed and either refrigerated for use within 48 hours or frozen for later use. Milk must be transported to the hospital in its refrigerated or frozen state, labeled with the name, date, and time. Mothers should be instructed to pump their breasts every 2 to 3 hours during waking hours and one to two times at night. Once lactation is established, the night pumping may be discontinued. The practice of random culturing of milk samples has not been found helpful in reducing contamination. Instead, rigorous attention to handwashing and sterile pumping technique is stressed. If an infection is suspected, a culture of that infant's mother's milk is appropriate. Mothers need continued support and encouragement to sustain lactation in the absence of a nursing infant. Support groups, as well as periodic visits with a lactation specialist, may help accomplish this.

Once enteral feedings are initiated, the infant's own mother's milk should be given in the order in which it was expressed. Continuous feeding is not optimal for the administration of human milk, as much of the lipid component will precipitate in the tubing and be lost to the infant. If it is attempted, tubing should be changed every 4 hours to avoid bacterial contamination.

Feeding at the breast may be initiated once the infant has been judged capable of tolerating oral feeds (usually around 33 to 34 weeks gestation). Preliminary data[2] have shown that feeding at the breast is no more stressful to the LBW infant in terms of oxygenation, heart rate, respiratory rate, and temperature than are bottle feedings. Therefore, mothers should be encouraged to breastfeed as often as possible. When the mother is unavailable, milk can be offered via cup, dropper, or finger feeding to avoid the development of nipple confusion. This approach has been very successful in the third world, and instruction should be offered to both mothers and the staff of the neonatal intensive care unit in its application. If the mother's milk supply is low or the infant is inefficient at removing milk from the breast (or both situations exist), supplementation may be offered at the breast with the use of a supplemental nurser, as described previously. In the absence of direct suckling, the milk supply often falters at 4 to 5 weeks postpartum but can be managed with support and encouragement and, if necessary, galactagogic medication.

An innovative approach to breastfeeding in the neonatal intensive care unit has been developed in the third world and Europe. It is called kangaroo care. After stabilization, the infant is held skin to skin against the mother's chest inside her clothing and nurses in this position on demand. Physiologic stability and temperature are maintained without compromise in this manner. In the third world, kangaroo care has been used in conjunction with early discharge of the stabilized infant and close outpatient follow-up. In industrialized nations, it usually has been used as an adjunct to neonatal intensive care unit care, with the parent providing kangaroo care for parts of the day.

Once the infant is ready for discharge, the mother should be instructed to continue pumping her breasts after feedings. This will ensure adequate stimulation even if the infant is inefficient at the breast.

TABLE 1. Breast Infection and Treatment

	ENGORGEMENT	CLOGGED DUCTS	MASTITIS	RECURRENT/ CHRONIC MASTITIS	ABSCESS
Patient Characteristics					
Fever	–	–	+	+	+
Lactation	Bilateral or unilateral	Bilateral or unilateral	Unilateral focal	Unilateral focal	Unilateral focal
Pain	Diffuse, mild	Diffuse, mild	Severe	Severe	Severe
Signs (warmth, erythema, tenderness)	–	–	+	+	+*
Treatment					
Frequent feeds	+	+	+	+	+†
Warm soaks	+	+	+	+	
Alternate breastfeeding position	+	+	+	+	+
Antibiotic (duration)	—	—	1–2 wk	3–4 wk	3–4 wk
Bedrest	—	—	+	+	+

*Drainage and a palpable mass may be present.
†If there is no drainage or if abscess is not near the infant's mouth.

Breastfeeding the LBW infant offers mothers an opportunity to provide the best nutrition possible and to offer care to their infants that not even the highest technology can match. In this way, it encourages bonding and provides a sense of some control to the parents in an otherwise overwhelming situation. The parents will have done their best for their infant and given him or her the best start possible.

MATERNAL PROBLEMS

Breast Infection

Infection of the breast can be seen as a continuum, ranging from engorgement to clogged ducts to bacterial mastitis to recurrent or chronic mastitis to abscess formation. Characteristics and treatment are summarized in Table 1.

In addition to bacterial infection, fungal infection is common in the breastfeeding dyad. It is usually manifest in the infant in the form of oral thrush or candidal diaper dermatitis or both. Nipple thrush in the mother is characterized by severe, bilateral, burning pain that continues after the feeding ends. Treatment consists of applying clotrimazole or nystatin to the nipples after each feed and to the diaper area four to six times a day. In addition, oral nystatin is given to the infant after feeds. Candidal vaginitis in the mother should be treated with clotrimazole vaginal suppositories. Infection often recurs and can become chronic if not treated aggressively. Treatment should continue for at least 1 week after all symptoms have disappeared in both mother and infant. If conditions predisposing to candidal infection are present and the infection has been recurrent, consideration should be given to prophylaxis with a single daily dose to both mother and infant. Routine treatment of oral thrush in a breastfed infant should include treatment of the mother as well.

Drugs

Although almost all drugs pass into human milk, they are usually well tolerated by the infant. Delivery to the infant is dependent on maternal dose, timing of medication with respect to feedings, half-life of the drug, volume of distribution, and acidity. Maternal medications should be avoided when possible, but only a few are contraindicated, including bromocriptine, ergotamine, lithium, antimetabolites, phenindione, and drugs of abuse. Radionuclides and iodides used for diagnostic tests require temporary cessation of breastfeeding.

Medical Conditions

Postpartum depression is not an uncommon complication of childbirth and is not prevented by breastfeeding. It should be remembered that treatment with certain antidepressants, tricyclics in particular, may not preclude breastfeeding. Precipitous weaning may, in fact, worsen the mother's symptoms.

Maternal insulin-dependent diabetes mellitus is also consistent with successful breastfeeding. Careful attention should be paid to increasing the mother's caloric intake. In addition, there is often a decrease in insulin requirement seen immediately after birth. All these factors emphasize the need for careful metabolic monitoring during lactation. It should be remembered that lactosuria is normal during lactation, and specific glucose testing is, therefore, necessary. The infant of a diabetic mother may be prone to hypoglycemia, congenital malformations, and feeding problems. These will need careful attention to ensure successful lactation.

Maternal breast cancer is considered a contraindication to breastfeeding, as lactation may delay initiation of treatment.

SUMMARY

A unique symbiosis exists for the breastfeeding dyad, with each dependent on the other. This relationship offers the infant the best nutrition possible and protection from infection, allergy, and other illness while helping the mother return quickly to her prepregnancy state of health. The closeness between a breastfeeding mother and infant cannot be quantified but surely represents a uniquely supportive start to family life.

REFERENCES

1. American Academy of Pediatrics Committee on Drugs: Transfer of drugs and other chemicals into the human milk. Pediatrics 93:137–150, 1994.
2. Meier P, Anderson GC: Responses of small preterm infants to bottle and breastfeeding. Matern Child Nurs 12:92–105, 1987.
3. World Health Organization and UNICEF: Protecting, Promoting and Supporting Breastfeeding: The Special Role of Maternity Services. Geneva, Switzerland, author.

FLUID AND ELECTROLYTE THERAPEUTICS

STEPHEN BAUMGART, M.D.
ANDREW T. COSTARINO, JR., M.D.

Abnormalities in water and electrolyte balance in the neonate result from (1) developmental immaturity in renal function and its humoral control, (2) changing proportions of extracellular and intracellular fluid and solutes associated with the transition from the in utero to the extrauterine environment, and (3) environmental adaptation to the increased insensible water losses. Additionally, extreme prematurity and cardiorespiratory failure in the critically ill newborn and the therapies necessary for these conditions can cause further disruptions of fluid and electrolyte homeostasis.

NEONATAL RENAL FUNCTION AND THE NEONATAL KIDNEY

In comparison to older infants and children, the newborn baby has a lower glomerular filtration rate (GFR). Glomerular filtration increases in the first few hours of life, leading to an acute rise in GFR that continues throughout the first postnatal week. These acute postnatal changes are followed by a slower renal maturation throughout infancy. In premature infants <33 weeks gestation, the magnitude of these changes at birth are reduced because of the diminished numbers of nephrons.

Tubular structure and function are similarly immature in the newborn, resulting in a decreased ability to both concentrate urine and excrete excess water. In full-term infants, the impaired concentrating ability is primarily a result of low interstitial urea concentration and a shortened loop of Henle. These developmental differences are exaggerated in premature infants, in whom the poor urine-concentrating ability is further impaired by a distal tubule and collecting system that is poorly responsive to arginine vasopressin. As a result, urine concentration >600 mOsm/L is unlikely to occur in premature infants during the first week of life. In contrast to the proximal tubule and loop of Henle, the functional development of the distal tubules occurs early in gestation. Thus, even very premature infants can produce a dilute urine.

The primary cause for limitation in excretion of water and salt for both term and preterm infants is the low GFR. In term infants, there is an additional bias toward sodium resorption associated with a high circulating level of aldosterone maintained by a blunted feedback response to renin production. This bias toward sodium reabsorption ensures sodium retention necessary for postnatal growth and contributes to the term infant's inability to excrete an excess load of salt and water. Premature infants, in contrast, manifest a high basal excretion of sodium, which is primarily due to a less mature proximal tubule. Whereas the inability to concentrate urine renders the preterm infant particularly vulnerable to extracellular water (ECW) contraction and hypertonicity, the decreased ability to excrete water and salt loads renders them more susceptible than older children and adults to fluid overload. This apparent impaired ability for the neonate's renal tubules to modify resorption and excretion of filtered water and solute has been interpreted by some authors as indicating a developmental glomerular-tubular mismatch. However, under normal conditions and during moderate stress, the neonatal kidney is capable of retaining the necessary amounts of water and solute required for growth while also eliminating nitrogenous wastes.

Potassium balance is also a problem for the newborn infant, particularly the preterm infant. Not only is the GFR lower than normal (in all newborn infants), but also in very immature kidneys, aldosterone's effect may be insufficient to suppress potassium secretion, resulting in potassium retention and sodium wastage. As a result, very low birth weight (VLBW) infants can develop life-threatening hyperkalemia in the first week of life.

FUNCTION OF HUMORAL MODULATORS ON FLUID BALANCE IN NEONATES

Renin-Angiotensin-Aldosterone System

The renin-angiotensin-aldosterone system (RAAS) matures early in gestation, and the combined effects of an expanding capacitance of the extracellular fluid compartment (associated with growth), blunted negative feedback on renin production, and poorly responsive renal tubules sustain the high level of plasma renin activity (PRA) that is characteristic of infants after birth. As the infant matures, physiologic stimuli to the RAAS slowly decrease, reducing all measures of RAAS activity. Angiotensin and aldosterone production parallel PRA response, and angiotensin-converting enzyme (ACE) decreases with gestation, with higher levels appearing in premature babies with respiratory distress. Respiratory illness, mechanical ventilation, and salt restriction are associated with increases in RAAS activity.

Arginine Vasopressin (Antidiuretic Hormone)

Fetal arginine vasopressin (AVP) levels increase during early gestation, and by midgestation, the AVP response to both osmotic and baroreceptor stimulation is functional. Hypothalamic AVP production then plateaus at the end of the second trimester. Thus, in viable human neonates, urinary AVP excretion does not vary with gestational age during the immediate newborn period. High neonatal plasma AVP levels present at parturition fall rapidly during the first 24 hours of life, then more slowly thereafter. However, the distal nephron response to AVP (reabsorption of filtered water) is blunted in neonates, limiting the ability to concentrate urine.

Vaginal delivery, birth asphyxia, and meconium aspiration are associated with higher AVP levels, whereas maternal anesthetic is associated with lower levels. These observations suggest that pain, hypoxia, and intracranial pressure may be part of the stimulus for AVP release at the time of birth. Similarly, postnatally high AVP levels have been observed with hypoxia, mechanical ventilation, pneumothorax, and intracranial hemorrhage, suggesting nonosmotic release of AVP. The finding of high AVP levels in these situations suggests that the syndrome of inappropriate antidiuretic hormone (SIADH) may contribute to the hyponatremia frequently seen in these infants.

In summary, production and release of AVP are intact in neonates despite premature birth and may cause SIADH in some distressed subjects. However, AVP's effect on water conservation is limited by tubular immaturity and a low renal medullary concentration gradient, resulting generally in a dilute urine production in babies.

Atrial Natriuretic Peptide

Atrial natriuretic peptide (ANP) levels are significantly higher after birth than in older children and adults. Infants who receive a sodium-supplemented formula will maintain high ANP levels, allowing them to excrete the excess salt. A blunted natriuretic response to ANP may be present in premature infants.

BIRTH, TRANSITION, AND REDISTRIBUTION OF BODY WATER

Intrauterine growth during the latter half of gestation is characterized by an increase in both cell number and cell size. During this time, as the absolute amount of total body water increases, the proportion of water in the intracellular compartment expands more rapidly than the extracellular volume. At 16 weeks of fetal life, 90% of body mass is water, distributed as one-third intracellular and two-thirds extracellular (Fig. 1). By term gestation, only 80% of total body mass is water, and the ratio of intracellular water/extracellular water is approximately 1:1. Postnatally, the distribution of total body water remains relatively stable, and whereas increasing cell mass with growth results in an absolute increase in total body water by adulthood, only 60% to 70% of body weight is water.

In addition to these gradual changes occurring during gestational and postnatal life, a sudden efflux of volume from the intracellular to the extracellular compartment occurs at birth. This event is followed by cardiovascular and renal responses that result in a diuresis of salt and water during the first 48 to 72 hours of life. Contributions to the observed expansion of the extracellular compartment in the first hours of life may come also from placental transfusion and the resorption of fetal lung fluid. The end result is that the systemic circulation is primed during the transition period, and in the hours to days that follow, total body water is reduced by 5% to 7% (more fluid is lost from the extracellular compartment, whereas the intracellular space is relatively preserved).

Premature babies have a relatively large extracellular water and salt pool, which in the healthy infant, will contract quickly after birth due to larger than normal insensible water losses from the immature skin and dilute urine production by the immature kidney. If this tendency is allowed to occur, the resultant increase in extracellular osmolality will promote a concurrent contraction in the intracellular water compartment. In critically ill premature infants, diuresis may

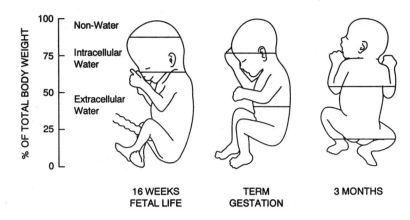

FIGURE 1. Changes in the composition of body fluids occurring during normal fetal and neonatal development. (From Costarino AT, Baumgart S: Modern fluid and electrolyte management of the critically ill premature infant. Pediatr Clin North Am 33:153–178, 1986.)

be delayed in association with the renal and hormonal influences described previously. This results in a tendency toward fluid retention and edema in these patients that occurs even if exogenous fluid administration is restricted. Usually, however, by 1 to 2 weeks of age, premature babies equilibrate at a relatively dry weight and body fluid composition, similar to that observed in more mature infants. Thereafter, growth begins primarily from expansion of intracellular mass.

NEONATAL ENVIRONMENT AND WATER EVAPORATION

Water metabolism and energy metabolism are closely linked. Metabolic wastes are eliminated from the skin (heat), respiratory system (CO_2), kidney (urea and fixed acids), and gastrointestinal tract (solid, insoluble). Water is obliged to accompany each of these processes and may be readily measured in the urine and stool. Obligate evaporative losses from the skin (separate from perspiration) and respiration are termed insensible water loss and are not as easily measured. In the premature neonate exposed to the extrauterine environment without adequate physiologic and anatomic preparation, water losses will be markedly increased and will exceed that necessary for the function of waste elimination.

Net Insensible Water Loss

Total net insensible water loss comes from the combination of ventilatory and transcutaneous evaporation. Early investigations of term neonates conducted in metabolic chambers indicated that 23% of an infant's metabolic energy production at rest may be dissipated through insensible water loss (approximately 40 ml/kg/d). More recent studies have concluded that in an individual infant, evaporative heat loss may comprise an even greater proportion of the metabolic energy generated.

Ventilatory Water Loss

Hydration is linked to ventilation because of the evaporation of water from the respiratory tract. At room temperature and moderate (40%) relative humidity, the term infant at rest loses between 0.6 and 0.8 ml/kg/h during spontaneous breathing. This volume usually accounts for 30% of net insensible water loss.

A variety of conditions alter respiratory water loss. For example, in LBW infants nursed in incubators or breathing artificially humidified gas, any disturbance from the resting, steady state (e.g., respiratory distress) leads to an increase in metabolic rate that requires an increase in minute ventilation. As a result, respiratory water loss may increase three-fold as ventilation increases. Infants warmed in nonhumidified incubators and supplemented with dry inspired gases (e.g., oxygen) will experience increased respiratory water loss >2 ml/kg/h (>50 ml/kg/d). Humidification of inspired gas will reduce evaporative loss from breathing. However, >80% relative humidity may be required to significantly affect these losses. Endotracheal intubation and ventilation with gases completely saturated with water at body temperature will eliminate respiratory water loss. However,

particulate condensation within such ventilation systems must be avoided to prevent waterborne bacterial infection, as well as pneumonitis due to inadvertent water aspiration.

Transcutaneous Water Loss

Skin insensible water loss is a passive process, whereby water (free from solute) is lost directly from exposed epidermal epithelium. This should be distinguished from sweating, where sweat glands actively secrete water and solute onto the skin surface. Sweat contributes little to transcutaneous water loss and heat dissipation in neonates, since apocrine function is immature and an integrated sweat response to heat stimulation is blunted. Transcutaneous evaporation in preterm infants, therefore, remains predominantly insensible and cannot be viewed as a fixed proportion (i.e., 23%) of metabolic heat dissipation.

Hammerlund et al. reported their findings of transcutaneous water loss in premature infants.[4] They found that transepidermal water loss increased in infants of shorter gestation and younger postnatal ages (Fig. 2). Rates of water evaporation increase geometrically in the smallest, most immature subjects. Additionally, they found that although incubator humidification (≤60% relative humidity) reduced large evaporative losses in VLBW infants (≤27 weeks gestation), transepidermal evaporation always remained much greater than that found in infants ≥28 weeks. These results are not surprising, considering the thinner, more permeable skin in premature babies and their larger surface/body mass ratio.

In Table 1, body surface area/body mass ratio is represented for an adult and for premature babies weighing 1.5 and 0.5 kg. The higher relative proportion of neonatal body weight comprised of water is demonstrated in Figure 1, and the immaturity of the very premature infant's skin as a barrier to insensible water evaporation is described in Figure 2. These comprise the three major factors contributing to the geometrically higher insensible water loss in very premature infants when compared with more mature babies.

Environmental Effect on Evaporative Water Loss

The convection-warmed incubator is the most commonly used device for warming premature infants. Air temperatures are raised within an enclosed hood (to in excess of 10.0°C above the 25°C room air temperature) to maintain LBW neonates isothermally at 36.5°C body temperature. If not humidified (to avoid bacterial contamination), air water vapor pressure decreases inside the incubator and promotes increased evaporation. Compared with bundled term infants, naked premature babies inside incubators experience an increased transepidermal evaporation that is more than that necessary for heat dissipation. Circulation of the air inside the incubator by forced convection may further disturb evaporative gradients near the infant's skin and thereby increase water losses.

Open exposure of critically ill LBW infants while they are nursed under radiant warmers leads to a similar vapor pressure gradient that favors evaporation. The cool, dry air passing over the infant at room temperature is warmed and humidified at the patient's skin surface

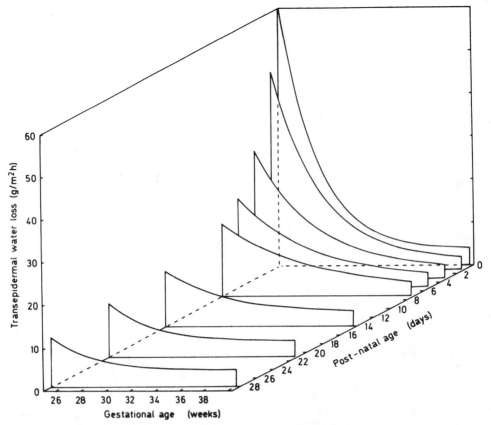

FIGURE 2. Relationships between transepidermal water loss (g/m²/h), gestational age, and increasing postnatal age. Note the geometrically higher levels of insensible water loss in small, very premature infants, early in life. (From Hammerlund K, Sedin G, Stromberg B: Transepidermal water loss in newborn infants: VIII. Relation to gestational age and post-natal age in appropriate and small for gestational age infants. Acta Paediatr Scand 72:721–728, 1983, with permission.)

and then carries water away as it rises by convection. Minor turbulence in the nursery air may worsen the evaporative process under radiant warmers.

A variety of clear plastic films and hoods have been advocated to reduce transepidermal evaporative exposure. The degree to which these films are effective in achieving this goal varies with each application. Other infant environmental factors influencing insensible water loss have been reviewed and include skin blood flow, phototherapy, clothing, and artificial skinlike membranes.

PREVENTION OF NEONATAL FLUID DISORDERS

Respiratory Distress Syndrome

Premature infants with surfactant deficiency demonstrate low lung compliance, high pulmonary vascular and peripheral airways resistance, abnormal pulmonary lymphatic drainage, and atelectasis. Increased capillary permeability to protein and water and low serum oncotic pressure due to a lower serum albumin concentration promote water movement into the pulmonary interstitium. Accumulation of

lung water further worsens lung compliance. Treatment with high inspired oxygen and mechanical ventilation may produce more lung injury, resulting in worsening pulmonary edema. The diuresis that normally occurs with transition to the extrauterine environment is delayed. The diuresis is associated with an increased GFR, natriuresis, and an increased free water clearance. Figure 3 illustrates changes in observed urine volume, renal functions, and lung function (PAO₂ – PaO₂) before, at the onset, during, and after diuresis in premature infants with RDS. Respiratory improvement occurs only after diuresis occurs. Although diuretics may produce a diuresis, they have had mixed results in hastening pulmonary recovery and have not been shown to reduce the incidence of bronchopulmonary dysplasia.

We recommend not replacing all fluid losses to maintain body weight within 5% to 10% of birth weight (the traditional concept of maintenance) but instead to permit body water to contract (10% to 20% weight loss over the first 3–5 days of life) (Table 2). Such a fluid restriction during the acute phase of RDS may prevent later development of pulmonary edema, patent ductus arteriosus with congestive heart failure, and severe bronchopulmonary dysplasia.

The end of spontaneous diuresis can be recognized by a fall in urine flow to <2 ml/kg/h and a reduction in the sodium content (<3% fractional excretion). At this point, liberalization of volume intake may be pursued with caution, and sodium intake may be increased to avoid hyponatremia at the end of the first week of life.

Bronchopulmonary Dysplasia

High pulmonary hydrostatic pressure, low capillary oncotic pressure, and impaired pulmonary lymphatic drainage are present in infants with bronchopulmonary dysplasia (BPD) and result in chronic

TABLE 1. Body Surface Area/Body Mass Ratio

WEIGHT	BODY SURFACE AREA	BODY MASS
70 kg adult	1.73 m²	250 cm²/kg
1.5 kg premature infant	0.13 m²	870 cm²/kg
0.5 kg micropremature infant	0.07 m²	1400 cm²/kg

lung water retention. Scarring with distortion of lung anatomy also occurs as BPD develops. Excessive fluid volume administration often worsens the pulmonary water accumulation, decreases lung compliance, and contributes to airway obstruction. Poor nutrition coupled with increased energy demands in infants with BPD further complicate the situation by causing hypoalbuminemia, poor capillary integrity in damaged tissues, and diminished growth.

High fluid volume intake over the first 3 to 5 days of life, patent ductus arteriosus, and failure of a diuresis to occur before 2 weeks of age have all been associated with the development of BPD. However, despite these observations, fluid restriction, indomethacin, and diuretics may not always prevent development of BPD or reduce its severity. The more important factors associated with the occurrence of BPD are probably the degree of lung maturation and the need for mechanical ventilation and supplemental oxygen. It is important to remember, however, that modest water restriction and provision of adequate nutritional substrates (>80 kcal/kg/d) are important ad-

junctive components in the treatment of children with BPD. Calorically dense premature formula or parenteral therapy with dextrose concentration and lipid infusion may allow the clinician to achieve these ends.

In addition to fluid restriction and caloric supplementation, sparing use of diuretics has been demonstrated to be useful in the management of this disease. Unfortunately, chronic diuretic therapy (e.g., furosemide or thiazides) may result in chloride, sodium, and potassium depletion, dehydration, and urinary calcium wasting, causing bone demineralization and renal calculus formation. Chronic diuretic therapy with chlorothiazide and spironolactone or every other day furosemide may reduce the incidence of complications. Periodic assessment of serum electrolytes and bone mineralization (by roentgenograms and alkaline phosphatase assays) and renal ultrasound examination for calculae are part of the routine care of infants with BPD.

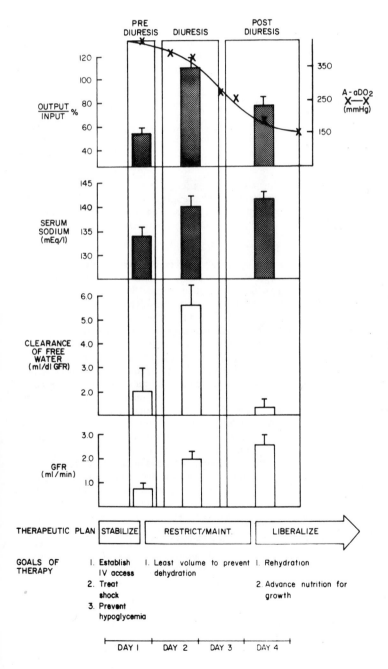

FIGURE 3. Diagram outlining the clinical course of respiratory distress syndrome (A-aDO₂, x–x) in conjunction with a diuresis (percent urine output/input fluid volume). Rises in renal filtration (GFR) and serum sodium concentration are observed during the first week of life. Free water clearance appears to constitute the main physiologic event during diuresis, with improved lung function. Serum sodium concentration usually rises by 3 to 5 mEq/L, and a significant natriuresis occurs as well. At the bottom of this figure a therapeutic schema is presented in three phases: (1) initial stabilization, (2) maintenance with parenteral fluid volume restriction, and (3) careful liberalization of fluid volume administered only after a diuresis has been observed. (From Costarino AT, Baumgart S: Modern fluid and electrolyte management of the critically ill premature infant. Pediatr Clin North Am 33:162, 1986.)

TABLE 2. Recommendations for Water and Electrolyte Administration in Preterm Newborn Infants

1. *Expect weight loss* during the first 3–5 d of life.
2. *Maintain normal serum electrolyte concentrations*
   Sodium   135–145 mmol/L
   Potassium   3.5–5 mmol/L
   Chloride   98–108 mmol/L
3. *Avoid oliguria:* <0.5–1 ml/kg/h for 8–12 h

Phase 1: Transition* during the first 3–5 d of life is characterized by (1) large transcutaneous water evaporation and (2) renal diuresis of a large surfeit of extracellular salt and water.

Birth Weight (g)	Expected Weight Loss (%)	Water Intake† (ml/kg/d)	Sodium Intake‡ mmol/kg/d	Chloride Intake‡ (mmol/kg/d)	Potassium Intake‡ (mmol/kg/d)
<1000	15–20	90–140	0	0	0
1000–1500	10–15	80–120	0	0	0

Phase 2: Stabilization at euvolemic weight for ≤10–14 d. Weight gain is not a priority as parenteral and enteral nutrition are cautiously advanced. Transcutaneous water evaporation is diminishing as the neonatal epidermis cornifies.

Birth Weight (g)	Weight Change (%)	Water Intake (ml/kg/d)	Sodium Intake (mmol/kg/d)	Chloride Intake (mmol/kg/d)	Potassium Intake (mmol/kg/d)
<1000	0	80–120	2–3	2	1–2
1000–1500	0	80–100	2–3	2	1–2

Phase 3: Established Growth >2 weeks of postnatal life in all weight categories to match intrauterine growth rate is the objective. Oral enteral intake is eventually ad libitum.

Weight Gain (g/kg/d)	Parenteral Volume (ml/kg/d)	Enteral Volume (ml/kg/d)	Sodium Intake (mmol/kg/d)	Chloride Intake (mmol/kg/d)	Potassium Intake (mmol/kg/d)
15–20	140–160	150–200	3–5	3–5	2–3

*The end of transition is recognized by (1) urine volume <1 ml/kg/h and urine osmolality > serum osmolality, (2) fractional excretion of sodium diminished from >3% to ≤1%, and (3) urine specific gravity above 1.012
†Water intake volume should be 10%–20% less with humidified incubator or artificial plastic shielding placed over the infant to conserve insensible water evaporation.
‡Often 0.5–1.5 mmol/kg/d sodium is administered to these infants inadvertently with transfusions, medications, and line infusions.

The Very Low Birth Weight Baby

The extremely premature infant (<750 g, <25 weeks gestation) has a watery, gelatinous skin devoid of keratin and a body surface area/body water mass ratio that is six times greater than that of an adult (Table 1). As a result, transepidermal evaporation is geometrically higher than in larger premature infants (Fig. 2), leading to large free water losses (5 to 7 ml/kg/h), hypernatremia, hyperglycemia, and hyperkalemia. Dehydration of the intracellular compartment will occur as the osmotic pressure falls in the extracellular space. This phenomenon has been implicated in the pathogenesis of neurologic injuries sometimes seen in this population. Renal immaturity results in an inappropriately high urine output with high sodium content (fractional excretion often exceeds 10%), further worsening the acute dehydration. Electrolyte aberrations, particularly hyperkalemia, occur at 48 to 72 hours of age and may be associated with shock and dysrhythmias. Fully replacing water loss at volumes of 150 to 200 ml/kg/d or more will lead to intravascular fluid overload and may result in patent ductus arteriosus, congestive heart failure, pulmonary edema, and intraventricular hemorrhage. We believe that fluid therapy in these infants is best approached by infusing the least amount of water volume required to maintain the serum sodium concentration in a high-normal range (145 to 150 mEq/L) during the first 24 to 72 hours (Table 2). No sodium or potassium should be administered (if possible), and a 15% to 20% weight loss should be tolerated. The clinician caring for these infants must be watchful for inadvertent administration of sodium and other solutes, which occurs with bicarbonate infusion, blood product transfusion, and medication administration.

In the face of high insensible water losses (120 to 170 ml/kg/d), maintaining relative fluid restriction often may be achieved only by reducing transcutaneous water loss through the use of thin plastic shields. Humidification of incubators to control water loss by reducing the evaporative gradient near the skin is effective but risks promoting contamination by waterborne bacteria.

After the first 3 to 5 days of life, the stratum corneum matures, and transcutaneous water loss is reduced. If sodium restriction is continued at this point, hyponatremia may occur. Therefore, sodium and potassium chloride must be supplemented (Table 2). In the second to third week, nutrition (parenteral, enteral, or both) to promote growth (~15 g/kg/d) becomes the priority for fluid therapy.

Late Onset Hyponatremia of Prematurity

Infants recovering from premature birth frequently manifest mild or moderate hyponatremia at 2 to 6 weeks of age, with serum sodium concentrations ranging between 124 and 130 mmol/L. By this age, cardiorespiratory failure usually has resolved, phototherapy for hyperbilirubinemia has ceased, and the infant has begun enteral feedings. Whereas the GFR has increased substantially by 2 to 6 weeks of age, maturation of tubular function progresses more slowly, leading to distal nephron delivery of sodium at a rate greater than the immature kidney can accommodate. Thus, urinary output and urinary sodium losses remain high. Enteral feedings at this juncture may be barely sufficient to sustain nutrition, and feeding intolerance or risk for bowel injury may necessitate using dilute formulas. Inadvertent sodium restriction may also result from the use of breast milk or a formula with a low salt content. Since new tissue growth, particularly bone, requires that the infant incorporate sodium at a rate of 1.2 mmol/kg/d, a further loss of sodium from the extracellular compartment will occur. Late onset hyponatremia of prematurity usually resolves spontaneously as water and sodium regulatory responses mature. In the meantime, however, treatment must include a liberalized sodium chloride intake (3 to 5 mmol/kg/d) (Table 2).

Fluid Intake To Promote Nutrition and Growth

After the first 2 weeks of transition and stabilization, new tissue growth becomes the primary goal of fluid intake therapy. Fortunately, maturation of neonatal kidney function permits a more liberal approach. Fluid intakes in excess of 150 to 200 ml/kg/d may be needed to meet increased energy requirements, to replete protein loss from damaged tissues, and to achieve catchup growth (Table 2).

Accretion of body mass at 15 to 20 g/kg/d requires 0.75 ml of water for each gram of lean mass acquired. Sodium, potassium, and chloride requirements of 3 to 5 mmol/kg/d must be provided to replete losses from earlier restrictions and to provide for new tissue growth (particularly bone growth). When considering the options for providing these fluid requirements, one should note that human milk has a relatively low protein content (1.5 g/100 kcal) and somewhat higher osmolality (40 mOsm/100 kcal) than 24 kcal/30 ml premature infant formulations (protein 2.4 to 3 g/100 kcal and 21 to 27 mOsm/100 kcal). Renal solute load (urea and excess minerals) with any formula should not exceed 30 mOsm/kg/d (while providing 120 to 150 kcal/kg/d). A urine osmolality between 100 and 500 mOsm/kg is required for solute load excretion if the urine volume ranges between 60 and 120 ml/kg/d.

Concentrating premature formulas to 27 to 30 kcal/oz (400+ mOsm/kg) to restrict fluid intake in BPD babies (at ≥150 kcal/kg/d) may result in solute waste excretion requirements that exceed the concentrating capacity of the immature kidney. Preliminary investigations to test specialized lipid-supplemented formulas are underway. These preparations are especially designed to meet the hypercaloric substrate demands of babies with BPD while limiting protein and other renal solute loads.

CONCLUSIONS

Fluid and nutritional therapy in the critically ill neonate is an important component in the effective care of these patients. Advances in fluid regimens over the last 20 years have played an important role in improving the outcome of this population. Appropriate fluid therapy must consider gestational maturity, chronologic age, and the diseases affecting the infant. Thus, each patient will have unique fluid and nutritional requirements, but some general summary recommendations are appropriate.

During the acute phase of transition to extrauterine life, a relative fluid restriction (50 to 80 ml/kg/d) is recommended, and indices of fluid balance should be carefully monitored every 6 to 8 hours, including net fluid intake and urine volume output, body weight, urine specific gravity, urine reducing substance, and serum glucose, sodium and potassium concentrations. An increase in serum sodium of ≥10 mmol/L in 24 hours suggests that water dehydration is more likely than salt excess. Because of equipment attached to the baby and clinical imprecision of the instruments of body weight measurement over 24 hours, weight loss may not herald dehydration, but it may be useful in predicting trends over the first week of life. A 10% to 20% weight loss is commonly observed.

Following the first 3 to 5 days of life, fluids should be liberalized by 1 to 2 ml/h to optimize nutrition and to achieve a urine flow ≥0.5 ml/kg/h and a urine specific gravity between 1.012 and 1.016. Infants should be fluid restricted to prevent pulmonary edema. However, the desire to restrict must be balanced by the desire to maintain cardiac output, to sustain caloric intake, and to provide adequate systemic perfusion. Finding the proper balance between dehydration and fluid congestion requires close scrutiny throughout the critical period of neonatal transition.

REFERENCES

1. Costarino AT, Baumgart S: Modern fluid and electrolyte management of the critically ill premature infant. Pediatr Clin North Am 33:153–178, 1986.
2. Costarino AT, Baumgart S: Water metabolism in the neonate. In Cowett RM (ed): Principles of Perinatal-Neonatal Metabolism. New York, Springer-Verlag, 1991:623–649.
3. Costarino AT, Baumgart S: Water as nutrition. In Tsang RC, Lucas A, Uauy R, Zlotkin S (eds): Nutritional Needs of the Preterm Infant: Scientific Basis and Practical Guidelines. Baltimore, Williams & Wilkins, 1993:1–14.
4. Hammarlund K, Sedin G, Stromberg B: Transepidermal water loss in newborn infants: VIII. Relation to gestational age and post-natal age in appropriate and small for gestational age infants. Acta Paediatr Scand 72:721–728, 1983.

OSTEOPENIA OF PREMATURITY

JEFFREY L. LOUGHEAD, M.D.
REGINALD C. TSANG, M.B.B.S.

The improved survival of low birth weight (LBW) infants since the 1970s has resulted in an increased frequency of osteopenia and rickets in the preterm population. Osteopenia is a general diminution of bone mineral mass, and rickets is a specific decrease in the mineral/osteoid ratio of growing bone. Rickets of prematurity is most frequently a deficiency of calcium and phosphorus and differs from the vitamin D deficiency rickets commonly found in term infants and older children. The frequency of rickets of prematurity is directly related to the severity of illness and inversely related to the birth weight of the preterm infant. The incidence has been estimated to be as high as 30% in the very low birth weight (<1500 g) population and as high as 75% in the extremely low birth weight (<1000 g) population. The true incidence is difficult to measure because of the subtleness of clinical signs and the lack of readily available reliable laboratory indicators. The clinical signs of large anterior fontanel, lethargy, and weakness in term infants are frequently masked by the overall illness of the infant. Rachitic rosaries, frontal bossing, and limb deformities are late and unusual findings in rickets of prematurity. Commonly, the diagnosis is made by radiography, frequently after a fracture draws attention to the child's osteopenia. The most sensitive laboratory measure of osteopenia is by photon absorptiometry, a technique usually available only as a research tool.

The primary risk factor for osteopenia and rickets of prematurity is preterm birth. During the last trimester, the fetus receives 80% of its calcium and phosphorus supply, increasing its body weight by 300% and its length by 150%. During this trimester, the fetus receives up to 120 to 150 mg elemental calcium per kilogram per day and 80 to 100 mg elemental phosphorus per kilogram per day, rates difficult to achieve after birth, especially if full enteral nutrition is not tolerated. Additional risk factors include such diseases as neonatal hepatic and intestinal diseases, unsupplemented human milk feedings, and exposure to calciuric drugs. Reliance on parenteral nutrition places the LBW infant at markedly increased risk of osteopenia and rickets. Unlike rickets in the older child, vitamin D deficiency appears to contribute only in the uncommon instances of extreme maternal vitamin D deficiency.

Treatment of rickets of prematurity is limited by the same factors that lead to its development. Reducing or eliminating exposure to known risk factors, including calciuric drugs such as loop diuretics (possibly methylxanthines [caffeine, aminophylline] and in part glucocorticoids), and optimizing delivery of calcium and phosphorus are the goals of therapy. Until recently, delivery of adequate quantities of parenteral calcium and phosphorus was difficult due to precipitation of calcium and phosphorus salts. Newer amino acid formulations have improved the stability of calcium and phosphorus in hyperalimentation solutions, allowing for sufficient quantities of these minerals to prevent and even treat rickets. Delivery of 12.5 to 15 mmol/L of calcium and phosphorus in hyperalimentation solutions of 10% to 12.5% dextrose and 2% amino acids, in Ca:P molar ratios of 1:1 to 1.3:1 or weight ratios of 1.3 to 1.7:1, have been shown to be stable and will prevent demineralization.[1] Concentrations as high as 20 mmol/L have been used successfully but should be monitored closely for precipitation and metastatic calcifications. The use of calcium gluconate and a mixture of monobasic and dibasic phosphate salts appears to improve solubility. The physiologic vitamin D requirement for infants on parenteral nutrition is low, and 30 IU/kg/d has been demonstrated to maintain serum 25(OH)D concentrations (the storage component of vitamin D) in a normal range. The current recommendation of 160 IU/kg/d, up to a maximum of 400 IU/d, should be more than adequate to prevent vitamin D deficiency in infants receiving parenteral nutrition.

Full enteral nutrition provides the best opportunity to provide sufficient calcium and phosphorus to prevent or treat rickets of prematurity. Whereas the use of human milk for preterm infants has gained wide support over the past decade because of its known benefits, it appears to be inadequate in providing the preterm newborn infant with sufficient concentrations of calcium and phosphorus.[2] Consumption of 120 kcal/d of human milk can be expected to provide only 50 mg/kg/d of elemental calcium and 25 mg/kg/d of elemental phosphorus compared with intrauterine accretion rates of at least 100 mg/kg/d and 50 mg/kg/d, respectively. Supplementation of human milk with individual mineral components or commercially available preparations has been used to successfully treat and prevent osteopenia and rickets of prematurity. It is recommended that both minerals be used together as hypocalcemia has occurred when only phosphate has been supplemented. The optimal quantity of supplement is not known, but factoring in intestinal absorption, total intakes of 150 to 200 mg/kg/d of elemental calcium and 75 to 100 mg/kg/d of elemental phosphorus are recommended. The addition of 100 to 125 mg/kg/d of elemental calcium and 50 to 65 mg/kg/d of elemental phosphorus to human milk feedings (or term formula in countries without special preterm formulas) will supply calcium and phosphorus at recommended rates.

Commercial human milk additives for preterm infants have been developed to bolster the caloric, protein, vitamin, and mineral content of human milk. Both powder and liquid preparations are available, and they increase the overall provision of calcium and phosphorus to 145 to 225 mg/kg/d and 62 to 126 mg/kg/d, respectively, for infants receiving 120 kcal/kg/d. These preparations have the advantage of ease of use, but their solubility is less than that of commercially prepared preterm formulas. An alternative using calcium gluconate (9.4 mg/ml of elemental calcium) and a mixture of both monobasic and dibasic phosphate salts divided in six to eight daily doses appears to be successful. To improve tolerance, it is suggested that individual mineral therapy begin with one-half the goal dose, increased slowly over 5 to 10 days. When adding these minerals to milk, the phosphorus component should be added first and mixed well before adding the calcium supplement to minimize the formation of insoluble Ca-P salts.

The use of commercially prepared term formulas in preterm infants has diminished with the development and acceptance of specialized formulas for preterm infants. Thus, for preterm infants and infants with osteopenia or rickets, term infant formulas should be avoided, and preterm infant formulas should be provided. These specialized formulas are designed to provide the infant with 132 to 216 mg/kg/d of elemental calcium and 66 to 108 mg/kg/d of elemental phosphorus. Preterm formulas have the advantage of improved solubility and ease of use compared with supplementation of term formulas. Their use has markedly simplified the treatment of rickets and reduced the incidence of osteopenia.

Feeding techniques may also contribute to rickets of prematurity. Continuous feedings have been reported to decrease the delivery of calcium and phosphorus to the infant because of settling and binding to feeding tubes. This complication appears to be greater with powder supplements. These losses must, however, be weighed against the possible advantages of improved tolerance and lower metabolic costs of the continuous technique.

Alterations in vitamin D metabolism do not appear to be a major component of osteopenia and rickets in preterm infants. Low serum 25(OH)D concentrations have been reported in preterm infants supplemented with 400 IU/d of vitamin D and receiving the lower calcium and phosphorus concentrations commonly found in human milk or term formulas. The standard 400 IU/d appears adequate for infants on higher calcium and phosphorus intakes. Furthermore, the provision of as much as 2000 IU/d of vitamin D will not prevent the development of rickets if calcium and phosphorus intakes are inadequate. For treatment of rickets, the daily provision of 400 IU/d seems sufficient, and there is little support that provision of more than 400 to 800 IU/d is advantageous.

Soy formulas have been associated with a high frequency of rickets in preterm infants in the past. This is thought to be secondary to the high concentration of the phytate form of phosphate, which has poorer bioavailability. However, comparison studies in term infants have demonstrated identical bone mineral content measurements in newly formulated soy formula, human milk, and cow's milk formula-fed infants.[3] Despite this observation, we believe it is safer to avoid soy formulas in preterm and rachitic infants because there are insufficient bone mineral content data in the preterm population.

Treatment of fractures in rachitic newborns is conservative. In addition to minimizing manipulation of the affected area (including the occasional use of light splints), therapy is directed toward provision of adequate nutritional calcium and phosphorus.

Biochemical monitoring during institution of therapy for rickets should include at least every other day serum calcium and phosphorus concentration determinations until maximum calcium and phosphorus supplementation has been achieved. Thereafter, once or twice weekly monitoring should be sufficient. Serum alkaline phosphatase measurements may be helpful, and these should be monitored weekly. However, the usefulness of alkaline phosphatase measurements is diminished by wide variations in normal ranges and by contributions of alkaline phosphatase from sites other than bone. Serial alkaline phosphatase measurements, viewed in the context of the total patient, may give an early indication of successful therapy, with a steady decline in serum concentrations. Weekly monitoring of serum sodium, potassium, and creatinine will be helpful in early detection of side effects of therapy. Similarly, weekly urine calcium, phosphorus, and creatinine determinations are helpful in marking the success of therapy and detecting excessive mineral supplementation. Osteopenia of prematurity is associated with decreased to absent urinary phosphorus excretion and elevated calcium excretion. Adequate therapy will result in normalization of the urinary electrolytes and a fractional excretion of phosphorus of 3% to 5%. Radiographic changes are late and poorly sensitive to therapeutic changes. Studies at baseline and monthly to bimonthly may be helpful in confirming healing.

The duration of therapy is commonly 3 months. Failure to demonstrate significant improvement within 3 to 6 weeks may indicate an alternative uncommon diagnosis, such as vitamin D resistance, or the presence of a rare trace mineral abnormality, such as copper deficiency or aluminum toxicity.

Prognosis for even severely affected infants is good. Resolution of clinical rickets usually occurs by 6 months of age, and bone mineral content should be comparable to that of term infants by 1 year. Defects in primary dentition, including hypoplasia and hypomineralization, have been reported in former osteopenic newborns. Special attention should be directed toward ensuring good dental care in these infants.

In conclusion, osteopenia and rickets of prematurity are conditions related to a deficiency in the calcium and phosphorus supply during periods of rapid bone growth. Preventive measures ensuring adequate supply of these minerals should reduce the incidence of these diseases. The role of vitamin D appears minimal, but further study is necessary. Treatment is aimed at providing recommended rates of both calcium and phosphorus along with 400 IU of vitamin D daily. The outcome with adequate therapy appears to be good, with full resolution often by 1 year of age.

REFERENCES

1. Koo WWK, Tsang RC, Succop P, et al: Minimal vitamin D and high calcium and phosphorus needs of preterm infants receiving parenteral nutrition. J Pediatr 8:225–233, 1989.
2. Lemons JA, Moye L, Hall D, Simmons M: Differences in the composition of preterm and term human milk during early lactation. Pediatr Res 16:113–117, 1982.
3. Mimouni F, Campaigne B, Neylan M, Tsang RC. Bone mineralization in the first year of life in infants fed human milk, cow-milk formula, or soy-based formula. J Pediatr 122:348-354, 1993.

INFANTS OF DIABETIC MOTHERS

Michael K. Georgieff, M.D.

Advances in maternal and fetal care over the past two decades have improved the outlook for the infant born to a diabetic mother (IDM) to the point where the vast majority of pregnant diabetic women can expect to have a healthy child if they seek early prenatal care. Practitioners who treat pregnant women with diabetes and their offspring have learned to be more aggressive in prevention and treatment of conditions that complicate this disease. This is due in large part to a greater understanding of the causes of morbidity and mortality for the fetus and newborn during diabetic pregnancies. Much of the research effort has focused on the effect of maternal glycemia on the fetus, although not all the abnormalities encountered in the IDM can be attributed solely to lack of maternal glucose control.

This chapter focuses on the treatment of IDM in the newborn period. Understanding the pathophysiology on which each treatment is based is important and is discussed in each section before treatment recommendations are given.

FETAL PATHOPHYSIOLOGY DURING DIABETIC PREGNANCY

Although the etiology of fetal and neonatal sequelae of maternal diabetes is complicated and likely multifactorial, the majority of neonatal complications observed in infants of diabetic mothers appear to be related to the fetal response to lack of maternal glycemic control (Fig. 1). The Pederson hypothesis, in its simplest form, states that maternal hyperglycemia results in fetal hyperglycemia, since glucose readily traverses the placenta. Treatment of maternal hyperglycemia with insulin, however, does not relieve fetal hyperglycemia, since insulin does not cross the placenta from mother to fetus. As a result, the fetus is responsible for its own glucose homeostasis.

In the first half of pregnancy, fetal hyperglycemia appears to proceed relatively unchecked, since the islet cells of the fetus are not capable of responsive insulin secretion until well into the second trimester. Investigators have proposed two major fetopathies on the basis of early gestational hyperglycemia. The first is a higher prevalence of congenital anomalies of the brain, heart, kidneys, intestine, and skeleton. These anomalies occur during organogenesis and must, by definition, happen between the periconceptional period and 2 months gestation. The second is the effect of hyperglycemia without hyperinsulinemia on growth. Unlike the growth acceleration that occurs later in gestation, it appears that hyperglycemia alone reduces fetal growth. Serial ultrasonographic studies indicate that the most poorly controlled diabetics have the smallest fetuses before 20 weeks gestation.

During the second half of pregnancy, particularly late in the third trimester, many of the fetal events that are responsible for the characteristic pathophysiology of the newborn IDM take place. With the onset of islet cell hyperplasia late in the second trimester, the fetus of the poorly controlled diabetic is exposed to both hyperglycemia and hyperinsulinemia. This potent combination of a major metabolic fuel and a significant anabolic hormone causes a cascade of third trimester events that result in increased fetal and neonatal morbidity and mortality.

During late fetal life, chronic hyperglycemia and hyperinsulinemia result in fetal growth acceleration. The increased size of the IDM is not proportional, unlike fetuses who are genetically predisposed to large size. The predominant effect of hyperglycemia and hyperinsulinemia is increased fat stores, which result in weight gain, especially after 32 weeks gestation. Complications at the time of delivery can include shoulder dystocia and perinatal asphyxia. The rate of cesarean delivery is higher in IDM because of fetal macrosomia.

Intrauterine hyperglycemia and hyperinsulinemia also cause remarkable metabolic alterations in the fetus. Wide swings in maternal serum glucose concentrations result in an uneven delivery of glucose to the fetus, with the risk of alternating hyperglycemia and hypoglycemia. Repeated episodes of fetal hypoglycemia may occur as a consequence of high levels of circulating fetal insulin at a time of sudden reduction in maternal serum glucose and placental glucose delivery. These events have been implicated in the increased fetal mortality rate of diabetic pregnancies. In the newborn period, the sudden interruption of glucose delivery accompanied by high circulating insulin levels results in neonatal hypoglycemia.

Intrauterine hyperglycemia and hyperinsulinemia also affect the fetus's basal metabolic rate, with profound secondary effects on fetal oxygenation, erythropoiesis, and acid-base and iron status. Hyperglycemia and hyperinsulinemia have been shown independently and in consort to increase fetal oxygen consumption by up to 30%. The fetus increases its rate of substrate uptake and oxidation, yet the placenta has limited ability to increase oxygen delivery in the face of increased demand. The resultant fetal hypoxemia is believed to be in part responsible for the increased incidence of fetal death, metabolic acidosis, erythropoiesis, and alterations in fetal iron distribution. Accelerated erythropoiesis can result in polycythemia, which may contribute to the higher incidence of stroke, seizures, necrotizing enterocolitis, and renal vein thrombosis in newborn IDM. Furthermore, there may be long-term neurologic sequelae of prolonged fetal hypoxia or iron redistribution.

Fetal hyperinsulinemia is likely to be responsible for delayed functional maturation of fetal organs. The pathophysiology is not well understood, but it is thought that insulin blunts the maturing effect of cortisol on the lung and liver at 34 to 36 weeks gestation. The resultant immaturity may contribute to the higher incidence of respiratory distress syndrome (RDS) and hyperbilirubinemia in the newborn IDM.

Finally, fetal hyperglycemia and hyperinsulinemia may transiently affect organ function and structure in newborn IDM. Hypertrophic cardiomyopathy with intraventricular septal hypertrophy is thought to be such a case, where the increased mass of the heart is likely due to excessive glycogen deposition.

IMPLICATIONS OF FETAL PATHOPHYSIOLOGY ON PRENATAL MANAGEMENT

There is clear evidence that fetal and neonatal morbidity and mortality during diabetic pregnancy can be reduced by strict maternal glycemic control. Periconceptional glucose control appears to reduce the incidence of congenital anomalies. Fetal macrosomia can be averted by appropriate maternal control from 32 weeks gestation until term. Similarly, fetal hyperinsulinemia and its attendant metabolic abnormalities can be reduced by glycemic control after 28 weeks gestation.

Other fetal morbidities are not as clearly linked to maternal glycemia. These include fetal hypoxia, polycythemia, and neonatal hypoglycemia in the growth-retarded IDM. The etiology of these morbidities may be more dependent on advanced maternal diabetic vascular disease and decreased nutrient transport rather than fetal hyperglycemia and hyperinsulinemia. The pathophysiologies of neonatal hypocalcemia, hypomagnesemia, poorer neurodevelopmental outcome, and small left colon syndrome remain elusive. Thus, their relation to maternal glycemia is not as well understood.

PRENATAL DIAGNOSIS AND TREATMENT

Extensive reviews have been written about the management of maternal diabetes, and a detailed approach is beyond the scope of this section. Nevertheless, the physician who will care for the newborn IDM should be conversant with maternal therapy and should understand the results and implications of common fetal surveillance testing. In addition, management of the newborn IDM includes consultation with the delivering physician regarding plans for timing of delivery and expected neonatal complications.

Before the time of delivery, maternal hemoglobin A_{1c} results from the entire pregnancy should be reviewed. Particular attention should

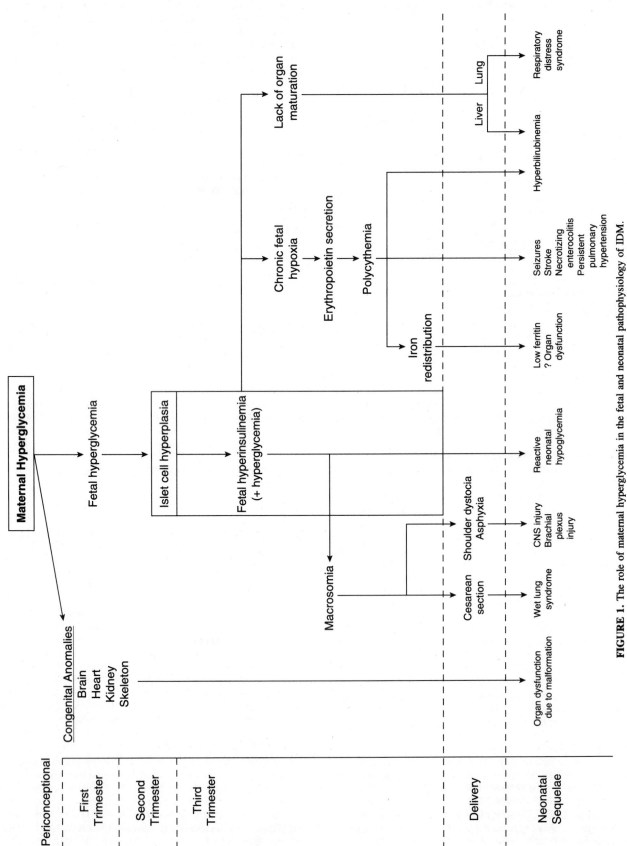

FIGURE 1. The role of maternal hyperglycemia in the fetal and neonatal pathophysiology of IDM.

be paid to values beginning at 32 weeks gestation, since values at that time have been correlated with neonatal macrosomia, polycythemia, and hypoglycemia. Hemoglobin A_{1c} values less than 7% reflect good control, whereas values greater than 8% reflect poor control. Infants born to mothers with late gestation hemoglobin A_{1c} values greater than 10% should be expected to present with neonatal complications.

The results of maternal serum alpha-fetoprotein levels measured at 16 to 18 weeks gestation and fetal ultrasound studies should be reviewed before attending the delivery of the IDM to ascertain whether an infant is likely to have congenital anomalies. Nonstress tests should be performed twice weekly starting at 32 weeks gestation. If the nonstress test becomes nonreactive, a contraction stress test should be performed. Information about the results of these tests, maternal reports of fetal movement, and quantitation of the biophysical profile will help the physician estimate the potential for perinatal asphyxia.

Finally, assessment of fetal lung maturity, particularly in insulin-dependent diabetics, is important. Gestational diabetic patients are now routinely delivered at term. However, many physicians still recommend that mothers classified as White class B or greater be delivered electively at 38 weeks. Many centers recommend an ultrasound-directed amniocentesis at 37 weeks gestation to determine lung maturity. The narrow time window between complete maturation of the lungs (as late as 37 weeks gestation) and the rise in the incidence of fetal death (after 38 weeks gestation) makes optimal timing of the delivery of the IDM born to a class B or greater diabetic mother difficult. Documentation of an L/S ratio of 3:1 with phosphatidylglycerol (PG) present is reassuring with respect to pulmonary maturity.

DIAGNOSIS AND TREATMENT OF ABNORMALITIES FOUND IN NEWBORN IDM

IDM are susceptible to metabolic, growth, and hematologic abnormalities in the neonatal period for the reasons discussed earlier. A general approach to screening for these abnormalities is presented in Table 1. In addition, IDM have higher incidences of congenital anomalies, respiratory disorders, cardiac dysfunction, and poor neurologic outcome compared with gestational age-matched infants born to nondiabetic mothers. The following sections outline the diagnostic and therapeutic approaches to each of these abnormalities.

METABOLIC ABNORMALITIES

Hypoglycemia

Diagnosis

Up to 40% of IDM experience significant hypoglycemia following birth. This is more common in macrosomic and growth-retarded IDM than in those whose size is appropriate for dates. Hypoglycemia is defined as a serum glucose <35 mg/dl in a term infant and <25 mg/dl in a preterm infant in the first 3 days after birth. After 72 hours, hypoglycemia is defined as a serum glucose <45 mg/dl.

Neonatal hypoglycemia in IDM is generally due to a combination of hyperplasia of the pancreatic islet cells and removal of an exogenous glucose source (maternal) following delivery. During gestation, the fetus is exposed to maternal glucose but not insulin, as the former crosses the placenta whereas the latter does not. In response, the fetus's islet cells become hyperplastic, with consequent fetal hyperinsulinemia. Thus, it is not surprising that the prevalence and severity of neonatal hypoglycemia in IDM are closely linked to lack of maternal glycemic control and that it is seen most commonly in macrosomic infants. Decreased hepatic glucose production due to low glucagon and catecholamine output contributes to the pathogenesis of neonatal hypoglycemia.

Reactive hypoglycemia in macrosomic IDM tends to occur within 2 hours of birth and is an exaggeration of the normal decrease in serum glucose observed following delivery. It frequently persists up to 72 hours and may require aggressive therapy. Occasionally, hypoglycemia will persist for up to 1 week. Symptoms include jitteriness, sweating, tachypnea (or apnea), seizures, agitation, and respiratory distress.

Neonatal hypoglycemia in IDM can also occur as a consequence of intrauterine growth retardation. This situation is encountered most often in infants born to mothers with advanced diabetic vascular disease. In growth-retarded IDM, the hypoglycemia is more often due to decreased hepatic glycogen stores (as seen in other forms of intrauterine growth retardation) rather than to neonatal hyperinsulinemia.

Treatment

Neonatal hypoglycemia can be **prevented** by maintaining tight glucose control during pregnancy, thus reducing islet cell hyperplasia. In addition, close monitoring of the maternal glucose status in the hours before delivery will prevent the about-to-be-born infant from being exposed to a large bolus of glucose.

The **asymptomatic IDM** should be watched closely for hypoglycemia, particularly if macrosomia is present. Serum glucose levels should be checked hourly until the first feeding occurs and preprandially for the next several feeds. Asymptomatic infants with normal serum glucose levels will not generally require parenteral dextrose therapy. Thus, prophylactic administration of intravenous dextrose is unwarranted. Early initiation of feedings (by 1 hour of age) is highly recommended, since such feedings result in higher serum glucose values in the early neonatal period. The slow rate of gastric emptying in newborn infants may effectively titrate glucose to the IDM, thus dampening wide swings in glucose delivery.

Asymptomatic IDM who develop low serum glucose levels within the first 3 hours of life (despite early initiation of feedings), IDM who are ill with cardiorespiratory illnesses, and IDM who are premature will require parenteral glucose therapy. These subpopulations should be started on intravenous dextrose before symptoms of hypoglycemia develop. It is not appropriate to push a bolus of intravenous dextrose to correct asymptomatic hypoglycemia, since this will stimulate the hypertrophied islet cells to release a large amount of insulin. Bolus infusion of dextrose will cause more severe hypoglycemia than that initially treated and is far more likely to cause symptoms. Instead, the proper approach is to start a steady infusion of intravenous dextrose as outlined in the section on symptomatic hypoglycemia.

The **symptomatic IDM** should be approached aggressively but carefully (Table 2). The goal of intravenous glucose therapy is to correct the hypoglycemic state. Nevertheless, rapid delivery of glucose will result in the release of additional insulin by the hyperactive islet cells and cause reactive hypoglycemia. The key to therapy is a continuous glucose infusion rather than administration of intermittent boluses.

A symptomatic infant may be given an initial dose of 200 mg/kg body weight of glucose as a $D_{10}W$ solution over 5 minutes, followed by a constant infusion of 4 to 6 mg/kg/min (Table 2). Serum glucose levels should be measured frequently until a normal value is achieved (>35 mg/dl). Persistent hypoglycemia should be treated by increasing the rate of the infusion by 2 to 4 mg/kg/min and repeating the serum glucose determination. It is not unusual for IDM to require 10 to 12 mg/kg/min to maintain serum glucose concentrations above 45 mg/dl in the first 3 to 5 postnatal days. Rates as high as 15 to 17 mg/kg/min may be required. As the infant recovers and maintains adequate serum glucose levels, the infusion rate may be decreased *slowly* by increments of 5% to 10% to the more standard 6 to 8 mg/kg/min. Glucagon, epinephrine, or glucocorticosteroid administration is usually not indicated in this disease, although these agents may be helpful in hypoglycemic growth-retarded infants.

The prognosis for hypoglycemic IDM who do not have seizures is excellent. Thus, the prompt recognition and treatment of hypoglycemia before the onset of seizures is important. The outcome of infants with neonatal seizures caused by hypoglycemia is less favorable, with some estimating the neurologic morbidity rate at 50%.

TABLE 1. Initial Assessment of IDM*

TIME	ASSESSMENT					
Prenatal	Ultrasound for size and anomalies					
	Biophysical profile					
	Maternal hemoglobin A_{1c}					
Delivery Room	Physical examination for					
	Congenital anomalies					
	Size for dates					
	Respiratory status					
Postnatal	*1–6 h*	*6–12 h*	*12–24 h*	*24–48 h*	*48–72 h*	*72–96 h*
Serum glucose	X2	X	X	X†	X†	
Calcium				X	X†	
Magnesium				X	X†	
Hemoglobin/hematocrit	X			X†	X†	
Platelet count	X					
Bilirubin			X‡	X†	X†	X†
Ferritin	X					

*These guidelines represent initial, minimal assessments. Abnormal parameters will need to be followed more closely.
†If previous value was abnormal.
‡If clinically jaundiced.

Hypocalcemia

Diagnosis

Hypocalcemia complicates the neonatal course in up to 50% of IDM and is of the early onset variety, occurring in the first 72 postnatal hours. IDM who have suffered perinatal asphyxia or are premature have the highest risk of neonatal hypocalcemia. Neonatal hypocalcemia is defined as a total serum calcium of <7 mg/dl or an ionized calcium of <4 mg/dl. Hypocalcemia rarely causes clinical symptomatology and is, therefore, frequently missed. Nevertheless, since calcium is an important messenger in multiple enzymatic processes, asymptomatic hypocalcemia must still be considered potentially harmful to the IDM.

The etiology of early neonatal hypocalcemia remains poorly understood, although it is likely related to a state of transient hypoparathyroidism. The fetus receives a high delivery rate of elemental calcium via the placenta. Parathyroid hormone (PTH), calcitonin, and most likely vitamin D do not cross the placenta, leaving the fetus responsible for its own calcium balance. With large amounts of calcium being delivered transplacentally, fetal PTH levels are low at the end of gestation. When the placental calcium delivery is abruptly discontinued at birth and feedings have not yet been established, the newborn infant must be able to increase PTH levels to maintain serum calcium concentrations in a normal range. IDM, as well as premature and asphyxiated infants, demonstrate a delay in PTH response, the pathophysiology of which is not well established. In the IDM, this delay in PTH regulation is independent of the presence or absence of birth asphyxia. An additional factor that may precipitate hypocalcemia in infants of insulin-dependent mothers is neonatal hypomagnesemia.

The signs and symptoms of neonatal hypocalcemia closely mimic those of hypoglycemia. They frequently present as abnormalities on neurologic examination and include jitteriness, sweating, tachypnea, irritability, and seizures. Symptoms generally occur 24 to 72 hours after delivery and, thus, may be distinguishable from the symptoms of hypoglycemia on the basis of their slightly later onset.

Treatment

Treatment of **asymptomatic hypocalcemia** with intravenous boluses of calcium gluconate is rarely indicated and can be dangerous. Prevention of symptoms can be ensured by placing the infant on a low-phosphorus enteral or parenteral formulation (calcium/phosphorus ratio of 1.5 to 2:1). Breast milk, as well as most commercial formulas, will achieve these goals.

IDM with **symptomatic hypocalcemia** should be treated, but one may find that large amounts of calcium are required. Treatment may appear futile, since the body acts as a large calcium sink. Thus, repeated boluses of calcium result in only transient increases in the serum calcium level. Nevertheless, intravenous 10% calcium gluconate, preferably administered through a central venous catheter, can be given slowly and cautiously to treat symptomatic hypocalcemia. The goal is to maintain serum calcium concentrations above 7 mg/dl. Therapeutic calcium is given as a 10% calcium gluconate solution 100 to 200 mg/kg (1 to 2 ml/kg) over 5 to 10 minutes (Table 2). Constant ECG monitoring is required, since rapid calcium infusion will induce recalcitrant bradycardia and hypotension. After the initial treatment, 10% calcium gluconate can be added to the maintenance intravenous solution in a concentration of 400 to 800 mg/100 ml of fluid. This concentration will provide 36 to 72 mg/kg day of elemental calcium. Generally, this amount will be needed only for the first 2 days of therapy, after which the dose can be halved (over the next 24-hour period) and then quartered. Treatment of hypocalcemia is rarely successful when hypomagnesemia is also present. Hypomagnesemia must be treated before or at the same time as hypocalcemia.

The prognosis following early neonatal hypocalcemia is excellent, provided that seizures are not present. Seizures associated with low calcium concentrations (<6.5 mg/dl) have been associated with an increased frequency of neurologic abnormalities.

Hypomagnesemia

Diagnosis

Hypomagnesemia is frequently found in association with hypocalcemia and, in many instances, must be addressed before the treatment of hypocalcemia will be successful. Up to 40% of IDM will have concurrent hypomagnesemia, defined as a serum magnesium level less than 1.5 mg/dl. The etiology of hypomagnesemia in IDM is not fully understood, but contributing factors include transient hypoparathyroidism in the newborn (see Hypocalcemia) and excessive urinary magnesium losses in insulin-dependent mothers during gestation. The latter has been postulated to impair magnesium transfer to the fetus.

The symptoms of hypomagnesemia appear within 24 hours of birth and are similar to those of hypoglycemia and hypocalcemia. Generally, magnesium levels must be less than 1.2 mg/dl for symptoms to occur. Hypomagnesemic infants can be irritable and jittery. In addition, they may have muscle fasciculations, hyperreflexia, and seizures.

Treatment

Asymptomatic hypomagnesemia is best corrected through the addition of magnesium sulfate to the parenteral solution (Table 2).

TABLE 2. Doses for Acute and Chronic Correction of Metabolic Abnormalities in Newborn Infants of Diabetic Mothers

| CONDITION | ACUTE CORRECTION | | | | | CHRONIC INFUSION | | |
	SOLUTION	VOLUME AMOUNT	DOSE	INFUSION RATE	ROUTE	SOLUTION	RATE	DOSE
Hypoglycemia	$D_{10}W$ (10 g/100 ml)	2–4 ml/kg	200–400 mg/kg	Over 5 min	Peripheral or central IV	$D_{10}W$	3–4 ml/kg/h (72–96 ml/kg/d)*	6 mg/kg/min
Hypocalcemia	10% calcium gluconate (100 mg calcium gluconate/ml)	1–2 ml/kg	100–200 mg/kg	Over 5–10 min†	Central IV preferable, never into umbilical artery catheter	400–800 mg of calcium gluconate added to 100 ml of IV maintenance solution	100 ml/kg/d	36–72 mg Ca^{2+}/kg/d
Hypomagnesemia	5% magnesium sulfate (50 mg $MgSO_4$/ml)	0.5–1 ml/kg	25–50 mg $MgSO_4$/kg (0.2–0.4 mEq Mg^{2+}/kg)‡	Over 1 h with ½ dose over first 15–20 min†	Central IV preferable	31–62 mg 5% magnesium sulfate in 100 ml of maintenance IV solution	100 ml/kg/d	31–62 mg $MgSO_4$/kg/d (0.25–0.5 mEq/kg/d)

*Initial recommended rate; may need to double to keep blood sugar normal.
†Requires continuous ECG monitoring and capability for ventilatory support.
‡Maximum dose is 1 mEq/kg/h; may repeat q8–12h.

The recommended dose is 0.25 to 0.5 mEq/kg/d. **Symptomatic hypomagnesemia** can be corrected by the slow IV administration of 0.5 to 2.5 ml/kg of a 5% solution of magnesium sulfate (10 mg $MgSO_4$/ml) over 1 hour. Half the dose may be given in the first 10 to 20 minutes (Table 2). As with the intravenous treatment of hypocalcemia, continuous ECG monitoring is mandatory because of the risk of heart block, refractory bradycardia, and hypotension. After initial treatment, further hypomagnesemia can be prevented by adding magnesium sulfate to the parenteral solution.

No specific studies have addressed the long-term outcome of IDM with hypomagnesemia. It is likely that, without seizures, the prognosis is as excellent as it is for IDM with hypocalcemia and hypoglycemia.

HEMATOLOGIC ABNORMALITIES

Polycythemia and Hyperviscosity

Diagnosis

Twenty percent to thirty percent of IDM are polycythemic at birth, with central hemoglobin concentrations greater than 20 g/dl and hematocrit levels greater than 65%. The majority of symptoms ascribed to polycythemia in the newborn are more likely due to accompanying blood hyperviscosity. However, blood viscosity is not routinely measured, whereas hemoglobin and hematocrit levels are. Thus, most physicians equate elevated red blood cell indices with the risk of hyperviscosity and its complications, although the correlation is not 1:1. When evaluating an IDM for polycythemia, reliance on heelstick hematocrit determinations is not appropriate, since the hematocrit is frequently elevated in such specimens and is generally much higher than centrally obtained values.

The etiology of polycythemia in the IDM has been elucidated over the past 15 years. The incidence and severity are related to lack of maternal glycemic control (Fig. 1). The process of red cell mass expansion is thought to be predominantly a third trimester phenomenon. Maternal hyperglycemia causes fetal hyperglycemia, which in turn results in islet cell hyperplasia and fetal hyperinsulinemia. Fetal hyperglycemia and hyperinsulinemia raise fetal oxygen consumption by up to 30%, increasing substrate uptake, activity, and heat production. The capacity of the placenta to increase oxygen transport under these conditions is relatively limited, rendering the fetus hypoxemic. Oxygen transport may be further complicated by placental vascular disease, particularly in women with more advanced diabetes.

The fetus attempts to maintain tissue oxygen delivery by increasing oxygen-carrying capacity. This is accomplished through erythropoietin secretion and augmented hemoglobin synthesis. In severe cases, the fetus becomes polycythemic.

The hematocrit should be followed on a daily basis, and a platelet count should be obtained at least once. Although severely polycythemic fetuses are at risk for intrauterine infarcts, their risk may further increase after birth with the free water diuresis and low fluid intake that occurs during the first 3 days in all newborns. An increase in hematocrit between birth and day 3 is not unusual. A falling platelet count in a polycythemic IDM is an indicator of significant microvascular sludging and thrombosis secondary to polycythemia.

The classic clinical picture of the polycythemic IDM is a plethoric infant who is sluggish and lethargic. The clinical symptoms are predominantly due to sludging of blood in the microvasculature of the brain, intestine, kidney, and lung. Neurologic symptoms range from jitteriness and a high-pitched cry to lethargy and seizures. Neuroimaging studies (cranial ultrasound, CT, MRI) may reveal the presence of a stroke or venous sinus thrombosis, although lesions associated with polycythemia are usually microscopic and not detectable on scan.

During the first few days of life, careful daily abdominal examinations are indicated. IDM may be poor feeders and demonstrate significant feeding intolerance, manifested as intestinal hypomotility, vomiting, and abdominal distention. The risk of necrotizing enterocolitis is increased due to microinfarcts of the intestinal circulation.

Renal vein thrombosis remains a major risk in polycythemic IDM. This should be suspected and evaluated in the polycythemic IDM who presents with any of the following findings: hematuria, thrombocytopenia, flank mass, or hypertension. A careful palpation of the abdominal flanks for renal masses, as well as testing the urine for hematuria, should be considered standard in the polycythemic IDM.

Sludging of the microvasculature of the lung may also occur in the polycythemic IDM. The increased pulmonary vascular resistance that accompanies this microthrombosis is likely an important contributor to the increased incidence of persistent pulmonary hypertension (persistent fetal circulation) seen in IDM. Neonatal polycythemia is transient, since it is a response to fetal hypoxia. With the onset of normoxemia following birth, the increased red cell mass is no longer required, and the red cells break down over a 60- to 120-day period.

Treatment

Clinical judgment must be used to decide whether to treat polycythemia in newborn IDM, since symptomatology, hematocrit, and blood viscosity may not intercorrelate in individual patients. Furthermore, neonatal blood can be hyperviscous at a hematocrit <65%, and renal vein thrombosis has been described in IDM with hematocrits of 60%. Therefore, treatment of IDM with symptomatic hyperviscosity is indicated despite hematocrits <65%.

Asymptomatic infants with hematocrits ranging from 65% to 70% should be hydrated with intravenous fluids (generally $D_{10}W$) at the rate of 100 ml/kg/d and have their hematocrits measured at least daily for the first 3 days of life (Table 1). If the infant becomes symptomatic or the hematocrit rises despite fluid therapy, a partial exchange transfusion should be performed.

All **symptomatic infants,** regardless of hematocrit and those infants whose central hematocrit is ≥70%, require immediate therapy in the form of a partial exchange transfusion. It is not appropriate to simply phlebotomize these infants, since the volume of blood removed might cause significant problems with hypovolemia. Adequate vascular access is important for properly performing a partial exchange transfusion. This is most easily accomplished if the infant has umbilical catheters in place. Other options include withdrawing blood from the central venous catheter and infusing the replacement solution through a peripheral venous catheter. The replacement fluid is generally plasmanate, although fresh frozen plasma or even normal saline can be used. The formula for calculating the volume of blood to withdraw and fluid to administer is

$$\frac{OH - DH}{OH} \times \text{Total blood volume in milliliters}$$

where OH = observed hematocrit
DH = desired hematocrit

The blood volume of newborn infants is approximately 85 ml/kg body weight. For a 4 kg IDM, the blood volume would be 340 ml. To decrease the hematocrit from 65% to 55%, 52 ml of blood should be withdrawn and replaced with plasmanate. Since this represents 15% of the infant's blood volume, plasmanate should be infused as the blood is withdrawn to avoid hypovolemic shock.

The outcome of IDM on the basis of the presence of polycythemia alone has not been evaluated. However, studies of newborn infants with polycythemia from a variety of causes suggest an increased rate of long-term neurodevelopmental handicaps in infants who are symptomatic in the newborn period.

Iron Redistribution and Iron Deficiency

Diagnosis

Recent studies have shown that up to 65% of all IDM and 95% of large for dates IDM demonstrate abnormalities of iron metabolism at birth. These abnormalities include decreased serum and storage iron (low ferritin concentrations), increased total iron-binding capacity, decreased transferrin saturation, and increased free erythrocyte protoporphyrin concentrations. A serum ferritin concentration <60 μg/L, a serum iron <100 μg/dl, or an iron-binding capacity saturation <33% at birth is abnormal.

The abnormal iron status in IDM results from a combination of increased fetal iron demand for erythropoiesis, redistribution of fetal iron into the red cell mass, and potential impairment of transplacental iron transport. The estimated increase in fetal hemoglobin mass ranges from 30% to 40%, resulting in a commensurate increase in iron need. The placenta appears to have a limited ability to upregulate iron transport, rendering the fetus dependent on accumulated fetal iron stores. The use of fetal stores is reflected in low ferritin concentrations at birth. Once fetal liver iron stores are depleted, nonstorage organs, such as the heart and brain, become compromised. An autopsy study of IDM demonstrated that liver, heart, and brain iron were reduced to 7%, 44%, and 61%, respectively, of control values.

In theory, once normoxemia is established postnatally, iron should be liberated from the expanded red cell mass over the first 2 months of life and be available for tissue repletion. However, a recent follow-up study supports the notion that these infants are iron deficient and

do not simply exhibit a redistribution of fetal iron. This study demonstrated significantly lower 6-month ferritin levels in IDM fed a low-iron formula when compared with infants born to nondiabetic mothers fed the same formula.

Treatment

There have been no controlled trials of iron supplementation of newborn IDM. Nevertheless, no infant should be fed a low-iron formula without providing an iron supplement during the first year because of the risk of iron deficiency and its attendant developmental sequelae. We recommend that all large and small for dates IDM have serum ferritin and hemoglobin concentrations measured in the newborn period. Those with abnormally low ferritin concentrations should have follow-up values determined at 2 months of age. If the values are persistently low, these infants would be candidates for iron supplementation, using the same supplementation regimen as for other iron-deficient children. One group of IDM that bears close observation for signs and symptoms of iron deficiency are those born with low ferritin concentrations and normal to low hematocrits. These infants are usually born to mothers with either advanced diabetic disease (White class ≥D) or significant hypertension during pregnancy. Their total body iron at birth appears to be low rather than normal, thereby increasing their risk of iron deficiency later in infancy.

Only one follow-up study of IDM has been performed. This study suggests a long-term risk of iron deficiency in IDM fed a low-iron formula. Neurodevelopmental outcome as a function of iron status at birth has not been evaluated, but iron-deficient IDM would be at equivalent to or greater risk of neurodevelopmental sequelae than iron-deficient infants born to nondiabetic mothers.

HYPERBILIRUBINEMIA

Diagnosis

IDM have a higher incidence of significant hyperbilirubinemia than have infants born to nondiabetic mothers. Since virtually all newborn infants demonstrate some degree of neonatal jaundice, incidence figures for IDM are not relevant. IDM are at increased risk of hyperbilirubinemia because of an enlarged red cell mass, increased ineffective erythropoiesis, and relative immaturity of hepatic bilirubin conjugation and excretion (Fig. 1). A larger red cell mass, as seen in polycythemic IDM, provides a greater source of bilirubin in need of conjugation and excretion. In addition, IDM have been shown to have a high degree of ineffective erythropoiesis, where red cell precursors are trapped in the reticuloendothelial system and destroyed, releasing bilirubin precursors into the circulation. Finally, as with the lung, the liver of the IDM is immature compared with the livers of gestationally age-matched controls. Specifically, glucuronyl transferase appears to be less effective in conjugating indirect bilirubin and preparing it for excretion through the biliary tree. This functional immaturity appears to be related to the increased exposure to insulin and decreased sensitivity to cortisol.

IDM will present with neonatal jaundice in the same manner as infants born to nondiabetic mothers. However, because of the increased bilirubin load and the decreased capacity for handling it, physicians should expect a sharper rate of rise and a peak at 4 to 5 days, as opposed to the normal 3 days. Large for dates IDM are particularly vulnerable as they are the ones most likely to be polycythemic as well as to demonstrate hepatic immaturity. The plethora accompanying polycythemia may make it more difficult to clinically appreciate jaundice. Therefore, we recommend measuring the serum bilirubin concentration at 24 to 36 hours of age and following it until there is a downward trend. This may occur after the infant ordinarily would have been discharged (4 to 5 days).

Treatment

Treatment of hyperbilirubinemia in IDM is similar to treatment of infants of nondiabetic mothers and includes hydration, phototherapy, and, in rare circumstances, double-volume exchange transfusion. The clinical threshold for instituting therapy is the same as in infants of nondiabetic mothers and is discussed elsewhere in this book. There are no outcome studies to suggest that IDM are particularly vulnerable to kernicterus.

RESPIRATORY COMPLICATIONS

Respiratory Distress Syndrome
Diagnosis

Infants of diabetic mothers are five to six times more prone to respiratory distress syndrome (RDS) than are gestational age-matched infants born to nondiabetic mothers and remain at higher risk until near 38 weeks gestation. The incidence of RDS has declined since its peak of 30% in the late 1960s, largely due to a change in obstetric management. That is, IDM are no longer being delivered before 38 weeks for fear of intrauterine death unless there are signs on biophysical profile to suggest otherwise.

RDS is defined as the respiratory sequelae of pulmonary surfactant deficiency and is characterized by loss of lung volume and microatelectasis. Infants generally present within 30 minutes of birth with tachypnea, grunting, and cyanosis. Their chest x-rays demonstrate a diffuse, low-volume reticulogranular pattern with air bronchograms. RDS occurs with higher frequency in IDM because of the later onset of maturity of the type II alveolar cells. Insulin blunts production of dipalmityl lecithin, most likely by antagonizing the maturing effect of cortisol on this system. IDM exposed to excessive endogenous insulin are thus at greatest risk for RDS.

Treatment

RDS is best **prevented** in the IDM by avoiding delivery while the lungs are immature. Because of the known delay in pulmonary maturation in infants whose mothers are White class A–D, IDM should be delivered when the L/S ratio exceeds 3:1 and phosphatidylglycerol (PG) is present in amniotic fluid samples.

Treatment of the IDM with established RDS is similar to infants born to nondiabetic mothers, and is discussed elsewhere in this book. Since IDM with RDS are frequently near-term infants, they are at increased risk to exhibit persistent pulmonary hypertension of the neonate, particularly if they are polycythemic. In those cases, care should be taken to ensure that the infant is well oxygenated (arterial oxygen saturations >95%) and ventilated. The management of infants with pulmonary hypertension is discussed in Chapter 5.

Transient Tachypnea of the Newborn (Wet Lung Syndrome)
Diagnosis

Because of the higher rate of cesarean delivery of infants of diabetic women, the physician should be vigilant for the respiratory symptoms of retained fetal lung fluid and be able to distinguish it from RDS. Transient tachypnea of the newborn is generally evident from birth and is characterized by tachypnea and wet-sounding lungs on auscultation. Grunting is rarely noted. The chest x-ray is distinguished from that of RDS by normal to increased lung volumes and coarse perihilar rather than fine generalized infiltrates. Unlike RDS, transient tachypnea improves over the first 24 to 48 hours of life and is rarely associated with CO_2 retention. It is unusual for an infant with transient tachypnea to require mechanical ventilation.

Treatment

Transient tachypnea in the IDM is approached in the same manner as in infants born to nondiabetic mothers. Supplemental oxygen should be administered early in order to maintain arterial oxygen saturations greater than 95% and ensure a smooth transition from the fetal to the neonatal circulatory pattern.

CARDIOVASCULAR ABNORMALITIES

The IDM is at increased risk for both structural and functional cardiovascular abnormalities. Structural abnormalities are discussed in the section on Congenital Anomalies.

Intraventricular Septal Hypertrophy
Diagnosis

This transient but potentially compromising lesion should be suspected in macrosomic IDM born to mothers with very poor glycemic control. Thirty percent of newborn IDM demonstrate evidence of cardiomyopathy, with up to 10% manifesting frank congestive heart failure. These abnormalities have been ascribed primarily to hypertrophic subaortic stenosis resulting from glycogen loading of the intraventricular septum. The amount of hypertrophy appears to be directly related to the degree of maternal (and fetal) hyperglycemia. Hyperinsulinemia is thought to play an important role in the cardiomegaly as well.

The lesion can be diagnosed on prenatal ultrasound and can be reversed with adequate maternal glycemic control. Postnatally, IDM with septal hypertrophy will exhibit similar physiology to adults with idiopathic hypertrophic subaortic stenosis, in that heart failure will be primarily due to left ventricular outflow obstruction. Unlike adults, however, this lesion is transient in IDM and will disappear over a period of weeks to months. Nevertheless, the lesion can compromise cardiorespiratory well-being in the newborn period and requires treatment if outflow obstruction is significant enough to cause heart failure.

Treatment

Digoxin and other inotropes are contraindicated in this disease because they increase contractility, thereby increasing the degree of end-systolic outflow obstruction. Hypovolemia may also worsen this condition. Therefore, diuretics are also contraindicated despite signs of heart failure. Therapy is aimed at maintaining an adequate intravascular volume through hydration and relieving the outflow obstruction with a beta-blocker. A consultation with a cardiologist is strongly suggested. The long-term outcome of septal hypertrophy is excellent, with spontaneous resolution and generally no long-term myopathic effects.

NEUROLOGIC ABNORMALITIES

IDM can manifest a wide spectrum of short-term and long-term neurologic abnormalities. These can be congenital (structural or functional), acquired at delivery, or occur as a result of postnatal complications. Structural abnormalities are discussed in the section on Congenital Anomalies. Short-term neurologic abnormalities seen in the newborn period include those related to perinatal asphyxia, brachial plexus nerve injuries, lethargy, and seizures. Later neurologic manifestations include delay in motor or cognitive development, or both.

Perinatal Asphyxia
Diagnosis

IDM are at increased risk for perinatal asphyxia. The increased incidence is related to the combination of fetal macrosomia, which places the infant at risk for shoulder dystocia during delivery, and chronic intrauterine hypoxia, which decreases the infant's tolerance to the hypoxic stress of labor and delivery. Cardiomyopathy, which occurs frequently in IDM independently of asphyxia, can complicate the management of and recovery from perinatal asphyxia in the IDM.

The neurologic signs and symptoms of perinatal asphyxia in the IDM are identical to those found in infants born to nondiabetic mothers. They include initial hypotonia or flaccidity, followed by increasing tone, jitteriness, and risk of seizures. Seizures due to perinatal asphyxia commonly occur between 12 and 48 hours after delivery. Neurologic symptoms that occur in the neonatal period due to prenatal asphyxia (chronic intrauterine hypoxia) may be difficult to distinguish from those due to events at the time of delivery.

Treatment

The treatment of the asphyxiated IDM is similar to that of the asphyxiated infant of a nondiabetic mother. Before delivery of an IDM with fetal distress, one should make preparations for resuscitation of a depressed infant. The physician should be skilled in the basics of administering neonatal life support, including establishing an airway, providing oxygen and mechanical ventilation, and supporting the circulation with volume expanders and pressors. Since term and near-term IDM are particularly prone to persistent pulmonary hypertension, liberal amounts of supplemental oxygen should be administered to ensure a smooth transition from the fetal to the neonatal circulatory pattern. Arterial oxygen saturation should be maintained >95%. IDM are also more likely to need circulatory support because of their myopathic hearts. Thus, volume expansion followed by institution of pressors may be necessary.

Following stabilization, relative free water fluid restriction (60 ml/kg/d) is indicated to reduce cerebral edema. Seizures secondary to perinatal asphyxia will frequently require an antiepileptic, such as phenobarbital. During the acute phase of cerebral edema, more than one drug may be needed. The prognosis of IDM with perinatal asphyxia is similar to that of infants with asphyxia born to nondiabetic mothers.

Brachial Plexus Injuries

Diagnosis

Brachial plexus injuries can complicate deliveries of IDM and are related to stretching of the neck during delivery of macrosomic infants. Brachial plexus nerve injuries most commonly result in Erb's palsy (roots C5–C7), which generally can be treated conservatively. The majority of infants recover function within 2 weeks. More extensive and serious nerve injuries may include Klumpke's paralysis (roots C7–C8), diaphragmatic paralysis due to phrenic nerve damage (roots C3–C5), recurrent laryngeal nerve damage, or Horner syndrome (roots T1–T2).

Clinical signs of Erb's palsy include an arm that hangs limply extended at the elbow and is internally rotated. The hand is relatively unaffected. Klumpke's paralysis presents with shoulder, upper arm, and hand weakness and eventually will result in the familiar claw hand position. It is usually the result of breech delivery and is more likely than Erb's palsy to result in lifelong disability. Diaphragmatic paralysis may be asymptomatic or may present with significant respiratory distress. Frequently, these infants are identified later following repeated episodes of lower lobe pneumonias on the affected side. IDM who exhibit a hoarse cry at birth should be evaluated for laryngeal nerve palsy.

Treatment

Erb's palsy can be treated expectantly, but persistent findings should be referred for evaluation by a neurologist, as well as physical and occupational therapy. Klumpke's paralysis, diaphragmatic paralysis, and recurrent laryngeal nerve damage are more extensive lesions that need attention in the immediate newborn period. The latter two injuries may compromise respiratory well-being. Diaphragmatic paralysis will lead to recurrent lower lobe atelectasis and pneumonia, and recurrent laryngeal nerve damage may result in recurrent aspiration syndromes due to failure to oppose the vocal cords. Both conditions may require surgical intervention to prevent pulmonary morbidity. Surgical consultation to help with management is strongly suggested.

Lethargy and Hypotonia

Diagnosis

IDM are commonly described as lethargic newborns, although exact prevalence figures are undocumented. These infants are fre-

quently poor feeders and exhibit paucity of movement. Lethargy is usually obvious within the first hours of delivery and may extend up to a week postnatally. Although the exact etiology of lethargy is unknown, the lethargic IDM is usually macrosomic, implying that poor maternal glycemic control is involved in producing the clinical picture. Perinatal asphyxia, glucose and electrolyte abnormalities, polycythemia, cardiomyopathy, and tissue iron deficiency may all contribute to the classic picture of a plethoric, sluggish IDM.

Treatment

Lethargy may improve after treatment of potential underlying causes, such as glucose and electrolyte abnormalities or polycythemia. If the infant is polycythemic, lethargy should be considered a neurologic symptom and is an indication for partial exchange transfusion (see Polycythemia). Similarly, lethargy accompanying a low serum glucose level should be considered a sign of symptomatic hypoglycemia and an indication for prompt treatment (see Hypoglycemia). There are no outcome studies assessing long-term developmental outcomes of IDM who were lethargic or hypotonic in the newborn period.

Jitteriness and Hypertonicity

Diagnosis

In addition to lethargy and hypotonicity, IDM commonly exhibit jitteriness and hypertonicity in the newborn period. Jitteriness is defined as extreme irritability or hypertonicity with tremulousness, which ceases with physical restraint. It must be distinguished from seizure activity, which is not controllable. As with lethargy, the cause of neonatal jitteriness in IDM is likely multifactorial and generally relates to either glucose and electrolyte abnormalities, which make the brain more irritable (i.e., hypoglycemia, hypocalcemia, hypomagnesemia), or to hypoxic events at delivery.

The time of onset of symptoms is related to the etiology. Thus, jitteriness due to hypoglycemia can be expected in the first 24 hours of life, whereas jitteriness secondary to hypocalcemia or hypomagnesemia will appear between 24 and 72 hours. Jitteriness following hypoxic insult generally occurs after 12 hours and coincides with the onset of cerebral edema.

Treatment

The treatment for jitteriness is directed at correction of the underlying disturbance. As with lethargy, jitteriness should be considered a significant neurologic symptom and an indication for immediate correction of any underlying metabolic abnormality. There are no outcome studies assessing long-term developmental outcome of IDM who were jittery in the newborn period.

Seizures

Diagnosis

IDM are at increased risk for seizures in the neonatal period because of the higher prevalence of hypoglycemia, hypocalcemia, hypomagnesemia, polycythemia, and perinatal asphyxia in that population. Neonatal seizures must be clinically and electrically distinguished from jitteriness. Seizures in the newborn infant can be overt (with either localized or generalized tonic-clonic motor activity) or subtle, with symptoms such as apnea, facial twitching, and rhythmic mouth movements. The diagnosis requires a high index of suspicion in the context of an infant with metabolic or hematologic abnormalities.

Treatment

Treatment always includes correction of any underlying metabolic or hematologic abnormality before initiation of anticonvulsants. As with lethargy and jitteriness, seizures should be considered a significant neurologic symptom when deciding whether to treat hypoglycemia, hypocalcemia, hypomagnesemia, or polycythemia. Frequently, treatment of the underlying disorder will terminate the seizure without recurrence. The physician may choose to observe the child off anticonvulsants at that point. Consultation with a pediatric neurologist regarding anticonvulsant therapy is advised in such instances.

The mainstays of first-line anticonvulsants in newborn infants are phenobarbital and phenytoin. We prefer phenobarbital because of its lower risk of acute toxicity. The initial loading dose of phenobarbital is 20 mg/kg. A second and third minibolus of 5 to 10 mg/kg often will be necessary to control the seizures and should be followed by a maintenance dose of 5 mg/kg/d. Serum phenobarbital levels are generally maintained between 20 and 40 μg/ml. The initial loading dose of phenytoin is 20 mg/kg. It must be given very cautiously, with constant ECG monitoring. Since phenytoin is not well absorbed orally during the first year of life, it is not recommended for long-term therapy. The maintenance dose is 5 mg/kg/d in two divided doses.

The prognosis of IDM with seizures in the newborn period varies with the etiology of the seizures. Infants who experience hypoglycemic or hypocalcemic seizures carry a 50% risk of subsequent neurodevelopmental abnormality. The prognosis following seizures from hypoxic-ischemic encephalopathy is worse, with up to 80% exhibiting developmental delays.

Developmental Outcome

Diagnosis

IDM are at increased risk for both motor and cognitive delay. Increased rates of motor delay documented in older studies were most likely due to perinatal-neonatal events, such as birth asphyxia. More recently, studies have demonstrated that infants of less well controlled diabetic mothers who had late or no prenatal care do less well on cognitive testing. The relationship of cognitive developmental outcome to maternal glycemic control suggests that consequences of fetal hyperglycemia and hyperinsulinemia (including chronic intrauterine hypoxia, hypoglycemia, and brain iron deficiency) may play a major role. Nevertheless, little work has been done to elucidate the etiology of cognitive differences in IDM despite a body of literature supporting the concept of neurodevelopmental risk in these infants.

Treatment

The physician needs to institute prompt treatment of underlying metabolic and hematologic abnormalities that can cause brain injury and result in long-term developmental sequelae. We recommend that a developmental assessment, such as the Bayley Scales of Infant Development, be performed at 1 year of age in all IDM who had prenatal or perinatal risk factors or are failing to track developmentally.

INTESTINAL ABNORMALITIES

Small Left Colon Syndrome

Diagnosis

Although neonatal small left colon syndrome is rare and may be asymptomatic, it has become almost synonymous with diabetes in pregnancy. The syndrome is defined by a uniformly small diameter of the descending and sigmoid colon and rectum. Unlike other congenital anomalies in IDM that occur early in gestation (Fig. 1), this anomaly most likely occurs during the second half of gestation, well after organogenesis is complete.

The etiology of small left colon syndrome is unclear, although investigators have proposed that hyperglucagonemia, in response to reactive fetal hypoglycemia, causes intestinal hypomotility and lack of induction of proper intestinal maturation and growth. Interestingly, a far greater number of IDM clinically demonstrate feeding intolerance due to intestinal hypomotility than are diagnosed with small left colon syndrome. It is possible that intestinal hypomotility and small left colon syndrome are two ends of a clinical spectrum with a common etiology.

The infants with small left colon syndrome generally present with signs of intestinal obstruction, including feeding intolerance, vomiting, and abdominal distention. The signs and symptoms may mimic meconium plug syndrome. Intestinal perforations have been reported.

Treatment

Management of small left colon syndrome includes having a high index of suspicion in the presence of an IDM with intestinal symptoms, and it is confirmed by water-soluble contrast enema. If identified early, abdominal distention can be minimized, and conservative expectant management can be pursued. This includes very slow advancement of hypocaloric feeds until the symptoms resolve and full feedings can be tolerated. Persistence of symptoms beyond 2 weeks warrants a more complete workup for Hirschsprung's disease.

GROWTH ABNORMALITIES

Macrosomia

Diagnosis

Infants born to diabetic mothers are at increased risk for abnormal fetal growth because of the intrauterine metabolic environment. Classically, IDM are thought of as being large for gestational age, as defined by a weight greater than the 95th percentile for their gestational age. Up to 60% of IDM have been reported to be macrosomic, although the prevalence is closer to 20%. In the modern era of obstetric diagnosis and therapeutics, the prevalence of macrosomia is decreasing and may soon approach that of nondiabetic populations.

Macrosomia is found predominantly in infants born to mothers with relatively early stages of diabetes (gestational diabetes and White class A–C). Macrosomia is directly related to maternal glycemic control, particularly during the second half of gestation. The fetus's increased size is due to the combination of increased levels of metabolic fuel (glucose) and a major fetal anabolic hormone (insulin) and predominantly reflects increased storage of fat, with only a modest (12%) increase in protein stores. Certain organs, such as liver, spleen, heart, and lung, are more affected than others, such as brain.

The macrosomic IDM is at greater risk for birth injury because of cephalopelvic disproportion. These injuries include perinatal asphyxia, subdural hemorrhage, brachial plexus injury, diaphragmatic paralysis, recurrent laryngeal nerve paralysis, and clavicular fracture. Proper evaluation before delivery includes knowledge of the status of maternal glycemic control and results of fetal ultrasonographic studies and biophysical profile assessments.

Evaluation of the newborn infant includes plotting the infant's weight, length, and head circumference on appropriate growth curves. Birth weights >95th percentile should be considered abnormal. Body proportion measurements, such as the ponderal index and the mid-arm circumference/head circumference ratio, have a better predictive accuracy for identifying infants at risk for metabolic abnormalities and can be used to target infants who should be watched more carefully in the newborn period for other sequelae of maternal diabetes, including hypoglycemia, hypocalcemia, and polycythemia. On physical examination, these infants appear to be disproportionately heavy for their length and head circumference. They have obviously increased fat stores.

Treatment

No treatment is indicated for the macrosomia per se. There is no convincing evidence that large for dates infants grow up to be fat children and adults. By and large, most appear to return to a genetically programmed growth curve well within the standards for the population. Treatment of birth injuries related to delivery of the macrosomic infant is discussed in the section on Neurologic Abnormalities.

Intrauterine Growth Retardation

Diagnosis

Not all infants born to diabetic mothers are at risk for macrosomia. A subgroup of infants, generally born to mothers with advanced diabetes (White class ≥D), are at risk for fetal growth deceleration, defined as a birth weight <5th percentile or abnormally low body proportion indices (i.e., ponderal index or midarm circumference/head circumference ratio). Although the prevalence of growth-retarded IDM is low (<5%), this group of infants appears to be at particularly high risk for perinatal asphyxia, prolonged intrauterine hypoxia with resultant polycythemia, and neonatal hypoglycemia. The growth retardation is likely due to placental vascular insufficiency secondary to a combination of maternal diabetic vascular disease and a higher incidence of maternal hypertension. Both impair growth by reducing transplacental nutrient and oxygen delivery.

Proper evaluation before delivery includes biophysical profile assessment and ultrasonographic estimation of fetal weight. Postnatally, the infant should be plotted on standard growth curves to assess the degree of growth retardation. Weight and length values below the 5th percentile indicate significant fetal growth deceleration. Signs on physical examination, such as decreased muscle and fat mass or a wasted body habitus, indicate growth retardation. Measuring the ponderal index or midarm circumference/head circumference ratio is a better way to predict which infants will suffer the metabolic sequelae of intrauterine growth retardation. Those with abnormally low body proportion ratios should be closely monitored for hypoglycemia, hypocalcemia, and polycythemia.

Treatment

There is no specific treatment for the growth retardation per se. Intense feeding regimens (hypercaloric feedings) have not proved useful. In fact, they may be dangerous in the early neonatal period, since these infants are at increased risk for necrotizing enterocolitis on the basis of perinatal asphyxia, sludging of intestinal microcirculation with polycythemia, and intestinal hypomotility. Growth-retarded IDM should be fed carefully in the neonatal period, starting with dilute, hypocaloric formula, until it is clinically obvious that the infant is tolerating feeds. These IDM should have the same growth and neurologic risks as growth-retarded infants born to nondiabetic mothers. Growth-retarded infants with severe wasting, particularly those born prematurely, are likely to remain small for age throughout childhood. Those with microcephaly are at increased risk of neurologic morbidity.

CONGENITAL ANOMALIES

Diagnosis

Multiple congenital anomalies in IDM are defined as structural abnormalities on physical examination or radiographic study evident before the tenth postnatal day. Defined in this manner, an increased rate of congenital anomalies of the cardiovascular, intestinal, renal, skeletal, and central nervous systems has been described in IDM. Greater than 50% of the anomalies affect the central nervous and cardiovascular systems. The overall rate of anomalies is reported to range from 6.4% to 10%, nearly quadruple the rate found in the general population. As the rates of perinatal morbidity and mortality from other causes in IDM decrease, congenital anomalies are emerging as the main cause of mortality in IDM.

Anomalies of the cardiovascular system include transposition of the great vessels, ventricular septal defect, and left-sided obstructive lesions, such as hypoplastic left heart syndrome, aortic stenosis, and coarctation of the aorta. Atrial septal defects also have been reported. The common neurologic abnormalities are related to failure of the neural tube to close and include meningomyelocele, encephalocele, and anencephaly.

The skeletal system appears particularly sensitive to periconceptional glycemic status. Anomalies include the caudal regression syndrome, which is almost synonymous with IDM, spinal anomalies, and syringomyelia. Interestingly, in experimental animal models, the caudal regression syndrome can be achieved through early gestational hyperglycemia. Renal anomalies include hydronephrosis, renal agenesis, and cystic kidneys. Intestinal anomalies include atresia anywhere along the gastrointestinal tract but more commonly in the duodenum and rectum.

Congenital anomalies are thought to be related to maternal factors, especially glycemic control at the time of conception and during early gestation. The pathophysiologic relationship between major anomalies and preconceptional and periconceptional glycemic control is poorly understood. However, a number of well-done epidemiologic studies consistently demonstrated a strong association. For example, the rate of major congenital anomalies for IDM can be predicted from maternal hemoglobin A_{1c} values at 14 weeks gestation. Mothers with hemoglobin A_{1c} values <7 have the same risk of producing an infant with congenital anomalies as has mothers from a nondiabetic population (<2%). The risk rises to 5% for hemoglobin A_{1c} values between 7 and 8.5 and increases further to 22% for hemoglobin A_{1c} values greater than 10. Infants of diabetic fathers do not have an increased risk of congenital anomalies.

Most congenital anomalies are noted either on prenatal ultrasound or on initial physical examination. Anomalies of the cardiovascular system may be obvious on the physical examination of the newborn (i.e., murmur, cyanosis), while others, such as renal anomalies, require a high index of suspicion, since they may be asymptomatic during the neonatal period. Many diabetic mothers are routinely screened with ultrasound at 28 weeks gestation. Those performing and interpreting the ultrasound study should pay particular attention to the integrity of the skeletal, central nervous, cardiac, and renal systems. They should alert the postnatal caregivers of any detected anomalies, particularly those that may affect management of the infant in the perinatal period. Likewise, it is important for the future caretaker of the IDM to be aware of the results of such prenatal tests, especially in the detection of lesions that may be clinically silent in the newborn period (i.e., hydronephrosis, cystic kidney, ventricular septal defect) but will manifest later in postnatal life.

A careful physical examination of the newborn IDM is essential. In particular, attention must be paid to the cardiovascular and genitourinary systems. On the other hand, it is not cost effective to presumptively screen all newborn IDM for congenital anomalies by ultrasound or x-ray if the newborn physical examination is normal.

Treatment

Treatment and outcome of congenital anomalies are dependent on the type of anomaly.

ACKNOWLEDGMENTS

I would like to thank Theodore R. Thompson, M.D., for his suggestions on the content and presentation of this chapter, Karen Hauff, Pharm.D., for pharmaceutical advice, and Ginny Lyson for her editorial assistance. I extend a special note of thanks to John Widness, M.D., who has taught me so much about diabetes in pregnancy through our long collaboration.

REFERENCES

1. Brody SA, Schroeder P, Ueland K: Protocols for the management of diabetic pregnancies. *In* Brody SA, Ueland K (eds): Endocrine Disorders in Pregnancy. East Norwalk, CT, Appleton & Lange, 1989:383–391.
2. Hare J, White P: Gestational diabetes and the White classification. Diabetes Care 3:394–399, 1980.
3. Itani O, Tsang RC: Calcium, phosphorus and magnesium in the newborn: Pathophysiology and management. *In* Hay WW Jr: Neonatal Nutrition and Metabolism. St. Louis, Mosby, 1991:171–202.

NEONATAL HYPOGLYCEMIA

Marvin Cornblath, m.d.

A number of definitions of significant neonatal hypoglycemia have been used in the past. These include response of clinical manifestations to glucose therapy, statistical norms, theoretical norms, and neurodevelopmental outcomes usually correlated with inadequate neonatal data. None, however, is totally relevant to current nursery populations. New data show correlations between concentrations of plasma glucose and changes in neurophysiologic function (brainstem auditory evoked response [BAER] or visual evoked response [VER]) and increases in cerebral blood flow, blood volume, and glucose utilization. Measurements of glucose transporters, hormones, and receptors, as well as alternate substrates, are beginning to provide leads in redefining neonatal hypoglycemia. As in all biologic phenomena, neonates show a range of low plasma glucose concentrations at which specific responses occur. Deviations from these biologic norms represent a continuum of abnormality.

DEFINITION

Hypoglycemia is defined as a (reliable) significantly low plasma or serum glucose value for a newborn infant at a specific postnatal age. This may be present without (asymptomatic) or with (symptomatic) clinical signs and symptoms.

- Minimal hypoglycemia: Plasma glucose values between 35 and 45 mg/dl
- Moderate hypoglycemia: Plasma glucose values between 25 and 35 mg/dl
- Profound hypoglycemia: Plasma glucose values less than 20 to 25 mg/dl

Whether plasma glucose concentrations from 25 to 45 mg/dl are of any significance or consequence remains unanswered at this time. The evidence does not support the conclusion that these plasma values alone correlate with impaired neurologic or intellectual outcome.

MANAGEMENT

Clinical management (Fig. 1) is based on four principles: (1) screening infants at high risk, (2) confirming that the plasma glucose is low, (3) demonstrating that the clinical manifestations are due to the low glucose and clear promptly after adequate therapy, and (4) carefully observing and documenting all these events.

Screening

Glucose oxidase strip tests whether read by meter or by eye are too variable and unreliable to determine initiation of therapy in the asymptomatic neonate or to establish the diagnosis in the symptomatic infant. Screening is indicated at any age in all infants with the following clinical manifestations: episodes of tremors, cyanosis, seizures, apnea, limpness, irregular respirations, lethargy, difficulty in feeding, hypothermia, exaggerated Moro reflex, irritability, high-pitched cry, change in mental status, and coma. Less common signs of hypoglycemia include vomiting, tachypnea, bradycardia, and eye-rolling.

Hypoglycemia frequently can be anticipated by screening infants known to be at risk.

1. Large for gestational age (LGA): >90th percentile
2. Small for gestational age (SGA): <10th percentile or smaller of discordant twins (>25% discordant)
3. Preterm (≤36 weeks) or postterm (≥42 weeks)
4. Infants of mothers with late, little, or no prenatal care
5. Polycythemia (Hb >22 g/dl, Hct >65%)
6. Hypothermia [≤36.4° C (97.5° F) rectally]
7. Infants of insulin-dependent mothers (IDM) or gestational diabetic mothers (IGDM) or of massively obese mothers
8. Apgar scores ≤5 at 5 minutes or later
9. Significant hypoxia or perinatal distress requiring major resuscitation (Ambu bag, 100% oxygen)

It is also important to screen those infants with (1) a microphallus or anterior midline defects and direct or persistent hyperbilirubinemia, (2) exomphalos, macroglossia, and gigantism, (3) severe erythroblastosis, and (4) isolated hepatomegaly. A positive family history of neonatal hypoglycemia or an unexplained death in infancy is another important indication for screening.

Routine screening is usually done on or shortly after admission to the nursery at ½ to 2 hours of age and repeated before feedings over the first 24 hours of life. If the infant is not feeding well or is NPO for any reason, glucose can be monitored at 4 to 6, 12, 18, and 24 hours of age or whenever clinical manifestations are present. For practical purposes, screening is usually discontinued after 3 or more normoglycemic values.

If the screening value is ≤45 mg/dl, a blood sample should be obtained to confirm the low value by a reliable laboratory method. Careful handling of the blood sample is necessary to prevent glycolysis. Therefore, the specimen should be kept on ice, collected with a glycolytic inhibitor, and analyzed promptly. If the laboratory value is low, appropriate therapy is indicated.

TREATMENT

Therapy should be instituted once a diagnosis has been confirmed. The following guidelines will successfully maintain glucose levels above the 40 to 50 mg/dl range. The method used depends on the concentration of the plasma glucose, the condition of the infant, and the results of follow-up monitoring.

During the first hours after birth, the asymptomatic infant should be given a feed, put back to nurse, or given glucose water (Table 1), and another plasma glucose should be obtained after 30 to 60 minutes. If the glucose level is still low, the guidelines found in Table 1 should be followed. If the infant is symptomatic, IV glucose should be provided at a rate of 6 to 8 mg/kg/min, using the concentration of glucose that provides the total daily fluid requirement for the infant being treated.

Blood glucose values should be monitored at 1- to 2-hour intervals to be sure that normoglycemia has been achieved.

If hypoglycemia recurs or persists, the amount of parenteral glucose should be increased by no more than 2 mg/kg/min at 1- to 2-hour intervals.

Sodium chloride (1 to 2 mEq/kg/d as a 40 mEq solution) should be added after 12 hours to prevent iatrogenic hyponatremia. After 24 hours, potassium (1 to 2 mEq/kg/d as KCl or buffered potassium phosphate) should also be added to the IV fluids.

Once the glucose values are stable, glucose monitoring should be continued at 4- to 8-hour intervals until adequate feeds and normoglycemia have been present for approximately 24 hours. The rate of glucose infusion should be decreased (again by no more than 2 mg/kg/min at 1- to 2-hour intervals) until the parenteral fluids are discontinued. Hypertonic glucose infusions should not be stopped abruptly, or a reactive hypoglycemia may ensue.

In infants in whom it is difficult to give parenteral glucose, glucagon (300 µg/kg *not to exceed 1 mg total*) may be given SC or IM while arranging the infant's transfer to a neonatal intensive care unit.

If the hypoglycemia persists despite glucose infusion rates of 10 to 12 mg/kg/min (or more), a plasma sample should be obtained for insulin, glucose, growth hormone, thyroid, and cortisol measurements, as well as ketone, lactate, uric acid, and alanine measurements, to rule out pathologic or recurrent causes of hypoglycemia (e.g., hyperinsulinism, hypopituitarism). In these refractory infants, prednisone 2 mg/kg/d PO or hydrocortisone 5 mg/kg/d PO or IV should be given until there is a definitive diagnosis. It is important at that

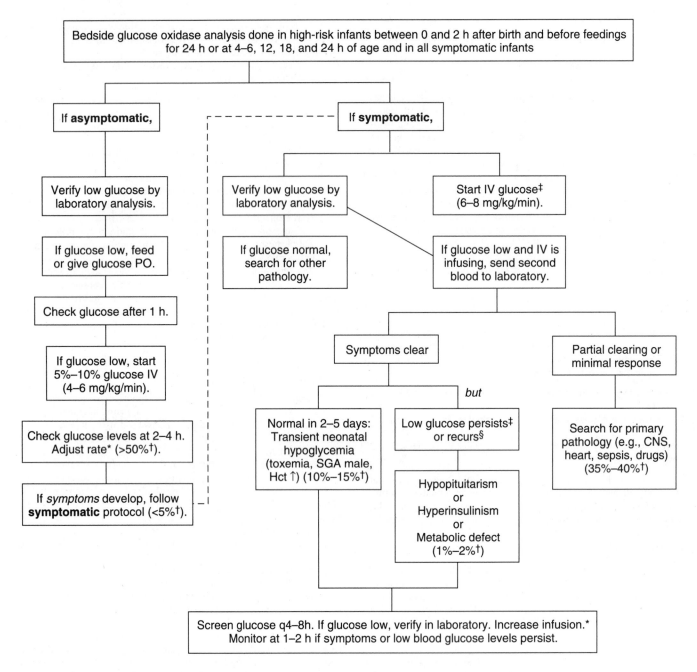

FIGURE 1. Management of neonatal hypoglycemia.

*↑↓ infusion rates by no more than 2 mg/kg/min at 1–2 h.
†Frequency among cases of neonatal hypoglycemia.
‡If glucose <25 mg/dl, give bolus of 1 ml/kg 25% dextrose or 2.5 ml/kg 10% dextrose at 1–2 ml/min.
§Give glucose at >12 mg/kg/min; get plasma levels for insulin/glucose ratio, growth hormone, steroids, etc. (see text).

time to obtain a consultation or transfer the infant to a neonatal intensive care unit for definitive diagnosis and care.

If the insulin/glucose ratio is >0.3 and the low blood glucose persists or recurs with parenteral glucose and steroids, one should consider using diazoxide 5 to 15 mg/kg/d in three divided doses until consultation or transfer occurs. If hypoglycemia alone is responsible for the abnormal signs, the clinical manifestations should subside within minutes to hours in response to adequate treatment with intravenous glucose. If the signs and symptoms persist, however, they may well be secondary to a variety of other neonatal problems. A systematic clinical and laboratory diagnostic evaluation is indicated in such cases to determine the primary disease. For these reasons, monitoring is indicated in infants with

1. Central nervous system pathology, including intrauterine or perinatal infections, congenital defects, hemorrhage, seizures, and changes in mental status
2. Hypoxia and/or asphyxia, especially with ischemia
3. Sepsis, especially bacterial, gram negative
4. Congenital heart disease, especially left heart abnormalities
5. Multiple congenital anomalies
6. Drugs taken by or given to mother
7. Adrenal hemorrhage
8. Hypothyroidism
9. Neonatal tetany
10. TORCH (toxoplasmosis, rubella, and cytomegalovirus and herpes infection) or other congenital infections

TABLE 1. Guidelines for Therapy of Neonatal Hypoglycemia

PLASMA GLUCOSE (mg/dl)	ASYMPTOMATIC OR NO IV	SYMPTOMATIC OR ON IV
35–45	Nurse, give formula feed, or oral glucose, 10 ml/kg 5% dextrose water by nipple or gavage	Start IV glucose, increase rate or concentration of glucose to 4–6 mg/kg/min
25–34	Start IV glucose 6–8 mg/kg/min as 5%, 10%, or 15% glucose in water depending on fluid needs and clinical condition	Increase to 6–8 mg/kg/min
<25	Minibolus of 0.25 g/kg as 2.5 ml/kg of 10% or 1 ml/kg of 25% glucose at rate of 1–2 ml/min; continue IV glucose at rate of 6–8 mg/kg/min	

Although support of the low plasma glucose level is indicated, the primary disease often is responsible for the morbidity or mortality in these infants.

Hypoglycemia requiring therapy may also occur after an exchange transfusion, postoperatively, with malposition of an umbilical artery catheter, and most commonly, following the abrupt cessation of hypertonic parenteral glucose (by infiltration or by choice).

PROGNOSIS

The prognosis for infants with hypoglycemia either alone or in combination with other perinatal problems remains to be established. Hypoglycemia of short duration (<12 to 18 hours), even if symptomatic, does not appear to have any proven or well-documented long-term sequelae. Thus, although not a medical emergency, the diagnosis and treatment of neonatal hypoglycemia should be carried out expediently.

If the hypoglycemia is profound, persistent, or recurrent, there may be long-term consequences. More often than not, however, the hypoglycemia is associated with or secondary to a multiplicity of problems ranging from CNS congenital anomalies to intrauterine infections. In these infants, the outcome is more likely to be related to the primary disease than the secondary hypoglycemia.

CONCLUSIONS

It is necessary to document in the chart every glucose value, the time, source, and method of analysis, and all clinical manifestations thought to be related to the hypoglycemia. Finally (*most important and most often neglected*), it is important to note the response of the clinical manifestations, as well as that of the plasma glucose value, to the therapy initiated. This is critical in establishing a diagnosis and measuring the effectiveness of therapy.

NEONATAL HYPERBILIRUBINEMIA AND KERNICTERUS

M. Jeffrey Maisels, m.b., b.ch.

Although jaundice in the newborn is a very common event, it creates considerable anxiety because bilirubin toxicity, although rare, may have devastating consequences. Our approach to the treatment of hyperbilirubinemia has evolved from the observed association between high bilirubin levels and kernicterus in infants with erythroblastosis fetalis. Newborns who develop kernicterus or acute bilirubin encephalopathy initially become lethargic and hypotonic and feed poorly. Subsequently, they develop opisthotonus and, if they survive, develop an athetoid form of cerebral palsy, sensorineural hearing loss,

gaze palsies, and dental dysplasia. Contrary to popular belief, classic kernicterus has occurred in otherwise healthy, breastfed, full-term infants with very severe hyperbilirubinemia (usually >35 mg/dl). The majority of studies, however, suggest that moderate elevations of serum bilirubin in otherwise healthy infants are not associated with a significant increase in serious neurologic abnormalities or low IQ scores.

FULL-TERM INFANTS

Full-term healthy newborns present a unique problem. In the past, most babies were bottle fed and remained in the nursery for several days. Bilirubin levels were lower and peaked while the baby was in the hospital, making the recognition and follow-up of jaundice a relatively simple matter. Today, neonatal jaundice is an outpatient problem. Full-term newborns are discharged from hospital at age 36 hours (and many earlier), and more than half of these babies are breastfed. As the peak bilirubin level in breastfed infants does not occur until age 3 to 5 days, previous guidelines for the management of jaundiced babies in hospital are now largely irrelevant.

Certain basic principles underlie the recommendations given in Table 1. First, the risks of toxicity from moderate levels of hyperbilirubinemia in full-term healthy infants are very small. Second, treatment in this population is not free of risk. Hyperbilirubinemia and phototherapy often lead to interruption or cessation of breastfeeding. Hospitalization is prolonged, or readmission is required. The negative effects of intervention on maternal behavior and the potential harmful effects on infants have been documented and suggest that we should be cautious about treating many thousands of babies in this manner when the benefits of the treatment may not outweigh the risks.

Table 1 provides guidelines for the management of hyperbilirubinemia in the healthy term newborn. Full-term refers to infants born at 37 or more weeks of gestation. The bilirubin levels refer to the total serum bilirubin. Direct bilirubin, if measured, is not subtracted from the total. These guidelines apply only to full-term healthy new-

TABLE 1. Management of Hyperbilirubinemia in the Healthy Term Newborn*†

AGE (h)				
≤24	Term infants who are clinically jaundiced at ≤24 h are not considered healthy and require further evaluation			
	Total Serum Bilirubin mg/dl (μmol/L)‡			
	Consider Phototherapy§	*Phototherapy*	*Exchange Transfusion if Intensive Phototherapy Fails‖*	*Exchange Transfusion*
25–48	≥12 (205)	≥15 (255)	≥20 (340)	≥25 (430)
49–72	≥15 (255)	≥18 (310)	≥25 (430)	≥30 (515)
>72	≥17 (290)	≥20 (340)	≥25 (430)	≥30 (515)

*Term refers to infants born at 37 or more weeks gestation.

†These guidelines apply only to healthy infants who are >24 h old and who do not have obvious hemolytic disease due to Rh or ABO incompatibility or glucose-6-phosphate dehydrogenase deficiency. It may be difficult to rule out ABO hemolytic disease as well as other, rarer causes of hemolysis. Diagnosis of glucose-6-phosphate dehydrogenase deficiency requires an awareness of genetic background and should be considered particularly in families from Greece, Turkey, Sardinia, China, and Nigeria and in Sephardic Jews from Kurdistan, Iraq, Iran, Syria, Turkey, and Buchara.

‡1 mg/dl ~ 17.1 μmol/L

§Phototherapy at these bilirubin levels is a clinical option, meaning that the intervention is available and may be used on the basis of individual clinical judgment.

‖Intensive phototherapy (see text) should produce a decline of serum bilirubin of 1–2 mg/dl within 4–6 h, and the bilirubin level should continue to fall and remain below the threshold for exchange transfusion. If this does not occur, it is considered a failure of phototherapy.

Modified from American Academy of Pediatrics, Provisional Committee on Quality Improvement: Management of hyperbilirubinemia in the healthy term newborn, Pediatrics 94:558–565, 1994. Reproduced by permission from *Pediatrics*.

TABLE 2. Use of Phototherapy in Full-Term Infants with ABO Hemolytic Disease

AGE (h)	TOTAL SERUM BILIRUBIN LEVEL	
	mg/dl	µmol/L
<12	10	170
12–17	12	205
18–23	14	240
≥24	15	255

From Osborn LM, Lenarsky C, Oakes RC, et al: Phototherapy in full-term infants with hemolytic disease secondary to ABO incompatibility. Pediatrics 74:371, 1984. Reproduced by permission of *Pediatrics,* Copyright 1984.

borns. Such conditions as sepsis, hemolytic disease, low serum albumin, and severe, persistent metabolic or respiratory acidosis appear to increase the risk of bilirubin toxicity. Depending on the infant's age and clinical condition and the presence of one or more of these risk factors, phototherapy or exchange transfusion may be indicated earlier or at bilirubin levels 3 to 7 mg/dl lower than those shown in Table 1.

Guidelines for the use of phototherapy in full-term infants with ABO hemolytic disease are given in Table 2.

JAUNDICE ASSOCIATED WITH BREASTFEEDING

Breastfed infants are three times more likely to have a serum bilirubin level >12 mg/dl during the first few days of life than are formula-fed infants. Early and frequent nursing (at least 8 times a day) may decrease bilirubin levels. Feeds should not be supplemented with water. In controlled trials, breastfed infants who received water or dextrose water supplements had higher serum bilirubin levels than unsupplemented infants.

If intervention becomes necessary in a breastfed infant, several options are available (Table 3). Although the maximal decline in bilirubin levels can be achieved by both discontinuing breastfeeding and administering phototherapy, *the vast majority of infants can continue to nurse while they receive phototherapy.* Newer fiberoptic devices make home phototherapy a reasonable option in many infants and make it much easier for the mother to continue nursing. When circumstances permit, parents should be given this information and the option of making an informed decision about which intervention they prefer. Mothers should be encouraged not to interrupt nursing if at all possible, and the option of doing nothing or providing phototherapy while nursing is continued should be offered.

LOW BIRTH WEIGHT INFANTS

Premature infants are generally believed to be at greater risk for developing bilirubin encephalopathy than are full-term infants exposed to similar bilirubin levels. Thus, low birth weight (LBW) infants are treated more aggressively than are full-term infants. Because phototherapy is a noninvasive and an essentially safe intervention, it is reasonable to use it rather liberally to treat jaundice in LBW infants. These infants stay in the nursery for weeks and often are very sick. Compared with the other interventions we inflict on neonates in our neonatal intensive care units, phototherapy is one of the more benign and, if used appropriately, will virtually abolish the necessity for exchange transfusion. Suggested guidelines for the use of phototherapy and exchange transfusion in LBW infants are given in Table 4.

PHOTOTHERAPY

Phototherapy is the most widely used method of treating hyperbilirubinemia. It effectively lowers the serum bilirubin concentration and reduces the need for exchange transfusion. As with any therapy, it is important that phototherapy be used in a therapeutic dose. This is particularly important when bilirubin levels approach the range at

which exchange transfusion might be indicated. When indicated, maximal efficacy can be achieved by one or more of the following maneuvers.

1. Use "special blue" fluorescent tubes in fluorescent phototherapy units. These narrow spectrum tubes carry the designation F20 T12/BB (not F20 T12/B, which are the standard blue tubes) and provide significantly more energy output in the blue spectrum than standard fluorescent tubes.
2. Place full-term babies naked (except for a diaper) in a basinette (not an incubator) and lower the fluorescent lamps as far as possible (to within 15 to 20 cm of the infant). This will increase the dose of phototherapy significantly. If warming of the infant occurs, the lamps can be elevated slightly, but this is generally not necessary. *Note that there are no data to indicate how close to the baby one can bring a halogen phototherapy lamp without incurring the risk of a burn. When halogen lamps are used, manufacturers' recommendations should be followed.*
3. Increase the surface area of the infant exposed to the light by placing the infant on a fiberoptic phototherapy blanket while using a standard phototherapy system. When necessary, diapers should be removed to increase the exposed surface area. Note that with light sources currently in use, it is not possible to provide an overdose of phototherapy. Fiberoptic devices have been an important addition to phototherapy. They allow better parent contact, do not require eyepatching, and permit easy administration of double phototherapy when necessary.

Although not clearly documented in clinical trials, continuous phototherapy should be more efficient than intermittent phototherapy. Continuous phototherapy should be used in infants who are admitted with very high bilirubin levels until a satisfactory decline has been achieved. On the other hand, for modest elevations of bilirubin, it is perfectly acceptable to interrupt phototherapy during feeding or for parental visits.

In most cases, it is not necessary to provide additional fluid to infants receiving phototherapy. Some full-term infants who are admitted with high bilirubin levels are also mildly dehydrated and should be supplemented with additional fluid (preferably a milk-based formula). Excess fluid does not affect the serum bilirubin concentration, but because the photo products of phototherapy are excreted both in urine and in bile, the efficacy of phototherapy can be improved by maintaining good urine output.

EXCHANGE TRANSFUSION

The technique for performing exchange transfusion is described in standard neonatal texts and is beyond the scope of this section.

PHARMACOLOGIC TREATMENT

Pharmacologic agents have been used to accelerate the normal metabolic pathways for bilirubin clearance (e.g., phenobarbital), inhibit the enterohepatic circulation of bilirubin (agar), and inhibit the production of bilirubin (synthetic metalloporphyrins). Recent research

TABLE 3. Approaches to Prevention and Treatment of Jaundice Associated with Breastfeeding

Prevention
1. Encourage frequent nursing (i.e., at least 8 to 10 times per day)
2. Do not supplement with water or dextrose water

Treatment Options
1. Observe, continue nursing
2. Temporarily discontinue nursing, substitute formula
3. Alternate feedings of breast milk and formula
4. Supplement breastfeedings with formula
5. Use phototherapy together with any of the above

TABLE 4. Approaches to Use of Phototherapy and Exchange Transfusion in Low Birth Weight Infants*

| BIRTH WEIGHT (g) | TOTAL SERUM BILIRUBIN IN mg/dl (μmol/L)† | |
	PHOTOTHERAPY‡	EXCHANGE TRANSFUSION§
<1500	5–8 (85–140)	13–16 (220–275)
1500–1999	8–12 (140–200)	16–18 (275–300)
2000–2499	11–14 (190–240)	18–20 (300–340)

*Note that these guidelines reflect ranges used in neonatal intensive care units. They cannot take into account all possible situations. In some units, prophylactic phototherapy is used for all infants who weigh less than 1500 g. Higher intervention levels may be used for small for gestational age infants, based on gestational age rather than birth weight.
†Consider initiating therapy at these levels. Range allows discretion based on clinical conditions or other circumstances that may increase the risk of bilirubin toxicity (see text).
‡Used at these levels and in therapeutic doses, phototherapy should, with few exceptions, eliminate the need for exchange transfusion. There are no data, however, to indicate that phototherapy used in this way will improve developmental outcome.
§Levels for exchange transfusion assume that bilirubin continues to rise or remains at these levels in spite of intensive (i.e., double) phototherapy (see text).
From Maisels MJ: Jaundice. *In* Avery GB, Fletcher MA, MacDonald MG (eds): Neonatology: Pathophysiology and Management of the Newborn. Philadelphia, JB Lippincott Company, 1994:688.

indicates that intramuscular tin mesoporphyrin (SnMP) is effective in decreasing bilirubin production and the need for phototherapy in ABO hemolytic disease, type I Crigler-Najjar syndrome, and premature infants. This agent is not available for clinical use.

The use of high-dose intravenous immunoglobulin 1 g/kg IV over 6 to 8 h will significantly reduce the need for exchange transfusions in infants with isoimmune hemolytic disease. This therapy has been used successfully in a controlled trial of 32 infants with Rh hemolytic disease, and the risks of IVIg are certainly less than the risks of an exchange transfusion.

REFERENCES

1. American Academy of Pediatrics, Provisional Committee on Quality Improvement: Management of hyperbilirubinemia in the healthy term newborn. Pediatrics 1994 94:558–565, 1995.
2. Maisels MJ: Jaundice. *In:* Avery GB, Fletcher MA, MacDonald MG (eds): Neonatology: Pathophysiology and Management of the Newborn. Philadelphia, JB Lippincott Co, 1994:630–725.

INFANTS OF DRUG-DEPENDENT MOTHERS

LORETTA P. FINNEGAN, M.D.

The prevalence of maternal substance abuse over the last quarter century has escalated at an alarming rate. The extent of drug use during pregnancy is often underestimated, as are the effects on the fetus and neonate. This lack of awareness is related in part to our tendency to minimize the existence of socially undesirable problems, especially among those of higher socioeconomic standing. Nevertheless, the sequelae of both licit and illicit substance abuse by the mother during pregnancy must be recognized and addressed in order to provide optimal medical care of the neonate. Stereotypic biases should not interfere with the diagnosis or treatment. Drug dependence in pregnancy crosses all socioeconomic and racial barriers. Therefore, the clinician should not rule out drug exposure in any neonate who is exhibiting symptoms at birth related to withdrawal or other known associated conditions.

Because of the extremely high-risk environment from which she comes, the pregnant drug-dependent woman predisposes her infant to a host of neonatal problems. In heroin-dependent women, a significant

part of the medical complications seen in their neonates is due to low birth weight and prematurity. Therefore, such conditions as asphyxia neonatorum, intracranial hemorrhage, hyaline membrane disease, intrauterine growth retardation, hypoglycemia, hypocalcemia, septicemia, and hyperbilirubinemia may be commonly seen. Because infants born to women who receive methadone maintenance are more apt to have higher birth weights and a decreased incidence of premature birth, medical complications generally reflect (1) the amount of prenatal care the mother has received, (2) whether she has suffered any particular obstetric or medical complications, including toxemia of pregnancy, hypertension, or infection, and (3) most importantly, multiple-drug use that may produce an unstable intrauterine milieu complicated by withdrawal and overdose. This last situation is extremely hazardous, since it may predispose to fetal distress, meconium staining, and subsequent aspiration pneumonia.

Neonatal opiate or CNS depressant abstinence syndrome is described as a generalized disorder characterized by signs and symptoms of hyperirritability, gastrointestinal dysfunction, respiratory distress, and vague autonomic symptoms, including yawning, sneezing, mottling, and fever. These infants generally develop tremors, which are initially mild and occur only when they are disturbed but which progress to the point where they occur spontaneously without any stimulation of the infant. A high-pitched cry, increased muscle tone, and irritability develop. The infants tend to have increased deep tendon reflexes and an exaggerated Moro reflex. The rooting reflex is increased, and the infants are frequently seen sucking their fists or thumbs, yet when feedings are administered, they have extreme difficulty and regurgitate frequently because of uncoordinated and ineffectual sucking reflexes. Opiate-addicted infants may develop loose stools and, therefore, are susceptible to dehydration and electrolyte imbalance.

At birth, most infants whether born to heroin-dependent or methadone-dependent mothers, appear physically and behaviorally normal. The time of onset of withdrawal signs ranges from shortly after birth to 2 weeks of age, but for most, signs appear within 72 hours. The type of drug used by the mother, the dose, the timing of the last dose before delivery, the character of the labor, and the maturity, nutrition, and presence of intrinsic disease in that infant may play a role in determining the time of onset and severity. Therefore, a variety of clinical courses may be delineated. The withdrawal syndrome may be mild and transient, be delayed in onset, have a stepwise increase in severity, present intermittently, or have a biphasic course that includes acute neonatal withdrawal signs followed by improvement and then the onset of a subacute withdrawal reaction.

Drug-exposed infants and their mothers experience a difficult early period during which both are less available for, less likely to initiate, and less responsive to social involvement than are comparison dyads. Although better adjusted at 4 months of age, the life stress and infant behavior findings indicate the importance for maternal addiction treatment programs to facilitate positive mother-infant interaction.

It is clear from numerous studies that despite the maternal choice of drug, the neonatal abstinence syndrome may persist in some infants for weeks and in others for months. Various investigators have found these infants to have hyperphagia, increased oral drive, sweating, hyperacusis, irregular sleep patterns, poor tolerance to holding or to abrupt changes of position, and loose stools. Therefore, the clinician not only must assess these infants in the neonatal period but also must realize that long-term follow-up will be essential.

ASSESSMENT OF NEONATAL ABSTINENCE

We have developed a Neonatal Abstinence Score that can be used to monitor the passively depressant-exposed neonate in a comprehensive and objective way. It is essential for assessing the onset, progression, and diminution of symptoms of abstinence. The score is used to monitor the infant's clinical response to and need for pharmacotherapeutic intervention and to achieve safe medical withdrawal from the in utero drug exposure.

The abstinence score lists 21 symptoms most commonly seen in the exposed neonate. Signs are recorded as single entities or in several categories if they occur in varying degrees of severity. Each symptom and its associated degree of severity have been assigned a score. Higher scores are assigned to symptoms found in infants with more severe abstinence who are at increased risk for morbidity and mortality. The total abstinence score is determined by adding the score assigned to each symptom observed throughout the entire scoring interval. The scoring system is dynamic rather than static; that is, all of the signs and symptoms observed during the 4-hour intervals at which infant symptoms are monitored are point-totaled for that interval. Infants are assessed 2 hours after birth and then every 4 hours. If at any point the infant's score is 8 or higher, scoring is done every 2 hours and continued for 24 hours from the last score of 8 or higher. If the 2-hour scores continue to be 7 or less for 24 hours, 4-hour scoring intervals may be resumed.

If pharmacotherapy is not needed, the infant is scored for the first 4 days of life at the prescribed 4-hour intervals. However, if pharmacologic intervention is required, the infant is scored at 2- or 4-hour intervals depending on whether the abstinence score is less than or greater than 8 throughout the duration of the therapy. Once therapy is discontinued, if there is no resurgence in the total score to 8 or higher after 3 days, scoring may be discontinued. If there is a resurgence of symptoms with scores consistently equaling 8 or higher, scoring should be continued for a minimum of 4 days following discontinuation of therapy to ensure that the infant is not discharged prematurely, with the consequent resurgence of abstinence at home.

The Neonatal Abstinence Score Sheet is shown in Figure 1. Symptoms are listed on the left, with their respective scores listed to the right. The time of each evaluation is given at the top, and the total score is shown for each evaluation. A new sheet should be started at the beginning of each day. The complete scoring system allows scoring as frequently as every 2 hours for a full 24-hour period on each sheet.

A *Comments* column is provided so that the nursing and medical staff can record important notes regarding the infant's scoring and treatment and can make reference to relevant progress notes recorded in the infant's chart. Some important points to remember when using the score sheet are

1. The first abstinence score should be recorded approximately 2 hours after the infant is admitted to the nursery. This score reflects all infant behavior from admission to that first point when the scoring interval is complete (this is the first time indicated on the score sheet). The times designating the end of the scoring intervals (whether every 2 or every 4 hours) have been left blank to permit the nursing staff to choose the most appropriate times for the scoring intervals in relation to effective planning and implementation of nursing care.
2. All infants should be scored at 4-hour intervals except when high scores indicate more frequent scoring.
3. All symptoms exhibited during the entire scoring interval, not just at a single point, should be included.
4. The infant should be awakened to elicit reflexes and specified behavior, but if the infant is awakened for the purpose of scoring, one should not score for diminished sleep after feeding. Sleeping should never be recorded for a scoring interval except under extreme circumstances when the infant has been unable to sleep for an extended period of time (i.e., 12 to 18 hours). If the infant is crying, he or she must be quieted before assessment of muscle tone, respiratory rate, and the Moro reflex.
5. Respirations are counted for 1 full minute.
6. The infant is scored if prolonged crying is exhibited, even though it may not be high pitched.
7. Temperatures should be taken rectally (mild pyrexia is an early sign indicating heat produced by increased muscle tone and tremors).
8. If the infant is sweating solely because of conservative nursing measures (e.g., swaddling), a point should not be given.

Before pharmacotherapy is initiated, other common neonatal metabolic alterations that can mimic or compound abstinence must be ruled out (e.g., hypocalcemia, hypomagnesemia, hypoglycemia, and hypothermia). Toxicologic examination of the urine immediately after birth is necessary to ensure an appropriate choice of pharmacotherapy. Urine collected after 24 or 36 hours of life is likely to be negative for qualitative toxicologic assessment. Maternal urine toxicology may be necessary if the infant's quantity is inadequate or initially discarded. Better information regarding in utero exposure can be obtained through meconium testing, although a lack of availability and costs may inhibit this technology in some centers.

The total scores have been categorized into ranges of scores indicating the severity of abstinence in relation to functional disturbances in various physiologic systems. The total abstinence scores dictate the specific dose of the pharmacotherapeutic agents used to medically withdraw infants. In the score-dose titration approach, the initial dose of a specific pharmacotherapeutic agent (i.e., paregoric or phenobarbital) and all subsequent doses are determined by and titrated against the total abstinence score. When phenobarbital is used, an initial dose of 20 mg/kg is administered in an attempt to achieve an expected therapeutic serum level with a single dose.

The need for pharmacologic intervention is indicated when the total abstinence score is 8 or higher for three consecutive scorings (e.g., 9–8–10) or when the average of any three consecutive scores is 8 or higher (e.g., 9–7–9). Once an infant's score is 8 or higher, the scoring interval automatically becomes 2 hours, so that the infant's symptoms are controlled within 4 to 6 hours. If the infant's total score is 12 or higher for two consecutive intervals or the average of any two consecutive scores is 12 or higher, therapy should be adjusted according to the schedule shown in Table 1.

In summary, it is important to remember that all infants who meet the scoring criteria for pharmacologic intervention should have the prescribed medication regimen started no later than 4 to 6 hours after loss of control. The more severe the abstinence, as reflected by the total score, the greater the need to initiate pharmacotherapy as soon as possible. Finally, the longer the delay in initiation of appropriate pharmacologic intervention, the greater the risk of increased infant morbidity.

GENERAL MEASURES IN TREATING NEONATAL ABSTINENCE

While the infant is being assessed with the Neonatal Abstinence Score for potential initiation of pharmacotherapy, general treatment measures should be considered. Overall comfort should be maintained by swaddling, use of a pacifier for excessive sucking, nasal aspiration when necessary, frequent diaper changes (exposure of hyperemic buttocks in severe cases for air drying), use of soft sheets or sheepskin to decrease excoriations, and positioning to reduce aspiration if vomiting is a problem. Consideration of weight change patterns is also a key issue and demand or reduced feeding is frequently recommended. Waterbeds have been found to be a useful adjunct to supportive care of narcotic-exposed neonates.

RECOMMENDED PHARMACOLOGIC AGENTS FOR NEONATAL DEPRESSANT ABSTINENCE

Many pharmacologic agents have been used in the treatment of neonatal abstinence, and some appear to be effective in relieving symptoms. The most effective have been paregoric (camphorated tincture of opium) and phenobarbital in treating and controlling symptoms of depressant abstinence. The advantages of paregoric use are (1) it can be administered orally, (2) it has no known adverse effects, and (3) there is a wide margin of error because of the low dose of opiate and a short half-life. Paregoric can also provide a level of sedation that inhibits bowel motility, thereby diminishing the loose stools frequently accompanying abstinence. Among paregoric-treated infants, nutritive sucking has been found to be much closer to normal than among those treated with phenobarbital. However, in comparison

Date: _____   Daily Weight: _____

System	Signs and Symptoms	Score	AM	PM	Comments
	Excessive High Pitched (other) Cry	2			
	Continuous High Pitched (other) Cry	3			
	Sleeps <1 hour after feeding	3			
	Sleeps <2 hours after feeding	2			
	Sleeps <3 hours after feeding	1			
	Hyperactive Moro reflex	2			
	Markedly Hyperactive Moro reflex	3			
	Mild Tremors Disturbed	1			
	Moderate-Severe Tremors Disturbed	2			
	Mild Tremors Undisturbed	3			
	Moderate-Severe Tremors Undisturbed	4			
	Increased Muscle Tone	2			
	Excoriation (specific areas)	1			
	Myoclonic Jerks	3			
	Generalized Convulsions	5			
	Sweating	1			
	Fever <101 (99-100.8F/37.2-38.2C)	1			
	Fever >101 (38.4C and higher)	2			
	Frequent Yawning (>3-4 times/ interval)	1			
	Mottling	1			
	Nasal Stuffiness	1			
	Sneezing (>3-4 times/ interval)	1			
	Nasal Flaring	2			
	Respiratory Rate >60/min.	1			
	Respiratory Rate >60/min. with retractions	2			
	Excessive Sucking	1			
	Poor Feeding	2			
	Regurgitation	2			
	Projectile Vomiting	3			
	Loose Stools	2			
	Watery Stools	3			

TOTAL SCORE _____

INITIALS OF SCORER _____

FIGURE 1. Neonatal Abstinence Score Sheet. Evaluator should place a check next to each sign or symptom observed at various time intervals, then add scores for total score. (From Finnegan LP: Neonatal abstinence syndrome: Assessment and pharmacology. *In* Rubatelli FF, Granati B, (eds): Neonatal Therapy: An Update. New York, Excerpta Medica, 1986.)

with other drugs, a paregoric regimen has the disadvantage of requiring larger doses and a longer duration of therapy.

Phenobarbital is especially effective in controlling two of the more commonly occurring symptoms of abstinence, irritability and insomnia, through a nonspecific CNS depression. The disadvantages of phenobarbital include considerable depression of sucking and less effectiveness in alleviating seizures secondary to narcotic abstinence.

Furthermore, loose stools are not prevented, and control of symptoms may not be fully accomplished, even at doses that produce plasma levels considered to be in the toxic range.

In our clinical research studies, we have investigated the effectiveness of paregoric and phenobarbital in the treatment of the neonatal abstinence syndrome. In assessing the number of days to control abstinence symptoms and the total length of treatment, paregoric was

TABLE 1. Titration Dosage Schedule According to Abstinence Scores

ABSTINENCE SCORE	PAREGORIC DOSE (ml/kg/d q4h)	PHENOBARBITAL DOSE (mg/kg/d q8h)
8–10	0.8	6
11–13	1.2	8
14–16	1.6	10
17 or above	2	12
	(continue at 0.4-ml increments until control is achieved)	

most successful when the infant was exposed to opiates only. When the infant was exposed to nonopiates, phenobarbital was most successful. There appeared to be no significant difference between phenobarbital and paregoric when the infants were exposed to both opiates and nonopiates.

PHARMACOTHERAPEUTIC REGIMENS

Score-Dose Titration Approach with Paregoric

Once the criteria are met to initiate pharmacotherapy (indicated by the total abstinence scores), the total scores dictate the dose of medication as prescribed in Table 1. Because steady-state levels of paregoric are not achieved, serum concentrations are not helpful in managing the infant.

Dose adjustments and timing of dose changes must be carefully monitored. An increase in dose is necessary at any time after the initiation of therapy when there have been three consecutive total scores of 8 or higher or an average of any three consecutive total scores of 8 or higher. When the change in dose is indicated, the time intervals for administration of the next dose should remain the same as the prescribed dosing schedule. For example, if the total withdrawal score indicates that an increase in dose is needed, the adjusted dose should be given on schedule (i.e., 4 hours after the previous dose) until the total abstinence scores consistently fall below 8.

Substantial changes in the infant's weight indicate a need to recalculate the base dose. This will necessitate weight-related dose adjustments during any phase of pharmacologic intervention (i.e., dose increases, maintenance doses, and dose reductions).

Once abstinence is controlled using the prescribed dose schedule, the following procedures should be implemented to maintain control for 72 hours, followed by lowering of the medication dose. The dose administered to achieve control should be maintained for 72 hours before a dose reduction schedule is initiated. When symptoms are controlled, the total daily dose is decreased by 10% every 24 hours. When dose levels reach 0.5 ml/kg/d, paregoric may be discontinued. If an infant's abstinence scores remain low (1 to 3) for a minimum of 72 hours after lowering the dose (usually a rare event), the rate at which the dose is tapered may be increased (with caution) to 15% to 20% (maximum).

If phenobarbital is used, the dose administered to achieve the phenobarbital serum level necessary to control abstinence should be noted. Serum levels of phenobarbital should be determined using micromethod blood samples every 24 hours throughout the treatment phase and until the serum concentration reaches a homeopathic level during administration. Phenobarbital (20 mg/kg) is initially administered in a quantity sufficient to achieve a serum level of 18 to 22 µg/ml. When an adequate serum level is achieved and the infant is controlled, a maintenance dose of 4 to 6 mg/kg/d is administered. After 72 hours of steady-state maintenance in a clinically controlled situation (verified by constant serum level determinations and total scores of less than 8), the dose should be lowered to 2 to 3 mg/kg/d, allowing the serum levels to decline at a rate of 10% to 20% per day. If serum phenobarbital levels indicate that the dose has been tapered too rapidly, (>20% decrease in the serum level in 24 hours), the maintenance dose should be increased slightly. If total abstinence scores escalate to 8 or higher, the phenobarbital dose should be increased to achieve the serum level at which the infant was previously controlled. This level should be maintained, assuming the infant is controlled again, for 48 hours before lowering the dose again. If the dose has been tapered too slowly (<10% decrease in the serum level in 24 hours), the maintenance dose should be decreased to 1 mg/kg/d. Once the serum level falls below 10 µg/ml and the total score is less than 8, the phenobarbital should be discontinued.

If appropriately assessed and treated with adequate medication, the drug-exposed infant should be entirely normal by 1 to 6 months of age. Long-term outcome is more dependent on environmental influences and other neonatal conditions than the occurrence of neonatal abstinence syndrome.

REFERENCES

1. Finnegan LP: Neonatal abstinence syndrome: Assessment and pharmacotherapy. *In* Rubatelli FF, Granati B (eds): Neonatal Therapy: An Update. New York, Elsevier Science Publishers, 1986:122–146.
2. Finnegan LP, Ehrlich SM: Maternal drug abuse during pregnancy: Evaluation and pharmacotherapy for neonatal abstinence. Modern Methods in Pharmacology. Vol. 6: Testing and Evaluation of Drugs of Abuse. New York, Wiley-Liss, Inc., 1990:255–263.
3. Finnegan LP, Kaltenbach K: The assessment and management of neonatal abstinence syndrome. *In* Hoekelman RA, Friedman SB, Nelson NM, et al. (eds): Primary Pediatric Care, 3rd ed, St. Louis, Mosby-Yearbook, 1990:1377–1378.
4. Finnegan LP, Kandall SR. Maternal and neonatal effects of alcohol and drugs. *In* Lowinson JH, Ruiz P, Millman RB (eds), Langrod JG (assoc ed): Substance Abuse: A comprehensive textbook, 2nd ed. Baltimore, Williams & Wilkins, 1992:628–656, 1992.
5. Kaltenbach K, Finnegan LP: Neonatal abstinence: Pharmacotherapy and developmental outcome. *In* Neurobehavioral Toxicology and Teratology, Vol. 8. ANKHO International Inc., 1986.

EFFECTS OF MATERNAL ALCOHOL INGESTION ON THE DEVELOPING FETUS

DENA HOFKOSH, M.D.

Behold, thou shalt conceive and bear a son: and now drink no wine or strong drinks.—Judges 13:7

References to the dangers of alcohol consumption during pregnancy can be traced back to biblical times. However, it was not until 1973 that Jones et al. described the specific features of children born to alcoholic women and introduced the term fetal alcohol syndrome (FAS) to describe the most severe expression of prenatal alcohol exposure.[1] Numerous subsequent studies have confirmed the teratogenic effect of alcohol, isolating it from the effects of other potentially confounding variables, such as maternal malnutrition and exposure to other potentially teratogenic substances.

DESCRIPTION

Fetal alcohol syndrome is a clinical diagnosis based on a history of maternal alcohol use during pregnancy and some or all of the following features: (1) characteristic craniofacial dysmorphology, (2) growth deficiency, often of prenatal onset, and (3) evidence of central nervous system (CNS) dysfunction. The diagnosis of FAS is made with confidence when all of these characteristics are present (Table 1). The term fetal alcohol effects (FAE) has been used to describe less severe manifestations of prenatal alcohol exposure or incomplete features of FAS.

The most easily recognized craniofacial features of FAS are microcephaly, short palpebral fissures, thin upper lip, elongated and flattened midface and philtrum, short nose, and narrow bifrontal diameter. Other characteristic features, seen in 25% to 50% of children with FAS, include cardiac anomalies, eye anomalies including ptosis,

TABLE 1. Fetal Alcohol Syndrome

History of Maternal Alcohol Use

Craniofacial Dysmorphology
Microcephaly
Short palpebral fissures
Thin upper lip
Elongated and flattened midface and philtrum
Short nose
Narrow bifrontal diameter

Growth Deficiency, Usually of Prenatal Onset

Central Nervous System Dysfunction
Mental retardation
Learning problems
Short attention span
High activity level
Impulsivity
Tremulous movements
Other behavior problems

Other Anomalies
Cardiac anomalies
Eye anomalies, including ptosis, myopia, and strabismus
Pectus excavatum
Dental malocclusion (in later childhood)
Sensorineural hearing loss

myopia, and strabismus, pectus excavatum, dental malocclusion (in later childhood), and sensorineural hearing loss. Prenatal growth is often affected, and 80% of children with FAS are small for gestational age.

Mental retardation is the most severe expression of CNS dysfunction among children with FAS. The degree of mental retardation is generally mild. The mean intelligence quotient is 65. Even among children with an IQ in the normal range, learning problems, short attention span, high activity level, impulsivity, and other behavior problems are common. Children with FAS are commonly described as having impaired judgment, poor memory, and difficulty with abstract thinking, characteristics that may persist into adulthood.

Infants exposed to alcohol prenatally may demonstrate behavioral disorganization, including poor state control, irritability, and tremulousness. These behaviors may be a manifestation of acute alcohol withdrawal in infants born to women who were intoxicated shortly before delivery. However, similar behaviors are also seen among infants exposed to alcohol earlier in pregnancy, in which case, they probably represent the behavioral manifestations of alcohol's teratogenic effects on the CNS.

In later childhood, the facial dysmorphology of FAS often becomes less noticeable, but affected individuals continue to be picky eaters who are difficult to feed and grow poorly. Although there may be modest catchup in head circumference, many children with FAS remain microcephalic. Vision, hearing, and dental problems, cognitive dysfunction, and behavior problems are the major concerns for older children and adults with FAS.

EPIDEMIOLOGY

The prevalence of FAS is estimated to be 1 to 2/1000 live births worldwide. FAE may occur in as many as 3 to 5/1000 live births in an unselected population. FAS is certainly the leading preventable cause of mental retardation.

PATHOPHYSIOLOGY

Alcohol and its metabolites (acetaldehyde) are thought to affect protein synthesis, influencing both growth and morphology of brain and other tissues. The specific mechanism by which alcohol exerts its teratogenic effect is not known.

Genetic variation, both maternal and fetal, in susceptibility to the effects of alcohol influences the expression of fetal alcohol exposure. Fraternal twins discordant in the severity of FAS have been reported.

The most severe manifestation of prenatal alcohol exposure, the complete FAS, has been reported in 30% to 40% of the offspring of women who are severe alcoholics (average ingestion of more than four to five drinks or 2 to 2.5 oz of absolute alcohol per day). FAS has also been reported among the offspring of women who engage in binge drinking: intermittent ingestion of large amounts of alcohol (five to seven drinks per occasion) to the point of intoxication. Less severe teratogenic effects, such as low birthweight or neurobehavioral disorganization in the absence of craniofacial dysmorphology, may be seen at lower levels of alcohol ingestion (two drinks per day). No safe level of alcohol consumption during pregnancy has been established.

Women who use alcohol may also use other substances that may exert independent teratogenic or toxic effects. Concomitant use of tobacco, for example, may magnify the impact of alcohol exposure on fetal growth. Infants born to women identified as cocaine users may demonstrate similar neurobehavioral characteristics to those with FAS. Although the specific effects of alcohol have been isolated from the effects of maternal malnutrition on fetal development, the nutritional status of the mother may modify the expression of alcohol exposure.

INTERVENTION

Although there is no specific treatment for FAS or FAE, the recommended approach to intervention consists of (1) early identification of affected children, (2) referral for appropriate developmental, special education, and behavior management services, (3) support for both adoptive and birth families, and (4) prevention through education.

IDENTIFICATION

Discussion about drug and alcohol use during pregnancy, as well as during child rearing, should be a routine component of obstetric and pediatric care, conducted in a sensitive and nonjudgmental manner. Although FAS can be difficult to recognize in newborns because the dysmorphology is subtle, the diagnosis should be considered in the neonate with growth retardation, microcephaly, unusual facial features, or evidence of neurobehavioral disorganization, such as irritability, tremulousness, or poor state control. Furthermore, any evaluation of an infant for developmental delay should include a careful examination for the dysmorphology and growth failure characteristic of FAS. FAS should be considered in the differential diagnosis of behavior problems, short attention span, impulsivity, learning problems, and mental retardation among preschoolers and schoolaged children.

REFERRAL FOR DEVELOPMENTAL SERVICES

Parents often find the behavioral disorganization of infants with FAS/FAE challenging. Therefore, emotional support, as well as specific suggestions for positioning, handling, and feeding, may be very helpful. Behavior problems, short attention span, impulsivity, and cognitive deficits may require educational and behavioral interventions during the preschool and schoolage years. Educational services for children with FAS/FAE should be based not on the diagnosis but on the individual child's strengths and needs as determined through appropriate psychoeducational evaluation. Pediatricians should refer children and families to resources for early intervention, behavior management, parenting support, and special education in their communities.

SUPPORT FOR FAMILIES

Families of children with mental retardation, behavior problems, and other developmental disabilities often experience relief when a specific diagnosis is made, finding themselves better able to advocate for therapeutic and educational resources for their children and move ahead through their own grieving process. This scenario is particularly true for adoptive families who may have suspected or known of a history of prenatal alcohol exposure. For birth families, the grief and guilt in response to the diagnosis of FAS may be so overwhelming that the pediatrician should consider referral for mental health counseling.

Alcoholism in a parent affects children after birth in ways that may be as profoundly impairing as the teratogenic effects of prenatal alcohol exposure. Pediatricians must recognize that alcoholism occurs more often than it is identified and that it is a disease requiring specific forms of treatment. Education and support are not adequate interventions for individuals addicted to alcohol. Women may be more willing to acknowledge and seek treatment for their addiction in the context of a diagnosis of FAS in their children. Therefore, pediatricians are in a unique position to facilitate referral for treatment and must be aware of resources for treatment of alcohol and other drug addiction in their communities.

PREVENTION

Prevention is the most powerful intervention for FAS/FAE. Women should be educated about the effects of alcohol on the developing fetus and counseled that there is no safe amount of alcohol. The most conservative recommendation is to avoid alcohol use during pregnancy. Women must also understand that several weeks often pass between conception and the recognition of pregnancy, during which time alcohol can have a significant effect on the fetus. Women who are contemplating pregnancy should be advised to stop drinking before conception. Teenagers and young adults who may engage in binge drinking and unprotected sexual activity should also understand the implications of fetal alcohol exposure. Pediatricians who have an established relationship with a family, who are trusted as an advocate for children, and who can obtain and provide information in a nonjudgmental fashion are in an excellent position to discuss the sensitive issue of alcohol and other drug use with the families of children under their care.

REFERENCES

1. Jones KL, Smith DW, Ulleland CN, Streissguth AP: Pattern of malformation in offspring of chronic alcoholic mothers. Lancet 1:1267–1271, 1973.
2. Streissguth AP, Randels SP, Smith DF: A test-retest study of intelligence in patients with fetal alcohol syndrome: Implications for care. J Am Acad Child Adolesc Psychiatry 30:584–587, 1991.

NEONATAL SEIZURES

MARK S. SCHER, M.D.

Definitions in the International Classification of Epileptic Seizures do not apply to newborns. Neonates are unable to sustain generalized tonic-clonic activity (as do older children), although independently, tonic and clonic movements can occur in the same patient. Behavioral seizure manifestations in this age group tend to be brief and subtle, and in many instances, the clinical behaviors are unusual or more difficult to recognize.

Electrographic seizures in the newborn indicate a disturbance of the central nervous system (CNS), suggesting a need for prompt and appropriate treatment. Neonatal seizures, however, are not disease specific and may be caused by a variety (or a combination) of medical conditions. The proper treatment of neonatal seizures depends on etiology. A transient metabolic disturbance that causes seizures, such as hypoglycemia, hypocalcemia, or hypomagnesemia, would, therefore, require correction of these underlying metabolic derangements as the primary course of action. Since the majority of neonatal seizures occur in the context of hypoxic ischemic encephalopathy and cerebrovascular lesions, many medical conditions may contribute to the initiation of seizures.

The diagnosis of neonatal seizures is quite challenging for the clinician. Five clinical categories of neonatal seizures have been described traditionally (i.e., subtle, focal clonic, multifocal clonic, tonic, and myoclonic); however, broader classifications now include electrographic seizures without clinical accompaniments, clinical accompaniments without electrographic seizures, and electroclinical dissociation (i.e., the same clinical events occurring with and without electrographic seizures). Although video electroencephalography can document coincidental electrical and clinical events, routine paper EEG recordings generally are used to document the seizure event. More than 50% of seizures are expressed only on an electrographic basis, particularly in neurologically depressed newborns, infants with pharmacologic paralysis for ventilatory control, or those with antiepileptic drug usage. In addition, the inability of the immature brain to propagate a seizure focus contributes to the lack of clinical expression. All these situations result in the underdiagnosis of seizures unless an EEG recording is promptly obtained. Guidelines for the identification and treatment of neonatal seizures, therefore, need to be continually clarified.

TREATMENT

If the correction of a transient metabolic disturbance cannot stop seizures from occurring, alternate treatment strategies must include the use of antiepileptic medication. It is generally assumed that neonates should be aggressively managed with one or more of these drugs to minimize the physiologic and metabolic abnormalities associated with seizures. Questions persist with respect to when, how, and for how long to treat neonates who have seizures. Some practitioners believe that neonates should be treated only when clinical seizures are recognized and that brief electrographic seizures do not necessarily require intervention. Others argue that this practice may be harmful in view of experimental evidence that electrographic seizures adversely affect brain metabolism and viability. Despite this disagreement, current practice usually involves emergent treatment of neonatal seizures. There is no consensus with respect to the necessity of treatment with minimal or absent clinical seizure phenomena.

Of the antiepileptic drugs prescribed for neonatal seizures, phenobarbital and phenytoin are the most widely used. Benzodiazepines, primidone, and valproic acid are effective adjunctive agents. In neonates, the half-life of phenobarbital ranges from 45 to 173 hours. The recommended initial loading dose is 20 mg/kg, with a maintenance dose of 3 to 4 mg/kg/d. Although no consensus on therapeutic levels has been reached, serum levels between 16 and 40 µg/ml are generally accepted as therapeutic. There is no consensus with respect to the maintenance of a drug regimen if only electrical seizures persist. The preferred loading dose of phenytoin is 15 to 20 mg/kg. Serum levels of phenytoin are difficult to maintain because of the rapid redistribution of the drug to body tissues. With either phenobarbital or phenytoin, continued treatment after cessation of seizures is decided on an individual basis.

Some centers have used diazepam to treat neonates with seizures. Like phenobarbital and phenytoin, the drug has a wide range of half-lives (18 to 54 hours) in the newborn population. Because diazepam is slowly and erratically absorbed after intramuscular injection, intravenous administration is recommended. The recommended IV dose for acute management of neonatal seizures is 0.05 mg/kg, although higher loading doses (up to 1 mg/kg) may be required following the loading dose. Diazepam can be given as a continuous infusion at a maintenance dose of 1 mg/kg/h. However, because of the relatively short half-life and a propensity to be deposited in muscle, diazepam is not generally used as maintenance antiepileptic therapy. Another benzodiazepine, lorazepam has been effective for controlling refractory seizures in neonates in a dose of 0.05 mg/kg. The side effects of lorazepam are similar to the side effects of diazepam.

Primidone is a rarely used medication in neonates with refractory seizures. A loading dose of 20 mg/kg yields a therapeutic plasma level. In neonates, the introduction of primidone after phenobarbital has been administered does not necessarily impair clearance of the latter, as the ability to metabolize primidone to phenobarbital is reduced in this age group.

EFFICACY OF TREATMENT

Published studies concerning the efficacy of phenobarbital report conflicting results. With conventional (20 mg/kg) loading doses, only one third of neonates with seizures respond to phenobarbital alone. With doses as high as 40 mg/kg, 85% may achieve control. However, these results are based on studies in which the cessation of seizure activity was monitored clinically. EEG studies to verify the resolution of electrographic seizures have not been performed.

Free or unbound drug fractions have been used to assess the efficacy and potential toxicity of antiepileptic drugs in pediatric populations. Such studies have demonstrated that phenobarbital is 50% protein bound and phenytoin is 85% protein bound, although binding can be altered significantly in a sick neonate with metabolic dysfunction. Biochemical alterations may cause toxic side effects by raising the serum concentration of the drug. To guard against untoward effects, evaluation of efficacy must take into account not only the total but also the free fractions. Serial drug determinations combined with continuous EEG recordings to document seizure cessation before toxic side effects ensue should improve the titration of antiepileptic drugs.

DISCONTINUATION OF DRUG USE

The decision to maintain or discontinue antiepileptic drug therapy is fraught with uncertainty. Discontinuation of drugs before discharge from the neonatal intensive care unit should be attempted in the infant who shows no demonstrable brain lesion on cranial imaging, who demonstrates age-appropriate findings on neurologic examination, and who has a normal interictal EEG background pattern. Some authors suggest cessation of antiepileptic pharmacotherapy even in patients at high risk for seizures beyond the newborn period, since only 15% to 20% of neonates ultimately develop epilepsy. If seizures recur in the first 2 years of life, they tend to be a seizure type (e.g., infantile spasms) that does not respond to conventional antiepileptic drugs. Moreover, a honeymoon period, lasting months to years, may elapse before seizures reoccur. Parents of infants at risk for subsequent epilepsy should, therefore, be instructed in the recognition of these clinical presentations.

NEONATAL INTRACRANIAL HEMORRHAGE AND ITS SEQUELAE

Evan Y. Snyder, m.d., Ph.d.
Ann R. Stark, m.d.

Intraventricular hemorrhage (IVH) remains a substantial problem in prematurely born newborn infants. Some degree of IVH occurs in approximately 27% to 45% of infants with birth weight less than 1500 g (Table 1). A combination of anatomic and physiologic factors contributes to the etiology of IVH. Factors related to prematurity include persistence of the germinal matrix—a vascular border zone with tenuous, poorly supported vasculature and high metabolic demands. In addition, premature infants have underdeveloped cerebral vascular autoregulation and an anatomically vulnerable venous drainage system. Events of the perinatal period, such as the stress of labor and delivery, or therapeutic interventions, such as mechanical ventilation, or both are superimposed on these developmental factors.

TABLE 1. Incidence of Intraventricular Hemorrhage (IVH)

	PERCENT OF INFANTS WITH ANY IVH	PERCENT OF INFANTS WITH SEVERE IVH
Gestational age (wk)		
<34	19–25	
<26	39	18
Birth weight (g)		
<1500	27–45	6–18
<1000	30	15
<750	53–63	17–32

The routine use of cranial ultrasound examination in preterm infants to diagnose IVH has resulted in increased detection of other intracranial abnormalities. Periventricular echolucencies (PEL) and periventricular echodensities (PED) are seen in 3% to 7% and 10% to 18%, respectively, of infants with birth weight less than 1000 g. These abnormalities are believed to correlate with the neuropathologic condition known as periventricular leukomalacia (PVL). Although PVL and IVH may share some common etiologies, for example, hypoxia-ischemia, and can occur together (75% in one autopsy series), each may be found independently of the other.

Infants with birth weight less than 1500 g or gestational age <32 weeks or those >32 weeks who have risk factors for hypoxic-ischemic injury should be routinely monitored with ultrasound examination (Table 2). Ninety percent of all IVH occurs within the first 3 days of life (50% on day 1, 25% on day 2, 15% on day 3), and 20% to 40% exhibit progression.

The head ultrasound examination (HUS) remains the modality of choice for screening. Each hemorrhage is described in terms of its location, the measured size of ventricles, and the extent and location of parenchymal involvement, if present (Table 3). This system has advantages over more subjective descriptions or "grades." It facilitates decision making and follow-up for an individual infant over time and enhances communication among physicians. It provides objective, quantifiable evidence for the success or failure of interventions. It allows evaluation and comparison of studies in different institutions, providing standardization for clinical research. Furthermore, the extent of parenchymal involvement and the size of ventricles most affect prognosis.

COMPLICATIONS

The major complications of IVH are blood loss and shock, seizures, apnea, unconjugated hyperbilirubinemia, motor or cognitive handicap (or both), and posthemorrhagic hydrocephalus.

Blood loss and shock are treated with standard interventions, including intravascular volume repletion, pressor support, and red blood

TABLE 2. Timing of Cranial Ultrasound Examinations

CONDITION	TIMING OF EXAMINATION
Premature infant, gestation <32 wk or birth weight <1500 g	Routine monitoring on days 1–3, 7–10, 21–28, and at 40 wk postconceptional age
Premature infant, gestation ≥32 wk with risk factors for hypoxia-ischemic injury	Same as routine monitoring
Premature infant, gestation ≥32 wk, who is healthy	40 wk postconceptional age or before discharge home or transfer to level II nursery (at a different hospital)
IVH present	Weekly until resolved; more frequently if clinical indications such as new bleeding or signs of posthemorrhagic hydrocephalus

TABLE 3. Three-Tiered System to Describe IVH Using Ultrasonography

Intraventricular Blood
Location is identified as right, left, bilateral, or germinal matrix

Degree of Ventricular Enlargement
Direct measurements of ventricular size are made from the ultrasonogram using the sagittal or coronal axis or both

Measurements Along Sagittal Axis for Infants >28 wk Gestational Age
This is the 45° line across the lateral ventricle that connects an imaginary 2 o'clock position on the thalamus with the white matter in the parietal lobe

Normal:	<5 mm
Mild ventriculomegaly:	10–15 mm
Moderate ventriculomegaly:	15–20 mm
Severe ventriculomegaly:	>20 mm

Measurements in Coronal Plane
Measured at level of foramen of Monro, which separates lateral ventricles from third ventricle; measurements along these axes are less affected by variations in technique from scan to scan
Biparietal distance (BP) = width between inner table of skull
Biventricular distance (BV) = width between outermost margins of ventricles at foramen of Monro

	BV/BP ratio
Normal:	0.25
Mild ventriculomegaly:	0.25–0.40
Moderate ventriculomegaly:	0.40–0.60
Severe ventriculomegaly:	>0.60

Parenchymal Blood
Size and location are identified on scan

---

cell replacement. Thrombolytic agents are avoided acutely, and underlying coagulopathies are treated. Because autoregulation of cerebral blood flow (CBF) is underdeveloped in the preterm infant, making the system pressure passive, cerebral perfusion pressure depends on systemic mean arterial blood pressure. Hypotension will cause a fall in CBF, and hypertension will cause an increase in CBF. Mean arterial blood pressure should be maintained in the normal range.

Seizures are treated with anticonvulsants. Hypoglycemia, hypocalcemia, hypomagnesemia, hyponatremia, hypoxia, acidemia, and other well-identified metabolic aberrations must be excluded as contributing factors to seizure frequency. If apnea is frequent or prolonged enough to produce hypoxia, hypercapnia, acidosis, bradycardia, or hypotension, assisted ventilation is provided. Even modest hypoxia, hypercapnia, or both may further impair autoregulation. Unconjugated hyperbilirubinemia is monitored and treated routinely.

Psychomotor outcome relates most directly to the degree of parenchymal involvement and usually is not altered by specific management after IVH has occurred. Parenchymal blood most likely represents hemorrhagic infarcts in the periventricular white matter rather than mechanical extension of intraventricular blood. Intraventricular blood, however, may cause compression and obstruct periventricular venous drainage, resulting in venous congestion, periventricular ischemia, and hemorrhagic infarction. Although infarcted tissue cannot be reclaimed, maintaining adequate systemic arterial blood pressure and, therefore, adequate CBF may prevent extension of infarction. Appropriate blood pressure can be achieved through the prompt but slow repletion of intravascular volume coupled with the judicious use of pressors. Cerebral hyperperfusion can be avoided by correcting hypoxia, hypercapnia, and acidosis and by preventing acute episodes of systemic hypertension by avoiding excessively rapid intravascular infusions. Antihypertensive drugs should not be used.

Most specific management following IVH has been directed toward preventing or treating posthemorrhagic hydrocephalus (PHH). This condition is most commonly the result of a blood-induced obliterative arachnoiditis. PHH must be distinguished from ventriculomegaly. Ventriculomegaly refers to the presence of enlarged ventricles following IVH. The term PHH is reserved for ventriculomegaly that is accompanied by the symptoms and signs of increased intracranial

pressure (ICP) (Table 4). Growth in occipital-frontal circumference (OFC) ≥2 cm/wk is an objective and sensitive clinical sign of increased ICP, especially when accompanied by widening sutures or bulging anterior fontanelle (AF), and can be measured easily. In cases of communicating hydrocephalus, the most common variety of PHH, a manometric measure of opening pressure (OP) during a lumbar puncture (LP) is equally sensitive, objective, and almost as easily obtained. Simple manometric readings taken with a 22-gauge spinal needle correlate well with transfontanelle pressure monitors or other more expensive devices.

The size of the ventricles measured on an ultrasonogram must be considered in the context of head growth and signs of increased ICP. Enlarged ventricles accompanied by minimal or very slow growth of OFC may be a sign of cerebral atrophy. Conversely, rapidly increasing OFC with normally sized ventricles may be a sign of catchup head growth. Ventricular size may increase without signs of increased ICP. The significance of this is not known, especially if the cortical mantle remains >0.5 cm thick. The British Ventriculomegaly Group found that they treated some infants unnecessarily if they relied solely on absolute ventricular size and not on change in OFC. The velocity of ventricular size change, as opposed to a single measurement of ventricular size, may prove useful but requires further research. Critical velocities of growth have not been established. Although ventricular enlargement may precede an increase in OFC by 2 weeks, the time course of ventricular enlargement may not be linear. It may occur in incremental jumps, thus complicating simple extrapolation. Ventricular measurements are often more valuable to exclude PHH, since a minimal increase over time makes PHH unlikely. These measurements, although not always diagnostic of PHH, may nevertheless aid in the management of these infants.

TABLE 4. Clinical Findings That Define Posthemorrhagic Hydrocephalus

Signs or Symptoms of Increased ICP*
Feeding intolerance
Apnea
Lethargy
Bradycardia

At least one of the objective findings below should also be present to attribute these nonspecific findings to increased ICP

Increase in OFC >2 cm/wk
This is usually accompanied by
  Bulging AF
  Widely spaced sutures
HUS showing enlarged ventricles in combination with accelerated growth of OFC will rule out catchup head growth
HUS showing enlarged ventricles but with slow growth of OFC may suggest cerebral atrophy

Increased OP on LP
Manometer reading from 22-gauge spinal needle ≥80–110 mm H_2O
OP does not reflect ICP in noncommunicating hydrocephalus; suspect this condition if <3 ml CSF can be obtained over a 5-min period in presence of other evidence of increased ICP

Velocity of Ventricular Growth as Measured on HUS
Increased 5–10 mm/wk, thus progressing from mild to moderate or moderate to severe ventriculomegaly
Critical velocities of growth have not been reliably established; if ventricles are rapidly growing but OFC is stable, measure OP by LP
Ventricles may enlarge without signs of increased ICP; significance of this not known, especially if cortical mantle remains >0.5 cm
Ventricles may increase before OFC increases; intervene for increased ICP when growth in OFC ≥2 cm/wk, bulging AF, increased OP, symptoms, or rapid crossing of measured severity categories within 1 wk

---

*OFC, occipital-frontal circumference; ICP, intracranial pressure; AF, anterior fontanelle; CSF, cerebrospinal fluid; HUS, head ultrasound examination; OP, opening pressure; LP, lumbar puncture.

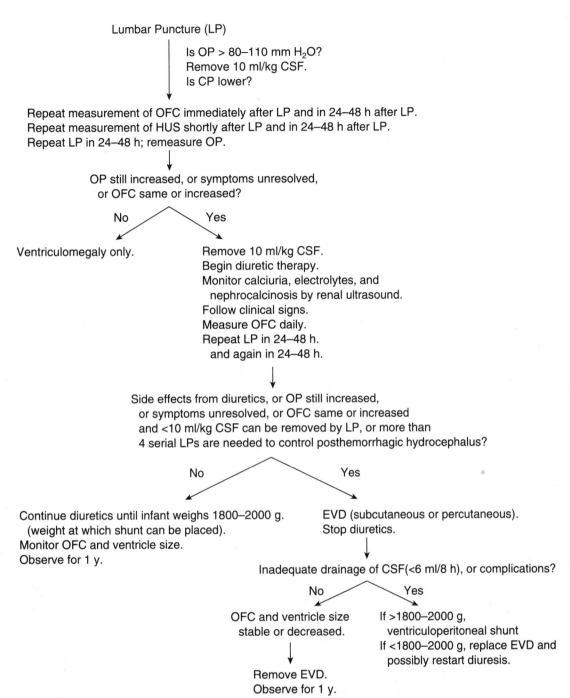

FIGURE 1. Algorithm for management of suspected posthemorrhagic hydrocephalus. EVD, external ventricular drainage; OFC, occipital-frontal circumference; ICP, intracranial pressure; AF, anterior fontanelle; CSF, cerebrospinal fluid; HUS, head ultrasound examination; OP, opening pressure; CP, closing pressure; LP, lumbar puncture.

Increased ICP that requires intervention usually will be manifested by growth in OFC ≥2 cm/wk, bulging AF, increased OP, and symptoms, such as apnea or lethargy (Table 4). However, if ventricular size increases rapidly at the rate of ~5 to 10 mm/wk or progresses within 1 week from one measured "severity category" to another (Table 4), even with stable head circumference, an LP is performed to measure OP and remove cerebrospinal fluid (CSF). A decrease in ventricular size on HUS, especially accompanied by a decrease in OFC, immediately following removal of 10 to 15 ml/kg of CSF and a lower closing pressure, will support the diagnosis of PHH. In noncommunicating hydrocephalus, OP does not reflect ICP. This condition may occur in very small preterm infants with severe bleeds and

is frequently the result of a clot in the aqueduct of Sylvius or the fourth ventricle. One should suspect noncommunicating hydrocephalus if CSF flow is very slow and meager (e.g., less than 3 ml/5 min) despite other evidence of increased ICP. In such a case, greater weight should be accorded the other three criteria for PHH (Table 4), including the rapid crossing of measured "severity categories" within 1 week (Table 3). The diagnosis of noncommunication will affect therapy, and early ventriculostomy may be appropriate. ICP can be measured directly from a ventriculostomy. Excluding babies with elevations of venous pressure, such as occurs with pneumothorax or during treatment with continuous positive airway pressure, a clinical estimate of ICP is the vertical distance between the AF and the level of the right atrium of the heart, measured at the point where the fontanelle flattens as the baby is tilted up from a supine position. The normal distance will be ≤50 mm, suggesting ≤50 mm H₂O ICP.

PHH usually develops 1 to 3 weeks after IVH. The data from Dykes et al.[1] on the natural history following IVH reflects the experience in most centers. Of 409 infants with IVH, only 13% developed progressive ventricular dilatation. In two thirds of this small percentage, ventricles either stopped growing or decreased in size without progressing to severe dilatation. The remaining third continued to progress to severe ventricular enlargement. Only 2 of these 18 babies, however, had increased ICP.

Although it is not clear which treatment is optimal, identification of which patient requires treatment is becoming more clear. No specific intervention is needed for asymptomatic ventriculomegaly, although the infant must be observed closely for the development of signs and symptoms of increased ICP. A comparison of infants with asymptomatic ventriculomegaly who were closely observed for signs and symptoms of increased ICP and those who received active intervention with serial lumbar punctures revealed no differences in neurodevelopmental outcome or eventual need for shunt.[1] Preliminary evidence obtained using near infrared spectroscopy indicates that lumbar punctures are effective when ICP is increased but not under other circumstances, even when ventricles are enlarged.

In cases of ventriculomegaly that is symptomatic (i.e., true PHH), the only effective intervention is to decrease ICP. Elimination of CSF achieves this most expeditiously. Placement of a ventriculoperitoneal (VP) shunt is the definitive long-term treatment. Short-term treatment includes serial lumbar punctures, diuretics, or external ventricular drainage (EVD), but these are temporizing measures. No one temporizing modality seems to alter the natural history more effectively than any other. Although no large, prospective, randomized study comparing modalities is available, in most series, ventricular size will stop enlarging or return to normal size in approximately two thirds of infants with PHH. Approximately one third will ultimately need VP shunts regardless of the type and timing of intervention. In general, PHH is more likely to develop following large hemorrhages with intraparenchymal involvement than after smaller hemorrhages. The greater the extent of bleeding or parenchymal involvement, the more likely that a shunt will be needed to treat the resulting PHH. Acquired noncommunicating hydrocephalus may progress quickly and resolve slowly, necessitating shunt placement before hospital discharge. However, it is difficult to predict the course of an individual infant. Furthermore, psychomotor developmental outcome depends most on the degree of parenchymal involvement and not on ventricular size, requirement for shunt placement, or gestational age.

A VP shunt, the definitive therapy for PHH, has many disadvantages. Placement and removal require surgical procedures. Shunts are difficult to place and maintain in small preterm babies who weigh less than 1800 to 2000 g and are prone to infection. Complications, which include ventriculitis, shunt obstruction, and shunt breakage, are difficult to assess in premature infants. Multiple revisions may be required either because of complications or because of rapid growth of the infant. Because it is difficult to predict which infants with PHH will require a permanent shunt, temporizing measures, including diuretic therapy, LPs, or EVD, are used to decrease ICP until it is clear whether PHH will resolve spontaneously.

ALGORITHM FOR DETECTING AND MANAGING IVH

Our approach to screening, monitoring, and management of IVH is summarized in Table 2 and Figure 1. Few infants with IVH develop PHH, and only infants with PHH require treatment. This approach enables identification of infants who need the volume of intracranial CSF reduced by diversion, removal, or decreased production while avoiding intervention when it is either not necessary or not beneficial. The therapies, with their attendant risks, need be directed to only the small number of babies who have evidence of increased ICP. Assuming that increased ICP is deleterious to the brain, only the effective removal of CSF will limit this damage. To be effective, an LP must remove at least 10 ml CSF per kilogram body weight. If ICP is increased and LPs are ineffective or unduly stressful, early institution of EVD is recommended for the effective removal of CSF. A temporizing ventriculostomy may be performed via surgical subcutaneous placement of an EVD and reservoir or can be placed percutaneously at the bedside. Both procedures are safe and effective.[2,4]

The diuretics acetazolamide (25 mg/kg/d PO up to 100 mg/kg/d prn) and furosemide (1–3 mg IV or PO b.i.d.) decrease production of CSF and, thus, may be useful interventions. Metabolic acidosis can be avoided by supplementing bicarbonate (Bicitra, 8 mEq/kg/d) to keep the serum bicarbonate level greater than 18 mEq/L. The urinary ratio of calcium/creatinine should be monitored. If this ratio becomes elevated, furosemide therapy should be discontinued to avoid nephrocalcinosis. Electrolytes must be followed closely.

CONDITIONS THAT MIGHT INFLUENCE IVH

Conditions associated with IVH and asphyxial damage include hypoxia and acidosis from pulmonary insufficiency, pulmonary air leak, and patent ductus arteriosus (PDA). These conditions should be avoided. Some interventions, including pancuronium for mechanically ventilated infants and indomethacin treatment, have been suggested as specific prophylaxis for IVH. However, because their selective effect on IVH is still unresolved, pancuronium and indomethacin use should be based on cardiovascular or pulmonary indications. Although indomethacin affects platelet function, it has not been shown to extend an existing IVH. However, in an infant known to have IVH who develops a clinically significant PDA, risks of indomethacin use should be weighed against those of operative ligation. Phenobarbital is ineffective as a prophylactic agent against IVH in preterm infants and may increase risk of IVH in mechanically ventilated infants. Phenobarbital should, therefore, be used only for its antiepileptic, sedative, or other well-established metabolic properties. No specific prophylactic agents have been identified. Ultimately, the prevention of preterm labor will be the most effective prophylaxis for IVH. Furthermore, transport of a mother in preterm labor to a high-risk obstetrical center is probably safer from the point of preventing IVH than transporting a premature newborn to a neonatal intensive care unit.

ACKNOWLEDGMENT

We thank Drs. Jane Stewart, Jeffery Garland, Walter Allan, and Joseph Volpe for suggestions regarding this material.

REFERENCES

1. Dykes FD, Dunbar B, Lazarra A, Ahmann PA: Posthemorrhagic hydrocephalus in high-risk preterm infants: Natural history, management, and long-term outcome. J Pediatr 114:611–618, 1989.
2. Marro PJ, Dransfield DA, Mott SH, Allan WC: Posthemorrhagic hydrocephalus: Use of an intravenous-type catheter for cerebrospinal fluid drainage. Am J Dis Child 145:1141–1146, 1991.
3. Ventriculomegaly Trial Group: Randomized trial of early tapping neonatal posthaemorrhagic ventricular dilatation. Arch Dis Child 65:3–10, 1990.
4. Volpe JJ: Intracranial hemorrhage: Germinal matrix–intraventricular hemorrhage of the premature infant. In Volpe JJ: Neurology of the Newborn, 3rd ed. Philadelphia, WB Saunders, 1995:403–463.

NEUROLOGIC BIRTH TRAUMA

André J. du Plessis, M.D.

Joseph J. Volpe, M.D.

Birth trauma occurs most commonly in the setting of a difficult labor or delivery or both. Although often imprecisely considered as any neurologic injury occurring during the birth process, the term *neurologic birth trauma* is used here to denote mechanical injury. Although the incidence of birth trauma in general is decreasing, the overall incidence of neurologic birth trauma is difficult to establish conclusively. Several factors influence the identification of neurologic birth trauma. First, birth trauma to the nervous system may occur in association with somatic injuries or with nonmechanical brain insults (such as hypoxia-ischemia), and the manifestations of such associated injuries may obscure the clinical recognition of traumatic injury. Second, recognition of the incidence and extent of neurologic trauma has increased with advances in diagnostic techniques. At the same time, advances in obstetric care, with improved techniques for monitoring fetal well-being and the progression of labor, have allowed earlier detection of complicated labor, more rational planning of delivery, and the selective use of cesarean section or instrumental delivery. In this section, neurologic birth injury is discussed according to anatomic locus, beginning rostrally and proceeding caudally.

INJURY TO THE SCALP AND CRANIUM

Cephalhematoma is a subperiosteal hemorrhage of the outer table of the skull. This lesion remains limited to individual skull bones (most often parietal) and does not cross sutures or fontanelles. Cephalhematoma occurs in 1% to 2% of overall births and in up to 33% of forceps deliveries. Spontaneous resolution occurs over weeks to months. An underlying linear skull fracture is present in 10% to 25% of cases. Rare complications include infection, hyperbilirubinemia, and meningitis.

Subgaleal hemorrhage is a more serious lesion, with a mortality of approximately 20%. Blood loss into the relatively unrestricted subgaleal space may be great enough to cause hypovolemic shock. Unlike cephalhematoma, this lesion may cross sutures and fontanelles, often accumulating dependently in the occipitocervical area. A strong association with instrumented deliveries exists, and approximately 50% of subgaleal hematomas occur following vacuum extractions (0.5% to 1% of vacuum extractions may be complicated by this lesion). Associated lesions include skull fracture and sutural diastasis, as well as other manifestations of intracranial trauma in the form of subarachnoid and subdural hemorrhage, tentorial tears, and cerebral laceration. Bleeding diatheses, such as hemophilia and vitamin K deficiency (delayed presentation at 2 to 3 days), may predispose to subgaleal hemorrhage. Conversely, a secondary consumptive coagulopathy may result. Acute management should include the prompt restoration of intravascular volume. Coagulopathies, primary or secondary, should be treated appropriately. Once the infant's condition is stable, intracranial traumatic injuries should be excluded by CT scan.

Skull fractures may be linear or depressed. Linear fractures occur most commonly in the parietal region and only rarely are associated with epidural or subdural hematoma or cerebral parenchymal injury. An underlying dural tear may predispose to the later development of a leptomeningeal cyst and a "growing" skull fracture, evident on palpation as an enlarging skull defect. Depressed skull fractures occur almost invariably following forceps delivery. Underlying intracranial lesions are unusual, and in their absence, neurologic symptoms or signs are rare. However, intracranial hemorrhagic lesions and displaced bone fragments should be excluded by CT scan. Depressed fractures may elevate spontaneously. Conservative methods, such as vacuum applied to the depressed area, have been advocated. However, when an infant is symptomatic, intracranial bone fragments are evident, or the fracture is associated with a hematoma (epidural or subdural), a surgical evaluation is indicated. Occipital *osteodiastasis* refers to displacement of the cartilaginous part of the occipital bone, usually in the setting of breech delivery. Underlying dural tears with venous (subdural) hemorrhage or cerebellar laceration may be associated.

INJURY TO INTRACRANIAL STRUCTURES

Intracranial trauma may be ischemic or hemorrhagic. Hemorrhage may be extraparenchymal (extradural, subdural, or subarachnoid), intraparenchymal (cerebral or cerebellar), or intraventricular. Ischemic brain lesions may occur secondary to a focal vascular disturbance.

Diffuse ischemic brain lesions are not related strictly to mechanical injury but may occur secondarily if associated with hypotension and, as a consequence, impaired cerebral blood flow.

Epidural hematoma is a subperiosteal hemorrhage of the inner skull table. The lesion is rare in the neonate, representing only 2% of all intracranial hemorrhages. Associated injuries include skull fracture and cephalhematoma, although one or both may be absent. The clinical presentation may include seizures and signs of raised intracranial pressure. Surgical evacuation is recommended, particularly in patients with focal signs or evidence of intracranial hypertension. More conservative measures have been described, such as needle aspiration of an overlying cephalhematoma, with subsequent resolution of a contiguous epidural hematoma.

Subdural hematoma (SDH) occurs most commonly in the setting of breech and instrumented (forceps or vacuum) deliveries, which can cause sufficient cranial distortion to result in excessive tensile stress on the dural structures and venous rupture into the subdural space. Major venous sinus rupture due to laceration of the tentorium (more commonly) or the falx (less commonly) or due to occipital osteodiastasis may lead to major subdural hemorrhage, whereas rupture of the bridging veins over the cerebral or cerebellar convexities tends to cause less severe hemorrhages. Supratentorial SDH may remain clinically silent, present with focal signs, or develop into chronic subdural fluid collections. Posterior fossa SDH is more serious because of the limited expansile space and the proximity to vital brainstem structures. These hemorrhages may present with cranial nerve signs, respiratory abnormalities and opisthotonus. In this clinical setting, the risk of cerebellar herniation into the foramen magnum precludes lumbar puncture. The diagnosis should be made by CT or MRI, with a high index of suspicion. Management of SDH depends on the location and clinical course. Drainage of supratentorial SDH is indicated only in the presence of intracranial hypertension or excessive cranial growth, with the development of craniocerebral disproportion. In the posterior fossa, progressively symptomatic SDH mandates urgent neurosurgical evaluation. In the absence of parenchymal injury, supratentorial SDH is associated with a good prognosis. Large posterior fossa SDH with major tentorial or falx tears are nearly uniformly fatal. However, incidental asymptomatic SDH around the tentorium, detected by CT scan, have been described. Untreated, these infants have a normal outcome as the lesions gradually resolve.

Primary subarachnoid hemorrhage (i.e., not associated with intraventricular, intraparenchymal, or subdural hemorrhage) is a more common and often incidental finding, usually of little clinical significance. Occasionally, seizures develop, although both the infant and the EEG usually appear normal between seizures. Rarely, these infants show a catastrophic deterioration. Acute treatment is symptomatic. The risk of delayed posthemorrhagic hydrocephalus requires close monitoring of head circumference.

Of all term infants with *intraventricular hemorrhage,* approximately 50% have a history of difficult forceps or breech deliveries. Up to 30% of these infants may develop posthemorrhagic hydrocephalus requiring a CSF shunting procedure.

Intracerebellar hemorrhage in the term infant is usually associated with traumatic forceps or vacuum delivery. Occipital osteodiastasis may cause tentorial or falx rupture and, in severe cases, cerebellar laceration. By head ultrasound and CT imaging, these lesions may be contiguous with, and difficult to distinguish from, posterior fossa SDH. Clinical presentation may be delayed for up to 96 hours. The management of infants with posterior fossa hemorrhages traditionally has been surgical, with craniotomy and evacuation of the hematoma. Earlier series reported 85% survival in infants treated surgically. In cases of clinical deterioration, especially with brainstem signs, surgery should be an emergency consideration. More recently, successful conservative management of cerebellar hemorrhage with dexamethasone and close clinical and CT vigilance has been reported. Survivors of cerebellar hemorrhage may be left with hypotonia, ataxia, and significant developmental delay.

Focal cerebral infarction in a vascular territory may occur in association with traumatic intracranial lesions. Putative mechanisms include (1) vascular (intimal) stretch injury with thrombosis or distal embolic infarction or both, (2) arterial compression by a hematoma, (3) brain herniation with arterial compression on the margins of the falx or tentorium, and (4) vasospasm caused by extravasated blood.

INJURY TO THE SPINAL CORD

The incidence of spinal cord injury (SCI) occurring at birth is unknown. However, a decrease in the incidence of SCI appears to have accompanied improvements in obstetric management. Longitudinal and torsional forces on the neck during delivery may result in direct trauma to the cord or to the vertebral arteries, with resulting cord ischemia. The level of SCI is usually cervical or cervicothoracic, depending on the fetal presentation. Cervicothoracic junction (C8–T1) injury occurs during vaginal breech delivery, and upper cervical cord injuries (C1–6) occur during difficult cephalic delivery. Vaginal breech delivery accounts for up to 70% of cases. Particularly dangerous is the "star-gazing" breech presentation (with hyperextended neck), and vaginal delivery of these infants carries a 25% risk for cervical SCI. Fetal hypotonia may result in fetal malposition and the loss of muscle tone required to resist the traction forces of delivery. This mechanism may be an important contributing factor in the depressed (e.g., asphyxiated) term infant and in the normally hypotonic preterm infant. Other risk factors include forceful extraction, brow and face presentations, and shoulder dystocia. Ischemic SCI following traumatic delivery may result from vertebral artery injury or birth asphyxia. Mechanical and ischemic SCI have different topographies. Traumatic injury occurs in the cervical-upper thoracic region, and ischemic injury occurs in the more caudal (watershed) regions of the thoracolumbar cord. The former is much more common than the latter.

Following a complicated (especially breech) delivery, certain signs should raise the possibility of SCI. Flaccid extremity weakness with areflexia and retained facial activity, particularly in the setting of a sensory level, is highly suggestive of a cord lesion. Paradoxical breathing, poor anal tone (and loss of the anal wink reflex), and a passive urinary bladder with priapism may be present. Unusual upper extremity and hand positions have been described, presumably due to incomplete injury to the cervical segments supplying the arms and hands.

Plain radiographs of the spine are usually normal in the presence of SCI, only rarely showing fracture-dislocation. Ultrasound diagnosis through the incompletely ossified posterior cervical spine has been described. This technique allows repeated bedside studies in critically ill newborns and has been recommended as an initial investigation in suspected SCI. The value of CT myelography lies in its ability to demonstrate CSF block due to epidural hematoma, a finding that mandates urgent neurosurgical intervention. Magnetic resonance imaging (MRI) with its excellent soft tissue resolution is superior to CT myelography in several ways, particularly in distinguishing between intramedullary and extramedullary injury. However, in the acute setting, transport of a critically ill infant may not be feasible. Bedside electrophysiologic studies, such as somatosensory evoked potentials (SEP), may localize a functional SCI, even in the absence of structural injury by CT myelography or MRI.

Prompt recognition is the cornerstone of SCI management. At the earliest suspicion of SCI, the infant's neck and trunk should be immobilized, as movement of the unprotected cervical spine may lead to inadvertent extension of SCI. Intubation for respiratory support should be performed with extreme, expert care. Once the infant's condition is stable, cord compression (e.g., by epidural hematoma) should be excluded by CT myelogram or MRI. Loss of normal autonomic regulation may result in hemodynamic and temperature instability. Any source of pain or discomfort (such as a distended bladder) may precipitate hypertensive crises via massive spinal reflexes. Regular bladder emptying may be achieved by passive bladder Credé maneuvers. The value of newer pharmacologic agents to prevent or reduce the extent of SCI, such as steroids, monosialogangliosides, calcium channel blockers, and excitatory amino acid antagonists, re-

mains unresolved, although data from experimental animals and adult humans appear promising.

Prognosis in SCI depends largely on the spinal level and the predominant mechanism of injury (transection, ischemia, or compression). Upper cervical SCI has the worst outcome, particularly in terms of spontaneous breathing. Issues of withdrawal of life support commonly arise in this setting, and for this reason, clinical prognostic guidelines have been suggested. Based on the expected time required for spinal shock to resolve, failure of spontaneous respiratory efforts and limb movements at 3 weeks, and almost certainly by 3 months, are likely to predict permanent ventilator dependence and severe quadriparesis. More caudal SCI occur less commonly but may have a better functional outcome, particularly with lesions below the fourth thoracic segment, when independent living with crutches may be possible.

INJURY TO PERIPHERAL NERVES

Brachial Plexus Injuries

Following an earlier decrease in incidence, brachial plexus injuries (BPI) have occurred at a steady rate of 0.37 to 0.87 per 1000 live births for several decades. Improved rates of recovery, from an earlier 13% to 18% to the current 70% to 95%, suggest that the severity of injury may be decreasing. BPI occur after difficult deliveries, and risk factors include large infants, infants of diabetic mothers, prolonged labor, abnormal fetal presentations, and instrumented midpelvic delivery. Parity is a more controversial risk factor, and both primiparity and multiparity have been implicated. Recurrence of BPI in subsequent pregnancies may be as high as 14%. In the term cephalic delivery, prolonged second stage of labor, particularly with shoulder dystocia, is a high-risk situation for development of BPI. In the premature infant, lower plexus injury may occur during precipitous breech delivery. The loss of protective muscle tone in premature and asphyxiated infants may predispose the plexus to extreme traction injury during difficult delivery. The severity of nerve injury may range from neuropraxia to root avulsion, depending on the degree of traction injury. Severe root avulsions may be associated with localized spinal cord hemorrhage. Neuropraxia, the mildest form of injury, results from functional disruption of anatomically intact neural elements. Neuropraxic injury tends to recover fully, whereas root avulsion has no potential for spontaneous recovery. Intermediate grades of injury may result in partial structural nerve disruption, with subsequent scarring and residual functional deficit. The distribution of injury within the plexus may depend on the fetal presentation. Upper plexus (C5, C6) injuries tend to occur with cephalic presentations, whereas involvement of the lower plexus (C8, T1) tends to follow breech deliveries. Root avulsion is rare with upper plexus injuries, tends to occur at the C8 and T1 levels, and may be accompanied by Horner's syndrome. This variety of injury has a particularly poor prognosis for recovery. Upper plexus (C5, C6) and Erb-Duchenne palsies are the most common types (58% to 87%), with complete plexus involvement occurring in 10%. Lower plexus (C8–T1), or Klumpke's, palsies rarely occur in isolation and are almost invariably associated with C5, C6, and C7 involvement. Bilateral (often asymmetric) BPI occurs in 2% to 23% of cases, most commonly after breech delivery. BPI may be associated with other peripheral nerve lesions (discussed subsequently).

Most BPI are sustained during complicated delivery, when such associated injuries as birth asphyxia and fractures may obscure the signs of plexus injury. Injury to the right brachial plexus is more common, probably because of the higher incidence of left occipitoanterior fetal presentation. In the more common upper plexus (C5, C6) palsy, the arm hangs limply at the side, in adduction and internal rotation at the shoulder, and extension and pronation at the elbow. Reduced spontaneous movement and an asymmetric Moro response are present on the affected side. Sensation and intrinsic muscle function in the hand are retained, preserving the grasp reflex. Biceps and brachioradialis reflexes are depressed. Lower plexus (C8, T1) injury is manifested additionally by loss of distal muscle function and weak intrinsic hand muscles. The triceps tendon reflex may be depressed. Sensory and sweating function may be lost in the arm, with absence of the grasp reflex. In severe lower plexus injuries involving T1, a Horner syndrome with ipsilateral miosis, ptosis, and facial anhidrosis may be present. BPI may occur in association with other soft tissue, skeletal (humeral and clavicular fractures), and neural injuries. Phrenic nerve (C4) injury may occur in 5% to 9% of BPI, and 75% of all phrenic nerve injuries occur in this setting. The diaphragmatic paralysis (usually unilateral) may cause respiratory distress and be mistaken for more common respiratory illnesses. In the presence of BPI, respiratory distress may necessitate fluoroscopy to exclude diaphragm paralysis. Phrenic injury is usually neuropraxic, and 50% to 60% of patients recover in 2 to 4 weeks. Persistent diaphragmatic paralysis beyond this period may require diaphragmatic plication or prosthesis or phrenic nerve pacing. Rare cases of higher cervical, laryngeal, and hypoglossal nerve involvement have been described following traumatic delivery. In general, these lesions have a good prognosis for recovery.

The diagnosis of BPI is essentially clinical. Once it is diagnosed, prognostic information may be gained by differentiating proximal (often severe and inoperable lesions) from more distal plexus lesions. Winging of the scapula, diaphragmatic paralysis, and Horner's syndrome are all suggestive of proximal or root lesions. The value of electromyography (EMG) and nerve conduction studies in the management of BPI is controversial. Proponents suggest that EMG delineates the extent and pattern of involvement and distinguishes axonal from neuropraxic lesions and preganglionic from postganglionic lesions. Electrodiagnostic studies may assist in the planning of and intraoperative monitoring of surgical procedures. Myelography may be useful in delineating surgical options, since pseudomeningoceles may be noted at the site of root avulsion, with the leakage of contrast into the root sleeve. This technique positively identifies root avulsions in up to 90% of cases. MRI has been used, mainly in older patients, to identify root avulsions and to distinguish proximal distal plexus lesions. Following the diagnosis of BPI, associated problems, such as fractures and diaphragmatic paralysis, should be excluded.

Management begins with conservative measures. For the first 7 to 10 days, painful traumatic neuritis is likely, and the affected arm should be rested. Thereafter, range of motion exercises should commence. Previous splinting practices (in abduction and external rotation, i.e., Statue of Liberty) are discouraged. Complete recovery of BPI occurs in 70% to 92% of cases. BPI that resolve totally usually start recovery within 2 weeks, and there is normal function by 5 months. Other infants show significant but subtotal improvement over the first 12 months, and after 24 months, no further improvement is likely. Some infants are left with considerable deficits and may be candidates for new reconstructive neurosurgical techniques. Operative results are best in those undergoing early surgery. Guidelines for the selection of surgical candidates have been developed. For infants with upper plexus injury, biceps recovery at age 3 months is used as a guideline: no biceps recovery by 3 months is an indication for surgery, whereas significant biceps recovery suggests that a conservative approach be followed. For infants with slight but definite improvement at 3 months, reassessment at 6 months is recommended. Surgery postponed later than 6 months is unlikely to be beneficial. Good functional recovery can be expected in 65% to 80% of infants undergoing upper plexus surgery. For infants with complete plexus or lower plexus palsies (especially with Horner syndrome), the absence of hand movement at 3 months indicates that spontaneous recovery is unlikely, and surgery is recommended.

Facial Nerve Injuries

Facial nerve injury, occurring in 7.5/1000 live births, is the most common peripheral nerve birth injury. Risk factors include prolonged second stage of labor and midforceps delivery. These lesions are thought to result from pressure against the maternal sacral promontory. Infants present with hemifacial weakness, a flattened nasolabial fold,

widened palpebral fissure, and an asymmetric facial grimace on the ipsilateral side. Outcome is usually excellent, with full recovery in most cases over the first 3 weeks.

REFERENCES

1. Gilbert A, Rabazoni R, Amar-Khodja S: Indications and results of brachial plexus surgery in obstetrical palsy. Orthop Clin North Am 19:9, 1988.
2. Laurent JP, Shenaq S, Lee R, et al: Upper brachial plexus birth injuries: A neurosurgical approach. Concepts Pediatr Neurosurg 10:156, 1990.
3. Painter MJ, Bergman I: Obstetrical trauma to the neonatal central and peripheral nervous system. Semin Perinatol 6:89, 1982.
4. Volpe JJ: Perinatal trauma. *In* Neurology of the Newborn, 3rd ed. Philadelphia, WB Saunders, 1994:767.

HEMOLYTIC DISEASES OF THE NEONATE

ROSITA S. PILDES, M.D.
SUMA P. PYATI, M.D.

Accelerated destruction of erythrocytes in the fetus and newborn infant may be due to maternal immunization and transplacental transfer of antibodies, hereditary defects of the neonate's red blood cells (RBCs), or acquired disorders (Table 1). This chapter is limited to discussion of hemolytic diseases due to isoimmunization (erythroblastosis fetalis), with the emphasis on prevention and early identification of sensitization in the mother at risk and on the current approach to management of the fetus and neonate.

Rh HEMOLYTIC DISEASE

Rh hemolytic disease in the neonate was the most common cause of kernicterus before the introduction of high-titer anti-D immunoglobulin in 1968 (RhIg, RhoGAM, anti-D immunoglobulin) for the prophylaxis of perinatal maternal sensitization. The incidence of Rh hemolytic disease varies among different populations based, in part, on the prevalence of the Rh-negative antigens. The Rh (D)-negative genotype is present in approximately 15% of Caucasians, 5% of African Americans, and less than 1% of Asians. With appropriately administered RhIg, the incidence of hemolytic disease should be 3/10,000 births. Unfortunately the documented incidence is 10.6/10,000 births. Thus, many pregnant women do not receive adequate preventive therapy and continue to deliver affected infants.

Pathogenesis

Rh incompatibility exists when the fetus is Rh(D) positive (D/d) and the mother is Rh(D) negative (d/d). In the commonest scenario, a woman becomes sensitized from the transplacental passage of antigen on fetal red cells during a current or previous pregnancy or abortion. In rare circumstances, sensitization occurs following the transfusion of mismatched blood. Fetal RBC can be found in maternal sera as early as the first trimester. The volume is usually small and not sufficient to produce primary immunization unless there are repeated episodes of fetomaternal transfusion. Larger fetomaternal hemorrhages usually take place late in pregnancy or at delivery. As little as 1 ml of fetal blood is sufficient to sensitize the mother.

Once the mother is immunized, IgM and IgG anti-D antibodies are produced, the indirect Coombs' test becomes positive, and the IgG anti-D antibodies cross the placenta and coat the fetal erythrocytes, leading to agglutination, trapping, and subsequent destruction of the erythrocytes in the spleen of the fetus and newborn. The rate of destruction is proportionate to the amount of antibody coating the erythrocytes. Extramedullary hematopoiesis and reticuloendothelial clearance of sensitized cells lead to enlargement of the liver and spleen. The resulting spectrum of disease is wide. Approximately 50% of the neonates have clinically indiscernible or mild disease, resulting in exaggerated physiologic anemia at approximately 12

TABLE 1. Hemolytic Anemia in the Neonate

Immune Disorders
Hemolytic disease in the newborn
  Rh incompatibility: anti-D, anti-CD, anti-DE
  ABO incompatibility: anti-A, anti-B, anti-AB
  Other incompatibility: anti-C, anti-E, anti-Kell, and other IgG antibodies
Maternal autoimmune disease, e.g., systemic lupus erythematosus
Drug induced, e.g., by penicillin

Membrane Defects of the Red Blood Cell
Hereditary spherocytosis, elliptocytosis, stomatocytosis, pyropoikilocytosis
Enzymatic deficiency: glucose-6-phosphate dehydrogenase, pyruvate-kinase, others
Hemoglobinopathies: alpha- and gamma-thalassemia syndromes
Galactosemia
Hereditary 5′-nucleotidase deficiency
Congenital erythropoietic porphyria

Acquired Disorders
Syphilis, toxoplasmosis, cytomegalovirus infection, herpes simplex infection
Bacterial infection
Disseminated intravascular coagulation (DIC)
Localized intravascular coagulation
Sequestered blood

weeks of age, and 25% have moderate hemolysis and require treatment. The remaining 25% have severe hemolysis that can manifest as profound anemia, hydrops fetalis, congestive heart failure, or fetal death. However, the overall risk of maternal sensitization is low for the following reasons.

1. The father may be Rh (D) negative (d/d) or heterozygous (D/d), resulting in an Rh (D)-negative fetus.
2. Associated ABO incompatibility confers protection, since fetal cells entering the mother are destroyed before they can elicit an antibody response.
3. Fetomaternal transfusions occur in less than 50% of pregnancies.

Although the disease is usually more severe in successive pregnancies, 1% of women develop antibodies before delivery of their first infant. Early identification of the sensitized mother and advances in fetal therapy have dramatically decreased the incidence and severity of Rh hemolytic disease. Nevertheless, the presence of hydrops, anemia, or hyperbilirubinemia at or shortly after birth should alert the pediatrician to a possible underlying hemolytic process requiring prompt diagnostic and therapeutic intervention. Early discharge policies and current trends of allowing bilirubin values to reach levels higher than previously recommended introduce the potential for failure to identify the infant with hemolytic disease who may be at risk for kernicterus.

Management of Mother

All pregnant women should be screened at the first antepartum visit for ABO, Rh type, and antibodies. A complete history of abortions, stillbirths, previous sensitized pregnancies, or blood transfusions should be obtained.

Rh (D)-Negative Unimmunized Mother

RhIg Antepartum Prophylaxis. RhIg destroys the fetal RBC entering the maternal circulation before the maternal immune system can recognize the invading cells and develop an antibody response. Prompt treatment with RhIg as outlined below is 98% to 99% effective in preventing sensitization of the Rh-negative mother to the Rh antigen.
1. Repeat antibody screen at 28 weeks, and if serum is still negative, administer RhIg routinely (300 μg IM).
2. Administer RhIg in the following circumstances.
   a. Chorionic villus sampling at 10 to 12 weeks (50 μg)

   b. Spontaneous or induced abortion <12 weeks (50 μg), >12 weeks (300 μg)
   c. Antepartum bleeding (300 μg every 12 weeks until delivery)
   d. Ectopic pregnancy
   e. Abdominal trauma (300 μg)
   f. Amniocentesis (300 μg)

RhIg Postpartum Prophylaxis. All neonates born to Rh (D)-negative women *must be tested* at birth, and management of the mother should be jointly coordinated by the perinatologist, the pediatrician, and the blood bank. *If the neonate is Rh (D) negative,* there is no need to administer RhIg to the mother. *If the neonate is Rh (D) positive,* RhIg (300 μg) *must* be administered to the mother within 72 hours of delivery. If administration is inadvertently omitted, RhIg can be given up to 4 weeks after delivery. If the neonate is anemic at birth and the estimated fetomaternal transfusion exceeds 30 ml (Betke-Kleihauer test), 10 μg RhIg per milliliter estimated transfusion should be administered at a rate of 1200 μg IM every 12 hours until the total dose is given.

In the future, other preparations may become available, such as monoclonal RhIg or ion exchange-prepared RhIg for intravenous use (currently available for use in Canada). Advantages of these preparations include greater purity, the need for a smaller dose, and less reaction, discomfort, and cost.

Rh (D)-Negative Immunized Mother

Serial Antibody Titers

FIRST IMMUNIZED PREGNANCY. Starting at 18 to 20 weeks of pregnancy, antibody levels of all immunized women should be monitored at 2- to 3-week intervals. If antibody titers remain below the critical level for a given laboratory (e.g. 1:16), the prognosis is favorable, and amniocentesis can be avoided. If levels exceed the critical level, amniocentesis and ultrasound should be performed to assess fetal well-being.

SUBSEQUENT IMMUNIZED PREGNANCY. Monitoring serial antibody titers alone is not adequate. Amniocentesis and ultrasound are warranted regardless of antibody titers.

Serial Amniocentesis. Timing of initial amniocentesis is based on the antibody level and on the outcome of previous pregnancies. The initial amniocentesis is generally performed at 28 weeks but may be performed as early as 18 to 22 weeks gestation. Bilirubin pigment in amniotic fluid can be quantitated accurately by spectrophotometric scan and measurement of the deviation in optical density (ΔOD) at 450 nm, which is the wavelength absorbed by bilirubin (Fig. 1). Values are interpreted using prognostic zones on Liley's three-zone chart (Fig. 2). Serial amniotic fluid analyses are performed at 1- to 3-week intervals depending on previous ΔOD at 450 nm to determine the trend. Fetal lung maturity is determined concomitantly.

The Rh(D) genotype of the fetus can be determined rapidly in amniotic fluid or chorionic villus cells using the polymerase chain reaction (PCR). The test can be available in any laboratory using molecular biology techniques. Determination of the Rh type of the fetus early in pregnancy offers the opportunity to identify the fetus who requires no further investigation, thus eliminating the need for serial amniocentesis.

Fetal Sonography. Sonography and two-dimensional Doppler measurements are useful in assessing fetal heart size, ascites, movement, or death.

Management of Fetus
Evaluation and Monitoring

Management is individualized based on the gestational age of the fetus, the Liley zone, and the trend of amniotic fluid ΔOD at 450 nm. Current recommendations are as follows.
1. Zone 1: mild or not affected; safe to deliver near term
2. Low zone 2: amniotic fluid should be tested every 2 to 3 weeks

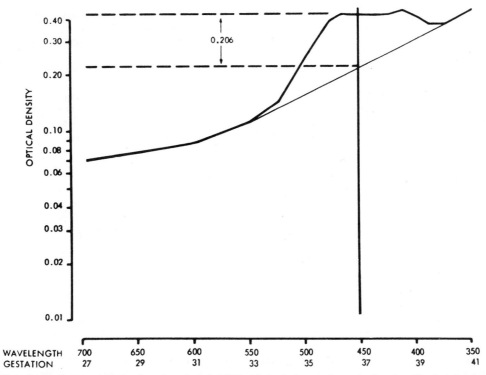

FIGURE 1. Spectrophotometric estimation of amniotic fluid bilirubin levels from an immunized mother. The deviation in optical density is calculated by subtracting the projected optical density from the measured optical density at 450 nm (0.206 in this illustration).

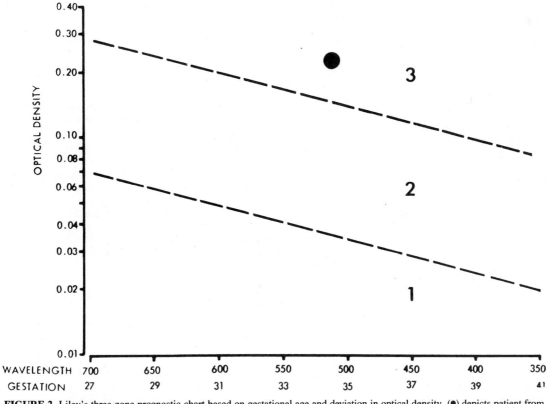

FIGURE 2. Liley's three-zone prognostic chart based on gestational age and deviation in optical density. (●) depicts patient from Figure 1. Zone 1 indicates a normal or mildly affected infant; zone 2, intermediate; zone 3, severe disease or impending fetal death.

a. If the ΔOD readings fall: prognosis is favorable; safe to deliver near term
b. If the ΔOD readings remain the same or rise: fetus may be in jeopardy
c. >32 weeks: deliver preterm; exact timing may be based on lung maturity
d. 23 to 32 weeks: consider intrauterine intraperitoneal transfusion (IUPT) or intrauterine intravascular transfusion (IUIVT).
3. High zone 2 or zone 3: severe disease
a. >33 weeks: deliver preterm
b. 23 to 33 weeks: IUPT or IUIVT
c. 18 to 22 weeks: IUIVT with repeated transfusion may offer the only chance for survival.

Plasmapheresis has been employed to decrease levels of anti-D antibodies in maternal serum until the fetus reaches a size when transfusion is possible. Antenatal steroids are usually administered for 48 hours before delivery (if time permits) to enhance fetal lung maturity.

Intrauterine Transfusion

Intrauterine transfusion (IUT) is usually limited to fetuses between 18 and 33 weeks gestation. Although relatively safe, IUT is not without risk. Hence, if the fetus is 33 weeks or older, determination of pulmonary maturity, administration of prenatal steroids, and premature delivery are recommended. IUT may be given through the intraperitoneal or the intravascular route, using frozen, deglycerolized, and irradiated, group O, Rh-negative RBCs that are compatible with the mother's serum.

Intrauterine Intraperitoneal Route (IUPT). Packed cells with a hematocrit of approximately 90% are injected into the fetal peritoneal cavity, and 85% of these cells are absorbed through the lymphatic channels and survive in the fetus.

Volume of transfusion =
(Weeks gestation − 20) × 10 ml packed RBC

Direct Intrauterine Intravascular Transfusion (IUIVT). This is superior to IUPT transfusion in skilled hands and has dramatically improved the survival of the fetus with hydrops.

Volume of transfusion = 50 ml packed RBC/kg
injected at rate of 5–10 ml/min directly into umbilical vein

This procedure is repeated weekly depending on the level of the fetal hemoglobin determined through cordocentesis.

Combination of IUPT and IUIV. A combination of IUPT and IUIV may be used to transfuse the required amount of erythrocytes and prolong the interval between transfusions.

Prenatal Pharmacologic Agents

The following agents have been used in an effort to decrease hemolysis even though the benefits are controversial.

1. Promethazine, an immunosuppressive drug
2. Oral antigen: Rh-positive membrane in an enteric-coated capsule, used in an effort to induce tolerance to the antigen in the mother
3. Immune serum globulin
4. Phenobarbital given for at least 1 week before delivery to increase conjugation and excretion of bilirubin by the fetal liver

Neonate of Immunized Mother
Clinical Features

Symptoms may be absent, mild, moderate, or severe. Anemia is often the presenting finding at birth and reflects the severity of the hemolytic process. Hemoglobin values may continue to fall rapidly, but with use of phototherapy, the degree of anemia generally will not correlate with the degree of hyperbilirubinemia. Jaundice is not visible at birth, as unconjugated bilirubin produced by the fetus is lipid soluble and freely transported through the placenta and metabolized by the

mother. Jaundice usually becomes apparent in the first 24 hours of life, beginning as early as a half-hour of age in some infants. The pediatrician should be vigilant and anticipate a rapid rise in bilirubin after birth.

Severely affected neonates may present with marked pallor, edema, pleural and pericardial effusions, ascites, tachycardia, and hepatosplenomegaly at birth. Petechia and purpura due to thrombocytopenia and possibly due to anoxic injury to the capillaries may be present in association with severe anemia. Hypoglycemia may occur secondary to hyperplasia of the islet cells in the pancreas. The causes of the beta cell hyperplasia are unknown.

Laboratory Features

1. Direct Coombs test is positive even when the anemia is mild.
2. Peripheral blood counts show decreased hemoglobin concentration, increased reticulocyte count, increased number of nucleated red cells, marked polychromasia, and anisocytosis. Spherocytes are not present in the blood smear (unlike ABO incompatibility).
3. Leukocytocis and immature white blood cells may be present.
4. Thrombocytopenia and clotting defects are not uncommon.
5. Unconjugated bilirubin may rise rapidly after birth, and conjugated bilirubin may be found in instances of severe intrauterine hemolysis.
6. Hypoproteinemia, particularly in hydropic infants, can be more significant than anemia.
7. Blood volume is not significantly elevated, even in hydrops. Elevations in central venous and aortic pressures are likely due to fetal asphyxia and acidosis. Elevated umbilical venous pressure probably reflects abdominal distention rather than congestive heart failure.

Laboratory Features in Neonates Delivered Following IUT. The pediatrician should be aware that the findings at birth may be misleading in these severely affected neonates. The following features may be present.

1. Normal hematocrit at birth
2. Negative direct Coombs test
3. Relatively normal peripheral smear
4. Low levels of hemoglobin F
5. Rapid increase in bilirubin after birth despite the low number of fetal erythrocytes.

The absence of fetal Rh-positive erythrocytes may be due to suppression of erythropoiesis or destruction of cells by anti-D antibodies. In addition, the Rh test may be falsely negative because the red cells are completely coated by anti-D antibodies.

Management

Delivery Room. A pediatrician skilled in resuscitation and partial exchange transfusion should be in the delivery room when an infant at risk for severe disease is expected. Group O, Rh-negative RBCs compatible with the mother's serum should be readily available at delivery.

Resuscitative measures include establishment of adequate ventilation and perfusion and correction of acid-base balance. In hydropic infants, high peak inspiratory pressures may be required to achieve adequate ventilation. Paracentesis and thoracentesis are indicated if ascites and pleural effusions preclude ventilation. A central hematocrit should be obtained if the infant is pale, and a partial exchange transfusion using packed RBC (PRBC) is performed if the hematocrit is less than 30% (or the hemoglobin concentration is less than 10 g/dl) in term infants. Treatment should be initiated at higher values in preterm or very sick neonates.

Transfusion volume = BW (kg) × 80
$$\times \frac{\text{desired hematocrit} - \text{observed hematocrit}}{\text{PRBC hematocrit} - \text{observed hematocrit}}$$

The technique of partial exchange transfusion is similar to that of exchange transfusion.

Hydropic infants may have increased total body water and extracellular fluid, but the blood volume is generally normal or reduced. Hence, PRBC (20 to 40 ml/kg) or partial exchange is helpful in correcting shock and restoring the oxygen-carrying capacity.

Nursery or NICU

EVALUATION AND MONITORING. A detailed obstetric history of the mother must be obtained, and a thorough physical examination must be performed. The infant with evidence of hemolysis should be closely monitored. The following laboratory tests should be obtained.

1. Maternal and neonatal blood group and Rh type; direct Coombs test
2. Central hematocrit or hemoglobin level (cord and neonatal samples)
3. Conjugated and unconjugated bilirubin level (cord and neonatal samples)
4. White blood cell count and reticulocyte count
5. Peripheral blood smear for erythrocyte morphology
6. Plasma glucose, serum albumin, and liver function tests as indicated

Precise serum bilirubin and hemoglobin or hematocrit values are monitored every 4 to 6 hours or more frequently depending on the levels and the predicted rate of hemolysis.

PHOTOTHERAPY. Exposure of the neonate to phototherapy should effectively reduce serum bilirubin levels and, in most cases, prevent the evolution of hazardous levels of hyperbilirubinemia. In previous years, the rate of bilirubin rise was used as a guide to predict the need for an exchange transfusion. These rigid guidelines are no longer applicable when phototherapy is used, as bilirubin values may plateau despite an early rise. We start prophylactic phototherapy on the first day of life in all infants with evidence of hemolysis, using a standard phototherapy unit with four daylight and four special blue fluorescent lamps. Other kinds and combinations of fluorescent lamps, including fiberoptic blankets, are available for use. A shield of the corrective type of Plexiglas should be used to screen out the ultraviolet light. For a further discussion of phototherapy see discussion of hyperbilirubinemia and kernicterus.

REPLACEMENT PACKED RED CELL TRANSFUSION. A replacement transfusion may be necessary for correction of anemia despite prevention of significant hyperbilirubinemia by phototherapy. This is still a better alternative to a double volume exchange. We transfuse infants whose hemoglobin values fall rapidly below 10 g/dl (hematocrit <30%). Symptomatic infants are transfused at higher values. Approximately 10 ml/kg of packed RBC are transfused.

EXCHANGE TRANSFUSION
Objectives

1. Reduce the serum bilirubin concentration before neurotoxic levels are achieved.
2. Correct the associated anemia.
3. Curtail further hemolysis by removing both the antibody-coated neonatal red cells that are destined to be hemolyzed and the maternally derived anti-D antibody circulating freely in the plasma.

Indications. Guidelines for exchange transfusion that are followed in our nursery are listed in Table 2, and the potential complications are shown in Table 3. In general, the bilirubin level at which exchange transfusion is performed depends on the birth weight and the general condition of the infant. Recently, the bilirubin/albumin ratio has been suggested as a possible adjunct to the criteria shown in Table 2 when deciding about the need for exchange transfusion. Bilirubin values fall precipitously in the presence of developing kernicterus. Hence, clinical signs, such as lethargy or sudden unexplained poor feeding, should be considered indications for exchange transfusion. In asymptomatic, full-term, healthy neonates with hemolytic disease, our criteria for blood transfusion and exchange transfusion do not differ

TABLE 2. Suggested Guidelines for Exchange Transfusion in Infants with Hemolytic Disease

	MAXIMUM *TOTAL* BILIRUBIN VALUES (mg/dl) ALLOWED BEFORE EXCHANGE TRANSFUSION	
BIRTH WEIGHT (g)	UNCOMPLICATED COURSE	COMPLICATED COURSE*
<1000	10	10
1000–1249	13	10
1250–1499	15	13
1500–1999	17	15
2000–2449	18	17
>2500	20	18

Complicated course:
History of previous child with severe hemolytic disease.
History of intrauterine transfusion.
Hydrops, hypoalbuminemia, metabolic acidosis.
Clinical deterioration, lethargy, poor feeding, or symptoms compatible with kernicterus.
Modified from Gartner LM, Lee K-S: Jaundice and liver disease. *In* Fanaroff AA, Martin RJ (eds). Neonatal-Perinatal Medicine, 5th ed. St Louis: Mosby–Year Book, 1992:1075–1104.

(even on the first day of life) from criteria used for term infants with anemia and unconjugated hyperbilirubinemia due to other etiologies.

Amount and Type of Blood. A two-volume exchange (160 ml/kg) replaces 85% to 90% of the sensitized red cells and eliminates 55% of the intravascular bilirubin. However, only 25% to 35% of the total bilirubin pool is eliminated, and this may result in a rapid postexchange influx of bilirubin into the intravascular space. Although some of the anti-D antibody is also removed, residual anti-D antibodies in the extravascular pool may contribute to subsequent hemolysis of Rh-positive cells. Bilirubin may, therefore, continue to rise and postexchange values must be monitored closely until a safe plateau is established. The blood should be compatible with both the mother and the infant's serum and free of the antigen corresponding to the antibody responsible for the hemolysis. Thus, the erythrocytes are

1. Rh (D) negative if maternal antibody is anti-D
2. Group O if mother and infant are of different ABO groups
3. Group specific if mother and child have the same ABO group

Whole Blood or Blood Components

1. Whole blood: Heparinized fresh whole blood is metabolically superior but has a short shelf life and is not readily available. The time required for identifying a suitable donor and performing the required screening of fresh blood may be more than 24 hours, thus precluding its use in neonates requiring urgent exchange transfusions.
2. Reconstituted blood components: Erythrocytes reconstituted with fresh frozen plasma and restored to a hematocrit of 45% to 50% are generally used. These erythrocyte preparations include
   a. Fresh (<7 days old) erythrocytes collected in CPDA-1
   b. Saline-washed erythrocytes stored 7 days
   c. Frozen and deglycerolized erythrocytes

One of the disadvantages of reconstituting erythrocytes with fresh frozen plasma is that the infant is usually exposed to a minimum of two donors. To avoid exposure to additional donors, the actual volume to be exchanged in larger neonates should be approximated to the nearest packed red cell unit. In very low birth weight infants, only a portion of a unit is required, and the rest should be preserved by the blood bank for future use in the same infant.

Irradiation of the erythrocytes is indicated when transfusing infants who have been treated with an intrauterine transfusion, in infants with a suspected cellular immunodeficiency or malignancy, and when blood is donated by a first-degree relative.

Method. The procedure must be supervised by experienced personnel. Respiratory, acid-base, and cardiovascular status should be

TABLE 3. Potential Complications of Exchange Transfusion

Blood Components Related
Transmission of infection
  Hepatitis
  Human immunodeficiency virus
  Cytomegalovirus, malaria, syphilis
  Bacterial
Metabolic
  Hypoglycemia
  Hypocalcemia, hyperkalemia
  Acidosis, alkalosis
Bleeding
  Thrombocytopenia
  Excessive heparinization
Hemolysis of transfused blood: sickle cell hemoglobin
Graft-versus-host disease

Umbilical Venous Catheter Related
Air embolism
Thrombosis, embolization
Necrotizing enterocolitis
Vessel perforation, intravascular catheter loss
Accidental hemorrhage
Bacterial infection
Cardiac arrhythmia

closely monitored. The transfusion is generally performed through an umbilical venous catheter placed through the ductus venosus into the inferior vena cava, near but not in the heart. Ideally, the location of the catheter tip should be documented radiographically before initiating the exchange. A rule of thumb is to insert the umbilical venous line 1 cm beyond the area where good blood return is obtained. Free flow of blood must be assured before starting the exchange.

Only end-hole catheters should be used, as the dead space near the tip of side-hole catheters promotes thrombus formation. Before insertion, the umbilical venous catheter must be filled with heparinized saline (1 U of heparin per milliliter of saline) and connected to a syringe. It should *never* be left open to air, since negative intrathoracic pressure may result in an air embolism. The catheter should be secured with suture, and the insertion site should be visible at all times to avoid accidental hemorrhage.

Exchange transfusions can be accomplished using a discontinuous or an isovolumetric technique. In the discontinuous or push-pull method, blood is alternately removed and replaced through a single vascular access in aliquots that are tolerated by the infant. Usually, this is 5 ml per pass for infants weighing under 1500 g, 10 ml for infants weighing 1500 to 2500 g, 15 ml for infants weighing 2500 to 3500 g, and 20 ml for infants over 3500 g. With a single syringe connected to a special four-way stopcock (a commercially available, disposable kit), the predetermined aliquot of blood is gradually withdrawn from the baby and discarded into a waste container. The replacement blood for transfusion is then withdrawn from the buretrol and gradually infused into the baby. The stopcock is rotated in a clockwise sequence to avoid errors, and the entire procedure is completed in a relatively closed system. Each push-pull cycle may be completed in 2 to 4 minutes (total time, 1 to 2 hours). Care should be taken to minimize abrupt hemodynamic changes, especially in preterm neonates at risk for intraventricular hemorrhage.

The isovolumetric exchange transfusion may be less stressful for preterm and sick newborn infants. This method requires two persons who concurrently and continuously remove blood through an umbilical arterial catheter and replace it through an umbilical venous catheter. Automated syringe pumps may be used if the venous and arterial catheters are of the same caliber. Donor blood must be gently agitated every 15 minutes, as sedimentation of the RBCs may result in blood with a reduced hemoglobin concentration toward the end of the procedure. Blood is warmed in an in-line blood warmer to a maximum of 37°C and infused through a standard blood filter. The practice of routinely using supplemental calcium or albumin or both before or

during an exchange is controversial. It may be prudent to monitor serum levels of ionized calcium and albumin and treat only if necessary.

AFTER EXCHANGE TRANSFUSION. Rebound of bilirubin is common in the immediate postexchange period. Hence, bilirubin values need to be followed closely. Indications for repeat exchange transfusion are the same as for the first exchange. Hypoglycemia is common in the first 1 to 2 hours after the exchange transfusion. Glucose should be measured whenever signs compatible with hypoglycemia appear. Electrolytes and calcium should be determined shortly after the exchange transfusion and repeated thereafter as needed.

The catheter may be kept in place if a repeat exchange transfusion in the next several hours is contemplated.

After Discharge. Late anemias are commonly observed in infants with erythroblastosis fetalis. Infants who have and who have not been exchanged are both at risk for this complication. In some circumstances, the anemia can be severe and lead to cardiac failure or death. Furthermore, infants treated with multiple intrauterine transfusions can develop bone marrow hypoplasia and demonstrate late anemia with low or absent reticulocyte counts and low erythropoietin levels despite hematocrit readings as low as 15%. These infants may require repeated transfusions, although a recent pilot study suggests that erythropoietin 200 μL/kg SC given three times a week may have a role in shortening the duration of the postnatal anemia and decreasing the number of postnatal transfusions required by infants with Rh hemolytic disease.

Experimental Therapies. Tin-protoporphyrin, a synthetic heme analog, inhibits the activity of heme oxygenase and thereby limits the degradation of heme to bile pigment. Administration of this agent to experimental animals has been shown to decrease bilirubin. The usefulness of tin-protoporphyrin and other protoporphyrins and mesoporphyrins in neonatal hemolytic disease is undetermined.

ABO HEMOLYTIC DISEASE

Hemolytic disease can also occur when the major blood group antigens of the fetus are different from those of the mother. Anti-A

TABLE 4. Clinical and Laboratory Features of Rh and ABO Incompatibility

	Rh INCOMPATIBILITY	ABO INCOMPATIBILITY
Mother	Rh (D) negative	O group
Neonate	Rh (D) positive	A or B group
Antenatal screening	Mandatory	None
Antenatal prophylaxis	RhIg routine at 28 wk, delivery, other special indications	None
Antenatal fetal treatment	May be necessary	None
First pregnancy affected	Rare (<5%)	Often (40%–50%)
Subsequent pregnancies	Increasing severity	Not predictable
Stillbirths, hydrops	Yes	None, rare
Severe anemia at birth	Common	Unusual
Late anemia	Frequent	Rare
Hepatosplenomegaly	+++	+
Jaundice in first 24 h	Yes	Yes
Direct Coombs test (baby)	+++	Weak; cord blood more likely to be positive
Indirect Coombs test	Always +	+
Spherocytes	None	++
Nucleated RBC	+++	+
Reticulocytosis	++	+
Need for exchange transfusion	60%–70%	10%
Selection of blood for transfusion	Rh(D) negative Group specific	Group O only

or anti-B antibodies in the serum of an O group mother can enter the fetal circulation and react with erythrocytes of a group A or B fetus. Unlike Rh hemolytic disease, ABO incompatibility does not require previous sensitization because of naturally occurring anti-A or anti-B antibodies in the mother. Hence, ABO incompatibility can be seen in first pregnancies and cannot usually be predicted. The incidence is significantly higher in African Americans than in Caucasians and occurs with equal frequency in newborns of primipara and multipara mothers. Subsequent pregnancies are not more severely affected.

Forty-five percent of the U.S. population have O blood group, 41% have A, 10% have B, and 4% have AB blood group. In approximately 20% of pregnancies, maternal serum contains anti-A or anti-B antibodies, and the fetal erythrocytes bear the respective antigen. Yet only 3% of pregnancies have evidence of ABO incompatibility disease, and exchange transfusion is required in only 1:1000 to 1:4000 pregnancies. Well-known differences between ABO incompatibility and RH incompatibility are shown in Table 4. Hemolysis in ABO incompatibility is usually not severe, the direct Coombs test is only weakly positive, and the RBCs have only a slightly decreased life span for the following reasons.

1. The newborn erythrocyte has a sparse distribution of A or B antigenic sites, which limits binding of anti-A and anti-B antibodies.
2. The presence of the A or B antigen in all the neonatal body tissues permits widespread neutralization of maternal antibody.
3. Placental antigens neutralize maternal antibody, thereby decreasing the amount of antibody transplacentally transported.

Clinical and Laboratory Features

1. The direct Coombs test is weakly positive or negative and is more likely to be positive in cord blood. For this reason, cord bloods are saved in our nursery and examined whenever the possibility of ABO incompatibility is present. In addition, naturally occuring anti-A IgG is an incomplete antibody that agglutinates well in 20% albumin but poorly in normal saline. It is important to note that a positive Coombs test does not always mean that the neonate has hemolytic disease. The diagnosis of ABO hemolytic disease is one of exclusion.
2. The predominant sign is unconjugated hyperbilirubinemia during the first 24 hours of life.
3. Conjugated hyperbilirubinemia, sometimes severe, can be present at birth. Therefore, an extensive and unnecessary workup should be avoided when the diagnosis of ABO incompatibility is considered. A decrease in conjugated bilirubin is usually observed within the first 2 weeks of postnatal life.
4. Anemia is generally mild and supports the diagnosis. The reticulocyte count is elevated.
5. A distinguishing feature of ABO hemolytic disease is the presence of an abnormal number of microspherocytes in the peripheral blood smear. Antibody-coated erythrocytes lose a portion of their membrane during passage through the spleen and liver, leading to a reduced red cell membrane/volume ratio and formation of microspherocytes with increased osmotic fragility. The microspherocytes are best demonstrated and quantitated by the glutaraldehyde-fixed preparations.
6. Physical examination may be normal, or there may be hepatosplenomegaly secondary to extramedullary erythropoiesis.

Treatment

Treatment is directed at lowering bilirubin levels. Exchange transfusion for the sole purpose of removal of antibody or sensitized red cells is not necessary. Although the disease is usually mild, we have seen many infants with severe disease who require repeated exchange transfusion. With phototherapy, bilirubin levels may plateau despite rapidly rising levels in the first 24 hours after birth. Occasionally, anemia may be sufficiently severe to require a simple transfusion. Late anemia does not occur because anti-A and anti-B antibodies

disappear from the newborn's circulation, presumably due to antibody uptake by A or B substance.

MINOR GROUP HEMOLYTIC DISEASE

The majority of minor group antibodies are anti-C, anti-E, and anti-Kell. Hemolytic disease is infrequent because of the low potency of the corresponding antigens. The diagnosis and therapeutic intervention in these disorders are similar to those described for Rh hemolytic disease.

NEONATAL POLYCYTHEMIA AND HYPERVISCOSITY

VIRGINIA DELANEY-BLACK, M.D.

DIAGNOSIS

Neonatal polycythemia represents a significant increase in newborn hematocrit from the normal range at term (40% to 60%) to levels of 65% or greater. Identifying the polycythemic newborn is complicated by variations in the venous hematocrit during the immediate newborn period. Studies have suggested that the hematocrit at term will rise from cord levels to a peak at 2 hours of age and then drop slowly over the next several hours. It is important to recognize this natural variation in diagnosing polycythemia. The infant whose hematocrit level makes him or her polycythemic at 2 hours of age may, without any intervention, have a normal level at 6 to 8 hours following delivery. Routine hematocrit screening in the well infant has been reviewed recently by the American Academy of Pediatrics Committee on Fetus and Newborn. The Committee does not recommend universal screening, although screening for high-risk infants may be appropriate. In the child with distress, the timing of initial hematocrit screening should be determined by the signs.

One of the most common pitfalls in defining polycythemia is to use a heelstick or fingerstick hematocrit without a confirming venous sample. Peripheral sampling overestimates the venous hematocrit in newborns. The difference between the two sites may be minimal if the extremity is warm and peripheral perfusion is good. However, in the immediate newborn period or even later in the infant with problems, there may be very poor correlation. Although the peripheral hematocrit level may suggest polycythemia, confirmation by venous (or arterial) sampling is necessary.

NEONATAL HYPERVISCOSITY SYNDROME

The major contribution to whole blood viscosity in newborns is hematocrit value. Hence, most infants with elevated viscosity will also be polycythemic. Infants with altered plasma proteins or lipids or abnormal red blood cell deformability may have hyperviscosity without polycythemia. Considerable variance in the frequency of hyperviscosity without polycythemia has been reported. Because viscosity is not measured in the clinical setting, a high index of suspicion may be required.

ETIOLOGY AND COMPLICATIONS

It is commonly believed that cord blood hematocrits are higher than normal adult hematocrits because of the lower arterial oxygen concentration to which the fetus is exposed during intrauterine life. Increasing the fetal hematocrit increases the oxygen-carrying capacity. Factors that may interfere with placental oxygen concentration have all been associated with increased newborn hematocrits to varying degrees. For example, high altitude, maternal diabetes, and intrauterine growth retardation have all been associated with an increased risk of neonatal polycythemia, whereas maternal smoking typically results in only a small but measurable increase in hematocrit.

Even under these adverse intrauterine conditions, not all infants will develop polycythemia. At sea level, as few as 1% to 2% of infants will have elevated hematocrit values, and at 5000 feet, as many as 4% to 5% may be affected. Conversely, not all newborns with neonatal polycythemia have been exposed to prolonged oxygen deprivation. Acute or chronic placental transfusions may also result in polycythemia. The earliest descriptions of neonatal polycythemia were in monozygotic twins with arteriovenous anastomoses. The donor twin on the arterial side was anemic, and the recipient twin on the venous side was polycythemic. Because the transfusion was chronic, both twins probably had relatively normal blood volumes. Infants with more acute placental transfusions following delayed cord clamping or fetal distress may have an increased blood volume at delivery and may have tachypnea as a result. In most infants with polycythemia, there is no obvious cause identified.

A variety of newborn problems have been associated with neonatal polycythemia (Table 1). Fortunately, even when these problems appear, most polycythemic infants do well. Careful observations and symptomatic treatment for hypoglycemia, feeding difficulties, and cardiorespiratory problems usually suffice. If signs persist or if the signs are serious, treatment with partial plasma exchange transfusion may be warranted to reduce the neonatal problems. It is important to use caution in determining who should undergo this procedure, which has its own inherent risks. There is no convincing evidence that postnatal treatment of polycythemia, particularly if it has been present for some time before delivery, will eliminate sequelae. Furthermore, if sequelae do occur, they may be related to the cause of the polycythemia, rather than to the polycythemia itself.

TREATMENT

When a partial plasma exchange transfusion is warranted by the child's condition, appropriate preparations will reduce the risk. To calculate the volume of exchange, the following formula may be used.

$$\frac{\text{Estimated blood volume} \times (\text{current Hct} - \text{desired Hct})}{\text{current Hct}}$$

or in a term infant

$$\frac{\text{Weight (kg)} \times 80 \text{ ml/kg} \times (\text{current Hct} - 50\%)}{\text{current Hct}}$$

A typical volume of exchange for a 3-kg term infant would range from 48 ml (initial hematocrit of 65%) to 80 ml (initial hematocrit of 75%).

Plasmanate is often the diluent used because it will remain within the intravascular space. Unless mitigating factors exist, fresh frozen plasma, because of its coagulation factors, should not be used. The initial procedure is similar to a two-volume exchange transfusion and requires a warmer bed, a monitor, a sterile exchange tray, and an individual to supervise and record. The infant should be restrained. The stomach can be aspirated if the infant has fed or if secretions are present. The umbilical site should be prepared and draped. A slow pull-push procedure through the umbilical vein is the technique most commonly used. Other techniques use one or more peripheral sites to avoid the potential adverse effects of the procedure on gastrointestinal blood flow. Even when peripheral sites are used, signs of bowel ischemia may occur. Following the exchange, the infant should be given nothing by mouth (NPO) until stable. Vital signs should be monitored until the infant is clinically well. Careful observation for hypoglycemia is needed, especially if the infant is to be without feedings for several hours. With appropriate calculation of the volume for exchange, the need for a second procedure is extremely unlikely.

REFERENCE

1. American Academy of Pediatrics Committee on Fetus and Newborn: Routine evaluation of blood pressure, hematocrit, and glucose in newborns. Pediatrics 92:474–476, 1993.

NEONATAL SKIN DISORDERS

LAWRENCE M. SOLOMON, M.D.
STEVEN W. NEUBAUER, M.D.

Normal skin care should include gentle washing with a mild antibacterial soap, such as chlorhexidine gluconate 4% solution, after temperature stability is achieved. Vernix need not be completely removed. Baby products should be avoided, and a fragrance-free hydrophilic ointment or cream can be used for lubrication. What is trivial trauma in an adult may cause skin injury in the neonate, and adhesives, such as those in tape, should be avoided. The umbilical cord is often treated with triple dye and then cleaned daily with alcohol. Antibacterial ointments may be used when outbreaks of staphylococcal disease occur.

TRANSIENT CUTANEOUS LESIONS

Physiologic Desquamation

This normal phenomenon begins in the first few days of life and consists of very superficial scaling that resolves spontaneously. It does not require treatment except for appearance, which may improve with lubricants.

Milia

Milia occur normally in term infants as yellow or pearly white, 1-mm papules on the face, scalp, and, rarely, the penis. When they occur in the mouth, they are referred to as Epstein's pearls. No treatment is required, and they resolve spontaneously in the first few weeks of life.

Miliaria

Miliaria result from obstruction of the sweat gland ducts and occur in a warm, humid environment. Tiny superficial vesicles without redness (miliaria crystallina) and with redness (miliaria rubra) may occur. A less warm, dry environment is the only treatment necessary.

Sebaceous Hypertrophy

Sebaceous hypertrophy is seen as a profusion of very tiny (0.1 to 0.2 mm) white or yellow lesions over the nose and malar region. These hyperplastic sebaceous glands fade spontaneously over the first few weeks of life.

Sucking Blisters

Sucking blisters occasionally are found at birth on the upper extremity as small intact or ruptured bullae. No treatment is required.

TABLE 1. Neonatal Findings and Diagnoses Associated with Neonatal Polycythemia

Cardiorespiratory	**Hematologic**
Tachypnea	Hyperbilirubinemia
Cyanosis	Disseminated intravascular
Apnea	coagulation
Cardiomegaly and increased pulmonary	Thrombocytopenia
vascularity	
	Metabolic
Gastrointestinal	Hypoglycemia
Poor feeding	
Regurgitation	**Neurologic**
Abdominal distention	Lethargy
Diarrhea	Hypotonia
Necrotizing enterocolitis	Seizures
Pneumatosis intestinalis	Tremulousness

Lesions Due to Birth Injury

Petechiae, abrasions, ecchymoses, and, in the extreme case, skin necrosis may occur on the presenting part. These all generally heal without serious sequelae. Mechanical injury due to laceration, burns, forceps, or scalp electrodes also may occur and should be treated conservatively with antibiotic ointment. Viral or bacterial infection should be ruled out.

Caput Succedaneum

Caput succedaneum is a diffuse edematous swelling of the presenting portion of the scalp. The boggy swollen skin may display a few ecchymoses, and this may occur also on the perineum. The swelling generally resolves after a few days to a week.

Cutis Aplasia

This localized congenital absence of the skin is a relatively rare developmental anomaly that occurs most frequently on the scalp. The lesions are sharply marginated, 1 to 2 cm in size, atrophic and hairless, or ulcerated. They may be associated with an underlying skull defect or, rarely, with other malformations. Conservative treatment with antibiotic ointment leads to healing in a few months. Biopsy or surgical procedures generally are not necessary, although a skull film may be appropriate.

Erythema Toxicum

Erythema toxicum is an extremely common, benign, self-limited eruption in term infants. Firm, discrete, 1- to 3-cm, pale yellow or white papules and pustules occur on an erythematous base, or erythematous macules, up to 3 cm in diameter may occur alone. Lesions typically appear between 24 and 48 hours of age but may appear up until 2 weeks of age. They typically last less than 1 week. Individual lesions occur most often on the trunk but may appear anywhere except on the palms or soles.

A smear of the contents of a pustule will reveal many intraepidermal eosinophils, and peripheral eosinophilia may be present. The cause is unknown, and there are no associated complications. Treatment is not required. An infant with this eruption should be observed for other possible diagnoses, such as a bacterial or viral infection.

Transient Neonatal Pustular Melanosis

This is another common, self-limited, benign dermatosis of the neonatal period that presents at birth as a spectrum of lesions varying from pigmented macules (encircled by a fine scale) to superficial vesicopustules. As the vesicles rupture, they often leave hyperpigmented macules that may be present for months. New lesions usually do not develop after birth. There is very little or no erythema, and a smear of the lesional contents reveals mostly polymorphonuclear leukocytes. Dark-skinned infants are most often visibly affected, and as in erythema toxicum, the cause is unknown. A search for other possible diagnoses should be made in an ill infant, most notably bacterial or viral infection.

NEVI

Nevi are described elsewhere and are discussed here only to outline appropriate therapy during the neonatal period.

Vascular Nevi

Most vascular lesions, whether flat, capillary (strawberry), cavernous, or mixed, require no treatment during the neonatal period except as outlined. With very large vascular malformations or diffuse neonatal hemangiomatosis, there may be associated involvement of organs other than skin and there may be cardiovascular compromise. Large hemangiomas may be associated with thrombocytopenia (Kasabach-Merritt syndrome). Port-wine stains in the region of the first branch of the trigeminal nerve may be associated with Sturge-Weber syndrome and require CNS and ocular examination. Hemangiomas that completely obstruct vision or compromise the airway require

immediate intervention. A short intensive course of corticosteroids may be effective in such cases.

Pigmented Nevi

Congenital pigmented nevi may be observed in 1 of 22 newborn infants. It is important to differentiate between nevocellular nevi, epidermal nevi, cafe au lait macules, lentigines, and a dermal melanosis such as Mongolian spot. All these lesions are pigmented and may be seen at birth. During the neonatal period, attention should be directed at those lesions associated with extracutaneous involvement. Extensive and midline congenital nevocellular nevi may be associated with leptomeningeal melanocytosis. Large and small congenital nevocellular nevi are associated with malignant transformation and should be evaluated for excision. Epidermal nevi are linear hyperpigmented (scaly) lesions that are often present at birth. They are associated with central nervous system, skeletal, ocular, and renal anomalies.

DIAPER DERMATITIS

PAUL J. HONIG, M.D.

Diaper dermatitis is a significant problem for pediatricians and family physicians. The incidence of the problem in the United States is unknown. However, 20% of skin consultations for infants and young children in Great Britain are because of diaper dermatitis.

Although the causes of diaper dermatitis are many, the diaper seems to be the essential element. Infants raised in cultures where diapers are not used rarely have problems in the diaper area. Additionally, the skin area covered by a diaper is rarely inflamed in toilet-trained children.

The common categories of diaper dermatitis include primary irritant dermatitis, monilial diaper dermatitis with or without id, atopic diathesis, seborrheic diathesis, or a combination of these (mixed diaper dermatitis). Knowledge of the factors that contribute to inflammation of the skin in the diaper area (Fig. 1) in all the conditions mentioned allows one to make sensible treatment decisions.

Occlusion (trapping of moisture) and friction are responsible for most of the changes seen in the diaper area. The diaper area should be kept as dry as possible. Therefore, the frequency of washing should be decreased, and mild soaps (e.g., Dove, Tone, Caress) should be recommended. Adding more moisture to wet skin makes no sense. Removal of diapers for as long as is practical [not after feeding (gastrocolic reflex) or drinking a large volume of fluid] is very helpful. Avoidance of airtight occlusions is important. Infants with an atopic diathesis do worse with frequent cleansing, and therefore a mother's urge to cleanse must be restrained. Diaper wipes should be avoided. Moisturizers can be used as cold cream cleansers to clean and deodorize the diaper area after urination. Soap and water should be used only after bowel movements. Friction can be reduced by avoiding tightly fitting diapers. Petrolatum decreases friction but traps moisture and potentially causes further maceration of the skin. Although diaper area ointments are used to reduce friction, most have not been tested. Cornstarch is an excellent agent for reducing friction and has the added benefit of absorbing moisture.

Once maceration of skin occurs, overgrowth of *Candida albicans* and bacteria occurs on the skin surface of the diaper area. Many of the topical antifungals, such as clotrimazole and econazole, will clear *C. albicans,* as well as *Staphylococcus aureus.* If thrush is present, oral nystatin 200,000 U (2 ml) 1 ml into each cheek four times per day for 7 days is advisable. This medication may help those infants who are seeding *C. albicans* from their gastrointestinal tracts onto the skin of the diaper area.

Topical application of a broad-spectrum antibiotic cream is necessary to eliminate gram-negative bacteria. Eradication of these organisms is vital because of the enzymes they can produce. These enzymes (ureases) break down urea, releasing ammonia, which raises

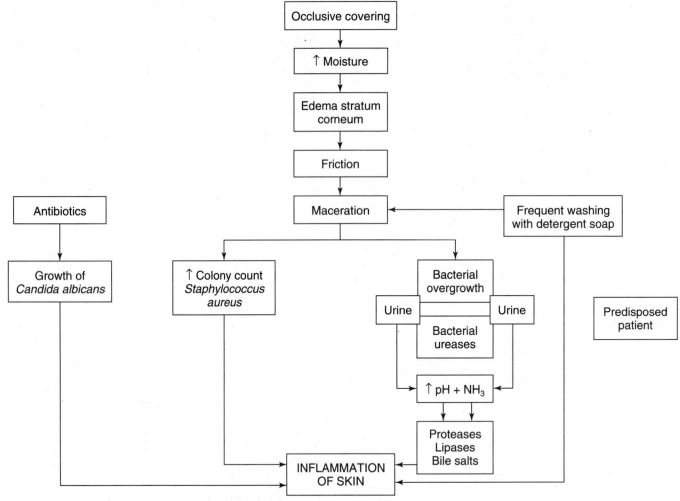

FIGURE 1. Factors that contribute to inflammation of the skin in the diaper area. (From Honig PJ: Dermatitis. In Textbook of Pediatric Emergency Medicine. Baltimore, Williams & Wilkins, 1993.)

the pH of the environment. At a high pH, the activity of proteases and lipases from the intestine (i.e., from the pancreas and intestinal flora) is increased and, in association with bile salts, further accentuates inflammation and skin damage. Acidification of the environment with oral cranberry juice or tea will reduce the activity of these harmful enzymes. Barrier creams, such as triple paste, afford added protection to the skin from the proteases, lipases, and similar enzymes.

Hydrocortisone cream 1% is an appropriate topical steroid for control of inflammation in the diaper area of any of the various types of diaper dermatitis. Fluorinated steroids should never be used under occlusion of the diaper. Combination creams that include steroids stronger than 1% hydrocortisone (e.g., Lotrisone, Mycolog) should be avoided in children.

Parents should not be made to feel guilty about the presence of a diaper rash. In many instances, individual predispositions (e.g., atopic eczema) make individual infants prone to recurrences. Psychologic support is important for families in these circumstances. One must stress that when all else fails to cure the rash, toilet training will not (toilet training should not be advised, however, until an infant is 18 months of age or older).

Other diagnoses to consider if a rash in the diaper area does not respond to treatment include histiocytosis X, acrodermatitis enteropathica, mucocutaneous candidiasis, psoriasis, scabies, and allergic contact dermatitis. These entities may look very similar to routine diaper dermatitis, but routine therapy will not clear the condition in

a reasonable period of time. Therefore, diaper dermatitides recalcitrant to therapy should be referred to a pediatric dermatologist for further evaluation.

APNEA OF PREMATURITY

MONA SHEHAB, M.D.
RICHARD J. MARTIN, M.D.

Apnea is an extremely common disorder of prematurity that if left untreated, has the potential of compromising the well-being of any infant. Apnea is most common in the very immature infant, with 25% of infants under 2500 g and 84% of infants under 1000 g exhibiting apneic episodes during the neonatal period. The onset of apnea typically occurs during the first week of life or after termination of assisted ventilation. Thereafter, the frequency and duration of apnea decrease as postconceptional age approaches term.

Infants who exhibit frequent apnea of more than 10 to 15 seconds duration, accompanied by clinically significant bradycardia or oxygen desaturation, require medical intervention. In many of these infants, bradycardia is the presenting symptom and is thought to be a consequence of obstructed or ineffective inspiratory efforts that fail to trigger an apnea alarm. An infant can be presumed to have idiopathic apnea of prematurity only if a precipitating cause of the apnea, such as infection, intracranial pathology, metabolic disorder, such as hypoglycemia, or impaired oxygen delivery (secondary to hypoxemia or anemia) cannot be identified. Careful clinical judgment, following a good history and physical examination, is needed to determine how aggressively such a specific etiology for neonatal apnea should be sought before starting symptomatic therapy.

The pharmacologic agents most widely used for the treatment of apnea of prematurity are the methylxanthines, theophylline, and caffeine. Pharmacologic data in infants have demonstrated a markedly prolonged elimination half-life for theophylline in premature newborns when compared with more mature newborns, children, or adults. Because the usual metabolic pathways for theophylline elimination, via hydroxylation or demethylation, are undeveloped, elimination progresses by a slow but available pathway of methylation to caffeine, which is itself biologically active. Both agents are very effective, have their various advocates, and have been widely used for nearly 20 years. Theophylline is typically administered as an initial loading dose of 5 to 6 mg/kg, followed by a maintenance dose of 1 to 2 mg/kg every 8 hours. The intravenous route is typically used at the start of therapy, and the oral route is then substituted. When intravenous administration is needed, and IV theophylline is not available, aminophylline (theophylline ethylenediamine, 79% theophylline by weight) may be given at doses that are 20% higher. Serum concentrations of theophylline should be monitored whenever aminophylline or theophylline is used. Therapeutic concentrations of 5 to 10 μg/ml are desirable, and concentrations above 15 μg/ml should be avoided. The therapeutic effect of theophylline may include the additional effect of its caffeine metabolite, which is commonly found in serum at 30% of the concomitant theophylline concentration. When caffeine is used therapeutically, it is given orally, usually as caffeine citrate. A loading dose of 10 mg/kg caffeine is followed by 2.5 mg/kg caffeine once daily to achieve serum concentrations from 5 to 20 μg/ml. For both agents, the most commonly observed toxic effects are tachycardia, feeding intolerance, and hyperexcitability. No serious long-term sequelae have been reported.

Presumably, the methylxanthines stimulate central neural output to the respiratory muscles, although the precise mechanisms whereby they decrease apnea have not been determined. The decision about when this therapy should be discontinued may be more difficult than deciding when to begin treatment. The most common clinical practice is to stop xanthine therapy as soon as possible after 35 weeks postconceptional age has been reached and apnea has ceased. The infant should then be monitored closely for approximately 7 days to ensure that clinically significant apneic episodes do not recur. Another pharmacologic agent, doxapram, has been proposed for infants in whom xanthines are ineffective, but its use has not gained broad acceptance, and concerns about its safety have not been resolved.

For recently extubated preterm infants or those not responding readily to xanthine therapy, continuous positive airway pressure (CPAP) delivered by nasal prongs at 2 to 5 cm H_2O pressure is a safe and effective way to treat apnea of prematurity. CPAP is thought to decrease the frequency of apnea by splinting the upper airway with positive pressure. Therefore, CPAP may be most effective in infants whose apneic episodes are precipitated or prolonged by pharyngeal obstruction. Some infants on CPAP develop abdominal distention related to feeding difficulties, and irritation of the nose also may occur. When prolonged apnea persists in spite of these therapeutic efforts, endotracheal intubation and artificial ventilation should be initiated at minimal ventilator settings to allow for spontaneous ventilatory efforts and minimize the risk of barotrauma. Meanwhile, a review of the history and physical examination is appropriate, for it is possible that an underlying, potentially treatable cause of such severe persistent apnea may be found.

REFERENCES

1. Aranda JV, Turmen T: Methylxanthines in apnea of prematurity. *In* Soyka LF (ed): Clinical Perinatology, Philadelphia, WB Saunders Co, 1979:87–108.
2. Brouard C, Moriette G, Murat I, et al: Comparative efficacy of theophylline and caffeine in the treatment of idiopathic apnea in premature infants. Am J Dis Child 139:698–700, 1985.
3. Miller MJ, Martin RJ: Apnea of prematurity. *In* Hunt CE (ed): Clinical Perinatology. Philadelphia, WB Saunders Co, 1992:789–808.

INTRAUTERINE DIAGNOSIS AND APPROACH TO THE MALFORMED INFANT

Deborah A. Driscoll, M.D.

Advances in prenatal diagnosis enable the obstetrician and geneticist to identify many congenital malformations, chromosomal abnormalities, and gene defects antenatally. Specific indications for prenatal genetic testing are well established (Table 1). Although routine ultrasound screening of all pregnancies is still controversial, the diagnostic capacity of ultrasonography has increased significantly and permits the reliable detection of many structural abnormalities during the second trimester of pregnancy (Table 2). Once an anomaly is detected, a comprehensive fetal evaluation is essential to establish a diagnosis, provide the family with an appropriate prognosis, and formulate a realistic management plan.

FETAL EVALUATION

When an anomaly is detected during routine sonographic examination, referral to a prenatal diagnostic center with expertise in the evaluation, diagnosis, and management of fetal malformations is recommended. A team approach that includes a geneticist, perinatologist, neonatologist, pediatric surgeon, pediatric subspecialists, and genetic counselor is often used to arrive at a diagnosis and an accurate assessment of prognosis and treatment options. This approach provides parents with the information and support they need to make important decisions regarding the evaluation and treatment of their fetus.

History

A complete history, including an extended family history, is obtained to determine if the pregnancy is at risk for an identifiable genetic disorder, if similar or related anomalies are present in relatives, or if there was known exposure to teratogens or infectious agents associated with congenital anomalies.

Ultrasonography

A very detailed sonographic examination is performed to confirm the presence of a fetal anomaly, judge the severity of the defect, and evaluate other organ systems for associated abnormalities. It is important to differentiate single, isolated malformations from multiple anomalies. Certain kinds of anomalies may occur together either as a nonrandom association of findings, such as the VATER (vertebral,

TABLE 1. Indications for Prenatal Genetic Evaluation

Advanced maternal age
Previous child with a chromosomal abnormality
Parent is carrier of a balanced translocation
Parents are known carriers of an autosomal recessive gene
Parent is carrier of an X-linked or autosomal dominant gene
Previous child with a congenital malformation
Previous stillbirth or multiple spontaneous abortions
Fetal congenital malformation

TABLE 2. Congenital Malformations That May be Detected by Ultrasonography

TABLE 2. Congenital Malformations That May be Detected by Ultrasonography

Neural tube defects
  Anencephaly
  Spina bifida
Hydrocephalus
Cystic hygroma
Ventral wall defects
  Omphalocele
  Gastroschisis
Genitourinary anomalies
  Renal agenesis
  Hydronephrosis
  Polycystic kidney disease
Heart defects
Cleft lip and palate

anal atresia, tracheoesophageal fistula, renal or radial defects) association, or as part of a well-defined genetic disorder due to a single gene defect. Alternatively, they may occur as a result of a chromosomal abnormality. The identification of a particular pattern of anomalies often provides us with clues to the diagnostic possibilities, enabling us to provide the family with prognostic information.

This is accomplished by screening the entire fetus, with particular attention to known associated findings. For example, cardiovascular and genitourinary abnormalities and neural tube defects are frequently seen in association with an omphalocele. Therefore, in addition to a sonogram to evaluate the spine, intracranial anatomy, kidneys, and bladder, a fetal echocardiogram should be performed to evaluate the fetal heart.

Ultrasonography can also be used to visualize more subtle abnormalities, such as hypertelorism or hypotelorism, cleft lip and palate, abnormal ear position, and micrognathia. These findings may be suggestive of a known genetic syndrome or chromosomal abnormality, such as trisomy 13. However, it is important to realize that there are technical limitations because of the fetal position, maternal body habitus, and amniotic fluid volume that may influence the ability of the ultrasonographer to detect minor anomalies. Furthermore, the presence of some features may be dependent on the gestational age of the fetus.

Fetal Echocardiography

Cardiac defects are the most common type of congenital malformation (4 to 8 per 1000 liveborn infants) and frequently occur in association with extracardiac malformations and chromosomal abnormalities. Indications for fetal echocardiography are listed in Table 3. A fetal echocardiogram is generally performed after 18 weeks gestation to define cardiac position and to evaluate the four chambers, ventricular outflow tracts, aortic arch, venous connections, heart rate, and rhythm.

Cytogenetic Studies

In most instances when a fetal anomaly is detected by ultrasonography or echocardiography, it is advisable to obtain fetal cells for cytogenetic analysis. Numerical and structural chromosomal abnormalities may result in malformations that may be seen sonographically. For example, trisomy 21 is associated with endocardial cushion defects, duodenal atresia, cystic hygromas, and more subtle findings, such as nuchal skin thickening and hypoplasia of the middle phalanx of the fifth digit. Multiple malformations are frequently seen in association with trisomy 18 and 13 as well.

The presence of a fetal chromosomal abnormality may dramatically alter the obstetric as well as neonatal management. In a previable fetus with a severe congenital anomaly or a cytogenetic abnormality, such as aneuploidy or an unbalanced translocation, a couple may wish to electively terminate the pregnancy. If the fetus is viable and has a cytogenetic abnormality, such as trisomy 18 or 13, which is considered lethal and is usually not compatible with extrauterine survival, the obstetrician and neonatologist may consider performing a cesarean section only for maternal indications, withholding resuscitative efforts at delivery and refraining from postnatal or in utero surgical intervention. When there is uncertainty about the prognosis, close monitoring of the pregnancy and postnatal evaluation of the infant are recommended.

As in utero fetal therapy becomes more widely used for the treatment of congenital malformations, cytogenetic analysis should be considered essential in the evaluation of a fetus as a potential candidate for this type of intervention.

PROCEDURES FOR OBTAINING FETAL CELLS

Amniocentesis

Amniocentesis is the most widely used technique for obtaining a fetal sample for cytogenetic analysis in the second and third trimesters. The fluid and cells may also be used for metabolic studies, DNA testing, and alpha-fetoprotein testing when indicated. Amniocentesis refers to the removal of amniotic fluid transabdominally under sonographic guidance. The procedure is performed after 15 weeks gestation and is considered a relatively safe procedure. There is approximately a 0.5% procedure-related risk of miscarriage. The cells must be cultured before analysis, and it may require 7 to 14 days for a cytogenetic diagnosis.

Chorionic Villus Sampling

Chorionic villus sampling (CVS) is an alternative method that may be used to obtain a sample of the fetal trophoblast tissue for fetal cytogenetic, biochemical, and molecular analysis. It is performed earlier in pregnancy, at 10 to 12 weeks, and is more likely to be used when a fetus is predicted to be at high risk for a genetic defect based on the family history. However, it cannot be used to evaluate a pregnancy at risk for a neural tube defect, since alpha-fetoprotein levels cannot be determined by CVS. Fragments of chorionic villi are aspirated either transabdominally or transcervically under sonographic guidance. The rate of fetal loss is approximately 1% higher than with amniocentesis. Occasionally, a placental biopsy may be performed later in pregnancy when severe oligohydramnios precludes the performance of amniocentesis.

Percutaneous Umbilical Blood Sampling

Fetal blood may be obtained for prenatal diagnosis of cytogenetic abnormalities, congenital infections (such as toxoplasmosis and parvovirus infection), immunodeficiencies, and thrombocytopenia by ultrasound-guided aspiration of blood from the umbilical vein. This technique may be used when obstetric circumstances or advancing gestational age necessitates a rapid diagnosis. Peripheral blood lymphocytes may be cultured and karyotyped within 48 to 72 hours, in contrast to amniocytes, which require 7 to 14 days. Percutaneous umbilical blood sampling (PUBS) is usually performed by experienced perinatologists or geneticists, and there is a reported loss rate of 1% to 5%.

MANAGEMENT OF PRENATALLY DIAGNOSED FETAL MALFORMATIONS

After extensive antenatal evaluation of the fetus with a congenital anomaly, the parents are counseled about the nature and extent of the defect, the possible diagnoses, potential outcomes, and management issues. Neonatologists, pediatric subspecialists, and pediatric surgeons often are included in these discussions to provide the couple with prognostic information as well as to discuss the medical and surgical interventions that may be required postnatally. The possibility of in utero medical or surgical intervention may be reviewed with the family in selected situations. Fetal surgery for the correction of congenital diaphragmatic hernia, cystic adenomatoid malformation of the lung,

TABLE 3. Indications for Fetal Echocardiography

Family history of congenital heart disease
Maternal disease (i.e., diabetes)
Maternal exposure to teratogens (i.e., lithium)
Fetal extracardiac malformations
Fetal chromosomal abnormality
Fetal arrhythmia

and obstructive uropathies has been successfully performed at a few centers that specialize in fetal therapy. Fetal cardiac arrhythmias have been successfully treated with the administration of antiarrhythmic agents to the mother or directly to the fetus. The decision to offer treatment in utero is dependent on the overall evaluation of the fetus and the risks and benefits of in utero versus postnatal therapy.

The management plan and options for the pregnancy are dependent on the gestational age of the fetus, fetal viability, severity of the defect, and diagnosis, as well as consideration for the parents' wishes. In the event that a couple elects to terminate a pregnancy, every effort should be made to confirm the diagnosis and provide the family with an accurate assessment of the recurrence risk. Confirmatory cytogenetic studies, autopsy, and a genetic evaluation are recommended. Posttermination counseling is provided to review the findings, diagnosis, recurrence risk, and availability, accuracy, and limitations of prenatal testing in subsequent pregnancies. It is often a good time to address the parents' emotional needs.

When a couple chooses to continue the pregnancy and the prognosis is reasonable or uncertain, we recommend close monitoring of the pregnancy, with delivery at a tertiary care center prepared to evaluate the infant and provide the appropriate care. A timed delivery may be necessary to ensure that the essential personnel (neonatologist, pediatric surgeon, specialist) are available.

The time before delivery is used to prepare the couple for the birth of a child who may require intensive medical or surgical therapy (or both) and, ultimately, special medical and educational attention. It is an emotionally difficult time for the family, which is often helped by trained counselors, religious personnel, social workers, and psychologists, who can provide the family with emotional support.

FOLLOW-UP OF THE HIGH-RISK INFANT

JUDY C. BERNBAUM, M.D.

After hospital discharge, many of the special care needs of the high-risk infant continue. Although they still require well child care, many of these infants have needs that are far from routine. Special attention must be given to their growth and nutrition and the sequelae of any illnesses experienced during the neonatal period. Although premature infants are more likely to develop long-term problems and experience continuing medical problems, many of the same issues apply to term infants as well.

GROWTH EXPECTATIONS

The pattern of growth is a valuable indicator of an infant's well-being. Aberrant growth may reflect the presence of chronic illness, feeding difficulties, poor nutrition, or social-emotional difficulties. Preterm infants are at particular risk for growth disorders. It is crucial to monitor nutritional intake closely and to interpret growth rates with a complete understanding of the infant's past history, current problems, and expectations for growth.

Many factors affect the growth of a preterm infant, including gestational age, birth weight, severity of neonatal illness, caloric intake, current illnesses, environmental factors in the home, and heredity. Caloric requirements for a healthy preterm infant generally exceed those of a normal term infant, especially during periods of rapid catchup growth. Chronic illnesses that increase caloric expenditure add to an infant's daily requirements. Malabsorption after necrotizing enterocolitis and chronic emesis from gastroesophageal reflux (GER) may impair growth because of increased losses. In contrast, decreased intake may be caused by fatigue, hypoxemia, oral motor dysfunction, or esophagitis from GER. Finally, infants with intrauterine growth retardation caused by congenital infections, chromosomal abnormalities, or other syndromes may never achieve normal growth.

PATTERNS OF GROWTH

When evaluating the growth of a low birth weight (LBW) infant, the gestational age should be taken into consideration. Growth parameters should be plotted on standard curves or, preferably, on recently available growth curves for preterm infants[4] according to the infant's adjusted age until approximately 2 ½ years of age, when the difference becomes insignificant. Various patterns of growth emerge from different groups of patients.

Healthy LBW, appropriate for gestational age (AGA) infants generally experience catchup growth during the first 2 years of life, with maximal growth rates between 36 and 40 weeks postconception. Little catchup growth occurs after 3 years. Head circumference usually is the first parameter to demonstrate catchup growth and often plots at a higher percentile relative to weight and length. Increases in weight are followed within several weeks by increases in length. Rapid catchup head growth must be distinguished from pathologic growth associated with underlying hydrocephalus. An imaging study may be necessary if the infant's history or symptoms suggest increasing intracranial pressure. A head circumference that falls more than 3 standard deviations (SD) below the mean is often associated with significant developmental disabilities.

It is helpful to evaluate an infant's weight gain in comparison with gains in length. Low weight for length or a decline in all growth parameters is suggestive of inadequate nutrition. Weight percentiles significantly greater than length percentiles indicate obesity. Obesity may occur in a preterm infant whose parents overfeed their previously underweight baby. It is common to see an infant who was formerly failing to thrive rather abruptly become obese when the medical problems resolve but the diet remains high in calories.

Growth of the small for gestational age (SGA) infant is strongly influenced by the cause of the intrauterine growth retardation. Overall, LBW SGA infants demonstrate less catchup growth than do LBW AGA infants, but when they do, it occurs by 8 to 12 months adjusted age. Approximately 50% of SGA infants have a weight that is below average at age 3 years, whereas only 15% of LBW AGA infants remain below normal weight at the same age. SGA infants with symmetric growth retardation (i. e., the birth head circumference and weight were in a similar percentile) are less likely to demonstrate catchup growth than are those SGA infants whose birth head circumference was at a significantly higher percentile than their weight. As with AGA infants, head circumference is normally the first parameter to demonstrate catchup, followed by weight and then length.

Because of the wide range of growth considered within the normal range for preterm infants during the first several years of life, it is best to analyze trends rather than make assumptions based on single measurements. When abnormalities are noted in growth trends, an investigation should be undertaken to identify a possible cause.

NUTRITIONAL REQUIREMENTS

Although somewhat controversial, the traditional goal for preterm infants is to achieve a growth rate approximating the expected fetal growth rate at the same postconceptional age. Since weight gain is suboptimal during acute illness, all efforts should be made to promote catchup growth once the medical condition is stable. The nutritional needs of the preterm infant during the first few months of life exceed those of a term neonate, but by 40 weeks postconception if there are

TABLE 1. Selected Caloric Supplements

SUPPLEMENT	CALORIC DENSITY	ADVANTAGES	DISADVANTAGES
Carbohydrates			
Polycose	2 kcal/ml	Well tolerated, less sweet	
Karo syrup	4 kcal/ml	Well tolerated; readily available; inexpensive	May cause loose stools
Fats			
Microlipids	4.5 kcal/ml	Well tolerated	Limited availability; high cost
Medium-chain triglyceride oil	7.6 kcal/ml	High caloric density; usually well tolerated	May cause diarrhea; does not mix well with formula
Vegetable oil	9 kcal/ml	Easily available and low cost	Does not mix well with formula
Avocado (pureed; ½ avo-cado/26 oz formula)		High caloric density; well tolerated	Season availability; expensive; more preparation needed
California variety, brown	Adds 7.4 kcal/oz		
Florida variety, green	Adds 5.7 kcal/oz		
Dry baby cereal	10 kcal/Tbsp	Readily available; inexpensive; may help with gastro-esophageal reflux	Low caloric density; may cause constipation
Proteins			
Powdered skim milk	27 kcal/Tbsp	Readily available; mixes well with formula	

no exceptional medical problems or feeding difficulties, the dietary needs are similar. At that time, most preterm infants will grow normally receiving either breast milk or formulas designed for term infants. Some infants, however, will continue to require more highly concentrated formula or breast milk because of increased caloric requirements or feeding dysfunction. For these children, either a more concentrated formula can be used or caloric supplements can be added to formula or breast milk (Table 1). Infants given such feedings should be monitored for symptoms of intolerance, such as vomiting and diarrhea.

Healthy preterm infants generally require 110 to 130 kcal/kg/d to achieve adequate growth, but infants with chronic disease may require up to 150 to 175 kcal/kg/d. Caloric intake should be increased as tolerated until weight gain is satisfactory. Caloric requirements needed for catchup growth can be calculated for infants after 40 weeks postconceptional age by using the following formula.

$$\text{kcal/kg required} = 120 \text{ kcal/kg} \times \frac{\text{ideal weight for actual height}}{\text{actual weight}}$$

When using caloric additives or concentrating formula, care should be taken to maintain an appropriate caloric distribution of nutrients with a ratio of carbohydrates/fats/protein of approximately 40:50:10 (Table 1).

FEEDING PROBLEMS

Although unusual in term infants, feeding disorders are relatively common in preterm infants. Most feeding problems occur in the neonatal period, but many infants demonstrate recurrent or chronic problems with sucking and swallowing. If these problems remain unrecognized, they may lead to significantly impaired nutritional intake and have a negative impact on the parent-infant relationship. Infants at risk for developing feeding problems include those in whom oral feedings were delayed during the neonatal period and those with immature oral motor skills related to prematurity. Furthermore, infants with transient or more permanent neurologic deficits are at very high risk for feeding abnormalities. Additional risk factors for the development of feeding dysfunction include chronic lung disease, tracheostomy, GER, and inconsistent feeding techniques by multiple caregivers.

Oral reflexes that allow normal feeding and protect the airway from aspiration may be hypoactive or hyperactive in preterm infants. Abnormal reflexes, such as the tonic bite reflex, abnormal tongue thrust, and hyperactive gag, can further destroy any hope for successful and pleasurable feeding. The hyperactive gag is particularly troublesome because the child may develop oral hypersensitivity and

not be able to tolerate the nipple or spoon on the tongue and may resist any oral stimulation. Other causes of hypersensitivity or tactile defensiveness include prolonged intubation and repeated suctioning or passage of nasogastric feeding tubes.

The evaluation of a possible feeding disorder should include a detailed history of feeding behaviors and nutritive intake, a physical examination including assessment of oral motor reflexes, and observation of a feeding. If an infant with chronic lung disease desaturates during feeding, increasing the supplemental oxygen during feeding can improve feeding behavior. Evaluation of the type of nipple and the size of its hole may reveal that the hole is too small, causing fatigue, or too large, making it difficult to control the flow. Indications for radiologic evaluation include suspected aspiration during feeding or an anatomic abnormality, such as a tracheoesophageal fistula or delayed gastric emptying.

All of these conditions are amenable to therapy if they are identified early enough. A pediatric speech pathologist or occupational therapist trained in feeding techniques often can be helpful in assessing a feeding problem and developing an appropriate feeding program once the problem has been defined.

IMMUNIZATIONS

Most preterm infants should receive the same immunizations as the term infant and on similar schedules without correcting for their prematurity. The AAP Committee on Immunization Practice recommends that full doses of DTP vaccine be administered to prematurely born infants at the appropriate postnatal (chronologic) age. A large percentage of preterm infants demonstrate inadequate protection if given a reduced dose of DTP vaccine at the standard intervals. Similarly, the AAP recommends that full dose oral polio vaccine (OPV) be administered at the appropriate chronologic age, but only after discharge from the hospital. Inactivated polio vaccine (IPV) should be given to any child who remains hospitalized beyond 2 months of age, is immunocompromised, or lives with an immunodeficient individual. Measles, mumps, and rubella, *Haemophilus influenzae* type b, and hepatitis B vaccines should be given at the same chronologic age as recommended for full-term infants.

Influenza Vaccine

Infants with chronic pulmonary disease (BPD) or cardiac disease with pulmonary vascular congestion are at high risk for developing serious illness if they are infected with an influenza virus. To protect vulnerable infants, immunization with influenza vaccine is indicated for household contacts, including siblings, primary caretakers, and home care nurses, as well as hospital personnel. For infants more than

6 months of age, two dose of split virus vaccine should be given 1 month apart between October and December, followed by one annual dose. Adults and older siblings with natural immunity or who have received previous immunizations need only one yearly dose.

SPECIALIZED CARE

Retinopathy of Prematurity

According to 1992 recommendations in the AAP Guidelines for Perinatal Care, all infants who have a birth weight of less than 1500 g and require oxygen therapy during the neonatal period should have an ophthalmologic examination to rule out retinopathy of prematurity (ROP). The initial examination should not occur before 4 to 6 weeks of age, as a vitreous haze may interfere with visualization of the retina. If only one examination is possible, it should take place at 7 to 9 weeks of age to coincide with the peak period of occurrence of ROP. A schedule of follow-up visits is based on the initial findings. All infants with immature fundi or any state of ROP require close monitoring until the eyes have matured or the ROP has completely resolved. Thereafter, routine follow-up visits to assess for refractive errors should be scheduled at 1 year of age and before kindergarten begins unless abnormal clinical signs appear sooner.

Hearing Problems

The incidence of sensorineural hearing loss in preterm infants is generally reported to be between 1% and 3%. Several factors place preterm infants at particular risk for hearing loss, including hypoxia, hyperbilirubinemia, infections, unstable blood pressure, environmental noise, and ototoxic drugs. According to the American Academy of Pediatrics Joint Committee on Infant Hearing, infants with any of the risk factors listed in Table 2 should receive auditory screening, preferably by brainstem auditory evoked response (BAER), before 3 months of age. Passing an initial hearing screening does not preclude the possibility of an acquired hearing loss later in life. Absent or abnormal responses to auditory stimulation, delays in speech development, poor articulation, or inattentiveness should raise the suspicion of a hearing loss that requires a more thorough evaluation. All infants who fail an initial hearing screening should be referred to an audiologist for further testing and intervention.

Periventricular Leukomalacia

Periventricular leukomalacia (PVL) is ischemic infarction of the white matter adjacent to the lateral ventricles, frequently leading to cyst formation in the involved areas. The reported incidence of PVL in infants with birth weights <1500 g varies from 2% to 22%. Infants at risk for PVL are those whose perinatal course was complicated by severe hypoxia, ischemia, or both. Infants of early gestational age are particularly susceptible to the development of PVL because of their inability to regulate cerebral blood flow.

In the weeks that follow a major insult leading to PVL, phagocytosis of the necrotic material occurs, with development of fluid-filled, periventricular cysts. The documentation of cyst and estimation of size can be done most easily using cranial ultrasonography. However, CT or MRI scans are just as informative. Resolution of the cysts is highly variable, and some never completely resolve. Beyond the neonatal period, screening for the presence of PVL should be considered in any child with cerebral palsy without an apparent cause. Since there are no symptoms associated with the development of PVL, it can be easily missed during the neonatal period.

If PVL is not associated with residual cysts, few if any sequelae develop. If PVL is associated with the loss of vital areas of neural tissue and formation of cysts >3 mm in diameter, the infant so affected is at an increased risk for cerebral palsy, developmental delay, and visual or auditory impairments. When cysts persist, an infant's motor development is most often affected. Cerebral palsy, manifested as moderate to severe quadriplegia or diplegia, is reported to develop in 90% to 100% of these children. The intellectual capacities of children with PVL and cyst formation is more variable. Mental retardation is more common in infants with residual cysts but ranges from mild to severe. If the cysts develop in the occipital region, visual impairment may result.

All infants with PVL, especially those with cysts, should be closely monitored for neurodevelopmental sequelae. Periodic cranial imaging studies, preferably head ultrasonography, will determine stability or resolution of the cysts. Parents of infants with PVL should be counseled on the importance of periodic neurodevelopmental assessments for early detection of any sequelae and intervention when appropriate.

Chronic Lung Disease

Bronchopulmonary dysplasia (BPD) is the most frequently diagnosed chronic lung disease in preterm infants, usually developing as a sequel to the acute lung injury experienced during the first few weeks of life. Infants with mild or minimal residual lung disease will usually be brought to the primary care provider with their first viral respiratory tract infection. Those with more severe disease often will be discharged with medication requirements, nebulizer treatments, and supplemental oxygen. Clinical manifestations are similar to those in the nursery and include tachypnea, tachycardia, retractions, rhonchi, bronchospasm, and poor air movement into the lungs bilaterally. More subtle signs of chronic respiratory distress include poor weight gain, feeding intolerance, decreased activity and a reduced tolerance to exercise. The discussion of the medical management of infants with BPD earlier in this chapter focuses on the use of supplemental oxygen.

TABLE 2. Criteria for Hearing Screening

Risk Criteria: Neonates (Birth–28 d)

The factors that identify neonates who are at risk for sensorineural hearing impairment include the following:

1. Family history of congenital or delayed onset of sensorineural impairment in childhood
2. Congenital infection known or suspected to be associated with sensorineural hearing impairment, such as toxoplasmosis, syphilis, rubella, cytomegalovirus, and herpes
3. Craniofacial anomalies, e.g., morphologic abnormalities of the pinna and ear canal, and absent philtrum
4. Birth weight <1500 g (~3.3 lb)
5. Hyperbilirubinemia at a level exceeding indication for exchange transfusion
6. Ototoxic medications, including but not limited to the aminoglycosides used for more than 5 days (e.g., gentamicin, tobramycin, kanamycin, streptomycin) and loop diuretics used in combination with aminoglycosides
7. Bacterial meningitis
8. Severe depression at birth, which may include infants with Apgar scores of 0 to 3 at 5 min after birth, those who fail to initiate spontaneous respiration by 10 min after birth, or those with hypotonia persisting to 2 h of age
9. Prolonged mechanical ventilation for a duration ≥10 d (e.g., persistent pulmonary hypertension)
10. Stigmata or other findings associated with a syndrome known to include sensorineural hearing loss (e.g., Waardenburg or Usher's syndrome)

From American Academy of Pediatrics Joint Committee on Infant Hearing: 1990 position statement. ASHA (Suppl 5):3, 1991.

Supplemental Oxygen

The decision to continue an infant on supplemental oxygen relates to the severity of the underlying lung disease. However, the need for supplemental oxygen should not necessarily interfere with hospital discharge. Some of the more common indications for the use of supplemental oxygen include evidence of desaturation while breathing room air, poor oral feeding due to air hunger, apnea or bradycardia associated with hypoxia, poor growth associated with borderline hypoxia, poor exercise tolerance, lethargy, and tachycardia or tachypnea that improves with the use of supplemental oxygen. If possible, it is best to determine the adequacy of oxygenation during sleep, feedings, and periods of activity. Pulse oximetry readings should be maintained ≥95%. This level of saturation is recommended to preclude the development of pulmonary hypertension and resultant right heart strain. Although many centers begin weaning infants with lower oxygen saturations, studies have shown that infants with chronic lung disease who are optimally oxygenated demonstrate better weight gain, attain corrected age-appropriate milestones more readily, and have fewer intercurrent respiratory illnesses than do infants with lower saturations.

Before weaning from supplemental oxygen, the infant's medical stability must be assured, as must adequacy of weight gain, exercise tolerance, and caloric intake. It is preferable to wean a child off oxygen slowly and in a stepwise fashion. A period of several weeks to a month should pass between each step, during which the infant must remain medically stable, gain adequate weight, demonstrate good exercise tolerance, and maintain adequate oxygen saturations. Many home care services can perform intermittent oximetry in the home to assist management. It is easier to wean an infant off oxygen if the infant is kept maximally bronchodilated with supplemental medications. During an illness, it is common to have to increase the amount of supplemental oxygen or to restart it temporarily if the child has recently been weaned from it.

To compensate for increased energy expenditures, the infant with BPD often requires a higher than normal caloric intake (120 to 150 kcal/kg/d). Increased caloric needs complicated by poor nutritional intake often result in poor growth. Poor nutritional intake in this population may be caused by hypoxemia, anorexia, tachypnea, exercise intolerance, oral motor dysfunction, or GER. In addition, it is often difficult to maximize caloric intake in the face of fluid restriction and feeding (exercise) intolerance. Caloric intake can be maximized by adding supplements, concentrating formulas, or using isocaloric formulas.

Even with supplemental calories, there are times when growth is not adequate because the infant either tires easily or refuses any additional increased oral intake. It is then that supplemental nasogastric feedings should be considered, either after each bottle feeding or continuously during the night. Each method has its own advantages and disadvantages and must be considered within the context of individual family and patient needs. It is crucial to offer sucking opportunities routinely to any child who is tube fed to stimulate the development of the sucking reflex. A feeding therapist may be needed in these instances to help prevent the poor quality of sucking frequently encountered in these children.

Intercurrent Illnesses

Many infants with BPD will develop bronchospasm during viral or bacterial respiratory illnesses. If the infant is not already on main-

TABLE 3. Examples of Medication Changes for Infants with Chronic Lung Disease Who Have Increased Bronchospasm Associated with Acute Illness

MAINTENANCE REGIMEN	REGIMEN DURING ACUTE ILLNESS WITH BRONCHOSPASM
No medication	Begin beta$_2$-agonist (oral or inhaled) ± methylxanthine.*
Beta$_2$-agonist	Change to nebulizer (if on MDI† or oral formulation) and consider increasing frequency of treatments.
Beta$_2$-agonist and cromolyn	Increase frequency of beta$_2$-agonist (q3–4h). Do not give cromolyn more than four times per day. If no response, consider a short course of steroids.
Methylxanthine	Check level and adjust if subtherapeutic or supplement with beta$_2$-agonist (oral or inhaled), or both and adjust frequency as needed.

*Example, theophylline.
†Metered dose inhaler

tenance therapy, bronchodilators can be initiated during acute illnesses. If the infant is on maintenance bronchodilator therapy, synergistic medications can be added during acute exacerbations and withdrawn as the acute symptoms resolve. Examples of treatment regimens are given in Table 3.

Minimizing the exposure of infants with BPD to environmental irritants and communicable diseases will help decrease the frequency of intercurrent episodes of bronchospasm and allow more time for the lung to heal. Some environmental irritants are cigarette or fireplace smoke, pet fur or dander, kerosene heaters, paint, and infectious agents. The less irritation the lung is exposed to, the quicker the recovery process will be.

Rehospitalization is a common occurence in children with BPD, especially during the first year of life. Parents of these infants should be advised of this possibility before initial hospital discharge. Every effort should be made to treat the infant with intercurrent illnesses and associated bronchospasm as an outpatient, but if the child does not readily respond, hospitalization is appropriate for more aggressive treatment.

Managing infants with BPD is a major clinical challenge for the practicing physician. The many facets of their care require a complete understanding of how their lung disease affects their physical well-being. Fortunately, the majority of their medical problems occur during the first 1 or 2 years of life, and improvement can be expected in each subsequent year.

REFERENCES

1. Ballard RE (ed): Pediatric Care of the ICN Graduate. Philadelphia, WB Saunders Co, 1988.
2. Bernbaum J, Hoffman-Williamson M: Primary Care of the Preterm Infant. St. Louis, Mosby-Year Book Medical Publishers, 1991.
3. Hack M, Fanaroff AA: Growth pattern in the ICN graduate. *In* Ballard RE (ed): Pediatric Care of the ICN Graduate. Philadelphia, WB Saunders Co, 1988.
4. IHDP growth percentiles for LBW premature infants. Ross Products Division, Abbott Laboratories, Columbus, Ohio, 1994.

22

Special Problems in the Adolescent

GYNECOLOGY

Marc R. Laufer, M.D.
Joan Mansfield, M.D.

THE ADOLESCENT PATIENT

Adolescence is a period of transition in the patient-doctor relationship. The pediatric office visit usually focuses on the concerns of the parent about the health and needs of the child. As the girl enters adolescence, she becomes a patient in her own right, with concerns that she may have difficulty sharing completely with her parents. It is important for the physician to encourage communication between the parents and the teen about sexuality and, at the same time, to provide the opportunity for her to bring her sexual concerns to her physician for advice and adult guidance in confidence. The physician who is not able to counsel the adolescent confidentially on issues of sexuality and contraception may prefer to refer the patient to a setting where these services are available. Since patient and parent often have different perspectives on the medical problem at hand, it is important for the teen to be seen alone at some point during the visit, usually during the physical examination. The physician can then address any confidential concerns and, together with the patient, develop a plan that can be shared with the parent. Frequently, the adolescent will present with a minor complaint unrelated to gynecologic issues when she is, in fact, concerned about pregnancy or contraception. The review of systems, therefore, becomes a valuable tool for uncovering the real reason for the visit and for teaching the adolescent the variety of health-related concerns that can be addressed during a visit with a physician. An examination of the external genitalia to rule out congenital abnormalities should be included in the physical examination of the adolescent female.

Counseling begins early in adolescence with basic information on the expected course of pubertal growth and development and reproductive function. This patient population requires extensive education, counseling, and support in addressing the importance of contraception in preventing unplanned pregnancy and the use of condoms to reduce the risk of sexually transmitted infection. Two thirds of teens have had at least one exposure of sexual intercourse by age 18. One in ten adolescent women becomes pregnant each year. Sexually transmitted infections are of epidemic proportions in this age group. Many teens are unaware of the risks of sexual activity, including unwanted pregnancy, sexually transmitted infection, and loss of self-esteem. It is appropriate to review these risks in an objective, nonjudgmental fashion. The patient may be reminded that many teens choose not to be sexually active for these reasons. If she chooses to be sexually active, she may be encouraged to act responsibly to reduce the risks by using contraception effectively and getting regular gynecologic care. This care includes having a pelvic examination with a Papanicolaou (PAP) smear to detect cervical dysplasia at least annually and testing of asymptomatic sexually transmitted infections at 6-month intervals.

DISORDERS OF MENSTRUATION

Amenorrhea

Amenorrhea is often divided into categories of primary and secondary amenorrhea. Individuals with primary amenorrhea are defined as not having had a menstrual period by age 16 in the presence of female secondary sexual maturation, or by age 14 in the absence of secondary sexual maturation. Secondary amenorrhea is the cessation of menstrual periods. There is considerable overlap in the differential diagnosis of these two types of amenorrhea. However, it is important to obtain an extensive history and physical examination in order to begin the workup to determine the etiology.

Primary Amenorrhea

Primary amenorrhea may result from delayed puberty, interrupted puberty, hormonal imbalance causing anovulation, or an anatomic abnormality preventing menstruation. Delayed puberty, that is, the absence of secondary sexual development by age 13.5 in girls, is discussed in Disorders of Puberty in Chapter 9.

A patient who has not had menarche within 4 years of breast development has delayed menarche. Evaluation of this patient should consist of a careful history, including symptoms or signs suggestive of chronic disease interrupting the progression of puberty, hormonal imbalance, such as hypothyroidism, androgen excess, or hyperprolactinemia, timing of breast and body hair development, athletic activity, and dietary intake. A history of cyclic lower abdominal pain suggests an obstructed uterus. Review of height and weight charts is very helpful, since chronic disease, malnutrition, or endocrinopathy is often present with abnormalities of growth.

The physical examination in the patient with primary amenorrhea and secondary sexual development should include height and weight measurements. Skin should be examined for evidence of endocrinopathy or excessive body hair. Quantitation of secondary sexual development should be done by the Tanner staging of breast and pubic hair development and measurements of areolae and glandular breast tissue dimensions. An attempt should be made to express galactorrhea, suggesting the diagnosis of hyperprolactinemia. A neurologic examination, including visual fields by confrontation, is useful, since pituitary and hypothalamic mass lesions may interrupt the progression of puberty. The external genitalia should be examined for signs of estrogenization (pale pink vaginal mucosa, developed labia minora, fimbriated hymen), and evidence of hymenal patency. Hyperandrogenism may be evidenced by hirsutism, and in extreme cases of virilization, clitoromegaly may be present.

An assessment of internal pelvic structures should be done with the patient in the lithotomy position. If the vaginal opening comfortably admits a single finger, a thin Huffman speculum may be used to visualize the cervix. A vaginal bimanual examination of the uterus and adnexae should also be performed. If the hymeneal opening does not admit a finger, the depth of the vagina can be assessed using a saline-moistened cotton swab, and the pelvic structures can be assessed by rectoabdominal examination. A pelvic ultrasound study may be helpful for assessment of pelvic structures.

Laboratory evaluation may be focused by the differential diagnoses suggested by the history and physical examination. A complete blood count (CBC), erythrocyte sedimentation rate (ESR), luteinizing hormone (LH), follicle-stimulating hormone (FSH), prolactin, thyroid function tests, and radiograph of the left hand and wrist for bone age are useful initial screens. A quantitative assessment of estrogen effect on the vagina using a vaginal smear for maturation index is also helpful.

Secondary Amenorrhea

The adolescent who had established menstrual cycles and who then ceases menstruation for 3 months or more is said to have secondary amenorrhea. Since the most common cause of adolescent amenorrhea is pregnancy, any teen who expresses concern about a period that is even slightly delayed warrants prompt attention. She should be interviewed alone and given a chance to discuss her concerns privately. Many teens will not acknowledge that they are sexually active, even when carefully questioned. A urine screen for hCG is, therefore, a fundamental part of the evaluation of any teen with a delayed menstrual period. The focus of the history and physical examination is the same as with the patient who presents with primary amenorrhea, since the diagnostic possibilities overlap. A pelvic examination is appropriate to assess the estrogen effect on the vaginal mucosa and to assess the size of the uterus and ovaries.

The adolescent who has persistent oligomenorrhea and who has not established a pattern of regular menstrual cycle within 4 years of menarche often has a hormone imbalance causing chronic anovulation. Some of these patients have chronic ovarian androgen excess (polycystic ovary syndrome) and may show the classic triad of obesity, slowly progressive hirsutism, and oligomenorrhea. Not all patients with this hormonal pattern have obvious signs of androgen excess on examination. Other patients may have partial disruption of the hypothalamic pituitary ovarian axis due to intense exercise, stress, chronic illness, or limitation of food intake. Some have no apparent reason for their persistent anovulatory state. Since women with chronic anovulation have an endometrium that is chronically exposed to unopposed estrogen, they are at risk for developing endometrial hyperplasia, dysfunctional bleeding, and even endometrial cancer. Therefore, patients who do not have what appears to be an ovulatory period at least every 3 months should be cycled with medroxyprogesterone acetate or oral contraceptives.

The initial laboratory tests for the patient with secondary amenorrhea include a urine pregnancy test and LH, FSH, prolactin, and thyroid function tests. If the pregnancy test is negative, a progestin challenge is a useful way to assess the estrogen state of the patient. Medroxyprogesterone (Provera) 10 mg is given daily for 10 days. If this is followed by a withdrawal bleed, the patient is producing estrogen. A medroxyprogesterone challenge not followed by a withdrawal bleed demonstrates a hypoestrogenic state. A low estrogen state may be the result of low levels of LH and FSH because of hypothalamic or pituitary dysfunction or because of an inability of the ovary to respond to high levels of gonadotropins. If LH and FSH are elevated into the menopausal range, the patient has ovarian failure as a cause of her low estrogen state. If the initial LH and FSH are elevated, the tests are usually repeated to confirm the diagnosis. A karyotype and measurement of antiovarian antibodies can help to determine whether a chromosomal abnormality or autoimmune process underlies the ovarian failure.

An androgen excess state requires evaluation of ovarian and adrenal androgens. Polycystic ovary syndrome describes a constellation of symptoms associated with androgen excess. The pathophysiology of this disease process is not entirely understood. The LH/FSH ratio may be reversed in a 3:1 or greater fashion, and the patient may be

obese and hirsute and have insulin resistance. All of these findings may be present, or they may be absent. A total testosterone test and determination of adrenal androgens should be done.

Treatment. If the patient does not have cyclic menses on her own, she should be cycled with medroxyprogesterone 10 mg/d for 12 to 14 days every 1 to 3 months to prevent endometrial hyperplasia. If she is sexually active, it is preferable to use oral contraceptives to avoid exposure to medroxyprogesterone early in an undiagnosed pregnancy. The patients should return to the office 2 to 3 weeks after her initial visit to discuss her response to the progestin challenge and the results of her initial laboratory evaluation.

Patients with polycystic ovary syndrome usually have adequate to high estrogen levels and should be cycled to prevent endometrial hyperplasia. Oral contraceptives are the treatment of choice, since they usually can lower free androgen levels and prevent progression of hirsutism. A pill containing a nonandrogenic progestin, such as desogestrel, norgestimate, or norethindrone, is preferable. Desogen or Ortho Cept (both ethinyl estradiol 30 mg with desogesterol 0.15 mg), Ortho-Cylen (ethinyl estradiol 35 μg with norgestimate 0.25 mg), or Ortho Tri-Cylen (ethinyl estradiol 35 μg with norgestimate 0.18, 0.215, 0.25 mg) may be used, and Modicon (35 μg ethinyl estradiol with 0.5 mg norethindrone), Ovcon-35 (35 μg ethinyl estradiol with 0.4 mg norethindrone), Ortho-Novum 1/35, Norinyl 1/35, and Demulen 1/35 are alternatives. If the patient is opposed to or is not a candidate for oral contraceptives, cycling with medroxyprogesterone 10 mg for 12 to 14 days a month can give regular menses and prevent endometrial hyperplasia in these patients. However, hirsutism and acne may progress. For those patients in whom hirsutism is a major concern, the combination of the oral contraceptive agent with an end-organ antiandrogen can be most helpful. Spironolactone 100 mg twice daily is effective in inhibiting new terminal hair formation. If a sexually active individual is started on spironolactone, she must be on an oral contraceptive agent, as spironolactone is teratogenic. If using this combination therapy, the adolescent needs to be informed that this therapy takes approximately 3 months for full effect. She may thus choose to hold off on waxing or electrolysis until after the 3-month period to minimize the number of mechanical hair removal treatments required.

The optimum dose of estrogen for estrogen replacement in adolescents has not been clearly established. The usual menopausal dose of conjugated estrogens (Premarin 0.625 mg/d) may not be adequate to allow the normal adolescent increase in bone density to take place. If growth is not yet complete, estrogen replacement is begun at low doses to maximize the growth response. One regimen is to begin at 0.3 mg Premarin and increase to 0.625 to 1.25 mg as growth slows in the second year of treatment. Once the dose of Premarin has reached 0.625 mg/d, the replacement is given cyclically on days 1 to 25 each month, and medroxyprogesterone 10 mg/d is added initially 5 days per month for 3 months, increasing to 12 to 14 days per month. Low-dose oral contraceptives containing 30 to 35 μg ethinyl estradiol are alternative approach to estrogen replacement once breast development is satisfactory. Other forms of estrogen replacement include ethinyl estradiol 30 to 35 μg, transdermal beta-estradiol patches (Estraderm), or micronized estradiol (Estrace) 2 mg. All are used with cyclic progestin for 12 to 14 days per month.

Pregnancy

Pregnancy is the most common cause of secondary amenorrhea in adolescents. As mentioned earlier, any teenager who expresses concern about a period being slightly delayed should have a urine pregnancy test, since many teens who are at risk for pregnancy will deny sexual activity. Often, the alleged reason for the office visit is a minor physical complaint, such as sore throat or fatigue, and the delayed period is discovered only on review of systems. The newer urine hCG office pregnancy tests, such as ICON hCG (Hybritech), use monoclonal antibodies to hCG and enzyme-linked radioimmunoassay. The detection level varies with the kit. The ICON hCG is positive above

20 to 50 mIU/ml hCG. The urine specific gravity should be 1.015 or above for greatest sensitivity. Thus, pregnancy can usually be diagnosed 7 to 10 days after conception, even before the period is due.

The pregnancy should be dated by sizing of the uterus by pelvic or rectoabdominal examination, as well as date of last menstrual period. The 8-week uterus is the size of an orange, and the 12-week uterus is the size of a grapefruit. Adolescents are at increased risk for complications of pregnancy, including premature births and eclampsia.

Abortion

The pregnant teenager should be counseled about her options for continuing or terminating the pregnancy. Laws vary from state to state, but in most cases, the physician is required not to reveal the diagnosis of pregnancy to the family without the patient's consent. The patient may be encouraged to involve her parents in her decision. Many teens continue their denial despite an office visit confirming the pregnancy and do not follow through with either obtaining obstetric care or making a decision to terminate the pregnancy in the first trimester when medical risk of pregnancy termination are lowest. Several visits are often necessary to ensure that the patient makes a decision and follows through with appropriate medical care.

Elective pregnancy termination can be safely performed in an outpatient environment. The procedure can be performed by an experienced gynecologist, with the patient receiving a paracervical block, intravenous sedation, or general anesthesia.

Following an elective termination, the patient can be given prophylactic antibiotics for 3 to 5 days (e.g., doxycycline 100 mg twice daily). The patient should use nothing per vagina (tampons, douching, or sexual intercourse) for 2 weeks. A 2-week postabortion checkup is necessary, at which time the patient should be examined to confirm that the uterus is small and that the beta-hCG is negative. If there is any question about whether the uterus is empty, the pathology specimen should be reviewed to confirm the presence of the complete products of conception. In addition, ultrasonography can be helpful to rule out retained products of conception.

Confirmed products of conception rule out an ectopic pregnancy unless the rare case of a heterotopic pregnancy exists. If the pathologic specimen fails to reveal chorionic villi, the quantitative beta-hCG should be followed to zero. If the beta-hCG does not fall to zero and remains elevated, the patient must be evaluated to rule out an ectopic pregnancy.

Teen Pregnancy

Should the patient elect to continue the pregnancy, the importance of proper nutrition and avoiding cigarette smoking, alcohol, and drug use should be reviewed. The social consequences of teen pregnancy are considerable both for the adolescent, who faces social isolation, interruption of schooling, and economic difficulties, and for her child, who is at risk for abuse, neglect, and inappropriate behavioral expectations from his or her young parent. The provider may consider referral of the pregnant adolescent to a teen parent program where some of these needs can be addressed. Postpartum contraception is important, since repeat pregnancy is very common.

Ectopic Pregnancy

Ectopic pregnancies have become increasingly frequent in young women and now comprise 0.5% of all pregnancies under age 25. Irregular vaginal bleeding is the most common symptom in patients with an ectopic pregnancy. Abdominal pain and amenorrhea should suggest consideration of this diagnosis. A pelvic examination may reveal an adnexal mass, but most ectopic pregnancies are not palpable on bimanual examination. If an ectopic pregnancy is suspected, a quantitative serum hCG should be obtained and repeated in 48 hours if the diagnosis remains in question. The normal doubling time of serum hCG levels is approximately 2.3 days at 5 to 8 weeks gestation. In ectopic pregnancy, hCG levels usually are lower than normal, and

the rate of rise is slower. Thus, the quantitative serum hCG should increase by 68% every 48 hours. If the serum hCG is greater than 6000 mIU/ml (IRP) (about 5 to 6 weeks gestation), an intrauterine gestational sac should be visible on abdominal ultrasound. Transvaginal ultrasound may detect a gestational sac at 1000 to 2000 mIU/ml hCG. Absence of the gestational sac on ultrasound examination suggests a possible ectopic pregnancy.

Treatment. A patient with a suspected ectopic pregnancy should be referred immediately to a gynecologist. The pregnancy can be removed surgically by operative laparoscopic salpingostomy with preservation of the fallopian tube. A patient with a hemoperitoneum is a candidate for an operative laparoscopic approach as long as she is not hypotensive. If the patient is hemodynamically unstable, a laparotomy is performed with a salpingostomy or salpingectomy if the tube is unable to be saved. Even if a ruptured fallopian tube is unsalvageable, the ovary is conserved for steroid function and the possible future use for in vitro fertilization if the other tube should be nonfunctional.

Medical treatment of ectopic pregnancies with methotrexate followed by citrovorum factor has been used in some centers as an alternative to surgical treatment. The methotrexate can be given on an outpatient basis 1 mg/kg/IM on days 1, 3, 5, and 7, alternating with calcium leucovorin 0.1 mg/kg PO on days 2, 4, 6, and 8, or as an inpatient IV with 100 mg/m² IVB at time 0, 200 mg/m² over 12 hours given at 30 minutes, followed by calcium leucovorin 15 mg PO at 24, 36, 48, and 60 hours. There are centers treating with a single IM dose of methotrexate 50 mg/m² without calcium leucovorin treatment. Methotrexate given by any of these protocols requires close follow-up and compliance. The beta-hCG should be measured twice weekly. The methotrexate dose is repeated if the beta-hCG drops less than one log in 18 days, plateaus, or increases. No further follow-up is needed after two consecutive normal beta-hCG titers. An ectopic pregnancy can rupture even if the quantitative serum beta-hCG is falling. Thus, patients should report any changes in symptoms immediately. Poorly compliant adolescents are not candidates for methotrexate therapy.

Abnormal Vaginal Bleeding

Abnormal vaginal bleeding may be due to pregnancy, hormonal abnormalities, blood dyscrasia, infection, local lesion, anatomic abnormality, or local trauma. Since adolescents frequently have anovulatory cycles in the first 2 years after menarche, painless cycles at irregular intervals are frequent. Patients who have bleeding at intervals of less than 22 days, whose menses last longer than 7 days, or who have heavy bleeding with clots are considered to have excessive bleeding. Despite the fact that the majority of adolescents are initially anovulatory after menarche, they usually do have cyclic variations in estrogen levels, resulting in cyclic vaginal withdrawal bleeding at variable intervals between 28 and 39 days. The teens whose anovulation is characterized by an acyclic pattern, often with intervals of amenorrhea followed by prolonged bleeding, are said to have dysfunctional uterine bleeding as a cause of their prolonged heavy menses. This is a common cause of excessive vaginal bleeding but remains a diagnosis of exclusion.

Evaluation

Evaluation usually begins with a careful history of the character and time course of the bleeding, past menstrual history, and history of prior difficulty with bleeding tendencies in the patient or family members. A physical examination should include postural vital signs and careful attention to findings that might suggest clotting abnormality (such as bruising or petechiae) or endocrine abnormality (such as hirsutism or thyroid disease). Whether or not the patient is actively bleeding, a pelvic examination with visualization of the cervix and vagina should be performed. Initial laboratory tests include a urine and serum beta-hCG and a CBC. Clotting studies, including a platelet count, PT, PTT and bleeding time, are usually obtained if significant menorrhagia occurs with a fall in the hematocrit or if the abnormal bleeding started at menarche. If the patient is bleeding heavily, a typing and crossmatching should be done since transfusion is sometimes necessary. Cervical cultures for gonorrhea and *Chlamydia* are performed in the adolescent who might possibly be sexually active. Endocrine tests, such as LH, FSH, prolactin, and thyroid function tests, may be included if the patient has a history of apparent anovulatory bleeding.

Treatment

Treatment of dysfunctional bleeding varies with the severity of the problem.

Mild Bleeding. Patients with mild dysfunctional bleeding, that is, patients who have a normal hemoglobin and monthly menses lasting more than 7 days or cycles of less than 21 days for 2 months or more with only moderately increased flow, may be asked to keep a menstrual calendar and be given iron supplements to prevent anemia.

Moderate Bleeding. Patients with moderately severe dysfunctional bleeding have moderate to heavy flow and menses every 1 to 3 weeks, often with bleeding lasting more than 7 days. Mild anemia is often present. In these patients, treatment may be with either medroxyprogesterone or oral contraceptives. Medroxyprogesterone 10 mg once or twice a day for 10 to 14 days may be started on the 14th day after the period began or on the day of the visit. Repeat cycles of medroxyprogesterone 10 mg for 12 to 14 days each are begun either beginning on day 14 after the first day of withdrawal bleeding or for the first 12 to 14 days of each calendar month. This latter method is simpler for patients to remember. If the patient begins to have bleeding even before she reaches the 14th day of the cycle, medroxyprogesterone may be started on day 12, or she may be switched to oral contraceptives. If patients do not tolerate medroxyprogesterone, the dose may be decreased temporarily to 5 mg/d. Norethindrone acetate (Norlutate) 10 mg daily for 10 to 14 days may be used as an alternative to medroxyprogesterone. Cycling should be continued for 3 to 6 months. If the patient does not begin to cycle on her own within 2 months after stopping the treatment, she should again be treated with medroxyprogesterone or oral contraceptives to prevent further dysfunctional uterine bleeding. It must be remembered that cyclic medroxyprogesterone is not a form of contraception and may be teratogenic. Thus, it is not the therapy of choice for the sexually active female.

Severe Bleeding. If the patient has a history of prolonged or heavy dysfunctional bleeding, or if she has milder irregular bleeding and is in need of contraception, oral contraceptives should be used as the initial treatment. Ovral, Lo/Ovral, or Norinyl (Ortho-Novum) 1/50 or 1/35 may be chosen. Ovral is the most effective in stopping heavy bleeding, since it is comprised of a strong progestin norgestrel coupled with 50 μg of ethinyl estradiol. Initially, the patient takes one Ovral twice a day for 3 days until the bleeding stops, and then continues one pill a day to complete a 21-day cycle. Lo/Ovral is often the choice for younger adolescents, since the estrogen dose is lower than that in Ovral. Lo/Ovral may have to be given three or four times a day initially until the bleeding stops, then decreased to once a day. It should be remembered that high doses of combination estrogen-progestins are associated with severe nausea. Thus, if oral contraceptives are given twice, three, or four times daily, an antiemetic should be prescribed.

If the bleeding is initially quite heavy and the patient is mildy anemic (Hgb 9 to 11 g/dl), Ovral may be begun four times a day. Bleeding should slow promptly and stop within 24 to 36 hours. Ovral may be continued four times a day for 4 days total, then three times a day for 3 days, then twice a day for 2 weeks. The patient is continued on cyclic oral contraceptives for 3 to 6 months. Patients who initially require a pill containing 50 mg of ethinyl estradiol usually can be switched to a pill containing 35 mg of ethinyl estradiol after the first cycle. The physician must be in close contact with the patient during the initial phase of the treatment to be sure that the bleeding is slowing and the patient understands how to taper the medication. After the first month, it is convenient to switch the patient from 21-day to 28-day pill packages. The proper use of 28-day packages should be reviewed to avoid confusion. Oral iron and folic acid (1 mg/d) should be given to treat the anemia.

The patient who has a history of prolonged heavy bleeding with a hemoglobin less than 9% is considered to have severe dysfunctional bleeding. She may have clinical signs of blood loss. If the initial hemoglobin is less than 7 g/dl, or if she is orthostatic this heavy bleeding and a hemoglobin of less than 10 g/dl, she should be admitted to the hospital. Clotting studies and a pregnancy test should be done. A transfusion occasionally is necessary. Ovral is given every 4 hours until the bleeding stops (four to eight tablets), then four times a day for 4 days, three times a day for 3 days, and twice a day for 2 weeks. Norinyl (Ortho-Novum) 1/50 may be used in a similar regimen. In patients with acute severe hemorrhage, Premarin 25 mg IV has been used every 4 hours for two to three doses. Intravenous estrogen increases clotting at the capillary level, which is quite effective at stopping the hemorrhage. However, this method carries a higher risk of blood clots. Ovral is begun at the same time, since the effect of the intravenous estrogen is short lived. The Ovral also adds the progestational agent needed to stabilize the endometrium and avoid an estrogen withdrawal bleed after stopping the intravenous estrogen. Antiemetics are used to reduce nausea in all these high-dose estrogen regimens.

If estrogen is contraindicated, norethindrone acetate (Norlutate) 5 to 10 mg or medroxyprogesterone 10 mg can be given every 4 hours and decreased to four times a day for 4 days, three times a day for 3 days, and twice a day for 2 weeks.

If hormone tablets given every 4 hours do not control bleeding within 24 to 36 hours, an examination under anesthesia and dilatation and curettage may be necessary. Withdrawal flow should begin 2 to 4 days after the last hormone tablet is taken, and the patient should be given Ovral 28 for 3 to 6 months after an interval of 4 to 7 days from the last pill of the initial cycle. Replacement of iron and folate is begun in the first cycle.

Patients with low platelet counts, leukemia, or aplastic anemia may require prolonged therapy to suppress menses. Continuous Lo/Ovral 21 may be used for several months but may cause breakthrough bleeding. Oral contraceptive agents may also affect liver function tests. Diagnostic confusion may result, since the etiology of the abnormal liver function tests may be the cancer itself, chemotherapy, or oral contraceptive effects. Medroxyprogesterone 10 mg may be given daily for months. When platelet counts improve, the patient should be cycled with a low-dose progestin-dominant pill such as Lo/Ovral. Another alternative for the cancer patient is induction of amenorrhea with the use of a GnRH agonist. These medications can be given intramuscularly or intranasally with good result. It has been well described that the first menses on GnRH agonists can be excessive and is then followed by amenorrhea. The heavy first period should be appropriately timed so as not to come at a time of thrombocytopenia. The GnRH agonist should be continued until the patient is no longer thrombocytopenic and resumption of menses is considered safe. The use of GnRH agonists for longer than 6 months is associated with hypoestrogenic side effects, the most significant being the risk of osteoporosis.

Contraception

Contraceptive information is a basic part of health education for the adolescent. Confidentiality has been shown to be an important factor in determining whether the sexually active adolescent obtains and uses contraception. The physician who elects to provide oral contraceptives for adolescents in his or her practice should also perform pelvic examinations, including Papanicolaou smears, screening for asymptomatic gonococcal and chlamydial infections, and treatment of sexually transmitted infections.

Oral Contraceptives

Oral contraceptive pills containing estrogen and a progestin remain the most popular and most effective form of contraception for adolescents. Although the theoretical failure rate of oral contraceptive pills containing estrogen and progestin is 0.3 to 0.5 pregnancies per 100 women years of use, the actual failure rate in adolescents is much higher, since many teens use the pills incorrectly or sporadically or discontinue use within a few months.

Absolute contraindications to estrogen-containing oral contraceptives include undiagnosed abnormal vaginal bleeding, pregnancy, active liver disease, cyanotic congenital heart disease, a history of thromboembolic disease, and hypertension. Relative contraindications to pill use include lipid disorders, collagen vascular disease, migraine with focal neurologic deficits, sickle cell disease, diabetes mellitus, and depression. In these cases, the risks of pregnancy should be weighed against the risks of pill use, and the patient may be encouraged to consider the alternative of barrier methods of contraception. Many sexually active teens are also cigarette smokers. Although the risk of thromboembolism in teen pill users who smoke is small, the patient should be encouraged to discontinue cigarette use if possible. There is controversy about whether pill use is associated with an earlier presentation of breast cancer, and patients with a family history of early onset breast cancer should be advised that this remains an unanswered question. Multiple studies, however, show no lifetime increased risk of breast cancer in pill users.

Oral contraceptive pills containing 30 to 35 μg of ethinyl estradiol are appropriate for most adolescents. A fixed-dose pill using 35 μg of ethinyl estradiol in combination with 1 mg norethindrone (Norinyl or Ortho-Novum 1/35) is one commonly used oral contraceptive. Triphasic combinations with ethinyl estradiol and norethindrone (Ortho-Novum 7/7/7) or levonorgestrel (Triphasil, Tri-Levlen) are similar in efficacy. Levonorgestrel triphasics have less breakthrough bleeding.

In recent years, new progestational agents have become available in oral contraceptive agents in the United States. These new progestins have been available in the European markets for many years. Desogestrel, gestodene, and norgestimate have been found to be effective as contraceptive agents, and studies suggest that these progestins have less androgenic properties and long half-lives. Effects on weight, lipids, and glucose tolerance are minimized, and breakthrough bleeding is less frequent. Formulations available in the United States include those with desogestrel and norgestimate. Examples of these new products include Ortho-Cept or Desogen (0.15 mg desogestrel with 0.03 mg ethinyl estradiol), Ortho-Cyclen (0.25 mg norgestimate with 0.035 mg ethinyl estradiol), and Ortho Tri-Cyclen (0.18 mg, 0.215 mg, and 0.25 mg norgestimate with 0.035 mg ethinyl estradiol). In the near future, a triphasic formulation of desogestrel will become available. Within the group of pills containing 30 to 35 μg ethinyl estradiol, some are relatively more progestin dominant and some more estrogen dominant. An estrogen-dominant pill, such as Modicon or Demulen 1/35, is a good choice for a patient who has hirsutism, acne, or polycystic ovary syndrome. A pill containing 30 μg ethinyl estradiol with norgestrel 0.3 mg (Lo/Ovral) can be useful when breakthrough bleeding is a problem, as can short courses (3 months) of pills containing 50 μg of mestranol (Ortho-Novum, Norinyl 1/50). Prolonged use of pills containing 50 μg of estrogen is avoided when possible in adolescents. A 28-day packet is preferred to a 21-day packet to increase compliance. Pills containing 20 μg of ethinyl estradiol are associated with more breakthrough bleeding and less efficacy if pills are omitted and are, therefore, reserved for patients who are unable to tolerate 30 to 35 μg doses of estrogen.

A complete physical examination with blood pressure, weight, breast examination, pelvic examination, Papanicolaou smear, and cervical cultures, should be undertaken before the pill is prescribed. Oral contraceptives may be prescribed in the young adolescent who has not yet established regular ovulatory cycles, since the risk of pregnancy in this patient is significant. A basic laboratory evaluation of menstrual irregularity (FSH, LH, prolactin, TSH, urine pregnancy test) is appropriate before starting oral contraceptives in the patient with a history of irregular cycles. In the patient with amenorrhea who has a negative pregnancy test and who has not been sexually active within 2 weeks, medroxyprogesterone 10 mg PO for 10 days can be used to induce withdrawal bleeding before beginning oral contraceptives.

The patient who has started oral contraceptives should return within 3 months for a repeat weight and blood pressure determination and review of any side effects. If compliance is likely to be a problem, it is appropriate to have the patient return monthly initially to reinforce teaching about contraceptive use and address any concerns or minor side effects the patient may be experiencing. Pelvic examinations for cultures at 6-month intervals and annual Papanicolaou smears are recommended in any sexually active adolescent woman.

Common side effects of pill use are mild nausea, breakthrough bleeding, and breast tenderness. Weight gain is a major concern of adolescents considering oral contraceptive use, but in most cases, there is no weight change in patients taking the pills. Patients who are on an anticonvulsant metabolized by the liver may require 50 μg of ethinyl estradiol. Oral contraceptives should be discontinued before surgery requiring immobilization.

All teens using oral contraceptives to prevent pregnancy should be strongly encouraged to use condoms as well to reduce the risk of acquiring sexually transmitted infections.

Miniprogestin-Only Pills. Oral contraceptives containing small amounts of progestins alone, such as Ovrette (norgestrel 0.075 mg) or Nor-Q.D. or Micronor (norethindrone 0.35 mg) are an alternative for patients who have a medical contraindication to estrogen. Menstrual irregularities, both amenorrhea and irregular bleeding, are very frequent side effects of these pills. Since pregnancy rates are higher on minipills, particularly if pills are omitted, periodic pregnancy tests often become necessary for these patients.

Implantable Contraceptives

Norplant, a contraceptive device consisting of six small Silastic rods containing levonorgestrel that are implanted in the skin of the arm under local anesthesia and sterile conditions, has recently become available in the United States. The implant provides 5 years of contraception. This appears to be an attractive option for patients who have demonstrated poor compliance with oral contraceptives (especially teen parents). The expense of the initial implantation and the frequency of menstrual irregularity as a side effect may limit the usefulness of this method. The rods must be removed after 5 years.

Depot medroxyprogesterone acetate 150 mg IM every 3 months is now an approved contraceptive method in the United States. It may be an alternative to consider in patients who are unable to comply with oral methods because of poor compliance, mental retardation, or mental illness. Amenorrhea is common. Long-term effects on bone density have not been adequately studied.

Barrier Methods

Barrier methods of contraception have become an attractive approach for teens as concerns about sexually transmitted diseases have increased in recent years. Latex condoms containing nonoxynol 9 spermicide provide the best protection against sexually transmitted infection. Both male and female teens should be counseled explicitly on proper condom storage and use. Adolescent women should be encouraged to use additional nonoxynol 9 preparations in case of condom breakage. Vaginal spermicidal foams, creams, vaginal contraceptive film, and contraceptive sponges all provide additional protection when used with a condom. The methods are all available in pharmacies without prescription. Contraceptive sponges may be inserted for up to 24 hours and should be left in place for 8 hours after intercourse. Although condoms provide considerable protection against pregnancy and infection, it should be stressed that the protection is incomplete, and there is no such thing as completely safe sex. Careful selection of partners, reducing the number of partners, and using the condom throughout each episode of sexual intercourse reduces the risk further. The diaphragm is another barrier method of contraception and must be fitted and prescribed by a physician. It is used most successfully by motivated women who are comfortable with their anatomy, especially those who have had experience using tampons. The diaphragm is filled with spermicidal jelly and left in place for 8 hours after intercourse. The diaphragm is initially fitted by the provider, and the patient practices inserting and removing it during the office visit and returns for a second visit wearing the diaphragm to be sure that it is being correctly inserted. Since the diaphragm provides less protection against sexually transmitted infection than the condom, patients using this method are advised to have their partners use condoms.

Postcoital Contraception

Postcoital contraception has been shown to be 96% effective in preventing pregnancy if given within 48 to 72 hours of intercourse. Two Ovral (ethinyl estradiol 50 µg, norgestrel 0.5 mg) tablets are taken immediately, and two more are taken 12 hours later. Nausea is a frequent side effect. Intrauterine devices are seldom used in adolescents because of concerns about the increased likelihood of pelvic inflammatory disease, with resulting infertility, in this patient population. Natural family planning is of little use in adolescents, who frequently have variable menstrual cycles and who have difficulty complying with the periodic abstinence required by the method. Withdrawal or coitus interruptus is likewise unreliable, partially due to the presence of sperm in the preejaculate fluid.

Abstinence

Abstinence should be encouraged as the only truly reliable method of preventing pregnancy and avoiding sexually transmitted infection. Many teens who have experimented with sexual activity decide to return to abstinence. They should be supported in their decision but advised that if they again resume sexual activity, they should be sure to use contraception immediately and continually.

GYNECOLOGIC INFECTIOUS ABNORMALITIES

Vulvovaginitis

Physiologic Leukorrhea

Physiologic leukorrhea, a white, mucoid, homogeneous, nonirritating desquamation of squamous cells, begins before menarche in all pubertal adolescent females. Squamous cells alone are seen on saline wet-mount slide. Patients can be reassured that this is a normal part of adolescent development.

Candidal Vulvovaginitis

Candidal vulvovaginitis may occur in sexually active or virginal females in adolescence, although it is more common in sexually active teens. It occurs frequently in patients on broad-spectrum antibiotics, in diabetics, in patients on glucocorticoids, in obese patients, and in pregnant patients. The discharge is pruritic, and the vulva and vagina are inflamed with red papular satellite lesions on the vulva and a lumpy white vaginal discharge, revealing candidal hyphae and buds on potassium hydroxide preparation.

Treatment. The imidazole medications are the basis of the multiple treatment regimens of candidal vaginitis. Vaginal suppositories are less messy than creams but may not treat vulvar involvement as well. Recommended treatment regimens include the following.

- Butoconazole 2% cream 5 g intravaginally for 3 days*
- Clotrimazole 1% cream 5 g intravaginally for 7–14 days†
- Clotrimazole 100 mg vaginal tablet for 7 days†

---

*These creams and suppositories are oil based and may weaken latex condoms and diaphragms.
†Over-the-counter preparations.

- Clotrimazole 100 mg vaginal tablet, two tablets for 3 days
- Clotrimazole 500 mg vaginal tablet, one tablet single application
- Miconazole 2% cream 5 g intravaginally for 7 days*†
- Miconazole 200 mg vaginal suppository, one suppository for 3 days*
- Miconazole 100 mg vaginal suppository, one suppository for 7 days*†
- Terconazole 0.4% cream 5 g intravaginally for 7 days
- Terconazole 0.8% cream 5 g intravaginally for 3 days
- Terconazole 80 mg suppository, 1 suppository for 3 days*
- Tioconazole 6.5% ointment 5 g intravaginally in a single application*

Although a longer course of treatment is required, nystatin is an alternative if patients develop an allergic vaginal irritation on imidazole preparations. Imidazoles should be avoided in the first trimester of pregnancy.

Bacterial Vaginosis

Bacterial vaginosis is another cause of vaginal discharge. Although it has been associated with the presence of the bacterium *Gardnerella vaginalis*, it probably represents an overgrowth of mixed anaerobic bacteria. Normal lactobacilli are absent. It occurs more commonly in sexually active adolescents. The discharge is gray, white, or yellow and homogeneous, adhering to the vaginal walls and usually malodorous. Saline preparations reveal squamous cells coated with bacteria. The vaginal pH is above 4.5.

Treatment. Treatment is with metronidazole 500 mg PO or clindamycin 300 mg PO twice daily for 7 days. The side effects of metronidazole are nausea, headache, metallic aftertaste, and, rarely, blood dyscrasias. The patient should be instructed to avoid alcohol use during treatment, since alcohol in the presence of metronidazole causes emesis. The side effects of clindamycin include nausea, loose stools, and rash. Single-dose metronidazole 2 g PO has been shown to be as effective as the longer courses of therapy.

Recently, intravaginal antibiotics have shown good resutls for bacterial vaginosis. Metronidazole gel 0.75% one full applicator (5 g) intravaginally twice daily for 5 days or clindamycin cream 2% one full applicator (5 g) intravaginally once daily for 7 days is associated with clinical cure rates similar to those for oral therapy.

If the infection recurs repeatedly, it may be helpful to treat the partner of the sexually active patient as well. The health care provider must be aware that recurrent vaginal infections may be the initial presenting symptom of women with HIV disease.

Trichomoniasis

Trichomoniasis is a sexually transmitted infection presenting with a yellow, frothy vaginal discharge, sometimes with dysuria. The cervix may appear inflamed and friable. Saline preparation shows many polymorphonuclear leukocytes and active wriggling trichomonads.

Treatment. Treatment is with metronidazole 2 g PO in one dose. The sexual partner should be treated simultaneously. Alcohol should be avoided during treatment, and intercourse should be postponed until the partner is also treated. The single-dose treatment is effective in 86% to 95% of patients. If the infection recurs more than once, a 7-day course of metronidazole 500 mg twice daily may be used. Metronidazole should be avoided during pregnancy. Clotrimazole (Gyne-Lotrimin, Mycelex) 1% cream or 100-mg vaginal tablets for 7 nights may be used in the pregnant patient.

Nonspecific Vulvitis

Nonspecific vulvitis may be caused by heat, nylon underpants, poor hygiene, or sand. Hydrocortisone cream 1% may be applied three times daily to the vulva. The precipitating causes should be eliminated.

Chlamydia trachomatis Cervicitis and Urethritis

Chlamydia trachomatis is present in 5% to 18% of asymptomatic sexually active teenage women, 40% to 50% of patients with a vaginal discharge, and about half of patients who have gonorrheal infection. Although the infection frequently is asymptomatic, the classic presentation is a mucopurulent cervical discharge with white cells present on wet preparation. Symptoms often include a vaginal discharge, dysuria, and the abdominal pain and systemic symptoms of pelvic inflammatory disease (PID). *C. trachomatis* is also a common cause of perihepatitis, presenting with right upper quadrant pain and tenderness as a complication of PID. Symptomatic or asymptomatic pyuria in the adolescent female may be caused by *Chlamydia* or *Neisseria gonorrhoeae,* and sexually transmitted infection should always be considered in the adolescent female with these findings.

Endocervical *Chlamydia* cultures have a specificity of 100% but a sensitivity of only 80% to 90%. A dacron swab is used for culture. A number of less expensive screening tests for *Chlamydia* based on laboratory examination of direct smear with fluorescein-labeled antibody (MicroTrak), enzyme immunoassays (Chlamydiazyme, CellTech), DNA probes, and office-based tests (Testpack CHLA-MYDIA) are practical alternatives to culture with somewhat lower sensitivities. Since *Chlamydia* is an intracellular organism, proper techniques must be used in obtaining the specimens to maximize yield. The symptomatic patient with a purulent discharge should be treated immediately at the time of testing, and treatment should be completed even in the absence of a positive test result.

Treatment. Regimens for cervical and urethral infections include the following.

- Doxycycline 100 mg PO b.i.d for 7 days
- Azithromycin 1 g PO in a single dose
- Ofloxacin 300 mg PO b.i.d. for 7 days
- Tetracycline 500 mg PO q.i.d. for 7 days
- Erythromycin base or stearate 500 mg PO q.i.d. for 7 days
- Erythromycin ethylsuccinate 800 mg PO q.i.d. for 7 days

Tetracycline or doxycycline should not be used in the pregnant patient. The recommended regimen for pregnant women is erythromycin base 500 mg PO four times a day for 7 days. Alternative regimens for pregnant women include the following.

- Erythromycin base 250 mg PO q.i.d. for 14 days
- Erythromycin ethylsuccinate 800 mg PO q.i.d. for 7 days
- Erythromycin ethylsuccinate 400 mg PO q.i.d for 14 days

Erythromycin estolate is contraindicated during pregnancy because of drug-related hepatotoxicity. If erythromycin cannot be tolerated, the treatment of choice is amoxicillin 500 mg PO three times a day for 7 to 10 days.

Partners should also be treated. Rescreening in 3 to 6 weeks is useful in the adolescent sexually active patient who is at high risk for reexposure.

Gonococcal Cervicitis and Urethritis

Neisseria gonorrhoeae is another frequent cause of a purulent vaginal discharge in teens. Like *Chlamydia,* colonization with *N. gonorrhoeae* may be asymptomatic, and sexually active teenage women from high-risk populations should be screened with endocervical culture on Thayer-Martin medium at least twice a year. Patients with gonorrheal infection often have *Chlamydia* as well, and treatment should cover both organisms. Cervical gram stain may reveal intracellular gram-negative diplococci within polymorphonuclear leukocytes, but this finding is less common and less sensitive than in males with *N. gonorrhoeae* urethritis. Urethral infection with *N. gonorrhoeae* may be asymptomatic or may cause urinary frequency, dysuria, and pyuria. A Bartholin gland abscess may be caused by *N. gonorrhoeae, Chlamydia,* or other organisms and presents with labial pain and swelling. Treatment should include both antibiotic treatment covering *N. gonorrhoeae* and *Chlamydia* and, in most cases, surgical drainage.

Treatment. Treatment of asymptomatic infection, cervicitis, urethritis, or sexual contacts of patients with *N. gonorrhoeae* infection should include coverage for *Chlamydia,* since the organisms fre-

quently coexist. Penicillin-resistant *N. gonorrhoeae* have been identified with variable frequency throughout the United States. Chromosomally mediated resistance to penicillin may include resistance to tetracycline. The currently recommended treatment of gonorrhea cervicitis or urethritis follows.

1. Ceftriaxone 250 mg IM once plus doxycycline 100 mg PO two times a day for 7 days. The ceftriaxone may be mixed with 1% lidocaine without epinephrine to reduce the pain of injection.
2. In the patient with a history of immediate or anaphylactic reaction to penicillin, spectinomycin 2.0 g IM plus doxycycline 100 mg PO two times a day for 7 days should be used as an alternative, although cross-reactivity between third-generation cephalosporins and penicillin is uncommon.

Ofloxacin has been approved recently for treatment of gonococcal infection. Ofloxacin 400 mg can be given PO once, followed by doxycycline 100 mg twice daily for 7 days or ofloxacin 300 mg four times a day for 7 days. Other regimens with less data available on efficacy include ciprofloxacin, 500 mg PO once with 1 g probenecid, norfloxin, 800 mg PO once, cefuroxime axetil 1 g PO with 1 g probenecid, cefotaxime 1 g IM, and ceftizoxime 500 mg IM, all followed by doxycycline. Ciprofloxacin and norfloxin should not be used in patients who are pregnant or who are less than 17 years of age. Amoxicillin 3 g PO with 1 g probenecid given in the office is an alternative if the gonorrheal strain is known to be penicillin sensitive. This should be followed by doxycycline. Tetracycline 500 mg PO four times a day is a less expensive alternative to doxycycline, but compliance is likely to be less complete. The pregnant patient should receive erythromycin base or stearate 500 mg PO four times a day or erythromycin ethylsuccinate 800 mg four times a day for 7 days instead of doxycycline. If vomiting results, erythromycin base may be given 250 mg PO four times a day for 14 days.

A serologic test for syphilis should be sent at the time of treatment. Sexual partners should be treated. A test of cure should be done 7 to 10 days after completion of treatment regimens other than ceftriaxone-tetracycline. Rescreening 1 to 2 months after treatment is of value in all cases, since reinfection is common.

Gonococcal Pharyngitis

Gonococcal pharyngitis is diagnosed by pharyngeal culture on Thayer-Martin medium and treated with ceftriaxone 250 mg IM. Nonpregnant patients who are at least 17 years of age may be treated with ciprofloxacin 500 mg PO once if they cannot tolerate ceftriaxone. They should be recultured after treatment. Penicillin-sensitive gonorrheal pharyngitis may be treated with ampicillin 3.5 g PO with 1 g probenecid, followed by ampicillin 500 mg PO four times a day for 2 days.

Gonococcal Proctitis

Gonococcal proctitis may present with discharge of blood and purulent material or, less acutely, with pain on defecation. Gonococcal proctitis may be diagnosed by culture of rectal swab on Thayer-Martin medium. Treatment is the same as for cervicitis.

Gonococcal Arthritis

Gonococcal arthritis is often associated with asymptomatic gonococcal infection or with mild cervicitis or pharyngitis. The mild form is associated with migratory polyarthralgias, tenosynovitis, fever, and skin lesions consisting of papules sometimes progressing to purpuric vesicopustular lesions. Fluorescent antibody staining of biopsies reveal *N. gonorrhoeae* infection in half of these patients. Blood cultures may be positive if taken within 2 days of the onset of symptoms. The late form consists of a monarticular arthritis often in the knee. Synovial fluid culture is positive in 20% to 50%, although blood cultures are negative and systemic symptoms are not present. Patients who are unreliable or who have purulent joint effusions should be hospitalized.

Treatment. Regimens for gonococcal arthritis include the following.

- Ceftriaxone 1 g IM or IV q.d.
- Ceftizoxime 1 g IV q8h
- Cefoxatime 1 g IV q8h

Ampicillin 1 g IV every 6 hours may be used if the *N. gonorrhoeae* is documented to be penicillin sensitive. In patients who are allergic to cephalosporins, spectinomycin 2 g IM every 12 hours may be used.

The patient should be cultured for *Chlamydia* as well. The joint should be immobilized, and repeated aspirations of the joint may be necessary. Hip arthritis requires open drainage. Parental treatment should be continued until the patient has been asymptomatic for 24 to 48 hours, and the patient may then be discharged to complete 7 days of antibiotic treatment with oral cefuroxime axetil 500 mg twice a day, amoxicillin 500 mg with clavulanic acid three times a day, or ciprofloxin 500 mg twice a day if not pregnant and over age 16.

Pelvic Inflammatory Disease

Pelvic inflammatory disease (PID) refers to infection of the upper genital tract, including the fallopian tubes. One million women are treated each year for acute salpingitis, and 16% to 20% of these cases occur in adolescents. Adolescents are at higher risk of PID than are adults because of the high prevalence of gonococcal and chlamydial infection in the adolescent age group. One third to one half of patients with PID have positive endocervical cultures for *N. gonorrhoeae*. The prevalence of positive chlamydial cultures in acute PID is similar. Patients with repeated episodes are less likely to be culture positive for these organisms. Other associated organisms are coliforms, *Gardnerella vaginalis*, *Haemophilus influenzae*, group B streptococci, *Bacteroides* species, *Peptostreptococcus*, *Peptococcus*, and *Mycoplasma hominis*.

The patient with PID classically presents with lower abdominal pain, vaginal discharge, and fever, often within 7 days of the onset of menses. Irregular vaginal bleeding may also be a symptom of PID. Symptoms of chlamydial PID may be somewhat less acute. The diagnosis of PID is often difficult to make, since many patients do not have a classic presentation. The diagnosis is likely if the patient has the following symptoms and signs: a history of lower abdominal pain and cervical motion tenderness or uterine tenderness with adnexal tenderness, along with either purulent cervical discharge, elevated sedimentation rate >15 mm/h, white blood cell count above 10,500/mm³, or pelvic abscess by bimanual examination or ultrasonography. The differential diagnosis includes acute appendicitis, ectopic pregnancy, ovarian abscess, ruptured corpus luteum, and endometriosis. It is important to remember that cervical motion tenderness is caused by any disease process that causes peritoneal irritation. Laparoscopy may be necessary if symptoms are acute and the diagnosis is in doubt. Complete evaluation should include a pregnancy test, a complete blood count, sedimentation rate, serologic test for syphilis, and cultures for *N. gonorrhoeae* and *Chlamydia*.

Treatment. Incomplete or delayed treatment and recurrent PID are associated with tubal occlusion, future ectopic pregnancy, infertility, and chronic pelvic pain. Since compliance with oral antibiotic therapy is often poor in teens and the risk of subsequent infertility is high, some centers admit all adolescents with PID for intravenous antibiotics. Patients with an uncertain diagnosis, suspected tuboovarian abscess, right upper quadrant pain suggesting perihepatitis (Fitz-Hugh-Curtis syndrome), peritoneal signs, temperature greater than 38°C, vomiting, pregnancy, or a history of poor compliance should be admitted to the hospital for treatment. PID during pregnancy is extremely rare. Thus, if a patient is having acute abdominal pain and is pregnant, other diagnoses need to be ruled out.

Many regimens have been used for the treatment of PID. The current CDC guidelines for inpatient treatment of PID are either of the two following regimens.

1. Cefoxitin 2 g IV q6h or cefotetan 2 g IV q12h plus doxycycline 100 mg PO or IV q12h for at least 48 hours after the patient clinically improves. The patient is continued on doxycycline 100 mg PO b.i.d. for 10 to 14 days. Ceftizoxime, cefotaxime, and ceftriaxone are acceptable alternatives to cefoxitin.
2. Clindamycin 900 mg IV q8h (or 600 mg IV q6h) plus gentamycin 2 mg/kg IM or IV, followed by 1.5 mg/kg every 8 hours (if renal function is normal). Tobramycin may be substituted. This regimen should be continued until 48 hours after the patient's symptoms have improved. The patient should then be continued on doxycycline 100 mg b.i.d. for 10 to 14 days. Clindamycin 450 mg q.i.d. is an alternative.

Although we strongly recommend inpatient treatment for all adolescents with PID, in the less acutely ill patient with a history of good compliance, an outpatient treatment regimen is ceftriaxone 500 mg IM (or cefoxitin 2 g IM with probenecid 1 g PO), followed by doxycycline 100 mg PO two times a day for 10 to 14 days. Erythromycin 500 mg four times daily is an alternative for patients who cannot take doxycycline. An alternative outpatient regimen is ofloxacin 400 mg PO two times a day for 14 days plus either clindamycin 450 mg PO four times a day or metronidazole 500 mg PO two times a day for 14 days. The patient should return in 48 to 72 hours for a repeat pelvic examination to determine whether symptoms are improving. The patient's partner should be treated, and the patient should not have intercourse for 3 to 4 weeks. A discussion of safe sex and the use of condoms should be undertaken.

Sexually Transmitted Viral Infections

Human Papillomavirus

Human papillomavirus (HPV) has become an increasing concern to those providing health care to adolescents. HPV infection is common in sexually active teens. HPV is a DNA virus with more than 50 subtypes. Hand and common warts are of the subtypes 1, 2, 4, 7, 26, 27, 28, and 29. Genital warts are caused by HPV DNA subtypes 6, 11, 16, 18, 30–35, 39, 42–44, 48, and 51–55. Subtypes 6 and 11 are associated with the typical cauliflower-like genital warts found on the vulva, vagina, cervix, urethra, and anus. These lesions are associated with a high rate of spontaneous regression and low rate of persistence and not associated with invasive squamous cell carcinoma. Subtypes 16 and 18 are flat condylomas and are associated with cervical dysplasia and genital cancers. HPV subtypes 16 and 18 are seen in 70% of invasive cervical carcinomas. Regression of these lesions is uncommon, and persistence and progression are the rule. HPV subtypes 31, 33, and 35 are associated with 15% of invasive cervical cancers. Genital warts typically appear within 4 to 6 weeks of exposure, but the incubation period is up to 8 months or more. Findings may be subclinical and detectable only by typical HPV changes on Pap smear (koilocytes or cervical intraepithelial neoplasia, CIN) or on biopsy using DNA probes.

Treatment. Exophytic warts are treated in the office with the application of locally destructive agents to the warts. Trichloroacetic acid (TCA) is used in strengths from 25% to 85%; 85% TCA must be applied just to the lesions to avoid burns. Normal saline may be applied after TCA to reduce the burning sensation. TCA is reapplied weekly. This regimen appears to be less problematic and more effective than using 25% podophyllin. If the lesions fail to respond, the patient may be referred for cryocautery or laser treatment. Carbon dioxide laser treatment requires general anesthesia and is associated with considerable posttreatment discomfort and sometimes with scarring or bleeding. New experimental treatments of genital warts include 5-fluorouracil cream and injections of interferon alfa-2b. The effectiveness of these regimens is being evaluated.

Patients with abnormalities on Pap smear consistent with HPV infection should be referred for colposcopy and biopsy. If the biopsy reveals cervical dysplasia, cryotherapy, laser, and cone biopsy are commonly used therapies. Follow-up at 3 months is required, with subsequent Pap smears at frequent intervals. Patients whose biopsy reveals HPV without dysplasia may be treated with locally destructive therapies or observed closely with repeated Pap smears, since the natural history of this infection in the adolescent and the likelihood of subsequent dysplasia or genital cancer in this population are not known.

Partners of patients with HPV should be examined for genital warts. Wrapping the penis in a cloth soaked with vinegar (acetoacid) or 5% TCA before examination improves the chances of detecting warts.

Human Immunodeficiency Virus

Human immunodeficiency virus (HIV) infection is discussed in detail elsewhere. Adolescents currently account for only 1% of cases with AIDS, with considerable geographic variation in prevalence. However, many of the women who present with AIDS as adults presumably acquired their infection in adolescence. This is of special concern, since they may pass the infection on to their child before they themselves develop symptoms. The HIV virus may be more easily acquired by patients with genital lesions of other sexually transmitted infections. Adolescents with multiple partners are at increased risk. Condom use, reducing the number of sexual partners, and abstinence should be encouraged to reduce the likelihood of acquiring HIV infection. Voluntary testing for HIV infection is an option that should be considered carefully and accompanied by supportive counseling in the adolescent, since considerable anxiety and depression may result.

Genital Herpes Infection

Genital herpes infection is usually associated with herpes simplex type 2, although up to 15% of primary genital infections are type 1. Sixty percent of patients with HSV-2 will have recurrence of symptoms over the year following their first episode. Recurrence occurs in 14% of HSV-1 genital infections. In primary infections, vesicles appear on the vulva, labia, or cervix, rupturing to produce painful ulcers associated with burning, dysuria, inguinal adenopathy, and often systemic symptoms of fever, headache, and malaise. Urinary retention due to dysuria is a possible complication. Symptoms improve in 10 to 21 days. Recurrences are generally milder and last 3 to 5 days. Itching or burning sensations may precede the appearance of vesicles. Viral culture of the vesicle or ulcer is often used to confirm the diagnosis.

Treatment. Treatment with acyclovir 200 mg PO five times a day for 10 days can reduce symptoms and shorten the course of primary herpes infection. Local treatment measures include sitz baths in tepid water or Burow's solution, dry heat from a hairdryer set on low, and lidocaine jelly 2% applied to genital lesions. If dysuria is severe, voiding in a shower or sitz bath may help to avoid urinary retention. *Candida* vaginitis may accompany herpes. Severely ill patients may require hospitalization and intravenous acyclovir. Recurrences of genital herpes usually can be treated with local measures. Acyclovir 200 mg five times a day for 5 days can be begun with the first sign of symptoms but is usually not necessary. Patients should not have intercourse while genital herpes lesions are present. Although condoms can help to prevent transmission of herpes, they do not provide complete protection. Transmission is most likely when active lesions are present and during the prodromal period. However, viral shedding in asymptomatic patients may also transmit the virus to sexual partners.

Pediculosis Pubis (Crabs)

Pubic lice are usually transmitted by sexual contact, although they may be acquired by contact with infected blankets, towels, and clothing. The primary symptom is pruritus. Adult lice may be visible on the pubic hair. Nits appear as small white bumps firmly attached to pubic hair.

Treatment. Treatment is with 1% lindane (Kwell) shampoo lathered into hair and left on for 5 minutes. Repeat treatment in 1 week may lessen the likelihood of recurrence. Clothing, sheets, and blankets should be laundered in hot water or set aside for 2 weeks. One percent permethrin creme rinse (Nix) applied for 10 minutes is newer and very effective alternative treatment. Other pyrethrin preparations (RID, A-200 Pyrinate) also may be used.

Vulvar Ulcers

The most common causes of vaginal ulcers are herpes simplex virus, syphilis, and chancroid. Primary syphilis presents as a painless hard ulcer. The rapid plasma reagin (RPR) is usually positive by the seventh day. Therapy is discussed in Chapter 18. Chancroid, although still rare in the United States is increasing in prevalence. Multiple purulent irregular ulcers are seen with tender inguinal adenopathy.

Treatment. Patients with ulcers associated with tender adenopathy who do not have syphilis or herpes may be treated with erythromycin base 500 mg PO four times a day for 7 days or ceftriaxone 250 mg IM for suspected chancroid. Nodes may require drainage if they become fluctuant. Other causes of genital ulcers are inflammatory bowel disease, Behçet's disease, lymphogranuloma venereum, and mononucleosis.

PELVIC PAIN

Primary Dysmenorrhea

Primary or physiologic dysmenorrhea is characterized by pelvic pain on the first day or two of menses. The pain may be related to increases in prostaglandin secretion. Associated systemic symptoms related to prostaglandins include nausea and vomiting, dizziness, syncope, and diarrhea. Patients who have mild symptoms on the first day of menses should have a general physical examination, including examination of hymenal patency. These patients usually respond well to mild over-the-counter analgesic regimens, such as ibuprofen 200 to 400 mg. A pelvic examination should be performed in the patient with severe dysmenorrhea, since uterine anomalies leading to partial obstruction and endometriosis may be the underlying causation.

Treatment. Nonsteroidal anti-inflammatory drugs (NSAID) are usually quite effective in primary dysmenorrhea. Many different regimens exist for NSAID treatment of dysmenorrhea, including naproxen sodium (Anaprox) 550 mg at the start, then 275 mg every 6 hours, naproxen sodium (Anaprox DS) 550 mg twice a day, naproxen (Naprosyn) 250 to 375 mg two to three times a day, ibuprofen 800 mg, followed by 400 mg every 4 to 6 hours up to 800 mg three times a day, mefenamic acid (Ponstel) 500 mg to start, then 250 mg every 6 hours, and flurbiprofen (Ansaid) 50 mg every 6 hours or 100 mg every 12 hours.

If the patient does not respond to intensive NSAID therapy, oral contraceptives may be prescribed for 3 to 6 months. Pills with 30 to 35 μg ethinyl estradiol, such as Desogen, Ortho-Cept, Norinyl 1/35, Ortho-Novum 1/35, Triphasil, Tri-Levlen, Tri-Norinyl, and Ortho-Novum 7/7/7, are usually prescribed. If the pain is not relieved with the combination of NSAID and oral contraceptive agents, further evaluation is needed.

Endometriosis

Endometriosis is a common cause of chronic pelvic pain in adolescents. Most severe symptoms are typically just before and during menses, but acyclic pain is also a common presentation. Pain tends to increase with time. In contrast to functional dysmenorrhea, the pain of endometriosis persists and gradually increases despite treatment with oral contraceptives and NSAID. Most adolescents with endometriosis have normal findings or only mild or moderate tenderness on pelvic examination, without detectable masses or nodularity. Patients whose symptoms persist or increase on this regimen should be referred to a gynecologist for operative laparoscopy to diagnose and treat the endometriosis.

Treatment. Multiple treatment regimens of endometriosis have been used. Initial treatment is surgery at the time of diagnosis. Endometriosis can be vaporized with laparoscopic laser therapy or with fulguration with the use of laparoscopic cautery therapy. Medical therapy as an adjuvant to the surgical therapy can be used. All medical regimens are directed toward suppression of ectopic endometrial tissue in hopes of eliminating pain and preventing fertility. Regimens include

TABLE 1. Comparison of Hormonal Therapies for Endometriosis

THERAPY	RESULTANT HORMONAL STATE			SIDE EFFECTS
	ACYCLIC	HYPOESTROGENIC	HYPERANDROGENIC	
Progestins	+	+	−	Breakthrough bleeding, depression, bloating, decreased libido
Noncyclic OCPs*	+	−	−	Those routinely listed for oral contraceptives, nausea, breakthrough bleeding
Methyltestosterone	±	−	+ +	Virilization, masculinization of a female fetus
Danazol	+	+	+ +	Weight gain, acne, hirsutism, voice changes
GnRH agonist	+	+ +	−	Vasomotor symptoms (hot flushes), bone loss, vaginal dryness
GnRH agonist plus steroid add back (Premarin and Provera or OCPs)	+	?	−	Possible decreased vasomotor symptoms, bone loss, vaginal dryness
Mifepristone (RU 486)	+	±	−	Anorexia, nausea, dizziness, somnolence

*GnRH, gonadotropin-releasing hormone; + +, extremely effective; +, effective; ±, sporadically effective; −, not effective; ?, questionably effective; OCP, oral contraceptive pills.
Adapted from Laufer MR: Endometriosis in adolescents. Curr Opin Pediatr 4:582–589, 1992.

treatment with progestins, such as daily or depot medroxyprogesterone acetate, treatment with androgens, such as danazol, continuous oral contraceptive use with a progestin-dominant pill, such as Lo/Ovral, and most recently, the use of GnRH analogs to suppress ovarian function completely. All of these regimens have frequent side effects, some of which are poorly tolerated by adolescents. Table 1 lists the commonly available medical therapies with their associated side effects.

Pelvic Masses

A pregnant uterus is a common cause of a lower abdominal mass in an adolescent, even in the absence of a reported history of sexual activity. The differential diagnosis of the patient with a positive urine test for hCG and a pelvic mass includes intrauterine pregnancy, ectopic pregnancy, miscarriage, gestational trophoblastic neoplasia (choriocarcinoma, molar pregnancy), and some ovarian tumors contain germ cell elements that secrete hCG.

Etiology. Causes of adnexal masses include ectopic pregnancy, benign persistent follicular or corpus luteum cysts of the ovary, dermoid cysts, hydrosalpinx, endometriomas, and ovarian tumors. An ovarian tumor, although rare in an adolescent, can occur and is often discovered as an asymptomatic pelvic mass or as a cause of enlarging abdominal girth. Ovarian masses may be associated with chronic pelvic or periumbilical pain. Severe pain similar to that associated with appendicitis may represent torsion of an ovarian mass, infarction, or perforation of a cyst or tumor. Granulosa cell tumors or ovarian cysts that secrete estrogen may present as irregular vaginal bleeding or amenorrhea in the adolescent. Corpus luteum cysts secreting estrogen and progesterone may also present with amenorrhea or with vaginal bleeding as they degenerate and hormone levels fall. A congenital anomaly of the uterus or vagina that obstructs menstrual flow presents with pain and a pelvic mass consisting of the obstructed uterus or uterine horn.

Diagnosis. Pelvic ultrasonography is helpful in the diagnosis of the pelvic mass, although findings may occasionally be misleading. Physiologic developing ovarian follicles reaching a size of 1 to 3 cm are a normal finding, and small amounts of fluid may be seen in the cul-de-sac with ovulation. Fluid can also be a sign of bleeding, infection, or a ruptured cyst. Simple ovarian cysts are generally 3 to 6 cm in diameter and unilocular. It should be remembered that primary solid masses, such as dermoids, that are palpable on bimanual examination may be missed on ultrasound. Thus, a bimanual or rectoabdominal examination should not be omitted in the adolescent with pelvic pain. Transvaginal ultrasound provides greater detail in evaluation of the adnexal region than abdominal ultrasound. CT and MRI scans are also used in the evaluation of pelvic masses when the diagnosis has not been established by pelvic examination and ultrasound. MRI has become the gold standard for the evaluation and identification of pelvic anatomy in patients with mullerian anomalies.

Treatment. If a simple ovarian cyst of less than 6 cm in size is documented by bimanual examination or ultrasound in an adolescent, the patient may be followed by monthly pelvic examination or ultrasound films until the cyst resolves. Monophasic oral contraceptive pills are often prescribed for 3 months to suppress the hypothalamic-pituitary-ovarian axis and prevent the formation of new cysts. If the cyst has developed on triphasic pills, many physicians will switch to monophasic pills. If the cyst is greater than 6 cm in size or is causing symptoms, the cyst may be aspirated or removed laparoscopically, and the fluid and cyst wall should be sent for cytologic-pathologic study. The patient is frequently given oral contraceptives to suppress further cyst formation. Attempts should be made to preserve as much ovarian tissue as possible and minimize periovarian adhesions. Solid or mixed cystic and solid ovarian masses are generally approached surgically.

SEXUALITY EDUCATION AND CONTRACEPTION

PAMELA J. MURRAY, M.D., M.H.P.

SEXUALITY EDUCATION

Sexuality and the role of sexuality education are best understood in a life-span perspective. Both are processes that have a place at all stages of human development. However, as adolescence approaches, the concerns and anxieties surrounding sex education focus on sexual behaviors and the negative outcomes of sexual intercourse. As a consequence, inadequate attention is paid to promoting a positive and self-accepting sexuality for all persons. Ideally, accurate and comprehensive knowledge of sexuality and reproductive health issues should precede the onset of sexual intercourse. Parents, teachers, health practitioners, and other community resources may provide this education.

Our culture promulgates many conflicting messages about sexuality. For example, it unrealistically glamorizes sexuality in the media yet heavily values premarital virginity as morally correct individual behavior. The confusion that results from these inconsistent messages inhibits quality sexuality education. There is inadequate portrayal of responsible sexual behavior in the media. Education curricula rarely discuss specific sexual behaviors or feelings. Public discussion of all but sensationalized sexual issues is limited by personal anxieties and concerns about repercussions. Young people are usually well aware of the direct and indirect messages conveyed by the media about sexual issues. An awareness of the media can provide many opportunities for discussion and education when combined with a willingness to listen and respond.

The factors that contribute to adult sexual identity are described in the discussion that follows in this chapter. In the home setting, family values, behavior, and verbal communication all contribute to the individual's sexual development and education. In addition to parents and other family members, the peer group, an individual's sexual partners, health practitioners, teachers, and nonparenting adults may all play a role in this educational process. The content and values communicated outside the family may be different from the previous parent-child discussions. An atmosphere of nonjudgmental openness and a level of comfort on the part of the parents will encourage young people to share their questions and ask for parental clarification of both content and values.

The discussion by parents of intimacy, affection, romance, and relationships should be encouraged. Acceptance and endorsement of developmentally appropriate self-exploration, including masturbation, should be supported as a normal expression of one's sexuality. Parents themselves often benefit from access to sexuality education programs and resources. Civic, health, educational, and religious institutions can contribute to this effort by discussing sexuality in a manner that is compatible with their own values and role in the community.

Improved training and preparation in sexuality teaching is needed for teachers, health practitioners, and parents. Peer educators have been shown to be effective in conveying knowledge and simultaneously providing role modeling of desirable values and behaviors, such as postponing sexual involvement. The older teen peer educators themselves benefit from their preparation and participation in these programs. Access to correct information and role models that promote the delay of sexual intercourse should be available before the majority of teens consider sexual exploration and experimentation if they are to be effective at delaying sexual behaviors and minimizing some of the negative consequences.

Comprehensive school-based sexuality education beginning in the earliest primary grades exists in Sweden and other countries. It is one of the factors that contribute to very low pregnancy and birth rates in the presence of more sexually experienced teenagers than are found in other industrialized countries.

Conclusions from the field of sexuality and pregnancy prevention education can help plan the content and methods of new sexuality curricula. Explicit discussion of reproduction and contraception does not accelerate initiation of sexual intercourse. In some circumstances, curricula containing such material is associated with both postponement of intimate sexual involvement and better subsequent contraceptive use. Comprehensive sexuality education needs to be of sufficient duration to allow for thorough communication of the content, reflection, discussion, and review.

CONTRACEPTION

Adolescents are initiating sexual intercourse at younger ages. At each teenage year, a higher percentage of both recent and "ever" sexual experience is reported. For females, 58% have had intercourse by the age of 18; for males, 67% report intercourse by their eighteenth birthday.

It is estimated that 1 of every 8 young women between the ages of 15 and 19 becomes pregnant each year. This translates into more than 1 million pregnancies annually in 15- to 19-year-olds, even with the general increase in the use of both condoms and other contraceptive methods. It is estimated that 50% of teen pregnancies occur within 6 months of initiating intercourse because contraception may be used less often, less consistently, and improperly.

A sexual health history is an essential component of the routine adolescent health maintenance visit and may be indicated at episodic visits, depending on the complaint. This interview should be conducted in private with the adolescent alone. Guidelines for consent, confidentiality, and financial obligation should be established and discussed with the patient. The sexual history provides a unique op-

portunity to educate the adolescent about normal reproductive anatomy and physiology and the strong sexual and romantic feelings that emerge in adolescence and to assess the patient's concerns about these issues. Information gathered by a trained nursing staff or in response to written questionnaires may identify important sexual health care needs. Sexual responsibility, including pregnancy and sexually transmitted disease (STD) prevention, should be emphasized. Pamphlets and posters displayed in the waiting area can provide further education for the adolescent and his or her parents. Adolescents or their parents, guardian, or caretakers may initiate the request for a "pelvic exam," a "VD" or "STD" checkup, or a contraceptive method or education. Such requests should always be addressed or referred.

Individual and family religious and moral belief systems, popular myths and misinformation, and conflicts or uncertainties about sexual activity and relationships influence sexual behaviors. Developmentally normal risk taking and peer pressure may interfere with compliance with STD protection and contraceptive use. Drugs, and alcohol in particular, may alter judgment about sexual involvement and impair coitally related prevention activities. Some adolescents have misconceptions about how pregnancy risks vary within the menstrual cycle. If they have not conceived during a period of unprotected sex, they may have generalized their experience and come to doubt their fertility. Nonjudgmental exploration of these issues will help the adolescent and the practitioner choose a contraceptive method that best meets the patient's needs. Counseling about contraceptive options should involve a nondirective discussion reviewing potential contraceptive choices, including their use, risks, side effects, and benefits. The decision to choose a particular method of contraception must include consideration of the adolescent's ability, as influenced by age and developmental stage, to correctly use and comply with recommended follow-up.

Contraceptive Options

Abstinence

Abstinence from sexual intercourse is practiced by many teenagers. It is the most effective way of avoiding pregnancy and is an essential component of any contraceptive options counseling. Some adolescents limit their sexual intimacy or select behaviors without risk of pregnancy, such as manual, oral, or anal-genital contact. Identification of these sexual practices is important to ensure detection of and to discuss protection from STDs. Supporting adolescents in their choices and providing information to plan knowingly about future sexual activities are essential.

Withdrawal

Withdrawal, or coitus interruptus, is practiced frequently by adolescents at their first and subsequent sexual encounters. Many teenagers who say that they are not using any contraception will specify, if asked, that the male partner regularly "pulls out" before ejaculation. Although recent studies suggest that there is no sperm in preejaculate, it is often difficult for the male partner to withdraw completely in sufficient time. Additional factors limiting the effectiveness of this method include unfamiliarity with one's own and one's partner's sexual response and the often clandestine and rushed nature of adolescents' sexual encounters. Withdrawal offers no protection against STDs.

Periodic Abstinence, Fertility Awareness Methods

Fertility awareness methods, such as the rhythm method, cervical mucus testing, and basal body temperature charting, are rarely used correctly by adolescents. It is a very rare teenager who meticulously documents her menses, basal body temperature, and cervical mucus quality and quantity for the suggested 1 to 2 years needed to predict ovulation accurately. For some mature 18- or 19-year-old adolescents in stable relationships, fertility awareness methods may be a reasonable contraceptive choice when adequate initial education, ongoing support, and a committed partner are available.

Barrier Methods

Condoms. Condoms are essential for protection from most STDs and can be a highly effective contraceptive method when used consistently at every intercourse with a vaginal spermicide. As with other contraceptive choices, proper detailed instruction about use should be given.

Lubricated condoms made from latex are widely used, inexpensive, and reliable. For individuals allergic to latex, natural-membrane condoms provide contraceptive benefit but less protection from STDs. Condoms are intended for one use only, and it is recommnded that they be stored where they are not exposed to excessive heat. A recent trial found no change in condom reliability if carried in a wallet for 3 months in varied climates. They are widely available without prescription and are found in pharmacies, supermarkets, and 24-hour convenience stores and may be available in some schools. Condoms treated with the spermicide nonoxynol-9 are available, as are extra-large condoms and more durable condoms intended for anal intercourse. Oil-based lubricants (e.g., petroleum, mineral oil) and vaginal medications (e.g., clindamycin cream) should not be used with condoms as they damage latex condoms and make them more likely to tear or leak.

Spermicides. Spermicides, when used with condoms provide highly effective contraception, approaching that of combined oral contraceptives (COC). Nonoxynol-9, the active ingredient in most spermicidal preparations, may also decrease the risk of transmission of some bacterial and viral STDs. Spermicides are safe and available without prescription. Vehicles include foams, gels, creams, tablets, suppositories, and vaginal contraceptive film. Each preparation of spermicide has instructions that specify the proper insertion technique and the onset and duration of effectiveness. Spermicides must be reapplied with each act of intercourse. Spermicide use near the time of conception has not been associated with adverse fetal outcomes. Some individuals are sensitive or allergic to either the spermicide or the base. Changing brands or preparations may avoid further irritation.

Diaphragm and Cervical Cap. These barrier methods, in conjunction with spermicide, provide effective contraception. Older adolescents who are comfortable with touching their own genitals and handling the devices and who have personal or medical reasons for not choosing hormonal contraception may select these methods. Each must be fitted by a trained practitioner who can verify that the young woman can successfully place and remove the contraceptive device. A 1- or 2-week trial of use at home is recommended before a final decision is made.

Female Condom. A female condom is now available. A tubular polyurethane condom that has an inner circular rim with a diaphragm-like fit and an outer ring that is positioned externally against the labia can be purchased without a prescription. The anticipated higher unit cost, limited availability, and complexity of this item may deter teens from trying it.

Combined Oral Contraceptives

The COC pill is the most common contraceptive choice among sexually active adolescents. When taken properly, it provides very effective contraception by suppressing ovulation and by altering the physiology of the female reproductive tract by the effects of both its hormonal components, estrogen, and a progestogen. It also offers numerous noncontraceptive benefits that may appeal to young women. Nevertheless, teenagers using the COCs experience a failure rate higher than in the general population because of the multitude of factors that influence compliance with any medication regimen. The higher failure rate applies to all reversible contraceptive choices.

Concern that COCs should not be started until after 6 to 12 months of regular menses have occurred has not been substantiated. The young newly postmenarcheal girl who is sexually active is at high risk for unintended pregnancy. The consequences of accelerated closure of epiphyses, a small theoretical risk at best, must be weighed against the many real consequences of an unintended pregnancy.

The absolute contraindications to starting COCs are relatively rare in adolescents and include the following conditions: a history of clots (cerebrovascular accident, myocardial infarction, pulmonary or thromboembolism, or phlebitis), cancer of estrogen-influenced tissues (breast or reproductive regions), cholestasis (of pregnancy, liver tumors, or impaired liver function), complicated migraines with an associated neurologic deficit, or conception (pregnancy). Strong relative contraindications likely to be found in adolescents include severe headaches, particularly migraines exacerbated by COCs, severe hypertension confirmed on repeated examination, hepatitis (proven infection or acute mononucleosis), cyanotic heart disease, hospitalization (major surgery requiring immobilization in the next 4 weeks or serious injury and immobilization), or the presence of undiagnosed abnormal vaginal bleeding that could have a hematologic cause.

In young females with chronic medical problems, careful consideration of contraceptive choices should be presented and weighed against risks of pregnancy. Cognitive, behavioral, or psychiatric difficulties that may interfere with compliance with contraception present additional challenges to the practitioner.

Noncontraceptive benefits of COCs include relief of menstrual cycle problems, including dysmenorrhea, Mittelschmerz, and some premenstrual symptoms. Other indications include endometriosis and ovarian hyperandrogenism. The COC may be indicated for therapy after appropriate diagnostic measures have been taken in young women with abnormal vaginal bleeding or irregular menses. Overall, COC users experience less risk of severe pelvic inflammatory disease (PID), decreased risk of ovarian and endometrial cancer, fewer functional ovarian cysts, fewer nonmalignant breast cysts and fibroadenomas, fewer ectopic pregnancies, and less iron deficiency anemia. Other benefits include improvement in acne and manipulation of the timing of menses when it would pose unusual personal inconvenience. Menstrual regulation can be used to decrease the frequency of menses to only three or four times a year in young women with developmental delay and hygiene problems associated with menstrual flow.

Many formulations of low-dose COCs are available. Young women should be started on one of these preparations. The most commonly used low-dose COCs contain between 30 and 35 μg ethinyl estradiol, available as a fixed-dose or triphasic preparation. Progestational agents and doses vary among pill formulations. New progestogens in COCs include norgestimate, desogestrel, and gestodene. These compounds have been formulated to better simulate natural progesterone and are reported to cause less androgenic side effects, such as acne, weight gain, and amenorrhea than other progestational agents. They appear to be good COC choices for both contraceptive and medical indications. Access to *Contraceptive Technology*[2] is recommended for any practitioner prescribing contraception.

Minor side effects, including physical discomfort (nausea and breast fullness and tenderness), mood changes, and breakthrough bleeding, are common in the first cycles and tend to diminish over the initial three cycles of pill use. Lower progestogen doses are associated with an increased risk of breakthrough bleeding and very scant (or even absent) menstrual flow. Persistent side effects of nausea, mood changes, and headaches may be dose related. Some individuals are more bothered by either the estrogenic or progestogenic side effects. Changing the pill formulation or time of day that the pill is taken may minimize these unpleasant symptoms.

With the lower-dose formulations, the risk of accidental pregnancy following one or more missed pills increases. A single missed pill that just precedes or follows the normal 7-day hormone-free week (days 22 to 28) carries a significant increase in the risk of ovulation. Therefore, 28-day pill packages, rather than 21-day packages, are strongly recommended to maintain the pill-taking habit. An alternate barrier and spermicide method should be explained and prescribed, to be used as backup for the entire first month's cycle of pills and when pills are missed for any reason. When antibiotics are prescribed, backup protection is recommended, although the risk of decreased contraception appears to be primarily theoretical. In contrast, medications that alter liver metabolism, including rifampin and the most commonly used anticonvulsants, can decrease the effectivensss of COCs. For these drugs, backup protection and COC dose or regimen adjustments are necessary.

Ideally, a complete physical evaluation, including pelvic and breast examinations, is performed before COCs are initiated. At the same time, a Papanicolaou (Pap) smear, gonococcal culture, *Chlamydia* determination, rapid plasma reagin (RPR), and wet preparation of vaginal vault secretions should be obtained. Attention should be given to the need for human immunodeficiency virus (HIV) testing. Immunization against hepatitis B should be initiated. In the case of not yet sexually active adolescents or adolescents who refuse to have a pelvic examination but want to begin COCs, a plan should be made and documented to perform the examination after not more than 6 months on the pill. In nonsexually active teenagers, the STD evaluation is not needed. In teenagers who continue to refuse to have a pelvic examination but who are sexually active, the relative risks of pregnancy should be balanced against the recommended regimen.

Written instructions, including the routine for starting pills and procedures for missed pills, should be reviewed with the patient. Either Sunday-start or flexible-start regimens are acceptable as long as the instructions are clear and understood. Pills may be started at other times in the menstrual cycle if one can be certain that the patient is not pregnant and is prepared for additional menstrual cycle disturbances initially. Return visits may be scheduled after one full cycle of pills to address any problems, encourage compliance, and reeducate about alternative methods if needed. A pill check appointment at 3 months is scheduled to review weight and blood pressure changes and assess any side effects. At the same time, the practitioner can evaluate the patient's satisfaction with and understanding of COC use. Three months later, a 6-month follow-up appointment can reinforce the previous issues. In most sexually active adolescents, a repeat examination and STD evaluation are routine at 6-month intervals, as sexual partners often change as frequently.

Common misconceptions that may need to be addressed include the belief that the pill causes cancer, impairs fertility, or is bad for one's health if taken for too long. These issues need to be reviewed at initial educational and follow-up sessions. The risk of cardiovascular complications in teens due to COCs is very small whether or not they smoke. More importantly, the long-term risks of smoking deserve mention, and intervention can be offered to encourage abstinence from tobacco use. At all visits, the necessity of additional barrier protection to decrease exposure to STDs should be emphasized.

Postcoital Contraception or "Morning-After Pill." Contraceptive education for all teens should include information about postcoital contraception. Neither contraception nor human behavior is perfect. Events such as rape, broken condoms, missed pills, and poor judgment may place a woman at risk of an unwanted pregnancy. In such emergencies, postcoital or emergency contraception initiated within 72 hours of unprotected sex can decrease the risk of pregnancy about 75%. The Yuzpe regimen consists of 100 mg of ethinyl estradiol and 1 mg of norgestrel (two tablets of Ovral) taken by mouth and repeated 12 hours later. This therapy is most effective if initiated within 24 hours of intercourse. Other COC combinations have been suggested that supply at least equivalent doses of levonorgestrel and ethinyl estradiol (e.g., four tablets of Lo-ovral, Nordette, or Levlen initially and again in 12 hours). Although nausea and, occasionally, vomiting are reported side effects, the Yuzpe protocol is much better tolerated than the previously recommended 5-day course of high-dose estrogen. A menstrual period usually will occur within 21 days. However, all patients should be seen for follow-up in 3 weeks. This provides a prime opportunity to reinforce ongoing contraceptive plans. RU 486, still not approved for any clinical indications in the United States, is a highly effective postcoital contraceptive.

Progesterone-Only Pills, or Minipills. These pills consist of a small dose of progesterone and are taken every day without a hormone-free interval. Even under ideal conditions, progesterone-only pills are less effective than other hormonal methods and produce irregular

bleeding patterns. They are most often used for lactating women, older women of reproductive age, and individuals with unacceptable side effects from estrogen or higher-dose pills. They may be prescribed when COCs are contraindicated because of hypertension, migraine, or other conditions.

Depo-Medroxyprogesterone

Medroxyprogesterone acetate (Depo-Provera) may be given as a 150-mg IM injection every 12 weeks and provides extremely effective contraception. Initially, it is often accompanied by irregular menstrual bleeding. Most young women develop amenorrhea after a series of injections. The most commonly reported side effects include mood changes, weight gain, and nausea. Diminished estrogen levels temporarily decrease bone density maturation, a process that resumes when Depo-Provera use is discontinued. Depo-Provera users do not report other common symptoms of hypoestrogenism (e.g., hot flashes or insufficient vaginal lubrication), but estrogen supplementation may be used to control prolonged or heavy menstrual bleeding caused by this contraceptive hormone. After injections are stopped, it may take up to 2 years until fertility returns. Depo-Provera has been approved by the FDA for contraceptive use since 1992 and has gained acceptance among teens because of its reliability and convenience.

Norplant Implants

Norplant, which has been licensed in the United States since 1990, consists of six Silastic-coated capsules of levonorgestrel that are implanted subcutaneously in the upper arm. It provides 5 years of highly effective contraception through a continuous delivery of an ultra-low dose of progestin. The effect is reversible, but only by removal of the capsules by a minor surgical procedure. Both irregular menstrual bleeding and amenorrhea occur in Norplant users. Despite the lower dose of progestin, weight gain has been a problem for some adolescents. The risk of an accidental pregnancy is greater than with Depo-Provera. Indications include those mentioned for both the minipill and medroxyprogesterone and difficulties with compliance with other regimens in women who desire long-term contraception. Norplant appears to be well accepted and tolerated by already parenting adolescents. It may be used in some young women in whom the COC is contraindicated. It offers an attractive option for some adolescents and their families when medical conditions, psychiatric illness, or cognitive disabilities contraindicate pregnancy or parenthood.

Pre-Norplant counseling, insertion, and removal should be provided by a practitioner with specific training. Regular gynecologic evaluation for STDs should be scheduled as for all adolescents. Recent data suggest that Norplant had decreased efficacy in women on medications that increase liver enzyme activity (e.g., anticonvulsants, particularly phenytoin [Dilantin], and rifampin).

Intrauterine Devices (IUDs)

The IUDs currently available in the United States include the TCu-380A and the progesterone T device. IUDs are absolutely contraindicated in women with active, recent, or recurrent pelvic infection or suspected pregnancy. They are strongly not recommended for individuals at high risk for future STDs, including women with multiple sexual partners or with partners who have multiple partners. Thus, the IUD is rarely a preferred contraceptive choice for adolescents because they, in general, continue to change partners and have a high incidence of STDs. Recent data from the Alan Guttmacher Institute suggest that unmarried adolescents have roughly the same number of sexual partners a year that unmarried persons in their twenties have.[1] A skilled counselor and trained practitioner are required to obtain informed consent and perform the insertion and removal procedures.

Sterilization

An option sometimes requested by parents of developmentally disabled adolescents and by teenage mothers with several offspring is sterilization. Although voluntary surgical contraception, including tubal ligation and vasectomy, provides contraception for many older women and men, it has little place, if any, in the choices for adolescents. Federal and state funds usually cannot be used to support sterilization in individuals younger than 21 years of age. The use of these funds usually requires informed consent, documentation of mental competence, and a 30-day waiting period. When there are extenuating medical reasons to consider sterilization in an adolescent, legal counsel and court involvement are advised. Medical alternatives may include continuous COC use, endometrial ablation, Norplant, Depo-Provera, or Depo-Lupron, depending on the patient's family's concerns and underlying problems.

Impending Developments

New developments in contraception include other progestin-containing implants, injections and vaginal rings, male oral contraceptives, new COC formulations, hormone-releasing transdermal patches, and variations in barrier contraceptives and spermicide delivery options. Adolescents are often eager to try these new products. Practitioners should be prepared to offer them accurate information about reliability and efficacy with respect to the adolescent lifestyle.

REFERENCE

1. Alan Guttmacher Institute: Sex and America's Teenagers. New York, The Institute, 1994.
2. Hatcher RA, Trussell J, Stewart F, et al: Contraceptive Technology, 16th ed. rev. New York, Irvington Publishers, 1994.

SEXUAL ORIENTATION AND GENDER IDENTITY

ROBERT J. BIDWELL, M.D.

For many health practitioners, sexual orientation and gender identity are issues that provoke feelings of uncertainty, anxiety, and sometimes disapproval. For youths becoming aware of their lesbian, gay, bisexual, or transsexual (transgender) identities, the feelings are even more tumultuous and compounded by growing up in a society that often views this important part of who they are as sick or sinful. In the past 20 years, the health professions have begun to change their attitudes to reflect increased knowledge about the origins and nature of sexual orientation and gender identity. In 1973, The American Psychiatric Association accepted homosexuality as a part of the spectrum of human sexuality. In 1993, the American Academy of Pediatrics reaffirmed its position on the responsibility of pediatricians to recognize and address the special experience and needs of gay and lesbian adolescents.[1] Transsexualism continues to be classified in the American Psychiatric Association's *Diagnostic and Statistical Manual-IV* (DSM-IV) under the heading of gender identity disorder.

DEFINITIONS

Sexual orientation and gender identity are complex concepts not easily described, especially when applied to the childhood and adolescent years, with their dramatic developmental changes. In simplistic terms, however, human sexuality can be considered as having three components: core morphologic identity (the personal sense of being male or female), gender role behavior (the degree of meeting society's expectations for male or female behavior), and sexual orientation (the pattern of affectional and sexual attraction to those of the same or opposite sex). *Transsexual (transgender)* individuals have a core morphologic identity that is opposite from their biologic sex (i.e., the biologic male who feels like a woman trapped in a man's body). *Homosexual* individuals have a core identity consistent with their biologic sex but have a gay or lesbian sexual orientation, being attracted to members of the same sex. *Bisexuals* are attracted to people of both sexes. *Transvestitism* (or dressing in the clothes of the opposite

sex for sexual gratification) is technically a fetish. However, many transsexual and a few gay youths crossdress for identity rather than erotic reasons.

DEMOGRAPHICS

The percentage of the population that is heterosexual, bisexual, or homosexual is uncertain. Alfred Kinsey, in his famous studies of male and female sexuality in the 1930s and 1940s, found that about 10% of males and 5% of females were predominantly homosexual in their behaviors for a least 3 years during adulthood.

More recently, a 1992 large-scale study of Minnesota secondary school students found that nearly 9% of 18 year olds reported being "unsure" of their sexual orientation.[2] Although only 2.8% of males reported homosexual activity, 6% reported predominantly homosexual attractions. Sexual orientation is a complex phenomenon, and especially in the adolescent years, self-identification as straight (heterosexual) or gay and reported sexual behavior may be unreliable indicators of present or future identity. Some gay and lesbian teenagers have been only heterosexually active, and many have not been sexually active at all. Bisexuality may be even more prevalent than homosexuality. Transsexualism is thought to be much less common, perhaps in the range of 1 in 30,000 males and 1 in 100,000 females. Whatever their present prevalences, heterosexuality, homosexuality, bisexuality, and transsexuality have coexisted in most cultures and historical periods.

HOMOSEXUALITY

Origins of Sexual Orientation

Debate continues over the determinants of sexual orientation. Some theories suggest a biologic explanation (genetic, prenatal hormones, or brain anatomy), whereas others suggest environmental influences (family patterns, personal experiences, the influence of societal labeling). Perhaps nature and nurture are both at play. Nevertheless, there is growing agreement that sexual orientation is established by early childhood, is not a choice, and is not amenable to change. Furthermore, there is growing acceptance that homosexuality is not a matter of "something gone wrong" but is a natural developmental outcome for a certain proportion of any population.

The Nontraditional Child

Some children and youths will come to health providers' attention because of nontraditional gender behaviors, that is, the very effeminate boy or masculine girl. Research is limited but suggests that although nontraditional children may as adults lie anywhere along the spectrum of sexual orientation, a significant percentage (perhaps 50% or more) will, in fact, be homosexual or bisexual. Smaller percentages may be transsexual or heterosexual. Treatment of nontraditional children has ranged from psychotherapy or behavior modification to counseling that validates a child's unique identity and helps the child and family adjust to a world not always accepting of differences.

Growing Up Lesbian and Gay

Most gay, lesbian, and bisexual adolescents are invisible, not fulfilling society's stereotypic expectations of these orientations. They are ordinary teenagers and face the same developmental tasks as other adolescents. Nevertheless, their experience is special in that they grow up in an environment that is often unaccepting of an integral part of who they are. There are few adolescents as isolated as the gay, lesbian, or bisexual teenager. They have little access to accurate information about sexual orientation and almost no access to supportive counselors, peer groups, or visible adult role models. They often experience a deep sense of guilt, believing they are somehow flawed or responsible for their sexual orientation. They live with a daily fear that their terrible secret will become known to family or friends. They have heard the myths concerning homosexuality and fear that these will come to describe their own futures as well. The threat of violence is a daily reality for many. Some experience physical and verbal abuse when their sexual orientation is discovered or assumed. Many more, including those who are invisible, experience the psychic damage of witnessed violence, "fag" jokes, and disapproving comments that sometimes come even from those they love and respect.

Like other youths who are alone, fearful, and subjected to violence, gay and lesbian adolescents are at increased risk of a variety of self-destructive behaviors. Many will have school problems and have increased withdrawal from or conflict with their families. Some are forced to run away from home because of parental rejection and turn to the streets for survival. This often includes involvement in prostitution, dealing drugs, and other illegal activities. Whether living on the streets or at home, many will become involved with substance use. Because there is no safe place to explore their sexuality through such approved dating rituals as those of heterosexual teenagers, they are forced to have sex in circumstances that are often degrading and place them at high risk for HIV and other STDs. The risk of suicide is exceptionally high among these youths.

Most gay, lesbian, and bisexual teenagers do not engage in high-risk behaviors but decide to put a hold on their sexual development and expression, focusing instead on their studies, sports, or other activities. This may be adaptive behavior for a period of time but eventually leads to great psychic distress in many teenagers and adults.

Health Status of Lesbian and Gay Youth

Little research has been done on the health status of lesbian and gay youths. Information on adult gays and lesbians may or may not be descriptive of the adolescent population. Certainly, some gay and lesbian adolescents, like other alienated youths, may be more likely to engage in high-risk behaviors that could have an impact on their health. Furthermore, gay and lesbian teenagers are less likely to receive health information specific to their sexual orientation. They are also less likely to reveal their sexual orientation to health providers and, therefore, to receive appropriate care.

Lesbian adolescents face health risks related to their status both as women and as lesbians. Lesbian teenagers are subject to the same gynecologic concerns as heterosexual teenagers, including dysmenorrhea, dysfunctional uterine bleeding, and malignancy. Some lesbian teenagers are bisexually active and are, therefore, at risk for unintended pregnancy and sexually transmitted diseases (STDs), including HIV. HIV is also a potential risk through contact with menstrual blood. Exclusively homosexual lesbians have a very low incidence of STDs (if their partners are not bisexually active), although vaginitis due to *Gardnerella vaginalis, Candida* organisms, *Trichomonas* organisms, and herpes virus has been reported in this group. Lesbians may also be subjected to physical and sexual violence because of their sexual orientation.

Gay male youths, like lesbian teenagers, may be homosexually or heterosexually active or may not be sexually active at all. If homosexually active, gay youths are prone to a variety of STDs, including gonorrhea, syphilis, HIV, hepatitis B, genital warts, herpes simplex, and enteric pathogens. They may also experience trauma secondary to anal intercourse that can result in rectal fissures, hemorrhoids, fecal incontinence, allergic proctitis, and rectal foreign bodies. It should be noted that anal intercourse is not exclusive to gay males, and many gay males do not engage in this practice. Perhaps even more serious than STDs and trauma are the health consequences of violence, including such self-inflicted violence as substance abuse and suicide to which many alienated youths resort in their despair.

Approaching the Gay and Lesbian Teen

Most gay, lesbian, and bisexual adolescents are invisible, neither voluntarily disclosing their orientation nor identifiable by stereotypes. It has been said that health providers who believe they have no gay or lesbian patients simply have not made these invisible teenagers feel comfortable in discussing this important part of their lives. It is essential, therefore, that health providers not assume the heterosexuality of any patient and recognize the red flags of teenagers in distress, including acting-out behaviors, declining school

performance, substance use, increased *heterosexual* activity, and depression.

It is also important to recognize that the role of health providers is not to identify every lesbian or gay adolescent. Instead, it is to provide a clinical environment that facilitates discussion of sexual orientation among other sensitive issues. A first step can be to provide clear messages in waiting rooms and examination rooms, through brochures and posters, that sexual orientation is among several sensitive issues that can be discussed with the practitioner. The provider also should be able to offer objective information and appropriate medical screening and care and to connect teenagers to supportive community resources. It is also the role of the provider to give all adolescents the clear message that wherever they might be on the continuum of sexual orientation, heterosexuality, homosexuality, and bisexuality are all normal and healthy developmental outcomes.

Immunizations

In addition to receiving two doses of MMR by early adolescence and a Td booster at about age 15, all gay and lesbian adolescents should receive a hepatitis B immunization series before becoming sexually active or as soon after sexual debut as possible.

Counseling and Anticipatory Guidance

The counseling provided gay and lesbian youths is perhaps even more important than the medical screening and care they receive. The goal of counseling is to provide information and support, to promote health-enhancing behaviors, and to enhance their development into healthy, productive adults, no matter what their sexual orientation might be.

Many adolescents carry negative notions of what it means to be lesbian or gay. It is important that the practitioner provide the teenager information on sexuality in general and sexual orientation in particular. Adolescents should understand that sexual orientation is not a choice and that it is a normal developmental outcome for between 3% and 10% of the population. The adolescent's discomfort about the possibility of a lesbian or gay identity should be explored sympathetically. Nevertheless, they should be helped to understand that their futures can include loving, committed relationships, parenthood, rewarding careers, and community respect, although these may seem impossible to them during the early stages of gay or lesbian self-awareness. Visible gay and lesbian role models should be pointed out. Openly gay and lesbian health providers can also serve as role models for teen patients as rapport is established. It is important not to offer reassurance that the teenager with homosexual feelings is "just going through a phase," as this often is not the case and may lead to further distress. It is better to tell the teenager, "I cannot tell you whether you are gay/lesbian, bisexual, or straight. Only you can decide this for yourself. What I can do is provide you information and support as you sort through your feelings and what they mean. What I also can do is remind you that whoever you are in terms of sexual orientation is all right."

It is also important to discuss with teenagers who feel they are lesbian or gay the realities of a society that is not always accepting of their orientation. Specifically, providers should discuss how the teenager will address such issues as coming out (revealing their sexual orientation) to family or friends and the possibility of verbal or physical harassment and discrimination. Much of the isolation gay and lesbian youths experience can be lessened by referring them to local gay and lesbian teen support groups or supportive counselors. Information about these resources usually is available through local gay and lesbian community centers or youth service agencies. It is unethical and dangerous to refer any teenager to a counselor or therapist who claims an ability to change sexual orientation.

As some gay and lesbian teenagers may be engaged in high-risk behaviors, it is important to address each of these as well. Whether a teenager is sexually active or not, it is important to review contraception, pregnancy, STDs, and safer sex practices. The provider should also emphasize that abstinence is a reasonable and healthy option for any teenager, especially during early and middle adolescence.

Finally, the practitioner should examine carefully his or her own attitudes toward homosexuality. If these include significant discomfort or disapproval, a referral should be made to another practitioner comfortable in dealing with medical and counseling issues related to sexual orientation.

THE TRANSSEXUAL ADOLESCENT

The transsexual (transgender) teenager is perhaps the least understood and most isolated of adolescents. The DSM-IV refers to transsexualism under the heading of gender identity disorder. Four criteria apply to this designation. First, there must be a strong desire to be, or insistence that one is, of the opposite gender. Second, there must be a persistent discomfort with one's designated sex or with societal gender role expectations for that sex. One also must not have a physical intersex condition, such as testicular feminization syndrome or congenital adrenal hyperplasia. Finally, the individual must evidence significant distress in social, educational, occupational, and other settings.

Transsexual individuals are biologic males and females who "feel trapped in the body of the opposite sex." They are, therefore, distinct from transvestites, who most often are heterosexuals who derive erotic pleasure from dressing in the clothing of the opposite sex. They are also separate from the small minority of gay or lesbian youths who crossdress either to challenge society's gender role expectations or to fit their preconceived notions of how gay and lesbians dress and behave.

The origins of transsexualism are uncertain, though both biologic and environmental theories have been offered. It appears to be established by early childhood, when most transsexual individuals begin to show very feminine or masculine behaviors incongruent with their biologic sex.

The lives of gender-atypical children and transsexual adolescents are often difficult. Unlike gay and lesbian youths who can often hide their sexual orientation, transsexual youths are subjected to ridicule, harassment, and ostracism from an early age in almost every social setting, including schools, youth agencies, and within their own families. Many engage in varying degrees of crossdressing in an attempt to bring their physical self into congruence with their inner self. Because of harassment, many run away from home to street life for survival. In larger towns and cities, often there is an already established transsexual community on the streets that provides the teenager with support, validation, and survival skills. Unfortunately, this group may also provide an entry into prostitution and substance abuse. Some transsexual youths will shoplift in order to obtain clothing of the opposite sex. Many of these survival activities lead to involvement in the juvenile justice system, which may be as abusive as life on the streets. The gay and lesbian community may provide little outreach or support for transsexual youths, who are sometimes viewed as oddities. It is believed that the risk of exposure to HIV and other STDs is very high among these youths and that they are especially prone to suicide.

Health providers work with transsexual youths in a variety of settings. Many transsexual youths live at home and attend school and may be seen by providers in regular clinic visits. Issues of gender identity should be explored with any youth when red flags, such as crossdressing, appear. One should not label a teenager but should be able to provide support, information, and anticipatory guidance before crises occur. Conflicts with peers and family should be explored, as well as such risk behaviors as street life, sexual activity, substance use, and suicidal ideation. Appropriate medical screening should be performed.

More importantly, if gender identity is thought to be an issue, particularly if the teenager has experienced problems at home or school related to this, the health provider should take the lead in bringing together a multidisciplinary team to develop a unified plan of treatment and create a safety net of services. This team should include the patient and his or her primary health provider, psychiatrist, school counselor or teachers, and any youth agency personnel involved in the adolescent's life. Parents should also be involved if possible. The team's goal is to ensure that the school, the home, and the broader community are safe places for the adolescent. The goal is not to modify the teenager's gender-atypical behaviors, such as crossdressing, although mental health professionals can help the crossdressing teenager anticipate and plan for the consequences of crossdressing in an often unaccepting world. The team should ensure through policies and procedures that the home, school, involved agencies, and the community's streets are safe for the teenager, whether or not his or her actions or dress is gender typical. Such a plan is essential to prevent the teenager from turning to street life or suicide.

The primary health provider and psychiatrist should work closely together in creating a plan of treatment for the transsexual adolescent. The psychiatrist should determine whether the adolescent is, in fact, transsexual based on DSM-IV criteria. The goal of treatment is not to change gender identity, which is already well established by adolescence. Instead, it is to help the transsexual teenager learn survival skills to live in an often hostile environment. If the adolescent is transsexual, the psychiatrist and primary health provider should discuss the advisability of beginning hormone therapy, which is usually requested by these patients. Hormonal therapy consists of estrogens for biologic males and androgens for biologic females. For male-to-female transsexuals, a reasonable regimen is 1.25 mg to 2.5 mg of Premarin daily. The timing of the initiation of hormone therapy will vary with each patient. It should not be started before the patient has a sexual maturity rating (SMR) of V. Beginning hormonal therapy before the age of 18 requires parental consent. The dangers of postponing hormonal therapy should be seriously considered. These include the likelihood of a teenager accessing hormones on the street without medical monitoring and the possibility that if the teenager is told to wait, he or she may choose suicide instead. The health provider should also let the teenager know that when he or she is an adult and financially secure, sex change and other cosmetic surgeries are available. The expected physical changes resulting from hormone therapy, as well as its side effects, routes of administration (oral versus injection), and costs, should be discussed. Patients should be supported, and anticipatory guidance should be provided as they begin to assume the persona of the opposite sex through dress, name change, and hormone therapy.

It is especially important that the health provider maintain continuity of care, since hormonal therapy will not remove all the difficulties faced by transsexual adolescents. It is not uncommon for patients who have begun hormonal therapy to change their minds and discontinue it, only later to request it again. This ambivalence should be expected and accommodated.

PARENT ISSUES

Many parents will be devastated by the thought that their child may be dealing with issues of sexual orientation or gender identity and may experience varying degrees of guilt, anger, and repulsion. The health provider must consider carefully the consequences of breaching confidentiality to share this information with parents. Some parents may reject or respond violently toward a gay, lesbian, or transsexual child. Others will seek out therapy to change their child's orientation or identity. If parents know or are informed of these matters, the role of the health provider is to discuss their concerns and feelings, to provide information and correct misconceptions, and to connect the family to supportive community services and counseling. Parents/Friends of Lesbians and Gays has local chapters providing support groups and written materials in many communities (Parents/Friends of Lesbians and Gays, 1012 14th Street NW, Washington, DC 20005).

An emerging issue in pediatrics is the growing number of children and adolescents who have gay and lesbian parents, many growing up in two-mother or two-father families. Research shows that these young people are as emotionally healthy as youths growing up with heterosexual parents. Nevertheless, supportive counseling should be provided, particularly during the early adolescent years.

EDUCATION AND ADVOCACY

Health providers have an important role to play in improving the physical and emotional well-being of gay, lesbian, bisexual, and transsexual youths. By recognizing and addressing the special experience and needs of these young people, health providers can begin to undo the harm that comes from being isolated and stigmatized. Even more important, they can serve as educators and advocates within their communities by challenging misinformation whenever it appears and by ensuring that these adolescents grow up in communities that celebrate their existence and nurture their development into happy, healthy, and productive adults.

REFERENCES

1. Committee on Adolescence, American Academy of Pediatrics: Homosexuality and adolescence. Pediatrics 92:631–634, 1993.
2. Remafedi G, Resnick M, Blum R, Harris L: Demography of sexual orientation in adolescents. Pediatrics 89:714–721, 1992.

SUBSTANCE ABUSE

Laura F. McNicholas, M.D., Ph.D.
Charles P. O'Brien, M.D., Ph.D.

Substance use disorders have been primarily defined in adults as the problem use of illicit drugs, notably heroin (and other opioids) and cocaine. The only legal substances associated with abuse problems in the adult population are alcohol and nicotine (in the form of tobacco) and abuse of legal prescription drugs. Further, substance use disorders clearly fall into the category of chronic relapsing diseases. Adults with substance use disorders can be expected to have a prolonged course with remissions and exacerbations. In the adolescent, however, *no* drug use is legal (at least until age 18 or 21 for tobacco products and alcoholic beverages). Further, although it is generally recognized that adolescent substance abuse precedes and frequently proceeds to adult substance abuse and dependency, the issue of chronicity in adolescent substance abuse is not clear. Teens are frequently referred to treatment with very short histories of substance abuse or misuse. The issues of legality and chronicity have clouded the definition of adolescent substance abuse by altering the emphasis on the various factors used to define substance abuse. Further, many times the presentation of an adolescent with a substance abuse disorder is a symptom of family dysfunction, an issue that may or may not be addressed effectively in treating the identified patient. It is usually more efficient to deal with the substance abuse issue as a part of family dysfunction rather than a primary disease. A potential problem with the family approach is that it deemphasizes the seriousness and chronicity of the adolescent's drug use disorder and may give the adolescent permission to make someone (e.g., parent) other than himself or herself responsible for the drug-abusing behavior.

Adolescence is generally considered to be a stage of development when the person is testing limits and modifying social and cognitive skills and functions. It has been suggested that part of this development "may involve experimentation with a wide range of behaviors, attitudes, and activities" and that "this process of testing attitudes and behavior may include drug use."[6] Referring for treatment every adolescent who occasionally uses alcohol or marijuana is ineffective and trivializes the real problem of adolescents who have substance use disorders requiring treatment. Despite the issues of legality of any drug use and the chronicity of drug abuse, there are no special criteria for defining adolescent substance abuse that would set it apart from

adult substance abuse. The *Diagnostic and Statistical Manual of Mental Disorders,* 4th ed (DSM-IV) definitions of substance dependence and abuse are given in Table 1.

Patients who meet the diagnostic criteria should be considered for treatment of a substance use disorder. The treatment of an adolescent should not be used to avoid treating family dysfunction that may be brought to light by the use of drugs during adolescent development.

MAGNITUDE OF THE PROBLEM

The National Institute of Drug Abuse regularly surveys high school seniors for the use of illicit substances. In the 1990 survey, it was found that 18% smoked cigarettes daily, with over 10% using more than 10 cigarettes daily. Further, 90.7% of high school seniors reported the use of alcohol, and the number reporting daily use was 4.2%. Those reporting having had more than five alcoholic drinks in a row within the past 2 weeks, a frequent marker for adult problem drinking or alcohol abuse, was 33%. Marijuana had been used by 73% of high

TABLE 1. DSM-IV Criteria for Substance Dependence and Abuse

Criteria for Substance Dependence

A maladaptive pattern of substance use, leading to clinically significant impairment or distress, as manifested by three (or more) of the following, occurring at any time in the same 12-month period:

1. tolerance, as defined by either of the following:
   a. a need for markedly increased amounts of the substance to achieve intoxication or desired effect
   b. markedly diminished effect with continued use of the same amount of the substance
2. withdrawal, as manifested by either of the following:
   a. the characteristic withdrawal syndrome for the substance
   b. the same (or a closely related) substance is taken to relieve or avoid withdrawal symptoms
3. the substance is often taken in larger amounts or over a longer period than was intended
4. there is a persistent desire or unsuccessful efforts to cut down or control substance use
5. a great deal of time is spent in activities necessary to obtain the substance (e.g., visiting multiple doctors or driving long distances), use the substance (e.g., chain-smoking), or recover from its effects
6. important social, occupational, or recreational activities are given up or reduced because of substance use
7. the substance use is continued despite knowledge of having a persistent or recurrent physical or psychological problem that is likely to have been caused or exacerbated by the substance (e.g., current cocaine use despite recognition of cocaine-induced depression, or continued drinking despite recognition that an ulcer was made worse by alcohol consumption)

Criteria for Substance Abuse

A. A maladaptive pattern of substance use leading to clinically significant impairment or distress, as manifested by one (or more) of the following, occurring within a 12-month period:
   1. recurrent substance use resulting in a failure to fulfill major role obligations at work, school, or home (e.g., repeated absences or poor work performance related to substance use; substance-related absences, suspensions or expulsions from school; neglect of children or household)
   2. recurrent substance use in situations in which it is physically hazardous (e.g., driving an automobile or operating a machine when impaired by substance use)
   3. recurrent substance-related legal problems (e.g., arrests for substance-related disorderly conduct)
   4. continued substance use despite having persistent or recurrent social or interpersonal problems caused or exacerbated by the effects of the substance (e.g., arguments with spouse about consequences of intoxication, physical fights)
B. The symptoms have never met the criteria for Substance Dependence for this class of substance.

From American Psychiatric Association: Diagnostic and Statistical Manual of Mental Disorders, 4th ed. Washington, DC, The Association, 1994.

school seniors, with 17% reporting current use and 2.9% reporting daily use. All other drugs of abuse combined accounted for less than 9% of adolescent substance abuse. Because this survey captures only adolescents in school, there has been concern that specific subgroups of adolescents, who may be at a higher risk of drug abuse, were not being surveyed. In 1993 Kipke et al.[4] reported on a study of patients seen at a primary health clinic in Los Angeles, whose clientele consists primarily of youths aged 12 to 24, with a focus on nonhomeless, high-risk youth and runaway, homeless youth in the area. Of the 1121 patients evaluated, 62% were homeless. Homeless youth had a significantly higher prevalence of recent alcohol and drug use than did the nonhomeless youth. Homeless youth were more likely to report use of alcohol, marijuana, inhalants, stimulants, hallucinogens, and opioids, as well as injecting drug use. Findings such as these support the theory that specific subgroups of adolescents are at significantly higher risk of substance abuse than the general population and that health care workers need to be especially vigilant for substance abuse problems in these subpopulations.

TREATMENT MODALITIES

As with adult substance abuse treatment, there are a variety of treatment modalities and approaches for the adolescent substance abuser. In general, adolescent substance abusers are treated in the same facilities as adult substance abusers, and treatment is primarily based on a drug-free model. No matter which treatment setting is used for an adolescent, the basic components of treatment should include individual counseling; individual or group psychotherapy or both; self-help group participation; substance abuse education; education to provide an understanding of the disease model of drug abuse or dependence, including its chronic nature, diagnosis and treatment of any coexisting medical and psychiatric disorders; random urine or breath testing for illicit or abused substances; relapse prevention; and family therapy.

Inpatient Treatment

Probably the modality first thought of by parents and by the substance-abusing adolescent, the inpatient setting may not be the physician's referral of first choice for most patients. Inpatient hospitalization actually consists of two very different modalities, detoxification and rehabilitation. Inpatient detoxification usually lasts 3 to 7 days, depending on the drug(s) of abuse, and is reserved for medically complicated cases. Many patients express dissatisfaction with inpatient detoxification because of its short time period and the difficulty in arranging immediate outpatient follow-up. Inpatient rehabilitation is usually a 21- to 28-day program for the patient who has completed detoxification or who does not require medical management of his or her drug detoxification. Rehabilitation programs are generally more structured than other substance abuse treatment modalities. Most are based on the Alcoholics Anonymous (AA) model of assisting the patient to achieve a drug-free lifestyle, including the concepts of recognition of the drug abuse problem and admitting the need for help. However, they frequently do not recognize age differences or other psychiatric comorbidity. Those rehabilitation programs based on the AA model have four key elements.

1. The possibility of change
2. The disease concept
3. Abstinence and lifestyle changes as long-term goals
4. Acceptance of self-help group principles and traditions

The last two elements may be particularly difficult to accomplish in an adolescent population because of the patients' psychologic stage of development.

An alternative to the AA model of inpatient rehabilitation is the multidisciplinary approach. This model recognizes the multiple domains in which the substance-abusing adolescent may have problems, including family issues, psychosocial problems, school or employment issues, and comorbid psychiatric diagnoses. A multidisciplinary team of psychiatrists, social workers, drug counselors, and school or vocational counselors attempts to address all of the adolescent patient's issues associated with the drug abuse problems.

A problem with inpatient programs in general is the low rate of outpatient follow-up for the patient. This problem is due to a number of factors: the adolescent's perspective that his or her problem is cured after the inpatient stay, the difficulty in arranging timely follow-up because of the scarcity and overcrowding of appropriate programs, and frequently, the lack of internal family structure to encourage continued attendance in outpatient care. Additionally, some insurance programs do not cover outpatient aftercare, so that the needed follow-up may be a financial burden on the family resources.

Residential Treatment

Therapeutic communities and other residential treatment programs, including halfway houses, are designed to provide the adolescent patient with a long-term (usually longer than 6 months), structured, drug-free environment. These programs employ diverse approaches to treatment, with the therapeutic community likely to provide the most structure and be the more restrictive of the available programs. Although the focus of all residential treatment is the achievement of long-term sobriety, the focus of the individual program may be on intensive family therapy, on school or employment skills, or on team work and community skills in wilderness programs. Many judicial programs are using some of the residential program approaches in boot camp settings.

Although generally less expensive than inpatient hospital care, the overall cost of long-term residential care can easily exceed the cost of an inpatient 21- or 28-day program and is frequently not covered by insurance. They have the disadvantage or, in some cases, advantage of removing the adolescent from the home environment, which may make reintegration into that environment more difficult unless family therapy is an integral part of therapy.

Outpatient Treatment

The most used and most useful modality of treatment, outpatient programs can range in structure and services from drop-in services for on-the-spot counseling to intensive day hospital. Most programs have elements of individual, group, family, and vocational therapy, usually with an emphasis on AA-oriented groups. In adult populations, it has been shown that most alcoholics can be successfully detoxified on an outpatient basis. For rehabilitation, outpatient day hospitalization was equal to 28-day in-patient treatment at 7-month follow-up after discharge.[1] Comparable studies in the adolescent population have not been done. Outpatient treatment, particularly partial or day hospitalization, has an advantage in treatment of the adolescent who will be remaining in his or her home, as *both* the patient and family must learn to deal with the problems in that environment without the adolescent patient's returning to substance abuse. For this reason alone, good family therapy should be an essential part of the adolescent substance abuse treatment. Further outpatient treatment programs need to be structured so that the patient progresses through the program over a 1- to 2-year period, thus impressing on the adolescent the chronicity of the disorder and the importance of treating this as a chronic, relapsing disorder.

SPECIAL ISSUES IN THIS POPULATION

Dually Diagnosed Patients

There has been a great deal of research done on the incidence of comorbid psychiatric disorders in the adult substance-abusing population, with a high incidence of depressive symptoms and disorders being reported. The literature available concerning dually diagnosed adolescent patients is scarce but is one area where research is going forward. Stowell and Estroff stated that Hoffman reported signs and symptoms that relate to depression in up to 50% of adolescent substance abuse patients[7] but did not directly address the issue of psychiatric diagnosis in these patients. Stowell and Estroff, however, studied 226 consecutive adolescent patients admitted for inpatient substance abuse treatment. They found that 82% of their patients met DSM-III-R criteria for a psychiatric disorder, 61% for mood disorder, 43% for anxiety disorder, and 54% for conduct disorder (74% of the patients had more than one psychiatric disorder other than a substance abuse disorder). These data, if replicated, indicate an extremely high rate of dual diagnosis in the hospitalized adolescent substance abuse patient. There is no comparable study in adolescent patients in outpatient treatment. Whereas Stowell and Estroff[7] did not differentiate between primary psychiatric comorbid disorders (those independent of substance use disorders), Bukstein et al.[2] did. They also studied hospitalized adolescent substance-abusing patients and found a 51% incidence of affective disorders, with 30.7% meeting diagnostic criteria for a major depressive episode. Only 16.7% of the patients had a primary major depression diagnosis, however, and more than 60% of these diagnoses were secondary to the substance use disorder.

There are a number of reasons why it is important to diagnose comorbid psychiatric disorders in this population adequately. First, if there is a comorbid primary psychiatric disorder, that disorder must be treated independently of the substance abuse disorder, or it is likely to be a high risk factor for relapse to substance abuse. Second, the presence of one or more comorbid psychiatric disorders may dictate or limit the type(s) of treatment available to the patient, as many residential programs do not accept dually diagnosed patients. Finally, the presence of a comorbid psychiatric disorder may influence treatment outcome. There is evidence that patients who fail to complete inpatient treatment are more likely to have a conduct disorder diagnosis in addition to substance use disorder and that patients with a concurrent diagnosis of affective disorder are more likely to complete inpatient treatment.[3] These data are similar to adult data, which suggest that substance abuse patients with personality disorders do less well in treatment than those without personality disorders.

Homogeneous or Heterogeneous Age Groups in Treatment

Most adolescents with substance abuse disorders are referred to an adolescent treatment program if one is available. It has been assumed that issues specific to adolescents can be better addressed in an age-matched group of patients. Marshall and Marshall[5] have challenged this view with preliminary data showing that adolescents may have more stable recovery, measured by fewer relapses, when treated in a setting with a heterogeneous age group than when treated in an adolescent treatment setting. Issues concerning these conclusions arise from the methods used in this preliminary study: retrospective survey data collected from people who remain involved with recovery groups. This selection process necessarily leaves out those patients who maintain their sobriety without affiliation with a recovery group. Random assignment prospective studies, as pointed out by Marshall and Marshall,[5] will be difficult, especially with the needed long-term follow-up, but should be done to adequately answer the question of whether adolescent treatment programs should be maintained or combined with adult substance abuse treatment programs.

SUMMARY

As with many fields of pediatric and adolescent medicine, the treatment of adolescent substance use disorders remains a copy or adaptation of adult treatment programs. The epidemiology of substance abuse in the adolescent population is not measured well, except in those adolescents who remain in school—certainly not the group most heavily involved with substance abuse. Research methods need to be developed to study the adolescent population as a whole, as well as to study subpopulations of interest. The needs of some special populations, such as dually diagnosed patients, are beginning to be addressed, but other groups with special needs, such as homeless youths and pregnant teenagers, are not well served. Studies of how to engage these patients in treatment and then to measure the effectiveness of that treatment are badly needed. Further, despite general acceptance that most adults in substance abuse treatment began abus-

ing drugs in adolescence, we have no good measures to predict which adolescents will go on to have lifelong substance use problems.

Outcome studies in the adult substance abuse treatment programs are well underway, but equal time, again, has not been devoted to problems of adolescent substance abuse treatment programs. The issue of whether adolescent treatment programs should be separate from adult programs is raised by recent research.[5] Without decent outcome studies in adolescent programs, this question will remain unanswered, and in this day of medical cost-cutting, the adolescent program may have trouble justifying its existence. It is extremely tempting to support the position that adolescents are merely young adults, and, therefore, special programs are not necessary, without examining the aspects of adolescence that make it a unique developmental stage. The task facing providers of treatment for adolescent substance abuse disorders is to provide that treatment and to structure it in such a way as to allow adolescents to complete their development without the stagnating effects of abuse of mind-altering and mood-altering substances.

REFERENCES

1. Alterman AI, Droba M, McLellan AT: Response to day hospital treatment by patients with cocaine and alcohol dependence. Hosp Commun Psychiatr 43:930–932, 1992.
2. Bukstein OG, Glancy LJ, Kaminer Y: Patterns of affective comorbidity in a clinical population of dually diagnosed adolecent substance abusers. J Am Acad Child Adolesc Psychiatry 31:1041–1045, 1992.
3. Kaminer Y, Tarter RE, Bukstein OG, Kabene M: Comparison between treatment completers and noncompleters among dually diagnosed substance-abusing adolescents. J Am Acad Child Adolesc Psychiatry 31:1046–1049, 1992.
4. Kipke MD, Montgomery S, MacKenzie RG: Substance use among youth seen at a community-based health clinic. J Adolesc Health 14:289–294, 1993.
5. Marshall MJ, Marshall S: Homogeneous versus heterogeneous age group treatment of adolescent substance abusers. Am J Drug Alcohol Abuse 19:199–207, 1993.
6. Newcomb MD, Bentler PM: Consequences of Adolescent Drug Use: Impact on Lives of Young Adults. Newbury Park, CA, Sage, 1988:214.
7. Stowell RJAA, Estroff TW: Psychiatric disorders in substance-abusing adolescent inpatients: A pilot study. J Am Acad Child Adolesc Psychiatry 31:1036–1040, 1992.

EATING DISORDERS

Rebecca F. O'Brien, m.d.

Anorexia nervosa and bulimia nervosa are relatively common disorders among adolescent and young adult women, with a prevalence of clinically significant eating disorders from 1% to 3%. Males are affected less frequently (female/male ratio of 10:1). Anorexia nervosa is characterized by extreme weight loss to 15% or more below ideal body weight, intense fear of becoming fat, and a distorted body image. Bulimia nervosa is characterized by binge eating followed by purging behaviors, such as self-induced vomiting, fasting, exercise, and laxative or diuretic use. Bulimic symptoms can also occur as part of the anorexia nervosa syndrome.

A variety of theories have been proposed from virtually every biopsychosocial model of the pathogenesis of eating disorders. Starvation and malnutrition appear to be the most important biologic influences responsible for the symptoms seen in eating disorders. The most influential psychologic theories currently are those of the psychodynamic and cognitive theorists who view the central psychologic features to be a "pervasive sense of ineffectiveness," causing the individual to attempt to gain self-control through weight control and inaccuracy in identifying their bodily and emotional states.

Medical complications in eating disorders can be life threatening. The medical complications of anorexia nervosa are primarily the result of starvation and malnutrition. These include amenorrhea, estrogen deficiency, osteoporosis, euthyroid sick syndrome, hypercarotenemia, abnormal temperature regulation, bradycardia, hypotension, decreased left ventricular mass, cardiac arrhythmias, dehydration, reduced glomerular filtration rate, renal calculi, edema, decreased gastric emptying, constipation, elevated hepatic enzymes, anemia, leukopenia, and thrombocytopenia.

Patients with bulimia or binging and purging behaviors can have metabolic complications of hypokalemia and hypochloremic metabolic alkalosis, as well as parotid enlargement, dental enamel erosion, esophagitis, Mallory-Weiss tears, esophageal rupture, acute gastric dilatation or rupture, pancreatitis, aspiration pneumonia, cardiac arrhythmias, and colonic abnormalities from laxative abuse. Ipecac poisoning may occur from self-administration for the purpose of inducing vomiting. Mortality associated with eating disorders includes suicide as well as cardiac arrhythmias induced by electrolyte abnormalities. However, the cause of the terminal event may be unclear.

Optimal assessment and treatment of eating disorders should be provided by a multidisciplinary team, including the primary care medical provider, mental health professionals, and a nutritionist. Collaboration is essential in order to provide a unified front when recommendations are made to the patient and family, as their denial of the seriousness of the disorder and evading treatment can be problematic and dangerous to the patient.

MEDICAL ASSESSMENT

The initial medical assessment must include a detailed weight and nutritional history, including the presenting weight, maximum weight, weight before dieting, and perceived ideal body weight. Specific means by which the patient is controlling weight, including frequency and number of vomiting episodes, use of laxatives, diuretics, ipecac, diet pills, thyroid hormone, and exercise, should be determined. In diabetic patients, manipulation of insulin can be used as a method to control weight, and such a possibility should be considered. A history of substance abuse should be obtained, as alcohol and drug abuse may coexist with eating disorders, especially bulimia. Family history, with attention to psychiatric disorders, eating disorders, and obesity, should be obtained.

Psychiatric history should specifically address concurrent psychiatric disturbances, including personality and affective and anxiety disorders. Psychologic testing may be helpful. In the pediatric and adolescent population, it is crucial to involve the family in order to assess its contribution to maintaining the illness and to obtain its assistance in the patient's recovery.

A complete physical examination should include height and weight obtained in a hospital gown after voiding, postural vital signs, and attention to signs of dehydration. Commonly found signs with anorexia include lanugo hair, peripheral cyanosis, bradycardia, hypothermia, hypotension, generalized muscle weakness, and emaciation. Purging patients may have calluses of the dorsum of the hand, enlarged parotid glands, dental enamel erosion, or perioral irritation. Laboratory evaluation should be performed as indicated by the history both to rule out other disorders that may mimic an eating disorder and to assess medical complications. Such tests may include a complete blood count, erythrocyte sedimentation rate, electrolytes, blood urea nitrogen, creatinine, magnesium, phosphorus, calcium, carotene, albumin, liver function tests, amylase, urinalysis, stool guaiac, and electrocardiogram.

THERAPY

The goals of treatment are initially focused on nutritional rehabilitation in order to reverse the effects of malnutrition, which contributes to the biologic and psychologic disturbances. Many of the psychologic symptoms will reverse with refeeding, and complete psychologic evaluation may not be possible until weight is restored. In anorexia nervosa, the choice of initial treatment setting depends on the degree of malnutrition and the motivation of the patient and family. For those patients who are less than 20% below average weight for height with a short duration of symptoms, an initial outpatient treatment plan may be effective. However, for many patients who are more underweight or less motivated, an inpatient or partial day hospital program will be necessary. A staff that is experienced in dealing with patients with eating disorders is crucial for success. Many units use protocols and contracts that offer positive or negative reinforcers (or both) to help patients achieve weight gain.

A slow but steady weight gain is recommended, with particular care to avoid fluid retention and cardiac failure during the initial refeeding. A reasonable expectation for outpatient weight gain is ½ to 1 pound per week, with an inpatient weight gain of 3 pounds per week. The use of a nutritionist to prescribe a meal plan is helpful during the refeeding phase. Initially, a caloric intake of 30 to 40 kcal/kg/d is started, increasing during the weight gain phase as necessary to as much as 70 to 100 kcal/kg/d. A calorie intake of 40 to 60 kcal/kg/d in the weight maintenance phase is recommended. Nasogastric feeding or parenteral nutrition is rarely needed and then only in life-threatening situations. Limitation of exercise and bathroom privileges may be necessary during this phase. Outpatient follow-up should include regular monitoring of weight by the primary care physician. Those patients with chronic amenorrhea who fail to achieve weight gain and regular menses are at risk for osteoporosis, and hormonal replacement with estrogen and progestin should be considered in such individuals.

Individual and family psychotherapy generally is recommended. Initially, the focus may be on education about the disorder and the effects of starvation on the symptoms of anorexia. As the patient recovers physically, more insight-oriented therapy can be done. Controlled studies assessing the use of medications to treat children and adolescents with anorexia nervosa are lacking. However, if symptoms of depression persist after weight gain, consideration can be given for antidepressants as long as such medications are not contraindicated by the patient's cardiovascular status.

Hospitalization is rarely needed for those patients with uncomplicated bulimia nervosa. Occasionally, patients may be suicidal, have severe alcohol or substance abuse problems, or suffer from life-threatening medical problems, such as severe hypokalemia, and these patients require inpatient care. If outpatient therapy is unable to change the eating behavior, a short hospital admission to break the binge-purge cycle can be useful. A variety of psychotherapeutic approaches have been employed in bulimia nervosa, with cognitive-behavioral therapy being recommended as the most useful by the American Psychiatric Association. Antidepressant medications have been found to be useful in bulimia nervosa, including tricyclic antidepressants, MAO inhibitors, and fluoxetine.

REFERENCES

1. American Psychiatric Association: Practice guideline for eating disorders. Am J Psychiatry 150:212–228, 1993.
2. Herzog DB, Copeland PM: Eating disorders. N Engl J Med 313:295–303, 1985.
3. Yager J: The treatment of eating disorders. J Clin Psychiatry 49(suppl):18–25, 1988.

THE VERY YOUNG TEEN PARENT

ANN L. O'SULLIVAN, Ph.D, F.A.A.N.

A major task of adolescence is the development of healthy behaviors. The extent to which adolescent parents succeed in establishing healthy behaviors is associated with several important contextual factors, including how they behave as a daughter, student, sexual partner, and parent to their infant(s). There is increasing evidence that younger teenagers generally have more difficulty engaging in healthy behaviors than do older adolescents.

In 1979 when pregnancy in adolescence first became a listing in *Index Medicus*, the very young teen parent was an adolescent 17 years of age or younger. Today, a parent younger than 15 years of age is considered a very young teen parent (VYTP). The many developmental challenges that the younger adolescent faces, coupled with being a *parent*, may be too much for the less mature individual to handle. Yet, throughout our nation, the rise in births to teens under 15 is being seen in every rural, suburban, and urban area, and almost 50% of this very young group report having had five or more sexual partners. In addition, women who have had their first intercourse before 15 are much more likely than those who initiated sex at age 17 or older to have had recent sex with a risky partner (a bisexual, an intravenous drug user, or an HIV-infected man) and to have had a sexually transmitted disease (STD). Furthermore, a VYTP appears to be at more risk for future pregnancies than the 16- or 17-year old parent.

Adolescent males' responsiveness regarding pregnancy prevention varies less by age and apparently more by racial or ethnic group. Knowledge of a previous unplanned pregnancy does not impel young men to use contraceptives more consistently.[1]

Busy, hurried primary care providers for the VYTP or the infants of these parents should use a guide to interviewing that includes questions on school, sex, infant immunizations, safety, and psychologic adjustment. In other words, interviews must include questions based on the many roles these teens must perform (i.e., daughter or son, student, sexual partner, and parent).

Daughter

As a daughter, the VYTP usually denies her pregnancy for many months, most often 5 or 6 months, until it begins to show publicly. Her mother, the maternal grandmother, generally maintains the denial despite having heard her daughter vomit in the morning because of morning sickness or having noticed that the sanitary napkins in the house are not being used as usual. This silence and the potential anger that can build during this time must be addressed on a first visit to determine if the VYTP needs professional help in dealing with these feelings. Often, a provider hears from a maternal grandmother, "This was not the daughter I expected to get pregnant. She is quiet and stays to herself — she is not the hussy."

Once the baby is born, parental communication regarding sexuality, day care, smoking, drinking, and similar subjects is often a problem for the maternal grandmother and VYTP despite having the new baby in the household. In fact, a VYTP often is unsure exactly how she became pregnant but very often reports having had beer and wine coolers or smoked marijuana before her first—and sometimes only—sexual experience. Consequently, it is vital that the influence of alcohol and drugs on the new VYTP be discussed by the primary care provider in front of both the maternal grandmother and VYTP.

Loneliness and depression are reported by about 20% of VYTPs and does not represent postpartum blues. It is important, therefore, to monitor these feelings at primary care visits with such instruments as the Children's Depression Inventory (Kovacs) or Beck's Loneliness Instrument and Depression Inventory. Because VYTPs often have trouble remembering to take a contraceptive pill, vitamin, or depression medicine daily, mild depression is often best treated with what researchers call "talk therapy," either group or individual. Encouraging the VYTP to plan for weekly exercise is also a good therapy for mild depression. Moderate to severe depression needs referral to an appropriate specialist or program.

Student

Living in a household where no one has a high school diploma and where aspirations for higher education are neither fostered nor supported makes returning to school after the birth of a baby more problematic. Since the Graduate Equivalency Diploma is not recognized as a high school diploma by several branches of the Armed Forces and many states, it is essential that the VYTP receive the encouragement and support from someone to return to a traditional education setting. A discussion of how the teen performed in school before and during the pregnancy must include such questions as, "Did you repeat grade(s) in school?" and "Which grades?" in order for the provider to identify the level of resources necessary to ensure successful school reentry. Repeating several grades, especially the first and the fifth, often is an indication that the individual may have some type of learning disability that needs remediation. Failing in school is always upsetting to a VYTP whether it is "cool" to admit it or not. If the VYTP is having to change schools (from K-5 to a middle school or middle school to high school) because of age or address, it is very important to alert a gym teacher or counselor in order to gain some additional support for the teen. There is evidence that when a VYTP changes schools during a pregnancy or shortly thereafter, she is less able to establish herself as a student, is unknown by the teachers, and is more apt to be a poor attender or to drop out.[2]

Sexual Partner

Knowing whether the young teen has become a parent through an adverse sexual experience or via a spontaneous, though not adverse, sexual interaction is essential before discussing family planning and contraception. A preamble to very direct questioning, such as, "On the first visit, I always need to ask many questions that may sound like I am trying to get into your business, but I need this information to help me give you and your infant the best possible care" is important to set the stage for such invasive history taking. If the teen has had an adverse sexual experience, it is important to find the appropriate counseling to meet her needs.

A discussion of which method of contraception the teen chose in order to delay an immediate second pregnancy is an essential part of the care to a VYTP, whether you are delivering care to the teen or seeing her as part of your care for her infant. Since most teens have a great deal of difficulty remembering to take a pill each day, the newer forms of contraception, for example, Norplant or Depo-Provera, are often good methods for the VYTP. If a teen has not chosen a contraceptive method or has not stopped being sexually active, she is likely to have an additional unplanned pregnancy and must be presented with this reality. In addition, the teen must be reminded of the need *also* to prevent STDs in herself and her partners. Such teens may never have used a male or female condom and may be uncomfortable in purchasing condoms and in initiating the use of the condom. Some research has documented that white and nonwhite teens differ in their approaches as sexual partners, but all need instructions in how to initiate the use of condoms.

The primary care provider should concentrate on individualizing the education given regarding sexual behavior and the preparation necessary to prevent both STDs and pregnancy.

Parent

Over the past 10 years, researchers and advocates have debated whether a very young teen can parent while she is still a child or adolescent herself. The best-documented studies acknowledge that the infants of teens are advanced or appropriate in the areas of gross motor and personal-social skills but delayed in fine motor and language skills. Most recent research reaffirms that infants of teenage parents suffer more abuse than do infants of older parents.[3]

Because of the normal egocentrism of adolescence, the VYTP suffers from two phenomena called the *personal fable:* "It won't happen to me and my baby" and the *imaginary audience:* "I can't goo and coo to my baby in public because everyone is looking at me and I'll look silly." These normal feelings of adolescence pose immediate problems for the VYTP and her infant because one will find a VYTP taking her baby to inappropriate places at inappropriate times and not fearing for their well-being. In addition, it is very difficult to have a VYTP sit on the floor and play with her infant or toddler because she is embarrassed at what people will think of her. She fears that she will look foolish or childish now that she is a parent and wants to be treated as a woman rather than a girl. Because she is a provider, however, one must encourage the VYTP to stimulate her infant and toddler in a variety of ways.

Safety is an important area to discuss with the VYTP. Walkers have been documented as very unsafe for infants of VYTP, since the baby is often unattended while in the walker. An infant in a walker can get to the top of a staircase or grab a very hot curling iron in a matter of seconds. Thus, such as baby is much safer in a playpen or portable crib.

Spanking versus discipline must also be discussed. Often the VYTP has unrealistic expectations of a 9-month-old or 19-month-old child and must be educated about normal infant and toddler growth and development. Group parenting programs while they are at school are excellent opportunities for VYTPs to learn these most important developmental milestones. Neighborhood parenting programs may be very effective if they can be held at convenient times for school-attending teen parents. A VYTP needs to have the timeout technique for disciplining a young child explained and then demonstrated. Otherwise, she will likely return to your practice and say this technique did not work for her the first time she tried it. She will refuse to try it again because it made her feel foolish when her toddler did not immediately stay in the designated timeout place. Telling parents that five countries have prohibited spanking, including Finland, Sweden, Norway, Denmark, and Austria, gives an opening for the discussion of corporal punishment and spanking. Giving the message that not spanking takes more thinking and creativity and may teach the toddler or child something is very important. Acknowledging that all parents feel momentary rages and need to know how to handle such feelings is also important.

Sucking and feeding practices of the infant of a VYTP when not appropriate can become extreme. Overfeeding appears to be the most common problem of the young infant, and underfeeding seems to be the most common problem of older infants and toddlers. The importance of nonnutritional sucking for all infants must be discussed because of the many negative myths regarding pacifiers. Research supports the use of pacifiers over thumb, blanket, or favorite toy sucking as the most appropriate way to meet the normal sucking needs of infants. Teaching a VYTP how to choose a safe, one-piece pacifier is important. One must discuss and demonstrate the dangers of the two-piece plastic and rubber pacifier models.

Immunizations to prevent communicable diseases in both the VYTP and her infant is a tremendous challenge. Since the federal government suspended data collection on immunization rates among preschool children in 1985, we can only go by what experts believe in 1993. Depending on the community, complete immunization for infants by 2 years of age can vary from 30% to 70%. Approximately 50% of VYTPs have received the booster tetanus and measles, mumps, and rubella immunization. Because the VYTP typically has so many sexual partners as well as risky partners, it is important to consider her at high risk for hepatitis and, thus, an excellent candidate for the hepatitis B vaccine. Without extra outreach and follow-up on missed appointments, the infants of VYTP often will join other 2 year olds who are underimmunized and at risk for preventable diseases.

PRIMARY CARE PROVIDERS

In addition to delivering the primary care to a VYTP it is important for primary care providers to advocate for more resources for the VYTP family. With less family support in the 1990s, communities and especially primary care providers in those communities must demand more parenting courses, formally and informally, for the VYTP. More day care programs that concentrate on the weaknesses of infants of teens in their stimulation programs and more Head Start programs must be found for these infants.

In 1990, $25 billion was the single year public cost for all families started with a teen birth, yet only 2 cents out of each dollar is spent on preventing teen pregnancy. Primary care providers must advocate for doubling or tripling the amount spent on preventing these very young teens from becoming parents. Charles Dickens said in *Oliver Twist* "Children have to be taken care of and if nobody will do it, they will take care of themselves. They will re-create a family, come hell or high water." We must stop this cycle as primary care providers.

Support for the normal activities of the VYTP is essential as part of the primary care provider visit. Many more grandparents are unavailable to help their daughters than were available 15 years ago. Some maternal grandmothers are former teen mothers and are trying to get their own lives together. Others are those one reads about in the newspaper: 29 years of age, addicted to cocaine, and having their fifth, often low birth weight, infant. Without some scheduled fun, no parent, much less a VYTP, can withstand the daily responsibilities of parenting. Research supports the fact that a VYTP living with her parents does better than one living by herself, traveling from relative to relative or living in a shelter.

REFERENCES

1. Marsiglio W: Adolescent males' orientation toward paternity and contraception. Fam Plan Pers 25:22–31, 1993.
2. O'Sullivan A, Jacobsen B: A randomized trial of a health care program for first time adolescent mothers and their infants. Nurs Res 41:210–215, 1992.
3. Stier DM, Leventhal JM, Berg AT, et al: Are children born to young mothers at increased risk of maltreatment? Pediatrics 91:642–648, 1993.

UNDERSTANDING AND ASSESSING ADOLESCENT INFLUENCES AND RISK-TAKING BEHAVIOR

ERIC J. SIGEL, M.D.
S. JEAN EMANS, M.D.

Adolescents represent a unique and challenging patient population. Some practitioners may initially be hesitant to take care of teenagers. The key to adolescent health care is developing an appreciation for the dynamic process inherent in adolescence. A path exists from childhood to adulthood, and a clinician can positively affect the process, both medically and psychologically, if an understanding of adolescence is developed. Appreciating the powerful influences that the teen experiences in today's world is vital, including the variety of cultural and family backgrounds and the pressures from society and the media. Adolescence represents a time of experimentation, and a clinician should recognize the high-risk behaviors that teens may engage in, factors that may predispose a teen to such behaviors, and office interventions that can positively affect morbidity. Finally, to better treat teenagers, an understanding of how to make an office conducive to treating an adolescent population and guidelines about preventative screening should be developed.

PSYCHOLOGIC DEVELOPMENT

There are several psychologic tasks of adolescence that must be completed for a preteen to emerge as a healthy adult. Adolescents need to separate from parents or adult caregivers, establishing their own sense of identity and independence. Positive self-esteem is needed so the adolescent can deal confidently with the many challenges that exist. Although pubertal development usually occurs in early adolescence, the psychologic tasks may not be completed until the early 20s. A straight path to completing these goals is rare, as teenagers often experiment and sometimes deviate from their course toward adulthood. Appreciating that adolescent patients are constantly evolving and struggling with such issues will make it easier to understand and subsequently to treat them for any given condition.

Adolescent psychosocial development can be loosely divided into three stages—early (11 to 14 years), middle (15 to 17 years), and late (18 to 21 years). Each phase has particular characteristics. Early

Supported in part by project MCJ-MA 259195 from the Maternal and Child Health Bureau (Title V, Social Security Act), Health Resources and Services Administration, Department of Health and Human Services.

adolescence is highlighted by changing body image. Teens can be quite preoccupied with their bodies. They may be uncomfortable with their appearance, comparing themselves with their peers. They demonstrate increased interest in sexual anatomy and physiology, which can lead to anxieties and questions regarding menstruation, masturbation, and wet dreams. This interest provides the practitioner with an opportunity to address teens' concerns and allay their fears. The struggle for independence begins as teens typically become less interested in parental activity and more focused on their peers. Identity development starts to evolve as teens begin to move from concrete thinking to abstract thinking. They may begin to test authority in hopes of better defining their values. A lack of impulse control may be present that can lead to risk-taking behavior.

During middle adolescence, identity development continues, characterized by an increasing willingness to share feelings and an expanding intellectual ability. The teen may have completed pubertal development but may spend an inordinate amount of time adjusting his or her appearance, often conforming to peer culture. More time is devoted to peers and less to families. Teens, as well as adults, can have a sense of invulnerability in which negative consequences of their behavior may not be appreciated.

Once teens enter late adolescence, they have ideally become separate entities from their families, completing the struggle for independence, although there may be a period of regression when they move out of the home. They may be able to better appreciate and actually seek out advice from parents or caregivers. Ego development at this stage leads to a rational and realistic conscience and a sense of perspective, with the abilities to delay, compromise, and set limits. Practical goals for the future may be formed, and the adolescent may further refine his or her set of values.

CHANGING FAMILY STRUCTURE

Growing up today is different from the way it was two generations ago. A classic family structure consisting of two parents, one of whom may have been in charge of raising the children, exists less commonly. This change has important implications on how the adolescent may access the health care system and how he or she complies with medical therapy. Appreciating the framework of family structure will give the practitioner insight into the adolescent's perspective of the world and how multiple, sometimes competing forces may influence the teen. Understanding the teen's daily life can help tailor therapy and help the clinician determine whether intervention in the social realm may be necessary.

Diversity among family structure abounds. Roughly 50% of marriages end in divorce. In addition to the significant emotional impact this creates, the ease of accessing and interacting with the medical system is affected. Parental conflicts may occur around issues of medical care; for example, parents may not agree on the best clinician for their child. Health care may be splintered when a child spends summers and weekends with one parent and the rest of the time with the other. In these situations, adolescents may be more responsible for their own medical care, coming to the office alone. Parental input may be insufficient to assume compliance with medications or follow-up. When both parents need to be included in the planning, in addition to time constraints imposed on the clinician, disagreements on how to appropriately address immediate concerns may exist. Appreciating the dynamic triad between the adolescent and two separate caretakers can help greatly in formulating management plans, especially in those with a chronic illness.

Apart from divorce, single parent homes, especially in urban settings, are common. Most often, the head of the household is the mother or grandmother, as approximately two thirds of urban children are born out of wedlock, many to teen mothers. Often, the responsibility of raising the children is left to the grandmothers. Recognizing this family structure can help the clinician develop an alliance with the teen and help guide an appropriate intervention. Practitioners cannot assume that a father is present and need to be sensitive to such

possibilities while interviewing the adolescent. If no role model is present, the teen may rely heavily on a group of significantly older adolescents and be more likely to become involved in high-risk behaviors. If, as a practitioner, a lack of existing role models for the adolescent is recognized, it is important to encourage involvement with organized youth groups or Big Brother-Big Sister programs.

Some teenagers may live within the structure of a "wandering home." Extended families are often large, with aunts, grandmothers, godmothers, and older siblings playing a key role in adolescents' lives. For a variety of reasons, whether it be financial, work schedules, neighborhood safety, size of the household, presence of drugs or violence, or simply choice, teens may sleep in many different homes with different rules. This phenomenon has multiple implications, especially for the adolescent with chronic disease. For example, an asthmatic who is on chronic therapy needs to be responsible for having medication and knowledgeable about the regimen because each caretaker may not be familiar with the illness. In the office, histories may be of variable accuracy, since the caretaker may not be consistent. To provide quality medical care, the clinician needs to take such situations into account when designing a regimen and prescribing therapy. Another scenario that arises is involvement with social service agencies. Adolescents in foster care will appear in the office—sometimes with a foster parent, sometimes with a social worker. Asking open-ended questions about the circumstances is critical, as the information can reveal significant pathology, both emotional and physical. Past medical history and immunization records are often scant, even though follow-up and compliance are fairly complete.

Working parents, whether married or single, present a special nuance to understanding adolescents' daily schedules. Some public schools dismiss students in the early afternoon, allowing the adolescent a potential 5 hours of free time, often without adult supervision. Most teens will have responsibilities, but the more unsupervised time, the greater the potential to engage in high-risk activities. The practitioner should take this into account when assessing risky behavior and should also be able to help the teen develop some constructive activities to help reduce the chance of morbidity.

Obtaining a family structure history at each annual checkup and updating it at sick visits is essential. Having an active phone number in the chart is invaluable for follow-up. Understanding the adolescent's environment is critical to positively influence his or her health and well-being.

INFLUENCES ON THE ADOLESCENT

Aside from the family, many other groups exert influence on an adolescent's development. Peer groups play a key role in determining an adolescent's set of values. The media can have great impact on the way teens view society. In turn, society places great expectations on young people, which can be a source of motivation but also the root of great frustration. Whether an adolescent has hope for the future affects daily behavior. The threat of HIV infection remains a constant worry for many teens.

Recognizing the influence of a teen's peer group can provide vital information in helping to understand the teen. Peer groups can be institutional, usually set up by adults and defined by a sports team, the school paper, a church group, or informal groups that are initiated and chosen by the individual, such as cliques or fraternities. How peers influence individual teens is unclear. Adolescents may experience pressure to conform to the positive expectations of others, or they may model behavior (teens imitating peer behavior). During early adolescence, teens turn toward each other for guidance and support. High school students spend 29% of their time with peers and only 15% of their time with adults. Determining the degree of peer influence is difficult, since peers usually reinforce, rather than contradict, parental values.

Peers can be quite a positive force, encouraging each other to perform scholastically and athletically while helping to reinforce a solid set of moral principles. An adolescent, though, may be in conflict, trying to choose between what he or she feels is right and what he or she thinks friends think is right. If a teen has low self-esteem, a peer group may be able to exert considerable influence. A teenager can be drawn into a "bad crowd," especially if support is missing at home, potentially leading to risk-taking behavior. Patients should be asked about their peer groups. "Who do you hang out with?" What do you and your friends do for fun?" "What organizations and school groups do you belong to?" An open discussion about peer pressure should be a part of annual examinations, especially during early and midadolescence.

Medical care can be affected directly by a teen's interaction with a specific peer group. An adolescent with diabetes may feel uncomfortable sharing the illness with peers and subsequently may participate in physical and social activities without taking the illness into account. Empowering patients with chronic illness to discuss their disease with peers, for both their medical and psychologic well-being, can be important in adolescent counseling.

The media has the potential to be both a positive and negative influence in teenagers' lives. Fifteen-year-olds spend, on average, 5 hours a day watching television. Campaigns targeting drunk driving in the teen population can have a positive influence on teen behavior. After 100 episodes of popular television shows addressed teen drinking, surveys in the subsequent months suggested that adolescents heard the message and planned to change behavior. In contrast, when teens are subjected to slim, athletic, sexy men and women throughout the visual media, self-esteem can suffer. Eating disorders have become increasingly prevalent in adolescents. The clinician needs to be sensitive to body image and weight issues in light of society's emphasis on what makes a person attractive.

The threat of HIV has affected adolescents' thoughts if not lifestyles. Virtually all teenagers have been taught about HIV in school. The presence of HIV has resulted in many school systems implementing a comprehensive sex education program, starting in the early grades. Although teens' knowledge of HIV transmission and prevention is relatively high, clinicians should review the facts, including prevention, with all patients. Unfortunately, knowledge does not necessarily translate into behavior. Just because teens know the facts does not mean they will abstain or practice safer sex. Assessing their risk factors while having an open dialogue can help the teen understand the consequences of risky behavior. Counseling and HIV testing may be appropriate for that teen (see next section). Reassurance, if the patient does not appear to be at risk, and further emphasis on prevention are imperative.

Societal and parental expectations have an impact on adolescent development. Cross-cultural variability also becomes a factor when analyzing developmental influences. Goals, such as outstanding grades and excellence in sports, are important and have the potential to motivate a child. Conversely, such expectations can be so overbearing that teens may perceive themselves as failures if they do not live up to parental expectations. This can be quite damaging to an adolescent's self-image. Education is not a priority in all families, and familial conflict can develop for the teen who desires higher education. Other responsibilities, such as providing income or helping to raise other children in the household, can be another source of frustration.

Defiant, antiparental behavior exhibited by risk taking vis-a-vis sexual and substance use experimentation can occur. Somatic complaints, such as headaches and abdominal pain, are frequent manifestations of many psychologic issues. A detailed social history needs to be obtained, including the adolescent's perception of what expectations are placed on them. The clinician's awareness of this issue becomes particularly important toward the end of tenth grade, when post-high school plans begin to evolve. Cultural subtleties abound. The question "What are your plans after high school?" provides valuable insight into the adolescent's ideas for the future. It is critical not to ask "Where are you going to college?" Automatically, the teen will feel like somewhat of a failure within the clinician-patient relationship if, in fact, the patient does not plan on college.

For certain teens, hope for the future does not exist. With the dramatic rise in violence and the continuing cycle of poverty, teens may not envision much of a life beyond their early 20s. This comes into direct conflict with societal expectations of having a job and starting a family. Developing a positive sense of self takes on a different form. Excelling on the basketball court, becoming the toughest in a gang, or rejecting authority can help the teen define himself or herself in the world he or she knows. Risk-taking behavior can stem from such an outlook. This represents an adaptation to what society is perceived to provide. Medical intervention can have an effect if it is done within the context of the adolescent's world.

Institutions also play a role in influencing today's teens. Sometimes they are self-selected by the teens, other times by adults. Religious affiliation can provide spiritual structure and numerous role models for teens to follow. Strong religious affiliation is associated with less risk-taking behavior.

Sports teams, whether community based or school based, also contribute to a teen's development. Adherence to a training regimen can provide a sense of discipline. Becoming a team player can help establish independence from parents, as well as enhance self-esteem. Obligations to teammates can help an adolescent reject experimenting with drugs and cigarettes that are harmful to the body, although highly competitive sports, especially football and wrestling, can put athletes at risk for anabolic steroid use. Belonging to other school groups, scout groups, and community organizations plays some role in a teen's development. Jobs can influence teens as they evolve into adulthood. A combination of all these forces contributes to the makeup of the developing adolescent. Understanding the influences on an individual basis can greatly enhance the practitioner-patient relationship and help the practitioner in developing a health care strategy that will benefit the patient through adolescence and beyond.

ADOLESCENTS AT RISK

Every adolescent today has the potential to engage in high-risk behavior. Surveys have shown that 54% of high school students have had sexual intercourse and 90% have tried alcohol. Within the last 30 days, 35% have been drunk, 36% have used tobacco, and 4% have carried firearms. The leading cause of death among urban teens is homicide. Over 1 million teenage girls become pregnant each year. Clinicians need to be able to recognize adolescents at risk and identify those already involved in risk-taking behavior. An adolescent visit should focus on keeping or making adolescents safe as they enter this experimentation phase in their lives.

Identification

Practitioners have a variety of approaches to identify high-risk behavior. Initially, one can interview the parents alone, providing them the opportunity to express their concerns. The concept of confidentiality and the importance of interviewing the teenager alone should be explained, so parents can begin to understand and respect the relationship between their adolescent and the clinician. The majority of the visit should be spent alone with the patient to gather further history and perform the physical examination. The interaction can be initiated with discussion of confidentiality: whatever is talked about remains between the practitioner and the patient, unless a serious life-threatening issue arises. Explaining that all the questions that will be asked are asked of all teenagers and that they are relevant to the teen's general health often will put the adolescent at ease.

A good organizational approach to collecting information is the HEADSS (Table 1) outline, suggested by Goldenring and Cohen, which provides a framework for a social history inventory. It can certainly be adjusted for the individual based on age and previous history. The outline can key the clinician in to whether the patient may be at risk for engaging in harmful behavior or whether, in fact, the patient has already participated in high-risk behavior.

Often, asking questions about peer group behavior makes it easier for adolescents to communicate with the practitioner. "Do any of your

TABLE 1. HEADSS Interview

Home Who lives with patient? Where? What are relationships like at home? Change in relationships? Recent death or divorce? New people at home? Discipline at home? Own room? Recent moves? Running away? What do parents and relatives do for a living? Ever institutionalized? Incarcerated? (patient or family) **Education and Employment** Grade level? School performance? Recent change in grades? Ever had to repeat? Favorite subjects/worst subjects Suspensions/expulsions/dropping out School/employment attendance Future education/employment goals Any current or past employment? Relations with teachers, employers? Recent change of schools? **Activities/Affect/Anger** What do you do for fun? Do you have friends? Sports/exercise, hobbies, favorite music Church attendance, membership in clubs/gangs? TV—how much? Reading for pleasure? Does patient have car? Use seatbelts? Use a bicycle helmet? History of arrests/acting out? Frequency of fighting? Ever carry a weapon?	**Drugs (Include Alcohol and Tobacco)** Use by peers? Use by patient? Use by family members? Amounts, frequency, patterns of use? Driving while using? Source? How paid? **Sexuality** Is patient in relationship? Orientation? Degrees and types of sexual experience? Number of partners? Masturbation? (normalize) History of pregnancy/abortion? STDs—knowledge and prevention? Contraception? Frequency of use? Comfort with sexual activity, enjoyment? History of sexual/physical abuse? **Suicide/Depression** Feelings of "boredom"? Appetite/eating behavior change Sleeping difficulties? Feelings of withdrawal/social isolation Feelings of hopelessness/helplessness History of past suicide attempts/depression Preoccupation with death Suicidal ideation History of suicide/attempts in peers/relatives

Adapted from Goldenring JM, Cohen E: Getting into adolescents' heads. Contemp Pediatr 5:75, 1988.

friends carry a gun or knife?" or "Do people drink beer at the parties you go to?" is much less threatening than asking directly. Once the history is elicited about peers, more direct questions are possible: "Have you ever felt the need to carry a weapon?"

Clinicians may not ask questions because of uncertainty about what to do with a positive response. The following section separates high-risk behaviors and offers some interventional strategies. Multiple high-risk behaviors often occur in the same teen.

Violence

The 1990s have witnessed an incredible rise of violence. Homicide is now the leading cause of death in the black male population age 15 to 24 years. In the 1990 National School-Based Youth Risk Behavior Survey, 4% of all high school students and 21% of black male students had carried a gun in the last 30 days. Studies in Baltimore revealed that almost one half of the boys in high school had carried a gun previously. The incidence of violence is highest in urban centers but also affects suburban and rural populations. Young children often have witnessed violent behavior or experienced it directly in the form of physical or sexual abuse. Since one fourth of girls and one sixth of boys will be victims of sexual abuse by the age of 18, teens need to be asked about the possibility in a sensitive manner. If abuse is detected, victims often need counseling support, and social service agencies need to be notified.

The spectrum of violence in the teen population ranges from verbal arguments to physical fights to the use of weapons. As with most primary care, prevention needs to be the ultimate goal. Discuss with patients their approach to situations of conflict. Prepare them by having them think about what they would do in a tense situation. Encourage them to talk with the adversary about the conflict instead of fighting, and reassure them that walking away certainly may be the safest way out, even if they lose face. Role play with them so they can practice. Determine why the adolescent needs to carry a weapon. Knowing the community can help one guide the teen to counselors, support groups, or after school activities that can help the adolescent

stay away from threatening situations. Acknowledge pressures that exist to join gangs, and help the patient work out alternatives. Discussing the risk of having a gun, emphasizing the relationship between alcohol use and violent acts, and encouraging them to relinquish firearms to a higher authority is appropriate. Gun safety should also be addressed to help prevent complications from accidents.

Substance Use

Substance abuse is highly correlated with younger age of initiation of drinking, decreased school performance, and associating with people who are >3 years older. These factors should be red flags when taking the psychosocial history, warning the clinician that the patient is at risk. Using the association of alcohol use and violent acts—almost 50% of homicides involve alcohol—and the association between alcohol use and sexual risk taking—condoms are often forgotten when under the influence—can help the adolescent develop an appreciation for the consequences of substance use. (See Substance Abuse for detailed discussion.)

Sexual Behavior

Adolescence represents a time of budding sexuality. Teens begin to discover their bodies and the associated sexual urges. This normal maturational process has the potential to produce negative consequences.

The average age, as of 1990, of initiation of sexual intercourse is 15 for males and 16 for females, and it is substantially younger for urban populations, especially males. By 18, 72% of males and 70% of females have had sexual relations. Although condom use has increased in the past decade (58% have used condoms, with 30% reporting regular use), more education is necessary. Every year, 2.5 million U.S. teens are infected with a sexually transmitted disease (STD), which correlates to one sixth of sexually active teens. Among innercity sexually active youth, 25% of black and 20% of white females have been pregnant, and 14% black and 10% white males report that they have impregnated a partner.

The onus is on the provider to detect which adolescents are having sexual relations and the degree of risk taking involved—the number of partners and the use of protection. One can ask directly or initiate the discussion by asking about peer behavior. When talking with a teen, never assume a heterosexual relationship. "Have you ever had a romantic or sexual relationship with, or romantic interest in, either guys or girls?" An open-ended, nonjudgmental questioning style will let the adolescent know that the provider is open to discussing issues of homosexuality. In addition to inquiring about sexual abuse and date rape, the question, "Have you ever traded sex for drugs or money?" is pertinent, since 600,000 teens are prostitutes at any given time.

Adolescent males (female screening is discussed elsewhere) should be screened if they have had anal or vaginal intercourse or if they report urinary symptoms. Dipsticking a first-catch urine for leukocyte esterase is valuable in detecting STDs, especially asymptomatic *Chlamydia* infections. If the urine is positive for leukocyte esterase or a patient is symptomatic (discharge or dysuria), the clinician should test for *Chlamydia* with either a urethral swab (EIA or culture) or a urine specimen using new PCR technology and for gonorrhea by culturing a spun urine sample. In addition, a wet preparation to look for *Trichomonas* and a careful physical examination searching for genital warts should be done. Although treatment guidelines change, most STDs can be treated orally. It is important to treat symptomatic individuals for both *Chlamydia* and gonorrhea, since they often occur concomitantly. It is also imperative that partners seek medical attention, since any partner of the infected individual needs screening and treatment.

Additional screening for STDs includes a serologic test for syphilis, either yearly or with any new STD. High-risk teens, defined by the CDC as having three or more partners in the last 6 months, should be screened for hepatitis B and, if negative, immunized against hepatitis B. Although official recommendations are to vaccinate only high-risk teens, many clinicians believe that all adolescents deserve the hepatitis vaccine regardless of their degree of risk.

The question of HIV testing arises in many clinical situations. For example, the teen may be engaging in high-risk behavior, and the practitioner recognizes a legitimate possibility that the patient may be HIV positive, although the patient does not raise it as a concern. The practitioner has a responsibility for the well-being of the patient, and HIV should be introduced as a concern both for prevention counseling and medical implications. Another possibility may be that a teen has had intercourse once and becomes concerned that HIV may have been contracted, and testing is demanded. There are no strict criteria to determine who should be tested. The practitioner should help each individual through stepwise, comprehensive counseling that ideally should span at least three visits. It is essential to assess why the teen wants to be tested, what support systems are in place, and how the teen will respond if he or she tests positive. The degree of suicidality should be assessed. Issues of test confidentiality also need to be clarified. A second visit for follow-up questions and testing, if appropriate, should be scheduled, folowed by a test result appointment, encouraging the teen to bring a support person. Results should never be given over the phone, and the physician should be aware of where to refer individuals if they do test positive.

Being open to the possibility of homosexual thought or behavior is essential. Although society has slowly become more cognizant and accepting, with some high schools even having gay-lesbian support groups, it continues to be an extremely difficult issue for adolescents. The emotional struggle and isolation that teens can experience puts them at high risk for destructive behavior. The suicide rate among gay teens is three to five times higher than among heterosexual teens. Substance use can be quite significant, as can other high-risk behaviors. By keeping questions open-ended, the clinician can provide the opportunity for a teen to discuss this issue, with potential lifesaving interventions.

Steroid Use

Although practically speaking anabolic steroid use falls into the category of drug use, many practitioners do not view it as such. Indeed, many of the factors that contribute to high-risk behavior are not found in the steroid-using group. Roughly 6% of males and 2.5% of females use steroids, either injected or taken orally. Use can be broken down generally into two categories: to enhance athletic performance and to change body image. Screening questions directed toward all athletes is appropriate, especially wrestlers and football players, again inquiring first about use among teammates. Detection can be difficult. Body builder physiques, small testes, and newly acquired aggressive behavior in males and well-defined musculature, hirsutism, acne, and deepened voices in women may raise clinical suspicion. Discussing long-term side effects is important when counseling steroid-using teens. In addition, feelings of pressure that may come externally from coaches and teammates and internally from the desire to excel or improve appearance should be recognized and addressed.

Tobacco Use

Tobacco use has remained prevalent in the teen population despite well-known adverse health consequences. According to the Youth Risk Behavior Survey, roughly 36% of high school students have used tobacco in the last 30 days: 32% have smoked cigarettes, and 10% have used smokeless tobacco. Almost 18% of seniors use tobacco on a regular basis. White students are more than twice as likely to use tobacco as are black students. Smoking has been significantly correlated with other high-risk behavior, such as drinking and early initiation of sexual activity.

Prevention should be the goal. Though teens may acknowledge the risks inherent in smoking, they see it as remote and irrelevant. Adolescent visits should focus on the influence of peers and the role of advertising in persuading young people to smoke. Immediate negative consequences of tobacco use, such as increased heart rate, addiction, bad breath, and stained teeth, should be emphasized.

When the physician is confronted with a regular user, issues that affect smoking cessation should be discussed, such as the readiness to quit and the obstacles to quitting. A schedule should be developed with a target date to quit agreed on. Close follow-up should be arranged to provide support for the patient. Alternatives to smoking should be offered, including nicotine gum. The nicotine patch can be used in older adolescents as long as it is used in conjunction with a cessation intervention.

Suicide

Suicide is the third leading cause of death among 15 to 19-year-olds. Many teens who commit suicide never have been evaluated for psychiatric illness or suicidal ideation. Males are three times more likely to complete a suicide, although females are three times more likely to attempt suicide. The risk increases with age, with teens in midlate adolescence 21 times more likely to commit suicide than during early adolescence. Suicidal ideation is relatively common, with some studies indicating that 40% of adolescents think about it, whereas 5% actually attempt suicide. The best predictors of completed suicide are depression or other psychiatric disorder(s), substance abuse, and previous suicide attempts. Disruption in significant relationships, persistent desire to be dead, and deteriorating school performance are all warning signs that are correlated with suicide behavior.

In addition to the psychosocial history, specific questions can include "Have you ever thought about trying to hurt yourself?" or "Some people your age think about suicide—have you ever considered or attempted suicide?" If there is a positive response, a clinician needs to assess the immediate threat, which includes whether the teen has a specific plan and what support systems are available to keep the teen safe. Psychiatric referral may be necessary, or even hospitalization if the threat is imminent. It is vital that the patient agree to a no-harm contract. Serious suicidal ideation is a clear-cut instance in which confidentiality needs to be broken to enlist the support of family.

DELIVERING ADOLESCENT CARE SUCCESSFULLY

To provide quality adolescent care in the office setting, the clinician needs to develop a collaborative partnership with the adolescent. Sev-

TABLE 2. Recommended Frequency of GAPS Preventative Services

	STAGE OF ADOLESCENCE		
	EARLY 11–14 y	MIDDLE 15–17 y	LATE 18–21 y
Health Guidance			
Parenting	O*	O	Opt
Adolescent development	Y	Y	Y
Safety practices	Y	Y	Y
Diet and fitness	Y	Y	Y
Healthy lifestyles (sexual behavior, smoking, substance abuse)	Y	Y	Y
Screening			
Hypertension	Y	Y	Y
Hyperlipidemia	HR-1†		O
Eating disorders	Y	Y	Y
Obesity	Y	Y	Y
Tobacco use	Y	Y	Y
Alcohol and drug use	Y	Y	Y
Sexual behavior	Y	Y	Y
Sexually transmitted diseases			
Gonorrhea	Y‡	Y‡	Y‡
Chlamydia	Y‡	Y‡	Y‡
Genital warts	Y‡	Y‡	Y‡
Syphilis	HR-2§	HR-2	HR-2
HIV	HR-2	HR-2	HR-2
Cervical cancer	Y‡	Y‡	Y
Depression/suicide risk	Y	Y	Y
Physical, sexual or emotional abuse	Y	Y	Y
Learning problems	Y	Y	Y
Tuberculosis	HR-3‖	HR-3	HR-3
Immunizations			
Measles, mumps, rubella	Patients who have only had one MMR		
Diphtheria/tetanus	10 years after previous Td booster		
Hepatitis B	Adolescents at high risk for infection		

*O, once per time period; Y, yearly.
†HR-1, If family history of cardiovascular disease <55 years old, or with family history of high cholesterol.
‡If the adolescent is sexually active.
§HR-2, Adolescents at high risk—more than one sexual partner in last 6 months, having exchanged sex for drugs, being a male who has engaged in sex with other males, having used intravenous drugs (HIV), having had other STDs, having lived in an area endemic for infection, and having had a sexual partner who is at risk for infection.
‖HR-3, Adolescents who have been exposed to active TB, have lived in a homeless shelter, have been incarcerated, have lived in an area endemic for TB, or currently work in a health care setting.
Adapted from the American Medical Association Guidelines for Adolescent Preventative Services. Chicago, AMA, 1990.

eral components contribute to creating such a relationship, by paying attention to physical details as well as personal interactions.

Ideally, a waiting room separate from infants and toddlers should be created so the teens can have a sense that it is their space. Posters on the wall, pamphlets directed specifically at teen issues, and videos about different aspects of adolescent health are important in creating such an atmosphere. Specific topics, such as teen pregnancy and homosexuality, can be displayed, conveying the message that this is the place to talk about such issues. Even a small practice can devote one session a week to adolescent medicine and transform the waiting room into a teen space.

To help facilitate information gathering, questionnaires can be given to adolescents while they wait. Some teens feel less threatened answering personal questions on a survey form. Since adolescent visits can be labor intensive, this method can help screen for high-risk behaviors along the line of the AMA's *Guidelines for Adolescent Preventative Services* (GAPS) recommendations. The clinician can incorporate the questionnaire into the record, and the answers can help the clinician direct the discussion to the adolescent's foremost concerns. This should not take the place of talking with the patient but should be used as an adjunct.

Medical staff need to be sensitized to the needs of adolescents. Health care personnel need to provide teenagers with a sense of respect and help them feel comfortable in their surroundings. Neither comments about patients nor discussion about their medical issues should be made in any common area. Ideally, an adolescent should be interviewed initially with his or her clothes on to make the interaction between patient and provider more comfortable. Staff should be versed in the concept of confidentiality and understand why the clinician sees the patient alone to be able to communicate this to parents.

Developing a logical approach to the adolescent visit is helpful to the clinician as well as the patient. Preventive and proactive care should be sought so that adolescents end up healthier and more interested in taking care of themselves. The AMA has developed *Guidelines for Adolescent Preventative Services* (GAPs) (Table 2), which detail what issues around health promotion need to be addressed at each annual visit. The use of seatbelts, bicycle helmets, nutrition, and exercise need to be discussed. GAPS also details when to administer immunizations, cholesterol screening, tuberculosis screening, and blood pressure checks. This can all be used to develop a cohesive method of delivering comprehensive health care to the adolescent.

REFERENCES

1. American Medical Association: Guidelines for Adolescent Preventative Services. Chicago, AMA, 1993.
2. Bradford B: Don't let our youth go down Tobacco Road. Contemp Pediatr 9:96, 1992.
3. Brent D: Suicide and suicidal behavior in children and adolescents. Pediatr Rev 10:269, 1989.
4. Brown B: Peer groups in peer cultures. *In* Feldman SS, Eliot GR (eds): At the Threshold: The Developing Adolescent. Cambridge, Harvard University Press, 1990.
5. Coupey S, Klerman L (eds): Adolescent sexuality: Preventing unhealthy consequences. Adoles Med State Art Rev 3:165, 1992.
6. Neinstein L: Adolescent Health Care: A Practical Guide. Baltimore, Urban & Schwartzenberg, 1991:39–44.
7. Stringham P, Weitzman M: Violence counseling in the routine health care of adolescents. J Adolesc Health Care 9:389, 1988.

Index

Note: Page numbers in *italics* refer to illustrations; page numbers followed by t refer to tables.

ISBN 0-7216-5016-3